BREAST ULTRASOUND

BREAST ULTRASOUND

A. THOMAS STAVROS, MD, FACR

Radiology Imaging Associates / Invision–Sally Jobe Breast Centers
Englewood, Colorado

With contributions by

Cynthia L. Rapp, BS, RDMS, FAIUM, FSDMS

Invision / Radiology Imaging Associates
Greenwood Village, Colorado

Steve H. Parker, MD, FACR

Sally Jobe Breast Center
Greenwood Village, Colorado

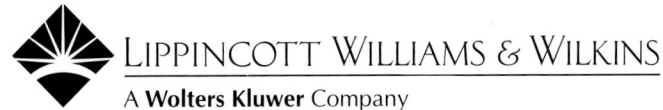

LIPPINCOTT WILLIAMS & WILKINS
A **Wolters Kluwer** Company

Philadelphia • Baltimore • New York • London
Buenos Aires • Hong Kong • Sydney • Tokyo

Acquisitions Editor: Lisa McAllister
Developmental Editor: Keith Donnellan
Production Editor: Steven P. Martin
Production Editor: Richard Rothschild, Print Matters, Inc.
Manufacturing Manager: Benjamin Rivera
Cover Designer: David Levy
Compositor: Compset, Inc.
Printer: Edwards Brothers

Library of Congress Cataloging-in-Publication Data
Stavros, A. Thomas.
    Breast ultrasound / A. Thomas Stavros.
      p. ; cm.
    Includes bibliographical references and index.
    ISBN 0-397-51624-X
      1. Breast—Ultrasonic imaging. 2. Breast—Diseases—Diagnosis. 3.
    Breast—Cancer—Ultrasonic imaging. I. Title.
    [DNLM: 1. Ultrasonography, Mammary. WP 815 S798b 2003]
    RG493.5.U47S73 2003
    618.1′907543—dc22

                                                    2003060296

Care has been taken to confirm the accuracy of the information presented and to
describe generally accepted practices. However, the authors, editors, and publisher are
not responsible for errors or omissions or for any consequences from application of the
information in this book and make no warranty, expressed or implied, with respect to the
currency, completeness, or accuracy of the contents of the publication. Application of
this information in a particular situation remains the professional responsibility of the
practitioner.

The authors, editors, and publisher have exerted every effort to ensure that drug selection
and dosage set forth in this text are in accordance with current recommendations and
practice at the time of publication. However, in view of ongoing research, changes in
government regulations, and the constant flow of information relating to drug therapy
and drug reactions, the reader is urged to check the package insert for each drug for any
change in indications and dosage and for added warnings and precautions. This is
particularly important when the recommended agent is a new or infrequently employed
drug.

Some drugs and medical devices presented in this publication have Food and Drug
Administration (FDA) clearance for limited use in restricted research settings. It is the
responsibility of the health care provider to ascertain the FDA status of each drug or
device planned for use in their clinical practice.

                                        10 9 8 7 6 5 4 3 2 1

CONTENTS

PREFACE

I have written *Breast Ultrasound* for radiologists, breast surgeons, breast pathologists, sonographers, and mammography technologists who perform diagnostic breast sonography. While this book is officially the first edition, it unofficially represents the third edition. During the nearly 10 years that I have been writing this book, ultrasound technology and our ability to demonstrate breast anatomy and pathology has changed so dramatically and rapidly that it has continually altered our ideas of possibilities and limitations. Each of the first two times I neared completion of the book, new developments made earlier writings seem obsolete, requiring significant rewriting and replacement of older images. Ultrasound transducer frequencies have climbed, bandwidths expanded, and dynamic ranges increased. Coded harmonics and real-time spatial compounding have suppressed speckle artifact and improved contrast resolution. Far more is possible today than was possible 10 years ago.

Sonographic resolution has increased beyond the ability to identify zones of the breast and tissue types to being able to identify several orders of mammary ducts and the functional unit of the breast, the terminal ducto-lobular unit (TDLU). Most benign and malignant breast pathology arises within the TDLU. Breast cancer enlarges and distorts the lobules from which it arises and the ducts through which it spreads. We now have the potential to recognize these changes at earlier stages, increasing sonographic sensitivity for early breast carcinoma and improving our ability to determine extent of malignant disease. Many benign processes also arise in the TDLU, some causing characteristically benign sonographic findings, improving our negative predictive ability.

This book has been written with a strong emphasis on how the gross histopathologic morphology of both benign malignant processes alters sonographic anatomy and how to use this information to improve our ability to characterize cystic and solid lesions of the breast. It is influenced greatly by the teachings of Laszlo Tabar and Michel Teboul.

Dr. Tabar has pioneered the teaching of mammography based upon subgross histologic alterations of anatomy. Dr. Teboul has pioneered the anatomic approach to breast imaging. The anatomic and pathologic bases for sonographic evaluation of the breast should be of interest to all subgroups of the targeted audience.

The algorithms that we employ to assess breast lesions sonographically were designed to comfort mammographers who might otherwise feel uncomfortable with sonographic characterization. To the greatest extent possible, we have tried to avoid reinventing the wheel. We have used as much of the information gleaned from mammography over the years as possible. We use mammographic ACR BIRADS categories to classify sonographic lesions. The risk of malignancy for a sonographic lesion in any given BIRADS category is the same as the risk of malignancy for a mammographic finding of the same category. Thus, management rules used every day by a mammographer for any given mammographic BIRADS category can be used to manage a sonographic finding in the same BIRADS category. The sonographic algorithm, like the mammographic algorithm, requires multiple suspicious findings in order to take into account the heterogeneity of breast cancer. We also use as many mammographic findings as possible in our sonographic algorithms. Six of the nine suspicious sonographic findings that we use to characterize solid breast nodules are simply suspicious mammographic findings applied directly to sonography. Similarly, about half the benign findings that we use for sonographic assessment of complex cysts are mammographic findings applied directly to sonography. Finally, the algorithm that we use for sonographically evaluating solid nodules and complex cysts is very similar to the mammographic algorithm. Both the mammographic and sonographic algorithms involve looking for suspicious findings first, and if any suspicious findings are found, an action is required. The sonographic algorithm goes one step further, requiring specific identification of benign findings before a nodule can be characterized as probably benign. Because the sonographic algorithms are based so heavily upon the algorithms with which all US mammographers are familiar, the mammographer should be comfortable with the sonographic algorithm that we present. The mammographer should conclude after reading this book that sonographic characterization beyond cyst vs. solid is not at all a wild and crazy scheme—it is merely the mammographic algorithm with extra steps of conservatism built into it.

This text was designed to be a reference text. Thus, each chapter was designed to stand alone. Some information has been presented more than once, and therefore, appears in several different chapters.

This book emphasizes the diagnostic role of sonography in characterizing and managing palpable and mammographic abnormalities rather than its role as a screening modality. However, other roles—such as evaluating nipple discharge and mammary implants—have also been presented in detail. The important roles of sonography in assessing extent of malignant disease and regional lymph nodes and in assessing the breast after breast cancer treatment have also been presented.

Diagnostic imagers are visual learners. Seeing lots of images facilitates visual learning. Thus, this book has been extensively illustrated. The images included should be useful as frames of reference within the readers' own departments.

We sincerely hope that the emphasis on how breast pathology affects the underlying anatomy and the employment of familiar mammographic findings, algorithms, and management rules helps readers achieve a comfort zone with diagnostic breast ultrasound that they may not have had before reading the book.

I would like to offer thanks for all those who have inspired, encouraged, and helped me to finally complete this task. I have been inspired by my partner and mentor Bill Jobe (Jobee-wan-Kanobe) and my partner and co-conspirator Steve Parker, who has written the chapter on ultrasound-guided intervention and who has encouraged me to speak and to write about breast ultrasound. I would like to thank Dr. Hanne Jensen and Dr. Laszlo Tabar for granting me permission to use some of their magnificent subgross 3D pathology images in this book. I would also like to thank: Maureen Biffinger, who made sure that I received copies all the breast biopsy reports over a period of about 15 years; Mary Mucilli and Charlie Winger, who helped manage the database of tens of thousands of sonography and breast biopsy reports and sonographic-pathologic correlations; and Jon McGrath, who helped manage and catalogue the database of thousands of sonographic, mammographic, and pathologic images. I would like to thank Cindy Rapp, RDMS, and Dr. David Harshfield for helping to edit multiple versions the book and Dr. Terry Giezinski, who helped proofread the galley proofs. Finally, I thank my wife, Margaret, and my children, Becca, Sarah, Charles, and Anne, for putting up with me and my absences during the long and winding journey to completion.

INTRODUCTION TO BREAST ULTRASOUND

GOALS AND INDICATIONS

Ultrasound (US) evaluation of the breast can be categorized as either diagnostic or screening. Breast imaging requires detection and characterization of breast abnormalities. The relative importance of detection and characterization is different for screening and diagnosis. The primary goal of screening is to detect breast cancer in large populations of asymptomatic patients. On the other hand, the primary goal of diagnostic breast ultrasound is to characterize either abnormalities that have already been detected by screening mammography or palpable abnormalities.

Breast ultrasound (BUS) was evaluated as a breast cancer–screening tool early in its development. It was an attractive alternative to mammography because it did not use ionizing radiation. Furthermore, because the mechanism by which ultrasound showed anatomy and pathology was different from that of mammography, it enabled one to "see through" mammographically featureless dense tissue and to show breast anatomy and pathology that mammography could not demonstrate. To capitalize on these advantages, automated whole breast ultrasound scanning devices were built and evaluated. Unfortunately, breast cancer–screening studies performed with these dedicated whole breast ultrasound scanners showed US to be less effective than mammography. Because of this, BUS is not recommend or widely used for primary breast cancer screening in the United States. Instead, it is used for diagnosis, after mammography has been performed in most cases. In our practice, 90% of all patients who undergo BUS have had mammography first. Of the 10% who do not undergo mammography before sonography, almost all are younger than 30 years of age, pregnant, or undergoing short-interval sonographic follow-up for lesions that are visible only by sonography. A few others have developed a new palpable mass with last screening mammogram less than 6 months earlier.

The early failure of BUS as a replacement for mammography in breast cancer screening does not diminish its value as a diagnostic tool. Its use in selected patients as a diagnostic adjunct to clinical and mammographic evaluation can be invaluable. The remainder of this book addresses the use and interpretation of BUS in a diagnostic role.

General Goal of Diagnostic Breast Ultrasound

The general goal of diagnostic BUS is to make a more specific noninvasive diagnosis in patients who have clinical or mammographic abnormalities than could be achieved with mammography and clinical findings alone. The use of BUS in appropriately selected patients (those who have clinical or mammographic findings that are not clearly malignant) should increase the certainty of a benign diagnosis in a large number of patients and should increase the suspicion of carcinoma in a small number of patients. Sonographic demonstration of suspicious findings appropriately leads to biopsy, even when mammographic findings are negative. On the other hand, sonographic demonstration of definitively benign findings obviates biopsy. Consequently, appropriately used BUS should lead to biopsy in some patients but should prevent unnecessary biopsy in most.

Ultrasound has a greater ability than mammography to differentiate among types of normal tissues and to characterize complex cysts and solid nodules. Mammography is capable only of showing four different densities (air, fat, water, and metal or calcium) and can further distinguish between different water-density tissues only by differences in thickness and compressibility and by whether the tissues contain some fatty or calcium density. Ultrasound, on the other hand, can distinguish among many different types of normal breast tissue. Like mammography, ultrasound can identify air, fat, and metallic or calcium densities. However, unlike mammography, ultrasound can also distinguish among different types of normal water-density tissues by echogenicity as well as thickness and compressibility. Sonographic breast anatomy is discussed in detail in Chapter 4.

Furthermore, the method of image acquisition differs between mammography and ultrasound. The mammographic image is a three-dimensional summation of anatomy and pathology resulting in superimposition of water-density tissues that tends to obscure anatomy and pathology. The ultrasound image, on the other hand, is essentially a tomographic slice through the breast. The mammographic density of breast tissues elsewhere within the breast, outside the slice of tissue within the ultrasound beam, is thus irrelevant to ultrasound. Because ultrasound can identify different echogenicities of various normal water-density tissues, and because superimposition of densities is not the problem that it is for mammography, ultrasound is more capable of showing the breast ductal and lobular anatomy and pathology than is mammography. Additionally, ultrasound can distinguish cystic from solid pathology of the breast. Mammography cannot. Unfortunately, many mammographers in the United States have advocated limiting ultrasound's role to distinguishing cystic from solid masses, a serious mistake. Properly used, ultrasound is clearly capable of much more and should be used at least as aggressively in patient management as is diagnostic mammography.

Mammographic Experience and American College of Radiology Lexicon and Categories

It is useful to think of sonographic characterization of breast lesions as occurring on two different levels. Level 1 characterization includes what even the least enthusiastic mammographers will credit ultrasound with being good at: distinguishing cystic from solid. However, level 1 characterization goes further than just assessment of cystic versus solid masses. There are really five separate categories that palpable lumps and mammographic densities can be placed into by level 1 characterization:

1. Normal tissue
2. Simple cystic lesion
3. Complex or complicated cystic lesion
4. Indeterminate cystic or solid lesion
5. Solid lesion

Level 2 characterization goes further, placing each sonographic finding into a risk category for malignancy. These categories were developed for mammography rather than sonography by the American College of Radiology (ACR) to help standardize and improve the quality of mammographic reporting and data analysis within the United States and are referred to as Breast Imaging Reporting and Data System (BIRADS) categories. Although the BIRADS categories were developed for mammography, not ultrasound, we believe that they can and should be applied directly to ultrasound with only minor modifications.

Classification of mammographic findings into BI-RADS categories was instituted to force radiologists to standardize terminology, commit themselves in the official report, prevent unclear reports, and reduce variability between radiologists in reporting of mammographic findings. Additionally, it was hoped that this would enable easy entry of data into databases for analysis of efficacy. Finally, assignment of an ACR BIRADS category was intended to standardize management decisions based on mammographic findings. In our opinion, although not perfect, the ACR BI-RADS categorization has generally been successfully used in mammography. Table 1–1 shows the mammographic ACR BIRADS categories, the descriptive term and risk for malignancy, and management suggestions for each category.

In the United States, characterization of mammographic findings into ACR BIRADS categories is mandatory to achieve Mammography Quality Standards Act (MQSA) accreditation. It is unwise to expect any less from sonography. All complex cystic, indeterminate cystic versus solid, and solid nodules shown on sonography should undergo level 2 characterization into ACR BIRADS categories. Such lesions may be characterized as BIRADS category 2 through category 5. Normal anatomy can be characterized as BIRADS category 1, and simple cysts may all be characterized as BIRADS category 2. Only by rigorously classifying all ultrasound examinations with BIRADS codes and performing long-term follow-up on hundreds or thousands of cases can the true value of showing normal anatomy for palpable lumps or the real risk for malignancy of various types of complex cysts be established. Those of us who have performed breast ultrasound for years feel we have a good subjective feeling for the value of ultrasound in predicting these things, but our subjective feelings to date have been verified only in very small groups of patients. Categorization of every sonographic finding into a BI-RADS category, entry of the finding and its BIRADS category into a database, and either biopsy or long-term sonographic or mammographic follow-up (3 years or more) will be necessary to prove the negative predictive value of sonographically normal findings in large groups of patients.

There is every reason to expect that sonographic BI-RADS categorization will be as successful as it has been mammographically. In fact, we have been prospectively assigning BIRADS risk categories to sonographic findings for several years, accumulating the findings in a database, and correlating with the data histologic findings, and we are now managing patients based on these correlations. For ultrasound, we have adopted a slight variation of the ACR BIRADS categories. We have broken the BIRADS 4 category into two groups: 4a and 4b. We have done this because we feel that the concept of "probable" is important medicolegally. The term probable implies a risk of 50% or greater and is useful to patients and referring physicians in making management decisions as well as being a common legal concept. Thus, our category 4a includes risks from at

TABLE 1–1. AMERICAN COLLEGE OF RADIOLOGY BREAST IMAGING REPORTING AND DATA SYSTEM (BIRADS) MAMMOGRAPHIC RISK CATEGORIES

BIRADS Category	Description	Risk of Malignancy (%)	Management[a]
0[b]	Incomplete, needs additional evaluation	Uncertain	Diagnostic mammograms, ultrasound, etc.
1	Normal	0	Return to routine screening
2	Benign finding	0	Return to routine screening
3	Probably benign	≤2[c]	Patient choice: follow-up versus biopsy
4	Suspicious	>2 and <90	Biopsy
5	Malignant	≥90	Biopsy

[a]Generally suggested management, not rigid requirement.
[b]Typical classification for palpable lump with negative or nonspecific mammograms.
[c]The level of risk for probably benign classification is ≤2% in the United States, a highly litigious society. Elsewhere in the world, in less litigious countries, ≤5% might be a more reasonable risk category for probably benign.

greater than 2% to less than 50%, and category 4b includes risks from at least 50% to less than 90% (Table 1–2). One additional difference between the ACR BIRADS categories and our modified sonographic BIRADS categories is that we rarely use category 0 with ultrasound. We feel that after diagnostic ultrasound, an adjunct to screening or diagnostic mammography in most cases, some definitive management decision is required, not additional imaging. The only time that we use ACR BIRADS category 0 in breast sonography is in young, pregnant, or lactating patients with palpable abnormalities who underwent ultrasound without first undergoing mammography. In such cases, when ultrasound shows a lesion requiring biopsy, we always request mammography before biopsy to make sure that there are not additional lesions requiring diagnosis. Table 1–2 summarizes our variation of the ACR BIRADS risk categories for breast ultrasound.

Each individual sonographic finding should be characterized into a BIRADS category. It is common to have many different ultrasound findings or lesions in the same

TABLE 1–2. MODIFIED AMERICAN COLLEGE OF RADIOLOGY BREAST IMAGING REPORTING AND DATA SYSTEM (BIRADS) ULTRASOUND RISK CATEGORIES

BIRADS Category	Description	Risk of Malignancy (%)	Management[a]
1	Normal	0	Clinical lump follow-up and return to screening
2	Benign finding	0	Clinical lump follow-up and return to screening
3	Probably benign	≤2[b]	Patient choice: follow-up versus biopsy
4a	Mildly suspicious	>2 and <50	Biopsy (additional imaging?)
4b	Moderately suspicious	>50 and <90	Biopsy
5	Malignant	≥90	Biopsy

[a]Generally suggested management, not rigid requirement.
[b]The level of risk for probably benign classification is ≤2% in the United States, a highly litigious society. Elsewhere in the world, in less litigious countries, ≤5% might be a more reasonable risk category for probably benign.

breast. In such cases, the summary BIRADS category for the entire breast should always be the highest BIRADS category in that breast. In other words, if there is a palpable lump caused by sonographically normal-appearing fibrous tissue (BIRADS 1), two mammographic nodules caused by simple cysts (BIRADS 2), and one nodule caused by a probably benign solid nodule (BIRADS 3), the BIRADS category for the entire study should be BIRADS 3.

Each clinical and mammographic finding that is being evaluated has a sonographic finding causing it that needs to be assigned to a BIRADS category, even when the sonographic finding is normal tissue, such as a palpable fibroglandular ridge (BIRADS 1). This discourages the concept of a negative ultrasound. We believe that using the term negative ultrasound examination implies that we are unable to find an explanation for the presenting problem. That is rarely the case. In fact, ultrasound almost always reveals a specific explanation for a palpable lump or mammographic abnormality, and that explanation is frequently normal breast tissues. On the other hand, reporting a "positive ultrasound examination" showing a fibrous ridge to be causing a palpable lump imbues the patient and the referring physician with much more confidence than does a report of a "negative ultrasound examination." Patients and referring physicians are more likely to interpret negative examinations as inadequate and likely to have missed some-

thing and are therefore more likely to demand an unnecessary biopsy.

How BUS changes BIRADS categories can be shown by comparing BIRADS categories assigned by mammography (performed first) and sonography. This can be demonstrated graphically in patients with a combination of palpable lumps and mammographic abnormalities (Fig. 1–1). Note that the peak representing BIRADS categories 1 and 2 (normal and definitively benign findings) is higher after ultrasound is used. The difference in the size of the ultrasound and mammographic peaks for BIRADS 1 and 2 represents the percentage of cases in which ultrasound has made a more specifically benign diagnosis than mammography and in which BUS has likely prevented unnecessary biopsy. Note also that peak 5 (malignant) is increased after ultrasound. Within the difference in the sizes of the mammographic and sonographic peaks for BIRADS category 5 are palpable cancers found by ultrasound and either missed completely or undercharacterized by mammography alone. Note that the middle categories of 3 and 4 (probably benign and suspicious), the least specific categories, for which positive biopsy rates are lowest, are reduced by ultrasound compared with mammography and clinical findings. Within these two peaks are most of the patients who undergo biopsy for benign conditions for whom sonography can potentially obviate unnecessary biopsy. In summary, after

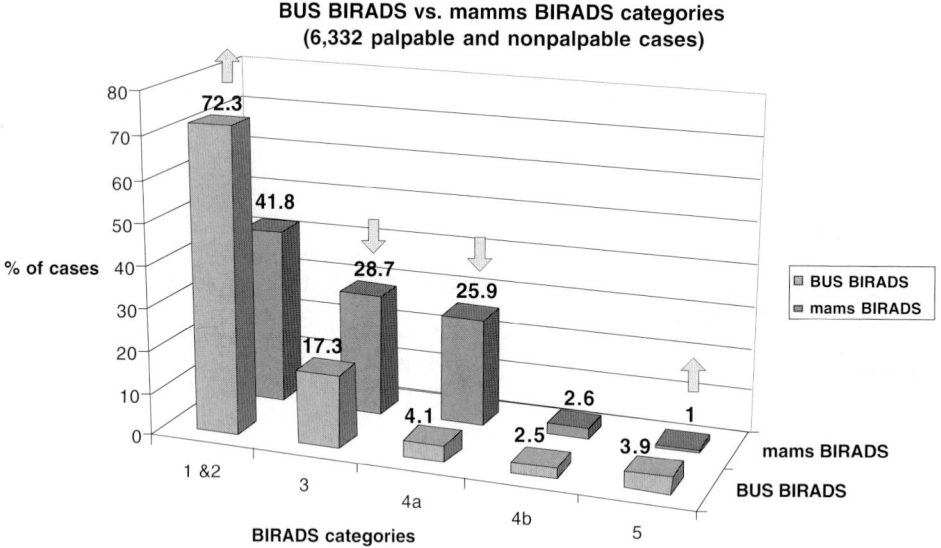

FIGURE 1–1 Comparison of breast ultrasound (BUS) and mammographic BIRADS codes in 6,332 cases that presented to ultrasound because of palpable lumps or mammographic abnormalities. The general goal of diagnostic breast ultrasound is to achieve a more specific diagnosis than can be obtained with mammography and clinical findings alone. Note that ultrasound places more patients into normal or definitively benign categories (BIRADS 1 and 2) than does mammography. Within the difference in the percentage of cases in categories 1 and 2 between ultrasound and mammography are the biopsies potentially prevented. Note also that there are more cases in the definitively malignant category 5 after ultrasound than after mammography alone. The percentage difference between ultrasound and mammography in BIRADS category 5 represents the palpable cancers found by ultrasound that mammography misses. Although the number of definitively benign and definitively malignant findings increases after ultrasound, the number of cases in the intermediate categories, BIRADS 3 and 4a, are reduced. This is especially important in the mammographic BIRADS 4a group (mildly suspicious), in which the positive biopsy result rate is only 10%.

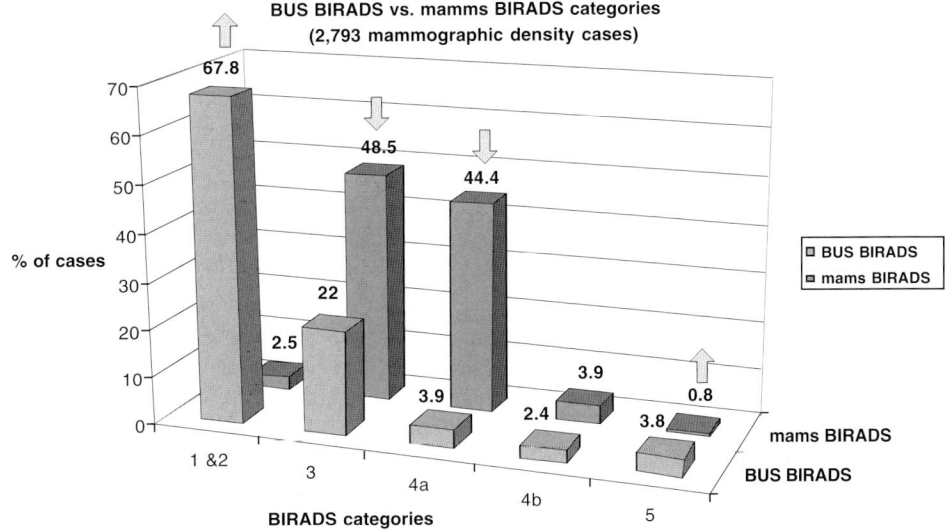

FIGURE 1–2 Comparison of breast ultrasound (BUS) and mammographic BIRADS categories in 2,793 cases that presented to ultrasound for evaluation of nonpalpable mammographic abnormalities shows an even more pronounced trend to more specific diagnoses than are shown in Figure 1–1. After ultrasound, the number of cases in the definitively benign (BIRADS 1 and 2) and definitively malignant (BIRADS 5) categories are greatly increased, and the number of cases in the intermediate-risk categories (BIRADS 3 and 4a) are markedly reduced (mams density = all mammographic abnormality types).

diagnostic breast ultrasound, cases are shifted out of the middle peaks into the more definitively benign (BIRADS 1 and 2) and definitively malignant (BIRADS 5) categories.

Figure 1–2 shows a comparison of the ultrasound and mammographic BIRADS categories when the indication

for BUS is a mammographic abnormality. Note that the effect for mammographic lesions is similar to that for a combination of palpable and mammographic lesions; cases are shifted out of the middle-risk BIRADS 3 and 4 categories into the more definitively benign BIRADS 1 and 2 or more

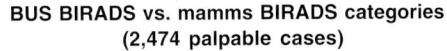
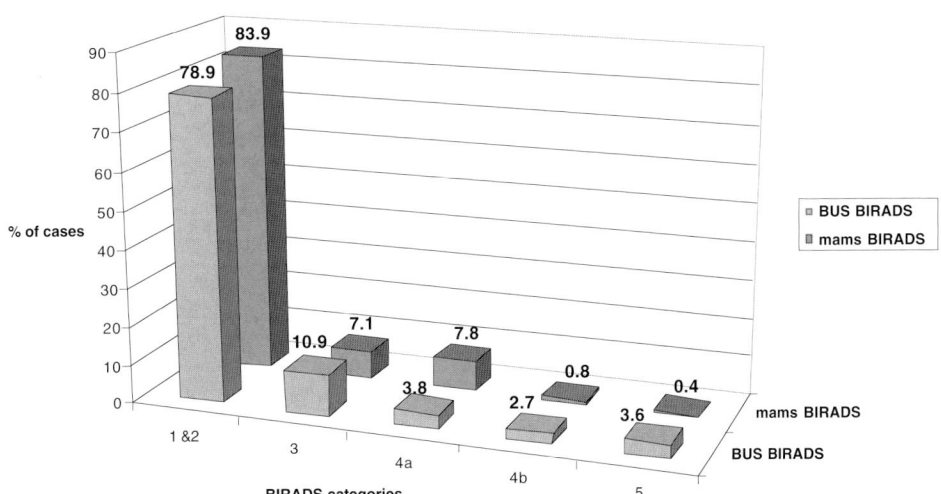

FIGURE 1–3 Comparison of breast ultrasound (BUS) and mammographic BIRADS categories in 2,474 cases that presented with palpable abnormalities shows much less difference in BIRADS categories between ultrasound and mammography than seen with nonpalpable abnormalities. This is largely because the mammogram results are negative in a large percentage of patients who are referred to ultrasound for evaluation of palpable lumps. Comparison of BUS BIRADS categories to all mammographic BIRADS categories together underestimates the difference in BIRADS categories that actually exists in individual cases. To see the magnitude of such differences, it is necessary to compare the BUS BIRADS codes between ultrasound and individual mammographic BIRADS categories one at a time, as shown in Figures 1–4 through 1–8.

definitively malignant BIRADS 5 categories. Figure 1–3 shows a similar comparison of sonographic and mammographic BIRADS categories for palpable lumps only. Note that the shift of cases to BIRADS 1 and 2 categories is unapparent because so many cases of palpable lumps are associated with normal but radiographically dense mammograms. However, this underestimates how different the ultrasound information is from the mammographic information.

If ultrasound BIRADS categories are compared with individual mammographic BIRADS categories one at a time, it can be seen that the ultrasound BIRADS category is dramatically different from the mammographic BIRADS category in a large percentage of cases (Fig. 1–4). Figure 1–5 shows the percentage of cases in which the ultrasound BIRADS code for palpable lesions is different from the mammographic BIRADS category by individual mammographic BIRADS categories for mammographic and palpable abnormalities. The effect on BIRADS category is greatest for BIRADS 3 and 4a lesions, the desired result. Figure 1–6 shows that the effect of BUS on BIRADS category is about the same for palpable and nonpalpable abnormalities, despite the similar appearance of mammographic and sonographic BIRADS categories in Figure 1–3. Figure 1–3 suggests that BUS does not affect BIRADS code for palpable lesions as much as it does for mammographic lesions in Figure 1–2. The reasons for the appearance in Figure 1–2 is that the mammogram is so fre-

quently negative in patients with palpable lumps and that the lump is so frequently caused by fibroglandular tissue that the bars for BIRADS 1 categories overwhelm those of other categories, both for mammography and for BUS. Note also that ultrasound gives the most "bang for the buck" in mammographic categories 3 and 4, especially category 4a, in which targeted ultrasound changed the BIRADS category in most cases for both palpable and mammographic abnormalities.

The importance of BUS showing a lower BIRADS category finding in cases that are characterized as BIRADS 4a by mammography must be emphasized. The positive biopsy rate in BIRADS 4a cases is only 10%. Thus, if a mammographic BIRADS 4a finding can be downgraded to BIRADS 1 or 2 by ultrasound, both biopsy and short-interval follow-up can be avoided. If ultrasound downgrades a mammographic 4a category to BIRADS 3, biopsy can be avoided, but short-interval follow-up will be necessary. Ultrasound has the least value in BIRADS category 5, in which the BIRADS code is the same for mammography and sonography in almost all cases (Fig. 1–4). The role of ultrasound in such cases has been largely to guide needle biopsy, but its role in determining extent of disease in such lesions should not be underestimated. This is especially true when high-resolution three-dimensional magnetic resonance imaging (MRI) is not available. Ultrasound can show unsuspected multifocal and multicentric disease,

(text continued on page 10)

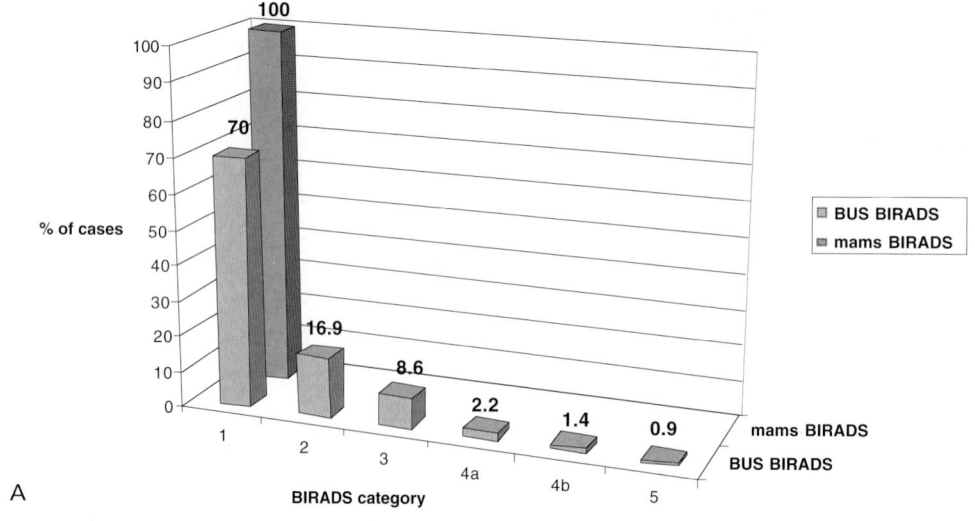

FIGURE 1–4 A: The breast ultrasound (BUS) BIRADS code differs from the mammographic BIRADS category 1 in 30.2% of 2,060 cases that presented to ultrasound for evaluation of palpable lumps with negative mammogram results. *(Continued.)*

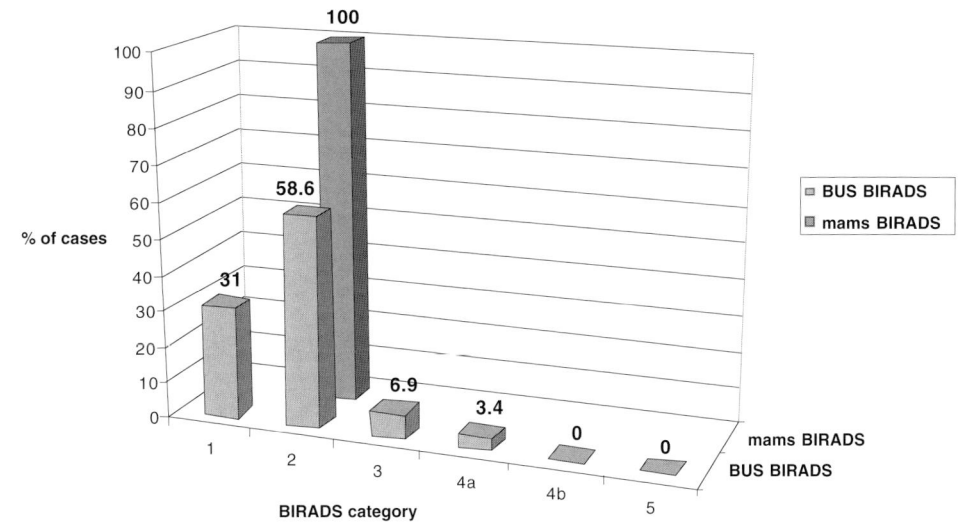

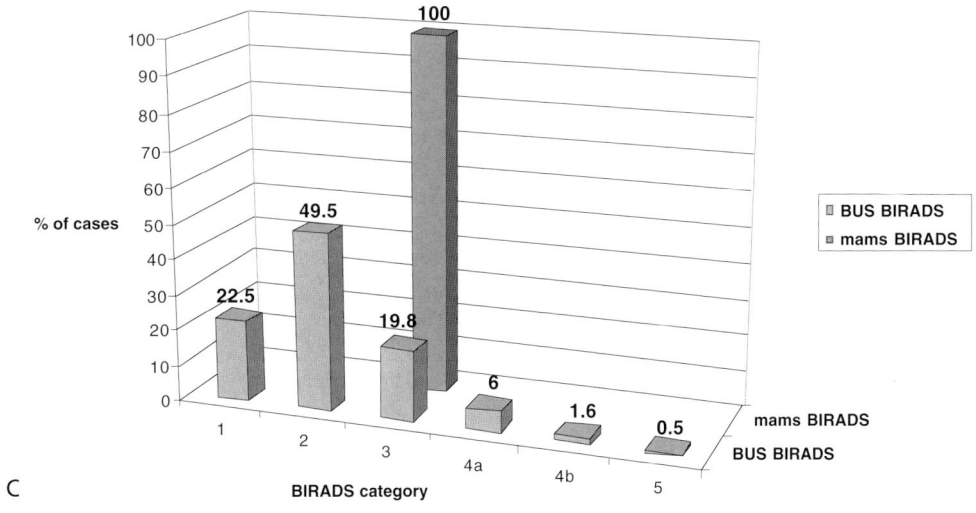

FIGURE 1–4 *(continued)* **B**: The BUS BIRADS code differs from the mammographic BIRAD category 2 in 41.4% of 29 cases that presented to ultrasound for evaluation of palpable lumps and had benign mammographic findings. In most cases, this was not because a lesion had been mischaracterized by mammography; rather, it was because BUS had shown a different lesion from the one classified as benign by mammography. **C**: The BUS BIRADS code differs from the mammographic BIRAD category 3 in 80.2% of 364 cases that presented to ultrasound for evaluation of palpable lumps with mammographic findings classified as probably benign. This graph shows the distribution of BIRADS categories by BUS for all palpable lesions characterized as BIRADS 3 by mammography. *(Continued.)*

BUS BIRADS vs. mamms BIRADS category 4a
(BUS BIRADS different in 87.7% of 332 palpable lumps)

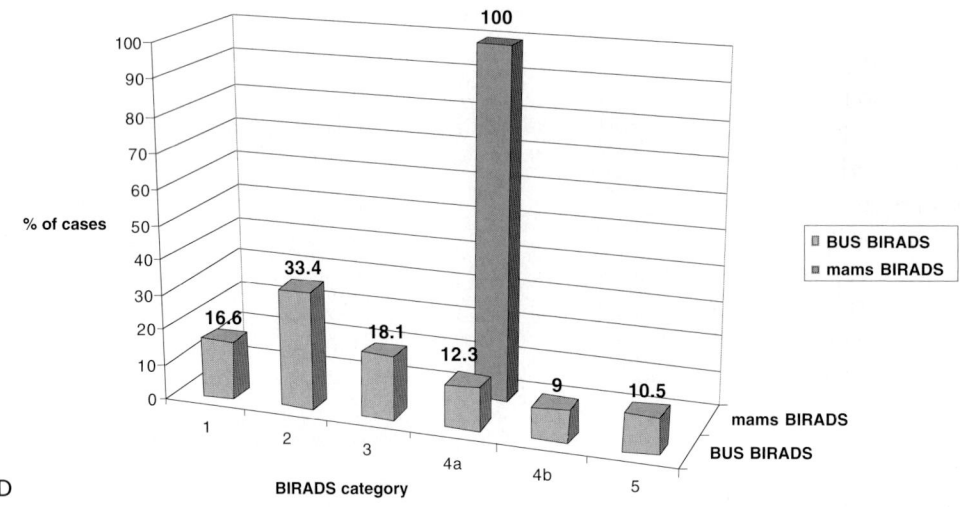

BUS BI-RADS vs. mamms BI-RADS category 4b
(BUS BI-RADS different in 29/7% of 37 palpable lumps)

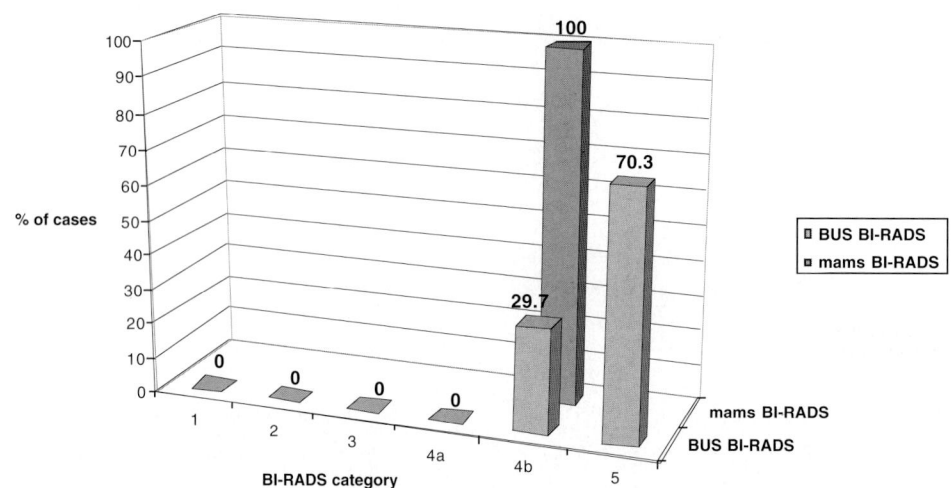

FIGURE 1–4 *(continued)* **D:** The BUS BIRADS code differs from the mammographic BIRAD category 4a in 87.7% of 332 cases that presented to ultrasound for evaluation of palpable lumps with mammographic findings classified as mildly suspicious. **E:** The BUS BIRADS code differs from the mammographic BIRAD category 4b in 29.7% of 37 cases that presented to ultrasound for evaluation of palpable lumps with mammographic findings classified as moderately suspicious.

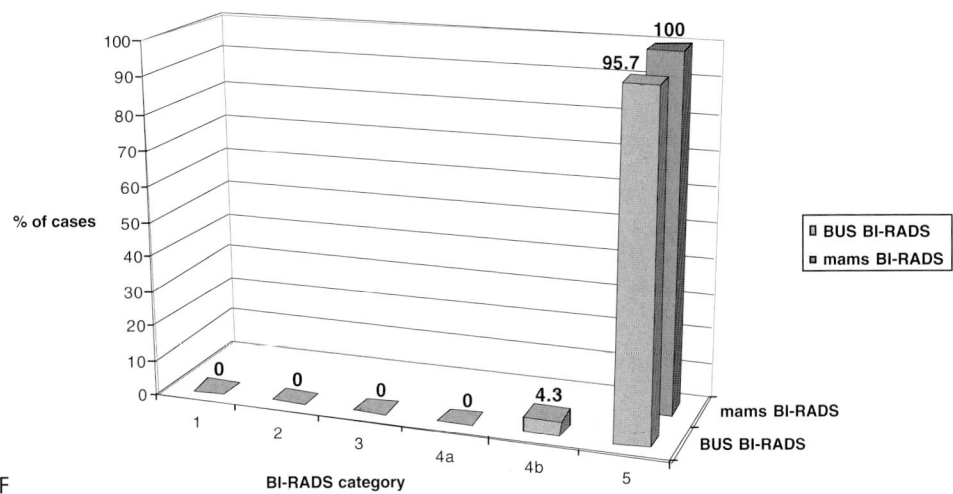

BUS BI-RADS vs. mamms BI-RADS category 5
(BUS BI-RADS different in 4.3% of 23 palpable lumps)

F

FIGURE 1–4 *(continued)* **F:** The BUS BIRADS code differs from the mammographic BIRAD category 5 in only 4.3% of 23 cases that presented to ultrasound for evaluation of palpable lumps and also had mammographic findings classified as malignant.

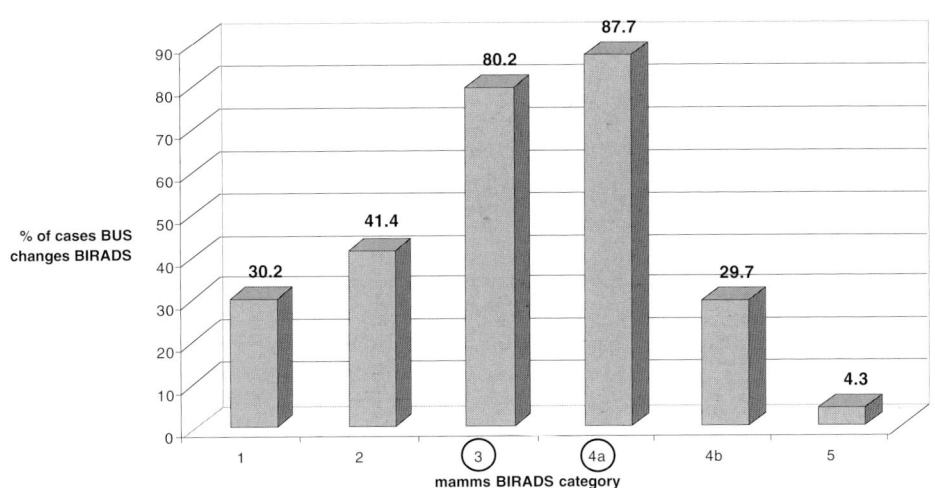

% of times BUS BIRADS differs from mamms BIRADS by BIRADS category
(2,845 cases of palpable lumps)

FIGURE 1–5 This graph shows the percentage of time the BUS BIRADS code differs from the mammographic BIRADS code. This graph summarizes Figures 1–1 through 1–4. Note that, despite the suggestion in Figure 1–3 that BUS and mammographic BIRADS codes are not greatly different, for patients presenting with palpable lumps as a group, they do differ greatly when assessed by individual mammographic BIRADS category. The greatest change in BIRADS categories occurs for mammographic BIRADS 4a cases, in which the category is changed 87.7% of the time; and it has the least effect in the mammographic BIRAD category 5, in which the risk category is changed in only 4.3% of 23 cases.

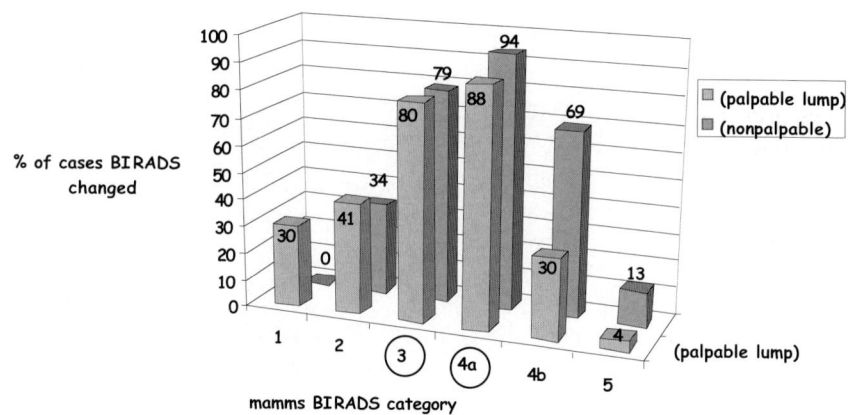

% of cases where BUS BIRADS differs from mamms BIRADS by mamms BIRADS category

FIGURE 1–6 This graph compares the percentage of the time that the BUS BIRADS category differs from the mammographic BIRADS category for each individual BIRADS category in patients presenting with palpable and mammographic abnormalities. Note that, despite the apparently little effect of BUS on the BIRADS codes for palpable abnormalities shown Figure 1–3, BUS actually changes the BIRADS code for palpable abnormalities almost as much as it does for mammographic abnormalities. BUS changes the BIRADS code and gives the most "bang for the buck" when used to evaluate abnormalities classified in intermediate-risk BIRADS categories 3 or 4a, regardless of whether the presenting abnormality is palpable or mammographic.

extensive intraductal components extending out from the invasive portion of the lesion, and nodal metastases in many cases, altering both the diagnostic and therapeutic algorithms.

Specific Goals of Breast Ultrasound

Although the general role of BUS is to make a more specific diagnosis than could be made with clinical and mammographic findings, there are also more specific goals for BUS (Table 1–3), which are described in the following sections.

TABLE 1–3. SPECIFIC GOALS OF DIAGNOSTIC BREAST ULTRASOUND

Prevent unnecessary negative biopsies

Prevent unnecessary short-interval follow-up

Guide interventional procedures

Improve clinical skills

Improve mammographic interpretive skills

Find cancer that was missed or underclassified by mammography

Stage cancers; determine extent of malignant disease

Preventing Unnecessary Biopsy

Ultrasound can help prevent biopsy in almost all cases when it shows BIRADS 1 or 2 findings causing a palpable or mammographic abnormality and in most cases when it shows BIRADS 3 findings as the cause. Figure 1–1 shows that, after ultrasound, the number of cases characterized as BIRADS 1 or 2 increases for both mammographic and palpable abnormalities. The only time BIRADS 1 or 2 findings on ultrasound may not be reassuring in the presence of a higher mammographic BIRADS category is when they are used to evaluate isolated mammographic calcifications characterized as BIRADS category 4a or higher. In such cases, stereotactically guided mammotomy is performed regardless of ultrasound findings. Thus, the use of ultrasound to avoid biopsy is limited to its evaluation of palpable lumps and mammographic soft tissue densities, not isolated calcifications on mammography.

Several studies have now shown the negative predictive value of sonographic BIRADS 1 studies to be between 99% and 100%, although all of these studies have evaluated relatively small groups of patients.

Preventing Unnecessary Short-Interval Follow-Up Examinations

The usual management of BIRADS 3 findings is to offer the patient a choice between biopsy and short-interval follow-up until long-term stability of the finding can be established, at which time it can be downgraded to BIRADS 2. The usual management of a BIRADS 1 or 2 finding is a return to routine screening. Short-interval follow-up mammography can be prevented by ultrasound in cases in which mammographic findings are characterized as BIRADS 3, but ultrasound shows the cause to be more definitively benign BIRADS 1 or 2 findings. How often ultrasound can achieve this in patients presenting with mammographic abnormalities or palpable lumps is shown in Figures 1–4c and 1–7, respectively. In patients with mammogram results classified as BIRADS 3, ultrasound often shows BIRADS 1 or 2 findings, and short-interval follow-up can be avoided in 72% of patients presenting with a palpable abnormality and in 74.9% of patients presenting with nonpalpable mammographic abnormalities. The use of ultrasound to evaluate mammographic BIRADS 3 findings has been controversial. However, by obviating the need for short-interval follow-up in almost three-fourths of patients, we feel justified in performing targeted diagnostic breast ultrasound in patients with BIRADS 3 findings on mammography, regardless of whether the indication is a palpable or a mammographic nodule or soft tissue density.

Guiding Needle Procedures

Ultrasound is used to guide the following needle procedures:

- Cyst aspiration
- Abscess drainage
- Biopsy [fine-needle aspiration biopsy, large core biopsy (also called ABBI: Advanced Breast Biopsy Instrumentation), mammotomy]

- Needle localization for surgical excision
- Galactography
- Sentinel node procedures
- Treatment of malignancies (radiofrequency, laser, cryotherapy, thermal)

Ultrasound-guided interventional procedures are discussed in detail in Chapter 17.

Improving Clinical Examination Skills by Palpating while Scanning Palpable Lesions

Palpating all palpable lesions while simultaneously scanning them will eventually improve clinical skills in anyone performing breast ultrasound. This is discussed in greater detail in Chapter 5.

Improving Mammographic Skills by Correlating Mammographic and Sonographic Findings

Mammographic skills will be improved by carefully correlating the following mammographic and sonographic findings for every nonpalpable mammographic abnormality evaluated:

- Size
- Shape
- Location
- Surrounding tissue density

Sonographic–mammographic correlation is discussed in greater detail in Chapter 6.

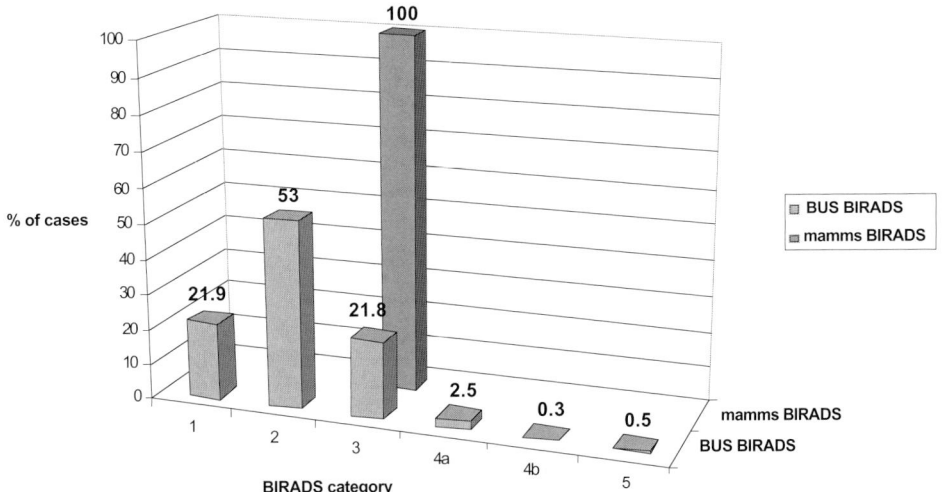

BUS BIRADS vs. mamms BIRADS category 3
(BUS BIRADS different in 78.2% of 1,373 nonpalpable mammographic lesions)

FIGURE 1–7 This graph demonstrates that BUS shows BIRADS 1 or 2 findings 78.2% of the time in patients who present with mammographic BIRADS 3 findings. Short-interval follow-up can be averted.

Detecting Some Palpable Cancers Missed By Mammography

Those who perform diagnostic BUS should routinely find carcinomas that are missed or undercharacterized by mammography. Most of these will be palpable carcinomas that are surrounded and obscured by dense tissues on the mammogram. Figure 1–8 shows sonographic versus mammographic BIRADS categories for palpable carcinomas. Note that 26% (34 of 132) of palpable carcinomas were missed mammographically and that another 4% (5 of 132) were undercharacterized as BIRADS 3 by mammography. That ultrasound routinely shows carcinomas missed by mammography should not be surprising. It is well known that mammographic sensitivity is reduced in women with dense breast tissue because dense tissue that surrounds a cancer may obscure it on mammograms. What our data indicate is that, in a carefully selected subset of all mammographic patients (i.e., those who have palpable lumps in areas of the breast that contain dense tissues on mammography), sonography can find cancers that are missed mammographically. Additionally, in all cases that were undercharacterized as BI-RADS 3 by mammography, the lesion was partially obscured by dense tissues. Thus, sonographic detection of carcinomas missed or undercharacterized by mammography does not represent a condemnation of mammography; rather, it demonstrates proper selection of a subset of patients in which mammographic sensitivity is known to be reduced.

BUS used in a targeted mode finds carcinomas that are neither palpable nor mammographically visible in only a small percentage of cases for the simple reason that the indications for targeted diagnostic BUS usually include the presence of either a palpable lump or a mammographic abnormality. Thus, we should not expect to find carcinomas that are neither palpable nor mammographically visible often when using BUS in a targeted diagnostic mode. (Secondary screening BUS is a completely different situation.) In our series, 8% of carcinomas that were found by targeted diagnostic BUS were neither palpable nor mammographically visible. In all cases, these incidental carcinomas were "second" lesions that existed in addition to normal tissue or to the benign lesion that caused the palpable or mammographic abnormality.

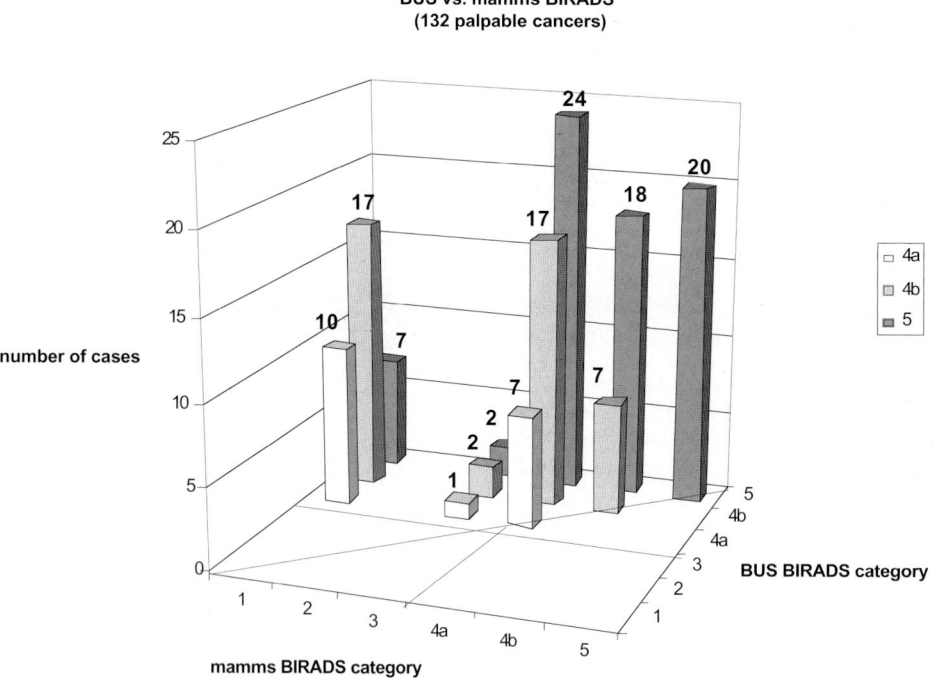

FIGURE 1–8 This figure compares breast ultrasound (BUS) and mammographic BIRADS categories for 132 palpable breast carcinomas. It demonstrates cancers found by ultrasound but either missed or underclassified by mammography. There are 34 cases (26%) in which the ultrasound showed BIRADS 4a or higher category and the mammogram result was negative. The three peaks along the left side of the graph represent cases with mammographic false-negative results. There were also five cases (4%) in which the mammogram was characterized as BIRADS 3 and BUS showed 4a or higher category. Note that these cases represent a highly selected subset of all cancers. These are cases in which there is a palpable lump as well as water-density tissue in the area of the lump on mammography that could obscure a noncalcified benign or malignant nodule; that is, these cases are preselected for ultrasound because there is a relatively high risk for false-negative mammography results.

Staging BIRADS 4b and 5 Lesions

Sonographic assessment of the extent of malignant disease, detection of multifocal and multicentric disease, detection of extensive intraductal components, and assessment of regional lymph nodes can be valuable. In our experience, contrast-enhanced MRI with the RODEO (rotating delivery excitation off-resonance) sequence is the best locoregional staging tool we have (positron emission tomography is best for assessing distant metastases); however, second-look sonography is usually necessary for ultrasound-guided biopsy mapping of extent of disease and preoperative localization. During the initial diagnostic BUS exam, there is an opportunity to obviate staging MRI and sentinel lymph node procedures. Sonographic assessment of extent of disease is discussed in detail in Chapter 14, and assessment of regional lymph nodes is discussed in Chapter 19.

Targeted Indications for Breast Ultrasound

The two main classes of BUS indications are nontargeted and targeted. Nontargeted examinations are usually screening examinations but occasionally may be used diagnostically when lesions are so numerous that only whole breast ultrasound can be used to evaluate them or when a structure (such as a breast implant) is so large that it encompasses virtually the entire breast. Targeted ultrasound examinations are always diagnostic and are used to evaluate palpable abnormalities and mammographic abnormalities that are classified as probably benign or suspicious (BI-RADS categories 3, 4a, and 4b). Category 5 mammographic lesions are also often scanned for purposes of staging when high-quality MRI is not available or for ultrasound-guided needle localization, sentinel node injection, or ultrasound-guided biopsy.

Most BUS examinations are performed for one of the above two reasons. This is appropriate because ultrasound is best at evaluating focal breast problems. In our practice, 90% of all BUS examinations are targeted toward improved diagnosis of either a palpable or mammographic abnormality or an area of focal pain. Another 6% of the scans are performed for follow-up of lesions previously shown on ultrasound, and 2% are targeted to evaluation of nipple discharge. Only 2% are nontargeted examinations. Table 1–4 shows a list of indications for a consecutive series of the last 11,433 BUS studies performed in our department.

Breast Ultrasound Targeted Toward Palpable Abnormalities

The mammographic density of the tissues in the area of the palpable abnormality should be taken into account before performing BUS. If the entire breast is replaced by fat, there is little or no chance that the mammogram will miss an abnormality that the sonogram will show, and therefore, BUS need not be performed to evaluate the lump if the lump is larger than pea-sized. The lump will invariably be due to a palpable fat lobule (sometimes called *nodular adiposity*) or a lipoma, neither of which requires evaluation other than mammography. On the other hand, if the breasts are mammographically dense, there is a good chance that the dense tissues will have obscured the cause of the palpable abnormality and, therefore, a good chance that sonography will demonstrate a cause of the lump that mammography has not been able to demonstrate. Even in patients who have mixed breast density—those whose breasts are not entirely fatty or entirely dense—the decision about whether to perform diagnostic targeted BUS should be based on the density of tissue in the vicinity of the palpable lump. Sonographic evaluation of palpable abnormalities is discussed in greater detail in Chapter 5.

Breast Ultrasound Targeted Toward Further Evaluation of Mammographic Abnormalities

BUS should also be done to evaluate lesions characterized mammographically as probably benign or suspicious (BI-RADS 3, 4a, or 4b). BUS of probably benign lesions may obviate biopsy, aspiration, or short-interval follow-up when the lesion is sonographically characterized as BI-RADS 2. Mammographic management of BIRADS 3 cases is either short-interval follow-up or intervention. Management of BIRADS 2 findings is return to routine screening. Thus, ultrasound may obviate the need for intervention or short-interval follow-up when it shows BIRADS 2 findings in a case that was characterized as BIRADS 3 mammographically. On the other hand, BUS of BIRADS 3 lesions may occasionally show a solid nodule with malignant or atypical features that would be characterized as BIRADS 4a, 4b, or 5 and that would require biopsy in a patient who might otherwise be recommended for follow-up, thus expediting the definitive diagnosis of malignancy. Sonographic assessment of and correlation with mammographic abnormalities is discussed in detail in Chapter 6.

TABLE 1–4. INDICATIONS FOR A CONSECUTIVE SERIES OF 11,433 BREAST ULTRASOUND STUDIES

Palpable abnormality	5,282 cases (46.2%)
Mammographic abnormality	3,681 cases (32.2%)
Mammographic and palpable abnormalities	606 cases (5.3%)
Follow-up of known ultrasound lesions	697 cases (6.1%)
Pain	686 cases (6.0%)
Secretions	252 cases (2.2%)
Nontargeted whole breast ultrasound	229 cases (2.0%)
TOTAL	11,433 cases (100.0%)

Role of Nontargeted Whole Breast Ultrasound

On occasion, nontargeted unilateral or bilateral whole breast ultrasound may be indicated. The following is a list of potential indications:

- Unilateral spontaneous bloody or serous secretions
- Evaluation of silicone implants in patients without palpable or mammographic abnormalities to detect implant rupture
- Patient refusal to undergo mammography because of radiation phobia
- Known metastases of breast origin, but radiographically dense, negative mammograms
- Known breast cancer, but question of multicentricity or tumor extent before conservative surgical treatment (staging)
- Follow-up of numerous sonographic lesions
- Secondary adjunct to screening mammography in patients with strong family history or *BRCA1* gene and radiographically dense but negative mammogram results

Nontargeted whole breast ultrasound is discussed in detail in Chapter 7. Nontargeted assessment of nipple discharge is discussed in Chapter 8, and nontargeted assessment of implants is discussed in Chapter 9.

SUMMARY

BUS has not proved efficacious as a primary screening tool for breast cancer. Nevertheless, it is an effective and invaluable diagnostic modality for evaluation of breast disease. The general goal of diagnostic BUS is to make a more specific diagnosis than could be made with clinical and mammographic findings alone in carefully selected patients. This involves not only detecting some cancers missed by clinical or mammographic examination, but also, far more commonly, preventing unnecessary biopsy by showing normal tissue or definitively benign lesions. Furthermore, sonography is an excellent tool for guiding needle procedures to diagnose, localize, or treat lesions found by ultrasound. Careful correlation of clinical and mammographic findings with sonographic findings in all patients eventually improves the examiner's clinical and mammographic interpretive skills. BUS is most effective when targeted toward a palpable abnormality or a focal mammographic abnormality, which constitute most indications for breast sonography. It may also be helpful in some patients with secretions or silicone implants. There are some indications for nontargeted whole breast ultrasound, but contrast-enhanced MRI or sestamibi studies may supplant BUS for most of these indications. Because MRI is sensitive but has a high false-positive result rate, BUS may still be useful in evaluating focal areas of abnormal contrast enhancement demonstrated by MRI and in

guiding either localization or biopsy of the MRI-demonstrated lesions, so-called second-look ultrasound.

Mammography remains the only imaging modality of proven value in primary screening for breast cancer. However, the role of breast sonography as an adjunct to mammography in secondarily screening women with mammographically dense tissue (in whom the sensitivity of mammograms is lower) is being reexplored with newer, high-resolution real-time equipment and improved scan techniques and looks promising.

SUGGESTED READINGS

Bassett LW, Kimme-Smith C. Breast sonography: technique, equipment, and normal anatomy. *Semin Ultrasound CT MR* 1989;10: 82–89.

Bassett LW, Kimme-Smith C, Sutherland LK, et al. Automated and hand-held breast US: effect on patient management [published erratum appears in *Radiology* 1988;167:582]. *Radiology* 1987; 165:103–108.

Bird RE, Wallace TW, Yankaskas BC. Analysis of cancers missed at screening mammography. *Radiology* 1992;184:613–617.

Cole-Beuglet C, et al. Ultrasound mammography: a comparison with radiographic mammography. *Radiology* 1981;139:693–698.

DeVere C. Current status of ultrasonic breast scanning. *Appl Radiol Ultrasound* 1980;Nov-Dec:145–149.

Egan RL, Egan KL. Detection of breast carcinoma: comparison of automated water-path whole-breast sonography, mammography, and physical examination. *AJR Am J Roentgenol* 1984;143:493–497.

Egan RL, Egan KL. Automated water-path full-breast sonography: correlation with histology of 176 solid lesions. *AJR Am J Roentgenol* 1984;143:499–507.

Farria DM, Mund DF, Bassett LW. Evaluation of missed cancers using screening mammography. *AJR Am J Roentgenol* 1995;126: 1645[abst].

Fletcher SW, Black W, Harris R, et al. Report of the international workshop on screening for breast cancer. *J Natl Cancer Inst* 1993; 85:1644–1656.

Giusseppetti GM, Rizatto G, Gozzi G, et al. Role of ultrasonics in the diagnosis of subclinical carcinoma of the breast. *Radiol Med* (Turin) 1989;78:339–442.

Guyer PB, Dewbury KC. Ultrasound of the breast in the symptomatic and x-ray dense breast. *Clin Radiol* 1985;36:69–76.

Heywang SH, et al. Advantages and pitfalls of ultrasound in the diagnosis of breast cancer. *J Clin Ultrasound* 1985;13:525–532.

Hilton SV, et al. Real-time breast sonography: application in 300 consecutive patients. *AJR Am J Roentgenol* 1986;147:479–486.

Jackson VP, et al. Automated breast sonography using a 7.5-MHz PVDF transducer: preliminary clinical evaluation. Work in progress. *Radiology* 1986;159:679–684.

Kaizer L, et al. Ultrasonographically defined parenchymal patterns of the breast: relationship to mammographic patterns and other risk factors for breast cancer. *Br J Radiol* 1988;61:118–124.

Kimme-Smith C, Bassett LW, Gold RH. High frequency breast ultrasound. Hand-held versus automated units: examination for palpable mass versus screening. *J Ultrasound Med* 1988;7:77–81.

Kolb TM, Kichy J, Newhouse JH. Occult cancer in women with dense breasts: detection with screening US—diagnostic yield and tumor characteristics. *Radiology* 1998;207:191–199.

Kopans DB, Meyer JE, Lindfors KK. Whole-breast US imaging: four-year follow-up. *Radiology* 1985;157:505–507.

Ma L, Fishell E, Wright B, et al. Case control study of factors associated with failure to detect breast cancer missed by mammography. *J Natl Cancer Inst* 1992;84:781–785.

Madjar H, et al. Value of high resolution sonography in breast cancer screening. *Ultraschall Med* 1994;15:20–23.

Maturo VG, et al. Ultrasound of the whole breast utilizing a dedicated automated breast scanner. *Radiology* 1980;137:457–463.

McCaffrey JF, et al. The abnormal mammogram—what to do. *Aust Fam Physician* 1991;20:1431–1435.

McSweeney MB, Murphy CH. Whole-breast sonography. *Radiol Clin North Am* 1985;23:157–167.

Rothschild P, Kimme-Smith C, Bassett LW, et al. Ultrasound breast examination of asymptomatic patients with normal but radiodense mammograms. *Ultrasound Med Biol* 1988;1:113–119.

Rubin E, et al. Hand-held real-time breast sonography. *AJR Am J Roentgenol* 1985;144:623–627.

Sickles EA, Filly RA, Callen PW. Breast cancer detection with sonography and mammography: comparison using state-of-the-art equipment. *AJR Am J Roentgenol* 1983;140:843–845.

Smart CR, Hendrick RE, Rutledge JH III, et al. Benefit of mammography screening in women ages 40 to 49 years. *Cancer* 1995; 75:1619–1626.

Vilaro MM, Kurtz AB, Needleman L, et al. Hand-held and automated sonomammography: clinical role relative to x-ray mammography. *J Ultrasound Med* 1989;8:95–100.

2

BREAST ULTRASOUND EQUIPMENT REQUIREMENTS

The intention of this chapter is to present only enough ultrasound physics and engineering concepts to help the user choose appropriate ultrasound systems and transducers for performing breast ultrasound (BUS).

The technical requirements for high-quality BUS are as great as or greater than those for any other tissue in the body. High-quality BUS requires excellent resolution very close to the skin (in the near field). The ultrasound transducer must also be specifically designed to perform *high-resolution, near-field imaging*. An electronically focused, linear array configuration with nominal center frequency of 7 MHz or higher is a minimum requirement (accreditation by the American College of Radiology, the American College of Surgeons, and the American Institute of Ultrasound in Medicine requires a minimum center frequency of 7 MHz). A short-axis plane (elevation plane) focal length close to the skin is also required. Most 5-MHz linear and curved array transducers are designed for imaging tissues that lie deeper than normal breast tissues, are focused too deeply in the short-axis plane, and therefore do not perform adequately in the breast.

Breast sonography requires both excellent spatial and excellent contrast resolution (Table 2–1).

SPATIAL RESOLUTION

Spatial resolution depends on both lateral and axial resolution. Lateral resolution is the resolution in the X and Y planes, whereas axial resolution is the resolution in the Z (depth) plane. Thus, there are three axes (long axis and short axis of the transducer and depth) and two planes (lateral and axial) that must be considered when discussing spatial resolution (Fig. 2–1).

Lateral Resolution (Long-Axis Electronic Focusing)

To achieve high-quality BUS, resolution in the two axes of the transducer—along the long and the short axes (elevation axis)—must be maximized. In an electronically focused linear array transducer, the individual transducer elements are placed side by side along the long axis of the probe and oriented perpendicular to the long axis (Fig. 2–2). When multiple elements transmit or receive together in an array, the beam can be electronically steered to focus along the long axis of the transducer. The more elements in the array that can be activated simultaneously while transmitting or receiving, the larger the aperture of the transducer, the tighter the focus, and the narrower the beam width that can be achieved. In general, each transducer element requires a channel. Thus, systems with more hardware channels can generally use more elements simultaneously to create a larger sonographic aperture and better long-axis lateral resolution. However, by using elegant multiplexing schemes, it is possible to transmit or receive on multiple different elements simultaneously while using a single hardware channel. Such multiplexing algorithms enable some systems that have fewer hardware channels to achieve apertures and beam widths that are quite competitive for high-resolution BUS with systems that have more hardware channels.

B-mode imaging ultrasound is pulsed ultrasound. A pulse is transmitted for a brief period of time, and the transducer then "listens" for a period of time. Most manufacturers do an excellent job of electronically and dynamically focusing during the listening period ("focusing on receive") along the long axis of the probe. The returning echoes can be focused at several different depths along the beam. When the focal depths are numerous and close enough together that they overlap, the return-

TABLE 2–1. NEAR-FIELD IMAGING RESOLUTION

Spatial resolution
  Lateral resolution
    Long-axis plane
      Electronic receive focus
      Electronic transmit focus
    Short-axis plane (elevation plane)
      Fixed acoustic lens
      Two-dimensional or 1.5-dimensional array
  Axial resolution

Contrast resolution

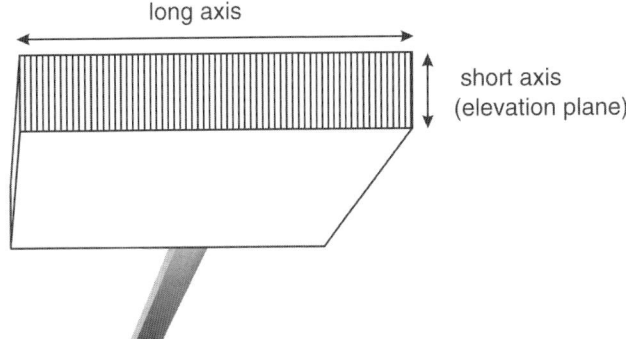

FIGURE 2–2 The elements of a conventional 1-D linear array transducer are arranged side by side along the length of the transducer, which is only one element wide. Electronic focusing along the long axis is achieved by electronically steering or phasing the beam and requires multiple elements. By using complex algorithms and multiple transmit zones, the beam can be focused electronically over a wide range of depths simultaneously (i.e., can be continuously dynamically focused). The more elements involved in focusing, the larger the aperture and the tighter the focus achievable. Because conventional 1-D linear arrays are only one element wide, they cannot be electronically focused in the short axis and require a fixed acoustic lens focused at a single depth.

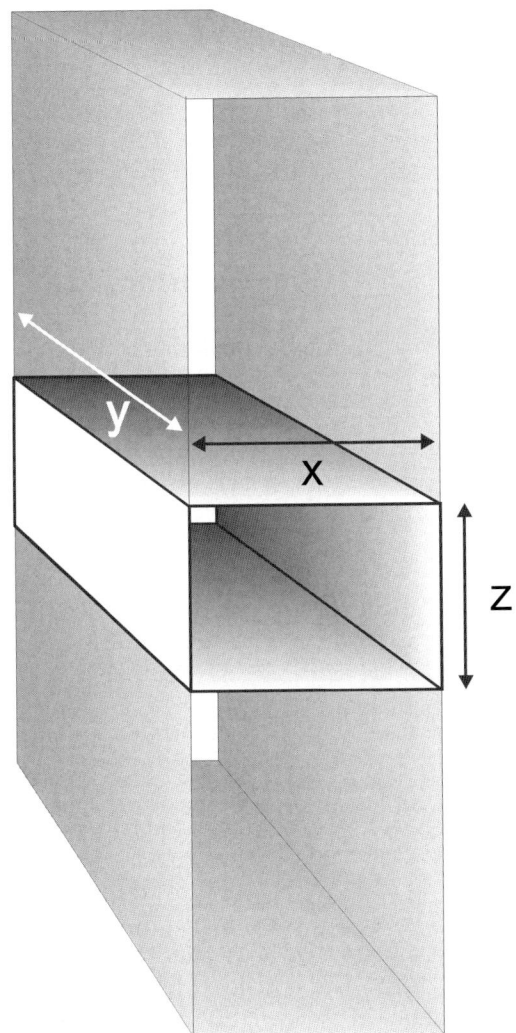

FIGURE 2–1 High-resolution ultrasound must have good spatial resolution in three planes: the Y plane, representing the lateral resolution parallel to the long axis of the transducer; the X plane, representing lateral resolution in the axis parallel to the short axis (elevation axis) of the transducer; and the Z plane, representing the axial resolution. The long-axis lateral resolution is related to aperture size, element size, number of channels and elements, and electronic focusing in both receive and transmit modes. The short-axis lateral resolution depends mainly on depth and focal length of the acoustic lens in conventional 1-D arrays. It depends somewhat on electronic focusing and complex lens shapes in 1.5-D arrays. The axial resolution depends on frequency of the transducer and bandwidth of the beam. Bandwidth is controlled by the transducer material and pulse length.

ing acoustic signal essentially becomes continuously focused on receive. In fact, most manufacturers now offer "continuous dynamic electronic focusing on receive" (Fig. 2–3). Continuous focusing on receive maximizes the lateral resolution and minimizes the beam width both closer to the skin and at depth than do other focus-on-receive algorithms.

Most manufacturers provide additional "focusing on transmit" in one or more zones. There can also be continuous electronic focusing through the area of interest during transmission ("dynamic electronic focusing on transmit"). Adding electronic focusing on transmission to dynamic electronic focusing on receive improves beam width slightly—probably in the range of 10% to 15%. In general, the more transmit focal zones that are used, the greater the depth over which long-axis lateral resolution can be optimized. However, the number of transmit focal zones is limited by frame rates because frame rate drops as the number of transmit zones is increased. In our experience, once frame rates slow to 10 or 12 frames per second (Hertz), no additional focal zones can be used. Depending on the depth of field, most systems limit the user to three or four transmitted focal zones before the frame rate becomes unacceptably slow. However, a few currently available systems can maintain a frame rate of 12 frames per second or higher, with many more than four transmit focal zones. Of course, when the number of focal zones during transmission is limited, it is important for the user to adjust the depth of the focal zones to the specific area of interest. It is not unusual to have to move transmit focal zones several times during the course of a BUS study as the depth of the area of interest changes.

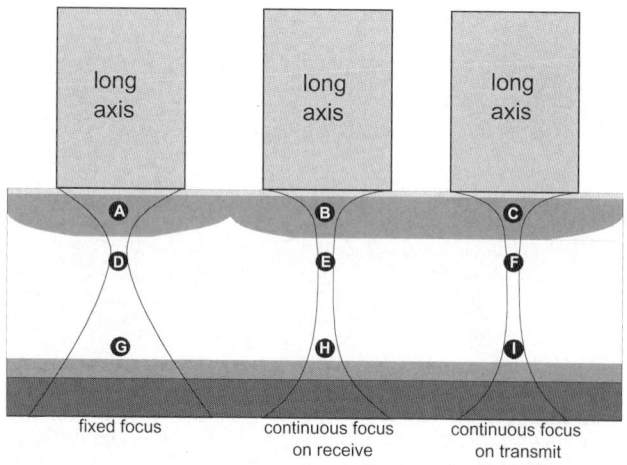

fixed focus   continuous focus on receive   continuous focus on transmit and receive

FIGURE 2–3 This figure illustrates the long-axis focusing characteristics of various transducer configurations. On the **left** is a fixed-focus transducer. Such transducers are obsolete and have been replaced with the **middle** or **right** configuration. Fixed focusing in the long axis must be distinguished from a fixed focal length in the short axis. All conventional 1-D linear transducers have a fixed focal length in the short axis. The **middle** configuration represents the long-axis beam profile of a beam that is dynamically focused on receive. The beam has a narrow profile at a wide range of depths, although the beam width is wider in the very near field before the beam has had time to become focused and in the far field where aperture size, scatter, and attenuation limit the degree of focusing. The configuration shown on the **right** represents continuous dynamic focusing on both transmit and receive. The beam width is improved by a small percentage, and the depth over which this happens is determined by the number of focal zones used on transmission. The rate-limiting step is the frame rate. As the number of transmission focal zones is increased, the frame rate decreases. Once the frame rate drops below 10 to 12 Hz, the image assumes a windshield wiper–like and unacceptably slow frame rate.

Most manufacturers offer excellent electronic focusing during both transmit and receive along the long axis of the transducer. Although there are some differences in long-axis focusing algorithms between various systems, most are quite adequate, in this respect, for performing diagnostic BUS. However, there are significant differences in the capabilities of various transducers and systems between their short-axis focusing capabilities, axial resolution, and contrast resolution.

Lateral Resolution (Short-Axis Focusing)

Electronic focusing is possible in the long axis but is not possible in the short axis (elevation axis) for conventional transducers that are only one element wide (in the short axis). When the short axis of the transducer is only one element wide, beam steering cannot be employed to allow electronic focusing in that plane. Rather, short-axis focusing requires a fixed acoustic lens that must be installed on the transducer at the time it is constructed and before it is delivered to the end-user. For any given transducer, the manufacturer must decide what the most common applications will be in order to determine the appropriate focal

length (depth) of the short-axis acoustic lens. The 5-MHz linear probes are built to perform peripheral vascular Doppler, which requires the fixed acoustic lens to be focused at about 3 to 4 cm (the depth at which the carotid, femoral, and popliteal arteries commonly lie). A focal depth of 3 to 4 cm is too deep for BUS in most patients, who when scanned in the supine position, have breasts that are 3 cm or less in thickness. The short axis focal zone of 5-MHz transducers falls within the chest wall deep to the breast tissues rather than within the breast in most patients. Within breast tissues, which lie superficial to the short-axis focal length of 5 MHz transducers, the ultrasound beam is too wide, resulting in volume averaging (slice thickness artifact) of surrounding breast tissues with small near-field pathologic lesions (Fig. 2–4). Volume aver-

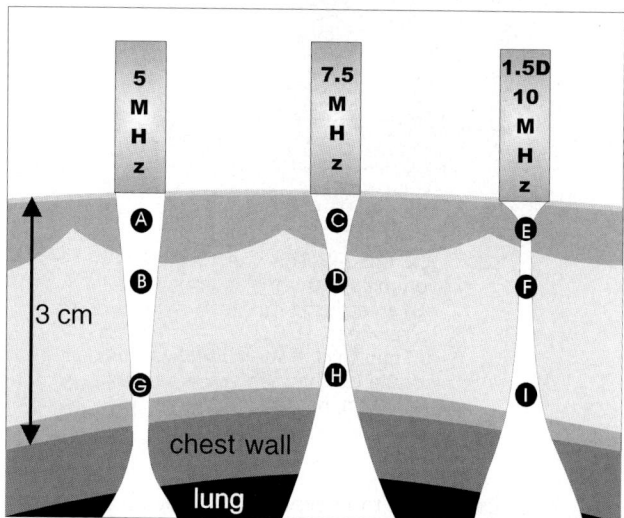

FIGURE 2–4 This figure shows short-axis beam profiles for various transducer configurations. On the **left** is the beam profile of a typical 5-MHz linear transducer designed to perform peripheral vascular ultrasound. Most transducers designed for peripheral vascular applications have an acoustic lens that focuses them in the short axis between 3 and 4 cm of depth. This is too deep for breast tissue and, in most patients scanned in the supine position, lies within the chest wall, not the breast. Because of this, small lesions in both the near and middle fields (**A**, **B**) may be subject to volume averaging with surrounding normal breast tissue that can falsely make cystic lesions appear solid and can make subtle isoechoic solid lesions difficult or impossible to perceive. The **middle** short-axis beam profile is that of a typical high-resolution, 7.5- to 12-MHz, small-parts transducer. The acoustic lens is focused at 1.5 to 2.0 cm, good depths for real-time breast ultrasound. The same small middle-field lesion (**D**) that was subject to volume averaging with the 5-MHz transducer will not be volume-averaged with this beam profile. However, even with good high-resolution small-parts transducers, there may be volume averaging in the very near (**C**) and very far fields (**H**). For near-field small lesions, use of an acoustic standoff of gel or a standoff pad may be necessary to avoid volume averaging. The **right** short-axis beam profile is that of a 10-MHz 1.5-D array transducer that has eight elements in the short axis. The beam is narrower in the near field because of electronic and complex lens focusing, but the beam is still wide in the far field because the short-axis aperture is too small to focus tightly electronically in the far field. With the 1.5-D array transducer, an acoustic standoff is rarely needed for near-field problems, but volume averaging continues to be a problem in the far field.

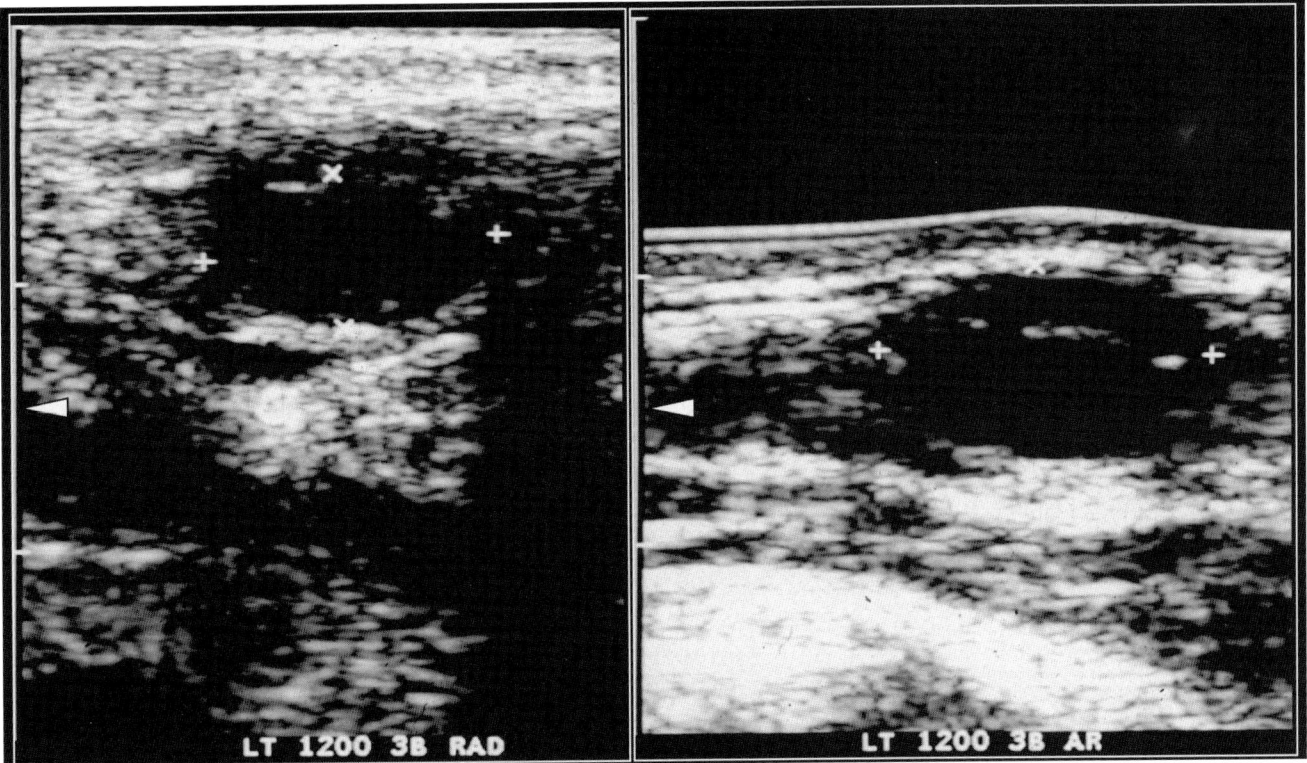

FIGURE 2–5 This is an example of a cyst mischaracterized as partially solid because of near-field volume averaging. This pea-sized palpable lump lies within 1 cm of the skin when scanned without an acoustic standoff. With a good 10-MHz transducer with a short-axis focal length of 1.5 cm (*arrowhead*, **left**), the lump appears to be caused by a mixed cystic and solid nodule (**left**). Using a 7-mm thick standoff pad and the same transducer as in the **left** image, the pea-sized palpable nodule can be seen to be a thinly septated but otherwise simple cyst. The cyst now lies deeper than 1 cm, near the optimal short-axis focal length of 1.5 cm (*arrowhead*, **right**).

aging resulting from a too deeply focused acoustic lens can cause small cystic lesions to be mischaracterized as solid (Fig. 2–5) and can even cause small cystic and solid lesions to become isoechoic with surrounding normal tissues and, therefore, to be missed (Figs. 2–6 and 2–7). Short-axis focal length is just one of the reasons that 5-MHz linear probes should not be routinely used for BUS. Other reasons are suboptimal axial resolution and contrast resolution. Elevation plane focal length may be a problem even for some multipurpose 7- to 7.5-MHz transducers. In such cases, the manufacturer may have compromised on the elevation plane focal length in order to enable both peripheral vascular and small-parts work to be performed with the same transducer. An acoustic standoff of gel or an acoustic standoff pad may be necessary to minimize this problem in certain cases, even when 7.5- to 10-MHz transducers are being used.

Although 5-MHz linear probes should generally be avoided when performing BUS, there are some exceptional circumstances in which the use of such transducers may be advantageous, usually when breast size and thickness greatly exceed 3 cm. These circumstances include evaluation of (a) the lactating breast, (b) the patient with mastitis or question of inflammatory carcinoma, (c) the patient with large silicone implants who has capsular contracture, and (d) the patient with severe macromastia. However, there will be only a very small percentage of women (less than 2%) whose breasts are so thick in the supine position that a 5-MHz probe will be necessary for penetration and adequate deep focusing.

In contrast to 5-MHz linear probes, most 7- to 12-MHz linear probes are designed to image superficial soft tissues and have elevation plane focal lengths ranging from 1.5 to 2.0 cm. This optimum focal length falls within the center of the mammary zone in most women who are scanned in the supine position. The more optimal short-axis focal depth results in a narrower beam width within the breast and decreases the problem of volume averaging, maximizing the chances of accurately characterizing cystic lesions and minimizing the chances of missing small, solid lesions that are located near the skin. The shallower short-axis focal length also improves our chances of showing normal breast structures such as mammary ducts and lobules.

Although using a 7- to 12-MHz probe with an appropriate shallow short-axis focal length will minimize the chances of mischaracterizing small, near-field cystic lesions as solid or completely missing a small superficially located solid lesion, some lesions are so small and so near

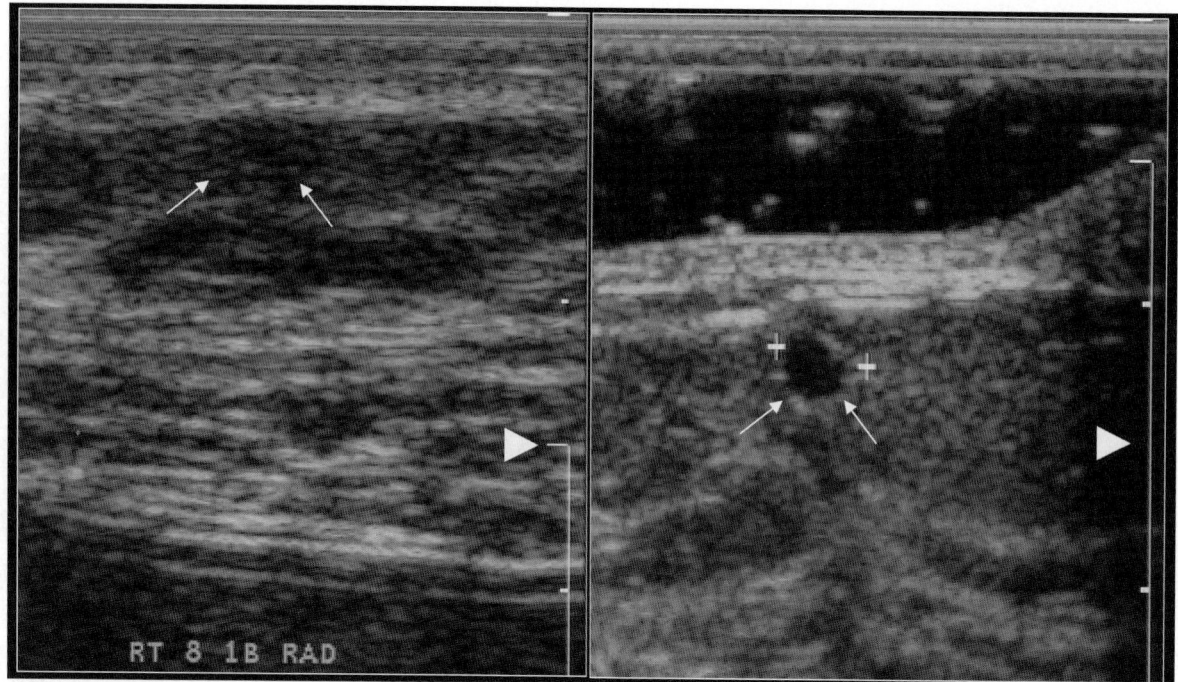

FIGURE 2–6 This BB-sized palpable lump (*arrows,* **left**) was invisible sonographically without a standoff. Note that the lesion lies far superficial to the 1.5-cm short-axis focal zone of the transducer (*arrowhead,* **left**). In our experience, volume averaging is a problem for any small lesion less than 7 to 8 mm in depth. Note also that the transmit focal zones (*white bar* in lower right corner of **left** image) is set too deeply, contributing further to volume averaging along the long axis of the transducer. When an acoustic standoff of gel was used and the transmit zones were adjusted, the BB-sized palpable lump was shown to be a superficially located simple cyst (*small arrows,* **right**). Because of the gel standoff, the depth of the cysts is now nearer the 1.5-cm short-axis focal zone of the transducer (*arrowhead,* **right**). Note that the long-axis transmit focal zones have now appropriately been moved to the same depth as the area of interest.

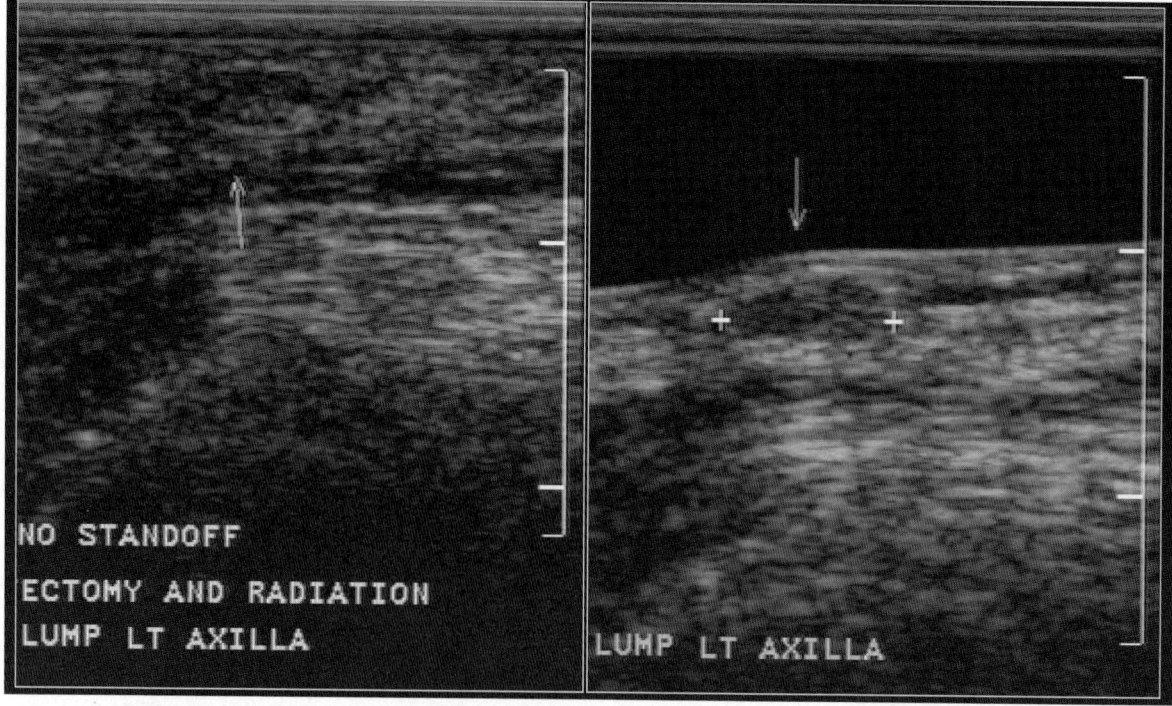

FIGURE 2–7 This is an example of a solid nodule that falsely appears to be isoechoic with surrounding tissue because of near-field volume averaging. This BB-sized nodule is caused by a very superficially located solid nodule that appears isoechoic to surrounding subcutaneous fat (*arrow,* **left**). It is visible only because of the thin, echogenic, fibrous pseudocapsule on its anterior and posterior margins that is evident primarily because of axial resolution. When scanned through a thin acoustic standoff pad, the nodule now lies nearer the 1.5-cm short-axis focal length of this 10-MHz transducer and is clearly hypoechoic to surrounding tissue (*arrow,* **right**).

the skin that even optimally focused high-frequency probes may have difficulty imaging and accurately characterizing them. Additionally, near-field reverberation and side-lobe artifacts may "fill-in" shallow lesions that lie within 6 to 7 mm of the skin, even when optimally focused near-field imaging probes are used. For lesions that are at least partially within the shallowest 6 to 7 mm of depth, an acoustic standoff of a thick layer of acoustic gel or an acoustic standoff pad may be necessary to define and characterize the lesion accurately (Figs. 2–5 to 2–7). Such superficial lesions include mammographic lesions that appear to lie very near the skin and very small, palpable lesions. Generally, palpable lesions that are pea-sized or smaller almost always lie very close to the skin—too close to be adequately evaluated sonographically without the use of an acoustic standoff.

The advantages of a thick layer of gel standoff are that it is quick to apply, the depth may be adjusted, and a lesion may be more easily palpated while it is scanned. The disadvantages are that some gels are too runny, having a tendency to slide off the patient as they warm; air bubbles are sometimes trapped within the gel, creating artifactual shadowing; and the lack of breast compression when using a gel standoff sometimes results in critical angle shadowing from obliquely oriented or curved tissue planes within the breast. The advantages of conventional standoff pads are that air bubbles can be avoided and that some compression may be used, pushing tissue planes within the breast parallel to the probe surface. Disadvantages of using standoff pads are their use is more time consuming, the thickness of the pad is fixed, it is more difficult to palpate lesions while scanning them with a standoff pad, and needle guidance while using a standoff pad is difficult.

Because the image is most severely compromised in the superficial 6 to 7 mm, the ideal standoff pad or layer of gel would be about 7 mm thick. Acoustic standoff pads of 2 or 3 cm are too thick and should not be used for BUS. When such pads are used, the short-axis focal length lies within the standoff rather than within the breast. Breast structures and lesions would then be scanned with a wide and rapidly diverging beam. This would create even worse beam width and volume averaging problems than would be present with no standoff pad at all. The acoustic standoff should be used only for evaluating the shallowest 1 cm of breast. The standoff should be removed when evaluating the more deeply located layers of breast tissue in the targeted area of interest (Fig. 2–8).

The 1.5-dimensional (1.5-D) array transducers that allow electronic focusing in the short axis as well as along the long axis of the probe are now available. A full implementation of two-dimensional (2-D) array would require nearly equal numbers of elements along both long and short axes of the probe and therefore a square rather than rectangular transducer footprint. At the present time, this is not practical because it would require thousands of chan-

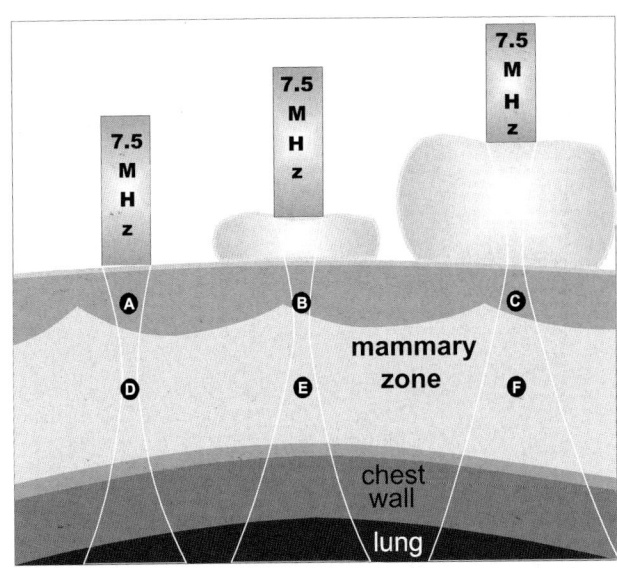

FIGURE 2–8 This figure illustrates the short-axis beam profile of a 7.5-MHz linear transducer with a short-axis fixed acoustic lens focal length of 1.5 cm with various acoustic standoffs. On the **left**, no standoff pad is used. Nodule *D*, which lies at 1.5 cm, is accurately characterized because the beam is narrower than the nodule. However, nodule *A* is so superficial that the beam has not yet become tightly focused in the short axis and is wider than the nodule, resulting in volume averaging. In the **middle** figure, a thin standoff pad has been used. Nodule *B*, which lies at the same depth as nodule *A*, now lies near the optimal short-axis focal point of the transducer. The volume averaging that occurred without a standoff pad no longer occurs. However, nodule *E*, which lies at the same depth as nodule *D* and now lies deeper than the short-axis focal length, is being scanned with a diverging beam and is subject to volume averaging that does not occur for nodule *D* when scanned without a standoff. Most lesions will lie within the middle or deep third of the breast and will be better evaluated without a standoff; hence, an acoustic standoff should be used only when necessary to evaluate small superficial lesions that lie within 1 cm of the skin. The **right** figure shows the effects of using a standoff pad that is too thick. The short-axis focal length of 1.5 cm now lies within the acoustic standoff, and the entire breast is being scanned with a diverging beam. Nodules *C* and *F* are both subject to severe volume averaging.

nels. Even with the use of synthetic apertures, the cost, size, and weight of such a machine would be prohibitive. Additionally, the footprint of such a probe would be too large for many everyday ultrasound applications, and the cable would be too heavy, thick, and stiff. However, a limited implementation of 2-D array (1.5-D array) is feasible. A 1.5-D array transducer contains elements that have been linearly etched in a plane parallel to the long axis of the transducer to create between three and eight separate elements in the short axis (Fig. 2–9). By phasing these multiple short-axis elements, and in combination with complex acoustic lens shapes, a limited degree of electronic focusing can be achieved in the short axis. The electronic short-axis focusing narrows the beam width in the near field, improving both spatial and contrast resolution in the near field. In our experience, both spatial and contrast resolution between about 5 and 12 mm of depth are improved in most

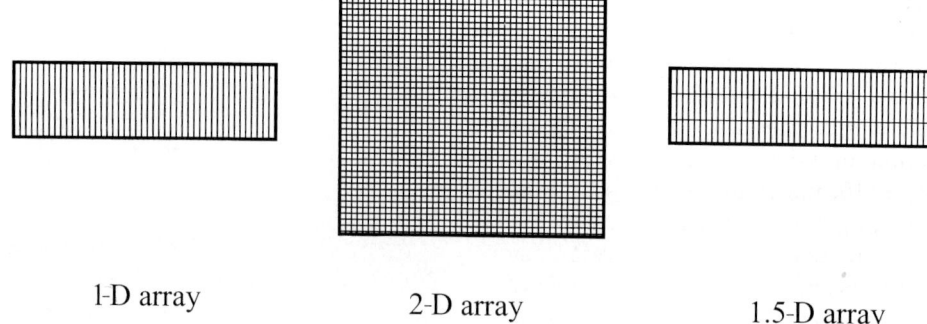

1-D array   2-D array   1.5-D array

FIGURE 2–9 "Footprints" of electronic linear array transducers include the conventional 1-D array transducer on the **left**, the full 2-D array transducer in the **middle**, and the 1.5-D array transducer on the **right**. Most commercially available linear array transducers used in breast ultrasound are 1-D arrays—one element wide, with individual elements oriented perpendicular to the long axis and arrayed parallel to the long axis. Because 1-D arrays are only one element wide, they cannot be electronically focused in the short axis and require an acoustic lens of fixed focal length. A full 2-D array has an about equal number of elements in both axes. This would create a beam width equally small in both axes. To our knowledge, there are no full 2-D arrays in existence. The 1.5-D array is a compromise between the 1-D and full 2-D arrays. The elements of the transducer are scored parallel to the long axis of the transducer to create between three and eight elements in the short axis. This allows a limited degree of electronic focusing. The limited number of short-axis elements and the relatively small aperture in the short axis limit electronic focusing power; thus, in addition to increasing the number of elements in the short axis, complex lens shapes are usually required to aid in focusing at different depths. Even the limited 1.5-D array configuration requires up to 1,028 channels, some of which are created by multiplexing. The 1.5-D array improves short-axis lateral resolution in the near and middle fields but does not help much in the far field because aperture of the short axis is too small for deep electronic focusing.

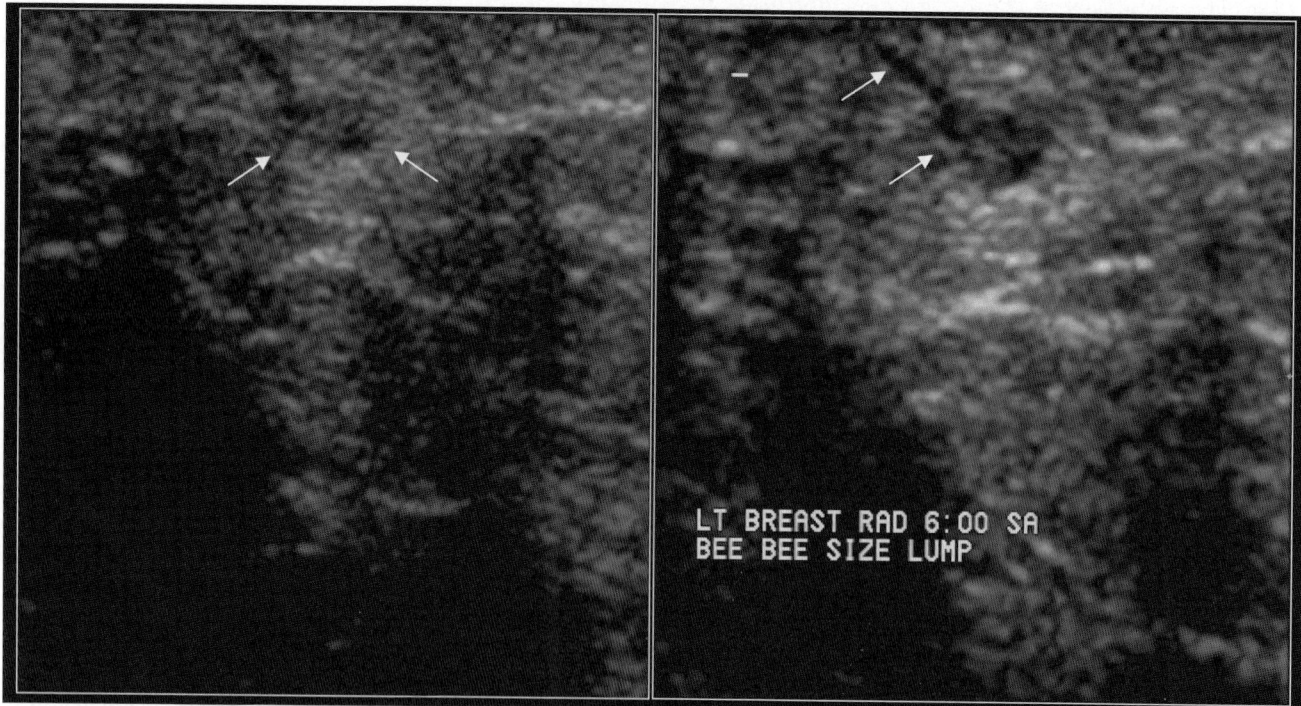

FIGURE 2–10 This figure shows the benefit of using a 1.5-D array transducer in identifying the site of origin of a BB-sized palpable nodule. When scanned with a conventional 1-D array transducer, the nodule appears solid and just deep to the skin (arrows, **left**). When the same nodule shown was scanned with a 1.5-D array transducer, the nodule appeared more hypoechoic and better defined, and the hair follicle into which the sebaceous gland of origin drained was clearly shown (arrows, **right**). This appearance is one of three classic appearances of benign complex cysts of skin origin (see Chapter 10 for details). The smaller beam width in the near field provided by the 1.5-D array transducer minimized volume averaging, allowing the hair follicle to be better demonstrated (**right**).

cases. This is of great benefit in breast imaging for any lesion that lies within the near field, especially for lesions arising from the skin (Fig. 2–10), and in evaluation of the portion of the mammary ducts that lie within the nipple in patients who present with nipple discharge (Fig. 2–11). Sonographic evaluation of skin lesions is discussed in greater detail in Chapter 10, and evaluation of ducts within the nipple is discussed in greater detail in Chapter 8. The benefits of 1.5-D array are more limited in the far field of the breast because the small aperture in the short axis limits the degree to which the beam can be electronically focused deeply within the breast (in the far field) (Fig. 2–4).

AXIAL RESOLUTION

Axial resolution is very important in BUS. Axial resolution is related to three parameters: transducer frequency, bandwidth, and pulse length (Table 2–2).

Axial resolution is inversely proportional to the wavelength of the ultrasound beam. The shorter the wavelength of the beam, the better is the axial resolution. Higher-frequency probes have shorter wavelengths and therefore better axial resolution than lower frequency probes. Im-

TABLE 2–2. AXIAL RESOLUTION

Axial resolution improves with:
- Higher transducer frequency
- Broader bandwidth
- Shorter pulse length

proved axial resolution is another reason that 7- to 12-MHz probes are superior to 5-MHz probes for BUS.

Axial resolution is also related to the pulse length of the transmitted sound. A short pulse is transmitted into the tissues, and then the transducer listens for the returning echoes. The transmission pulse length varies from system to system. For any given transducer frequency, the shorter the pulse length, the better the axial resolution.

Axial resolution is also better for wider bandwidth ultrasound beams than for narrower bandwidth beams. Ultrasound beams are not composed of a single frequency but rather of a spectrum of frequencies. The center of this range of frequencies is the center frequency of the beam. The width of this spectrum at a defined limit is the bandwidth. Ultrasound beams with equal center frequencies may have different bandwidths. Thus, a beam with a

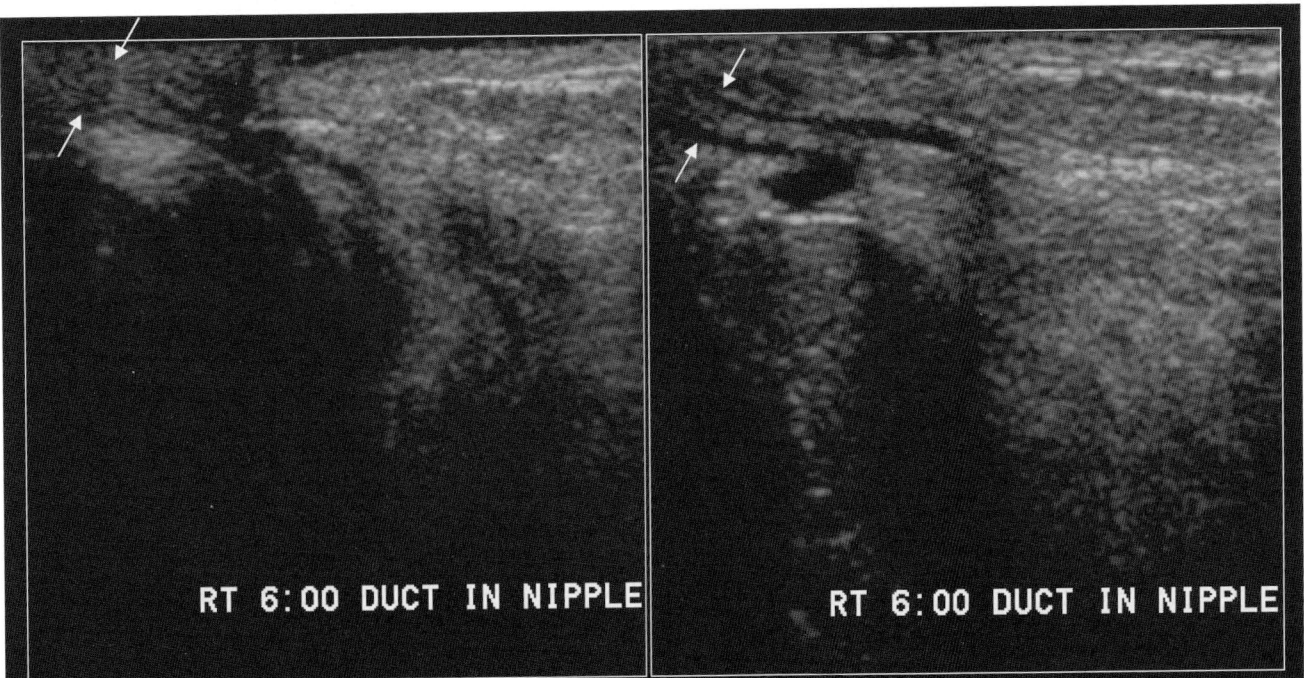

FIGURE 2–11 This figure shows the advantage of a 1.5-D array transducer in demonstrating the mammary ducts within the nipple. The **left** image shows the ducts within the nipple during a rolled-nipple maneuver (discussed in Chapter 8), as shown by a conventional 1-D array transducer. Note that the ducts are not visible near the tip of the nipple (*arrows*) because they are obscured by near-field volume averaging with the surrounding nipple tissue. The **right** image shows the ducts within the nipple in the same patient during the rolled-nipple maneuver, as demonstrated with a 1.5-D array transducer. Because of the narrower beam in the near field, volume averaging is minimized, and the ducts within the nipple are shown to be completely normal all the way to their orifices on the tip of the nipple (*arrows*).

7.5-MHz center frequency may have a frequency bandwidth from 5 to 10 MHz, and its bandwidth would be wider than an ultrasound beam, which has a 7.5-MHz center frequency but a bandwidth from 6 to 9 MHz. Ultrasound beam bandwidth is related to transducer bandwidth, but it is important to realize that the bandwidth of the ultrasound beam generated from the transducer is not necessarily identical to the transducer bandwidth. The transducer bandwidth merely defines the potential maximum bandwidth of an ultrasound beam that it generates. How much of that potential transducer bandwidth actually is incorporated into an ultrasound beam depends on the front-end design of the machine and the pulse length of the ultrasound beam. The potential transducer bandwidth depends on transducer composition and design. Composite transducer materials usually improve transducer bandwidth. As a practical matter, most manufacturers are producing composite transducers that have similarly wide bandwidths. However, because these similarly wide bandwidth transducers may be connected to ultrasound systems that have widely different front-end designs and use different pulse lengths, they may produce ultrasound beams with different bandwidths. Thus, despite identical potential transducer bandwidths, two different systems may generate beams that have very different bandwidths. For any given ultrasound beam center frequency, the broader the bandwidth, the better is the axial

resolution. The ultrasound system that employs a short pulse length will generate an ultrasound beam with wider bandwidth and will have better axial resolution. Equipment that uses short pulse lengths will show normal mammary ducts and tissue planes and capsules around benign breast lesions better than will equipment that uses long pulse lengths. Therefore, a machine with a short pulse length performs better than one with a longer pulse length for BUS.

Axial resolution is important in defining normal tissue planes and anatomic structures within the breast that lie in a plane parallel to the skin line and transducer face and perpendicular to the ultrasound beam, such as mammary ducts. Axial resolution is also very important in defining the pseudocapsule that surrounds benign simple and complex cysts and fibroadenomas. The importance of this capsule in characterizing breast lesions is discussed in detail in Chapters 10 and 12 (Fig. 2–12).

To summarize, excellent spatial resolution requires excellent axial as well as excellent lateral resolution. Probes with shallow (1.5 cm), fixed short-axis focal length and 2-D array probes improve short-axis lateral resolution. Higher-frequency, broad-bandwidth probes that are fired with short pulse lengths offer better axial resolution. Thus, for high-quality BUS, one must seek these characteristics to ensure optimal spatial resolution.

CONTRAST RESOLUTION

In addition to spatial resolution, BUS requires excellent contrast resolution to distinguish between different types of tissues and to improve the conspicuity of lesions. This is especially important when distinguishing subtle solid lesions from surrounding normal fatty or glandular breast tissues. Contrast resolution is a very complex phenomenon. First, it is very dependent on spatial resolution. The better the spatial resolution, the less volume averaging there will be, and the more accurately the returning echoes will reflect the true echo characteristics of the tissue at the center of the beam (Figs. 2–5 to 2–7, 2–10, and 2–11). In addition, suppression of side-lobe artifacts also improves contrast resolution. Finally, for a given spatial resolution, the contrast resolution is better for higher-frequency and broader-bandwidth transducers than for lower-frequency, narrower-bandwidth transducers.

As we have pushed the limits upward on transducer frequency, bandwidth, and dynamic range, we have improved inherent contrast resolution and decreased volume averaging, but we also have increased some other artifacts that degrade contrast resolution, such as clutter, reverberations, and side lobes. This is exacerbated by having to use higher transmit power to penetrate to the chest wall and higher gain settings to display the deep findings. Thus,

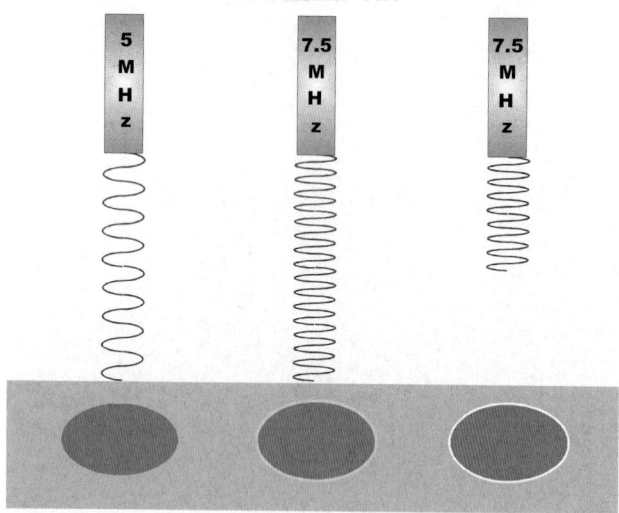

FIGURE 2–12 Axial resolution is better the higher the frequency, the broader the bandwidth, and the shorter the pulse length. Thus, the beam generated by a 5-MHz transducer **(left)** has poorer axial resolution than that from a 7.5-MHz transducer **(middle** and **right)**. The **right** image illustrates a 7.5-MHz transducer that uses a shorter pulse length than does the 7.5-MHz transducer in the **middle** image. This creates wider bandwidth and improves axial resolution over that of the **middle** transducer. Because the **right** transducer has better axial resolution, it shows the thin, echogenic capsule that surrounds a fibroadenoma better than does the **middle** transducer of the same frequency.

there is tradeoff between using the highest frequency and broadest bandwidth possible and in the amount of artifact introduced into the image.

The single most important way to improve contrast resolution is to minimize volume averaging by improving spatial resolution throughout the depth of interest. However, manufacturers are also employing other methods to improve contrast resolution for high-frequency, wide-bandwidth, and high-dynamic-range applications such as BUS.

RECENT TECHNICAL DEVELOPMENTS IN BREAST ULTRASOUND

Automatic Tissue Optimization

Dynamic image processing to remap gray scale over the range of gray shades actually present within the image is helpful in many cases and can decrease the appearance of gray haze in the image introduced by using high-dynamic-range settings (Fig. 2–13). This has been termed *automatic tissue optimization* (ATO) by one manufacturer. ATO is a technique that has long been used in photoediting software. Its application in ultrasound is unique in that it is performed in real time rather than as a postprocessing function on a single captured freeze-frame digital image.

High-Frequency Digitally Encoded Tissue Harmonics

A more robust approach to improving contrast resolution while using high-frequency, broad-bandwidth, high-dynamic-range settings is harmonic tissue imaging. In harmonics tissue imaging, the beam is transmitted at one frequency and received at a multiple of the transmitted frequency. This is advantageous because much of the artifact within the image that degrades its contrast resolution is generated by side lobes or backscatter from lower-frequency elements of the beam. By receiving only higher-frequency components and excluding the lower-frequency components of the returning echoes, much of the artifact is eliminated from the image while preserving the real information. At the high frequencies needed for BUS, only the first harmonic, which is received at twice the transmitted frequency, can be used. Thus, a beam is transmitted at one frequency and received at twice the transmitted frequency. Harmonic tissue imaging can be achieved by filtering the lower-frequency elements of the returning signal. However, simple filtration has two severe limitations. First, because the high-frequency components of the transmitted beam do not penetrate as deeply as the low-frequency elements, penetration and sensitivity for deep structures are decreased. By simple filtration of the returning beam, we are unable to use more than 4 MHz for the transmitted frequency and 8 MHz for the received frequency. Second,

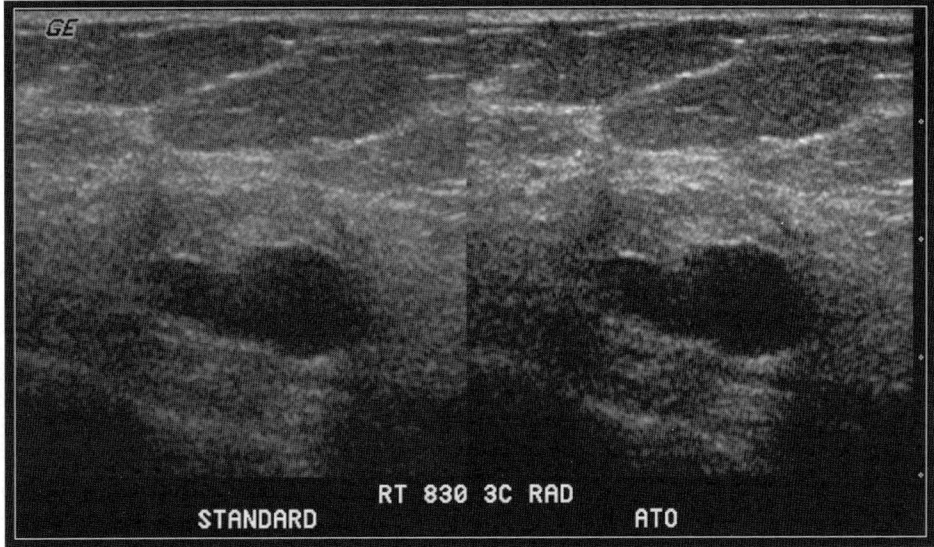

FIGURE 2–13 This split-screen image of a complex cyst near the chest wall illustrates the value of automatic tissue optimization. Automatic tissue optimization (ATO) algorithms remap the gray scan to expand the shades of gray over the range of grays actually present within the image. The **left** and **right** images are identical in all parameters except for ATO, which is not used in the **left** image and is used in obtaining the **right** image a few seconds later. Note that there is a gray haze throughout the **left** image that is absent from the **right** image after ATO.

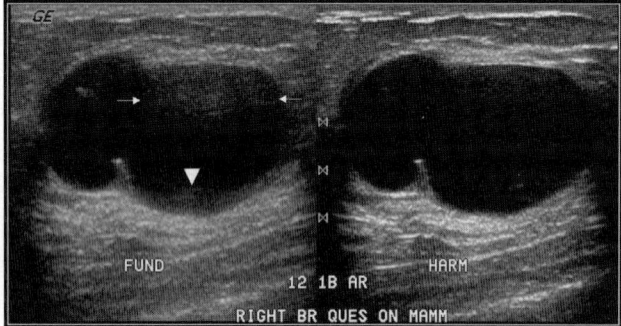

FIGURE 2–14 Coded harmonics reduces reverberation and clutter echoes from breast cysts. This split-screen image shows the same complex breast cyst shown with fundamental imaging on the **left** and coded harmonic imaging on the **right**, imaged only a few seconds apart without moving the transducer. All other parameters are identical. With fundamental imaging, there are prominent reverberation echoes in the near field of the cyst (*arrows*) and clutter echoes in its far field (*large arrowheads*). The artifactual echoes are significantly reduced but not completely eradicated from the cyst with coded harmonic imaging (**right**).

filtering out all lower frequency results in a narrow bandwidth, which markedly reduces axial resolution and decreases our ability to define normal anatomic structures such as duct walls and the thin, echogenic fibrous pseudocapsules that help us distinguish benign from malignant lesions. Thus, implementation of tissue harmonic imaging with a simple filtration results in narrow bandwidth of the received beam, even when the transmitted beam has a broad bandwidth and carries all the limitations imposed by narrow bandwidth.

A better approach to high-frequency tissue harmonics in the breast is digital encoding of the beam. This improves signal-to-noise ratios, allows better penetration

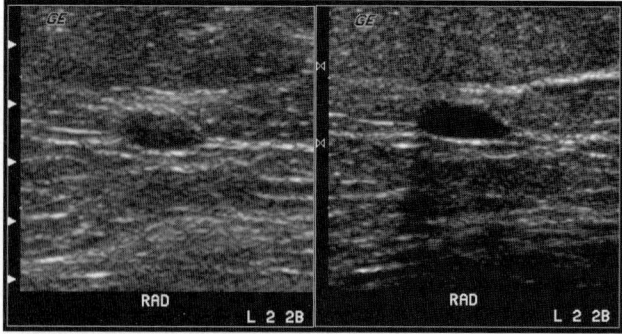

FIGURE 2–16 The **left** image shows a radial (RAD) view of a nodule in the left breast that was obtained with fundamental imaging and that appears to be solid. Radial views of the same nodule obtained a few seconds later with the same transducer using coded harmonic imaging show a simple cyst with all of the internal artifactual echoes suppressed (**right**).

with high frequencies, and enables us to receive the doubled frequency of the returning echoes at a broad bandwidth rather than the narrow bandwidth imposed by simple filtration techniques. With coded harmonics, the beam can be transmitted at a center frequency of 6 MHz and received at a center frequency of 12 MHz, with adequate penetration to the chest wall achieved in 94% of cases. Low-frequency artifacts are excluded from the beam while axial resolution is maintained or, in some instances, even improved over fundamental imaging. Reverberation, side-lobe, clutter, and speckle artifacts are all reduced, improving contrast resolution. Most cysts appear more hypoechoic (Fig. 2–14) or anechoic (Fig. 2–15) when imaged with coded harmonics than with fundamental imaging. Even lesions that contained so many echoes that their cystic versus solid nature was uncertain may become

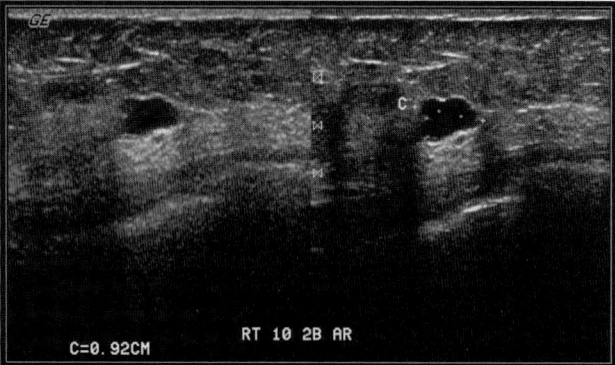

FIGURE 2–15 Coded harmonics completely clears all artifactual echoes from this small simple cyst. These split-screen images have been obtained with the same transducer and with identical parameters except for coded harmonic imaging. The **left** split-screen image was obtained with fundamental imaging and shows internal echoes along the edges of the cyst. The **right** split-screen image was obtained with coded harmonic imaging using the same transducer a few seconds later and shows the cyst to be completely anechoic. All of the internal echoes shown with fundamental imaging were artifactual and were completely suppressed by harmonic imaging.

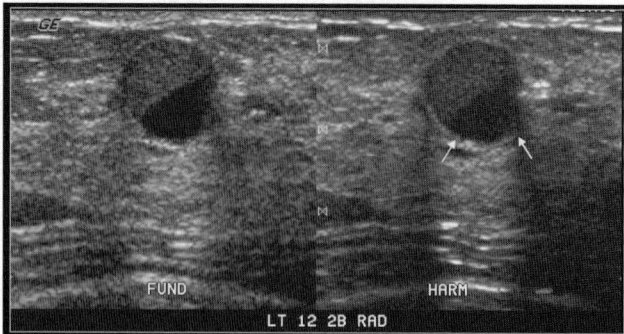

FIGURE 2–17 Coded harmonics does not decrease the echogenicity of cyst fluid in comparison to fundamental imaging in all cases. This "acorn" cyst contains a fat–fluid level. The echogenic fat layer is floating on the dependent fluid layer. Note that the dependent fluid layer appears more echoic (*arrows*, **right**) with coded harmonics than with fundamental imaging (**left**). The increased echoes shown with coded harmonics are real and caused by emulsified fat globules within the fluid level that have not yet separated into the fat layer. Thus, coded harmonics accentuates real echoes in addition to suppressing artifactual echoes.

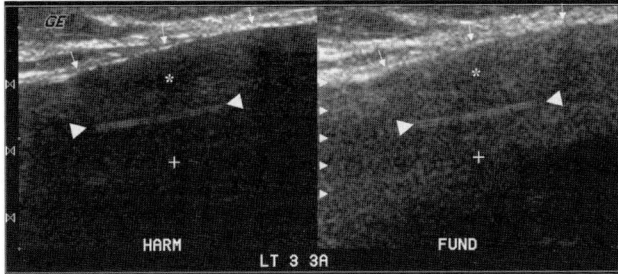

FIGURE 2–18 Coded harmonics (**left** split-screen image) decreases near-field reverberation and clutter echoes within breast implants in comparison to fundamental imaging (**right** split-screen image). This case demonstrates intracapsular rupture with only partial collapse of the implant. The implant shell (*arrowheads*) has abnormally separated from the fibrous capsule (*arrows*). In the **left** image, the extravasated silicone gel that lies between the implant shell (*) and the capsule has become slightly more echogenic than the gel that remains within the implant (+). Abnormally increased echogenicity of chronically extravasated silicone gel is one of the important findings that help to distinguish periimplant fluid lying between the capsule and shell from intracapsular rupture. With fundamental imaging (**right**), the artifactual echoes in the near field obscure the abnormally increased echogenicity of the extravasated gel, preventing definitive distinction of radial fold from intracapsular rupture.

clearly cystic when scanned with coded harmonics (Fig. 2–16). Furthermore, cysts that appear to become more echogenic with coded harmonics than with fundamental imaging have real echoes within them (Fig. 2–17). Thus, coded harmonics helps distinguish artifactual internal echoes within cysts from real internal echoes. The near-field reverberation artifacts that obscure implants are improved dramatically, allowing us to better identify abnormally echogenic extravasated silicone gel that lies between the fibrous capsule and the implant shell (Fig.

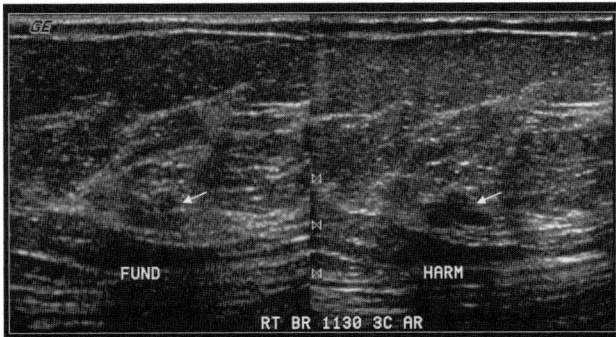

FIGURE 2–19 The ability of coded harmonics to suppress speckle artifact and other artifacts and to make solid nodules appear more hypoechoic and more conspicuous than they are with fundamental imaging is demonstrated. This lobulated solid nodule that presented as a circumscribed mammographic nodule could not be identified with certainty with fundamental imaging (**left** split-screen image) but was readily identified and distinguished from surrounding tissue with coded harmonics (**right** split-screen image). Note that coded harmonics also makes the fat appear more echogenic than solid nodules, which helps to define less echogenic solid nodules.

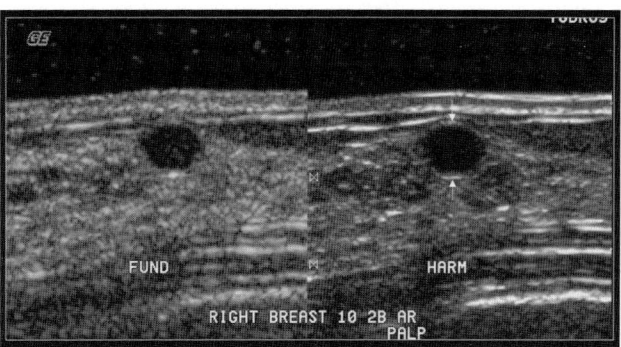

FIGURE 2–20 Coded harmonics helps to define the thin, echogenic pseudocapsule that surrounds most benign solid and complex cystic lesions within the breast because it improves rather than degrades axial resolution. Because the parts of the capsule we show best with ultrasound are thin and are parallel to the transducer face and perpendicular to the beam, we rely heavily on axial resolution to demonstrate them. Coded harmonics makes the capsule appear thinner, more echogenic, more sharply defined, and more complete (**right** split-screen image) than it appears to be with fundamental imaging (**left** split-screen image).

2–18). Additionally, a larger percentage of solid nodules appear hypoechoic compared with surrounding breast tissues with coded harmonics than with fundamental imaging, making them easier to perceive and less likely to be missed (Fig. 2–19). Because coded harmonics maintains the broad bandwidth of the ultrasound beam, it makes the thin, echogenic fibrous pseudocapsule that surrounds most benign cystic and solid breast lesions appear to be thinner, more echogenic, and more complete than with fundamental imaging. This is true even when the lesions are surrounded by hyperechoic fibrous tissues that are nearly as echogenic as the capsule (Figs. 2–20 and 2–21). Similarly, the shell of mammary implants and the fibrous capsule that surrounds the shell are better defined and appear thinner and brighter with coded harmonics imaging

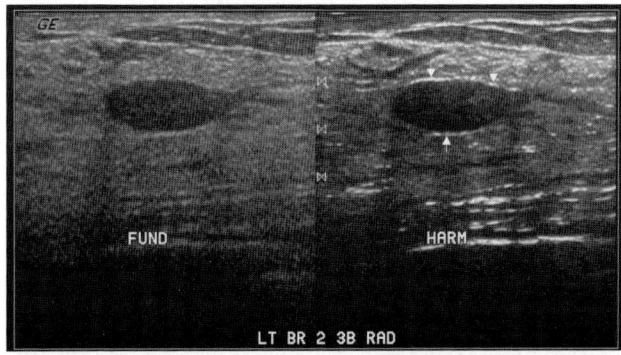

FIGURE 2–21 This classic, elliptically shaped, mildly hypoechoic, thinly encapsulated fibroadenoma is surrounded by echogenic fibrous tissue. The nodule appears more hypoechoic, and its pseudocapsule (*arrows*) appears to be thinner, more echogenic, and better distinguished from the surrounding echogenic fibrous tissue with coded harmonics (*arrows*, **right**) than it is with fundamental imaging (**left**).

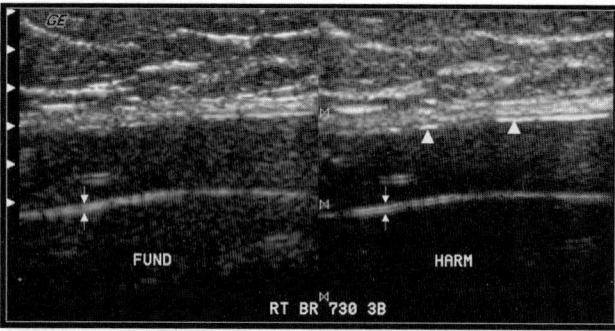

FIGURE 2–22 Coded harmonics (**right** split-screen image) shows the fibrous capsule around breast implants (*arrowheads*) and the double echogenic line that represents the inner and outer surfaces of the implant shell better than does fundamental imaging (**left** split-screen image). Note that the two echogenic lines that represent the leading and trailing surfaces of the implant shell are much thinner, brighter, and more clearly defined from each other with coded harmonic imaging than they are with fundamental imaging (*arrows*).

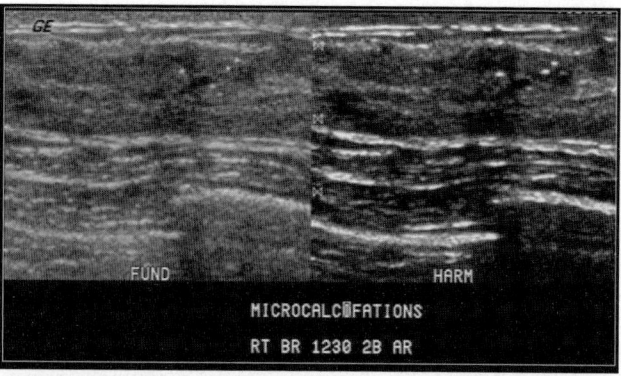

FIGURE 2–24 Speckle artifact prevents sonography from showing microcalcifications as well as they could be shown without speckle. Note how much more echogenic and easy to distinguish these calcifications are with coded harmonics (**right** split-screen image) than with the fundamental imaging (**left** split-screen image).

than they do with fundamental imaging (Fig. 2–22). With coded harmonics, the echotexture of normal breast structures and breast lesions appears to be finer and more uniform because of marked reduction in speckle artifact. Much of what we have come to accept as echotexture is not really texture at all, but speckle artifact (Fig. 2–23). Preliminary results suggest that because of speckle reduction that occurs with coded harmonics, calcifications may be more apparent sonographically (Fig. 2–24).

There are three main limitations to the use of coded harmonics. The first is reduced penetration. Coded harmonics will penetrate adequately in 94% of all patients, but in 6% of cases, usually women with large breasts composed primarily of fibrous tissue, fundamental imaging will still be required to obtain adequate penetration (Fig.

2–25). The second limitation is a reduction in frame rate that is acceptable as long as color or power Doppler is not used simultaneously. When Doppler is required, the image that is interlaced with Doppler must be constructed at fundamental rather than harmonic frequencies. The third limitation is minor. It is that the benefits of coded harmonics occur mainly in middle and far fields, and there is less noticeable benefit in the near field.

We believe that coded high-frequency harmonics is one of the most important developments in breast imaging since the advent of 10 MHz or higher imaging frequencies and that it is so important in breast imaging that it will become virtually mandatory if the costs can be reduced enough to make it generally affordable or if reimbursement for BUS improves.

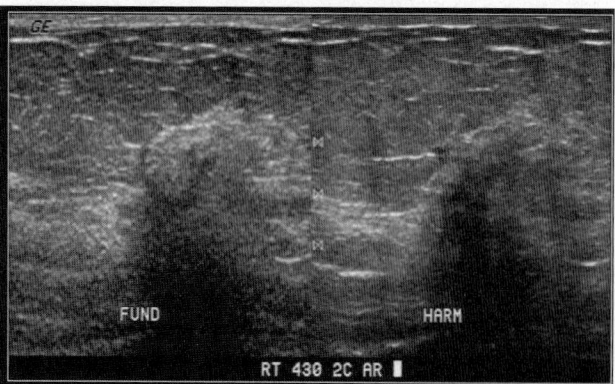

FIGURE 2–23 Suppression of speckle artifact and clutter in the far field with coded harmonics (**right** split-screen image) allows us to better define the margins of this shadowing desmoplastic invasive lobular carcinoma than can be defined with fundamental imaging (**left** split-screen image).

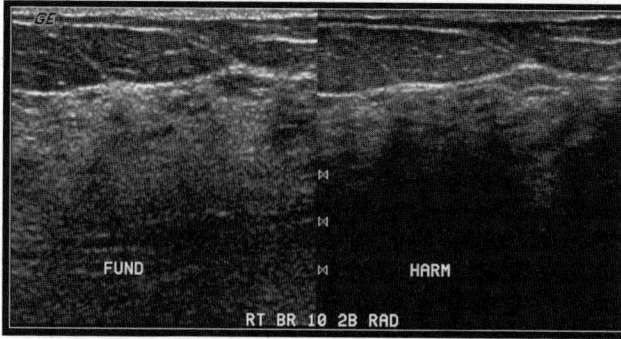

FIGURE 2–25 The most important limitation of coded harmonics is decreased penetration of breast tissues. Penetration is decreased in all patients, but adequate penetration to the chest wall is possible in 94% of our patients. However, in 6% of cases, penetration to the chest wall is not possible (**right** split-screen image) with coded harmonics, and we must rely on fundamental imaging (**left** split-screen imaging) in such cases. Patients in whom coded harmonics does not penetrate adequately usually have large breasts composed largely of hyperechoic fibrous tissues.

Real-Time Spatial Compounding of Images

Spatial compounding of the image is another recent development that improves both contrast and spatial resolution. In conventional real-time imaging, each frame is created by a single sweep of the beam, transducer element by transducer element, from one end of the transducer to the other at a 90-degree angle to the long axis of the transducer. In the image constructed with spatial compounding, each frame may be constructed of three or nine sweeps of the beam from one end of the transducer to the other. Using beam steering, all sweeps except the first sweep are created from different angles of incidence, creating a spatially and temporally compounded image that is obtained from multiple different angles over time (Fig. 2–26). Compounding the image builds up real echoes and averages out artifactual echoes both temporally and spatially, as long as the transducer position is held constant. Compounded images show reduction in artifactual echoes within cysts (Fig. 2–27), implants (Fig. 2–28), and solid nodules (Fig. 2–29) in comparison to conventionally obtained images. Because each image is obtained at multiple angles of incidence, the fibrous pseudocapsule around benign lesions is shown better and more completely, especially on the lateral edges, where critical angle phenomena normally prevent its demonstration with conventional imaging (Figs. 2–30 and 2–31). Other obliquely oriented thin structures, such as

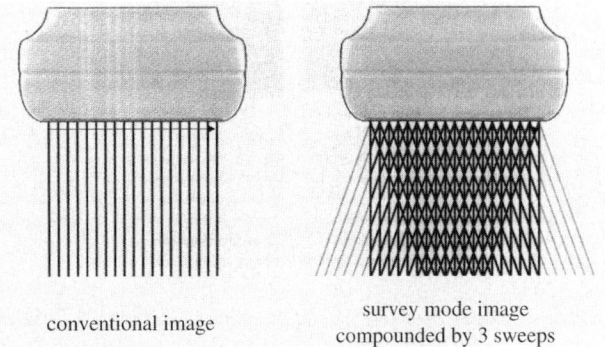

conventional image   survey mode image
                            compounded by 3 sweeps

FIGURE 2–26 This figure illustrates the differences between a conventional beam (**left**) and a real-time spatially compounded beam (**right**). The conventional image is constructed with a single sweep of the beam from one end of the image to the other. The beam is generated at 90 degrees to the surface of the transducer. The real-time compounded image is constructed with multiple sweeps of the beam from one end of the transducer to the other. The first sweep, as in conventional imaging, is generated at 90 degrees to the surface of the transducer. However, subsequent sweeps are electronically steered from the left and right, respectively. Either three or nine separate sweeps may be used to generate each frame of the real-time image. This compounds the image both spatially and temporally, averaging out artifactual echoes and building up real echoes.

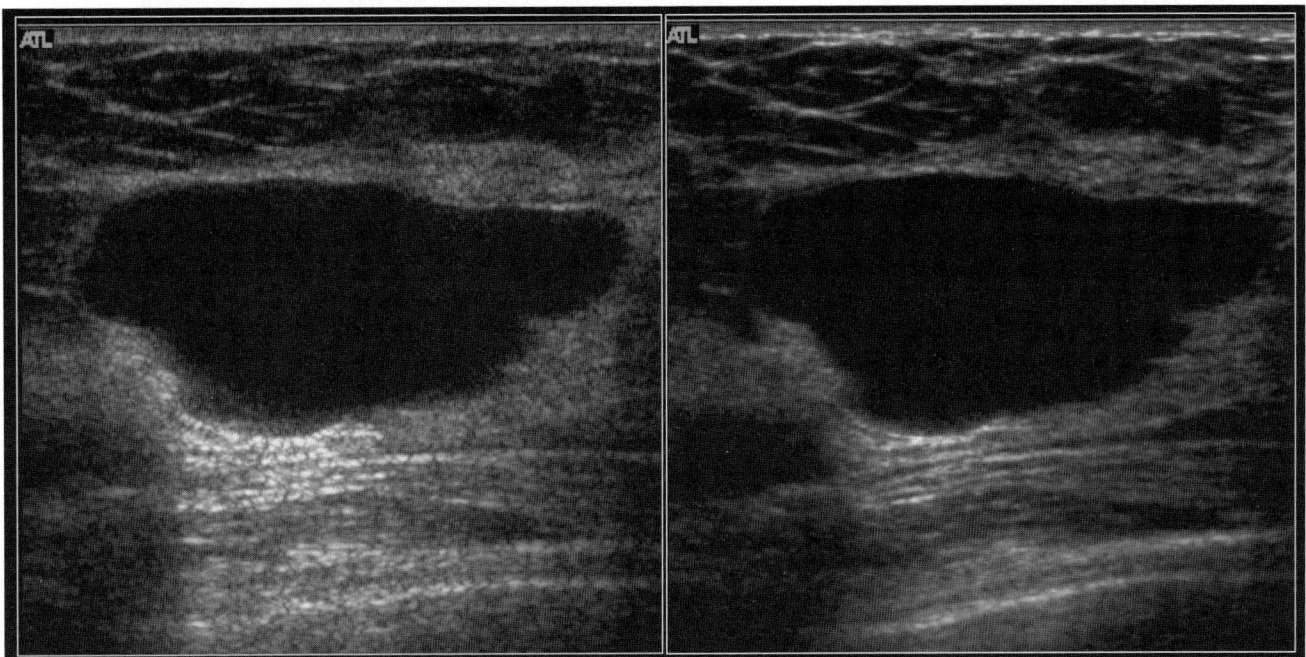

FIGURE 2–27 This case illustrates the effectiveness of spatial compounding in suppressing artifactual echoes. The **left** image shows a large, simple cyst that was scanned with conventional imaging and shows clutter artifact in both near and far portions of the cyst. The **right** image shows the same large cyst imaged with the same transducer using real-time compounding. Note that the artifacts in both near and far portions of the cyst are markedly reduced.

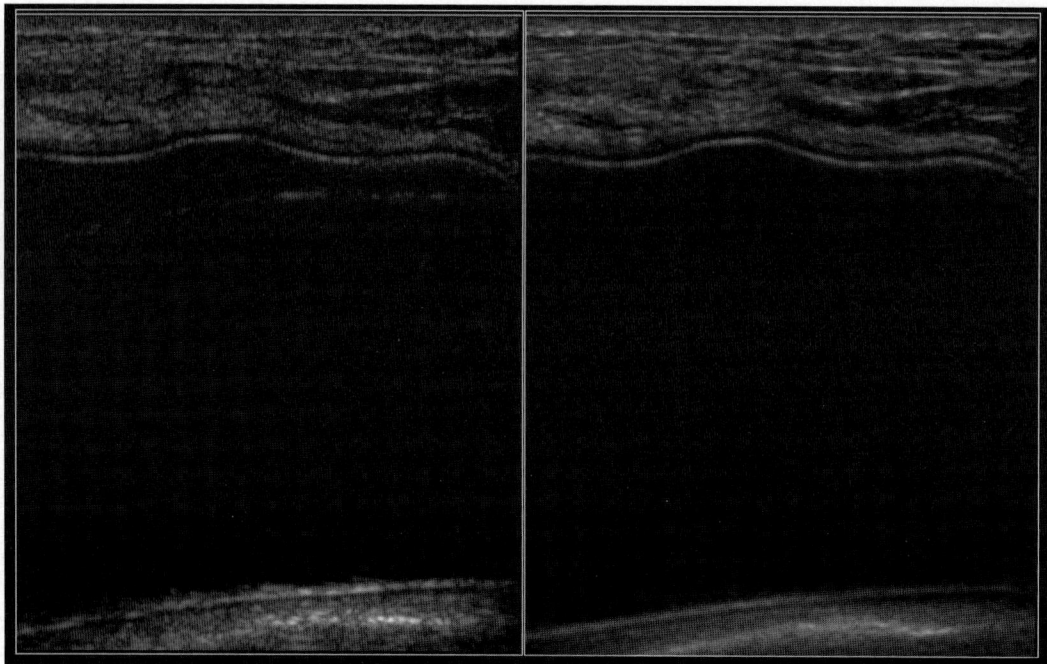

FIGURE 2–28 This case illustrates the value of spatial compounding in evaluating breast implants. The **left** image was obtained using conventional imaging and shows reverberation artifacts in the near field and some fuzziness of the posterior implant shell. The **right** image was generated with the same transducer and real-time compounding of the image. Note that the near-field artifacts are gone and that the posterior implant shell is more clearly defined.

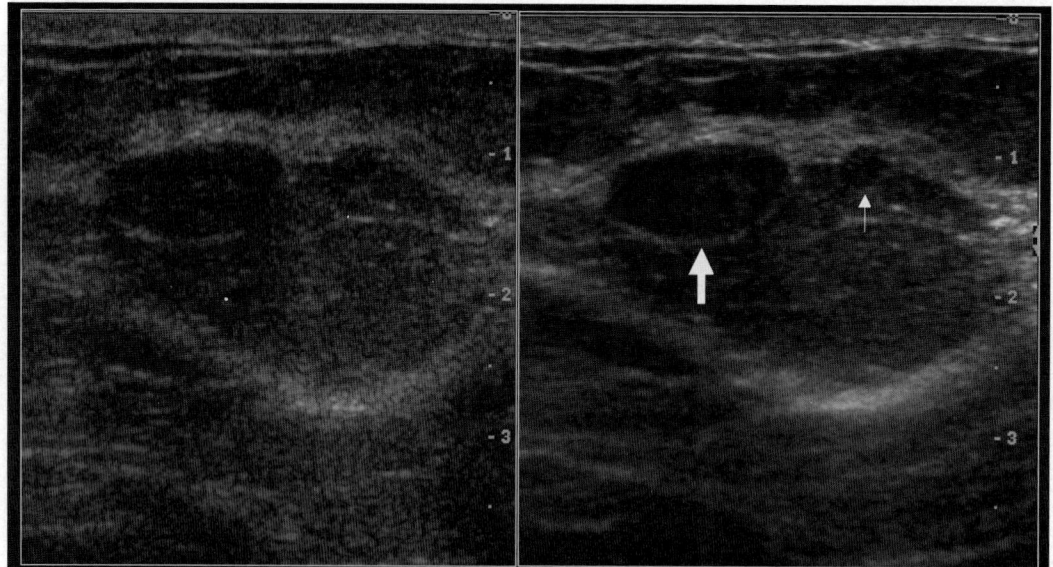

FIGURE 2–29 This case illustrates the value of spatial compounding in identifying and distinguished solid nodules from surrounding tissues. The **left** image shows an image of a classic, elliptically shaped, mildly hypoechoic, thinly encapsulated fibroadenoma surrounded by isoechoic fat generated by conventional imaging. The image of the fibroadenoma generated with spatial compounding (**right**) shows the nodule to be slightly more hypoechoic compared with surrounding tissues. It also shows that the pseudocapsule surrounding the lesion is thinner, better defined, and more complete than it was with conventional image. The compounded image also shows a second lesion (*small arrow*) that was not appreciated on the conventional image. The second nodule was more easily appreciated with real-time compounding because it appears slightly more hypoechoic and because the surrounding echogenic pseudocapsule is more completely defined.

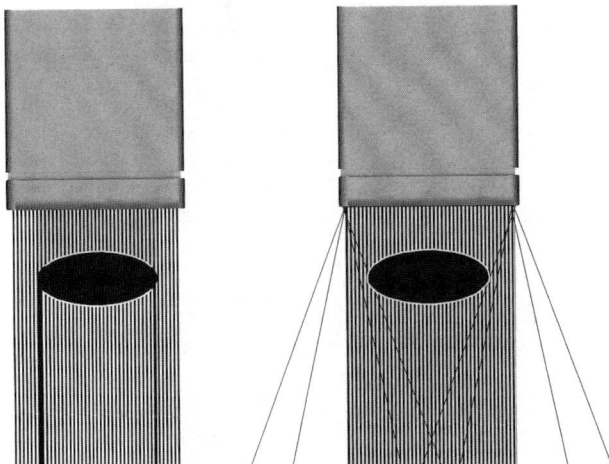

normal Cooper's ligaments and malignant spiculations, are shown better with compound imaging than with conventional imaging (Fig. 2–32). However, enhanced through-transmission deep to cystic lesions is less pronounced with compounding than with conventional imaging. In large cysts, the enhanced through-transmission may merely be triangular and narrower than with conventional imaging because of the angles of the steered beams (Figs. 2–33 and 2–34). In smaller cysts, the enhanced through-transmission seen with conventional imaging may be completely absent with real-time compounding (Fig. 2–35). Additionally, acoustic shadowing deep to desmoplastic carcinomas is decreased, but this actually may be helpful in better demonstrating the posterior border of the lesion (Figs. 2–36 and 2–37). Ultimately, much like coded harmonics, real-time compounding is a robust method of reducing speckle artifact (Fig. 2–38). Initially, we subjectively felt that the images obtained with real-time compounding appear smeared in comparison to conventional images because we had become accustomed to seeing speckle artifact in our images. We have incorrectly interpreted uniform dot size as representing good resolution when it merely represented uniform speckle noise. In fact, the spatial resolution and detail are better with spatial compounding than with

FIGURE 2–30 The conventional linear array ultrasound beam interrogates the surface of benign nodules from only one angle. Thus, along the lateral edges of the nodule, where the angle of incidence with the surface of the nodule is near 0 degrees, critical angle phenomena prevent demonstration of the thin, echogenic pseudocapsule and create the thin edge shadows deep to the edges of the lesion (**left**). Because the real-time compounded beam interrogates the surface of nodules from multiple angles, critical angle phenomena at the edges of the nodules are decreased. There are no thin edge shadows, and the capsule is more likely to be shown along the lateral edges as well as on the front and back surfaces of the nodule (**right**).

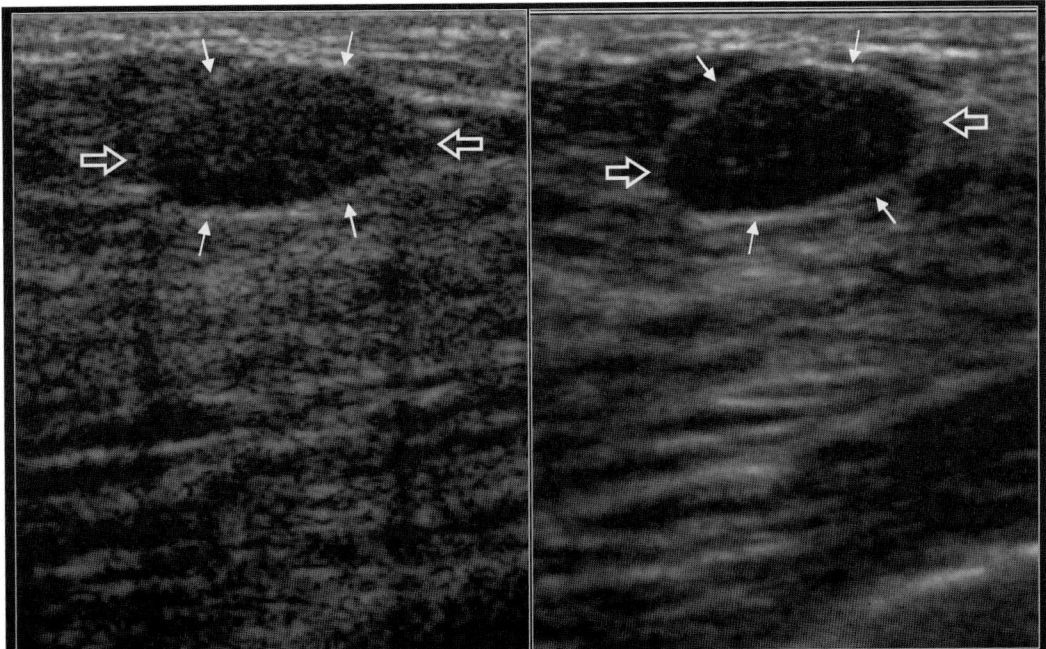

FIGURE 2–31 This classic, elliptically shaped fibroadenoma, when scanned conventionally (**left**), has a well-defined pseudocapsule along the anterior and posterior edges of the nodule (*small arrows*), where it is nearly perpendicular to the beam. However, along the lateral edges of the nodule, where the pseudocapsule lies at an angle nearer 0 degrees to the beam, it is not demonstrated (*open arrows*). Additionally, deep to the edges of the nodule, there are thin edge shadows (*arrowheads*). When the same nodule is scanned with spatial compounding (**right**), the capsule is better demonstrated on all surfaces of the nodule, including the edges (*open arrows*).

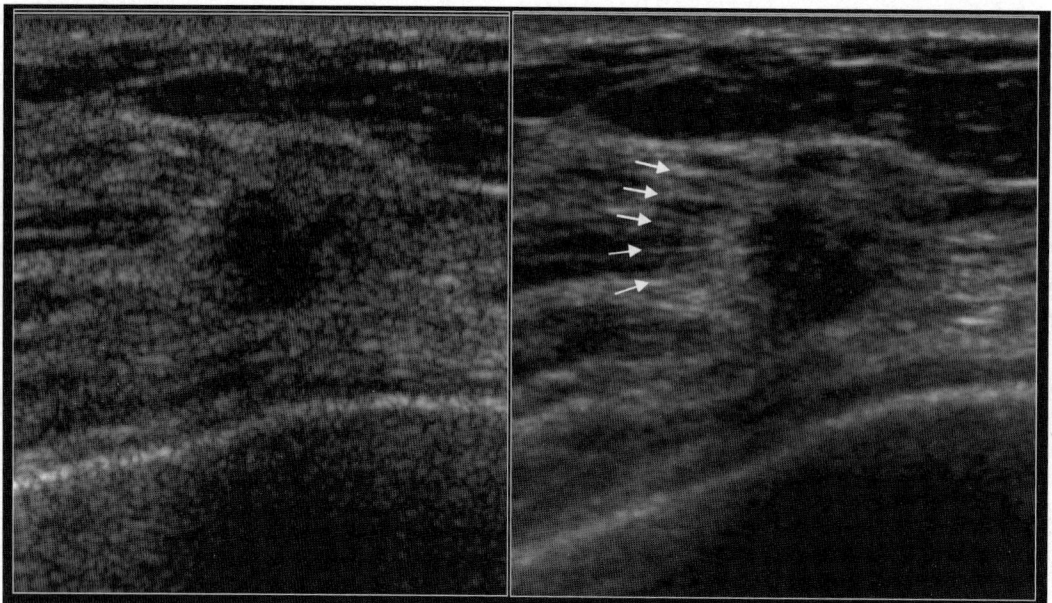

FIGURE 2–32 Spatial compounding better defines the margins of malignant nodules and shows malignant characteristics such as angular margins and spiculations more clearly. This malignant nodule has ill-defined margins when scanned with a conventional beam (**left**). When the same small malignant nodule was scanned with real-time compounding, frank spiculations that were obscured by speckle artifact during conventional imaging are now visible along the left edge of the nodule (*arrows,* **right**).

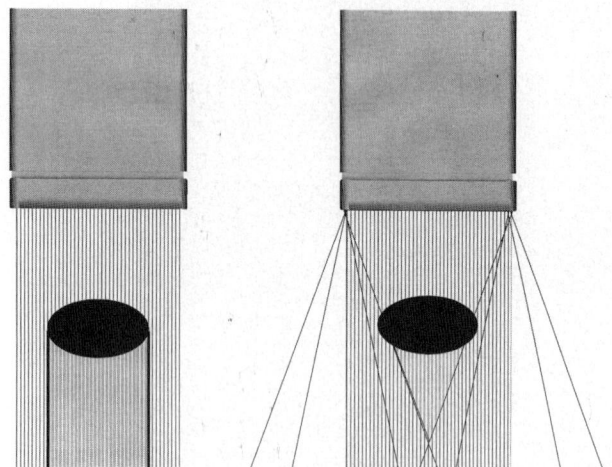

FIGURE 2–33 This figure shows that because of the multiple beam angles, enhanced through-transmission and thin edge shadows deep to cysts are decreased. A rectangular area of enhanced through-transmission with thin edge shadows is seen deep to a cyst using convention linear beams (**left**). Real-time compounding reduces the intensity of enhanced through-transmission and ablates thin edge shadows. Additionally, the enhanced sound transmission that persists is triangular rather than rectangular and does not extend as deeply with real-time compounding as with conventional imaging (**right**).

conventional imaging because the superimposed speckle artifact is removed.

Limitations or real-time compounding include a potential decrease in frame rate or high persistence and sensitivity to motion artifact during construction of the image. Unacceptable slowing of frame rate is prevented by continuously updating the frame as each steered sweep is performed, but this creates a high persistence, which, in turn, gives rise to sensitivity to hand movements during scanning. The degree of persistence depends on the number of image sweeps per frame. Persistence is less when only three sweeps are used to create the image, but the benefits of compounding are also less. The three-sweep mode is used for surveying the breast in real time. Persistence is increased markedly in the nine-sweep mode; hence, it is more useful for targeted evaluation of structures or pathology previously identified in survey mode. Persistence in the target mode can be a severe limitation in patients with pronounced respiratory motion.

Coded harmonics and spatial compounding achieve similar benefits by different mechanisms and therefore theoretically could be used simultaneously, for even greater improvement in image quality. However, the limitations are also similar; thus, slow frame rates, high persistence, and computer speed limitations might prevent simultaneous application of these technologies.

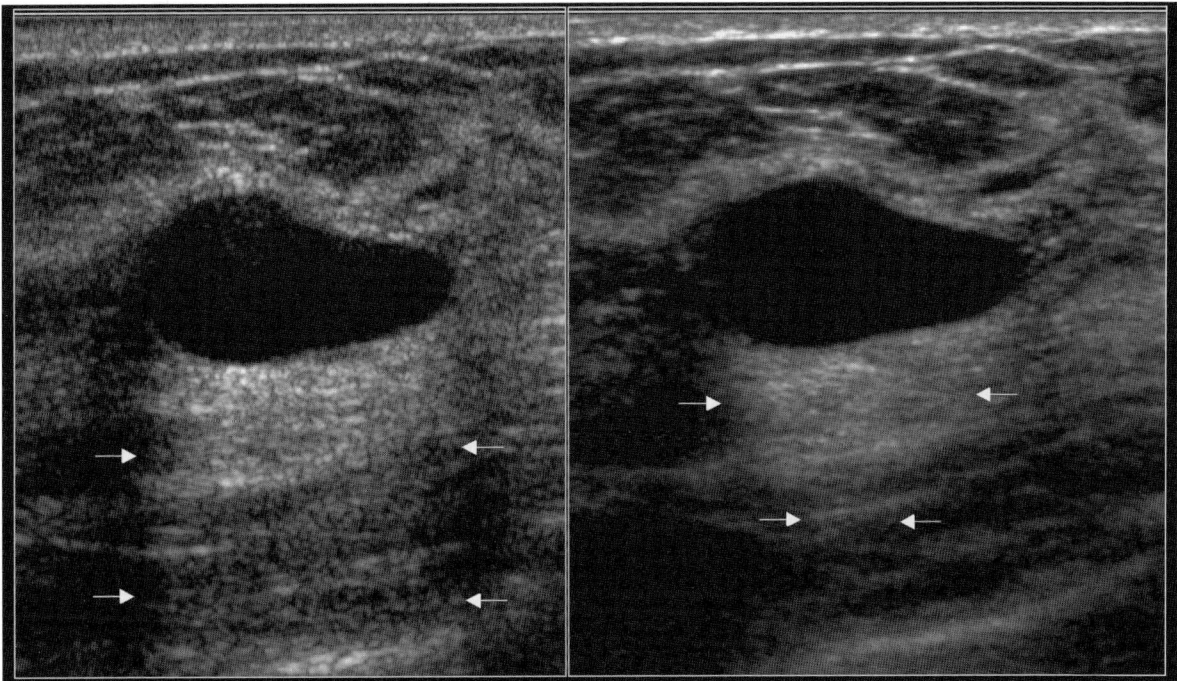

FIGURE 2–34 This cyst shows a rectangular area of strongly enhanced through-transmission and has thin edge shadows when scanned with a conventional linear array beam (*arrows,* **left**). When scanned with real-time compounding, the internal artifacts within the cyst are decreased, but the enhanced sound transmission is less intense, is triangular, and does not extend as deeply as it does with conventional sonography (*arrows,* **right**). Additionally, the thin edge shadows that were seen with the conventional beam are not present in a compounded beam.

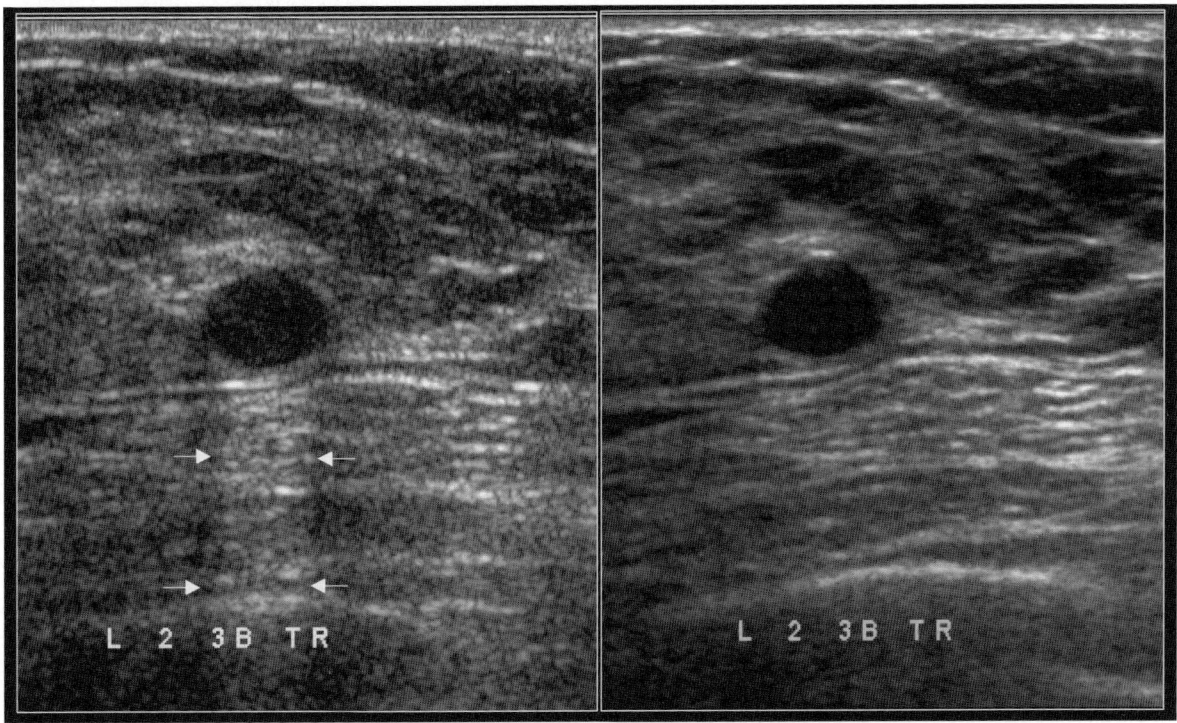

FIGURE 2–35 This small, complex cyst shows enhanced through-transmission and thin edge shadows when scanned with a conventional linear array beam (*arrows,* **left**). The same small, complex cyst when scanned with real-time compounding does not demonstrate enhanced through-transmission and does not cause thin edge shadows. Real-time compounding tends to decrease enhanced through-transmission only deep to large cysts but can completely eradicates it deep to small cysts (**right**).

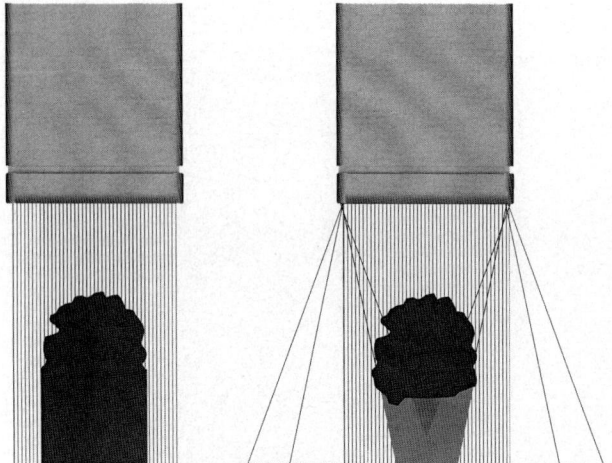

FIGURE 2–36 Spatial compounding decreases acoustic shadowing caused by certain carcinomas with desmoplasia. The **left** image shows intense shadowing from a carcinoma that obscures the posterior border of the lesion. With spatial compounding, the intensity of the acoustic shadowing is decreased, the shape of shadowing is triangular, and it extends less deeply than it does with conventional imaging (**right**). The posterior border of the lesion, however, may be better demonstrated with spatial compounding.

Split-Screen Imaging

It is very useful for equipment used in BUS to have split-screen imaging capabilities. Split-screen imaging can be important in the breast in several circumstances. First, it is useful for comparing mirror-image locations in the right and left breast when it appears that either a mammographic or palpable abnormality is caused by asymmetric breast tissue. It is also useful in evaluating foreign structures such as implants and subtle lesions such as lipomas. Split-screen imaging is also useful in documenting dynamic events that would normally require videotape or a stored cine loop to demonstrate. Finally split-screen images can be combined to create a field of view twice the width of the long axis of the transducer in cases in which the structure or lesion of interest is wider than the standard 37- or 38-mm small-parts transducer (Fig. 2–39). The uses of split-screen imaging in BUS are discussed and illustrated in detail in Chapter 3.

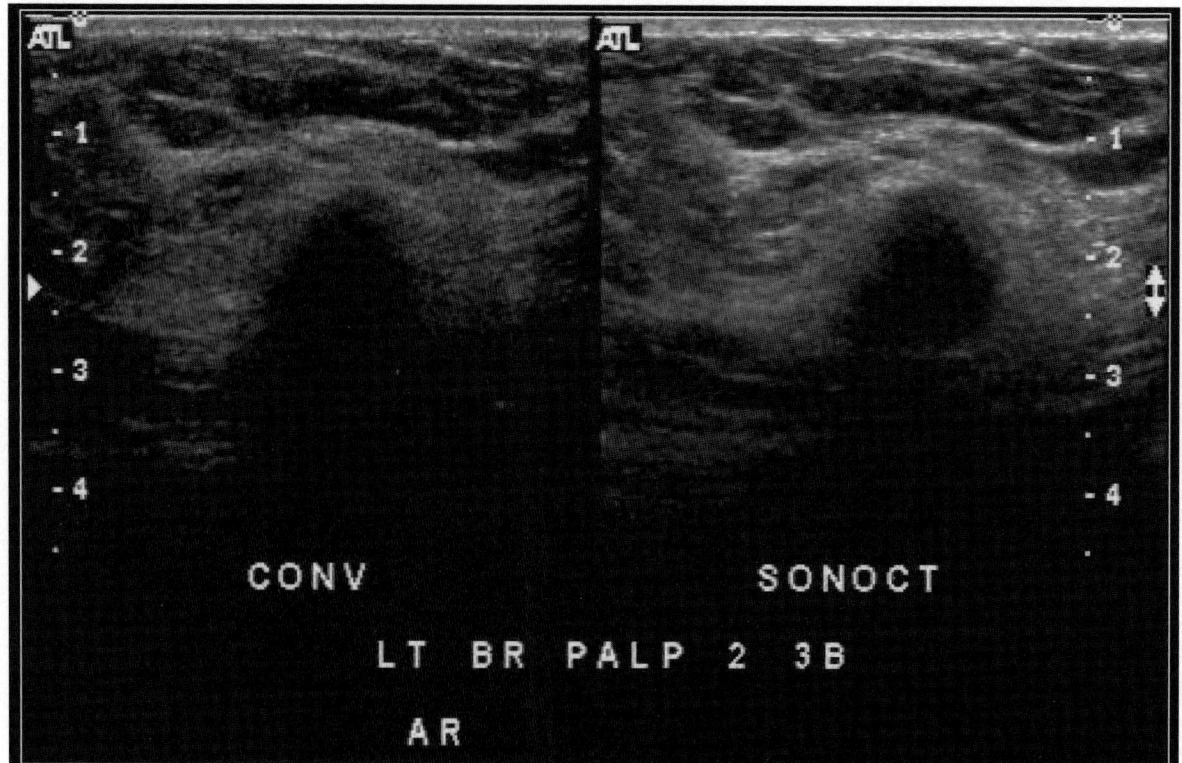

FIGURE 2–37 This 1.5-cm tubular carcinoma caused such intense acoustic shadowing when scanned with a conventional linear array 12-MHz beam that the posterior margin of the tumor was obscured (**left** split-screen image). When the same nodule was scanned with real-time compounding, the acoustic showing was decreased enough that the posterior margin of the tumor and the chest wall deep to the tumor could be defined (**right** split-screen image).

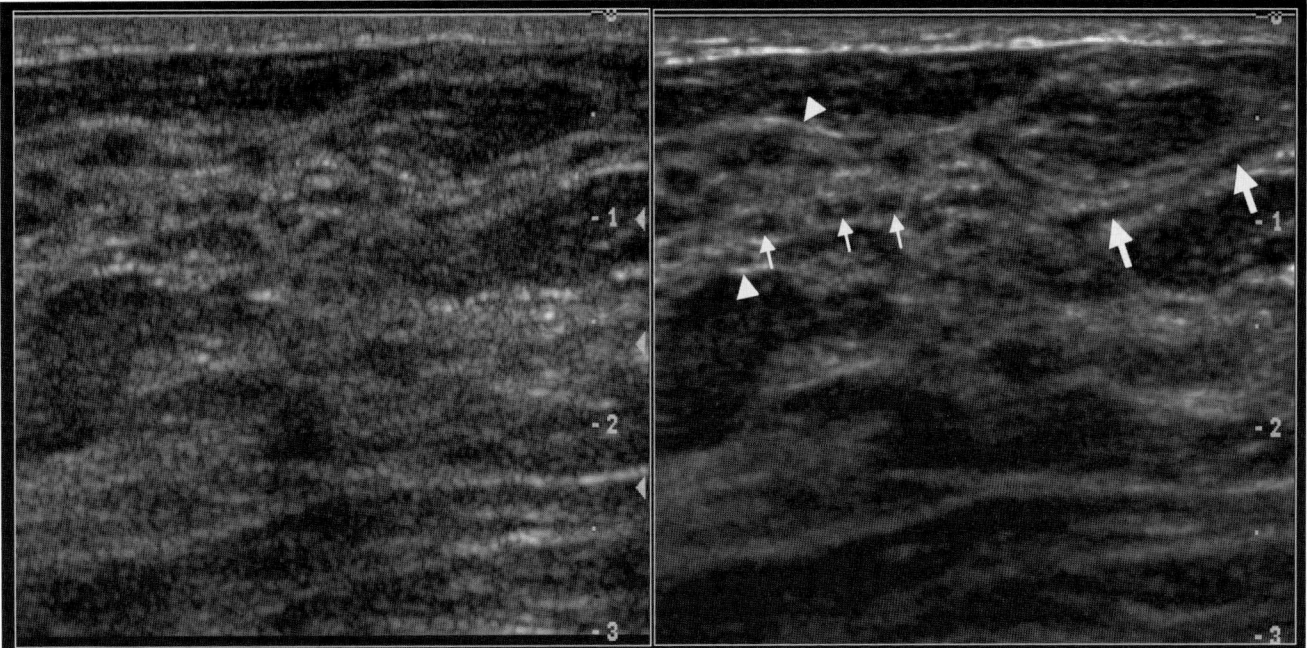

FIGURE 2–38 The most consistent benefit of real-time compounding is suppression of speckle that is evident in every image. The **left** image shows normal fibroglandular tissue surrounded by premammary and retromammary fat scanned with a convention linear array beam. Note the "salt-and-pepper" stippled pattern at all levels of the image. The **right** image shows the same tissue imaged with real-time compounding. The echotexture is much smoother, and there is less salt-and-pepper stippling than when scanned with conventional imaging. At first glance, a sonographer or sonologist may have the impression that the image is blurred because we have become accustomed to seeing speckle in ultrasound images and may misinterpret the absence of speckle as blurring of the image. When closely inspected, however, the detail is actually higher in the compounded image because speckle does not obscure it. Note how much thinner and brighter the anterior mammary fascia and retromammary fascia appear with real-time compounding (*arrowheads*). Also note the targetoid short-axis appearance of several small ducts that appear as tiny echogenic dots surrounded by gray, loose, periductal, fibroelastic tissue (*small arrows*) with compounding, but not with conventional imaging. Also note how much more clearly the long axis of the lobar duct is shown with compounding than it is with conventional imaging (*large arrows*).

Curved Arrays, 5-cm Transducers, Virtual Convex Imaging, and Extended Field of View

In addition to combined split-screen images, there are other methods of obtaining a larger field of view. This can be important in demonstrating large lesions, large structures such as implants, very large masses, long intraductal components of breast cancer, and multifocal or multicentric lesions. Several hardware and software approaches have been developed to deal with this problem.

First, a 5- to 7-MHz curved linear transducer can be used. This is usually the least desirable choice because the frequency is less than optimal and the short-axis focal length is about 5 cm, usually too deep for breast imaging. However, in certain circumstances, such as postpartum mastitis, inflammatory carcinomas, and capsular contracture around implants, a lower-frequency curved linear transducer may be necessary (Fig. 2–40).

Second, the length of the transducer may be increased. In Germany, for example, a 50-mm long transducer is mandatory for BUS. At least two manufacturers have specifically addressed this problem by building 50-mm long high-frequency transducers. The 50-mm long transducers also speed bilateral whole breast ultrasound for either diagnostic or screening purposes. To maintain the lateral resolution of such elongated probes, the number of transducer elements and the effective number of channels must be increased without increasing element size (Fig. 2–41). Elongating the transducer by enlarging elements would degrade the lateral resolution. Unfortunately, some lower-frequency long linear transducers have employed larger elements to achieve their length.

Third, elements at the end of a linear small-parts transducer can be steered or phased to create a "virtual convex" or trapezoidal image that is composed of a typical linear image centrally with phased images on either end (Figs. 2–42 and 2–43). The lateral resolution in the center

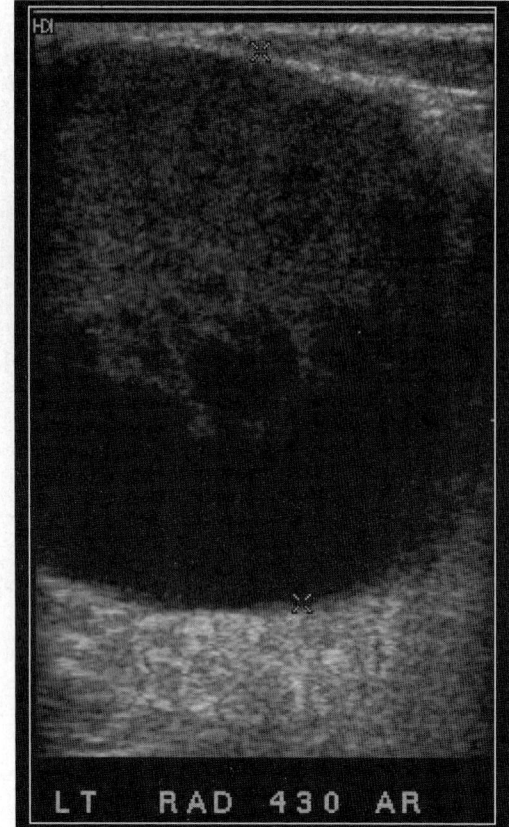
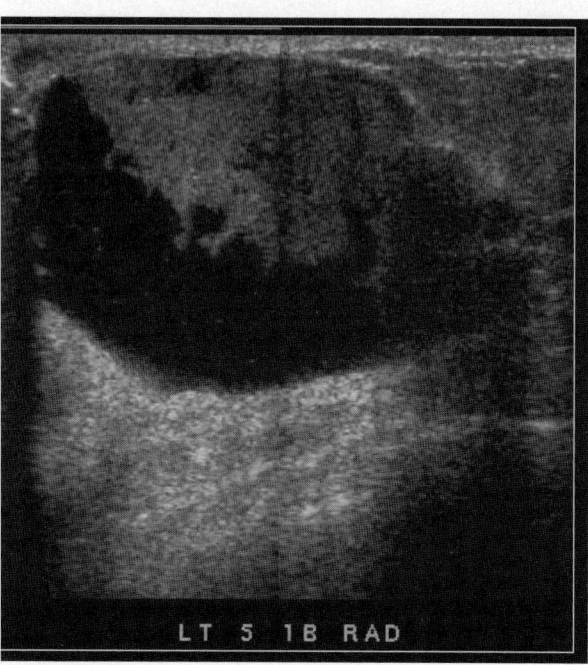

FIGURE 2–39 A: This large, intracystic, papillary carcinoma is too large to demonstrate with the standard 38-mm wide, 12-MHz linear array transducer. **B:** By using split-screen imaging and combining the left and right image into a single fused image, we can now show the entire intracystic tumor, creating a wider field of view than we were able to obtain without split-screen imaging.

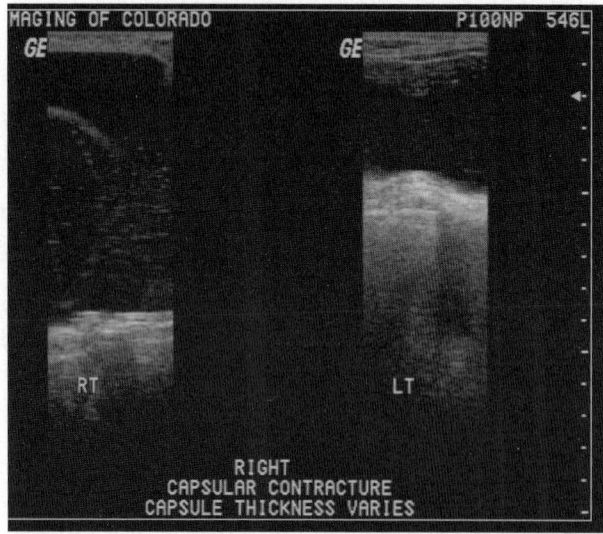
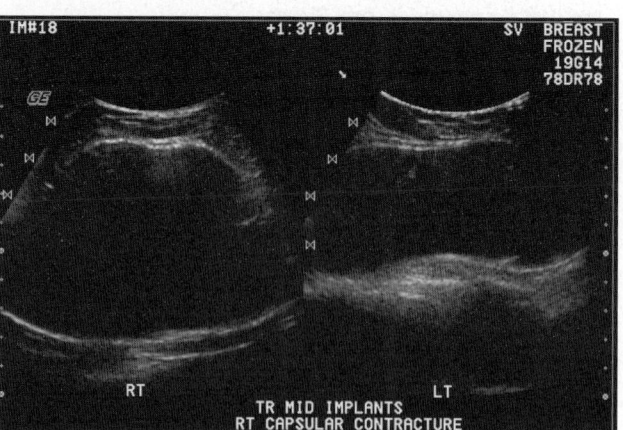

FIGURE 2–40 A: These split-screen images show the right implant to be thicker than the left because of capsular contracture. However, the field of view is so small that we cannot appreciate the abnormal spherical shape of the right implant and the convex outward posterior border that define capsular contracture sonographically. From these images alone, we cannot be sure whether the anteroposterior (AP) dimension of the right implant is too large or the AP dimension of the left implant is too small because of partial rupture. **B:** Using the large field of view of a convex, 7-MHz linear array transducer, we can appreciate the abnormally spherical shape and convex outward posterior border of the right implant that typify capsular contracture (**left**). The implant on the patient's left side shows a normal convex inward shape of the posterior wall (**right**).

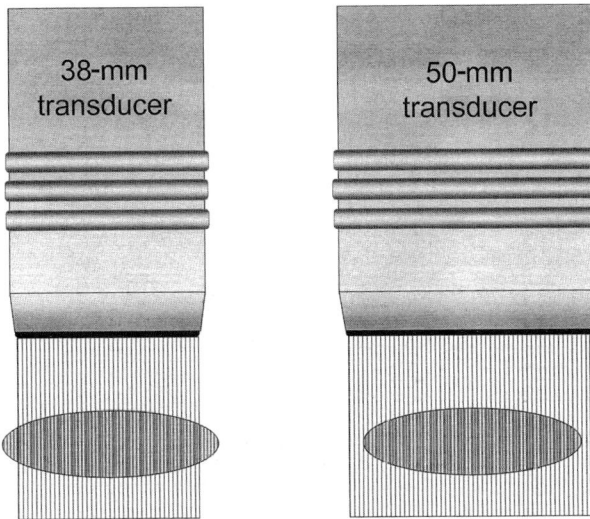

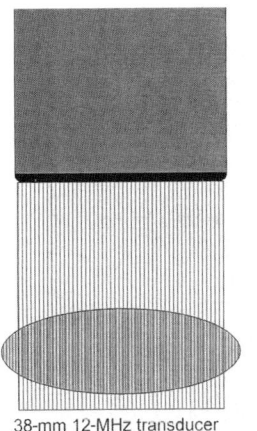
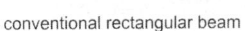
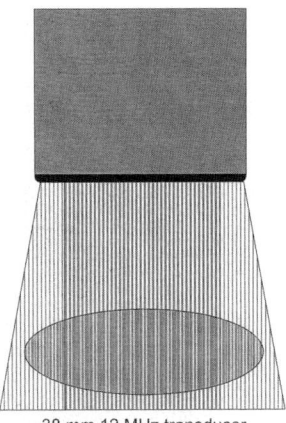

FIGURE 2–41 Lesions larger than 38 mm but smaller than 50 mm in the largest transverse measurement may be most optimally imaged with a 50-mm long, high-frequency transducer.

FIGURE 2–42 Another way to expand the field of view with a standard 38-mm long, 12-MHz transducer is to phase the beam on either end, creating a trapezoidal shaped or virtual convex beam. This approach is less effective for very superficially located lesions and more effective for deeper lesions because the beam diverges as it passes more deeply.

rectangular portion of the beam is similar to that of the linear transducer when the ends of the beam are not phased, but the lateral resolution in the triangular ends of the field of view are reduced by phasing and divergence of the beam.

Finally, certain equipment is capable of constructing an image larger than the rectangular shape of the ultrasound beam by linear translation along the long axis of the transducer to actually create an extended field of view (Fig. 2–44).

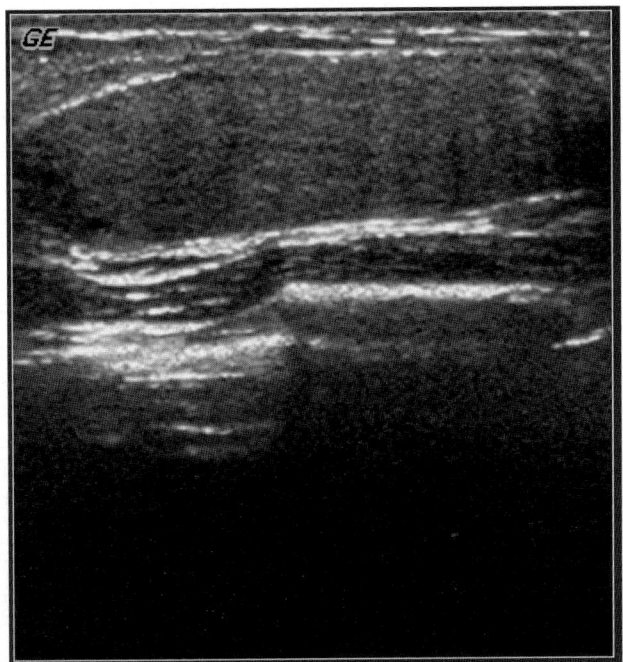

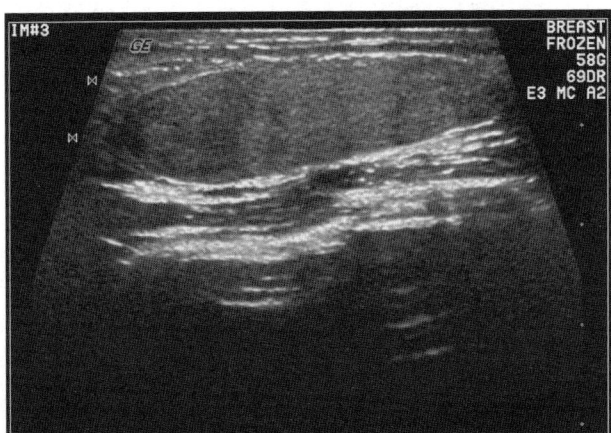

FIGURE 2–43 A: This large fibroadenoma was longer than the 38-mm, 12-MHz linear array transducer and wider than the width of the conventional linear array beam. Its largest dimension could not be accurately measured, and both lateral margins of the lesion could not be evaluated on a single image. **B:** The entirety of the nodule was visible when scanned in virtual convex mode. Both lateral margins of the lesion are well demonstrated on a single image, and the largest dimension of the lesion can be accurately measured.

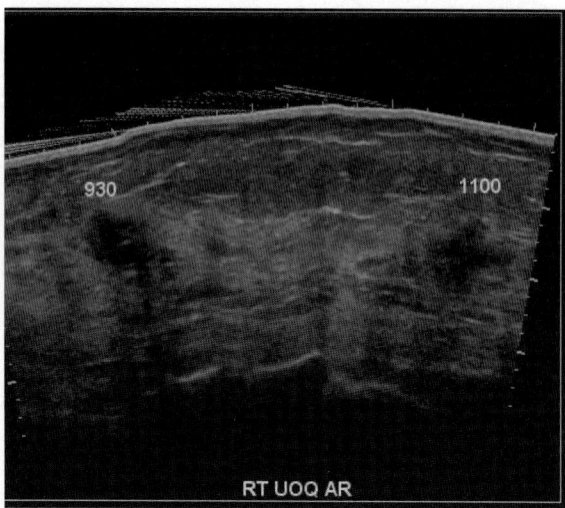

FIGURE 2–44 Extended field-of-view applications allow "painting" of an indefinite length of tissue. An entire longitudinal, radial, or transverse view of the breast can be obtained, and even both breasts may be included in the same image. This obliquely oriented, extended field of view of the upper outer quadrant of the right breast shows two widely separated malignant solid nodules.

THE CHANGING CONCEPT OF NOMINAL TRANSDUCER FREQUENCIES

The frequency label placed on a transducer by a manufacturer has been termed its *nominal frequency*. Traditionally, the center frequency of an ultrasound transducer had been used as its nominal frequency. For example, two different transducers might both have 7.5 MHz center frequencies. However, one might have a relatively wide bandwidth from 4.5 to 10.5 MHz. The other might have a narrower bandwidth from 6 to 9 MHz. Both would have been considered 7.5-MHz transducers. The disadvantage of the traditional method of selecting a nominal transducer frequency is that it does not convey any information about the transducer bandwidth. Partly to convey information about bandwidth, and partly to gain marketing advantages, the old convention used in selecting a nominal transducer frequency has become less predictable.

In some instances, the ends of the transducer frequency bandwidth rather than center frequency are used as its nominal frequency. The configuration of the probe is stated first as a letter (C for convex or curved array, or L for linear), followed by the upper end of the bandwidth, and completed with the lower end of the bandwidth. Thus, a linear 7.5-MHz center frequency probe with a bandwidth from 10 to 5 MHz is labeled an L10–5 MHz probe. Other manufacturers label the nominal probe frequency with the upper end of the bandwidth. Thus, the transducer with a bandwidth from 10 to 5 MHz is labeled an L10 transducer. Yet others have used various filtering schemes to shift the

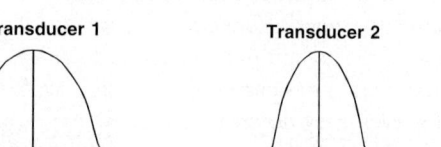

convention	nominal transducer frequency	
classical	L7.5 MHz	L7.5 MHz
bandwidth	L10-5	L9-6
upper end	L10	L9

FIGURE 2–45 Different nomenclature conventions are used to convey the transducer frequency and bandwidth. The oldest convention uses the center of the bandwidth as the transducer frequency. Thus, a transducer with a center frequency of 7.5 MHz and a bandwidth of 5 to 10 MHz would be termed a 7.5-MHz transducer. Unfortunately, a narrower-bandwidth transducer with a bandwidth of 6 to 9 MHz and a center frequency could also be termed a 7.5-MHz transducer with this convention, even though it would be a much less suitable transducer for breast ultrasound. To identify bandwidth as well as frequency, a more recent convention is to use the upper and lower ends of the bandwidth to define the transducer. The transducer with a bandwidth of 5 to 10 MHz would be termed a linear 10–5. One other frequently used convention is to use the upper end of the bandwidth to define the transducer frequency. Thus, the transducer with a bandwidth of 5 to 10 MHz would be termed a 10-MHz transducer. The use of different conventions for nominal frequency can be confusing to the end user in some cases. A 7.5-MHz transducer from one manufacturer may have the same frequency and bandwidth as a 10-MHz transducer produced by a different manufacturer.

center frequency higher. Thus, the center frequency might be shifted to 8 MHz from 7.5 MHz. The nominal frequency of such a transducer might be L8 MHz. Recent changes in the convention for selecting nominal transducer frequency have, in some cases, conveyed additional information on bandwidth to the end user. However, more often, the variability in the definition of nominal transducer frequency has been confusing to the end user and has made it difficult to compare the true frequencies and bandwidths of various transducers (Fig. 2–45).

INTERPRETIVE DIFFICULTIES PRESENTED BY IMPROVED RESOLUTION

Although there are great advantages to higher spatial and contrast resolution in BUS, some new interpretive difficulties can be encountered. Cysts that appear to be simple cysts on older, lower-resolution equipment may appear to have internal echoes on newer, higher-resolution equipment. In many cases, these are not artifactual echoes but rather real echoes that represent proteinaceous debris, cholesterol crystals, floating foamy macrophages, or floating papillary apocrine metaplasia cells. Such findings are not worrisome to the pathologist, who merely classifies all of these findings as part of the spectrum of fibrocystic change. However, they do create potential problems for the sonographer or sonologist, who has been taught that any cyst with internal echoes must be classified as a complicated or complex cyst and that all complex cysts are worrisome. Thus, higher-resolution equipment shows findings that require the sonologist or sonographer to learn more about breast pathophysiology and to develop algorithms to deal with the extra information provided. The algorithm we have developed for complex cysts is discussed in greater detail in Chapter 10.

Additionally, high-resolution ultrasound equipment can show more and smaller normal breast structures than did older equipment. It can clearly show normal ducts and lobules [terminal ductolobular unit (TDLU), the functional unit of the breast] in many patients. It can also show abnormally enlarged TDLUs caused by a variety of benign fibrocystic or benign proliferative changes. Most breast malignancies arise within and ultimately enlarge the TDLUs. The enlarged TDLUs resulting from benign fibrocystic change and benign proliferative changes may be difficult or even impossible to distinguish from enlarged malignant TDLUs sonographically, thus creating interpretation difficulties for the sonographer or sonologist. Benign, mildly enlarged TDLUs did not cause difficulty when older, lower-resolution equipment was used because they were not routinely visible with such equipment. The range of normal and fibrocystic and benign proliferative variants is discussed in greater detail in Chapter 4, and algorithms for distinguishing them from malignancy are discussed in greater detail in Chapter 12.

Finally, high-resolution ultrasound equipment can show enlarged, solid-appearing ducts (due to either inspissated secretions within ectatic ducts or periductal isoechoic fibroelastic tissue). Some malignancies may arise in larger ducts, and many others spread through the larger central ducts. It may be difficult or even impossible to distinguish enlarged ducts containing viscous, echogenic inspissated secretions of chronic duct ectasia from ducts distended with neoplasm and necrotic debris on ultrasound. Once again, this causes interpretive difficulties for the sonographer or sonologist that rarely occurred with older, lower-resolution equipment that either did not show the ectatic ducts or made them falsely appear anechoic. Algorithms for evaluating enlarged ducts are discussed in greater detail in Chapters 8 and 12.

Until recently, ultrasound equipment that offered excellent spatial resolution in both axial and lateral planes and that also demonstrated excellent contrast resolution was available only on top-of-the-line, very expensive equipment. The cost of such equipment is frequently in the $150,000 to $250,000 range and has generally been available only in inpatient diagnostic imaging departments or in large, multimodality outpatient imaging facilities. However, much of the mammography done in the United States is performed in stand-alone breast centers or geographically separate areas of a radiology department. The combination of a low BUS volume and relatively low reimbursement for BUS examinations has meant that most of these mammography centers could not afford high-quality near-field imaging equipment. However, ultrasound equipment manufacturers have recently begun to recognize that BUS is an important niche market, and they have begun to build dedicated, high-quality, near-field imaging machines that have only one or two high-frequency transducers for a price that such centers can better afford (about $100,000).

Summary of Imaging Requirements and Options

In summary, high-quality BUS requires superb near-field imaging equipment. Transducers with center frequencies within the 7- to 12-MHz range, short-axis focal zone of about 1.5 cm, continuous electronic focusing on transmit and receive, broad bandwidth, and short pulse lengths give the best combination of spatial and contrast resolution for BUS. When this type of equipment is used, many more normal structures and more alterations caused by proliferative and fibrocystic change become visible within the breast, therefore requiring a more thorough knowledge of breast anatomy and pathology for proper interpretation of findings. Such equipment is absolutely essential for BUS to realize its tremendous diagnostic potential.

Current developments offer to make BUS even more valuable. Coded harmonics and spatial compounding improve contrast resolution while maintaining or improving spatial resolution, allowing us to make specific benign and malignant diagnoses in a larger percentage of cases. Various methods of extending the field of view can be helpful in selected cases.

COLOR DOPPLER AND PULSED DOPPLER SPECTRAL ANALYSIS

Like imaging of the breast, color and pulsed Doppler analysis of the breast requires high-frequency ultrasound. In most cases, the Doppler frequency is the same as or slightly lower than the center frequency of the transducer. Thus, transducers with 7.5 MHz (center frequency) and a bandwidth from 5 to 10 MHz would have a Doppler frequency in the 6.5- to 7.5-MHz range. On some systems, Doppler frequency may be independently selectable. In such cases, the manufacturer of the system usually offers the option of downshifting the Doppler to a frequency near the lower end of the bandwidth. Thus, the Doppler frequency on a probe with a bandwidth from 5 to 10 MHz may be downshifted to 5 MHz. This enables the color and pulsed Doppler to be steered better and allows better penetration to structures deeper than 3 cm.

Although Doppler steering may be advantageous in peripheral vascular work, where vessels being studied are nearly parallel to the skin, steering is not necessary, and often counterproductive, in evaluation of the breast. There are several reasons for this. First, steering the Doppler beam reduces Doppler sensitivity. Second, it is often necessary to downshift the Doppler frequency in order to steer the Doppler beam. Decreasing Doppler frequency also decreases Doppler sensitivity for superficially located vessels such as tumor vessels in the breast. The increased sensitivity to flow deeper than 3 cm gained by downshifting the Doppler frequency is not necessary in breast tumors that are usually less than 3 cm deep. Finally, the vessels of interest in the breast, tumor vessels, do not course parallel to the skin, as do large vessels such as the carotid and femoral arteries. Rather, tumor vessels usually form a random net of small vessels in and around the tumor nodule. The tumor vessels from which the best Doppler signals are obtained are usually those that are oriented parallel to the ultrasound beam and perpendicular to the skin and transducer face. Doppler steering is not necessary to obtain optimal signals from such vessels.

Doppler modes available include color Doppler, power Doppler, and pulsed Doppler with spectral analysis. Color and pulsed Doppler spectral analysis have been advocated for distinguishing benign from malignant solid nodules, but we have found imaging algorithms more valuable for this. We do not use color Doppler for characterizing solid nodules, except in rare case. However, we do use color and power Doppler for several niche applications in the breast and currently would not order equipment for BUS that did not have at least power Doppler capability.

Doppler shows blood flow best when it is coursing at and angle of incidence of 0 degrees to the beam. This is true for all three Doppler modes, but power Doppler is the least sensitive to angle of incidence of the three. Color and pulsed Doppler spectral analysis is based on detection of phase shift of red blood cells and therefore shows direction of flow, but is highly angle dependent and relatively insensitive to slow flow or small vessels. Power Doppler is based on detection of amplitude of flow and is more sensitive to slow flow and small vessels, but cannot show direction of flow. Power Doppler is more subject to motion artifact, a shortcoming that can be exploited when evaluating vocal fremitus or other intentionally induced vibration in the chest.

Doppler sensitivity is generally much better on high-end ultrasound equipment than it is on low-end equipment, but as for imaging, the expense of high-end equipment can be prohibitive for BUS.

Summary of Doppler Requirements and Options

In summary, color, pulsed, and power Doppler evaluation of the breast, like sonographic imaging of the breast, requires a high-frequency transducer and Doppler frequencies near the center frequency of the transducer rather than downshifted frequencies, and does not require Doppler beam steering. Doppler evaluation of the breast is discussed in greater detail in Chapter 20.

SUGGESTED READINGS

Bassett LW, Kimme-Smith C. Breast sonography: technique, equipment, and normal anatomy. *Semin Ultrasound CT MR* 1989; 10(2):82–89.

Dempsey PJ. The importance of resolution in the clinical application of breast sonography. *Ultrasound Med Biol* 1988;14(1):43–48.

Fishell EK, et al. Clinical performance of a cone/annular array ultrasound breast scanner. *Ultrasound Med Biol* 1990;16(4): 361–374.

Goldstein A. Instrumentation of digital gray-scale US. *Radiographics* 1993;13:1389–1395.

Hayashi N, et al. Breast masses: color Doppler, power Doppler, and spectral analysis findings. *J Clin Ultrasound* 1998;26(5):231–238.

Kelly-Fry E, et al. Variation of transducer frequency output and receiver band-pass characteristics for improved detection and image characterization of solid breast masses. *Ultrasound Med Biol* 1988;1:143–161.

Kimme-Smith C, et al. Ultrasound mammography: effects of focal zone placement. *Radiographics* 1985;5(6):955–969.

Kimme-Smith C, et al. Ultrasound artifacts affecting the diagnosis of breast masses. *Ultrasound Med Biol* 1988;1:203–210.

Kossoff G, Jellins J. The physics of breast echography. *Semin Ultrasound CT MR* 1982;3(3):5–12.

Kremkau FW. Multiple-element transducers. *Radiographics* 1993;13: 1163–1176.

Lagalla R, et al. Image quality control in breast ultrasound. *Eur J Radiol* 1998;27[Suppl 2]:S229–233.

Landini L, Sarnelli R, Squartini F. Frequency-dependent attenuation in breast tissue characterization. *Ultrasound Med Biol* 1985;11(4): 599–603.

Martinoli C, et al. Power Doppler sonography: clinical applications. *Eur J Radiol* 1998;27[Suppl 2]:S133–140.

Moshfeghi M, Waag RC. In vivo and in vitro ultrasound beam distortion measurements of a large aperture and a conventional aperture focussed transducer. *Ultrasound Med Biol* 1988;14(5): 415–428.

Moskalik A, et al. Registration of three-dimensional compound ultrasound scans of the breast for refraction and motion correction. *Ultrasound Med Biol* 1995;21(6):769–778.

Ritchie WGM. Axial resolution. *Ultrasound Q* 1992;10(2):80–100.

Rubin E, et al. Hand-held real-time breast sonography. *AJR Am J Roentgenol* 1985;144(3):623–627.

Samuels TH. Breast imaging: a look at current and future technologies. *Postgrad Med* 1998;104(5):91–94, 97–101.

Shankar PM, et al. Advantages of subharmonic over second harmonic backscatter for contrast-to-tissue echo enhancement. *Ultrasound Med Biol* 1998;24(3):395–399.

Smith SW, Trahey GE, von Ramm OT. Two-dimensional arrays for medical ultrasound. *Ultrason Imag* 1992;14(3):213–233.

Tenekeci AN, et al. Sonographic pitfall in diagnosing breast cysts: pseudomural projections. *J Clin Ultrasound* 1998;26(3):181–182.

Teubner J, van Kaick G, Junkermann H. 5MHz realtime sonography of the breast. 1. Technical equipment studies. *Radiologe* 1985; 25(10):449–456.

Trahey GE, et al. The impact of acoustic velocity variations on target detectability in ultrasonic images of the breast. *Invest Radiol* 1991;26(9):782–791.

Ueno E, et al. Current status of ultrasound examination of the superficial organs (breast and thyroid). *Rinsho Byori* 1993;41(1):15–25.

Venta LA, et al. Sonographic evaluation of the breast. *Radiographics* 1994;14(1):29–50.

Wright IA, et al. Power Doppler in breast tumors: a comparison with conventional colour Doppler imaging. *Eur J Ultrasound* 1998; 7(3):175–81.

Zhu Q, Steinberg BD. Wavefront amplitude distribution in the female breast. *J Acoust Soc Am* 1994;96(1):1–9.

3

BREAST ULTRASOUND TECHNIQUE

The actual technique of breast ultrasound (BUS) is just as important to high-quality diagnostic BUS as the ultrasound equipment used. The technique varies between patients and with scan locations, indications, and lesion type. It is important to customize the scan technique to the clinical circumstances.

TRANSDUCER AND ACOUSTIC POWER SETTINGS

In general, we use the highest probe frequency that adequately penetrates to the chest wall to evaluate the breast. The 7.5- to 12-MHz transducers achieve adequate penetration in the majority of women. However, women who have unusually thick breast tissue while in the supine position may require use of a lower-frequency transducer to penetrate the breast. Circumstances requiring a lower-frequency transducer include very obese patients or very large-breasted women; women with very large silicone implants, especially when there is capsular contracture; patients with puerperal mastitis; and patients with severe lymphedema of the breast caused by a variety of conditions, including inflammatory carcinoma and recurrent carcinoma metastatic to axillary lymph nodes. Equipment requirements are discussed in greater detail in Chapter 2.

Most ultrasound systems boot up at low power settings by default for safety reasons. However, in some patients, low power may result in inadequate sound penetration to the chest wall. In such cases, the acoustic output power should be turned to maximum before switching to a lower-frequency transducer.

PATIENT POSITIONING

The patient is scanned in supine or contralateral posterior oblique positioning (Fig. 3–1). In other words, for the oblique position, the breast to be scanned should be elevated somewhat relative to the opposite breast. The degree of obliquity varies, depending on breast size, pendulousness, and the location in the area of interest within the breast to be scanned (Fig. 3–2). Generally, the larger or more pendulous the breast and the farther lateral the area of interest, the greater the degree of contralateral obliquity that is required. In patients with very large or pendulous breasts or lesions located very far laterally, a contralateral lateral decubitus position may be necessary. When the area of interest is located far medially, supine positioning is usually best. The patient is asked to bring her ipsilateral arm above her head and to place her ipsilateral hand behind her head. This positioning, in combination with some degree of compression of the breast with the transducer, accomplishes two important things. First, it thins the area of the breast being scanned to the greatest degree possible, ensuring that the 7- to 12-MHz probes used for BUS will adequately penetrate to the chest wall. Second, it pulls the normally conically shaped tissue planes of the breast into a horizontal orientation that is nearly parallel to the transducer surface and perpendicular to the ultrasound beam. This positioning technique minimizes the amount of image degradation and critical angle shadowing that result from reflection and refraction by obliquely oriented tissue planes within the breast.

Occasionally, if a lesion is palpable only when the patient is in an upright position, at least part of the examination should be performed with the patient in the upright position. This technique is especially helpful if the lesion is superficially located. However, the breast is thicker in the upright than in the supine position, and deeper lesions may be missed completely if only upright scan positions and high-frequency transducers are used. A breast that is only 3 cm thick when the patient is placed in the contralateral posterior oblique position described previously can be as much as 10 cm thick with upright positioning. The 7- to 12-MHz probes we normally use for BUS usually will not penetrate to the chest wall in the upright position if the area of interest is in the inferior portion of the breast. (The

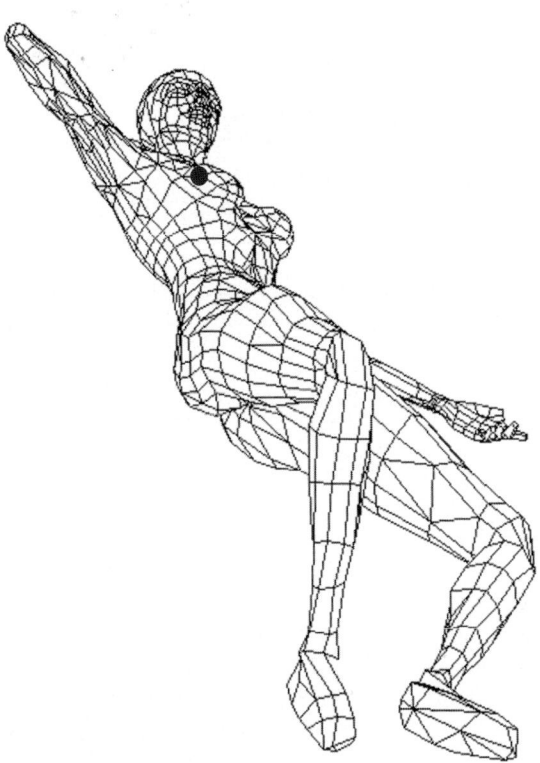

FIGURE 3–1 The patient is usually scanned in a contralateral posterior oblique position with the ipsilateral arm abducted and the hand placed under the head in order to thin and flatten the breast. This positioning helps ensure adequate penetration to the chest wall with high-frequency transducers and minimizes critical angle effects caused by tissue planes in the breast that are steeply obliquely oriented in upright or prone positions. Additionally, this positioning stretches the wrinkles out of the skin, minimizing trapping of air bubbles during sonographic survey, and stretches Cooper's ligaments, facilitating compression of the area of interest between the transducer and chest wall.

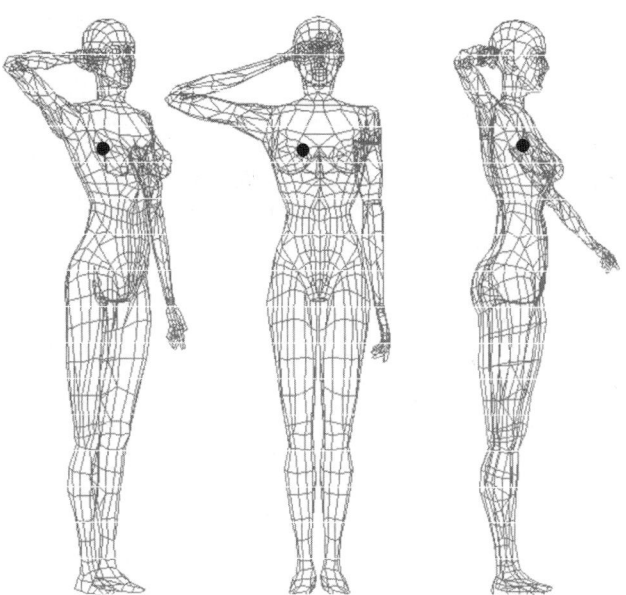

FIGURE 3–2 The degree of posterior obliquity is varied in order to thin and flatten the portion of the breast being sonographically evaluated. When evaluating the upper outer quadrant, the most frequent area of concern in most patients, the patient is usually placed into a 30- to 45-degree contralateral posterior oblique position (**left**). For lesions that are located medially, a supine position is usually preferable (**middle**). For lesions that are located very near the lateral edge of the breast or in patients with very large and pendulous breasts that hang laterally in the supine position, a contralateral lateral decubitus position is usually the most effective (**right**).

superior portion of the breast may actually become thinner when the patient is in the upright position.) Furthermore, tissue planes are more steeply oblique in the upright than in the supine position, and the obliquely oriented tissue planes will further degrade the image. If a lesion is found in the upright position, its location should be noted and then subsequently scanned with the patient placed in the usual supine or contralateral posterior oblique position. In this way, the lesion can be characterized more accurately, and the surrounding tissues can be better evaluated. Occasionally, when large, central ducts are the targets for evaluation, scanning in the upright position may be helpful, especially if the ducts are in the upper part of the breast. Ducts that are too tortuous to be adequately evaluated in the supine position may become straighter and more easily evaluated in the upright position. The technique for evaluating subareolar ducts in patients presenting with nipple discharge is discussed and illustrated in greater detail in Chapter 8.

In cases in which there is dependent or floating debris within complex cysts, it may be helpful to scan while the patient is in different positions in order to demonstrate movement of debris. Generally, supine and left lateral positions can be used to document movement while scanning in the transverse plane, and supine and upright positions can be used to document movement while scanning in the longitudinal plane. We routinely employ these maneuvers to document definitively benign findings such as milk of calcium (Fig. 3–3) and fat–fluid levels within cysts (Fig. 3–4). Evaluation of complex breast cysts is discussed in greater detail in Chapter 10.

COMPRESSION OF THE BREAST WITH THE ULTRASOUND TRANSDUCER

A variable degree of compression can be applied with the transducer. This further thins the breast tissue being scanned and also tends to force normal breast tissues into a plane parallel to the transducer surface and perpendicular to the ultrasound beam, improving penetration and image quality. Greater compression pressure can be useful for small, deeply located lesions that lie near the chest wall, especially when fibrous tissue lies superficial to the lesion. Sometimes, a superficial structure, such as an obliquely oriented Cooper's ligament within the subcutaneous tissue, creates an acoustic shadow, preventing evaluation of deeper

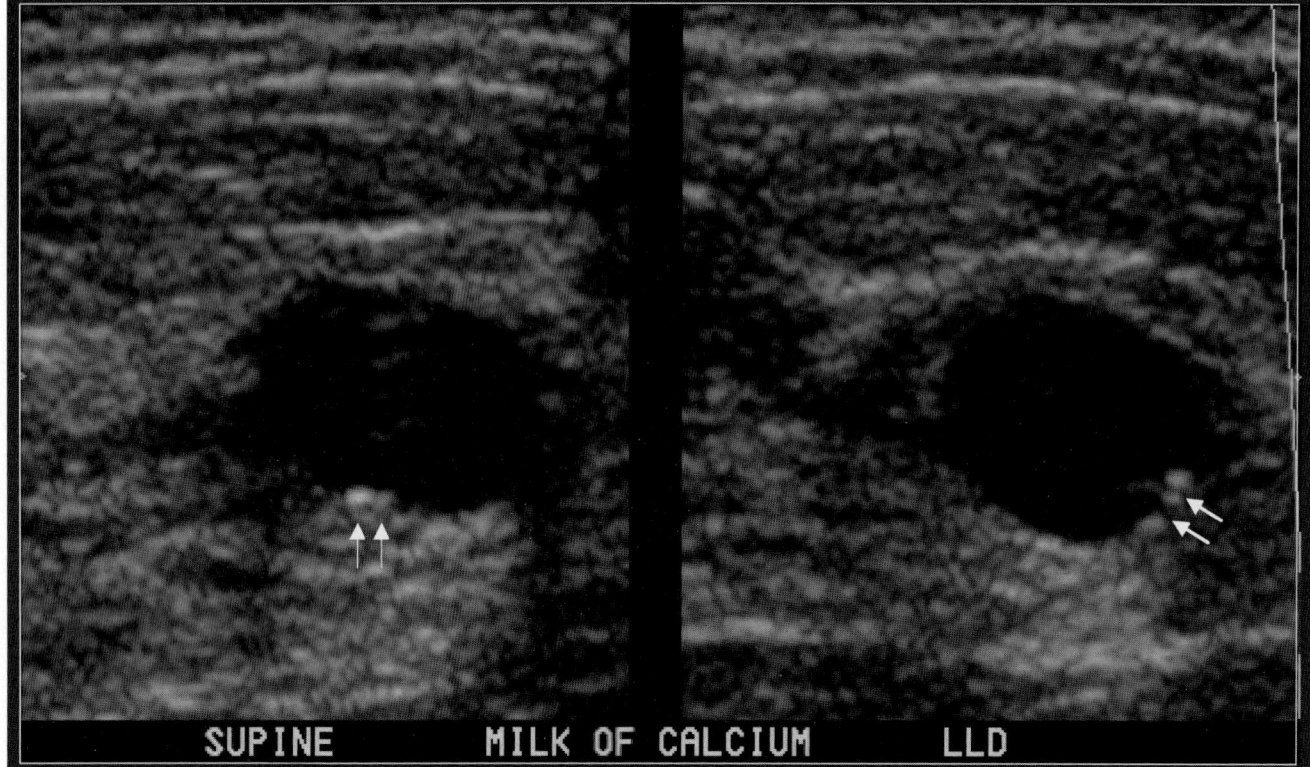

FIGURE 3–3 Changes of patient position during an examination can be used to document motion of complex cyst contents. In this case, supine (**left** split-screen image) and left lateral decubitus (LLD) images are compared while scanning transversely, in order to demonstrate the movement of milk of calcium (*arrows*) within this complex cyst. Milk of calcium is a definitively benign finding, both mammographically and sonographically.

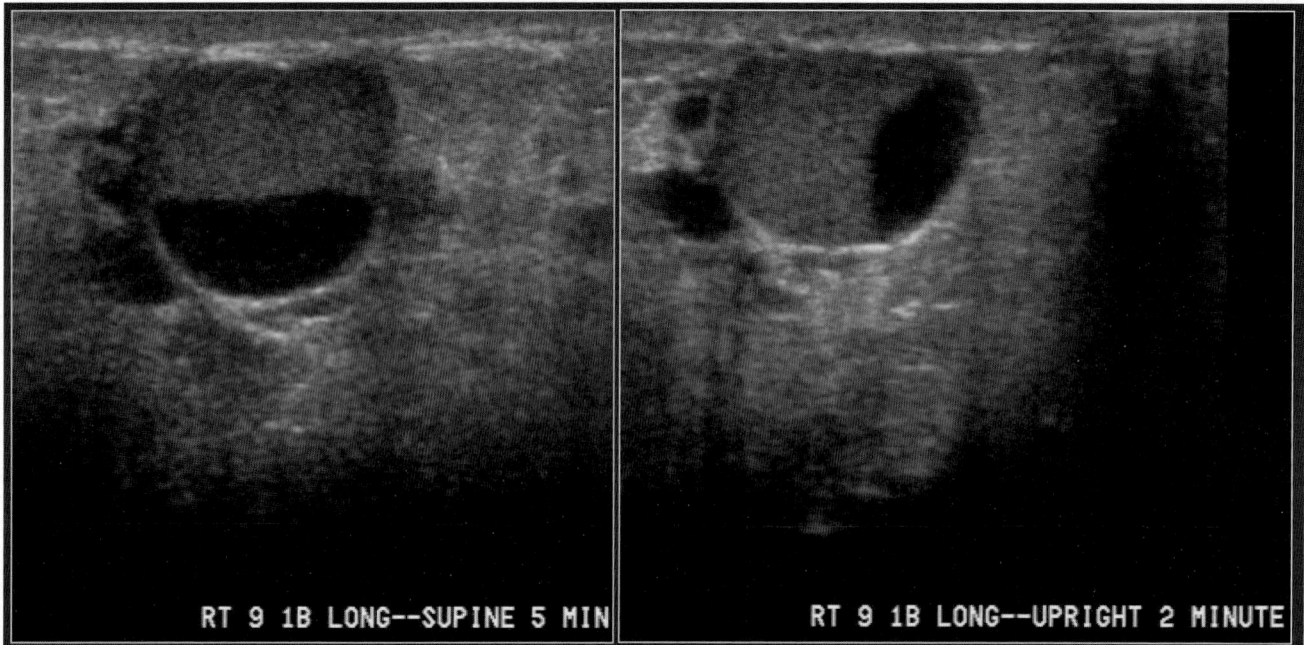

FIGURE 3–4 In this case, longitudinal images obtained in the supine (**left**) and upright (**right**) positions document the movement of echogenic lipid material to the nondependent position within this complex cyst. This is a useful maneuver to document a fat–fluid level, a definitively benign finding.

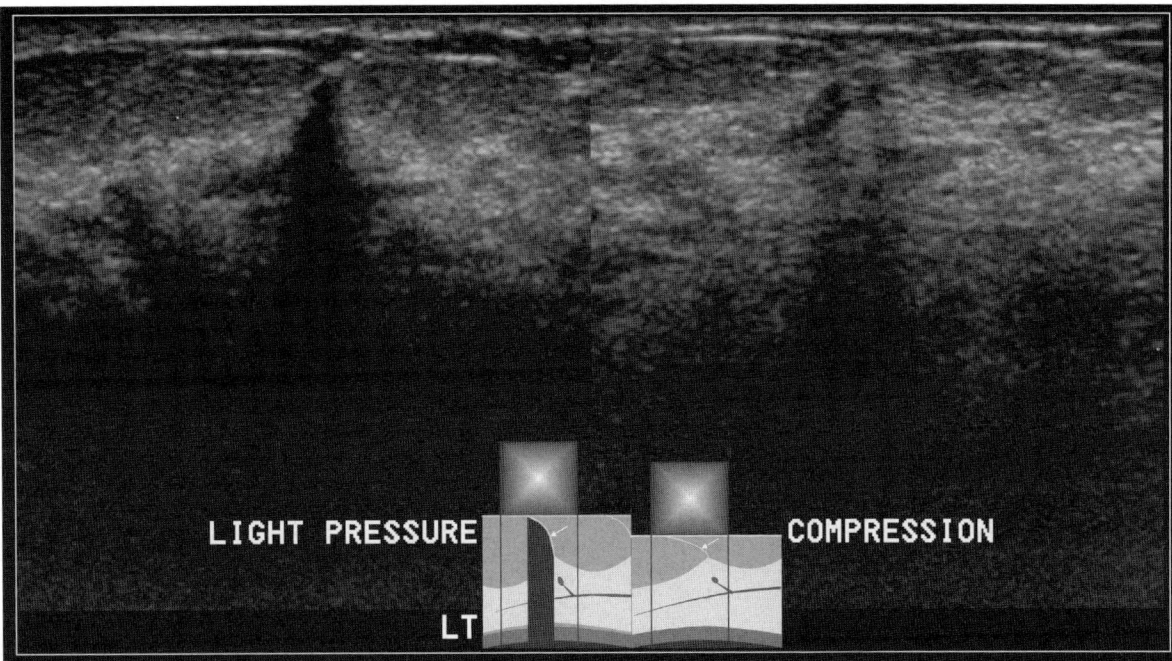

FIGURE 3–5 This split-screen image shows artifactual shadowing arising from Cooper's ligament within the premammary zone when too little compression is used (**left**). More vigorous compression pushes the ligament into a horizontal orientation, ablating critical angle shadowing arising from it (**right**).

structures. Moderate compression with the transducer can push such a Cooper's ligament into a plane that lies parallel to the transducer surface and eradicate the artifactual acoustic shadowing it causes (Fig. 3–5). Shadowing arising from Cooper's ligaments can simulate shadowing caused by the desmoplastic reaction associated with invasive malignan-

cies. Another method of dealing with critical angle shadowing is to scan the same area of interest with the transducer angled cranially, caudally, to the left, or to the right in order to change the angle of incidence of the beam to one more nearly perpendicular to the anatomic structure causing shadowing (Fig. 3–6).

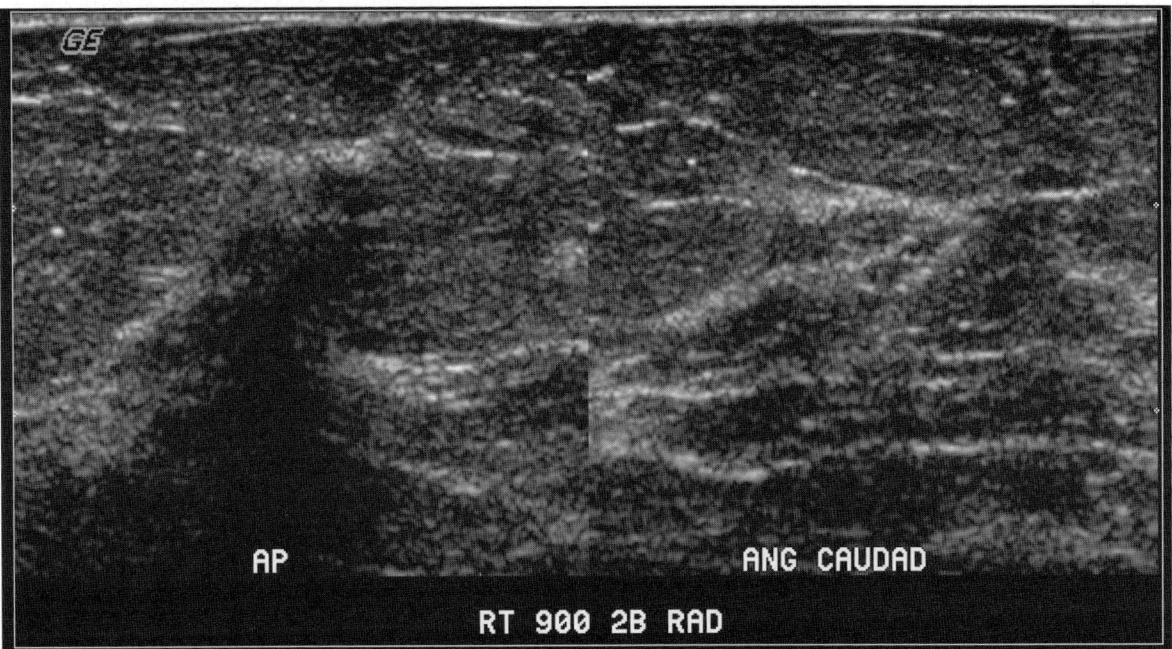

FIGURE 3–6 This split-screen image shows artifactual shadowing arising from an obliquely oriented area of fat-surrounded fibroglandular tissue (**left**). With angulation of the transducer so that the ultrasound beam strikes the tissue more nearly perpendicularly, the critical angle shadowing is eradicated (**right**).

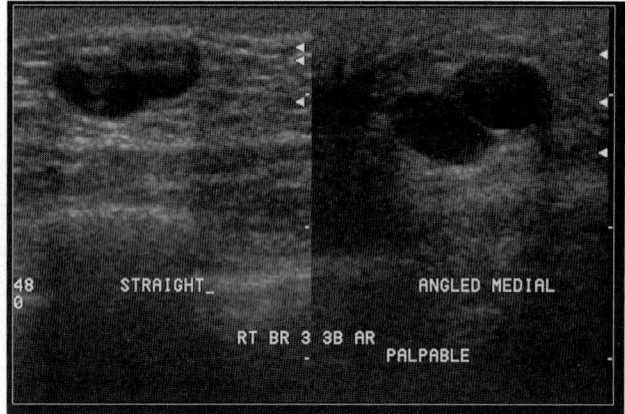

FIGURE 3–7 This split-screen image shows that using too much scan pressure can also cause problems in some cases, especially within cysts that lie in the near field. The **left** image shows near-field reverberation echoes within a superficially located cyst that has been scanned with vigorous compression. The **right** image was obtained with less compression and with the transducer angled slightly, markedly decreasing near-field reverberation echoes.

Heavy compression with the transducer does not always improve image quality. Using vigorous compression and scanning in a scan plane exactly perpendicular to near-field tissue planes can push near-field reverberation echoes and side-lobe artifacts deeper into the breast, especially interfering with evaluation of near-field cysts. The net effect may be to deepen the zone of suboptimal spatial and contrast resolution from the usual 5 to 7 mm to 10 mm or more. Some superficial lesions may be better seen if scan pressure is consciously lightened by lifting the probe slightly so that contact with the skin is barely maintained or by angling the transducer slightly so that the beam traverses through near-field tissues obliquely rather than perpendicularly to superficial tissue planes (Fig. 3–7). Near-field imaging problems and the use of acoustic standoff are discussed in Chapter 2.

SCANNING PLANES

Longitudinal and transverse scan planes may be sufficient for a generalized ultrasonographic search of a region and for specific evaluation of simple and complex breast cysts. However, demonstration of normal ductal anatomy requires scanning in the radial scan planes because the normal mammary ducts are generally radially oriented away from the nipple. Scanning the breast along normal anatomic-lobar planes improves understanding of the site of lesion origin and helps narrow the differential diagnosis. For example, radial and orthogonal antiradial scan planes can be useful in evaluating solid breast nodules for evidence of intraductal or periductal invasive tumor spread. The need for radial orientation of scan planes is also discussed in Chapters 9 and 12.

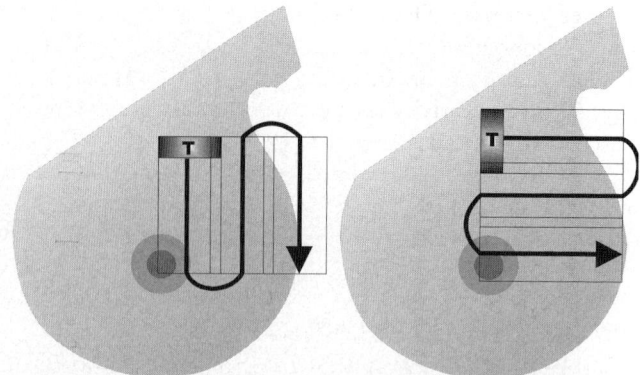

FIGURE 3–8 The breast may be surveyed sonographically using a "lawnmower" pattern in longitudinal and transverse planes. Longitudinal and transverse planes are not parallel to the long axis of the underlying lobar anatomy, however, and make interpretation of abnormal findings more difficult. If this style of survey is used, as soon as pathology is identified, the scan lane should be adjusted to radial and orthogonal antiradial planes.

Real-time ultrasound survey of the breast using a hand-held linear probe can be time consuming and tedious, but need not be. Scanning may be done longitudinally, transversely, or in both directions and can be likened to mowing the lawn (Fig. 3–8). One should overlap the previous scan path slightly with each strip of breast scanned. Whole breast survey can also be performed radially, antiradially, or in both directions (Fig. 3–9). However, regardless of the survey method chosen, once detected, a lesion is always scanned in radial and antiradial axes. Our preference for targeted diagnostic ultrasound examinations is to survey the breast in a radial fashion of the breast because this is roughly parallel to long axis of breast lobes. For whole breast ultrasound survey of the breast, scanning in an antiradial fashion from peripheral to central is efficient and minimizes interference of the examination by wrinkles and air bubbles. The chances of geographically missing a lesion increase as the area to be

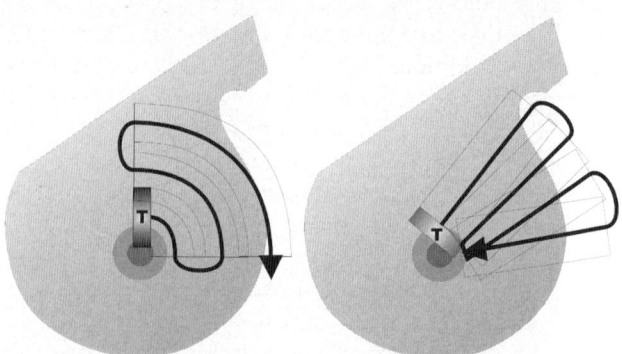

FIGURE 3–9 A better survey pattern uses a radial and an orthogonal antiradial pattern. Scanning the breast in an antiradial plane from peripheral to central minimizes tissue wrinkles, most consistently keeps Cooper's ligaments under tension, and speeds the examination. All positive findings are evaluated in the radial plane as well as the antiradial plane.

scanned increases. The risk of missing a lesion is one reason why sonography has not been found to be as useful as mammography in breast cancer screening. (Mammography's greater sensitivity for microcalcifications is the main reason.) In our experience, however, ultrasound is better than mammography for almost everything except detecting isolated calcifications of low- to intermediate-grade ductal carcinoma *in situ*.

SIMULTANEOUS PALPATION AND SCANNING OF PALPABLE ABNORMALITIES

When the indication for targeted diagnostic BUS is a palpable abnormality, sonography is targeted to the area of the palpable abnormality. In such cases, it is essential to palpate while scanning, especially if it appears that a definitively benign structure such as a simple cyst or an area of fibrosis is the cause of the palpable abnormality. The importance of palpating the lesion while scanning it is discussed in further detail in Chapter 5.

AREAS OF THE BREAST SCANNED FOR MAMMOGRAPHIC ABNORMALITIES

When the indication for targeted diagnostic BUS is a mammographic abnormality, the total area of breast tissue scanned will vary somewhat, depending on the location of the abnormality. Generally, lesions that are near 12:00 or 6:00 on mammography lie exactly where expected, and therefore, a smaller area can be scanned to find and characterize the lesion because there is little rotation of the breast or obliquity of the x-ray beam on the craniocaudal (CC) view of the mammogram. However, it is more difficult to predict the actual location of a lesion if it appears to be near 3:00 or 9:00 on the mammogram. The obliquity of the x-ray beam on routine mediolateral oblique (MLO) mammographic views causes lesions to project higher or lower than their true positions during supine scanning for ultrasound. Additionally, the compression and rotation of the breast tissues that occur during performance of the routine MLO view can displace lesions superiorly or inferiorly from their anatomic location during ultrasound scanning. Mammographic lesions that appear to be at 3:00 or 9:00 may actually lie much higher or lower than expected. Therefore, successful identification of lesions that appear to lie near 3:00 or 9:00 on mammograms usually requires that a wider segment of breast tissue be scanned to find the lesion at sonography than is necessary for lesions that lie near 6:00 or 12:00. Generally, a scan area the size of a breast quadrant, a 90-degree wedge, will suffice for most lesions that appear to be near 3:00 or 6:00, whereas lesions that lie near 6:00 or 12:00 can usually be found by scanning as little as a 30-degree wedge of tissue.

When a lesion is visible on only one view of the routine mammogram, it may be necessary to scan an entire hemisphere of the breast to find the lesion sonographically. A lesion that is seen in the lateral aspect of the breast on the CC view, but that is not visible on the MLO view, may require scanning the entire lateral half of the breast. A lesion seen in the upper half of the breast on the MLO view, but not visible on the CC view, may require scanning the entire upper half of the breast. Sonography for evaluation of mammographic abnormalities is discussed in greater detail in Chapter 6.

Scanning the Subareolar–Nipple Complex

Ultrasound of the nipple–areolar complex requires special consideration. The ease with which sound passes through the nipple and areola varies not only from patient to patient but also with scan environment and technique. When a lesion lies near or deep to the areola, it is important to use warm jelly and scan in a warm room. Cold room temperature and cold jelly cause the smooth muscle elements in the nipple and areola to contract, wrinkling the areola, increasing critical angle shadowing, and degrading the image of subareolar tissues. This approach is especially important when the indication for sonography is nipple discharge and attempted galactography has failed. Lesions that appear on the mammogram to be directly retroareolar are usually found slightly to the side of the nipple during sonography. Because it is difficult to determine where the lesion would lie in the absence of mammographic compression, it may be necessary to scan all around the areola to find the lesion. In some cases, it is useful to angle the beam so that the area directly deep to the nipple is scanned.

The scan technique for evaluation of secretions is unique. A large amount of warm jelly should be placed around the nipple and areola. The periareolar area is scanned radially in a clockwise fashion from 12:00 to 12:00. There are several special compression maneuvers that can be used to better demonstrate the ducts deep to the areolar–nipple complex. These maneuvers are discussed and illustrated in much greater detail in Chapter 8.

IDENTIFICATION OF SCAN PLANE AND LESION LOCATION

It is important that there be a brief and very reproducible method of reporting where a lesion lies sonographically. The method we use has three descriptors: a clock face location, similar to that of the American College of Radiology (ACR) lexicon; a description of how far from the nipple the lesion lies; and a description of the depth of the lesion (Fig. 3–10). We use a descriptor with five components to indicate the precise location of a scan plane location within the breast:

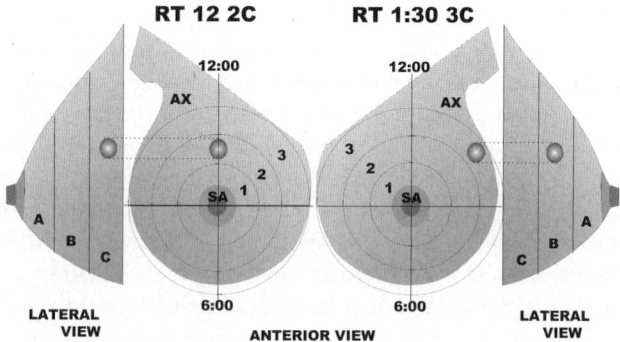

FIGURE 3–10 The locations of scan planes are documented by five descriptors. The first descriptor is the abbreviation for the right or left side. The second descriptor is the clock-face position of the lesion. The third descriptor is the abbreviation for the distance from the nipple. We use five zones: SA for subareolar; 1, 2, and 3 for equal width rings extending from the areolar margin to the edge of the breast; and AX for the axillary segment of the breast. An alternative used by many is the distance from the nipple in centimeters. The fourth descriptor is the depth of the lesion. We use A, B, and C to divide the breast into thirds in depth. A represents the superficial third of the breast; B, the middle third; and C (for chest wall), the deep third of the breast. Alternatively, depth in centimeters from the skin can be used, but this may vary with the degree of compression and scan position. The fifth descriptor is the abbreviation for the transducer orientation. We use radial (RAD), antiradial (AR), longitudinal (LONG), transverse (TR), and occasionally, oblique (OBL) scan orientations.

1. The first descriptor is the side, right or left, abbreviated *R* or *L*.
2. The second descriptor is a clock face position. We use positions halfway between the hours when necessary.

Thus, a lesion lying half way between the 1:00 and 2:00 positions would be termed 1:30.

3. The third descriptor defines the distance from the nipple of a lesion or anatomic structure. In our system, the distance description includes five locations: 1, 2, 3, subareolar (SA), and axillary (A). The numbers 1, 2, and 3 define equal-width rings extending from the areolar margin to the periphery of the breast. The ring labeled *1* is most central, and the ring labeled *3* is most peripheral. Another acceptable alternative for describing distance from the nipple is to measure the actual distance from the nipple in centimeters. Some have painted centimeter markers on the transducer to facilitate this. The trend is to use actual distances from the nipple in centimeters rather than zones because the distance from the nipple appears to vary much less than do the distances from the chest wall and periphery of the breast with changes in compression or patient position.

4. The fourth descriptor is the depth of the lesion or anatomic structure of interest. The depth description includes A, B, and C. These letters divide the breast into equal thirds in depth. The A zone is most superficial. The C zone is the deepest third and can be remembered as *C* for near the chest wall. The B zone, the middle zone, is where most pathologic lesions arise. An acceptable alternative is to use the depth in centimeters for this descriptor.

5. In addition to the four location descriptors, a scan plane orientation descriptor is used. This may be transverse (tr), longitudinal (lo), radial (rad), antiradial (ar), or oblique (obl) (Fig. 3–11).

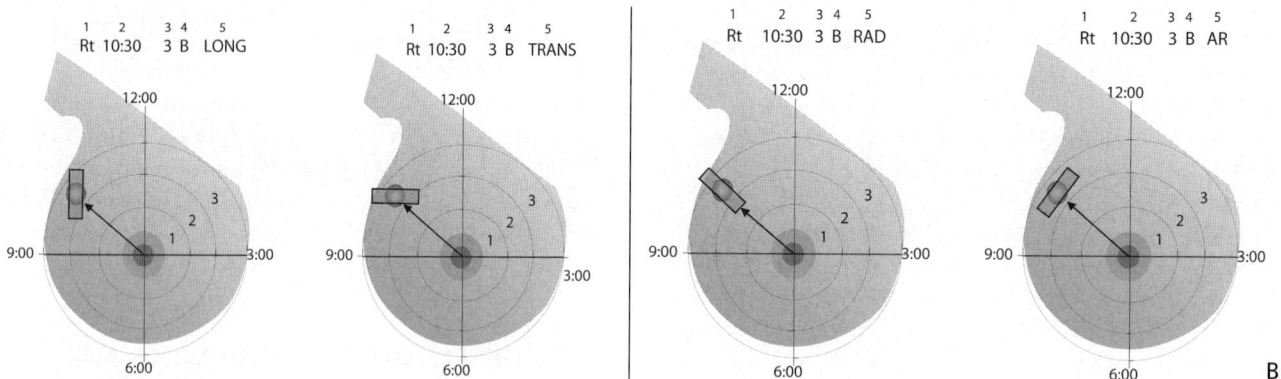

FIGURE 3–11 A: Longitudinal and transverse scan planes are obtained parallel to the long and short axes of the thorax. Although such scan planes are useful in most body parts scanned with ultrasound, they are less useful in the breast than elsewhere. The anatomy planes of the breast are not oriented longitudinally or transversely with respect to the thorax, except exactly at 12:00, 3:00, 6:00, and 9:00. In the upper outer quadrants of the breast, most breast tissue and lesions lie at oblique angles to the longitudinal and transverse planes. **B:** The radial scan plane extends out from the nipple, as would the spoke from the hub of a wheel. The antiradial plane lies at 90 degrees to the radial plane. The radial plane is parallel to the longitudinal plane at 6:00 and 12:00 and parallel to the transverse plane at exactly 3:00 and 9:00. The antiradial plane is parallel to the longitudinal plane at exactly 3:00 and 9:00 and parallel to the transverse plane at exactly 12:00 and 6:00. The major lobar ducts extend out from the nipple in radial fashion. Thus, radial scan planes roughly parallel the long axis of the lobar ducts. The true radial plane is the starting point of assessment of lesions. To assess the relationship of a lesion to the ductal system, the scan plane may need to be adjusted slightly off the true radial plane, because of tortuosity of the central ducts or the location of peripheral lesions in branch ducts.

In the American Institute of Ultrasound in Medicine (AIUM) and ACR BUS accreditation programs, descriptors 1, 2, 3, and 5 are mandatory, but descriptor 4, the depth of the lesion, is not.

The method that we use for describing the sonographic location is important for two reasons. First, it is highly reproducible and enables us to find a lesion again easily for later ultrasound-guided needle procedures or for follow-up studies. Second, it represents a cryptic, easy-to-type, shorthand method for annotating a lesion location while scanning the patient. Anything that can be done to reduce keystrokes while scanning is helpful. For example, it is much easier to type 10 keystrokes—"L {space} 3 {space} 2 B {space} rad"—than it is to type "left breast at 3:00 about halfway from the areolar margin to the periphery of the breast, about midbreast in depth, and scanned in a radial scan plane."

SPLIT-SCREEN IMAGING

Split-screen imaging is invaluable in BUS and can be routinely used in several different circumstances. First, split-screen images of mirror-image locations in the right and left breasts should be used to confirm that a mammographic or palpable abnormality is caused by asymmetric fibroglandular elements rather than a cystic or solid mass (Fig. 3–12). One of the main strengths of mammography is that bilateral imaging is usually performed, establishing the contralateral breast as a normal standard with which to compare. By using mirror-image split-screen sonographic imaging, one of mammography's greatest strengths can be emulated. This concept is discussed and illustrated further in Chapter 6. Second, split-screen imaging with and without compression can be used to capture a summary of dynamic events occurring during the ultrasound study on

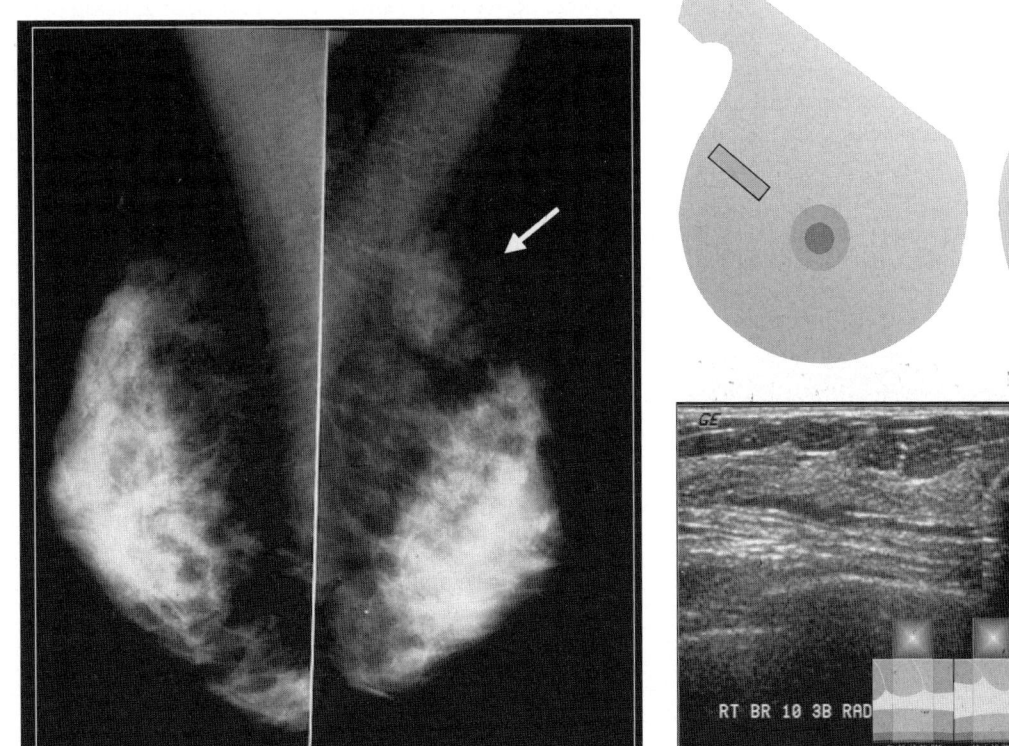
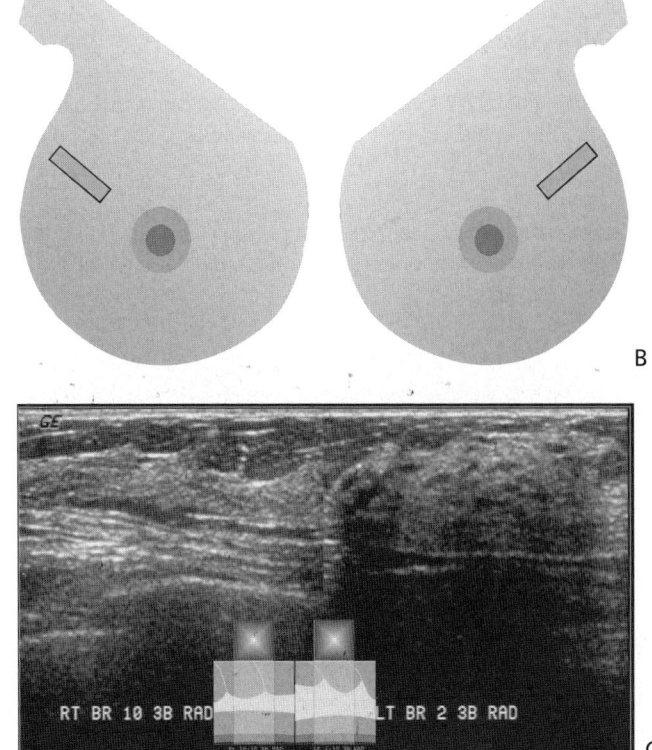

FIGURE 3–12 A: There is a focal mammographic asymmetry in the axillary segment of the left breast (*arrow*). This may merely represent accessory breast tissue, a mass in the axillary segment, or an occult mass within accessory breast tissue. Targeted ultrasound was used to further evaluate this focal asymmetry. **B:** Split-screen mirror-image scanning of right and left sides is reassuring when focal mammographic asymmetries appear to be caused by fibroglandular elements at sonography and no pathologic lesion can be found sonographically. **C:** Sonography revealed no mass, nodule, cyst, or architectural distortion in the axillary segment of the left breast, but did show the presence of prominent fibroductal tissues. Split-screen mirror-image scans of the right and left axillary segments show much thicker fibroglandular tissue on the left than on the right, accounting for the increased density in that area mammographically and confirming the presence of accessory breast tissue in the axillary segment of the left breast.

single hard-copy, freeze-frame images. Split-screen imaging with and without compression can be used as an alternative to storing cine loops or videotaping examinations for documenting dynamic events during the examination. Split-screen imaging can be used to document several different types of dynamic events occurring during the BUS examination:

- Compressibility of a lesion and the effect of compression on tissues adjacent to the lesion
- Rotation of a lesion
- Mobility of echoes within an enlarged echogenic mammary duct
- Compressibility of an enlarged echogenic duct
- Movement of necrotic debris in early immature abscesses
- Eradication of artifactual critical angle shadowing caused by Cooper's ligaments

To demonstrate the degree of compressibility of a structure or lesion, we store the image obtained without transducer compression on the left side of the split screen and the image obtained with compression on the right side of the screen. When documenting compressibility, it is important to scan very lightly for the left noncompressed image—so lightly that we are barely touching the skin—and to compress vigorously for the right-sided compressed image. Using a light scanning technique is especially important when the object being compressed is a fat lobule or lipoma. Some advocate using compressibility in the characterizing solid nodules as benign or malignant because fibroadenomas are generally more compressible than are malignant nodules (Figs. 3–13 and 3–14). However, some fibroadenomas do not compress much, and high-grade and

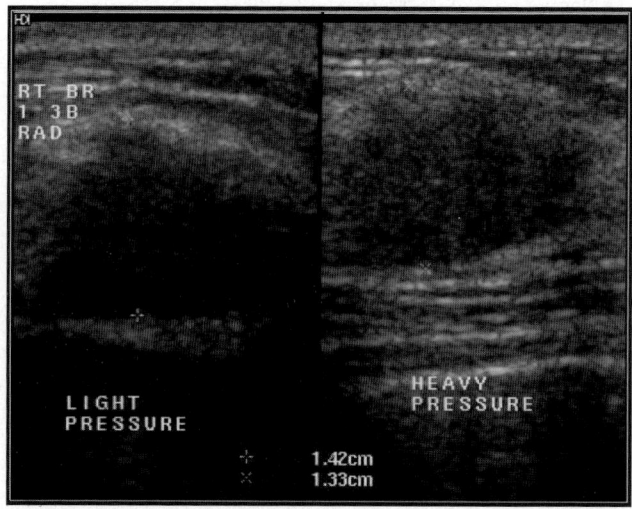

FIGURE 3–14 This high-grade invasive ductal carcinoma is mildly compressible, less than 10% (1.42–1.33)/1.33, less than the usual fibroadenoma and much less than a normal fat lobule or a lipoma.

special-type tumors that lack much desmoplasia may be moderately compressible. We have elected not to use assessment of compressibility for distinguishing benign from malignant, but we do use it for distinguishing fat lobules and lipomas from other solid structures and lesions in the breast. If we are evaluating compressibility, we can compare anteroposterior measurements of the lesion with and without compression. Fat lobules and lipomas are much softer than any other solid structures and usually can be compressed 30% or more. Demonstrating lesion compressibility of 30% or greater is strong evidence that the lesion contains only fat (Fig. 3–15). Furthermore, fat lobules and lipomas are softer than surrounding normal tissues and do not indent normal tissues during vigorous compression maneuvers. For example, during the compression maneuver, a fat lobule or lipoma would never indent the pectoralis muscle, whereas a fibroadenoma or carcinomas often would (Fig. 3–16). This is discussed and illustrated further in Chapters 4, 5, and 13. Split-screen images with and without compression can be used to check the rotational mobility of fibroadenomas. Fibroadenomas often rotate when compressed, whereas invasive carcinomas, which are fixed to surrounding breast tissues, do not rotate (Fig. 3–17). Rotation of lesions is also discussed in Chapter 12.

Split-screen imaging with and without compression is also valuable in evaluating enlarged subareolar ducts that contain echogenic, inspissated debris. Alternating compression and compression release, ballottement with the transducer, can cause secretions to move back and forth within the duct lumen, proving that the echoes are not caused by tumor. Movement can be documented on real time as well as with either color or power Doppler (see Chapter 20 and color images in Fig. 20–36). The color or power Doppler signal created by ballottement of the duct

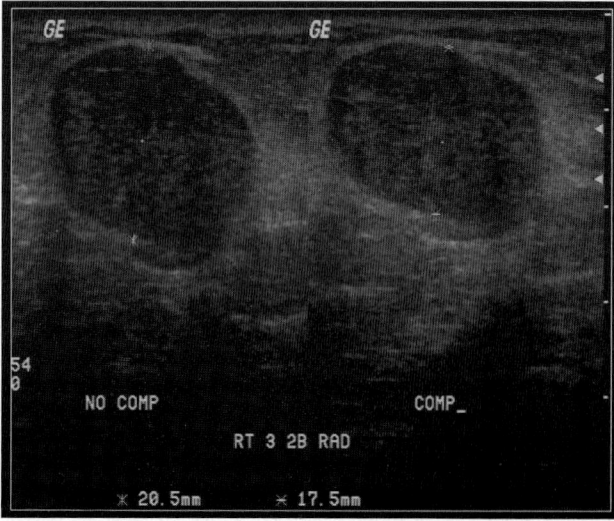

FIGURE 3–13 These split-screen images were obtained with and without compression of a solid nodule that later proved to be a fibroadenoma. This lesion compressed 15% (20.5–17.5)/20.5. This is quite typical for fibroadenomas, which may be as much as 20% or 25% compressible if myxomatous.

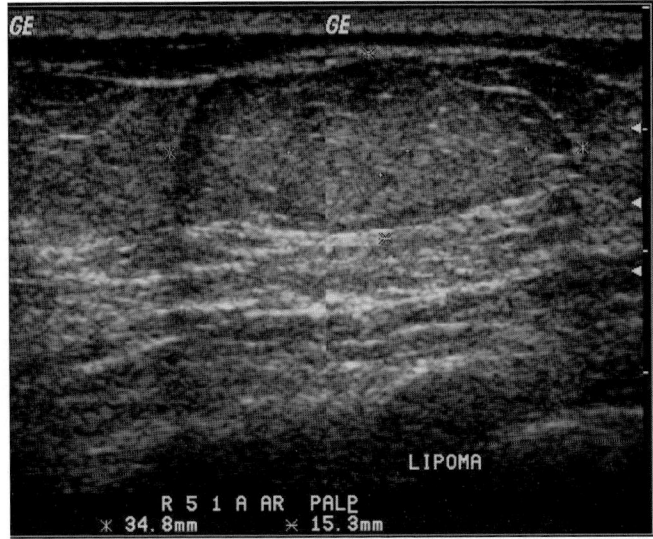
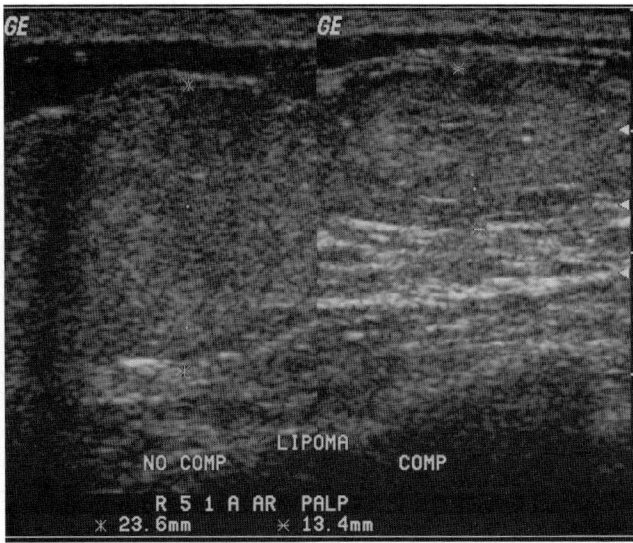

A

B

FIGURE 3–15 A: This solid, well-encapsulated, isoechoic, and homogeneous nodule presented as a new palpable lump. **B:** Split-screen images obtained without compression (**left**) and with vigorous compression (**right**) show the lesion to be very soft and compressible, 43% (23.6–13.4)/ 23.6. Although some fibroadenomas and even a few malignant nodules that contain little desmoplasia or represent special-type tumor are mildly to moderately compressible (as shown in Figures 3–13 and 3–14), they do not compress as much as 30% or more. We feel that compressibility of 30% occurs for solid nodules only when the nodule represents either a fat lobule or a lipoma. We use compressibility to document entrapped fat lobules or lipomas but do not use compressibility to try to distinguish between benign and malignant nodules because they overlap too much in the degree of compressibility.

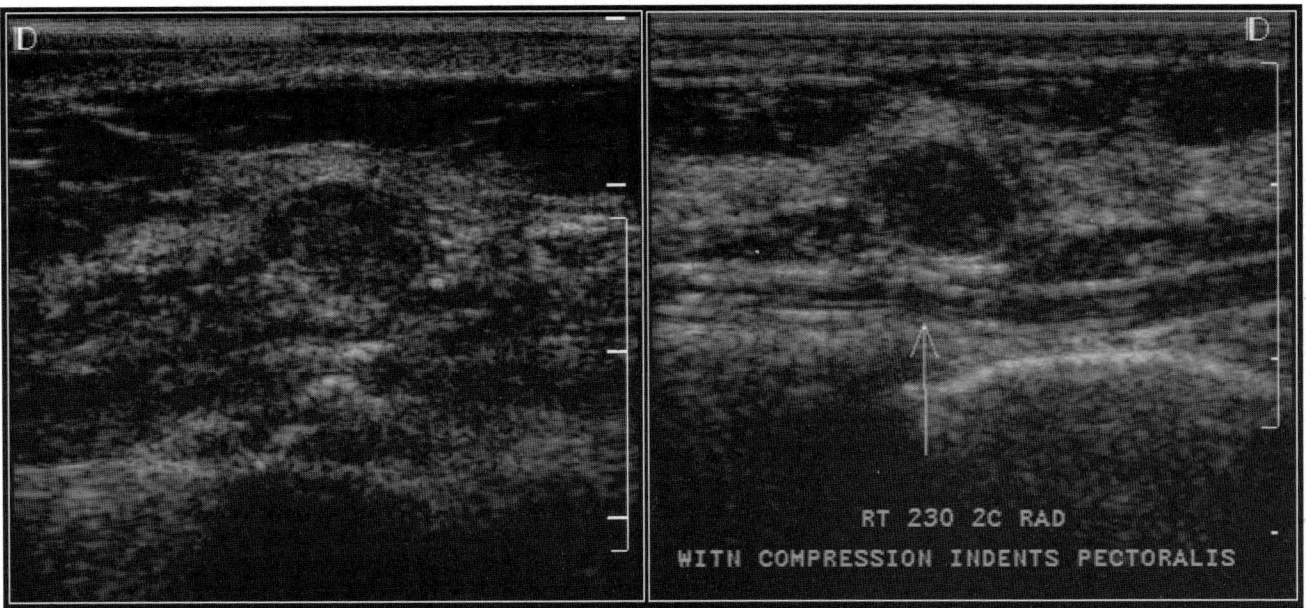

FIGURE 3–16 Split-screen images obtained with and without compression can be used not only to evaluate the compressibility of a lesion but also to assess the effect of the compressed nodule on the surrounding tissues. The oval-shaped, isoechoic, circumscribed lesion shown in the **left** image presented as a palpable lump. Without compression, we were uncertain whether this was a fat lobule entrapped within a fibrous ridge or a solid nodule such as a fibroadenoma. This lesion was less than 30% compressible. However, some fat lobules that are entrapped within surrounding firm fibroglandular tissue will be buttressed by the surrounding tissue and, therefore, will be relatively incompressible. However, the compressed nodule severely indented the pectoralis muscle, indicating that it was much firmer than the muscle. This excluded a fat lobule or lipoma because neither would be firm enough to indent muscle, and it indicated that the lesion represented a firm nodule, such as a fibroadenoma.

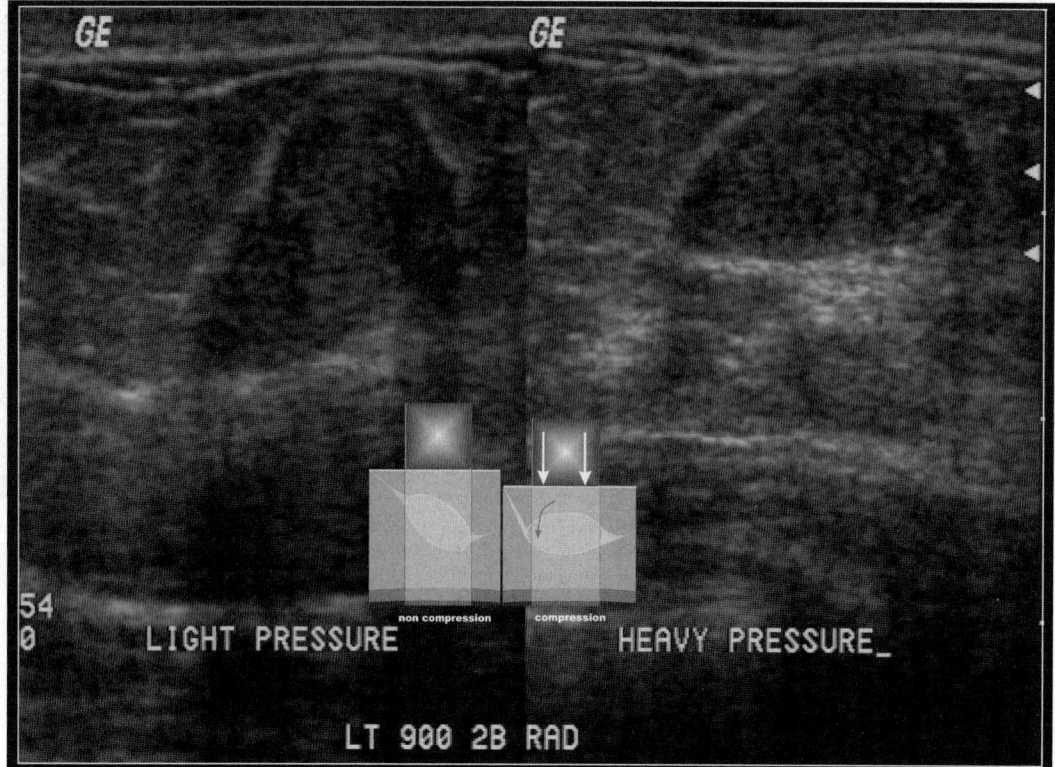

FIGURE 3–17 This fibroadenoma lies in an oblique plane and appears larger in the anteroposterior dimension than in its horizontal dimension (taller than wide) when scanned with light pressure (**left**). However, when imaged with vigorous compression (**right**), the nodule rotates into a horizontal plane and now appears clearly larger in horizontal than vertical dimension (wider than tall).

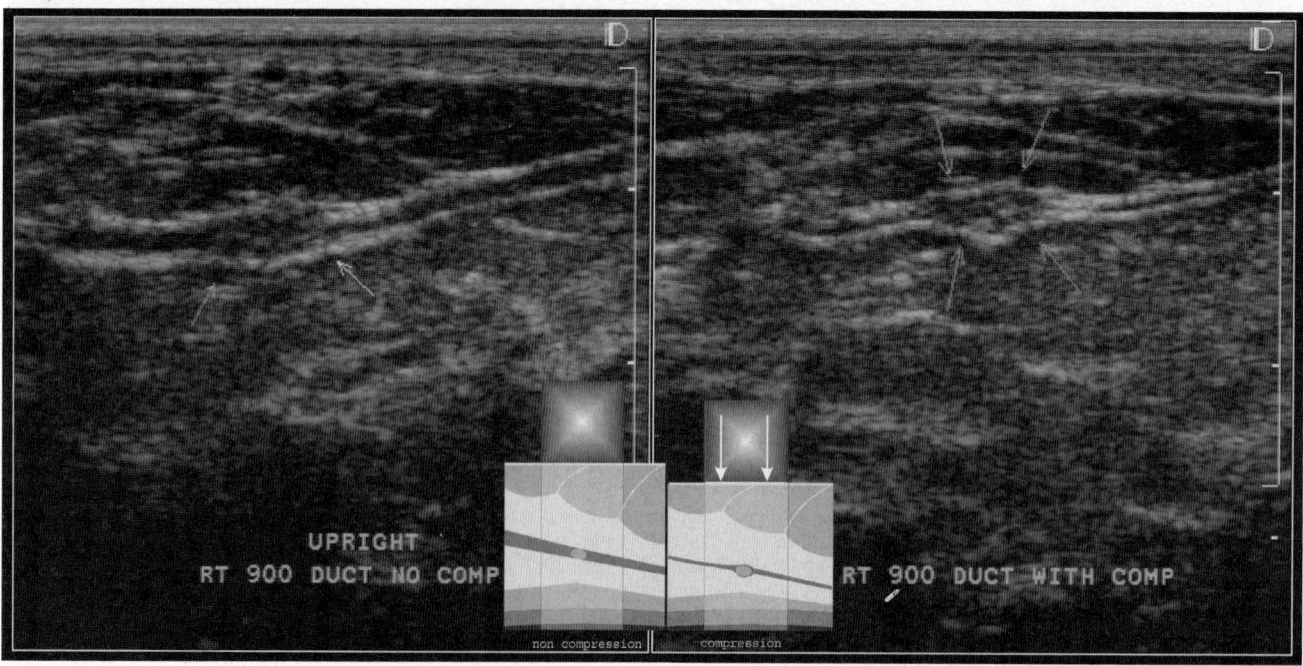

FIGURE 3–18 These split-screen images obtained with compression (**right**) and without compression (**left**) were obtained in a patient who presented with nipple discharge. The part of the duct that appears wider in the noncompressed view is also much less compressible. The incompressible segment of the duct is the site of the papilloma that has caused echogenic secretions that fill the more compressible segments of the duct (histology indicated benign, large duct papilloma).

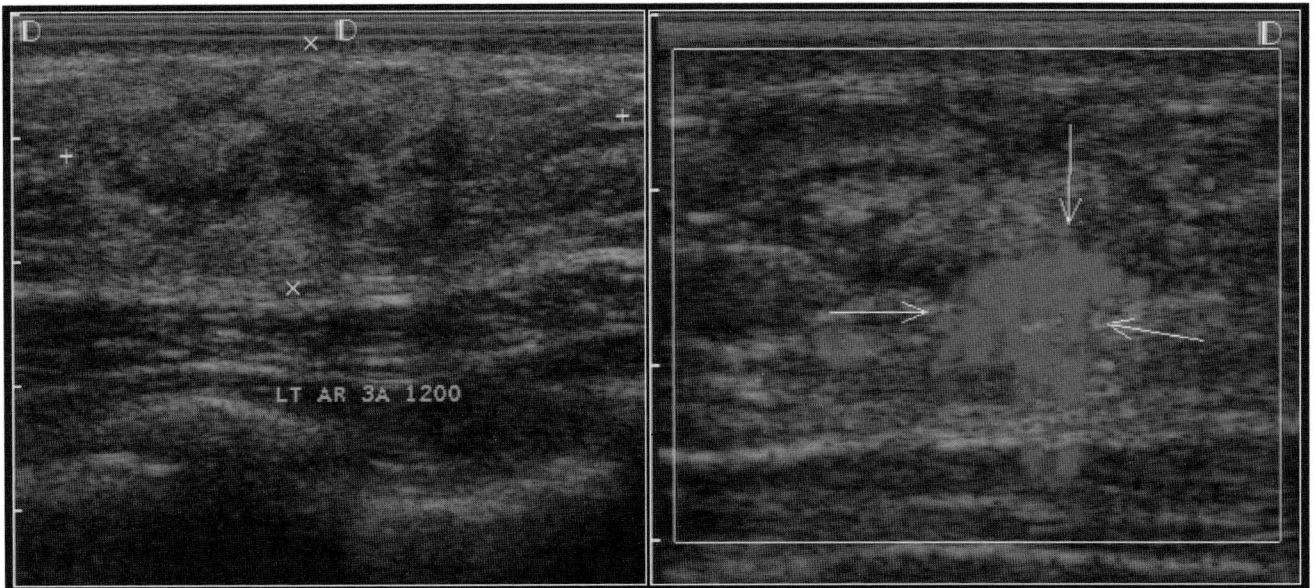

FIGURE 3–19 The real-time B-mode image shows an immature puerperal breast abscess that appeared solid because the necrotic tissue within the developing abscess had not completely lique-fied. A color Doppler image obtained during the compression-release phase of ballottement shows a color signal (*arrows*) deep within the breast in an area that appeared to be inhabited by normal breast tissue. However, the Doppler signal indicated the presence of liquefied devital-ized tissue sloshing back and forth within the developing cavity of an immature breast abscess. Identifying this focus of echogenic, but liquefied, sloughed tissue enabled early ultrasound-guided aspiration for culture and sensitivity and establishment of drainage.

has been termed the "color swoosh" and is discussed in detail in Chapters 8 and 20. Split-screen imaging can document which parts of a large echogenic duct are compressible and which are not. Intraductal papillary lesions can cause bloody secretions to fill the duct, and the secretions may be equal in echogenicity to the intraductal papillary lesion, obscuring it. When the duct is compressed, the softer, blood-filled portion of the duct compresses, but the segment of duct containing the less compressible papillary lesion does not, allowing the lesion causing the bloody secretions to be identified and localized for ultrasound-guided vacuum-assisted needle biopsy (Fig. 3–18). This concept is discussed and illustrated in detail in Chapter 8. Ballottement of the breast with alternating compression and compression release can cause necrotic debris within an abscess to move, proving that the lesion is filled with echogenic necrotic debris rather than representing a solid nodule or edematous, infected breast tissue. The earlier that liquefactive necrosis can be identified, the earlier that aspiration, culture, and placement of drainage catheters can be instituted. This is discussed and illustrated further in Chapter 11 (Fig. 3–19).

Split-screen images obtained with and without compression can be used to demonstrate that certain types of shadowing are caused by critical angle shadowing from a steeply oriented Cooper's ligament rather than from a scirrhous carcinoma (Figs 3–5 and 3–6). This is discussed fur-

ther in Chapters 12 and 21.

Split-screen images obtained with and without compression can also be used to help distinguish between recurrent tumor and chronic hematoma within an irregularly shaped lumpectomy cavity. The noncompressed cavity may be indistinguishable from recurrent tumor, but compression usually flattens the fluid-containing cavity into a linear configuration (Fig. 3–20).

Finally, split-screen images with and without compression can be used in the breast exactly as they are in peripheral venous evaluations. Normal breast veins are soft and compressible and superficially located. Abnormal veins, such as those in venous malformations or hemangiomas, also compress if not thrombosed (Fig. 3–21). Superficial thrombosis of breast veins causes pain and a palpable cord and makes these normally compressible veins noncompressible (Fig. 3–22).

SUMMARY

In conclusion, it is essential that the technique for BUS be optimized and standardized at any given institution. Patient position, transducer pressure, and concomitant palpation and scanning schemes all contribute to the quality of the ultrasound. Those who perform BUS should become

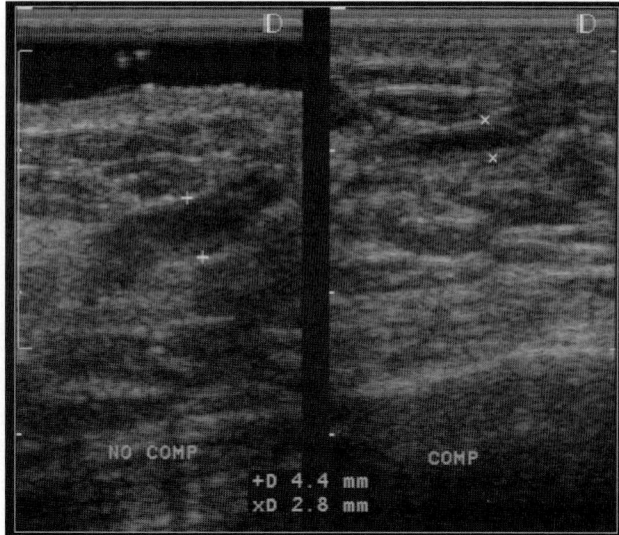

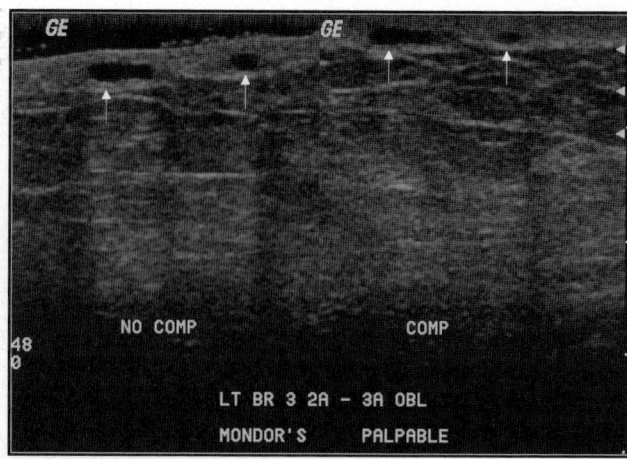

FIGURE 3–20 Split-screen images obtained in short axis relative to a lumpectomy scar obtained without (left) and with (right) compression show an angular hypoechoic structure that is more than 30% compressible, indicting that it was a chronic hematoma or seroma within the lumpectomy cavity, not recurrent tumor. The cavity was much more worrisome in appearance in the scan plane parallel to the cavity. Distinguishing recurrent tumor from other abnormalities within the lumpectomy site is discussed in detail in Chapter 18.

FIGURE 3–22 These split-screen images of a palpable abnormality showed the superficially located, multilocular cystic structure to be incompressible. Additionally, color Doppler showed no blood flow within the structures. Long-axis views, however, showed the structures to be continuous with patent venous channels, indicating that they represent superficial venous thrombosis, or Mondor's disease. The palpable abnormality was elongated and cordlike, typical of Mondor's disease. Superficial thrombosis of breast veins is discussed in detail in Chapter 11.

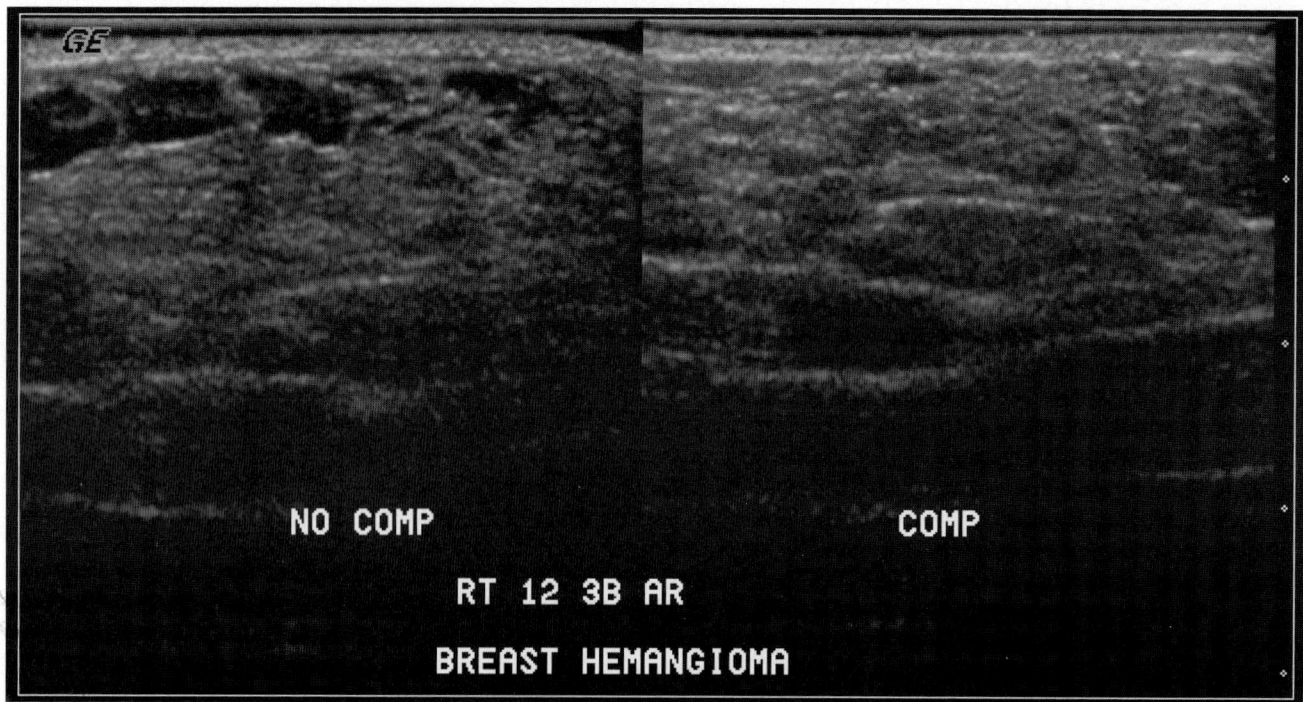

FIGURE 3–21 These split-screen images of a palpable abnormality in the right breast obtained without (left) and with (right) compression show the cystic multilocular structure to be virtually 100% compressible. Additionally, color Doppler showed venous blood flow within the cystic structures that could be augmented by transducer compression, indicating the presence of a nonthrombosed venous malformation or cavernous hemangioma of the breast.

familiar with these techniques in order to provide optimal breast diagnostic services.

This chapter is meant only as an introduction to imaging techniques. Techniques for evaluating specific clinical problems [normal anatomy (Chapter 4), nipple discharge (Chapter 8), implants (Chapter 9), complex breast cysts (Chapter 10), solid breast nodules (Chapter 12)] are discussed in greater detail elsewhere in this book.

SUGGESTED READINGS

Bassett LW, Kimme-Smith C. Breast sonography: technique, equipment, and normal anatomy. *Semin Ultrasound CT MR* 1989; 10(2):82–89.

Baum G. Labeling of meridional and radial scans of the breast. *J Ultrasound Med* 1982;1(4):105–110.

Brem RF, Gatewood OM. Template-guided breast US. *Radiology* 1992;184(3):872–874.

Conway WF, Hayes CW, Brewer WH. Occult breast masses: use of a mammographic localizing grid for US evaluation. *Radiology* 1991;181(10):143–146.

Di Vito J Jr, Rossmann MD. Breast sonography: technique to mimic mammographic position. *J Ultrasound Med* 1994;13(1):33–36.

Edde DJ. Whole-breast compression ultrasonography with the patient in the sitting position. *Can Assoc Radiol J* 1994;45(4): 324–326.

Lunt LG, Peakman DJ, Young JR. Mammographically guided ultrasound: a new technique for assessment of impalpable breast lesions. *Clin Radiol* 1991;44(2):85–88.

Richter K. Technique for detecting and evaluating breast lesions. *J Ultrasound Med* 1994;13(10):797–802.

Rosensweig R, et al. Radial scanning of the breast: an alternative to the standard ultrasound technique. *J Clin Ultrasound* 1982;10(4): 199–201.

Rubin E, et al. Hand-held real-time breast sonography. *AJR Am J Roentgenol* 1985;144(3):623–627.

Sickles EA. Breast imaging: a view from the present to the future. *Diagn Imaging Clin Med* 1985;54(3–4):118–125.

Venta LA, et al. Sonographic evaluation of the breast. *Radiographics* 1994;14(1):29–50.

BREAST ANATOMY: THE BASIS FOR UNDERSTANDING SONOGRAPHY

BREAST ANATOMY

The breast is composed of 15 to 20 lobes in most women during their reproductive years. Each lobe consists of numerous lobules and small branch ducts that join to form larger ducts progressively until there is only one main subareolar duct draining the whole lobe. A widened portion in each major lobar duct just deep to the nipple, where milk accumulates during lactational letdown, is called the *lactiferous sinus* (Fig. 4–1). There are usually fewer duct orifices on the nipple than there are lobes because some of the major ducts join just below the nipple. Although central ducts draining each lobe course in a radial pattern away from the nipple, individual segments of ducts may not be truly radially oriented owing to tortuosity. Additionally, smaller peripheral ducts may have their long axes oriented radially (Fig. 4–2). Breast lobes vary greatly in size and often overlap other lobes, making attempted surgical segmentectomy difficult and susceptible to error.

Lobar ducts tend to lie nearer to the chest wall than the skin, within the posterior half of the lobe. According to Teboul, there are usually five rows of lobules that arise circumferentially from each lobar duct. One row of lobules lies anteriorly, two lie anterolaterally, and two lie posterolaterally. The anterior and anterolateral lobules are more numerous than are posterior lobules and have longer extralobular terminal ducts, accounting for the tendency of the lobar duct to be located posteriorly within the lobe. The orientation of the anterior and anterolateral lobules is probably responsible for the taller-than-wide shape of most small breast carcinomas (see Chapter 12).

The functional unit of the breast, the terminal ductolobular unit (TDLU), is composed of a lobule and its terminal duct (Fig. 4–3). Hundreds or even thousands of lobules may be present within the breasts of certain patients. Lobules arise from smaller, more peripheral branch ducts, but a few may arise from larger central ducts. How-ever, rarely do TDLUs arise from the lactiferous sinus portion of main lobar ducts within 5 cm of the nipple. The number of TDLUs in the breast varies from patient to patient, with age, and with hormonal influences. Certain times in life are characterized by rapid proliferation of TDLUs—the postovulatory phase of each menstrual cycle, during pregnancy and lactation, and in late adolescence and the early 20s. TDLU proliferation may also occur during use of exogenous hormones, either birth control pills or postmenopausal hormone replacement therapy (HRT). Regression of lobules due to atrophy or sclerosis also tends to occur rapidly at certain times—following each pregnancy and after menopause. The presence of fully developed TDLUs after menopause is uncommon unless the patient is on HRT and is associated with increased risk for developing carcinoma. Regression is not necessarily uniform from right to left or from one part of the breast to another, and uneven regression can create clinical, mammographic, and sonographic asymmetries.

Breast tissue can be classified histologically as either stromal or epithelial-myoepithelial. Stromal elements include fat and fibrous tissue (including Cooper's ligaments). There are two types of stromal fibrous tissue: dense *inter*lobular stromal fibrous tissue and loose stromal fibrous tissue that surrounds ducts (periductal) and lies within lobules (*intra*lobular). A large portion of stromal fibrous tissue is composed of extracellular matrix, which, in turn, is composed of variable amounts of fibroblasts, collagen, and hyaluronic acid. Dense interlobular stromal fibrous tissue is high in collagen and low in hyaluronic acid, whereas loose intralobular and periductal stromal tissue is high in hyaluronic acid and contains less collagen. Hyaluronic acid is a huge hydrophilic molecule that facilitates passive diffusion into and out of epithelial cells and is soft and pliable, allowing for easy expansion and contraction of ducts and lobules under hormonal influences. Loose stromal fibrous tissue is also more vascular and contains more inflamma-

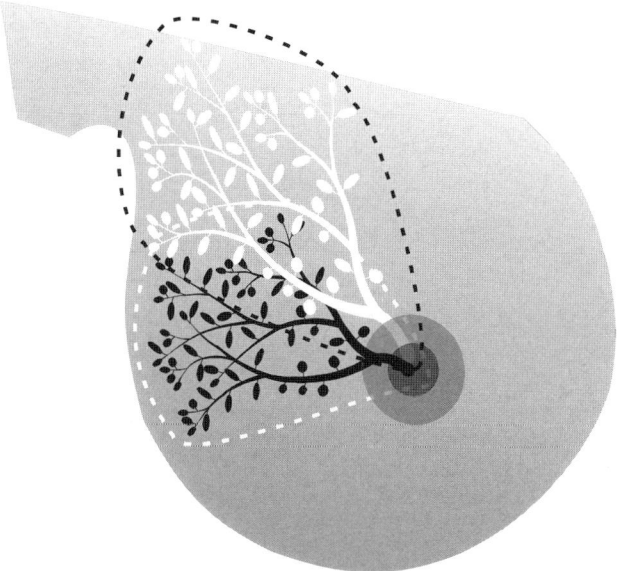

FIGURE 4–1 The lobar ducts drain to the nipple in a generally radial fashion that is similar to the arrangement of the spokes of a wheel. More peripheral portions of the ductal system, however, may lie in planes other than the radial plane. The peripheral portions of lobes often overlap, and it is usually not possible to identify the edge of a breast lobe on ultrasound.

tory cells than does dense interlobular stromal fibrous tissue. The differences between the loose and dense stromal fibrous tissues are not very important for mammographers because both are of about equal water density mammographically. However, the tissue differences are important for sonographers because the loose and dense stromal fibrous elements have markedly different echo textures. The epithelial and myoepithelial elements of the breast (excluding the skin) line the ducts of all sizes and the ductules (acini) within the TDLU as well as the terminal duct. Each TDLU contains variable numbers of ductules (usually 30 to 50) and loose intralobular stromal fibrous tissue. Epithelial cells line each ductule and are surrounded by more widely spaced myoepithelial cells that likely contract during breast-feeding, expressing milk from the lobule into the ductal system. The squamous epithelium that covers the nipple extends for a short way into the terminal end of the terminal ducts within the nipple, and desquamated squames create keratin plugs that help prevent bacterial colonization of the ducts under normal circumstances.

Most breast pathology arises within the TDLUs. Most ductal carcinomas are thought to arise within the terminal duct near its junction with the lobule, then spreading

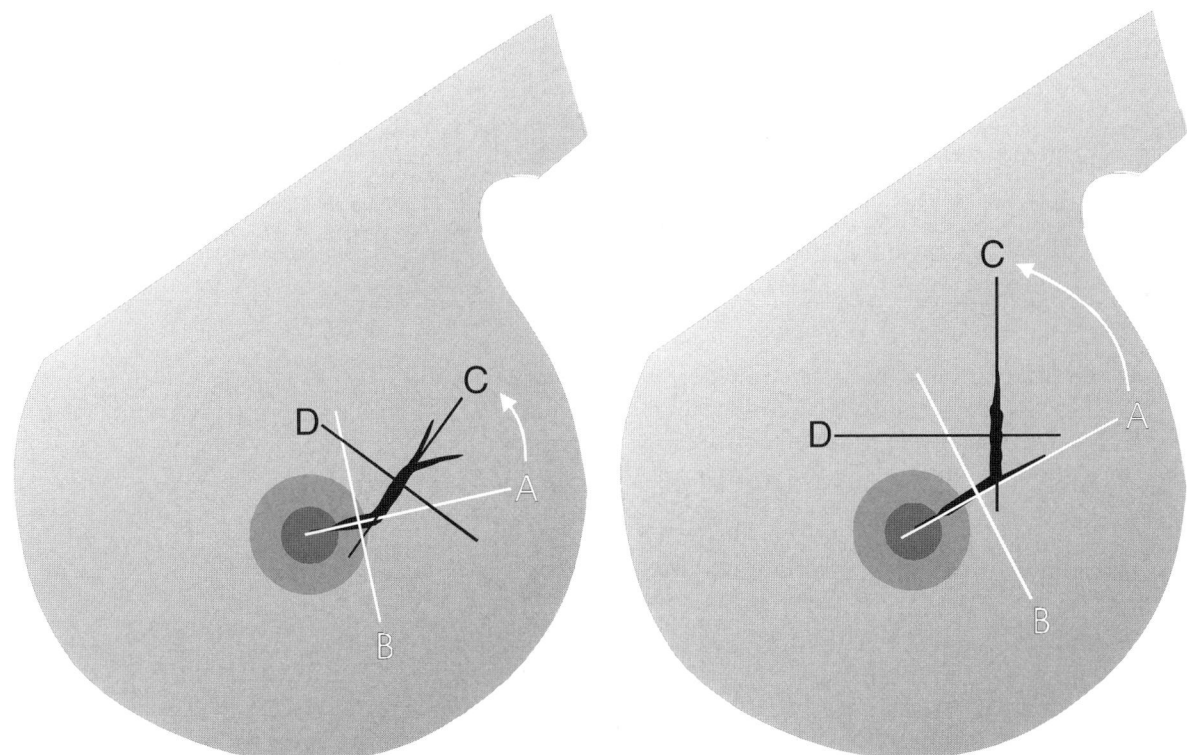

Tortuous duct   Branch duct

FIGURE 4–2 Central lobar ducts may be tortuous, so that portions of the duct lie in a plane other than *(C)* the true radial plane *(A)* **(left)**. Additionally, peripheral ducts may lie in planes other than *(C)* the true radial plane *(A)* **(right)**. Sonography of all lesions should begin in the true radial plane in order to demonstrate the relationship of the lesion to the ductal system, but because of ductal tortuosity or location of the lesion in a peripheral branch duct, slight adjustments off the true radial plane may be necessary to best accomplish this. B, antiradial plane; A, true radial plane; C, plane of tortuous central duct or peripheral branch duct.

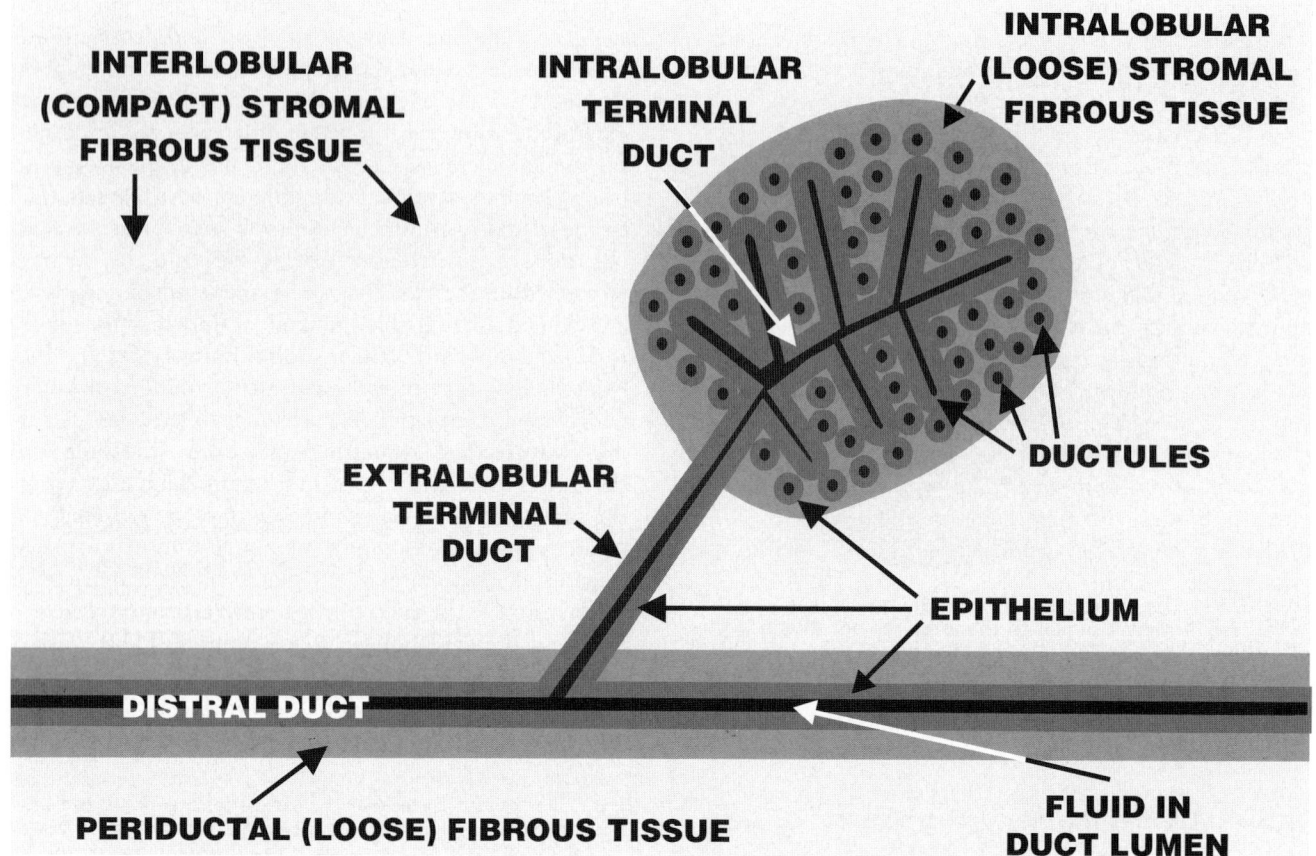

FIGURE 4–3 The functional unit of the breast is the terminal ductolobular unit, which consists of the intralobular and extralobular portions of the terminal duct and the lobule. The lobule is composed of the intralobular terminal duct, ductules (acini), and intralobular stromal fibrous tissue. The larger ducts may be collapsed or ectatic to variable degrees. The walls of ducts and ductules are composed of epithelium, myoepithelium, and basement membrane. Surrounding the ducts is a loose, fibroelastic stromal tissue that is similar to the intralobular stromal tissue but that differs greatly from the less elastic, more compact interlobular stromal fibrous tissue.

intraductally through the extralobular terminal duct to large ducts and retrogradely into intralobular ductules. Larger central ducts generally give rise only to intraductal papillomas and the duct ectasia–periductal mastitis complex. Under certain circumstances, the subareolar ducts may present an avenue for infection to enter the breast. Cancers that arise in central ducts probably evolve from preexisting papillomas or from uncommon centrally located lobules. However, central ducts are commonly secondarily involved by ductal carcinoma *in situ* elements that grow centrally from peripherally arising cancers.

The lumina of ducts and intralobular ductules often contain variable amounts of fluid, protein, and cellular debris.

The breast is roughly circular in shape from anteriorly, but has an extension of tissue toward the axilla called the *axillary segment* or *tail of Spence*. The nipple lies slightly medial and inferior to the center of the breast, accentuating the portion of breast tissue that lies within the upper outer quadrant.

Thus, the greater number of breast lesions that arise in the upper outer quadrant is at least partially due to the greater tissue volume in that quadrant and the slower regression of tissues in that quadrant with age than in other quadrants.

Each mammary lobe is encased within a fascial sheath. The fascia that lies on the anterior surface of the lobe and that separates it from the subcutaneous fat (premammary zone) is called the *anterior* or *premammary fascia*. The fascia that lies on the posterior surface of the lobe and that separates the lobe from the retromammary fat is termed the *retromammary fascia*. Between the anterior and posterior mammary fascia lies the mammary zone, within which lie most of the ducts and lobules of the breast. The anterior mammary fascia is not a smooth, continuous structure. Rather, it is scalloped, pointed toward the skin at each point at which it is continuous with a Cooper's ligament. Each Cooper's ligament may be thought of as two leaflets of closely apposed anterior mammary fascia that separate posteriorly as they course horizontally along the anterior surface of the mammary zone. Although most TDLUs lie within the mammary zone, a few may extend into Cooper's ligaments and lie anterior to the mammary zone within the more superficially located subcutaneous fat (Fig. 4–4). Most breast carcinomas arise within the mammary zone because the TDLUs from which they arise lie within the mammary zone. However, a few cancers may arise within unusually superficially located TDLUs.

The nipple and areola are covered by pigmented squamous epithelium. Both the nipple and the areola contain smooth muscle, which has an erectile function when stimulated or exposed to cold. Cold-induced contraction of smooth muscle with the nipple and areola is important sonographically because the areolar becomes wrinkled and the nipple becomes longer. Muscular contraction contributes to critical angle acoustic shadowing, which interferes with sonographic evaluation of the subareolar and intranipple regions of the breast. To minimize cold-induced smooth muscle contraction, the room and acoustic gel temperatures should be warm. The areola also contains sebaceous glands that lubricate it during lactation. Occasionally, these glands can become obstructed or inflamed. Techniques for evaluating the nipple–subareolar complex are discussed in detail in Chapter 8.

Lymphatic Drainage of the Breast

The breast lymphatics drain primarily to the axilla, with less extensive drainage to the internal mammary and infraclavicular systems. Much of the breast drains first superficially toward a rich layer of lymphatics just superficial to the anterior mammary fascia, then to the periareolar plexus, and finally to the axilla. The axillary lymph nodes are the most common site of involvement for lymphatic metastases of breast cancer.

The presence, level, and number of axillary lymph nodes that are involved by tumor are key prognostic indicators for breast cancer; thus, evaluation of axillary lymph nodes by surgical and imaging techniques is important.

Axillary lymph nodes are divided into levels by the pectoralis minor muscle. The lowest axillary lymph nodes, level I nodes, are lateral and inferior to the pectoralis minor muscle. Level II nodes are deep to the pectoralis minor muscle, whereas level III or apical nodes lie medial and superior to the pectoralis minor muscle. Axillary dissections usually involve only level I and II axillary nodes. Sentinel node evaluation involves only the lowest of level I nodes. Modified radical mastectomy and radical mastectomy address level II axillary lymph nodes, but these procedures are infrequently performed today in the United States.

Internal mammary lymph nodes lie within the second through fourth intercostal spaces beside the deep edge of the sternum along the course of the internal mammary artery and veins. Breast lymphatic drainage reaches the internal mammary lymph nodes by vessels that penetrate

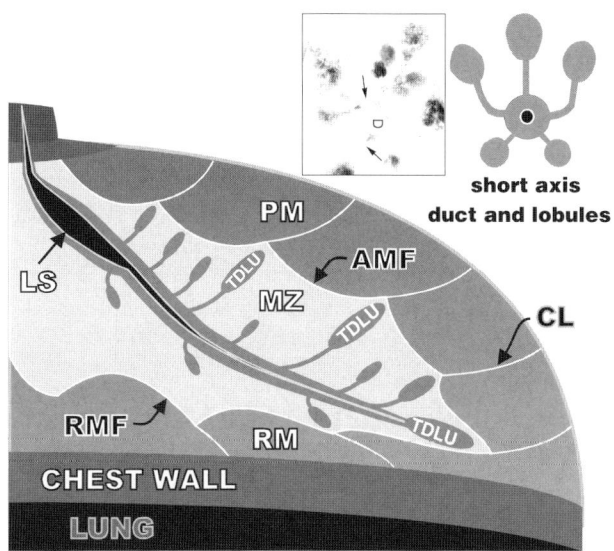

FIGURE 4–4 There are three major zones within the breast. The most superficial is the premammary zone *(PM)* or subcutaneous fat. The premammary zone contains subcutaneous fat, Cooper's ligaments *(CL)*, and in some cases, a small minority of peripheral ducts and lobules. Most processes arising in the premammary zone are of skin or subcutaneous fat origin (e.g., sebaceous cysts, lipomas, venous thrombosis). The premammary zone, however, may be involved secondarily by malignant or inflammatory conditions arising more deeply within the mammary zone. The middle zone is the mammary zone *(MZ)*. It contains all of the central ducts and most of the peripheral ducts and lobules. Most breast pathology arises within the mammary zone. The deepest of the three zones is the retromammary zone. It generally contains only fat and ligaments and is rarely the site of origin of breast pathology. However, like the premammary zone, processes arising from the more superficially located mammary zone may secondarily involve the retromammary zone. The premammary zone is separated from the mammary zone by a tough layer of fascia, the premammary fascia that is continuous with Cooper's ligaments. The retromammary zone is separated from the mammary zone by a similar layer of fascia, the retromammary fascia. Thus, the mammary zone is enveloped between the layers of the premammary and retromammary fascia. The lobar duct has an ampullary or dilated segment in the subareolar area termed the lactiferous sinus *(LS)*, which is easy to see sonographically and may be several millimeters in diameter when distended with milk or fluid. Terminal ductolobular units arise from the major lobar ducts in rows. There are generally five rows of ducts, three extending anteriorly and two posteriorly, an anatomic feature that affects the sonographic appearance of small, malignant nodules. (Subgross histology courtesy of Hanne M. Jensen, MD, University of California at Davis.)

through the chest wall into the intercostal spaces. In some cases, there are superficial medial intramammary lymph nodes that mirror the internal mammary lymph nodes. The far medial and deep medial parts of the breast drain to the internal mammary chain.

Lymphatic drainage of the breast can reach the supraclavicular nodes only after first passing through the subclavian or deep jugular chains.

A significant percentage of patients have lymph nodes that are imbedded within the substance of the breast—

intramammary lymph nodes. These intramammary nodes are most common in the axillary segment or far lateral aspects of the breast. Intramammary lymph nodes also occur in the far medial aspect of the breast and are occasionally sonographically demonstrable. Intramammary lymph nodes may occur in any quadrant of the breast, but locations other than upper outer quadrant and far medial area of the breast are rare.

Sonographic assessment of lymph nodes and breast carcinoma lymph node metastases are discussed in greater detail in Chapter 19.

Blood Supply and Drainage of the Breast

The arterial supply of the breast is carried by perforating branches of the internal mammary arteries that lie along the medial aspect of the breast, intercostal perforators, and by lateral thoracic and thoracoabdominal branches of the axillary artery. Knowledge of the arterial anatomy of the breast is important to surgeons and also for continuous-wave Doppler evaluation of the breast when color Doppler guidance is not available.

Anatomically, the venous drainage of the breast is more variable than is the arterial inflow. Although arteries usually accompany deep breast veins, arteries do not accompany the superficial breast veins. Veins draining the breast represent an avenue for hematogenous metastases. Lymphatic drainage often parallels venous drainage, so that color Doppler demonstration of a large vein leading away from a tumor may offer clues about where sentinel lymph node metastasis is most likely to occur.

Doppler evaluation of the breast is discussed in greater detail in Chapter 20.

Embryologic Development of the Breast

The breasts arise embryologically from the ventral streaks. These streaks develop into the mammary ridges that extend from the precursor of the axilla to the precursor of the groin along the "milk line." Normally, most of the mammary ridge regresses and disappears, leaving only a small portion in the upper third to form the breast bud. Abnormal persistence of portions of the mammary ridges can result in a spectrum of accessory breast variants, including accessory breast with nipples, accessory nipple alone, and accessory breast tissue without an accessory nipple. Accessory breast tissue can occur anywhere along the milk line but is most common in the axillary segment of the breast. Accessory breast tissue is a common cause of focal mammographic asymmetries.

Early in embryogenesis, cords of epithelium grow from the remaining portion of the mammary ridge into the underlying dermis. During the second and third trimesters, these cords grow deeper into underlying subcutaneous fat until, at birth, there is a network of branching ducts. Lob-

ules do not begin to develop until adolescence. These ducts tend to be more prominent at birth than later in childhood because of the residual stimulation from maternal hormones. Stimulation from maternal hormones may even cause secretions from the newborn breast called "witch's milk."

Changes in Breast Anatomy Over Time

The anatomy of the breast varies greatly, not only from patient to patient but also with time and complex hormonal influences during the lifetime of individuals. The prepubertal breast has only minimal duct development in the immediate vicinity of the nipple.

As previously discussed, newborns can have some ductal development owing to maternal hormonal influences. After a few weeks to months, when maternal hormone effects abate, the ductal tissue regresses. From the newborn period to the onset of thelarche, when the ovaries begin production of estrogens, the breasts are inactive.

With the onset of estrogen secretion by the ovaries, the breasts begin to develop (thelarche). This early breast development precedes menarche by months to years. The first change is increased fluid retention of the stromal support elements in the immediate subareolar locations. This fluid retention is followed by proliferation of the ducts and their associated periductal stromal fibrous tissue, resulting in a visible and palpable disk of tissue deep to the nipple. There is growth in length and branching of the ducts, but only minimal lobular development until later in adolescence and in the early 20s. Asymmetric development may simulate a subareolar nodule that should not be excised because excision will prevent development of a breast on that side. Interestingly, the clinical, mammographic, and sonographic features of asymmetric thelarche are virtually identical to those of asymmetric gynecomastia in males.

Ductal growth is stimulated by estrogen production, whereas full lobular development requires both estrogen and progesterone stimulation. The ovaries begin production of estrogen during thelarche, long before menarche and before the establishment of regular menses. Production of progesterone does not occur until well after menarche and requires the establishment of regular menses. Progesterone production requires normal corpus luteal development during the postovulatory phase of the menstrual cycle. In the first few months to years after menarche, a large percentage of cycles may be anovulatory and therefore unassociated with normal corpus luteal development and progesterone production. Thus, although early breast development due to estrogen production by the ovaries begins with the onset of puberty (11 to 14 years of age), lobular proliferation and maturation often do not occur until progesterone production stabilizes in the late teenage years or early 20s. Of course, early full-term pregnancy will accelerate development of lobules because during the second and third trimesters, there is abundant production of progesterone. On the other hand, early pregnancy that ends in the first trimester because of either spontaneous or therapeutic abortion will result in a marked estrogenic stimulation without the subsequent progesterone effect. This situation results in marked ductal proliferation without full development of the lobules and has been associated with an increased risk for breast cancer development later in life.

During the second and third trimesters of pregnancy, there is proliferation in both the number and size of TDLUs. Lobular enlargement is caused by both an increase in numbers of acini (ductules) within individual lobules and an increase in the amount of intralobular stromal fibrous tissue. Lobular proliferation and enlargement occur at the expense of the denser interlobular stromal fibrous tissue, which is compressed between the enlarging lobular units. If the TDLUs and ducts are considered glandular and the interlobular stromal fibrous and fatty elements are considered fibrous, the fibrous tissues become smaller and less extensive, and the glandular elements expand to occupy a greater percentage of the breast as pregnancy progresses. Ultimately, at some point during pregnancy, virtually all of the fibrous tissue is replaced by glandular tissue, and only glandular tissue and ducts are visible within the breast. This glandular predominance persists from the third trimester throughout the period of lactation. During the last trimester of pregnancy, the acini begin to secrete, and their lumina fill with fluid, a change that continues during lactation. Occasionally, secretory change may occur unusually early and asymmetrically within the breast, resulting in palpable abnormalities. Usually, such areas of palpable premature lactational change usually become clinically inapparent later in pregnancy as surrounding tissues also undergo lactational change. However, an asymmetric area of lactational change may lead to formation of a lactating adenoma, and obstruction of lobules undergoing lactational change may lead to galactocele.

After each pregnancy and lactational period, there is subsequent regression of the lobules. There is a tendency for the intralobular stromal fibrous tissue to undergo hyalinization and to become sclerotic as the acini atrophy. The number of ductules within each TDLU decreases, and the number of lobules also decreases. Either fat or sclerosis replaces the atrophic lobules. After menopause, very few mature lobules remain within the breast. In general, prominent lobules persisting into the postmenopausal period are worrisome. However, the effect of postmenopausal HRT must be taken into account. Simple estrogen (Premarin) replacement will not result in persistence of fully developed lobules but may slow their regression. However, combined estrogen-progesterone HRT, which is currently given to try to minimize hyperstimulation of endometrium, may result in postmenopausal persistence or development of mature lobules.

Fibrocystic Change and Benign Epithelial Proliferation

Unfortunately, the border between normal and abnormal breast anatomy is not clearly demarcated histologically (or sonographically). There is a spectrum of fibrocystic and proliferative changes that can be found in women who do not have clinical evidence of breast disease. Such changes have been termed *aberrations of normal development and involution* (ANDIs) and frequently alter the size and histologic constituents of ducts and TDLUs.

Some of the histologic entities associated with enlarged mammary ducts include lactation, ductal ectasia, florid duct hyperplasia or atypical ductal hyperplasia, and various types of *in situ* carcinoma. The contents of distended ducts may vary widely even within a single histologic entity. For example, in ductal ectasia, the lumen may be distended with fresh secretions, chronic inspissated secretions, acute inflammatory exudates, or intraductal fibrosis. Furthermore, it is not uncommon for two or more conditions, such as florid duct hyperplasia and ductal ectasia, to exist simultaneously within an enlarged duct.

Likewise, a variety of histologic entities may distend lobules. Both the size and number of lobules are increased by pregnancy, lactation, and adenosis. Microcysts, fibrosclerosis, papillary apocrine metaplasia, florid ductal hyperplasia, atypical ductal hyperplasia, and various types of *in situ* carcinoma may also distend lobules. As is the case for ductal enlargement, a mixture of different histologic entities may combine to enlarge the lobule. For example, in fibrocystic change, it is common to have microcysts, hyalinization of the intralobular stromal fibrous tissue, apocrine metaplasia, and florid usual ductal hyperplasia occurring together within a single, enlarged lobule.

SONOGRAPHIC BREAST ANATOMY

Structurally, the breast has three main sonographically identifiable zones from superficial to deep: the subcutaneous zone, the mammary zone, and the retromammary zone (Fig. 4–4). The subcutaneous zone is also called the premammary zone. This zone is the most superficial of the three and lies between the skin and anterior mammary fascia. Within the premammary zone lie fat and suspensory (Cooper's) ligaments, which are virtually always demonstrable, as well as blood vessels, which are occasionally sonographically demonstrable. Small, ectopic ducts and lobules may form within Cooper's ligaments and, therefore, may lie within the premammary zone. With increasing age, there is a tendency for the fibroglandular elements between Cooper's ligaments to regress, leaving progressively greater percentages of the residual fibroglandular elements trapped within Cooper's ligaments (Figs 4–5 to 4–8). A breast carcinoma can arise from TDLUs that lie

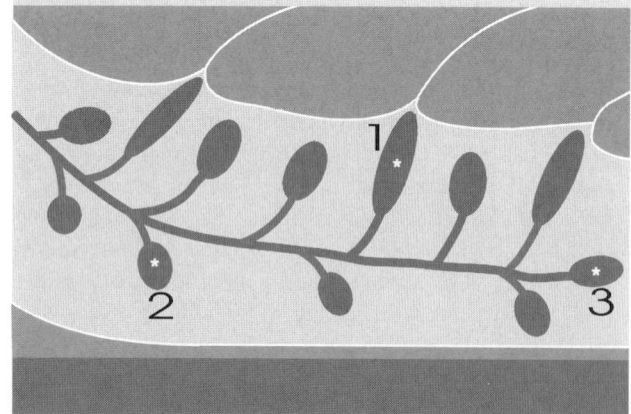

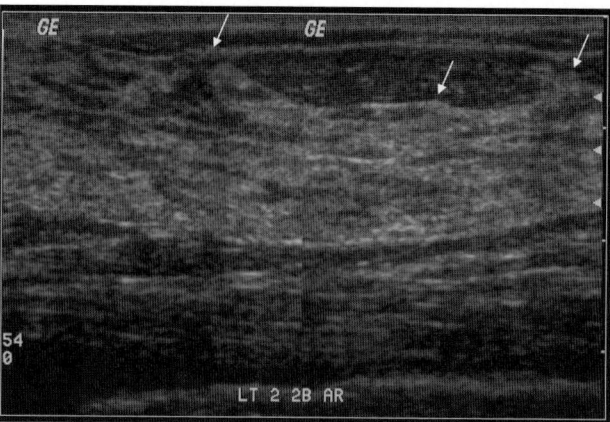

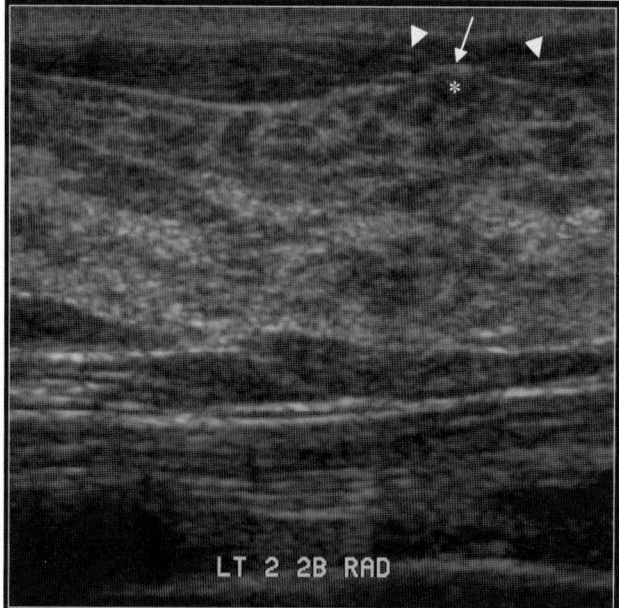

FIGURE 4–5 A: The configuration of the terminal ductolobular units (TDLUs) that arise from the lobar duct vary, depending on the location relative to the duct. The rows of lobules that lie anterior to the lobar duct *(1)* tend to be longer than the posterior rows of lobules *(2)* because the extralobular terminal duct is longer in the anterior TDLUs. There are more anterior rows of lobules, and each anterior row generally has more lobules than the posterior rows; thus, there are generally more lobules anterior to the lobar duct than there are posterior to the duct. A few lobules are terminal lobules *(3)* and are oriented horizontally rather than vertically. In early adulthood, the mammary zone is full of glandular tissue (TDLUs), ducts, and interlobular stromal fibrous tissue, with only slight indentations between Cooper's ligaments. Anterior TDLUs that lie immediately deep to Cooper's ligaments tend to be larger than those that lie between Cooper's ligaments. **B:** This is an example of the mammary zone before atrophy has begun to deepen the indentations between Cooper's ligaments. At each anterior point in the anterior mammary fascia *(arrows)*, the fascia is continuous with a Cooper's ligament. Before atrophy has begun, few of the TDLUs lie within Cooper's ligaments anterior to the mammary zone. **C:** This is an example of the mammary zone before atrophy has begun to deepen the indentations between Cooper's ligaments. At the anterior point in the anterior mammary fascia *(arrow)*, the fascia is continuous with Cooper's ligaments *(arrowheads)*. Before atrophy has begun, very few of the TDLUs lie within Cooper's ligaments anterior to the mammary zone. Note that the lobule at the base of Cooper's ligament *(*)* is larger and more prominent than the surrounding lobules that lie between Cooper's ligaments.

within Cooper's ligaments or may secondarily invade Cooper's ligaments and thus may lie completely or partially within the premammary zone. However, most sonographically identifiable processes that lie entirely within the premammary zone arise from skin and subcutaneous fat rather than breast tissue. Such subcutaneous lesions are not specific to the breast and can occur anywhere in the body and include lipomas, epidermal inclusion cysts, hemangiomas, lymphangiomas, and sebaceous cysts. Processes that cause skin thickening usually also affect the subcutaneous fat: infection, postsurgical scars, fat necrosis, radiation dermatitis, and fibrosis (Table 4–1).

The mammary zone lies between the superficial premammary zone and the deeper retromammary zone and is encompassed within mammary fascia. Almost all of the mammary ducts and TDLUs lie within the mammary zone (Fig. 4–4). Because most breast pathology arises within

TABLE 4–1. PATHOLOGY OF THE SKIN AND SUBCUTANEOUS FAT (PREMAMMARY ZONE)

Common
Sebaceous cyst, epidermal inclusion cysts
Lipoma, "nodular adiposity"
Edema, infection, mastitis
Hematoma, fat necrosis, scar tissue
Radiation fibrosis
Skin "moles," keratoses
Invasion, retraction of Cooper's ligament by deeper carcinoma

Uncommon
Carcinoma arising from terminal ductolobular unit lying within Cooper's ligaments

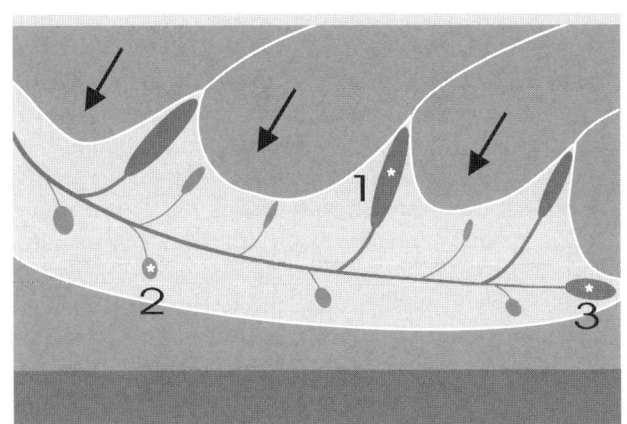
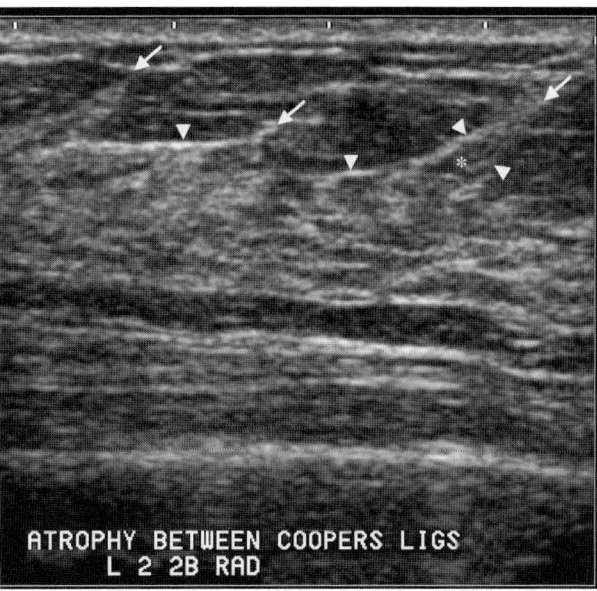

A   B

FIGURE 4–6 A: With the onset of parenchymal and stromal atrophy that usually begins after full-term pregnancies, there is progressive thinning of the mammary zone. This stromal and parenchymal atrophy is most pronounced in the area between Cooper's ligaments *(black arrows)*. The terminal ductolobular units (TDLUs) that lie between Cooper's ligaments *(2)* atrophy faster and to a greater extent than do the TDLUs that lie at the bases of Cooper's ligaments *(1)*. The pattern of atrophy in terminal TDLUs is more variable. The reason for slower atrophy in TDLUs near Cooper's ligament is uncertain but may be due to high levels of estrogen in fat lobules that lie adjacent the ligaments. **B:** This is an example of early atrophy between Cooper's ligaments. Note that the indentations between the points *(arrows)* at which the anterior mammary fascia *(arrowheads)* is continuous with Cooper's ligaments have deepened. Also note that the isoechoic tissue that represents glandular tissue and lobules is more prominent in the base of Cooper's ligaments than elsewhere because TDLUs that lie at the base of Cooper's ligaments atrophy more slowly than do TDLUs between Cooper's ligaments.

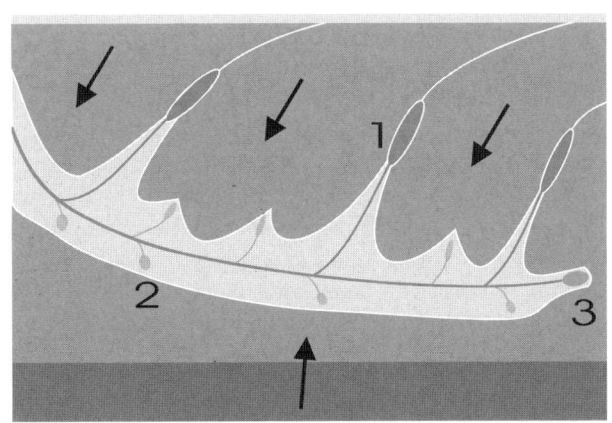
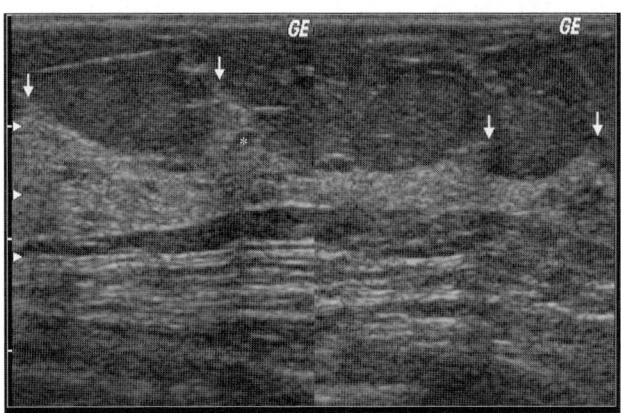

A   B

FIGURE 4–7 A: With greater degrees of atrophy (often after subsequent full-term pregnancies), there is a greater degree of atrophy and greater indentation between the points of continuity of the anterior mammary fascia with Cooper's ligaments *(black arrows)*. Terminal ductolobular units (TDLUs) between Cooper's ligaments *(2)* atrophy further. Some TDLUs that lie at the bases of Cooper's ligaments earlier in life may become entrapped within Cooper's ligaments *(1)* as the surrounding stroma atrophies. From these TDLUs that are entrapped within Cooper's ligaments may arise the entire spectrum of benign and malignant breast processes, explaining how cysts, fibroadenomas, and cancers that are completely surrounded by fat can occur. The effect of atrophy on terminal TDLUs *(3)* is more variable and less predictable. **B:** In this combined split-screen radial image, a greater degree of atrophy between the points of attachment of Cooper's ligaments *(arrows)* is evident. The TDLUs have atrophied too much to be sonographically visible, except for one *(*)* at the base of a Cooper's ligament. In this case, no TDLUs entrapped within Cooper's ligaments are visible.

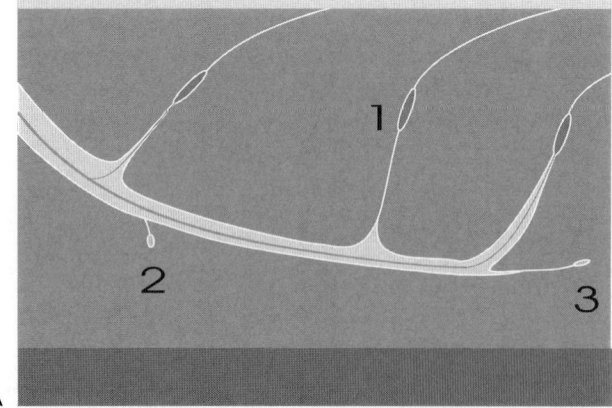

A

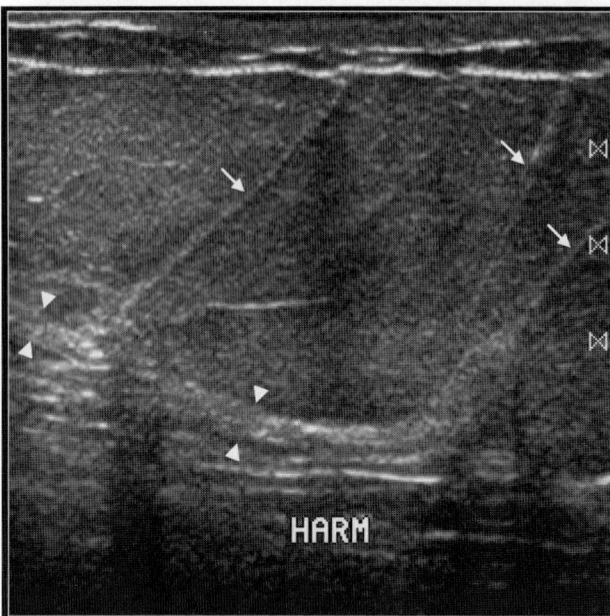

B

FIGURE 4–8 A: In the end stages of atrophy, the residual hyperechoic mammary zone may be very thin or even absent, leaving only fat, ducts of variable prominence, and Cooper's ligaments. Virtually all of the remaining TDLUs are entrapped within Cooper's ligaments (1). Most will be too atrophic to be sonographically visible. **B:** This patient has undergone a great deal of atrophy. The residual hyperechoic interlobular stromal fibrous tissue within the mammary zone *(arrowheads)* is very thin. Neither ducts nor TDLUs are sonographically demonstrable. Only interlobular stroma, fat, and Cooper's ligaments *(arrows)* are sonographically visible.

TDLUs or ducts, most significant breast pathology arises within the mammary zone. In some cases, particularly cases of invasive malignancy, pathologic processes may extend out of the mammary zone into either the premammary or the retromammary zone. Various amounts of stromal fat or fibrous tissue also lie within the mammary zone. Extensions of Cooper's ligaments cross from front to back and subdivide the mammary zone in an unpredictable fashion.

The retromammary zone lies between the mammary zone and the pectoralis muscle and other chest wall structures (Fig. 4–4). This zone virtually always appears to be much thinner in the anteroposterior (AP) dimension on sonograms than on mammograms because it is compressed between the mammary zone and the chest wall during sonography when the patient is scanned in a supine position. The retromammary zone may be so compressed that it is not even visible sonographically. Pathologic lesions that actually lie within the posterior half of the mammary zone and that may appear to be several centimeters from the chest wall on routine mammograms can appear immediately adjacent to (or even indent) the pectoralis muscle and chest wall during sonography. On the other hand, the retromammary fat is readily visible and accentuated on mammograms because it is pulled away from the chest wall and elongated during standard mammographic compression.

The retromammary zone contains mainly fat and a few suspensory ligaments. Most of the pathologic processes involving the retromammary zone arise within the mammary zone and only secondarily involve the retromammary zone. Because the retromammary zone is so compressed during sonography, it can be difficult to be certain whether a lesion involves the retromammary zone.

The mammary zone is encompassed within mammary fascia that appears sonographically as a thin, echogenic line. The premammary fascia separates the mammary zone form the premammary zone. The retromammary fascia separates the mammary zone from the retromammary zone. How well we can demonstrate the mammary fascia depends on the echogenicity of the breast tissue within the mammary zone that lies adjacent to the fascia. When breast tissues lying just deep to the premammary fascia are isoechoic, the fascia appears to form a well-defined, thin, echogenic line. However, when the tissue just deep to the anterior mammary fascia is as echogenic as the fascia, the premammary fascia cannot be identified. Also, in older women and individuals with extensive fatty involution of the breast, the premammary fascia may be incomplete and therefore may not be sonographically identifiable. The premammary fascia is a dense and tough structure that presents a relative barrier to direct extension of invasive malignancy into the premammary zone. However, the premammary fascia has gaps where it is continuous with Cooper's ligaments. At each of these points, the premammary fascia continues into the ligament, attaches to the skin, then comes back down the other side of Cooper's ligament and continues on as anterior mammary fascia. Thus, in effect, two layers of anterior mammary fascia form each Cooper's ligament. At the base of each Cooper's ligament, there is a triangular space where the layers of premammary fascia separate from each other. This is important because it represents a path of lower resistance for the growth of invasive malignancy that affects the shapes and surface characteristics of malignant nodules that lie in the anterior aspect of the mammary zone. How this affects the appearance of malignant nodules is discussed in greater detail in Chapter 12 (see Figs. 12–23 to 12–25).

The retromammary fascia is often more difficult to demonstrate than is the premammary fascia because of its depth and because it is compressed against the equally echogenic capsule surrounding the chest wall muscles. The retromammary fascia is usually more apparent near the lateral edges of the image and less apparent in the center of the image because the retromammary fascia is most tightly compressed against the chest wall where the curving chest wall comes closest to the probe, in the center of the image. At the edges of the image, where the chest wall curves away from the transducer, the retromammary zone is less compressed, and the retromammary fascia can separate from chest wall musculature and therefore can be better demonstrated.

Deep to the retromammary zone is the chest wall. In the upper part of the breast, the most superficial chest wall structure is the pectoralis major muscle, with intercostal and serratus anterior muscles, ribs, and costal cartilages lying more deeply. In the inferior segments of the breast, the pectoralis muscle is not present, and upper abdominal musculature and serratus anterior muscles may be the first encountered. In the axillary segment, the pectoralis minor muscle may be seen deep to the pectoralis major and is an important landmark for determining the level of axillary lymph nodes.

Deep to the chest wall lie the pleura and lung.

Recognizing the three separate sonographically visible zones of the breast forms the foundation of sonographic breast anatomy. However, full understanding depends on two additional important components of sonographic breast anatomy: echogenicity and morphology. By becoming familiar with the important characteristics of each, one can begin to differentiate between the different types of tissues within the breast and the lesions that arise from those tissues.

Echogenicity

The premammary zone has a similar appearance in all patients: the typical isoechoic appearance of fat with interspersed thin, echogenic curvilinear structures that represent Cooper's ligaments. In patients who are scanned in the supine position with vigorous transducer compression, Cooper's ligaments are pushed into an axis nearly parallel with the skin and transducer face. The lighter the compression used, the more steeply oblique the course of Cooper's ligaments becomes. When too little compression pressure is used, the steeply obliquely oriented ligaments can cast acoustic shadows that can simulate shadowing from an invasive malignant lesion. In such cases, compressing more

firmly forces the shadowing ligament more nearly parallel to the transducer face, which can eradicate this artifactual shadowing (see Chapter 3, Fig. 3–5).

Unlike the sonographic appearance of the premammary and retromammary fat, the sonographic appearance of the mammary zone varies greatly from one individual to another, and even from one part of the breast to another within an individual patient, depending on the relative amounts and distribution of hyperechoic fibrous elements and more isoechoic fatty or glandular elements.

The echogenicity of both normal and pathologic anatomic structures must be compared to a known standard. There are difficulties in interpreting the results of previously published sonographic studies about pathologic breast lesions. The standard against which the echogenicity of breast lesions were being compared varied or were not well defined. For instance, if a lesion was described as "hypoechoic," to what was it being compared? In many cases, any lesion that appeared to be more hypoechoic than the intensely echogenic normal interlobular stromal fibrous tissue of the breast was considered to be hypoechoic. As can be seen from the schematic gray-scale spectrum in Fig. 4–9, normal interlobular stromal fibrous tissue is at the echogenic end of the gray-scale spectrum, and only calcifications and needles are more echogenic. Therefore, virtually every other normal anatomic breast structure and all pathologic lesions except isolated microcalcifications would be hypoechoic compared with fibrous tissue. To state that a lesion is hypoechoic compared with the most echogenic tissue in the breast, interlobular stromal fibrous tissue, carries very little useful discriminating information.

Table 4–2 shows the spectrum of echogenicities of normal beast tissues and pathologic lesions of the breast using fat as the frame of reference against which echogenicity is compared.

It is far more useful to use a normal structure or tissue that is near the center of the gray-scale spectrum as a standard against which we compare other anatomic tissues and pathologic lesions. Additionally, the normal tissue whose echogenicity is to be used as the standard should be present in virtually all patients. Figure 4–9 shows that normal tissues that have echogenicities very near the center of the gray-scale spectrum include fatty breast tissues, TDLUs (containing epithelium and loose intralobular stromal fibrous tissue), and ducts (consisting of lumen, epithelium, myoepithelium, and loose periductal stromal fibrous tissue). However, TDLUs and ductal and periductal tissues are not sonographically demonstrable in all patients. Therefore, these tissues cannot reliably be used as the frame of reference for comparison in all patients. On the other hand, there is fat, at least within the subcutaneous zone, in virtually every woman's breast, even in women who have mammographically dense breasts. For these reasons, the echogenicity of normal breast fat is the standard against

loose stromal fibrous tissue = intralobular and periductal

dense stromal fibrous tissue = interlobular and Cooper's ligaments

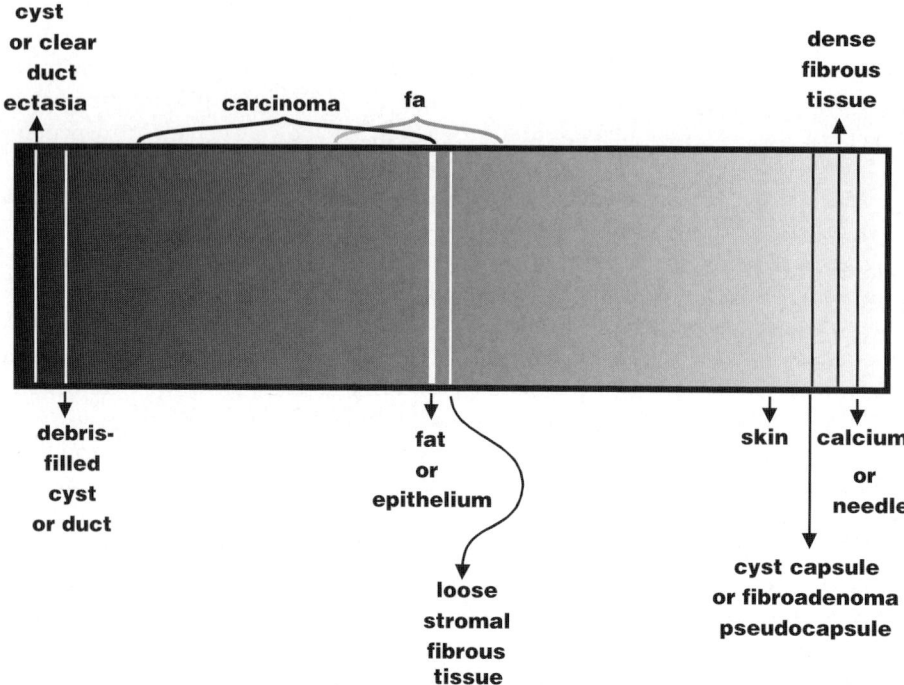

FIGURE 4–9 Having a frame of reference for echogenicity is essential. The frame of reference should (a) be near the center of the gray scale spectrum of tissues within the breast, and (b) be a normal structure that is present in the most normal individuals. The normal tissues in the breast that have echogenicities near the center of the gray scale spectrum include fat, epithelial tissues within ducts and lobules, and loose periductal and intralobular stromal fibrous tissue. Epithelial and loose periductal and intralobular stromal tissues are not sonographically demonstrable in most normal individuals. Fat, however, is present within the subcutaneous or premammary zone in most patients, regardless of how dense the tissues within the mammary zone appear to be mammographically. Thus, fat is the tissue to which echogenicity of other tissues and pathologic lesions should be compared. If fat is used as the frame of reference, it should be made to appear a midlevel gray, not black or hypoechoic, as the older ultrasound literature suggests. Note that most lesions are less echogenic than fat. Their conspicuity will be reduced if fat is made hypoechoic rather than isoechoic. Thus, structures and lesions similar in fat to echogenicity are termed *isoechoic*. Structures and lesions less echogenic than fat are termed *hypoechoic*, and those more echogenic are considered to be *hyperechoic*. Note that virtually all normal breast tissue and pathologic lesions of the breast are markedly hypoechoic to interlobular stromal fibrous tissue, which is more echogenic than anything but calcifications and needles. Thus, there is little differential diagnostic value in using intensely echogenic fibrous tissue as the frame of reference against which lesion echogenicity is compared. To term a lesion hypoechoic in comparison to the most echogenic tissue in the breast, as has unfortunately been done extensively in the older ultrasound literature, is not useful.

which all other normal anatomic tissues and pathologic lesions should be compared. Tissues and lesions that are blacker than normal breast fat should be considered hypoechoic, tissues and lesions that are whiter than fat should be considered hyperechoic, and tissues that have echogenicity identical to fat should be considered isoechoic. Lesions that have no internal echoes are anechoic. These definitions of hypoechogenicity, isoechogenicity, and hyperechogenicity will be used as the framework for all discussions of echogenicity in this book.

Furthermore, for solid nodules, it is useful to distinguish between mildly and severely hypoechoic and between mildly and severely hyperechoic. This lexicon is discussed in greater detail in Chapter 12.

If the echogenicity of normal breast fat is to be used as the standard against which everything else is compared, it is important to set up scan parameters such as total gain and time–gain curve (TGC) so that fat appears to be a midlevel gray. Additionally, the fat within the subcutaneous tissues, the fat in the mammary zone, and

TABLE 4–2. ECHOGENICITY AND PATHOLOGY OF BREAST TISSUES

Normal Breast Tissues	Echogenicity of Neoplasms

♦ Isoechoic normal breast tissues
• Fat
• Epithelium—ductules within terminal ductolobular unit
• Loose stromal fibrous tissue
  • Periductal stromal fibroelastic tissue
  • Intralobular stromal fibrous tissue
 	
♦ Hyperechoic normal breast tissues
• Skin
• Cooper's ligaments
• Interlobular stromal fibrous tissue
 	
♦ Hypoechoic normal breast tissue
• Nipple
• Blood in veins
	♦ Isoechoic or nearly isoechoic
	• Fibroadenoma
	• Papilloma
	• About one-third of carcinomas
	• Small, special-type tumors
	  • Colloid carcinomas
	  • Tubular carcinomas
	• Hyperechoic
	  • Central scars in some carcinomas
	  • Echogenic halo around spiculated carcinomal
	  • Needle tract through any solid nodule after core needle biopsy
	• Markedly hypoechoic
	  • About one-half to two-thirds of carcinomas
	  • Medullary carcinoma
	• Anechoic or nearly anechoic
	  • Areas of cystic necrosis in carcinomas
	  • Lymphoma
	  • Medullary carcinoma
	  • Some intensely shadowing desmoplastic carcinomas
	  • Metastases to intramammary lymph nodes

Fibrocystic and Benign Proliferative Epithelial and Myoepithelial Conditions

♦ Isoechoic—epithelial and myoepithelial proliferations
• Floral or papillary usual duct hyperplasia
• Atypical duct hyperplasia
• Papillary apocrine metaplasia
• Adenosis
• Debris and floating cells in complex cysts

♦ Appear isoechoic due to volume averaging with microscopic fluid-filled spaces, although expected to appear hyperechoic
• Fibrosclerosis
• Pseudoangiomatous stromal hyperplasia

♦ Hyperechoic
• Cyst wall
• Pseudocapsule of compressed tissue around fibroadenomas
• Focal fibrosis
• Fibrosclerosis (some cases, others isoechoic)
• Edema of fat
• Fibrosis of fat

♦ Anechoic
• Cyst fluid
• Duct fluid
• Dilated lymphatics

♦ Hypoechoic
• Cyst fluid containing cells or debris (including blood or pus)
• Duct fluid containing cells or debris (including blood or pus)

the fat in the retromammary zone should all demonstrate the same midlevel gray echogenicity (Fig. 4–10). This requires appropriate TGC settings (Fig. 4–11). Achieving a uniform level of echogenicity for fat at all depths in the breast usually requires a mildly sloping TGC. Using a TGC that is too flat is one of the more frequent technical errors. It makes the subcutaneous fat appear too echogenic, the fat in the mammary zone isoechoic, and the fat in the retromammary zone hypoechoic. On the other hand, a TGC that is set too steeply will result in fat ap-

pearing to be hypoechoic in the near field but hyperechoic in the far field.

Normal fat must not be demonstrated as being hypoechoic. About one-third of breast cancers and most fibroadenomas are only *mildly* hypoechoic with respect to fat, and these very subtle, mildly hypoechoic lesions are more likely to be indistinguishable from fat if fat is not displayed as a midlevel gray. A TGC setting resulting in "medium-gray fat" throughout the breast improves lesion conspicuity and sonographic sensitivity for subtle mildly

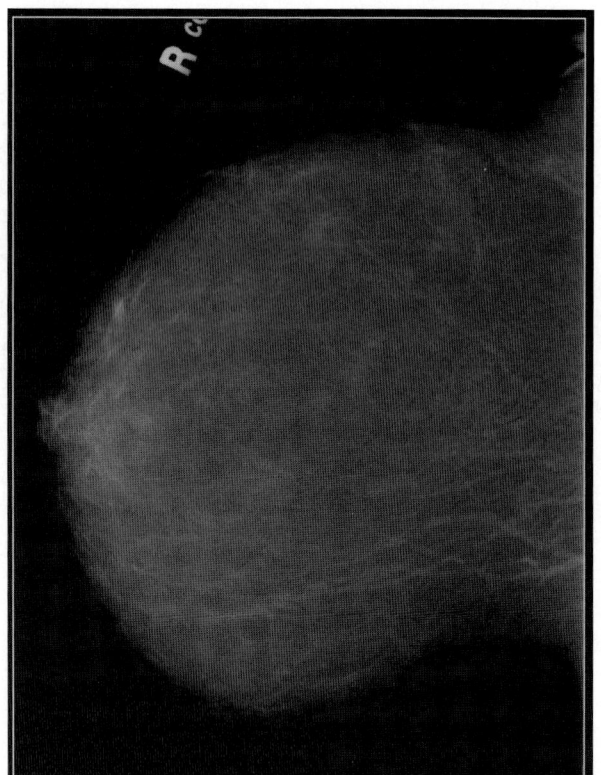

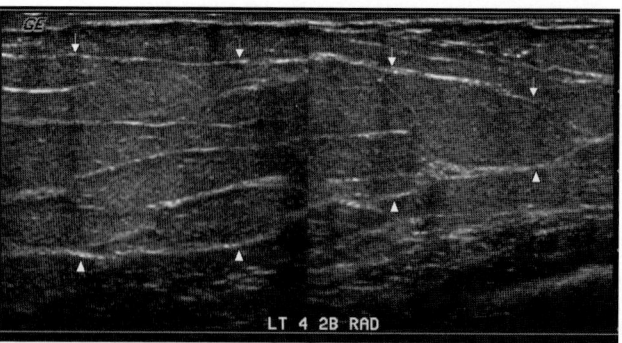

FIGURE 4–10 A: This is a craniocaudal (CC) view of the right breast in a woman whose breast has undergone extensive atrophy of parenchymal and stromal fibrous elements and is now composed entirely of fat. Few lesions will be missed by mammography in such fatty breasts, but small, palpable abnormalities that are pea-sized or smaller may still benefit from sonographic evaluation because they usually lie near the skin, which is "burned out" with currently used film-screen mammographic techniques. **B:** These split-screen combined images show the lateral aspect of the left breast in a patient who has undergone extensive atrophy and whose breasts are now composed entirely of fat. Note that total gain and time–gain curve settings appropriately make the fat in the near, middle, and far field appear a midlevel echogenicity. Note that the mammary zone *(MZ)* contains only isoechoic fat and Cooper's ligaments and demonstrates no visible ducts or lobules. The anterior mammary fascia *(arrows)* and the retromammary fascia *(arrowheads)* that envelop the mammary zone, however, are preserved.

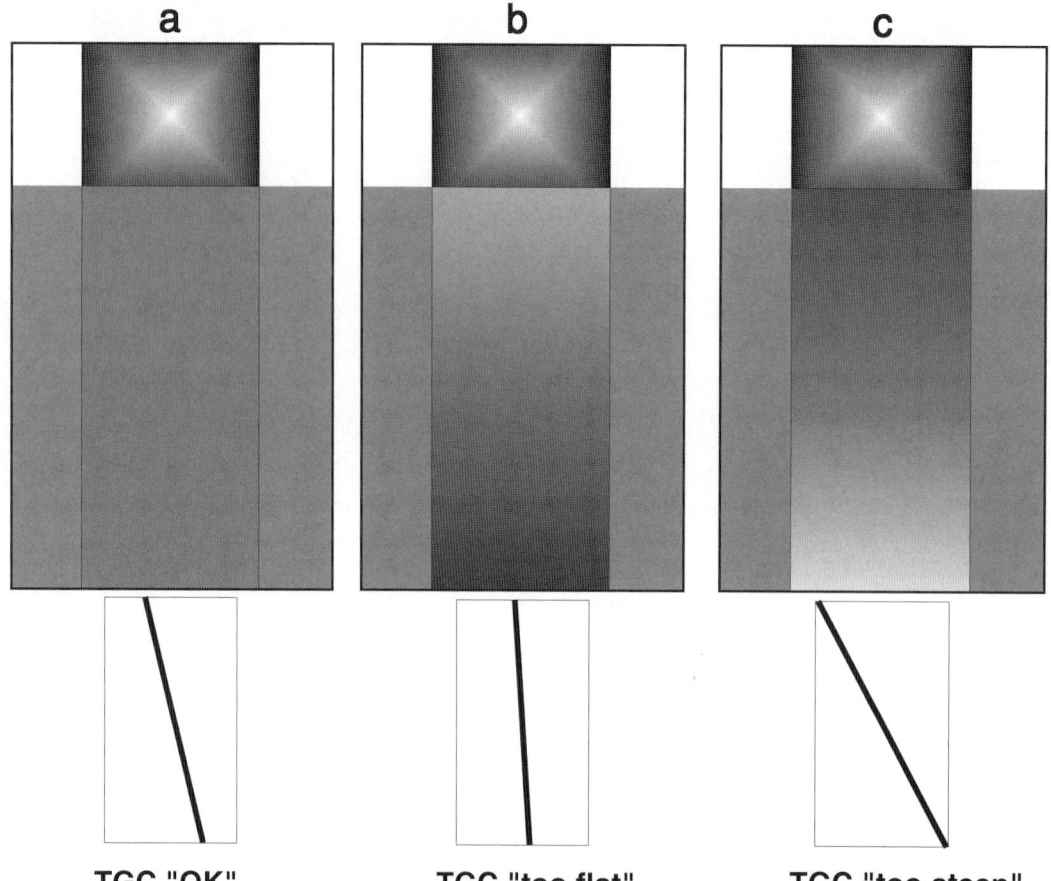

FIGURE 4–11 A: The time–gain curve (TGC) should be set so that fat is the same midlevel echogenicity in the near, middle, and far fields. A TGC slope that is too steep may result in the near-field fat appearing too hypoechoic, and a slope too flat may make the far-field fat appear too hypoechoic.

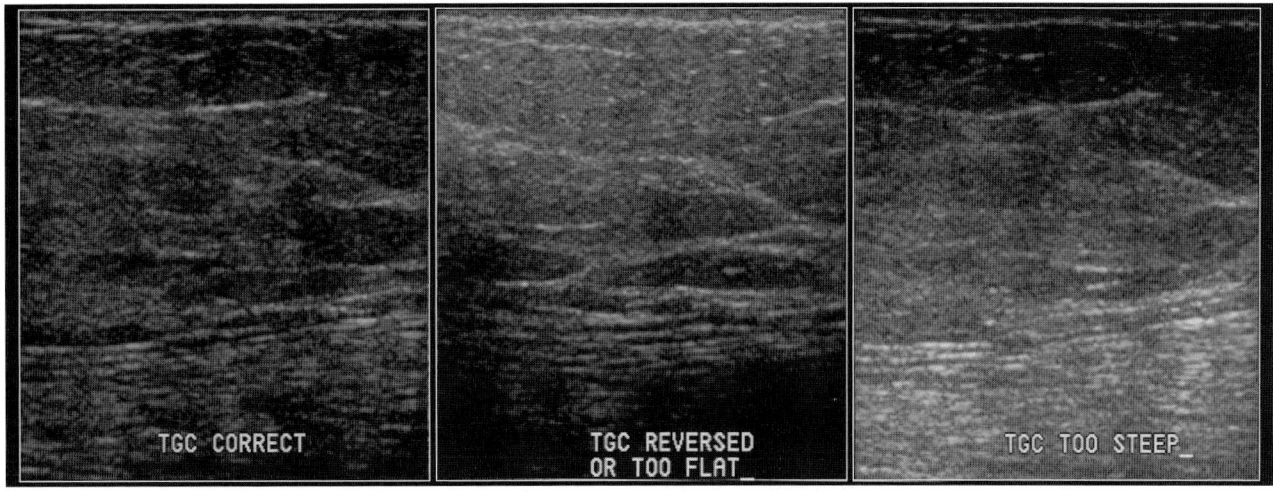

B

FIGURE 4–11 *(continued)* **B:** These figures show a fatty breast with different TGC slopes. The **left** image shows an appropriate slope that causes the fat in the near, middle, and far fields to be a midlevel echogenicity (isoechoic). The **middle** image shows the effects on echogenicity of a TGC that is too flat or even reversed (higher gain in near field). The fat in the near field is too echogenic, and the fat in the far field is too hypoechoic. The **right** image shows the effect of a TGC slope that is too steep. The near-field fat is now too hypoechoic, and the far-field fat is too echogenic.

hypoechoic lesions, whereas a TGC setting resulting in "black fat" reduces lesion conspicuity and sonographic sensitivity (Fig. 4–12). Using a high-frequency (10 MHz or higher), broad-bandwidth transducer that has high contrast resolution facilitates distinguishing these subtle lesions from surrounding fatty tissue. Coded harmonics and real-time compounding also help (see Chapter 2).

Mammographically dense (water density) areas of the breast can be caused by two very different types of tissue sonographically: dense, echogenic interlobular stromal fibrous tissue and isoechoic glandular and ductal elements (Fig. 4–13). There is a continuous spectrum from purely hyperechoic fibrous breast tissue to purely isoechoic glandular tissue (Fig. 4–14). Pure fibrous, pure glandular, and mixed fibroglandular breast tissues all have the same dense mammographic appearance (Figs. 4–15 to 4–17).

Breasts that are completely glandular and isoechoic are more likely to occur during the late teenage years and early 20s when there is rapid proliferation of lobules, during anovulatory cycles or in association with other ovulatory disorders, when there is an imbalance between endogenous estrogen and progesterone production, during the last two trimesters of pregnancy (adenosis of pregnancy), and during lactation. The echogenicity of glandular elements relative to fat varies slightly between early pregnancy and later stages of pregnancy and lactation. Glandular tissues are likely to be isoechoic during early pregnancy, but become slightly hypoechoic as lactational change fills the intralobular acini with secretions. Occasionally, lactational change can affect the breast asymmetrically during earlier phases of

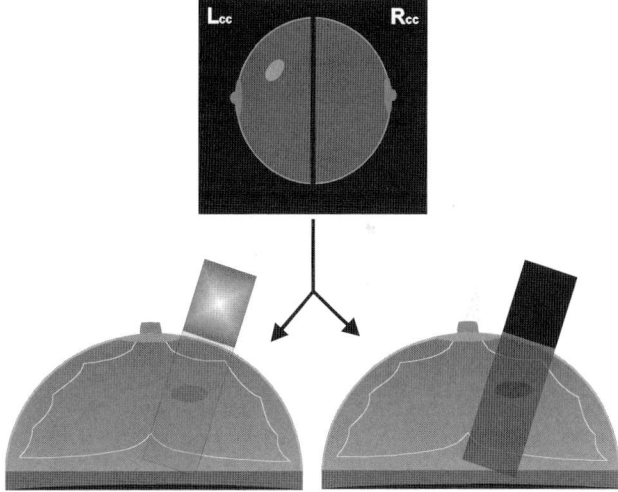

gray fat -- adequate gain   **black faat -- too little gain**

FIGURE 4–12 When fat is used as the frame of reference for echogenicity, the total gain and time–gain curve settings should be used to make the fat appear a midlevel gray. Although some lesions are isoechoic with fat, most pathologic lesions for which we search are mildly or moderately hypoechoic with respect to fat. By establishing a midlevel echogenicity for fat, we maximize the percentage of lesions that are conspicuously more hypoechoic than fat **(left).** On the other hand, if fat is made too hypoechoic by using too little gain, many lesions that are mildly hypoechoic with respect to fat may be less conspicuous and more difficult to identify **(right).** Thus, the percentage of all lesions that appear hypoechoic to fat will be minimized rather than maximized.

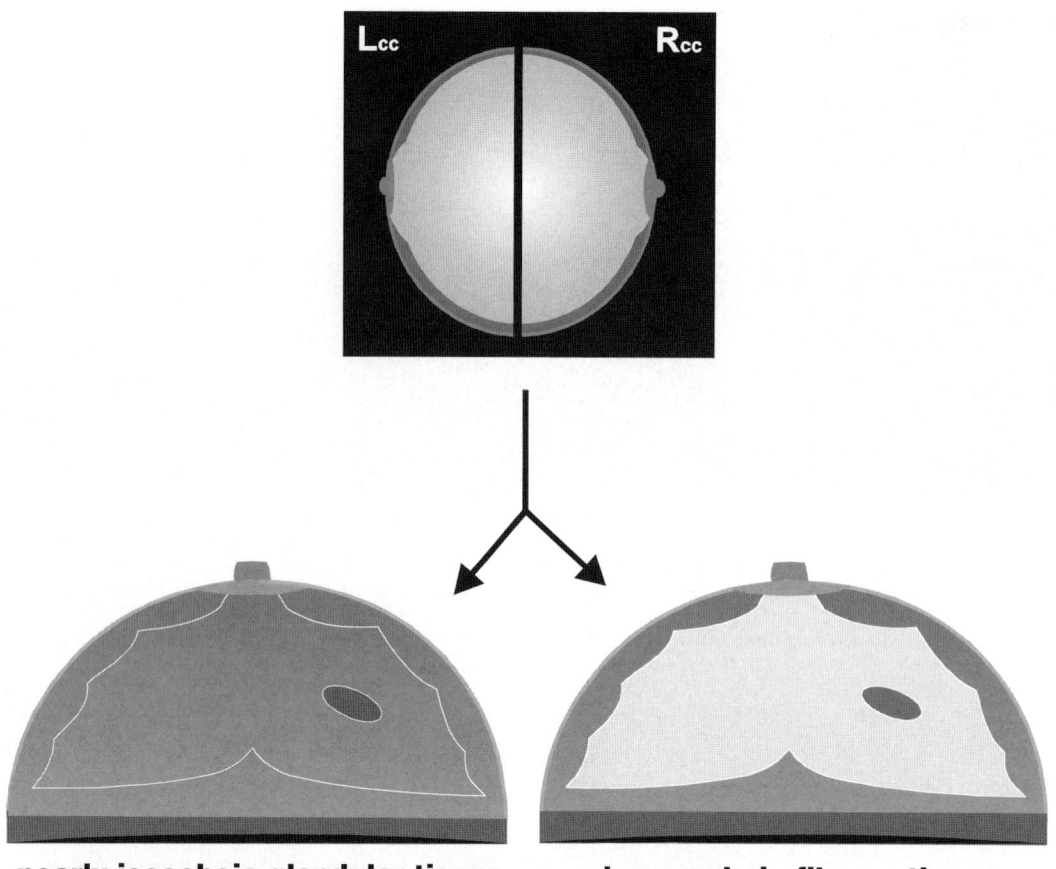

A   **nearly isoechoic glandular tissue   hyperechoic fibrous tissue**

B

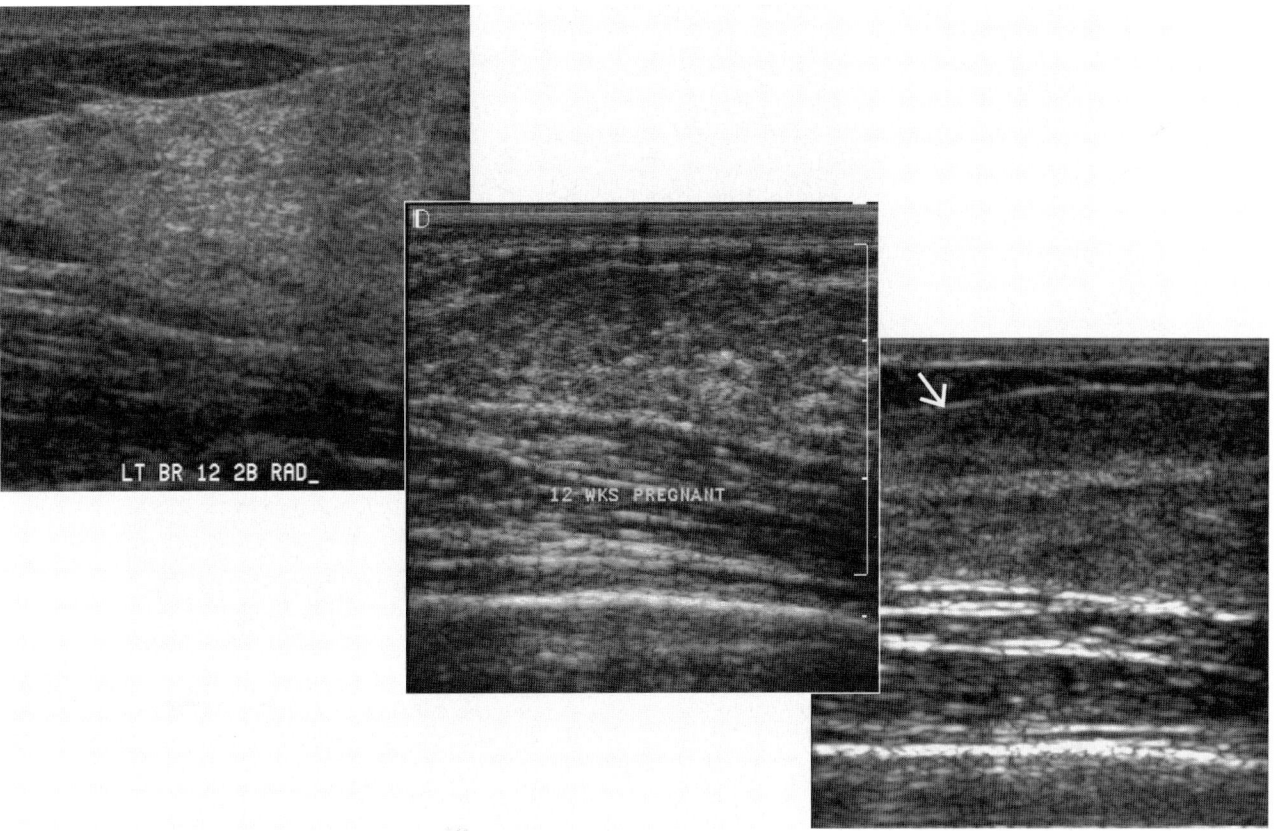

FIGURE 4–14 There is a continuous spectrum of echogenicities within the breast from purely hyperechoic interlobular stromal fibrous tissue (**left upper**) to purely isoechoic glandular tissue (**right lower**). Most patients have a mixture of the two tissue types (**middle**) rather than purely hyperechoic or purely isoechoic mammary zones. In patients with mixed echogenicity, the isoechoic tissues are generally present in the anterior half of the mammary zones because the isoechoic tissues represent the lobular elements of the breast, which are most numerous anterior to the lobar duct.

pregnancy, causing localized lumps or tenderness and foci of hypoechogenicity sonographically. Such foci can simulate masses and are sometimes diagnosed as secretory adenomas or lactating adenomas histologically (Fig. 4–18). Asymmetric foci of premature lactational change usually become inapparent clinically and sonographically as the surrounding tissues also undergo lactational change and become equally hypoechoic.

Secretory breast tissue can occasionally be seen in women who are not pregnant or lactating. The secretory change in such patients usually appears hypoechoic but may appear hyperechoic if the secretions or milk contained within the dilated acini are inspissated or "curdled" (Fig. 4–19A). Tissues undergoing focal secretory change are usually softer and more compressible than surrounding tissues

(text continued on page 74)

FIGURE 4–13 A: Two different types of tissues imaged with ultrasound. Hyperechoic, interlobular, stromal fibrous tissue and isoechoic glandular tissue (or mixtures of the two) can cause mammographically dense (water-density) tissue. The sensitivity of ultrasound for isoechoic and mildly hypoechoic lesions varies depending on the echogenicity of background tissues. Sensitivity is reduced in a background of isoechoic glandular tissue and increased in a background of hyperechoic fibrous tissues. This is analogous to the variation of mammographic sensitivity with background tissue density. Sensitivity is reduced in radiographically dense background tissue and increased in fatty density background tissues. **B:** This figure shows a typical mammogram in a patient with class 4 mammographic density (>75% dense). A mammogram such as this could be caused by either hyperechoic fibrous tissue (**right lower**) or isoechoic glandular tissue (**left lower**) throughout the entire mammary zone. An isoechoic solid nodule would be easier to miss in the equally isoechoic glandular background than in the markedly hyperechoic fibrous background.

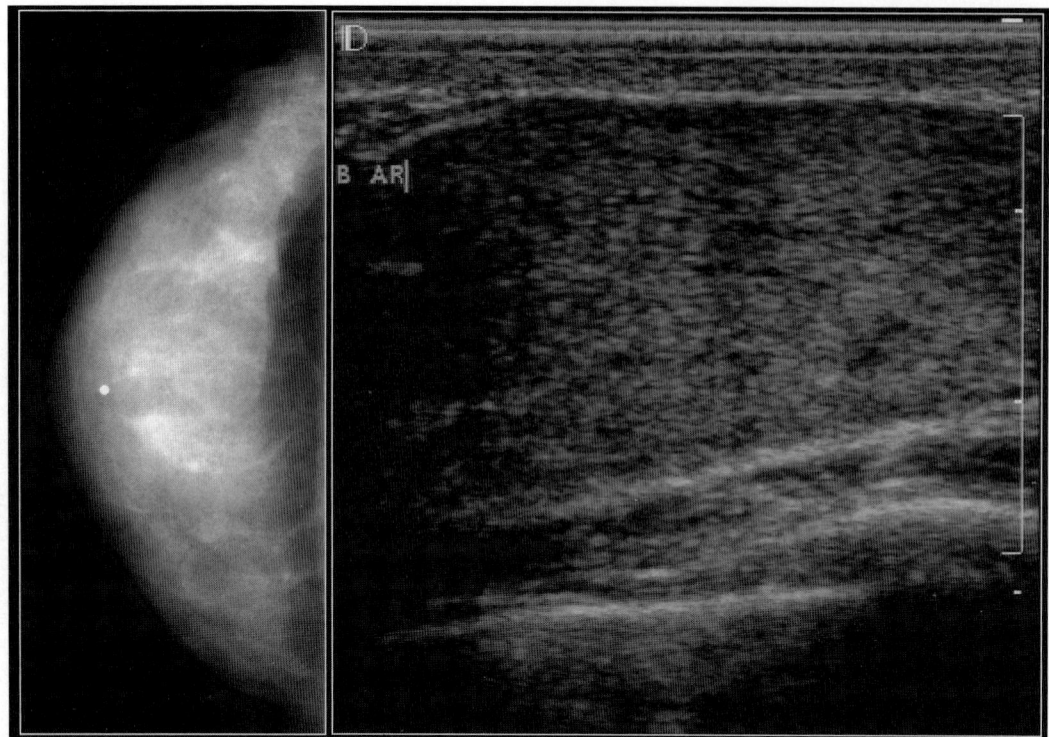

FIGURE 4–15 This patient had a homogeneously dense class 4 mammogram caused by purely isoechoic glandular tissue. Such an appearance is most likely to occur in patients who are in their late teens or early 20s and undergoing a phase of rapid lobular proliferation, during the last trimester of pregnancy, during lactation, or while undergoing replacement hormone therapy with high progesterone components. Occasionally, a patient, such as this 54-year-old, may have a purely isoechoic glandular breast composition with none of the above underlying causes to explain it. Isoechoic solid nodules would be relatively difficult to see and easy to miss when lying within such background tissue.

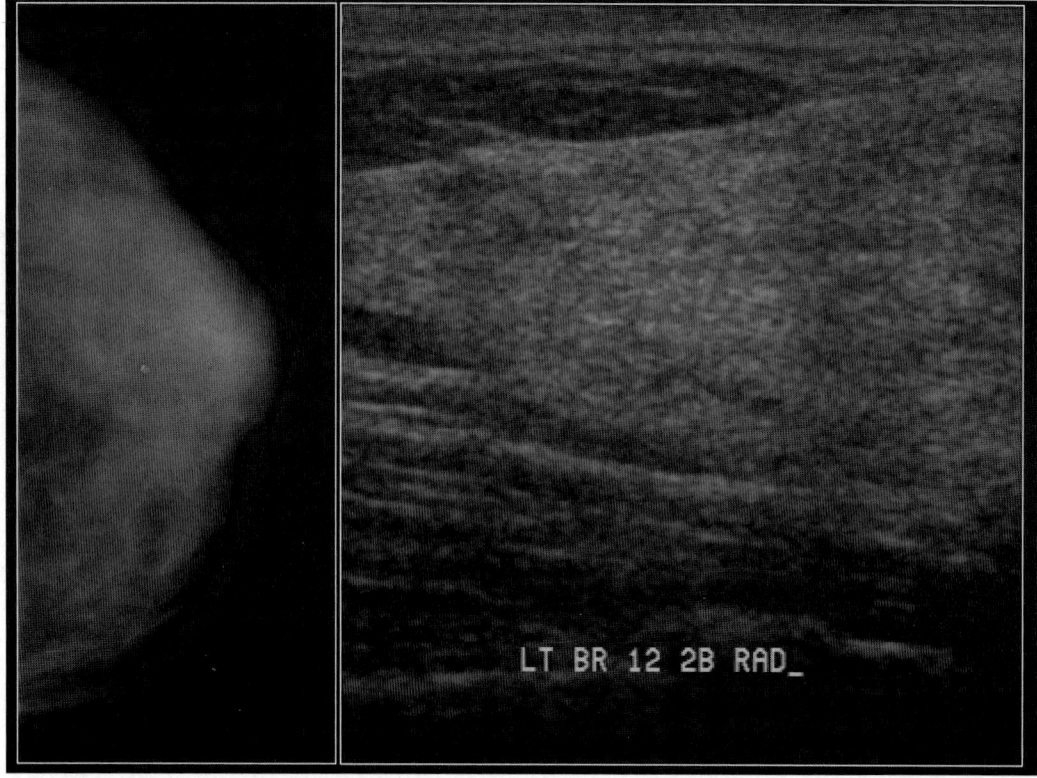

FIGURE 4–16 This patient had a homogeneously dense class 4 mammogram caused by purely hyperechoic fibrous tissue. Such an appearance is much more common than is the appearance of purely isoechoic glandular tissue. In most cases, there is no identifiable underlying cause, and this is simply a manifestation of the patient's genetic makeup. This appearance becomes less likely with age but can be maintained or even made to reappear after menopause by hormone replacement therapy. Little except isolated microcalcifications caused by low- to intermediate-grade ductal carcinoma *in situ* could be missed sonographically in a patient with such background tissue.

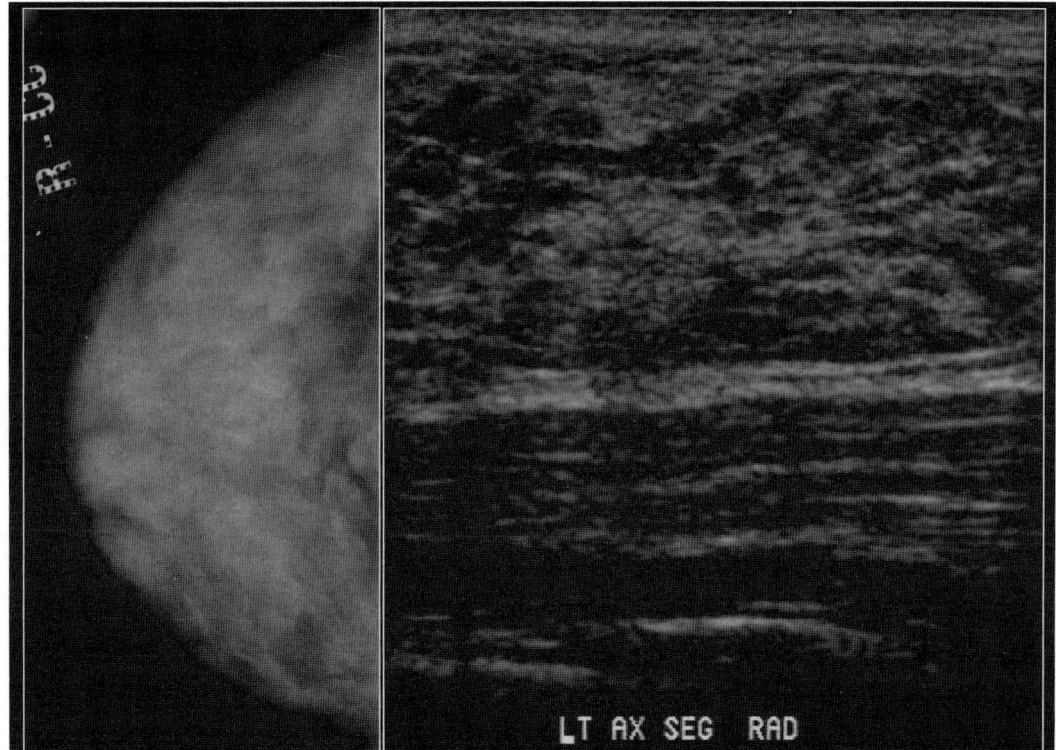

FIGURE 4–17 This patient had a homogeneously dense class 4 mammogram caused by a mixture of hyperechoic fibrous tissue and isoechoic lobular or glandular tissue. Such an appearance is more common than is the appearance of either purely isoechoic glandular tissue or purely hyperechoic fibrous tissue. The sensitivity for subtle isoechoic, small nodules will lie between the high sensitivity of purely hyperechoic fibrous tissue and the lower sensitivity of purely isoechoic glandular tissue and will also depend on the size of the lesion.

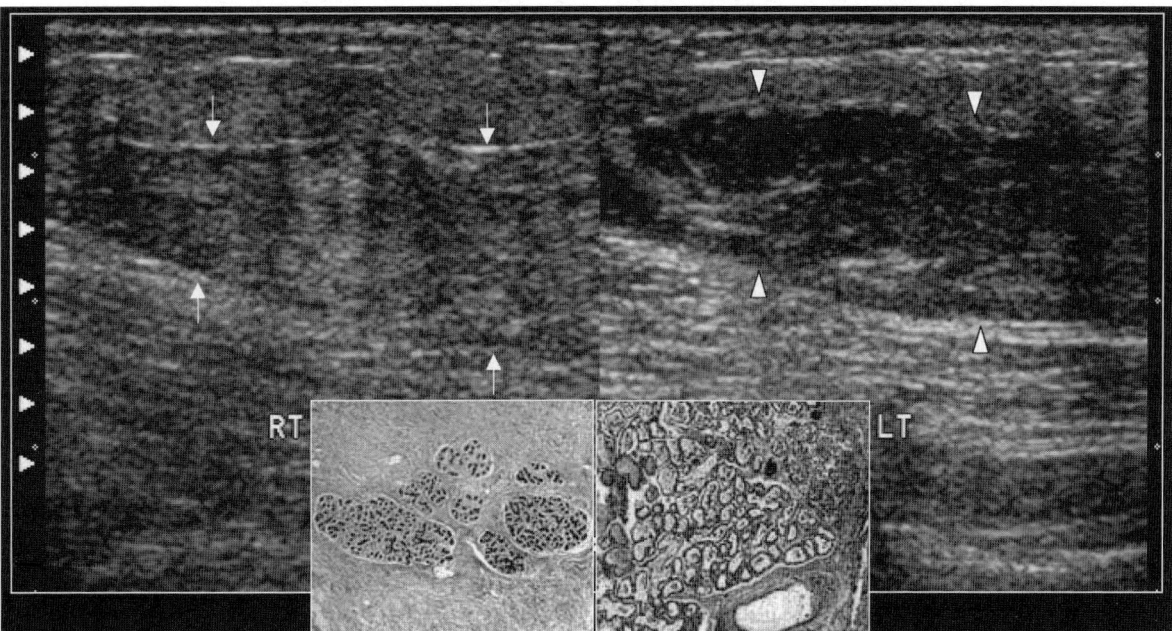

FIGURE 4–18 These split-screen images show mirror images of the upper inner quadrants of the right (**left**) and left (**right**) breasts in a patient in the third trimester of pregnancy. Note that the lobular tissue has enlarged at the expense of echogenic fibrous tissue that was present earlier in pregnancy to fill the entire mammary zone (**left**, *between arrows*). In the mirror-image location of the left, however, the tissue appears thicker and more hypoechoic (**right**, *arrowheads*). The patient complained of a nontender thickening in this area. The isoechoic tissue in the right upper inner quadrant represents adenosis of pregnancy, where both the number of lobules and the size of the lobules increase until they coalesce into a continuous isoechoic, glandular sheath. The more hypoechoic appearance on the patient's left side represented premature lactational change within preexisting adenosis of pregnancy. The secretions retained within individual lobular acini cause the hypoechogenicity. Premature lactational change is common during pregnancy and can occur even in the first or second trimester. It can cause a tender or nontender lump and, if focal, can be difficult to distinguish from a secretory or lactating adenoma both sonographically and histologically on needle biopsy. The natural history is for the lump and tenderness to become less apparent as the surrounding tissue also undergoes lactational change, but often the patient is too concerned to avoid biopsy. Unfortunately, both focal lactational change and lactating adenomas may be soft, compressible, and vascular, so that compressibility and Doppler are not helpful in making the distinction.

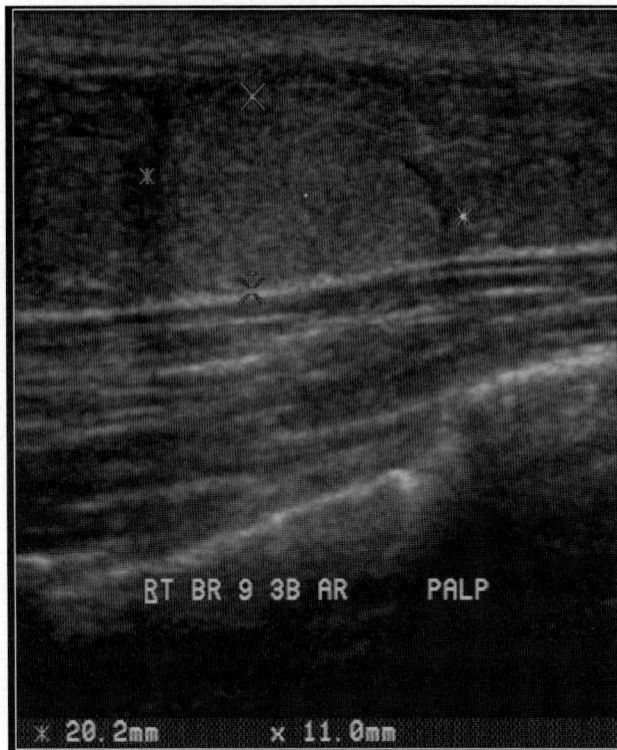

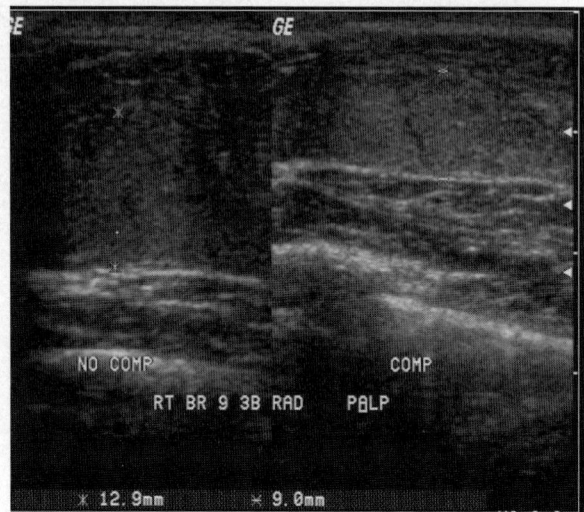

A   B

FIGURE 4–19 A: Although focal lactation change is most common in pregnancy, it can occur at times other than pregnancy or lactation, as in this patient. If the secretions become inspissated, the echogenicity of the involved glandular tissue may actually become mildly hyperechoic rather than hypoechoic. **B:** Even areas of focal lactational change that contain inspissated, hyperechoic secretions may be soft and compressible. Note that this area is more than 30% compressible, similar to many fat lobules. Although the echogenicity of the surrounding tissues is isoechoic with fat, and some lipomas may be mildly hyperechoic, we knew with certainty that this was not a fat-surrounded lipoma because the patient's mammogram was uniformly dense. Thus, correlation with the mammogram, as usual, was critical to proper diagnosis.

that have not undergone secretory change (Fig. 4–19B) and also tend to be more vascular. In a small percentage of patients, focal secretory change may be severe enough to cause cystic dilation of peripheral ducts and lobules (Fig. 4–20). Additionally, secretory change may cause dilation of peripheral lobar ducts rather than TDLUs in association with hypoechoic (Fig. 4–21) or hyperechoic (Fig. 4–22) glandular sonographic appearance. Focal lobular or ductal secretory changes can occur anywhere in the breast but most commonly occur within accessory breast tissue in the axillary segment of the breast. Focal secretory change can also occur in preexisting tubular adenomas (Fig. 4–23) and fibroadenomas (Fig. 4–24).

Secretory change that occurs within a preexisting tubular adenoma during pregnancy results in what has been termed a *secretory* or *lactating adenoma* that can be difficult or impossible to distinguish from focal secretory change sonographically. Even on ultrasound-guided core needle biopsy, the distinction may be difficult. It is our impression that lactating adenomas are overdiagnosed and that many cases histologically diagnosed as lactating adenomas actually merely represent focal secretory change in glandular tissue that will become clinically inapparent later in pregnancy. However, concerns about false-negative diagnoses of cancer and the rapid growth of neoplasms that can occur during pregnancy as a result of hormonal stimulation continue to result in virtually all areas of focal secretory change undergoing image-guided biopsy.

Between breasts that contain purely hyperechoic interlobular stromal fibrous tissue and breasts that contain purely isoechoic glandular tissue lies a continuous spectrum of breasts that contain various mixtures of fibrous and glandular elements. The distribution of fibrous and glandular elements is often asymmetric from right to left and may also be nonuniform within an individual breast (Fig. 4–25). Because isoechoic glandular tissues are manifestations of prominent lobules, and because lobules are more numerous in the anterior half of the mammary zone,

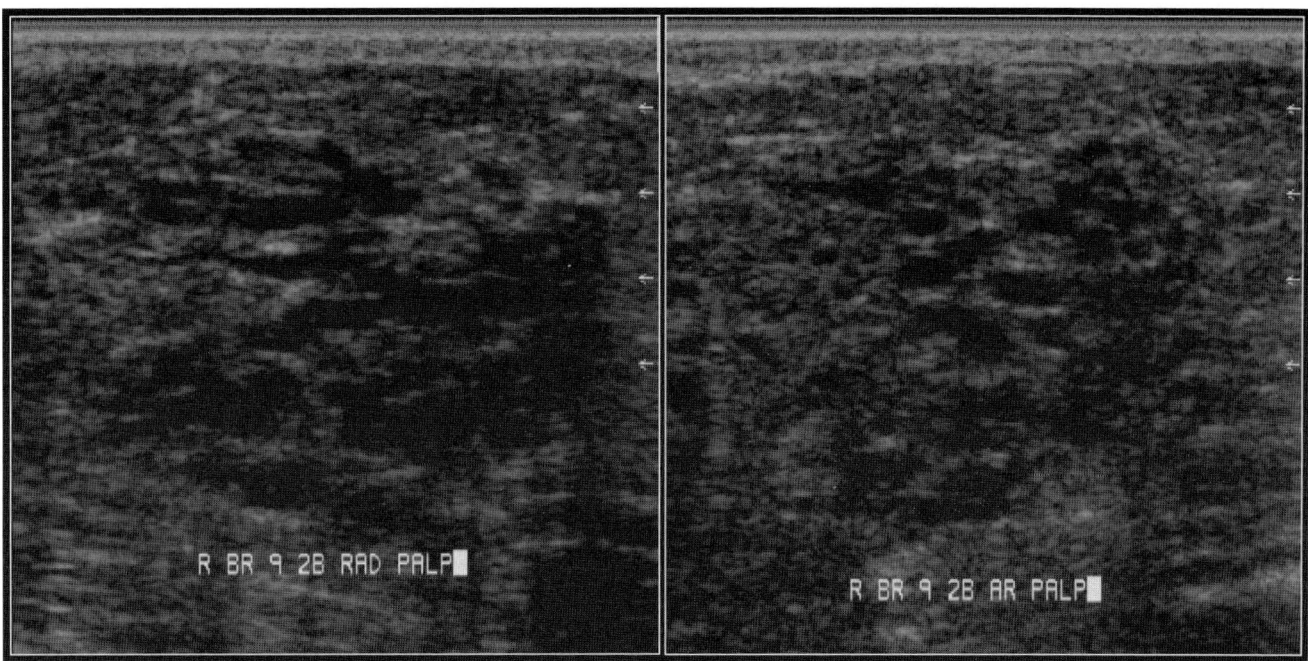

FIGURE 4–20 Radial (**left**) and antiradial (**right**) scans of the focal area of severe secretory change causing peripheral ductal and lobular dilation. Dilated ducts and lobules are shown parallel (**left**) and perpendicular (**right**) to their long axis.

isoechoic tissues are more commonly and more extensively seen in the anterior half than the posterior half of the mammary zone (Figs. 4–26 to 4–28).

The composition of the mammographically dense portions of the breast is important because it tells us about the reliability of a negative sonographic study. Sonography is used to "look through" mammographically dense tissues. If the mammographically dense tissue is caused primarily by dense, hyperechoic interlobular stromal fibrous elements, virtually all macroscopic pathologic lesions (except calcifications) will be highly conspicuous because virtually all macroscopic breast pathology is hypoechoic compared

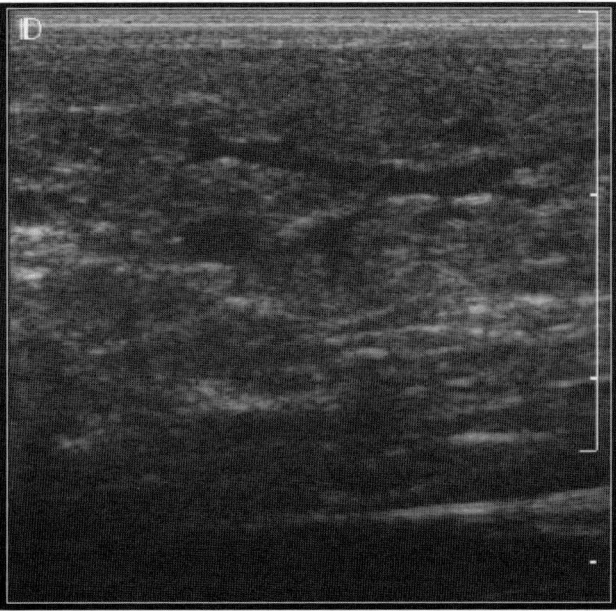

FIGURE 4–21 In this patient, a focal area of secretory change within accessory breast tissue is associated with peripheral duct ectasia and hypoechoic glandular tissue.

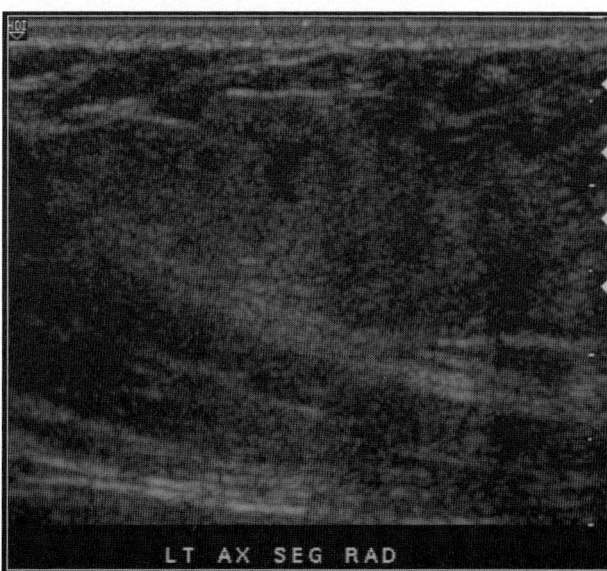

FIGURE 4–22 In this patient with focal secretory change, a dilated peripheral duct is associated with hyperechoic glandular tissue caused by inspissated secretions within the lobules.

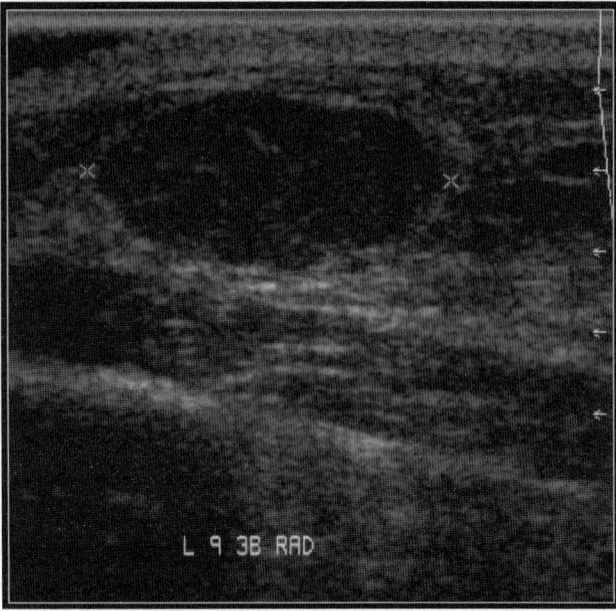

FIGURE 4–23 Secretory change has occurred within this preexisting tubular adenoma owing to hormonal stimulation from pregnancy, creating a secretory or lactating adenoma. During pregnancy, it may be difficult to distinguish between a focal area of glandular secretory change and a lactating adenoma by ultrasound alone. It may also be difficult for the pathologist to distinguish between the two entities from a core needle biopsy.

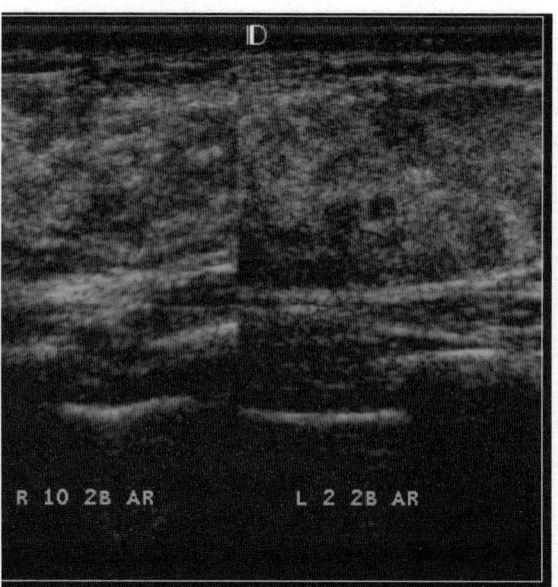

FIGURE 4–25 The size and number of lobules and thus the relative proportion of isoechoic glandular and hyperechoic fibrous tissue vary not only from patient to patient but also from right to left, as in this patient, and between different parts of the same breast. These split-screen images show mirror-image locations in the upper outer quadrants of the right (**left**) and left (**right**) breasts. Note that there is much more prominent glandular tissue on the **left** than in the mirror-image location on the **right**.

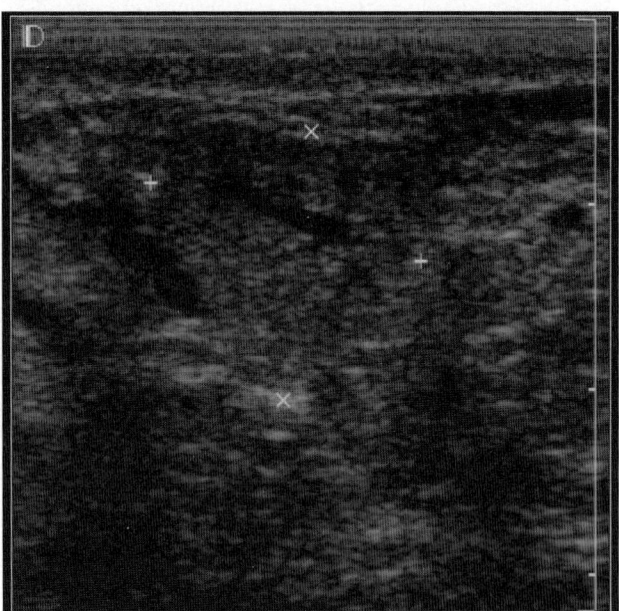

FIGURE 4–24 Secretory change has occurred within this fibroadenoma and led to a dilated duct within the nodule. The fibroadenoma presumably preexisted the onset of secretory change.

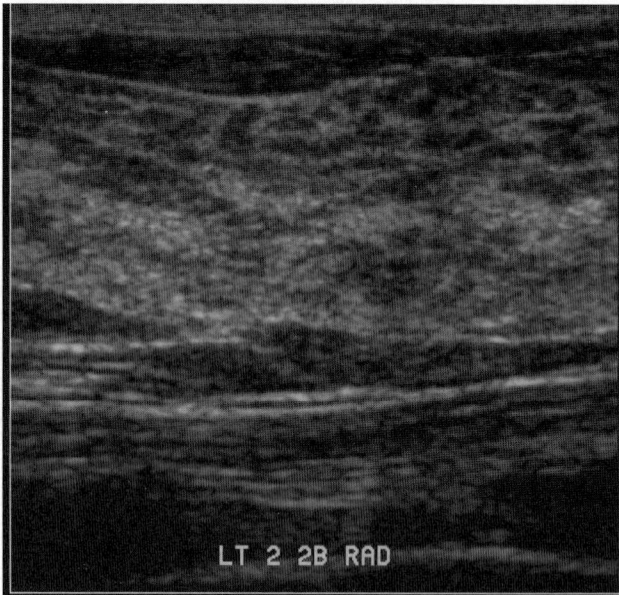

FIGURE 4–26 Some isoechoic lobules are visible in the posterior half of the mammary zone, but as usual, they are far more numerous and larger in the anterior half of the mammary zone just deep to the anterior mammary fascia. There are more rows of anterior lobules than there are rows of posterior lobules. Additionally, each anterior row has more lobules than each posterior row. Thus, there are many more lobules in the anterior half of the mammary zone than in the posterior half.

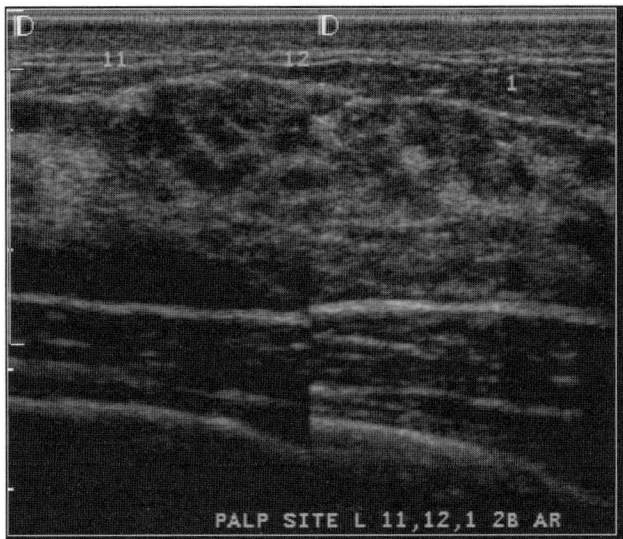

FIGURE 4–27 The lobules are larger and more numerous than in the patients shown in Fig. 4–26. The lobules in the far anterior aspect of the mammary zone, just deep to the anterior mammary fascia, are larger and more numerous than those in the posterior half of the mammary zone.

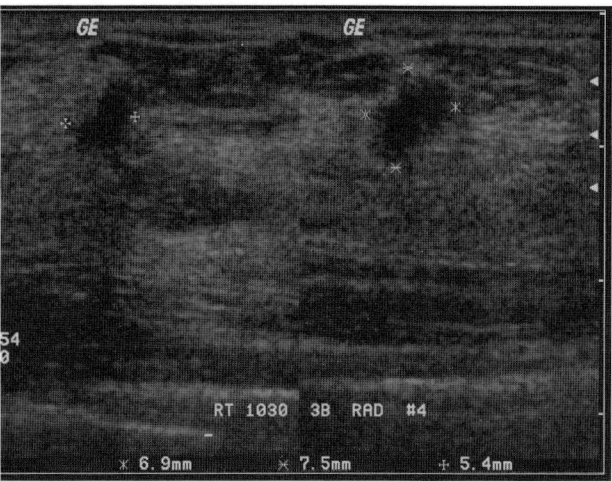

FIGURE 4–29 This small, 8-mm isoechoic solid nodule is highly sonographically conspicuous because it is almost completely surrounded by hyperechoic fibrous tissue.

with fibrous tissue (Fig. 4–29). This is analogous to the situation for mammography, where the negative predictive value is very high for fatty breasts.

On the other hand, sensitivity of ultrasound for some lesions will be significantly reduced when there is a large amount of isoechoic glandular tissue that demonstrates a midlevel (gray) echogenicity. The presence of isoechoic

glandular tissue does not adversely affect our ability to identify cysts and solid nodules that are hypoechoic with respect to glandular tissue and fat but will decrease the conspicuity of most fibroadenomas (Fig. 4–30) and about one-third of carcinomas (Fig. 4–31) that are only minimally nearly isoechoic with glandular tissue. The reduced conspicuity of some lesions when there is abundant isoechoic tissue on sonography is analogous to mammography's decreased sensitivity in dense breasts.

Knowing how the type of breast tissue affects negative predictive value is most important in patients with palpable lumps and dense tissue in the area of the palpable lump

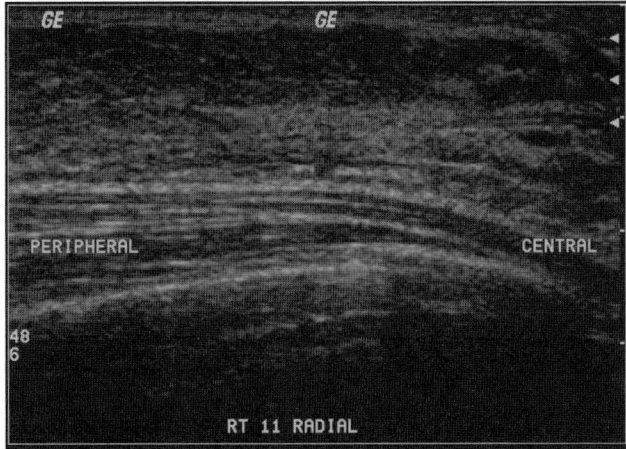

FIGURE 4–28 In this patient, the anterior lobules are so large and numerous that they have coalesced into a continuous sheet of isoechoic, glandular tissue in the anterior half of the mammary zone. The larger and more numerous the lobules and the more confluent they are, the more difficult it is to identify individual lobules. Thus, as seen in Figs. 4–26 and 4–27, there is a continuous spectrum of lobular prominence and a continuous spectrum in sensitivity for small, isoechoic solid nodules.

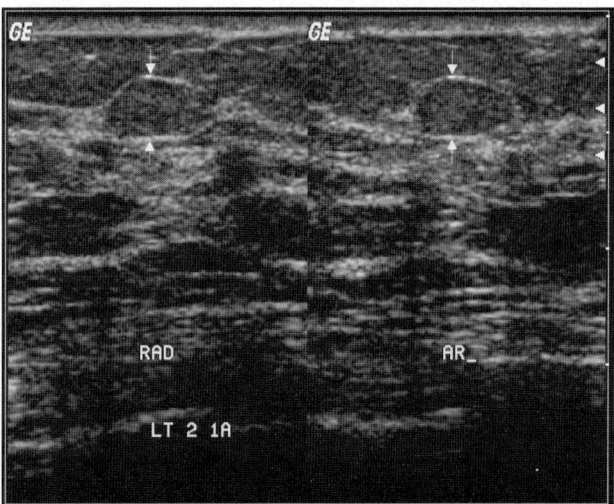

FIGURE 4–30 Within this anterior band of isoechoic glandular tissue is a small, relatively inapparent isoechoic fibroadenoma. The sensitivity for such nodules is reduced because they are indistinguishable in echogenicity from the background glandular tissue within which they lie.

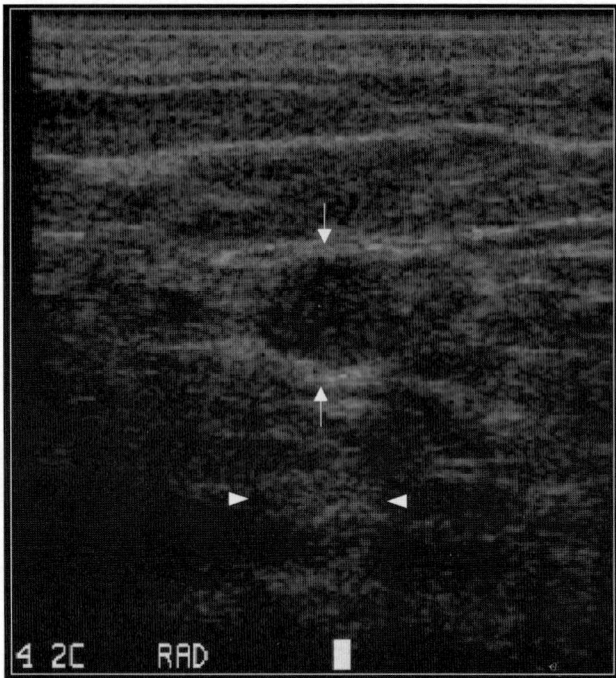

FIGURE 4–31 This small colloid carcinoma is difficult to identify because it is isoechoic to surrounding isoechoic fat. It is apparent only because of its echogenic capsule *(arrows)* and the enhanced through-transmission deep to it *(arrowheads)*. Small colloid carcinomas that are less than 1.5 cm in maximum diameter are the most likely to be missed, but small, intermediate-grade invasive ductal cancers, small medullary carcinomas, and small tubular carcinomas may all be isoechoic with fat or glandular tissue.

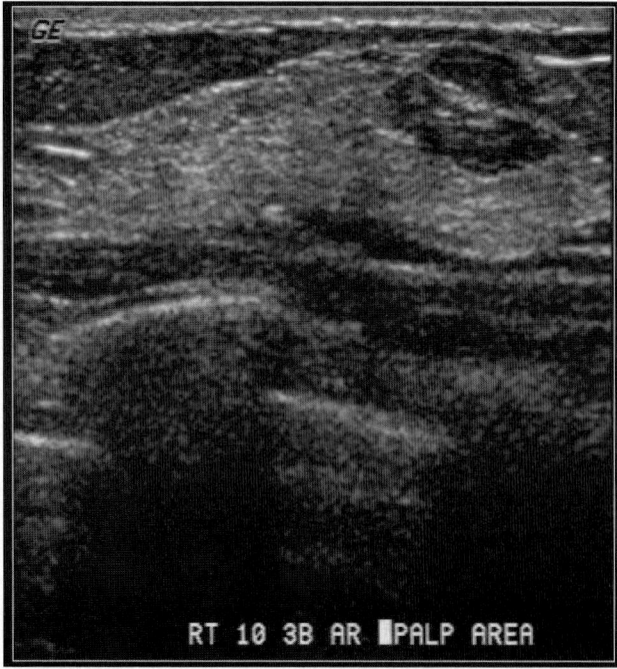

FIGURE 4–32 Sonographic and clinical correlation showed that the palpable lump about which the patient complained was caused by a purely hyperechoic fibrous ridge. The negative predictive value for a palpable, purely hyperechoic fibrous ridge approaches 100%. Thus, no biopsy or follow-up is necessary as long as mammography shows no calcifications within the ridge.

on mammography. A biopsy would be unnecessary in a patient with a palpable lump and negative mammograms in whom sonography showed purely hyperechoic fibrous tissue to cause the palpable lump (Fig. 4–32). On the other hand, in a similar patient, sonographic demonstration that the lump was caused by isoechoic glandular tissue would be less reassuring, and the referring physician might opt for biopsy (Fig. 4–33). Power Doppler vocal fremitus can be helpful in excluding occult isoechoic lesions (see Chapter 20).

As noted earlier, most patients have a mixture of hyperechoic fibrous and isoechoic glandular elements. The sensitivity in a breast composed of a mixture of hyperechoic fibrous tissues and isoechoic glandular tissues will be less than in a purely hyperechoic fibrous breast and higher than in a purely isoechoic glandular breast. The

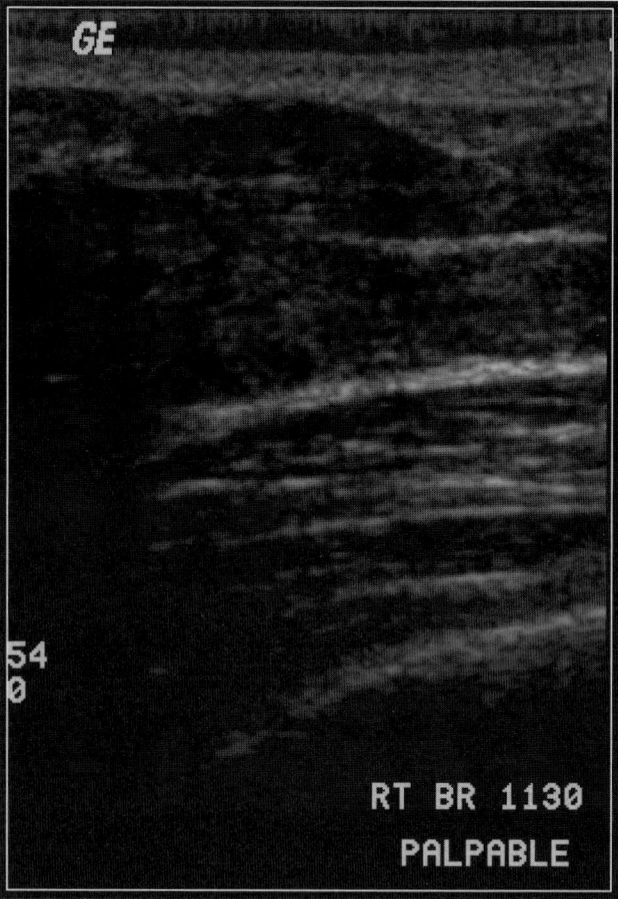

FIGURE 4–33 Sonographic and clinical correlation in this patient showed that the palpable lump about which the patient complained was caused by an isoechoic, glandular ridge. The negative predictive value is less than it is for the purely echogenic fibrous ridge shown in Fig. 4–32. Fremitus might further improve the negative predictive value by showing normal vibration of the entire ridge. However, because there is a slight chance that a small, isoechoic nodule could be obscured by surrounding gray glandular tissue, close clinical follow-up and a repeat sonogram in 6 months may be warranted. If the palpable abnormality were very suspicious, some surgeons would perform biopsy even though the ultrasound showed only isoechoic, glandular tissue.

greater the percentage of the breast that is composed of isoechoic tissue, the lower will be the sensitivity. One should not assume that sonography is completely insensitive for lesions when there is abundant isoechoic tissue. Rather, the sensitivity is relatively lower than in the purely hyperechoic breast. The sensitivity in glandular breasts may still be as high as the mid-90 percentile but is lower than the nearly 100% sensitivity in purely hyperechoic breasts.

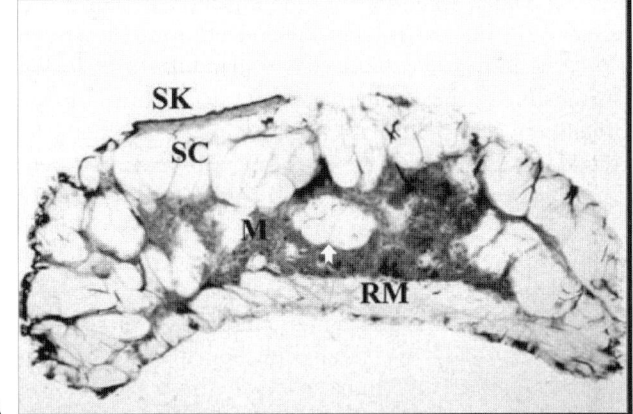

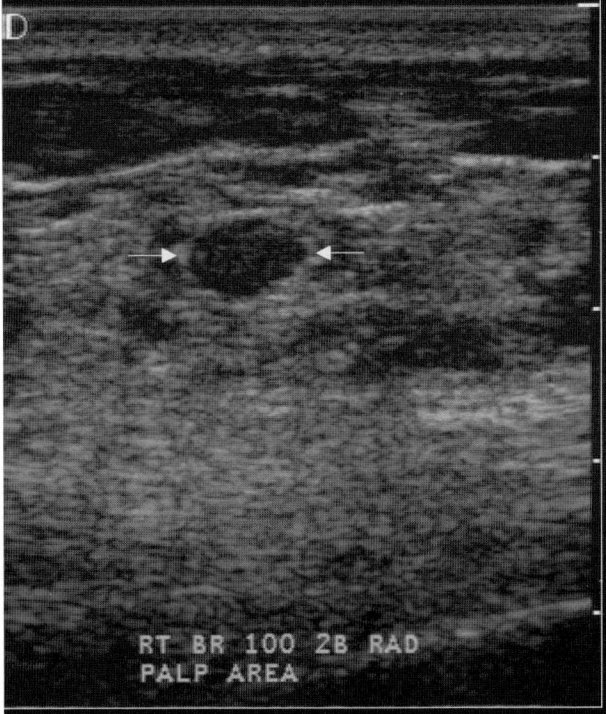

FIGURE 4–34 **A:** This section of an involutional breast shows a mixture of fibroglandular *(dark)* elements and fatty lobules *(arrow)*. (Whole mount pathology courtesy of Hanne M. Jensen, MD, University of California at Davis.) **B:** Some fat lobules are completely surrounded by echogenic fibrous tissue in all planes *(arrows)*. In such cases, orthogonal views are not helpful, and additional techniques are necessary to distinguish the structure from a solid nodule such as a fibroadenoma (see Fig. 4–36).

Morphology

Most breasts also have involuted fatty lobules interspersed with fibrous and glandular elements (Fig. 4–34). Each fat lobule is, in effect, a normal solid breast nodule. A fat lobule can be a cause of either a false-positive or a false-negative diagnosis. An isoechoic solid breast nodule may mistakenly be interpreted as a fat lobule, resulting in a false-negative diagnosis, or a fat lobule may be misinterpreted as a pathologic solid breast nodule, creating a false-positive diagnosis. Because fat lobules are potential causes of errors, having methods of distinguishing fat lobules from pathologic solid breast nodules is important.

There are several evaluations that help distinguish fat lobules from solid breast nodules. First, the structure must be evaluated in many planes. Most fat lobules are continuous with other fat lobules within a broad sheet of fatty tissue that is continuous with either retromammary or premammary fat. Thus, images obtained in a short-axis plane through the fat lobule may show a nodular appearance, but images obtained in an orthogonal long-axis plane may show a sheet of tissue continuous with either the premammary or retromammary zone (Fig. 4–35). Second, fat lobules are the most compressible structures in the breast. Split-screen images with and without compression in which the AP dimension of a fat lobule is measured often show compressibility of 30% or more (Fig. 4–36). Although some fibroadenomas and a few carcinomas may be partially compressible, neither is as compressible as are fat lobules. Thus, compressibility of 30% or more is strong evidence that the structure is fatty, either a fat lobule or lipoma, both definitively benign. The effect of compression on adjacent structures

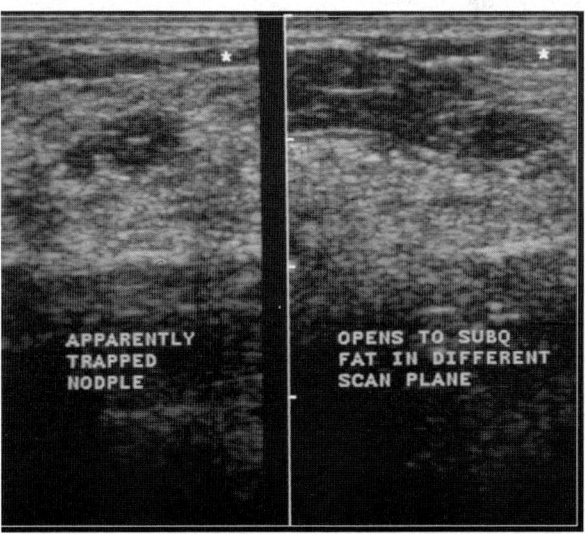

FIGURE 4–35 The first technique for distinguishing entrapped fat lobules from pathologic solid nodules is to scan in orthogonal planes. Most fat lobules that appear to be completely surrounded by echogenic fibrous tissue in one plane (**left**) actually communicate with either premammary or retromammary fat in the orthogonal view (**right**).

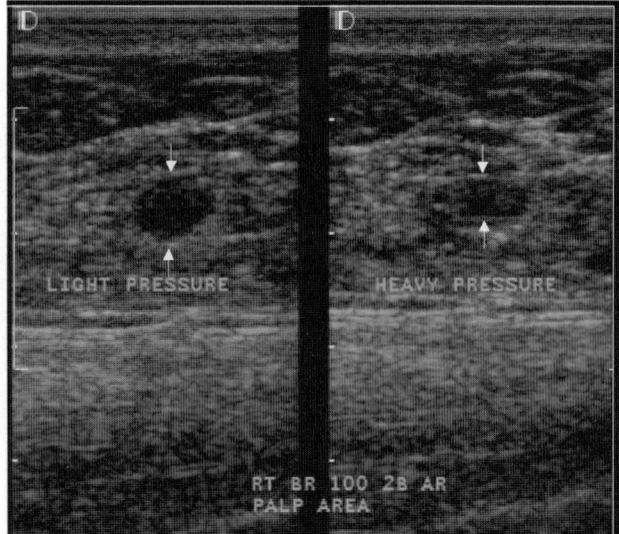

FIGURE 4–36 Split-screen images of the entrapped fat lobule show it to be more than 50% compressible, indicating that it is composed of fat and is either a fat lobule or a lipoma, not a fibroadenoma or carcinoma. Some fibroadenomas compress as much as 15% to 25%, but we have not seen fibroadenomas that compress more than 30%. We have not seen malignant nodules that compress more than 15%. This is the entrapped fat lobule shown in the image at the **right.**

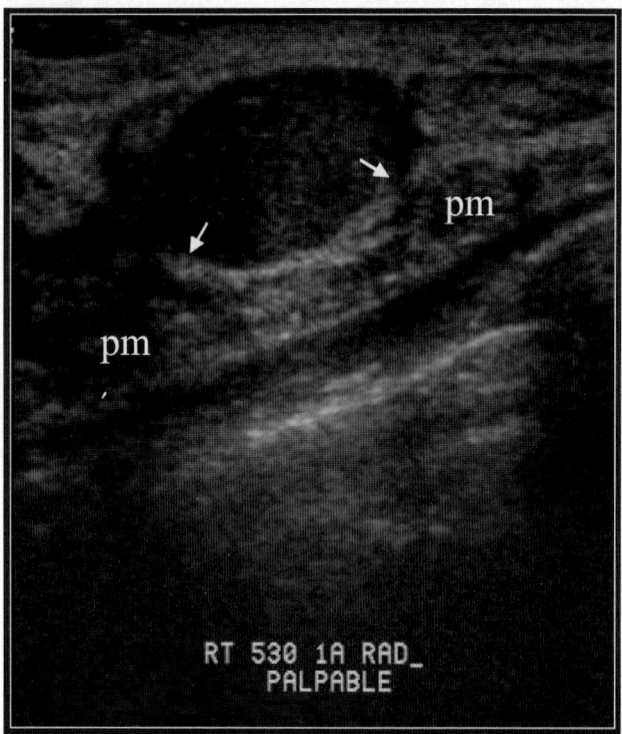

FIGURE 4–37 Another technique for distinguishing entrapped fat lobules from solid nodules such as this fibroadenoma is to observe the effects of compression on adjacent structures. Note that this lesion indents *(arrows)* the pectoralis muscle *(pm)* during compression, indicating that it is firmer than the muscle. Fat lobules are softer than muscle and will not indent the muscle during compression.

can also be evaluated. Because fat lobules are softer than surrounding chest wall, fibrous, or glandular elements, fat lobules will not indent these structures when compressed with the transducer. True solid nodules such as fibroadenomas and carcinomas, however, will frequently indent adjacent structures such as the pectoralis muscle (Fig. 4–37). Finally, most fat lobules are subdivided into smaller fat lobules by fibrous septa that appear sonographically as thin, straight echogenic lines bisecting the fat lobule horizontally (Fig. 4–38). Slight adjustments of the transducer position, scan angle, and degree of compression may be necessary to demonstrate optimally this thin, echogenic septation. In the absence of transducer compression forces, the septations can be too curved to be well demonstrated. However, when compressed with the transducer, these septations are pushed into a plane perpendicular to the ultrasound beam and parallel to the transducer face, creating a straight, well-circumscribed, thin, echogenic line through the center of the fat lobule (Fig. 4–39). Fibroadenomas occasionally have sonographically demonstrable internal fibrous septations that simulate the septations within fat lobules and that have been documented in the magnetic resonance imaging literature (Fig. 4–40). Such straight echogenic lines are not seen in carcinomas in the absence of core needle biopsy tract. An echogenic "vapor trail" of microbubbles may be seen through a solid nodule in the needle tract immedi-

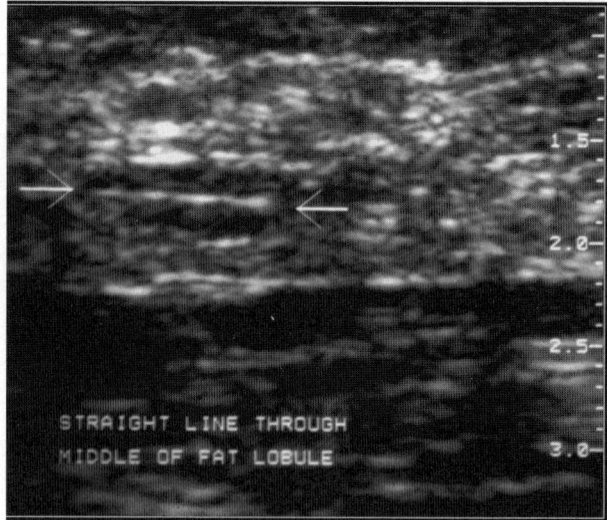

FIGURE 4–38 The final technique for distinguishing entrapped fat lobules from solid breast nodules is to look for the fibrous septation that subdivides fat lobules into smaller fat lobules. This gently curved septum is usually not well seen during routine scanning because its gentle curvature makes a poor specular reflector. However, during compression, it is pushed flat and into a horizontal plane perpendicular to the beam, making it a good specular reflector. We have never seen such a structure in malignant nodules. However, occasionally a septum may be seen within fibroadenomas. The nonenhancing septum is a well-established magnetic resonance imaging finding of fibroadenoma.

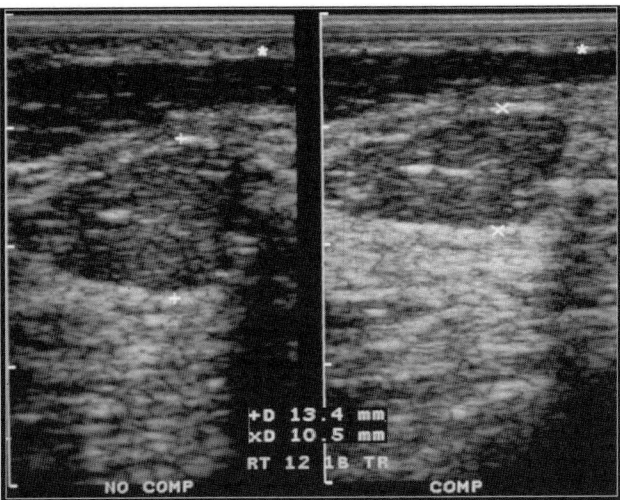

FIGURE 4–39 Note that the subdividing septation through this fat lobule is much better seen during compression (**right**) than it is when compression is not used (**left**). When not compressed, the septum is too curved to create a strong specular reflector. When compressed, it is straightened and forced into a horizontal plane that is more nearly perpendicular to the beam and thus better demonstrated.

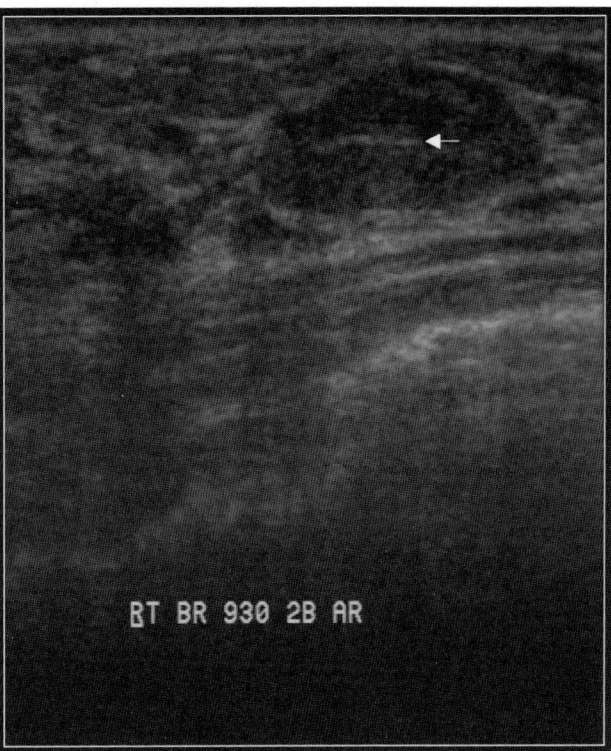

FIGURE 4–40 These split-screen images show a fibroadenoma that has an internal septum *(arrow)*, the same septum that has been described as the nonenhancing septum in the breast magnetic resonance imaging literature. This could make the fibroadenoma difficult to distinguish from a fat lobule, but it would be less compressible.

ately after core needle biopsy but is one-dimensional (1-D), linear, and only as wide as the needle (Fig. 4–41). A septation through a fat lobule, on the other hand, is a two-dimensional sheet of fibrous tissue nearly as wide as the fat lobule.

Once one is certain that the structure of interest is not a fat lobule, but a true nodule or mass, evaluation of its morphology becomes important. Characterization of these morphologic characteristics is discussed in detail in Chapter 12.

Sonography not only can distinguish general types of tissue from each other (i.e., fatty from fibrous from glandular) but also can identify individual mammary ducts in most patients and individual TDLUs in some patients. Mammary ducts and TDLUs are more sonographically apparent when surrounded by hyperechoic interlobular stromal fibrous tissue.

Ducts are hypoechoic to isoechoic linear structures extending out from the nipple radially like the spokes of a wheel from its hub. The central ducts have a vertical course anteriorly to posteriorly immediately deep to the nipple (without special compression maneuvers), but gradually curve into a more horizontal course farther from the nipple (Fig. 4–42). Several orders of branching ducts can be demonstrated (Fig. 4–43). The sonographic appearance of mammary ducts is highly variable, depending on the amount of loose periductal stromal fibrous tissue surrounding the duct, the degree of distention of the duct lumen by secretions, and the echogenicity of the secretions. Peripheral ducts may appear to be several millimeters in diameter, which is larger than the actual size of the peripheral

mammary ducts at pathology. The apparent larger sonographic size of ducts is a manifestation of the isoechoic appearance of the looser fibroelastic periductal stroma surrounding the duct. As noted earlier, this stromal fibrous tissue differs from hyperechoic tissue because it contains more hypoechoic hyaluronic acid and less echogenic collagen than does dense, hyperechoic interlobular stromal fibrous tissue. The looser tissue exists around ducts to enable them to distend greatly during lactation and letdown. Were the ducts surrounded tightly by dense interlobular stroma fibrous tissue, they would be relatively nondistensible. Under ideal circumstances, the duct wall may be seen as a thin, echogenic line down the center of the more isoechoic periductal elastic tissue on long-axis views and as a small, central circular or linear target-like echo on short-axis views in patients who do not have ductal ectasia (Fig. 4–44).

The lumen of a mammary duct may be collapsed or distended to various degrees by secretions. Dilation of ducts is common and is virtually a variant of normal, affecting up to 50% of women older than 50 years of age. However, the term *duct ectasia* describes not only the physical appearance of the dilated, fluid-filled duct but also a

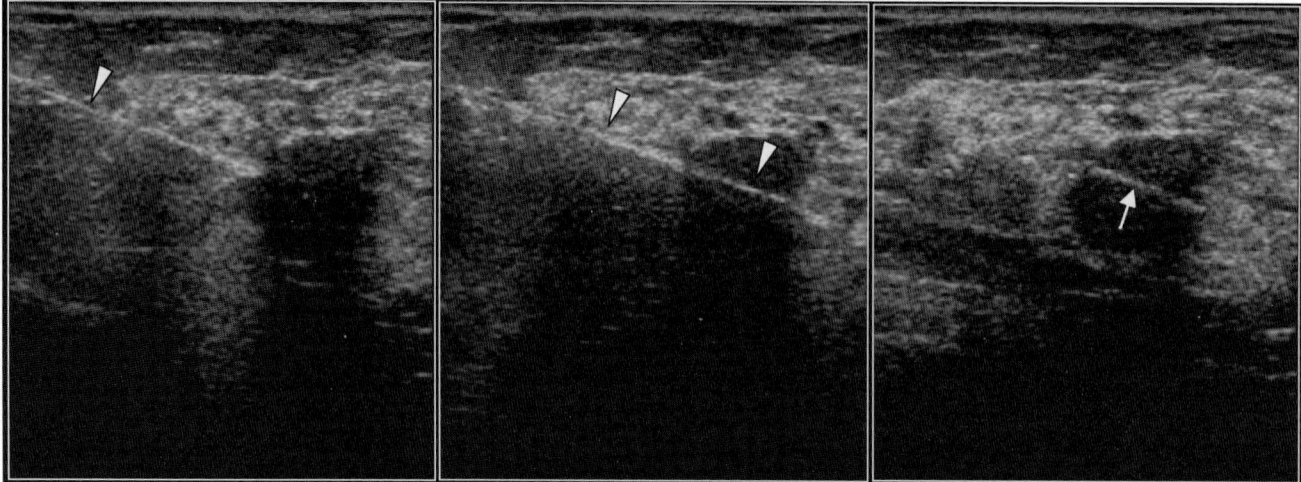

FIGURE 4–41 This malignant nodule is shown before core biopsy **(left)**, after firing with needle passing through the lesion **(middle)**, and after removal of the needle **(right)**. Note the persistent thin, echogenic line *(arrows)* marking the tract through which the core needle passed. This is the echogenic "vapor trail" of microbubbles created by passage of the needle through the lesion. The vapor trail is temporary, existing only a few minutes, but is useful in documenting that the needle actually passed through the lesion. It is punctate in short axis, indicating that it is a 2-D line rather than a 3-D sheet, as is the fibrous septation through fat lobules and occasional fibroadenomas *(arrowheads* indicate needle).

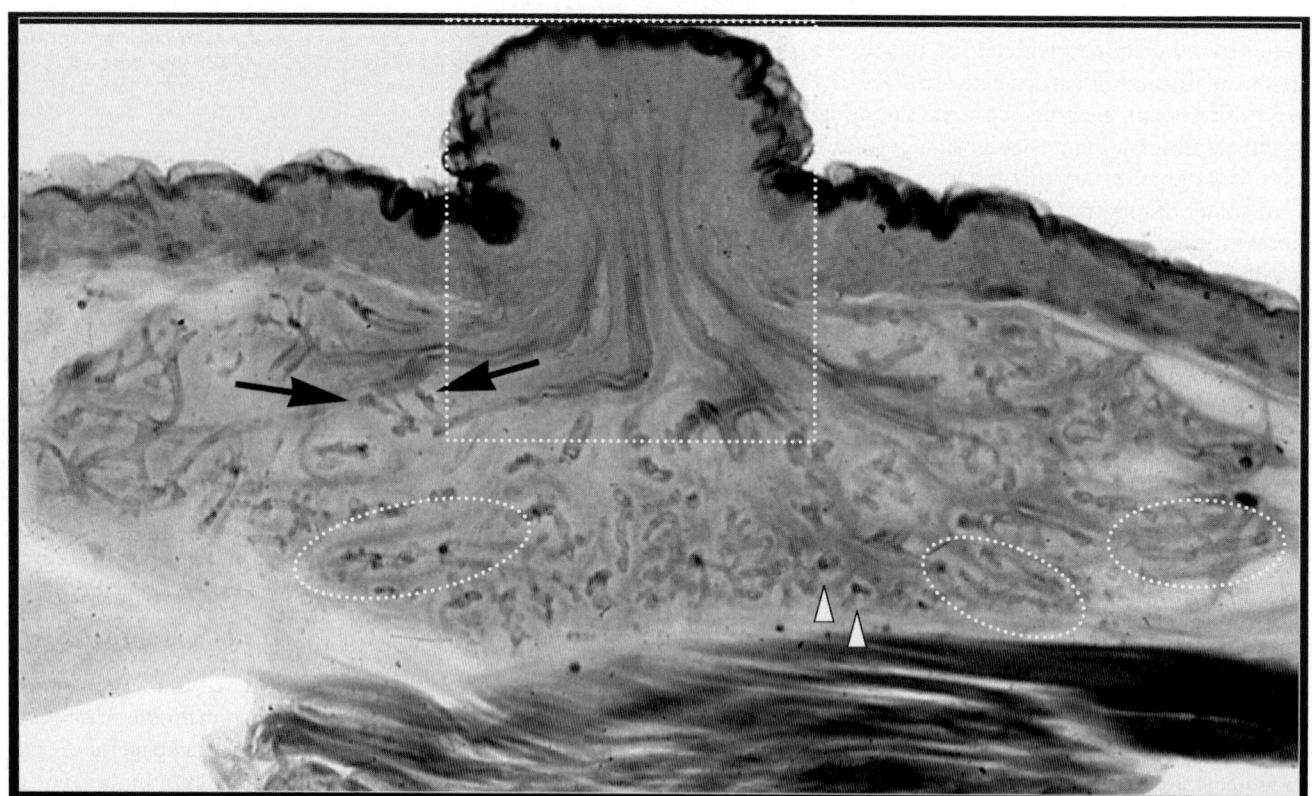

FIGURE 4–42 This subgross pathologic specimen shows that the ducts within the nipple and within the immediate subareolar region of the breast are oriented nearly perpendicular to the skin and parallel to the ultrasound beam when scanned from anteriorly *(white rectangle)*. Note that the periductal stromal tissue is lighter in color and less dense than is the interlobular dense stroma *(white oval* indicates parallel to long axis of duct; *white arrowheads* indicate perpendicular to long axis of duct). Note that the degree of duct dilation varies. Lobules only occasionally arise from main ducts within 5 cm of the distal orifice *(black arrows)*. (Courtesy of Hanne M. Jensen, MD, University of California at Davis.)

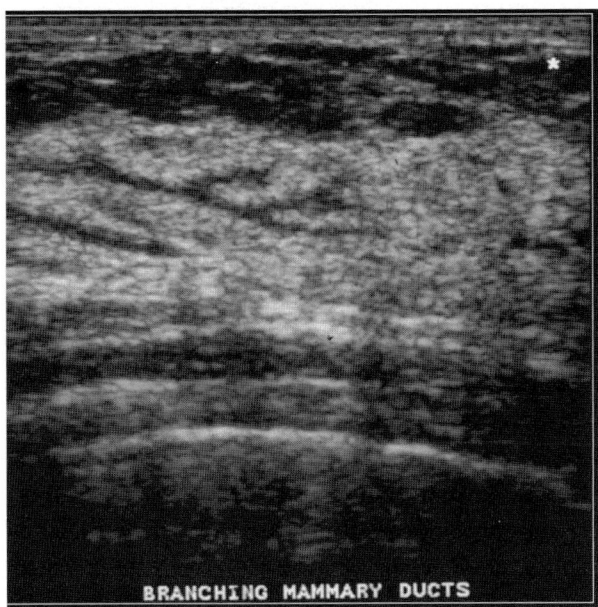

BRANCHING MAMMARY DUCTS

FIGURE 4–43 In this patient, several orders of mammary duct branches are visible within the background of hyperechoic fibrous tissue (nipple to left). Note that the ducts appear to be 2 to 3 mm in diameter, larger than their true size.

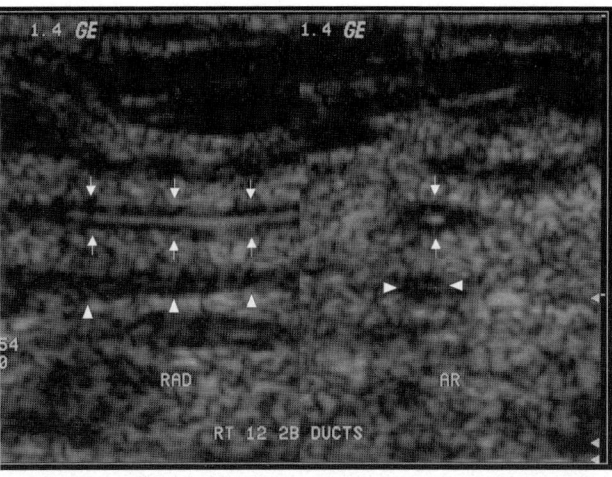

FIGURE 4–44 This split-screen image shows a nonectatic mammary duct and its enveloping periductal stroma *(arrows)* in its long axis (**left**) and short axis (**right**). A thin, echogenic line in the long axis and an echogenic dot in the short axis represent the collapsed duct, where the duct has a target-like appearance. Note that the duct that courses parallel and just deep *(arrowheads)* to the previously mentioned duct does not have a well-demonstrated central echo representing the duct. In the long-axis image, the central duct echo is poorly seen because the beam is slightly off-center and passes only through the periductal stromal tissue. In the short-axis image, the central duct echo of the more deeply located duct is not well seen because the beam does not intersect it at exactly 90 degrees. Thus, the periductal stromal fibrous tissue is much easier to demonstrate than is the central echo that represents the duct itself.

pathologic inflammatory condition of the duct and periductal tissues. This condition results in loss of duct wall elasticity and eventually progresses to intraductal and periductal fibrosis. Duct ectasia will be discussed in greater detail in Chapter 8.

In cases of mild duct ectasia, the duct wall may be seen as a thin, echogenic line between the fluid in the lumen of the duct and the surrounding isoechoic periductal elastic tissue (Figs. 4–45 and 4.46). As the degree of duct ectasia increases, the loose periductal stromal tissue becomes thinner. In cases of severe duct ectasia, the periductal loose stromal fibrous tissue becomes too compressed to be sonographically visible, and only the echogenic wall of the duct is seen. The number of ectatic ducts varies. Duct ectasia may involve only one duct or all of the ducts in the subareolar area. The echogenicity of the fluid within ectatic ducts varies, depending on the luminal contents. Chronic inspissated secretions and secretions containing large numbers of inflammatory or foam cells tend to be echogenic. When multiple ducts are ectatic, the degree of ectasia and echogenicity of secretions they contain can vary. Additionally, the degree of right-to-left asymmetry in the degree of ductal dilation can vary. In cases of severe chronic duct ectasia, intraductal and periductal fibrosis can result in obliteration of duct lumina by isoechoic tissue and can be accompanied by isoechoic periductal tissue as well. The variable appearances and complications are discussed and illustrated in greater detail in Chapters 8 and 11.

The anatomy of the ducts is best seen when the ducts are dilated. In areas of the breast other than the immediate

subareolar area, major lobar ducts tend to course through the posterior half of the mammary zone (Fig. 4–47). The ductal anatomy is the most consistently visualized anatomic structure in the breast, persisting even after all of the surrounding lobular and interlobular stromal fibrous elements have completely regressed, regardless of whether the ducts are ectatic (Fig. 4–48) or not (Fig. 4–49).

Demonstration of the mammary ducts is important in patients who present with nipple discharge and in patients who have sonographically demonstrable intraductal papillary lesions in the periareolar area. There is a widely held misconception that the nipple and areola do not transmit sound well and that the subareolar ducts are difficult or impossible to demonstrate, diminishing the role of ultrasound in such patients. We strongly disagree with that view. Although it is true that both the nipple and areola contain muscular fibers that, when contracted, can decrease sound transmission by making the nipple stand erect and by causing the areola to wrinkle, it is possible to use various techniques and maneuvers to minimize critical angle shadowing and maximize sonographic demonstration. Cold can stimulate muscular contraction within the nipple and areola; therefore, using warm jelly and scanning in a warm room are keys to minimizing muscular contraction. Additionally, the tissue planes within the nipple course in an AP direction, parallel to the long axis of the

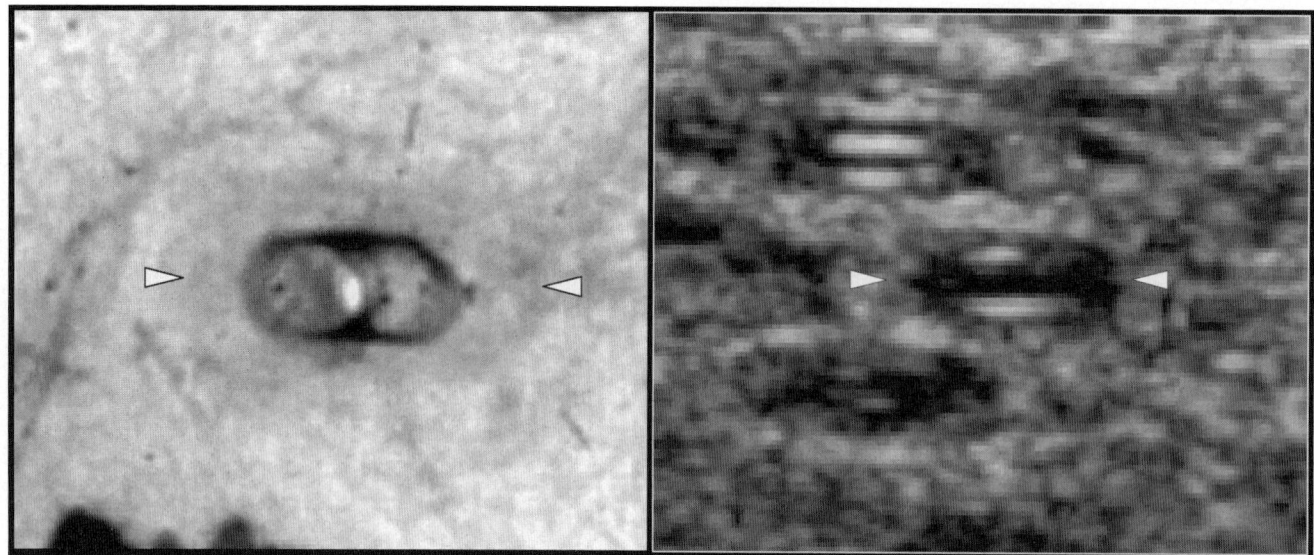

FIGURE 4–45 The **left** image is a short-axis slice through a mildly ectatic mammary duct, and the **right** image is a short-axis sonographic view through several ectatic mammary ducts. The middle duct on the sonogram *(arrowheads)* is dilated to a degree similar to the degree of ectasia on the histologic slice. The fluid-filled central lumen is clear on the histologic image and anechoic on the ultrasound. A thin, echogenic line represents the black duct wall on histology sonographically. The isoechoic tissue surrounding the ectatic duct on ultrasound represents the light gray periductal stromal fibroelastic tissue on histology (between arrowheads). Because of critical angle effects, only the anterior and posterior duct walls make bright specular reflectors on the short-axis ultrasound image. The lateral walls of the duct lie at angles of incidence that prevent them from being seen as echogenic lines. (Subgross histology courtesy of Hanne M. Jensen, MD, University of California at Davis.)

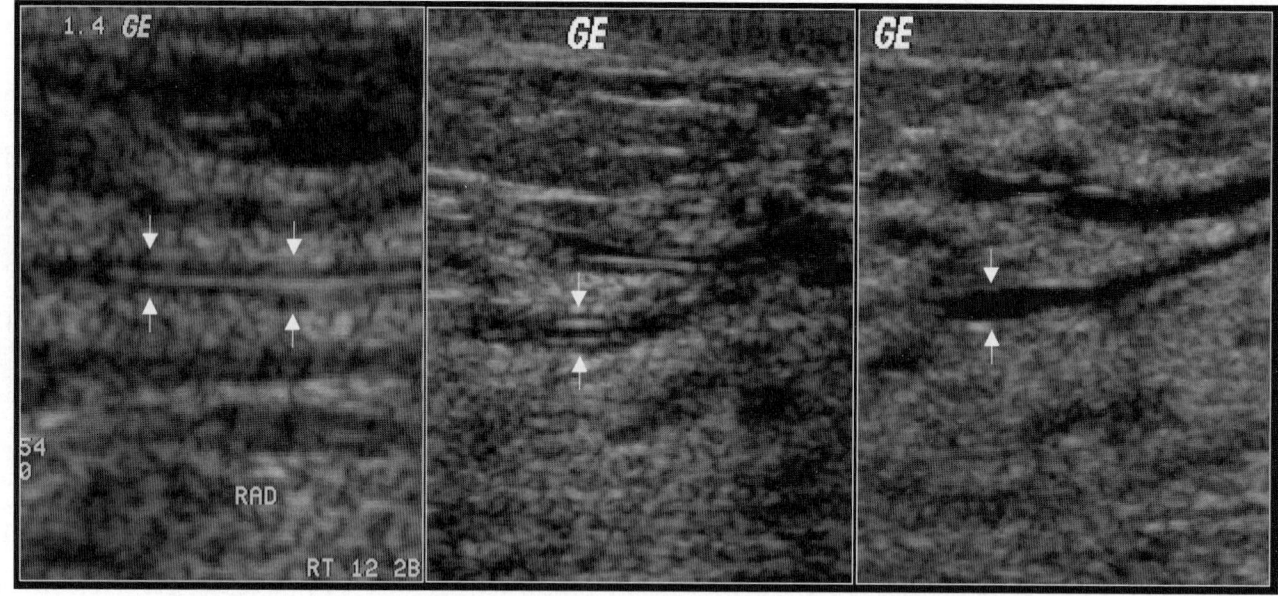

FIGURE 4–46 A: The sonographic appearance of mammary ducts varies with the degree of ductal dilation or duct ectasia. These three images show long-axis views of mammary ducts. The **left** image shows a duct that is not ectatic *(arrows)*. The collapsed lumen and two duct walls appear as a single echogenic line within the center of the isoechoic periductal stromal fibroelastic tissue. The **middle** image shows two mildly ectatic ducts *(arrows)*, with a small amount of anechoic fluid within the center of the duct. The anterior and posterior duct walls are now separated enough that they appear as separate echogenic lines surrounding the anechoic fluid-filled lumen. Note that the thickness of the isoechoic loose periductal stromal fibroelastic tissue in the **middle** image is less than it is in the **left** image because it has been compressed by the mildly ectatic duct. The **right** image shows a duct that is more severely ectatic *(arrows)*. The lumen has expanded enough that the periductal stroma is completely compressed and is no longer sonographically visible. The duct is represented by anechoic fluid in the lumen and thin, echogenic lines representing the anterior and posterior duct walls.

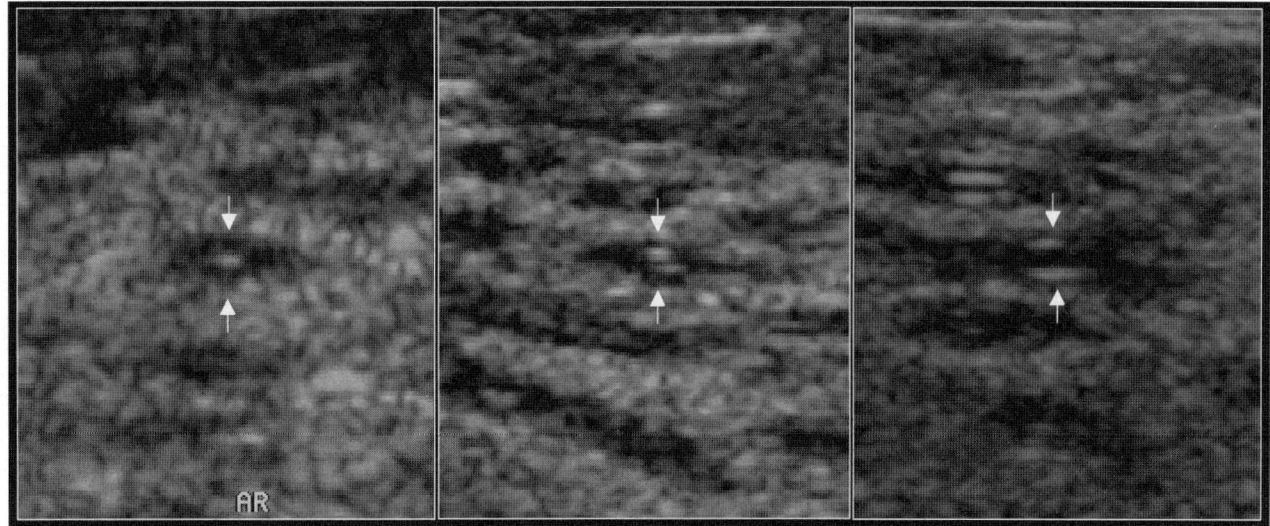

B

FIGURE 4–46 *(continued)* **B:** The sonographic appearance of mammary ducts varies with the degree of ductal dilation or ectasia. These three images show short-axis views of the same three ducts shown in part **A.** The **left** image shows a nonectatic duct in short axis *(arrows)*. A single central echo surrounded by a thick isoechoic band of loose periductal stromal fibroelastic tissue represents the collapsed duct. The **middle** image shows a mildly ectatic duct *(arrows)* in short axis. The anterior and posterior duct walls are separated by a small amount of fluid and are represented by separate thin, hyperechoic lines. The periductal stroma is compressed and thinned slightly by the mildly ectatic duct. The **right** image shows a more severely ectatic duct *(arrows)*. The anechoic fluid in the lumen more widely separates the echogenic lines representing the anterior and posterior duct walls, and the thickness of the periductal stroma is decreased further because it is being compressed by the ectatic duct. Note that only the anterior and posterior duct walls lie nearly perpendicular to the beam and make bright specular reflectors. The curving lateral walls lie nearly parallel to the beam and are well demonstrated sonographically.

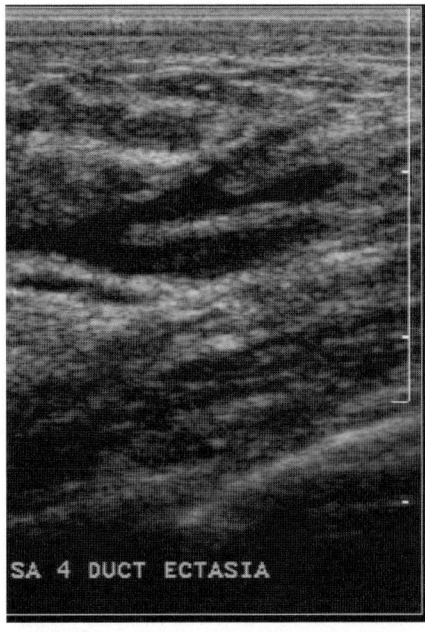

FIGURE 4–47 Duct anatomy is best seen in ectatic ducts. Most lobar ducts lie in the posterior half of the mammary zone, as did this one.

nipple. The tissue planes are parallel to the ultrasound beam and therefore poorly demonstrated sonographically when scanned from straight anteriorly. However, no structure, in any part of the body, will be well demonstrated when its long axis lies parallel to the ultrasound beam. Structures form strong specular reflectors and are best shown when scanned so that the ultrasound beam is perpendicular to their long axes. The challenge in demonstrating the subareolar and intranipple ducts, therefore, is simply to maneuver the subareolar and intranipple ducts into scan planes that are more nearly perpendicular to the ultrasound beam. To accomplish this, we have developed several maneuvers. Scanning from straight anteriorly may result in acoustic shadowing and obscuration of the intranipple and subareolar ducts (Fig. 4–50). The peripheral compression technique improves the angle of incidence with the subareolar ducts and can demonstrate parts of the subareolar duct that were obscured by shadows when scanned from straight anteriorly (Fig. 4–51). The two-handed compression technique is designed to better demonstrate the duct from the lateral edge of the areola to the point at which the duct enters the base of the nipple and to assess compressibility of echogenic contents within the

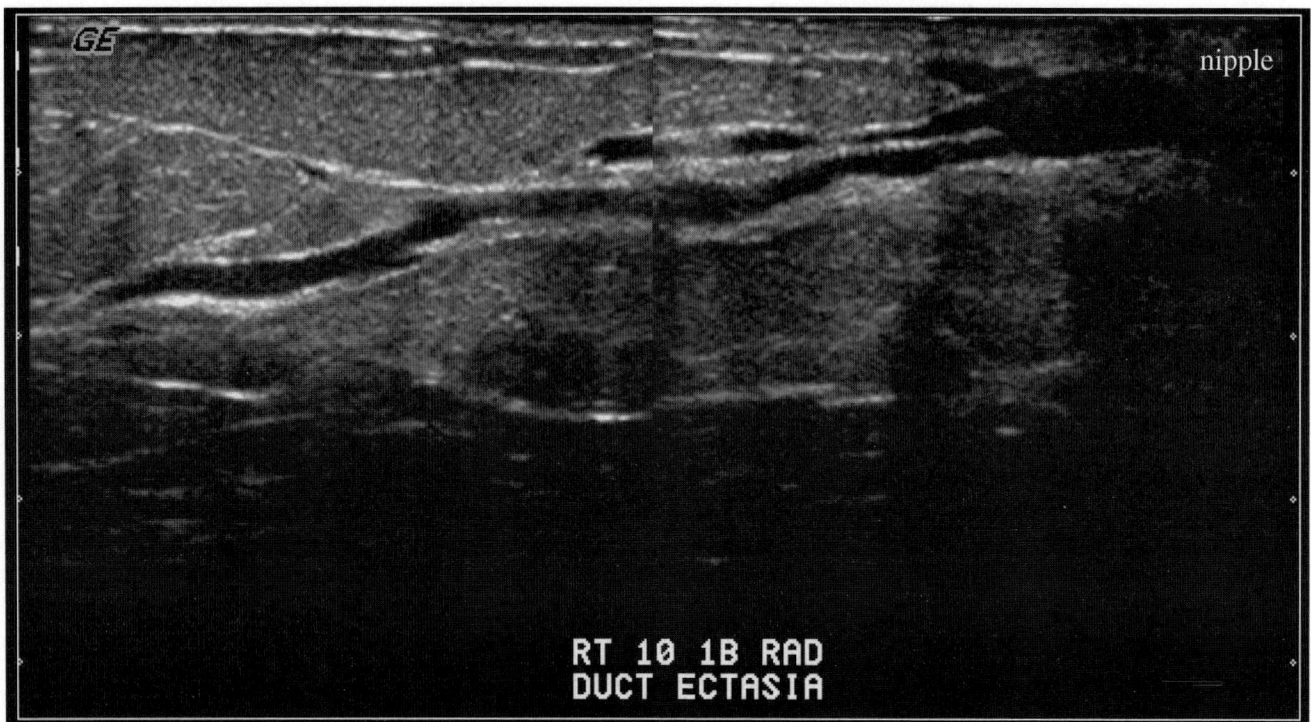

FIGURE 4–48 Mammary ducts are the most consistently demonstrable structures in the breast after fat lobules and Cooper's ligaments. Even when all of the hyperechoic stromal fibrous elements and all of the isoechoic lobular elements have atrophied, residual ducts may be visible in the breast. In this patient with complete fatty involution of fibrous and glandular elements, a prominent ectatic duct is seen extending into the upper outer quadrant of the right breast.

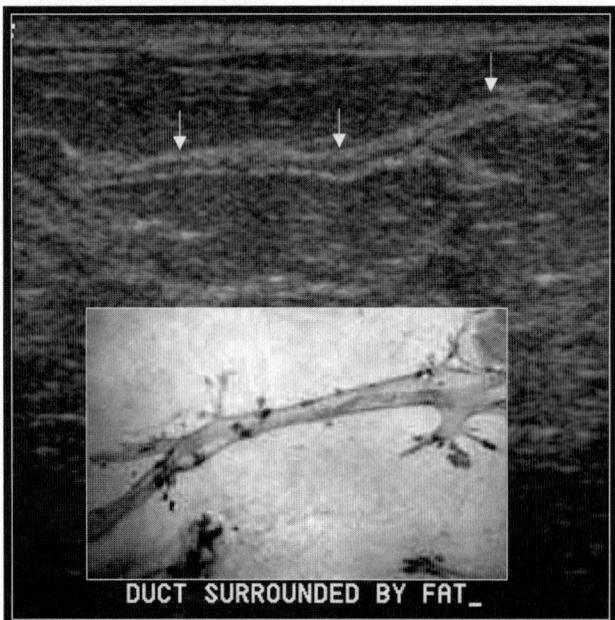

FIGURE 4–49 Even nonectatic ducts *(arrows)* may persist in breasts where the fibrous and lobular elements have been completely replaced by fat. (Histology image courtesy of Hanne Jensen, MD, University of California at Davis.)

duct lumen, facilitating distinction between echogenic secretions and solid intraductal papillary lesions (Fig. 4–52). The two-handed compression maneuver, however, usually does not demonstrate the duct within the nipple well. To best demonstrate the portion of the mammary duct within the nipple, we employ the rolled-nipple technique (Fig. 4–53). The rolled-nipple technique works best with a 1.5-dimensional (1.5-D) array transducer that can electronically focus closer to the skin in the short axis because it causes less volume averaging than a 1-D transducer that is focused more deeply.

Demonstrating the entire duct is critical when evaluating patients with nipple discharge or intraductal papillary lesions because an intraductal papillary lesion can lie anywhere along the course of the duct and its location is generally not predictable. Involvement of the nipple affects the method of biopsy and treatment used. Lesions that lie within the nipple are not accessible to ultrasound-guided core needle biopsy or ultrasound-guided mammotomy and require surgical biopsy and extirpation. On the other hand, if the nipple is spared and the papillary lesion is isolated to the subareolar ducts, the lesion can undergo ultrasound-guided mammotomy. Papillary lesions can involve the

(text continued on page 89)

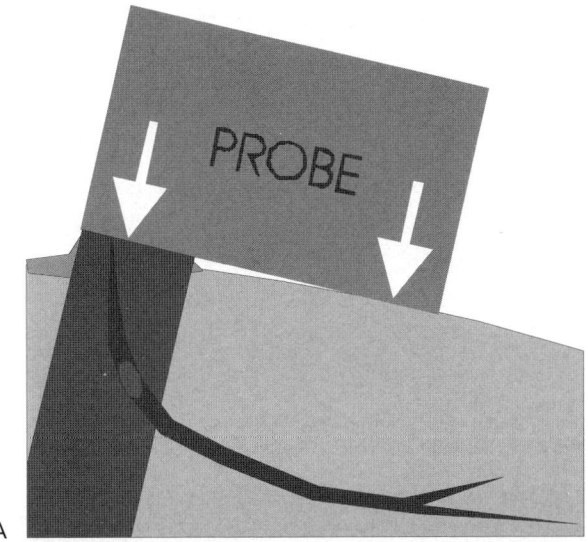

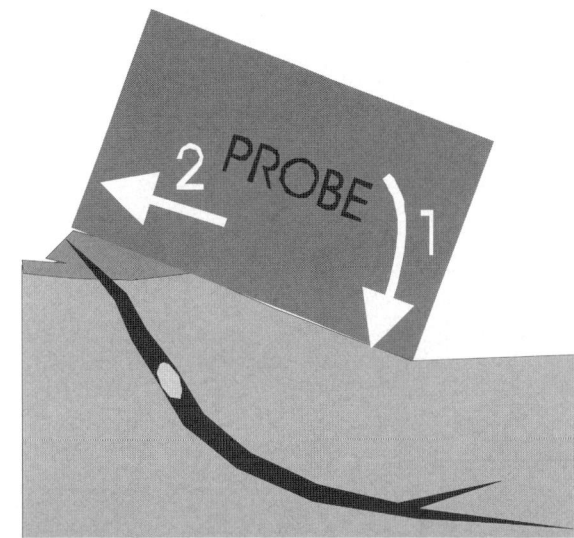

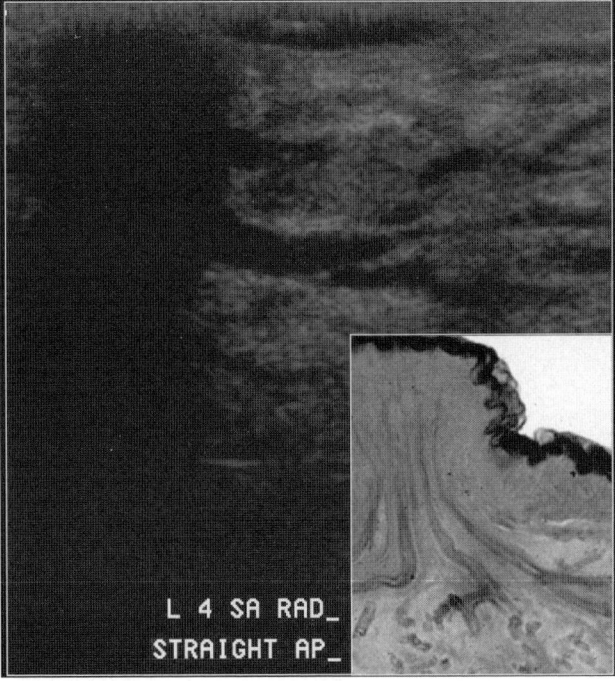

FIGURE 4–50 A: For several reasons, the ductal system within the nipple and immediate subareolar area may be difficult to demonstrate and may be completely obscured by acoustic shadowing in some cases. First, the tissue planes within the nipple and the ducts in the subareolar area lie more nearly parallel to the beam rather than perpendicular to it; they make poor specular reflectors. Wrinkles caused by contraction of muscular fibers in the areola may cause it to wrinkle, creating critical angle shadowing. The nipple may absorb and refract sound in some patients. It is important to demonstrate the entire ductal system when sonographically evaluating patients who present with nipple discharge or who have proven intraductal papillary lesions. Thus, it is important to develop techniques for demonstrating the entire ductal system, including the portions of the duct within the nipple and immediate subareolar area. **B:** A scan from a straight anterior approach in this patient failed to demonstrate the intranipple and subareolar ducts because of shadowing arising from the nipple. The sonographic evaluation for nipple discharge using the anterior approach is incomplete because about the last 1.5 cm of the distal duct cannot be evaluated using this approach. (Subgross histology courtesy of Hanne M. Jensen, MD, University of California at Davis.)

FIGURE 4–51 A: One way to improve visualization of the subareolar portion of the duct is to alter the angle of incidence of the beam with the steeply obliquely oriented duct. This can be accomplished with the peripheral compression technique. This technique is begun with the transducer oriented radially, paralleling the visualized duct's long axis. Compression is then applied to only the peripheral end of the transducer, forcing it into a plane more nearly parallel to the subareolar duct. Finally, the probe is slid centrally, pushing the nipple over onto its side. **B:** This is the same duct shown in Fig. 4.50 as it is being scanned with the peripheral compression technique. Note that the subareolar portion of the duct as far centrally as the edge the nipple is better demonstrated than it was with the straight anterior scan technique. However, the portions of the duct immediately deep to the nipple and within the nipple are still obscured by shadowing arising from the nipple. (Subgross histology courtesy of Hanne M. Jensen, MD, University of California at Davis.)

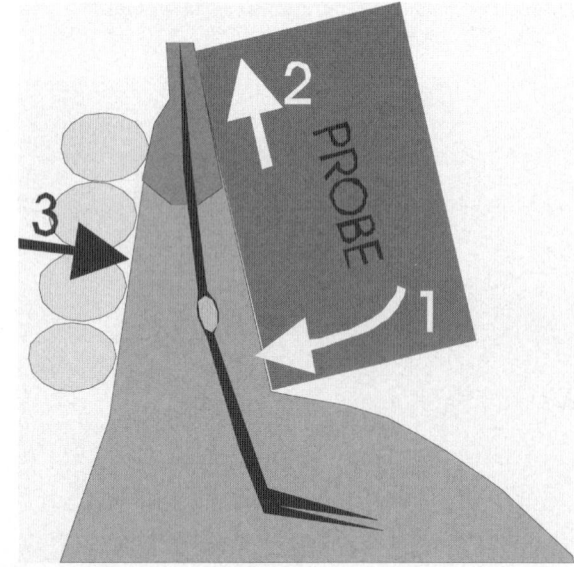

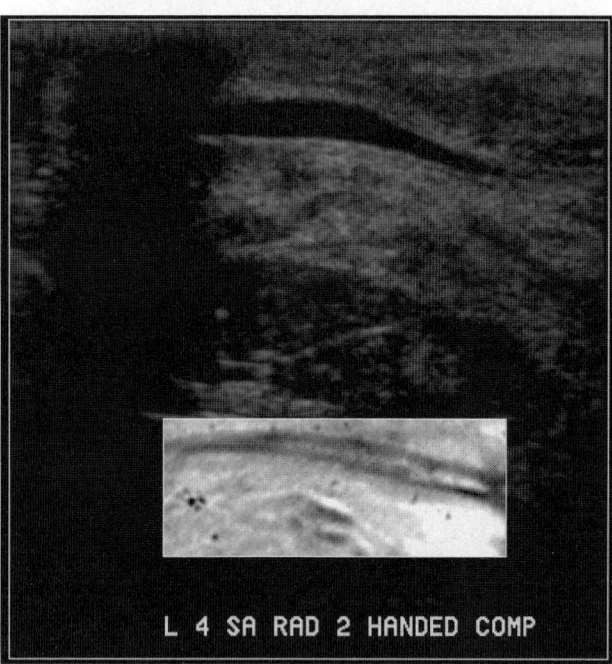

A

B

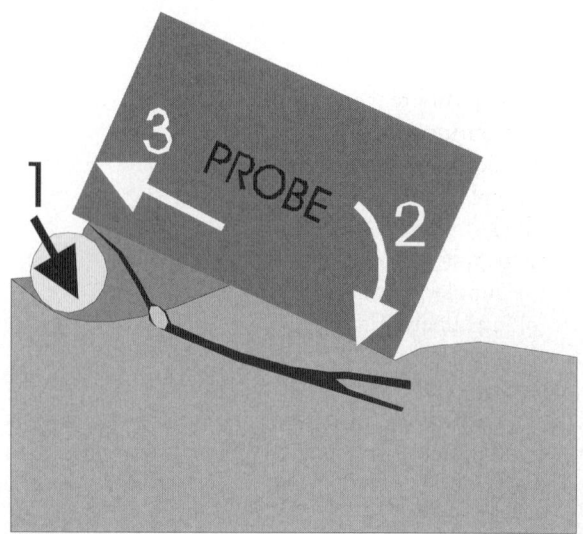

A

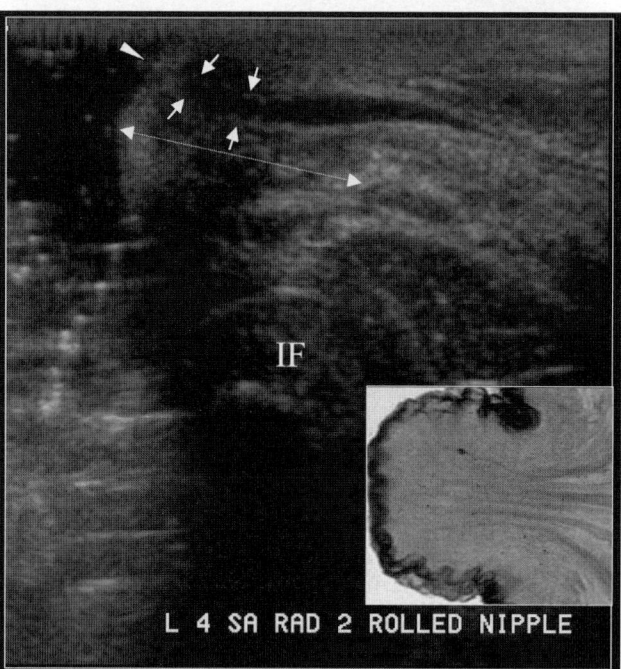

IF

B

FIGURE 4–52 A: This figure illustrates performance of the two-handed compression technique. This technique is begun with the transducer oriented radially along the long axis of the duct being visualized. The portion of breast through which the duct of interest courses is then compressed between the nonscanning hand and the transducer while the transducer is slid distally to include the nipple. This places nearly the entire length of the subareolar portion of the duct parallel to the transducer and perpendicular to the beam. This maneuver also compresses the duct, which is beneficial in patients who have echogenic secretions that could obscure an intraductal papillary lesion that is producing the secretions. Intraductal papillary lesions are less compressible than echogenic secretions and cause a focal bulge within the duct when the duct is compressed. **B:** This is the same duct shown in Figs. 4–50B and 4–51B. Note that the duct is now nearly parallel to the transducer face and perpendicular to the beam throughout the field of view. The hyperechoic duct wall and anechoic fluid within the lumen of the duct are well demonstrated. The compressed duct is also smaller in diameter than it was with the anteroposterior and peripheral compression scanning techniques. Note, however, that the portion of the duct within the nipple is still not well seen. (Subgross histology courtesy of Hanne M. Jensen, MD, University of California Davis.)

FIGURE 4–53 A: This figure illustrates the rolled-nipple technique. The technique is begun with the transducer placed at the edge of the nipple in a radial plane parallel to the long axis of the duct of interest. The index finger of the nonscanning hand is placed on the opposite side of the nipple from the transducer. The transducer is then slid distally on the nipple, forcing it onto its side, while the index finger opposite the transducer is depressed into the areolar tissue and under the nipple. Essentially, the transducer is used to "roll" the nipple onto its side over the index finger. The compression pressure used is light rather than heavy in order to prevent collapse of the intranipple ducts and to minimize near-field volume averaging problems. The 1.5-D array transducers offer a distinct advantage in minimizing the adverse effects of near-field volume averaging when using this technique. It is also necessary to have a foot pedal for freezing the image because the technique requires the use of both hands. **B:** This image demonstrates the rolled-nipple technique for viewing the ducts within the nipple. Note the nonscanning index finger deep to the nipple *(IF)*. The duct *(arrows)* is now well demonstrated through the nipple *(double-headed dotted arrow)* to the duct orifice on the surface of the nipple *(arrowhead)*. Demonstration of the entire nipple is necessary to exclude intraductal papillary lesions that (a) lie entirely within the nipple, (b) are long and extend into the nipple from the subareolar ducts, or (c) are multiple, one in the nipple and additional lesions more deeply within the same duct. (Subgross histology courtesy of Hanne M. Jensen, MD, University of California at Davis.)

nipple in three different ways. First, the entire lesion may lie within the nipple and can be missed unless the rolled-nipple technique is used. Second, a long lesion may extend into the nipple from its site of origin in the subareolar ducts. Finally, a single ductal system may contain more than one papillary lesion. Thus, there can be a lesion within the nipple as well as within the subareolar ducts. Sonographic evaluation of nipple discharge and intraductal papillary lesions is discussed in much greater detail in Chapter 8.

TDLUs are visible in a smaller percentage of patients than are the mammary ducts. The TDLU consists of the lobule and the extralobular terminal duct and is the functional unit of the breast and the site of origin of most breast pathology. Within the lobule lie the intralobular terminal duct, the ductules, and the intralobular stromal fibrous tissue (Fig. 4–3). All three components of the lobule are normally isoechoic and indistinguishable from each other. The extralobular terminal duct is also isoechoic. Thus, normal TDLUs are homogeneously isoechoic structures than have no sonographically identifiable internal structure and are shaped like tennis or badminton rackets, with the handles representing the extralobular terminal duct and the head representing the lobule (Fig. 4–54). Only when the ductules become cystically dilated and the intralobular stromal fibrous tissue becomes fibrotic or sclerotic and abnormally echogenic are we able to identify internal structure within the TDLU. Because the TDLUs are nearly isoechoic with fat, they generally are visible only in a background of

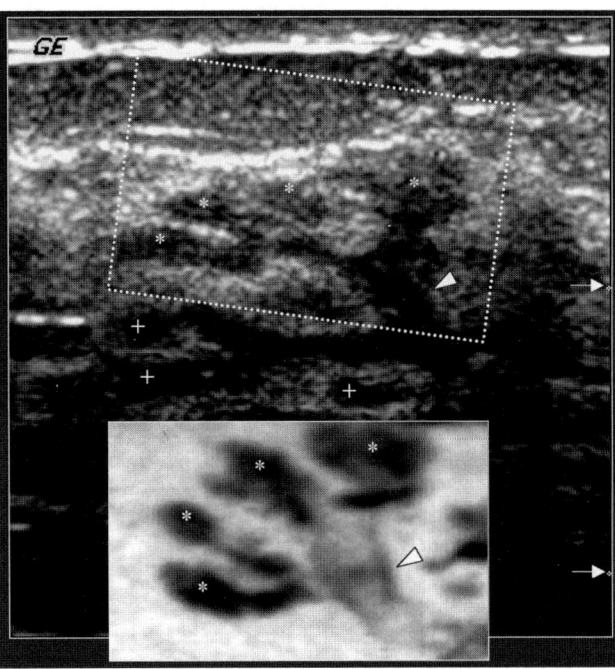

FIGURE 4–55 This sonogram shows mildly enlarged distal ducts *(arrowheads)* and lobules *(*)* of a breast lobe. Other lobules are visible *(+)*. Note the 1-cm marker along the right side of the image *(thin arrows)*. These sonographically visible lobules are about 2 mm wide. The hyperechogenicity of the background interlobular stromal fibrous tissue makes the isoechoic terminal ductolobular units more apparent. (Subgross histology courtesy of Hanne M. Jensen, MD, University of California at Davis.)

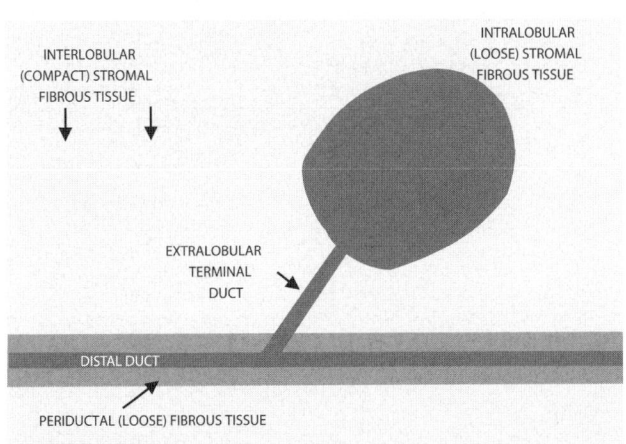

FIGURE 4–54 Although current ultrasound equipment with high-frequency near-field transducers can resolve the lobule as an isoechoic structure when it is surrounded by contrasting hyperechoic interlobular stromal fibrous tissue, these machines are not able to distinguish intralobular structures from each other unless the lobule has undergone cystic change. The epithelial and myoepithelial elements within the walls of ductules and the intralobular terminal duct and the loose intralobular stroma fibrous tissue are all equally isoechoic and sonographically indistinguishable from each other. The extralobular terminal duct also appears isoechoic. Thus, the sonographic appearance of the terminal ductolobular unit is that of a tennis racket–shaped isoechoic structure that is homogeneously gray in texture.

echogenic fibrous tissue (Fig. 4–55). However, occasionally even fat-surrounded TDLUs can be demonstrated sonographically (Figs. 4–56 and 4–57).

The length of the extralobular terminal duct varies, depending mainly on the position of the lobule relative to the major lobar duct. As a general rule, TDLUs that lie anterior to the main lobar ducts tend to have longer extralobular terminal ducts than do those located posteriorly (Fig. 4–56). However, the relative length of the terminal duct can vary from quite short (Fig. 4–58) to markedly elongated (Fig. 4–59) even for anterior TDLUs. The reason that anterior TDLUs are usually longer than posterior TDLUs is uncertain. The greater length of anterior TDLUs is probably at least partially responsible for many small cancers having a greater AP dimension than transverse dimension (i.e., being taller than wide, which is discussed in Chapter 12). Most TDLUs lie within the mammary zone, but some TDLUs extend into Cooper's ligaments where the ligament intersects the mammary zone (Fig. 4–60). Other intraligamentary TDLUs are stranded in the ligament as surrounding tissues atrophy. Most intraligamentary TDLUs are atrophic and therefore are usually not sonographically visible unless enlarged by fibrocystic change (Fig. 4–61), benign proliferative disorders (Fig. 4–62), or neoplasm (Fig. 4–63). Lesions that

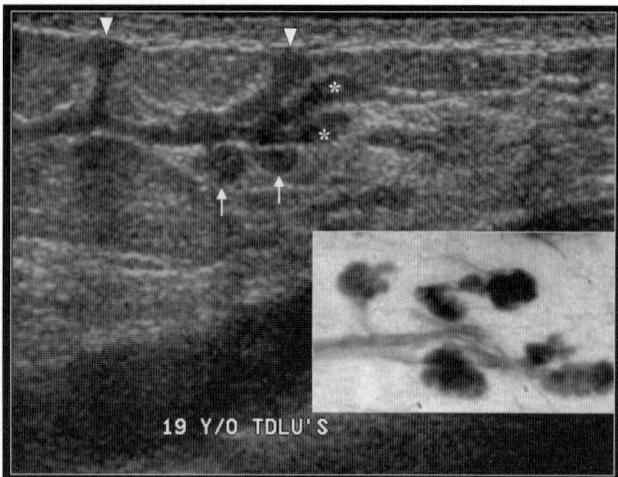

FIGURE 4–56 This patient is an example of the exception to the rule that terminal ductolobular units (TDLUs) are seldom demonstrable when surrounded by fat of equal echogenicity. There are several sonographically demonstrable TDLUs. The long axis of the anterior and posterior lobules is oriented in the anteroposterior (AP) axis. Note that the anterior TDLUs *(arrowheads)* have long, extralobular terminal ducts, and are thus "taller" than posterior lobules *(arrows)*. Note also that some of the lobules are terminal lobules *(*)* that lie at the end of the duct. Terminal lobules lie in a horizontal plane and are wider than tall. Most breast cancer arises within the lobule, and the shape of the lobule in which the cancer arises affects the shape of the cancer early in its course. The effect of lobular shape on the shape of cancers is discussed in greater detail in Chapter 12. (Subgross histology courtesy of Hanne M. Jensen, MD, University of California at Davis.)

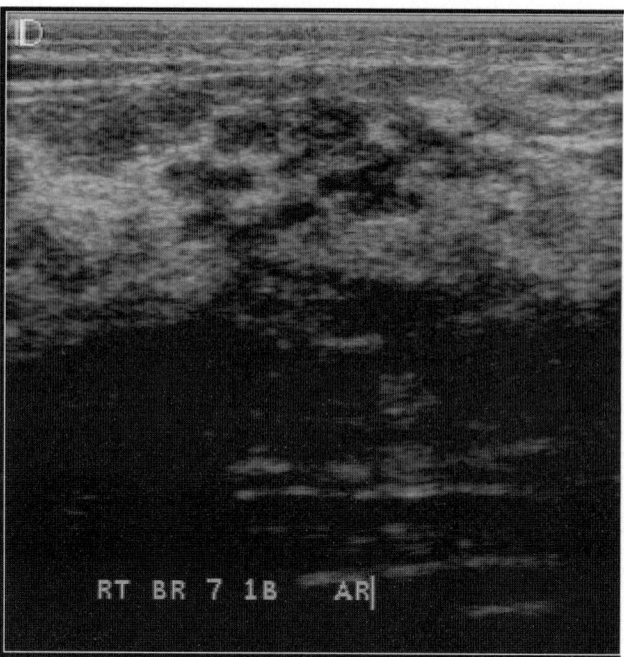

FIGURE 4–58 The shape of terminal ductolobular units (TDLUs) varies greatly from patient to patient, from breast to breast, and even within different parts of the same breast. Some TDLUs have short, extralobular terminal ducts and thus have a rounded appearance.

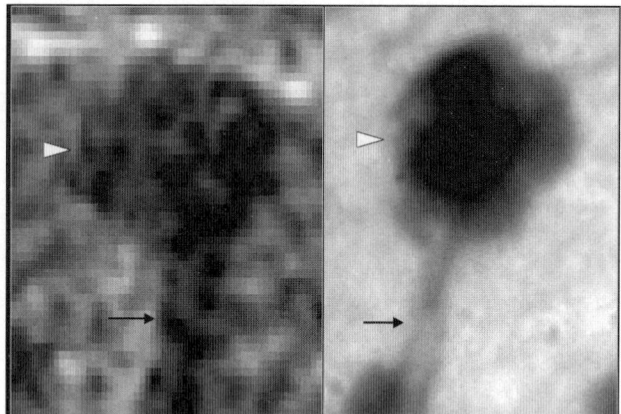

FIGURE 4–57 The left anterior terminal ductolobular unit shown in Fig. 4–56 is magnified in the **left** image and compared to a 3-D histopathologic image of a lobule on the **right** *(arrow* indicates extralobular terminal duct; *arrowheads* indicate lobule). (Subgross histology courtesy of Hanne M. Jensen, MD, University of California at Davis.)

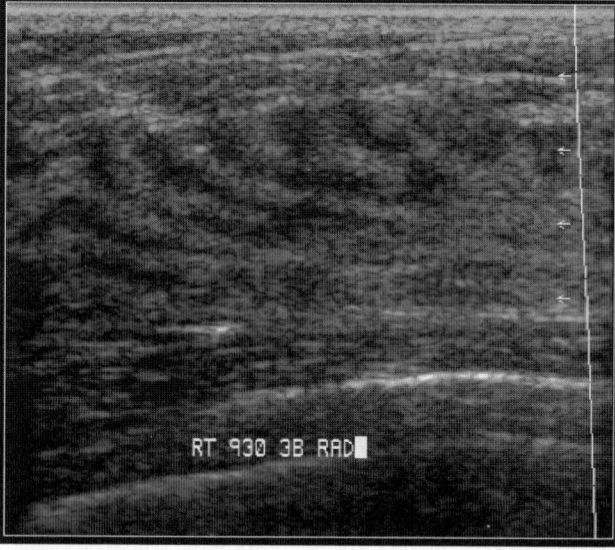

FIGURE 4–59 Other terminal ductolobular units have very long extralobular terminal ducts and therefore have a very elongated shape.

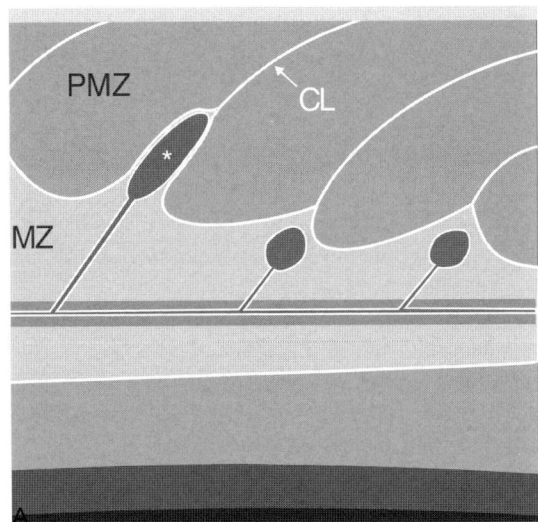

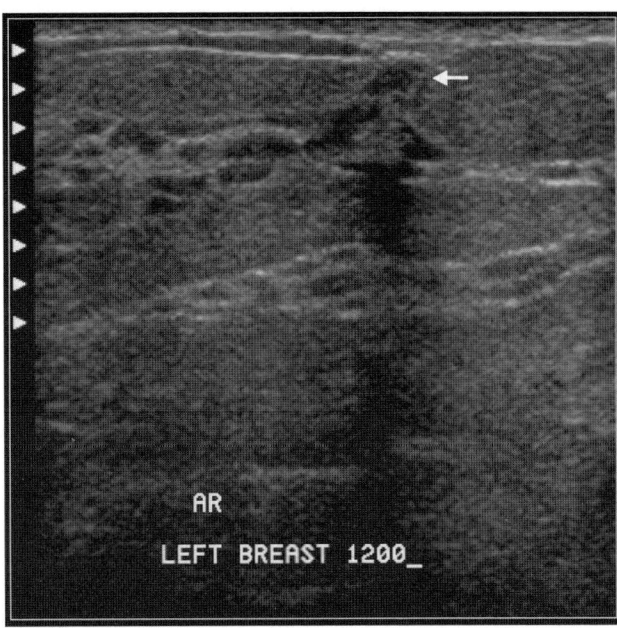

FIGURE 4–60 A: As the breast atrophies, the stromal and lobular elements regress more quickly between Cooper's ligaments than they do within the areas immediately deep to the ligament's attachment to the anterior mammary fascia. As the surrounding interligamentous tissue regresses, the more slowly regressing terminal ductolobular units (TDLUs) under the ligaments *(*)* may persist and become entrapped within the ligament, where they become completely surrounded by fat. It is within such entrapped TDLUs that completely fat-surrounded cysts, fibroadenomas, and carcinomas arise. **B:** A TDLU lies completely within a Cooper's ligament *(arrow)*. Whether it arose there or has been stranded there by regression of surrounding tissues is uncertain. There are numerous other isoechoic and mildly hypoechoic TDLUs within the mammary zone.

are completely fat surrounded must arise from ducts or lobules that lie within suspensory ligaments.

Normal TDLUs are usually 1 to 2 mm in diameter, but the size of TDLUs varies greatly from patient to patient, with age, and with the phase of the menstrual cycle. TDLUs affected by ANDIs may achieve diameters of 5 to 7

mm. The size of TDLUs even varies from one part of the breast to another (Fig. 4–64). In fact, TDLUs are in a constant state of change, with new ones forming, others enlarging or maintaining size, and still others regressing or disappearing. Within a single lobe of the breast, TDLUs in all phases and of all sizes may be seen. In general, the larger

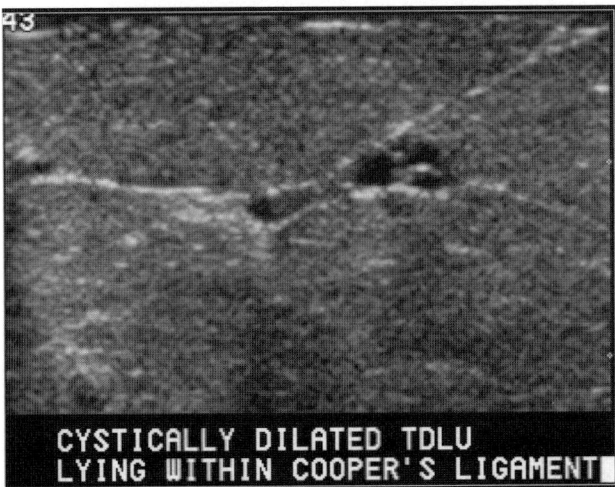

FIGURE 4–61 This small cluster of cysts lies at the intersection of a Cooper's ligament with the anterior mammary fascia. It arose from a terminal ductolobular unit that was entrapped within the ligament as the surrounding tissue regressed.

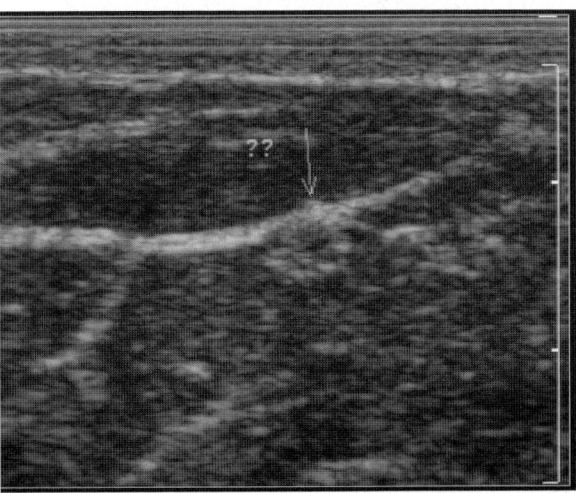

FIGURE 4–62 This small, solid nodule that presented as a subtle mammographic asymmetry lies within a Cooper's ligament. It arose from an entrapped terminal ductolobular unit. Biopsy revealed fibrocystic change.

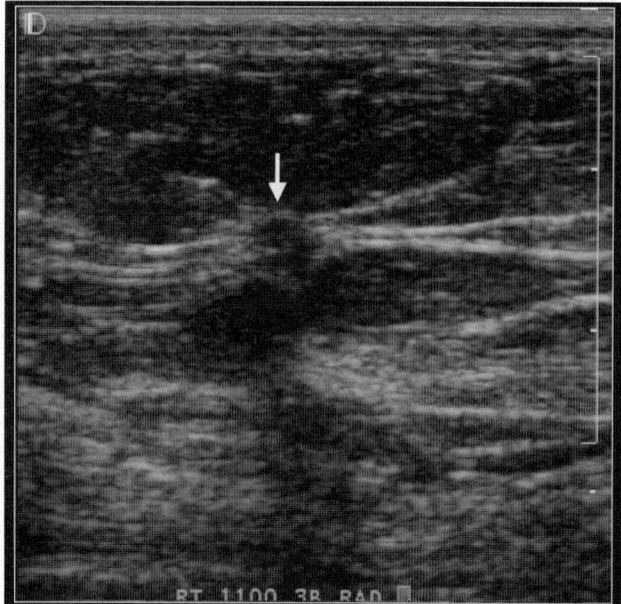

FIGURE 4–63 This small, 6-mm tubular carcinoma lies within a Cooper's ligament and is completely surrounded by fat. It presumably arose from a terminal ductolobular unit that was entrapped within the ligament when surrounding tissues atrophied and regressed.

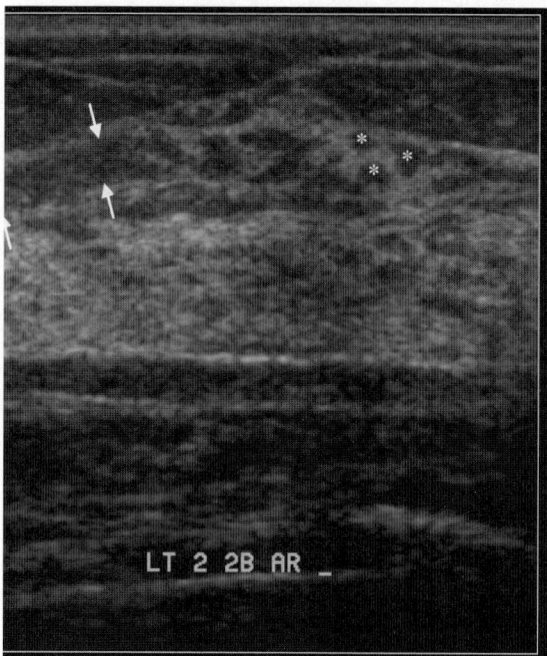

FIGURE 4–64 The size of terminal ductolobular units (TDLUs) varies not only from patient to patient and from right to left but also from one part of the breast to another. Note that on the left side of this image, the TDLUs have increased in size and number enough to have coalesced to form a continuous sheet of isoechoic glandular tissue *(arrows)*, whereas on the right side, multiple, normal-sized lobules are present *(*)*.

the TDLU, the more likely it is to be seen sonographically. When TDLUs are small, about the same size as the adjacent ducts, it may be difficult to distinguish short-axis images of ducts and their surrounding isoechoic loose periductal stromal tissue from those of TDLUs (Fig. 4–65).

TDLUs may not be sonographically demonstrable for several reasons:

1. TDLUs may be atrophic and too small to be identifiable sonographically.
2. TDLUs may be isoechoic and indistinguishable from surrounding isoechoic fatty or conglomerate lobular tissue.
3. The normally loose, isoechoic intralobular stromal fibrous tissue may become hyalinized and sclerotic, hyperechoic, and so similar in echogenicity to that of surrounding extralobular stromal fibrous tissue that it cannot be distinguished from it.

In breasts with extensive fatty involution, the ducts and TDLUs are less likely to be sonographically visible because the midlevel echogenicity of the ducts and TDLUs is nearly the same as that of the surrounding fat. Additionally, when atrophy has caused regression of supporting echogenic stromal fibrous elements, there is usually an associated regression and atrophy of small ducts and TDLUs. On the other hand, as noted earlier, even when TDLUs are atrophic and inapparent, larger central mammary ducts

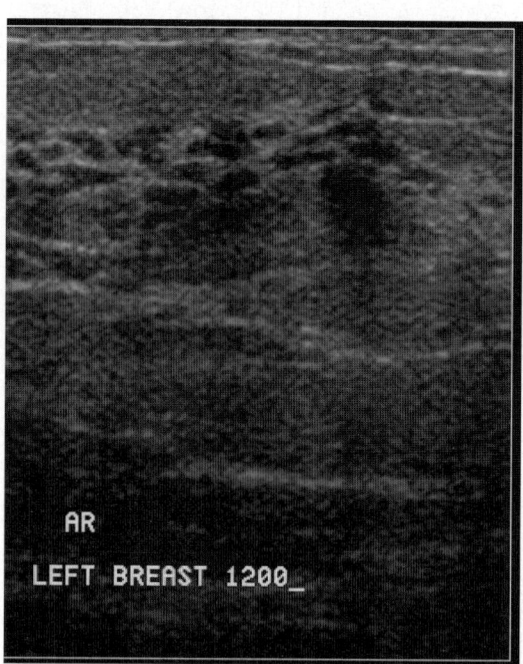

FIGURE 4–65 In some cases, it may be difficult to distinguish terminal ductolobular units from peripheral ducts in the short axis. Identifying the short-axis target-like appearance of the duct and its periductal loose stromal tissue (Fig. 4–44) will facilitate the distinction between short-axis ducts and lobules.

that are ectatic and filled with anechoic or nearly anechoic secretions may be sonographically visible, even when surrounded by fat (Fig. 4–49).

Most benign and malignant pathologic processes of the breast arise within the TDLU. Physiologic causes of sonographically visible TDLU enlargement include all causes of hormonal stimulation—pregnancy, lactation, functional ovarian cysts, and HRT. Fibrocystic and benign proliferative causes of sonographically visible TDLU enlargement include florid usual duct hyperplasia (papillary duct hyperplasia), apocrine metaplasia, stromal sclerosis, and microcysts. Lobular hyperplasia and adenosis cause an increase in not only the size of lobules but also their number. Of course, atypical hyperplasia and malignancy can also cause sonographically visible enlargement of TDLUs. Although sonography can demonstrate TDLU enlargement from any of the above causes, in most cases, the histologic cause of sonographic enlargement cannot be determined. Thus, the significance of TDLU enlargement must be viewed in the context of surrounding lobular prominence. If enlargement of TDLUs is bilateral and diffuse, it must be assumed that the lobular prominence is caused by one or more of the myriad ANDIs. However, when lobular prominence is isolated or markedly asymmetric, especially in postmenopausal patients, one should be more suspicious that the enlargement is caused by atypia or malignancy (Fig. 4–66).

TDLUs vary in size not only in association with fibrocystic change and benign proliferation of epithelial elements but also because of cyclical physiologic changes. In the postmenstrual and early follicular phases of the menstrual cycle, lobules tend to regress and become smaller and less sonographically apparent. However, in the late luteal phase of the menstrual cycle, particularly in the immediate premenstrual phase, stromal loosening and edema, secretions, and venous congestion can enlarge TDLUs. Thus, the sensitivity of ultrasound for small or subtle isoechoic solid nodules is theoretically better in the early proliferative phase of the menstrual cycle, when TDLUs are least prominent. This could be very important when sonography is used for bilateral whole breast screening and may even be important for targeted examinations when the clinical or mammographic indications for sonography are subtle. The variation in sensitivity with the menstrual cycles is common knowledge and widely suspected but, to the best of our knowledge, has not been proved. As a practical matter, it is difficult to schedule all patients who are to undergo breast ultrasound in the early preovulatory phase of their menstrual cycles. Many patients who discover a palpable abnormality are far too nervous and distraught to wait until the optimal time in the menstrual cycle to have ultrasound performed.

The importance of recognizing enlargement of TDLUs sonographically is not to try to make a definitive histologic

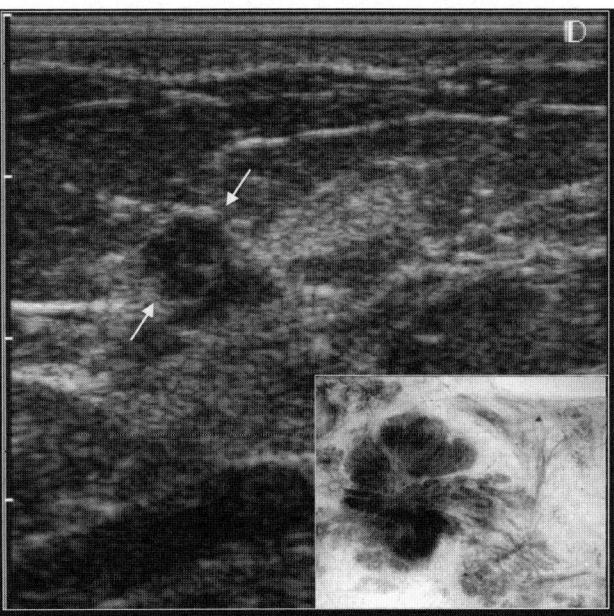

FIGURE 4–66 Because sonography is generally unable to distinguish the various causes of lobular enlargement from each other, the pattern of enlargement becomes important in assessing its significance. When lobular enlargement is generalized, bilateral, and roughly symmetric, the prudent assumption is that the cause is benign fibrocystic change or a benign proliferative disorder, even though any individual terminal ductolobular unit may contain atypia or ductal carcinoma *in situ* (DCIS). On the other hand, if lobular enlargement is isolated or markedly asymmetric, particularly in a postmenopausal patient, the risk of atypia or DCIS is much higher, and biopsy should be considered. In this postmenopausal patient, only one cluster of enlarged lobules was present and caused a mammographic density. Biopsy revealed atypical ductal hyperplasia superimposed on underlying florid usual duct hyperplasia and sclerosing adenosis. (Subgross histology courtesy of Hanne M. Jensen, MD, University of California at Davis.)

diagnosis of the underlying causes but rather to recognize that lobular prominence causes an intermediate sensitivity state. The sensitivity of detecting small, isoechoic solid nodules in patients with enlarged TDLUs lies between that of purely hyperechoic fibrous breast tissue and completely isoechoic glandular breast tissue. The sensitivity also depends on the degree of TDLU enlargement as well as the number and proximity of enlarged TDLUs. In essence, when there is diffuse and bilateral enlargement of lobules, the size of the largest lobules present in the breast creates a sliding "size floor," below which an isoechoic nodule cannot be detected. Thus, if the largest sonographically demonstrable nodules in the breast are 2 mm, a 3-mm nodule is potentially sonographically detectable. However, if adenosis has caused TDLUs to enlarge to 5 or 6 mm each, even a 5-mm isoechoic nodule cannot be distinguished from TDLUs enlarged by adenosis. An isoechoic nodule would have to be at least 7 mm to be large enough to be distinguished from lobules affected by adenosis. Additionally, the

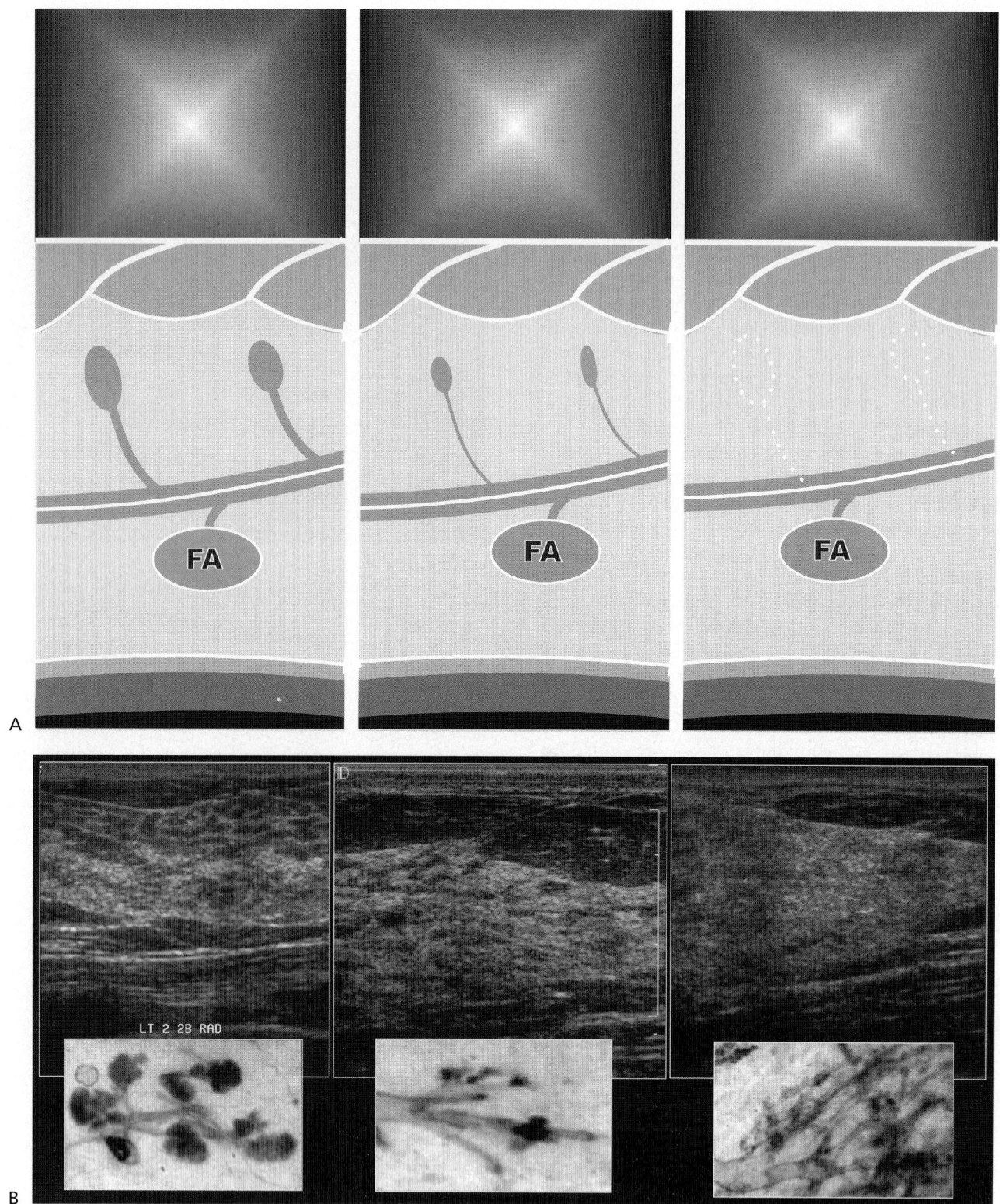

FIGURE 4–67 A: The size of the terminal ductolobular units (TDLUs) in the area of interest affects the sensitivity of sonography for small, isoechoic solid nodules. When TDLUs are normal in size (**left**), atrophic (**middle**), or hyalinized and echogenic, regardless of size (**right**), the sensitivity of sonography for smaller than 5-mm, solid, isoechoic nodules is high. **B:** This figure shows examples of normal-sized (2 mm or smaller) TDLUs (**left**), atrophic TDLUs (**middle**), and hyalinized TDLUs (**right**) that are indistinguishable in echogenicity from the background hyperechoic interlobular stromal fibrous tissue. All three tissue types represent highly sensitive backgrounds in which to detect small cystic or solid lesions, regardless of echogenicity. Only isolated microcalcifications might be missed in such background tissue, and this possibility is avoided by performing mammography before sonography in most patients. (Subgross histology courtesy of Hanne M. Jensen, MD, University of California at Davis.)

combined increase in the size and number of TDLUs can result in larger conglomerates of isoechoic tissue, as may occur in tumoral adenosis. If such a conglomerate of iso-echoic enlarged TDLUs achieved a diameter of 10 mm, it would be difficult to identify isoechoic nodules smaller than 11 mm, and so forth (Figs. 4–67 and 4–68). It is especially important to exercise caution when a large, isoechoic area of tumoral adenosis is identifiable because small, isoechoic fi-broadenomas (Fig. 4–69) or malignant nodules may be ob-scured by the surrounding adenosis (Fig. 4–70). Power Doppler vocal fremitus can help in this assessment and is discussed in Chapter 20.

Although the sonographic sensitivity for isoechoic solid nodules is diminished in the presence of large amounts of glandular tissue or enlarged TDLUs, the sensi-tivity is not reduced to zero. Furthermore, the presence of enlarged TDLUs affects the sensitivity for benign isoechoic solid nodules such as fibroadenomas to a much greater de-gree than for malignancies. Most fibroadenomas are nearly isoechoic with epithelium and loose intralobular stromal fibrous tissue of which enlarged TDLUs are composed. On the other hand, about two-thirds of malignant nodules are hypoechoic with respect to surrounding glandular tissue and will, therefore, be sonographically more obvious even in a background of enlarged isoechoic TDLUs. Only about one-third of malignant solid nodules are nearly isoechoic with surrounding glandular tissue and therefore more likely to be obscured by it. Additionally, many of these

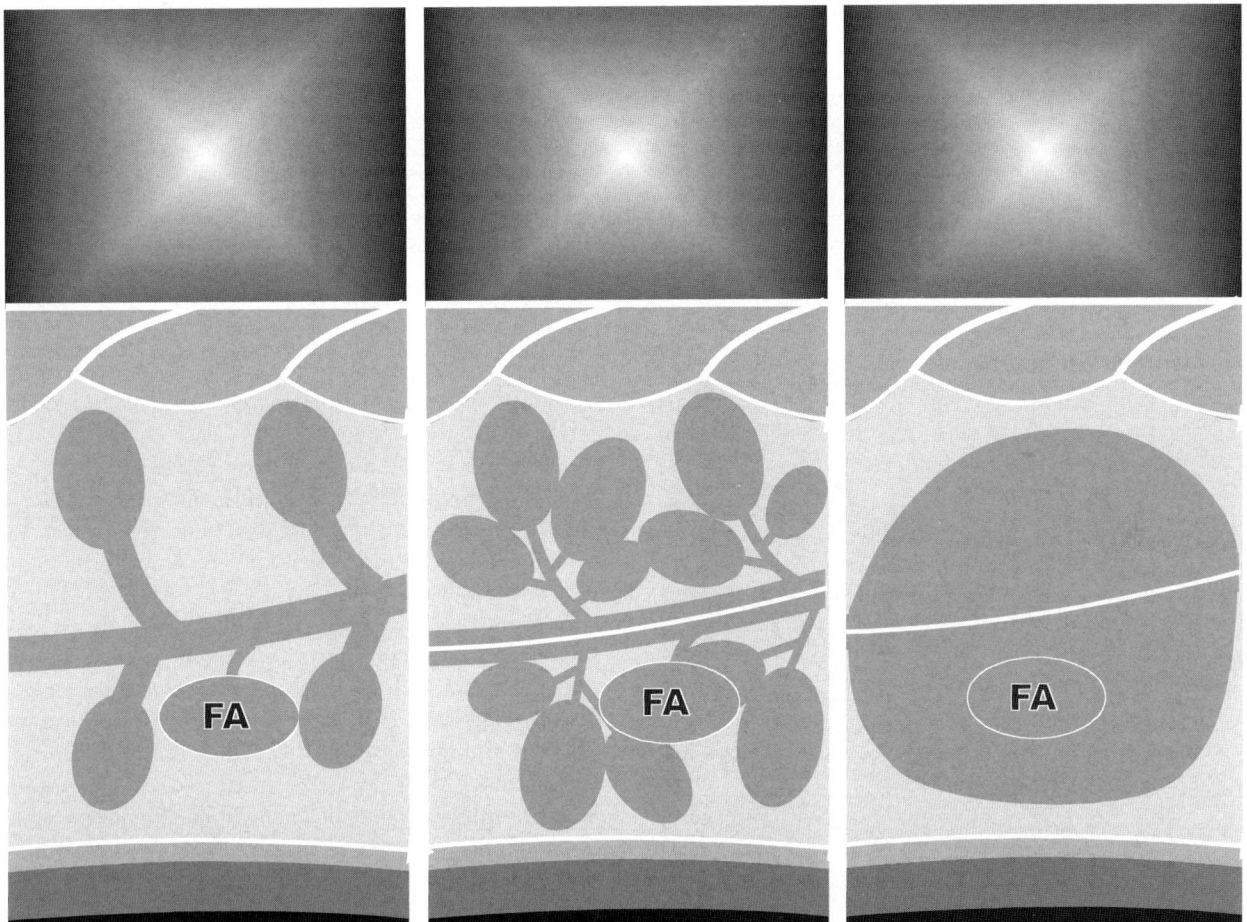

A

FIGURE 4–68 A: The size of the terminal ductolobular units (TDLUs) in the area of interest af-fects the sensitivity of sonography for small, isoechoic, solid nodules. The larger and more nu-merous the lobules in the area of interest, the lower the sensitivity. In benign fibrocystic change or benign proliferative disorders such as papillary apocrine metaplasia or florid usual duct hy-perplasia, individual TDLUs may be enlarged to 5 mm **(left)**. In adenosis, the number of ductules with TDLUs is increased, the number of TDLUs is increased, and the TDLUs are enlarged **(middle)**. In tumoral adenosis, a cluster of enlarged lobules may form an isoechoic mass of several cen-timeters **(right)**. The sensitivity of sonography for small, isoechoic, solid nodules decreases from left to right. Nodules smaller than 6 mm may be completely obscured by surrounding tissue of equal echogenicity. Identifying the echogenic pseudocapsule that surrounds a solid nodule may be the only means of identifying it. *Continued.*

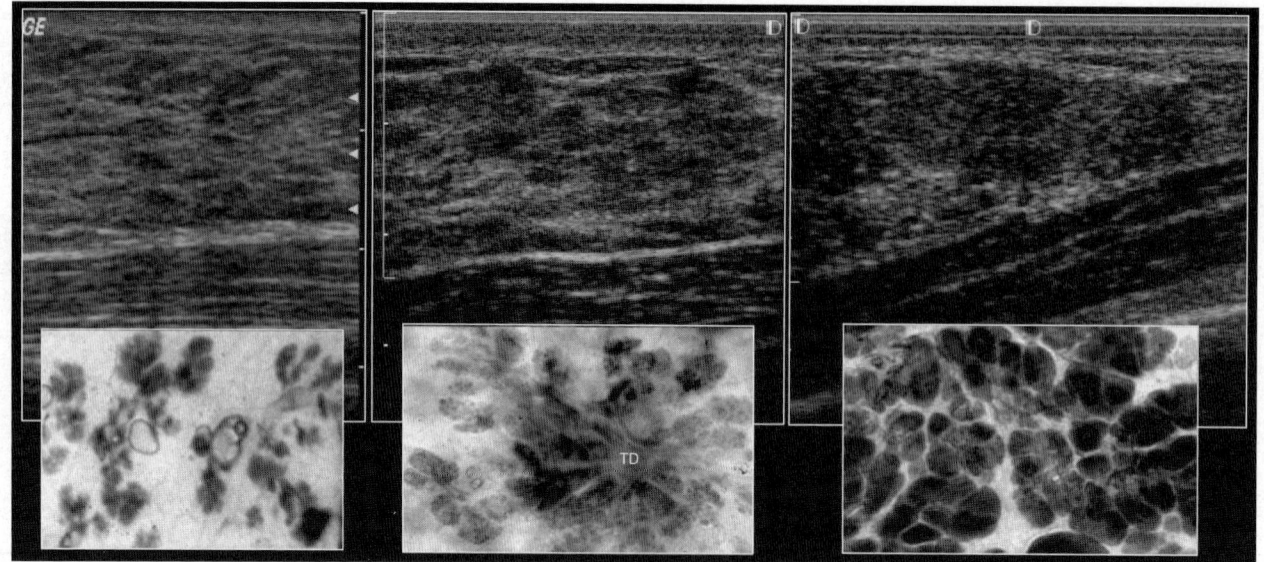

B

FIGURE 4–68 *(continued)* **B:** These images show a progression in the size and number of the TDLUs from left to right. In the **left** image, individual anterior TDLUs have reached 5 mm. In the **middle** image, the TDLUs not only are enlarged but also increased in number. In the **right** image, TDLUs are so large and numerous that they have coalesced to form a large, isoechoic mass of tissue. The importance of lobular size is not to attempt to make a histologic diagnosis by sonography, but to realize that the size of TDLUs in the area of interest creates a moving threshold beneath which it becomes more difficult to identify an isoechoic solid nodule. As the lobules become larger and more numerous from left to right, the sensitivity for small solid nodules decreases. (Subgross histology courtesy of Hanne M. Jensen, MD, University of California at Davis.)

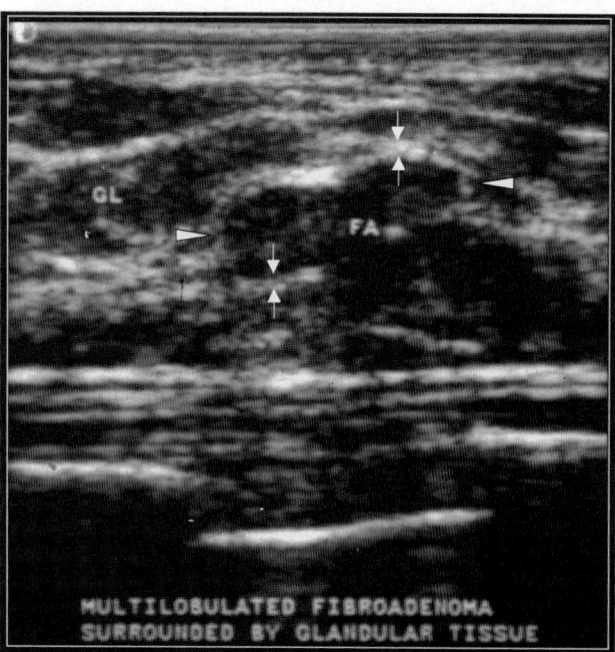

FIGURE 4–69 This bilobed fibroadenoma is almost 2 cm in diameter *(between arrowheads)* but is virtually indistinguishable from the background of isoechoic, glandular tissue except for the presence of a thin, echogenic pseudocapsule *(between small arrows)* of compressed tissue that surrounds the lesion. Identifying echogenic pseudocapsules of varied thickness becomes the key to detecting small, isoechoic, solid nodules in backgrounds of isoechoic, glandular tissue.

isoechoic malignancies have other malignant features that help distinguish them from glandular tissue and enlarged TDLUs.

It is also important to understand that fibrocystic and benign causes of enlarged TDLUs not only reduce the chances of detecting some solid nodules but also, in some cases such as sclerosing adenosis, can simulate malignancies, resulting in false-positive diagnoses (Fig. 4–71).

Fibrocystic change is a virtual variant of normal and is present to some degree in most women after the age of 35 years. Fibrocystic change may cause cystic enlargement and cystic dilation of TDLUs to various degrees. In cases of early or mild fibrocystic change, when the scan plane is exactly parallel to the long axis of the TDLU, a multiloculated complex cyst may be sonographically recognizable as cystic dilation of a single TDLU. In most cases, however, the scan plane will not be exactly parallel to the long axis of the TDLU, and the cystic dilation will appear as an amorphous collection of small cysts interspersed with echogenic tissue representing stromal fibrosclerosis. Each small cyst represents a severely dilated intralobular ductule. As the degree of cystic dilation of ductules increases, the number of ductules decreases, and the lobule enlarges further. Further cystic dilation results in lobulated cysts. The lobulations represent residuals of the dilated intralobular ductules. With still further distention of the lobule and the cystic development under tension, the lobulations become com-

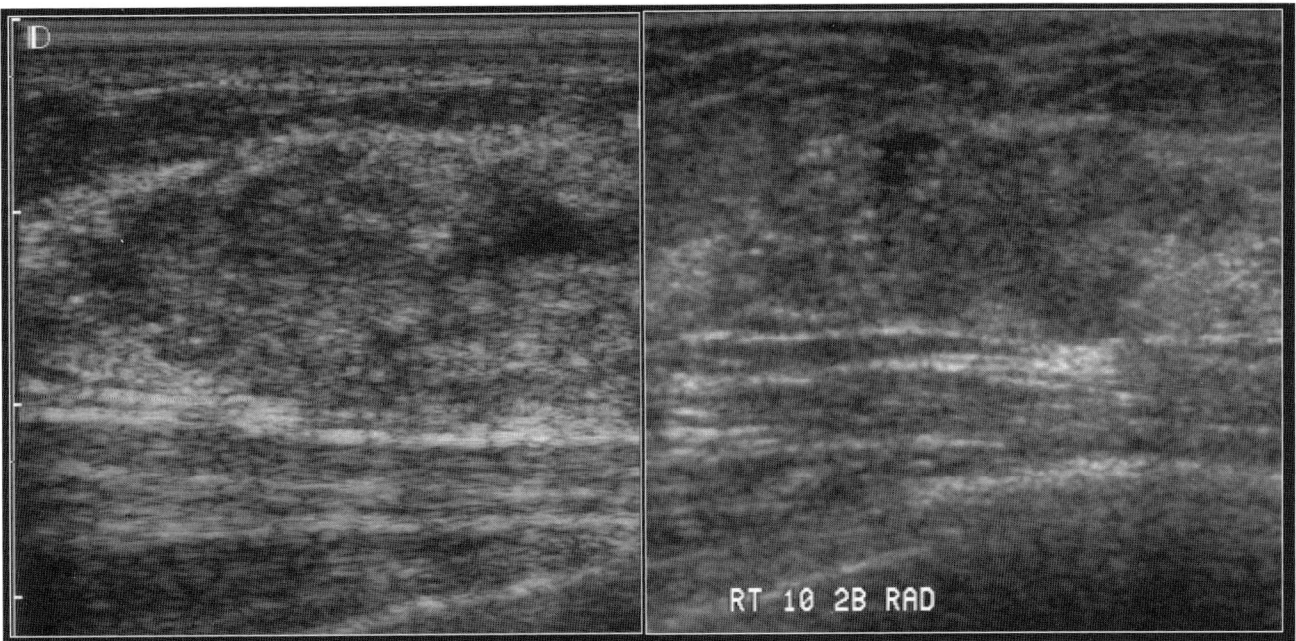

FIGURE 4–70 This figure illustrates the difficulty posed by large areas of isoechoic glandular tissue. The patients whose scans are shown in the **left** and **right** images both presented with palpable lumps and diffuse amorphous calcifications bilaterally classified as probably benign (BIRADS 3) and likely caused by fibrocystic change or adenosis. Targeted diagnostic ultrasound of both patients showed large, isoechoic areas containing punctate echoes interpreted as microcalcifications. Biopsy of the area shown on the **left** revealed sclerosing adenosis within a focus of tumoral adenosis. Biopsy of the area on the **right** showed extensive, low-nuclear-grade ductal carcinoma *in situ* (DCIS). Large areas of isoechoic glandular tissue decrease sonographic sensitivity, can be difficult to distinguish from noninvasive malignancy such as low-nuclear-grade DCIS, particularly when palpable and associated with calcifications, and are not as reassuring as would be purely echogenic tissue.

pletely effaced as the cyst assumes the spherical or elliptical shape typically associated with simple cysts.

TDLUs affected by fibrocystic change often contain benign proliferative conditions or other solid components of fibrocystic change of the breast, such as papillary apocrine metaplasia, fibrosclerosis, or papillary duct hyperplasia. The presence of these solid proliferative processes within the affected lobule creates internal echoes that require these cyst lesions to be classified as complex cystic. In fibrocystic change, the cystic components may be dominant, the solid proliferative components may predominate, or there may be any mixture of cystic and solid components. When solid proliferative components predominate, the affected TDLU may have the sonographic appearance of a worrisome solid microlobulated lesion rather than appearing cystic. This appearance explains why we sometimes obtain a nonspecific benign diagnosis such as fibrocystic change when a solid nodule undergoes biopsy. In some cases, the cystically dilated ductules are so small (microcysts) that they cannot be resolved with sonography. These anechoic but unresolved microcysts undergo volume averaging with the intervening hyperechoic fibrosclerotic stroma, appearing isoechoic and creating a solid appearance. Systematic sonographic evaluation of complex breast cysts is discussed and illustrated in greater detail in Chapter 10.

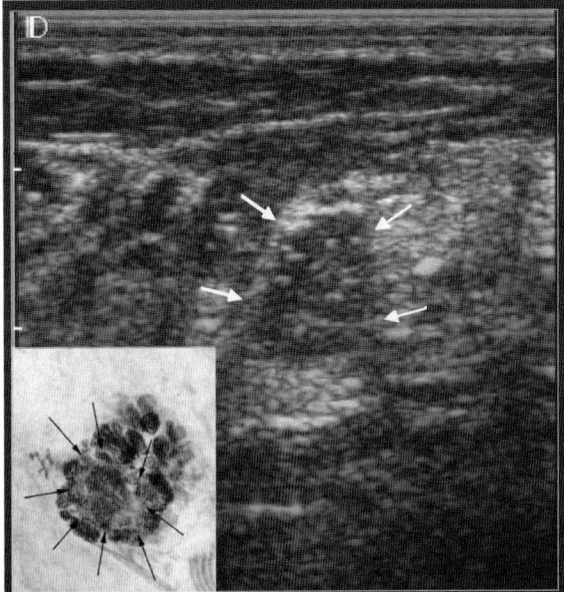

FIGURE 4–71 Focal areas of lobular enlargement caused by benign proliferative disorders such as sclerosing adenosis not only can reduce sonographic sensitivity for small isoechoic solid nodules but also can be causes of false-positive results. This taller-than-wide, microlobulated, isoechoic nodule *(arrows)* containing calcifications was characterized as BIRADS 4b (between 50% and 89% risk for malignancy). Biopsy revealed sclerosing adenosis with no atypia or malignancy. (Subgross histology courtesy of Hanne M. Jensen, MD, University of California at Davis.)

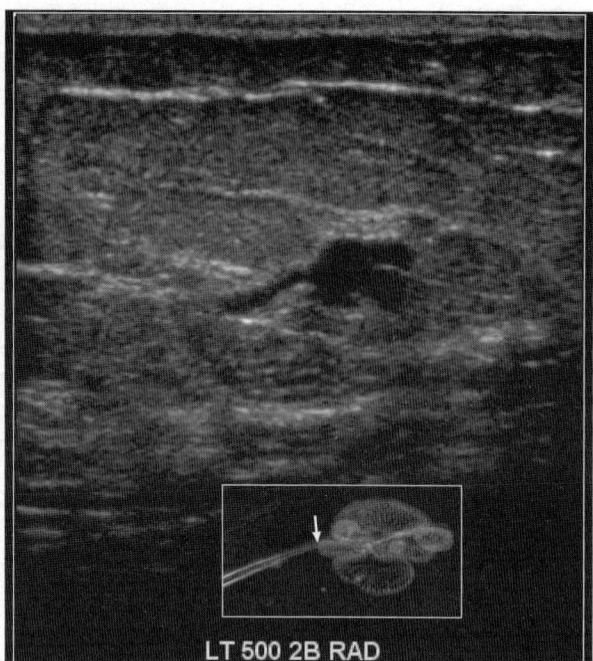

FIGURE 4–72 Occasionally, atrophic terminal ductolobular units (TDLUs) are cystic *(arrow)*. In such cases, the residual atrophic cystic lobules are little wider than the ectatic ducts *(arrowhead)* with which they are often associated. Note that all other lobules and stromal tissue around the atrophic cystic TDLUs has atrophied, leaving the lobules completely surrounded by fat.

With age, most TDLUs atrophy and regress. Atrophic TDLUs are generally not sonographically demonstrable unless the atrophic lobule has a cystic appearance (Fig. 4–72).

Accessory Breast Tissue

A significant minority of patients has accessory tissue that is often asymmetric from right to left. The axillary segment is most commonly involved, but accessory breast tissue can occur anywhere along the milk line, including axillary segment, upper outer quadrant, 6:00 position in the breast, or on the anterior abdominal wall inferior to the breast (Fig. 4–73). Accessory breast tissue may cause mammographic asymmetry (Fig. 4–74) or a palpable lump (Fig. 4–75) at any time during life but is most likely to cause a palpable abnormality when the breast tissues are stimulated by the hormones of pregnancy or lactation or when rapid weigh loss results in a decrease of surrounding fat. The accessory breast may not drain to the nipple through a major duct; thus, under hormonal stimulation, the accessory breast tissue can develop secretory change and severe duct ectasia that contribute to both its mammographic density and palpability (Fig. 4–76). Like breast tissue in the remainder of the breast, accessory breast tissue may be purely glandular or fibrous or may be com-

(text continued on page 101)

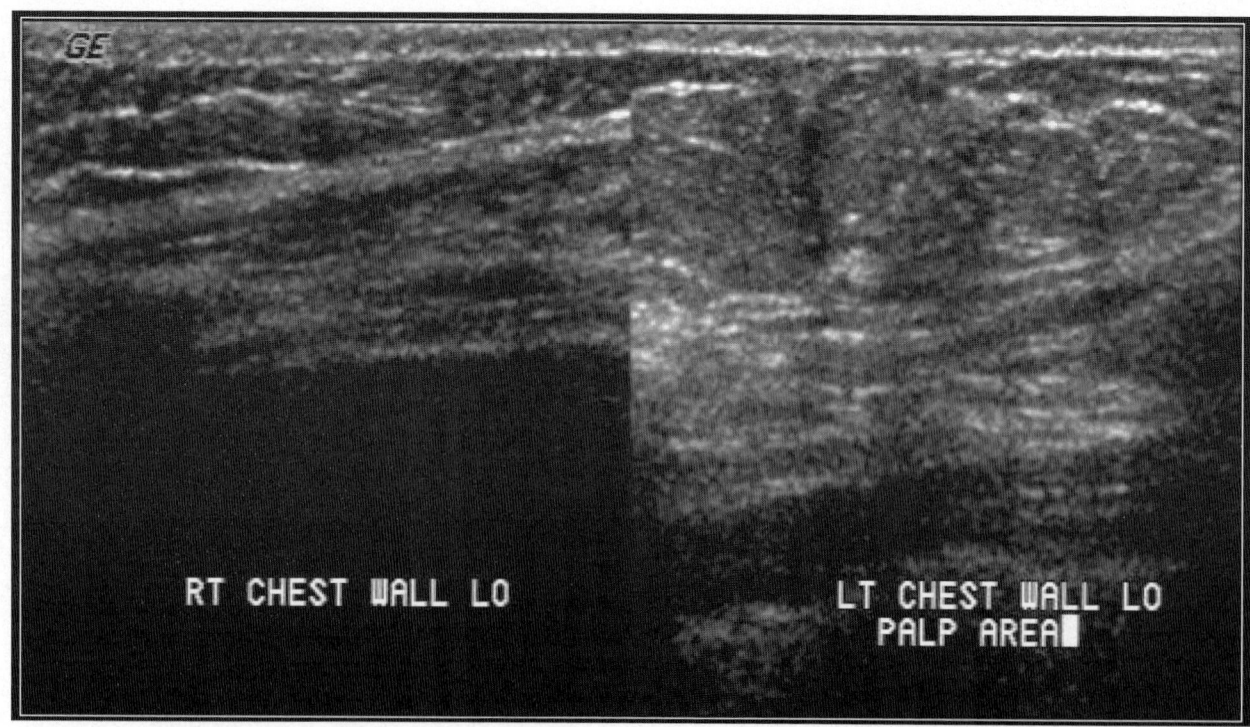

A

FIGURE 4–73 A: This split-screen image shows mirror-image locations on the right and left chest wall just inferior to the 6:00 position in each breast. The patient presented with a new palpable lump on the left during the first trimester of her first pregnancy. Note that the tissues are thicker on the left in the area of the palpable lump than on the right. This represents accessory breast tissue located along the "milk line" just below the breast that has been stimulated by the hormones of pregnancy.

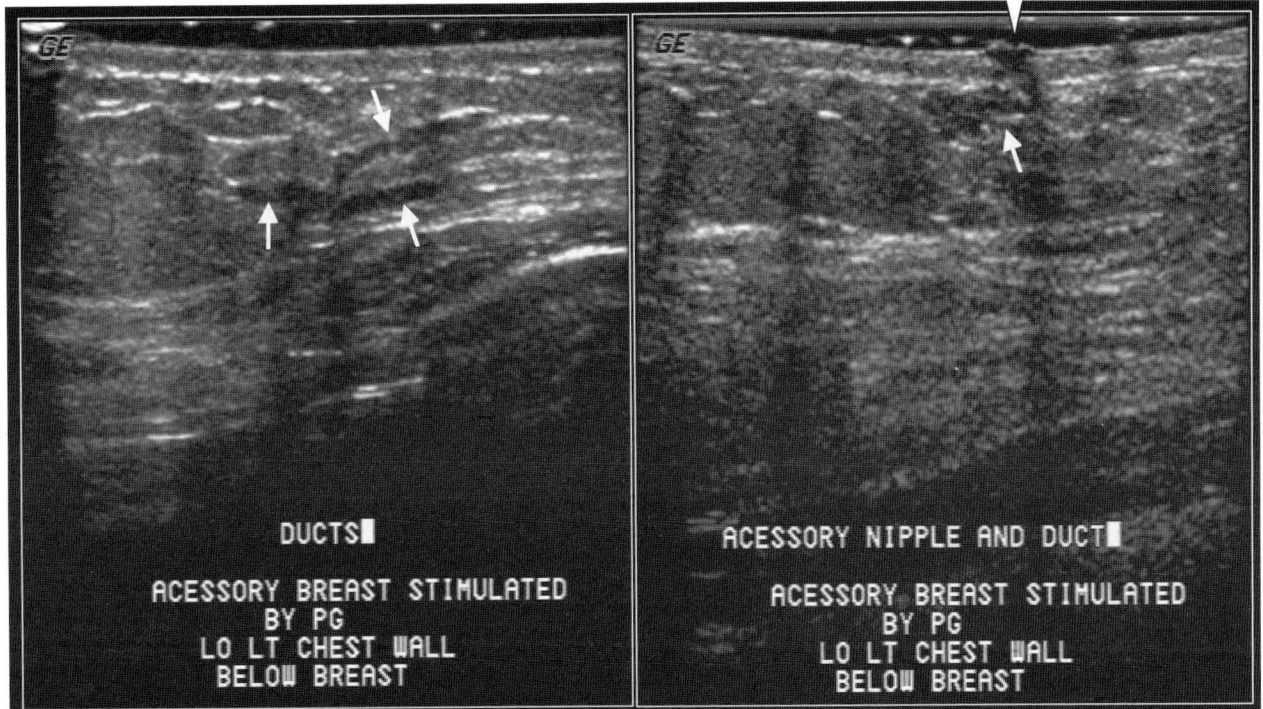

B

FIGURE 4–73 *(continued)* **B:** Additional scans through the palpable lump on the left chest wall just below the 6:00 position of the left breast show ducts *(arrows)* within the asymmetric thickening **(left)**. The **right** image shows an accessory nipple *(arrowhead)* with a prominent duct extending through the skin into the accessory breast tissue *(arrows)*. The patient had previously misinterpreted the accessory nipple as a skin mole until this time. Accessory breast tissue often first becomes clinically apparent when hormonally stimulated by pregnancy, with anovulatory cycles perimenopausally or perimenarchally, or with exogenous hormone therapy.

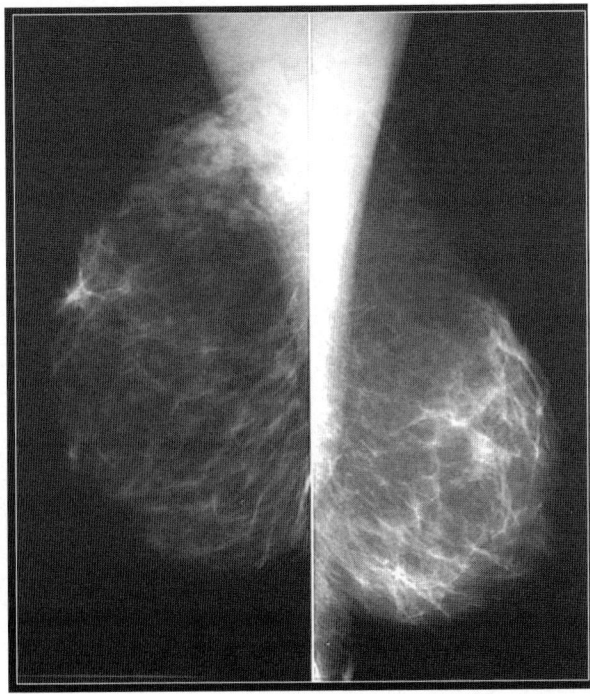

A

FIGURE 4–74 A: Routine screening mediolateral oblique (MLO) mammograms show marked asymmetric density in the axillary segment of the right breast. This is most likely merely accessory breast tissue, but in the absence of old films documenting stability, ultrasound was used to confirm the suspected diagnosis and to exclude an occult solid lesion within the asymmetry. *Continued.*

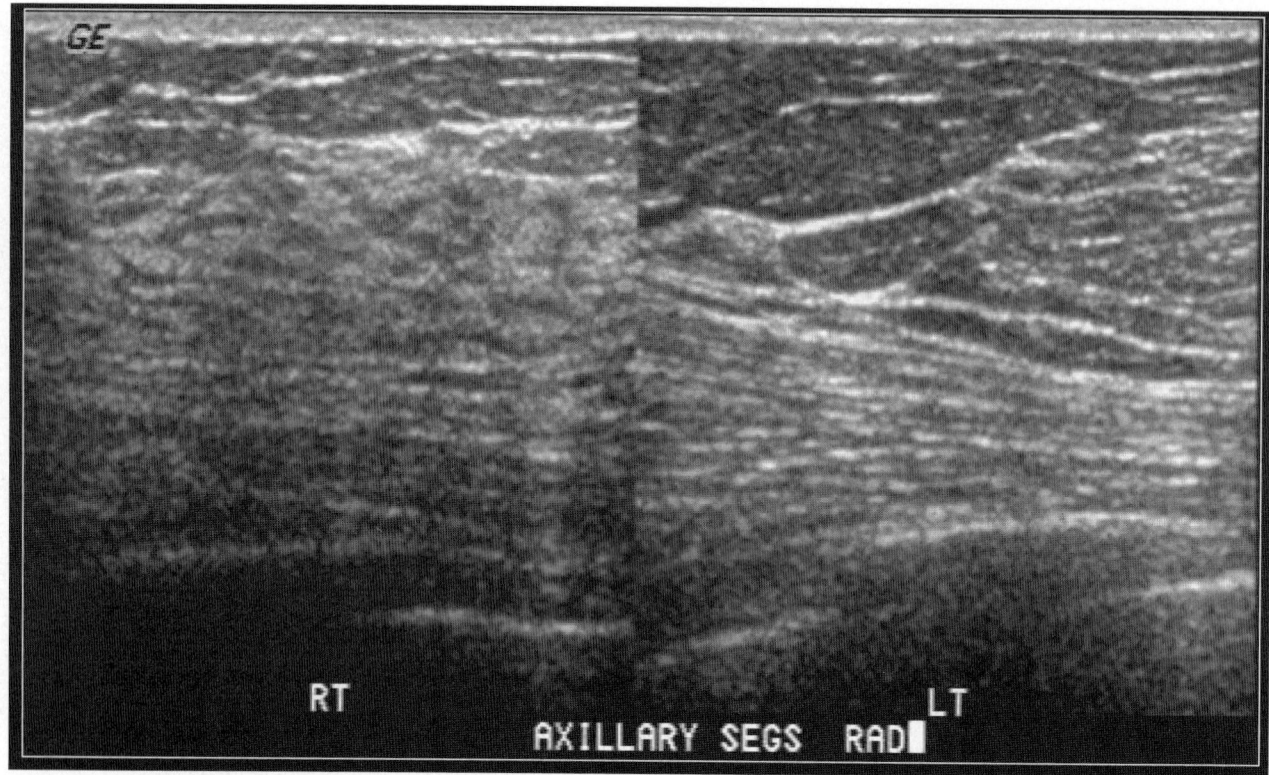

B

FIGURE 4–74 *(continued)* **B:** Split-screen mirror-image scans of the right and left axillary segments obtained in a radial plane show much thicker fibroductal tissue on the right, in the area of mammographic asymmetric density, than in the mirror-image location on the left. Split-screen mirror-image scanning is important when mammographic asymmetries are believed to be caused by normal breast tissue. The axillary segment of the breast is the most common location for accessory breast tissue.

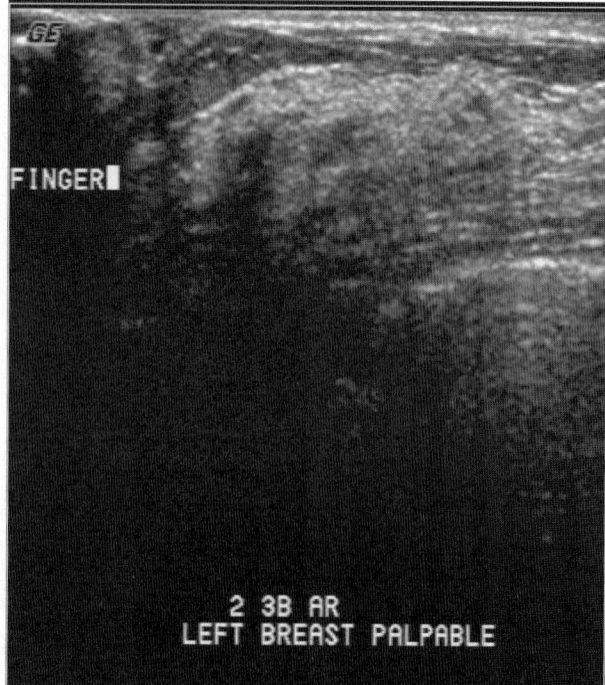

A

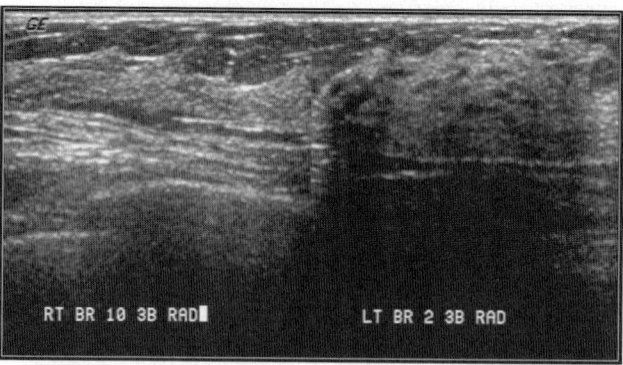

B

FIGURE 4–75 A: This patient presented with a palpable abnormality in the far upper outer quadrant of the left breast just medial to the axillary segment. A scan documenting that hyperechoic fibrous tissue was causing the palpable abnormality was obtained. The upper outer quadrant is the second most common location for accessory breast tissue after the axillary segment of the breast. **B:** Split-screen mirror-image scans of the upper outer quadrants confirm that the palpable, hyperechoic fibroductal tissue on the left is asymmetrically thickened compared with that on the right, explaining why it was palpable, whereas the fibroductal tissue in the right upper outer quadrant was not.

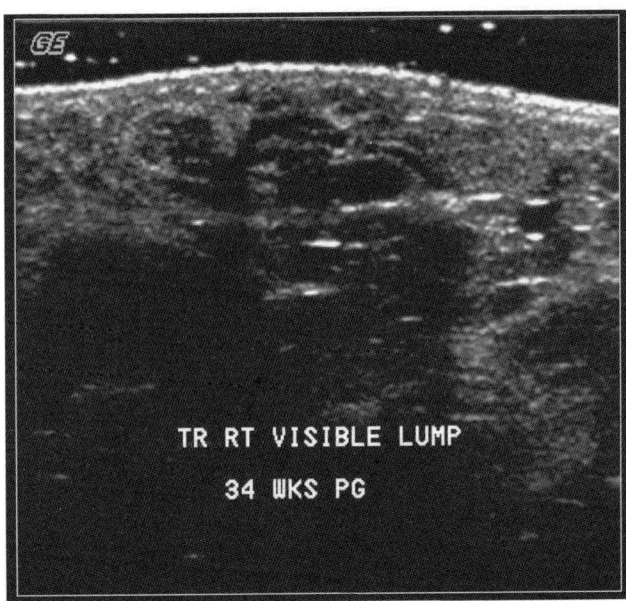

FIGURE 4–76 This patient developed a visible and palpable lump in the axilla during the third trimester of her first pregnancy. Sonography showed duct ectasia and secretory changes with accessory breast tissue. In many instances, there is no drainage from the accessory breast tissue; thus, secretions accumulate until back pressure causes secretory change to stop.

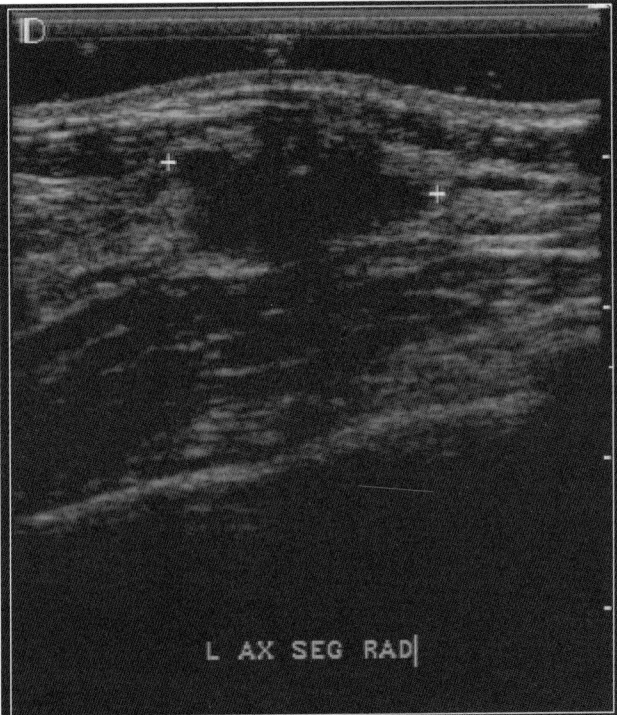

FIGURE 4–77 One must not automatically assume without sonographic confirmation that all palpable abnormalities or mammographic asymmetries in the axillary segment of the breast are merely caused by accessory breast tissue. Accessory breast tissue is subject to all the same fibrocystic, proliferative, and malignant changes that the breast tissue in the remainder of the breast is subject to. Thus, malignancy can occur within accessory breast tissue, as in this case.

posed of a mixture of fibrous and glandular or fatty elements. The tissue within accessory breast tissue is subject to all of the same benign fibrocystic and proliferative processes as the tissue in the remainder of the breast. Malignancy can also develop within accessory breast tissue (Fig. 4–77); hence, it cannot automatically be assumed that any mammographic density or palpable lump in the axillary segment is merely accessory breast tissue. The mammographically dense tissues that lie within the accessory breast tissue can obscure small malignant nodules. Thus, ultrasound should be used aggressively to investigate mammographic asymmetries and palpable lumps in the axillary segments or axilla.

Breasts of Infants and Perimenarchal Adolescents

Newborns may have some ductal development induced by maternal hormones that may even result in some secretion from the nipples (witch's milk). The involvement of the subareolar ducts may be asymmetric. Sonography shows findings similar to gynecomastia, with symmetrically or asymmetrically prominent subareolar ducts (Fig. 4–78). After a few weeks to months, this secretion spontaneously ceases, and ducts become less prominent sonographically. From the newborn period to the onset of thelarche, when the ovaries begin production of estrogens, the breasts are inactive.

Hormonal stimulation during thelarche causes the ductal system of the breast bud to proliferate and enlarge, creating a visible bulge and palpable lump beneath the nipple. In some patients, this may initially occur asymmetrically, simulating a unilateral breast nodule. This asymmetry will soon resolve, and the breast buds will become symmetric in most patients. It is very important to recognize early asymmetric development of breast buds as a variant of normal development and not to remove the "nodule." Removal will prevent development of a normal breast on that side. The sonographic appearance of asymmetric breast buds is, peculiarly, virtually identical to asymmetric gynecomastia (Fig. 4–79).

For evaluation of a subareolar nodule in both newborns and adolescents, use of the two-handed compression maneuver is invaluable in demonstrating that the nodule represents developing ducts, not a mass. Straight anterior scan approaches are parallel to the axis of the ducts and therefore show only a hypoechoic nodule corresponding to the palpable abnormality. The two-handed compression maneuver, on the other hand, creates an angle of incidence nearer 90 degrees and shows the individual ducts that cause the palpable subareolar nodule to better advantage (Fig. 4–80). The principles of scanning the subareolar region in infants and adolescents are identical to the principles for scanning patients who present with nipple discharge and male patients with gynecomastia.

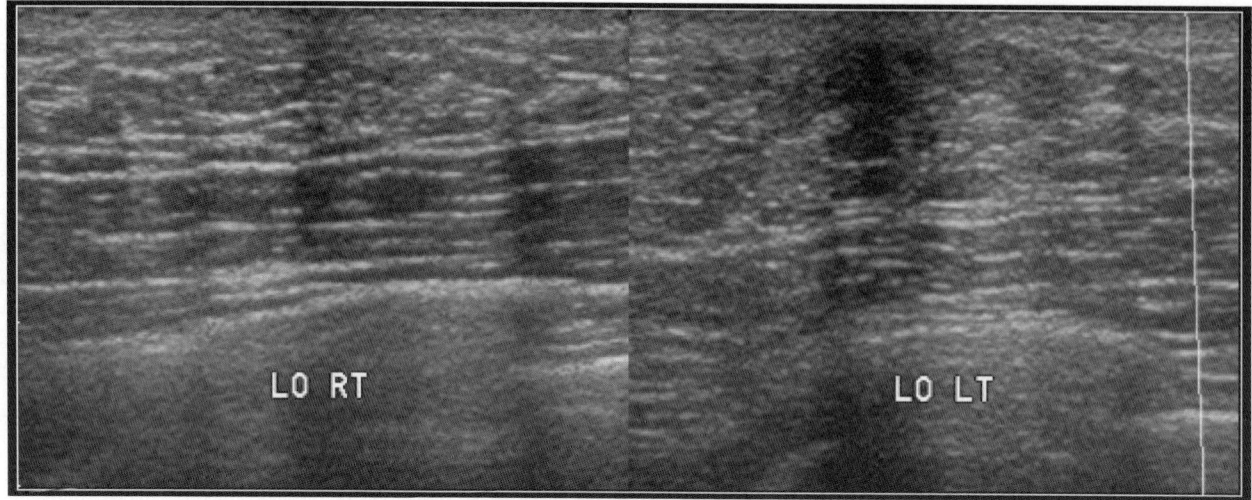

FIGURE 4–78 This figure shows stimulation of the subareolar ducts in a newborn girl who presented with a palpable lump in the left subareolar area and secretions from the left nipple ("witches' milk"). Split-screen mirror-image scans obtained in a longitudinal plane over the nipples show asymmetrically large ductal tissue on the left compared with the right. Images obtained with two-handed compression technique would have documented this better.

Chest Wall Problems

Costal cartilage can be of sonographic significance in thin, small-breasted women, in whom it may cause palpable abnormalities in the far medial aspect of the breast. The inexperienced sonographer or sonologist may mistake the palpable costal cartilage for a solid nodule when it is scanned in longitudinal planes, across the short axis of the costal cartilage (Fig. 4–81A). The location of the costal cartilage posterior to the pectoralis muscle and its characteristic rectangular shape when it is scanned in the transverse plane that lies parallel to its long axis will reveal the true nature of the palpable lump (Fig. 4–81B).

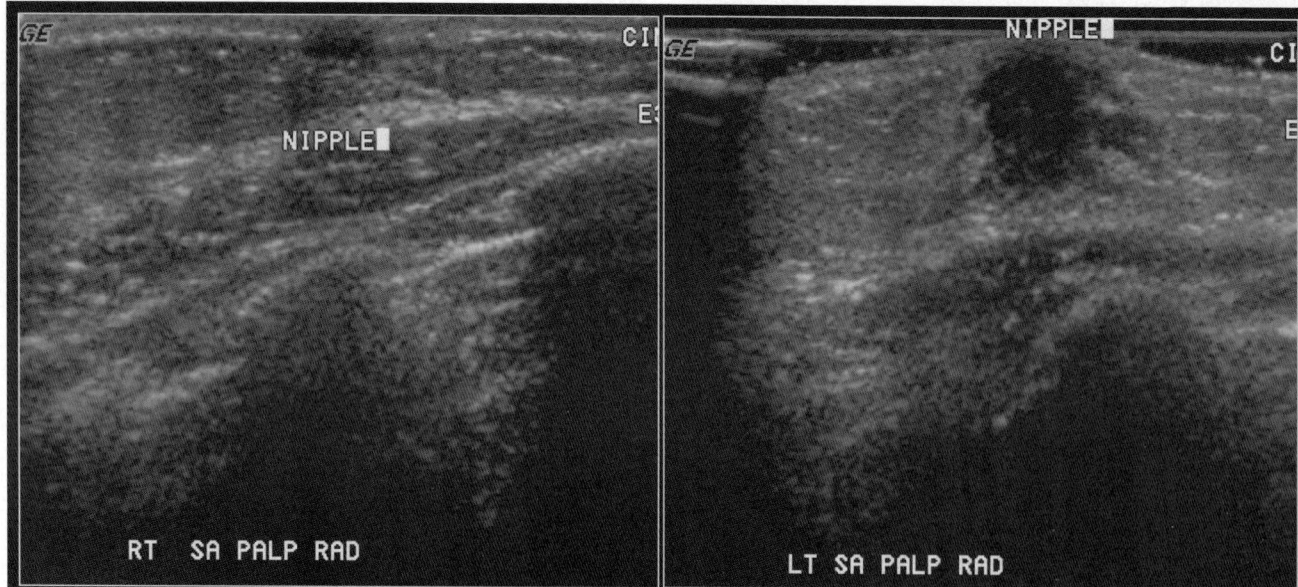

FIGURE 4–79 This 13-year-old girl presented with a palpable nodule in the left subareolar area, but no secretions. Split-screen images of the right and left nipple and subareolar areas show a hypoechoic, solid-appearing nodule on the left that actually merely represents asymmetrically developing ducts. Removal of this nodule would prevent development of a normal breast on the left side. Although the nodule is caused by developing subareolar ducts, their anatomy is not well seen because they course parallel to the beam and make poor specular reflectors. This makes it difficult to distinguish a true solid nodule from prominent subareolar ducts. Gynecomastia may have a similar sonographic appearance.

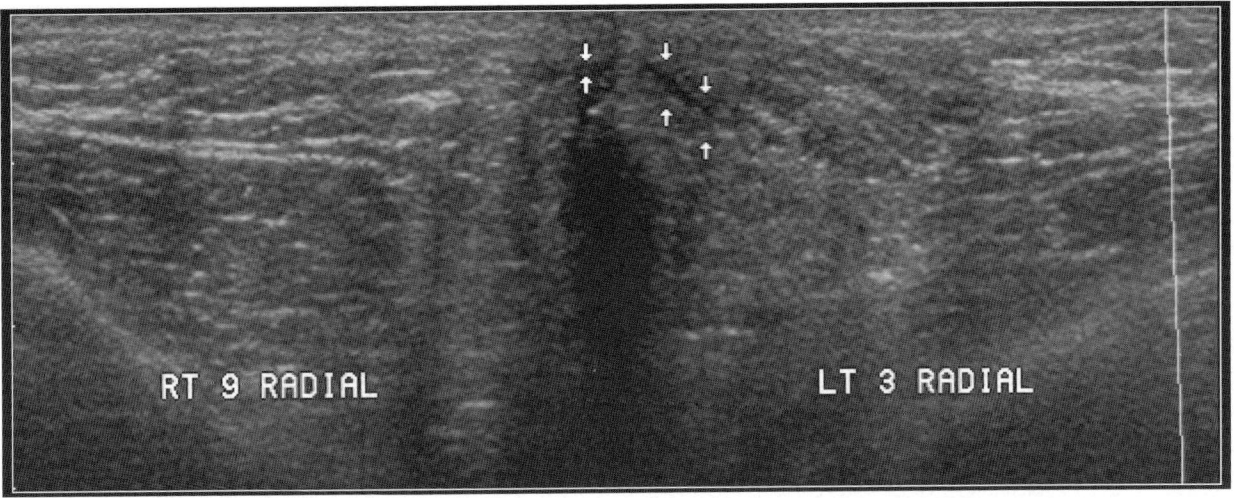

FIGURE 4–80 These images are obtained from the same patient shown in Fig. 4–79 using the two-handed compression technique. Note that the palpable nodule no longer has the sonographic appearance of a solid nodule and that individual ducts are now demonstrable because the angle of incidence of the beam with the ducts is improved by the two-handed compression technique (Fig. 4–52). Note that there are demonstrable ducts on the right, where developments is also occurring, but at a less advanced stage than on the left side. Asymmetric development of subareolar ducts is relatively common.

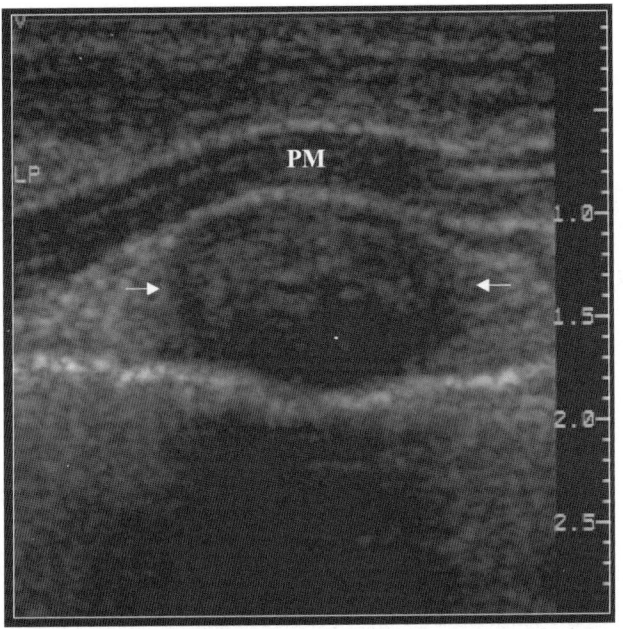

A

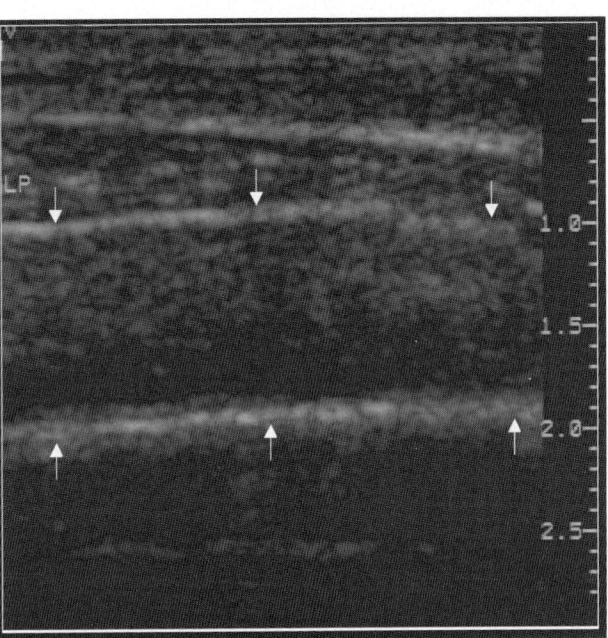

B

FIGURE 4–81 A: This thin, small-breasted patient presented with a palpable lump in the far medial right breast. Simultaneous palpation and scanning showed the lump to be caused by a prominent noncalcified costal cartilage. Inexperienced sonographers could mistake the short-axis view of a costal cartilage for a solid mass. However, this mistake should not be made because the costal cartilage lies within the chest wall musculature deep to the pectoralis muscle *(PM)*, not within the breast. **B:** The long-axis view through the costal cartilage *(arrows)* shows it to have a tubular or rectangular appearance in this axis. It appears ovoid and simulates a solid nodule only when scanned in its short axis.

Lymphatic System of the Breast

Intramammary lymph nodes are also of sonographic importance. These nodes may cause either mammographic or palpable abnormalities. The classic mammographic appearance of a well-circumscribed, isodense, ovoid or lobulated nodule with a fatty hilum is definitive. Nodules that fulfill these mammographic criteria do not require sonography for further evaluation. However, many intramammary lymph nodes are either not mammographically classic or are palpable but not mammographically visible. Still other intramammary lymph nodes are incidental findings. The classic sonographic appearance of intramammary lymph nodes is just as definitively benign American College of Radiology Breast Imaging Reporting and Data System (BIRADS) category 2, as is the

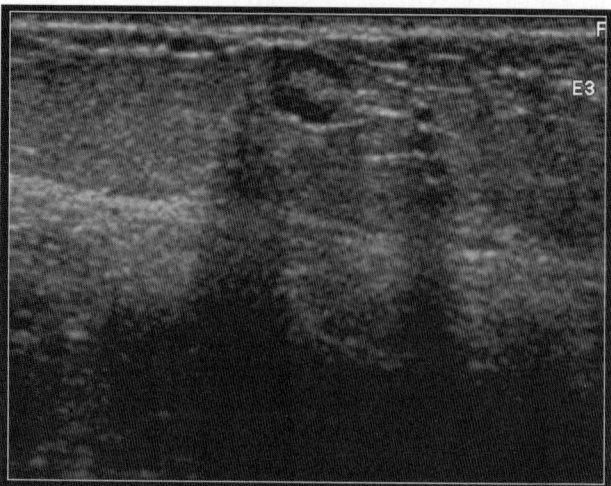

FIGURE 4–83 This figure demonstrates a normal intramammary lymph node shown in its short axis. Like the long-axis view, the normal lymph node has a sonographic appearance similar to a miniature kidney. The cortex is hypoechoic and C shaped; the thin echogenic capsule encompasses the cortex, but not the hilar opening; and the hilum is hyperechoic.

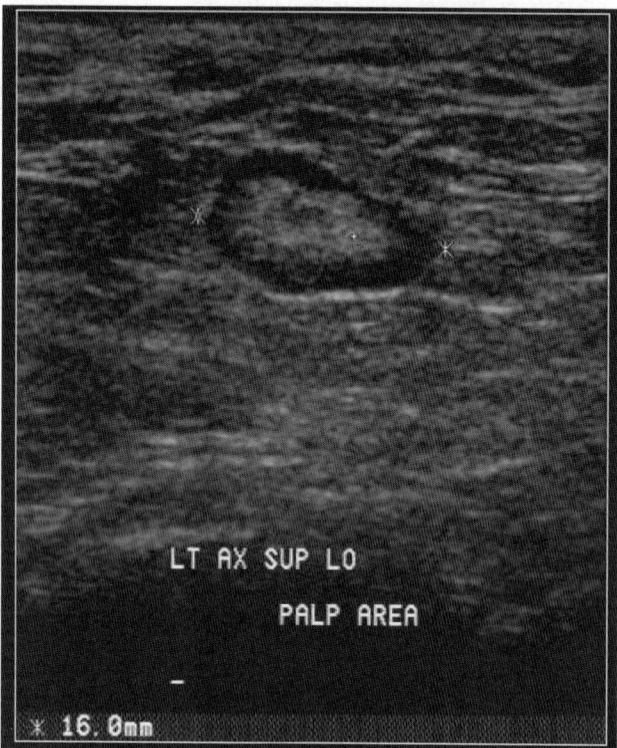

FIGURE 4–82 This figure shows a normal intramammary lymph node shown in its long axis. Note that it has a sonographic appearance similar to a miniature kidney. Normal intramammary lymph nodes are elliptical or gently lobulated in shape; are wider than tall; are encompassed in a thin, echogenic capsule (except at the hilum); and have a hyperechoic hilum. The sonographic appearance of a normal intramammary lymph node is just as characteristically benign as is its mammographic appearance. Size criteria are not as valuable as morphologic evaluation. Lymph nodes that have a maximum diameter larger than 1 cm are not abnormal. However, lymph nodes that have asymmetrically thickened cortex, a round shape, or a smallest diameter greater than 1 cm are more worrisome. Sonographic evaluation of lymph nodes is discussed in greater detail in Chapter 19.

classic mammographic appearance, and therefore obviates the need for biopsy or further imaging evaluation. An intramammary lymph node appears sonographically as an ovoid or gently lobulated, isoechoic, or hypoechoic solid nodule that contains a hyperechoic hilum or mediastinum encompassed by a thin, echogenic capsule (except at the opening of the hilum). In essence, the normal intramammary lymph node has a sonographic appearance similar to a normal kidney (Figs. 4–82 and 4–83). The hilum may be larger and the cortex thinner than usual in nodes with atrophy without being worrisome (Fig. 4–84). However, uniformly or eccentrically thickened cortex or convex indentation of the hilum from the periphery is worrisome. The range of normal sonographic appearances of lymph nodes is discussed in greater detail in Chapter 19.

Most intramammary lymph nodes lie in the upper outer quadrant of the breast, especially within the axillary segment of the breast, but they may occur anywhere in the breast. In our experience, the second most common location is far medially, superficial to the chest wall, in a location that parallels the internal mammary lymph nodes (Fig. 4–85). These superficial medial lymph nodes are more frequently shown sonographically than mammographically because they are so close to the chest wall that mammographic compression is unable to pull them far enough from the chest wall to make them mammographically visible.

Internal mammary lymph nodes lie along the deep edge of the sternum and lie in a chain that parallels the in-

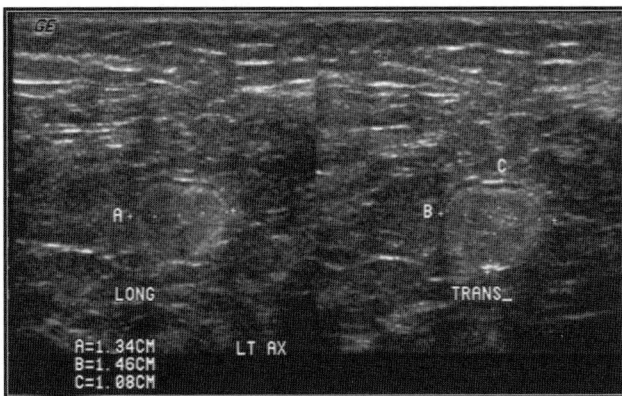

FIGURE 4–84 Lymph nodes that are enlarged by a prominent fatty hilum are also within the normal range. The cortex is thinned diffusely and less echogenic than in lymph nodes with smaller hila. The hilum tends to become less echogenic because the large amount of fat within it causes wider separation of the medullary cords and sinusoids, which are the source of the echoes within the hilum. Such nodes are variants of normal but are sometimes classified as lipogranulomatous. Lymphatic drainage enters through the cortex and drains through the hilum. Thus, metastases affect the cortex first, and only affect the hilum indirectly when metastatic deposits within the cortex thicken it enough to compress the hilum. Enlarged lymph nodes with thin cortex may harbor microscopic disease, but contain no gross metastatic deposits.

ternal mammary artery and veins on each side in the first three intercostal spaces. They drain the medial breast and may be a site for lymph node metastases for medially located breast cancer. Internal mammary lymph nodes may also be the site of metastases when lateral breast lesions have metastasized to axillary lymph nodes so extensively that axillary drainage becomes obstructed, forcing collateral lymphatic flow medially.

It is generally believed that normal internal mammary lymph nodes are not sonographically demonstrable and that only abnormally enlarged internal mammary lymph nodes can be demonstrated sonographically. This is not entirely true. Normal internal mammary lymph nodes can be seen in some patients, usually medial to the vessels and along the superior edge of the inferior cartilage in the interspace (Fig. 4–86), but much less often and reliably than can axillary and internal mammary lymph nodes. Color Doppler demonstration of the internal mammary vessels is helpful in identifying the internal mammary lymph nodes.

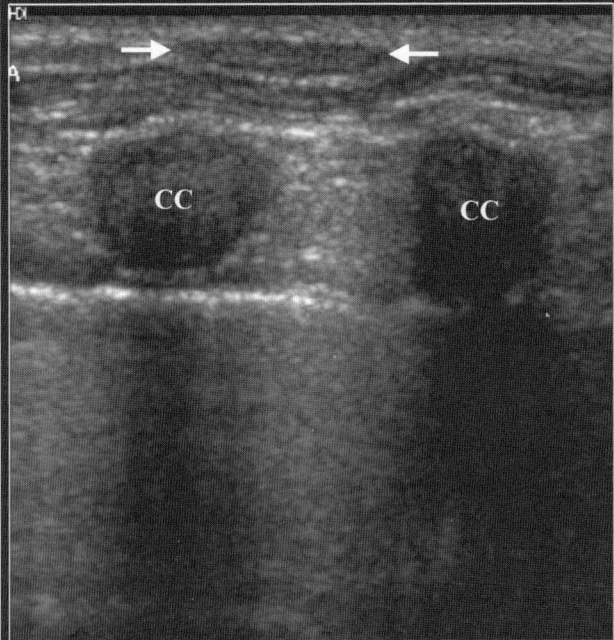

FIGURE 4–85 This medial "superficial" lymph node *(arrows)* presented as a palpable lump in a thin, small-breasted patient. Such palpable medial lymph nodes, although not common, are more frequently demonstrated sonographically than they are mammographically because they lie too close to the chest wall to be projected into breast tissue with routine mammographic compression. CC, costal cartilages.

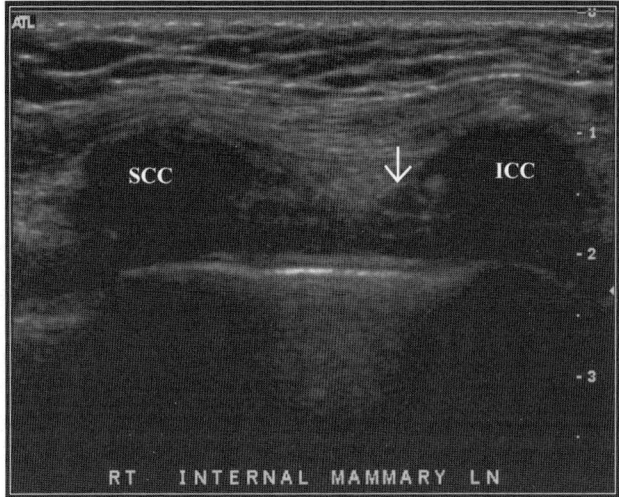

FIGURE 4–86 This is a normal internal mammary lymph node *(arrow)* shown in the longitudinal plane in a patient with no sonographic or mammographic abnormalities. Normal internal mammary lymph nodes are routinely smaller than axillary lymph nodes and are seldom more than 5 mm in diameter. It has been said that normal internal mammary lymph nodes are never visible. This not true. However, it is true that demonstration of internal mammary lymph nodes is less consistently achieved than is demonstration of axillary and intramammary lymph nodes and requires the highest-quality sonographic equipment. We have found that speckle artifact prevents demonstration of internal mammary lymph nodes and that techniques that suppress speckle, such as real-time compounding (shown above) and coded harmonics, greatly improve the success rate of sonographic demonstration. We have most consistently found internal mammary lymph nodes along the deep and upper surface of the more inferiorly located costal cartilage *(ICC)*. SCC, superior costal cartilage.

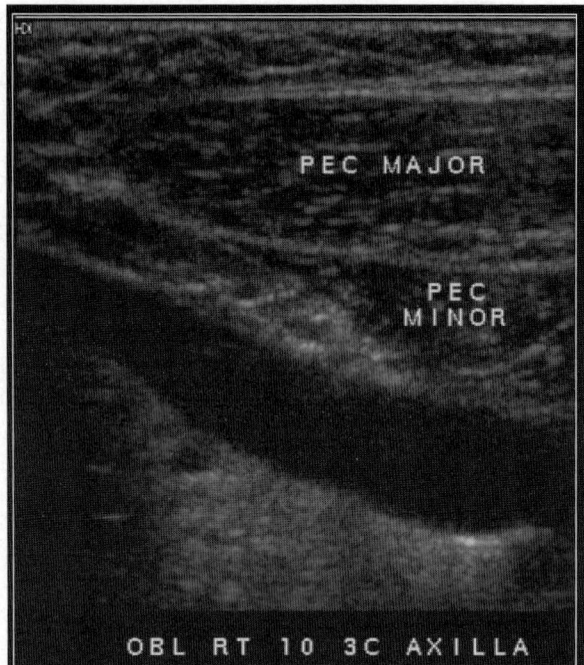

FIGURE 4–87 The pectoralis muscles are shown in the radial plane. The pectoralis minor muscle lies deep to the pectoralis major muscle and is smaller. The pectoralis minor is the landmark by which lymph node level is determined. Lymph nodes that lie peripheral to the edge of the pectoralis minor are considered level 1, or low, lymph nodes. Nodes that lie posterior to the pectoralis minor muscle are considered level 2, or midlevel, nodes, and nodes that lie above or proximal to the pectoralis minor are considered level 3, or high, lymph nodes. Sonography readily demonstrates level 1 lymph nodes. Level 2 lymph nodes are also usually well shown. Level 3 nodes, however, can be very difficult to demonstrate sonographically.

Evaluation of intramammary lymph nodes is important for the sonographer because they may cause both palpable and mammographic abnormalities that require sonographic evaluation. Evaluation of regional lymph nodes for metastases has become more important for staging because abnormal-appearing regional nodes can undergo ultrasound-guided biopsy and because of ultrasound's role in guiding sentinel lymph node biopsies. The pectoralis minor muscle is an important landmark for determining the anatomic level of visualized lymph nodes (Fig. 4–87). Sonographic evaluation of intramammary and regional lymph nodes is discussed in greater detail in Chapter 19.

Doppler Evaluation of Breast Vasculature

Superficial mammary veins are sometimes visible sonographically as anechoic tubular structures coursing roughly parallel to the skin when scanned with a very light touch. These superficial veins are especially prominent when vascularity of the breast is increased during pregnancy or lactation or by inflammation of any etiology. However, because of their superficial location and low turgor, superficial veins are easily collapsed, and thus obscured, using standard scanning technique. The more deeply located mammary veins are seldom seen without the aid of color Doppler.

A sonographically visible vein may be important to distinguish from a dilated, fluid-filled mammary duct or a dilated superficial lymphatic channel. This task is read-

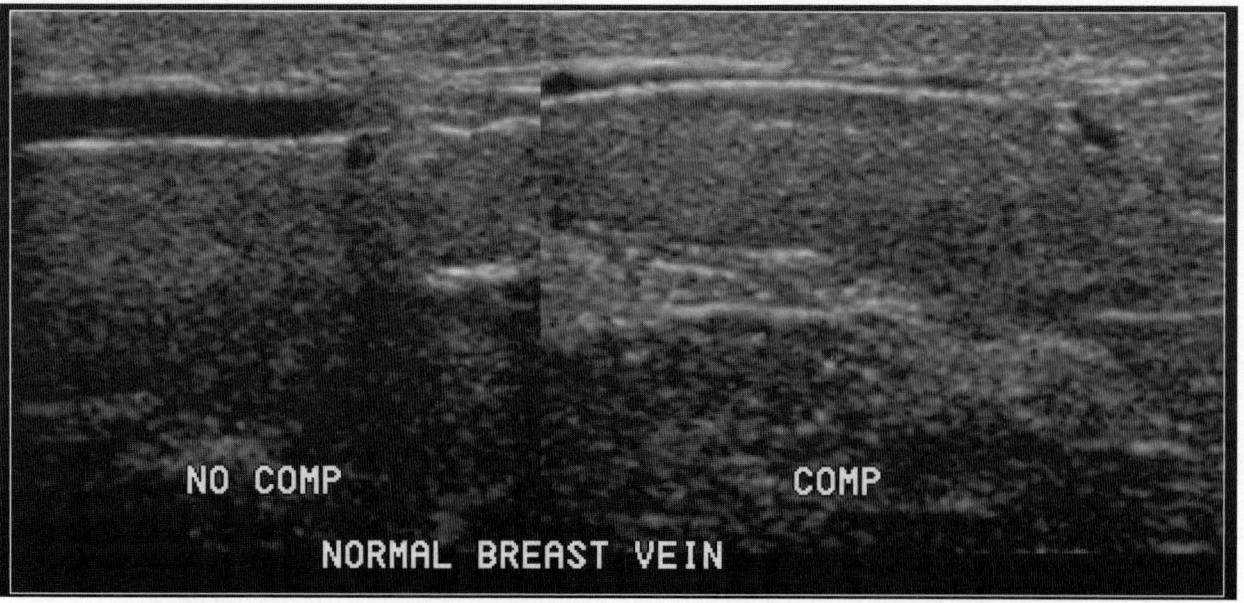

A

FIGURE 4–88 A: This figure shows a long-axis view of a superficial vein. The main significance is that the vein can be confused for a dilated duct (**left**). However, the superficial veins are very soft and easy to collapse completely with compression (**right**), even in comparison to ectatic ducts. In fact, they are so easily compressed that they are completely collapsed by routine scan pressures and therefore are seldom well seen unless very light scan pressure is used.

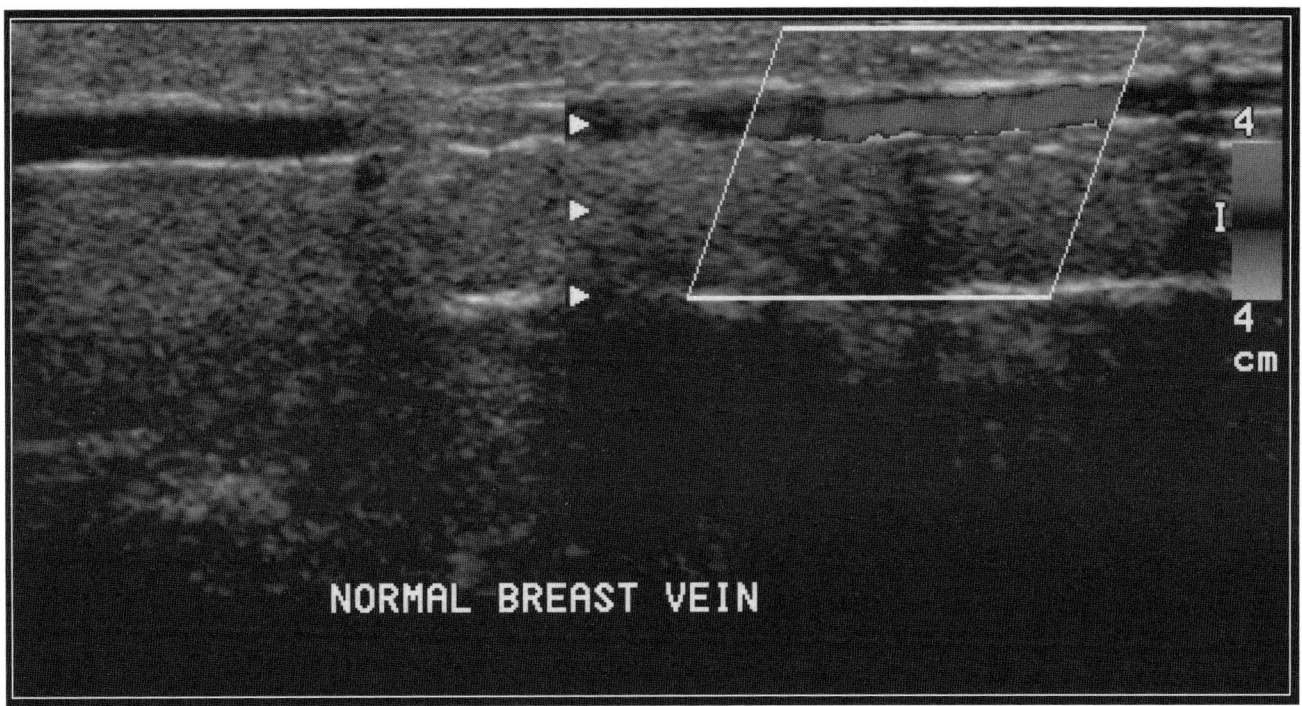

NORMAL BREAST VEIN

B

FIGURE 4–88 *(continued)* **B:** Color Doppler is helpful in distinguishing a normal superficial vein from an ectatic duct. However, it is important to scan with a steady, light scan pressure when making this distinction. Varying the scan pressure can cause secretions within ectatic ducts to move within the ducts and can cause a color signal that could be confused with flow in a vein.

ily accomplished using compression and color Doppler (Fig. 4–88).

A thorough knowledge of the vascular anatomy of the breast is very important to surgeons and to investigators using continuous-wave Doppler without image guidance. However, color Doppler–guided spectral analysis has allowed us to evaluate small arterial branches within the lesion and immediately surrounding tissues without having to know the artery from which these vessels arose. Thus, knowledge of the arterial anatomy has become less important to breast imagers who use color Doppler for guidance.

SUMMARY

A thorough understanding of breast anatomy and the broad spectrum of fibrocystic and benign proliferative change form the basis for evaluating breast pathology. Furthermore, being able to identify the normal anatomic structures of the breast on ultrasound is important to differentiate between the various normal tissues of the breast and the lesions that arise within these tissues. A thorough understanding of sonographic breast anatomy prevents the misclassification of normal anatomic structures as signifi-

cant pathology that would require biopsy. Finally, it is important to understand how the type of background breast tissue affects the sensitivity of breast ultrasound for certain types of pathology and how that might affect the need for additional evaluation or biopsy.

SUGGESTED READINGS

Bassett LW, Kimme-Smith C. Breast sonography: technique, equipment, and normal anatomy. *Semin Ultrasound CT MR* 1989; 10(2):82–89.

Blend R, et al. Parenchymal patterns of the breast defined by real time ultrasound. *Eur J Cancer Prev* 1995;4(4):293–298.

Gordenne W. Radiological anatomy of the breast. *J Belge Radiol* 1995;78(1):1–5.

Gordon PB, Gilks B. Sonographic appearance of normal intramammary lymph nodes. *J Ultrasound Med* 1988;7(10):545–548.

Gozzi G, et al. Causes of attenuation of the sound waves in neoplasms of the breast: histologic and echographic correlation study. *Radiol Med* (Torino) 1986;72(4):195–198.

Hefel L, et al. Internal mammary vessels: anatomical and clinical considerations. *Br J Plast Surg* 1995;48(8):527–532.

Malini S, Smith EO, Goldzieher JW. Measurement of breast volume by ultrasound during normal menstrual cycles with oral contraceptive use. *Obstet Gynecol* 1985;66(4):538–541.

Moriggl B, Steinlechner M. Ultrasono-anatomy for evaluation of the local lymphatic groups of the mamma. *Surg Radiol Anat* 1994; 16(1):77–85.

Ozdemir H, et al. Parasternal sonography of the internal mammary lymphatics in breast cancer: CT correlation. *Eur J Radiol* 1995; 19(2):114–117.

Picker RH, Fulton AJ. Maturational and physiological changes in the female breast. *Semin Ultrasound* 1982;3(3):34–37.

Scatarige JC, et al. Parasternal sonography of the internal mammary vessels: technique, normal anatomy, and lymphadenopathy. *Radiology* 1989;172(2):453–457.

Schneck CD, Lehman DA. Sonographic anatomy of the breast. *Semin Ultrasound* 1982;3(3):13–33.

Smith WL, Erenberg A, Nowak A. Imaging evaluation of the human nipple during breast-feeding. *Am J Dis Child* 1988;142(1): 76–78.

Spencer GM, Rubens DJ, Roach DJ. Hypoechoic fat: a sonographic pitfall. *AJR Am J Roentgenol* 1995;164(5):1277–1280.

Teboul M. Anatomy of the breast. In: *Atlas of ductal echography of the breast: the introduction of anatomic intelligence into the breast. Imaging.* Teboul M, Halliwell M, eds. Cambridge, MA: Blackwell Science, 1995:49–82.

Venta LA, et al. Sonographic evaluation of the breast. *Radiographics* 1994;14(1):29–50.

Yang WT, et al. Ultrasonographic demonstration of normal axillary lymph nodes: a learning curve. *J Ultrasound Med* 1995;14:823–827.

5

TARGETED INDICATION: PALPABLE ABNORMALITY

CORRELATING CLINICAL FINDINGS WITH ULTRASOUND FINDINGS

Diagnostic breast ultrasound (BUS) can be used to evaluate palpable abnormalities when the mammogram is dense and negative, when mammography shows probably benign findings, such as circumscribed nodules, and when mammographic findings are not specific. In general, BUS has not been used for diagnosis when the mammographic findings are probably or definitely malignant, but we are using ultrasound more, even in these cases for purposes of determining the extent of malignant disease and guiding interventional procedures.

In the United States, most patients with clinical abnormalities will have undergone mammographic evaluation before being considered for sonographic evaluation of palpable masses. In such cases, evaluation of the mammographic density of the tissue in the vicinity of the palpable lump is important. In a breast that is completely fatty, there will be little chance of the mammogram missing a significant lesion; therefore, there will be very little chance that sonography would add additional useful information, regardless of the position within the breast of the palpable abnormality (Fig. 5–1). The one exception to this rule is the palpable nodule that is pea-sized or smaller. To be palpable, such small lesions have to be very superficial in location. With current film-screen mammographic techniques, the skin and superficial portions of the subcutaneous fat may be "burned out" and difficult to evaluate mammographically. Thus, even in a breast that is entirely fatty on mammograms, we sonographically evaluate palpable nodules that are pea-sized or smaller, but not larger lumps. It is well known that lesions are more likely to be missed in mammographically dense breasts than in fatty breasts and that sonography is most likely to detect those findings missed by mammog-

raphy when the entire breast is composed of mammographically dense tissue. Thus, we should be aggressive about performing sonography to evaluate palpable abnormalities in women who have dense tissue on mammograms (Figs. 5–2 and 5–3).

The entire breast need not be radiographically dense in order for ultrasound to be helpful. There need only be enough mammographically dense tissue in the immediate vicinity of the palpable lump that it could obscure the cause of the palpable lump. For example, consider a patient with a lump in the upper outer quadrant of the breast. If there is fatty tissue in the lower outer, lower inner, and upper inner quadrants, but there is mammographically dense tissue in the upper outer quadrant, there is a high probability that the patient will benefit from ultrasound. On the other hand, if the palpable lump were in the lower inner quadrant, which is entirely fatty on mammograms, ultrasound would not add additional useful information (Fig. 5–4).

When the indication for BUS is a palpable abnormality, the precise location of the palpable abnormality is of utmost importance. An attempt should be made to palpate the lesion both before and during scanning of the lesion. For larger lesions, simultaneous palpation and scanning of the lesion is possible. This technique usually involves rolling a finger over the lesion and under the probe while centering the probe over the palpable abnormality (Fig. 5–5). For smaller palpable lesions or in cases in which breast tissue is very firm, rolling a finger under the probe while scanning the lesion may not be possible. When the examining finger is under the transducer, the ends of the transducer may not be in contact with the skin. In such a case, a better technique is to "trap" the palpable lesion between the index and middle fingers and then scan by placing the transducer longitudinally between the fingers (Fig. 5–6).

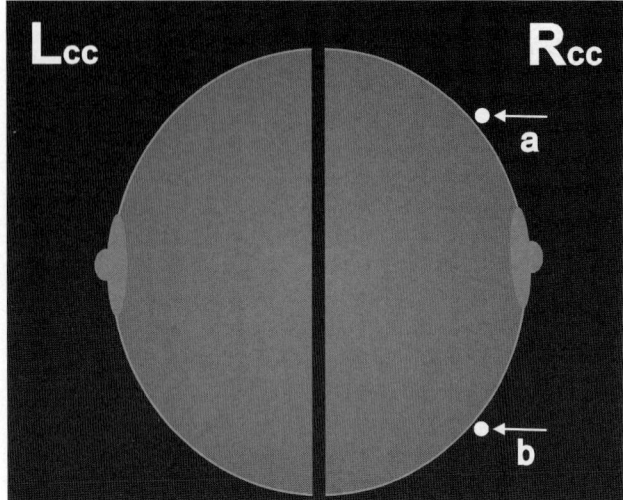

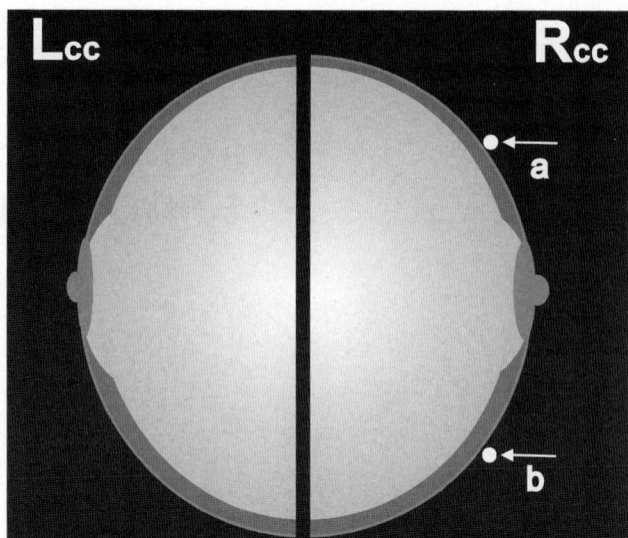

FIGURE 5–1 The density of mammographic tissue should be taken into account when deciding whether to perform ultrasound for evaluation of a palpable abnormality. When the breast is entirely fatty, as it is in this illustration, regardless of whether the lump is located laterally (*a*) or medially within the breast (*b*), there is little chance that sonography will show something missed by mammography. The lump must be caused by either a fat lobule or a benign lipoma. Thus, there will be little value to performing sonography.

FIGURE 5–2 The density of mammographic tissue should be taken into account when deciding whether to perform ultrasound for evaluation of a palpable abnormality. When the breast is entirely composed of dense tissue, there is a high probability that dense tissues are obscuring a lesion, and aggressive diagnostic ultrasound should be employed in evaluating the palpable abnormality, regardless of whether the lump is located laterally (*a*) or medially within the breast (*b*).

For very small lesions, trapping the lesion between two fingers may not even be possible. In these instances, a straightened paper clip can be rolled over the palpable lesion and under the probe in place of a finger (Fig. 5–7). The paper clip can be used to palpate indirectly and usually generates a shadow or ring-down artifact deep to it that in-

dicates its exact position relative to the suspected palpable abnormality (Fig 5–8). Recently, we switched from an opened paper clip to an empty metal ballpoint pen ink cartridge for three reasons. First, paper clips sometimes have rough ends that scratch the patient. Second, the empty ballpoint cartridge is larger and contains air that creates a

(text continued on page 113)

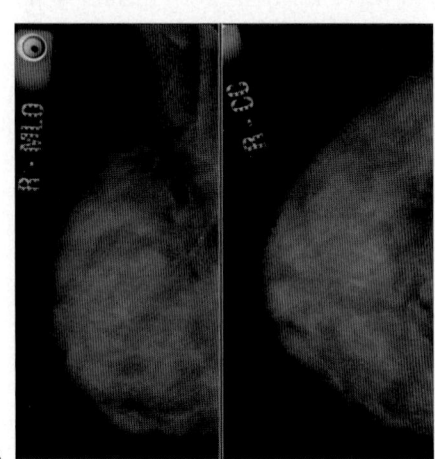

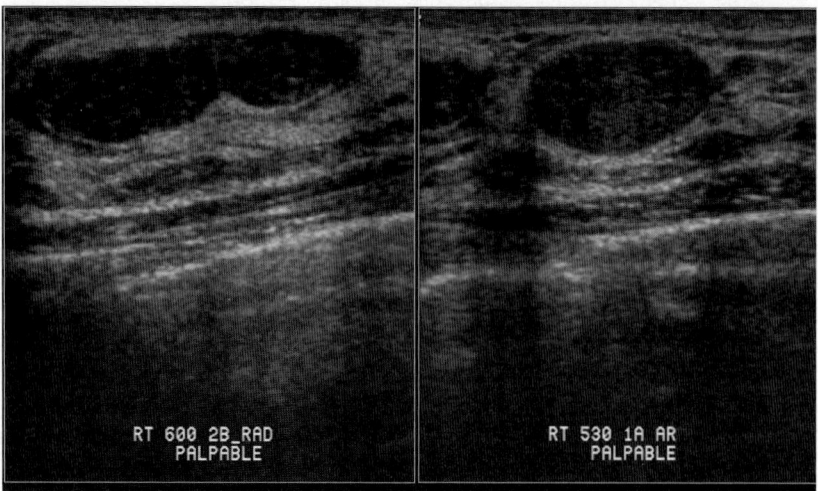

A   B

FIGURE 5–3 A: This mammogram shows a breast that is BIRADS density category 4 (>75% of breast volume is composed of dense tissues). The patient presented with two separate palpable lumps inferiorly in the right breast. The mammogram is normal, but because mammographically dense breast tissue can obscure masses of equal breast density, the patient underwent targeted sonography. **B:** Sonography of both palpable lumps showed them to correspond to BIRADS category 3 solid nodule, compatible with fibroadenomas. Neither solid nodule was shown mammographically because they were both obscured by the mammographically dense tissue that surrounds them.

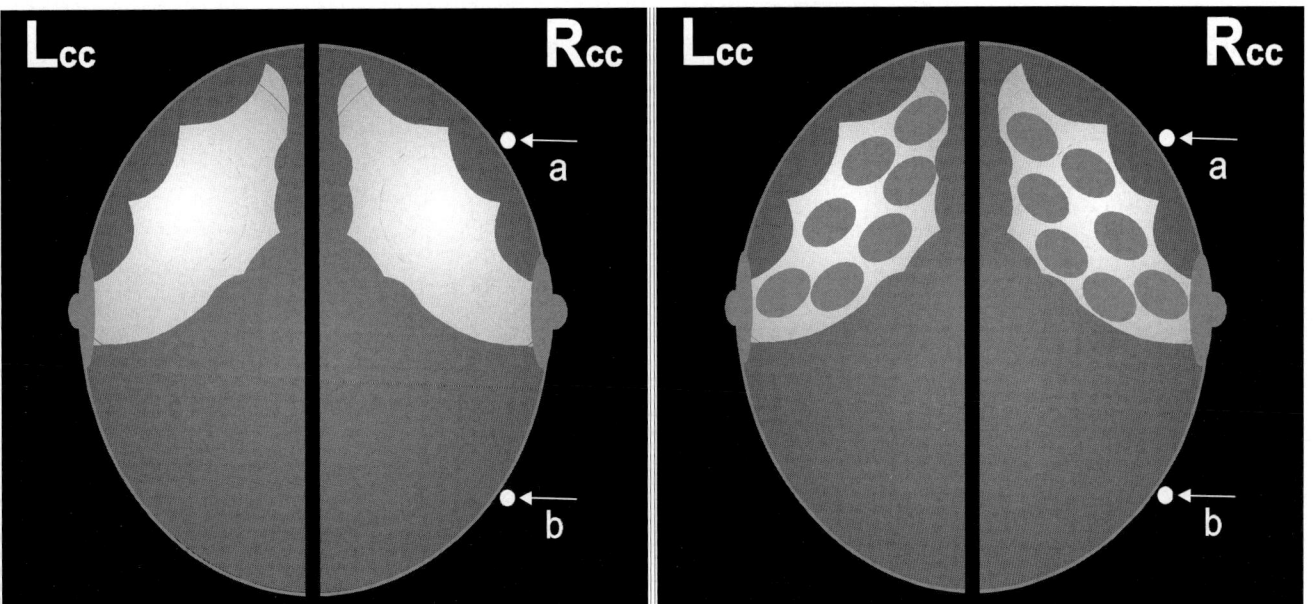

FIGURE 5–4 The breast density in the immediate vicinity of the palpable abnormality should be assessed in determining the need for sonography. Most patients do not have purely fatty or purely dense tissue on their mammograms. Most patients have a mixture of dense and fatty elements, with the dense elements most likely to lie within the upper outer quadrants, as shown in this illustration. In such cases, correlating the location of the lump with the distribution of dense tissue is critical in determining whether to perform ultrasound for evaluation of a palpable lump. In this case, a lump occurring in the location marked by *(a)* should be evaluated sonographically because dense tissue in the immediate vicinity could obscure a lesion mammographically. On the other hand, a lump in the location marked by *(b)* would be unlikely to benefit from sonography because there is only fat in the immediately vicinity and therefore little chance of sonography showing findings missed by mammography.

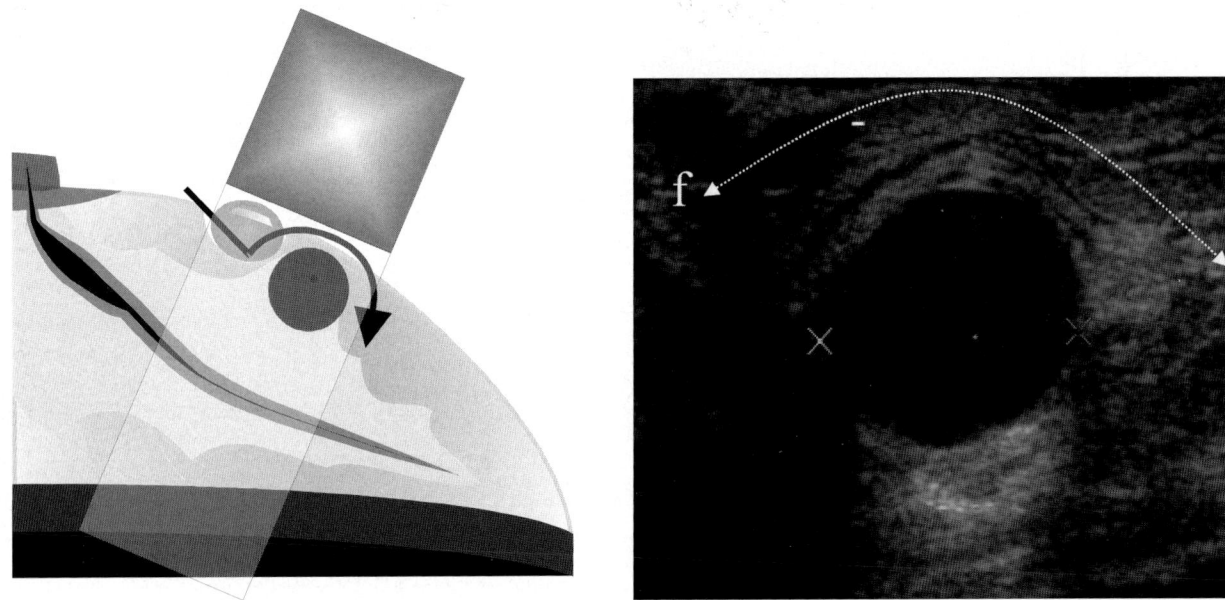

FIGURE 5–5 **A:** Palpating the lump while simultaneously scanning is critical in cases in which the palpable abnormality appears to be caused by normal breast tissues or definitively benign lesions such as simple cysts. For relatively large palpable abnormalities in soft, large breasts, it is usually possible to palpate the lesion with an index finger while scanning. **B:** That this definitively benign simple cyst is the cause of the palpable lump for which the patient presented is being documented by rolling the index finger *(f)* under the transducer and across the lesion *(arrow)* while simultaneously scanning.

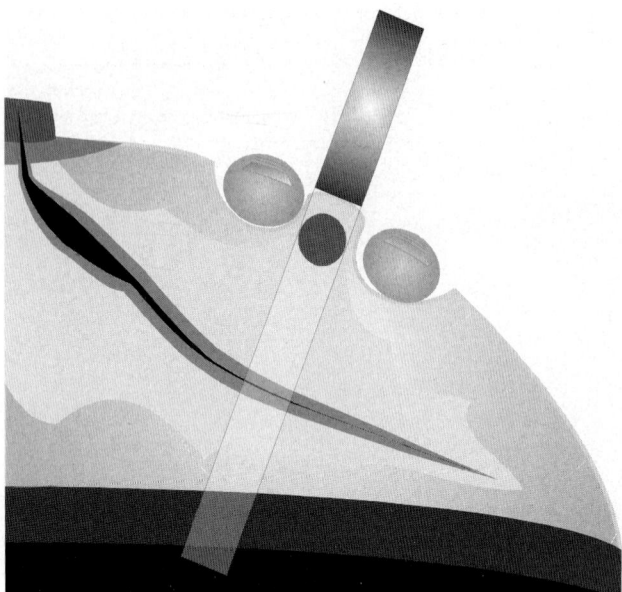

FIGURE 5–6 When the palpable lump is smaller or when the breast is smaller or firmer, it may not be possible to scan while palpating the lesion with the index finger because the ends of the transducer may lose contact with the skin. In such cases, the technique for simultaneous scanning and palpation is done with the lump trapped between the index and middle fingers of the nonscanning hand.

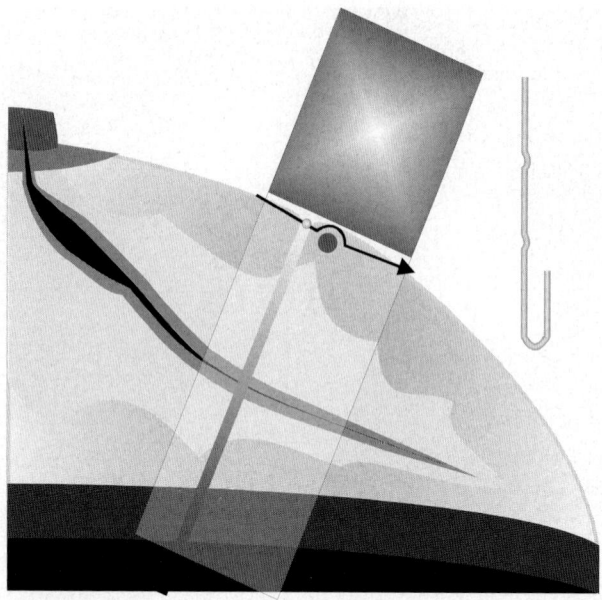

FIGURE 5–7 For very small, palpable lesions that feel pea-sized or smaller, neither rolling the index finger under the transducer nor trapping the lesion between the index and middle fingers is effective for confirming the etiology of the palpable lump. In such cases, it is usually possible to palpate the lesion with an un-folded paper clip or the empty ink cartridge from a ballpoint pen. A ring-down artifact is created that shows the location of the paper clip or ink cartridge. It is sometimes necessary to use a standoff of acoustic gel or a standoff pad when employing this technique.

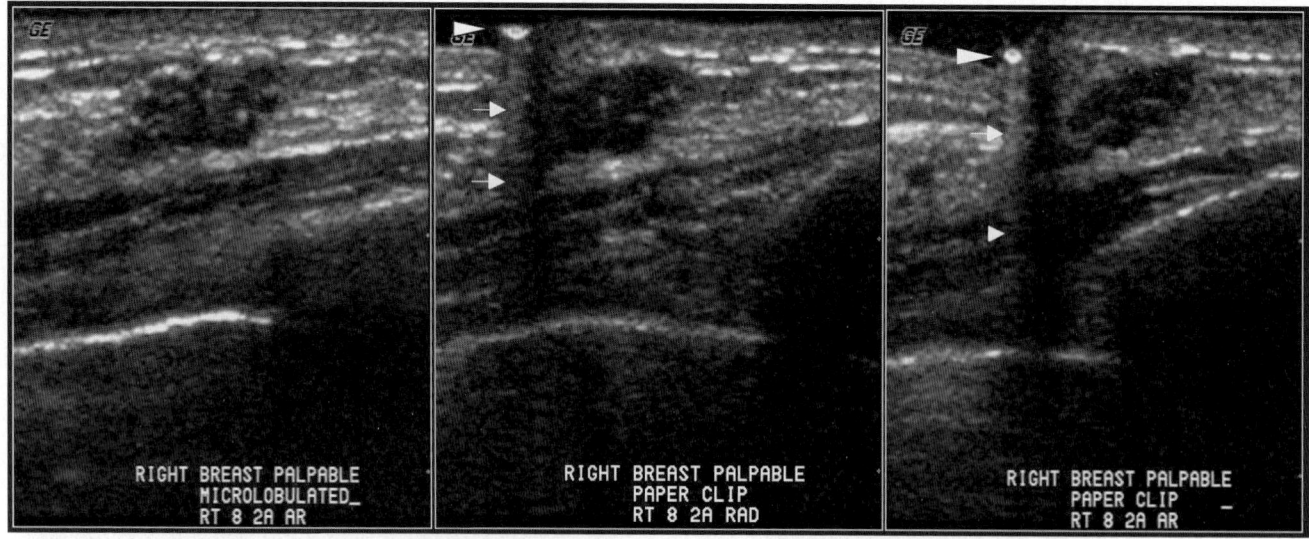

FIGURE 5–8 This palpable BB-sized lump is caused by a microlobulated solid nodule (**left**). To document this, a paper clip was used to palpate the lump while simultaneously scanning. Note that the clip *(arrowhead)* is better seen in the **right** image, for which a slightly thicker gel stand-off was used. The paper clip, which is closer to the skin in the **middle** image, appears wider and elliptical in shape because of near-field volume averaging. In the **right** image, with the clip slightly deeper within the field of view, the paper clip appears round. Note the faint ring-down artifacts created by the clip in the **middle** and **right** images *(arrows)*.

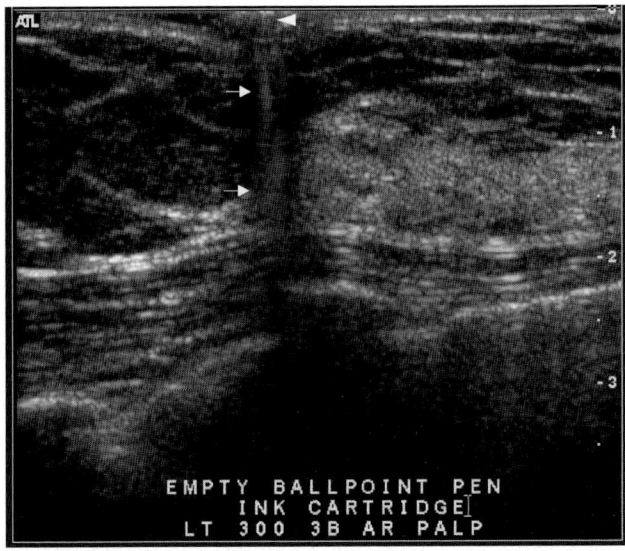

FIGURE 5–9 This patient's palpable lump is caused by a hyperechoic fibroglandular ridge. That the ridge is the cause of the lump is being documented by palpating it with an empty ballpoint ink cartridge while simultaneously scanning it. Near-field volume averaging interferes with demonstration of the cartridge *(arrowhead)*, but we know where the cartridge is because of the ring-down artifact created by the air within the cartridge.

better ring-down artifact. Third, the ballpoint ink cartridge is less flexible and better for indirectly palpating the lesion (Fig. 5–9).

Palpating while scanning the lump is important. One of the main goals of BUS is to demonstrate that the cause of a palpable or mammographic abnormality is definitively benign and does not require biopsy. However, the definitively benign causes of palpable breast abnormalities are so common that simply demonstrating that they exist in the same quadrant of the breast is insufficient to prove that they are causing the palpable abnormality. The two most common sonographically demonstrable, definitively benign causes of palpable breast abnormalities are purely hyperechoic interlobular stromal fibrous tissue and simple cysts. Fibrous tissue is present in some amount in most patients and will also be present in the same quadrant as palpable abnormalities in most patients. Simply demonstrating that fibrous tissue exists in the same quadrant as a palpable abnormality does not prove that it causes the lump. First, the technique of simultaneous palpation and scanning must be used to show that the fibrous tissue does, indeed, correspond to the palpable abnormality. Then, one must exclude the presence of any cystic or solid mass or nodule in the region as the cause of palpable abnormality.

Table 5–1 shows the various causes of palpable lumps as determined by simultaneous ultrasound and palpation in the last 1,867 consecutive patients seen in our department. Note that, including intramammary lymph nodes and ribs, normal structures account for most (1,214 of

TABLE 5–1 CAUSES OF PALPABLE LUMPS IN 1,867 CASES

Cause of Lump	No. of Cases	Percentage of Cases
Fibrous or fibroglandular tissue	590	32
Cysts	355	19
Fat lobules	330	18
Glandular tissue or adenosis	237	13
Fibroadenoma	185	10
Carcinoma	56	3
Lymph nodes	53	3
Miscellaneous	41	2
Rib	4	0.2

1,867, or 66%) of all palpable lumps found by patients or their referring physicians. That a lump is caused by a normal structure does not mean that the ultrasound should be considered negative.

In fact, reporting that the ultrasound is negative implies to the patient and the referring physician that we do not know the cause of the lump. It infers that we have not really solved the problem of what is causing the lump. The lack of confidence engendered by a negative ultrasound report is more likely to lead the patient or her physician to request a biopsy that usually is unnecessary. If targeted diagnostic BUS is to reach the intended goal of preventing unnecessary biopsies, more definitive reports on the cause of the palpable lump are necessary. Instead of merely reporting the results of ultrasound to be negative, clearly reporting that a normal structure (such as a fibrous ridge), not a cyst or cancer, causes the lump imbues both patients and referring physicians with more confidence that BUS has solved the problem of the palpable lump. For most patients and referring physicians, the knowledge that a normal structure gives rise to the palpable abnormality is reassuring and is more likely to dissuade them from requesting an unnecessary biopsy. Having the patient view the ultrasound monitor while simultaneously scanning and palpating the lump and pointing out its cause is even more reassuring than simply reporting the cause to the referring physician.

Two types of fibrous structures can lead to a palpable abnormality: a ridge of normal interlobular stromal fibrous elements that protrudes farther anteriorly into the softer subcutaneous fat than do the surrounding normal fibrous elements (Fig. 5–10); and an area of focal fibrosis (Fig. 5–11). Focal fibrosis has three possible etiologies: First, it can arise because surrounding tissues atrophy and regress, leaving an isolated collection of interlobular stromal fibrosis. Second, it can represent accessory breast tissue that is composed primarily of normal stromal fibrous elements

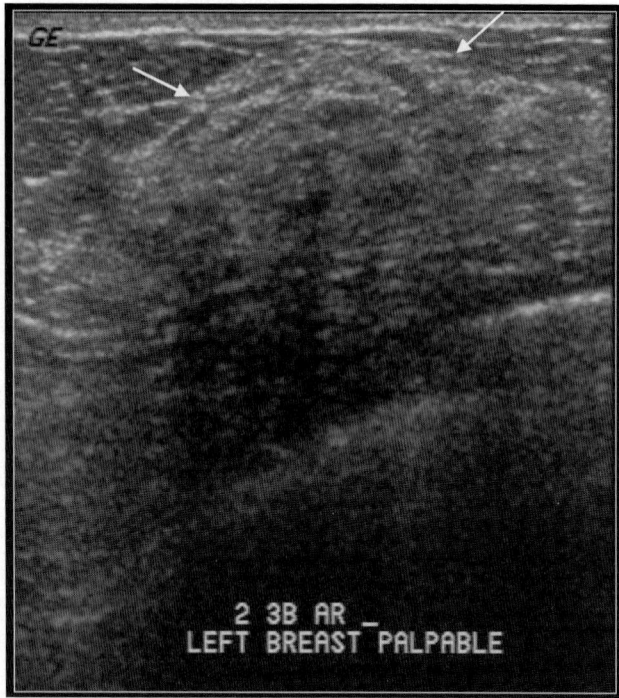

FIGURE 5–10 A hyperechoic, fibrous ridge (containing iso-echoic ducts) caused the palpable abnormality for which this patient presented. Hyperechoic, fibrous tissue is very firm to palpation and will be palpable when it protrudes farther into the soft subcutaneous fat than does surrounding tissue.

and can occur anywhere along the mammary line. Finally, it can arise as a pathologic fibrotic reaction to some unknown localized stimulus. The presence of sonographically demonstrable normal ducts or terminal ductolobular units (TDLUs) within the focal area of hyperechoic fibrous tissue favors residual normal tissue or accessory breast tissue. The presence of amorphous hyperechoic tissue without demonstrable ductal and lobular structure favors pathologic focal fibrosis.

Fibrous ridges, like mountain ridges, are often linear rather than round. When palpating across the ridge, the "steepness" of the edges is often different from one side to the other. In other words, a ridge at the 12:00 position may be very prominent when the finger moves from medial to lateral but barely perceptible when palpating from lateral to medial (Figs. 5–12 and 5–13). Such a ridge may not be palpable at all when the direction of palpation is parallel to the long axis of the ridge. For example, the ridge at 12:00 may not be palpable at all when the finger moves either superiorly or inferiorly in a craniocaudal direction. Palpation skills usually improve by correlating such palpable abnormalities with the real-time sonographic images.

Simple cysts are so common in 35- to 55 year-old patients that they must be considered variations of normal. As with palpable fibrous abnormalities, simply demonstrating that a cyst exists in the same quadrant of the breast

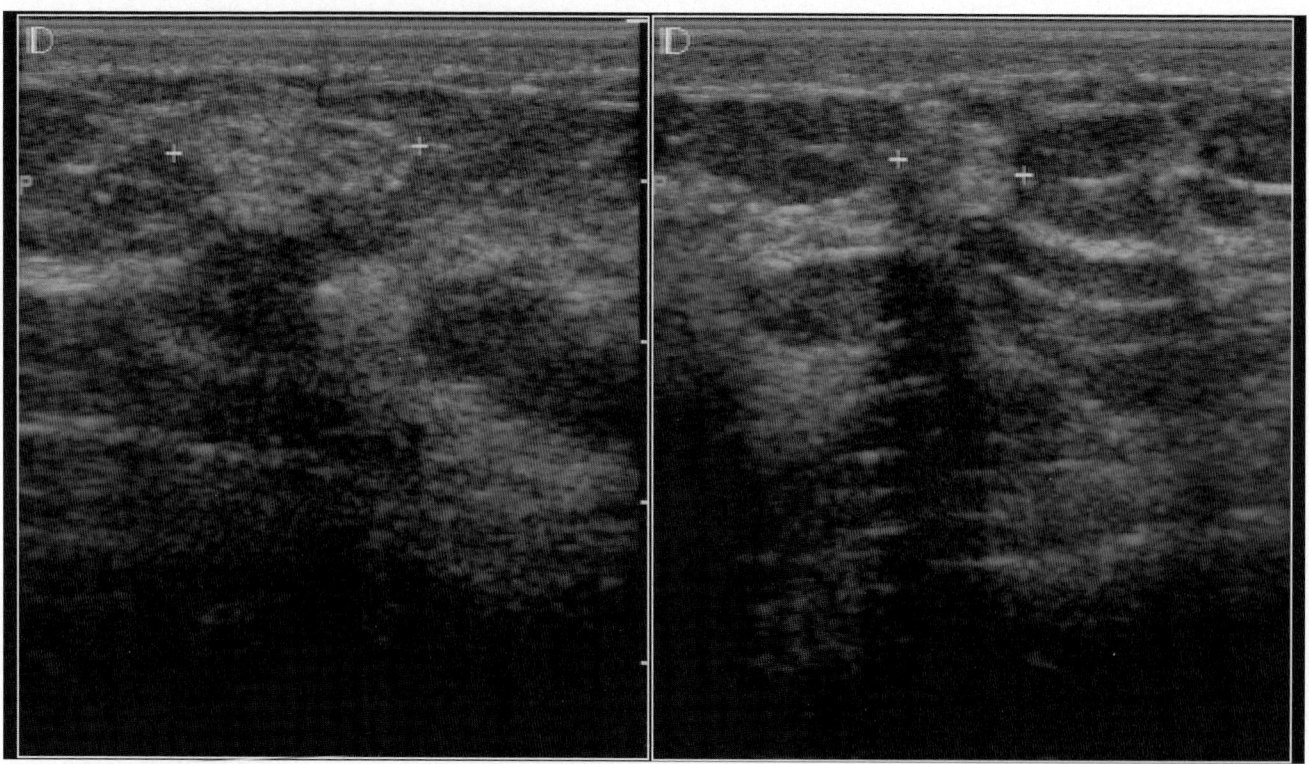

FIGURE 5–11 A focal area of hyperechoic, firm, fibrous tissue *(calipers)* surrounded by softer, isoechoic fat caused this small, palpable lump.

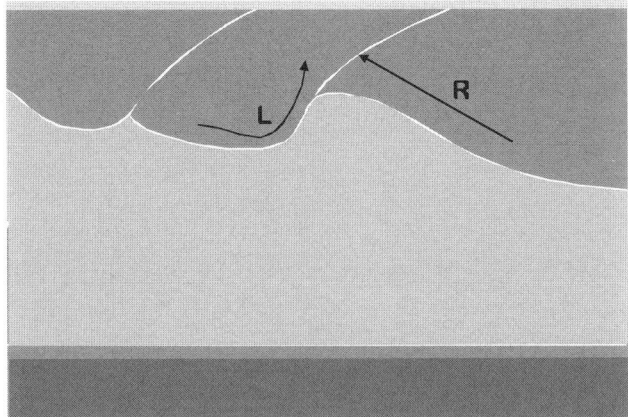

FIGURE 5–12 Fibroglandular ridges can feel different when palpated from different directions. When palpated from the right side of the image *(R)*, the ridge may not be discernible because the slope is gradual. However, when palpated from the left side of the image *(L)*, the edge of the ridge is much steeper and therefore much more apparent to palpation.

as a palpable abnormality is inadequate proof that it is the cause of a palpable abnormality. Palpating the cyst while scanning it in real time is essential in order to be sure that the cyst is, in fact, the cause of the palpable abnormality. The tissues surrounding the cyst should be assessed to exclude the possibility of an adjacent solid mass or nodule causing the palpable abnormality. A few times each year, we find a palpable solid mass lying immediately adjacent to

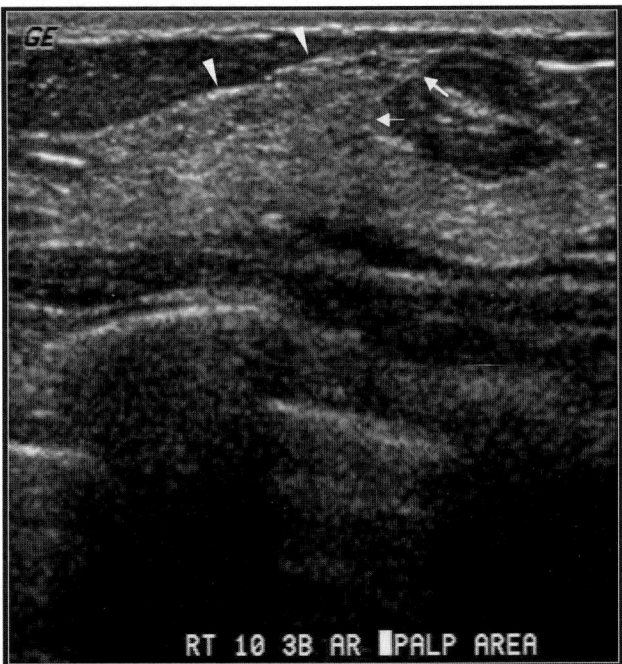

FIGURE 5–13 This ridge was palpable as a discrete lump when scanned from the right side of the image, where it has the appearance of an overhanging cliff *(arrows)*. However, when palpated from the left side of the image, the ridge did not cause a discrete lump because its slope was so gradual *(arrowheads)*.

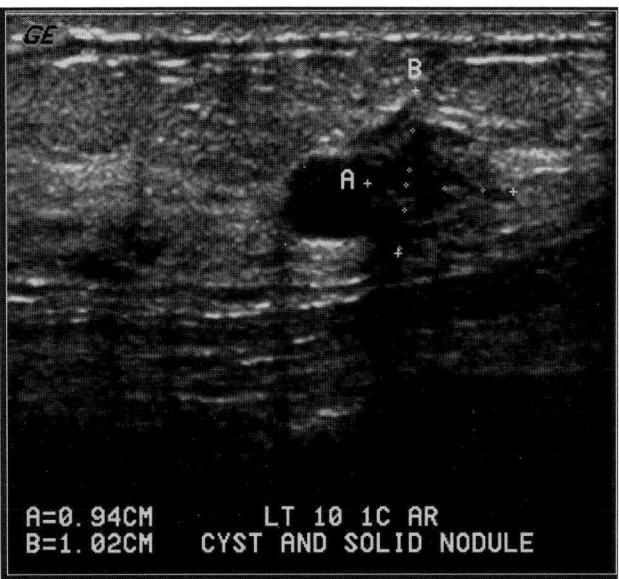

A=0.94CM   LT 10 1C AR
B=1.02CM   CYST AND SOLID NODULE

FIGURE 5–14 This patient presented with a palpable lump in the 10:00 location of the left breast. Although there is a simple cyst in this location, palpation while simultaneously scanning showed the lump to be caused by a solid nodule lying immediately adjacent to the cyst. Biopsy revealed the solid mass to be caused by intermediate-nuclear-grade ductal carcinoma *in situ*.

a nonpalpable cyst (Fig. 5–14). The danger in such cases is that the cyst will be seen, palpation during scanning will not be performed, the cyst will be assumed to be the cause of the palpable lump, and the cancer will be missed.

The firmness of cysts to palpation varies. Cysts that are firm to palpation are under tension and generally appear spherical at sonography. Confirming that such cysts are the cause of the palpable abnormality by palpating while scanning is usually quite easy (Fig. 5–15). However, many cysts are not under tension and are soft and compressible. These cysts typically appear elliptical or ovoid on sonograms—flattened in the anteroposterior direction. The flattest cysts are the least palpable. Thus, the palpability of a cyst is related to its tension, which is manifested in the anteroposterior dimension of the cyst. Many of these flat cysts are less firm to palpation than the surrounding fibrous or glandular elements. Sometimes, even cysts with very large maximum horizontal diameters are not palpable because they are soft and compressible (Fig. 5–16), whereas even very small, spherically shaped cysts are easily palpable because they are so tense (Fig. 5–17). In some cases, the layer of fibroglandular tissue that overlies or surrounds a cyst cannot be distinguished from the cyst during palpation, resulting in clinical overestimation of the size of the cyst (Fig. 5–18). Elliptically shaped, soft cysts are frequently surrounded by normal breast tissues that are firmer to palpation than the cyst. Thus, the tissues that surround the cyst, rather than the cyst itself, may be palpable.

In addition to cysts and fibrous tissue, isoechoic glandular tissue or adenosis can cause palpable abnormalities

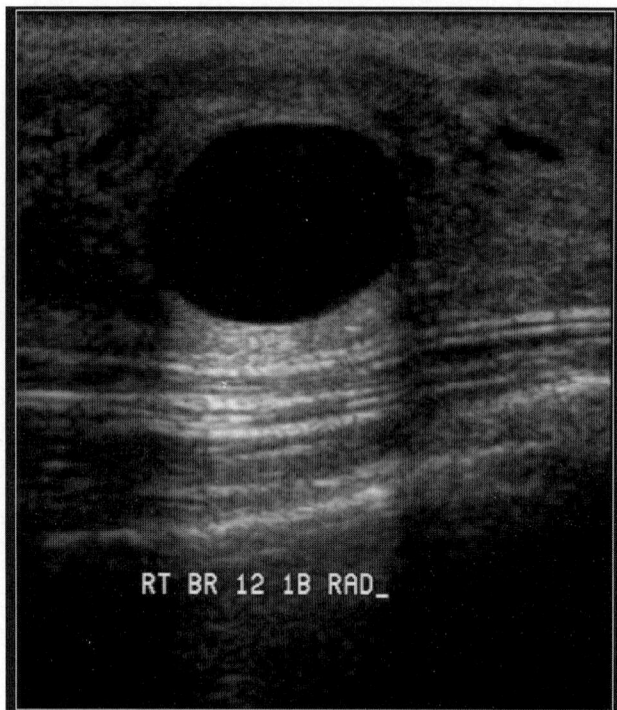

FIGURE 5–15 A spherically shaped simple cyst caused the palpable lump in this patient. The large anteroposterior dimension and spherical shape indicate that the cyst is under tension. Tense cysts are more likely than soft cysts to be tender and to require aspiration for symptomatic relief.

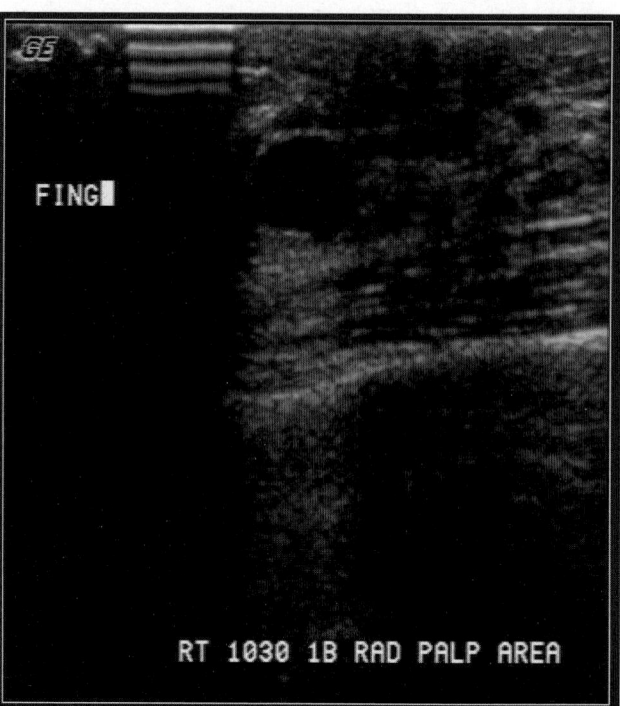

FIGURE 5–17 This small, 7-mm cyst caused a tender lump. Even though its maximum diameter was far smaller than the maximum diameter of the cyst shown in Fig. 5–16, it was clinically more evident because it was tense and noncompressible. The anteroposterior and horizontal dimensions are similar, and the lesion shape is spherical.

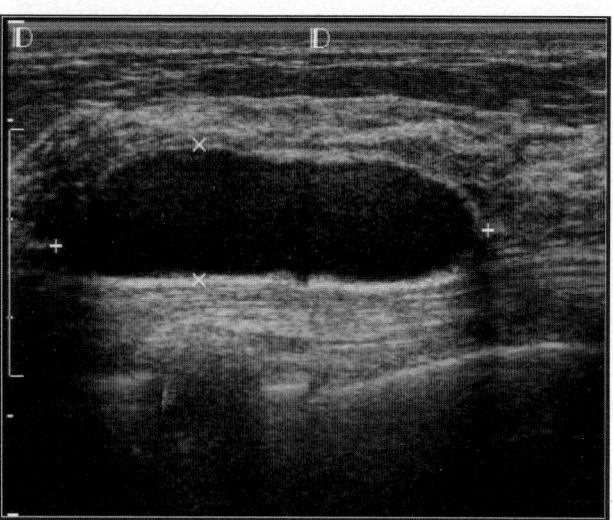

FIGURE 5–16 This large cyst was not initially palpated by either the patient or her physician. The cyst is so large in horizontal dimensions that split-screen combined images were necessary to demonstrate the entire cyst, but it is much smaller in the anteroposterior dimension, indicating that it is soft, compressible, and not under tension. Only after it was identified by sonography was it palpable.

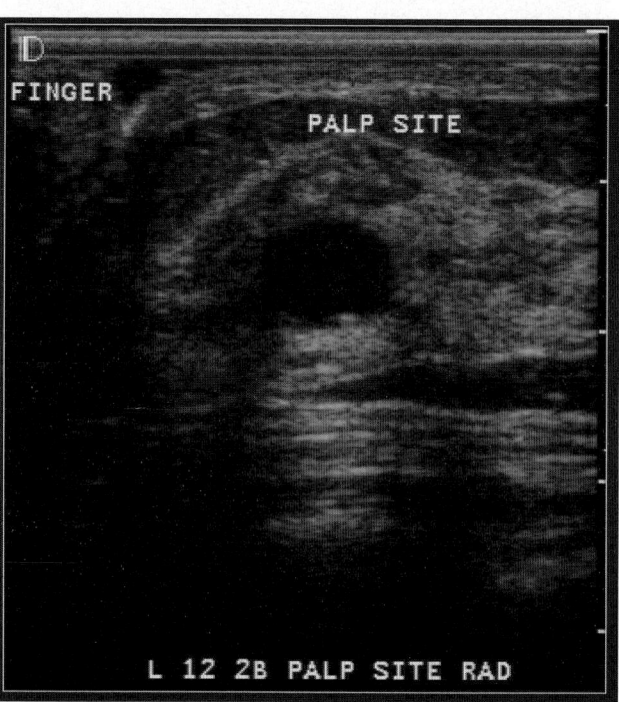

FIGURE 5–18 This small (8-mm), relatively deeply located, tense cyst presented as a much larger (2-cm), palpable lump. The overlying hyperechoic fibroglandular tissues contribute the apparent size of the lump at palpation.

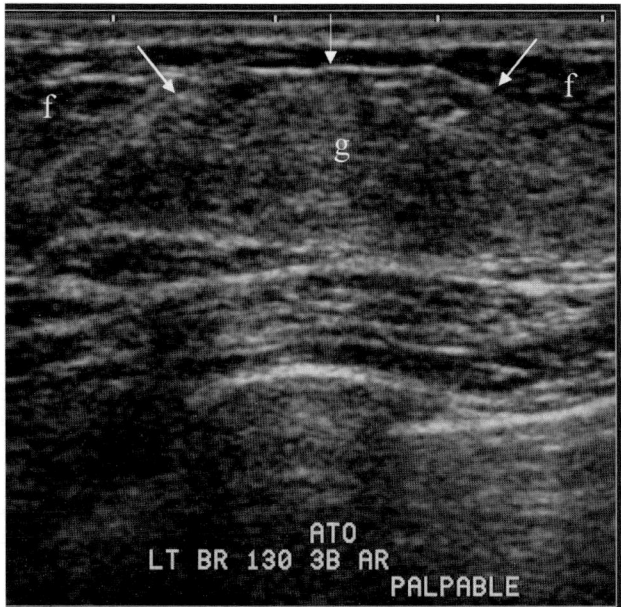

FIGURE 5–19 An isoechoic glandular ridge *(g)* caused the palpable lump in this patient. Although the echogenicity of the ridge is similar to that of surrounding subcutaneous fat *(f)*, the glandular tissue is much firmer to palpation.

(Fig. 5–19). Documenting that an area of isoechoic glandular tissue or adenosis causes the palpable abnormality by palpating while scanning is essential, just as it is for cysts and palpable fibrous tissue. However, documenting that isoechoic tissue causes a palpable lump is less reassuring than demonstrating that a cyst or hyperechoic fibrous tissue causes a palpable lump. The negative predictive value of palpable isoechoic glandular tissue is less than the nearly 100% negative predictive value of demonstrating either palpable hyperechoic fibrous tissue or a palpable simple cyst. Most fibroadenomas and about half of malignant solid nodules are nearly isoechoic with respect to glandular tissue and therefore are less conspicuous and easier to miss during sonography (Fig. 5–20). We are exploring the use of power Doppler vocal fremitus to help assess the significance of isoechoic tissue in patients with palpable lumps. The use of power Doppler vocal fremitus in such cases is discussed and illustrated in Chapter 20 (see Figs. 20–86 and 20–87). The negative predictive values of different tissue echogenicities are discussed and illustrated in Chapters 4 and 12.

One of the most common situations in which glandular tissue (adenosis of pregnancy) causes a palpable abnormality is during the first or second trimester of pregnancy. For reasons that are not completely understood, some

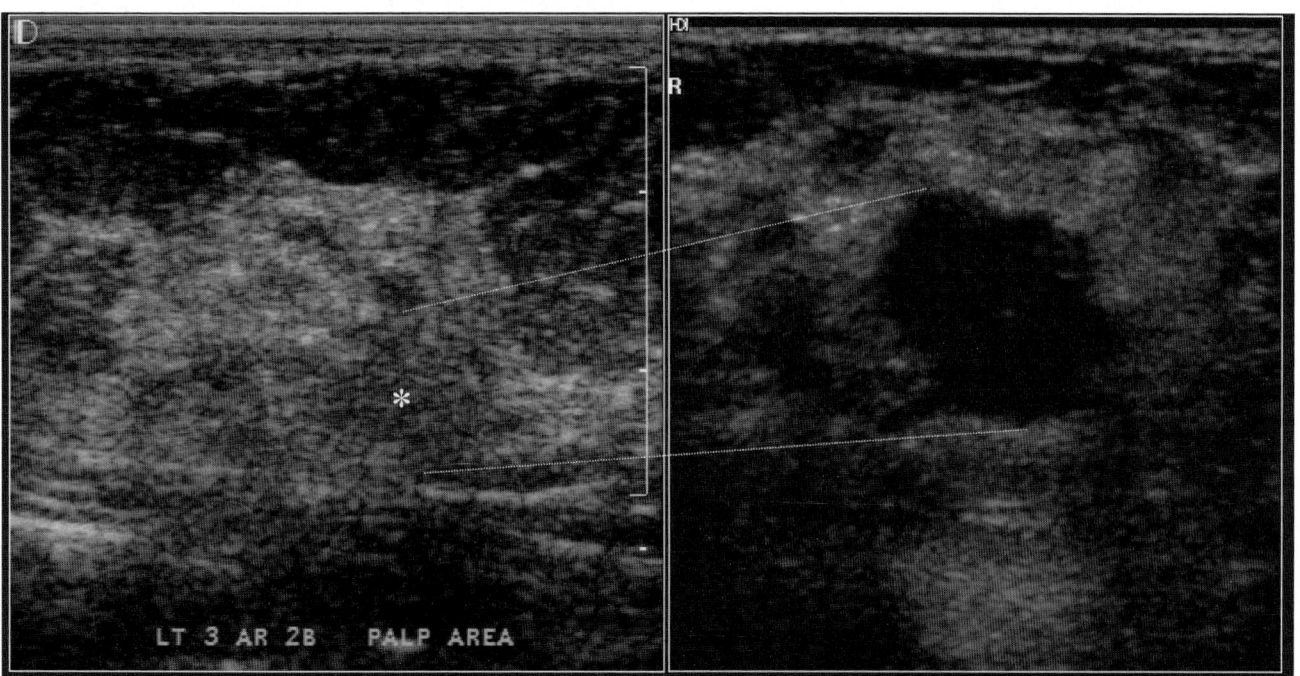

FIGURE 5–20 Palpable isoechoic tissue is not as reassuring as palpable hyperechoic tissue. About half of carcinomas are nearly isoechoic with glandular tissue and therefore hard to distinguish from normal glandular tissue. This patient presented with a palpable lump caused by a mixture of hyperechoic fibrous elements and what appear to be isoechoic glandular elements (*, **left**). The lump enlarged over 4 months. On follow-up sonogram, a large, hypoechoic mass that proved to be a high-grade invasive ductal cancer had arisen from the isoechoic area shown on the first examination (**right**).

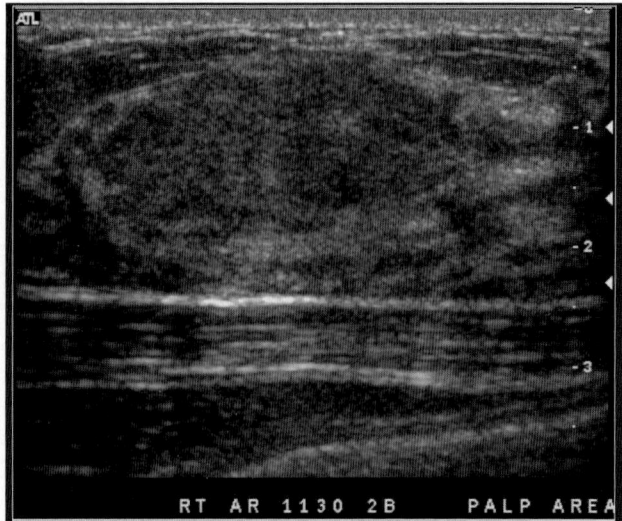

FIGURE 5–21 This pregnant patient presented early in the second trimester with a palpable lump in the upper central area of the right breast that ultrasound showed to be caused by isoechoic, glandular tissue that represents adenosis of pregnancy. The clinical lump became less apparent as the surrounding tissue "caught up" and also underwent physiologic change to adenosis of pregnancy.

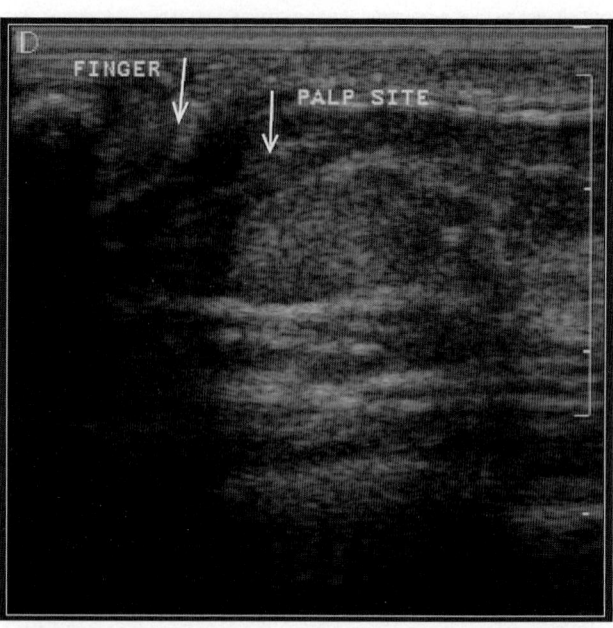

FIGURE 5–22 An isoechoic fat lobule caused the palpable lump for which this patient presented. She had recently lost 30 pounds. A period of rapid weight gain or weight loss contributes to the palpability of fat lobules in many patients.

TDLUs enlarge and coalesce with other enlarged TDLUs more rapidly and extensively than do surrounding TDLUs under the influence of the hormones of pregnancy, resulting in palpable foci of adenosis of pregnancy (Fig. 5–21). In some cases, these foci of adenosis can even undergo premature lactational change, which contributes further to palpability. In most instances, the surrounding TDLUs eventually "catch up," and the palpable abnormality becomes less prominent later in the pregnancy. Because the sensitivity of ultrasound for isoechoic solid nodules (including about half of malignant nodules) is decreased in the background of adenosis of pregnancy, and because malignant nodules may grow rapidly under the influence of the hormones of pregnancy, biopsy or very close clinical follow-up may be necessary. These patients should be advised that the palpable abnormality appears to be caused by glandular tissue stimulated by the hormones of pregnancy and will likely become less prominent in a few weeks as surrounding glandular elements enlarge. However, the patient should be instructed to examine the area closely, and if the area either does not decrease in prominence or becomes more prominent, the patient should return for repeat BUS and possible ultrasound-guided biopsy. Our experience has been that in most of such pregnant patients, the palpable abnormality regresses, and no further workup is necessary.

Fat lobules may also be a cause of palpable abnormalities. In a patient who, on mammography, has only fat in the quadrant of the breast in which the palpable abnormality lies, it should be apparent from the mammogram alone that fat or a lipoma is the cause of the palpable abnormality. In patients who have mammographically mixed breast density,

with residual dense fibrous or glandular elements interspersed with involuted fatty lobules, the cause of the lump may not be as apparent mammographically. In such patients, simultaneous palpation and real-time ultrasound scanning may conclusively demonstrate that the palpable abnormality is merely due to a prominent subcutaneous fat lobule that overlies deep fibrous or glandular elements (Fig. 5–22).

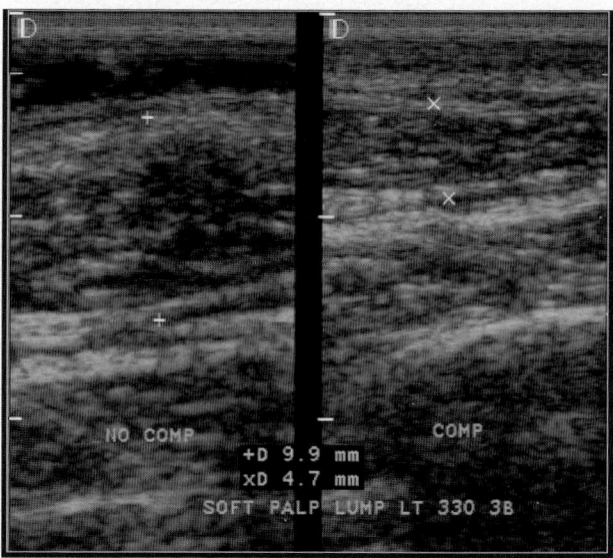

FIGURE 5–23 This palpable fat lobule was assessed with split-screen imaging, with very light scan pressure in the **left** image and vigorous compression in the **right** image. The anteroposterior dimension of the structure decreases by more than 30% with compression, indicating that it was either a fat lobule or lipoma.

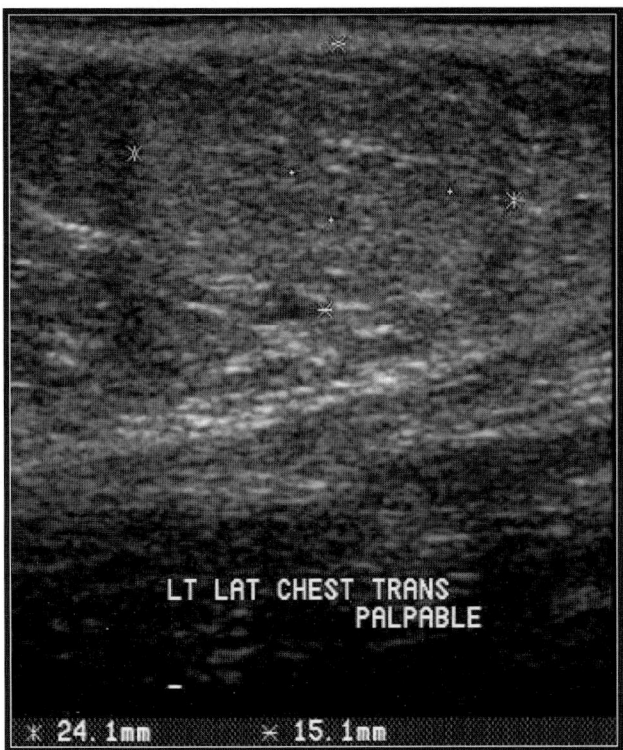

FIGURE 5–24 A mildly hyperechoic, subcutaneous lipoma caused the palpable lump for which this patient presented. It was more than 30% compressible. Its mild hyperechogenicity in comparison to surrounding subcutaneous fat helps distinguish it from a palpable normal fat lobule.

Palpable subcutaneous fat lobules are relatively soft and compressible in comparison to other causes of palpable abnormalities. As discussed and demonstrated in Chapters 3 and 4, split-screen ultrasound images done with and without compression frequently show compressibility in excess of 30% for fat lobules (Fig. 5–23), whereas similar-appearing fibroadenomas compress much less (see also Chapter 3, Fig. 3–13; Chapter 4, Figs. 4–36 and 4–39). Sonography may have difficulty distinguishing a palpable fat lobule from a lipoma. Subtle differences include that fat lobules often have a thin echogenic fibrous septum through them (see Chapter 4, Figs. 4–35, 4–38, 4–39, 4–40) and that small lipomas are often slightly hyperechoic in comparison to surrounding fat lobules (Fig. 5–24). (Fat lobules are discussed in Chapter 4, and lipomas are discussed in Chapter 13.) In our experience, palpable subcutaneous fat lobules are most commonly encountered immediately after a period of rapid weight gain or loss. Apparently, not all fat lobules increase or decrease in size at the same rate of speed during periods of rapid weight change.

In thin, small-breasted women, prominent costal cartilages may cause palpable lumps. In longitudinal scan planes that show the costal cartilage in short axis, the hypoechoic, oval costal cartilage may simulate a solid nodule (Fig. 5–25). However, this normal structure lies within the chest wall musculature rather than within the breast tissue and appears to be an elongated rectangular structure when scanned in transverse planes that are parallel to its long axis.

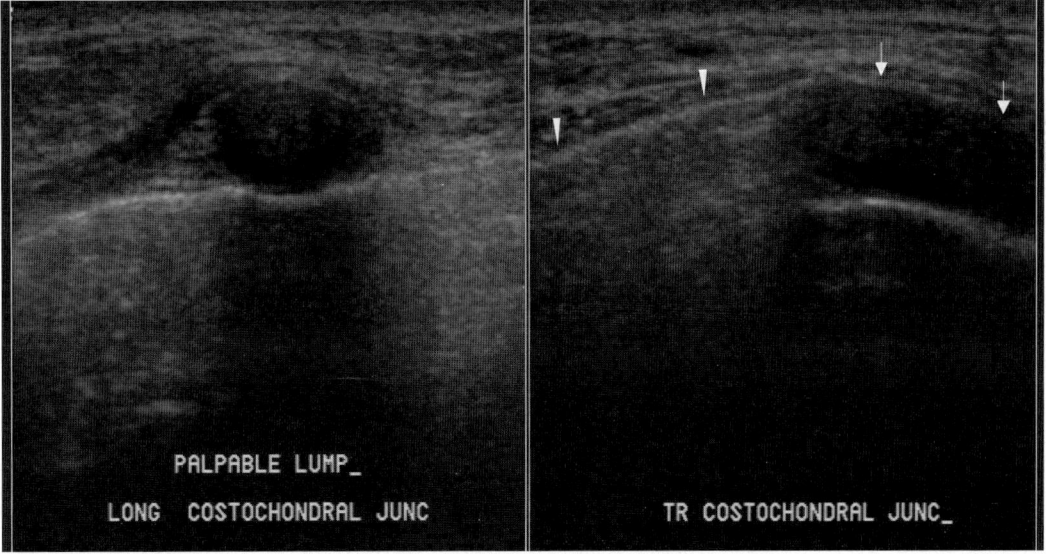

FIGURE 5–25 This patient presented with a palpable lump in the far medial breast. A longitudinal scan through the lump shows an apparent elliptically shaped nodule that is actually a noncalcified costal cartilage shown in its short axis **(left)**. The transverse view of the palpable lump is long axis to the costal cartilage and shows it to be tubular in shape rather than elliptical. Note that the lump is at the costochondral junction, with the shadowing ossified rib to the left of the image *(arrowheads)* and with the well-transmitting noncalcified, costal cartilage *(arrows)* shown to the right of the image. When costal cartilage is palpable, it is commonly at the costochondral junction, which may become inflamed and tender **(right)**. Note that it lies deep to the pectoralis muscle and within the chest wall, not within the breast. There is very little overlying breast tissue, explaining its prominent palpability. Patients who present with palpable costal cartilage are almost always very thin and have small breasts.

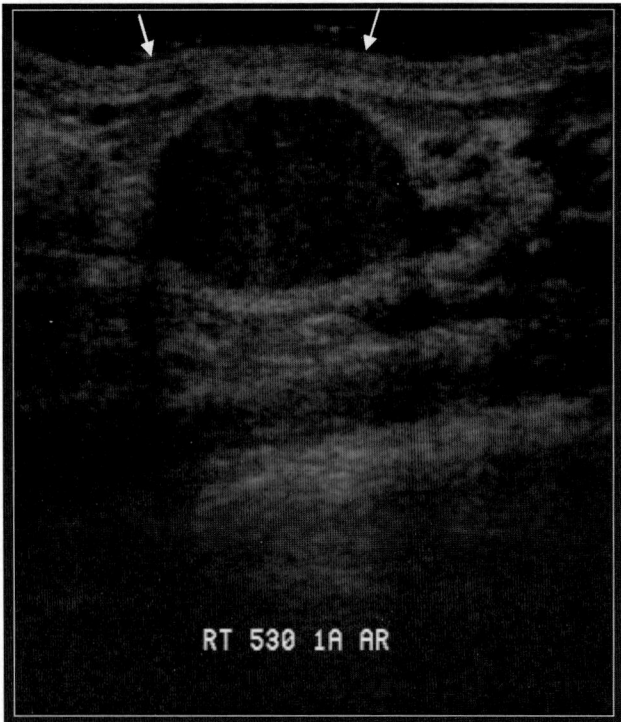

FIGURE 5–26 A benign fibroadenoma caused the palpable lump for which this patient presented. Note the bulge in the skin that it causes when scanned with a standoff of acoustic gel *(arrows)*.

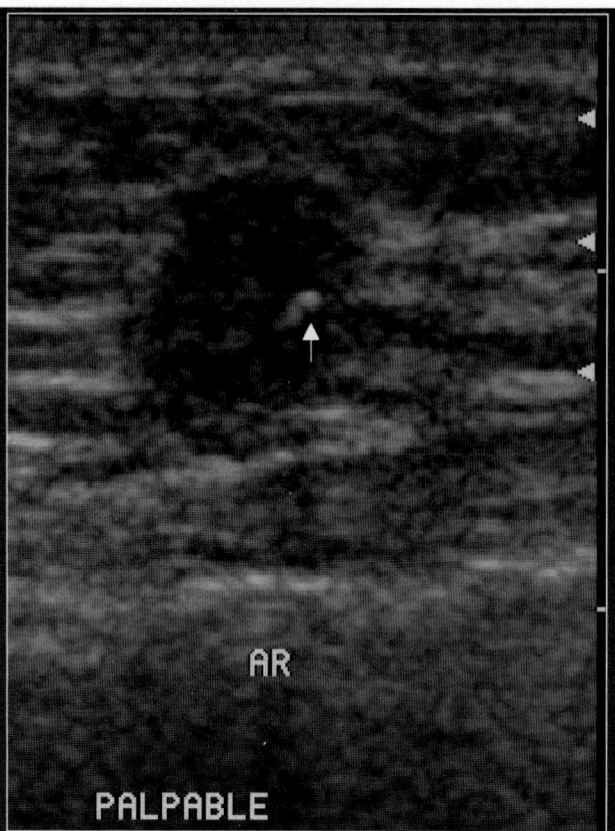

FIGURE 5–27 The palpable lump in this patient was caused by a small, hypoechoic malignant nodule that contained punctate calcifications *(arrow)* visible both mammographically and sonographically.

Finally, histologically benign or malignant solid nodules can cause palpable abnormalities (Figs. 5–26 and 5–27). Sonographically characterization of solid nodules is important in deciding how to manage such nodules and is discussed in detail in Chapter 12. However, keep in mind that the final decision about whether a solid nodule should undergo biopsy must be based on the wishes of the patient and her referring physician. In our experience, patients who have palpable solid breast nodules, even when sonographic features are classically benign, are more likely to choose biopsy than those with similarly benign-appearing, nonpalpable nodules.

Special consideration should be given to very small palpable abnormalities—those that are pea-sized or even BB-sized. Very small nodules must be in very close proximity to the skin to be palpable and to feel small. Pea- and BB-sized lesions usually lie well within 1 cm of the skin surface (Fig. 5–28). Because the elevation plane focal depth of most 7.5- to 12-MHz transducers is about 1.5 cm or deeper (deeper than the depth of the pea-sized or smaller nodule), the beam width at the depth of the nodule is usually wider than the diameter of the nodule. This limitation in short-axis focusing leads to volume averaging of the surrounding tissue with the nodule. Such volume averaging can lead to mischaracterization of cystic lesions as solid and can make solid lesions imperceptible or, at the very least, less well demonstrated. Additionally, reverberation echoes tend to "fill in" cysts that lie within 6 to 7 mm of the skin.

To avoid these problems, either a thick layer of acoustic gel or an acoustic standoff pad should be used. The standoff pad should be no more than 1 cm thick. Near-field imaging problems are discussed and illustrated in detail in Chapter 2 (see Figs. 2–5 to 2–7).

MUST ALL PALPABLE ABNORMALITIES UNDERGO BIOPSY?

Old dogma, based on outdated surgical literature, dictated that all palpable abnormalities must undergo biopsy, regardless of imaging findings. Some would still advocate such a position. However, because there is a spectrum of palpable abnormalities of the breast ranging from a generalized lumpiness to a hard, fixed, immovable mass, a means of differentiating between the different entities of this spectrum less invasive than biopsy should be and is available—sonography. Previously, this differentiation process and the decision to biopsy depended on many factors, including family history and self-history, other clinical findings, the experience of the examiner, the specialty of the referring physician, and the mammographic findings. Indeed, a negative mammogram that shows radiographically dense tissue in the area of the palpable lump might be falsely reassuring. With only a negative mammogram, a palpable abnormality might undergo either biopsy or short-interval clinical and mammographic follow-up. Now, with the advent of high-quality BUS, a better approach is available. Several studies have now been published showing a negative predictive value in excess of 99% when mammography is negative and sonography shows normal tissues to cause palpable abnormalities.

Sonographic evaluation of palpable lumps changes the American College of Radiology Breast Imaging Reporting and Data System (BIRADS) category initially assigned by mammography in a large percentage of patients whose in-

dication for targeted diagnostic BUS is a palpable lump. The significance of these changes is discussed and graphically illustrated in Chapter 1 (see Figs. 1–3 to 1–6).

In most cases, sonography will reveal a benign cause for the lump, but in certain cases, a worrisome or definitely malignant nodule is demonstrated. In such cases, sonography properly focuses attention on the need for expedient biopsy rather than clinical and short-interval mammographic follow-up. In many cases, sonography demonstrates malignant solid nodules that are not mammographically visible or that are undercharacterized into BIRADS 3 categories by mammography (see Chapter 1, Fig. 1–8).

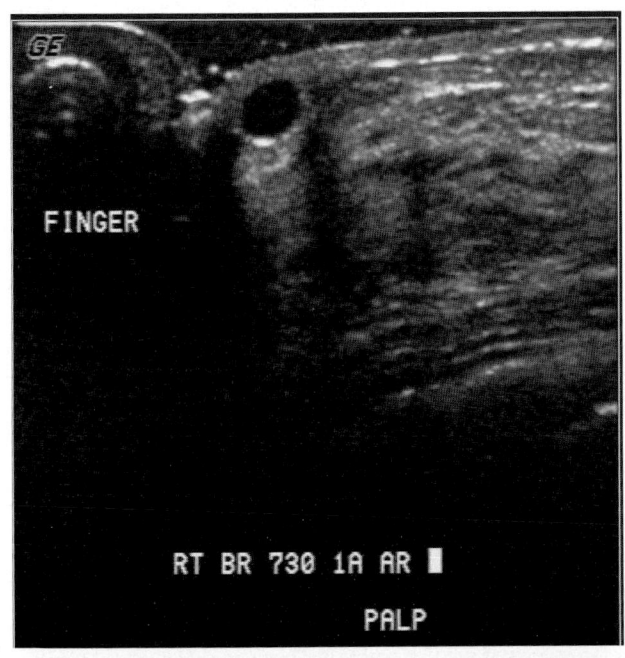

A

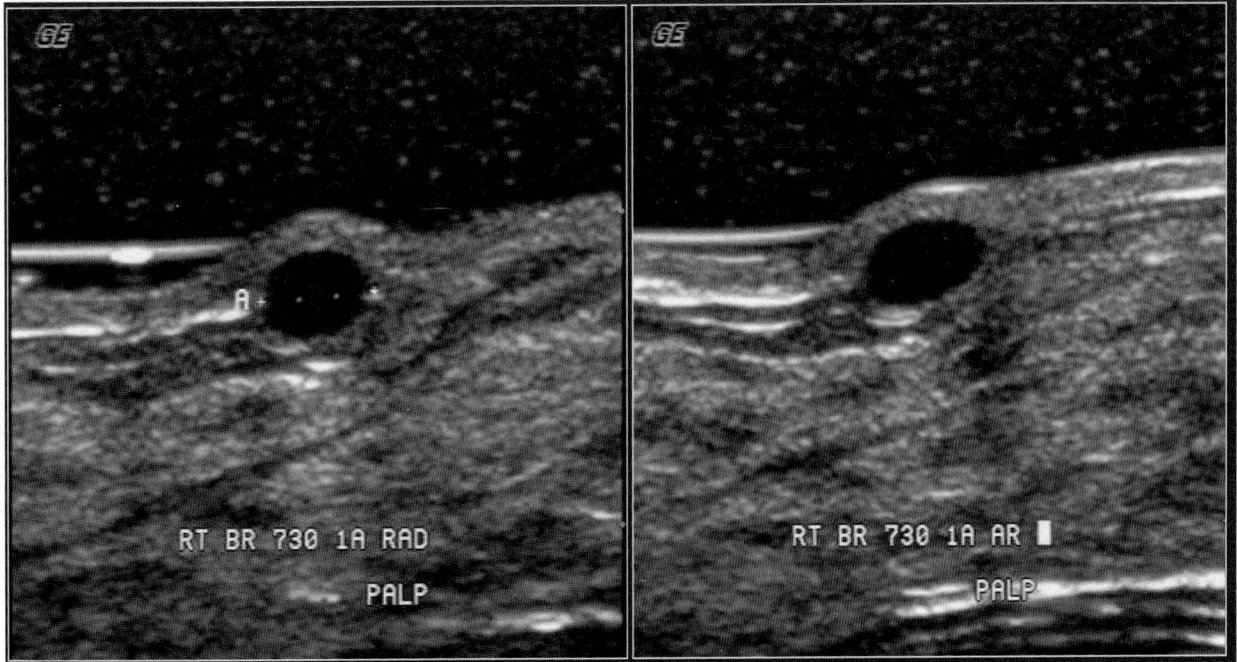

B

FIGURE 5–28 A: The BB-sized palpable lump for which this patient presented was caused by a small, very superficially located simple cyst. Such a small cyst would not be palpable if it lay deep within breast tissue. **B:** The same small cyst shown in A, when scanned through a standoff pad, pushes the skin outward into the standoff, demonstrating how tense it is. For a small lesion to be palpable, it must be (a) superficial in location, (b) surrounded by soft tissue, and (c) under tension. This small cyst meets all three criteria for small lesion palpability: it lies superficially, it is surrounded by soft subcutaneous fat, and it is tense.

That appropriately used targeted diagnostic BUS detects palpable carcinomas missed by mammography should not be viewed as an indictment of mammography, which is still the best available screening test for breast cancer. Instead, it indicates that *a highly selected subgroup* of all mammography patients in whom the risk for mammography missing carcinoma can be defined. By using BUS aggressively in such cases, we can find carcinomas that mammography misses. This highly selected subgroup of all mammography patients is defined by a palpable abnormality in association with the following:

- Negative or probably benign mammograms, but
- Radiographically dense tissue in the area of the lump that could obscure the cause of the palpable lesion, and
- Lack of worrisome calcifications in that same area

In patients meeting these criteria, sonographic demonstration of a solid mass with suspicious features requiring a BIRADS 4a or higher characterization is the key factor in biopsy appropriately being performed. Although we have emphasized the role of BUS in preventing biopsy, appropriate use of targeted ultrasound in patients with palpable abnormalities can clearly detect carcinomas missed or underclassified by mammography alone.

Any patient who is to undergo ultrasound for evaluation of a palpable abnormality should be questioned about additional palpable areas about which she might be concerned. In addition, the mammograms should be carefully inspected for additional areas that might require sonographic evaluation at the same time as the lump is evaluated. Although we target BUS to the area of the primary palpable lump, our threshold for evaluation of additional clinical and mammographic abnormalities is reduced when the patient is already on the table for evaluation of the palpable abnormality for which she presented. In such patients, only a few moments are required to evaluate a second or even third focal area of subtle mammographic or clinical abnormality that might otherwise be too minimal to evaluate on its own merits. About 8% of all the malignant lesions found at our institution sonographically were unsuspected clinically and mammographically before the patient underwent sonography. Most sonographically identified incidental carcinomas represent second or third lesions.

SUMMARY

In summary, ultrasound should be performed in patients with palpable abnormalities who have negative or nonspecific mammograms and radiographically dense tissues on mammography in the area of the palpable lump. Palpating while performing real-time sonography is important in documenting the precise cause of the palpable abnormality. About two-thirds of the time, a definitively benign cause for the palpable abnormality, such as a simple cyst, area of fibrous tissue, or fat lobule, is demonstrated. Occasionally, isoechoic glandular tissue causes the palpable abnormality. This is not quite as reassuring as fibrous tissue or a cyst, and at least short-interval clinical and mammographic follow-up is warranted in such patients. Power Doppler vocal fremitus may help in such cases. In certain patients with palpable abnormalities accompanied by negative or non-specific mammograms, sonography reveals a malignancy. In such cases, ultrasound is instrumental in expediting biopsy and treatment. Thus, BUS is an invaluable tool in the evaluation of a palpable abnormality, sparing most patients a biopsy and prompting expedient biopsies in those patients with suspected malignancy.

SUGGESTED READINGS

Bassett LW, Kimme Smith C. Breast sonography. *AJR Am J Roentgenol* 1991;156(3):449–455.

Burak Z, et al. Evaluation of palpable breast masses with 99Tcm-MIBI: a comparative study with mammography and ultrasonography. *Nucl Med Commun* 1994;15(8):604–612.

Cosmacini P, et al. Ultrasonographic evaluation of palpable breast masses: analysis of 134 cases. *Tumori* 1990;76(5):495–498.

Dennis MA, Parker S, Kaske TI, et al. Incidental treatment of nipple discharge caused by benign intraductal papilloma through diagnostic Mammotome biopsy. *AJR Am J Roentgenol* 2000;174:1263–1268.

Faulk RM, Sickles EA. Efficacy of spot compression-magnification and tangential views in mammographic evaluation of palpable breast masses. *Radiology* 1992;185(1):87–90.

Feig SA. The role of ultrasound in a breast imaging center. *Semin Ultrasound CT MR* 1989;10(4):90–105.

Feig SA. Breast masses. Mammographic and sonographic evaluation. *Radiol Clin North Am* 1992;30(1):67–92.

Guyer PB, Dewbury KC. Ultrasound of the breast in the symptomatic and x-ray dense breast. *Clin Radiol* 1985;36(1):69–76.

Guyer PB, et al. Direct contact B-scan ultrasound in the diagnosis of solid breast masses. *Clin Radiol* 1986;37(5):451–458.

Guyer PB, Dewbury KC. Sonomammography in benign breast disease. *Br J Radiol* 1988;61(725):374–378.

Hardy JR, et al. How many tests are required in the diagnosis of palpable breast abnormalities? *Clin Oncol (R Coll Radiol)* 1990;2(3):148–152.

Hayashi N, et al. Real-time sonography of palpable breast masses. *Br J Radiol* 1985;58(691):611–615.

Heywang SH, et al. Specificity of ultrasonography in the diagnosis of benign breast masses. *J Ultrasound Med* 1984;3(10):453–461.

Hilton SV, et al. Real-time breast sonography: application in 300 consecutive patients. *AJR Am J Roentgenol* 1986;147(3):479–486.

Jackson VP. The current role of ultrasonography in breast imaging. *Radiol Clin North Am* 1995;33(6):1161–1170.

Jokich PM, Monticciolo DL, Adler YT. Breast ultrasonography. *Radiol Clin North Am* 1992;30(5):993–1009.

Kimme-Smith C, Bassett LW, Gold RH. High frequency breast ultrasound: hand-held versus automated units; examination for palpable mass versus screening. *J Ultrasound Med* 1988;7(2):77–81.

Kimme-Smith C. Can quantitative ultrasound measurements help avoid breast biopsy? [Comment]. *AJR Am J Roentgenol* 1995;165(4):832–833.

Lee ME, Hashimoto B, Carter L. Role of direct contact, real-time breast ultrasound: one year's experience. *Ultrasound Med Biol* 1988;1:109–112.

Leonardi M, et al. The value of ultrasonography in benign breast diseases. *Minerva Ginecol* 1993;45(3):113–116.

Leucht W, et al. Improvement of preoperative evaluation of palpable, noncystic processes of the breast by echomammography. *Ultraschall Med* 1985;6(1):19–25.

Liberman L, et al. Imaging of pregnancy-associated breast cancer. *Radiology* 1994;191(1):245–248.

McCaffrey JF, et al. The abnormal mammogram—what to do. *Aust Fam Physician* 1991;20(10):1431–1435.

McNicholas MM, et al. Color Doppler sonography in the evaluation of palpable breast masses. *AJR Am J Roentgenol* 1993;161(4):765–771.

Muller JW. Diagnosis of breast cysts with mammography, ultrasound and puncture: a review. *Diagn Imaging Clin Med* 1985;54(3–4):170–177.

Mushlin AI. Diagnostic tests in breast cancer: clinical strategies based on diagnostic probabilities. *Ann Intern Med* 1985;103(1):79–85.

Otto RC. Value of ultrasound in breast diagnostics. *Bildgebung* 1993;60(4):263–266.

Pamilo M, et al. Ultrasonography of breast lesions detected in mammography screening. *Acta Radiol* 1991;32(3):220–225.

Perre CI, et al. Ultrasonographic study of the palpable breast tumor is very useful. *Ned Tijdschr Geneeskd* 1993;137(46):2374–2377.

Perre CI, et al. The value of ultrasound in the evaluation of palpable breast tumours: a prospective study of 400 cases. *Eur J Surg Oncol* 1994;20(6):637–640.

Potterton AJ, Peakman DJ, Young JR. Ultrasound demonstration of small breast cancers detected by mammographic screening [Comments]. *Clin Radiol* 1994;49(11):808–813.

Rubin E, et al. Hand-held real-time breast sonography. *AJR Am J Roentgenol* 1985;144(3):623–627.

Schepps B, Scola FH, Frates RE. Benign circumscribed breast masses: mammographic and sonographic appearance. *Obstet Gynecol Clin North Am* 1994;21(3):519–537.

Schoenberger SG, Sutherland CM, Robinson AE. Breast neoplasms: duplex sonographic imaging as an adjunct in diagnosis. *Radiology* 1988;168(3):665–668.

Shaw de Paredes E. Evaluation of abnormal screening mammograms. *Cancer* 1994;74[1 Suppl]:342–349.

Sickles EA, Filly RA, Callen PW. Benign breast lesions: ultrasound detection and diagnosis. *Radiology* 1984;151(2):467–470.

Stavros AT, et al. Solid breast nodules: use of sonography to distinguish between benign and malignant lesions [Comments]. *Radiology* 1995;196(1):123–134.

van Oord JC, et al. The value of ultrasound mammography in palpable breast masses. *Rofo Fortschr Geb Rontgenstr Neuen Bildgeb Verfahr* 1991;155(1):63–66.

Vega A, Garijo F, Ortega E. Core needle aspiration biopsy of palpable breast masses. *Acta Oncol* 1995;34(1):31–34.

Walsh P, et al. An assessment of ultrasound mammography as an additional investigation for the diagnosis of breast disease. *Br J Radiol* 1985;58(686):115–119.

Zonderland HM. Echography for palpable breast tumors. *Ned Tijdschr Geneeskd* 1993;137(46):2349–2350.

TARGETED INDICATION: MAMMOGRAPHIC ABNORMALITY

CORRELATING SONOGRAPHIC FINDINGS WITH MAMMOGRAPHIC FINDINGS

The second major targeted indication for breast ultrasound (BUS) is evaluation of a mammographic abnormality. Such mammographic abnormalities include discrete, well-circumscribed nodules; partially circumscribed nodules; indistinct nodules; developing densities; asymmetric densities (when present on both views); and subtle areas of architectural distortion within areas of dense breast tissue. Rarely, if ever, is BUS necessary for diagnosis when mammographic findings are strongly suggestive of malignancy. However, ultrasound can be useful in such patients for staging (detecting multifocality, multicentricity, extensive intraductal components, or abnormal regional lymph nodes) and for guiding needle biopsy and needle localization procedures. Ultrasound guidance is quicker and easier than stereotactic biopsy in almost all patients who have a nodule or mass, except in occasional patients who have small, deeply located lesions within large, fatty breasts.

The general goal of BUS in the evaluation of a mammographic lesion is to achieve a more specific diagnosis of the cause of the mammographic abnormality. Specific individual goals include preventing benign biopsies and finding carcinomas. Goals of BUS are discussed in detail in Chapter 1.

Some would argue that sonography is unnecessary in patients with completely circumscribed, round or oval, isodense nodules on mammography. Multiple studies have demonstrated that the chance of malignancy is 2% or less in this group—patients with American College of Radiology Breast Imaging Reporting and Data System (BIRADS) category 3 lesions. With such low risk, biopsy might be avoided. However, even with such a low risk for malignancy with BIRADS 3 findings, some further evaluation is usually necessary. Spot compression views are usually rec-

ommended. If diagnostic views show probably benign characteristics, short-interval follow-up is recommended. Diagnostic BUS is generally better than diagnostic mammographic views for BIRADS 3 water-density lesions when there are no calcifications, for several reasons:

1. First, sonography can show a definitively benign (BIRADS 2) finding, such as a simple cyst or homogeneously hyperechoic fibrous tissue to be the cause of the mammographic abnormality, obviating not only biopsy but also the need for short-interval follow-up. Sonography shows BIRADS 1 or 2 findings in cases that have been characterized as BIRADS 3 on mammograms 72% of the time. Thus, sonography can obviate short-interval follow-up in nearly three-fourths of cases in which mammography shows BIRADS 3 findings.
2. Sonography can unexpectedly show a solid indeterminate or solid malignant nodule, appropriately expediting biopsy rather than short-interval follow-up. Sonography upgrades mammographic BIRADS 3 findings less often than it downgrades them to BIRADS 2. Only 4% of the time does sonography upgrade BIRADS 3 mammographic findings to BIRADS 4 or higher, but in those cases, the sonographic findings might be life-saving.
3. There are problems with the concept of short-interval follow-up.
   a. First, patients should be informed that 2 to 3 years are required to distinguish slow-growing malignancies from benign lesions with certainty. Therefore, short-interval follow-up actually means that a unilateral mammogram should be performed at 6 months, followed by bilateral mammograms at 1, 2, and ultimately, 3 years. All during this short-interval follow-up, the patient will be uncertain of the outcome and under stress. The patient must be ap-

praised of and concur with the rationale for this approach.

b. During the 3 years of mammographic follow-up required to determine whether a mammographic lesion is benign or malignant, there is a chance that malignant lesions will grow and spread.

c. The ability to maintain a 2- to 3-year follow-up is being compromised by employers' "insurance shopping" and the anti–health care bias of the developing managed health care system. Most patients in the United States obtain health insurance through their employers. Employers frequently change insurance companies and health care providers based more on relatively small differences in annual insurance premiums than on quality of care. Employers and managed care companies, rather than patients, now often decide where the patient may or may not have mammography. The net result of the current managed care approach is that many patients undergo mammographic evaluation at a different mammography site each year. Patients seen in one mammography center this year are frequently forced to undergo mammographic evaluation at another center next year. Although radiologists make every attempt to obtain previous pertinent mammograms for comparison, this task is becoming more difficult, and the ability to obtain previous "outside" mammograms is much more difficult than obtaining previous mammograms from the same mammography center for comparison. Over 3 years, the chances of losing a patient to follow-up or picking up a patient already in follow-up from an outside center, but not being able to obtain the old films for comparison, are increasing dramatically. This current system so seriously compromises the ability to follow these patients for the necessary 2 or 3 years that, if a more immediate answer can be achieved by using sonography, it should be used very aggressively.

d. The patient should be informed that sonography has nearly an 80% chance of showing that the mammographic abnormality is caused by normal tissue or a benign entity for which neither biopsy nor short interval follow-up is necessary.

Despite all of its limitations, short-interval follow-up will be necessary in some patients. However, aggressive use of targeted diagnostic BUS can minimize the number of patients with mammographic densities who must undergo such follow-up.

Although the goal of aggressive sonographic evaluation of mammographic abnormalities should be to obtain immediate definitively benign or normal findings to prevent biopsy or suspicious findings to expedite biopsy, probably benign findings (BIRADS 3) that require short-interval

follow-up will be found in a small percentage of patients. Certain complex breast cysts and all solid nodules that do not undergo biopsy must be followed. Even solid nodules, for which histologic proof of benignity has been obtained by ultrasound-guided large core needle biopsy, must currently undergo short-interval follow-up.

The need for aggressive sonographic evaluation of mammographic densities that cannot be strictly characterized as BIRADS 3 is much less controversial. Mammographic nodules that are only partially circumscribed, nodules that are enlarging, focal asymmetries, architectural distortions, and density changes all warrant sonographic evaluation. We prefer to perform sonography as the first diagnostic examination in patients who have mammographic densities without associated calcifications. In some instances, additional mammographic views, including spot compression and magnification views, can solve the problem. However, BUS not only offers the advantage over mammography of being able to distinguish cystic from solid lesions but also can determine whether the partially obscured or indistinct borders of a lesion are due merely to surrounding fibrous tissue rather than infiltration of surrounding tissue by the nodule. If sonography does not reveal a definitive cause for the suspected mammographic abnormality, additional diagnostic mammographic views can still be obtained.

When sonography is used to evaluate a mammographic lesion further, one must confirm that the sonographic finding that is thought to explain the mammographic abnormality is, indeed, the same as the mammographic abnormality. In other words, it is necessary to be sure that the sonographic and mammographic abnormalities are not two different lesions. Ensuring that there are not two separate lesions—a mammographic lesion and a sonographic lesion—requires systematic, rigorous sonographic–mammographic correlation of the following:

- Size
- Shape
- Location
- Surrounding tissue density

Correlating all four of these imaging factors requires that the ultrasound plane be similar to the mammographic plane. In patients undergoing routine two-view mammography, sonographic–mammographic correlation is most easily accomplished by correlating the craniocaudal (CC) view of the mammogram with the transverse sonographic view. The CC view of the mammogram is easily reproduced sonographically by scanning in a straight transverse plane (Fig. 6–1). On the other hand, the orientation of the mediolateral oblique (MLO) view of the mammogram may lie between 30 and 60 degrees of obliquity. Because the exact degree of obliquity used for the MLO view of the mammogram is often unknown, reproducing the

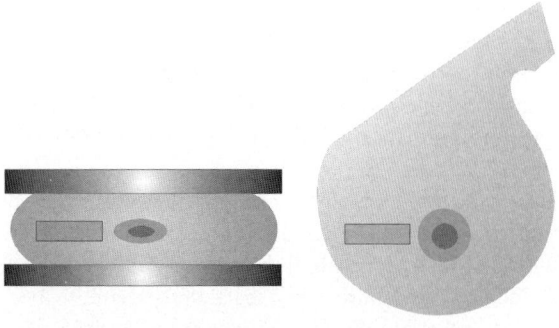

cc mammogram view   vs.   transverse US scan plane
US scan plane reliably reproduces mammographic compression plane

FIGURE 6–1 The easiest and most consistent way to correlate mammographic and sonographic findings is to compare the transverse sonographic plane with the craniocaudal view of the mammogram. The plane of the mammogram is consistently reproduced by scanning in a straight transverse plane.

corresponding plane sonographically can be difficult (Fig. 6–2). When a lesion is seen only on the CC view of the mammogram, correlating the sonographic and mammographic findings is easy. However, when a mammographic abnormality is visible only on the MLO view, the task is more difficult. In such cases, it is helpful to obtain a true mediolateral or lateromedial view to which a true longitudinal sonotomographic plane can be more easily correlated.

Size Correlation

To ensure that a sonographic finding corresponds exactly to the mammographic finding of concern, making sure that the sonographic and mammographic structures are the same size is the first concern. When comparing size, everything that is water density on mammograms must be accounted for and included in the sonographic measurements. Common mammographic water-density structures

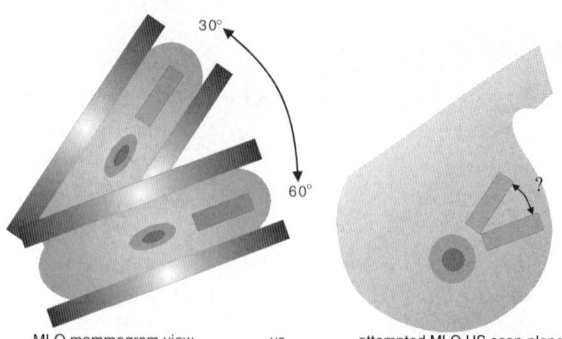

MLO mammogram view   vs.   attempted MLO US scan plane
scan plane less reliably reproduces mammographic compression plane

FIGURE 6–2 Correlating sonographic findings with the mediolateral oblique (MLO) mammographic view is difficult because the mammographic plane of obliquity can be between 30 and 60 degrees. The exact angle at which the MLO view was taken is not known in most cases and is therefore difficult to reproduce sonographically.

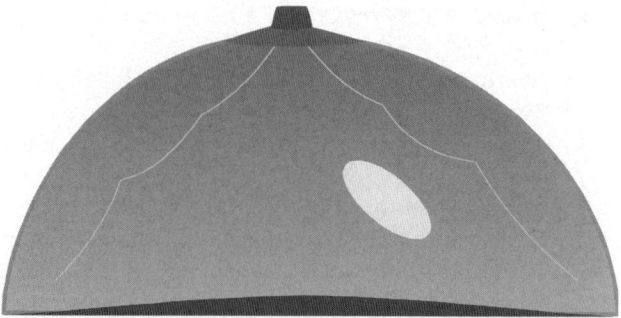

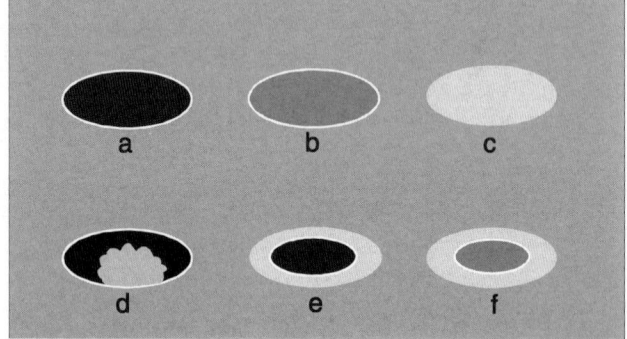

FIGURE 6–3 When correlating sonographic and mammographic sizes, everything that is water density and adjacent to the lesion must be included in the measurement. Thus, a 3-cm, oval-shaped, isodense, circumscribed mammographic nodule can represent a 3-cm cyst *(a)*, a 3-cm solid nodule *(b)*, a 3-cm area of focal fibroglandular tissue *(c)*, a 3-cm cyst containing a mural nodule *(d)*, a 1-cm cyst surrounded by 1 cm of fibroglandular tissue *(e)*, or a 1-cm solid nodule surrounded by fibroglandular tissue *(f)*.

that are identifiable sonographically include cysts, solid nodules, fibrous tissue, lobular tissue, adenosis, ducts, and the capsule around cysts or fibroadenomas (Fig. 6–3). The various water-density pathologic and anatomic structures cannot be distinguished from one another and can blend to form a single density on mammograms. This mammographic limitation makes the lesion appear larger mammographically than its actual size. Sonography can show a smaller lesion with adjacent or surrounding breast tissues. Therefore, a solid, elliptically shaped mammographic nodule (Fig. 6–4) can be caused by the following:

- A cyst or fibroadenoma surrounded by a thin, echogenic capsule
- A solid nodule surrounded by a thin, echogenic capsule
- A pseudomass of composed glandular, ductal, or fibrous tissue or any mixture of the three tissue types. Such tissues are equal in density to water and can produce mammographic densities or masses.
- A cyst that has an internal mural nodule. The mammogram will be unable to distinguish the mural nodule from the surrounding cyst fluid (although such cysts often also contain blood and are, therefore, of higher density on mammograms than are simple cysts).

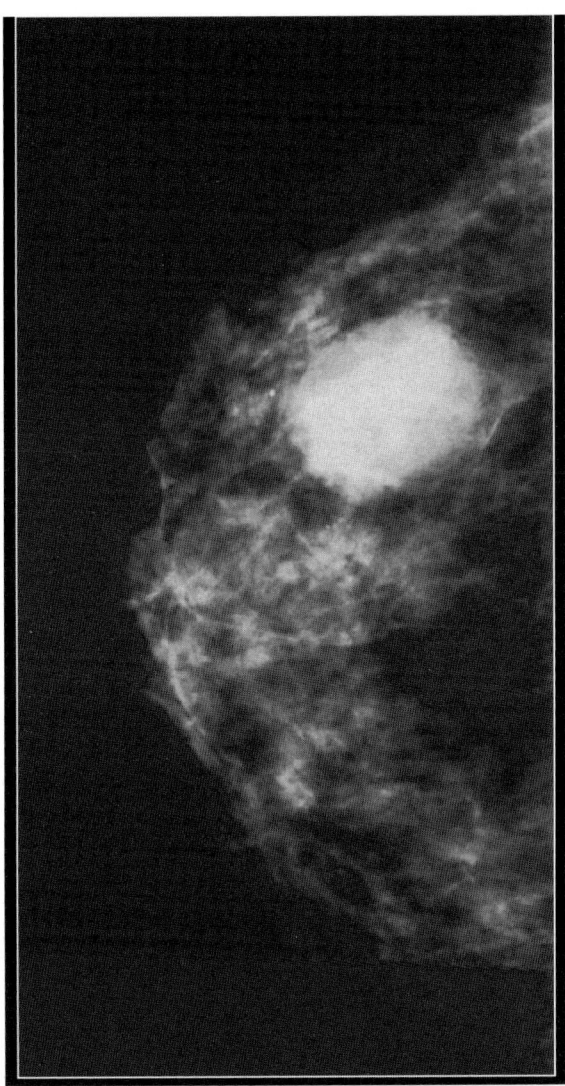

- A summation of a smaller cyst with surrounding water-density breast tissues, such as fibrous tissue or glandular tissue (adenosis). In such cases, including the cyst together with the surrounding breast tissue in the sonographic measurement is required to correlate best with mammographic size.
- A summation of a smaller solid nodule with surrounding water-density breast tissues, such as fibrous tissue or glandular tissue (adenosis). In such cases, the surrounding breast tissue should be included with the solid nodule in the sonographic measurement to correlate best with mammographic size.

When measuring lesion diameters, consistency should be maintained regarding whether the capsule that surrounds certain lesions is included in the measurement. If short-interval follow-up studies are performed and the capsule is excluded from the measurement on the first study, but included on the second, the false appearance that the lesion has enlarged could possibly lead to an unnecessary biopsy. On the other hand, if the capsule is included on the first study, but not on the second, the lesion may falsely appear smaller on the second study, when, in fact, the lesion

FIGURE 6–4 A: This craniocaudal mammographic view shows a 3-cm circumscribed nodule. **B:** All six of these lesions could correspond to the mammographic mass shown in part **A** in maximum diameter because we have appropriately taken into account everything that is water density in assessing how large the lesion will appear on mammograms. The mammographic mass could be caused by a cyst (**left upper**), solid nodule (**upper middle**), focal fibroglandular tissue (**upper right**), cyst containing a mural nodule (**lower left**), small cyst tightly enveloped in fibroglandular tissue (**lower middle**), or small solid nodule that is tightly enveloped in fibroglandular tissue (**lower right**).

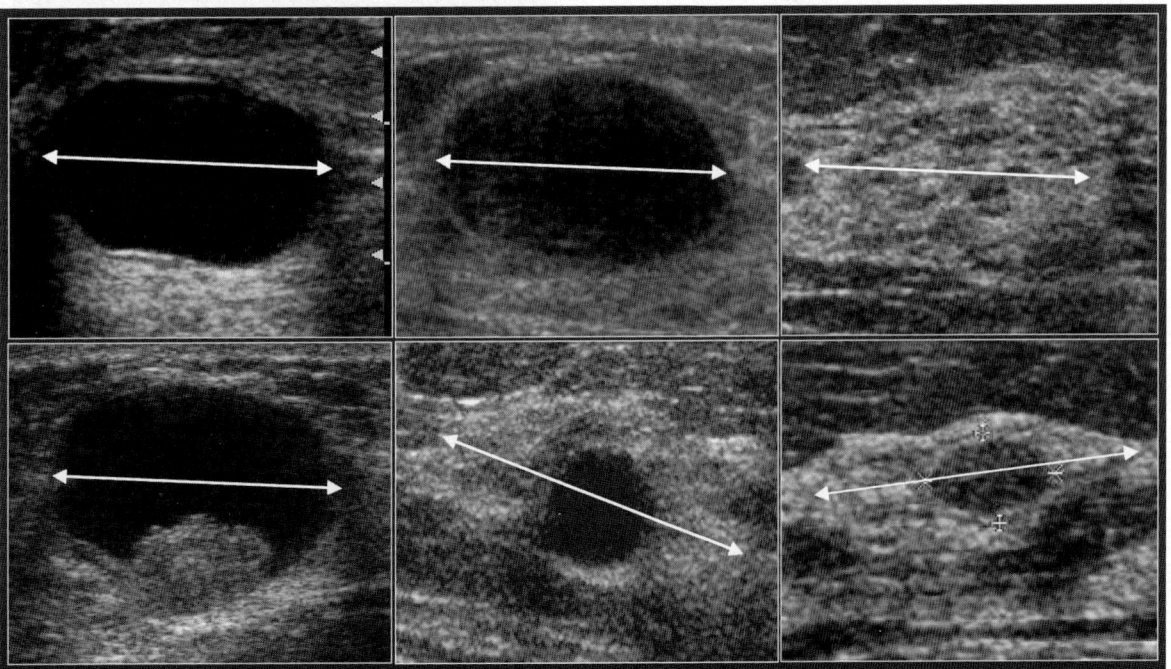

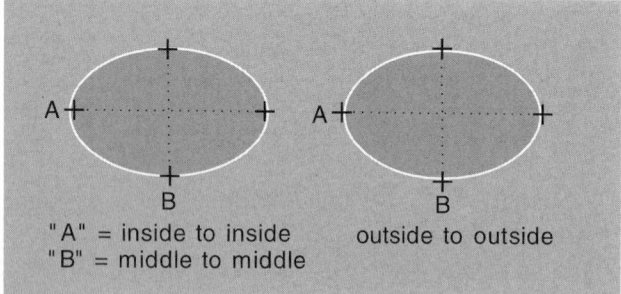

"A" = inside to inside   outside to outside
"B" = middle to middle

FIGURE 6–5 Measurement of breast lesions should be made outside to outside because the capsule that surrounds both benign and malignant lesions is water density, indistinguishable from the lesion mammographically, and therefore included in the mammographic measurement of the lesion. To obtain the best correlation between the sonographic and mammographic measurement of the lesion, it should be measured the way sonographically that it is mammographically. Other sonographic methods of measuring, such as leading edge to leading edge, inside to inside, and middle to middle, are less suitable for purposes of comparing with mammographic measurements. It is especially important to measure the same way on follow-up examinations as on the original examination. Measuring outside to outside on the first exam and inside to inside on the second exam may mask enlargement that has occurred. Conversely, measuring inside to inside on the first exam and outside to outside on the second exam will make a stable lesion falsely appear to have enlarged.

may be either unchanged in size or may have enlarged. Inconsistency in including the capsule will be especially problematic for lesions with relatively thicker capsules. To avoid such problems, the best approach is to include the capsule in the measurement of all lesions. The capsule, like the cyst or solid nodule it surrounds, is water density. Mammographically, the surrounding water-density capsule cannot be distinguished from the water-density lesion (unless the lesion is fat density) and therefore will be included in the measurement of the lesion mammographically. To obtain the best correlation between sonographic and mammographic measurements of size, the measurements should be made sonographically just as they are mammographically—by including the capsule (Fig. 6–5). Inclusion of the capsule within the measurement of a lesion is simply a corollary of the general rule to include all contiguous water-density structures when correlating the mammographic and sonographic size of a lesion.

Obviously, including the capsule within the measurement of the lesion will have the most effect when the capsule around the lesion is relatively thick, as with inflamed cysts (Fig. 6–6), or when the lesion is surrounded by water-density fibroglandular tissues, as shown in the lower middle and lower right lesions in Fig. 6–4. Including the

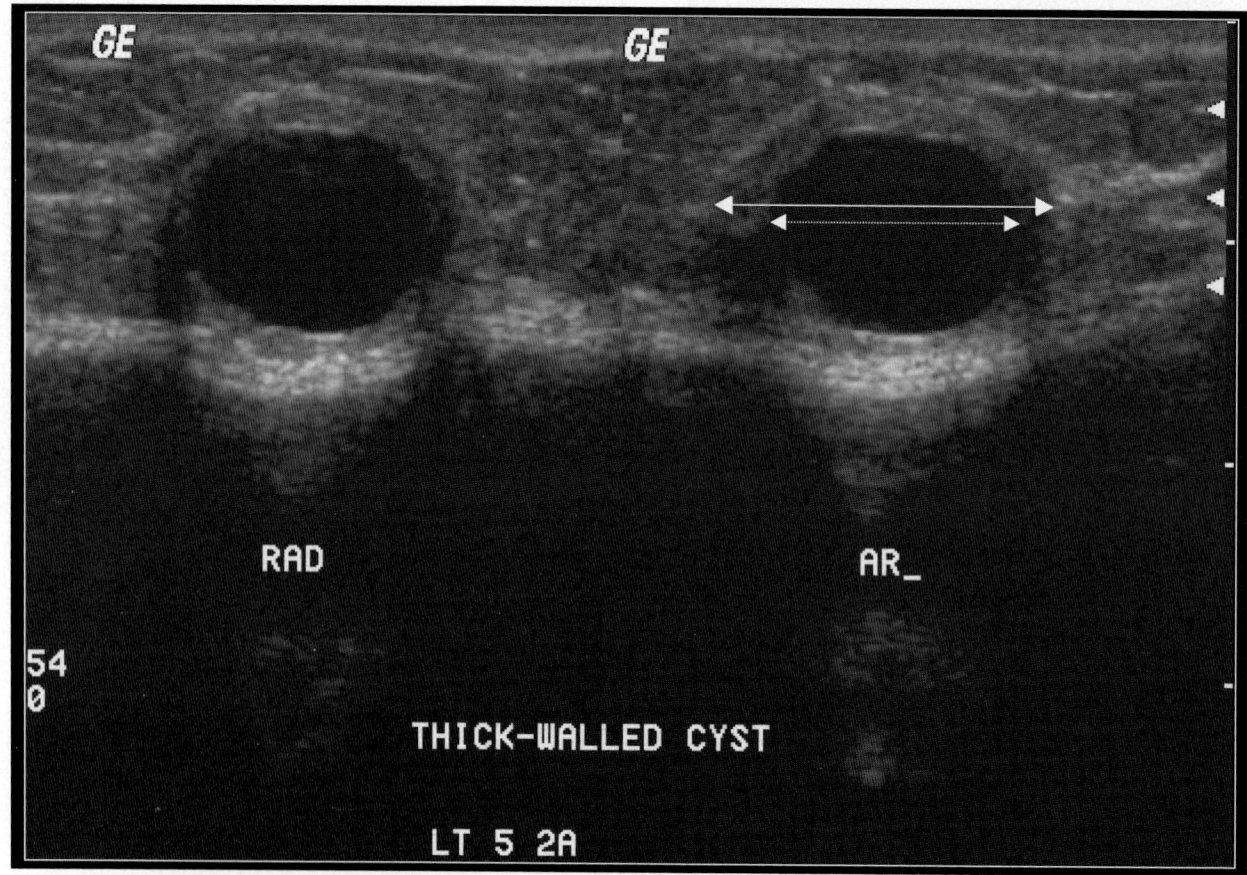

FIGURE 6–6 The method of measurement matters most when the lesion is small or when the wall of the lesion is thicker than usual. There is a significant difference in the inside-to-inside and outside-to-outside measurements of this thick-walled, inflamed cyst.

capsule within measurement of a lesion will also have a relatively large effect when the lesion is small. For instance, a 4-mm cyst cavity surrounded by a 1-mm thick capsule will measure 6 mm in diameter if the capsule is included, but only 4 mm in diameter if the capsule is excluded (Fig. 6–7, left). Exclusion of the capsule will cause a 33% undermeasurement of the lesion. However, if a cyst has a cavity of 18 mm and a 1-mm thick capsule, it will measure 20 mm if the capsule is included and 18 mm if the capsule is excluded. Exclusion of the capsule will result in undermeasurement of the lesion by only 10%, about the degree of measurement error in ultrasound (Fig. 6–7, right).

Either average or maximum diameters may be used for sonographic–mammographic size correlation. For firm, relatively noncompressible lesions, maximum and average diameters correlate equally well. However, for soft, compressible lesions (such as certain cysts, lipomas, or myxomatous fibroadenomas), maximum diameters obtained with ultrasound will correlate better with mammographic measurements than will average diameters. In such cases, the mammographic mean diameter will be larger than the sonographic mean diameter, even though the maximum diameters are similar. Such soft, compressible lesions have three axes: two that are long and oriented perpendicular to

the axis in which compression is applied, and one that is short and parallel to the axis of compression. The soft cyst is compressed in a plane perpendicular to its visible mammographic margins in both mammographic views (Figs. 6–8A and 6–9A). Therefore, each mammographic view shows only the two long axes of the cyst.

The short axis of the cyst is never visualized mammographically. The three dimensions that are mammographically visible are, therefore, long axes that all lie perpendicular to the axis of compression. If a mean diameter is calculated from these three long-axis measurements, it will be larger than the true mean diameter of the lesion because the compressed dimension is excluded. On the other hand, ultrasound will show the cyst in all three planes, including the shortest or compressed axis (Figs. 6–8B and 6–9B). A mean diameter of the compressible lesion obtained sonographically therefore will contain two long axes and one short axis, will more accurately reflect the mean diameter of the lesion, and will be less than the mean diameter obtained from mammography. Because many cystic and solid breast lesions are compressible to some degree, sonographic measurements of mean diameter will often be smaller than the mammographic mean diameter. However, long-axis measurements, maximum diameters that are perpendicular to the axis of

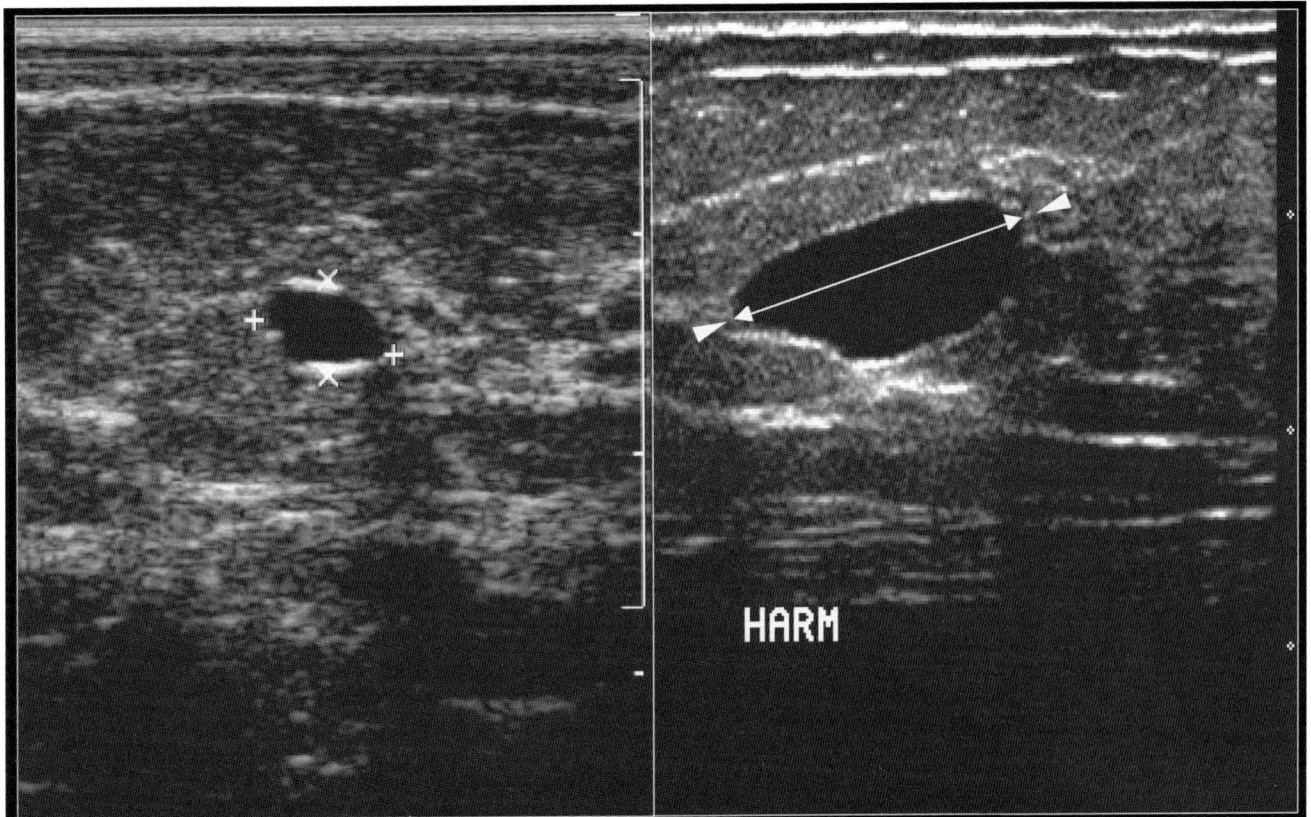

FIGURE 6–7 The method of measurement matters most when the size of the lesion is small because the capsule then comprises a greater percentage of the outside-to-outside diameter of the lesion, even when the capsule is thin (**left**). The larger the lesion, the smaller will be the relative contribution of a thin capsule to the maximum diameter of the lesion (**right**).

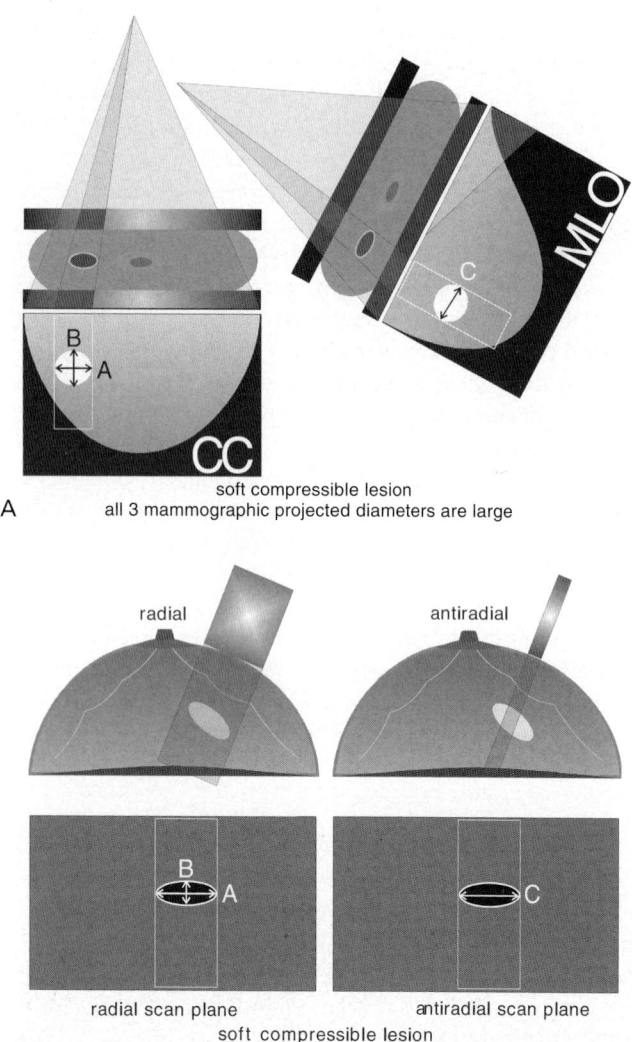

A

soft compressible lesion
all 3 mammographic projected diameters are large

radial   antiradial

radial scan plane   antiradial scan plane
soft compressible lesion
only 2 of 3 US diameters are large -- 1 of 3 is small

B

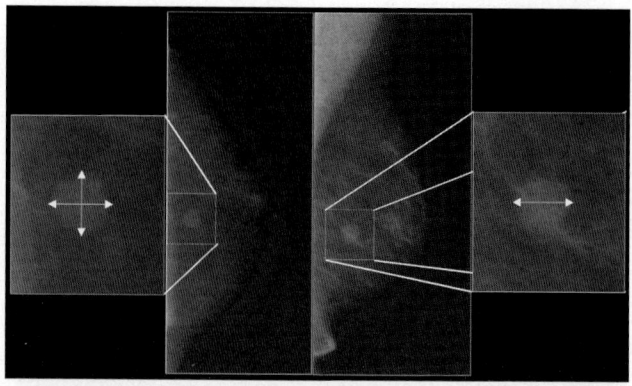

A

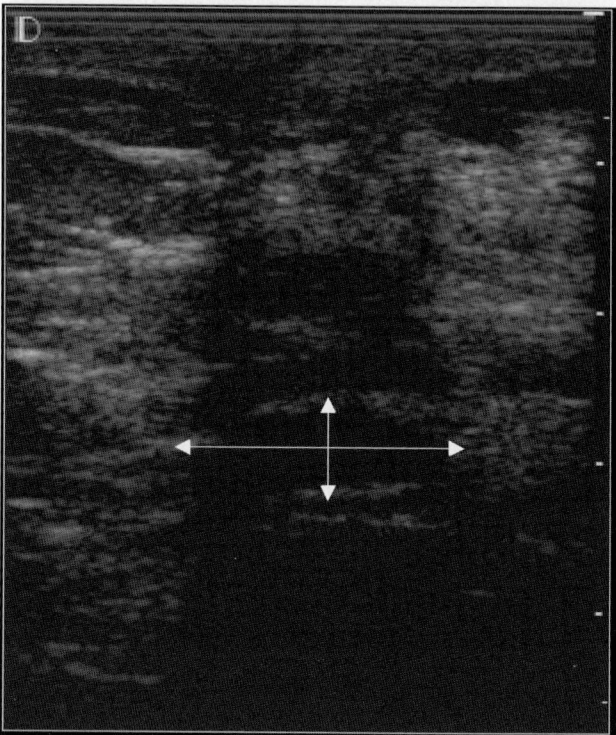

B

FIGURE 6–8 A: Although mean diameters are the best way to follow a lesion over time, maximum diameter correlates better with the mammographic measurement. This is because many breast lesions are partially compressible. To obtain three dimensions for a mean diameter calculation, measurements must be obtained from two mammographic views. Neither mammographic view shows the compressed dimension of the lesion. Thus, all three diameters used in mammographic measurement are obtained perpendicular to the axis of compression. The lesion tends to look spherical, and three large diameters are used in calculating a mammographic mean diameter. That the two mammographic views are not truly orthogonal to each other likely contributes to difficulties in obtaining accurate mean diameters. **B:** Sonography does show the compressed axis of the lesion as well as two axes that lie perpendicular to the axis of compression. Thus, the sonographic mean diameter contains one short and two long diameters, and the sonographic mean diameter is less than the mammographic mean diameter if the lesion is compressible. Only in completely incompressible lesions will the sonographic and mammographic mean diameters be identical. However, whether the lesion is compressible or not, the maximum diameters will correlate well between sonography and mammography.

FIGURE 6–9 A: Note that this compressible mammographic lesion appears to be spherical in shape and has three large and nearly equal diameters because the compressed dimension cannot be shown mammographically. Only the diameters perpendicular to the axis of compression are shown mammographically. **B:** The sonographic demonstration of the mammographic lesion in part **A** shows an elliptically shaped lesion because sonography can show the compressed dimension. The horizontal diameter, which is perpendicular to the axis of compression, is identical to the mammographic maximum diameter. The sonographic mean diameter includes two large diameters obtained perpendicular to the axis of compression and one short diameter obtained parallel to the axis of compression. Thus, the sonographic mean diameter is composed of two long and one short diameter and is consistently less than the mammographic mean diameter when the lesion is at all compressible. Compressibility also accounts for a consistent difference in the shape of the lesion on mammography and sonography. Compressible lesions that appear to be spherical in shape on mammography appear to be elliptically shaped on ultrasound. This consistent shape difference must be taken into account when correlating sonographic and mammographic shapes.

compression, will usually be nearly the same for mammography and sonography on nonmagnified views. Therefore, maximum diameters rather than average diameters should be used for sonographic–mammographic size correlations, especially if the lesion is compressible or has an ellipsoid rather than spherical shape at sonography (wider in the horizontal axes than the anteroposterior dimension). However, mean diameters are used when comparing measurements on serial ultrasound examinations.

Shape Correlation

To prove that a sonographic structure is the same structure that is visualized mammographically, the shape of the structure on sonography should be similar to the shape on mammography. As noted earlier, for mammographic lesions seen on both CC and MLO views, the correlation between transverse sonographic views and mammographic CC views is better than that between the mammographic MLO view and any oblique sonotomographic plane. Lesions that have lobulations or points on mammography should have lobulations or points sonographically (Figs. 6–10 and 6–11). The appearance of lobulations may be caused by breast tissue surrounding a cyst or nodule rather than by the nodule itself.

Apparent differences in shape between the mammogram and sonogram can be due to rotation of the lesion.

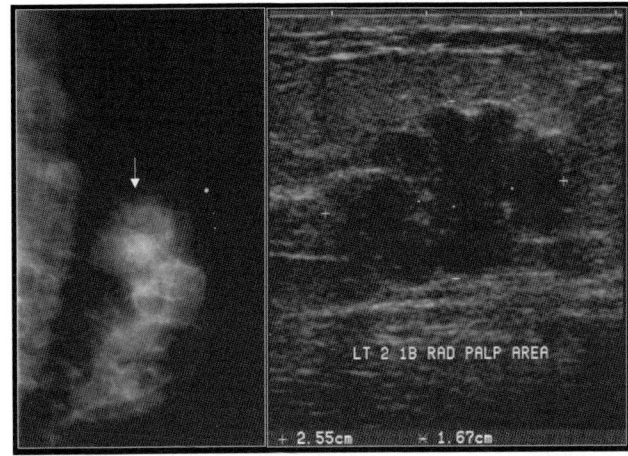

FIGURE 6–11 A multilobulated mammographic mass corresponds to a suspicious multilobulated solid nodule on sonography that proved to be intermediate-grade invasive ductal carcinoma.

Mammographic compression and sonographic compression place different rotational forces on breast structures. Mammographic compression pulls tissues away from the chest wall and rotates the long axis of a lesion perpendicular to the chest wall. Sonographic compression, on the other hand, pushes tissue planes toward the chest wall, and rotates the long axis of lesions parallel to the chest wall.

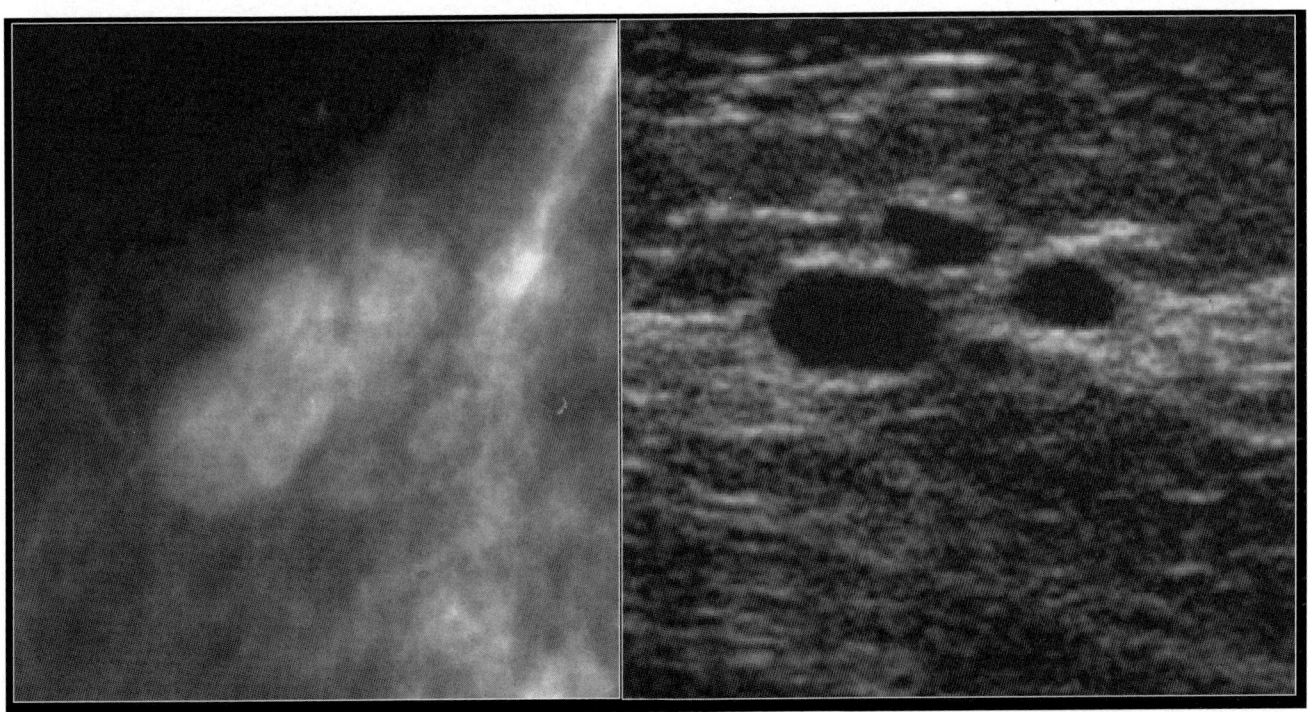

FIGURE 6–10 The mammographic shape should be similar to the sonographic shape. This trilobed mammographic nodule (**left**) corresponds to a cluster of cysts on sonography (**right**).

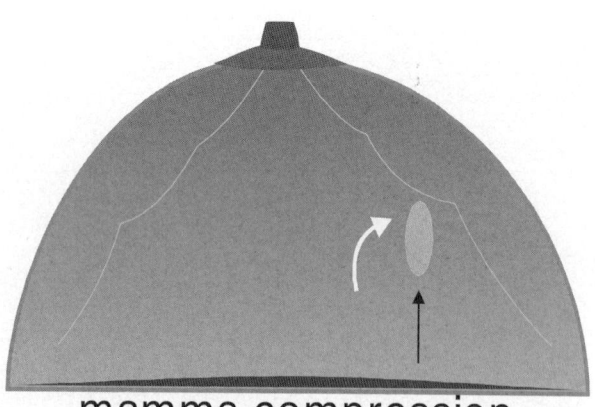

mamms compression

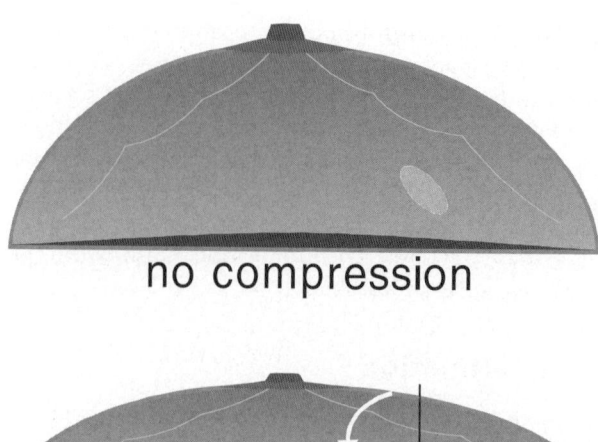

no compression

US compression

FIGURE 6–12 Consistent differences in mammographic and sonographic compression affect the position and shape of lesions. Mammographic compression pulls lesions away from the chest wall and generally rotates the long axis of the lesion perpendicular to the chest wall. Sonographic compression, on the other hand, pushes the lesion closer to the chest wall and generally rotates its long axis parallel to the chest wall. Thus, there is usually a 90-degree rotational difference in the direction of the long axis of a lesion relative to the chest wall. If this is not accounted for, it may mistakenly be concluded that the shape of the nodule at sonography differs from its shape on mammography.

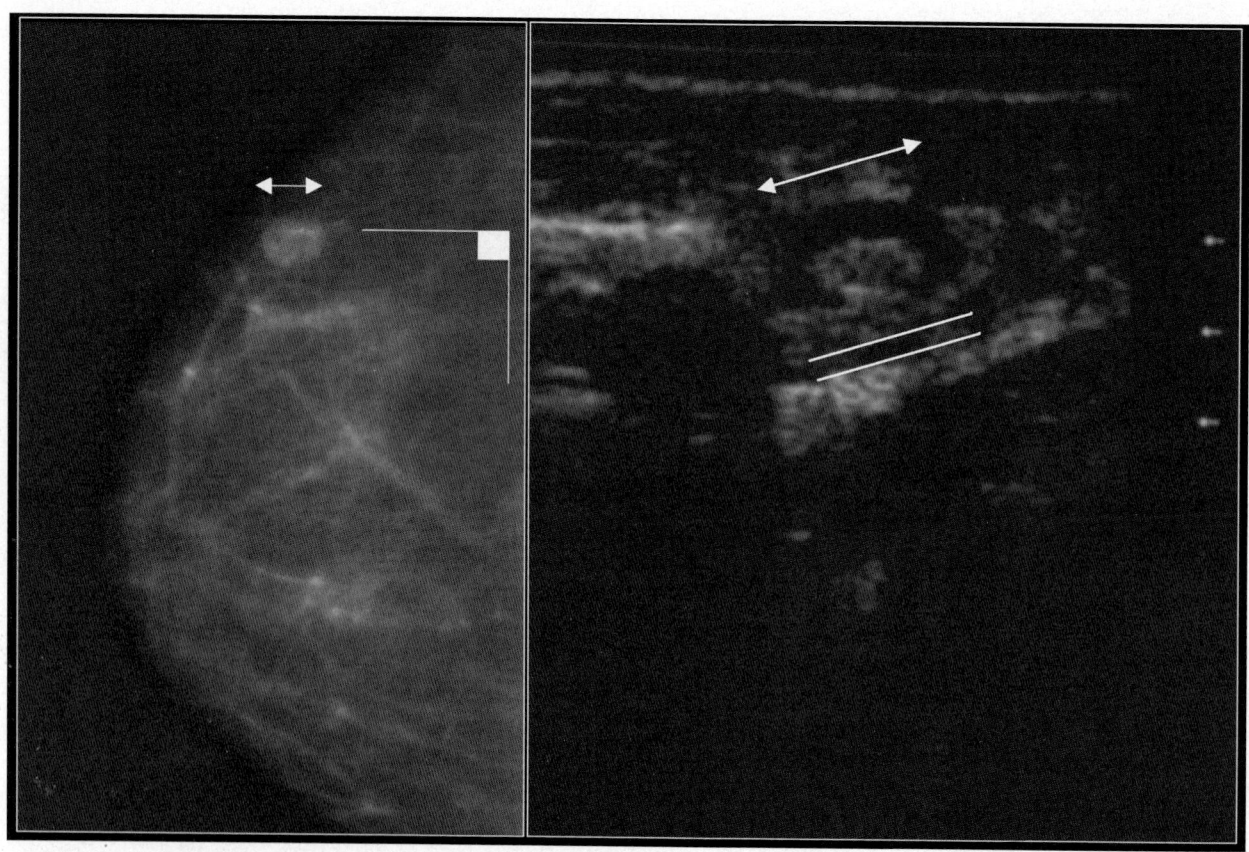

FIGURE 6–13 The long axis of this normal intramammary lymph node lies perpendicular to the chest wall on mammography because of the rotatory effects of mammographic compression (**left**). The same intramammary lymph node lies with its long axis parallel to the chest wall on ultrasound because of the effects of sonographic compression (**right**). Frequently, there is a 90-degree rotational difference in the orientation of the long axis of the nodule between mammography and ultrasound.

Thus, depending on the degree of rotation, there is often a 90-degree rotational difference in axis of the nodule between mammography and sonography (Figs. 6–12 and 6–13). If this rotation is not taken into account, the shape of the lesion may erroneously appear to be different on mammography and sonography.

Apparent differences in shape between a mammographic lesion and a sonographic lesion can also be caused by compression of a lesion, as discussed earlier. A soft, compressible structure, such as an incompletely distended cyst, may appear spherical on mammographic views but elliptical on sonographic views. As noted previously, such cysts have three axes: two that are long and oriented perpendicular to the axis in which compression is applied, and one that is short and parallel to the axis of compression. The soft cyst is compressed in a plane perpendicular to its visible mammographic margins in both mammographic views, each of which shows only the two long axes of the cyst, usually similar to each other. Because the short axis of the cyst is never viewed mammographically, these cysts will appear circular on both mammographic views, suggesting a spherical shape. On the other hand, ultrasound, which more accurately shows the cyst in all three planes (including the compressed dimension), appropriately demonstrates an elliptical shape (Figs. 6–8 and 6–9).

Location Correlation

The sonographic–mammographic location correlation requires evaluation of both mammographic views. The lesion location in the craniocaudal axis is more difficult to predict on the MLO views than is the location in the right-to-left axis on CC views. There are two reasons for this phenomenon. First, the exact degree of obliquity on the MLO view is uncertain, usually varying between 30 and 60 degrees. The distance above or below the posterior nipple line (PNL) at which a structure projects on the MLO mammographic view varies with the angle of obliquity and with the location of the lesion. Because the central plane through the posterior nipple line on MLO mammograms, unlike that of sonography, does not lie between the 3:00 and 6:00 positions, the projected location of medial and lateral lesions is different on MLO mammograms. Both medial lesions that lie superior to the nipple and lateral lesions that lie inferior to the nipple may project exactly at the level of the PNL on MLO mammograms (Fig. 6–14). On the other hand, medial lesions that lie at the level of the PNL will be projected to a location more inferiorly, and the farther medial the location, the farther inferiorly the medial lesion will project on the MLO view (Fig. 6–15). Lateral lesions that lie at the level of the PNL will be projected to locations more superiorly on MLO mammographic views. The farther laterally the lesion lies, the more superiorly it will be projected on the MLO view (Fig. 6–16). The effect

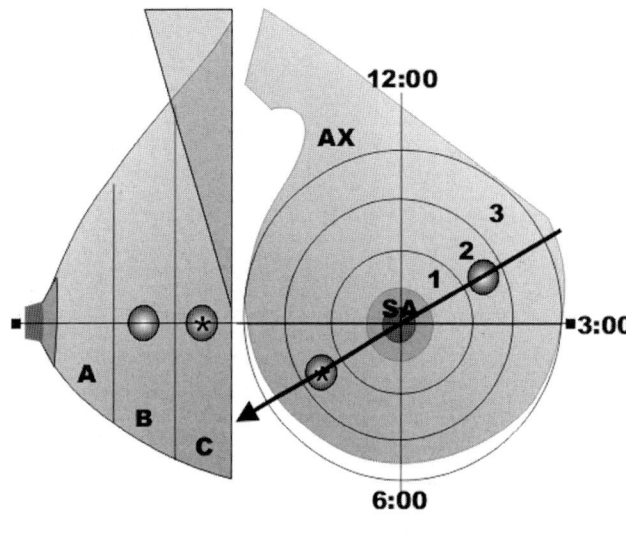

FIGURE 6–14 The x-ray beam passes from high medial to low lateral in performing a mediolateral oblique (MLO) mammographic view. Thus, lesions that appear to lie exactly at the level of the nipple on MLO views may actually lie within the upper inner quadrant or within the lower outer quadrant.

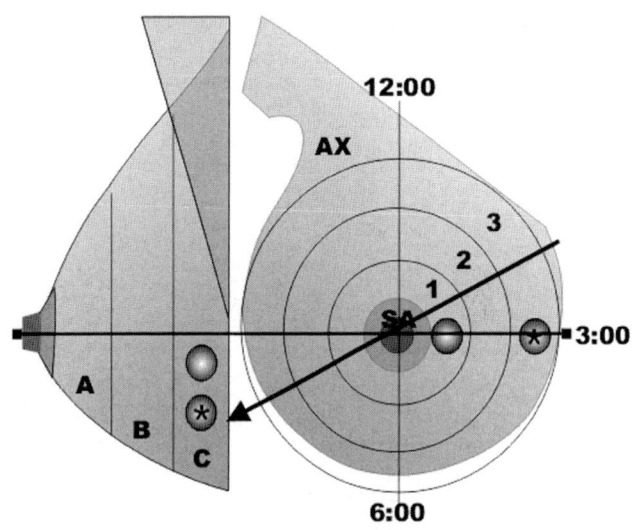

FIGURE 6–15 The x-ray beam passes from high medial to low lateral in performing the mediolateral oblique mammographic view. Thus, a medial lesion tends to project lower than its true location, and the farther peripherally a medial lesion lies, the lower it projects. Exceptions to this general rule can occur when a lesion lies near 12:00 or 6:00.

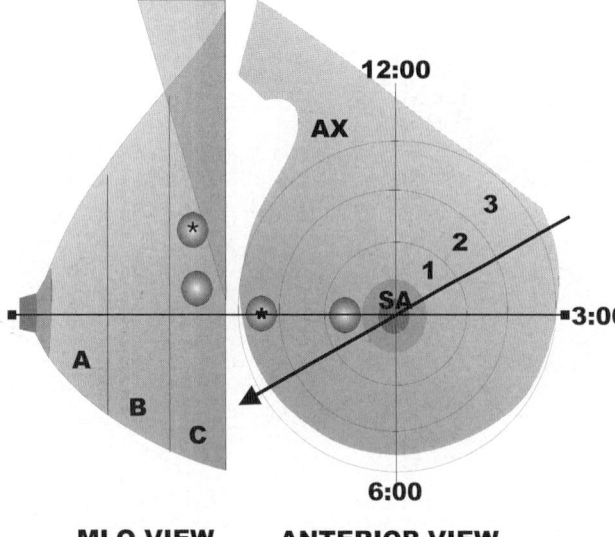

FIGURE 6–16 The x-ray beam passes from high medial to low lateral in performing the mediolateral oblique mammographic view. Thus, a lateral lesion tends to project higher than its true location, and the farther peripherally a lateral lesion lies, the higher it projects. Exceptions to this general rule can occur when a lesion lies near 12:00 or 6:00.

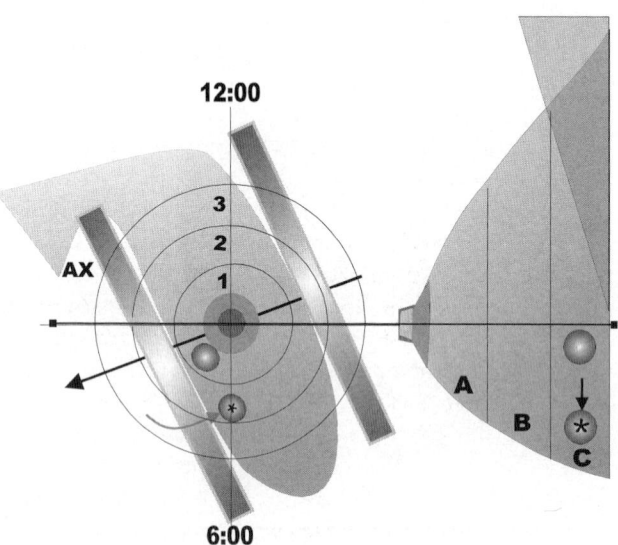

FIGURE 6–17 The application of mammographic compression while performing the mediolateral oblique view often has a strong rotatory component that can significantly displace a lesion upward or downward along the craniocaudal axis, creating greater uncertainty about the position of the lesion along the craniocaudal axis on that view.

of gravity and the rotatory forces used during compression affect the projected position of a lesion more on the MLO view than on the CC view (i.e., mammographic compression can move lesions farther cranially or caudally on the MLO view than compression can move lesions from right to left on the CC view) (Figs. 6–17 and 6–18). Therefore, a lesion that lies along the PNL on the mammographic CC view will usually lie very near 6:00 or 12:00 at sonography. On the other hand, a lesion that lies along the PNL on a mammographic MLO view (i.e., appearing to lie near 3:00 or 9:00) may actually lie several centimeters superior to or inferior to the 3:00 or 9:00 positions at sonography. The degree of movement superiorly or inferiorly with compression is greatest for peripherally located lesions and lesser for centrally located lesions. Understanding how the location of a nodule affects its projection on MLO mammographic views helps to better predict the area of the breast to evaluate sonographically. However, because of movement that occurs with compression and rotation of the breast during mammography, scanning a wider wedge of tissue may be necessary to find lesions that lie far medially or laterally on mammograms compared with those that appear to lie near

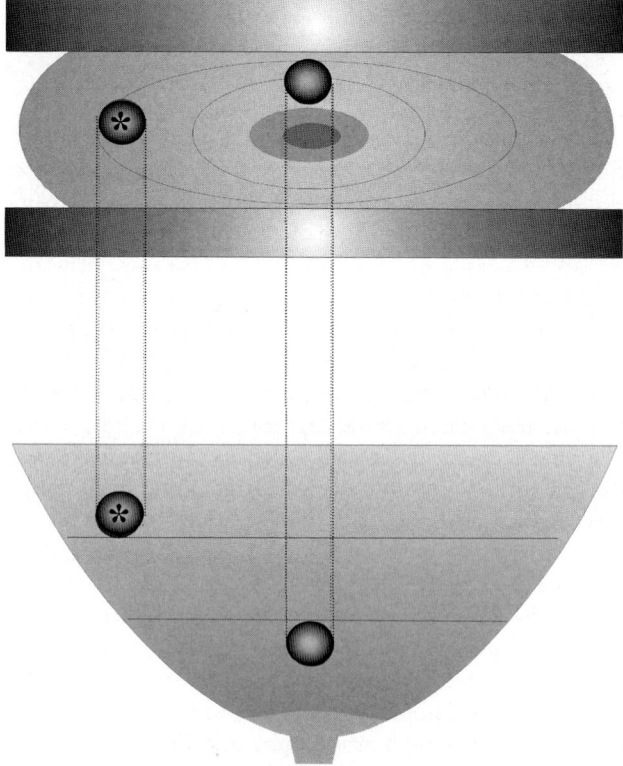

FIGURE 6–18 The application of mammographic compression on the craniocaudal (CC) view has a much smaller rotatory component than on the mediolateral oblique view that does not displace a lesion much to the left or right of its position in the breast relative to the nipple. Thus, a lesion projects along the mediolateral axis on the CC view near its true position, making it is easier to predict the location along the right-to-left axis than along the CC axis.

FIGURE 6–20 Compression applied during mammography affects the apparent location of a lesion relative to the chest wall as well as its apparent shape. When correlating location, the differences in mammographic and sonographic compression must be taken into account. Mammographic compression pulls a lesion away from the chest wall, whereas sonographic compression pushes a lesion closer to the chest wall. A lesion that appears to be several centimeters from the chest wall at mammography may actually indent the pectoralis muscle at sonography.

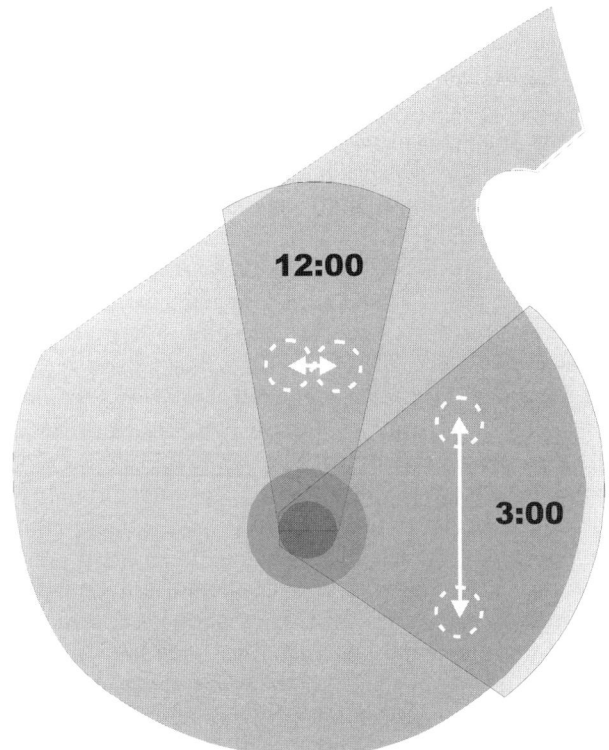

FIGURE 6–19 Angulation of x-ray beam on the mediolateral oblique (MLO) view and rotation of the breast that occurs during compression when performing the MLO view make it difficult to predict the location of lesions along the craniocaudal axis of the breast if they lie far medially or laterally. The location of lesions that lie near 12:00 or 6:00 is more predictable. Thus, lesions that appear to be near 12:00 or 6:00 can generally be found at sonography by scanning a narrow wedge of tissue. However, lesions that lie far medially or far laterally often require that a much larger wedge of tissue be scanned in order to find them.

12:00 or 6:00. Often, scanning can be initiated directly over the lesions that are located near 12:00 or 6:00 on the CC mammographic view, but scanning all the way from the 1:00 to 5:00 positions may be necessary to find lesions that project near 3:00 or 9:00 on the MLO mammographic view (Fig. 6–19).

The sonographic clock-face position of a lesion is more difficult to predict precisely if the lesion projects close to the nipple on mammograms than if it projects farther away. Interestingly, though, these periareolar lesions tend to project closer to their true position on MLO mammographic views than do peripheral lesions. Because of greater difficulty in predicting their location, periareolar lesions usually require that a wider-sector angle may have to be searched for lesions near the nipple. However, because the 2:00 and 4:00 positions are closer to each other nearer the nipple than they are when located farther from the nipple, the actual volume of tissue that requires scanning will not be greatly increased for lesions near the nipple.

Locating mammographic lesions at sonography becomes easier with experience. For mammographers who are inexperienced at sonographic detection and evaluation of mammographic lesions, this task may be very difficult in the beginning.

A few automated or semiautomated devices that scan the breast through compression plates similar to those used for mammography, in positions similar to those used for mammography, are available and can make sonographic correlation easier. Such equipment can enable fusion imaging. Having automated sonography built into a moving slit digital radiographic unit potentially can create automated sonographic–mammographic fusion imaging in the future.

When correlating lesion location on sonography and mammography, the distance that the lesion lies from the chest wall consistently differs. Mammographic compression devices pull lesions away from the chest wall and widens the retromammary fat zone. Sonography, typically performed with the patient supine, on the other hand, compresses the breast tissue and essentially obliterates the retromammary fat against the chest wall (Fig. 6–20). The net result of these differences between mammographic and sonographic compression is that mammographic lesions that appear to be several centimeters from the chest wall will appear much closer to the chest wall at sonography. For example, a mammographic nodule that appears to be several cm from the chest wall on mammograms may actually indent the pectoralis muscle at sonography (Fig. 6–21). This consistent difference in the portrayal of distance from the chest wall must always be kept in mind when comparing sonographic and mammographic locations.

Correlating Surrounding Tissue Density

Finally, taking into account the surrounding tissue density when comparing sonographic and mammographic structures is a necessity. A lesion that is completely fat surrounded

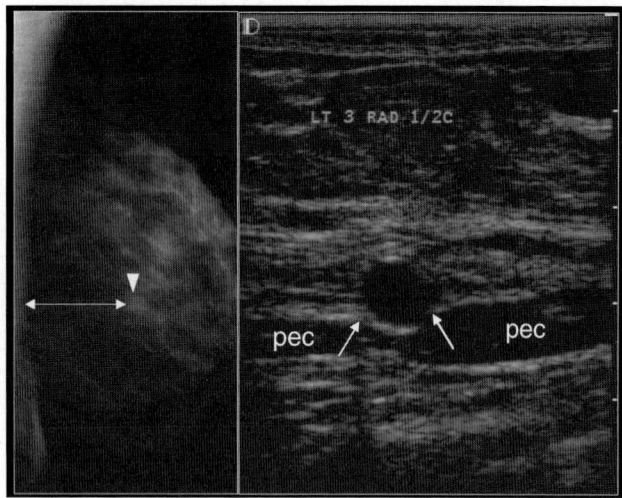

FIGURE 6–21 This small nodule appears to lie about 4 cm from the pectoralis muscle on the mediolateral oblique (MLO) mammogram because mammographic compression has pulled it away from the chest wall **(left)**. Sonography shows a cyst causing the nodule. The cyst appears to indent the pectoralis muscle on sonography (*arrows,* **right**), even though it appears several centimeters from the pectoralis on mammography. Sonographic compression consistently pushes lesions closer to the chest wall than they appear to be on mammography **(right)**.

on mammograms should be completely fat surrounded at sonography (Figs. 6–22). A lesion that appears to be completely surrounded by water-density tissue on mammography should be surrounded by hyperechoic fibrous or isoechoic glandular tissue sonographically. However, lesions encompassed with fibroglandular tissue must cause asymmetry, architectural distortion, or contain calcium to be visible mammographically (Fig. 6–23). A mammographic lesion that has a circumscribed anterior border but an obscured posterior border (a very common finding) should have fat around the anterior margin and either fibrous or glandular tissue around the posterior border sonographically (Figs. 6–24 and 6–25). A mammographic lesion that is partially obscured by adjacent fibroglandular tissue anteriorly should have hyperechoic fibrous tissue or isoechoic glandular tissue abutting it anteriorly (Fig. 6–26). The relationship of a lesion to a particular Cooper's ligament may be important. A mammographic lesion lying within and causing a focal widening of a Cooper's ligament should also lie with a Cooper's ligament sonographically (Fig. 6–27). An architectural distortion that is circumscribed anteriorly and obscured posteriorly may extend into a Cooper's ligament (Fig. 6–28). A mammographic lesion that projects superficial or deep to a band of water-density tissue should have a band of fibrous or glandular tissue in a corresponding superficial or deep position at sonography (Fig. 6–29).

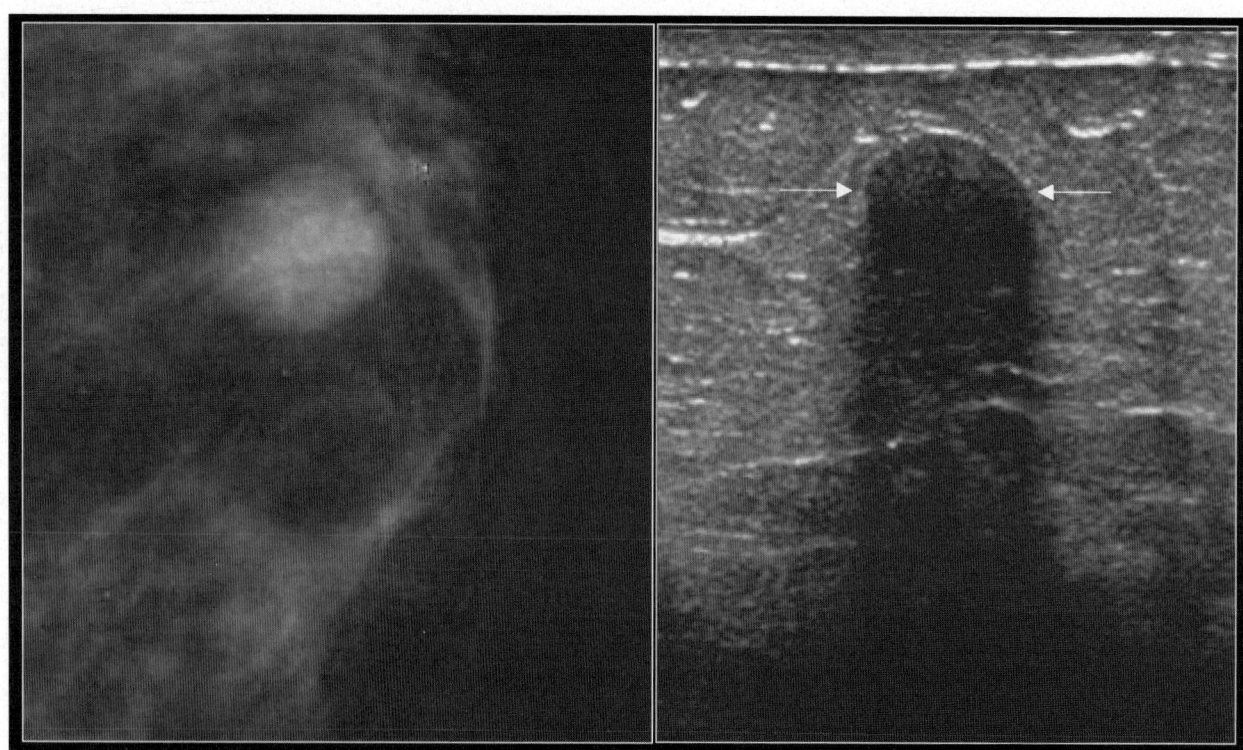

FIGURE 6–22 This circumscribed mammographic nodule is completely surrounded by fat.

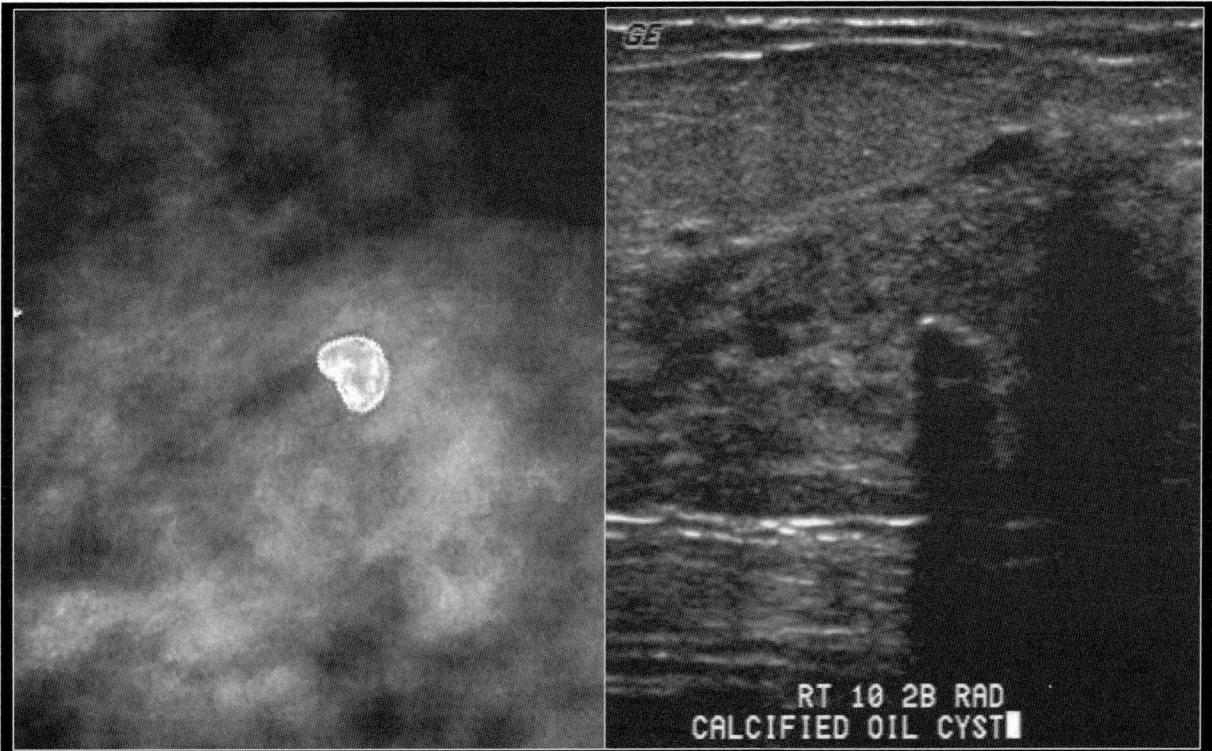

FIGURE 6–23 This mammographically definitively benign eggshell calcification that outlines the wall of an oil cyst is completely encompassed within mammographically dense tissue (**left**). Sonography shows the shadowing eggshell calcification to lie within an isoechoic, glandular area (water density on mammography) of the breast. The echogenicity of glandular tissue can be identical to that of fat; thus, it is necessary to know the density of tissue on mammography to distinguish isoechoic glandular from isoechoic fatty tissue in some cases. In others, compressibility is the key to the distinction (**right**). Sonography is not necessary to evaluate eggshell calcifications, which are BIRADS 2 on mammography. However, incidental eggshell calcifications noted during sonography can cause problems. Dense eggshell calcifications can cause acoustic shadowing that can appear falsely suspicious on sonography unless mammographic and sonographic correlation proves that the shadowing corresponds to a benign eggshell calcification on mammograms.

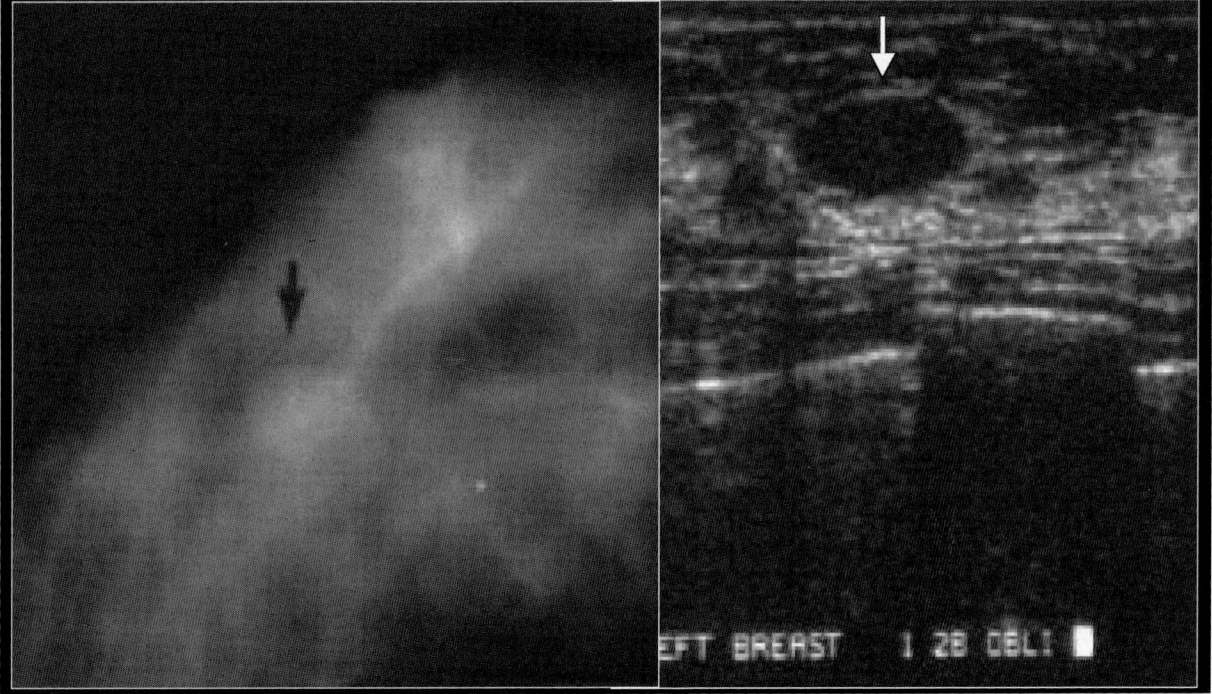

FIGURE 6–24 This mammographic nodule is circumscribed anteriorly (*arrow,* **left**) but obscured by dense tissue posteriorly. Sonography shows a BIRADS 3 solid nodule bordered by fat anteriorly (*arrow,* **right**), accounting for its circumscribed margin on the mammogram, and water-density fibrous tissue bordering on its deep surface, accounting for the obscured mammographic margin (**right**).

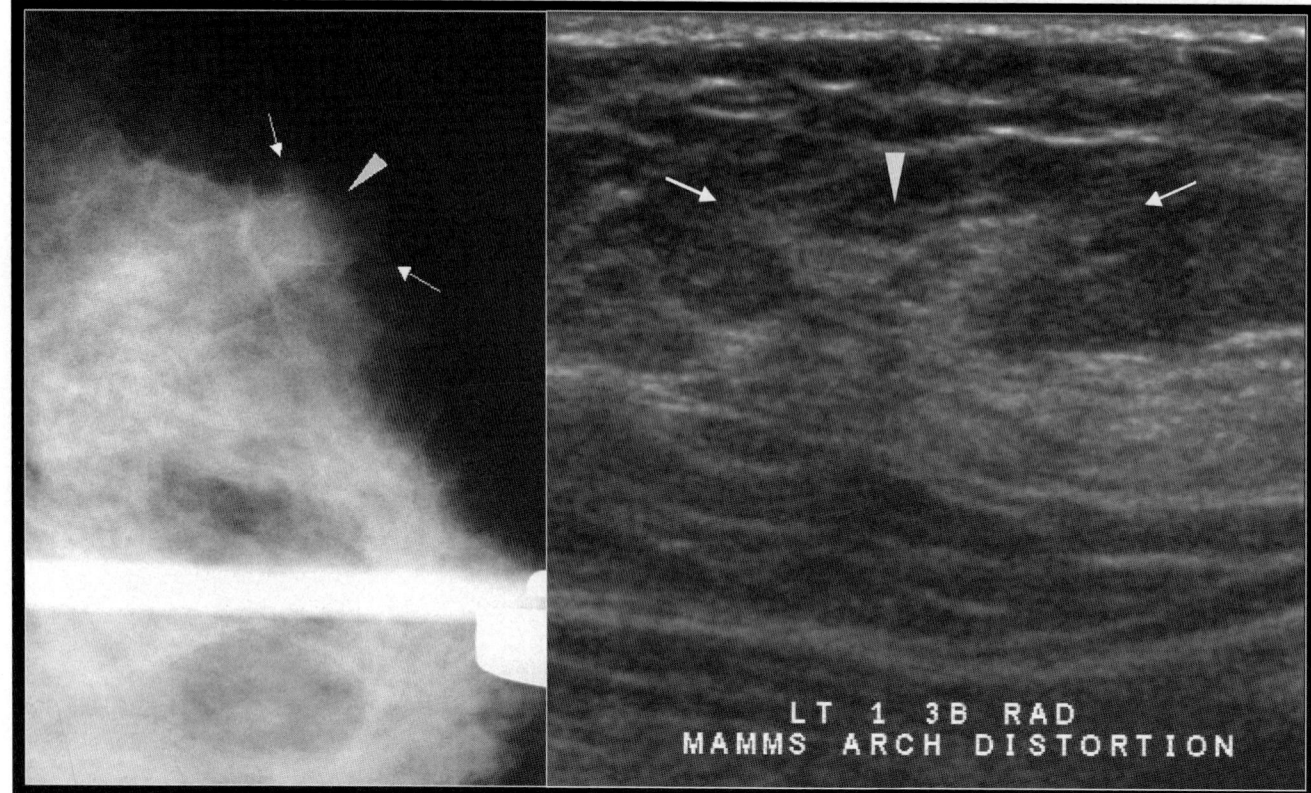

FIGURE 6–25 The sonogram shows that the mammographic architectural distortion *(arrow-head)* is caused by mixed isoechoic and hyperechoic fibroglandular tissue that protrudes anteriorly into the subcutaneous fat rather than the suspected malignant solid mass. The fat-surrounded collection of fibroglandular tissue is anvil shaped and surrounded by fat anteriorly, explaining its circumscribed anterior border at mammography. It is continuous with fibroglan-dular tissue posteriorly that is of equal water density, explaining its obscured posterior border on the mammogram. It is likely that architectural distortion is the result of atrophy and regres-sion of the surrounding fibroglandular tissue with age, leaving a peninsula of residual tissue in the bases of two Cooper's ligaments, one at each point on the "anvil" *(arrows).* Fibroglandular elements typically do regress more slowly when closely associated with Cooper's ligaments. The unusual and worrisome shape is created because of the underlying ligamentous anatomy. The sonographic findings are BIRADS 3, probably benign, preventing biopsy, but requiring short-in-terval follow-up. Were the tissue purely hyperechoic, without isoechoic glandular elements, the findings would be BIRADS 2, benign, preventing both biopsy and short-interval follow-up.

In correlating surrounding tissue density between mammography and sonography, remember that mammo-graphic compression tends to pull tissues away from the chest wall and to spread them apart, whereas sonographic compression tends to push lesions together along the an-teroposterior axis and against the chest wall. Therefore, a lesion that appears completely fat surrounded on mam-mography but has a band of fibroglandular tissue a few centimeters superficial to it on mammography may appear to abut or indent the band of fibroglandular tissue sono-graphically. Scanning with very light transducer pressure can allow the fat between the lesion and the overlying band of fibroglandular tissue to expand, confirming that the le-sion is really surrounded by fat at sonography, just as it is at mammography. Split-screen sonographic images per-formed with and without compression can be invaluable in documenting such anatomic features (Fig. 6–30).

In experienced hands, strict correlation of size, shape, location, and surrounding tissue density can successfully document that the sonographic findings and mammo-graphic findings represent the same structure in most cases. Occasionally, however, such correlation can be inconclu-sive in determining whether the mammographic and sono-graphic findings correspond or whether there are two separate lesions—one mammographic lesion and a separate sonographic lesion. In such cases, additional real-time sonographic survey should be performed to try to locate a structure that correlates better with the mammogram. Furthermore, the mammograms should be reevaluated or additional mammographic views (true lateromedial or

(text continued on page 141)

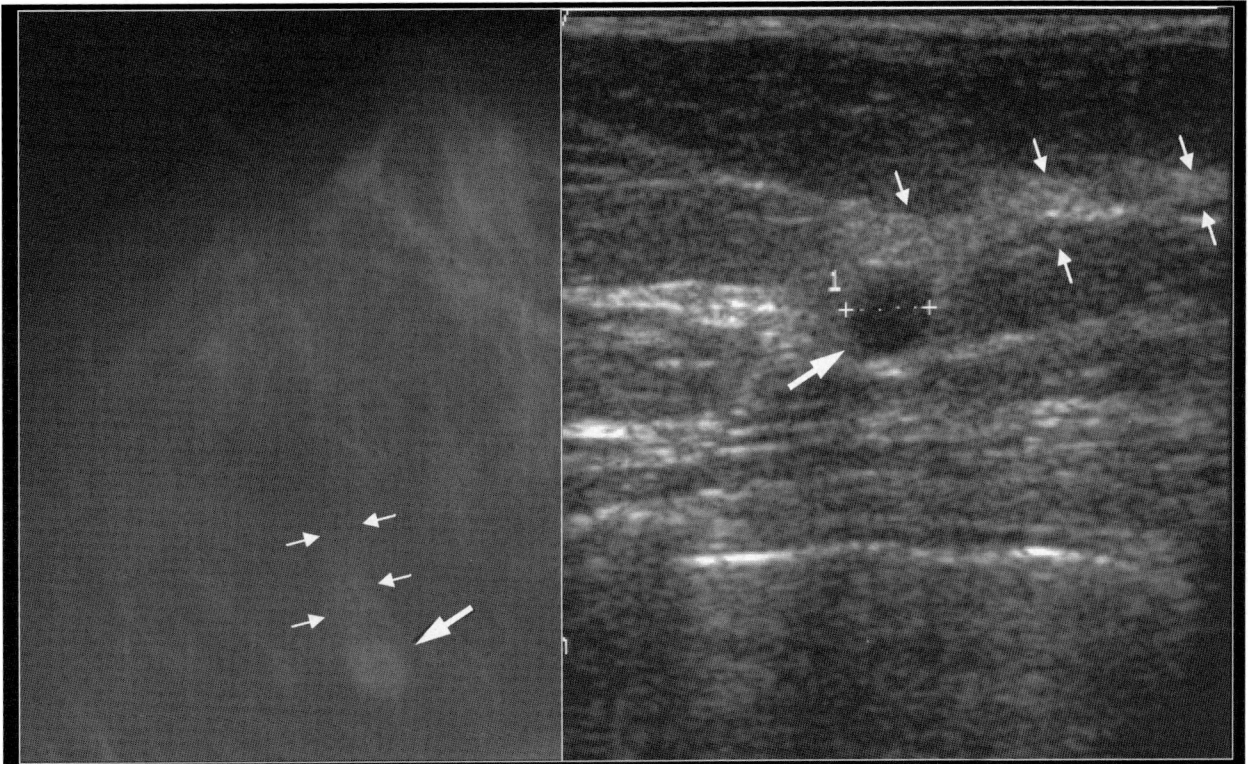

FIGURE 6–26 This small, elliptically shaped mammographic nodule (*large arrow,* **left**) is circumscribed by fat posteriorly and partially obscured by a "beard" of water-density tissue anteriorly (*small arrows,* **left**). Sonography shows a small cyst causing the nodule (*large arrow,* **right**) and a strand of hyperechoic fibrous tissue causing the anteriorly located soft tissue beard (*small arrows,* **right**). Note that the beard of fibrous tissue lies perpendicular to the chest wall on mammography and parallel to the chest wall on sonography.

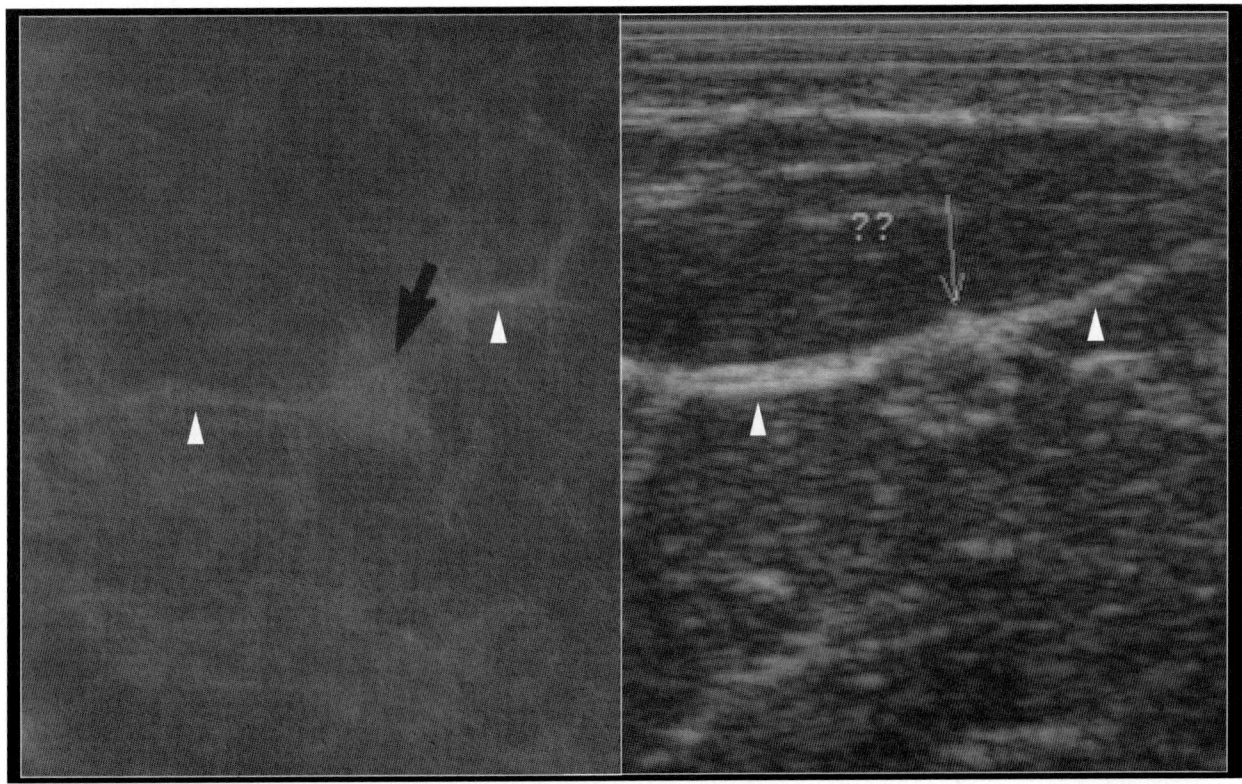

FIGURE 6–27 There is a mammographic architectural distortion resulting from a focal widening (*large arrow,* **left**) of the posterior aspect of a Cooper's ligament (*arrowheads,* **left**). Sonography shows an angular, suspicious solid nodule (*large arrow,* **right**) protruding from the deep surface of Cooper's ligament (*arrowheads,* **right**). On both mammography and sonography, the nodule is surrounded by fat, except along the anterior border, where it abuts a ligament.

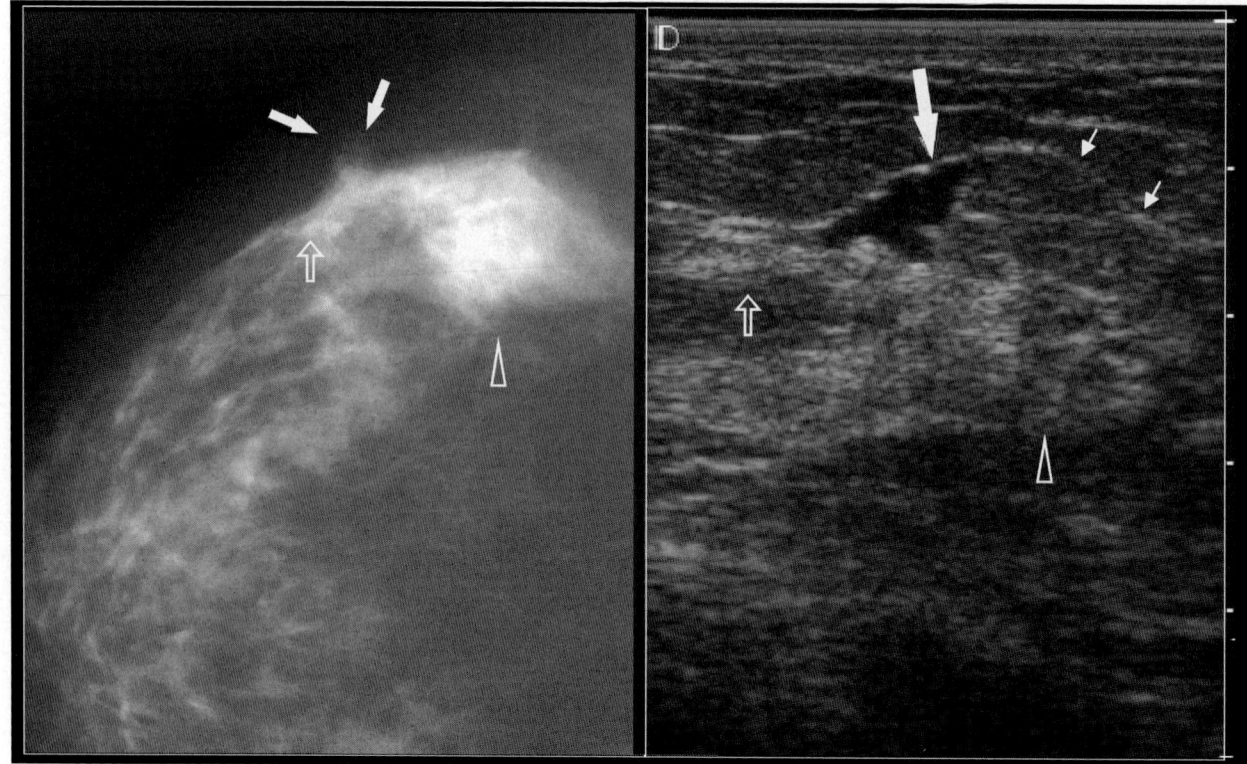

FIGURE 6–28 The craniocaudal mammographic view shows an angular architectural distortion (*large arrows,* **left**) arising at the junction of the mammary zone and subcutaneous fat protruding from the mammary zone superficially into a Cooper's ligament lying with the subcutaneous fat. Sonography shows the angular architectural distortion to be caused by a cystically dilated duct (*large arrow,* **right**) that lies within Cooper's ligament *(short arrow,* **right***)*. On both mammography and sonography, the distortion abuts a thin band of water density posteriorly (*hollow arrows*), and there is a thick collection of water-density tissue (*hollow arrowhead,* **left**) lying medially and deeper than the lesion. The mammographic finding is mildly suspicious (BIRADS 4a) because invasive breast cancers can create such an appearance when they invade the base of a Cooper's ligament but the sonographic findings are BIRAD 2, benign.

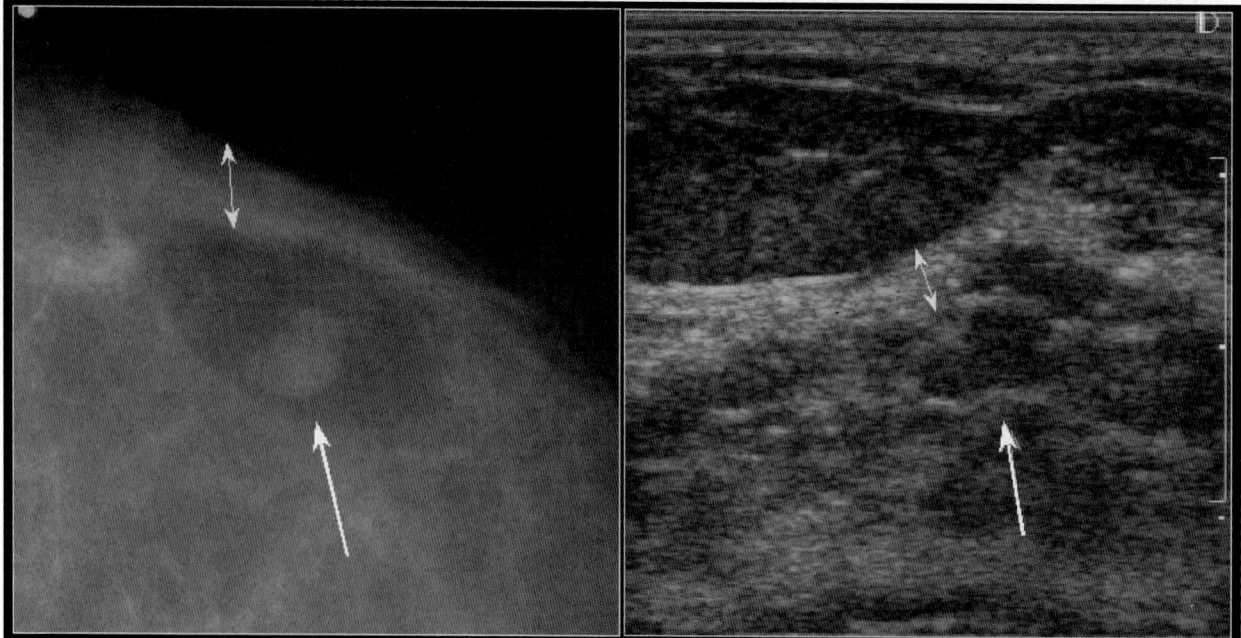

FIGURE 6–29 The craniocaudal mammographic view shows a lobulated, fat-surrounded nodule (*arrow,* **left**) that lies posterior to a band of water-density fibrous or glandular tissue (*double-headed arrow,* **left**). Sonography shows a lobulated solid nodule corresponding to the mammographic nodule (*arrow,* **right**), with a band of hyperechoic fibrous tissue lying anterior to it (*double-headed arrow,* **right**).

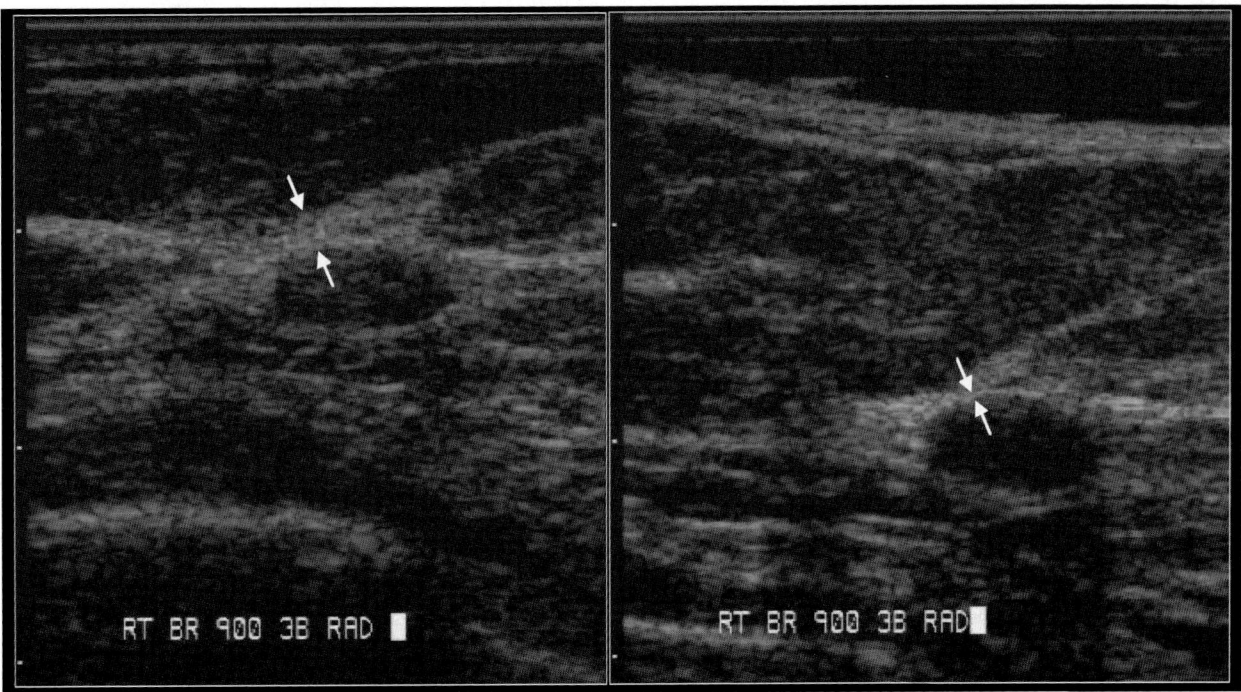

FIGURE 6–30 A sonogram performed with heavy compression has forced tissue planes closer together and makes the solid nodule appear to be encompassed within hyperechoic fibrous tissue anteriorly (*arrows,* **left**). A scan performed on the same nodule with very light compression shows the nodule to be surrounded by fat anteriorly (*arrows,* **right**). The lighter scan pressure has allowed the tissue planes to spread apart in the anteroposterior plane, giving a truer picture of the immediately surrounding tissues. Note that there is artifactual shadowing deep to the nodule.

mediolateral views) should be performed to determine whether the demonstrated sonographic lesion is, in retrospect, visible as a second mammographic lesion.

If the lesion is visible only on the MLO view, a true mediolateral view should be obtained. The position of the difficult-to-find lesion should be compared on the true mediolateral and mediolateral oblique films by placing the mediolateral and MLO views side by side (mediolateral on the left and MLO on the right) with the nipple at the same level on both views. If the nodule lies higher on the mediolateral view than on the MLO view, it usually lies medially. Because the beam passes from high medial to low lateral on the MLO view, medial lesions project lower than their true location on the MLO view. Thus, the medially located nodule will generally project higher on the true mediolateral view than it will on the MLO view. Conversely, if the nodule projects higher on the MLO view than on the true mediolateral view, it is usually located in the lateral half of the breast. If the CC view is placed next to the MLO view with the nipple at the same level, an arrow drawn through the nodule from the mediolateral to MLO view will usually point to the half of the breast in which the nodule lies (Figs. 6–31 and 6–32).

Occasionally, despite all efforts, sonographic–mammographic correlation can fail to determine whether the sonographically and mammographically demonstrated lesions are the same or whether, in fact, there are two different lesions. This problem arises most frequently either when (a) there are multiple mammographic lesions and there is a lack of certainty as to which lesion on the CC view corresponds to which lesion on the MLO view, or (b) when a density is seen on only one view of the mammogram. There are several possible approaches to solving this dilemma. First, the patient can be scanned through a Plexiglas plate that compresses the breast in a similar plane to that of the mammographic projection plane. This technique is usually performed in a manner similar to that used in obtaining CC mammograms and was described previously. Alternatively, the patient can be placed in the mammography compression device while the breast is scanned through a fenestrated mammographic compression plate with the hole directly over the lesion and is marked with a BB or an ink marker. Further, if sonography shows a cyst, but there is uncertainty about whether this cyst is the cause of a mammographic abnormality, the cyst can be aspirated under ultrasound guidance, and the mammogram can be repeated to make certain the mammographic nodule disappears (Figs. 6–33). Additionally, for solid nodules or complex cysts that cannot be completely aspirated, a needle with a retractable hookwire can be placed under ultrasound

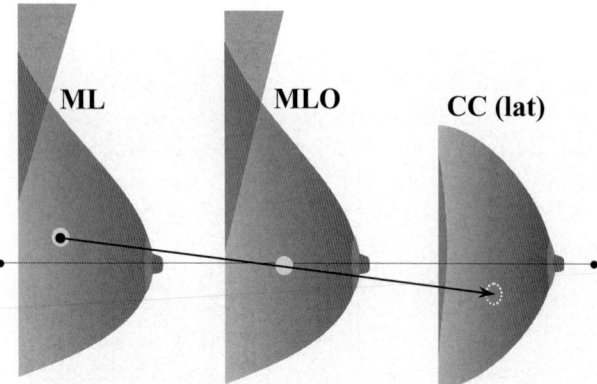

how to locate lesions seen only on MLO view

ML **MLO** **CC (lat)**

if lesion is lower on MLO than ML, it lies medially

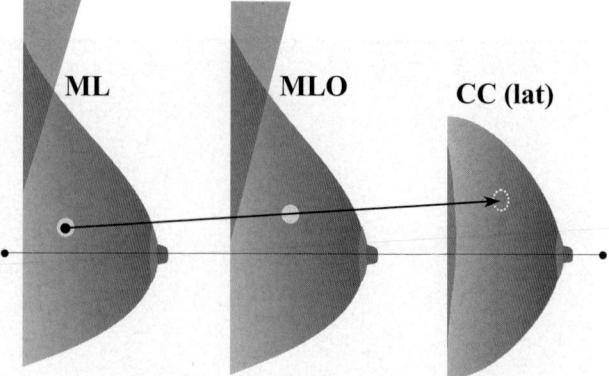

how to locate lesions seen only on MLO view

ML **MLO** **CC (lat)**

if lesion is higher on MLO than ML, it lies laterally

FIGURE 6–31 When a lesion is seen only on the mediolateral oblique (MLO) view, and when exaggerated craniocaudal (CC) views to the medial or lateral side also fail to show the lesion, a true mediolateral (ML) view may be helpful in determining whether the lesion lies in the medial or lateral half of the breast in order to facilitate targeted diagnostic breast ultrasound. If the true ML and MLO views are hung side by side with the nipple at the level and with the ML view on the left and MLO view on the right, the side of the breast in which the lesion lies becomes apparent in most patients. If the lesion is lower on the MLO view than on the ML view, it lies in the medial half of the breast because medial lesions usually project lower on the MLO view than their true CC axis positions (which is more accurately reflected by the true ML view). If the CC view is hung side by side with the ML and MLO views and placed to the right with the nipple at the same level as on the ML and MLO views, an arrow drawn through the nodule will point toward the half of the breast in which the nodule lies. Nodules that lie near 12:00 or 6:00 may violate this general rule.

FIGURE 6–32 When a lesion is seen only on the mediolateral oblique (MLO) view, and when exaggerated craniocaudal (CC) views to the medial or lateral side also fail to show the lesion, a true mediolateral (ML) view may be helpful in determining whether the lesion lies in the medial or lateral half of the breast in order to facilitate targeted diagnostic breast ultrasound. If the true ML view and MLO views are hung side by side with the nipple at the level and with the ML view on the left and MLO view on the right, the side of the breast in which the lesion lies becomes apparent in most patients. If the lesion lies more superiorly on the MLO view than on the ML view, it lies in the lateral half of the breast because lateral lesions usually project higher on the MLO view than their true CC axis positions (which is more accurately reflected by the true ML view). If the CC view is hung side by side with the ML and MLO views and placed to the right with the nipple at the same level as on the ML and MLO views, an arrow drawn through the nodule will point toward the half of the breast in which the nodule lies. Nodules that lie near 12:00 or 6:00 may violate this general rule.

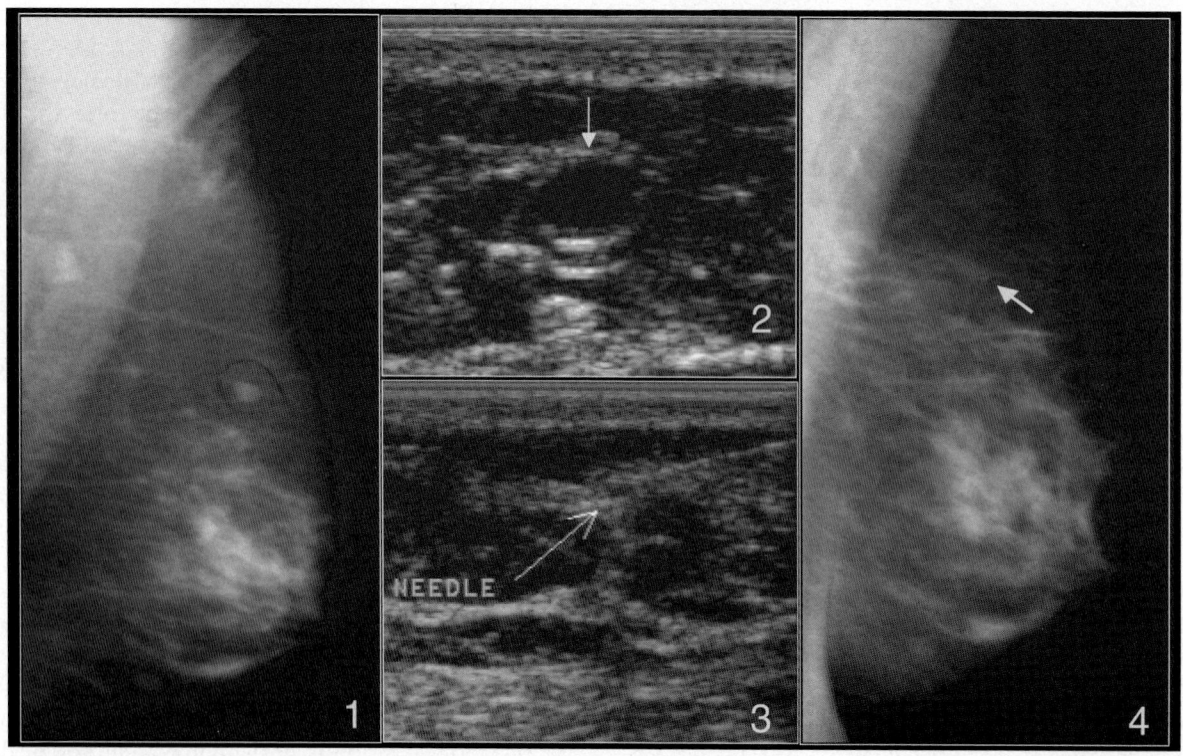

FIGURE 6–33 The mammogram showed a small fat-surrounded nodule in the upper outer quadrant of the left breast *(1)*. Sonography showed a cyst causing the nodule *(2)*. The cyst was aspirated under ultrasound guidance *(3)*. Repeat mammogram after aspiration showed no residual nodule, confirming that the aspirated cyst, indeed, did cause the mammographic nodule *(4)*.

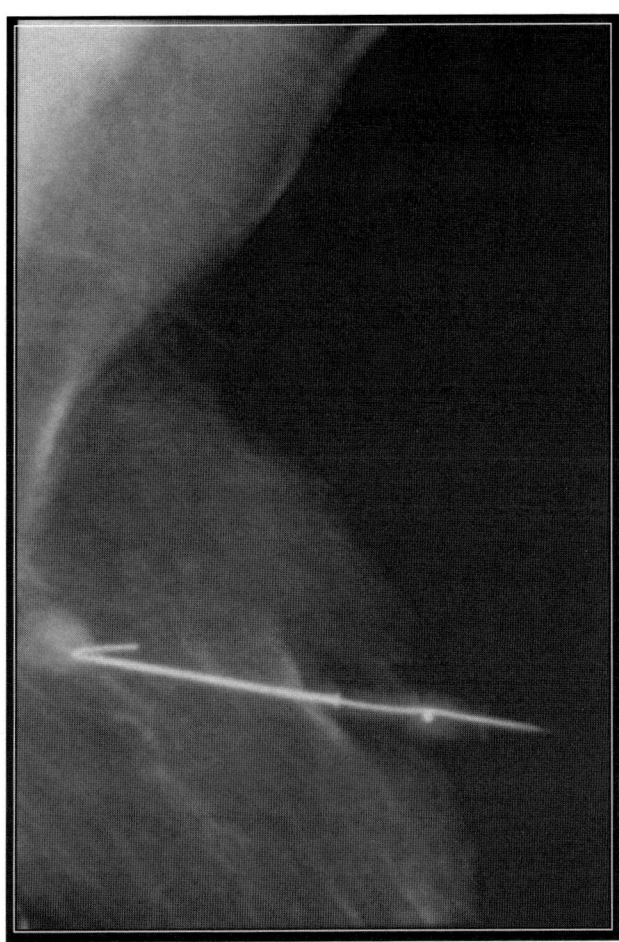

FIGURE 6–34 This mammographic nodule was caused by a subtle, deeply located, isoechoic, solid nodule that was identical in echogenicity to the surrounding fat lobules. Before performing ultrasound-guided core needle biopsy, it was necessary to document that the suspected lesion on ultrasound was, indeed, the cause of the mammographic nodule. A retractable hookwire was place under ultrasound guidance, and the postlocalization mammogram confirmed that the sonographically localized lesion was, in fact, the cause of the mammographic nodule. Ultrasound-guided core needle biopsy was then performed. Histology was determined to be colloid carcinoma.

guidance. A mammogram can then be taken to prove that the hookwire marks the mammographic lesion of concern (Fig. 6–34). Should aspiration or localization with retractable hookwire show definitively that the sonographic and mammographic lesions are different, additional effort should be made to find the second lesion sonographically. If necessary, both lesions can undergo imaging-guided aspiration or biopsy—the sonographically demonstrated lesion using ultrasound guidance, and the mammographically demonstrated lesion using stereotactic guidance.

In some cases, a completely fat-surrounded mammographic lesion will not be identifiable sonographically. Although sonography has been less successful than hoped in such cases, it has not been a total failure. We gain three im-

portant pieces of data when a real mammographic nodule seen in both views cannot be found sonographically. First, inability to identify a mammographic lesion sonographically is strong, indirect evidence that the lesion is solid. The sensitivity of ultrasound for cystic lesions is so high that the likelihood that a cyst could be missed sonographically is extremely low. Second, the solid nodule is virtually certain to be isoechoic with surrounding fatty breast tissues. Hypoechoic solid nodules would be readily visible, but lesions that are isoechoic with surrounding fat may be difficult or impossible to perceive. Third, it is apparent that the customary sonographic algorithm of looking for a hypoechoic lesion in a gray or white background has failed. However, virtually all breast lesions—cystic or solid and isoechoic or hypoechoic—are encompassed within an echogenic capsule. Benign lesions tend to have a thin, well-circumscribed capsule, and malignant lesions tend to have a thick, ill-defined capsule (halo). Because the algorithm of looking for a hypoechoic lesion has failed, altering the imaging algorithm to look for an echogenic capsule that has the shape of the mammographic lesion will facilitate detection of the lesion in many cases. The lesions most likely to be isoechoic to fat and missed sonographically are intramammary lymph nodes and fibroadenomas (Fig. 6–35), but occasionally small, circumscribed carcinomas can be isoechoic and difficult to perceive. This is especially true of pure ductal carcinoma *in situ* and small (<1.5 cm maximum diameter) colloid carcinomas (Fig. 6–36).

For lesions that are both palpable and mammographically visible, sonographic findings should be correlated with both the clinical and mammographic findings. A key point to remember is that the mammographic and palpable lesions might be either the same lesion or two different lesions. Sonographic–mammographic correlation is critical in making this determination (Fig. 6–37).

This rigorous exercise of correlating exact sonographic size, shape, location, and surrounding tissue density with mammographic size, shape, location, and surrounding tissue density when sonographically evaluating a mammographic lesion will, over time, improve both mammographic and sonographic skills.

SUMMARY

In summary, when a mammographic abnormality is evaluated by sonography, the size, shape, location, and surrounding tissue density should be the same on sonography as they are mammography in order to prove that the sonographic structure is the same structure as the mammographic structure. This approach is especially important if the sonographic findings indicate a benign cause for the mammographic abnormality, such as a simple cyst, that might not require biopsy. The original mammographic density may or may not be visible sonographically, but

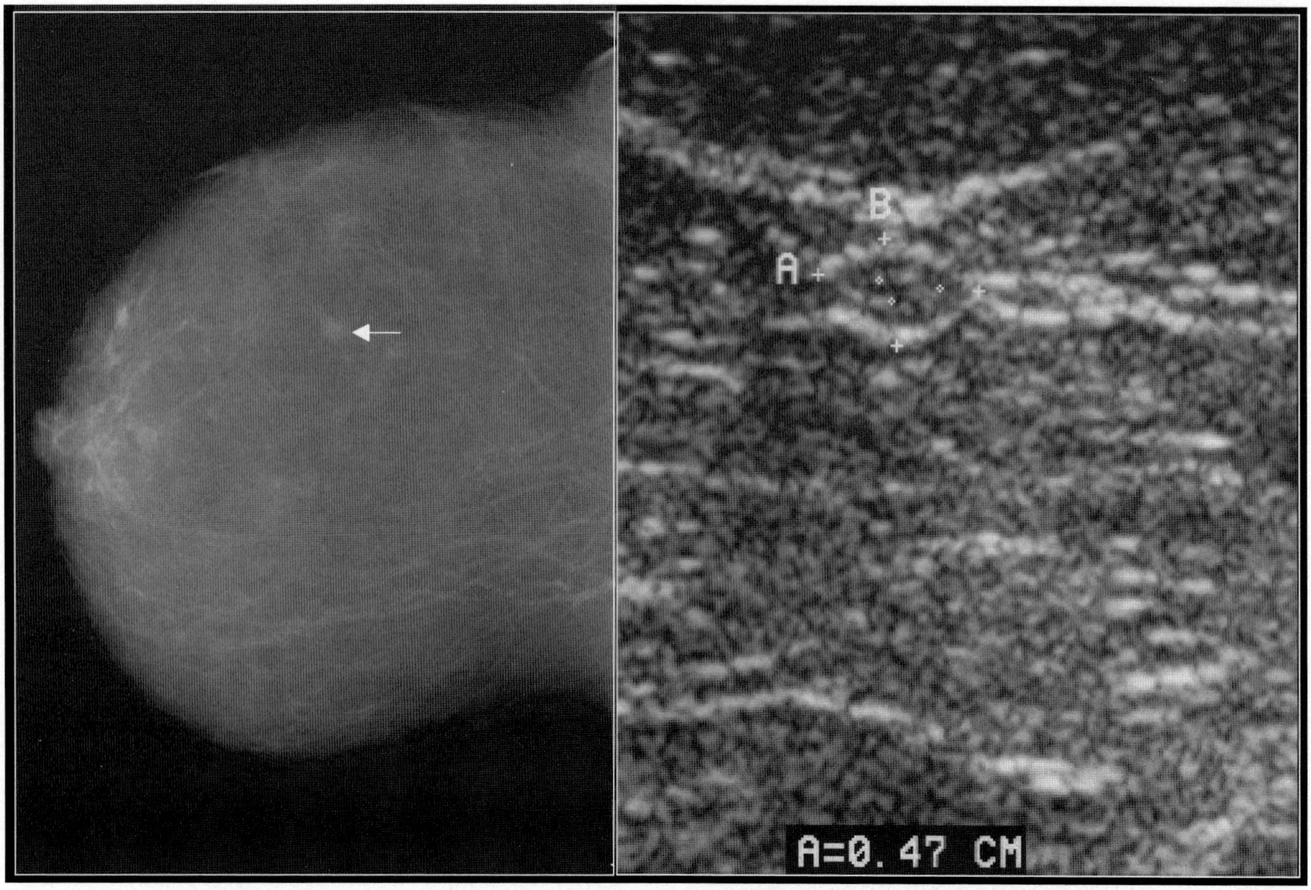

FIGURE 6–35 This small, oval-shaped, sharply circumscribed mammographic nodule (*arrow,* **left**) was present on both mammographic views. Ultrasound initially failed to demonstrate the lesion. This indicated that the lesion being sought was solid and isoechoic. It also indicated that the usual algorithm of looking for hypoechoic structures in an isoechoic background had failed. However, by looking for the hyperechoic capsule rather than a hypoechoic nodule, the lesion was found on sonography (*calipers,* **right**).

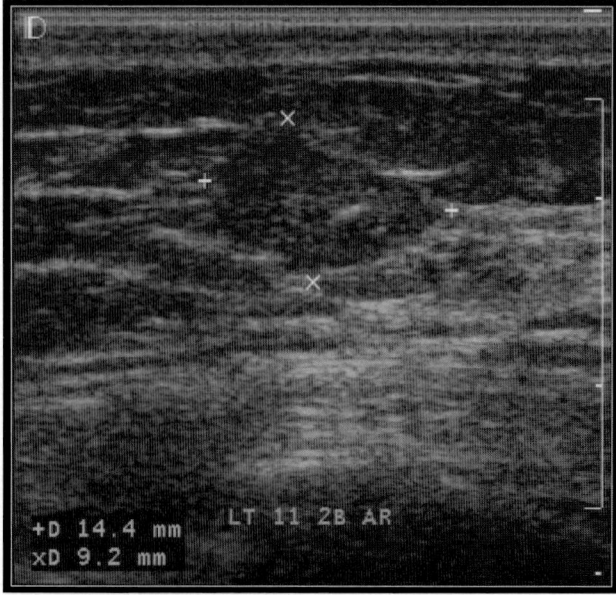

FIGURE 6–36 Most isoechoic, solid nodules that are hard to detect sonographically are benign fibroadenomas or normal intramammary lymph nodes. However, certain small, circumscribed, malignant nodules, such as this small colloid carcinoma, can be isoechoic with fat and difficult to detect sonographically.

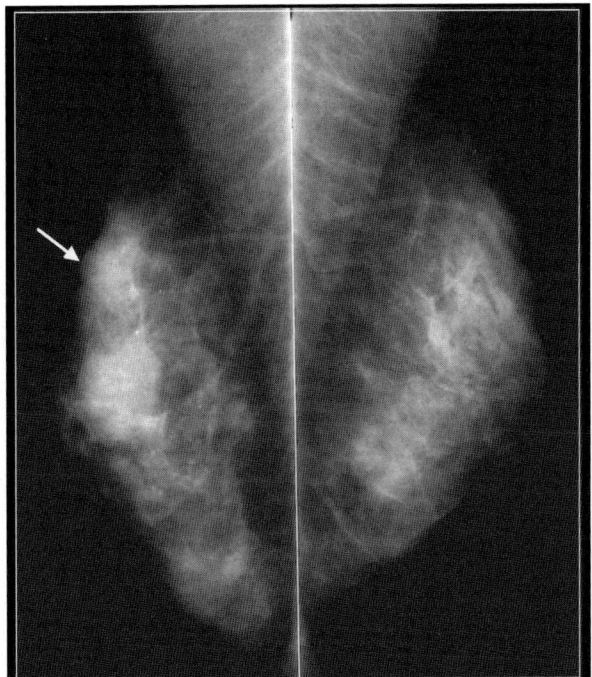

A

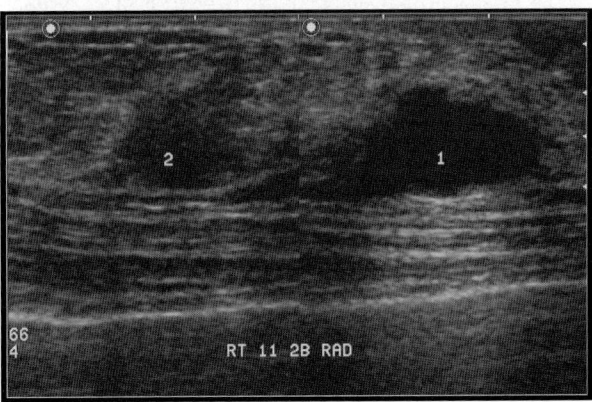

B

FIGURE 6–37 A: In patients who have both mammographic and palpable abnormalities, both mammographic–sonographic and clinical–sonographic correlation should be obtained. That there might actually be two separate lesions mammographically and sonographically, should always be kept in mind when correlating mammographic and sonographic findings. This patient presented with a palpable lump in the upper central left breast. Mammography showed an architectural distortion consisting of a bulge in the anterior mammary fascia *(arrow)*. **B:** Sonography showed a simple cyst *(1)* that initially was thought by the sonographer to explain both clinical and mammographic abnormalities. However, mammographic–sonographic correlation showed the cyst to lie too far inferiorly to explain the architectural distortion. Further correlation showed both the architectural distortion and the palpable lump to be caused by a more superiorly located malignant-appearing solid nodule *(2)*. There were two separate lesions. The malignant nodule was the cause of the suspicious mammographic abnormality and the lump, and the cyst was incidental.

further efforts to find the lesion and to characterize it sonographically are warranted. Additionally, reevaluation of the mammogram or obtaining additional mammographic views to better demonstrate the original mammographic finding or to find a second lesion that corresponds to the sonographic lesion may be helpful. If size, shape, location, and surrounding tissue density all correlate exactly, one can be sure that there is only one lesion and that the mammographic and sonographic findings represent the same structure. If sonographic and mammographic findings do not correlate, there are probably two lesions. Although the emphasis in this chapter has been on proving that the mammographic and sonographic lesions are one and the same, it is critical to remember that in a significant minority of patients undergoing sonography for evaluation of a mammographic abnormality, there will be two separate lesions—one sonographic lesion and one mammographic lesion. Strict adherence to this algorithm for every mammographic density evaluated with sonography will eventually improve both mammographic interpretive and sonographic skills and raise one's level of confidence in BUS.

SUGGESTED READINGS

Aitken RJ, Chetty U. Non-palpable mammographic abnormalities. *J R Coll Surg Edinb* 1991;36(6):362–371.

Brem RF, Gatewood OM. Template-guided breast US. *Radiology* 1992;184(3):872–874.

Brenner RJ. Follow-up as an alternative to biopsy for probably benign mammographically detected abnormalities. *Curr Opin Radiol* 1991;3(4):588–592.

Brombart JC. Breast echography. *J Belge Radiol* 1995;78(1):34–38.

Catarzi S, et al. A multicenter study for the evaluation of the diagnostic efficiency of mammography and echography in nonpalpable breast neoplasms [published erratum appears in *Radiol Med* (Torino) 1992;84(5):664]. *Radiol Med* (Torino) 1992;84(3):193–197.

Chetty U. Diagnosis of the impalpable lesion. *Br Med Bull* 1991;47(2):427–432.

Ciatto S, et al. Fine-needle aspiration cytology of nonpalpable breast lesions: US versus stereotaxic guidance. *Radiology* 1993;188(1):195–198.

Cole-Beuglet C, et al. Ultrasound mammography: a comparison with radiographic mammography. *Radiology* 1981;139(6):693–698.

Conway WF, Hayes CW, Brewer WH. Occult breast masses: use of a mammographic localizing grid for US evaluation. *Radiology* 1991;181(1):143–146.

Davies AH, et al. Ultrasound localization of screen detected impalpable breast tumours. *J R Coll Surg Edinb* 1994;39(6):353–354.

Dowlatshahi K, Snider H. Management of abnormal mammograms. *Admin Radiol* 1992;11:121–122.

Edelman B. Statistical analysis of US may cut breast biopsies. *Radiol Today* 1992;9:3.

Fornage BD, Toubas O, Morel M. Clinical, mammographic, and sonographic determination of preoperative breast cancer size. *Cancer* 1987;60(4):765–771.

Fung HM, Jackson FI. Clinically and mammographically occult breast lesions demonstrated by ultrasound. *J R Soc Med* 1990; 83(11):696–698.

Guyer PB, et al. Direct contact B-scan ultrasound in the diagnosis of solid breast masses. *Clin Radiol* 1986;37(5):451–458.

Hall FM. Probably benign breast nodules: follow-up of selected cases without initial full problem-solving imaging [Comment]. *Radiology* 1995;194(2):305.

Helvie MA, et al. Mammographic follow-up of low-suspicion lesions: compliance rate and diagnostic yield. *Radiology* 1991;178(1): 155–158.

Heywang-Kobrunner SH. Nonmammographic breast imaging techniques. *Curr Opin Radiol* 1992;4(5):146–154.

Lunt LG, Peakman DJ, Young JR. Mammographically guided ultrasound: a new technique for assessment of impalpable breast lesions. *Clin Radiol* 1991;44(2):85–88.

Matricardi L, et al. The use of echography and US-guided percutaneous puncture in addition to mammography for the detection of malignant breast tumors. *Radiol Med* (Torino) 1992;83(4):395–401.

McCaffrey JF, et al. The abnormal mammogram—what to do. *Aust Fam Physician* 1991;20(10):1431–1435.

McKenna RJ Sr. The abnormal mammogram radiographic findings, diagnostic options, pathology, and stage of cancer diagnosis. *Cancer* 1994;74[1 Suppl]:s244–255.

Meden H, et al. A clinical, mammographic, sonographic and histologic evaluation of breast cancer. *Int J Gynaecol Obstet* 1995; 48(2):193–199.

Pain JA, et al. Assessment of breast cancer size: a comparison of methods. *Eur J Surg Oncol* 1992;18(1):44–48.

Pearce RB. Ultrasound a useful adjunct to breast mammography. *Diagn Imaging* 1986;9:114–119.

Phillips G, McGuire L, Clowes D. The value of ultrasound-guided fine needle aspiration in the assessment of solid breast lumps. *Australas Radiol* 1994;38(3):187–192.

Reynolds HE. Sonographically guided breast intervention. *Appl Radiol* 1995;9:25–31.

Sailors DM, et al. Needle localization for nonpalpable breast lesions. *Am Surg* 1994;60(3):186–189.

Schepps B, Scola FH, Frates RE. Benign circumscribed breast masses: mammographic and sonographic appearance. *Obstet Gynecol Clin North Am* 1994;21(3):519–537.

Schlecht I, et al. Ultrasound detection of breast cancer with normal mammogram. *Aktuelle Radiol* 1995;5(5):297–300.

Schwartz GF, Feig SA. Management of clinically occult (nonpalpable) breast lesions. *Obstet Gynecol Clin North Am* 1994;21(4): 621–637.

Shaw de Paredes E. Evaluation of abnormal screening mammograms. *Cancer* 1994;74[1 Suppl]:342–349.

Sickles EA, Filly RA, Callen PW. Breast cancer detection with sonography and mammography: comparison using state-of-the-art equipment. *AJR Am J Roentgenol* 1983;140(5):843–845.

Smallwood JA, et al. The accuracy of ultrasound in the diagnosis of breast disease. *Ann R Coll Surg Engl* 1986;68(1):19–22.

Strasser K, et al. Sonography in breast diagnosis. *Radiologe* 1990; 30(3):130–134.

Urbanowicz Z, et al. Comparison of mammography and sonography in diagnosis of breast cysts. *Ginekol Pol* 1992;63(2):82–83.

Vetshev PS, et al. Ultrasound diagnosis of breast nodules. *Khirurgiia* (Mosk) 1995;(1):8–11.

Zaitsev AN, et al. Ultrasonography and mammography in breast cancer. *Vopr Onkol* 1994;40(1–3):87–90.

7

NONTARGETED INDICATIONS

Most of the diagnostic breast ultrasound (BUS) examinations that we perform are targeted to evaluation of either focal palpable or mammographic abnormalities. In targeted examinations, only a limited area of the breast in the immediate vicinity of the palpable lump or mammographic abnormality is scanned. The goal in such cases is to make a more specific diagnosis of the cause of the palpable or mammographic abnormality than could be made by mammography alone. On the other hand, in nontargeted BUS examinations, the entire breast (or both breasts) is scanned with the goal of finding lesions that are neither palpable nor mammographically visible.

It is important to distinguish whole breast sonography from screening sonography. Unilateral or bilateral whole breast sonography may be performed for screening purposes or for diagnosis. It is also important to distinguish primary from secondary screening sonography for breast cancer. In primary sonographic screening, sonography replaces mammography for breast cancer screening. In secondary sonographic screening, bilateral whole breast sonography is used as an adjunct to primary screening mammography. Secondary screening sonography is used in cases in which mammography is interpreted as negative [American College of Radiology Breast Imaging Reporting and Data System (BIRADS) category 1 or 2) and the risk for missing cancer or for the patient having cancer is higher than normal. Secondary screening might be performed in women with dense breasts, in which the sensitivity of mammography is lowered by mammographically dense tissue, or in cases in which the risk for developing breast cancer is very high because of a strong first-degree family history of breast cancer or presence of abnormal genes (such as *BRCA1, BRCA2, BRCA3*, or ataxia-telangiectasia genes).

To date, sonography has been shown to be inferior to mammography as a primary screening tool in virtually all published studies. Limitations of primary sonographic breast screening in comparison to primary mammographic screening include the following:

- Lower sensitivity for detection of small or pure ductal carcinoma *in situ* (DCIS) than mammography
- A large number of false-positive findings
- An unacceptably high operator dependence and reduced reproducibility in comparison to mammography

The lesions that are most likely to be detected by mammography but missed by ultrasound are small malignancies (<7 mm) that involve primarily a single terminal ductolobular unit (TDLU), and relatively small (<1.5 cm in maximum diameter) and circumscribed isoechoic carcinomas that are surrounded by isoechoic breast tissues. The small malignancies that involve primarily a single TDLU are likely to be low-nuclear-grade DCIS and to have calcifications that are mildly suspicious on mammograms. Such lesions may be visible by sonography but are difficult to distinguish from surrounding TDLUs that are mildly enlarged by fibrocystic change or other benign proliferative disorders unless associated suspicious calcifications can be detected. Although many calcifications can be detected sonographically, mammography has an advantage over sonography in detecting and characterizing such calcifications. Unfortunately, the types of lesions that are most likely to be missed by sonography, but detected by mammography, have the best prognosis of all malignant breast lesions for surgical cure; therefore, it is important that they not be missed. Because of mammography's superiority for detecting small subtle calcifications, mammography enjoys an advantage over sonography for detecting such small, curable lesions. The other type of lesion that may be missed by sonography but detected by mammography is the small, circumscribed isoechoic malignant nodule. Such nodules are water density and therefore easily distinguished from surrounding fat lobules mammographically, but they can be very difficult to distinguish from surrounding fat lobules sonographically. If mammography is performed first, such lesions will seldom be missed sonographically. However, in a primary screening mode, sonography can easily miss such lesions.

Because of the inferiority of sonography to mammography for detecting many small, curable breast carcinomas, primary sonographic screening for breast cancer cannot be advocated in the general population at this time. And despite the known limitations of mammography, it remains the only proven primary breast cancer screening modality.

The role of sonography for secondary breast cancer screening (i.e., whole breast ultrasound used as an adjunct after primary screening mammography) is more controversial and still evolving. Initial studies of secondary sonographic screening, like those of primary sonographic screening, found sonography wanting. However, more recently published secondary sonographic screening studies are far more encouraging. In four recent studies, bilateral whole breast sonography was performed in patients who initially had negative mammograms in which at least one-fourth of the breast was mammographically dense. In three of these studies, physicians, using state-of-the-art equipment, performed the examinations. In the other study, the initial evaluation was performed by a sonographer, with the radiologist scanning afterward when necessary. In all four studies, the sonographic detection rate of mammographically invisible and nonpalpable carcinomas was 3 per 1,000, less than would be expected in an initial mammographic screening population, but similar to the interval rate of mammographic cancer detection in populations heavily screened by mammography. The size and prognosis of the malignancies found only by sonography were similar to those found by primary interval mammographic screening. Furthermore, the time required for bilateral whole breast sonographic secondary screening in one of the studies was less than 6 minutes. Finally, the cost per cancer found was near that of primary screening mammography. Based on these encouraging studies, secondary screening sonography merits further evaluation in more widespread application (Fig. 7–1).

Despite these encouraging results, however, acceptance of secondary screening sonography by American radiologists will likely be slow and grudging. There are many problems that need to be overcome before secondary screening sonography becomes widespread in the United States. First, the number of radiologists in the United States skilled enough to achieve such results (and willing to try) is likely far too few. Sonography remains the most operator dependent of all imaging modalities, and skill levels of radiologists at performing diagnostic BUS vary widely. The ability to screen is likely to vary even more greatly than does the ability to perform diagnostic BUS. The recent published data are based on radiologists performing the ex-

amination in three of the four studies. However, most American radiologists rely on sonographers to perform the examination and do not perform entire examinations themselves. Radiologists who are skilled at performing BUS may not be able to perform the examinations as quickly as was done in the published studies. The economics of radiologist-performed screening sonography are poor compared with the economics of other radiologic imaging procedures, such as computed tomography (CT) or magnetic resonance imaging (MRI). The method of practice of most American radiologists would make physician-performed examinations difficult, if not impossible, to achieve. Most radiologists are responsible for supervising many different pieces of imaging equipment simultaneously. When the radiologist is physically present within an ultrasound room, performing sonographic examinations, he is unable to manage multiple other rooms simultaneously. This may result in decreased throughput on higher-cost, higher-profit equipment such as MRI and CT, a situation that both radiology groups and radiology administrators strongly discourage.

That there is now a severe shortage of radiologists in the United States exacerbates the problem. U.S. radiologists who are skilled in performing BUS may not feel that whole breast screening sonography is economically worth their efforts. The payment for sonography in the United States does not favor whole breast sonography. The payment for targeted BUS is low, often below the cost of performing even limited targeted examinations. In many centers, BUS and mammography are operated as "loss leaders" and are continued as a service to the population and as a tool for obtaining more profitable CT and MRI contracts. Furthermore, the insufficient payment is the same, regardless of whether sonography is targeted or nontargeted and regardless of whether the sonographic evaluation is unilateral or bilateral. Of course, the whole breast examination takes longer, and therefore has a higher cost that results in even greater losses for each study performed. Thus, in the United States, there is a real economic disincentive to extending the sonographic evaluation to include the whole breast and even more so toward evaluation the entirety of both breasts.

Additionally, there is also a strong medicolegal disincentive to whole breast sonography. Missed diagnosis of breast cancer is the number one cause of medical malpractice lawsuits in the United States. A significant percentage of American radiologists tend to "overcall" all lesions on targeted sonograms in order to avoid a medical malpractice suit for missed diagnosis of breast cancer. Radiologists within this subgroup actively avoid sonography anywhere other than the immediate area of interest in order to minimize their liabilities. The rationale behind this attitude is that a radiologist can be held liable only for a missed cancer that lies in the part of breast that was examined sonographically. It is reasoned that he or she cannot be held liable for

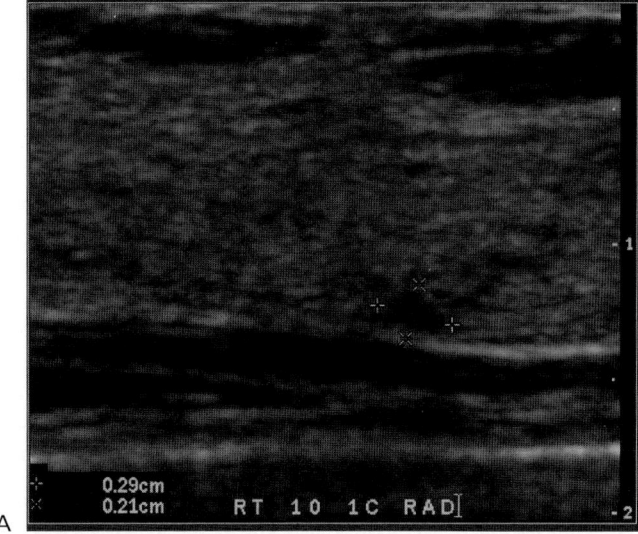

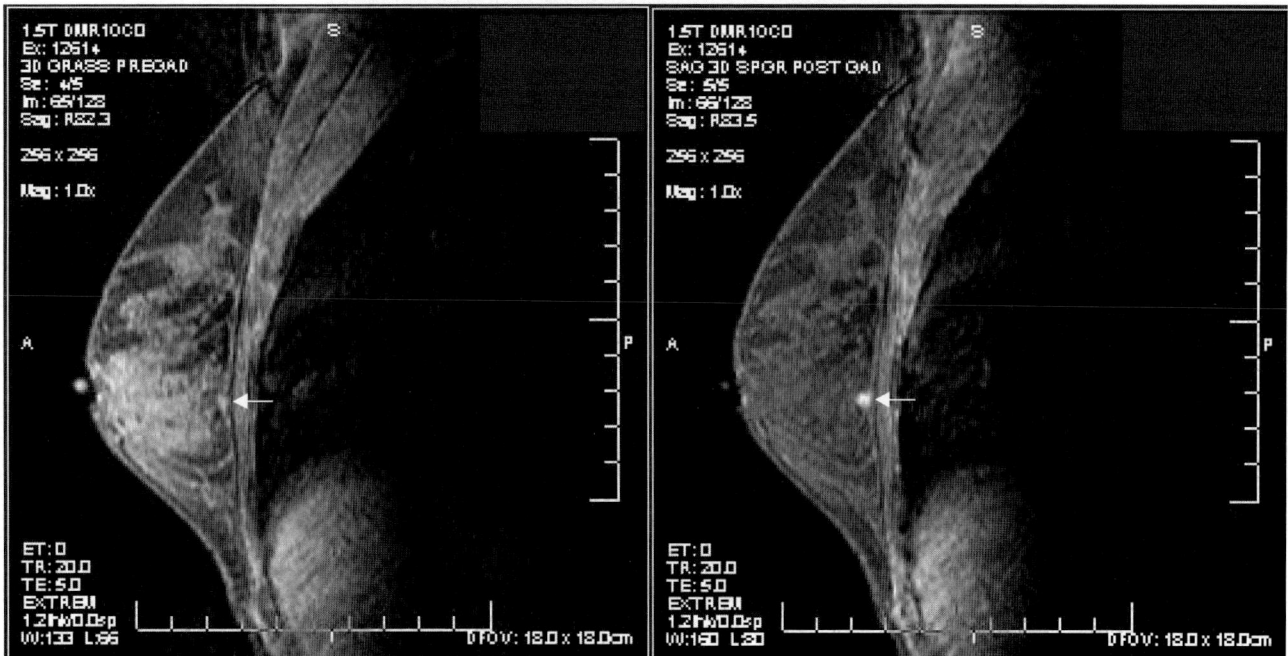

FIGURE 7–1 A: This patient had a positive self-history of breast cancer on the left side and had undergone left mastectomy. The left-sided breast cancer was palpable and had been shown by ultrasound but missed by mammography. For this reason, she insisted on routine whole breast ultrasound in addition to annual mammography for evaluation of her remaining right breast (secondary screening ultrasound). During this examination, mammography was negative, but BI-RADS category 4 in density (>75% of the breast tissue was water density). Screening ultrasound detected a 3-mm solid nodule *(calipers)* in the 10:00 position that is shown in the radial view above. **B:** Before and after gadolinium high-spatial-resolution magnetic resonance imaging scans (rodeo sequence) were performed to verify the sonographic findings and show abnormal enhancement of the lesion *(arrows)* that was shown by sonography. Ultrasound-guided mammotomy showed a small intermediate-grade invasive ductal carcinoma.

a missed cancer in a part of the breast that was not examined sonographically. Thus, in order to limit exposure to missed breast carcinomas, certain American radiologists have tended to avoid scanning areas other than the immediate area of clinical or mammographic concern. Finally,

the radiologists within the subgroup who tend to overcall all lesions on targeted examinations and who are unwilling to characterize lesions into BIRADS categories are likely to find many additional benign lesions during whole breast sonography that they will systematically overcharacterize, resulting in many additional unnecessary biopsies being performed. The net result in such cases might actually be an increase in biopsies of screening detected benign lesions that exceeds the number of negative biopsies prevented by aggressive targeted diagnostic BUS of palpable lumps and mammographic abnormalities. Thus, secondary screening whole breast sonography performed by radiologists unwilling to characterize lesions aggressively might cause diagnostic BUS to fail in its number one goal: prevention of unnecessary biopsies.

The ultimate fate of secondary sonographic screening in the United States is uncertain. Because of all the problems listed above, secondary sonographic screening for breast cancer is finding very slow acceptance in the United States. Within the United States, screening BUS may find so little acceptance among radiologists that it is only performed sporadically. Alternatively, secondary screening sonography might be performed by primary care physicians as part of an ultrasound-assisted physical examination outside of diagnostic radiology. Secondary screening bilateral whole breast ultrasound may readily be accepted and advocated by breast surgeons, gynecologists, and even family practitioners.

There is more willingness to assess the whole breast with sonography among physicians outside the United States. In countries where whole breast sonography is more widely employed, physicians usually perform the examinations themselves—a positive situation. Unfortunately, the physicians in certain countries do not appropriately distinguish between primary and secondary screening and often inappropriately use sonography for primary screening. It seems to us that such inappropriate use is often the result of "turf battles" between nonradiologists, who do not want to obtain mammography, and radiologists, who would prefer to use mammography for primary screening and sonography for secondary screening.

RADIATION PHOBIA WHEN MAMMOGRAPHY IS REFUSED AND ULTRASOUND MUST SUBSTITUTE

Periodically, there are patients who refuse mammography because of a fear of radiation. Often, this reaction is the result of a recent mass media talk show in which a nonmedical "expert" has stated that the radiation from routine screening mammography causes more breast cancers than can be cured by early mammographic detection. Such misinformation can create a temporary mass hysterical reaction in which many patients question the need or wisdom of mammography. However, only rarely does a patient flatly refuse mammography. Our approach is to discuss the risk-to-benefit ratio of mammography with the patient, explain its superiority over other methods for primary breast cancer screening, and strongly encourage the patient to un-

dergo mammography as scheduled. Even offering single-view mediolateral oblique (MLO) mammography rather than two-view mammography may aid in convincing some patients to undergo mammography. If, after conferring with the patient, she still refuses mammography, she can be offered nontargeted, whole breast sonography as an alternative to screening mammography. The underlying philosophy in offering this alternative is that evaluation with sonography, although inferior to mammographic evaluation for primary breast cancer screening, is better than no evaluation at all. More recently, we have encountered the rare patient who refuses mammography but agrees to undergo evaluation with contrast-enhanced MRI with the RODEO (rotating delivery of excitation off-resonance) sequence rather than ultrasound.

In cases in which patients refuse mammography, we offer sonography or MRI as an alternative only after advised consent. Recently, fewer patients have been refusing mammography. However, the next epidemic of refusals is probably only one talk-show interview about the dangers of mammography away. Therefore, an approach for handling this intermittently recurring problem is necessary.

WHOLE BREAST SONOGRAPHY PERFORMED FOR DIAGNOSIS RATHER THAN SCREENING

Nontargeted whole breast sonography can be performed for diagnosis rather than for primary or secondary screening. Mammography will almost always have been performed initially. Indications arise relatively infrequently, as seen from the data in Table 1–4, and include the following:

- Evaluation of nipple discharge and secretions
- Evaluation of silicone gel implants (for implant rupture)
- Known breast cancer metastases, but negative mammograms
- Known breast cancer, but multifocality, multicentricity, or extensive intraductal components and status of regional lymph nodes need to be assessed before definitive conservative therapy can be undertaken
- Follow-up of multiple bilateral ultrasound-detected lesions

Recent data suggest that contrast-enhanced MRI is superior to ultrasound for the last three indications, and special high-resolution, high signal-to-noise ratio, fat suppression sequences such as RODEO are superior for the second indication. MRI is very sensitive for both benign and malignant pathologic disorders of the breast and has a lower chance of a false-negative finding due to a geographic miss than does ultrasound. MRI has a high false-positive rate, however. The relative roles of ultrasound and MRI in patients with the previously listed nontargeted whole breast ultrasound indications have not been firmly established. In our practice, MRI is performed first for nontargeted indications. Second-look ultrasound, which has a lower false-positive rate (when used in a targeted fashion), is then used to evaluate abnormal areas on MRI or to localize such areas for percutaneous core, mammotomy, or excisional biopsy. Ultrasound is almost always used in conjunction with MRI to assist in localizing indeterminate lesions detected by MRI because there are still great difficulties in localization and biopsy of lesions MRI guidance while the patient is inside the magnet.

The whole breast can theoretically be evaluated more quickly and with less operator dependence with dedicated, automated whole breast ultrasound scanners than with real-time sonography. However, the theoretical advantages in speed and decreased operator dependence offered by automated whole breast scanners are nullified by the reduced spatial and contrast resolution of the lower-frequency transducers that dedicated whole breast scanners employ. Furthermore, the dynamic aspects of real-time sonography, which allow easy distinction of fat lobules from true lesions, are not possible with dedicated whole breast scanners. Thus, many fat lobules falsely appear to be lesions when using such equipment. Additionally, cyst versus solid determinations for small lesions are usually easier with real time, with which the location of the sonotomographic slice can be adjusted slightly to avoid volume averaging and a thin standoff can be used, when necessary, to achieve more optimal elevational plane focusing. Our experience with the available dedicated whole breast ultrasound scanners has been disappointing. We have tried several different dedicated whole breast scanners over the years and have found none to be competitive with high-resolution, near-field, real-time, electronically focused scanners.

DIAGNOSTIC WHOLE BREAST SONOGRAPHY

Nipple Discharge and Secretions

Sonographic evaluation of nipple discharge is discussed in detail in Chapter 8.

Silicone Gel Implants

Sonography of breast implants is discussed in detail in Chapter 9.

Known Breast Cancer Metastases but Negative Mammograms and Site of Primary Unknown

Occasionally, either distant metastases (Fig. 7–2) or axillary node metastases of breast cancer origin (Fig. 7–3) will be found in the absence of a clinically evident primary lesion.

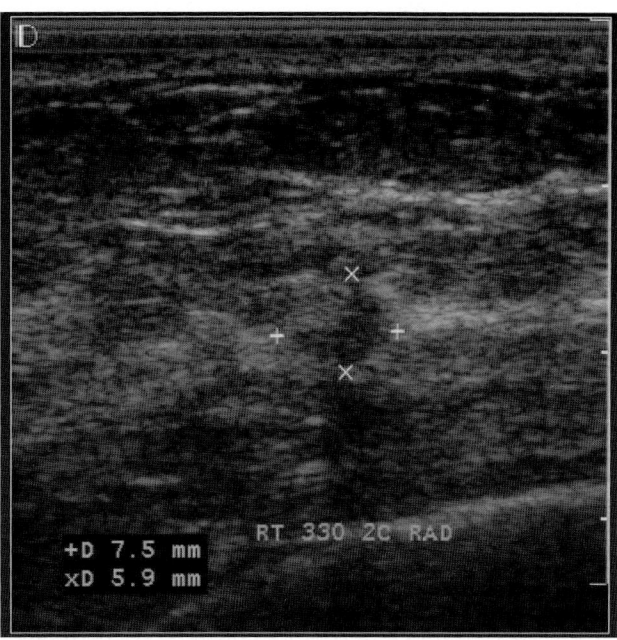

FIGURE 7–2 This patient presented with metastases to the spine of unknown origin. Biopsy of the spine suggested a likely breast origin. Bilateral whole breast ultrasound revealed a small, angular, solid nodule that biopsy revealed to be a primary breast carcinoma, the likely primary for spine metastases.

Mammography will be the first procedure performed but may not show the primary in certain cases. If the mammary zones are radiographically dense, nontargeted whole breast ultrasound can be used to evaluate the radiographically dense areas of the breast where dense tissue could potentially obscure the primary lesion. As in other cases for which whole breast diagnosis is desired, contrast-enhanced MRI may be used instead of whole breast sonography for this limited application. However, even when MRI detects a potential source of the primary lesion, sonography is the procedure of choice for confirming the presence of a solid nodule with indeterminate or malignant characteristics in the area of abnormal contrast enhancement of MRI as well as for guiding either needle biopsy or localizing the lesion for excisional biopsy.

Determining Extent of Malignant Disease

Although diagnostic BUS is usually targeted to the area of interest, a strong argument can be made for extending the examination to include the whole of one or both breasts and the regional lymph node basins when there is a finding that will require biopsy and is at high risk for malignancy (i.e., BIRADS 4b or higher). The goals of the extended examination are to detect multifocal and multicentric disease and extensive intraductal components, preoperative knowledge of which will likely alter the diagnostic and

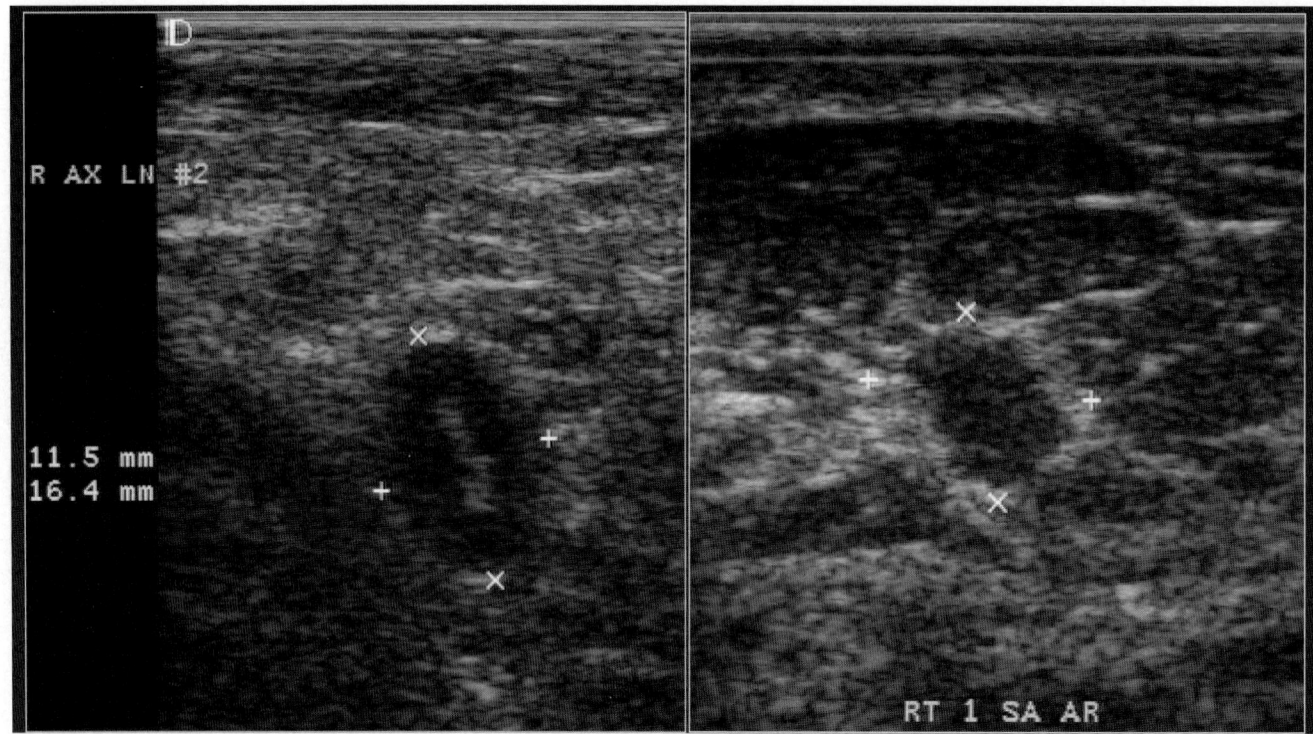

FIGURE 7–3 This patient presented with arm swelling. She had a history of ipsilateral breast cancer treated with lumpectomy 18 months earlier. She had not undergone axillary lymph node dissection, sentinel node procedure, postlumpectomy irradiation, or adjuvant chemotherapy. Sonography of the axilla showed an abnormal lymph node (*calipers,* **left**). Because of the presence of an abnormal axillary lymph node, whole breast sonography was performed, which revealed an angular, microlobulated, solid nodule with a thick, echogenic halo *(calipers).* Ultrasound-guided core needle biopsy of both the breast nodule and the lymph node revealed recurrent intermediate-grade invasive ductal carcinoma.

therapeutic algorithms. High-resolution three-dimensional contrast-enhanced MRI is probably superior to ultrasound for staging of breast cancer, but many institutions inside and outside of the United States are not equipped for such studies, and even in locations where MRI sequences such as the RODEO sequence are available, access to the MRI machine is limited, and the costs are high.

There is every reason to try to determine the extent of suspected malignant breast disease during the initial diagnostic BUS exam. If ultrasound shows no evidence of multifocal or multicentric disease, no evidence of extensive intraductal components, and sonographically normal axillary lymph nodes, staging MRI can still be performed. However, in a significant percentage of cases, ultrasound will show previously unsuspected multifocal (Fig. 7–4) or multicentric disease (Fig. 7–5) or extensive intraductal components (Fig. 7–6) of tumor. In such cases, ultrasound-guided needle biopsy can be used to map the extent of the disease, and staging MRI will not be necessary. Surgical treatment can be directed toward the most appropriate procedure for the extent of disease, the number or diagnostic and therapeutic procedures can be minimized,

and, when appropriate, induction chemotherapy can be used to try to reduce the extent of disease before surgery. Even abnormal axillary lymph nodes detected by sonography of regional lymph nodes can undergo ultrasound-guided biopsy. This can affect the interpretation of core needle biopsy results on the primary lesion in certain cases and can also obviate a sentinel node procedure in other cases (Fig. 7–7). A negative ultrasound of axillary lymph nodes does not exclude microscopic evidence of lymph node metastasis, of course, but a positive ultrasound can obviate a sentinel node procedure.

An argument might be made for extending the sonogram to include the entirety of both breasts whenever there is a lesion present that will undergo biopsy, even BIRADS 3 or BIRADS 4a lesions, that has less than 2% and 10% risk of being malignant, respectively. We have favored extending the examination to include the whole breast and the regional lymph nodes when lesions are characterized as BIRADS 4b or higher. Sonographic assessment of extent of malignant disease is discussed in detail in Chapter 14, and assessment of regional lymph nodes is discussed in detail in Chapter 19.

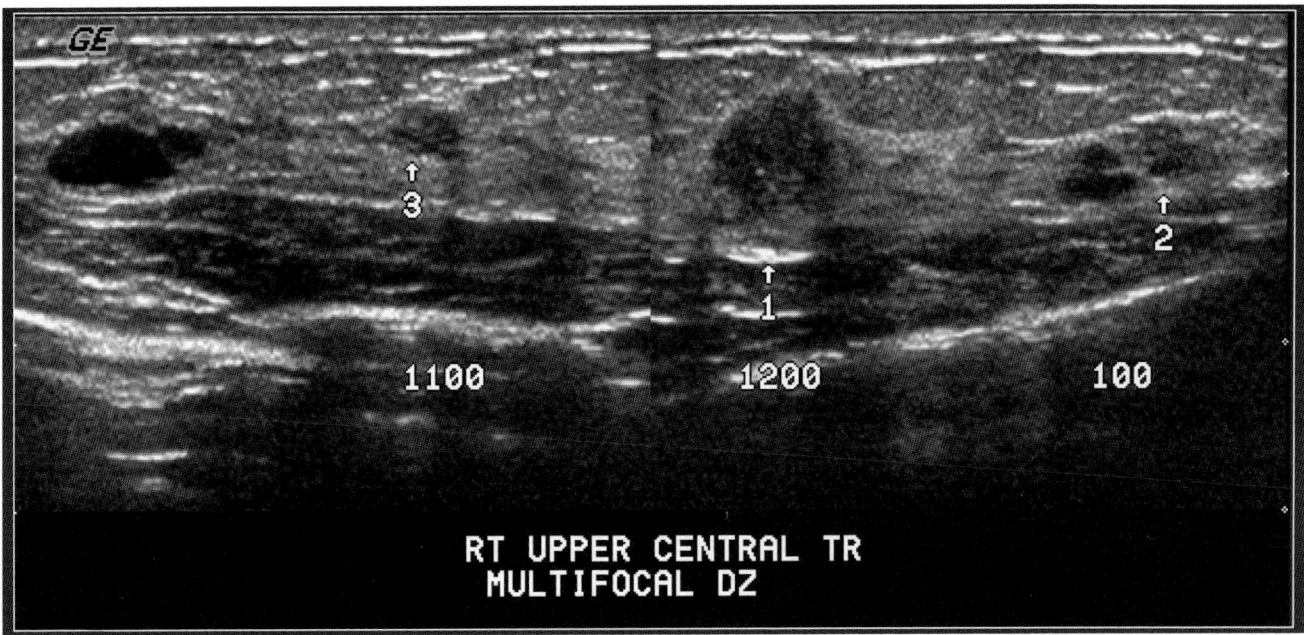

FIGURE 7–4 This split-screen combined transverse image through the upper central breast shows multifocal carcinoma. Three foci of tumor are shown *(arrows)*. All three lesions underwent ultrasound-guided core needle biopsy, which showed all three to be invasive ductal breast carcinoma. Because of the distance between lesion 3 and lesion 1, the patient underwent mastectomy rather than the scheduled lumpectomy that was to have been performed on lesion 1 in the 12:00 position.

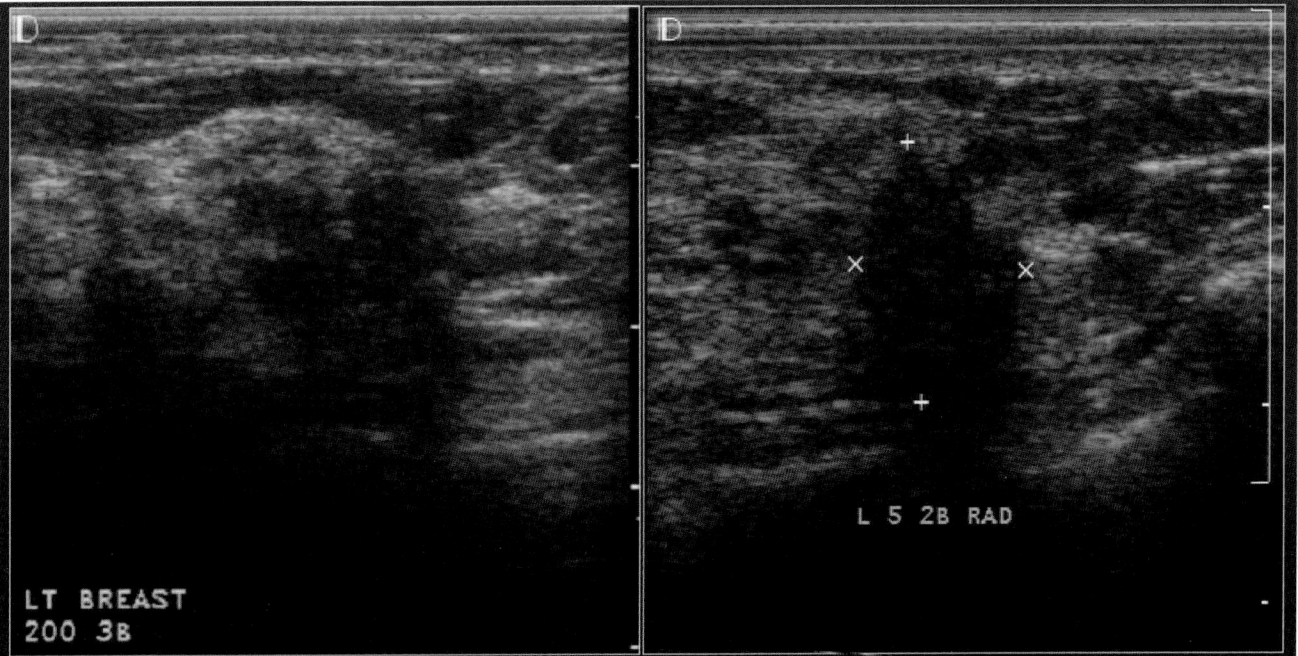

FIGURE 7–5 Targeted diagnostic sonography of a palpable lump in the upper outer quadrant of the left breast showed a solid nodule characterized as BIRADS 4b **(left)**. Because of the presence of a suspicious lesion requiring biopsy, whole breast sonography was performed and showed a second lesion in the lower quadrant at 5:00 **(right)**.

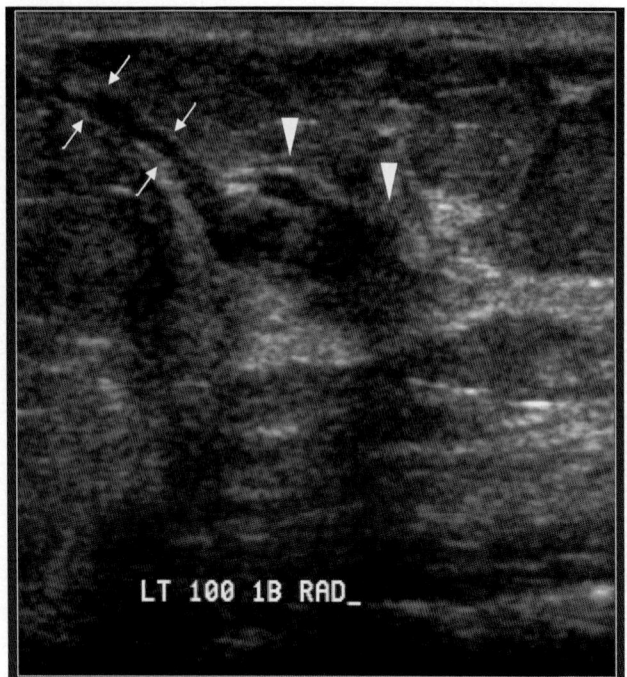

FIGURE 7–6 The indication for sonography in this case was a nonspecific mammographic asymmetry. Sonography showed a BIRADS 4b lesion with angular margins *(arrowheads)* and a long duct extension *(arrows)*. Ultrasound-guided large core needle biopsy of the main nodule and ultrasound-guided mammotomy of the duct extension showed high-grade invasive ductal carcinoma with an extensive intraductal component of tumor. The long duct extension was ductal carcinoma *in situ* extending away from the tumor toward the nipple within a major lobar duct. Because of the long ductal extension, the patient underwent segmentectomy rather than simple lumpectomy.

Follow-up of Multiple Bilateral Sonographically Detected Lesions

Some patients have multiple complex cystic or solid nodules bilaterally that can be characterized as BIRADS 3 but that require short-interval follow-up. The situation in such patients is frequently dynamic. The lesions tend to change in size and number. Some complex cysts are regressing as other new lesions are forming. In the case of multiple fibroadenomas, some lesions may enlarge or assume more suspicious characteristics over time, such as microlobulation, angularity, or shadowing, which would later precipitate biopsy. New solid nodules can develop. Because the new abnormalities often tend to occur in different areas of the breasts over time in these patients, whole breast ultrasound should be used for follow-up. Using whole breast ultrasound to follow patients with numerous lesions bilaterally is really a combination of diagnostic and screening ultrasound because the goal is not only to follow known lesions but also to detect new lesions that form in the interval.

SUMMARY

The greatest strength of diagnostic BUS is in evaluation of targeted clinical and mammographic abnormalities. Occasionally, however, nontargeted whole breast ultrasound may be useful. High-resolution contrast-enhanced MRI may replace ultrasound for some of these nontargeted indications. It is less operator independent but is expensive, re-

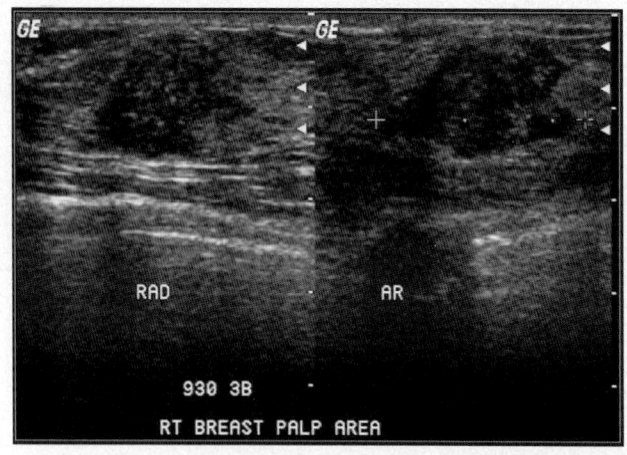

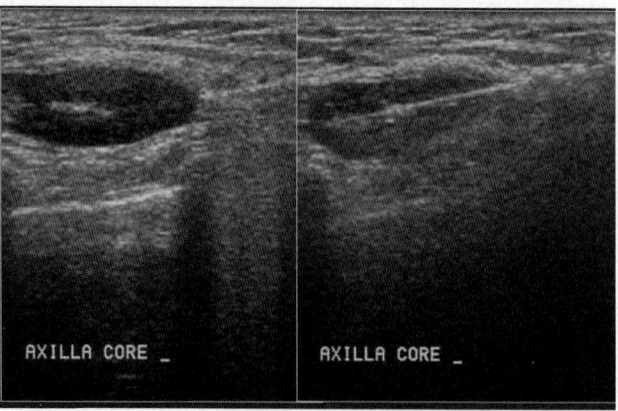

FIGURE 7–7 **A:** Sonography revealed an angular, hypoechoic, microlobulated, solid breast nodule containing calcifications causing the palpable lump. The lesion was characterized as BIRADS 5, and whole breast sonography and sonographic evaluation of axillary lymph nodes were performed. **B:** Whole breast sonography showed no evidence of multifocal or multicentric cancer, but sonographic evaluation of the axilla showed several morphologically abnormal axillary lymph nodes. The node shown **(left)** was the most abnormal appearing. Ultrasound-guided core needle biopsy of the primary tumor and lymph node showed intermediate-grade invasive ductal carcinoma. Documentation of a positive lymph node obviated an unnecessary sentinel node procedure and facilitated the decision to proceed straight to full axillary dissection.

quires contrast injection, and can require two different studies on two different days for bilateral evaluation. When MRI is used first, BUS may be confined to a second-look role and reserved for further characterization and localization of MRI-detected lesions in such patients. In locations where MRI is not available, whole breast ultrasound can be performed in place of MRI.

Whole breast ultrasound may be performed for screening or diagnosis. Breast ultrasound cannot replace mammography for *primary breast cancer screening*. However, the role of *secondary sonographic screening* performed as an adjunct to mammography is currently being reassessed; recent results appear encouraging, and its final status is yet to be defined.

When nontargeted whole breast ultrasound is performed, the limitations must be kept in mind. BUS requires high-resolution near-field imaging equipment. The encouraging data on whole breast screening are based on physicians scanning, not sonographers (ultrasound technologists). Ultrasound may miss cancers that present with calcifications only and lack a demonstrable nodule or mass. Whole breast ultrasound will detect many previously undetected complex cysts, indeterminate cystic versus solid lesions, and solid nodules. Most of these will be benign manifestations of fibrocystic change, fibroadenomas, or other benign proliferative disorders. One of the main goals of BUS, preventing unnecessary biopsies, will not be met if all unsuspected lesions found during whole breast ultrasound are not aggressively characterized sonographically and if all undergo biopsy.

The philosophy that all complex cysts and solid nodules are worrisome and must undergo biopsy is completely incompatible with performance of whole breast ultrasound. Physicians who employ that philosophy must limit the ultrasound examination to the area of clinical or mammographic concern. Their patients, however, would be better served by their physician better learning to characterize lesions sonographically. Any physician contemplating performing whole breast ultrasound for secondary breast cancer screening must first become adept at characterizing solid and complex breast lesions into risk categories (such as the BIRADS categories) to avoid unnecessary biopsies.

There are several indications for *diagnostic* whole breast ultrasound: nipple discharge, implant complications, evaluation of unknown metastasis, staging probable malignancies, and follow-up of multiple bilateral lesions.

Although galactography is the procedure of choice for evaluating nipple discharge, ultrasound is also quite effective for this purpose. The role of ultrasound in evaluation of nipple discharge is expanding because of the advent of ultrasound-guided vacuum-assisted biopsy, which can be used to avoid diagnostic and localizing galactography and excisional biopsy. Mammotomy not only is effective in definitively diagnosing intraductal papillary lesions but also

causes nipple discharge to cease in 90% of cases (see Chapter 8).

Despite the apparent superiority of MRI for implant evaluation, ultrasound is very effective for evaluation of implants, and more patients with implants will be evaluated sonographically because of lumps and mammographic abnormalities than will be evaluated by MRI for evaluation of implant rupture (see Chapter 9).

Sonographic assessment of extent of suspected malignant breast disease can obviate staging MRI and sentinel lymph node procedures when positive and is discussed in detail in Chapters 14 and 19.

SUGGESTED READINGS

Bassett LW, Manjikian VD, Gold RH. Mammography and breast cancer screening. *Surg Clin North Am* 1990;70(4):775–800.

Bick U. An integrated early detection concept in women with a genetic predisposition for breast cancer. *Radiologe* 1997;37(8):591–596.

Boetes C, et al. Breast tumors: comparative accuracy of MR imaging relative to mammography and US for demonstrating extent. Management of probably benign breast lesions. The limitations of breast cancer screening for first-degree relatives of breast cancer patients. Screening mammography and breast sonography. The effect of risk on changes in breast cancer screening rates in Los Angeles, 1988–1990. Periodic mammographic follow-up of probably benign lesions: results in 3,184 consecutive cases [Comments]. *Radiology* 1995;197(3):743–747.

Bohm-Velez M, Mendelson EB. Computed tomography, duplex Doppler ultrasound, and magnetic resonance imaging in evaluating the breast. *Semin Ultrasound CT MR* 1989;10(2):171–176.

Cross MJ, et al. New horizons in the diagnosis and treatment of breast cancer using magnetic resonance imaging. *Am J Surg* 1993;166(6):749–753; discussion, 753–755.

Dagan E, Gershoni Baruch R. BRCA1 and BRCA2—breast cancer susceptibility genes. *Harefuah* 1997;133(10):455–457.

DeMichele A, Weber BL. Recent advances in breast cancer biology. *Curr Opin Oncol* 1997;9(6):499–504.

den Otter W, et al. Exclusion from mammographic screening of women genetically predisposed to breast cancer will probably eliminate mammographically induced breast cancer. *Anticancer Res* 1993;13(4):1113–1135.

Fischer U, et al. MR-guided localization of suspected breast lesions detected exclusively by postcontrast MRI. *J Comput Assist Tomogr* 1995;19(1):63–66.

Frets PG, et al. Hereditary breast and/or ovarian cancer: consequences for family relations. *Oncologica* 1997;14(1):47–49.

Heywang-Kobrunner SH. Nonmammographic breast imaging techniques. *Curr Opin Radiol* 1992;4(5):146–154.

Hill AD, et al. Hereditary breast cancer. *Br J Surg* 1997;84(10):1334–1339.

Jackson VP. Sonography of malignant breast disease. *Semin Ultrasound CT MR* 1989;10(2):119–131.

Jackson VP. What is the role of sonographic breast imaging for detecting occult cancer in a patient with a strong family history of breast cancer and mammographically dense breasts without obvious masses? *AJR Am J Roentgenol* 1995;165(4):1004.

Jackson VP. Imaging the radiographically dense breast. *Radiology* 1993;188(2):297–301.

Kaizer L, et al. Ultrasonographically defined parenchymal patterns of the breast: relationship to mammographic patterns and other risk factors for breast cancer. *Br J Radiol* 1988;61(722):118–124.

Kolb TM, Lichy J, Newhouse JH. Occult cancer in women with dense breasts: detection with screening US—diagnostic yield and tumor characteristics. *Radiology* 1998;207(1):191.

Madjar H, et al. Value of high-resolution sonography in breast cancer screening. *Ultraschall Med* 1994;15(1):20–23.

Morrone D, et al. Diagnostic errors in mammography. I. False negative results. *Radiol Med* (Torino) 1991;82(3):212–217.

Otto RC. Discases of the female breast: screening, mammography, ultrasound. *Ther Umsch* 1993;50(5):323–333.

Pera A, Freimanis AK. The choice of radiologic procedures in the diagnosis of breast disease. *Obstet Gynecol Clin North Am* 1987; 14(3):635–650.

Polednak AP, Lane DS, Burg MA. Risk perception, family history, and use of breast cancer screening tests. *Cancer Detect Prev* 1991;15(4):257–263.

Reintgen D, et al. The anatomy of missed breast cancers. *Surg Oncol* 1993;2(1):65–75.

Roetzheim RG, Fox SA, Leake B. The effect of risk on changes in breast cancer screening rates in Los Angeles, 1988–1990. *Cancer* 1994;74(2):625–631.

Schlecht I, et al. Ultrasound detection of breast cancer with normal mammogram. Breast tumors: comparative accuracy of MR imaging relative to mammography and US for demonstrating extent: What is the role of sonographic breast imaging for detecting occult cancer in a patient with a strong family history of breast cancer and mammographically dense breasts without obvious masses? Breast sonography. *Aktuelle Radiol* 1995;5(5): 297–300.

Smallwood JA, et al. The accuracy of ultrasound in the diagnosis of breast disease. *Ann R Coll Surg Engl* 1986;68(1):19–22.

Stefanek ME, Wilcox P. First degree relatives of breast cancer patients: screening practices and provision of risk information. *Cancer Detect Prev* 1991;15(5):379–384.

Thompson WD. Genetic epidemiology of breast cancer. *Cancer* 1994;74(1 Suppl):S279–287.

Turney J. Public understanding of medical discovery. *Mol Med Today* 1995;1(8):359–363.

Unic I, et al. A review on family history of breast cancer: screening and counseling proposals for women with familial (non-hereditary) breast cancer. *Patient Edu Couns* 1997;32(1–2):117–127.

Yalow RS. Concerns with low level ionizing radiation: rational or phobic? *J Nucl Med* 1990;31(7):17A–18A, 26A.

8

NONTARGETED INDICATIONS: BREAST SECRETIONS, NIPPLE DISCHARGE, AND INTRADUCTAL PAPILLARY LESIONS OF THE BREAST

CLINICAL PROBLEM

Nipple discharge can be spontaneous, expressible, or both. It may be unilateral or bilateral and may emanate from single or multiple duct orifices. Discharge may be frankly bloody, serosanguinous, serous, greenish, or milky. Certain patients may not notice frank discharge but instead complain of crust on the nipple or stains on their bras or nightclothes. Multiple different pathologic conditions may cause nipple discharge, some serious enough to require surgical treatment, others less worrisome. Whether the discharge is spontaneous or present only when expressed is also an important factor. A relatively large percentage of normal patients can express secretions, and frequent squeezing or milking of the nipple can actually stimulate chronic discharge. Furthermore, secretions can be obtained from more than 80% of patients by using suction devices.

Clinical findings can be used to classify nipple discharge into high-risk or low-risk categories. Bilateral milky or greenish discharge from multiple different duct orifices of each nipple is generally a manifestation of fibrocystic change or duct ectasia and is not worrisome, especially if not spontaneous. On the other hand, discharge that is spontaneous, unilateral, emanating from a single duct orifice, and clear, serous, serosanguinous, or frankly bloody is of greater concern. Such discharge is more likely to be caused by a papilloma or carcinoma (Table 8–1).

Patients with clinically worrisome discharge require diagnostic evaluation and, in some cases, treatment. Palpability is not very helpful because 85% of patients with discharge have no palpable abnormality. Mammography generally also helps little, being normal more than 50% of the time even when a malignant lesion causes the discharge. Galactography has been the procedure of choice for evaluating most cases of clinically worrisome nipple discharge. However, sonography is also helpful in evaluating

nipple discharge, and in certain cases, it can replace galactography. In fact, the role of sonography in patients with nipple discharge has expanded rapidly since the advent of ultrasound-guided 11-gauge directional vacuum-assisted biopsy (DVAB).

In fact, we currently schedule patients with clinically worrisome nipple discharge for both sonography and galactography. We perform the sonogram first, and follow with galactography in cases in which sonography does not reveal a definitive cause for discharge. If the sonography shows a definitive cause for nipple discharge, such as an intraductal papillary lesion (IPL), we defer galactography and proceed directly to 11-gauge DVAB. However, if the sonogram is negative, we perform galactography as originally scheduled because galactography may demonstrate peripherally located papillary lesions and small lesions that lie within ducts that are not dilated and that sonography could miss.

HISTOLOGY OF SECRETIONS

Carcinoma, papillomas, duct ectasia, fibrocystic change, and hyperprolactinemia can all cause nipple discharge. Discharge is idiopathic in certain patients. In a review of multiple published galactographic series, including more than 1,600 cases with pathologic proof, Tabar and colleagues found large duct papillomas (intraductal papillomas) to be the most common cause of secretions (34%) (Table 8–2).

Fibrocystic change was the second most common cause, duct ectasia was the third, and carcinoma was the cause in only 10% of cases. However, the relative risk for carcinoma or papilloma varies tremendously between different published series, with the type of secretions, and with age. Bloody secretions increase the risks for both papillomas

157

TABLE 8–1. NIPPLE DISCHARGE

Worrisome (Papilloma or Carcinoma)	Not Worrisome (Fibrocystic, Duct Ectasia, Hyperprolactinemia)
Spontaneous	Expressible only
Unilateral	Bilateral
Single duct orifice	Multiple duct orifices
Serous or bloody	Milky or greenish

(mean, 61%; range, 3% to 78%) and carcinomas (mean, 13%; range, 5% to 28%). Serous secretions are associated with an intermediate risk for both papillomas (mean, 35%; range, 3% to 59%) and carcinomas (mean, 7%; range, 3% to 35%). Secretions caused by fibrocystic change or duct ectasia usually are greenish or milky but can be serous or frankly bloody in certain cases. These secretions are likely caused by hyperprolactinemia in at least some cases.

Papillomas

Intraductal papillomas (IDPs) are ductal epithelial proliferations that grow in an arborescent, frondlike pattern; they usually have central fibrovascular stalks and are covered by the normal double layer of epithelium and myoepithelium.

Papillomas can be divided into central and peripheral varieties. The approved American College of Radiology Breast Imaging Reporting and Data System (BIRADS) terminology for a central IDP is *large duct papilloma* (LDP). LDPs arise in the subareolar region in or near the lactiferous sinuses. The galactographic literature suggests that LDPs are usually single and occur most commonly in the perimenopausal period. However, the literature is based on galactography, which is generally performed only to evaluate a single duct. With ultrasound, on the other hand, we look at all of the central subareolar ducts and find that LDPs are multiple far more often than has been suggested in the galactographic literature. Sonography not only shows multiple papillomas within a single

TABLE 8–2. CAUSES OF NIPPLE DISCHARGE[a]

Cause	Percentage of Cases
Large duct papillomas	34
Fibrocystic change	25
Ductal ectasia	13
Carcinoma	10

[a]From Tabar et al. (1983).

duct (as does galactography) but also often demonstrates papillomas in multiple different lobar ductal systems. According to the galactographic literature, about 70% of LDPs cause nipple discharge. However, sonography shows a much higher percentage of asymptomatic LDPs than does galactography simply because it shows papillomas that lie within both secreting and nonsecreting ducts. Single LDPs are thought to have a much lower potential for malignant degeneration than do peripheral papillomas (PPs). Multiple LDPs likely carry a risk for malignant degeneration that lies somewhere between that of a single LDP and multiple PPs.

PPs that arise within the terminal duct of the terminal ductolobular unit (TDLU) are more often multiple than are LDPs. PPs tend to occur in younger patients and are frequently associated with diffuse epithelial proliferation of varying degrees in the affected and surrounding TDLUs, including atypical ductal hyperplasia (ADH) and ductal carcinoma *in situ* (DCIS), likely explaining the higher premalignant potential of PPs. PPs are less frequently a cause of nipple discharge (only about 20% of the time) and more frequently present as palpable or mammographic nodules than are LDPs. The term *papillomatosis* has been used to describe multiple PPs. Papillomatosis really represents a form of florid (papillary) usual duct hyperplasia and is discussed in detail in Chapter 15. Although we have been able to show PPs sonographically, we feel that sonography is less sensitive for PPs than for LDPs and that galactography may be more sensitive than sonography for detecting such lesions. Part of the rationale for scheduling both sonography and galactography is to try to avoid missing small PPs.

The papillomas most reliably detected by both ductography and sonography are centrally located LDPs rather than PPs. LDPs are often only 2 or 3 mm in diameter, but they may grow for considerable distances within the duct lumen, even extending into duct branches. Some LDPs grossly expand the duct and can become large enough to form palpable nodules.

LDPs contain highly variable histologic changes internally, including adenosis, sclerosing adenosis, apocrine metaplasia, usual duct hyperplasia, ADH, and even carcinomatous degeneration. Papillomas tend to secrete fluid into the ducts, leading to dilation of the duct and nipple discharge. LDPs frequently undergo partial infarction and necrosis, resulting in partial sloughing of the lesion, intraductal bleeding, and bloody discharge. Infarcted areas eventually become hyalinized and sclerotic, beginning in the stalk and then extending peripherally. Occasionally, by a combination of hypersecretion and obstruction of the duct, a papilloma will cause the duct around it to become cystically dilated, thereby becoming an intracystic papilloma (ICP). Evaluation of intracystic papillary lesions is discussed in detail in Chapter 10.

LDPs are very soft and friable. Careful surgical handling and pathologic fixation and mounting are necessary to preserve the diagnostic architecture. As is the case in many other pathologic conditions, the pathologist will more likely issue an accurate diagnosis if he is informed in advance that papilloma is the suspected preoperative diagnosis.

The variable histologic changes within papillomas and their variable locations result in histologic entities that are considered variants of the LDPs. Within the nipple, IDP variants include nipple adenoma and syringomatous adenoma. Within the subareolar ducts, subareolar sclerosing duct hyperplasia and duct adenomas are papilloma variants. Duct adenomas manifest peripheral sclerosis and central adenosis.

Duct Ectasia

In duct ectasia, the large subareolar ducts and intermediate-sized ducts become dilated and filled with thick, static secretions. The duct walls and periductal tissues are inflamed. Whether the duct dilation precedes early inflammatory changes or whether duct wall inflammation leads to dilation is uncertain. Chronic hyperprolactinemia and autoimmune mechanisms have been proposed as potential etiologies. However, regardless of the initiating etiology, fatty secretions within the ectatic duct ultimately exacerbate ductal and periductal inflammatory change and cause the condition to progress.

Duct ectasia evolves through many stages, including mild periductal inflammation with loss of normal periductal elastic tissue; periductal fibrosis and hyperelastosis; rupture of the duct wall with intense periductal inflammation (periductal mastitis); and finally, periductal and intraductal fibrosis and obliteration of the duct lumen. The histologic appearance varies greatly with the stage of development, accounting for the multiple different histologic terms used to describe this condition. *Duct ectasia* and *varicocele* tumor have been used to describe the early and often asymptomatic phases of this condition. *Comedomastitis* has been used to describe the thick, pasty or cheesy secretions that accumulate within the lumen of the dilated ducts in chronic duct ectasia. These grumous secretions are grossly similar to the necrotic debris that forms within the lumen of ducts involved with comedocarcinoma, accounting for the similar terminology. *Periductal mastitis* describes the phase in which duct rupture and release of duct contents into surrounding tissues leads to an acute inflammatory reaction around the duct composed primarily of lymphocytes, plasma cells, and macrophages. Plasma cell mastitis is merely a variant of periductal mastitis in which periductal plasma cells rather than lymphocytes predominate. *Mastitis obliterans* refers to fibrous obliteration of the duct lumen that represents the end stage of this disease. The fibrous oblitera-

tion can be homogeneous or occur in a garland pattern with a central nodule of fibrosis surrounded by multiple small lumina that resemble the pattern of recanalization of deep venous thrombosis.

The early stages of duct ectasia are usually asymptomatic, and uncomplicated duct ectasia is so common in the fifth and sixth decades of life that up to half of all women 60 years of age or older have duct ectasia histologically. However, up to 25% of patients with duct ectasia do have nipple discharge. This fluid is greenish or milky in about half of patients, but bloody in the other half. We have found bloody discharge to occur more frequently in patients with acute periductal mastitis because of marked inflammatory hyperemia in the ducts and erosion of the duct walls. The clinical findings of duct ectasia depend on the histologic stage of the disease. Acute periductal mastitis may cause sudden-onset localized pain, thickening, and skin erythema that resolves spontaneously. The patient may give a history of similar previous episodes in the same or different area of the ipsilateral or contralateral breast. Fibrosis in and around the subareolar ducts may cause nipple retraction that may clinically simulate infiltrating carcinoma in up to 30% of patients. Rupture of an acutely inflamed duct may lead to formation of nonpuerperal periareolar abscesses and fistulous tracts.

Fibrocystic Change

Fibrocystic change can cause secretions by various different mechanisms. In most cases, secretions probably originate peripherally within secreting and cystically dilated TDLUs that contain apocrine metaplastic changes. Such communicating cysts may intermittently become obstructed, leading to cessation of nipple discharge and formation of a tender, palpable lump. When the obstruction abates, discharge resumes, and the tender lump gradually resolves. Compression of the communicating cyst may express projectile secretions from the nipple (a "trigger point"). The trigger point of the communicating cyst is usually more peripherally located than that of central IDPs that cause discharge. Interestingly, the ducts between the secreting cyst and the nipple are not always dilated.

Hyperprolactinemia

Hyperprolactinemia can cause nipple discharge that is usually bilateral, milky, and from multiple duct orifices. A pituitary adenoma causes only a small percentage of prolactin-induced secretions. Other etiologies of hyperprolactinemia are more common. Many different types of medications can cause hyperprolactinemia, including birth control pills, phenothiazines, and certain antihypertensives. In other patients, no etiologic factor can be identified. The histologic changes found in the subareolar ducts in patients with hyperprolactinemia are similar to those associated with early duct ectasia. In fact, some researchers who believe that duct ectasia may be initiated by chronic hyperprolactinemia. In our experience, hyperprolactinemia also increases the risk for multiple central papillomas.

Florid or Papillary Usual Duct Hyperplasia

The distinction between florid usual ductal hyperplasia (papillary duct hyperplasia, PDH), which results in papillary excrescences from the duct walls, and true papillomatosis is largely semantic and somewhat subjective. True papillomas have a fibrovascular stalk through which they receive their blood supply, whereas PDH generally does not. However, papillomas are very friable and often fragmented during surgery or histologic preparation, making it difficult to distinguish between true papillomas and PDH from the small fragments. Most PDH occurs peripherally in the TDLUs, but PDH can also involve larger ducts that are more central. When PDH involves the central ducts, it often causes multiple tiny excrescences all along the wall instead of a single, large papillary lesion. Additionally, PDH may arise from the surface epithelium of a preexisting true papilloma. Our pathologists consider PDH in large ducts to represent a papilloma. PDH is discussed in further detail in Chapter 15, in conjunction with the discussion of ADH.

Atypical Ductal Hyperplasia

ADH may arise within the epithelium lining the surface of papillomas or from preexisting papillary usual duct hyperplasia. ADH arises from foci of underlying usual or florid duct hyperplasia, and the distribution, therefore, merely reflects that of usual duct hyperplasia. ADH is discussed in detail in Chapter 15.

Carcinoma

Most carcinomas arise peripherally within the TDLU. By the time there are symptoms, however, malignancy has typically involved multiple lobules and often has also spread centrally within the lobar ductal system for variable distances. A smaller percentage of carcinomas arise in the central ducts near the nipple, in locations similar to the sites of origins of central papillomas. Some of these malignant lesions arise in preexisting PDH, and a few may actually arise from the epithelium of preexisting LDPs. These centrally arising carcinomas are relatively uncommon but are far more likely to cause nipple discharge than are the more common, peripherally arising carcinomas. The discharge caused by these central malignancies is more likely to be bloody than the discharge associated with benign lesions. Centrally arising carcinomas may be pure DCIS, invasive, or mixed invasive and intraductal. Carcinoma is discussed in detail in Chapters 12 and 14.

CYTOLOGY OF NIPPLE DISCHARGE

The gross and cytologic analysis of nipple secretions is not conclusive for determining the cause. The false-negative rate is unacceptably high, and there are also many false-positive findings. Thus, negative cytology should not be considered reassuring in patients with worrisome nipple discharge. Furthermore, cytologic examination of discharge does nothing to localize the lesion for core biopsy, vacuum-assisted biopsy, or excision.

HISTOLOGIC DIAGNOSIS AND TREATMENT OF INTRADUCTAL PAPILLOMAS

The definitive treatment of papillary breast lesions causing nipple discharge has traditionally been surgical excision. Surgical treatment for nipple discharge has evolved over the years. Before the advent of galactography, limited excisional biopsy could be performed only if the lesion causing discharge was either palpable or mammographically visible. However, extensive resections were often performed—segmentectomy or mastectomy—if there was no palpable or mammographic abnormality. Next, subareolar ducts were ligated in order to stop discharge. Later, the suspected offending duct was cannulated during surgery to facilitate more limited surgical resection to the central ducts of the affected lobar ductal system. All of the aforementioned treatments had problems in the treatment of nipple discharge. First, mastectomy and segmentectomy are very radical procedures for a condition that has a benign etiology about 90% of the time. Second, although subareolar duct ligation was effective in stopping secretions, the offending lesion was not removed, a serious problem in the 10% or so of cases in which the cause of discharge was malignant. Finally, intraoperative cannulation did not always identify the correct duct and did not show the location within the duct of the offending lesion. This technique necessitated removal of the entire central portion of the duct.

In certain patients who desired definitive diagnosis, but did not care if discharge did not stop immediately, histologic proof of benign LDP could be obtained with ultrasound-guided large core needle biopsy. Core biopsy could also replace excisional biopsy in patients with sonographically demonstrated papillary lesions that did not cause nipple discharge. If core biopsy showed ADH or carcinoma, excision of the lesion was still necessary.

Use of 11-guage DVAB has dramatically altered the management of nipple discharge and IPLs. Under either ultrasound guidance or combined galactographic-stereotactic guidance, a definitive diagnosis can be obtained in all cases. Ultrasound-guided DVAB of papillary lesions is discussed in detail in the conclusion of this chapter.

MAMMOGRAPHIC FINDINGS IN PATIENTS WITH NIPPLE DISCHARGE

Routine mammography is usually normal in patients with nipple discharge caused by benign conditions. Benign conditions may cause the following mammographic findings: distended retroareolar ducts (Fig. 8–1), nodules (Fig. 8–2), periductal calcifications (Fig. 8–3), and nipple retraction (Fig. 8–4). All of these mammographic findings are nonspecific and therefore usually are not helpful in determining the exact cause of discharge. When the cause of discharge is malignant, the mammogram is more likely to be abnormal but is still negative about half of the time. A few patients with nipple discharge and abnormal mammograms may show classic findings of malignancy, but most, like patients with benign etiologies for discharge, have nonspecific findings.

GALACTOGRAPHY

Galactography was developed to circumvent problems with untargeted surgical treatment and has become the procedure of choice for evaluating clinically worrisome nipple discharge. Two galactograms were often necessary in pa-

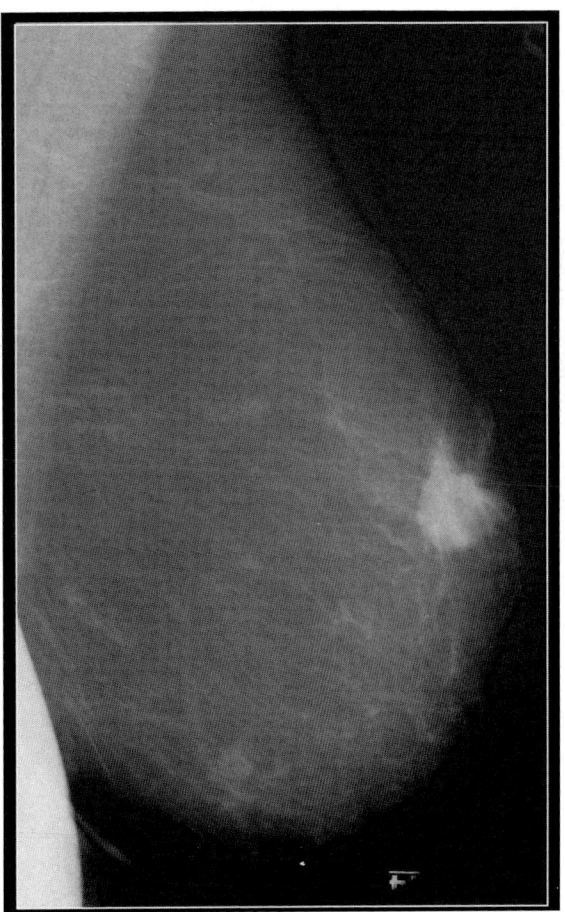

FIGURE 8–2 This patient with nipple discharge presented with a mammographic nodule that ultrasound showed to be caused by a malignant intracystic papillary lesion.

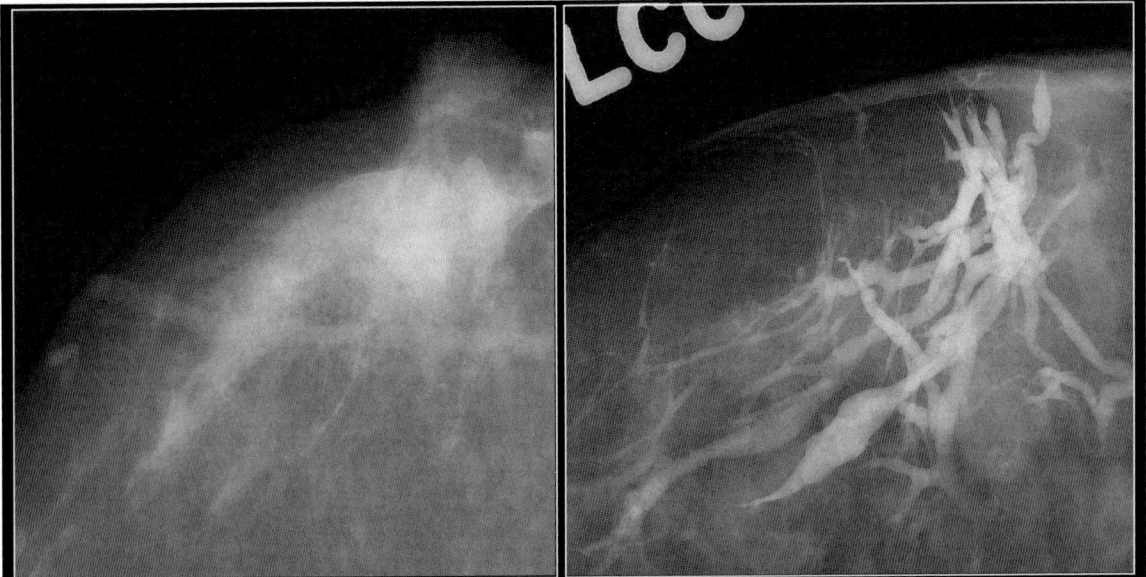

FIGURE 8–1 In this patient with a chief presenting complaint of nipple discharge, the mammogram shows only slightly prominent subareolar soft tissue density, a nonspecific finding that can be caused by dilated ducts with or without intraductal papillary lesions or by prominent periductal fibrous tissues. The galactogram, on the other hand, shows the subareolar prominence to be caused by duct ectasia without intraductal papillary lesions.

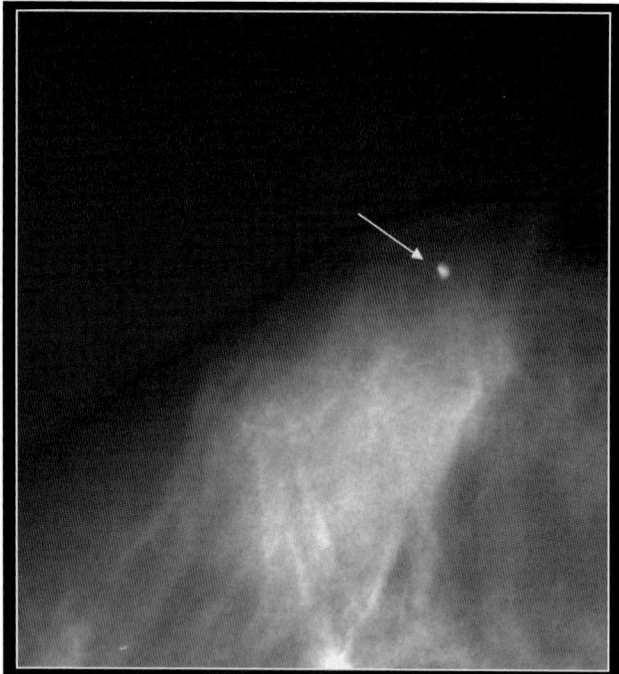

FIGURE 8–3 This patient with nipple discharge presented with a mammographically benign subareolar calcification *(arrow)* that ultrasound (see Fig. 8–46) showed to be a periductal calcification resulting from chronic duct ectasia.

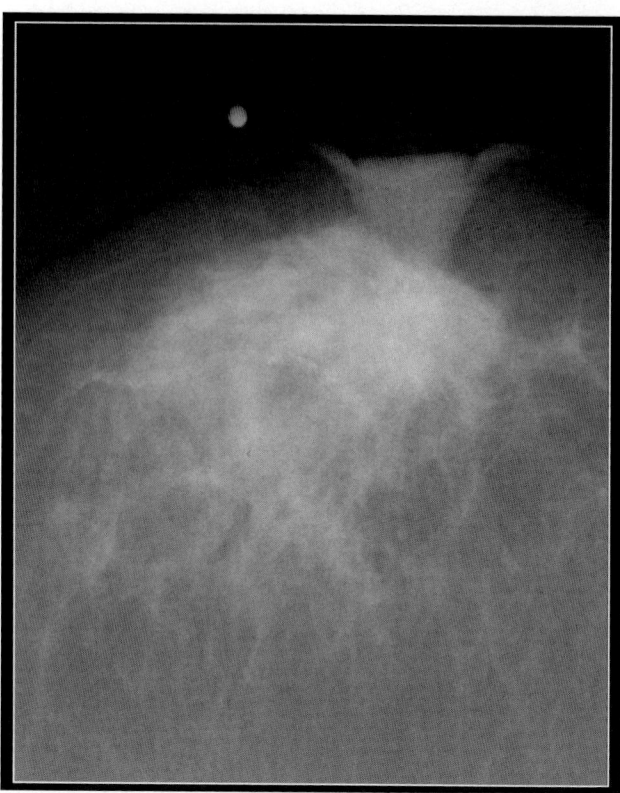

FIGURE 8–4 This patient with chronic "cheesy" nipple discharge has nipple retraction on the mammogram that could be caused by either malignancy or chronic duct ectasia. Biopsy showed invasive ductal carcinoma with intraductal carcinoma extending through the subareolar ducts and into the nipple.

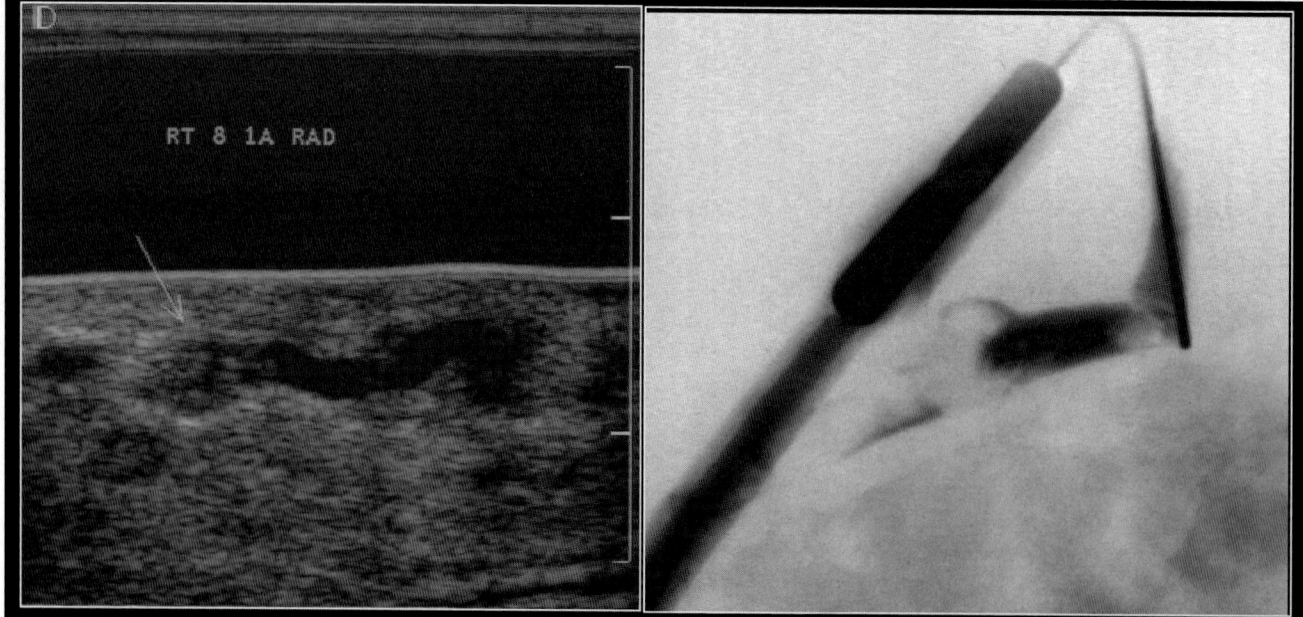

FIGURE 8–5 There are two different intraductal papillary lesions within this duct. The peripheral lesion expands the duct mildly and has duct dilation only between it and the nipple. The smaller, more centrally located lesion is round and short and does not expand the lumen. The duct is dilated both centrally and peripherally. The appearances are of #1 and #2 in Fig. 8–28.

tients who had IPLs: one for establishing the diagnosis and one for preoperative localization.

To perform galactography, the offending duct must be successfully cannulated, the duct injected with iodinated contrast, and craniocaudal as well as mediolateral oblique mammograms obtained. For successful identification and cannulation of the offending duct orifice, secretions generally must be expressible from the offending duct. Iodinated contrast (60%) is injected for the diagnostic galactogram. A mixture of half contrast and half methylene blue dye is injected for surgical localization. When the papillary lesion is small and located far peripherally, image-guided needle wire localization of the lesion may be necessary in addition to contrast and blue dye injection.

Galactographic findings in patients with nipple discharge vary with the causes of secretions. Papillomas and carcinomas cause similar findings, sessile polypoid filling defects (Figs. 8–5 and 8–6), or complete obstruction of a duct (Fig. 8–7). Cancer can also cause napkin-ring—type ductal narrowings. Malignant IPLs may predispose ducts to duct perforation and extravasation of contrast. The galactographic findings in duct ectasia vary with the phase of the disease. Early and intermediate phases cause only dilation and tortuosity of the ducts (Fig. 8–1). Thin secretions within the duct may dilute injected contrast, whereas in-

spissated secretions may cause filling defects that simulate papillary lesions. Later phases of duct ectasia, when periductal and intraductal fibrosis are extensive, cause galactographic findings similar to those seen with papilloma or malignancy. In fibrocystic change, galactography shows clusters of cysts that communicate with the ectatic or normal-sized ducts. Severe hyperprolactinemia manifests as dilation and tortuosity of multiple ducts similar to, but more severe than, the dilation and tortuosity caused by isolated duct ectasia. In some cases, hyperprolactinemia might cause multiple papillomas as well as duct ectasia (Fig. 8–10).

EVOLUTION OF THE ROLE OF SONOGRAPHY IN EVALUATING NIPPLE DISCHARGE

Galactography is usually scheduled as an elective procedure while the patient is actively secreting. However, the nipple discharge for which galactography is indicated is often intermittent because of periodic obstruction of the secreting duct within the nipple by keratin plugs. When the obstructing plug forms, spontaneous discharge ceases, and the patient is also unable to express secretions, preventing successful duct cannulation and galactography. Hot towels or ophthalmic atropine placed directly on the nipple may

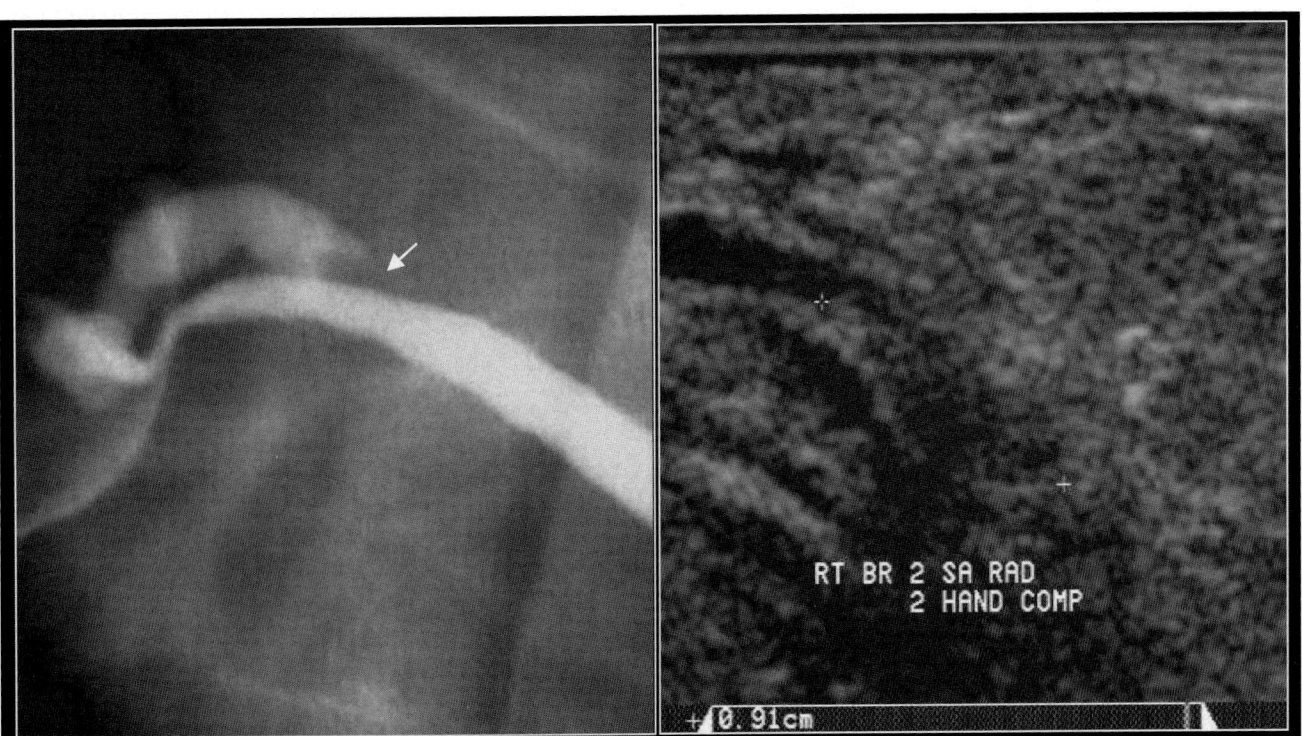

FIGURE 8–6 The diagnosis of an intraductal papillary lesion was made galactographically (*arrow,* **left**). The day of surgery, the patient was unable to express secretions, and galactography was not possible. The intraductal papillary lesion was easily identified (*between calipers,* **right**) and preoperatively localized sonographically. Note that sonography shows the true extent of the lesion far better than does galactography, which shows only obstruction of the duct.

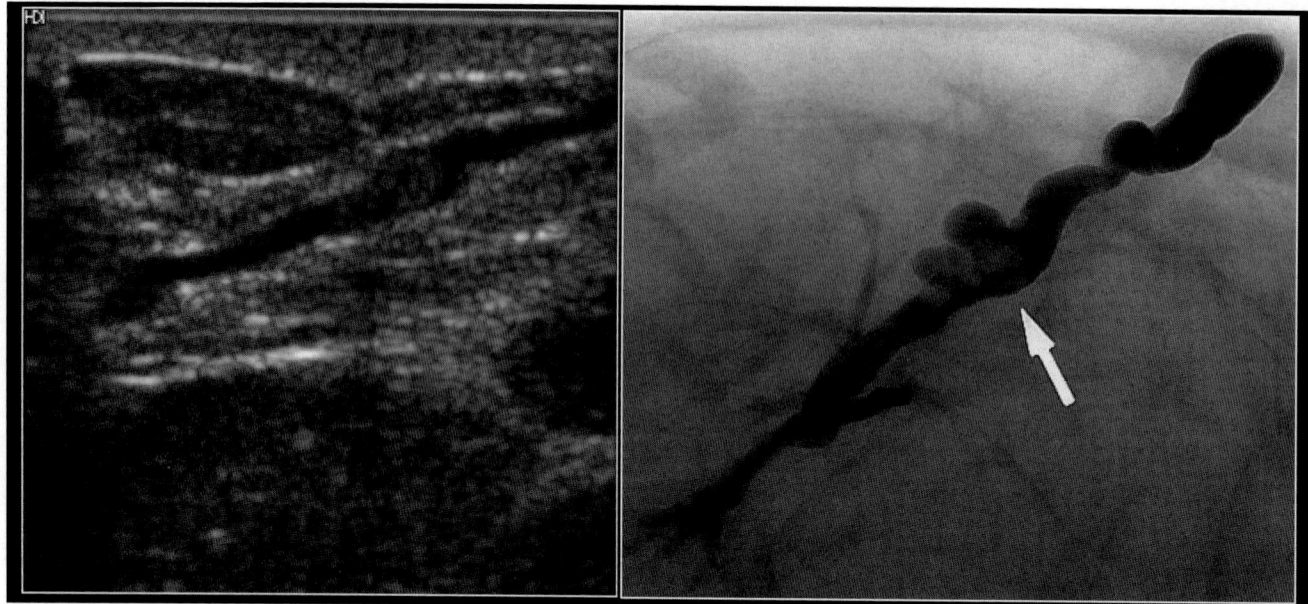

FIGURE 8–7 This short, round, intraductal papillary lesion mildly expands the duct. The lumen is dilated both centrally and peripherally. The diagnosis was made by sonography, and the galactogram was performed for preoperative localization.

relax the muscular sphincter around the duct orifice enough to allow the keratin plug to be expressed in some cases. However, in many cases, these techniques fail, and galactography must be rescheduled or an alternative procedure (ultrasound) performed.

The significance of rescheduling varies, depending on whether the purpose of the scheduled procedure is diagnosis or localization. Diagnostic galactograms can usually be rescheduled, but preoperative localization procedures are more problematic. Rescheduling surgery creates problems

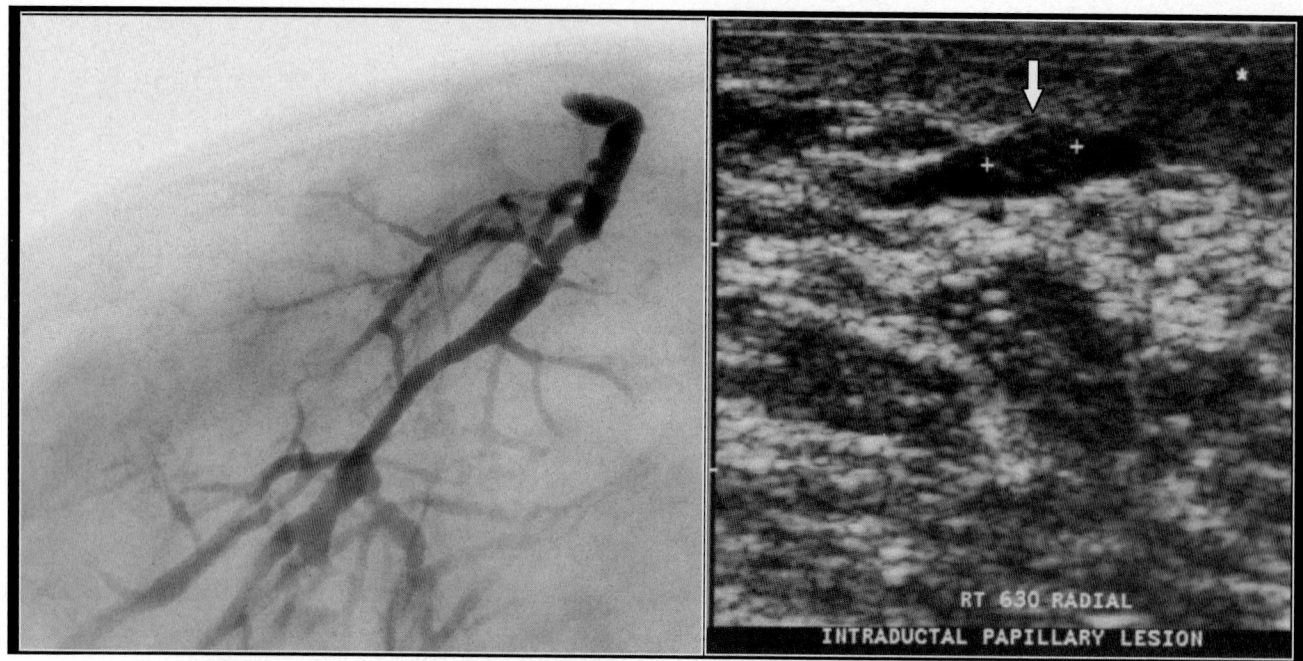

FIGURE 8–8 This patient presented with greenish nipple discharge from multiple different duct orifices, but bloody discharge from one. Galactographic cannulation and injection of the wrong duct was performed. The galactogram was normal **(left)**. Sonography performed immediately after the galactogram showed an intraductal papillary lesion missed by galactography. *(arrow).*

for the operating room, operating room nurses, anesthesia, radiology, pathology, and the surgeon. Without preoperative localization, the surgeon's choices are to perform a wide excision without localization or to reschedule surgery.

Attempted galactography might fail for other reasons. In certain patients, cannulating the duct may be technically impossible. Rarely, the wrong duct can be cannulated (Fig. 8–8). In other cases, successful duct cannulation and injection may lead to painful extravasation (Fig. 8–9). In certain cases, the affected duct may be so dilated and the contrast within the duct so dense that the contrast obscures small papillary lesions within the duct (Fig. 8–10). This is most likely to occur in patients who have bloody discharge from one duct orifice and greenish or milky discharge from multiple other duct orifices that enable them to be inadvertently cannulated. Finally, some patients may refuse galactography. Regardless of the reason for galactographic failure, ultrasound offers a viable alternative to galactography either for primary diagnosis or localizing an IPL for surgery.

Cases in which galactography was unsuccessful or suboptimal were the first cases in which ultrasound was employed to evaluate the etiology of nipple discharge. In fact, in cases in which galactography is not possible because of duct obstruction by a keratin plug, the obstructed duct dilates out of proportion to surrounding ducts and makes an ideal sonographic target within which even small IPLs can be easily detected. In fact, it was in exactly such a case that we first prospectively identified a papilloma and in subsequent similar cases that we developed our algorithm for evaluating the central mammary ductal system.

From the initial cases of intermittent discharge, we expanded the role of ultrasound to cases of unsuccessful cannulation, contrast extravasation, injection of the wrong ducts, and severely ectatic ducts. Ultrasound yielded a definitive diagnosis in most of these cases. Based on the success rate in these cases, we routinely began scheduling all patients whose chief complaint was nipple discharge for both sonography and galactography. We performed the sonogram first and followed with galactography in all cases. After a period of time, it became clear that when sonography showed a definitive cause for nipple discharge, the galactogram seldom contributed additional useful information, but when sonography failed to show a definitive cause, the galactogram occasionally demonstrated a definitive etiology such as a small IPL. This usually occurred in cases in which the central ducts were not ectatic and fluid filled and in cases in which papillomas were peripherally located. Based on these experiences, we gradually adjusted the role of sonography in the workup of nipple discharge in a step-by-step fashion to its current role. Before the advent of ultrasound-guided 11-gauge DVAB, ductal sonography could usually prevent one of the two galactograms. When the diagnosis was made with sonography, galactography was reserved for preoperative localization (Figs. 8–5 and 8–7). When the initial diagnosis was made with galactography, but galactography failed on the day of surgery, localization could be performed with sonography (Fig. 8–6).

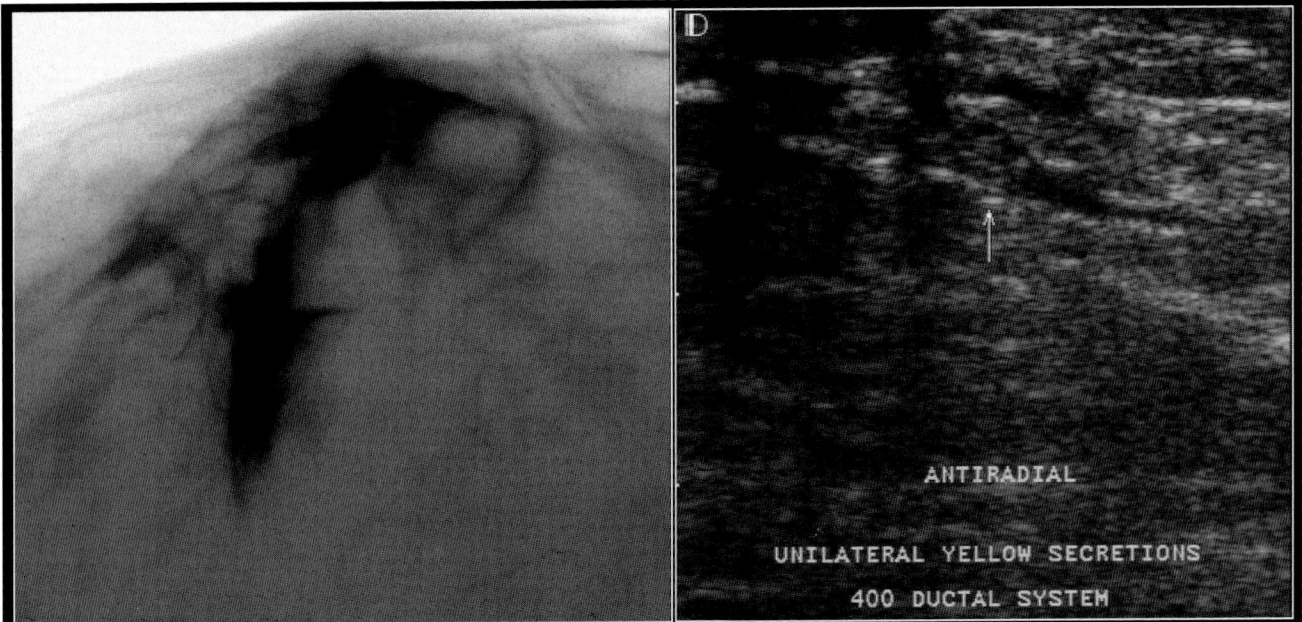

FIGURE 8–9 Galactographic cannulation of the offending duct was easily accomplished in this patient with nipple discharge, but injection of contrast resulted in immediate painful extravasation of contrast. Thus, the galactogram was a technical failure **(left)**. Sonography performed immediately after the failed galactogram, however, showed the intraductal papillary lesion (*arrow,* **right**) that caused the discharge.

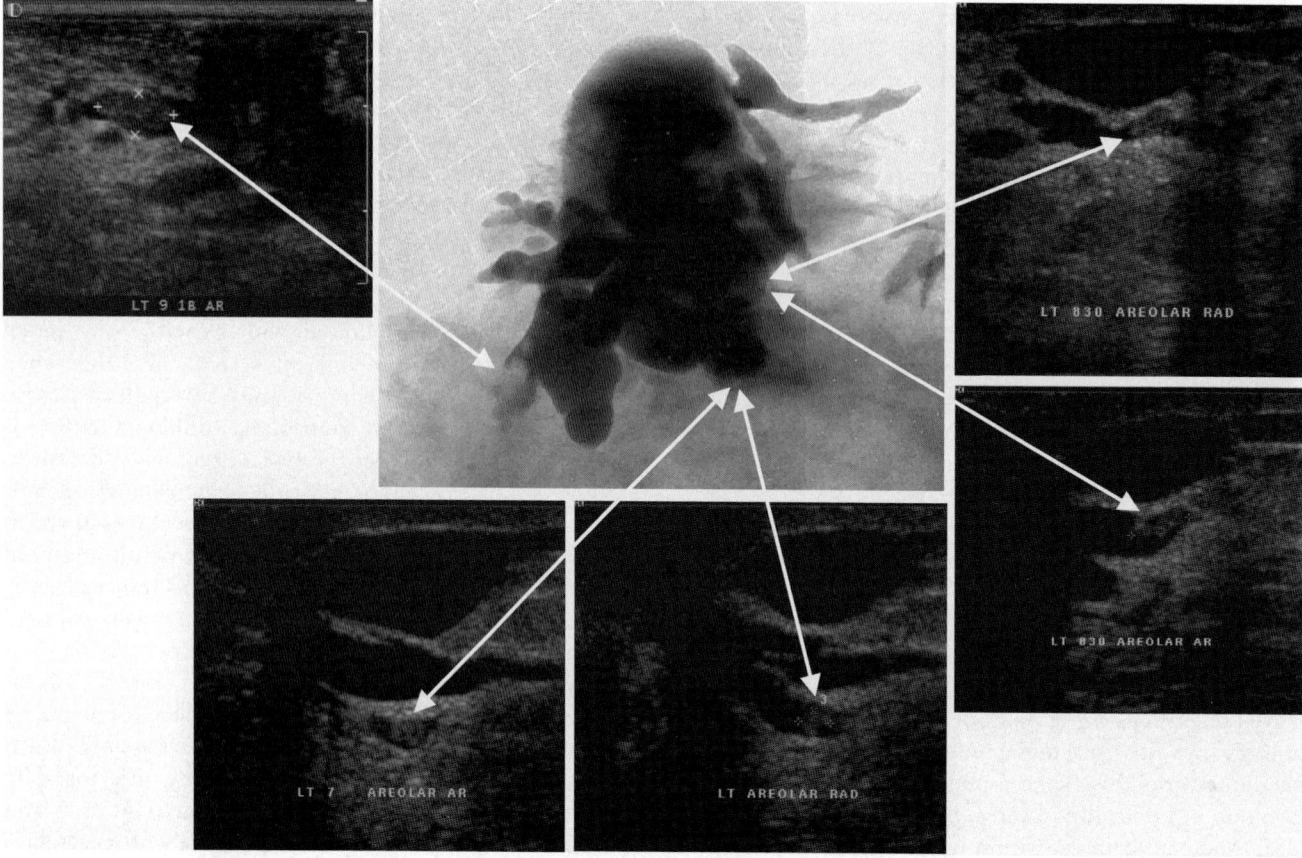

FIGURE 8–10 The density of the contrast within the severely dilated ducts nearly completely obscures two of the multiple intraductal papillary lesions within the ductal system (**upper middle**). The ultrasound shows two small, intraductal papillary lesions missed by galactography as well as one shown by galactography. This patient had severe hyperprolactinemia caused by a pituitary adenoma.

The current algorithm, developed since the advent of ultrasound-guided 11-gauge DVAB, is to schedule patients with nipple discharge for both sonography and galactography. We perform the sonogram first. If sonography shows an IPL, the galactogram is canceled, and the patient is offered ultrasound-guided DVAB. If the ultrasound does not show a definitive cause for nipple discharge, the galactogram is performed as scheduled. If the galactogram is normal or shows only duct ectasia or communicating cysts, no further workup is performed. If the galactogram shows an IPL, the sonogram is repeated using the galactogram as a guide with the expectation that ultrasound will be used to guide mammotomy. If postgalactogram ultrasound is not performed or fails to identify the IPL shown by galactography, either stereotactically guided mammotomy using galactography as a guide will be necessary or the duct will need to be injected with a mixture of blue dye and iodinated contrast to facilitate minimal surgical excision. When possible, sonographic guidance is far more efficient than either stereotactic guidance or surgical excision.

The development of ultrasound-guided core biopsy did not change the imaging algorithm for evaluation of nipple discharge very much. Even after documenting the diagnosis of benign IDP with core needle biopsy, surgical excision was usually still necessary to make nipple discharge stop. However, the more recent development of 11-gauge DVAB has changed the algorithm tremendously. Although the goal of ultrasound-guided mammotomy is simply to diagnose the lesion accurately, completely removing all sonographic evidence of the lesion and completely analyzing the removed tissue is the best way to make accurate diagnoses. (It must be remembered that sonographic evidence of complete removal is not the same as histologic evidence of complete removal. Thus, a localizing clip should be deployed in all cases in which all sonographic evidence of the lesion has been removed, in order to facilitate surgical excision in cases in which histology is atypical or malignant.) Even though we attempt to remove all sonographic evidence of the disease, we do so in order to make the most accurate histologic diagnosis possible, not to cure cancer. However, a fortunate side effect of completely removing all sonographic evidence of

IPLs under ultrasound guidance is the unexpected permanent disappearance of nipple discharge in 90% of patients whose lesions are benign IDPs. (Whether cessation of discharge is the result of removal of the papillary lesion, infarction of the lesion by interrupting the fibrovascular core, interruption of the duct, or a combination of all three is uncertain.) Thus, establishing the diagnosis of benign IDP with sonographically guided 11-gauge DVAB not only establishes accurate diagnosis in virtually all cases but also "cures" secretions in 90%. This means that when sonography shows an IPL, all sonographic evidence of the lesion is removed under ultrasound guidance, the histologic diagnosis of benign papilloma is established, nipple discharge stops, and diagnostic and localizing galactograms and surgical excision are no longer necessary. This dramatically decreases the complexity, cost, and time necessary for diagnosis and treatment of nipple discharge.

Performing sonography immediately after galactography is an excellent way of learning how to evaluate nipple discharge sonographically. Galactography shows the exact size, shape, and location of the duct of interest and any papillary lesion within it. Additionally, the offending duct is more distended immediately after the galactogram and therefore easier to evaluate sonographically (Fig. 8–11). Furthermore, postgalactogram sonography is invaluable and essential for any case in which ultrasound-guided DVAB will be used.

TECHNIQUE OF SONOGRAPHY FOR EVALUATING NIPPLE DISCHARGE

The IPLs causing nipple discharge are located in subareolar or periareolar segments of ductal system in most cases. Occasionally, a lesion lies within the nipple. Demonstrating the subareolar or intranipple ducts requires radial scan planes that lie parallel to the long and short axes of the ducts. However, true external radial plane scanning is merely the starting point for evaluation. There are varia-

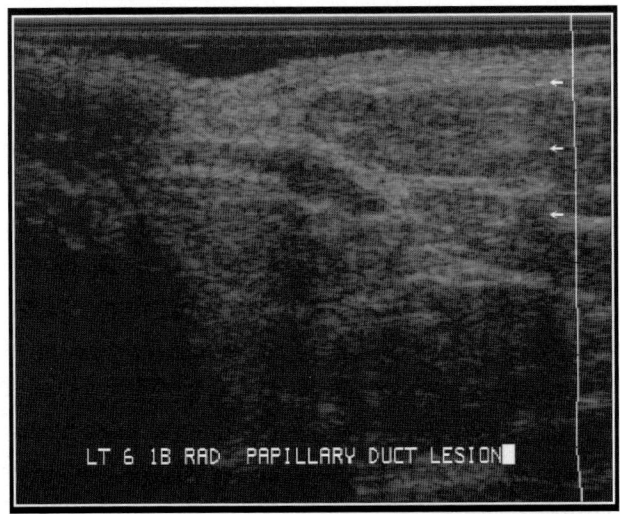

A

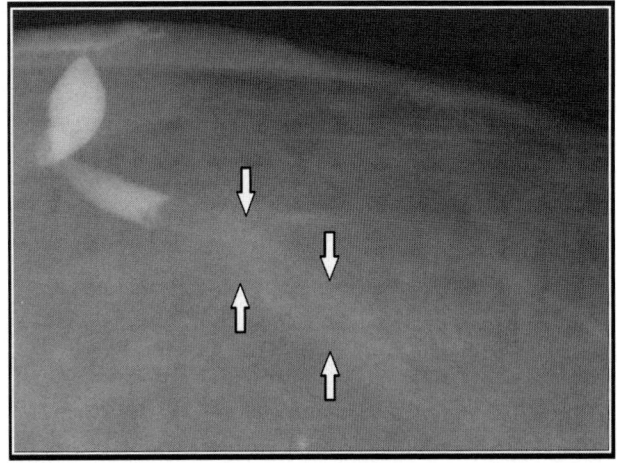

B

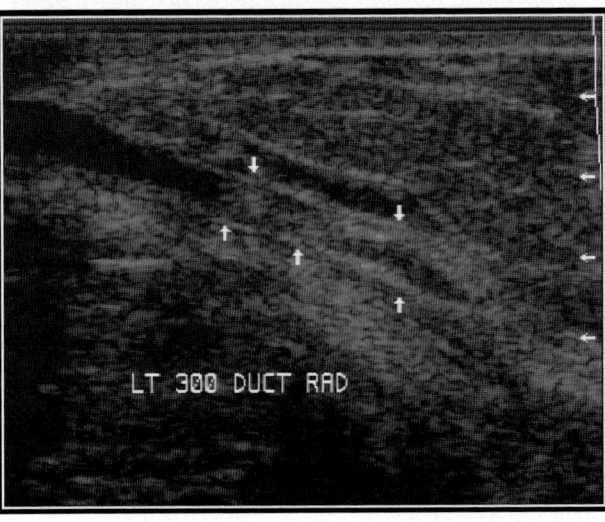

C

FIGURE 8–11 A: Sonography performed to evaluate nipple discharge showed a widened duct filled with low-level internal echoes. This appearance is nonspecific and could represent an intraductal papillary lesion, intraductal fibrosis, or inspissated secretions. **B:** Because the sonographic findings were nonspecific, galactography was performed and showed an intraductal papillary lesion. **C:** After galactography, the sonogram was repeated. The presence of fluid within the duct lumen and greater distention of the duct make the sonographic findings more specific. The duct between the nipple and the intraductal papillary lesion *(arrows)* is now dilated with contrast. Additionally, the postgalactogram study shows the sonographic appearance of the lesion so that ultrasound guidance for preoperative localization or directional vacuum-assisted biopsy later will be facilitated.

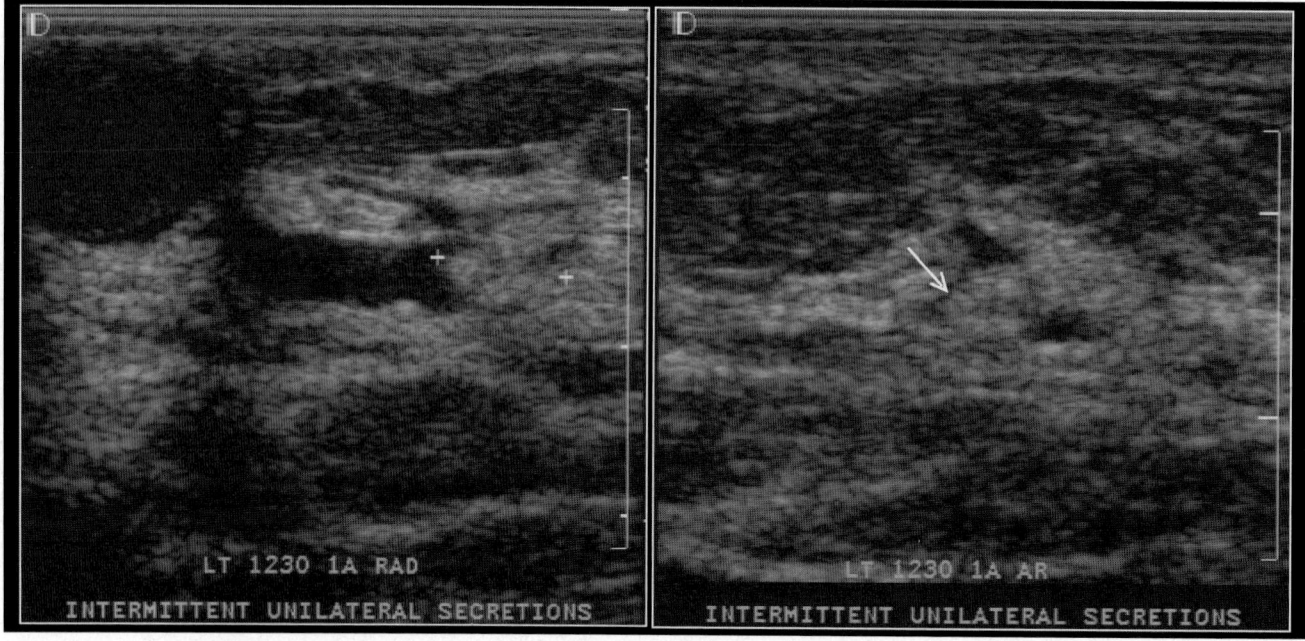

FIGURE 8–12 This apparent hyperechoic intraductal papillary lesion is merely interlobular stroma fibrous tissue lying between two peripheral tributaries and is thus a pseudolesion. The pseudolesion is as echogenic as the duct wall, a feature of interlobular stromal fibrous tissue, not that of an intraductal papillary lesion.

tions in the course of the duct that might require slight adjustments in order to scan ducts perfectly parallel to their long axes. The ducts of interest can be tortuous or can be branches of the main duct that are oriented in planes not perfectly radial to the nipple. In certain cases, changing patient position or breast compression can straighten ducts

that are too tortuous to evaluate otherwise. We usually perform ductal sonography in the supine position, but scanning in the upright position may straighten ducts that are too tortuous to image well in the supine position. In other cases, "pinching" the breast between the thumb and fingers of the nonscanning hand can straighten a tortuous duct.

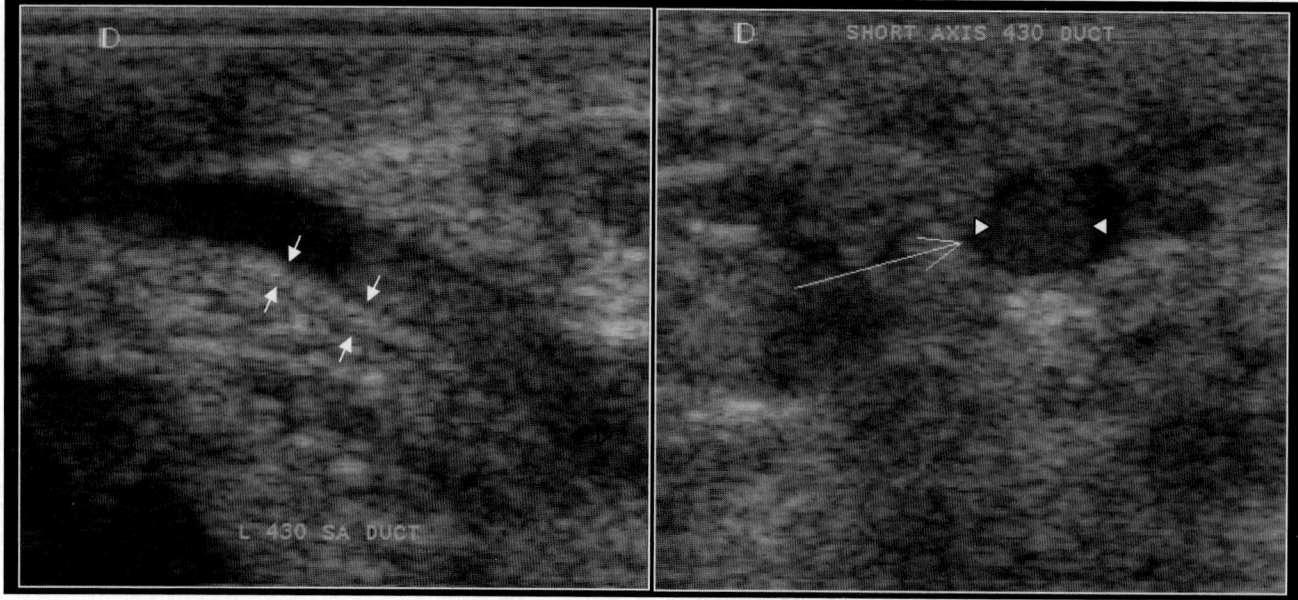

FIGURE 8–13 Intraductal papillomas are isoechoic with fat rather than echogenic or hyperechoic, as they have been described in the literature. The duct wall (*small arrows,* **left**) is hyperechoic and much more echogenic than the papillary lesion within the duct lumen (*between arrowheads,* **right**) (left = radial view; right = antiradial view).

An IPL must always be demonstrated in two orthogonal planes parallel (radial) and perpendicular (antiradial) to the long axis of the duct of origin. Echoes within the duct seen only on the long-axis view might only represent the wall of the duct in a tortuous curved segment or branch point. Duct wall echoes will not appear to be isoechoic solid lesions within the duct in the short-axis view but will appear hyperechoic, like the surrounding interlobular stromal fibrous tissue (Fig. 8–12). True IPLs, on the other hand, will appear to be isoechoic and intraductal on both long- and short-axis views (Fig. 8–13).

Having a warm room and using warm acoustic gel both minimize the contraction of the muscular fibers within the nipple and areola, minimizing wrinkling of the areola and cortical angle shadowing. We generally scan all of the subareolar ducts, starting in the 12:00 position and moving clockwise around the areola until we return to the 12:00 position. The locations of trigger points and of the discharging duct orifice on the nipple surface can be helpful in targeting the scan area of greatest interest. If a trigger point is demonstrable, scanning is begun in the area of the trigger point rather than at 12:00. Additionally, if the discharging duct orifice is near the periphery of the nipple, its clock-face position on the nipple usually, but not always, reflects the quadrant of the breast from which the secretions are originating. Therefore, scanning is begun at the clock-face position of the discharging duct orifice (Fig. 8–14). However, even when the beginning scan area is targeted to a location other than 12:00, the entire 360-degree arc around the nipple should be scanned because LDPs tend to be multiple

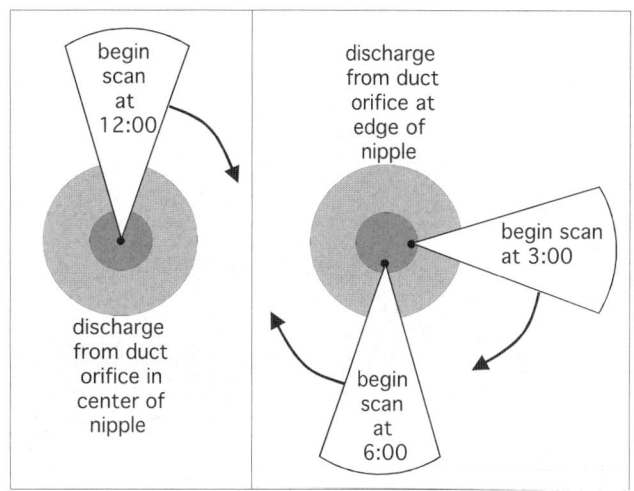

FIGURE 8–14 When the duct orifice from which the discharge is emanating is located in the center of the nipple or within a fissure, the quadrant of the offending duct is uncertain; thus, scanning is begun at the 12:00 position. However, when the offending duct orifice is located in the periphery of the nipple, the lobar duct from which the secretions are emanating usually lies in the same quadrant as the duct orifice; thus, scanning is begun at the clock-face position of the discharging duct orifice.

and to lie within multiple different ducts far more frequently than the literature would suggest (Fig. 8–15).

In certain patients, the nipple does not transmit sound well and may cast a shadow that interferes with visualization of the ducts within and deep to the nipple. Additionally, the ducts immediately deep to the nipple course into the breast directly away from the nipple at an angle nearly parallel to

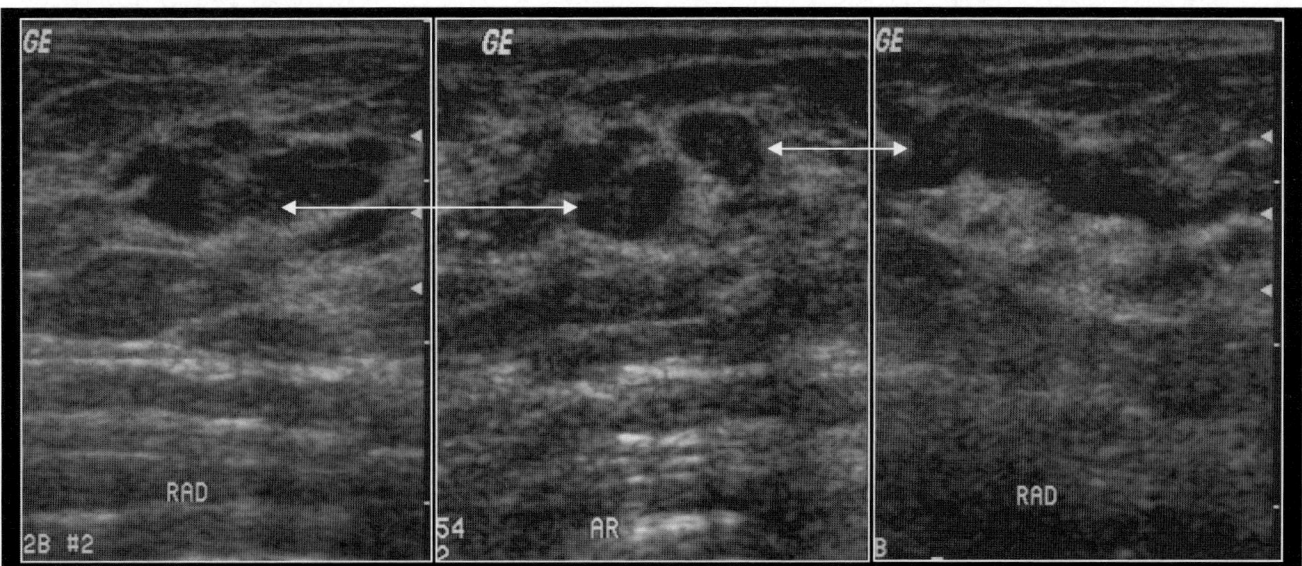

FIGURE 8–15 Multiple centrally located, large duct papillomas are more common than formerly believed, largely because ultrasound can evaluated multiple subareolar ducts, whereas galactography is generally used to evaluate only a single duct system. This patient had two separate papillary lesions lying within different branches of a lobar duct. **Left:** radial view of deeper lesion. **Middle:** antiradial view of both lesions. **Right:** radial view of more superficially located intraductal papillary lesion.

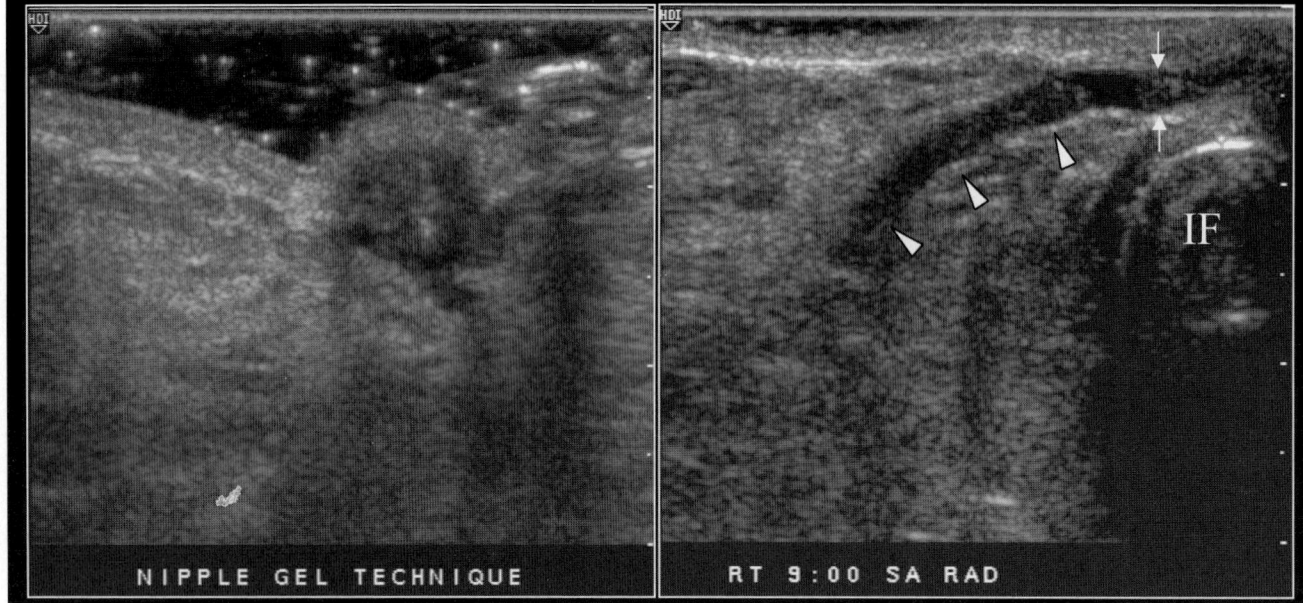

FIGURE 8–16 This patient who presented with nipple discharge had two intraductal papillomas within the same duct: one long lesion within the subareolar ducts *(arrowheads)* and a second short lesion entirely within the nipple *(arrows)*. The lesions were demonstrated with absolute certainty during the rolled-nipple maneuver **(right)** but could not be conclusively demonstrated with straight anteroposterior **(left)** compression, peripheral compression, or two-handed compression. IF, nonscanning index finger.

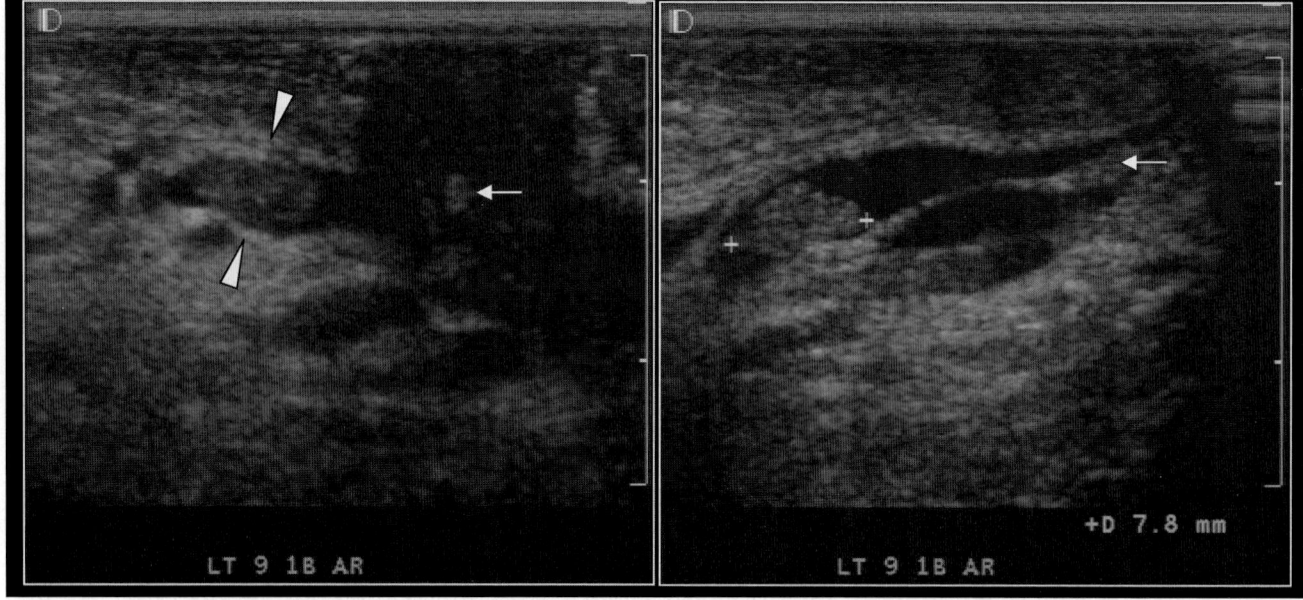

FIGURE 8–17 The **left** image obtained from a straight anterior approach shows a definite intraductal papillary lesion *(arrowheads)* and question of a second lesion *(small arrow)*. If there is only one peripheral lesion, it can be diagnosed with ultrasound-guided mammotomy, but if there is a lesion within the nipple, it is not accessible to mammotomy and requires surgical excisional biopsy. Because the ducts within the nipple are parallel to the beam, they are poorly shown. The *right* image shows the same duct during the rolled-nipple maneuver. The appearance of the peripheral lesion is unchanged. The questioned second lesion is now shown merely to represent normal nipple tissue lying between two separate ducts. The patient underwent ultrasound-guided mammotomy.

the ultrasound beam, leading to critical angle phenomena that further degrade their demonstration. Finally, branch ducts off the main duct also course at steep oblique angles to the ultrasound beam, making these tubular structures poor specular reflectors. Certain maneuvers can improve visualization of subareolar and branch ducts: (a) the peripheral compression technique, (b) the two-handed compression technique, and (c) the rolled-nipple technique. These special techniques for demonstrating the subareolar and intranipple ducts are discussed and illustrated in detail in Chapter 4 (see Figs. 4–50 to 4–53).

Both the two-handed compression maneuver and the rolled-nipple technique require either a foot pedal to freeze the image optimally or a long cine loop that can be rolled back to optimal frames after freezing. Demonstrating the ducts within the nipple requires extreme near-field focusing (within 0.5 cm of skin). Most high-frequency, small-parts transducers are focused at about 1.5 to 2 cm in the short axis, a bit too deep for this application, so that very little compression technique and a standoff of acoustic gel help. The 1.5-dimensional array transducers improve near-field focusing and allow better demonstration of the ducts within the nipple (see Chapter 2, Fig. 2–11).

These special techniques are important because lesions that lie entirely or partially within the nipple are not accessible to sonographically guided 11-gauge DVAB and require surgical excision. Involvement of the ducts within the nipple can occur in three ways. First, there may be multiple

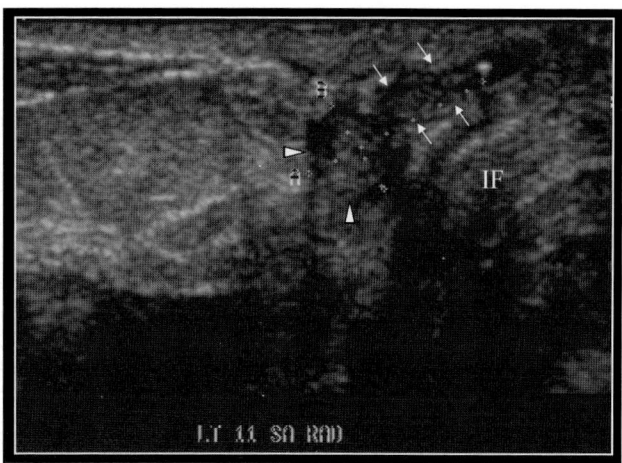

FIGURE 8–18 This patient who presented with nipple discharge had a papilloma arising in the subareolar duct but extending into the nipple shown on rolled-nipple technique. The extension into the nipple prevented performance of ultrasound-guided, vacuum-assisted large core needle biopsy and required that excisional biopsy be performed (*arrowhead* indicates subareolar portion of papilloma, *arrows* indicate intranipple portion of papilloma). IF, nonscanning index finger.

papillomas, one within the nipple and one deeper (Figs. 8–16 and 8–17). Second, a long, subareolar papilloma may extend superficially into the nipple (Fig. 8–18). Finally, the papilloma may lie entirely within the nipple (Fig. 8–19). In our experience, only by performing the rolled-nipple

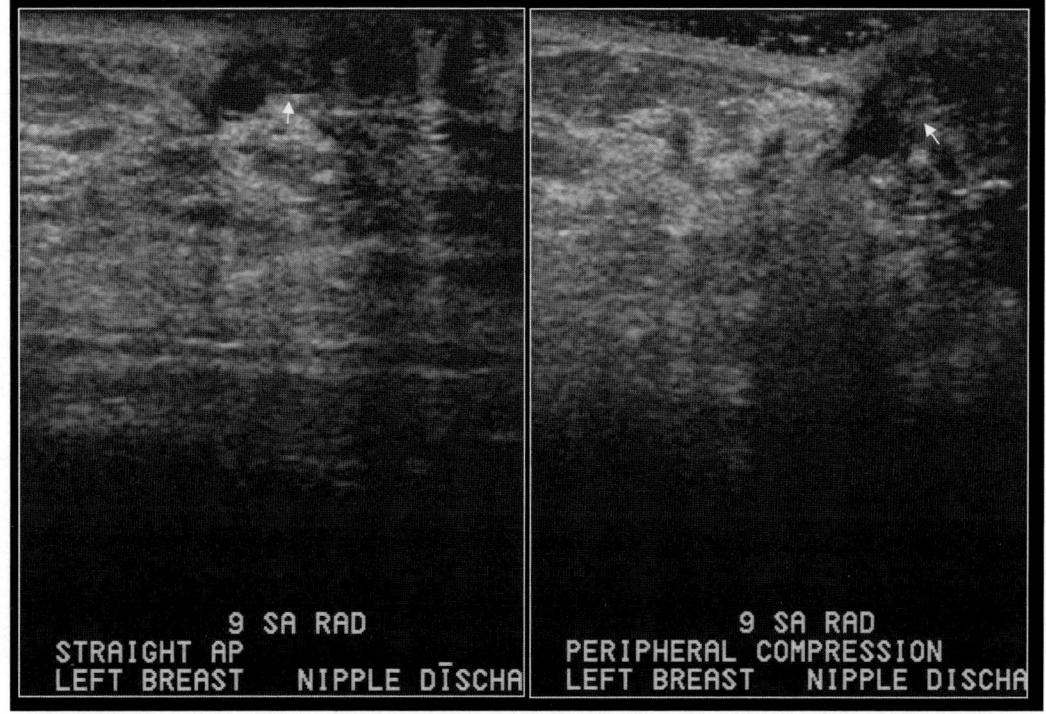

FIGURE 8–19 A, B: This patient with nipple discharge was evaluated with a straight anterior approach (**left**) and with peripheral compression (**right**). There is question of an intraductal papillary lesion, but it is not well shown. *Continued.*

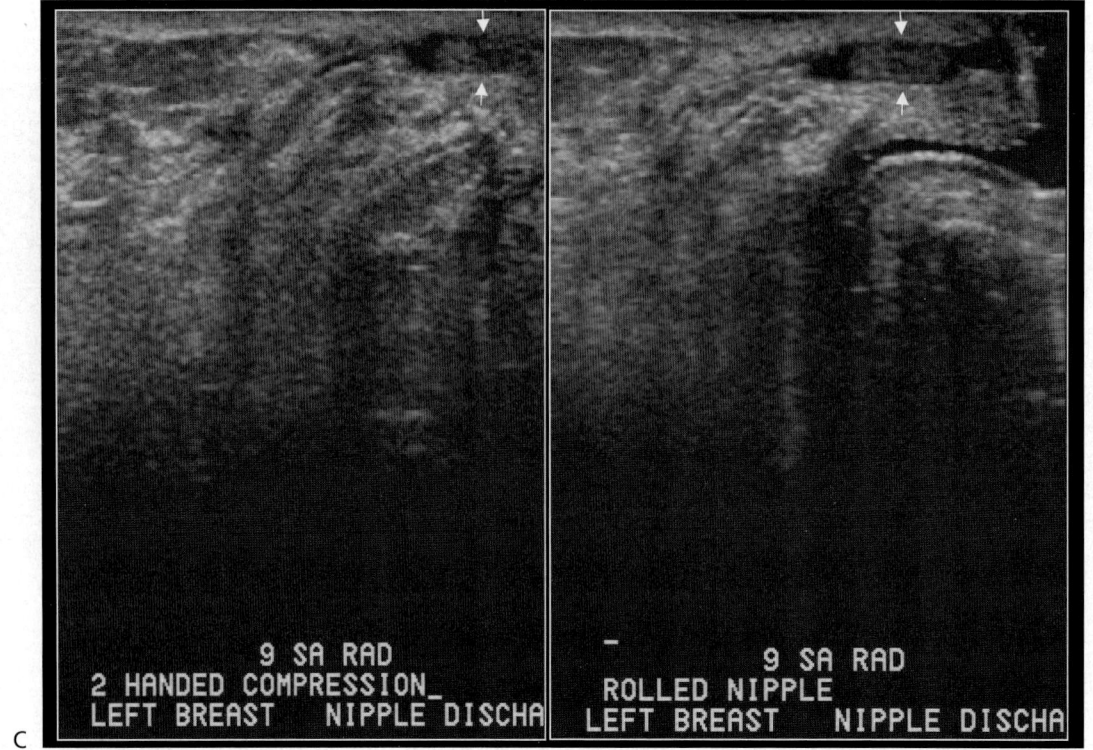

C

D

FIGURE 8–19 *(continued)* **C, D:** The same patient was scanned with two-handed compression (**left**) and rolled-nipple maneuver (**right**). Note how much more definitively the intraductal lesion lying within the nipple is shown with the rolled-nipple maneuver. The patient had to undergo surgical excision. Biopsy results indicated benign intraductal papilloma (nipple adenoma).

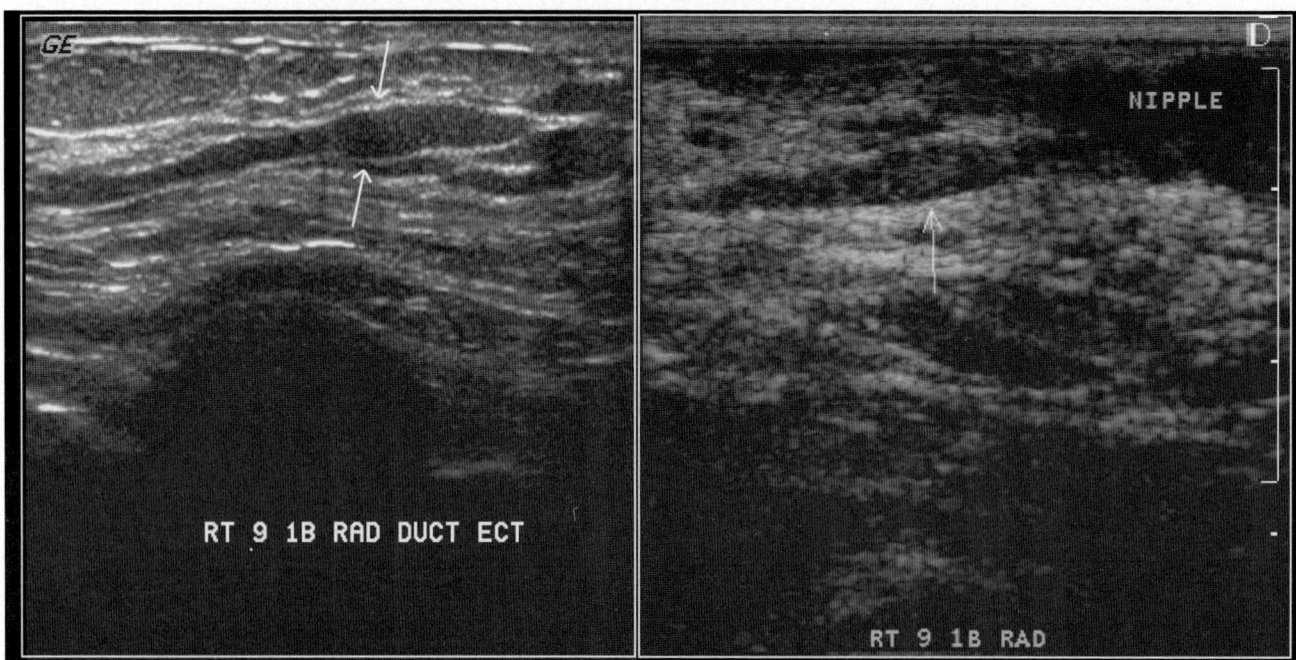

FIGURE 8–20 These radial views obtained in two different patients with nipple discharge show ducts that contain isoechoic material. The echoes within the duct shown on the **left** are caused by inspissated secretions. The echoes within the duct shown on the **right** are caused by intraductal fibrosis. A long papilloma can cause similar findings.

maneuver can nipple involvement be adequately shown sonographically.

Dynamic Maneuvers

In chronic duct ectasia, the secretions within the duct may become thick and cheesy and grossly and sonographically indistinguishable from the material within the ducts in comedo DCIS or from a long IDP (Fig. 8–20). However, dynamic maneuvers may help in this evaluation. Ballottement of the duct with the transducer may be useful in distinguishing between echogenic inspissated secretions and an IPL. Inspissated secretions slosh back and forth within the duct with alternating compression and compression release (Figs. 8–21 and 8–22). Papillomas, on the other hand, remain stationary during this maneuver. Doppler can also be used to distinguish echogenic secretions from DCIS or papilloma. The echoes produced by inspissated secretions moving back and forth during ballottement can generate a color or power Doppler signal called the "color swoosh" (Fig. 8–23; see also Chapter 20, Figs. 20–36 and 20–39). Some caution should be used in interpreting movement of debris within large mammary ducts because the necrotic debris associated with high-nuclear-grade DCIS will move back and forth during the ballottement maneuver in certain cases (Fig. 8–24).

Color or power Doppler can also be useful in distinguishing between inspissated secretions and IPLs by demonstrating the fibrovascular stalk (Fig. 8–25; see also Chapter 20, Fig. 20–38) that supplies IPLs. Papillary lesions are among the most vascular lesions that occur in the breast. Even tiny IPLs smaller than 5 mm usually have a fibrovascular stalk that is demonstrable with color or power

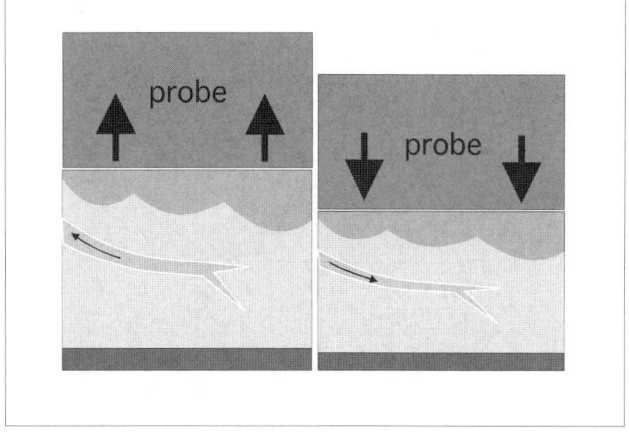

FIGURE 8–21 Ballottement of the duct can be useful in distinguishing between a solid intraductal tumor such as ductal carcinoma *in situ* or papilloma and inspissated secretions by forcing the secretions to "swoosh" back and forth within the duct lumen.

Doppler. If duct lumen that appears to contain echogenic material has a demonstrable fibrovascular stalk within it, the duct contains an IPL requiring biopsy in virtually all cases. As is always the case with Doppler, a positive study is worth more than a negative study. IPLs frequently undergo infarction and hyalinization and in such cases may not show any Doppler evidence of the presence of a fibrovascular stalk (Fig. 8–26). Inspissated secretions in chronic duct ectasia have no demonstrable fibrovascular stalk. In the presence of acute periductal mastitis, there may be blood flow within the wall of the duct, but there will be no blood flow within the lumen (see Chapter 20, Figs. 20–50 and 20–51, 20–52, and 20–54 to 20–56). Even when duct

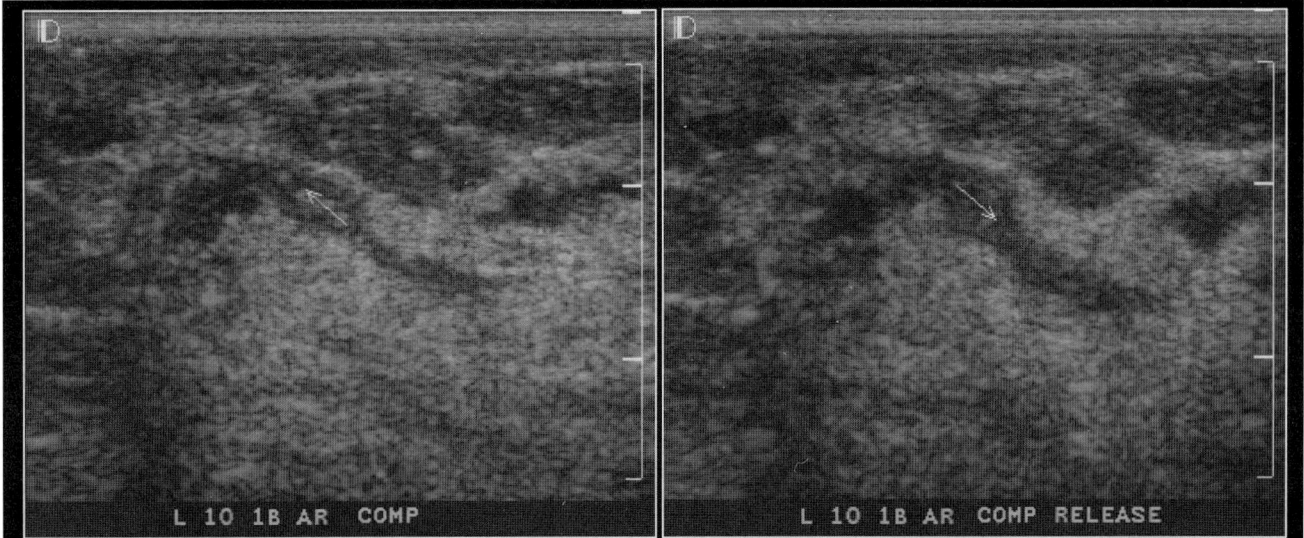

FIGURE 8–22 The back-and-forth movement of the echoes within the duct during ballottement was observed in real time. Such motion cannot be captured on freeze-frame images.

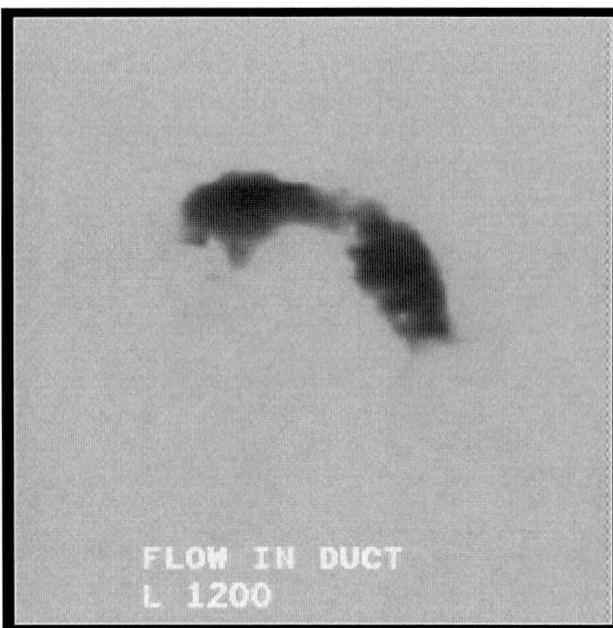

FIGURE 8–23 The motion of the echogenic blood within the duct shown in Fig. 8–22 was documented with a single freeze-frame image using power Doppler.

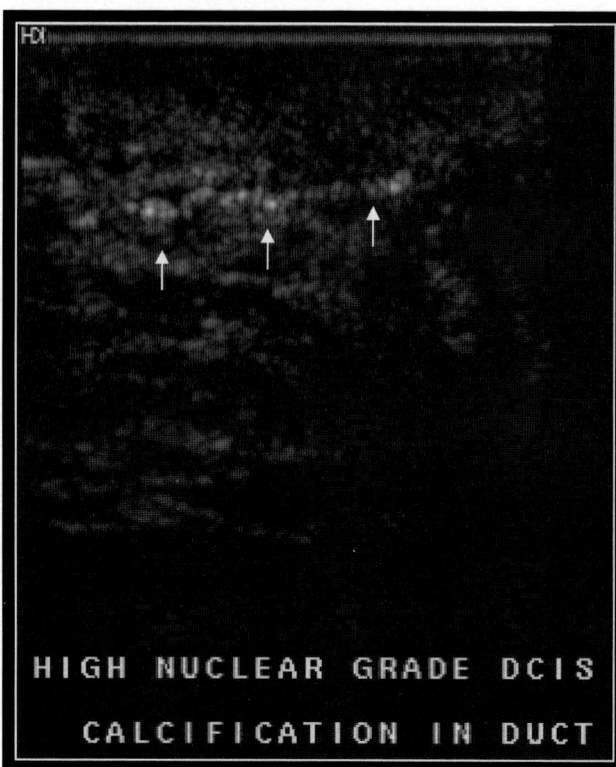

FIGURE 8–24 The calcifications in ductal carcinoma *in situ* occur within areas of necrosis in the center of the lumen. Because the calcifications lie within necrotic debris, even these calcifications can sometimes be made to move with ballottement. Thus, unless "color swoosh" fills the entire lumen, an associated intraductal papillary lesion cannot be excluded.

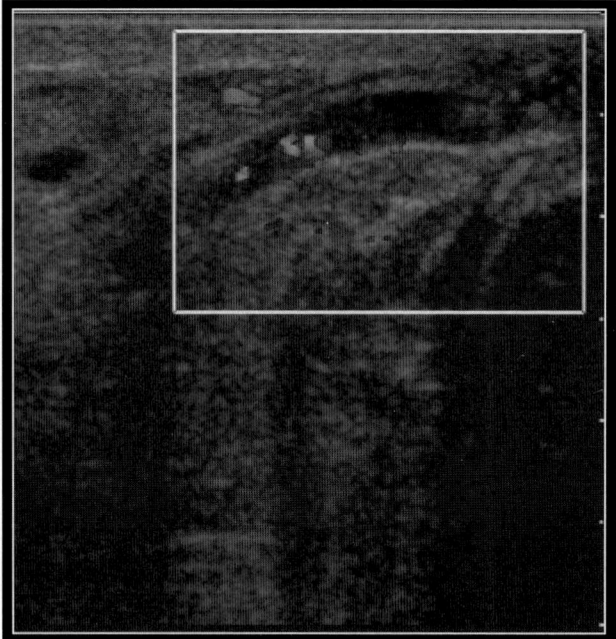

FIGURE 8–25 Intraductal papillomas have prominent fibrovascular stalks that can be demonstrated with color or power Doppler and that help distinguish them from echogenic inspissated secretions.

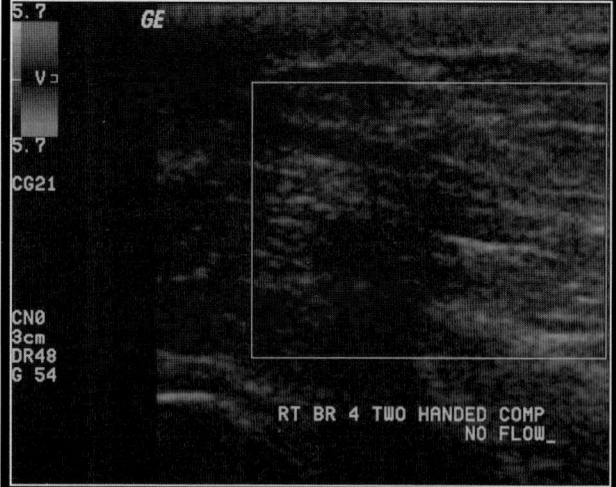

FIGURE 8–26 Although most intraductal papillary lesions have demonstrable fibrovascular stalks with color Doppler, some lesions, especially if small, may not have demonstrable flow.

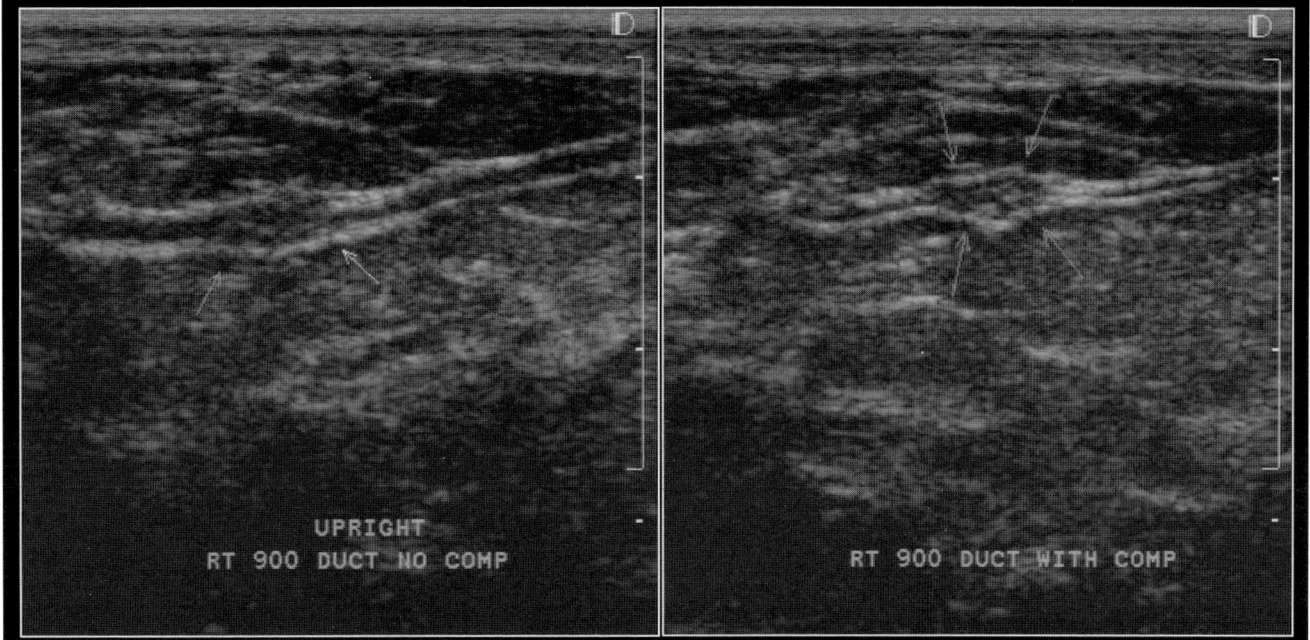

FIGURE 8–27 Radial view of a duct filled with internal echoes was scanned without compression (**left**) and with compression (**right**). The image obtained without compression shows a focal widening. The image obtained with compression shows the narrower portions of the duct to be soft and compressible, but the focally widened portion to be incompressible. This maneuver helps distinguish the less compressible portion of a duct containing a papillary lesion within its lumen from the more compressible parts containing only blood or echogenic secretions.

ectasia progresses to periductal and intraductal fibrosis, there is no sonographically demonstrable fibrovascular stalk. One additional caveat is that ducts that contain IPLs also often contain echogenic secretions or blood that can create a color swoosh. In fact, in such cases, the color swoosh is strongest at the point where the intraductal papillary narrows the lumen, causing a luminal stenosis that increases the velocity of moving secretions. Any variation in compression pressure while interrogating intraductal echoes with color or power Doppler can cause a localized color swoosh around the underlying papilloma that either obscures or is confused with a fibrovascular stalk (see Chapter 20, Fig. 20–39).

The secretions or blood associated with IPLs may be isoechoic with the lesion that caused them and thus may obscure the underlying lesion. In such cases, evaluating the compressibility of the duct with either the two-handed compression technique or simple transducer pressure can also be useful. Inspissated secretions and intraductal blood are soft, compressible, and mobile enough that segments of duct containing only inspissated secretions will almost completely collapse with transducer compression. Papillomas, although relatively soft compared with other solid breast nodules, are still firm enough to prevent complete collapse of the duct segment within which the lesion lies.

Thus, the echogenic inspissated secretions or blood within the duct will compress more than the IPL causing them, revealing the location of the offending lesion so that it can be targeted for DVAB. The effects of compression can be best demonstrated on split-screen images obtained with and without compression (Fig. 8–27).

SONOGRAPHIC APPEARANCE OF LESIONS CAUSING NIPPLE DISCHARGE

Papillomas, Florid (Papillary) Usual Duct Hyperplasia, and Carcinoma

There are several sonographic appearances of LDPs. The appearance varies, depending on the length of the papilloma, distribution of fluid within the duct, extension of papilloma into branches, whether the papilloma expands the duct, and whether the lesion is centrally or peripherally located (Fig. 8–28). The appearance also varies with the width of the papillary lesion, which can incompletely or completely span the duct or can even expand the diameter of the duct (Fig. 8–29).

Papilloma nodules not associated with dilated ducts or cysts present as solid nodules that are difficult to distinguish

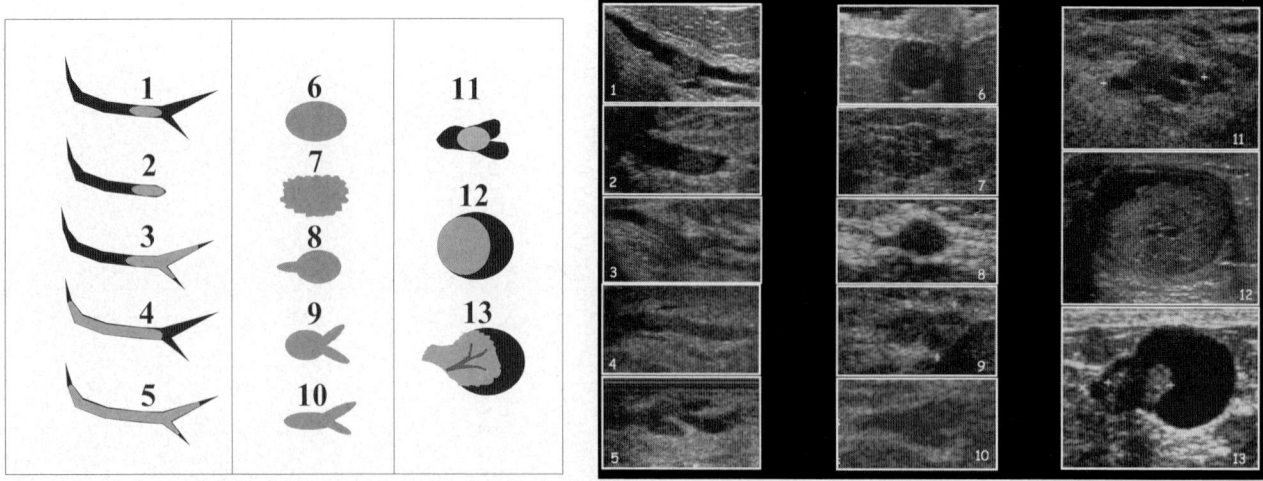

FIGURE 8–28 A: The appearance of intraductal papillary lesions varies greatly. Factors affecting the appearance include (1) the presence or absence of duct dilation and the distribution; (2) the length of duct involved; (3) involvement of branches of the duct; (4) expansion of the duct; and (5) encystment. **B:** The spectrum of appearances of large duct papillomas includes (1) small, ovoid nodule with duct ectasia proximally and distally; (2) small nodule with duct ectasia only distally; (3) long papilloma extending into two branch ducts; (4) long papilloma filling entire central duct; (5) very long arborizing papilloma. Papilloma without duct ectasia may appear as (6) round or ovoid nodule; (7) microlobulated nodule; (8) nodule with duct extension; (9) nodule with branch pattern; (10) "lazy Y." Nodule with duct extension and branch pattern may appear as (11) isolated minimal duct ectasia and small nodule; (12) intracystic papilloma; (13) intracystic papilloma with duct extension.

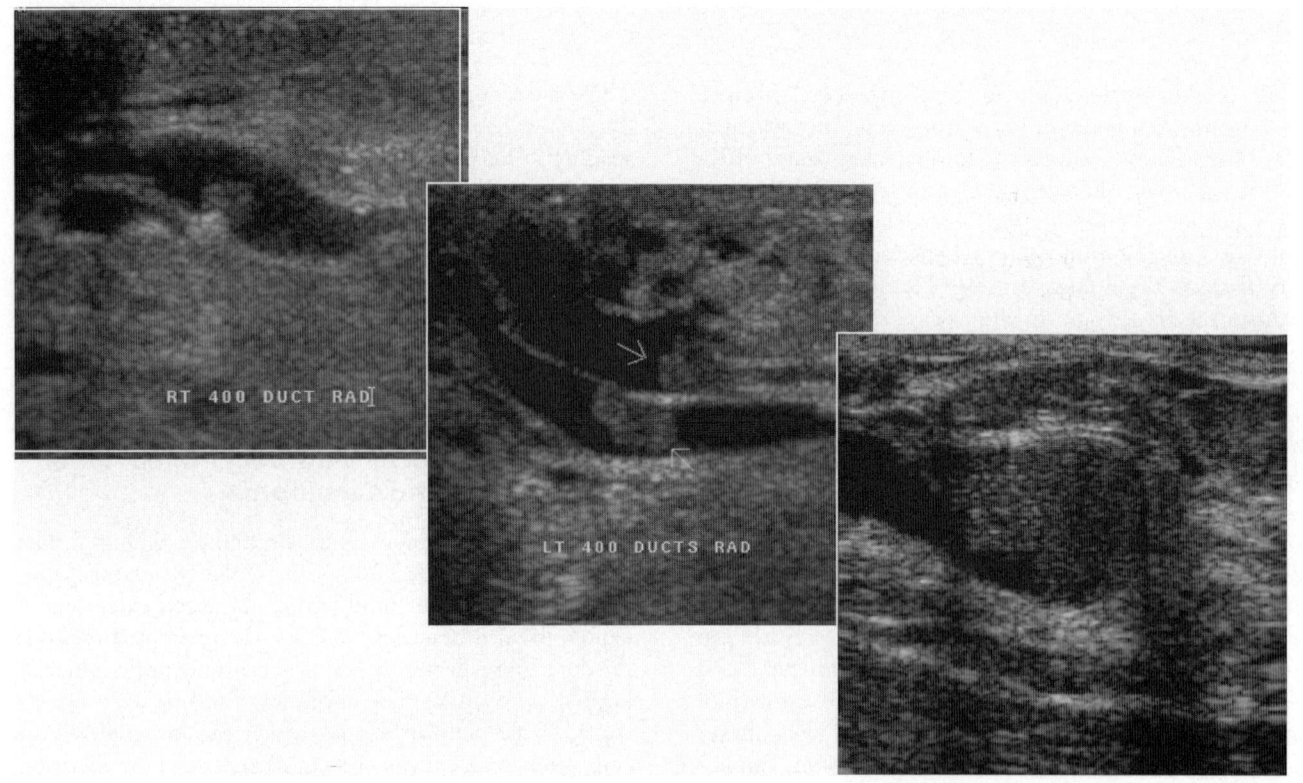

FIGURE 8–29 The width of the papilloma also affects its appearance. A few papillomas may be detected when they do not yet fill the lumen (**upper left**). Most are detected when they are equal in width to the ectatic duct in which they lie (**middle**). Some papillomas may greatly expand the duct (**lower right**).

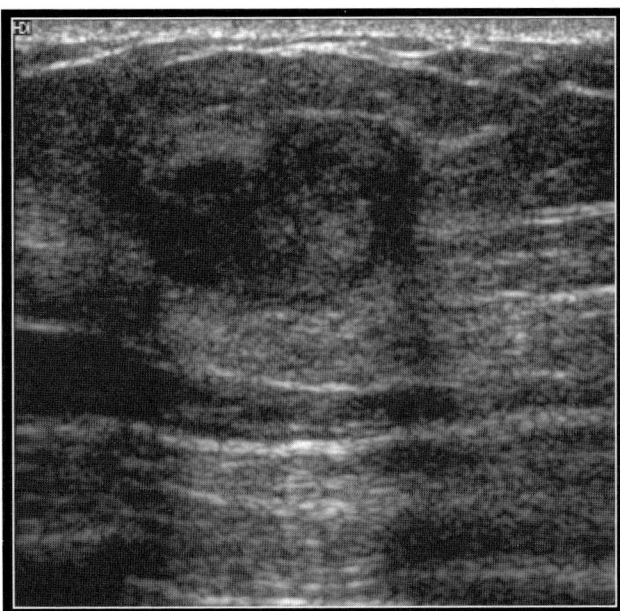

FIGURE 8–30 Most actively growing papillomatous nodules are associated with enhanced through-transmission of sound.

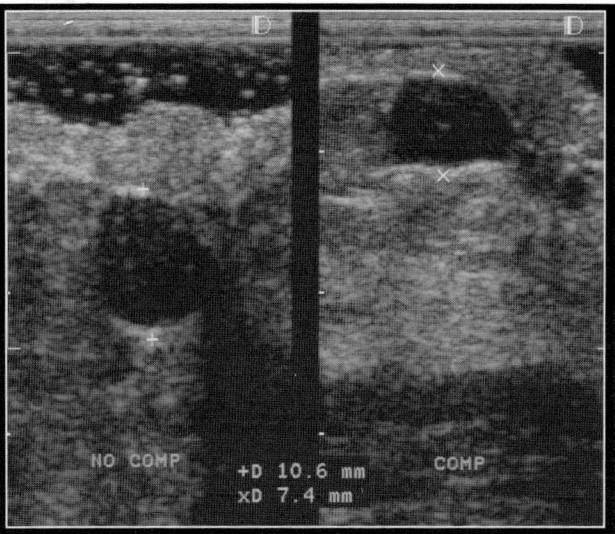

FIGURE 8–31 Papillomas that are associated with enhanced sound transmission are usually also soft and compressible.

from other common solid nodules, such as fibroadenomas and ductal carcinomas. Papillomatous nodules are usually relatively hypoechoic, are heterogeneous, and have markedly enhanced through-transmission while they are actively growing (Fig. 8–30). The hypoechoic heterogeneity reflects the heterogeneous texture and high fluid content of papillomas, with numerous individual papillae (fronds), each containing a fibrovascular core and separated from other papillae by fluid-containing spaces. The enhanced through-transmission is a manifestation of their high cellularity and lack of desmoplasia and the abundant fluid in the spaces between individual papillae. The factors that cause enhanced through-transmission also contribute to the softness and compressibility of papillomas (Fig. 8–31). With time, papillomas frequently undergo necrosis, hemorrhage, and hyalinization. This evolving process results in increased echogenicity, decreased sound transmission (Fig. 8–32), and in some instances, development of calcifications (Fig. 8–33).

Papillomas are usually encompassed by a thin, echogenic capsule that represents the wall of the duct from which they arise. The capsule can frequently be better shown when the nodule is scanned with very light compression (Fig. 8–31).

The surface of papillomatous nodules will frequently be lobulated or even microlobulated, similar to appearance 7 in Fig. 8–28. This appearance is caused by individual papillae or involvement of multiple branch ducts on the periphery of the lesion. Papillomatous nodules frequently have a less expansile component that grows down the duct in an antegrade fashion toward the nipple. Even

when the segment of duct between the papilloma nodule and the nipple is not distended with fluid, a portion of the duct may be distended by components of antegrade papillomatous growth. This phenomenon will be evident as a "duct extension" from the nodule oriented toward the nipple on radially oriented scan planes. When the duct exten-

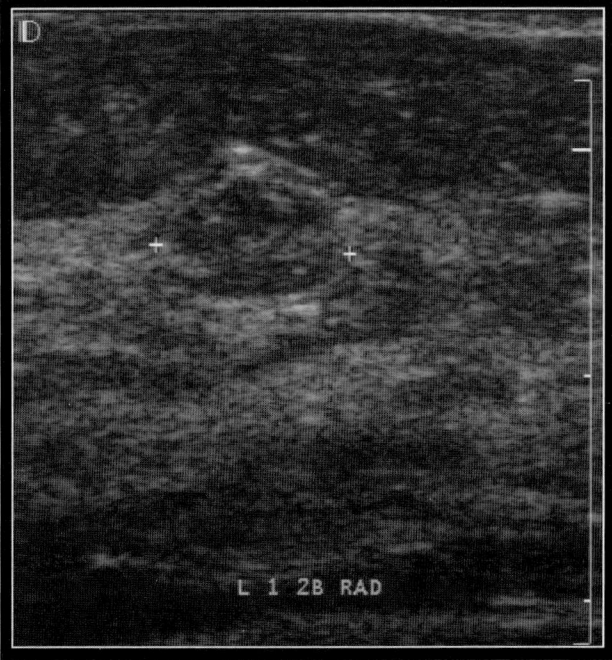

FIGURE 8–32 This benign papilloma has undergone repeated infarctions and has become hyalinized, resulting in heterogeneous areas of hyperechogenicity. Because of the hyalinization, it no longer has enhanced through-transmission. Such nodules are also firmer and less compressible than the typical nonhyalinized papilloma.

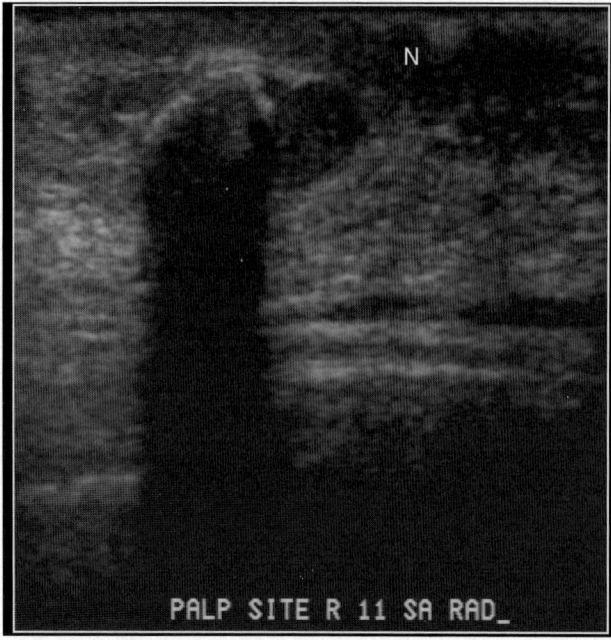

FIGURE 8–33 This infarcted intraductal papillary lesion has become densely calcified. It lies in the peripheral portion of the duct with the duct between it and the nipple *(N)* filled with inspissated echogenic secretions.

sion is short relative to the size of the nodule epicenter, the lesion has a "lazy keyhole" shape similar to appearance 8 in Fig. 8–28. This appearance is very characteristic for papilloma. In fact, in our experience, more than 90% of lesions having a keyhole-like shape represent benign LDPs.

Papillomatous nodules, like papillomas within dilated, fluid-filled ducts, can grow into branch ducts similar to appearance 9 in Fig. 8–28. Nodules with the "lazy Y" shape have both duct extension and branch pattern. The leg of the Y represents antegrade duct extension toward the nipple, whereas the arms of the Y correspond to retrograde growth into the peripheral branch ducts away from the nipple. The lazy Y shape is similar to that shown in appearance 10 in Fig. 8–28.

When a papilloma obstructs a duct and secretes fluid into the duct lumen distal to the obstruction, the duct can become so distended that it loses its ductal shape and assumes the shape of a spherical or an elliptical cyst. Such papillomas are said to be "encysted" or ICPs (appearance 12 in Fig. 8–28). ICPs do not differ histologically from smaller papillomas, except for their size and the degree of associated ductal distention. These papillomas can be difficult to distinguish from certain cases of fibrocystic change with papillary apocrine metaplasia. ICPs frequently grow into the ducts coursing away from the edge of the cyst, usually toward the nipple (appearance 13 in Fig. 8–28). Thus, duct extension helps distinguish between ICP and fibrocystic change. Sonographic analysis of complex cysts is discussed in detail in Chapter 10.

Making sonographic determination as to whether an IPL represents a benign LDP, ADH, or DCIS is impossible. The odds favor papilloma or PDH by about 9:1. However, for any purely IPL, there is a 6% to 13% risk for either atypia or malignancy. Therefore, any solid papillary lesion with duct extension or branch pattern indicating a location within the ductal system should undergo biopsy.

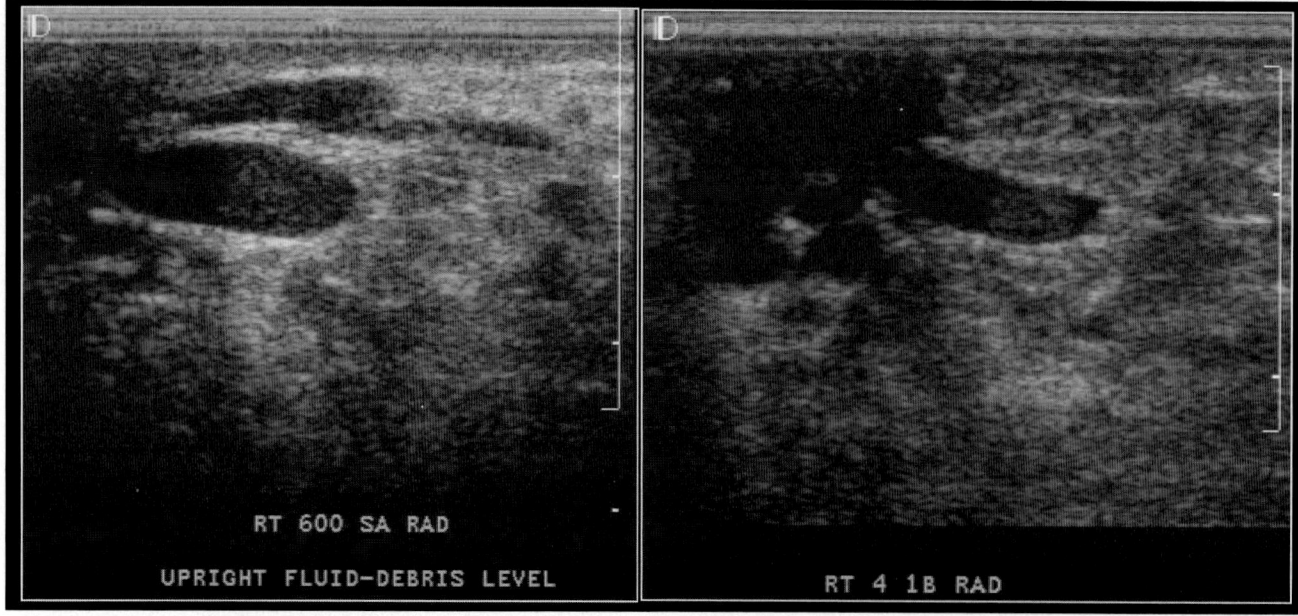

FIGURE 8–34 This fluid–debris level within an ectatic duct simulates an intraductal papillary lesion. The intraductal papilloma in the **right** image has a sonographic appearance similar to that of the fluid–debris level shown in the **left** image.

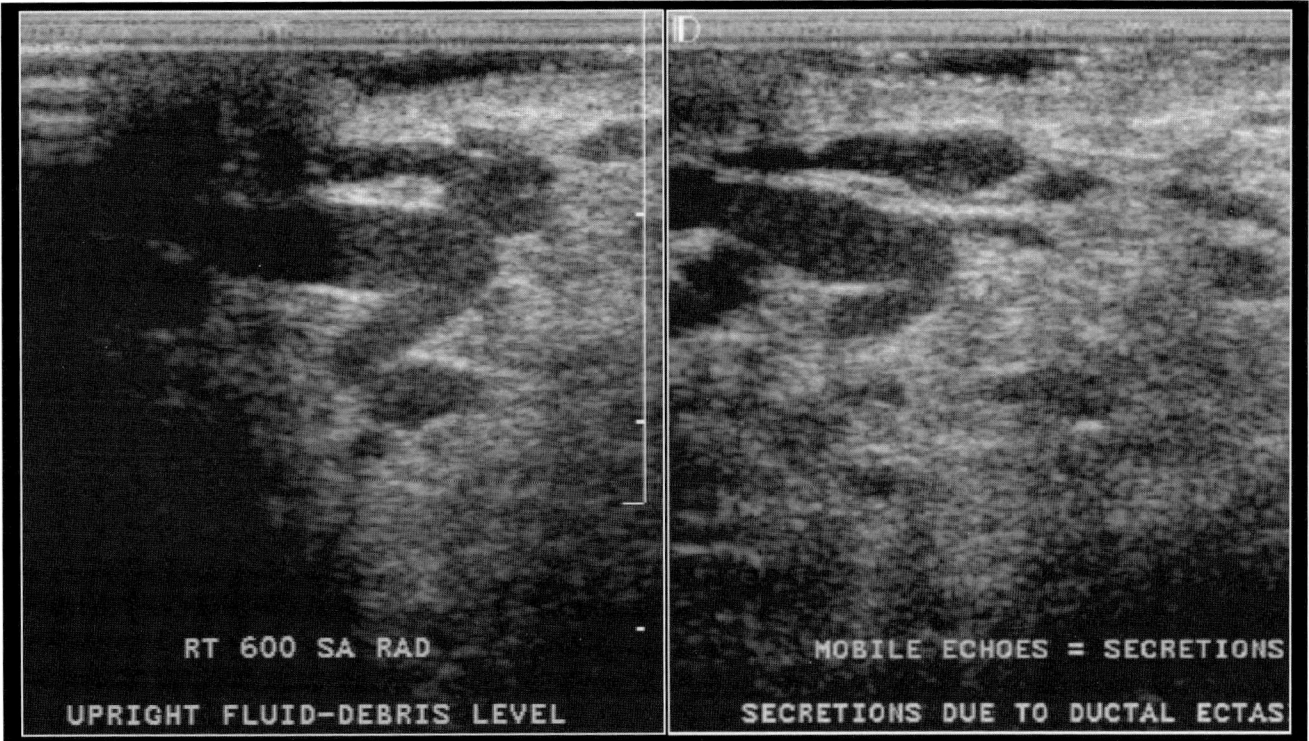

FIGURE 8–35 This fluid–debris level simulates the sonographic appearance of a long intraductal papillary lesion **(left)**. Ballottement of the duct with the transducer has caused the secretions to swirl within the ectatic duct fluid, distinguishing the debris from a true intraductal papillary lesion **(right)**. This could also be accomplished by placing the patient in a lateral decubitus or upright position and watching the debris change to the new dependent position within the duct.

The secretions associated with ductal ectasia may settle into a fluid–debris level that simulates a papillary lesion filling the dependent segment of the duct (Fig. 8–34). Changing the patient's position (left lateral decubitus or upright) or inducing sediment movement by percussing or ballotting the duct with the probe usually reveals the true nature of the echoes within the duct. Layering of intraductal echoes into a debris level implies that the supernatant fluid within the duct is relatively nonviscous. Swirling of the dependent debris within the duct fluid can be produced by these maneuvers (Fig. 8–35).

Malignant Causes of Nipple Discharge

The differential diagnosis of nipple discharge includes malignant etiologies: DCIS, invasive duct carcinoma, papillary carcinoma, and rarely, special-type tumors.

Both centrally located and peripherally arising DCIS can cause nipple discharge. Peripherally arising DCIS that originates within the TDLUs is far more common than is centrally arising DICS but is much less likely to present with nipple discharge. Central DCIS usually evolves from preexisting papillomas in the subareolar duct that can cause discharge even before malignant degeneration. The malignant lesions in such cases have the appearance of the underlying lesions from which they arose—papillomas. Small intraductal carcinomas cannot reliably be distinguished from IDPs sonographically because ADH and DCIS may develop within the epithelium covering the surface of a preexisting IDP. Central DCIS can also develop within centrally located TDLUs (Fig. 8–36). Peripheral DCIS that presents with nipple discharge usually is high nuclear grade and has extended aggressively into the subareolar ducts (Fig. 8–37). Peripherally arising DCIS more typically presents as mammographic calcifications.

Invasive carcinoma can also cause nipple discharge and, like DCIS, can arise centrally or peripherally. The histology of central invasive lesions tends to differ from that of peripherally arising invasive lesions. Peripherally arising lesions are usually invasive ductal carcinomas (invasive not otherwise specified), whereas central lesions are most likely to be invasive papillary carcinoma.

Peripherally arising invasive ductal carcinomas are usually mixed lesions, containing both invasive components and extensive intraductal components (DCIS). Such lesions typically have a sonographically malignant-appearing mass with hard findings corresponding to the invasive component of the lesion and a prominent duct extension toward the nipple with a fluid-filled dilated duct between the solid duct extension and the nipple (Fig. 8–38).

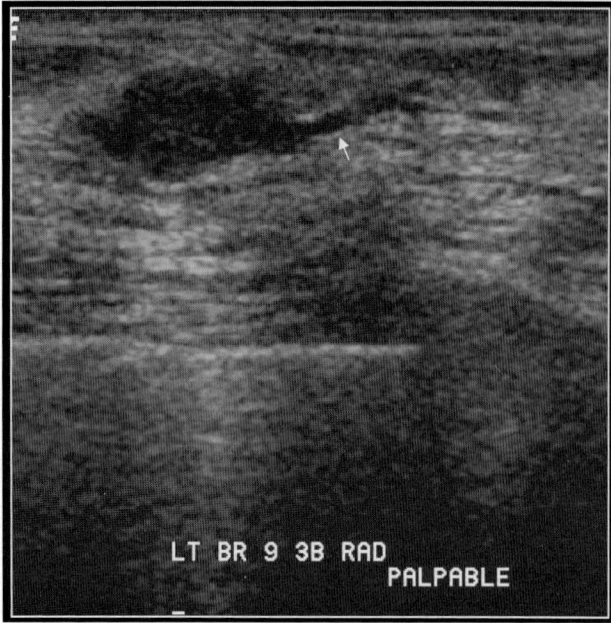

FIGURE 8–36 In this patient with nipple discharge, the offending lesion was ductal carcinoma *in situ* that arose centrally within a preexisting papilloma. The central-most portion of the duct was filled with secretions *(arrow)*.

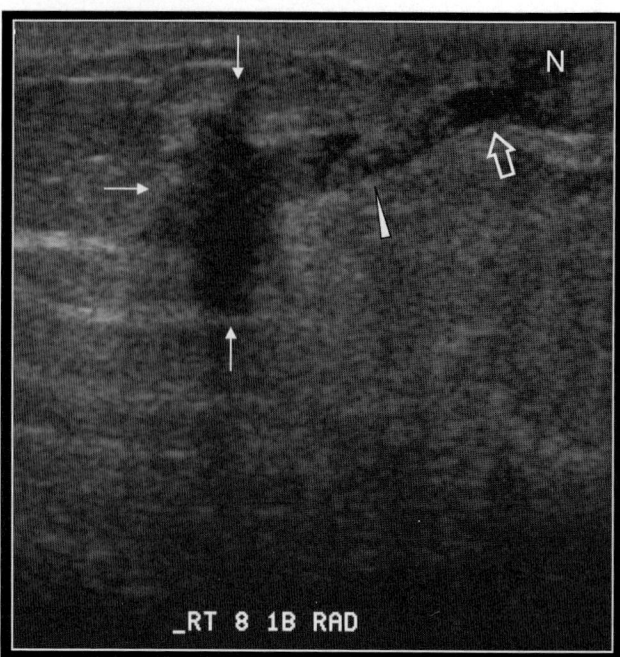

FIGURE 8–38 The nipple discharge in this patient was caused by a peripherally arising invasive ductal carcinoma *(small arrows)* with an extensive intraductal component growing within the duct toward the nipple *(arrowhead)*. The distal end of the duct is filled with secretions and blood *(hollow arrow)*. The invasive part of the lesion shows "hard" sonographic findings of angular margins and is taller than wide. N, nipple.

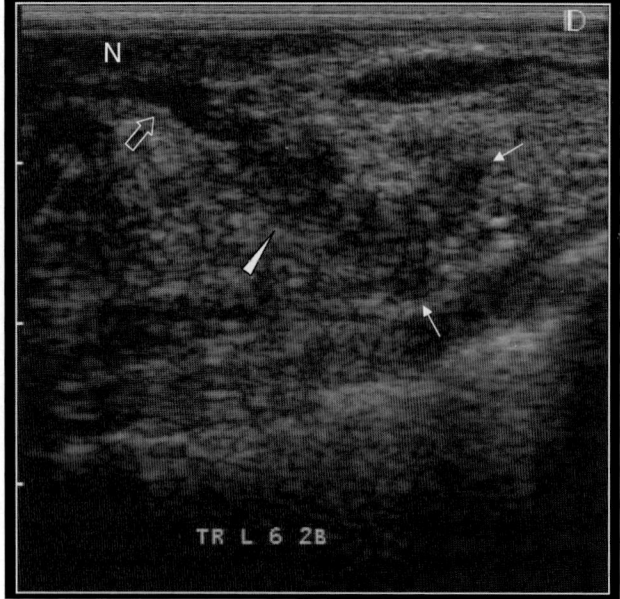

FIGURE 8–37 This patient's nipple discharge was caused by a peripherally arising ductal carcinoma *in situ* that has extended into the subareolar ducts. There is no nodule, just enlarged terminal ductolobular units *(arrows)* and an enlarged, solid-appearing subareolar duct *(arrowhead)*. The duct *(hollow arrow)* immediately deep to the nipple *(N)* is distended with secretions and blood.

Papillary carcinomas are often intracystic and present as palpable or mammographic masses rather than with nipple discharge. Evaluation of intracystic papillary breast lesions is discussed in detail in Chapter 10. Non-cystic invasive papillary carcinomas are usually bulky solid masses that show evidence of calcifications, microlobulation, duct extension, and branching pattern (Fig. 8–39) malignant findings that are discussed in greater detail in Chapters 12 and 14. Similar to benign papillomas from which they may arise, invasive papillary carcinomas often grow for long distances down the duct toward the nipple, making duct extension a very common finding. Like benign LDPs, invasive papillary carcinomas tend to be quite vascular and often have abundant flow on color Doppler (see Chapter 20, Fig. 20–2). Additionally, as is the case with benign papillomas, papillary carcinomas tend to be relatively soft and compressible. Thus, as for benign papillomas, excessive compression pressure with the transducer during color or power Doppler evaluation may obstruct flow through the lesion and create a false impression of absent flow (see Chapter 20, Fig. 20–14). Papillary carcinoma of the breast is discussed in detail in Chapter 14.

Occasionally, a centrally arising carcinoma of cell type other than papillary carcinoma may cause discharge (Fig. 8–40).

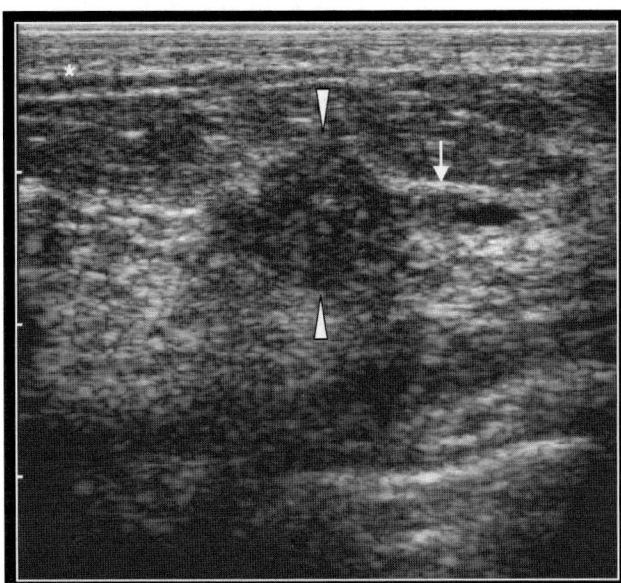

FIGURE 8–39 Most invasive papillary carcinomas arise centrally, probably from preexisting benign large duct papillomas. Such cases often show prominent duct extensions toward the nipple *(small arrow).*

Ductal Ectasia and Hyperprolactinemia

Ductal ectasia is the third most common cause of worrisome nipple discharge (the most common cause of nonworrisome discharge). Sonography is very effective in demonstrating duct ectasia as the cause of secretions. The

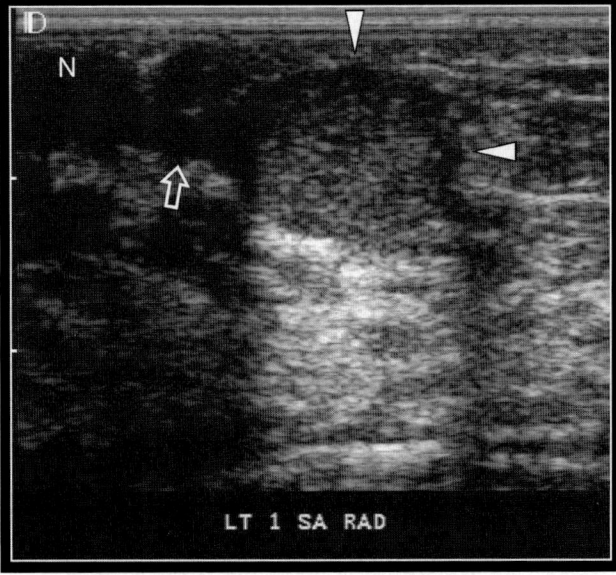

FIGURE 8–40 Not all intraductal malignant lesions causing nipple discharge are papillary carcinomas. The nipple discharge in this patient was caused by an intraductal, centrally located colloid carcinoma *(arrowhead)*, a very unusual occurrence. Colloid carcinomas are usually peripherally located and occur in older patients in whom the central ducts may be atrophic. The *hollow arrow* indicates secretions within the central duct lumen. N, nipple.

ductal dilation is usually bilaterally symmetric, but it may be markedly asymmetric (Fig. 8–41). Fluid within ectatic ducts may be completely anechoic, mildly echogenic, or so echogenic as to appear solid, depending on the age and viscosity of the secretions (Fig. 8–42). The distribution of involvement in ductal ectasia is not always uniform or symmetric. The age and activity of the inflammatory process in the duct walls and, consequently, the consistency and echogenicity of the secretions within the duct lumina vary from duct to duct. Thus, when several ducts in the subareolar area are ectatic, some may have nearly anechoic secretions, whereas others have relatively echogenic secretions (Fig. 8–43). In most cases, either color Doppler or one or more of the dynamic maneuvers described previously will enable characterization of echogenic, inspissated secretions from solid lesions filling the duct. The intraluminal echoes caused by inspissated secretions will be mobile during dynamic maneuvers, but the echoes caused by papilloma, carcinoma, and intraductal fibrosis will not (see Chapter 20, Fig. 20–36).

Duct ectasia has an inflammatory component that involves the duct walls and, during acute flare-ups, the periductal tissues. The sonographic findings of acute periductal mastitis are similar to those of puerperal mastitis, only more localized. Typically, the inflammation is periareolar, causing pain and occasional erythema of the skin. Sonographic findings include duct ectasia, localized edema of periductal tissues, isoechoic thickening of the walls of the affected duct, and localized hyperemia demonstrated by color duplex sonography within the duct wall and periductal tissues. The sonographic findings of all phases of the duct ectasia—periductal mastitis complex are discussed and illustrated in detail in Chapter 11 (see Figs. 11–47 to 11–80), and the Doppler findings are discussed and illustrated in greater detail in Chapter 20 (see Figs. 20–45 to 20–56).

Echogenic ducts in patients with ductal ectasia may be caused by viscous secretions or by the presence of obliterative intraductal and periductal fibrosis, a process that occurs in end-stage duct ectasia. Unlike the echogenicity caused by inspissated secretions, the echoes within ducts involved with end-stage fibrosis are not mobile. Such ducts appear solid and isoechoic and simulate the appearance of ducts distended with papillomas or DCIS (Fig. 8–44). Calcifications may be seen within the lumen of the involved ducts as well as in the periductal locations. The intraductal calcifications of duct ectasia sonographically are indistinguishable from those that form associated with necrotic debris within the center of the lumen in patients with DCIS (Fig. 8–45). However, the luminal calcifications of ductal ectasia (secretory calcifications) and DCIS are usually readily distinguishable mammographically. The periductal location of calcifications is quite typical of chronic ductal ectasia both mammographically and sonographically (Figs.

(text continued on page 184)

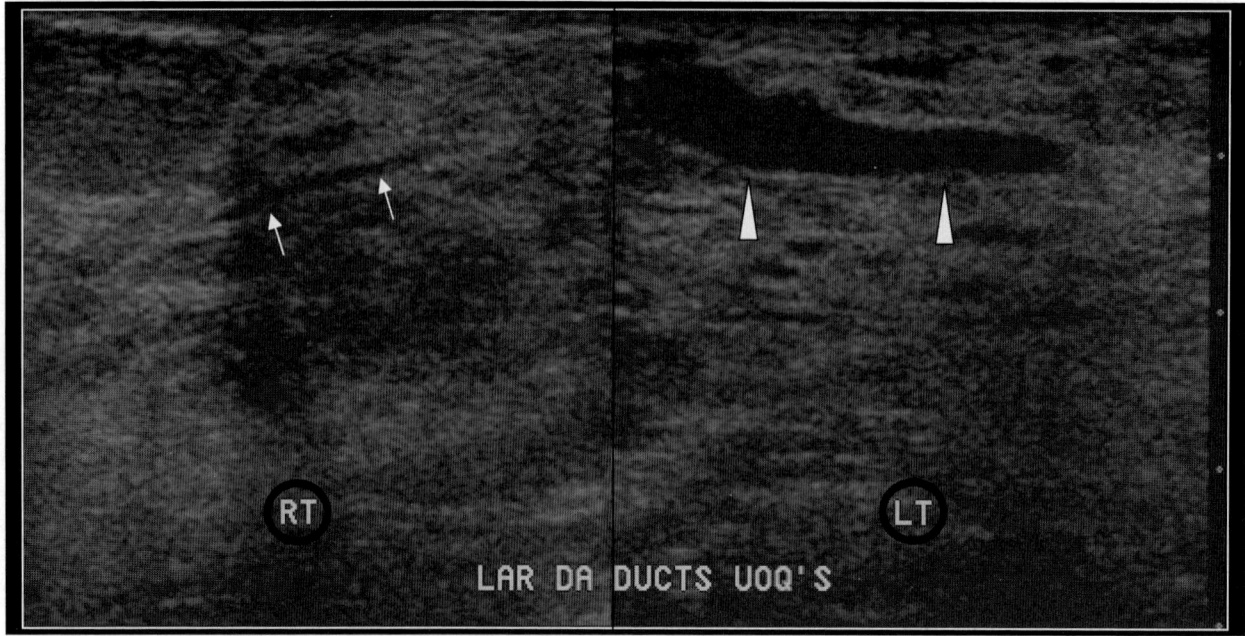

FIGURE 8–41 The unilateral left-sided nipple discharge in this patient was caused by markedly asymmetric duct ectasia. These split-screen mirror-image scans of the right and left subareolar ducts (obtained with two-handed compression technique) compare the size of the ducts on the two sides. Note that the ducts on the left side, where there is no nipple discharge, are small *(small arrows)*. The duct on the symptomatic side, however, is severely ectatic *(arrowheads)*.

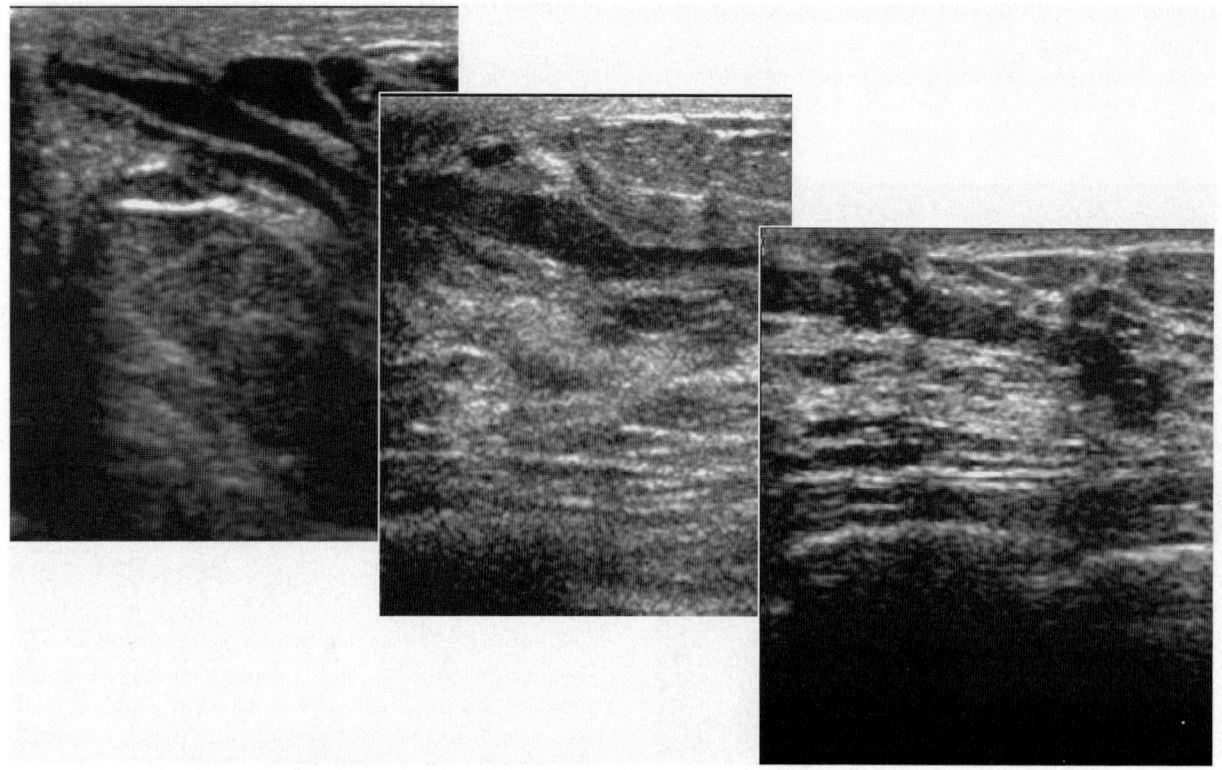

FIGURE 8–42 Upper left: The fluid within this ectatic duct is anechoic. This makes it easy to distinguish from tumor-filled duct and to exclude a coexisting intraductal papillary lesion. **Middle:** This ectatic duct contains mildly echogenic secretions. This makes it more difficult to exclude mildly hypoechoic intraductal papillary lesions within the duct. **Lower right:** The secretions within this ectatic duct are moderately echogenic, making it much more difficult to distinguish among inspissated secretions, blood, ductal carcinoma *in situ*, intraductal papilloma, and intraductal fibrosis caused by chronic duct ectasia. Ballottement and color Doppler evaluation for a fibrovascular stalk may be helpful in making the distinction.

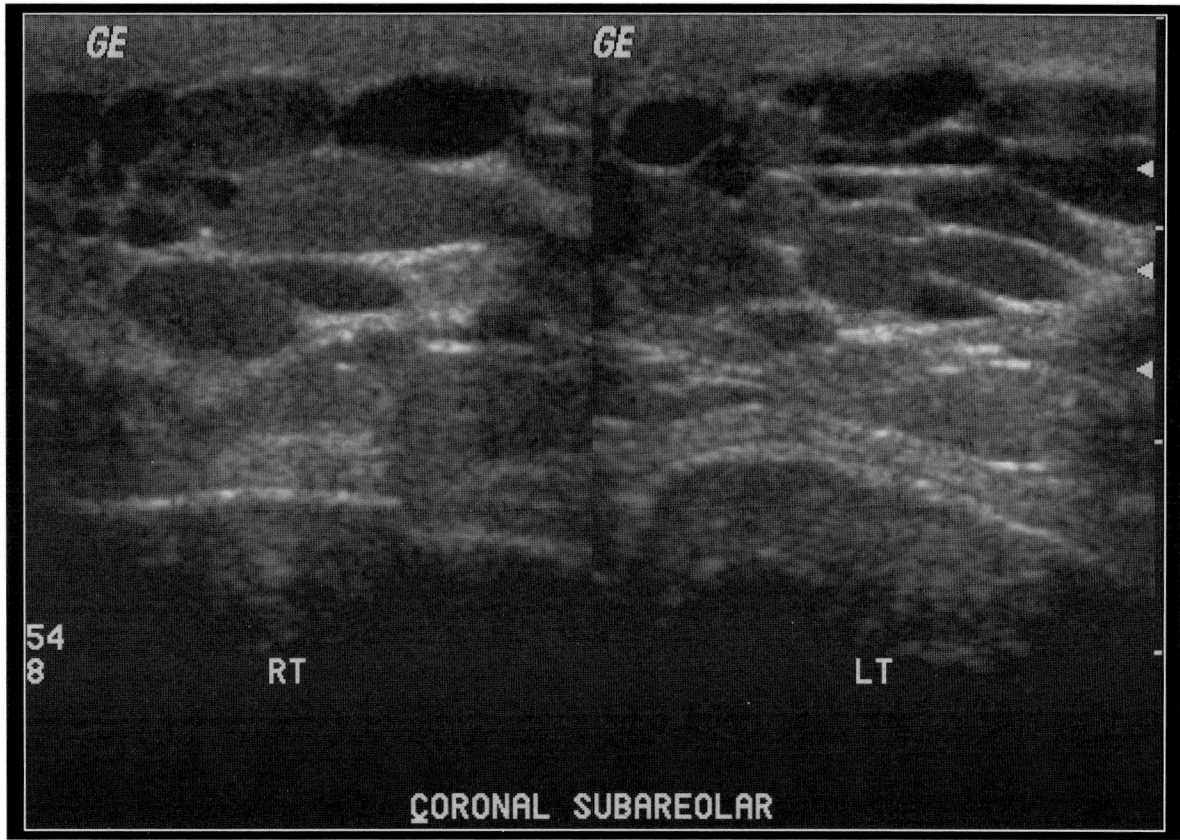

FIGURE 8–43 In patients with severe duct ectasia and multiple dilated ducts, the echogenicity of the secretions may vary from duct to duct, as in this patient.

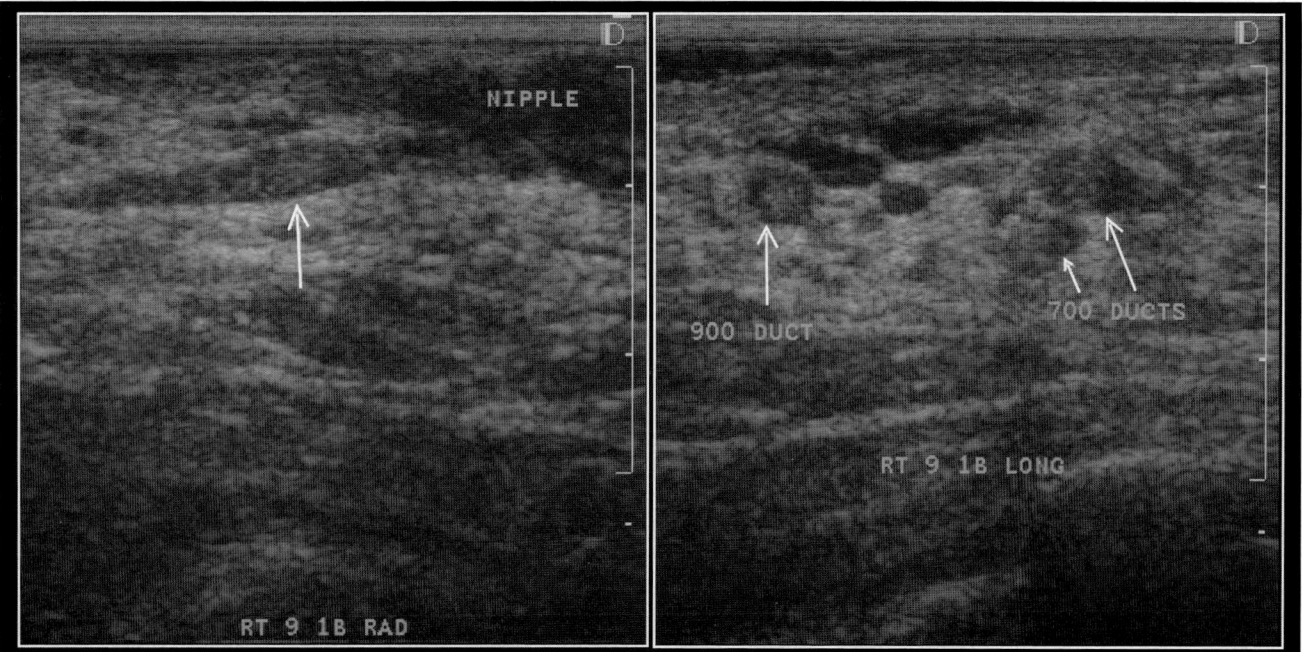

FIGURE 8–44 In end-stage duct ectasia, intraductal fibrosis may completely obliterate the lumen of the duct and simulate intraductal papilloma or ductal carcinoma *in situ* (DCIS). We cannot sonographically distinguish among fibrosis, intraductal papilloma, and DCIS, making biopsy necessary.

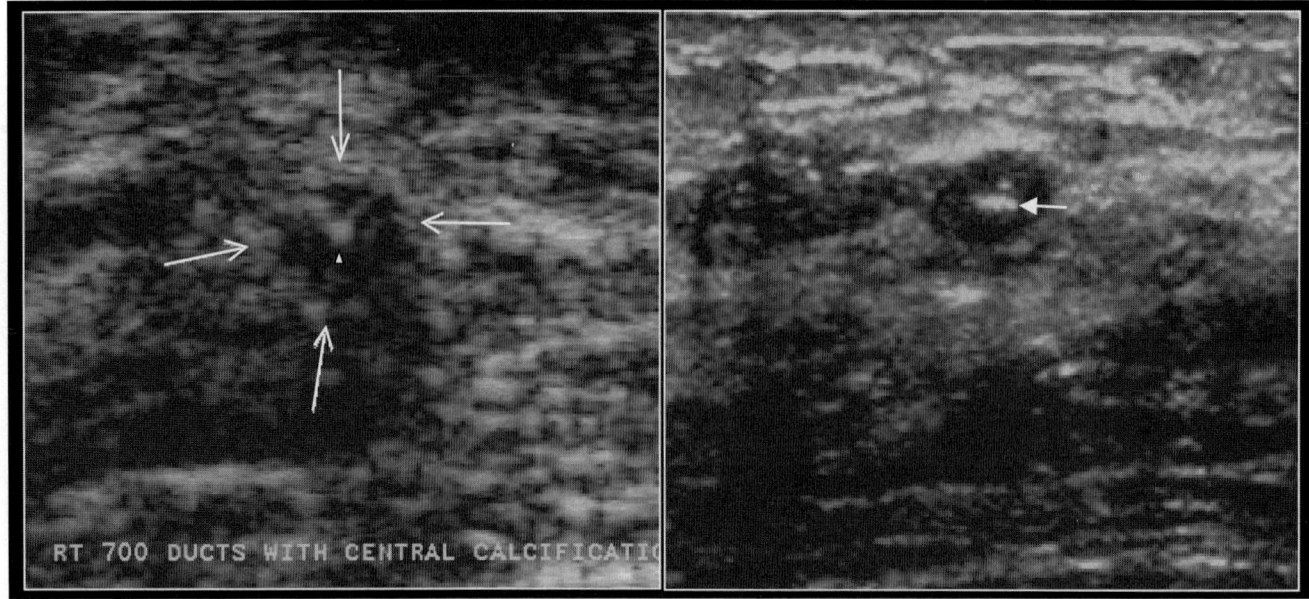

FIGURE 8–45 **Left:** The necrotic debris within the lumen *(arrows)* in chronic duct ectasia can calcify in a fashion similar to the calcification that occurs within the comedonecrosis in ductal carcinoma *in situ* (DCIS), as it has in this patient. The luminal calcifications in chronic duct ectasia and comedo DCIS cannot reliably be distinguished from each other sonographically but usually have different appearances and BIRADS classifications by mammography. **Right:** In this case, the luminal calcification *(arrow)* is caused by high-nuclear-grade DCIS with comedonecrosis. It is not distinguishable from the calcification within the duct lumen *(arrowhead,* **left)** caused by duct ectasia, shown in the **left** image.

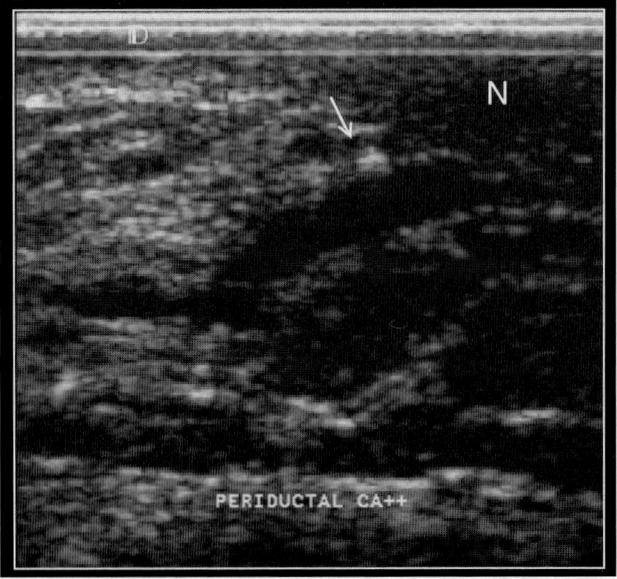

FIGURE 8–46 Unlike the intraluminal calcifications that can occur in chronic duct ectasia, the periductal calcifications *(arrow)* that can result from periductal mastitis are characteristic of duct ectasia and benign (BIRADS 2) lesions both mammographically and sonographically. Mammogram for this patient is shown in Fig. 8.3.

8–3 and 8–46). Intraductal fibrosis in end-stage duct ectasia may create a complex rosette pattern within the ducts. This pattern is similar to the cavernous transformation that can be seen in sites of venous thrombosis that recanalize to form into multiple small channels and can cause nipple retraction that is clinically indistinguishable from that caused by invasive carcinoma (Fig. 8–47). Ductal involvement by obliterative fibrosis due to chronic ductal ectasia may be quite extensive, potentially involving an entire lobe. In such cases, solid enlargement of numerous branch ducts, as well as the central duct, can be seen (Fig. 8–48). As with any other solid enlargement of the duct, this pattern is exceedingly difficult to distinguish from DCIS and usually requires histology for differentiation.

Hyperprolactinemia can cause duct ectasia and nipple discharge. Early in the course of hyperprolactinemia, before ducts become dilated, sonography may be normal. Later, the findings in patients become indistinguishable from those caused by duct ectasia of other causes. However, hyperprolactinemia tends to cause a greater degree of dilation and more uniformly involves all the subareolar ducts than does duct ectasia of other causes (Figs. 8–43 and 8–49). Some believe that virtually all cases of ductal ectasia are the result of hyperprolactinemia, with duct wall and periductal inflammation and fibrosis merely representing late sequelae.

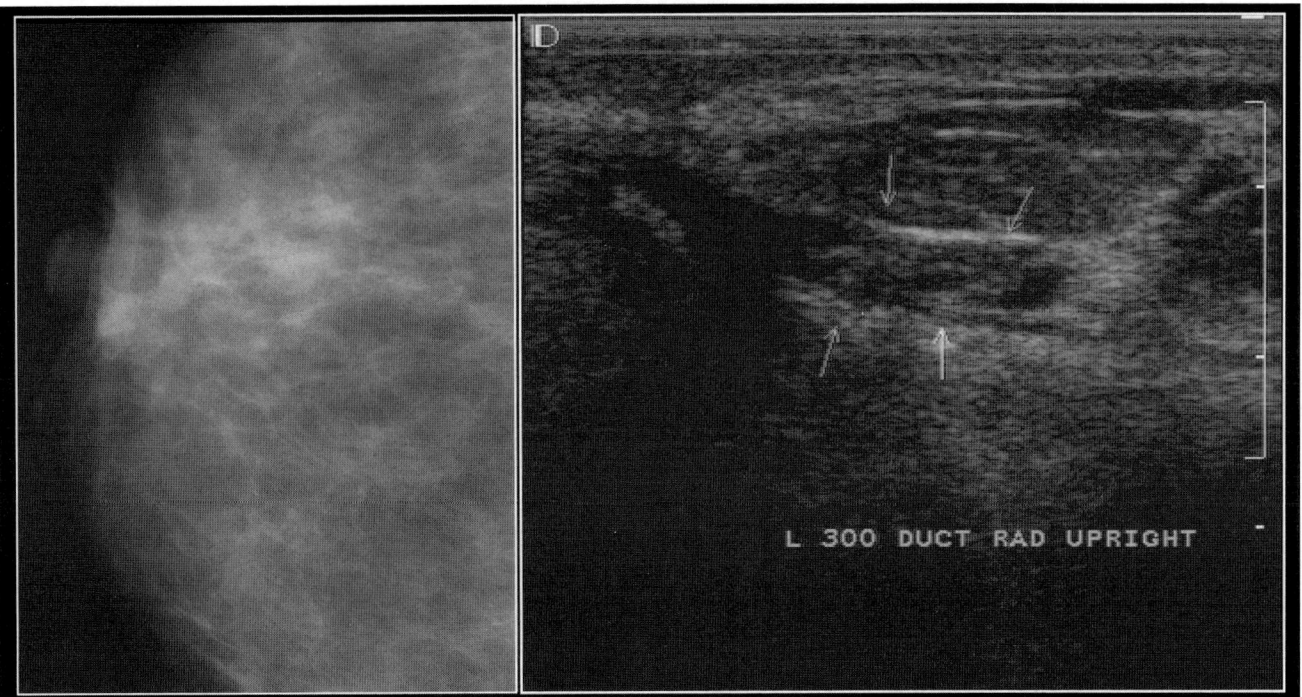

FIGURE 8–47 Although acute or subacute periductal mastitis can cause transient or intermittent nipple retraction, end-stage duct ectasia with intraductal and periductal mastitis can cause permanent nipple retraction that simulates that caused by malignancy. Note the multicanalicular appearance of the intraluminal fibrosis that simulates recanalized deep vein thrombosis (DVT). In cross section, this has a histologic appearance that has been likened to a rosette.

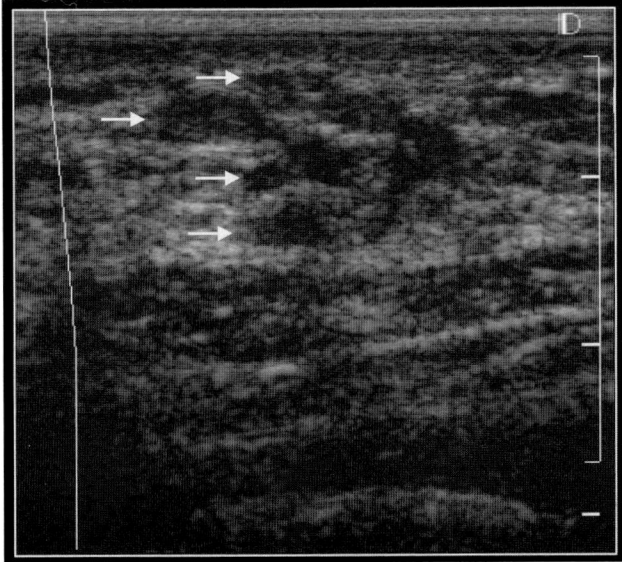

FIGURE 8–48 End-stage duct ectasia with intraductal fibrosis can involve many or all of the ducts within a breast lobe, as in this case. Note that at least four branches of duct are filled with solid material *(arrows)* that simulates extensive ductal carcinoma *in situ* (DCIS). The sonographic findings cannot reliably distinguish between intraductal fibrosis of chronic duct ectasia and DCIS, and biopsy is necessary. Increased blood flow on color or power Doppler would favor DCIS over intraductal fibrosis, which is usually avascular, but a negative Doppler cannot exclude DCIS.

It is important to recognize that only about 25% of all patients with ductal ectasia have nipple discharge. Ductal ectasia is very common and is asymptomatic in a large percentage of affected patients. Most often, ductal ectasia is simply an incidental finding in patients being evaluated for indications other than nipple discharge. Both the early and late phases of the process are typically asymptomatic.

Fibrocystic Change

Fibrocystic change is also a common cause of nipple discharge. In most cases, the diagnosis of fibrocystic change as the cause of secretions is made indirectly by exclusion of other causes. However, in certain patients, cysts that communicate with the duct system can be shown galactographically or sonographically and can then be assumed to be the cause of discharge (Fig. 8–50). This is especially true if there is a classic trigger-point history of alternating discharge and lump. The lump represents the communicating cyst that enlarges and becomes tender when its drainage into the ductal system becomes obstructed, simultaneously resulting in cessation of discharge. Eventually, the obstruction to drainage of the cyst abates, discharge resumes, the cyst decreases in size and tenderness as it is decompressed by drainage of fluid down the ductal tree and out through the nipple. During the nonobstructed phase, compression

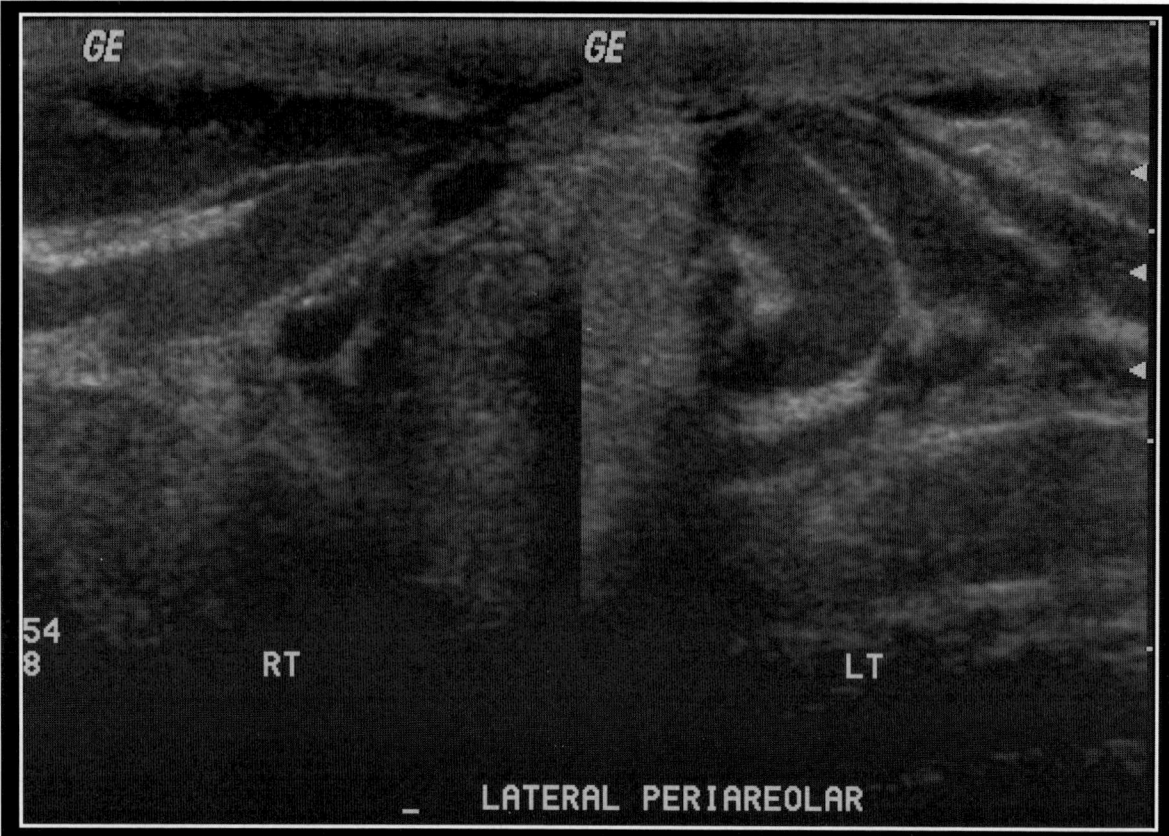

FIGURE 8–49 When duct ectasia is severe and uniformly affects all of the subareolar ducts, hyperprolactinemia should be suspected, and appropriate tests should be performed. These split-screen images in long axis of the right and left subareolar ducts in a patient with hyperprolactinemia caused by a pituitary adenoma show bilateral, uniform, and severe involvement of all of the ducts within the field of view. Note that the echogenicity of the secretions within the dilated ducts varies from duct to duct. This makes evaluation of the ducts for associated intraductal papillary lesions more difficult. The risk of having multiple intraductal papillary lesions is increased in patients with hyperprolactinemia. Figure 8–43 shows the short-axis views of these subareolar ducts.

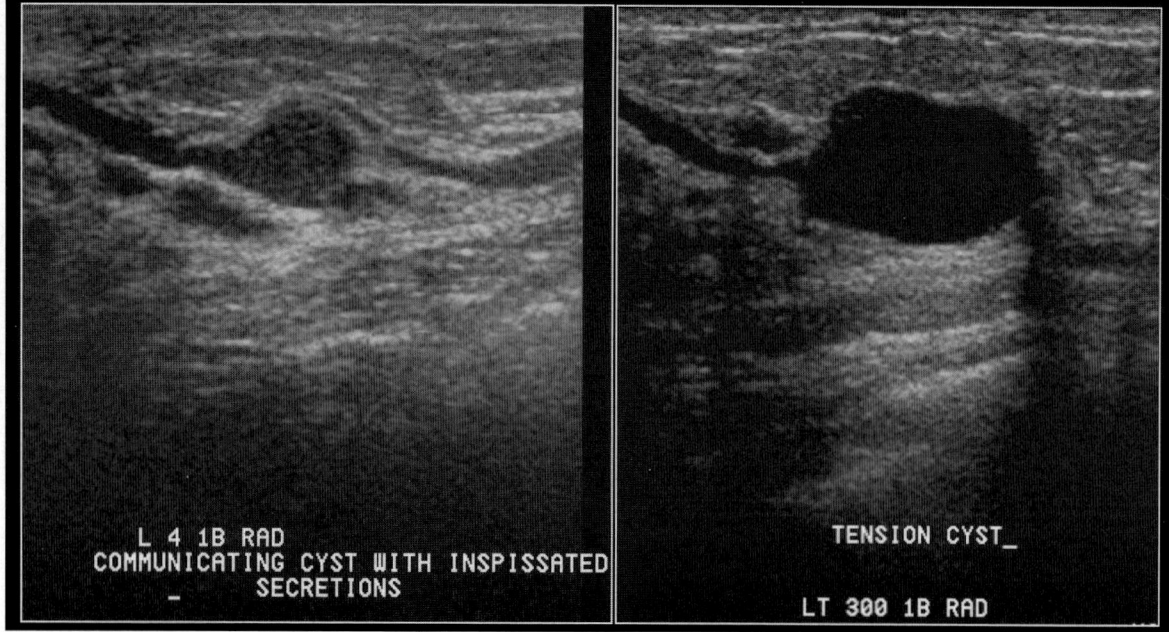

FIGURE 8–50 Nipple discharge can be caused by cysts that communicate with the ductal system. The cysts may be simple (**right**) or complex (**left**) by virtue of inspissated secretions, apocrine metaplasia, or both. The cysts often represent a trigger point, resulting in discharge when compressed. Communicating cysts may intermittently enlarge when obstructed, leading to temporary cessation of discharge. Later, when obstruction resolves, the cysts become smaller and less tense and tender.

of the cyst expresses discharge from the nipple, the trigger-point phenomenon. In some cases, the discharge may be projectile. When the cyst is compressed, a color swoosh toward the nipple can be shown, and when compression is released, a color swoosh back toward the cyst can be demonstrated (see Chapter 20, Fig. 20–37). Unfortunately, in most cases of discharge caused by fibrocystic change, the findings are not the classic findings listed above; instead, they are usually nonspecific—either multiple small peripheral cysts with sonographically difficult-to-demonstrate ductal connections (Fig. 8–51), small peripheral cysts without demonstrable connections to the duct system, or small peripheral cysts with no demonstrable sonographic abnormalities. Most communicating cysts that cause nipple discharge are affected by papillary apocrine metaplasia. The absence of duct ectasia or demonstrable papillary lesions within the subareolar and periareolar ducts represents indirect evidence that fibrocystic change is the cause of discharge, but is not definitive. In such cases, we perform

galactography because sonography may miss small papillomas in ducts that are not dilated or are located peripherally.

Multiple Different Causes of Nipple Discharge in a Single Patient

The sonographic demonstration of ductal ectasia or cysts certainly does not exclude the possibility of a coexisting papilloma or DCIS. Both duct ectasia and fibrocystic change are so common that they are virtual variants of normal. Because they are so common and so often asymptomatic, it should not be surprising that papillomas will coexist in certain patients, for in such cases, the papilloma, rather than duct ectasia or fibrocystic change, is the cause of nipple discharge.

Simply showing that a patient has a breast cyst that communicates with the ductal system does not prove that fibrocystic change is the cause of nipple discharge. An intracystic papillary lesion lying within a communicating

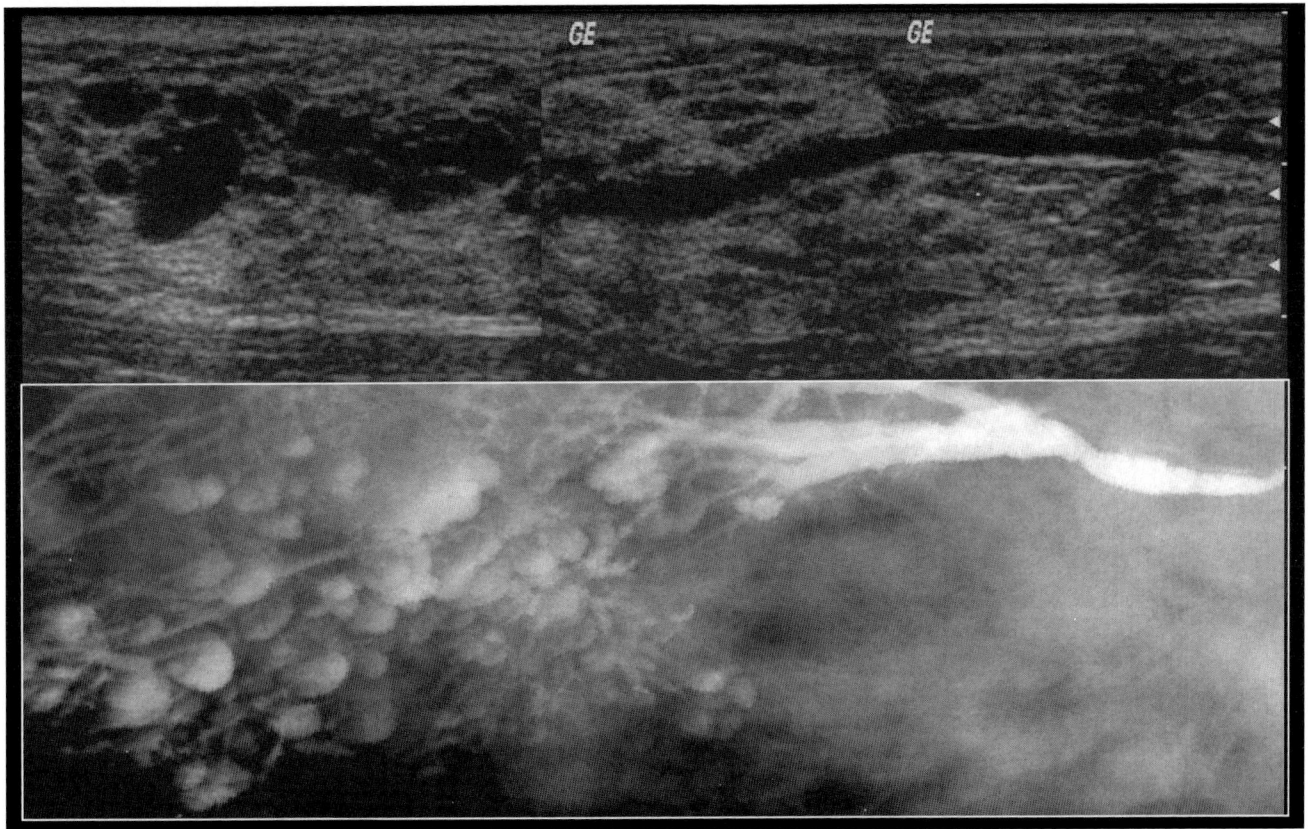

FIGURE 8–51 This 19-year-old girl presented with unilateral nipple discharge. Sonography of the subareolar ducts showed a single severely dilated duct coursing into the upper outer quadrant that appeared to contain no intraductal papillary lesions. The duct was followed peripherally into the axillary segment and low axilla, where it communicated with multiple cystically dilated lobules within accessory breast tissue. The involved duct was so long that a split-screen combined image was necessary to demonstrate the entire lobar ductal system. Because the actual communications between the numerous small cysts in the axillary segment and the dilated duct were difficult to demonstrate sonographically, galactography was performed to confirm the fibrocystic origin of secretions.

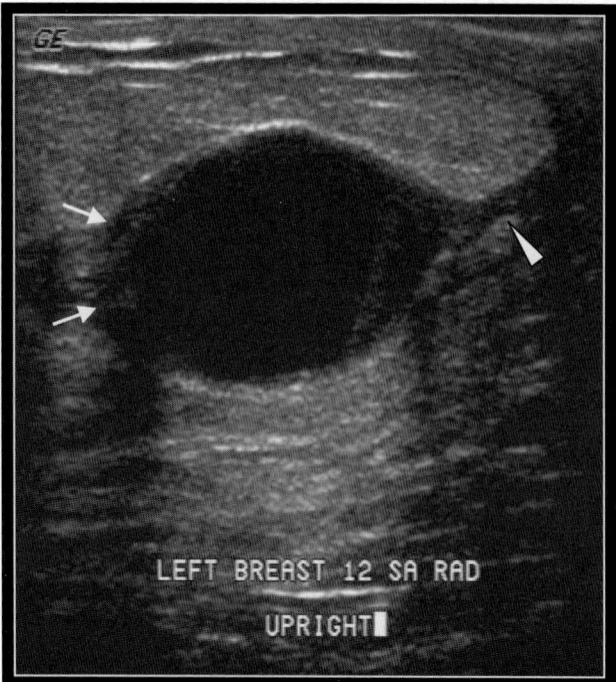

FIGURE 8–52 Nipple discharge may have multiple simultaneous etiologies. This patient had an intracystic papillary lesion within a cyst that communicates with the duct. There was also a fluid–debris level within the cyst. Because there may be multiple etiologies, all ectatic ducts and communicating cysts should be evaluated in their entirety for coexisting papillary lesions *(arrows)*.

cyst may be the cause of nipple discharge but will only be demonstrated if sought (Fig. 8–52). In certain cases, the papillary nature of the metaplastic apocrine cells will be difficult to distinguish from true ICPs or carcinomas. Such lesions must be characterized as suspicious, BIRADS 4, and must undergo either excisional or ultrasound-guided DVAB (with deployment of metal marker). Furthermore, even when a communicating cyst is found and does not contain an intracystic papillary lesion, the ducts in the entire subareolar region should still be scanned to exclude a coexisting IPL. The diagnosis of fibrocystic change and a communicating cyst as the cause of nipple discharge must be one of exclusion.

Likewise, simply showing the presence of duct ectasia does not prove that it is the cause of nipple discharge, nor that there are no associated IPLs. Duct ectasia, like communicating cysts, is an incidental asymptomatic finding in most patients, and not necessarily the cause of a chief complaint of nipple discharge. When duct ectasia is identified, it is still necessary to search the entire lumen of each ectatic duct looking for the presence of a coexisting IPL. In our experience, there is a correlation between severe duct ectasia and the presence of multiple central papillomas (Fig. 8–53), and patients with duct ectasia are more likely than other patients to have one or more IPLs. In fact, chronic

and severe hyperprolactinemia not only causes duct ectasia but also predisposes the patient to formation of multiple LDPs.

LIMITATIONS

False-Positive Results

Sonographic studies can be falsely positive for IPLs when the duct is tortuous or curved and part of the lateral wall is volume-averaged with the lumen of the curving duct. Sometimes, the dividing wall at a branch point in the duct will be mistaken for an intraductal lesion (Fig. 8–12). The branch point is usually more echogenic than true IPLs. Branch septae are usually similar in echogenicity to the hyperechoic interlobular stromal fibrous tissue, whereas papillary lesions in the duct are usually nearly isoechoic with fat and glandular tissue (Figs. 8–13). Additionally, IPLs are demonstrable in both long-axis and orthogonal short-axis views of the duct, whereas branch points simulate intraductal lesions only in the long axis (Figs. 8–12 and 8–13). Therefore, demonstration of IPLs in both long and short axes of the duct is very important. False-positive studies can also result from intraductal and periductal fibrosis in cases of severe end-stage chronic ductal ectasia (Fig. 8–44) and from adherent clots within the lumen when there is frank bleeding from either ductal ectasia or an IPL located elsewhere within the duct (Fig. 8–54). False-positive studies can also occur in ductal ectasia when the secretions are thick and inspissated, but movement of the secretions does not occur when using the dynamic maneuvers described previously.

False-Negative Results

Sonographic studies may be falsely negative when the duct containing the papillary lesion is not fluid filled and dilated. Although the discharging duct containing a papillary lesion usually becomes dilated, occasionally it does not. Sonography is less sensitive and more likely to miss a papillary lesion when ducts are not dilated. Sonography also becomes less effective the more peripherally a papilloma occurs. The peripheral ducts are smaller, far more numerous, and deeper, and they course at less optimal angles of incidence to the ultrasound beam. They are less likely to be dilated. For all of these reasons, the peripheral ducts are less completely and less well demonstrated than are the central ducts, making small, peripheral intraductal lesions or intralobular lesions harder to identify or distinguish from normal lobules. Additionally, the area of the breast that must be scanned is much larger if the peripheral ducts are to be evaluated. We usually limit our examination to the immediate subareolar and periareolar areas but follow each dilated duct peripherally until its lumen is no longer iden-

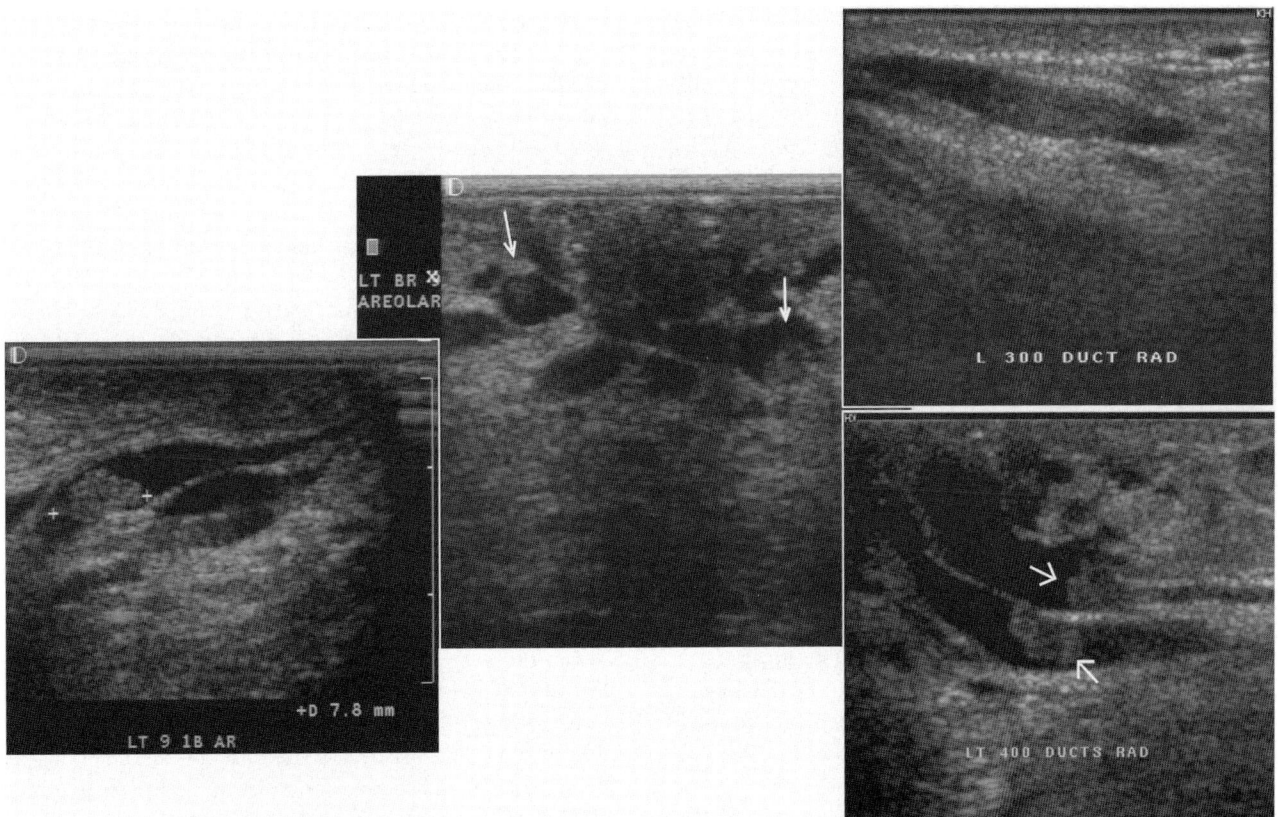

FIGURE 8–53 This collage shows long-axis views of four intraductal papillary lesions in four separate dilated ducts on the left side. The patient also had five intraductal papillary lesions within multiple dilated ducts on the right. We have seen this often enough to question whether chronic duct ectasia or hyperprolactinemia predisposes to formation of multiple papillary lesions.

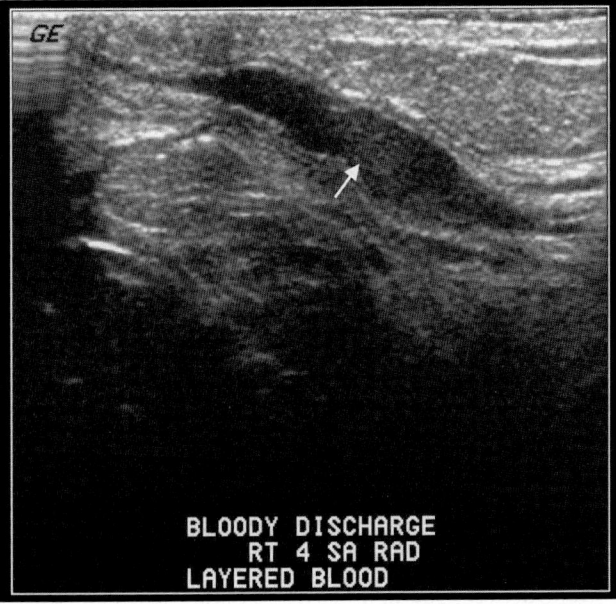

FIGURE 8–54 This patient presented with frankly bloody nipple discharge. The offending ectatic duct is acutely inflamed, as evidenced by isoechoic thickening of the wall. Adherent and layered echogenic clot simulates the presence of an intraductal papillary lesion, a potential cause of false-positive diagnosis. However, an underlying intraductal papillary lesion could also be obscured by the echogenic clot. Thus, echogenic clot within a bleeding duct can be a cause of both false-positive and false-negative diagnoses.

tifiable. Sometimes, ductal ectasia can be so severe that there are multiple layers of grossly distended tortuous ducts in the immediate subareolar location. The "tangle" of subareolar ducts in such patients is difficult to follow and evaluate, making it more difficult to identify deeper, smaller papillary lesions, especially if there is very commonly occurring echogenic debris within the duct lumen (Figs. 8–22, 8–34, 8–35, 8–42, 8–43, 8–49, and 8–54). The tortuosity of the ducts and associated intraductal and periductal fibrous reaction that occurs in these patients also makes the occurrence of both false-positives and false-negative findings more likely.

GALACTOGRAPHY VERSUS SONOGRAPHY FOR DIAGNOSIS AND LOCALIZATION

In a setting where ultrasound-guided DVAP is unavailable or cannot be performed, sonography may be necessary for preoperative localization in place of standard galactography under several different circumstances. First, localization galactography can be technically impossible the day of surgery because nipple discharge has spontaneously stopped, because the duct cannot be cannulated, or because the IPL does not cause discharge. Localization with sonographic guidance by percutaneous blue dye injection or needle lo-

calization of the papillary lesion itself may be performed (Fig. 8–55). When the duct is small, a 25-gauge 1.25-inch needle is used, and the duct is punctured using a subareolar needle course parallel to the duct to facilitate threading of the needle down the duct lumen and subsequent injection of blue dye into the duct (Fig. 8–56). When the affected duct is more severely dilated or the dilated segment is more peripherally located, radial approaches from peripheral to central may be used (Fig. 8–57). In patients who do not have nipple discharge but who do have a sonographically demonstrated ectatic duct with a suspected IPL, ultrasound-guided percutaneous galactography can be performed for either diagnosis (Fig. 8–58) or preoperative localization (Figs. 8–59).

Sonographic guidance for percutaneous galactography can be used when galactographic duct cannulation is not possible, regardless of the reason. As with standard localization galactography, 60% iodinated contrast is used for diagnostic studies, and a mixture of one-half 60% contrast and one-half methylene blue dye is used for localizing studies. When the duct is severely dilated, we usually aspirate about half of the duct fluid before injecting contrast or blue dye in order to minimize the chances of extravasation as well as to diminish patient discomfort. Because the sonogram alone is diagnostic in most cases, and because ultrasound-guided DVAB is now the definitive diagnostic procedure of choice,

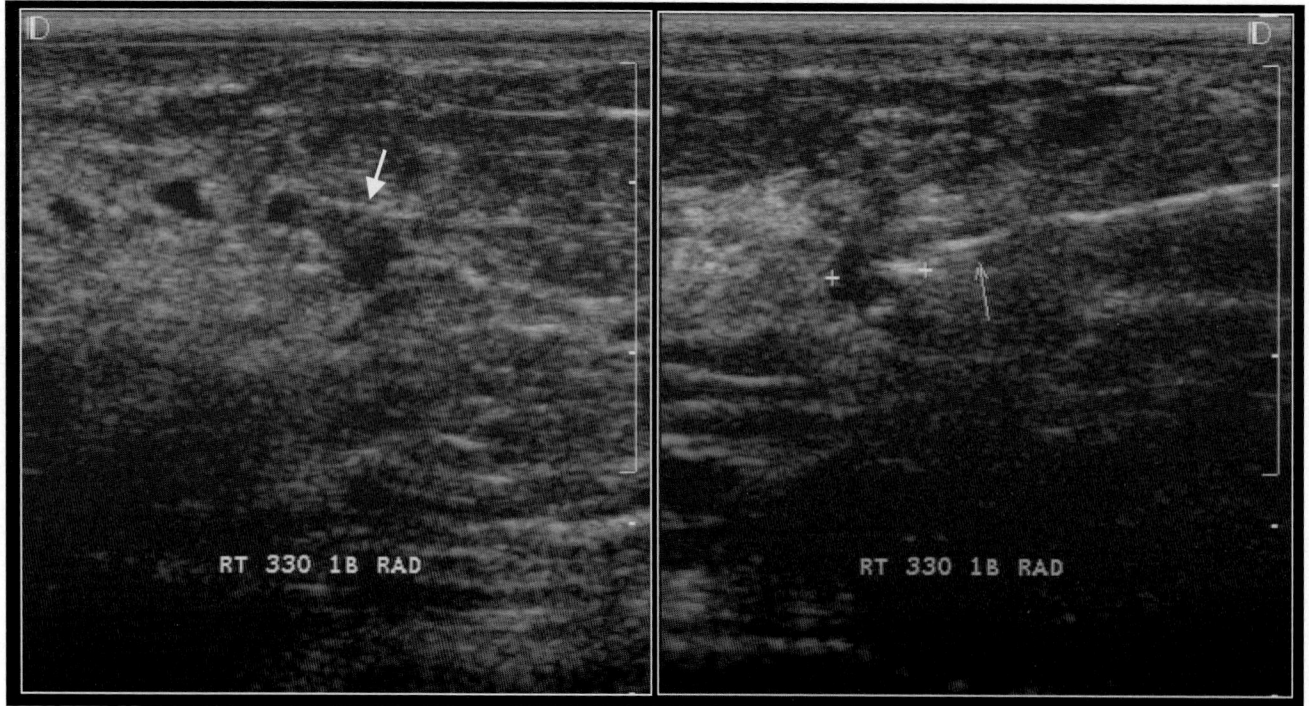

FIGURE 8–55 This small intraductal papillary lesion (*arrow,* **left**) lay within a mildly dilated peripheral duct. The dilation did not extend to the nipple, and the patient did not have nipple discharge; thus, standard galactographic localization for surgical excision could not be performed. Instead, ultrasound-guided needle localization was performed. Histology indicated benign large duct papilloma.

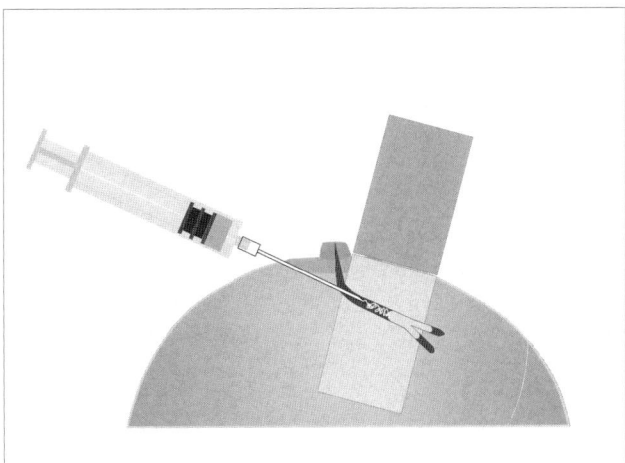

FIGURE 8–56 In patients who have an apparent intraductal papillary lesion demonstrated sonographically, but in whom cannulation of the duct orifice fails or in whom there is no expressible discharge, percutaneous galactography can be performed. For small ducts, a central subareolar approach with a 27-gauge needle is preferred. For more severely ectatic ducts, the peripheral approach shown for needle localization in Fig. 8–57 is preferred.

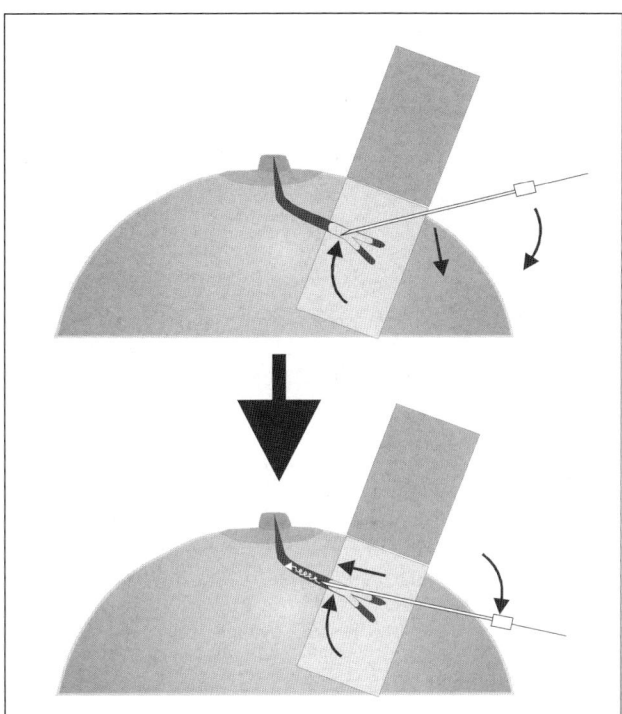

FIGURE 8–57 When there is no discharge or when cannulation of the duct orifice fails, and when the size of the ectatic duct is larger, a peripheral approach for injection of contrast and blue dye and needle localization can be used under real-time guidance. When the tip of the needle penetrates the duct wall and enters the lumen of the duct, the hub of the needle can be depressed and the needle threaded slightly toward the nipple within the duct lumen, similar to the method used for venipuncture. Once the tip of the needle is advanced a few millimeters central to the puncture site, a mixture of blue dye and iodinated contrast can be injected and the needle passed farther centrally within the duct lumen.

we have not used ultrasound-guided percutaneous galactography as much for diagnosis as we did in the past.

In cases in which the diagnostic galactogram demonstrates a small peripheral papillary lesion in an extensive ductal system, the surgeon may have difficulty removing the lesion without extensively resecting the entire blue-stained ductal system if only galactographic blue dye localization is used. Combined galactographic blue dye

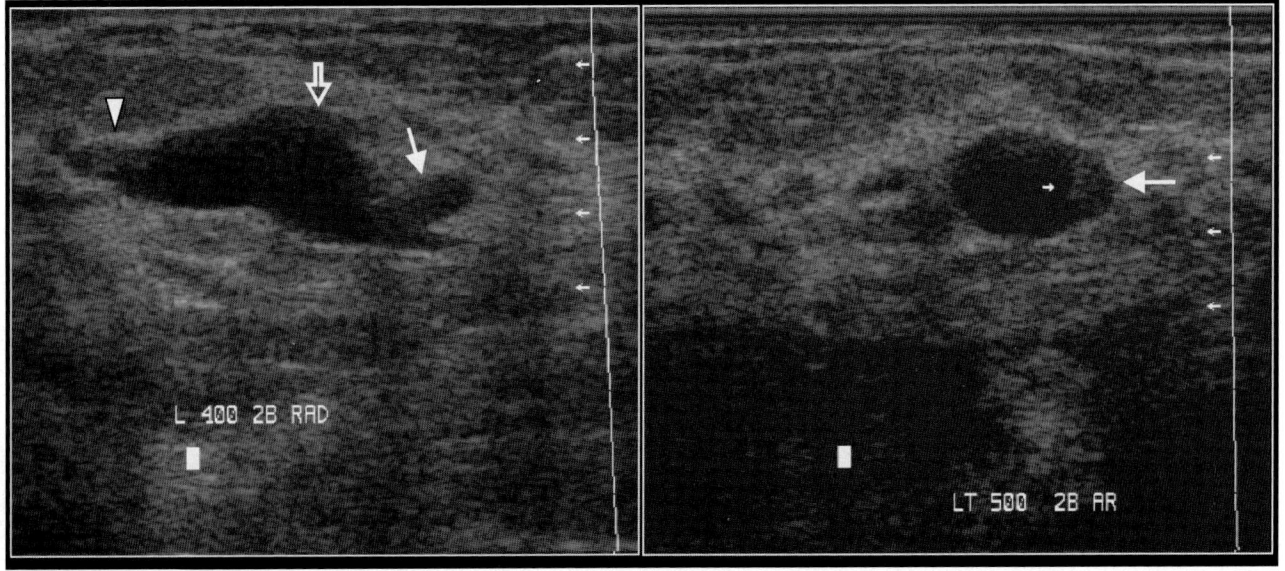

A

FIGURE 8–58 **A, left:** Long-axis view of an ectatic duct in a patient who presented with a mammographic asymmetric density but with no nipple discharge shows an obstructing intraductal papillary lesion centrally *(arrowhead)*, a subtle papillary lesion anteriorly *(hollow arrow)*, and a third papillary lesion in a branch duct *(arrow)*. **A, right:** Short-axis view in the same patient shows a fourth intraductal papillary lesion on the right lateral wall *(large arrow)* of the ectatic duct. *(Continued.)*

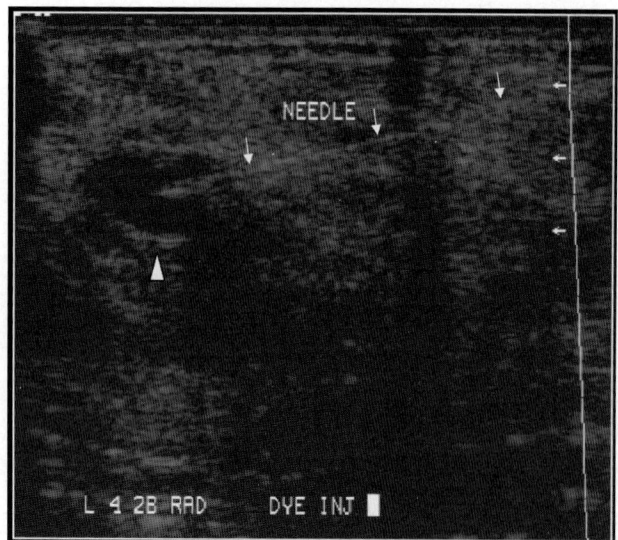

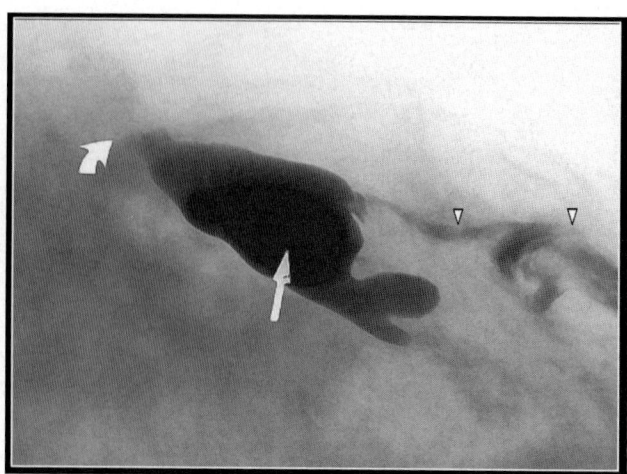

B

C

FIGURE 8–58 *(continued)* **B:** Because the patient did not have nipple discharge, standard galactography was not possible. Because the vacuum-assisted large core biopsy device had not yet been invented, percutaneous galactography was performed. The needle *(arrows)* was placed into the duct lumen *(arrowhead)* using a peripheral approach because of the large caliber of the lumen. **C:** The galactogram performed percutaneously shows the obstructing central papilloma well *(curved arrow)* but does not show the other three lesions *(large straight arrow)* as well as sonography because the diameter of the duct lumen and density of contrast obscure them. A small amount of contrast has leaked out along the needle tract *(arrowheads).*

injection of the duct system and sonographic direct needle localization of the papillary lesion may help the surgeon remove the lesion without having to resect the entire lobe.

Ultrasound-guided large core needle biopsy can be performed for confirmation of the suspected presence of a benign LDP when the lesion is an isolated nodule or when the papillary lesion lies within a duct that is not dilated to the nipple and is not causing a nipple discharge. This approach can be justified because the risk for malignant degeneration within histologically proven benign, central LDPs is very low. Liberman and associates have documented the accuracy of imaging-guided core needle

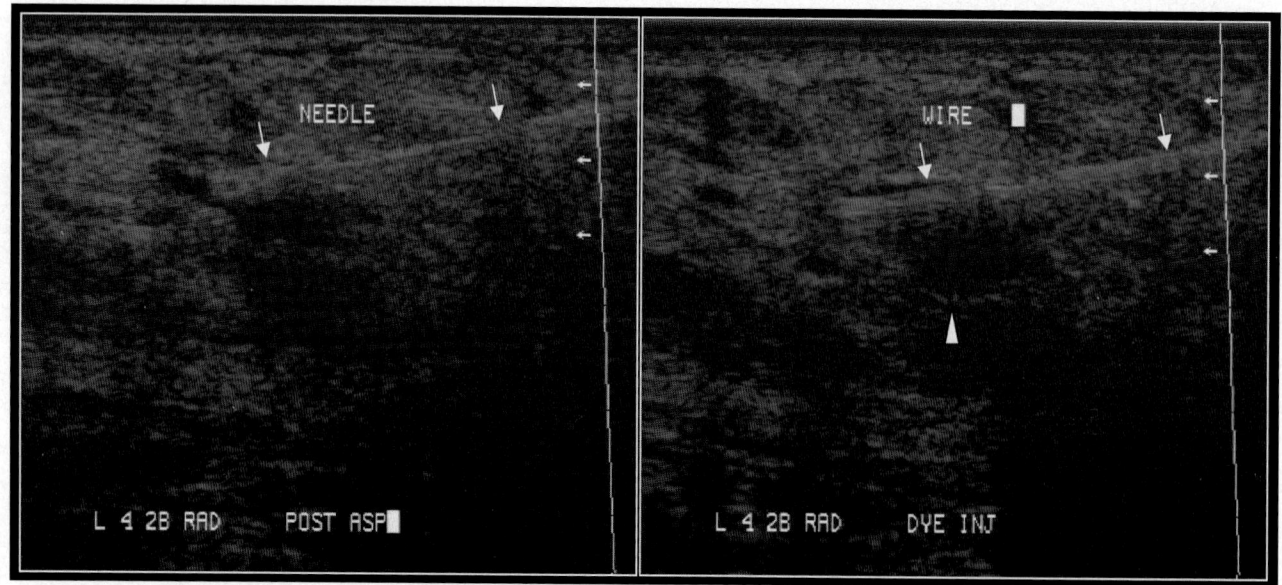

A

FIGURE 8–59 A, left: The day of surgery, a repeat percutaneous galactogram with injection of blue dye and iodinated contrast was performed *(arrows* indicate needle). **A, right:** Immediately after injection of the duct, a hookwire *(arrows)* was threaded through the injection needle and into the duct lumen. The needle was then removed, the wire was left in place, and the patient was moved to a mammography machine for confirmation *(arrowhead* indicates injected duct).

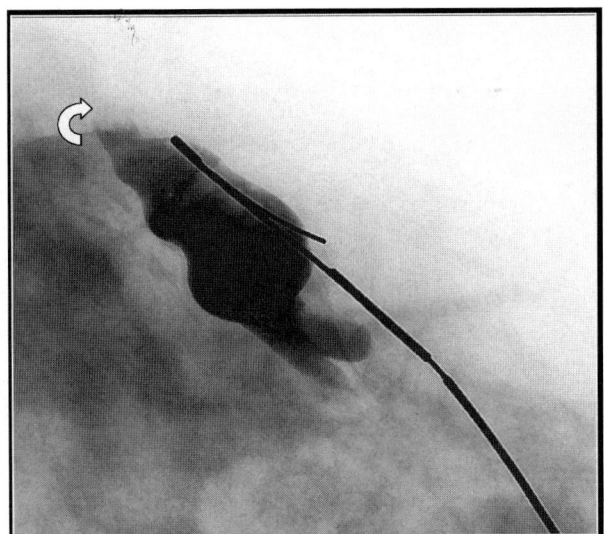

B

FIGURE 8–59 *(continued)* **B:** The confirming galactographic wire placement mammogram showed the localizing wire threaded centrally into the contrast-filled duct. The obstructing intraductal papillary lesion *(curved arrow)* was once again well demonstrated, but the additional papillary lesions were not. Histology indicated multiple benign intraductal papillomas.

FIGURE 8–60 Galactographic injection can be monitored by ultrasound. As contrast or blue dye is injected through the small galactographic needle, and sonographically visible echogenic microbubbles swirl within the duct that is being injected. This can be done if the mammography equipment is not operable, but preoperative localization is requested for surgical excision. However, we now more frequently monitor the galactographic injection to identify the duct of interest immediately before performing ultrasound-guided mammotomy (vacuum-assisted biopsy).

biopsy of IPLs. However, core needle biopsy is now seldom used in patients with nipple discharge because it generally does not stop the discharge. Such patients usually require and prefer excisional biopsy or ultrasound-guided mammotomy, which is more likely to stop the discharge.

Ultrasound can be used to guide galactography even when cannulation of the nipple is successful (Figs. 8–60 and 8–61). This technique is primarily of use in the operating room, immediately before surgery, but it can also be used to avoid postponing surgery when the mammography

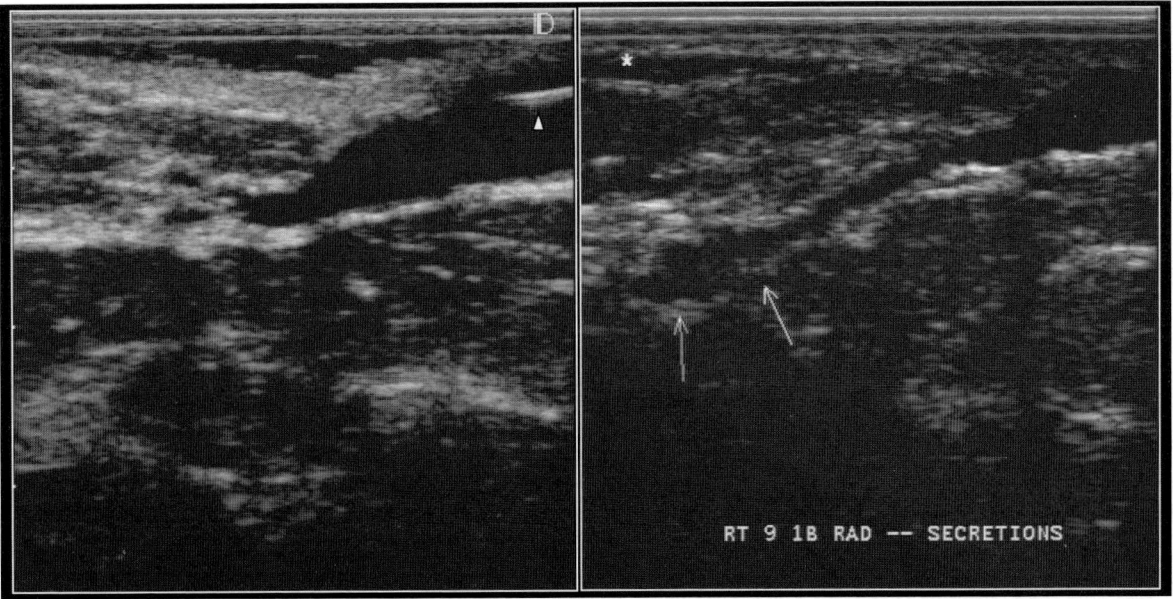

FIGURE 8–61 Left: After the needle is threaded into the discharging duct orifice, it is tilted to the side in order to increase its specular reflection *(arrowhead)*, and two-handed compression or rolled-nipple maneuver is performed to enable scanning of the nipple from its side. **Right:** During the injection of contrast and blue dye, the echogenic microbubbles swirl from central to peripheral within the duct lumen until they encompass the more peripherally located expansile intraductal papillary lesion *(arrows)*.

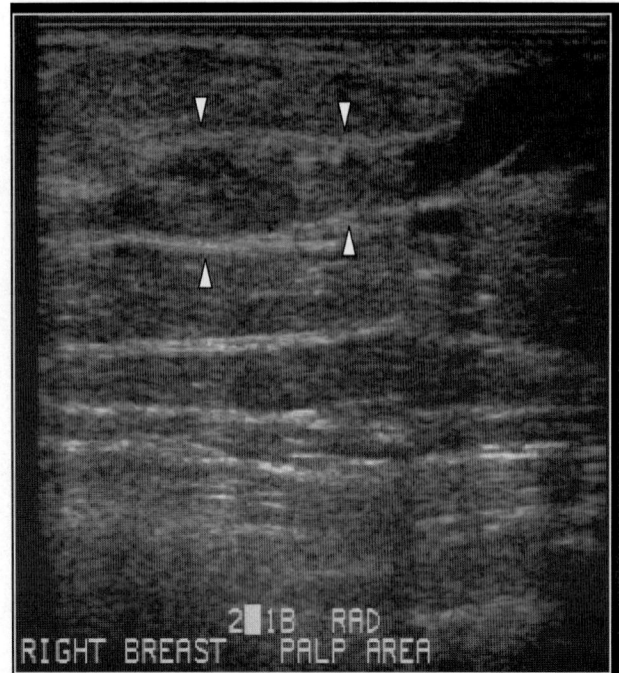

A

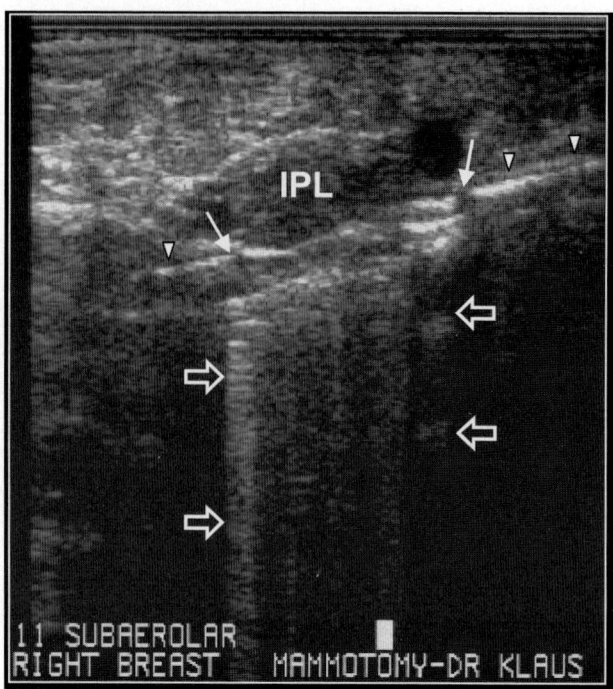

B

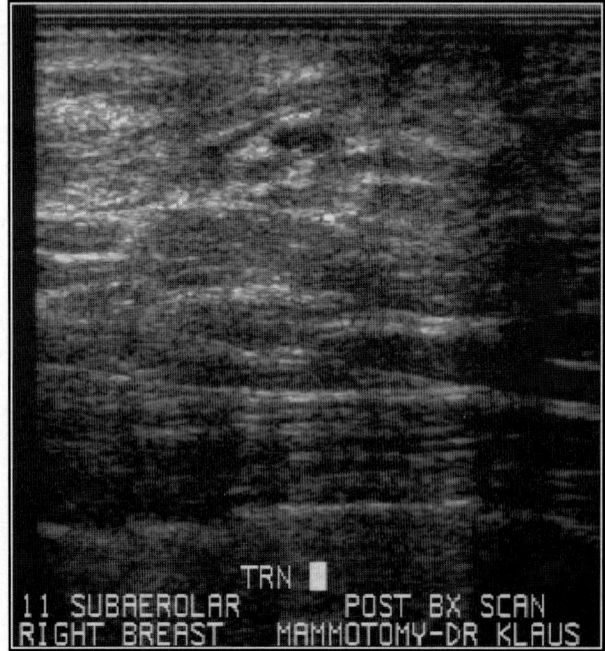

C

FIGURE 8–62 A: This patient, who presented with nipple discharge, had a large intraductal papillary lesion *(arrowheads)* well shown on the long-axis sonographic view of the offending duct. As in most current cases such as this one, ultrasound-guided mammotomy was the procedure of choice for obtaining histologic diagnosis. **B:** The mammotomy probe *(arrowheads)* is shown in long axis deep to the intraductal papillary lesion *(IPL)*. The precise location of the aperture *(arrows)* of the vacuum needle is readily apparent immediately deep to the lesion because of the ring-down artifacts *(hollow arrows)* that arise from the vacuum holes. **C:** Immediately after ultrasound-guided mammotomy, there is no residual intraductal papillary lesion. A localizing clip, as always, was deployed in case the histology was malignant and in case subsequent surgical excision was necessary. Histology, however, revealed benign large duct papilloma. Nipple discharge stopped immediately after the mammotomy, as it does in 90% of cases, and has not recurred in 2 years. Follow-up sonography over 2 years has also shown no recurrent lesion.

equipment is nonfunctional. We leave the needle in after we perform a galactogram to facilitate identification of the offending duct with ultrasound before performing ultrasound-guided DVAB far more frequently than for preoperative localization.

Finally, ultrasound-guided 11-gauge DVAB has become our favorite method of biopsy for sonographically or galactographically demonstrated IPLs (Fig. 8–62). In fact, in series of 75 cases of IPLs detected by galactography, ul-

trasound, or both, the lesion was found sonographically, and a definitive histologic diagnosis was made in all patients who underwent ultrasound-guided mammotomy. An unexpected benefit of the diagnostic mammotomy was cessation of the nipple discharge in 90% of the patients. At this point, it is still unclear whether the discharge stopped because of complete removal of the lesion, interruption of the communication of the affected duct with the nipple, or disruption of the fibrovascular core.

Regardless of whether the lesion is first shown by sonography or galactography, ultrasound guidance for biopsy can be provided in most cases. If the diagnosis is made sonographically, the patient proceeds straight to ultrasound-guided mammotomy. If the ultrasound does not show a definitive cause for nipple discharge, galactography is performed. The galactogram needle is left in position after injection of contrast during the mammographic filming. If there is an IPL shown by mammography that was initially missed sonographically, the patient is reexamined sonographically during reinjection of the duct. The microbubbles and swirling fluid of the injection are visible sonographically and reveal the duct of interest. The added distention of the duct created by the injection of additional contrast usually makes the intraductal lesion more readily apparent than it was before galactography. In the rare case in which sonography fails to show the lesion even after galactography, the biopsy can be performed under digital stereotactic guidance while contrast is still filling the ducts. Stereotactically guided DVAB using galactographic guidance is technically more difficult than using sonographic guidance, so that sonographic guidance is strongly favored whenever possible.

Under ultrasound guidance, all sonographic evidence of the lesion can be removed in a large percentage of cases when the maximum diameter of the IPL is 12 mm or less. However, even in cases in which the lesion is 13 mm or larger and sonography shows evidence of residual lesion after mammotomy, there is a high likelihood that definitive diagnosis of benign papilloma will be made and that nipple discharge will cease after completion of the procedure in a significant percentage of cases. In addition, of course, in a certain percentage of cases, the biopsy will reveal atypical hyperplasia or malignancy, and surgical excision of the area will be necessary for definitive treatment. Preoperative localization of the area in which the DVAB was performed will be necessary. Because all sonographic evidence of the lesion is removed in a large percentage of patients, the area will be difficult to relocalize later for excisional biopsy unless a metallic marker is deployed at the time of DVAB, which should be done in all cases.

BIRADS CHARACTERIZATION OF INTRADUCTAL PAPILLARY LESIONS

Until very recently, we have characterized all IPLs as BIRADS 4a, mildly suspicious, and recommended biopsy of all because of literature and our own findings suggesting a 13% risk for either atypia or malignancy within such lesions. However, our most recent study of ultrasound-guided DVAB has shown that 74 of 75 lesions were benign (less than a 2% risk for malignancy), potentially qualifying such lesions for BIRADS 3 classification. These findings are discrepant with our earlier findings. The reason for the

discrepancy is that the DVAB population of IPLs is a subset of the earlier population—a subset that is smaller and earlier in development.

Because the potentially BIRADS 3 population of IPLs is a subset of the entire IPL population, we have developed an algorithmic approach to characterizing them based on information available in the literature and our own data. The following IPL characteristics should be considered mildly suspicious, should result in BIRADS 4a characterization, and should indicate the need for biopsy:

- IPLs longer than 12 mm (Fig. 8–63) or involving branch ducts (Fig. 8–64) are more likely to be too long to be completely removed by the 11-gauge DVAB and therefore will be prone to sampling errors. Furthermore, extensive linear growth along the long axis of the ductal system suggests that the lesion is aggressive and more likely to be atypical or malignant.
- IPLs that focally expand the ectatic duct within which they lie also suggest that the lesion is more aggressive and more likely to be atypical or malignant (Fig. 8–65).
- IPLs that involve TDLUs should be considered to be of peripheral origin, regardless of the distance of the TDLUs from the nipple (Figs. 8–66 and 8–67). The literature strongly suggests a higher risk for malignancy in PPs.

Only IPLs that are ovoid, are 12 mm or less in length, involve only the central ducts or lactiferous sinuses, do not involve branch ducts or TDLUs, and do not expand the ducts may be characterized as BIRADS 3 (Fig. 8–68).

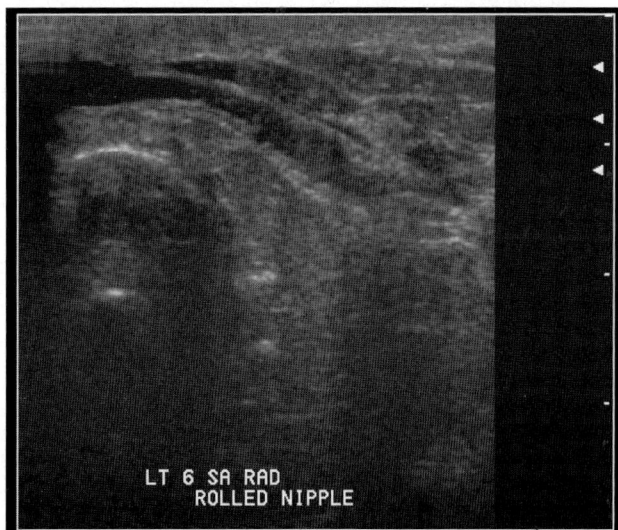

FIGURE 8–63 Intraductal papillary lesions longer than 12 mm are generally too long to be removed completely by ultrasound-guided 11-gauge directional vacuum-assisted biopsy and thus are prone to sampling errors. Such growth along the long axis of the duct also suggests that the lesion is more aggressive. Both of these factors are mildly suspicious and require BIRADS 4a characterization and biopsy.

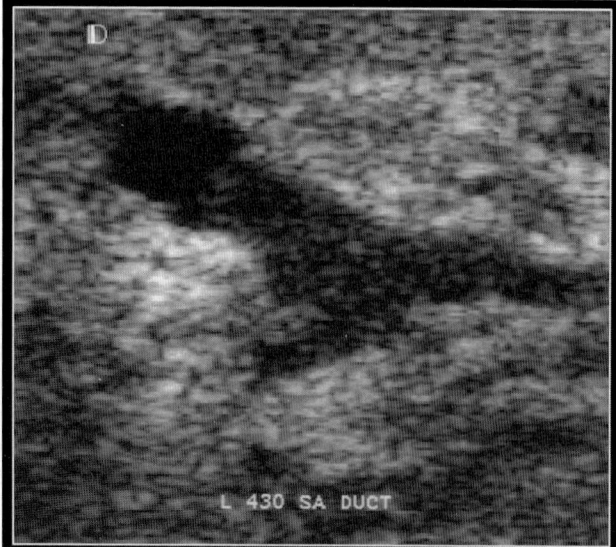

FIGURE 8–64 Intraductal papillary lesions (IPLs) that involve branch ducts tend to be more peripherally located and are more likely to have components that are difficult to remove completely using ultrasound-guided 11-gauge directional vacuum-assisted biopsy. Extension into branch ducts also suggests aggressive growth. Extension of IPLs into branch ducts should be considered mildly suspicious and demands a BIRADS 4a characterization and biopsy.

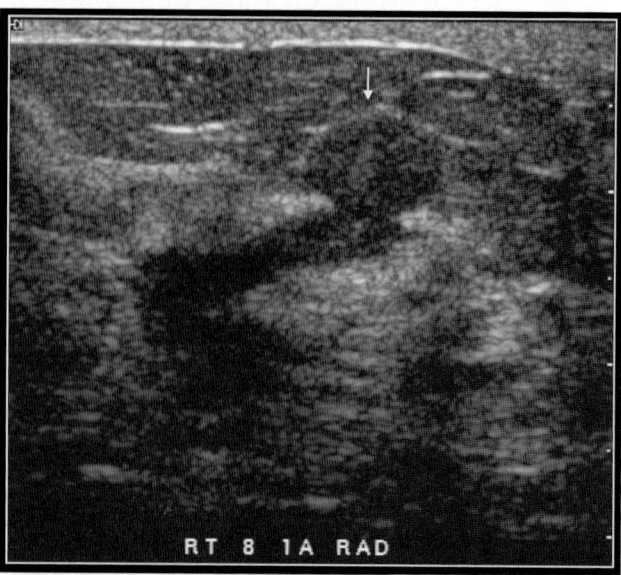

FIGURE 8–66 Peripheral papillary lesions arise from terminal ductolobular units (TDLUs), not from the subareolar duct lumina. This papillary lesion arose in a TDLU far from the nipple *(arrow)*. The literature strongly suggests that peripheral papillomas are at greater risk for malignant degeneration than are central lesions. Thus, peripheral papillomas should be considered mildly suspicious, should be characterized as BIRADS 4a, and should undergo biopsy.

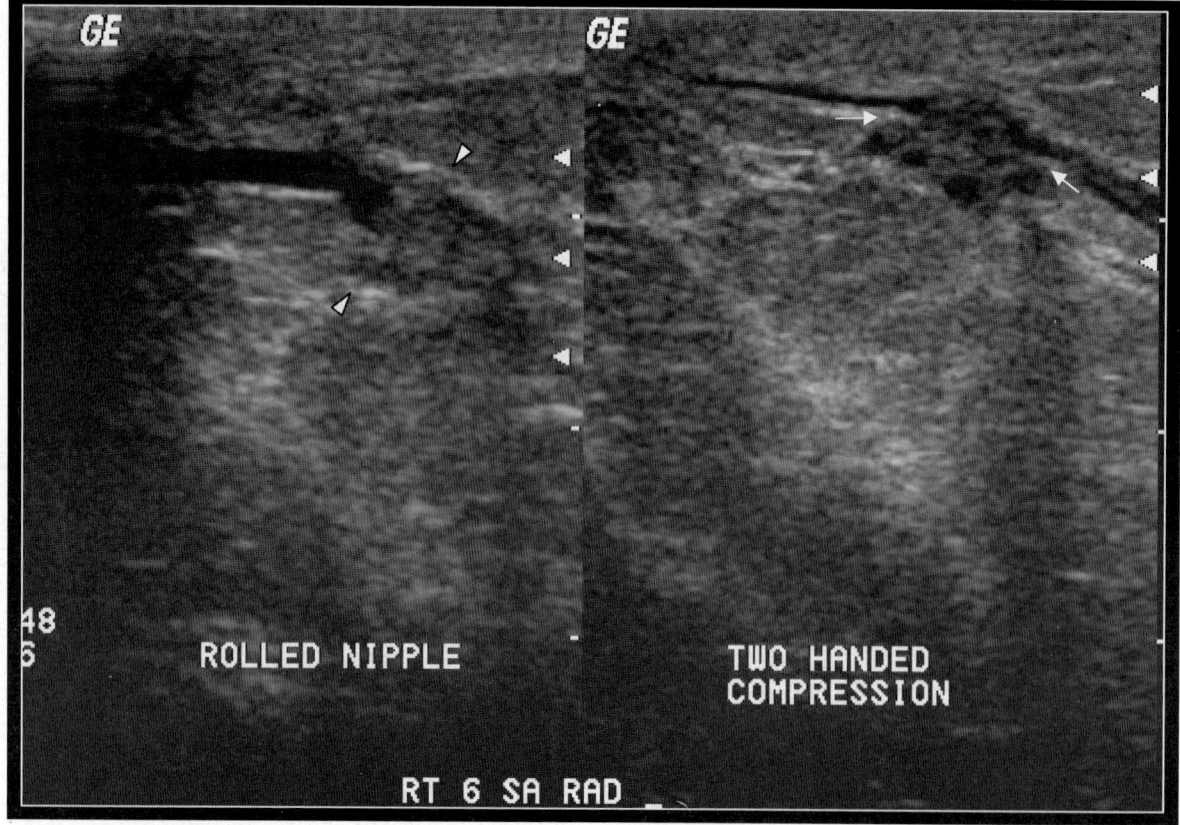

FIGURE 8–65 Focal expansion of the duct by an intraductal papillary lesion (IPL; *arrowheads,* **left**) suggests very aggressive growth, should be considered mildly suspicious, warrants BIRADS 4a characterization, and indicates the need for biopsy. Note that the expansile nature of this IPL is more apparent with compression **(right)**. With compression, it is evident that the lesion has eroded through the deep wall of the duct into the periductal tissues *(arrows)*.

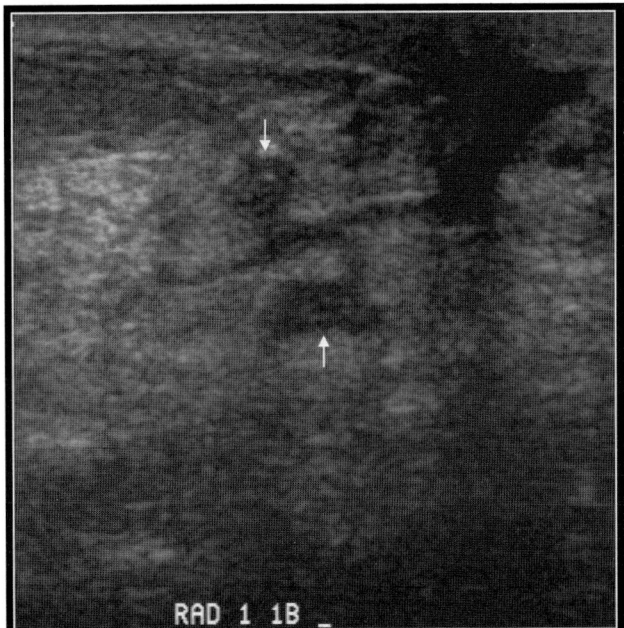

FIGURE 8–67 These discharge-producing lesions *(arrows)* should be considered peripheral papillary lesions not because they lie far from the nipple *(N)* but because they arise from terminal ductolobular units (TDLUs), not the periareolar main lobar duct. Although most TDLUs arise from peripheral branch ducts, a few, such as these, arise from the main lobar ducts. The literature strongly suggests a higher malignant potential for peripheral papillomas. Such lesions are also more likely to be multiple. Thus, lesions originating within TDLUs should be considered mildly suspicious (BIRADS 4a) and should undergo biopsy.

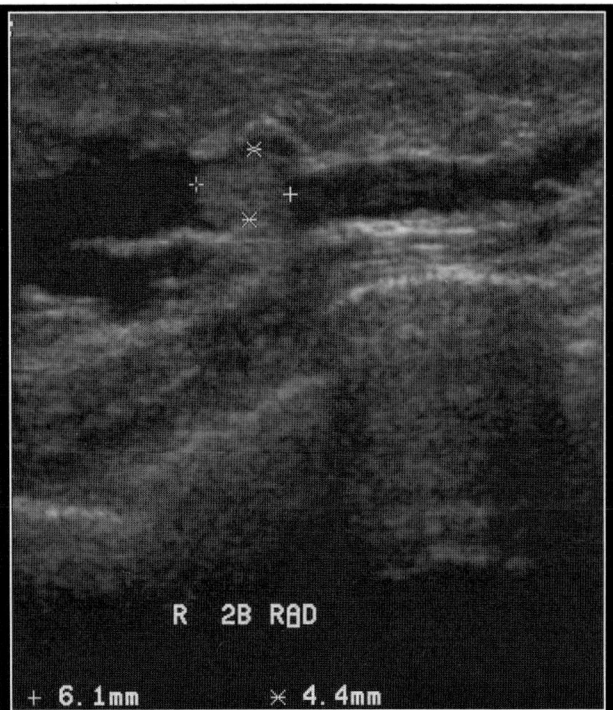

FIGURE 8–68 The subset of intraductal papillary lesions that have less than a 2% chance of being malignant and thus qualify for BIRADS 3 characterization includes small, short (less than 12 mm long), nonexpansile, round or oval lesions that lie within the subareolar and periareolar main lobar ducts and do not involve branch ducts or terminal ductolobular units.

As a practical matter, whether a lesion is characterized as BIRADS 3 or 4a is of little concern to a patient who presents with a chief complaint of nipple discharge. Such patients usually demand biopsy and removal of the offending lesion in order to stop the discharge. Only in asymptomatic patients will characterization of an IPL as BIRADS 3 have an effect on management.

SUMMARY

Although galactography has traditionally been the procedure of choice for evaluating the patient with suspicious secretions, the role of ultrasound is growing and evolving rapidly. Ultrasound can be used to demonstrate IPLs in patients in whom galactography is not possible because there is no nipple discharge and secretions are not expressible; duct cannulation fails; duct cannulation succeeds, but contrast extravasates; or the patient refuses galactography. Ultrasound can be used for both primary diagnosis of an IPL and for either preoperative localization for excisional biopsy or ultrasound-guided mammotomy. Ultrasound can be used to guide percutaneous galactography using iodinated contrast for diagnosis and a mixture of iodinated

contrast and blue dye for localization. Ultrasound-guided galactography can be performed in patients in whom IPLs are suspected but who have no expressible secretions.

Ultrasound can also be used to guide core needle biopsy of papillary lesions in patients who have no nipple discharge. However, core needle biopsy is usually insufficient in the patient who presents with a chief complaint of nipple discharge because, despite obtaining a definitive diagnosis, core biopsy will not stop the discharge. Our current preference after demonstrating an IPL has been to proceed straight to ultrasound-guided mammotomy. Mammotomy achieves a definitive diagnosis in most patients, removes the lesion completely in a slightly smaller percentage, and stops nipple discharge in about 90% of cases. A marker should always be deployed after ultrasound-guided DVAB of IPLs.

Ultrasound can occasionally demonstrate definitive causes of nipple discharge other than IPLs, including invasive malignancy, communicating cysts, and duct ectasia. However, unless findings are definitive, galactography is performed after sonography.

Caution should be used in characterizing IPLs into BIRADS categories. About 13% of IPLs are histologically atypical or malignant. However, a subset of smaller and earlier IPLs that meet criteria for BIRADS 3 (2% or less risk for malignancy) can be identified sonographically. Such lesions should be oval, short (12 mm or less), and nonexpansile and should neither involve branch ducts nor arise from TDLUs. Length greater 12 mm, involvement of branch ducts, focal expansion of ducts, or involvement of TDLUs excludes an IPL from BIRADS 3 characterization. The presence of any one of these findings is mildly suspicious, requires a BIRADS 4 characterization, and warrants biopsy.

SUGGESTED READINGS

Adler DD. Ultrasound of benign breast conditions. *Semin Ultrasound CT MR* 1989;10(2):106–118.

Cardenosa G, Doudna C, Eklund GW. Ductography of the breast: technique and findings. *AJR Am J Roentgenol* 1994;162(5): 1081–1087.

Carty NJ, et al. Prospective study of outcome in women presenting with nipple discharge. *Ann R Coll Surg Engl* 1994;76(6): 387–389.

Cilotti A, et al. Solitary intraductal papilloma of the breast: an echographic study of 12 cases. *Radiol Med* (Torino) 1991;82(5): 617–620.

Cilotti A, et al. The diagnostic imaging of complex breast nodules. *Radiol Med* (Torino) 1992;84(3):198–203.

Dennis MA, Parker S, Kaske TI, et al. Incidental treatment of nipple discharge caused by benign intraductal papilloma through diagnostic mammotome biopsy. *AJR Am J Roentgenol* 2000;174: 1263–1268.

Devitt JE. Management of nipple discharge by clinical findings. *Am J Surg* 1985;149(6):789–792.

Dunn JM, et al. Exfoliative cytology in the diagnosis of breast disease. *Br J Surg* 1995;82(6):789–791.

Estabrook A, et al. Mammographic features of intracystic papillary lesions. *Surg Gynecol Obstet* 1990;170:113–116.

Fajardo LL, Jackson VP, Hunter TB. Interventional procedures in diseases of the breast: needle biopsy, pneumocystography, and galactography. *AJR Am J Roentgenol* 1992;158(6):1231–1238.

Forest AM, Bremond A, Rochet Y. Cancer and nipple discharge. *J Gynecol Obstet Biol Reprod* (Paris) 1988;17(1):19–24.

Fung A, et al. Preoperative cytology and mammography in patients with single-duct nipple discharge treated by surgery. *Br J Surg* 1990;77(11):1211–1212.

Greenberg ML, Middleton PD, Bilous AM. Infarcted intraduct papilloma diagnosed by fine-needle biopsy: a cytologic, clinical, and mammographic pitfall. *Diagn Cytopathol* 1994;11(2):188–194.

Hirschman SA, et al. Intraductal carcinoma in a male breast: diagnosis by nipple discharge cytology. *Diagn Cytopathol* 1995;12(4): 354–356.

Johnson TL, Kini SR. Cytologic and clinicopathologic features of abnormal nipple secretions: 225 cases. *Diagn Cytopathol* 1991;7(1): 17–22.

Knight DC, et al. Aspiration of the breast and nipple discharge cytology. *Surg Gynecol Obstet* 1986;163(5):415–420.

Leveque J, et al. Nipple discharge without palpable tumor: apropos of 46 cases. *Rev Fr Gynecol Obstet* 1990;85(5):329–335.

Maluf HM, et al. Spindle-cell argyrophilic mucin-producing carcinoma of the breast: histological, ultrastructural, and immunohistochemical studies of two cases. *Am J Surg Pathol* 1991;15(7): 677–686.

Martorano MD, et al. Intracystic papilloma in male breast: ultrasonography and pneumocystography diagnosis. *J Clin Ultrasound* 1993;21:38–40.

Matricardi L, Lovati R. Ultrasonic appearance of a case of mammary duct ectasia. *J Clin Ultrasound* 1991;19(9):568–570.

Mendelson EB, Tobin CE. Critical pathways in using breast US. *Radiographics* 1995;15:935–945.

Mezi S, et al. The role of echography in the determination and monitoring of ductal ectasia in nipple discharge. *G Chir* 1993;14(7): 370–376.

Mori T, et al. Evaluation of an improved dot-immunobinding assay for carcinoembryonic antigen determination in nipple discharge in early breast cancer: results of a multicenter study. *Jpn J Clin Oncol* 1992;22(6):371–376.

Nishida M, et al. Usefulness of galactography for minimal noninvasive ductal carcinoma of the breast. *Nippon Geka Hokan* 1989; 58(2):250–256.

Paterok EM, Rosenthal H, Sabel M. Nipple discharge and abnormal galactogram: results of a long-term study (1964–1990). *Eur J Obstet Gynecol Reprod Biol* 1993;50(3):227–234.

Peters F, Schuth W. Hyperprolactinemia and nonpuerperal mastitis (duct ectasia). *JAMA* 1989;261(11):1618–1620.

Pignatelli V, et al. Galactographic features of the secreting breast. *Radiol Med* (Torino) 1989;77(6):643–649.

Ranieri E, et al. Male breast carcinoma in situ: report of a case diagnosed by nipple discharge cytology alone. *Anticancer Res* 1995; 15(4):1589–1592.

Rissanen T, et al. Ultrasound-guided percutaneous galactography. *J Clin Ultrasound* 1993;21(8):497–502.

Rubin E, et al. Hand-held real-time breast sonography. *AJR Am J Roentgenol* 1985;144(3):623–627.

Schild R, Fendel H. Doppler ultrasound differentiation of benign and malignant breast tumors. *Geburtshilfe Frauenheilkd* 1991; 51(12):969–972.

Schneider JA. Invasive papillary breast carcinoma: mammographic and sonographic appearance. *Radiology* 1989;171:377–379.

Sessa M, Cerroni L, Bertolotti A. Proliferative pathology of the mammary ducts: diagnostic value of ductogalactography and cytologic correlations. *Radiol Med* (Torino) 1991;81(5):597–600.

Srivastava A, et al. A safe technique of major mammary duct excision. *J R Coll Surg Edinb* 1995;40(1):35–37.

Tabar L, Dean P, Pentek Z. Galactography, the diagnostic procedure of choice for nipple discharge. *Radiology* 1983;149:31–38.

Van Steen A, Van Ongeval C, Veekmans P. Galactography. *J Belge Radiol* 1995;78(1):39–44.

Weiss H, et al. Sonographic detection of intracystic breast tumors. *Ultraschall Med* 1985;6(4):233–236.

Woods ER, et al. Solitary breast papilloma: comparison of mammographic, galactographic, and pathologic findings. *AJR Am J Roentgenol* 1992;159(3):487–491.

Wunderlich M. Mild, moderate and severe dysplasia in exfoliative cytological studies of breast secretions in connection with use of oral contraceptives. *Zentralbl Gynakol* 1994;116(11):622–627.

NONTARGETED INDICATIONS: MAMMARY IMPLANTS*

Patients with mammary implants may undergo sono-graphic evaluation for two main reasons: (a) evaluation of breast tissue (palpable or mammographic abnormality); and (b) evaluation of implant complications.

Recent studies comparing sonography with magnetic resonance imaging (MRI), mammography, and clinical findings have found sonography to be superior to mammography for detection for implant rupture but less sensitive than MRI. Therefore, patients *who are evaluated solely for implant integrity* usually undergo MRI rather than sonography. However, patients with implants, like those without implants, have palpable and mammographic abnormalities for which targeted sonography is the procedure of choice. Palpable lumps and mammographic abnormalities are far more common in patients with implants than is implant rupture; therefore, despite the apparent superiority of MRI for implant rupture, far more patients with implants will undergo sonography than MRI. The sonographer and sonologist, therefore, must have a thorough understanding of normal and abnormal implant appearances.

Sonographic evaluation of the patient with implants might show that the palpable or mammographic abnormality is caused by an implant complication or by common breast pathology. An implant abnormality may be an incidental finding during the targeted diagnostic examination.

TYPES OF MAMMARY IMPLANTS

Breast augmentation has been performed for more than a century. Many different substances have been used to augment the breast, including fat from lipomas, paraffin,

polyvinyl alcohol sponges, and free silicone injections. All have been associated with unacceptably high complication rates. Complications have included inflammation, granuloma formation, necrosis, hardening and deformity of the breast, migration of the implanted materials, and even embolization and death. In the early 1960s, surgeons began using silicone gel implants. Although silicone gel implants caused fewer and less severe complications than previous materials, many of the same complications still occurred. To improve the cosmetic results of implantation and to reduce the percentage and severity of complications, many different variations of breast augmentation have been developed and employed. The implantation site also varies. Implants can be placed in either subglandular or retropectoral locations. Finally, implants can be placed from inframammary, periareolar, and axillary routes, and they can also be placed endoscopically through paraumbilical incisions.

It is estimated that there are more than 200 different types and variations of mammary implants. Listing hundreds of implant types is impractical, but it is necessary to recognize a few broad classes of implants. Thus, the sonographer or sonologist who evaluates patients with implants must have a basic understanding of the multiple different types of implants and implantation. These classes are listed in Table 9–1. One must understand the great variation in the normal sonographic appearances of the various types of implants (Fig. 9–1) before one can hope to identify sonographic abnormalities.

In the United States, it is not possible to perform breast ultrasound without having to evaluate patients routinely with mammary implants because the prevalence of implants is so high. It is estimated that more than 2.5 million women in the United States have mammary implants. About 80% of these were performed to augment breast size, whereas 20% were performed to reconstruct the breast after mastectomy.

---

*This chapter was coauthored by Cynthia L. Rapp, R.T., R.D.M.S.

TABLE 9–1. TYPES OF MAMMARY IMPLANTS

Single-lumen silicone gel implant
- Smooth or nontextured shell
  - No fluorsilicone in elastomer membrane
  - Fluorsilicone added to elastomer membrane
- Textured shell
  - Polyurethane textured implant

Single-lumen saline implant
- Smooth shell
- Textured shell

Single-lumen fat-containing implant (textured)
- Soybean oil
- Peanut oil
- Triglyceride

Double-lumen (bilumen) implant
- Inner silicone gel compartment with smooth shell
- Outer saline compartment with textured or smooth shell

Double-lumen Becker expanders
- Inner saline compartment with fill port
- Outer silicone compartment

Single-Lumen Smooth Silicone Gel Implants

Single-lumen silicone gel implants are the prototype implants. First used in 1962, in use for more than 40 years, these single-lumen implants are composed of an outer silicone elastomer membrane ("shell") and are filled with silicone gel. Through most of the 1960s and 1970s, single-lumen silicone gel implants had relatively thin, smooth elastomer membranes. Use of such single-lumen smooth membrane silicone implants was associated with a relatively high rate of complications—rupture and especially contracture due to severe encapsulation.

The silicone elastomer shell is permeable to the oily components of the heterogeneous silicone gel that it envelops. Thus, over time, microscopic amounts of silicone can pass through the intact elastomer membrane to the outside. This phenomenon is known as "gel bleed." Silicone that passes outside the shell incites a foreign-body reaction that is thought to be responsible for the formation

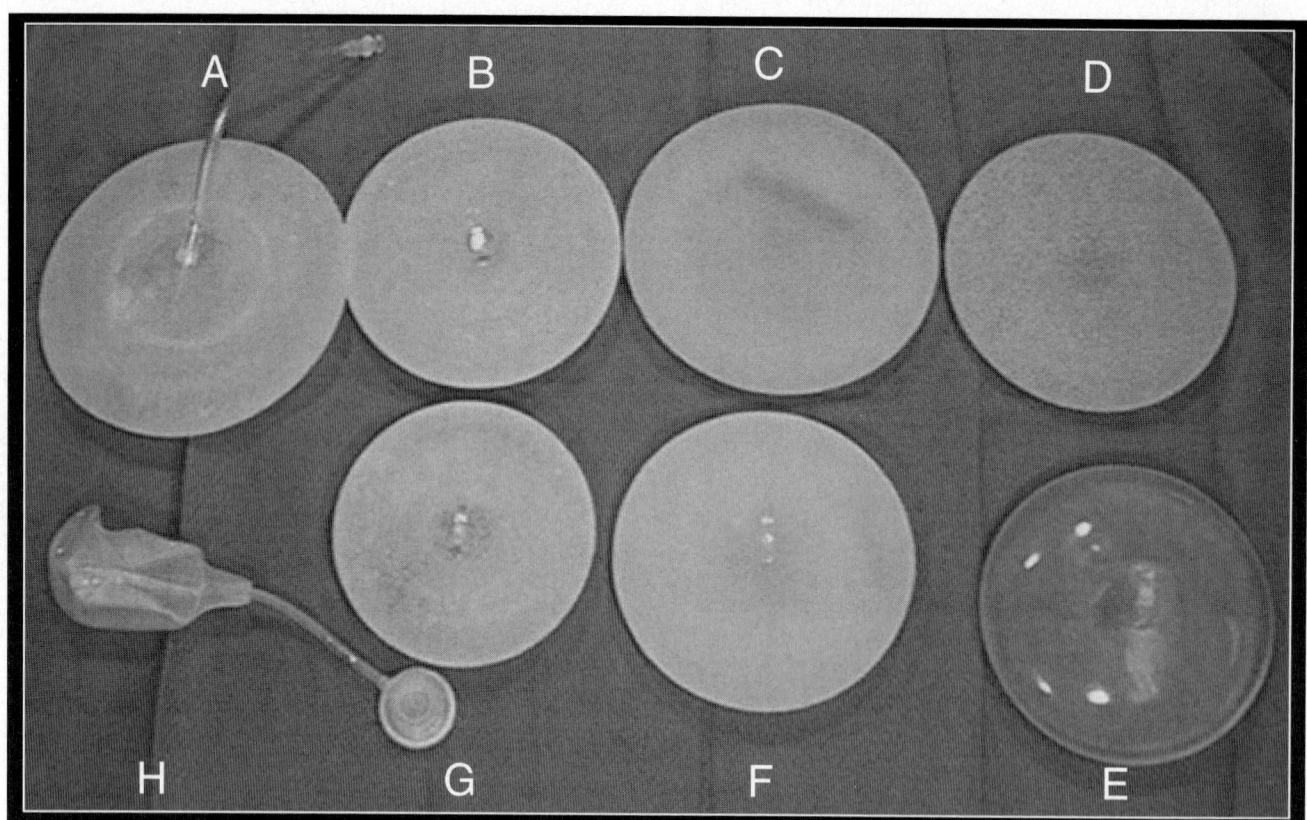

FIGURE 9–1 This figure demonstrates a small sample of the more than 200 types of different implants that have been used. **A:** A 400-mL, moderately textured single-lumen saline implant with needle inserted into diaphragm fill valve. **B:** A 300-mL, lightly textured single-lumen saline implant (with fill valve). **C:** A 400-mL, lightly textured single-lumen silicone gel implant. **D:** A 300-mL, heavily textured single-lumen silicone gel implant. **E:** A nontextured single-lumen saline implant. **F:** A 400-mL, lightly textured single-lumen saline implant. **G:** A 250-mL, moderately textured single-lumen saline implant. **H:** A collapsed double-lumen expander. Note that all of the saline implants and the expander have fill valves; the single-lumen silicone gel implants do not.

of a fibrous capsule that forms around the implant as a normal foreign-body reaction in all patients. The capsule is fibrous and is the body's response to the implant; thus, it must be distinguished from the shell, which is an elastomer membrane and part of the implant.

Although single-lumen, thin, smooth (nontextured) silicone gel implants were the predominant type of implant used during the 1960s and 1970s, they have been replaced by thicker and textured implants in recent years. However, single-lumen nontextured implants are still seen frequently today because the patients in whom they were placed 20 or so years ago are now within the mammographic screening cohort.

Addition of Fluorsilicone to the Elastomer Membrane

The addition of fluorsilicone to the elastomer membrane decreases its permeability to gel and is thought to help decrease problems with gel bleed and contracture. Fluorsilicone has routinely been used since the early 1980s.

Single-Lumen Textured Silicone Gel Implants

Textured silicone gel implants have shells whose outer surfaces have been roughened. Like nontextured single-lumen silicone gel implants, silicone gel fills the lumen. These implants have been found to incite less severe fibrous capsular reaction and therefore are less likely to cause capsular contracture. The random orientations of the fibers on the outer surface of the shell are thought to prevent the fibers within the capsule from developing parallel to each other, as they do in thickened, contracted capsules. Textured shells are also thicker than nontextured shells and, theoretically, more durable and less likely to rupture. Most single-lumen silicone gel implants placed since the early 1980s have had textured shells. Presently, textured single-lumen silicone gel implants can be used only in protocol studies, but textured single-lumen saline implants are still being widely used. Patients with textured implants placed in the early 1980s are now in the mammographic screening cohort; thus, textured implants are also frequently seen today.

Polyurethane Single-Lumen Textured Silicone Gel Implants

Polyurethane implants are textured single-lumen silicone gel implants to which a layer of polyurethane has been added on the outside surface. This polyurethane coating has been found to decrease capsule thickening and contracture even more effectively than does adding texture alone. Polyurethane also often stimulates the formation of an effusion around the implant, which is viewed as beneficial because it helps maintain space around the implant, pre-

venting contracture and thereby keeping the implant mobile, flexible, and less prone to traumatic rupture. The capsule around such effusions can undergo synovial metaplasia, essentially creating a bursa nearly identical to those around many joints. Unfortunately, fragments of polyurethane detach from the roughened surface of the shell and can be found within the periimplant effusion and also within the surrounding fibrous capsule. The sloughed polyurethane can degrade to 2,4-toluenediamine, which has been demonstrated to be carcinogenic in laboratory animals. Because of the potential risks, polyurethane implants were removed from the market in the early 1990s and are no longer used. However, many polyurethane implants placed in the 1980s are still in place and will be encountered in breast screening and diagnostic centers.

Other Materials Injected into Single-Lumen Implants

Over the years, all three types (nontextured, textured, and polyurethane coated) of single-lumen silicone gel implants have occasionally been injected with various materials by the surgeon at the time of implantation. Materials injected include saline, povidone-iodine (Betadine), antibiotics, and steroids. This practice continues for several reasons: (a) to improve the symmetry of the breasts, (b) to prevent infection, and (c) to decrease the thickness of the periimplant fibrous capsule and prevent contracture. The presence of pockets of such injected fluid within the silicone gel can create interpretive problems for both sonography and MRI.

Single-Lumen Saline Implants

Like single-lumen silicone gel implants, single-lumen saline implants have an outer silicone elastomer shell, but they are filled with saline rather than silicone gel. Single-lumen saline implants are the type most frequently implanted today in the United States. As has been the case for silicone gel implants, in recent years, most single-lumen saline implants have textured shells. Saline implants have the advantage over silicone gel implants of being implantable through smaller incisions because they can be placed while collapsed and inflated later. Thus, saline implants have fill valves that facilitate injections of saline to adjust implant size in order to achieve closer right-to-left symmetry. Saline implants are also less prone to capsular contracture than are silicone gel implants because they are not subject to the gel-bleed phenomenon that is thought to be responsible for capsular contracture. Finally, saline implants are less dense on mammograms and obscure less of the breast tissue than do silicone gel implants.

The disadvantages of single-lumen saline implants are that saline often gives a less optimal cosmetic result than does silicone gel and that saline implants are more prone to rupture with minor trauma. However, when saline implants do rupture, the saline is almost always rapidly resorbed and does not give rise to inflammation or granuloma formation. Prominent folds and wrinkles are also more common with saline implants than with silicone gel implants because saline implants are sometimes only partially filled and because saline is so much less viscous than silicone gel. The more numerous and deeper wrinkles and folds associated with saline-filled implants may be subject to fatigue fractures that account for at least some of their increased risk for sudden rupture. Since 1992, only saline implants have been used, except in cases in which patients have consented to participate in protocol studies.

Single-Lumen Soybean Oil Implants

Single-lumen soybean oil implants have an outer textured silicone elastomer membrane and contain soybean oil. Other fats used in implants are triglicerides and peanut oil. These oil implants are not yet in general use but are currently undergoing clinical trials. The chief advantage of fat- or oil-containing implants is that they are less radiographically dense and obscure less of the breast tissue during mammography than do either silicone or saline implants. The main disadvantage is that leakage of oils into surrounding tissues can cause an intense inflammatory reaction and fat embolism. Additionally, peanut products may cause anaphylaxis in certain patients. At this time, we have no sonographic imaging experience with such implants because little about them has been reported in the literature.

Double-Lumen (Bilumen) Implants

Double-lumen implants contain inner and outer compartments. The inner compartment is surrounded by a silicone elastomer membrane and contains silicone gel. The outer compartment is also surrounded by a silicone elastomer shell but contains saline. The outer saline-containing compartment has a fill valve, and its degree of filling varies. In most cases, only a small volume of saline is present within the outer compartment. The outer elastomer shell may be either smooth or textured. The advantages of double-lumen implants are that (a) like saline implants, double-lumen implants are somewhat smaller than single-lumen silicone implants when implanted but can subsequently be expanded using the outer saline compartment fill valves later; (b) like the saline implant, double-lumen implants are less likely to incite an abnormally thick, contracted capsule; (c) the inner silicone gel component gives a better cosmetic result than saline alone; (d) collapse of the outer saline compartment will not adversely effect the appearance of the breast in most patients because the center silicone gel component is mainly responsible for the implant size; and (e) rupture of the inner compartment and gel bleed will be contained within the outer saline compartment.

Double-Lumen Expander Implants (Becker Implants)

Double-lumen expander implants contain an inner saline-containing compartment and an outer silicone gel–containing compartment. As in other implants, a silicone elastomer membrane surrounds each compartment. The inner compartment has a fill port that may be removable. These expanders are used almost exclusively in the course of breast reconstruction after mastectomy. Like single-lumen saline and double-lumen implants, Becker expanders can be placed while deflated and subsequently expanded, usually by several small injections over time in order to stretch tissues gradually and to expand the space into which a permanent single-lumen saline implant will later be placed. Early on in the expansion process, the shell is extensively wrinkled and folded, but the wrinkles are gradually effaced as the expander enlarges. Recently, single-lumen saline expanders have been used in place of the double-lumen expanders.

Autologous Tissue Reconstructions

In addition to the types of implants mentioned previously, autologous implants may be used. Autologous implants usually involve swinging a flap from some other part of the body to the chest wall in stages. The most common of these reconstructions are (a) the transverse rectus abdominis myocutaneous (TRAM) flap, (b) the gluteus maximus flap, and (c) the latissimus dorsi flap. These implanted autologous tissues are usually grafted to the retropectoral space.

COMPLICATIONS OF MAMMARY IMPLANTS

Although 90% of patients profess satisfaction with the cosmetic result of their implants, there are numerous and relatively frequent complications, many of which are asymptomatic. Complications of mammary implants can occur immediately after surgery or months to years after implantation.

Acute complications include:

- Bleeding and infection
- Asymmetry
- Loss of nipple sensation
- Pain and tenderness

Long-term complications include:

- Encapsulation and capsular contracture
- Rupture (intracapsular or extracapsular)
- Migration
- Herniation
- Hematoma/seroma
- Infection

- Capsular calcifications
- Explantation or revision complications

   Possible long-term complications include:

- Autoimmune disorder (human adjuvant disease)
- Carcinogenesis

Acute Complications

Bleeding and Infection

The risk for bleeding and infection is similar to the risks of any surgery. Infection occurring in the acute phase may persist until the foreign body, the implant, is removed.

Asymmetry

Despite the best attempts of the surgeon, the right and left implants can be asymmetric in size, shape, or position. One advantage of saline and double-lumen implants is that the size of an implant can be adjusted in order to achieve better symmetry.

Loss of Nipple Sensation

There are several different surgical approaches available to the plastic surgeon for mammary augmentation: periareolar, inframammary, and axillary. Loss of nipple sensation occurs most frequently with the periareolar approach, occasionally with the inframammary approach, and rarely with the axillary approach. The axillary approach, however, is the most technically demanding approach.

Long-Term Complications

Encapsulation and Capsular Contracture

All implants become encapsulated by fibrous tissue; this is a normal host response to the implant, which is recognized as a foreign body. The periimplant capsule, which is part of the patient, must be distinguished from the elastomer shell, which is part of the implant. Capsule formation begins within weeks of implantation. Silicone droplets resulting from gel bleed (the passage of microscopic amounts of the oily components of silicone gel through the intact elastomer shell into surrounding tissues) or polyurethane granules become entrapped within the fibrous capsule, attracting giant cells and macrophages as a part of the foreign-body reaction.

   Normal periimplant capsules measure 1.0 to 1.5 mm in thickness, are usually soft and flexible, and encompass a space slightly larger than the implant. When the fibrous capsule becomes thicker than 1.5 mm, it begins to cause clinically detectable changes of capsular contracture. Pa-

tients who have microscopic amounts of silicone gel in the capsule tend to have thicker capsules and are more likely to have capsular contracture than are patients who do not have silicone gel within the capsule. Gel bleeds are associated with abnormal capsular thickening that occurs around single-lumen silicone gel implants, but not with single-lumen saline implants or with double-lumen implants that have intact outer shells. As the capsule becomes thicker, it pushes the implant into an abnormally spherical shape and makes the implant firm to palpation, eventually causing it to become tender. Eccentric capsular thickening can displace the implant and can also cause the implant to herniate superficially through thinner parts of the capsule.

   Baker and colleagues have proposed a system for grading the severity of implant capsular contracture. Baker grade 1 encapsulation is normal. The implant has a normal appearance and also feels normal. In Baker contracture grade 2, the implant appears normal but feels firm to palpation. In Baker grade 3, the implant is firm to palpation and appears mildly abnormal. In Baker grade 4 capsular contracture, the implant is very firm and tender, may have an abnormal position, and has a spherical rather than lenticuloform appearance. Patients with grade 4 contracture of the capsule usually require open capsulectomy with explantation, reimplantation, or both.

   In the past, severe contractures were treated with closed capsulotomy, in which the abnormal implant and its surrounding capsule were vigorously massaged in an attempt to relieve the contracture by traumatically rupturing the fibrous capsule around the implant. Although this led to decreased symptoms of capsular contracture in certain cases, it too often resulted in either localized tears in the fibrous capsule through which herniation of the intact implant membranes occurred or frank rupture of the implant. Today, closed capsulotomy is not recommended because of the high risk for rupturing the implant.

   Capsular contracture interferes with clinical evaluation and mammographic compression, particularly on push-back views, and can even make sonographic evaluation difficult.

   Implant shells and implantation techniques have been altered to minimize the risks for capsular contracture, which include (a) addition of fluorsilicone to the elastomer shell, (b) texturing of the outer surface of the elastomer shell, (c) addition of polyurethane to the textured outer surface of the elastomer shell, (d) use of saline implants, (e) use of double-lumen implants, and (f) changing the site of implantation from subglandular to retropectoral.

Retropectoral Implantation

Implants were first placed superficial to the pectoralis major muscle in the subglandular space but can also be placed deep to the pectoralis muscle within the retropectoral space. Retropectoral implantation is thought to minimize the risk for capsular contracture. The pectoralis muscles may massage the implant during normal physical activity in a manner similar to deep external massage, thereby preventing capsular thickening. Implants appear to incite a less severe foreign-body reaction within overlying muscle than they do within overlying breast tissues. Furthermore, retropectoral implants obscure less breast tissue during mammography than do subglandular implants during pushback (implant exclusion, or Eklund) views.

Rupture

Rupture of mammary implants is the second most common complication. There is a spectrum of ruptures ranging from microscopic rents too small for the surgeon to find at explantation surgery to complete collapse of the implant. Rupture can be caused by obvious trauma but can also occur spontaneously.

The silicone elastomer shell that envelops all implants weakens with age. Weakening is most severe where the radius of curvature is the smallest, at the edges of the implant and at the apex of radial folds, where fatigue fractures are most likely to occur. Saline implants are more prone to infolding because of lesser degrees of filling and the low viscosity of saline in comparison to silicone gel and thus are also more prone to sudden rupture than are silicone gel implants. Implants with thin, smooth elastomer shells are more prone to rupture than are implants with thick, textured shells. Most implants show some evidence of implant leakage by the time they have been in place for 15 years or more.

Silicone gel implant ruptures can be classified as intracapsular, extracapsular, or combined intracapsular and extracapsular. Intracapsular ruptures are more common.

Intracapsular ruptures result when the shell ruptures and silicone gel that leaks out of the implant remains confined within the periimplant fibrous capsule. The degree of leakage of silicone gel from the shell into the intracapsular space varies greatly. In early or mild cases, the amount of extravasation and the degree of shell collapse can be minimal. In such cases, all of the extravasated gel might lie within an individual radial fold. In other cases, all of the silicone gel escapes from the shell into the intracapsular space, and the shell collapses completely.

In extracapsular rupture, the fibrous capsule and the shell are both ruptured. Extravasated silicone gel no longer remains confined within the intracapsular space but extends into surrounding breast tissues. Theoretically, intracapsular ruptures precede all extracapsular ruptures. However, the intracapsular phase of the process can be difficult to detect on imaging studies. The extravasated silicone gel might escape from the implant directly through a coexisting rent in the fibrous capsule into surrounding

breast tissues without ever accumulating within the capsule in large enough amounts to be detectable.

Extravasated extracapsular silicone eventually incites an intense foreign-body inflammatory response that leads to formation of silicone granuloma, which may be palpable and tender. Intracapsular ruptures much less frequently incite formation of silicone granulomas.

Clinical findings associated with implant ruptures vary, depending on the type of implant, the severity of rupture, and whether the rupture is of the intracapsular or extracapsular type. Rupture of a single-lumen saline implant typically results in a complete collapse of both the implant and its capsule almost immediately after rupture, leading to marked asymmetry of the breasts. The distinction between intracapsular and extracapsular rupture is irrelevant for saline implants because the extravasated saline is rapidly absorbed into the body, regardless of its location inside or outside the capsule. Diagnostic imaging is not necessary for evaluation of implant rupture in such patients because the patient is immediately aware that the implant suddenly decompressed. Clinical findings alone are enough to establish the diagnosis. The role of mammography in patients with collapsed saline implants is primarily to exclude cancer before explantation or replacement of the implants. Additionally, the collapsed implant shell is readily apparent on mammograms as well as clinically. The role of ultrasound in such patients, as in patients without implants, is to evaluate palpable lumps and mammographic abnormalities to determine the need for concurrent biopsy at the time of explantation or reimplantation.

The clinical findings in rupture of single-lumen silicone gel implants or of double-lumen implants, on the other hand, are much more difficult to evaluate. Because of the very high viscosity and nonresorbability of silicone gel, leaks through defects in the elastomer shell are usually very slow, the leak may be limited by inflammatory response, and the shell does not usually rapidly decompress. The implant can remain almost fully expanded, having only a thin layer of sticky, extravasated silicone deposited along its outer surface as evidence of its rupture. Additionally, even in intracapsular ruptures in which all of the silicone gel extravasates from the shell and the shell collapses completely, the outer contour of the periimplant capsule can remain normal, the breast size will appear normal, and the rupture can be clinically inapparent. Likewise, rupture of the elastomer shell surrounding the inner silicone gel compartment of a double-lumen implant can allow mixing of saline and silicone gel within the intact outer compartment without affecting the overall size and outward appearance of the implant. Even rupture of the elastomer shell surrounding the outer saline compartment of a double-lumen implant may not be clinically obvious because the outer saline-containing compartment is so small in relation to the size of the inner silicone gel compartment.

The incidence of spontaneous implant rupture is uncertain because many cases are subclinical. The reported incidence varies greatly, depending on the patient population and the method of documenting rupture. Although initial studies suggested only about a 5% to 10% rate of rupture in asymptomatic patients based on clinical and mammographic findings, recent MRI studies have found that as many as 34% of implants may show evidence of rupture. Rupture of implants during mammography is rare but has been reported. Our more recent experience with ultrasound of implants is that intracapsular rupture is the rule, rather than the exception, in implants that are 15 years old or older.

Extracapsular extravasated silicone gel can migrate from the breast to other areas of the chest and abdominal wall. It can involve muscles of the chest wall or back or the axilla. Extravasated silicone may also be absorbed into lymphatic vessels and carried to the axillary lymph nodes. Microscopic amounts of silicone that are not detectable by imaging techniques can be found in these lymph nodes due to gel bleed even in the absence of rupture. However, macroscopic amounts of silicone gel that occur with extracapsular implant rupture and that migrate to axillary lymph nodes can be detected by mammography, ultrasound, and MRI. Silicone gel phagocytized by macrophages can be carried to remote parts of the body.

Migration

An implant can migrate from its normal implantation site, and even a small migration can create bothersome degrees of asymmetry.

Herniation

An intact implant can herniate through a rent in the fibrous capsule that surrounds it. This protrusion can result acutely from trauma or closed capsulotomy but can also occur gradually, most frequently because of uneven thickening of the capsule in patients with capsular contracture. The capsular disruption leading to implant herniation is usually localized. The increased pressure on the implant from the thickened segments of capsule causes the implant to bulge through thinner portions of the capsule. Clinically and mammographically, herniation may be apparent as a bulge in the contour of the breast, but such bulges are often difficult to distinguish from extracapsular silicone granulomas both clinically and mammographically. Sonography and MRI, however, can readily distinguish between extracapsular rupture with silicone granuloma and herniation of the implant.

Hematoma

Hematoma formation can occur long after implantation. This was often a complication of capsulotomy, when rupture of the fibrous capsule led to bleeding and hematoma formation. However, closed capsulotomy is rarely used today, and hematomas can occur both with other types of trauma and spontaneously. In patients with large retropectoral implants, the pectoralis muscle may be so stretched and attenuated that it is prone to tear and develop intramuscular hematoma with only minor trauma or intense exertion, even in the absence of trauma.

Infection

Infection complicates implants most frequently in the immediate postimplantation period. The findings of infection are the same as in patients without implants: mastitis and abscess formation. In rare cases in which infection is severe and persistent, chronic or acute capsulitis requires removal of the foreign body, the implant. In certain patients, implants can cause an intense chronic inflammatory response even in the absence of frank infection, and sterile abscesses do occur.

Capsular Calcifications

Focal or diffuse calcifications of the inner surface of the capsule commonly occur even in the absence of rupture, usually in reaction to microscopic gel bleed. Capsular calcifications tend to increase with the age of the implant. Capsular calcifications are considered to be of no clinical significance unless they simulate malignant calcifications on mammograms. Capsular calcifications that are mammographically visible in patients with intact implants are usually thin and closely applied to the surface of the implant and have a characteristically benign mammographic appearance. Dense calcification can create enough acoustic shadowing to prevent sonographic assessment of the implant for rupture. Calcifications can be troublesome in patients who have undergone explantation without capsulectomy. The calcifications in the unresected capsule can simulate malignancy, especially in cases in which there is associated intracapsular hematoma, seroma, or fat necrosis.

Possible Long-Term Implant Complications

Autoimmune Disease (Human Adjuvant Disease)

There have been reports of patients with implants developing nonspecific symptoms of fatigue, fever, generalized lymphadenopathy, weight loss, general malaise, breast and chest wall pain, and muscle and joint aches and pains.

These symptoms are indistinguishable from those of autoimmune disorders such as scleroderma, systemic lupus erythematosus, Sjögren's syndrome, rheumatoid arthritis, idiopathic thrombocytopenia, polymyositis, and dermatomyositis. Scleroderma-like symptoms have been the most commonly reported. Others have termed the constellation of findings *human adjuvant disease.*

That silicone implants cause such a condition seems unlikely. Medical-grade silicone is used in numerous other products in medicine besides breast implants, and there has been little suspicion of these other products causing autoimmune disorders. Silicone is used to coat catheters, pacemakers, and heart valves and is used in prosthetic joints, to coat needles and syringes, and in gastrointestinal medications. Additionally, silicone is used widely in the food, cosmetic, shaving cream, deodorants, and hair care products industries. Almost all Americans have already been exposed to silicone in everyday life, whether or not they have implants. Nevertheless, large, well-respected companies have been driven into bankruptcy by lawsuits for a condition whose existence is not only uncertain but also unlikely. Therefore, detection of implant rupture remains important for medicolegal reasons, even if not important for medical reasons alone.

Although it seems unlikely that silicone implants cause an autoimmune disorder and recent studies have found no evidence of this, no studies to date have had the statistical power to make this determination with absolute certainty. Because the autoimmune disorders that implants are said to cause are relatively uncommon, large, multicenter studies that include hundreds of thousands of patients and extend for more than 10 years may be necessary to determine with certainty whether there is a relationship between silicone gel implants and autoimmune disorders. Such multicenter, multiyear studies will be difficult to perform and very expensive.

Because the relationship of silicone gel implants to autoimmune disorders and the safety of such implants has been questioned, the U.S. Food and Drug Administration (FDA) has barred silicone gel implants from the market unless the patient and surgeon are willing to be part of a multicenter nationwide protocol study to assess their safety.

Carcinogenesis

There is no evidence that implants cause breast cancer. However, Handel et al. have shown that breast tumors in patients with implants are larger, have a higher stage, and have a poorer prognosis than those detected in women without implants. This situation is thought to be due to interference of the implant with the performance of mammography rather than a carcinogenic effect. Subglandular implants obscure between 22% and 83% (mean, 44%) of

the breast on routine mammographic views, depending on breast size and consistency. Even with pushback implant exclusion views, Silverstein found that 36% of the breast was obscured by subglandular implants. Retropectoral implants obscure less breast tissue than do subglandular implants—an average of 25% of the breast tissue on routine views and an average of 15% of breast tissue pushback views. Implants containing fat density (soybean or peanut oil) are being developed to try to minimize this problem. In addition, implants interfere with compression of the breasts, especially if very large implants have been placed or if the implant capsule is contracted and very firm, spherical in shape, and tender. Adequate compression is essential for optimal mammographic results. Because of these difficulties, aggressive use of special mammographic views (e.g., tangential, semireclining, cleavage) and diagnostic sonography is warranted for even minimal clinical findings if delay in diagnosis is to be avoided.

One potential advantage of implants is that nodules probably become palpable when they are smaller because they are displaced anteriorly and because surrounding breast tissues are compressed and thinned by the implants. However, the prognosis of palpable cancers is worse than the prognosis of nonpalpable cancers detected by mammographic screening alone.

IMAGING OF THE BREASTS IN PATIENTS WITH BREAST IMPLANTS

The goal of imaging in patients with breast implants is twofold: to evaluate breast tissues and to evaluate the implants for complications. The main roles for diagnostic sonography in patients who have implants are identical to the roles of sonography in evaluation of patients who do not have implants—to evaluate palpable and mammographic abnormalities. Studies have shown that MRI is more sensitive for implant rupture than sonography, which, in turn, is more sensitive than mammography. However, because far more patients with implants are evaluated for palpable lumps or mammographic abnormalities than for implant rupture, far more implant patients will undergo sonographic evaluation than will ever undergo MRI. Therefore, sonographers and sonologists must be familiar with both normal and abnormal sonographic appearances of implants.

Mammographic Findings

The type of implant present and the site of implantation can usually be determined mammographically. First, it is possible to distinguish between saline-filled and silicone gel–filled single-lumen implants. Saline within implants is less mammographically dense than is the silicone elastomer

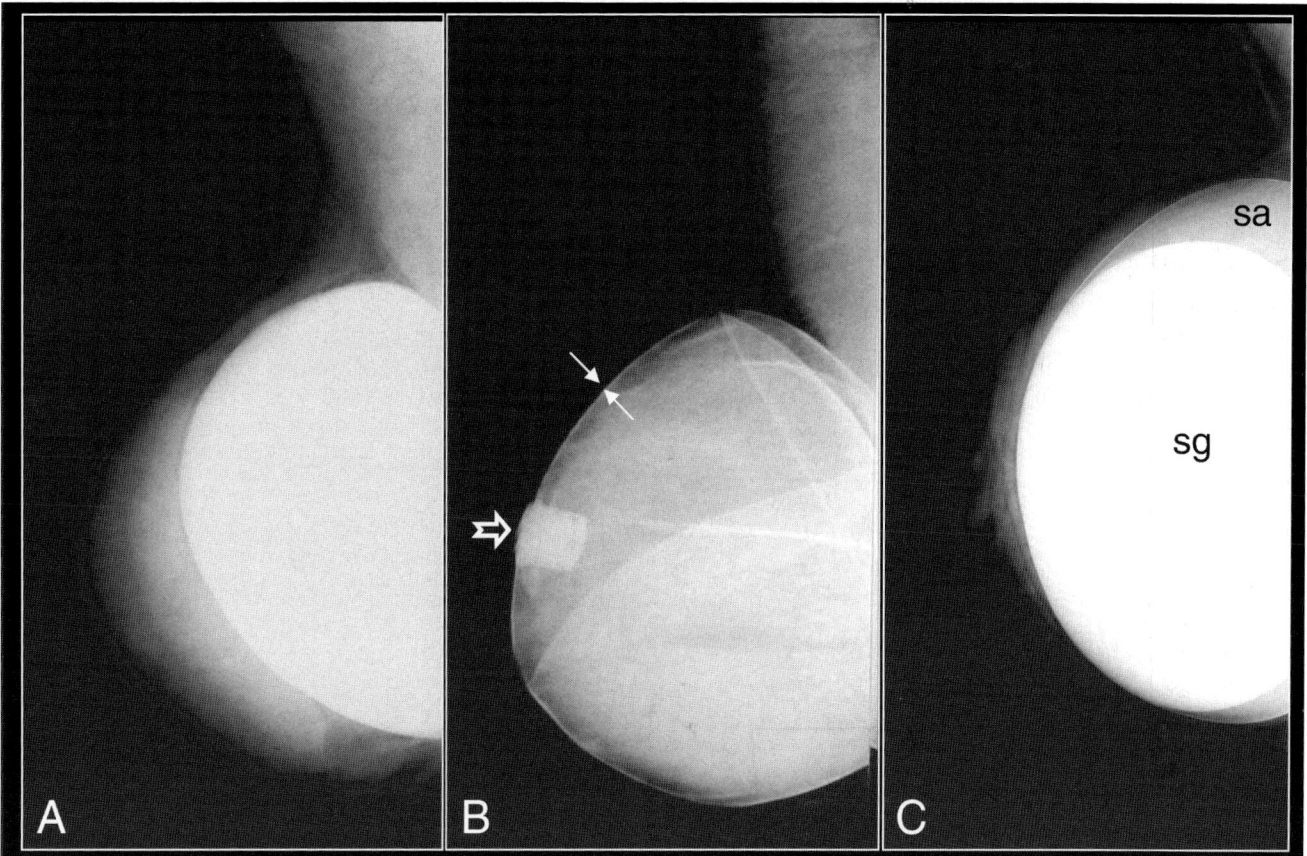

FIGURE 9–2 Mammography of a single-lumen silicone gel implant (**A**), a single-lumen saline implant (**B**); and a double-lumen implant (**C**). The single-lumen silicone gel implant is so opaque that the shell cannot be distinguished from the contents of the shell. On the other hand, the silicone elastomer shell *(small arrows)* of the single-lumen saline implant is more opaque than the saline that fills the shell. Only the outer shell of the double-lumen implant is visible because it contains less opaque saline. The inner shell is silhouetted by the equally dense silicone gel it contains. All three implants are subglandular in location.

membrane, whereas silicone gel is identical in density to the silicone elastomer shell and indistinguishable from it (Fig. 9–2). Second, it is possible to identify double-lumen implants that have silicone gel in the inner compartment and saline in the outer compartment (Fig. 9–2). Third, it is possible to determine mammographically whether the implant is retropectoral or subglandular in location (Fig. 9–3). This determination is always possible on the mediolateral oblique (MLO) views and sometimes possible on craniocaudal (CC) views that include the pectoralis muscle (Fig. 9–3). Finally, under ideal circumstances, it may be possible to determine mammographically whether the outer surface of the implant shell is textured or smooth (Fig. 9–4).

Mammography is sensitive for rupture of saline implants but is insensitive for detection of intracapsular implant rupture in patients with single-lumen silicone gel implants in comparison to sonography and MRI. Intracapsular ruptures are missed by mammography because the ra-

diographically dense extravasated silicone gel is contained within the fibrous capsule, which has the same shape as the intact implant. The extravasated silicone gel surrounds and obscures the equally dense, collapsed implant membranes (Fig. 9–5). Mammography is limited to evaluation of outline abnormalities of silicone gel implants and cannot depict internal abnormalities. Intracapsular ruptures do not disrupt the outline of the silicone density. When rupture of a single-lumen silicone gel implant is extracapsular and extravasated silicone gel has migrated away from the elastomer shell into the breast tissues, mammography can show extravasated gel only if it projects beyond the implant on the routine mammographic views (Fig. 9–6). Extravasated extracapsular silicone gel that lies too deep to be projected free of the implant on routine views will not be mammographically visible. Additionally, mammograms can show silicone within lymph vessels and lymph nodes. Thus, an abnormal mammogram more reliably predicts

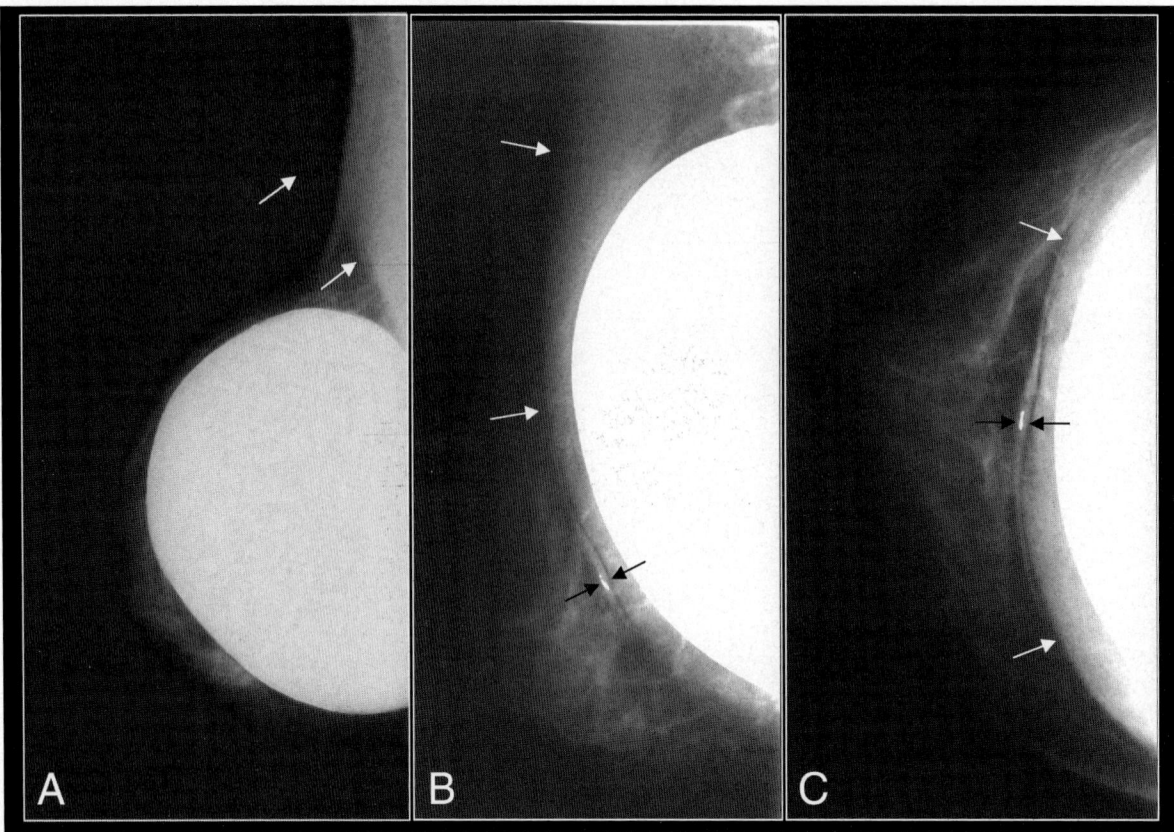

FIGURE 9–3 Mammography of subglandular (**A**) and retropectoral (**B**, mediolateral oblique view; **C**, craniocaudal view) implants. The *white arrows* outline the anterior aspect of the pectoralis major muscle. Note that there is a calcifying scar along the anterior edge of the pectoralis in both views of the retropectoral implant from a seat-belt injury incurred in a motor vehicle crash (*black arrows*). Both the subglandular and retropectoral implants are of the single-lumen silicone gel type.

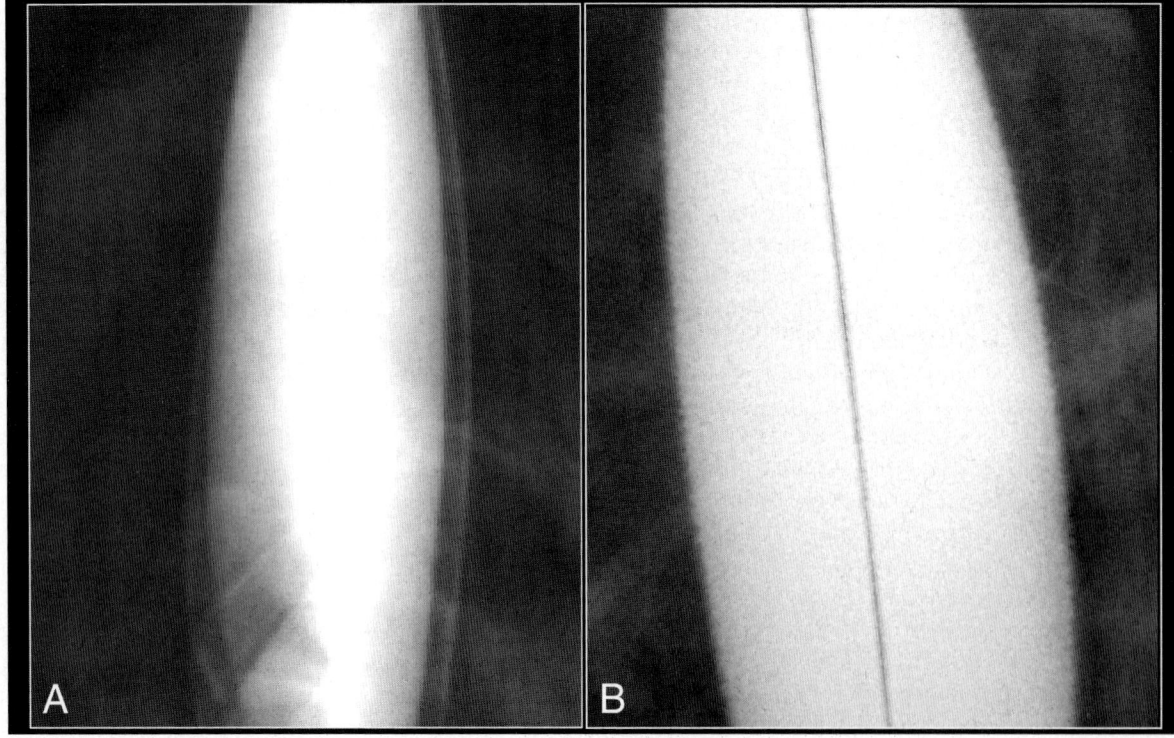

FIGURE 9–4 Magnified craniocaudal pushback views of nontextured double-lumen (**A**) and heavily textured single-lumen (**B**) silicone gel implants.

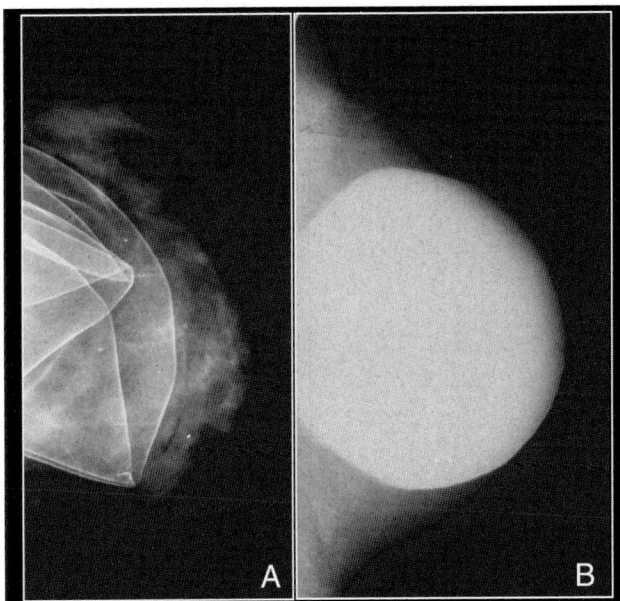

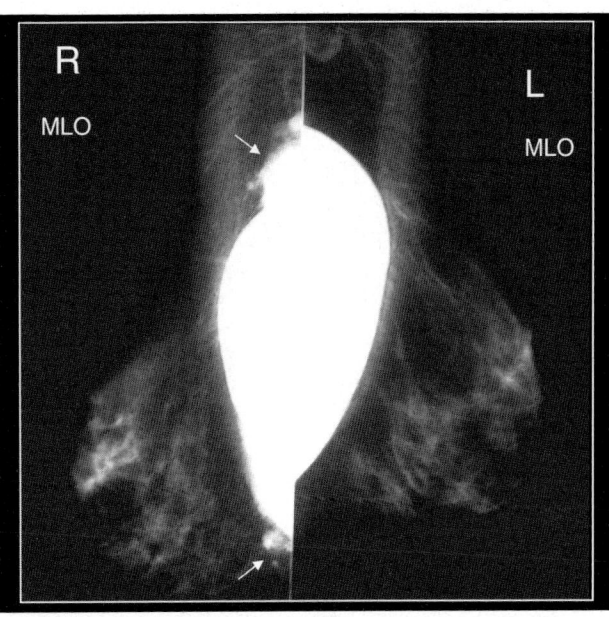

FIGURE 9–5 Mammography, although readily able to demonstrate rupture of single-lumen saline implants (**A**), is generally not useful for diagnosing intracapsular rupture of single-lumen silicone gel implants (**B**). The ruptured and completely collapsed shell of the single-lumen silicone gel implant shown in part **B** is silhouetted by the equally dense extravasated silicone gel that remains contained within the fibrous periimplant capsule.

FIGURE 9–6 Mammography can demonstrate extracapsular rupture of single-lumen silicone gel implants if the extravasated extracapsular gel *(arrows)* projects in tangent beyond the contour of the silicone gel that remains within the shell and periimplant capsule (retropectoral single-lumen silicone gel implants).

implant rupture than does a normal mammogram predict an intact implant.

Bulges, irregularities, or angulations in the outer contour of silicone implants on mammograms are nonspecific. They may correspond to herniation of the implant, silicone granuloma, or a combination of both (Fig. 9–7). If the bulge is angular rather than curved, it is more likely to represent extracapsular rupture than herniation. There is a spectrum from prominent or angular bulges to very mild or slight lobulation. Not all bulges or angles are related to implant herniation or rupture. Slight or mild lobulation of the contour of a silicone implant may merely represent wrinkles or folds in the surface of an intact implant.

Focal or diffuse calcifications may be seen along the surface of the implant and tend to increase with the age of the implant (Fig. 9–3). As noted previously, these calcifications are probably due to microscopic gel bleed through the capsule, usually lie along the inner surface of the capsule, do not indicate rupture of the implant, and are not thought to be of clinical significance.

Normal implants should be elliptical, conical, or discoid in shape on mammograms. A spherical shape suggests the presence of an abnormally thick, contracted capsule (Fig. 9–5). Such a capsule may be seen as a thickened band of soft tissue density paralleling the anterior aspect of the mammographically more dense silicone implant. It must be distinguished from the pectoralis muscle in patients

who have retropectoral implants (Fig. 9–3). In such cases, the pectoralis is much thicker in the upper outer quadrant, extends away from the implant toward the axilla, and becomes progressively thinner inferomedially. Because of these shape variations, an abnormally thick capsule can reliably be distinguished from the pectoralis muscle on MLO views, but the distinction can be difficult on CC views, where variations in thickness of the pectoralis muscle are more difficult to demonstrate.

Mammography is more effective in the evaluation of patients with single-lumen saline implants than it is in patients with single-lumen silicone gel implants. The saline within the implant is less opaque than the surrounding silicone elastomer membrane, allowing some demonstration of internal characteristics by mammography. Folds and lobulations are a normal mammographic finding in saline implants (Fig. 9–2). Rupture of saline implants is usually both clinically and mammographically obvious because virtually all ruptures are rapid and complete (with the exception of slow valve leaks) (Fig. 9–5).

Intact double-lumen implants are mammographically apparent. There is a dense inner component that represents the inner silicone gel compartment and an outer, less mammographically dense saline component (Fig. 9–2). Absence of a mammographically visible outer saline component suggests rupture of the outer saline shell (Fig. 9–8). However, rupture and complete collapse of the inner shell sur-

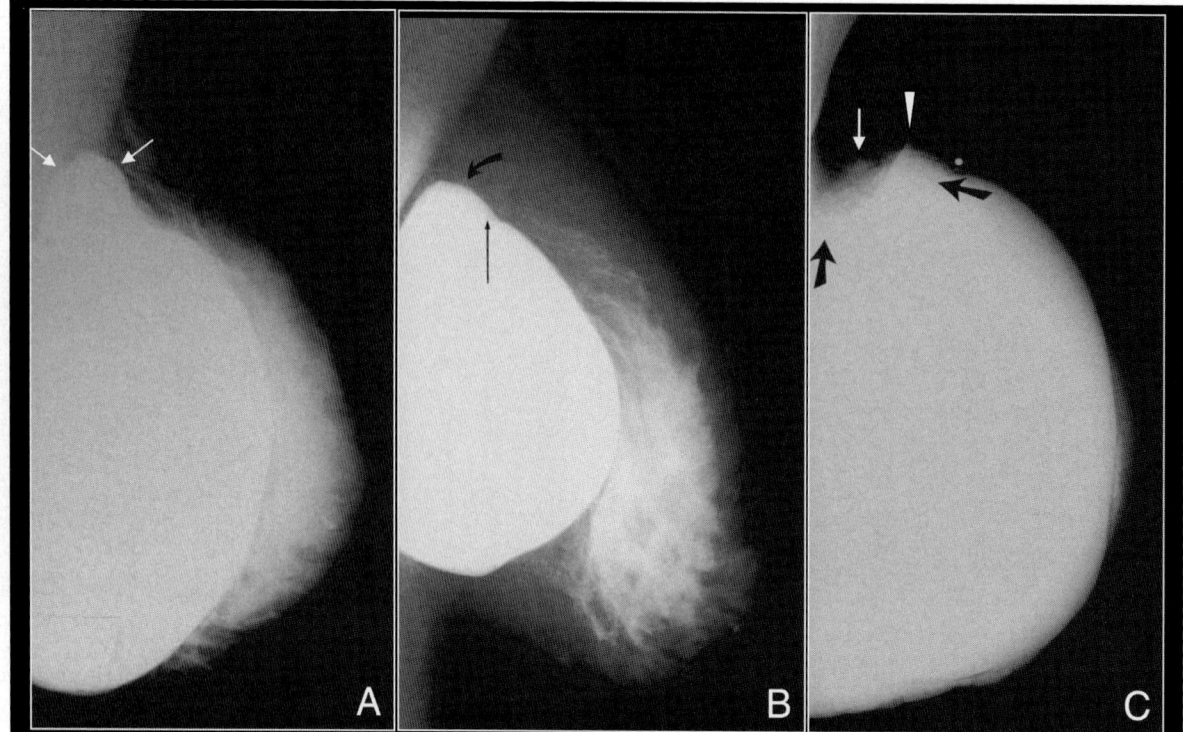

FIGURE 9–7 Mammographic findings in single-lumen silicone gel implants are limited to demonstration of contour abnormalities and can present difficulties in differentiating among wrinkles, herniations, and silicone granulomas. Extravasated silicone gel that does not project beyond the outer profile of the shell and capsule on routine views will be missed mammographically. The implant in part **A** has herniated through the periimplant capsule *(white arrows)*, but has not ruptured. The implant in part **B** was herniated and ruptured. The extravasated extracapsular silicone gel that was readily demonstrated by sonography was obscured mammographically by the silicone gel within the herniation *(curved arrow)*. The implant in part **C** is herniated and ruptured. In this case, however, the extravasated extracapsular silicone gel *(white arrow)* projects in tangent beyond the herniation *(white arrowhead)* and is mammographically visible.

rounding the silicone gel component of the implant may fill the saline compartment with silicone gel, making it appear that the saline compartment is absent. Ruptures of the inner shell without complete collapse may result in a mixing of water and silicone density within the inner and outer shells but is often undetectable on mammograms.

Sonographic Findings

Goals

Evaluation of implants may be either the primary or the secondary goal of sonography in these patients. In either case, both overlying breast tissues and the implant can be evaluated. If the patient has a palpable lump or mammographic abnormality for which sonography is indicated, the chief palpable or mammographic indication should be evaluated first. One must remember that patients with implants have all the same benign and malignant breast diseases as do patients without implants, and the problem for which the patient presented is likely to be unrelated to the

implant. The odds are greatly in favor of the presenting problem being caused by a common benign or malignant breast process, not by the implant. Only after the problem for which the sonogram is indicated is solved should evaluation for implant complications be undertaken. There is always the danger that assessment of the implant will distract the sonographer or sonologist from the real pathology for which the patient presented. On the other hand, if sonography is being performed primarily to evaluate implant problems, remember that, depending on the type, location, and complications of the implant, anywhere from 15% to more than 80% of the breast tissue may been obscured by the implants on mammograms, even on pushback views. Therefore, evaluating breast tissues in addition to evaluating the implants is important, especially in the tissues most likely to be obscured on mammograms (i.e., tissues that lie along the periphery of the implants posteriorly and in the axillary segment). Thus, after evaluating the implant for abnormalities, whole breast sonography should be performed to evaluate areas of the breast that may have been obscured by the implants on the mammograms.

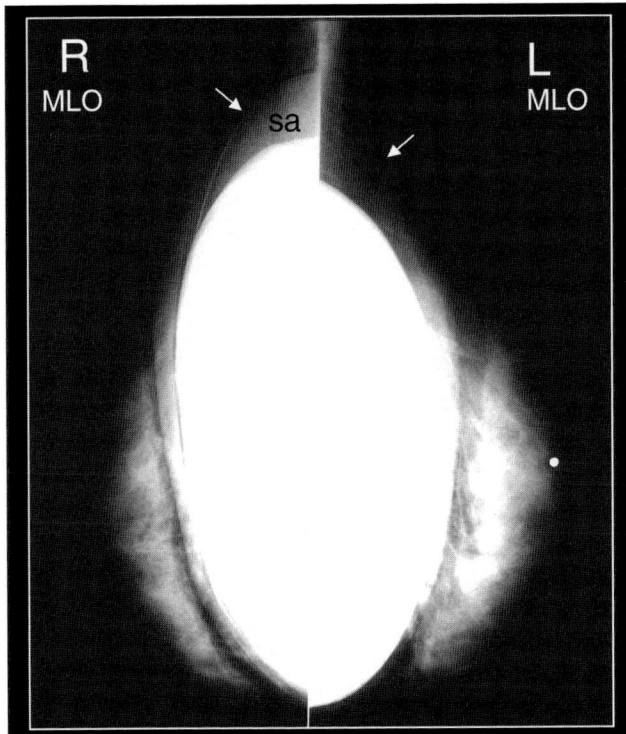

FIGURE 9–8 The outer saline compartment of the left retropectoral double-lumen silicone gel implant has ruptured and completely collapsed. The outer saline-containing shell *(sa)* of the right implant is intact.

Technique

Normally, patients with implants should be scanned in the same supine or contralateral posterior oblique position in which patients without implants are examined. However, certain patients may have palpable folds or wrinkles in the implant shell that are palpable only in certain positions. Such patients should be scanned in the position in which the abnormality is palpable as well as in the routine positions. Additionally, the axillary segment in patients with large implants may be thinner and easier to examine in the upright position.

The portion of the ultrasound examination that is targeted to palpable or mammographic abnormalities can be performed in a manner similar to targeted examinations in patients who do not have implants (described in detail in Chapter 3).

In most patients, the same 7- to 12-MHz linear, electronically focused probe that is used in patients without implants can be employed. However, in patients who have large implants or severe contracture, 5-MHz linear or even curved linear transducers may be necessary to demonstrate the deep portions of the centers of the implants.

Evaluation of the periphery of the implant is especially important because the shell is thinner along the edges, rupture is more common there, and extravasated extracapsular

silicone gel leading to silicone granuloma formation has a propensity to either occur in the periphery or migrate to the periphery of the implant. Assessing the periphery of the implant is also important in sonographic determination of the type of implant and in distinguishing the periimplant fibrous capsule from the implant shell. It is at the edges of the implant and at the bases of radial folds where the separation between the capsule and shell is greatest and easiest to demonstrate sonographically. Evaluation of the peripheral edges of the implant and the breast tissues superficial to the implant is usually possible with 7.5- to 12-MHz probes. Evaluation of the center of the implant is more likely to require lower-frequency, more deeply focused 5-MHz linear or curved linear transducers, especially in patients who have capsular contracture or intracapsular rupture in which the elastomer shell has completely collapsed and has fallen to the posterior aspect of the intracapsular space (Fig. 9–9).

We rely heavily on split-screen imaging of mirror-image locations in the right and left breasts, using the contralateral side as a control when evaluating implants. Split-screen mirror-image scanning is extremely helpful in most patients who do not have bilaterally symmetric implant complications. This approach is especially important in evaluating the alterations in internal echogenicity that can occur in patients with intracapsular rupture of single-lumen silicone gel implants, in which a subtle increase in echogenicity may be the primary clue to the presence of an intracapsular rupture.

Using very light compression during scanning of implants helps minimize reverberation echoes in the near field. The noncompressed shell maintains a slight curvature so that only a small segment of shell is perpendicular to the beam and can give rise to reverberation echoes. Heavy compression flattens the shell so that it is perpendicular to the beam along the entire length of the transducer. This results in very long and intense near-field reverberation echoes.

Normal Sonographic Implant Appearances

The normal sonographic appearances of implants vary greatly, depending on the type of implant and the implantation site.

Echogenicity of Implant Contents

The contents of both single-lumen silicone gel and single-lumen saline implants appear sonolucent. However, a variable amount of ring-down and reverberation artifact can be present in the near field (Fig. 9–10). These reverberations arise from mismatches between the implant shell and overlying breast tissues. These near-field artifacts can make evaluation of silicone gel implants for intracapsular rupture very difficult. Near-field artifacts can also increase the difficulty in evaluating the shell and capsule of the implant for

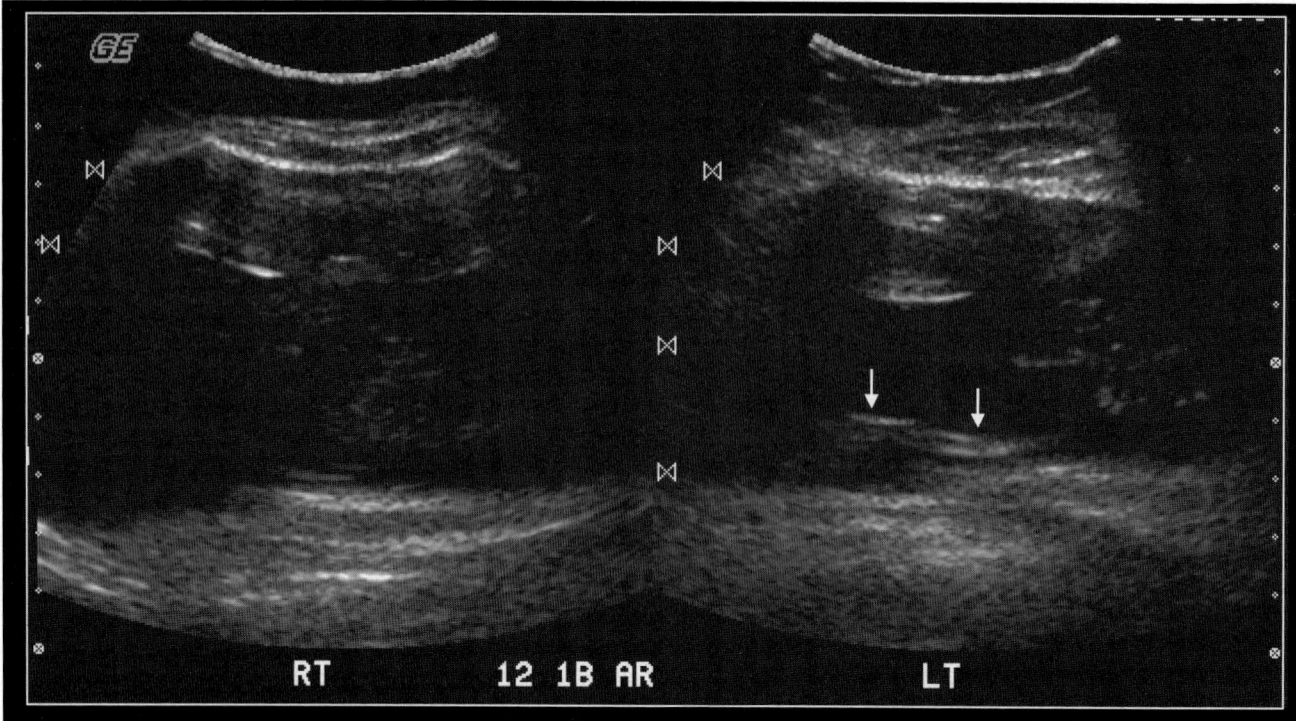

FIGURE 9–9 Curved linear 5-MHz transducers are particularly helpful in cases in which there is both severe capsular contracture and intracapsular rupture. The collapsed shell *(arrows)* may fall to the posterior aspect of the intracapsular space and may be too deep to demonstrate with standard high-frequency linear transducers.

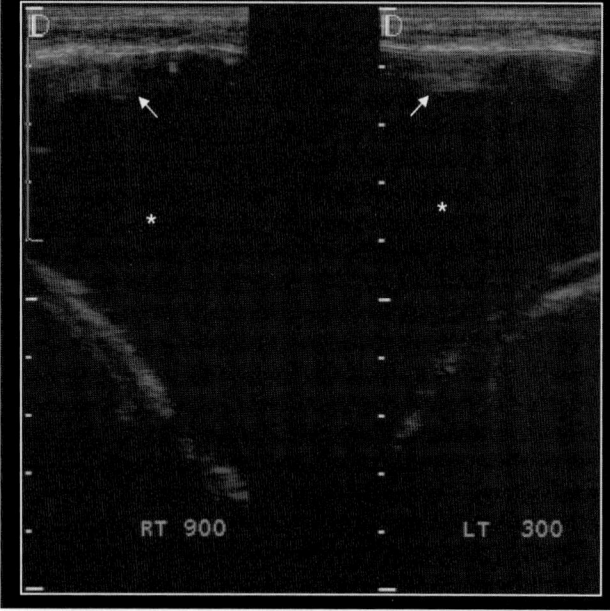

FIGURE 9–10 The silicone gel in most normal single-lumen saline and silicone implants appears anechoic *(*)* or nearly ane-choic. Split-screen mirror-image scans are helpful in demonstrating bilaterally symmetric echogenicity. In most cases, acoustic mismatches between breast tissue and the silicone elastomer implant cell cause some near-field reverberation artifacts *(arrows)*.

determining the type of shell (textured versus smooth) and whether the implant is single or double lumen. Recent technical developments that can significantly reduce near-field artifact in patients with implants include high-frequency coded harmonics (Fig. 9–11; see also Chapter 2, Fig. 2–18) and real-time compounding (see Chapter 2, Fig. 2–27). These developments have aided in identifying the type of implant and intracapsular rupture.

Surprisingly, many patients do not know the type of implants they have. In such patients, determining the type of implant from mammography is usually possible. However, mammograms are not available in some cases. In others, low-dose, high-contrast, film-screen combinations can make even saline implants appear so radiopaque that they are mammographically indistinguishable from silicone gel implants. When the patient does not know the type of her implants and when mammograms are either not available or are unhelpful, sonography can usually help determine the type of implants. This determination is not made from differences in the echogenicity of the filling material but rather by the presence or absence of a sonographic artifact created by the slower speed of sound through the silicone gel (997 m/s through silicone gel versus 1,540 m/s through soft tissues). Because of the slowing of sound in silicone, the chest wall deep to a silicone gel implant appears to be

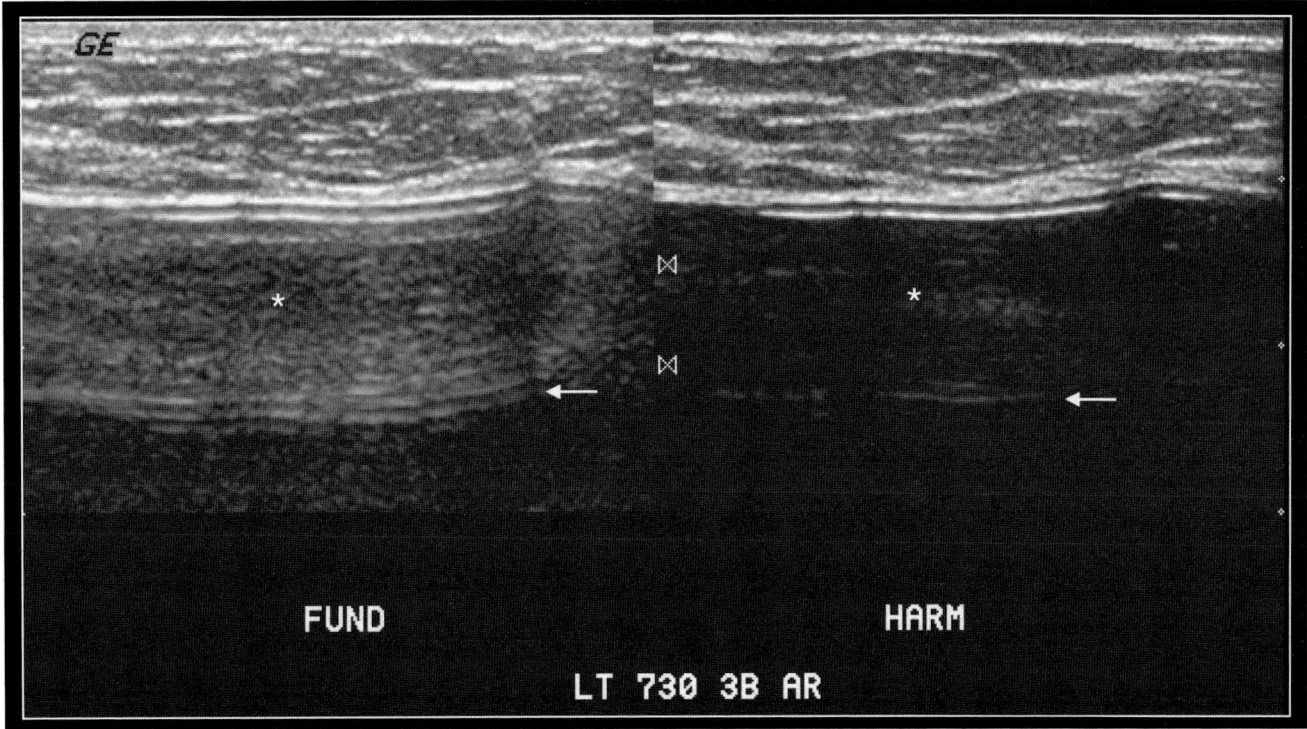

FIGURE 9–11 High-frequency coded harmonics (**right**) can greatly reduce the amount of near-field clutter *(*)* and reverberation artifacts *(arrow)* present on fundamental images (**left**) and can make sonographic evaluation of the implant capsule and shell easier and more accurate.

greater than it really is. By scanning the edge of the implant so that the implant extends halfway across the field of view, the apparent depth of the chest wall deep to the implant can be compared with the depth of the chest wall peripheral to the edge of the implant. If the implant is silicone, there will be a step-off in the chest wall at the edge of the implant, with the chest wall abruptly appearing deeper behind the implant than it is peripheral to the implant. On the other hand, if saline implants are scanned in the same fashion, there is no step-off in the chest wall (Figs. 9–12 and 9–13). If the edge of a double-lumen implant with saline in the outer compartment and silicone gel in the inner compartment is scanned, there will be no step-off in the chest wall behind the outer saline-filled compartment, but there will be a step-off behind the inner silicone gel–filled compartment (Fig. 9–14). This is true even though the shell surrounding the inner compartment is usually not visible because of critical angle phenomena.

The degree of step-off in the chest wall deep to the implant varies with the thickness of the silicone gel traversed by the ultrasound beam. Thus, the thicker the silicone gel compartment traversed, the greater the step-off. If a silicone gel–containing implant is soft and compressible, scanning the edge of the implant with excessive scan pressure may flatten the edge of the implant, decrease the

thickness of silicone gel traversed, and minimize or even completely obscure the step-off (Fig. 9–15). Therefore, it is important to use light scan pressure when evaluating the edge of an implant for determining whether the implant contains silicone gel or saline.

Differential central compression pressure is also important in demonstrating the artifactual step-off in the chest wall deep to silicone gel–containing implants. To best demonstrate the artifactual chest wall step-off, the ultrasound beam must be nearly perpendicular to the chest wall at the edge of the implant. This usually requires differential compression, with greater compression pressure being applied to the end of the transducer overlying the implant than is applied peripheral to the implant. If the angle of incidence with the chest wall is too steeply oblique, identifying the artifactual step-off is difficult (Fig. 9–16). Obtaining an angle of incidence nearly perpendicular to the chest wall at the edge of the implant can be difficult in patients who have severe capsular contracture and abnormally firm implants.

Although it is generally true that the same type of implant has been used on both sides, an occasional patient will be encountered who has a saline-filled implant on one side but a silicone gel–filled implant on the other side. In

(text continued on page 216)

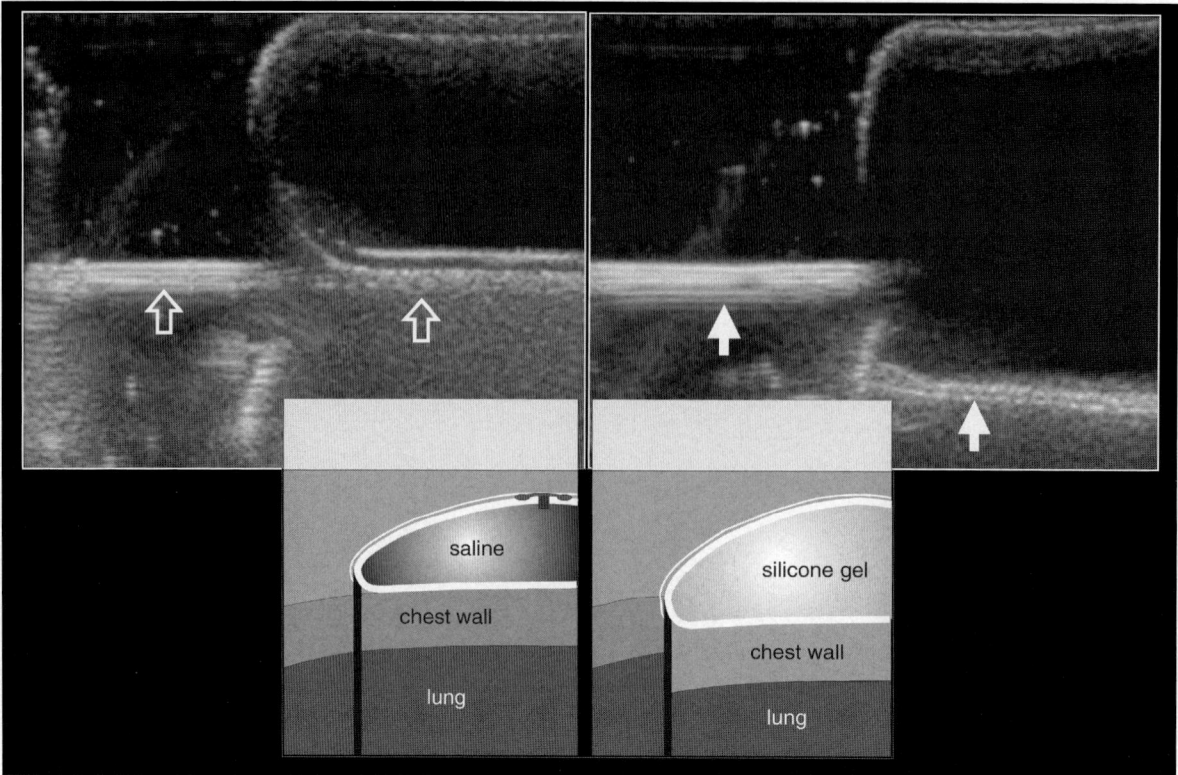

FIGURE 9–12 Single-lumen saline (**left**) and silicone gel (**right**) implants were scanned *in vitro* in a water bath. The bottom of the water pan forms a straight line (**left**, *hollow arrows*) with no step-off deep to the saline implant. There is an artifactual step-off in the bottom of the pan and posterior wall of the implant (**right**, *solid arrows*) deep to the silicone gel containing implant because of the slower speed of sound through silicone gel.

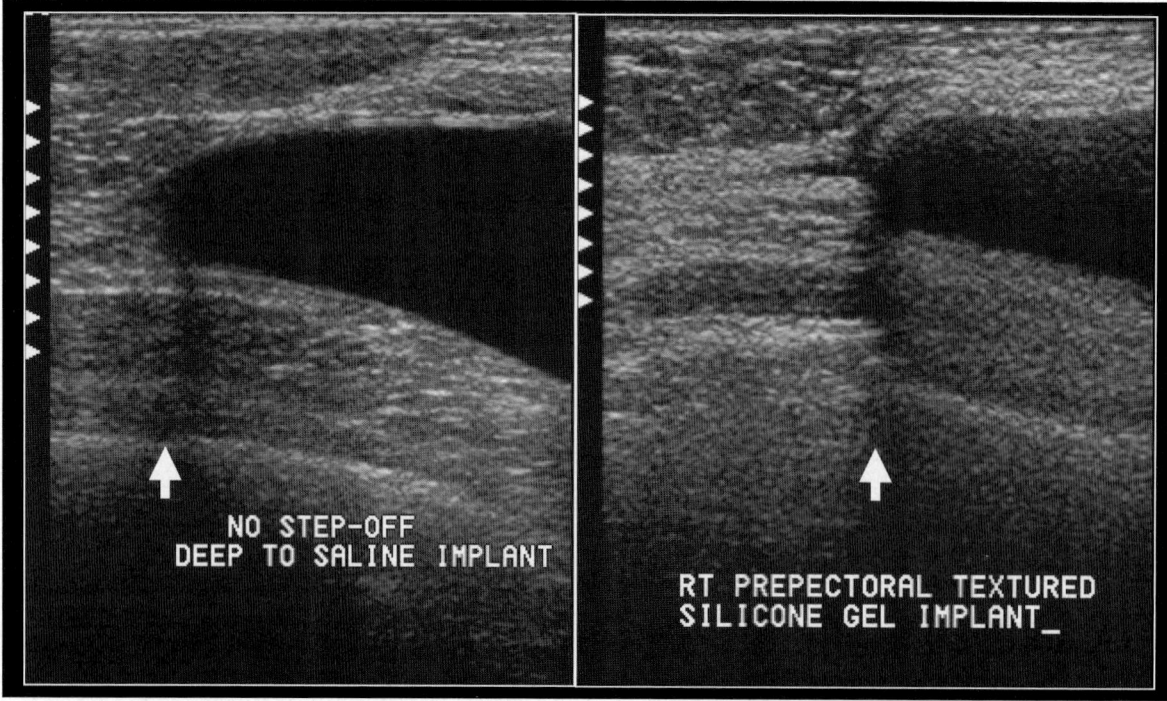

FIGURE 9–13 *In vivo* scans of subglandular single-lumen silicone gel (**left**) and single-lumen saline (**right**) in two different patients show a step-off in the chest wall at the edge of the silicone gel–containing implant (**right**, *arrow*), but no step-off at the edge of the saline-containing implant (**left**, *arrow*).

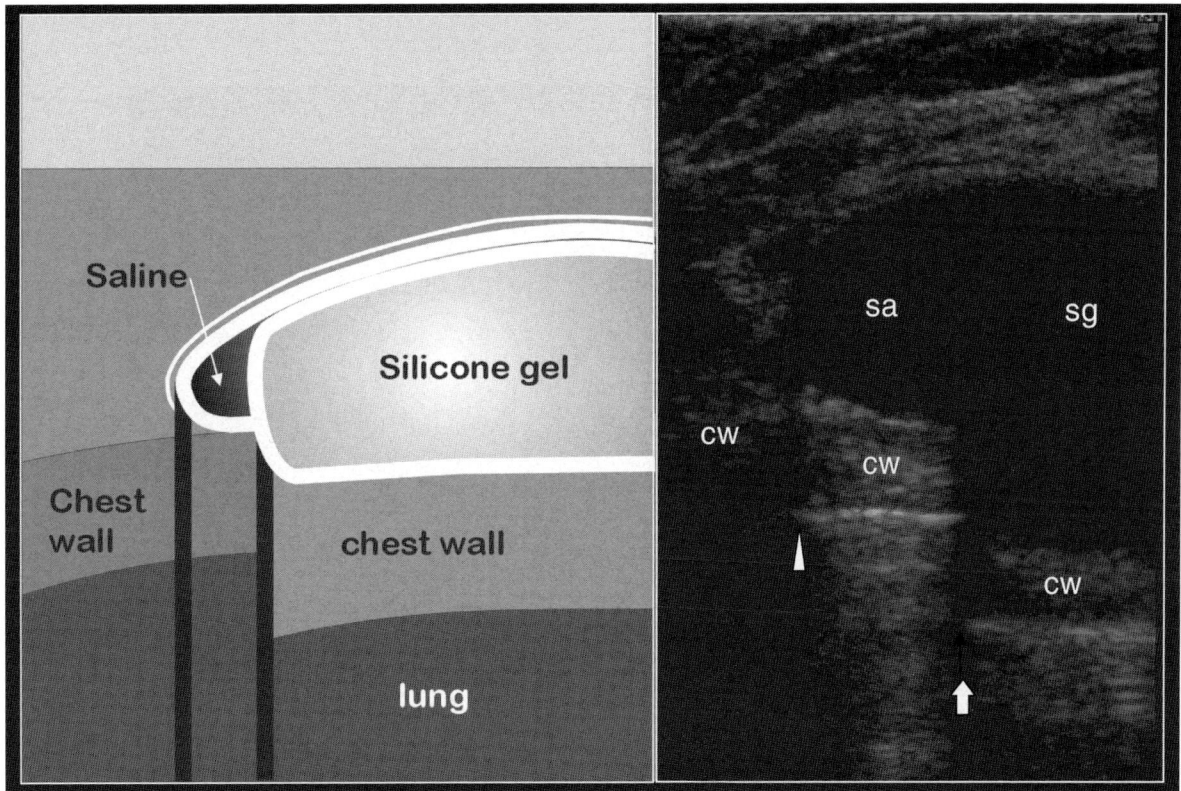

FIGURE 9–14 In double-lumen implants that have a saline-filled outer compartment and a silicone gel–filled inner compartment, there will be no step-off at the edge of the outer saline-containing compartment *(arrowhead),* but there will be a step-off at the edge of the inner compartment *(arrow).* sa, saline in outer compartment; sg, silicone gel in inner compartment; cw, chest wall.

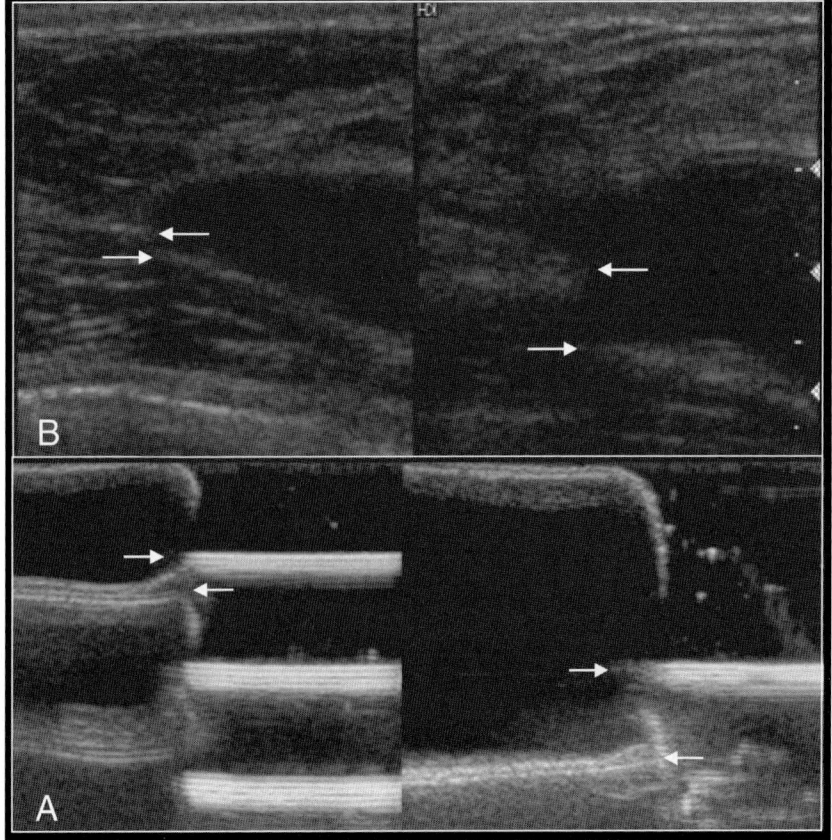

FIGURE 9–15 A: A single-lumen silicone gel implant scanned *in vitro* in a water bath with heavy compression (**left**) and light compression (**right**). **B:** A single-lumen silicone gel implant *in vivo* scanned with heavy compression (**left**) and light compression (**right**). Both *in vitro* and *in vivo,* heavy compression, by flattening the implant and minimizing the thickness of silicone gel that the ultrasound beam must traverse, minimizes the effects of the slower speed of sound through the implant and minimizes the artifactual step-off deep to the implant that enables us to determine that the implant is filled with silicone gel rather than saline. Using light compression improves our ability to distinguish between single-lumen saline and silicone gel implants.

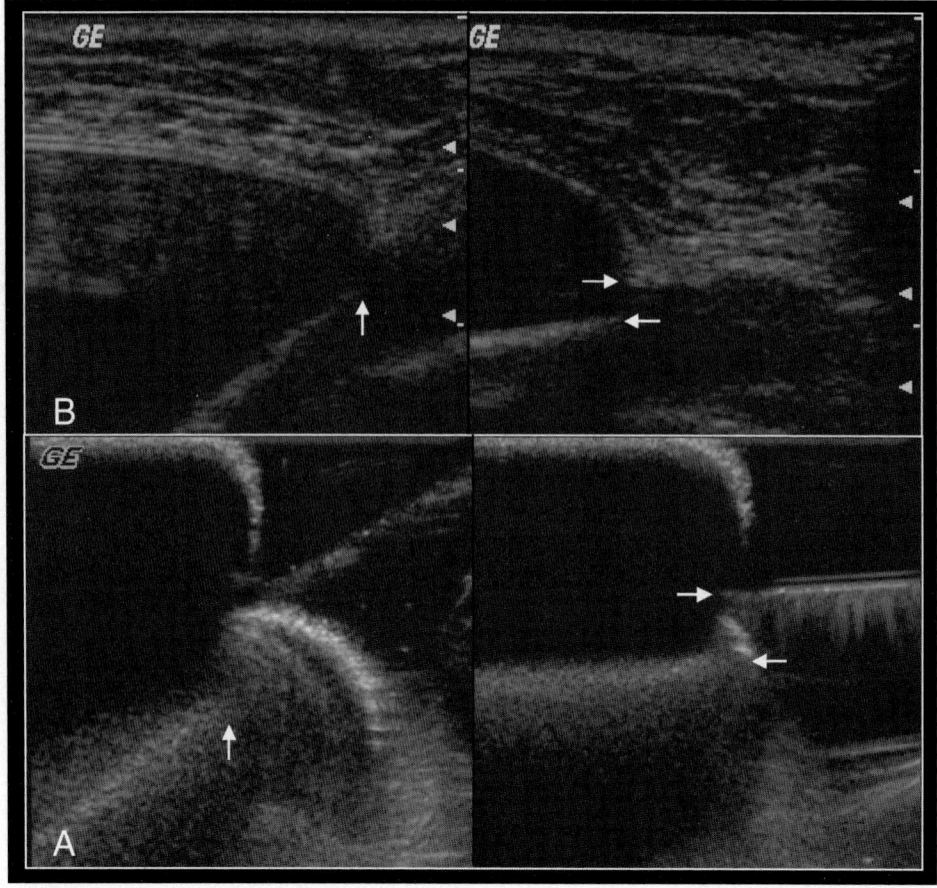

FIGURE 9–16 A: *In vitro* scans of the edge of a single-lumen silicone gel implant scanned at angle of incidence relative to the water bath that is oblique (**left**) and parallel (**right**). **B:** *In vivo* scans of the edge of a single-lumen silicone gel implant scanned at angle of incidence relative to the chest wall that are oblique (**left**) and parallel (**right**). Note that the images obtained at angles of incidence that are obliquely oriented with respect to the chest wall minimize the artifactual step-off deep to the implant. Scans obtained parallel to the water bath or chest wall maximize the artifactual step-off and improve our chances of correctly determining that the implants are filled with silicone gel.

such cases, there has usually been a previous unilateral rupture of a single-lumen silicone gel implant requiring explantation of the ruptured implant and reimplantation with a saline implant (Fig. 9–17).

Folds and Lobulations of the Elastomer Implant Membrane

The degree of wrinkling, folding, and lobulation in the implant membrane varies, generally being greater in saline than silicone gel implants. Wrinkles should be distinguished from folds. In wrinkles, the outer contour of the implant is lobulated, but the fibrous periimplant capsule and the elastomer shell remain parallel and tightly apposed to the shell throughout the course of the lobulation (Fig. 9–18, left). In radial folds, on the other hand, the outer contour of the implant may be maintained, but the elastomer shell invaginates and separates from the capsule, cre-

ating a potential space between the shell and capsule (Fig. 9–18, right).

Folds that are thin, that course into the implant contents nearly perpendicular to the outer membrane surface, and that do not contain significant space or fluid within them are radial folds that are considered variants of normal. These folds are generally of little immediate significance, except that they may be the cause of palpable abnormalities if they occur on the anterior surface of the implant shell (Fig. 9–19, left). Radial folds that lie on the posterior surface of the implant are never palpable (Fig. 9–19, right). Radial folds are dynamic structures and are not fixed in position and size. They occur because the relative size and position of the shell and capsule may vary in different patient positions and with different patient activities. Thus, a redundancy of the shell in a certain location that results in its in-folding may be present only in the

(text continued on page 219)

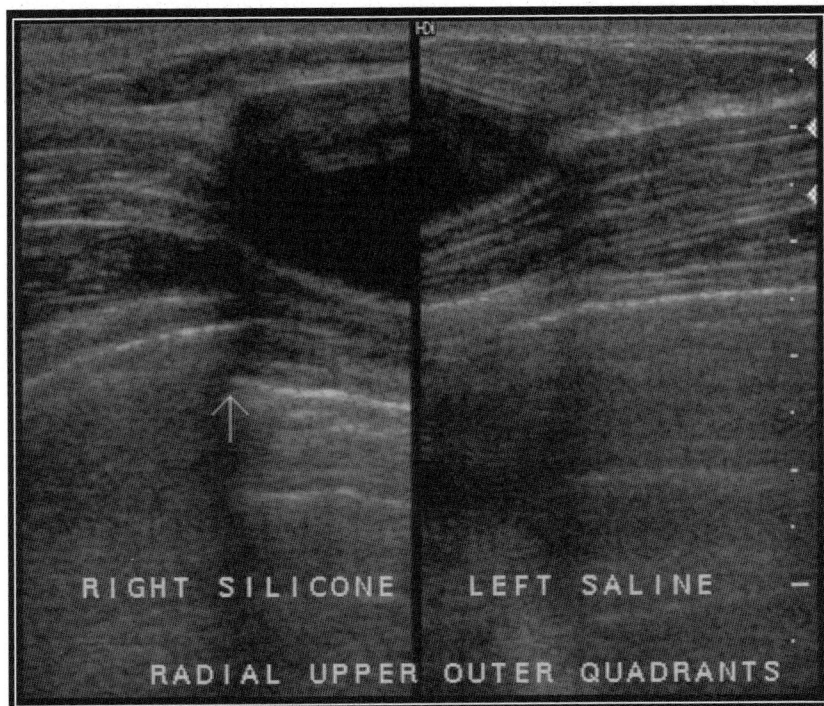

FIGURE 9–17 Sonograms of the edge of these implants show an artifactual step-off in the chest wall at the edge of the patient's right implant *(arrow)*, which is the original single-lumen silicone gel implant. There is no step-off in the chest wall at the edge of the newer, reimplanted single-lumen saline implant on the patient's left side.

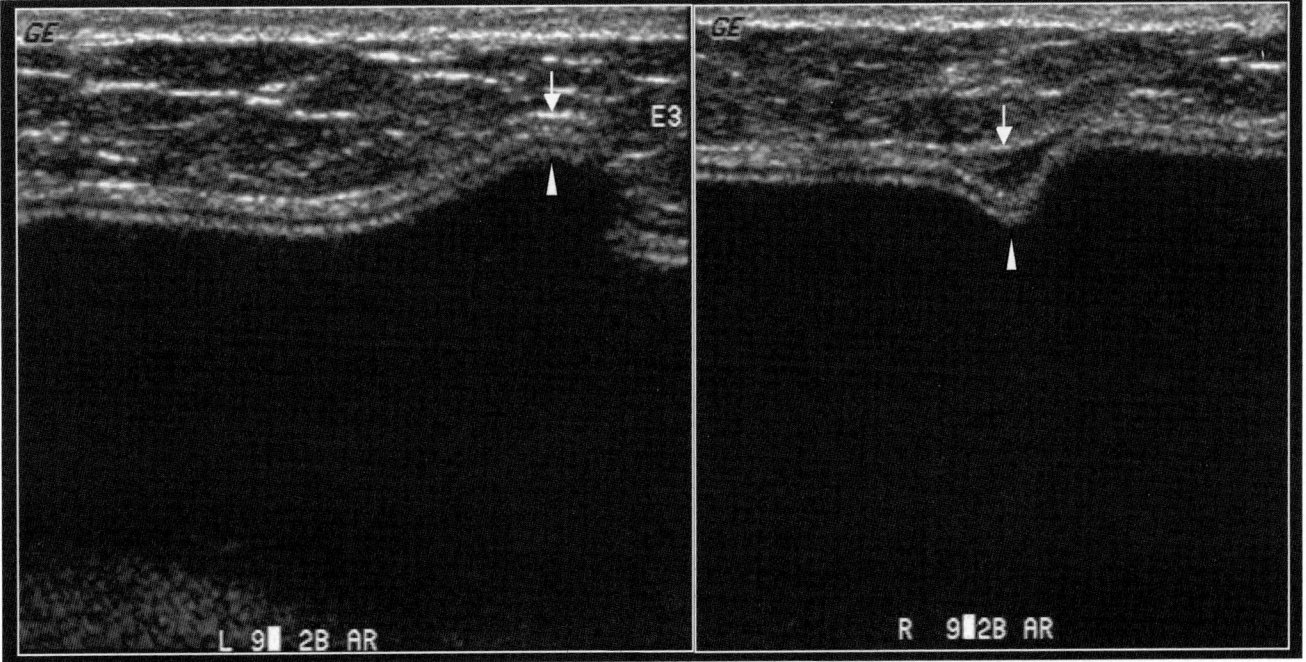

FIGURE 9–18 The **right** image demonstrates a short-axis view through a radial fold. The shell *(arrowhead)* has invaginated away from the capsule *(arrow)*, creating a potential space for either periimplant effusion or extravasated intracapsular silicone gel to accumulate. The **left** image shows a wrinkle in a different part of the same implant. The fibrous periimplant capsule *(arrow)* remains parallel to the silicone elastomer implant shell *(arrowhead)* throughout the course of the undulation.

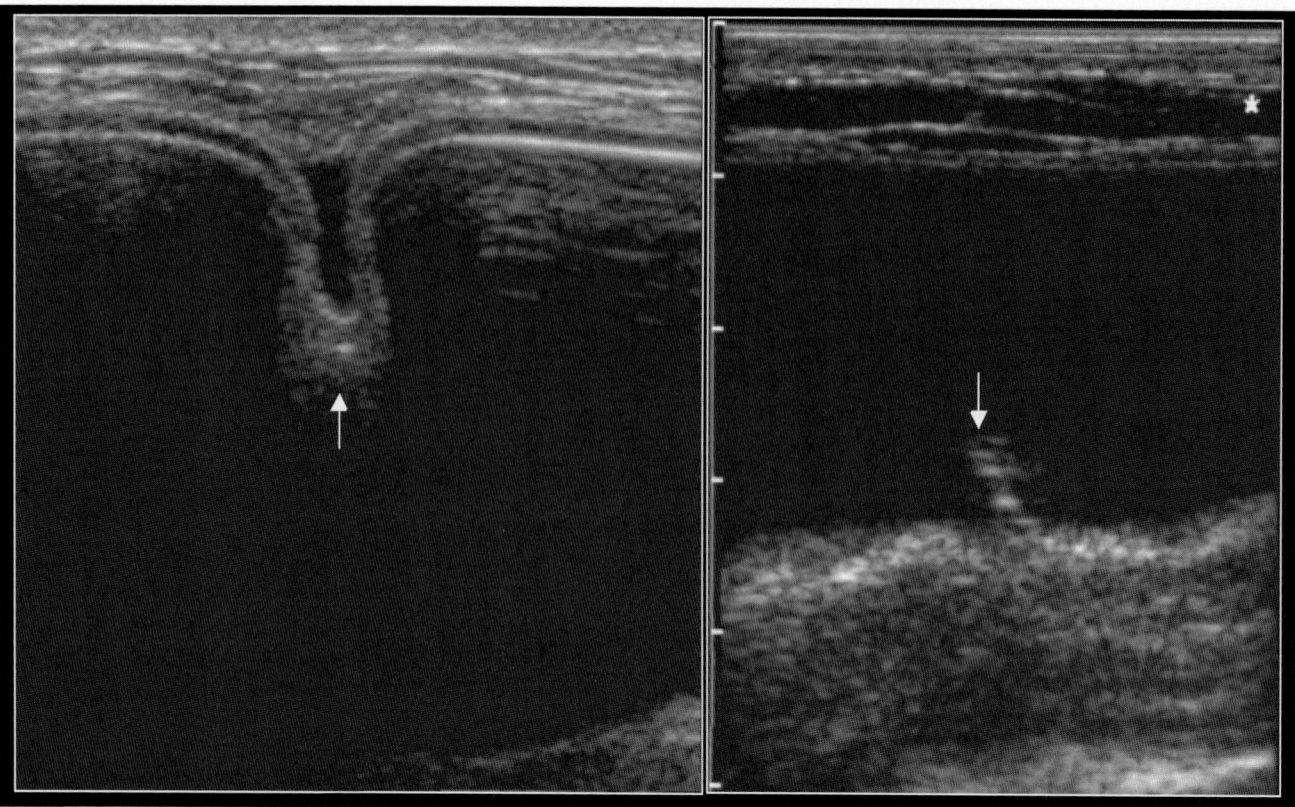

FIGURE 9–19 Radial folds that lie along the anterior aspect of implants may be the cause of palpable abnormalities, especially if there is little overlying breast tissue (**left**, *arrow*). Radial folds along the posterior aspect of the implant are not palpable (**right**, *arrow*)

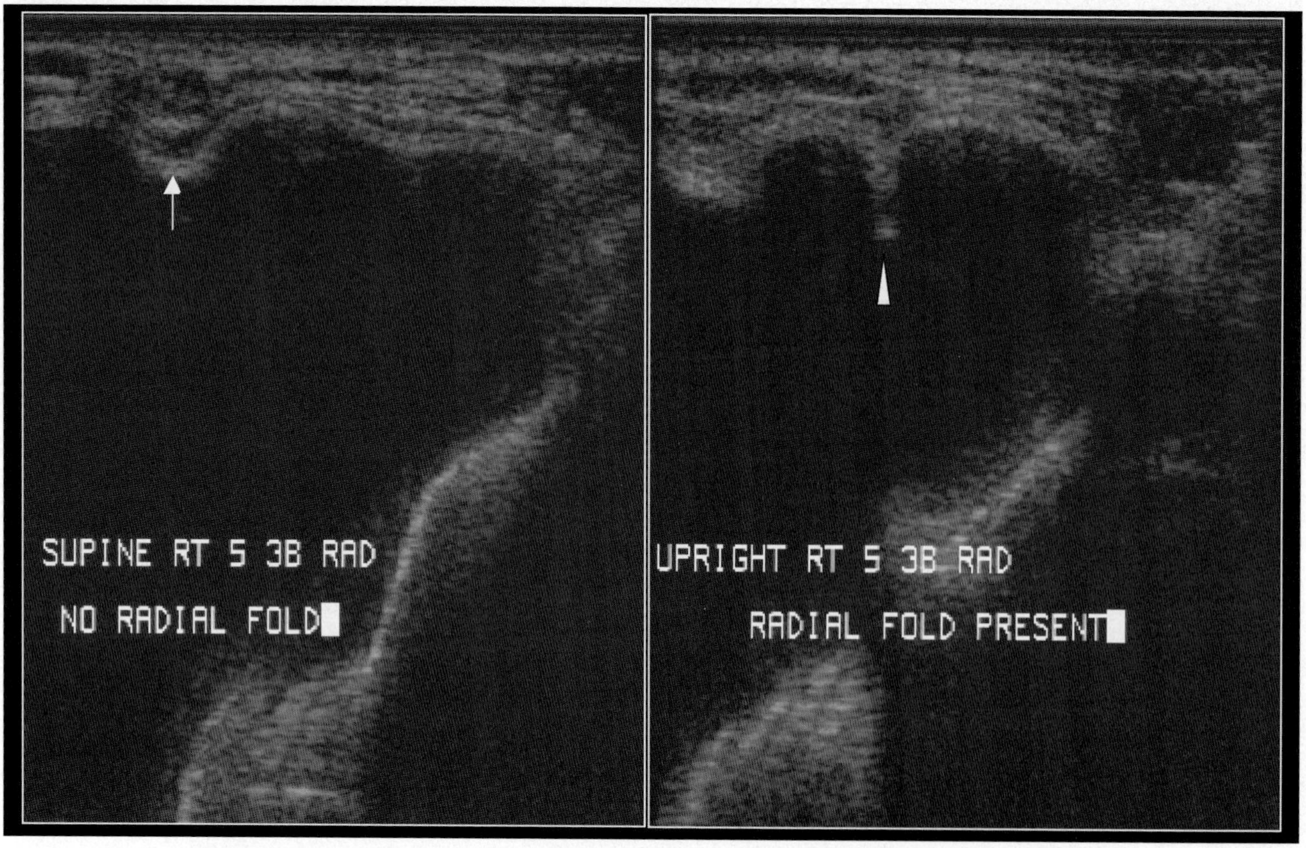

SUPINE RT 5 3B RAD
NO RADIAL FOLD▮

UPRIGHT RT 5 3B RAD
RADIAL FOLD PRESENT▮

FIGURE 9–20 Radial folds are dynamic and may be present only in certain positions. This radial fold formed and was palpable only in the upright position.

upright position, whereas a redundancy in the shell in a different part of the implant resulting in an in-folding may only be present in the supine position.

Because radial folds are dynamic, such a fold may be present and cause a palpable abnormality when the patient is in the upright position, but not when she is in the supine position in which patients are normally scanned. In such a case, scanning the patient in the supine position will fail to reveal the definitive cause of the palpable abnormality. For this reason, patients with implants who complain of palpable lumps that are present only in a certain position (upright) should be scanned in that position (upright) to maximize the chances of finding a definitive cause (Fig. 9–20).

Although radial folds likely have no short-term significance, they may be significant in the long term. The apices of these folds are probably subject to increased stress and fatigue fractures and may increase the risk for rupture. Distinguishing a radial fold that is a variant of normal from one that has undergone fatigue fracture and that is the site of localized intracapsular rupture can be difficult in certain cases and impossible in others and is discussed in more detail later in this chapter in the section on Intracapsular Rupture.

Implant Fill Valves or Ports

Saline implants, expanders, and certain double-lumen implants have fill valves or ports. There are various types and locations for fill ports. Two main classes of fill valves can be identified sonographically: diaphragm fill valves, which are by far the most frequently seen; and leaflet fill valves, which are less common. Diaphragm fill valves consist of the valve, an anchor on either end, and an elastomer strap that covers the outer surface of the valve (Fig. 9–21). The strap can be displaced to the side to allow the needle to enter the valve (Fig. 9–22). All of these parts are sonographically demonstrable *in vitro* (Fig. 9–23) and *in vivo* (Fig. 9–23B). The elastomer strap is the most difficult component to demonstrate and in some cases may not be demonstrable. There are different types of diaphragm fill valves. The second most common type of fill valve is discoid in shape rather than rectangular (Fig. 9–24). Leaflet fill valves lie internally and are unlikely to cause palpable abnormalities. Leaflet fill valves consist of an elastomer tube that extends internally into the implant from anteriorly that may be collapsed (Fig. 9–25, left) or distended with saline (Fig. 9–25, right). It is important not to confuse a leaflet fill valve with a collapsed implant shell in intracapsular rupture.

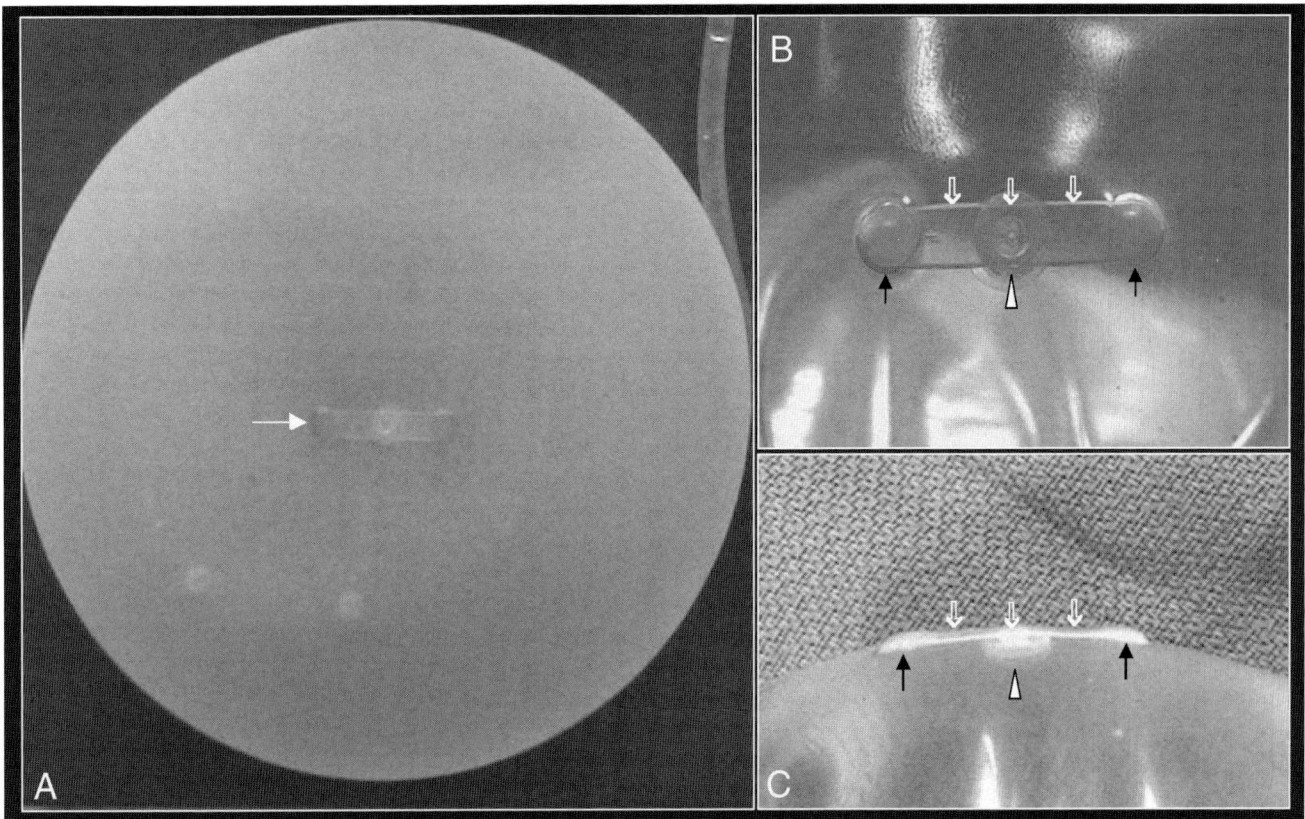

FIGURE 9–21 A: All single-lumen saline implants have a fill valve on the anterior surface *(arrow).* This is a diaphragm-type fill valve on the anterior surface of a lightly textured single lumen saline implant. The anterior **(B)** and side views **(C)** of a diaphragm fill valve on a nontextured single-lumen saline implant show several components: valve *(white arrowhead),* strap anchors *(black arrows),* and elastomer strap that covers the valve *(hollow white arrows).*

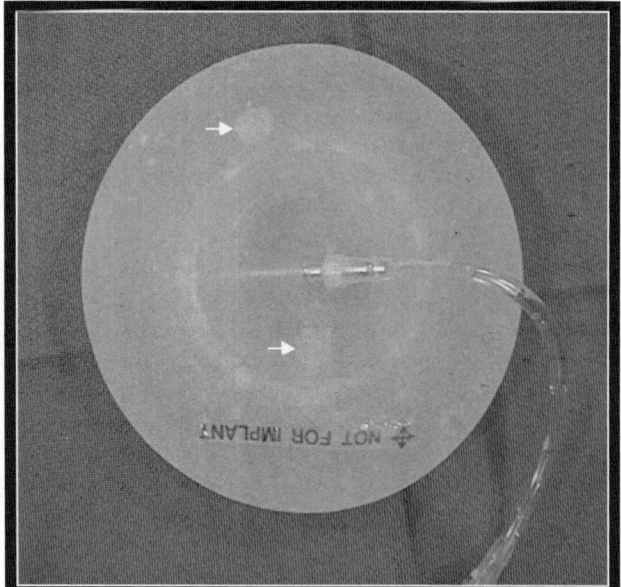

FIGURE 9–22 This is an anterior view of a lightly textured single-lumen saline implant with the special needle inserted through the diaphragm fill valve into the implant. Air bubbles *(arrows)* have been injected into the implant with the saline.

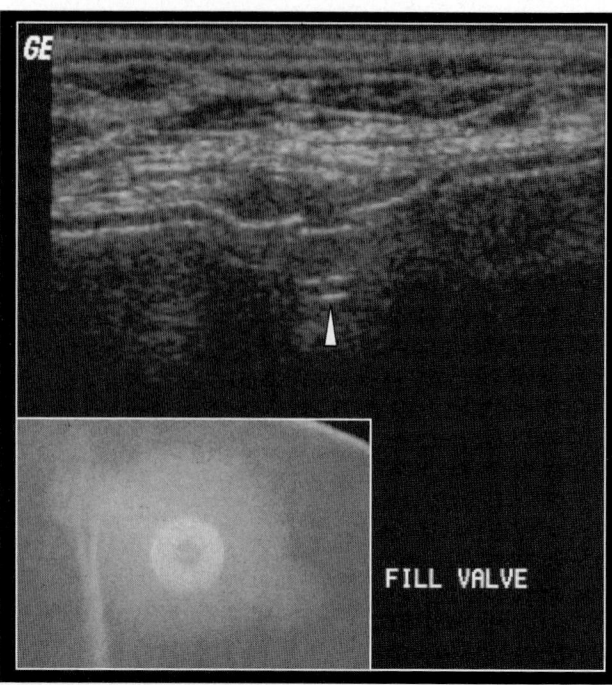

FIGURE 9–24 This discoid fill valve *(arrowhead)* is the second most common type seen.

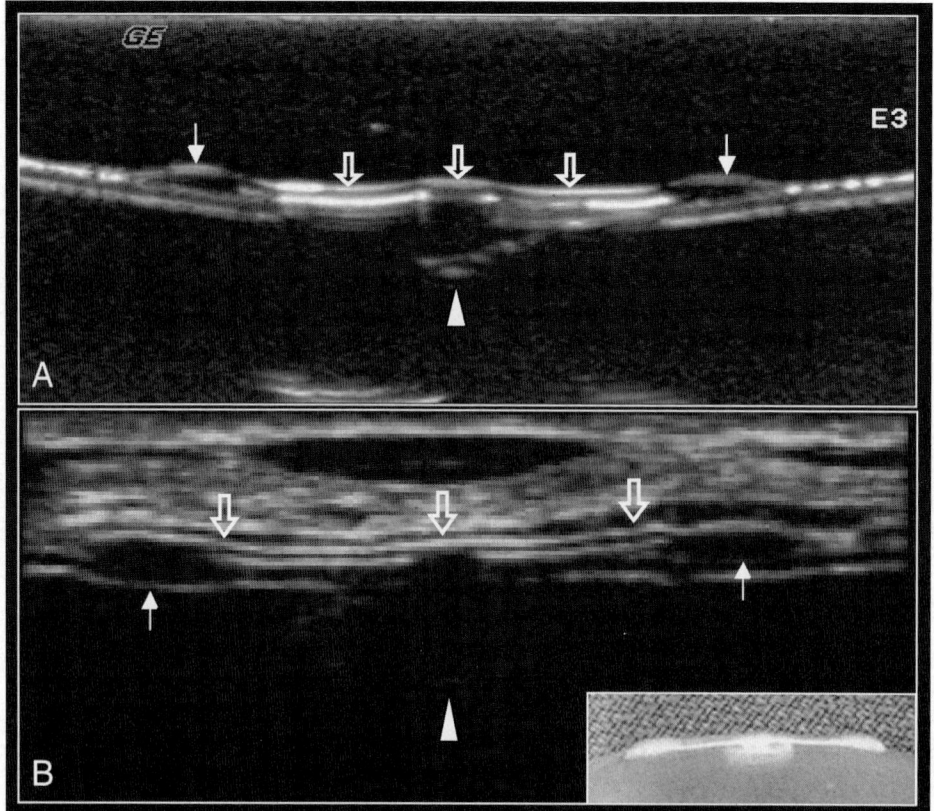

FIGURE 9–23 These are long-axis views of diaphragm fill valves on single-lumen saline implants obtained *in vitro* within a water bath (**A**) and *in vivo* (**B**). The *white arrowheads* point to the valves, the *hollow arrows* point to the elastomer strap that covers the outer surface of the valve, and the *white solid arrows* point to the anchors.

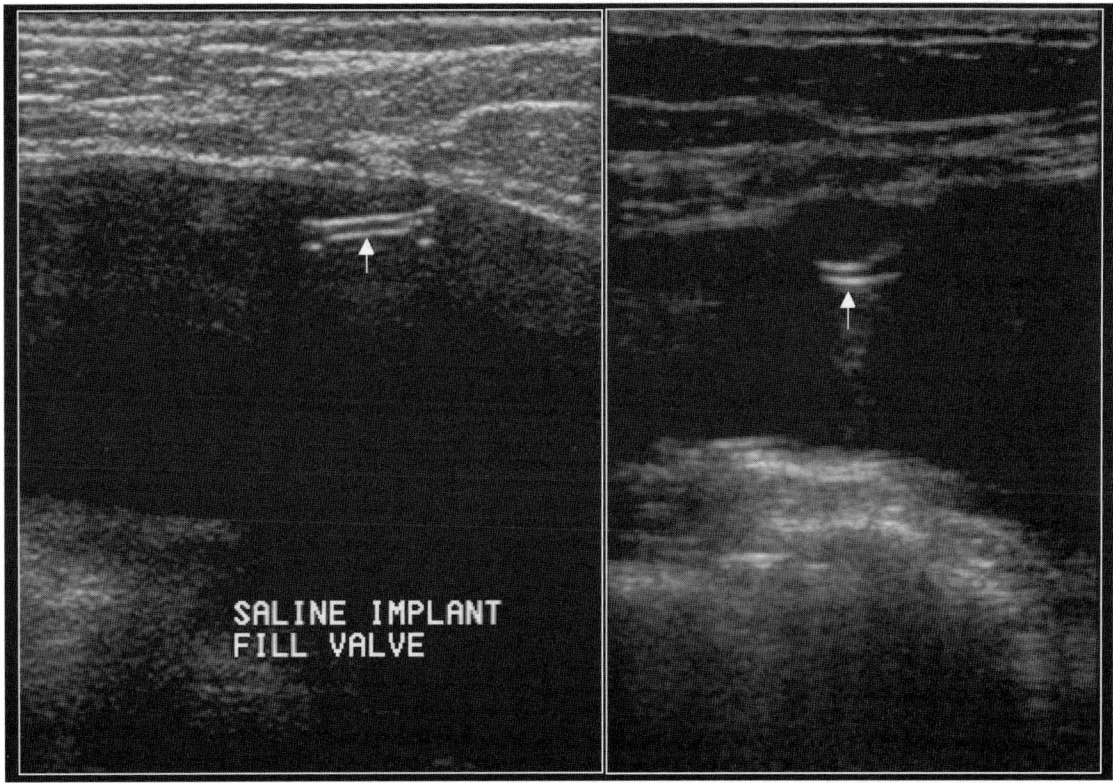

FIGURE 9–25 These are leaflet-type fill valves within a single-lumen saline implant. The leaflet fill valve on the **left** *(arrows)* is collapsed. The leaflet fill valve on the **right** *(arrows)* is distended with saline.

The valves are typically placed bilaterally symmetrically in the subareolar region, where they are sonographically visible, but not palpable. However, in some cases, a valve may not initially be placed subareolarly, and in other cases, it may migrate or rotate out from the subareolar reason as a result of asymmetric capsular contracture or capsular herniation. A valve that is not subareolar in location often has less breast tissue overlying it than does a subareolar valve and therefore may become palpable. That the valve causes the palpable abnormality for which the patient presents can be shown definitively by sonography, allaying patient and referring physician fears (Fig. 9–26). In other cases, a valve may become palpable because it has become everted owing to increased intraimplant pressure caused by capsular contracture. The eversion of the valve causes it to become palpable (Fig. 9–27).

Echogenicity of Silicone Gel

Normally, the silicone gel within single-lumen implants is anechoic except for near-field artifactual echoes. However, in certain patients who have neither intracapsular nor extracapsular rupture, heterogeneous echoes may be scattered throughout the gel (Fig. 9–28, left). These echoes might represent saline, povidone-iodine, antibiotics, or some other substance that was injected at the time of implantation, but in many cases, their cause is

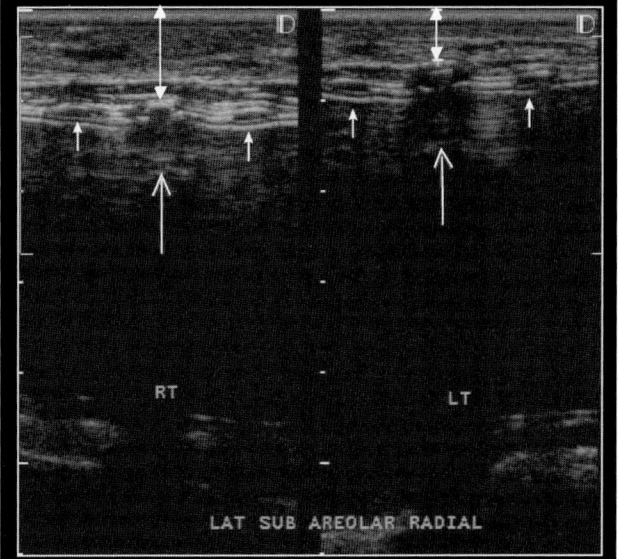

FIGURE 9–26 Valves are often placed directly behind the nipple, where they are not palpable. However, fill valves can cause palpable abnormalities in certain patients. This patient presented with a palpable lump on her left side that simultaneous scanning and palpation showed to be caused by a diaphragm fill valve *(long arrow)* that was asymmetrically placed medial to the nipple. The thickness of breast tissue overlying the left valve *(double-headed arrow)* is much less than on the right. The valve in her right implant lay in a normal position deep to the nipple *(short arrows* indicate anchors).

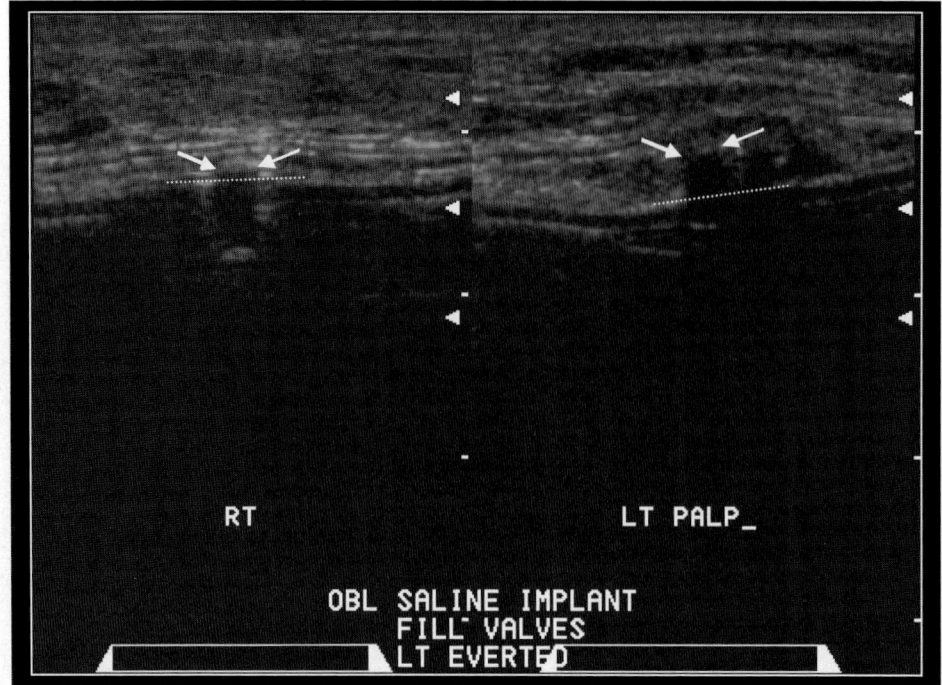

FIGURE 9–27 Fill valves on single-lumen saline implants can become palpable if the valve everts because of increased intraimplant pressure caused by chronic capsular contracture. Note that the nonpalpable normal valve on the **right** protrudes internally into the implant shell and that its outer surface of the valve (**left**, *arrows*) barely protrudes beyond the outer surface of the implant shell (**left**, *dotted line*). Note that the palpable valve on the left is abnormally everted and that the outer surface of the valve (**right**, *arrows*) protrudes well beyond the outer surface of the implant shell (**right**, *dotted lines*).

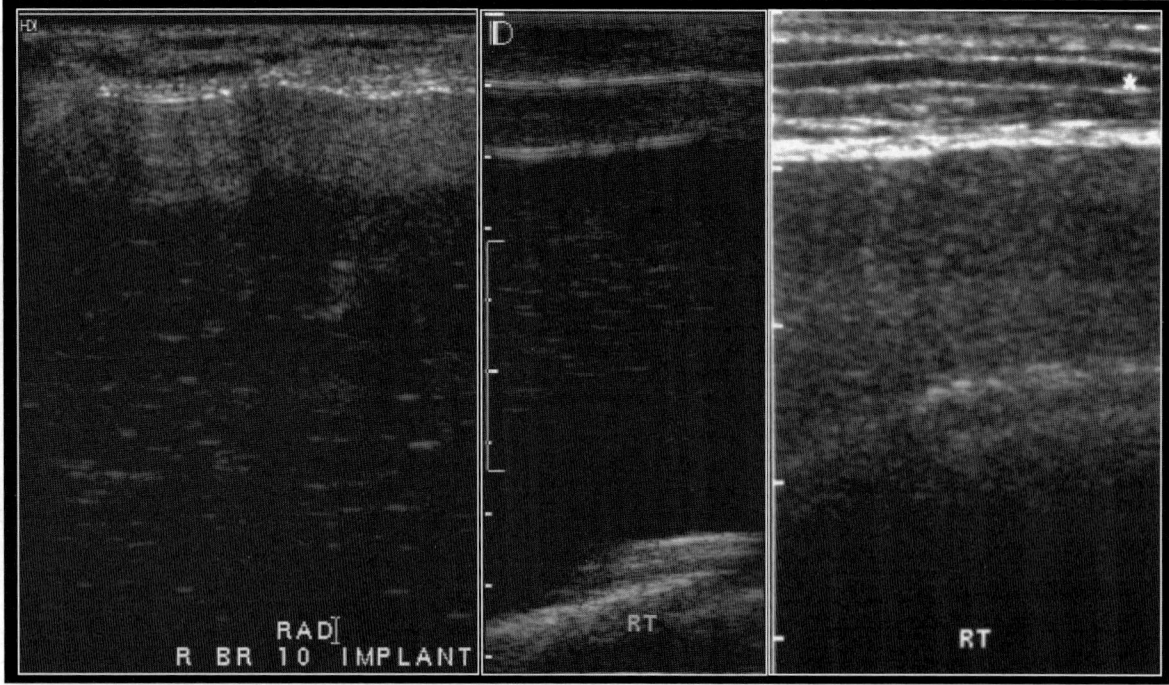

FIGURE 9–28 Although silicone gel normally is anechoic, in some patients with apparently normal implants, there are scattered heterogenous echoes within the gel. The cause of these normal echoes is usually unknown (**left**). In other cases, internal echoes may represent gas bubbles that have come out of the solution as a result of low barometric pressures at high altitude (**middle**). The increased echoes that occur within extravasated gel in cases of intracapsular rupture are smaller, more diffuse, and more homogeneous than are normal variant echoes (**right**).

unknown. In certain patients, these heterogeneous echoes appear to be gas bubbles that come out of solution under high-altitude, low-barometric pressure conditions (Fig. 9–28, middle). These normal variant echoes are more heterogeneous than the diffusely increased echogenicity that occurs within extravasated gel in intracapsular rupture (Fig. 9–28, right).

Sonographic Appearance of the Elastomer Implant Membrane

Implant shell types include smooth, lightly textured, heavily textured, and polyurethane textured (Fig. 9–29). In most cases, when proper equipment is available and proper technique is used, sonography can distinguish between the different types of implant shells. The appearance of implant elastomer shells will vary, depending on transducer frequency, bandwidth, depth of field, magnification, and angle of incidence. With 5- to 7.5-MHz narrow-bandwidth beams, depth of field in excess of 7 cm, and no magnification, the elastomer shell will usually be seen as a single echogenic line. In such cases, smooth implants are demonstrated as a thin, single echogenic line, whereas textured implants are seen as a thicker echogenic line, and heavily textured and polyurethane-coated shells appear as very thick echogenic lines (Fig. 9–30A, B). With 10- to 12-MHz broad-bandwidth beams, depth of field less than 5 cm, and magnification, the inner and outer surfaces of the shell each create echogenic lines that are separated by an anechoic space representing the thickness of the shell (Fig. 9–30C, D). The sonographic appearance of two parallel echogenic lines with an anechoic space between them is similar to that of an Oreo cookie that has been video-inverted—the "reverse Oreo cookie sign" (Fig. 9–31).

Only the outer surface of textured shells is textured. The inner surface, like the outer surface of nontextured shells, is smooth. Smooth shell surfaces are represented as thin, echogenic lines on ultrasound, whereas textured shell surfaces are represented by thick, ill-defined echogenic lines. Thus, both surfaces of nontextured shells are represented by thin, echogenic lines. The outer surface of textures shells is represented by a thick, less well-defined line,

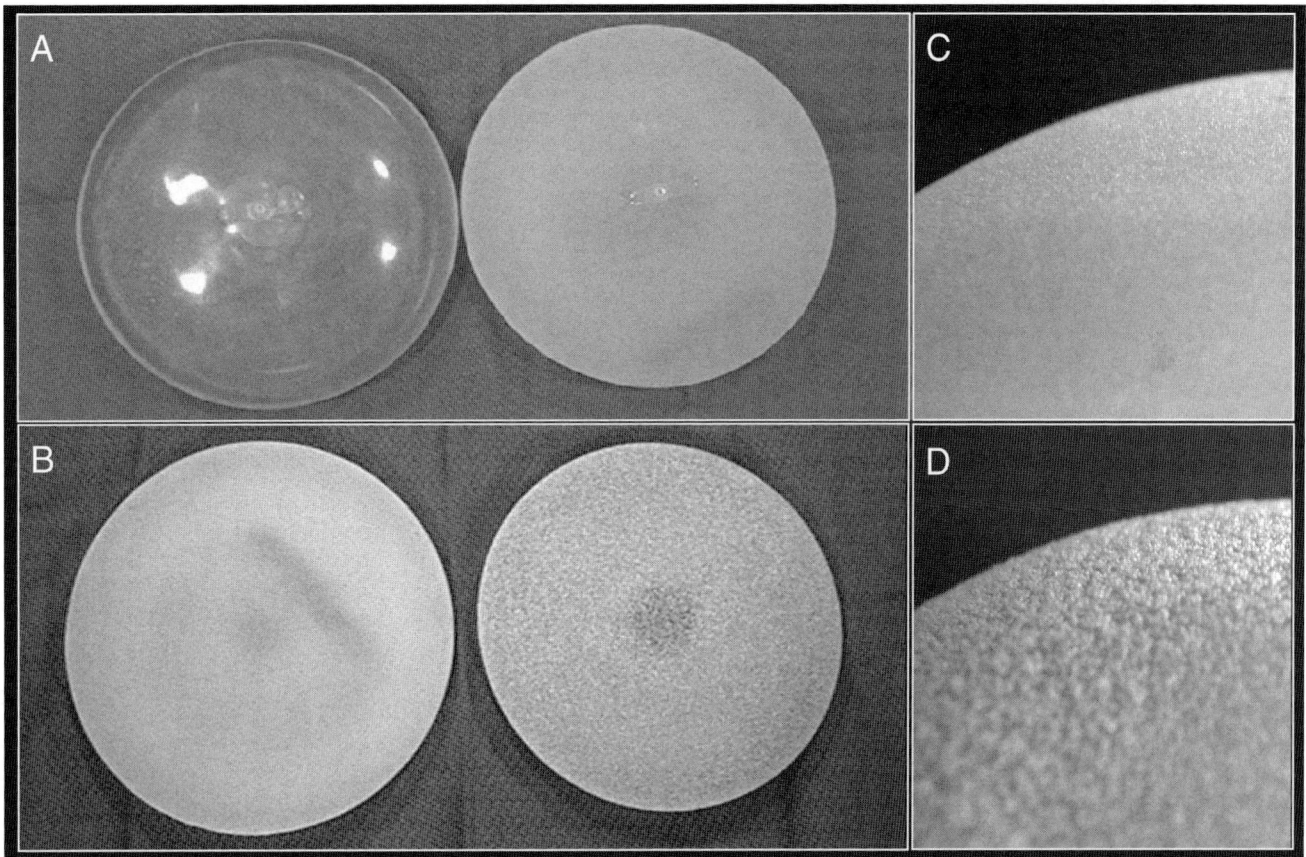

FIGURE 9–29 A: This is an anterior view of single-lumen saline implants, nontextured on the **left** and lightly textured on the **right.** Both have diaphragm type fill valves. **B:** This is an anterior view of two single-lumen silicone gel implants, lightly textured on the **left** and heavily textured on the **right.** Note that neither has a fill valve. **C:** This is a close-up view of the surface of a lightly textured implant. **D:** This is a close-up view of the surface of a heavily textured implant.

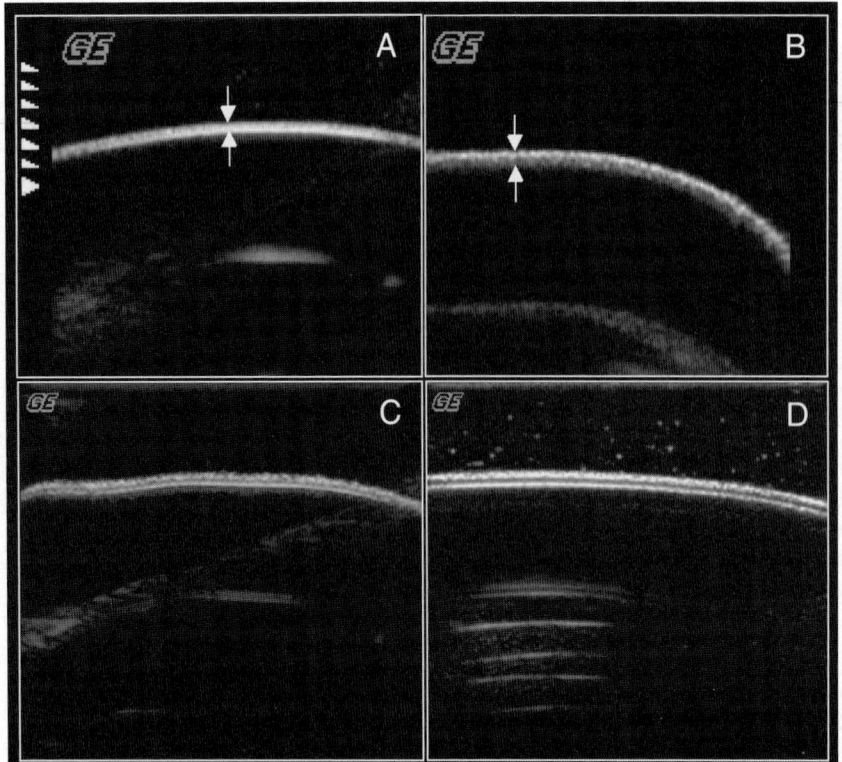

FIGURE 9–30 The *in vitro* images of lightly (**left**) and heavily (**right**) textured single-lumen silicone gel implants scanned in a water bath obtained with mid-transducer frequency (9 MHz) and large depth of field (7 cm) demonstrates only a single echogenic line *(arrows)* representing the shell of each implant. The echogenic line for the lightly textured implant (**A**) is thinner and better defined than that for the heavily textured implant (**B**). At higher transducer frequencies and lesser depths of field, however, the shell appears as a double echogenic line. The lightly textured shell (**C**) is thinner than the heavily textured shell (**D**).

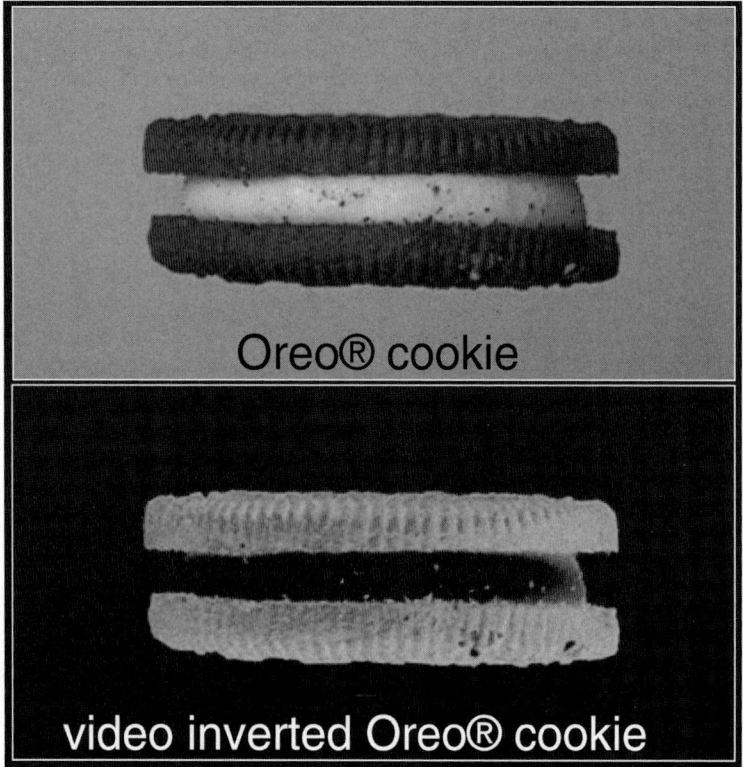

FIGURE 9–31 With proper equipment and technique, the sonographic appearance of the implant shell can be likened to a video inverted or reversed Oreo cookie. The anterior echogenic line represents the outer surface of the shell, the posterior echogenic line represents the inner surface of the shell, and the anechoic space between the echogenic lines represents the thickness of the shell.

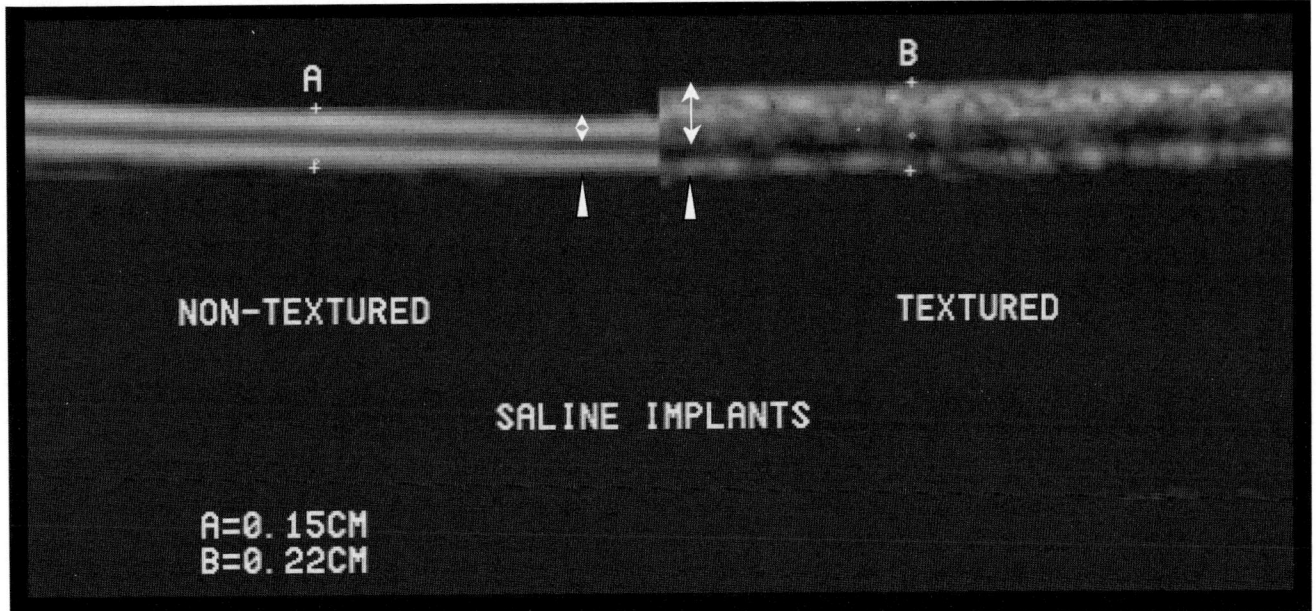

FIGURE 9–32 The overall thickness of textured shells (**right**) is greater than the thickness of nontextured shells (**left**). These *in vitro* images of nontextured (**left**) and lightly textured (**right**) implant shells scanned in a water bath were obtained with a 12-MHz transducer, a 5-cm depth of field, and write magnification. The inner surface of both nontextured and textured shells is smooth and represented by a thin, echogenic line *(arrowheads).* The outer surface of the non-textured shell is also represented by a thin, echogenic line (**left**, *double-headed arrow*). The outer surface of the textured shell is represented by a thick, ill-defined line (**right**, *double-headed arrow*).

whereas the inner surface is represented by a thin, echogenic line (Fig. 9–32). The shell of textured implants may actually be represented by three echogenic lines when scanned with very-high-frequency, broad-bandwidth transducers (12 MHz and higher). The two inner thin, echogenic lines represent the smooth inner and outer layers of the shell to which texture has been layered on the outer surface. The thicker, less well-defined outer layer represents the adherent texture. Heavily textured shells are thicker than lightly textured shells only in the outer texture (Fig. 9–33A). The echogenic line that represents the outer surface of heavily textured or polyurethane-coated shells may become so thick and ill defined and may absorb so much sound that it completely obscures the inner layer unless the shell lies precisely perpendicular to the beam (Fig. 9–33B).

The periimplant fibrous capsule is also represented by two echogenic lines representing its inner and outer surfaces. The isoechoic space between the two echogenic lines represents the thickness of the capsule (Fig. 9–34). However, because the echogenic lines that represent the inner surface of the capsule and the outer surface of the shell are in immediate contact with each other, they appear to be a single echogenic line. Thus, the capsule–shell complex of most implants is represented by three echogenic lines: the outer line representing the leading surface of the capsule,

the middle echogenic line consisting of the fused echogenic lines that represent the inner surface of the capsule and the outer surface of the shell, and the inner echogenic line representing the inner surface of the shell. The isoechoic or anechoic space between the outer and middle echogenic lines represents either the thickness of the capsule or the thickness of the capsule together with the periimplant effusion. The anechoic space between the middle and inner echogenic lines represents the thickness of the shell (Figs. 9–35 and 9–36).

The thickness of nontextured shells varies greatly. Most old nontextured implants implanted in the 1970s and early 1980s had very thin shells. Because of the high incidence of implant rupture after 12 to 15 years, new implants have been made with much thicker shells (Fig. 9–37). The middle echogenic line that represents a combination of the outer surface of the shell and inner surface of the capsule differs between nontextured and textured implants. It is thin when the implant is nontextured and thick or multilaminar when the implant is textured (Fig. 9–38A, B). It can be very difficult or impossible to demonstrate around heavily textured implants (Fig. 9–38C, D). The capsule is virtually never identified along the anterior surface of polyurethane-coated implants but usually can be

(text continued on page 228)

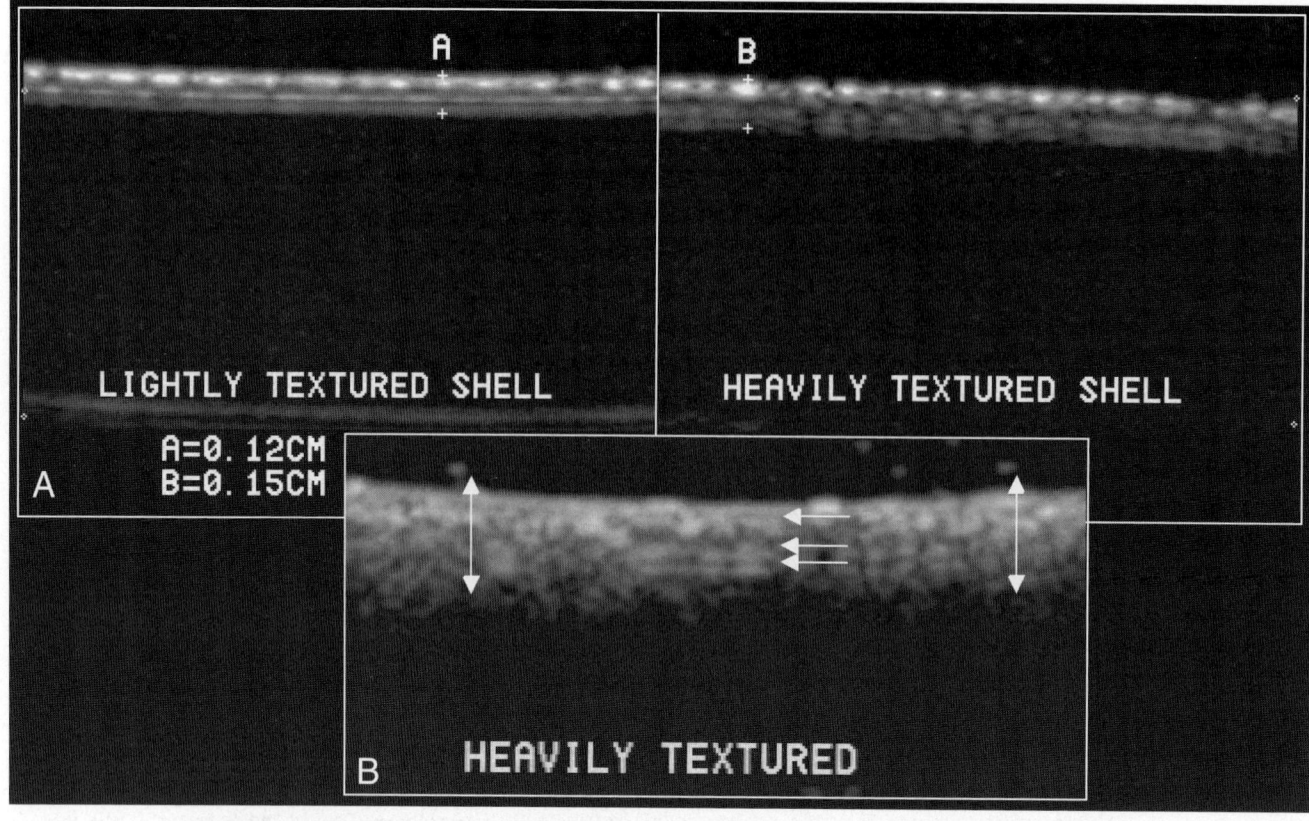

FIGURE 9–33 A: Both lightly and heavily textured implant shells may have a trilaminar appearance when scanned with very high frequency exactly perpendicular to the shell and at high levels of magnification. These *in vitro* images of lightly (**left**) and heavily (**right**) textured single-lumen silicone gel implants show the shells to be represented by three rather than two echogenic lines. The outer thicker and less well-defined echogenic line is caused by the texture on the outer surface of the shell. The middle echogenic line is the outer surface of the elastomer membrane to which the texture adheres. The posterior echogenic line represents the smooth inner surface of the elastomer membrane. The heavily textured implant shell is thicker overall than the lightly textured shell. The difference in the thickness between lightly and heavily textured shells is only in the superficial line that represents the texture. **B:** The outer surface of heavily textured shells may cause enough incoherence of the beam to obscure the echogenic lines that represent the inner surface of the shell. The shell will appear to be a single, very thick and very ill-defined line in the places where the shell is not exactly perpendicular to the beam *(double-headed arrows)*. Where the shell is precisely 90 degrees to the beam, the shell may appear multilaminar *(horizontal arrows)*.

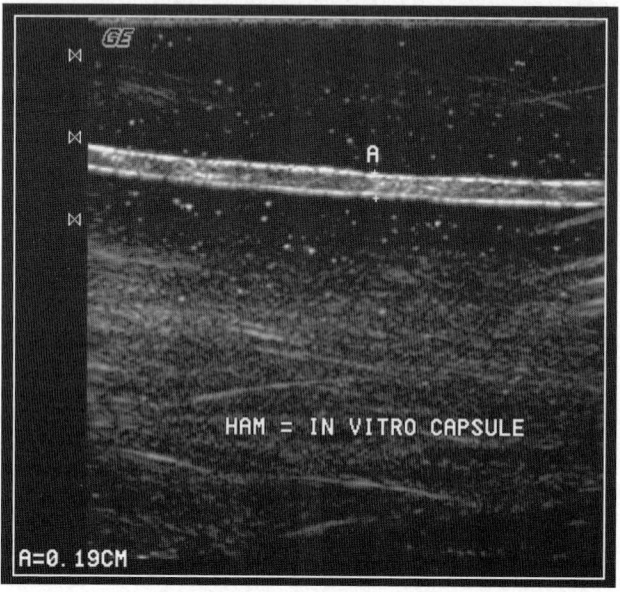

FIGURE 9–34 This is an *in vitro* image of thinly sliced ham scanned in a water bath with a 12-MHz transducer, shallow depth of field, and magnification. The thickness of this slice of ham is similar to the thickness of an abnormally thickened contracted periimplant capsule—between 1.5 and 2.5 mm. The anterior echogenic line corresponds to the outer surface of the capsule (ham), the posterior echogenic line corresponds to the inner surface of the capsule (ham), and the isoechoic space between the echogenic lines represents the thickness of the capsule.

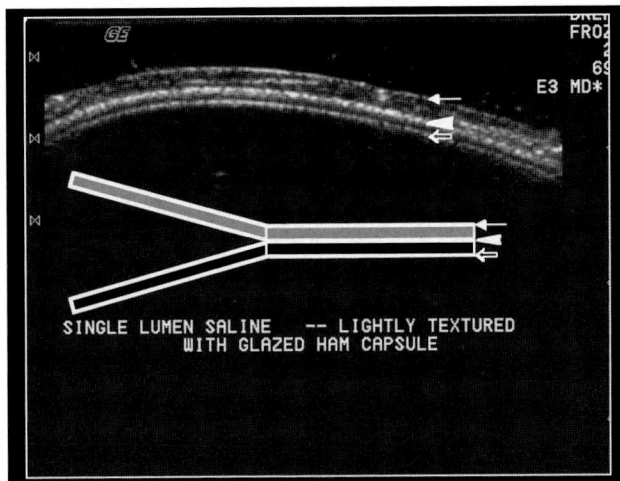

FIGURE 9–35 This *in vitro* image simulates the appearance of capsular contracture. A slice of ham was placed over the surface of a lightly textured implant, and the complex was scanned in a water bath with a 12-MHz transducer, shallow depth of field, and write magnification. Note that the capsule–shell complex is represented by three echogenic lines rather than four. The anterior echogenic line represents the outer surface of the abnormally thickened fibrous capsule *(arrow)*. The middle echogenic line represents a merger of the inner surface of the thickened capsule and the outer surface of the shell *(arrowhead)*. The inner echogenic line represents the smooth inner surface of the shell *(hollow arrow)*. The anechoic space between the middle and posterior echogenic lines represents the thickness of the shell.

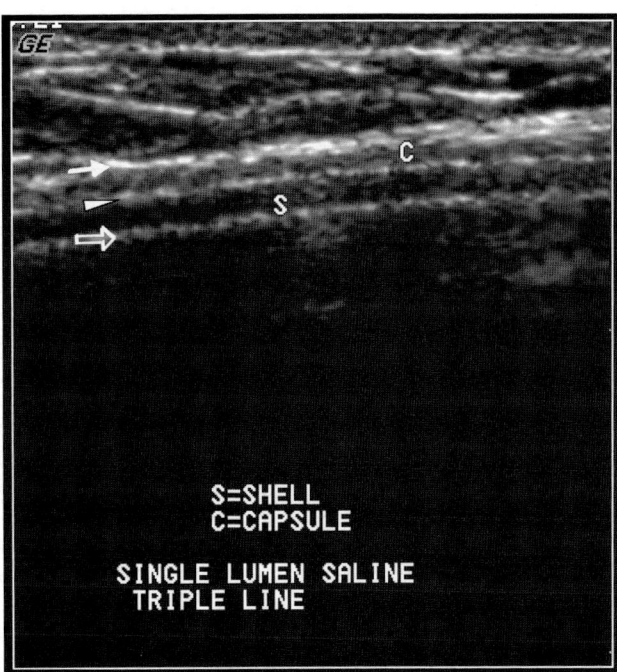

FIGURE 9–36 This *in vivo* image shows the capsule–shell echo complex in a patient who has a nontextured single-lumen implant and capsular contracture. The capsule–shell complex is represented by three echogenic lines. The anterior echogenic line is the outer surface of the capsule *(arrow)*, the middle echogenic line is the merged echo of the inner surface of the capsule and outer surface of the shell *(arrowhead)*, and the posterior echogenic line represents the inner surface of the shell *(hollow arrow)*. The space between the anterior and middle echogenic lines *(C)* represents the thickness of the capsule and is typically isoechoic. The space between the middle and posterior echogenic lines represents the thickness of the shell *(S)* and is anechoic.

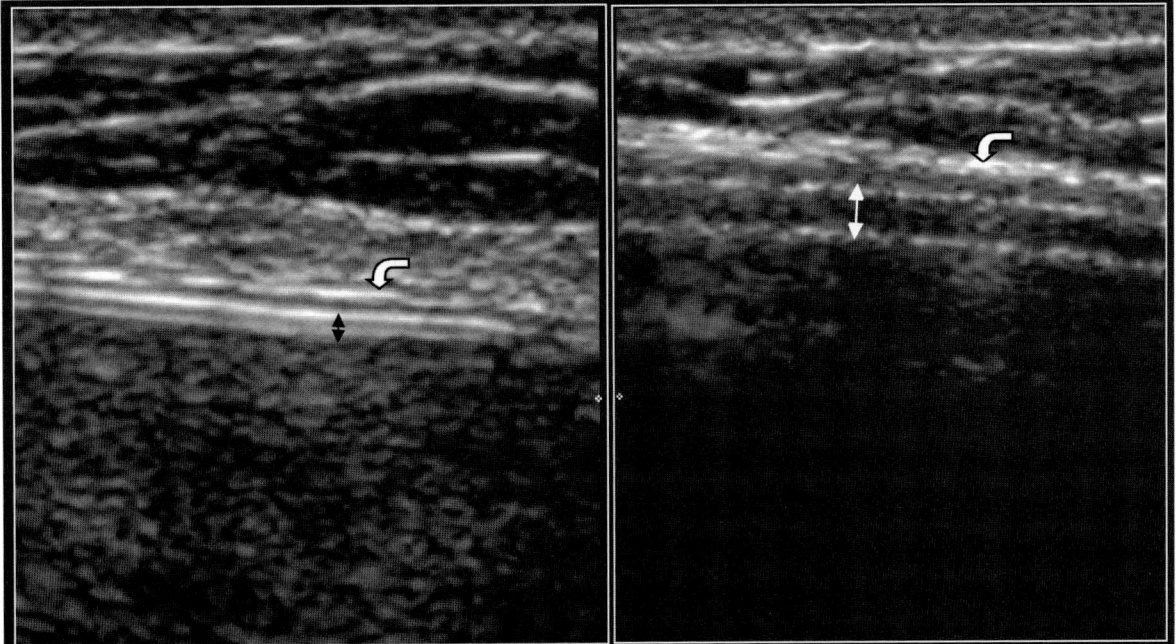

FIGURE 9–37 Note the difference in the thickness of the shells in these two nontextured single-lumen silicone gel implants. The implant on the **left** had a much thinner shell (black double-headed arrow) than the implant shown on the **right** (white double-headed arrow). The shell thickness on the left is typical of implants that were placed in the early 1970s, whereas the shell thickness on the right is more typical of implants placed since the 1980s. The *curved arrows* represent the outer surface of the fibrous periimplant capsule.

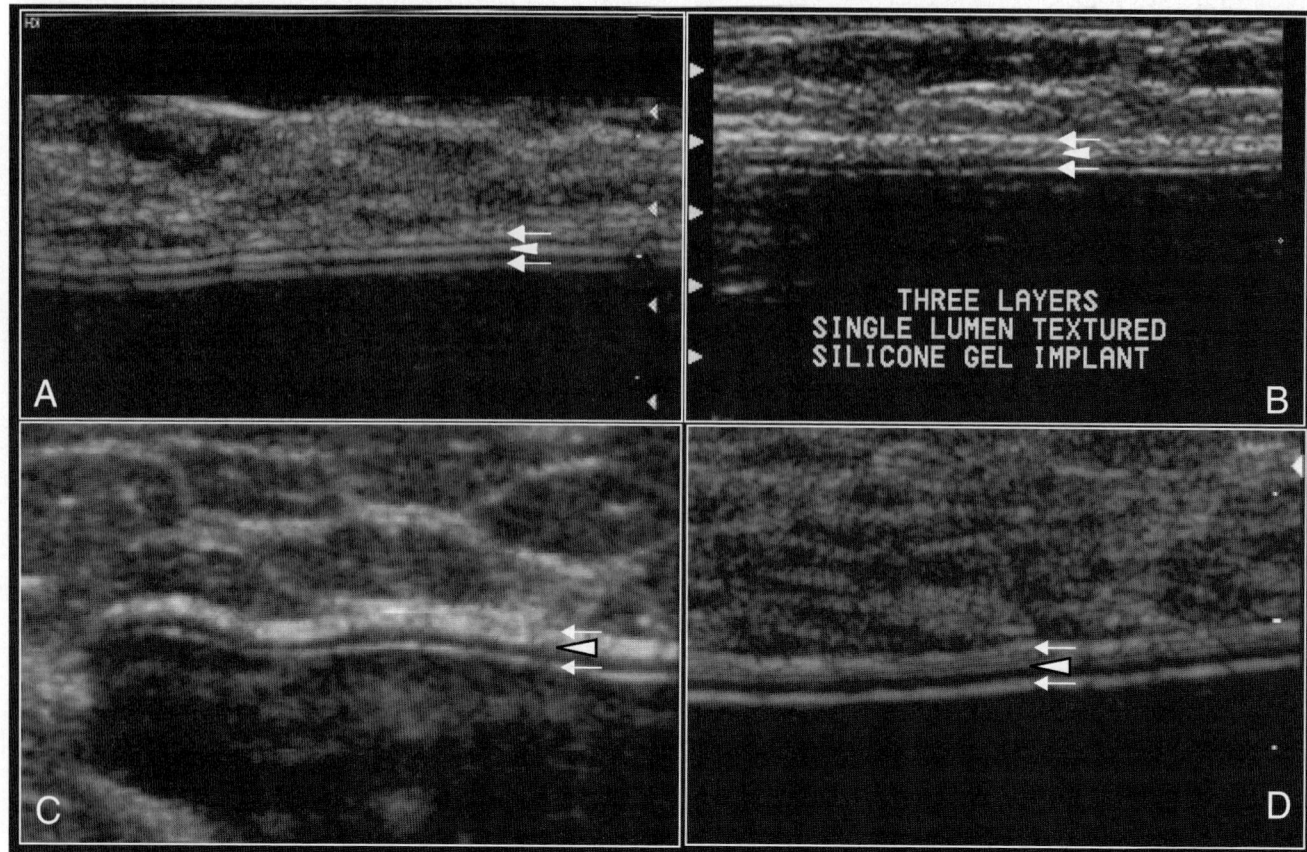

FIGURE 9–38 A: The three thin, equally spaced echogenic lines represent the capsule–shell echo complex in a patient who has a nontextured implant. **B:** This image shows three echogenic lines that represent the capsule–shell echo complex in a patient who has lightly textured implants. Note that the middle of the three echogenic lines *(arrowhead)*, the line that represents the merged echoes of the inner surface of the capsule and outer surface of the shell, is thicker than it is for the nontextured implant shown in part **A. C:** In this heavily textured implant, the capsule cannot be distinguished from the heavily textured outer surface of the shell. **D:** In this heavily textured implant, the outer surface of the shell appears multilaminar and is difficult to distinguish from the capsular echogenic line.

identified in such cases at the edge of the implant when there is an associated periimplant effusion (Fig. 9–39A). The capsule is also difficult to demonstrate in certain patients who have retropectoral implants, in whom the horizontal fibers of the pectoralis muscle may obscure the capsule (Fig. 9–39B).

Capsular Calcifications

Calcifications that form along the inner surface of the fibrous capsule are probably caused by microscopic gel bleed or fat necrosis. Light capsular calcification is considered a variant of normal and causes no technical problems (Fig. 9–40), but heavy and extensive capsular calcification may create enough acoustic shadowing and artifact to prevent adequate sonographic evaluation of the implant for rupture (Fig. 9–41).

Periimplant Fluid Collections

Periimplant effusions are normal findings. Normal effusions are small, are not under pressure, and are generally detectable only along the periphery of the implant or within radial folds (Fig. 9–42). Any type of implant may induce a surrounding fluid collection or effusion, but effusions are much more commonly associated with textured than smooth implants and are almost universally induced by polyurethane-coated textured implants because of sloughing polyurethane. These periimplant fluid collections are usually anechoic or nearly anechoic (Fig. 9–43, left). However, effusions tend to become more echogenic over time for a variety of reasons (Fig. 9–43, right). They tend to accumulate inflammatory cells, proteinaceous debris, and cholesterol crystals as a result of inflammation and foreign-body reaction. They also accumulate small

(text continued on page 231)

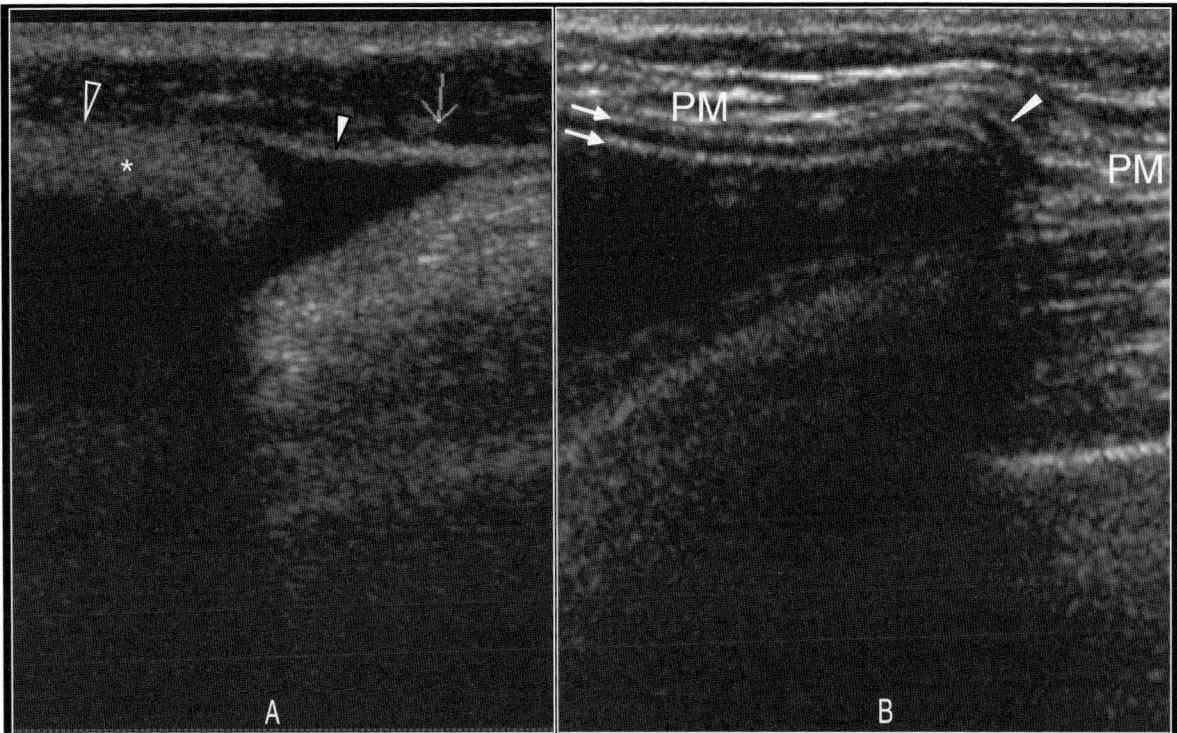

FIGURE 9–39 A: In heavily textured polyurethane-coated implants, only a single, very thick and ill-defined line *(hollow arrowhead)* represents the capsule–shell complex. The capsule can be identified separately only where it separates from the shell at the edge of the implant, where it surrounds a periimplant effusion *(arrowhead)*. **B:** The anterior echogenic line that represents the periimplant fibrous capsule can be particularly difficult to identify along the anterior aspect of a retropectoral implant. The fascicular pattern of the pectoral muscle *(PM)* creates multiple linear echoes parallel to the fibrous capsule that make the capsule difficult to identify. However, the fibrous capsule *(arrowhead)* can be identified at the edge of the implant where it separates from the implant shell *(arrowhead)*.

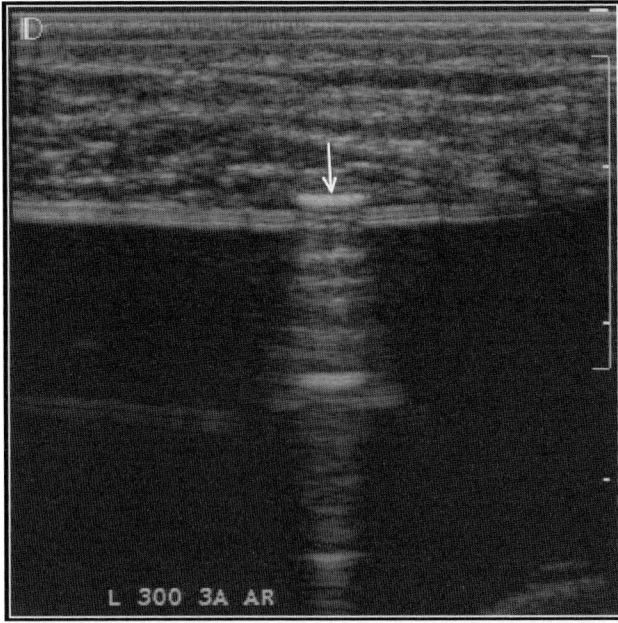

FIGURE 9–40 Capsular calcifications are usually of no significance. They typically lie within the inner surface of the capsule. Capsular calcifications create shadows that obscure the shell immediately deep to them. Calcifications that are not extensive do not interfere with sonographic evaluation of the implant shell.

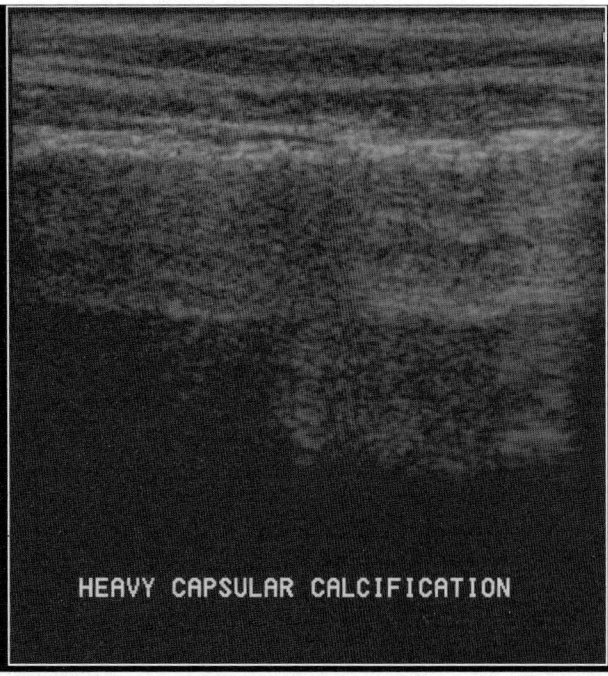

FIGURE 9–41 Occasionally, capsular calcifications can become so extensive and create so many artifacts that the shell is completely obscured by artifacts and can no longer be assessed sonographically. Such calcifications can simulate sheetlike collections of extracapsular silicone gel in patients who have extracapsular rupture.

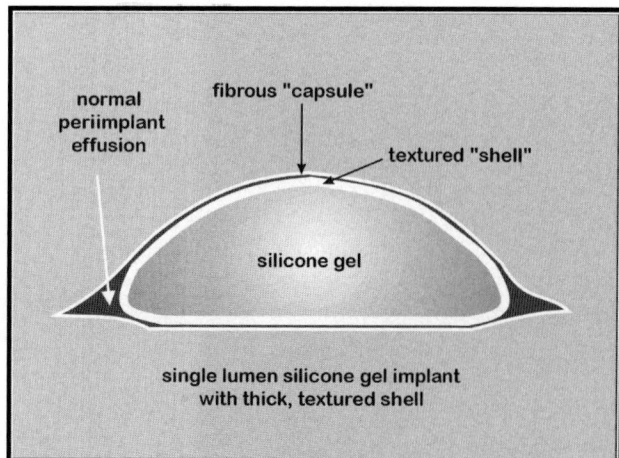

FIGURE 9–42 Periimplant effusions can accumulate between the implant shell and the surrounding periimplant fibrous capsule. Effusions are more common with textured silicone gel–filled implants than they are with nontextured saline-filled implants but can occur with any type of implant. Periimplant effusion tends to accumulate along the periphery of the implant and within radial folds. Polyurethane-coated implants invariably incite effusion formation.

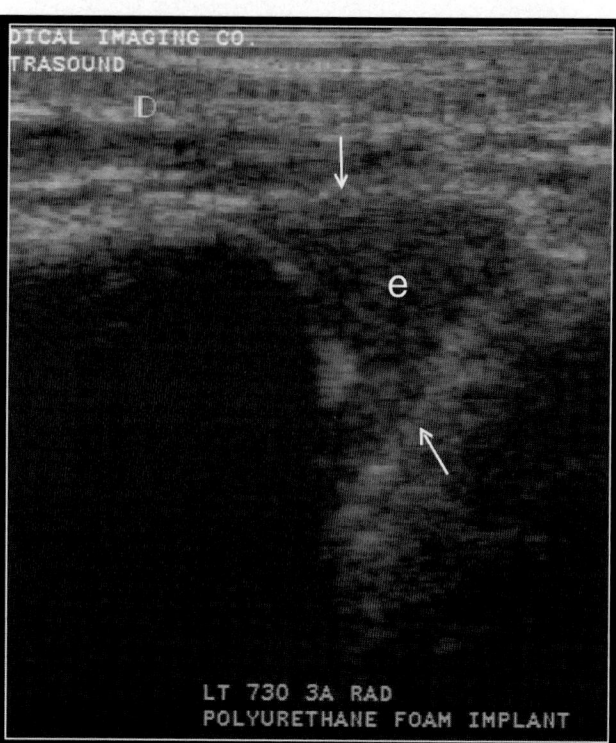

FIGURE 9–44 Effusions *(e)* surrounding polyurethane-coated implants are invariably echogenic because of sloughing of polyurethane particles from the surface of the implants into the effusion.

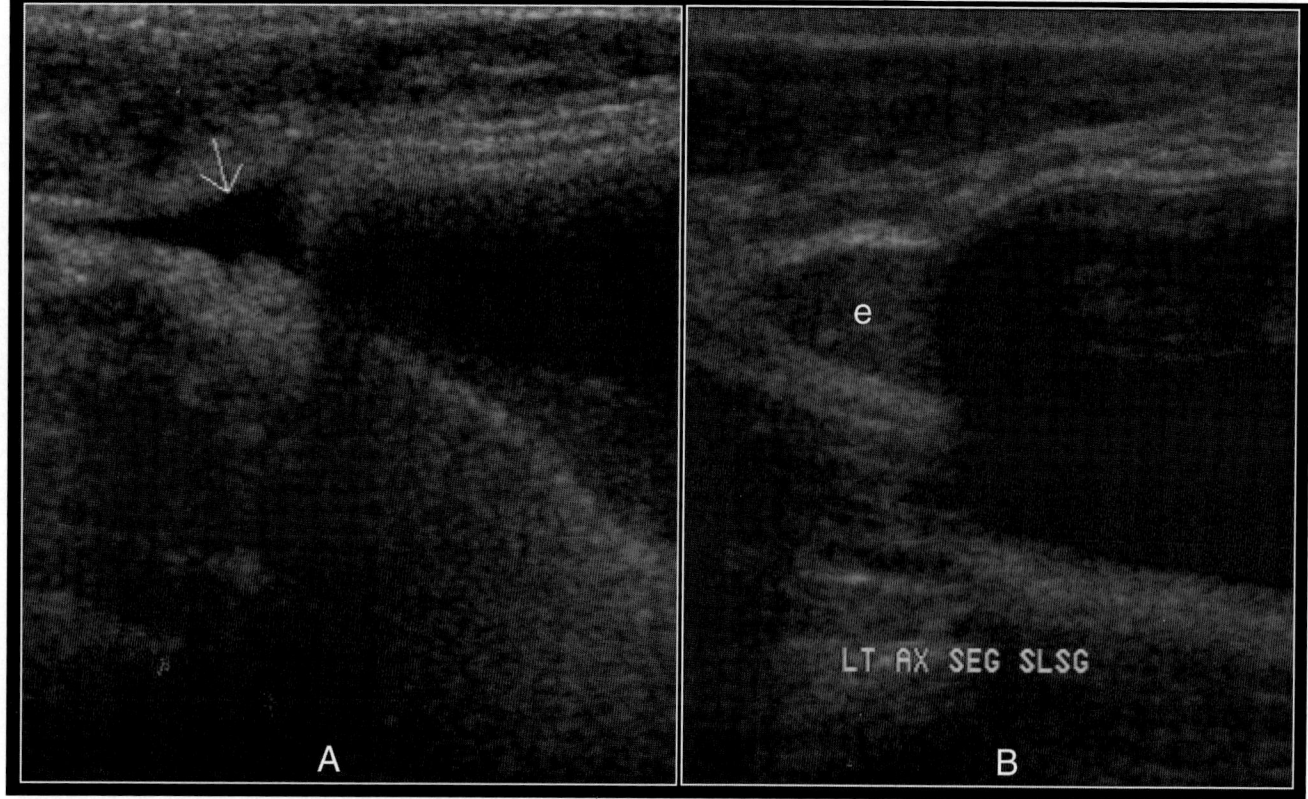

FIGURE 9–43 Most periimplant effusions are initially anechoic or nearly anechoic **(left,** *arrow***)** but can become echogenic **(right,** *e***)** over time for a variety of reasons.

amounts of silicone within the effusion because of gel bleed. The effusion may be echogenic from the start if there is hemorrhage into the periimplant space during or after surgery. Furthermore, polyurethane-coated textured implants may contribute to echoes within the effusion. The effusions around polyurethane-coated implants invariably become echogenic because of sloughing of polyurethane particles from the surface of the implant into the effusion (Fig. 9–44). In some cases, it can be difficult to distinguish between echogenic periimplant effusion and mildly echogenic or extravasated silicone associated with intracapsular implant rupture.

Using differential peripheral compression pressure while scanning the edges of the implant may improve the angle of incidence with the edge of the implant and may facilitate counting of echogenic lines to help distinguish between periimplant effusion and double-lumen implants (Fig. 9–45). Distinguishing a periimplant effusion from the outer compartment of double-lumen implant will be discussed in the section on double-lumen implants.

Implantation Site

In patients with subglandular or prepectoral implants, breast tissue and fibrous capsule lie superficial to the implant, whereas the pectoralis major muscle lies posterior to the implant (Fig. 9–46A). In patients with retropectoral implants, the pectoralis major muscle lies superficially, separating the glandular tissue from the implant and its capsule (Fig. 9–46B). The fascicular pattern of the pectoralis muscle can be difficult to distinguish from the horizontal striations within the shell of a textured implant directly anterior to the implant, but the pectoralis muscle extends away from the implant toward the axilla, whereas the multilaminar capsule–shell complex of the textured implant does not (Fig. 9–47). Remember that the pectoralis major muscle covers only the superior part of the implant in most patients, whereas the inferior part of the implant lies subglandularly. The pectoralis muscle is tapered along its long axis, being thickest in the axillary segment and gradually becoming thinner inferiorly and medially near its free edge (Fig. 9–48A). In general, the larger the retropectoral implant, the

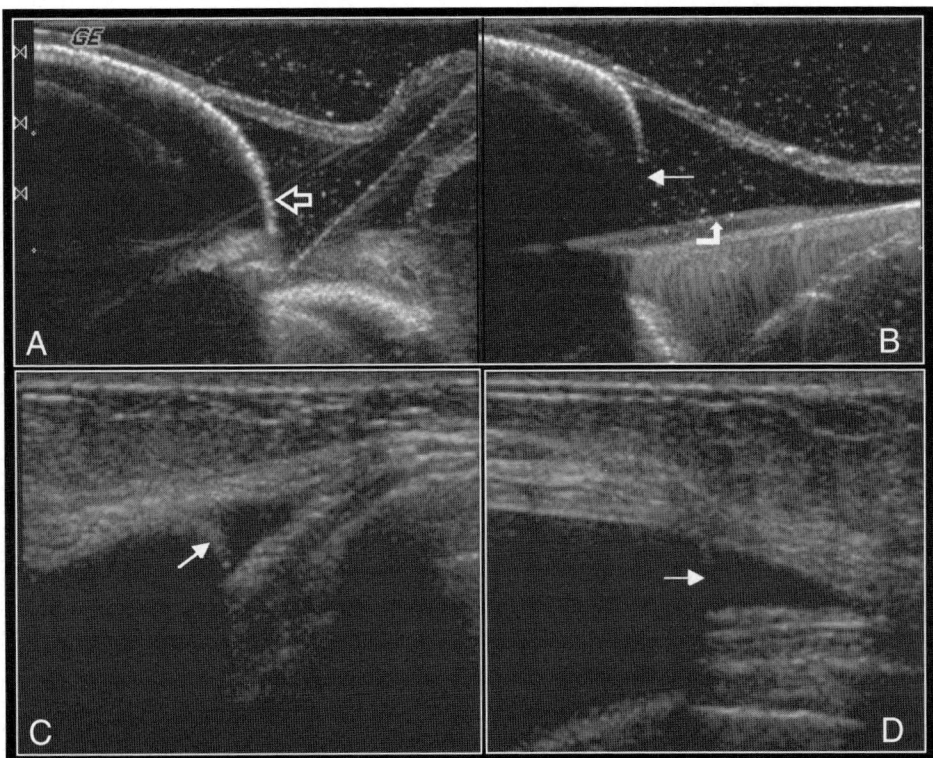

FIGURE 9–45 *In vitro* images of a simulated periimplant effusion were obtained by compressing the peripheral end of the transducer to a greater degree than the central end (**A**) and by using equal compression centrally and peripherally (**B**). Note that the shell at the edge of the implant is better seen with peripheral compression (**A**, *hollow arrow*) than with equalized pressure (**B**, *arrow*) owing to critical angle phenomena. By using differential peripheral compression pressure, the angle of incidence of the beam with the edge of the shell can be improved, and the shell can be better demonstrated. *In vivo* images of a periimplant effusion were obtained with peripheral compression (**C**) and equalized compression (**D**). The shell at the edge of the implant is better demonstrated with peripheral compression (**C**, arrow) than with equalized compression (**D**, arrow) owing to critical angle phenomena.

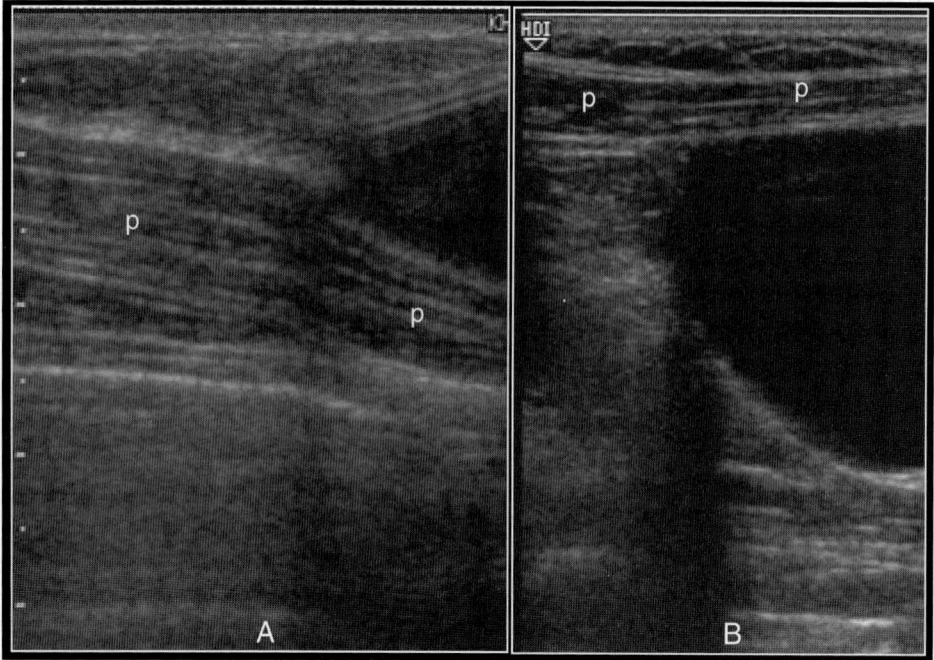

FIGURE 9–46 A: The pectoralis major muscle *(p)* passes posterior to a subglandular or prepectoral implant. **B:** The pectoralis *(p)* passes posterior to a retropectoral implant.

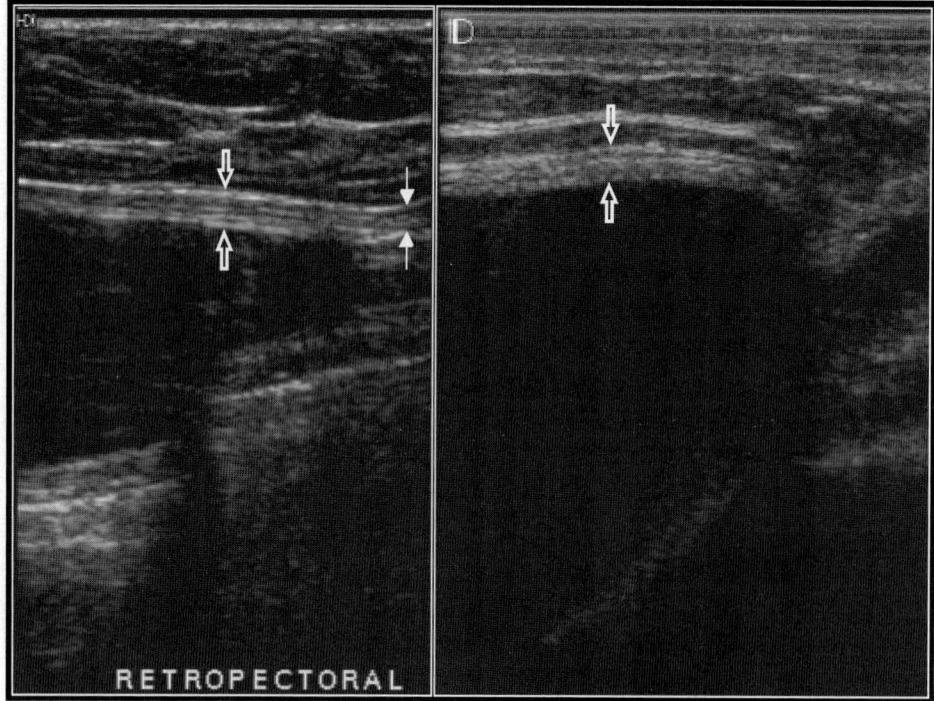

FIGURE 9–47 The echogenic striations of the pectoralis muscle (**left,** *hollow arrows*) can be difficult to distinguish from the multilaminar appearance of the capsule–shell complex of a heavily textured implant (**right,** *hollow arrows*). The distinguishing feature lies in the upper outer quadrant, where the pectoralis muscle will extend away from edge of the implant toward the axilla (*small arrows*).

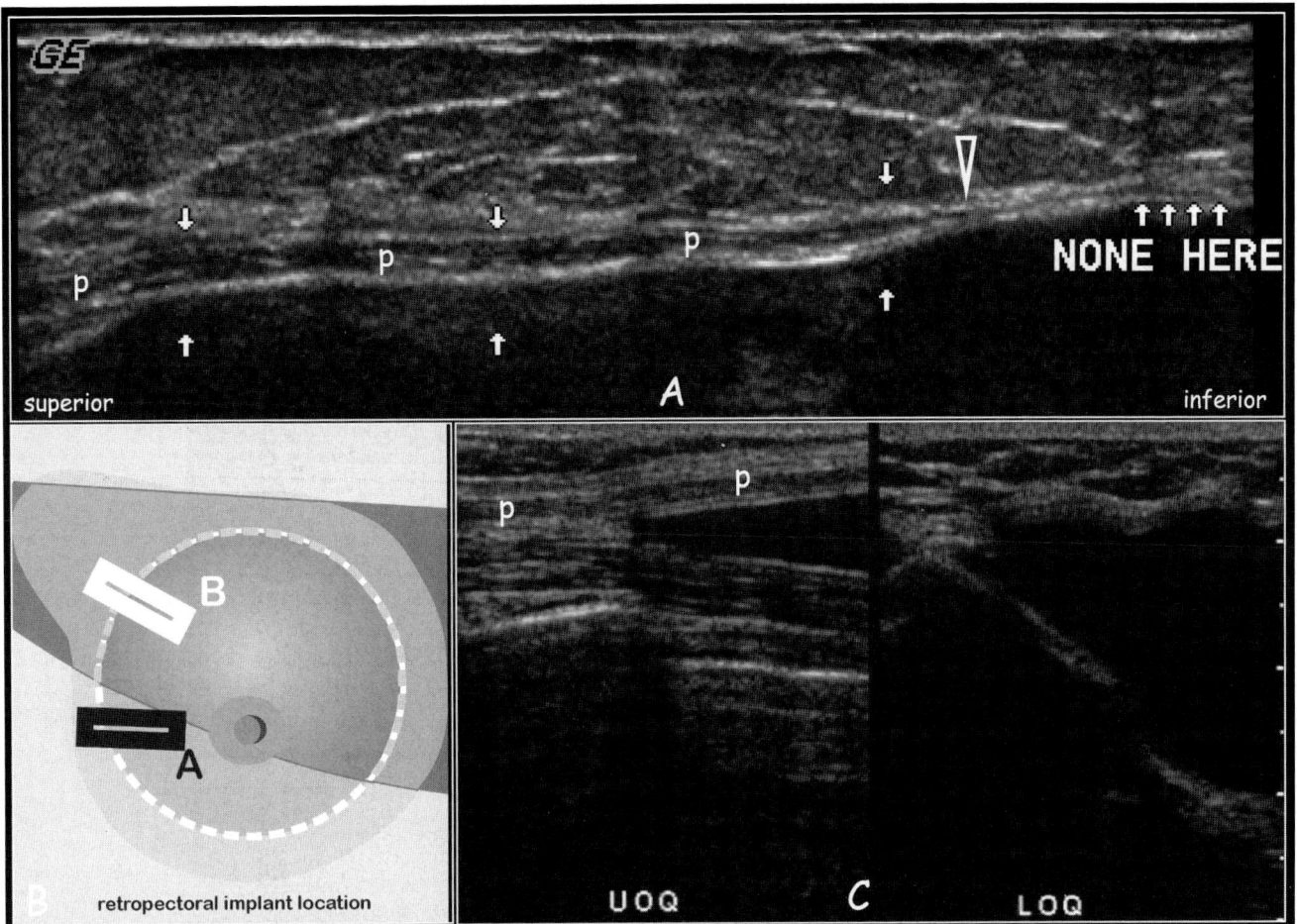

FIGURE 9–48 The pectoralis major muscle does not cover the entire retropectoral implant. In general, the larger the implant, the less of the implant is covered by the pectoralis muscle. **A:** The pectoralis gradually becomes thinner inferiorly, until it no longer covers *(hollow arrowhead)* the implant. **B:** Radially oriented scans in the upper outer quadrant will be able to show the pectoralis muscle coursing to the axilla *(plane B)*. Scans from the lower outer quadrant frequently will not *(plane A)*. **C:** Split-screen images of the upper outer quadrant (*UOQ*, corresponding to *plane B*) show the pectoralis muscle (p) coursing from anterior to the implant to the axilla, whereas a scan obtained through the lower outer quadrant (*LOQ*, corresponding to *plane A*) does not.

more stretched and thinned the muscle becomes, and the smaller the percentage of the implant that is overlain by the pectoralis muscle. Thus, when sonographically evaluating an implant to determine its implantation site, one must evaluate the axillary segment, where the muscle is thickest and where it courses away from the implant toward the axilla (Fig. 9–48B). If the inferior half of a retropectoral implant is scanned below the free edge of the pectoralis muscle, the sonographic appearance will be indistinguishable from that of a subglandular implant (Fig. 9–48C).

Abnormal Sonographic Implant Appearances

Capsular Contracture

The diagnosis of capsular contracture is made clinically, not by sonography. However, some patients with capsular contracture may need to undergo sonography for other in-

dications, and in such patients, there are demonstrable sonographic findings associated with capsular contracture. The sonographic findings that can be demonstrated include an abnormal shape, abnormal thickening of the capsule, and increased redundancy of the shell.

Split-screen mirror-image scans of the right and left sides in patients who have unilateral contracture nicely contrast the shape differences between capsular contracture and normal implants. The anteroposterior (AP) dimension is greater and the posterior wall of the implant has a convex outward shape on the side of the capsular contracture (abnormally spherical shape), whereas the AP dimension of the implant is smaller and the posterior wall of the implant is convex inward and lies parallels to the chest wall on the side without contracture (Fig. 9–49). The AP dimension may be so increased that 5-MHz linear or curved linear transducers and a large field of view are necessary to show the posterior

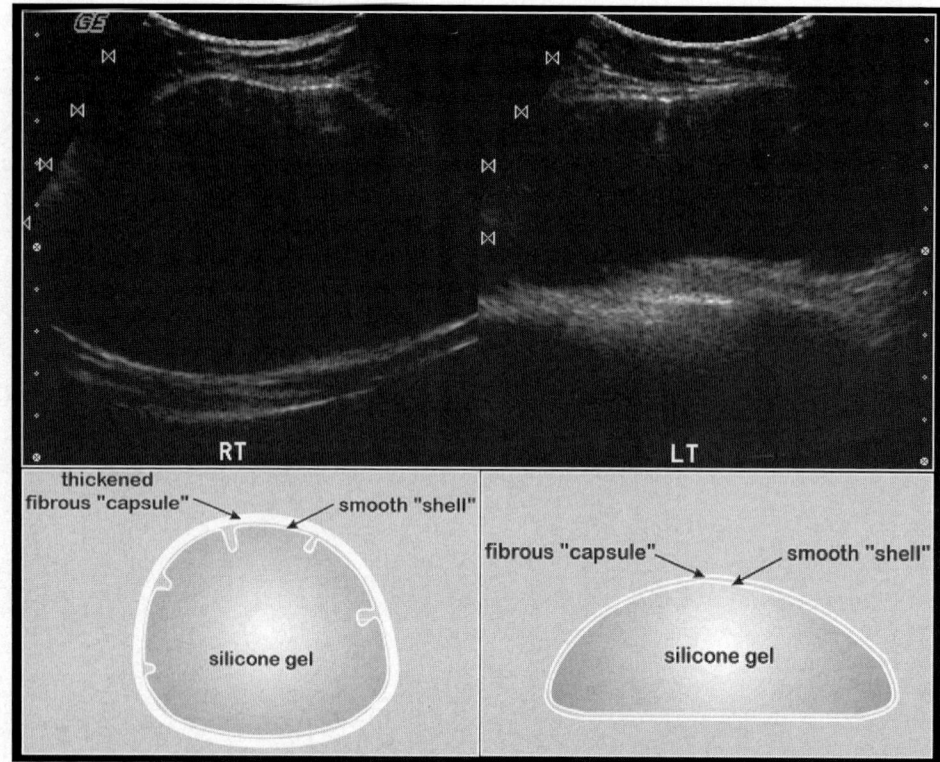

FIGURE 9–49 Split-screen mirror-image scans of the center of implants show a more rounded and spherical shape and much larger anteroposterior dimension for the contracted right implant than for the normal left implant. Note that the abnormally contracted implant has a posterior wall that is convex posteriorly because it is under pressure. Note that the soft normal left implant is convex anteriorly because it is soft enough to be indented by the chest wall deep to the implant. The larger field of view of the 5-MHz curved linear transducer improves the ability to assess implant shape in patients with capsular contracture.

wall of the implant. Demonstrating the posterior wall of the capsular space can be important in excluding intracapsular rupture in cases in which the shell collapses completely and falls to the posterior wall of the capsular space (Fig. 9–9).

The firmness of the contractured implants makes it difficult to scan the implant by preventing the transducer from being placed parallel to the chest wall at the edges of the implant. This can make assessing the type of implant and periimplant effusions technically difficult.

In patients with capsular contracture, the capsule is abnormally thickened (and usually isoechoic) to more than 1.5 mm. Instead of the thin, echogenic line seen in normal thin capsules, the thickened capsule presents as a double echogenic line with an isoechoic space between the lines. The capsular thickness is best demonstrated in regions where the capsule and shell are not in contact with each other—around the periimplant effusion at the edges of the implant (Fig. 9–50) or at the bases of radial folds (Fig. 9–51). Because the spherical shape of contracted capsules has a smaller volume than the normal lentiform shape, the shell becomes redundant, and the number of radial folds increases (Fig. 9–52). The thickness of contracted capsules

frequently varies from one part of the capsule to another (Fig. 9–52). Areas where there is less thickening of the capsule are prone to rupture and herniation of the implant, which will be discussed later in this chapter. Although the abnormally thick, contracted capsule is usually isoechoic, in a few cases, it can appear hyperechoic (Fig. 9–53).

Implant Herniation

The fibrous capsule that surrounds the implant shell can develop a rent through which the implant shell can herniate. This most commonly occurs in patients who have capsular contracture with very uneven thickening of the capsule. Herniations tend to occur through segments of capsule that are the thinnest. To diagnose herniation sonographically with absolute certainty, a focal defect in the fibrous capsule must be shown. The following sonographic findings are classic for implant herniation through a rent in the periimplant fibrous capsule:

1. Absence of the outer single, thin, echogenic line that represents the fibrous capsule localized to the area of bulging. In the herniated portion of the implant, there

(text continued on page 237)

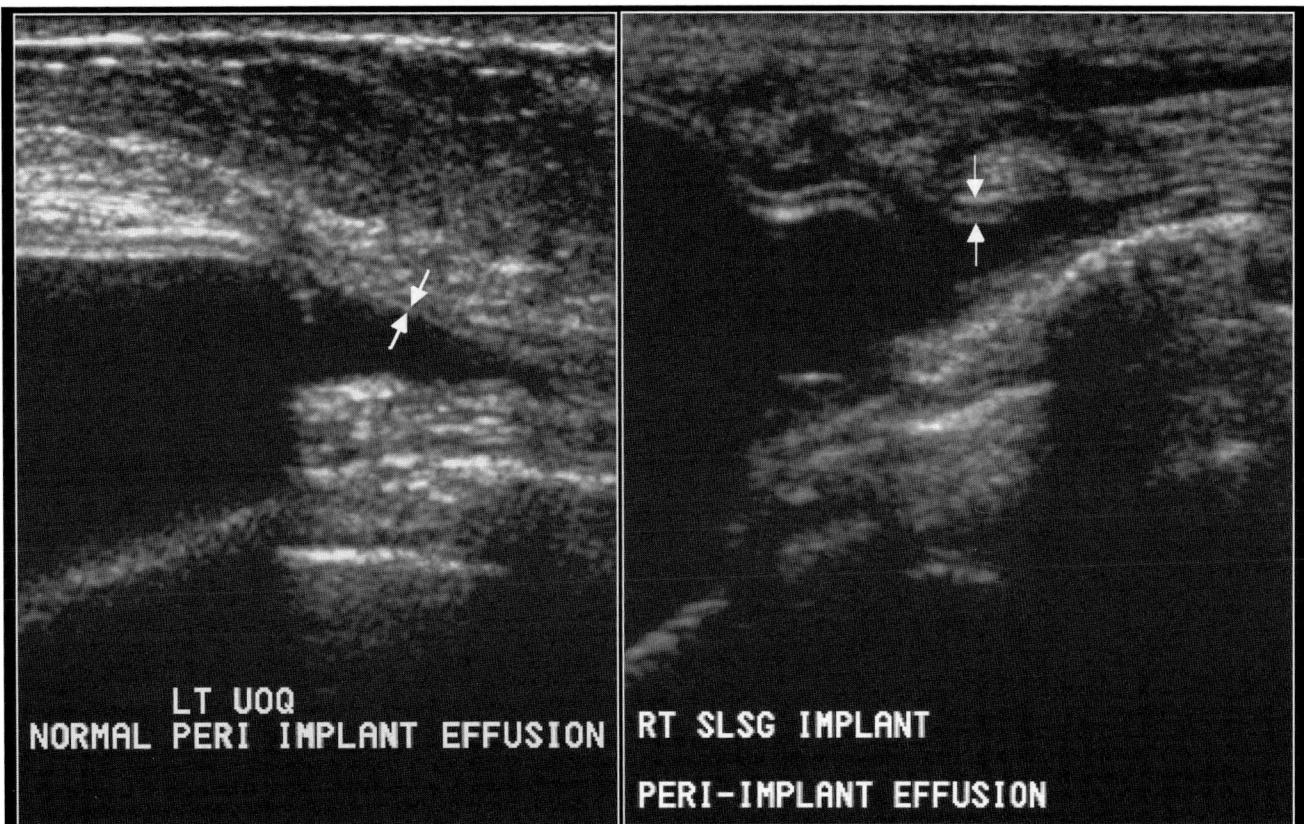

LT UOQ
NORMAL PERI IMPLANT EFFUSION

RT SLSG IMPLANT
PERI-IMPLANT EFFUSION

FIGURE 9-50 One of the places were the capsule and shell diverge from each other and one of the easiest places to assess capsular thickness is around periimplant effusions that occur along the edges of the implant. Capsules that are normal in thickness appear as a single thin, echogenic line (**left**, *arrows*). Abnormally thickened capsules appear isoechoic and bordered by thin, echogenic lines that define the anterior and posterior border of the capsule (**right**, *arrows*).

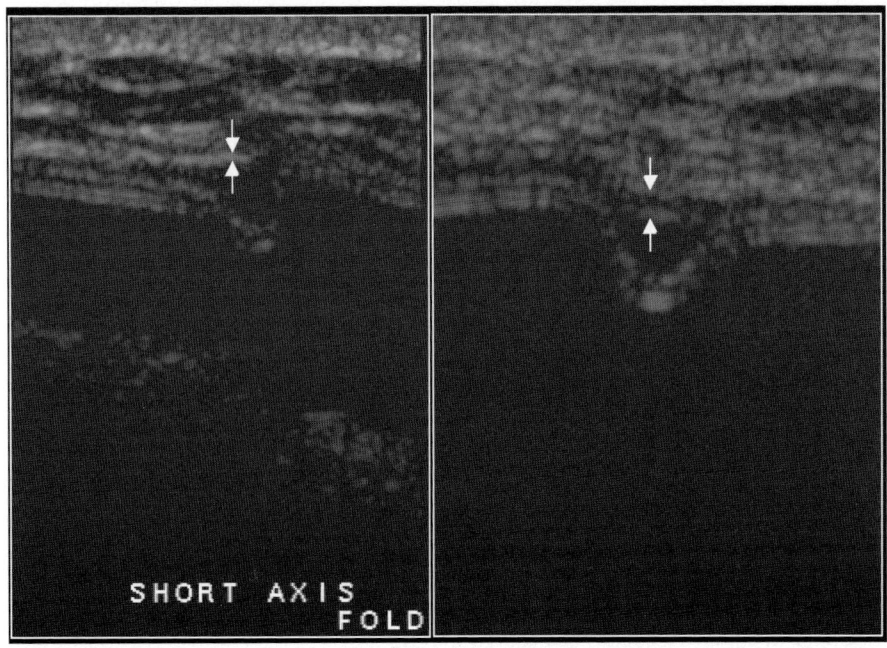

SHORT AXIS
FOLD

FIGURE 9-51 Another location where there is separation between the capsule and shell and where it is relatively easy to assess capsular thickness is on the anterior aspect of anteriorly located radial folds. The normal periimplant capsule is thin and sonographically represented by a single, thin echogenic line (**left**, *arrows*). The abnormally thickened and contracted capsule appears isoechoic and is bordered by thin, echogenic lines on both its anterior and posterior surfaces (**right**, *arrows*).

RT 2
3C RAD
E2

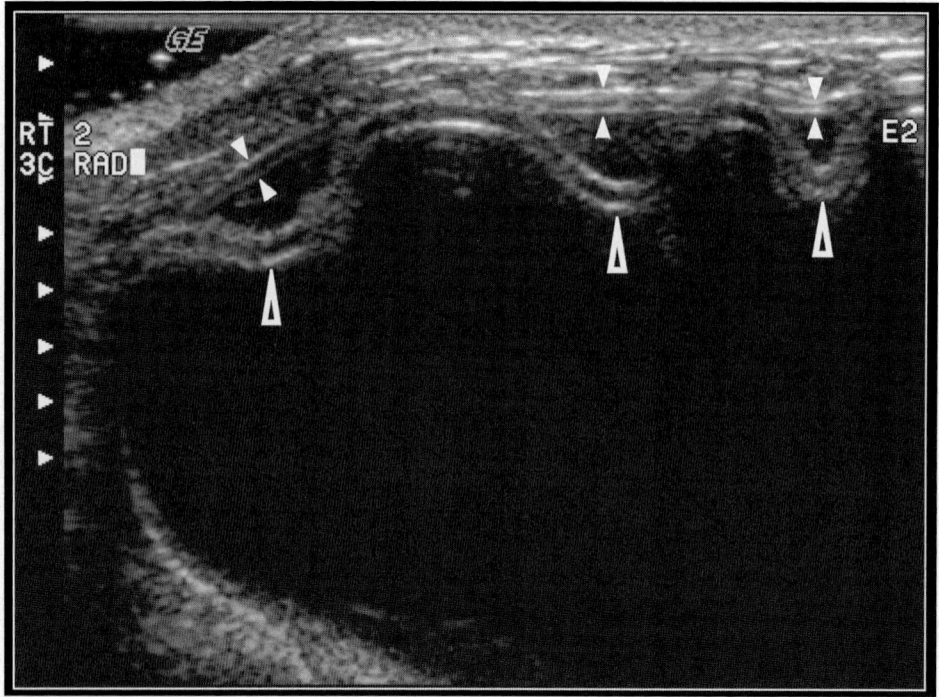

FIGURE 9–52 Capsular contracture, by pushing the implant into a near spherical shape, reduces the surface area relative to the volume of the implant. The shell of the compressed implant becomes redundant and develops more numerous radial folds *(large hollow arrowheads).* The thickness of the contracted capsule varies *(solid arrowheads).*

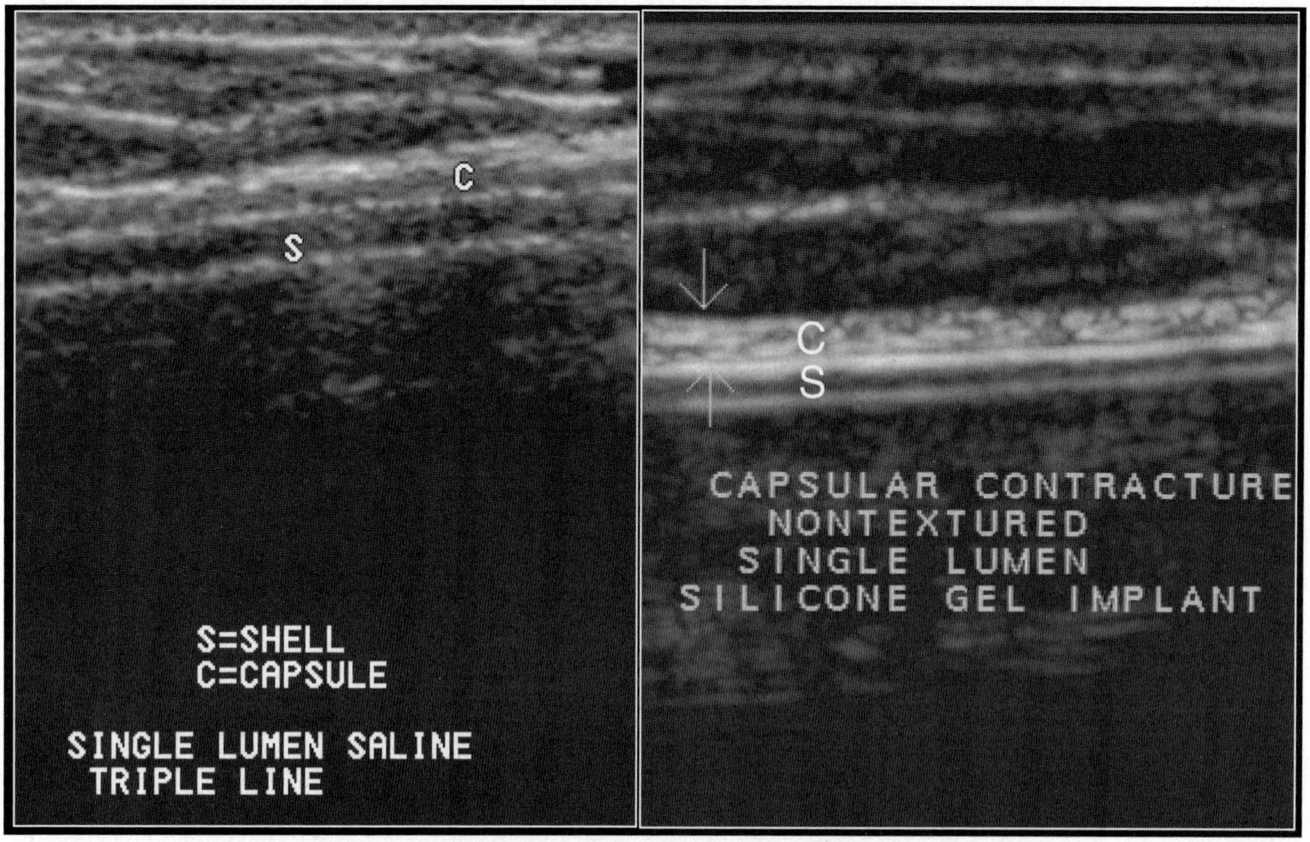

C
S
S=SHELL
C=CAPSULE
SINGLE LUMEN SALINE
TRIPLE LINE
C
S
CAPSULAR CONTRACTURE
NONTEXTURED
SINGLE LUMEN
SILICONE GEL IMPLANT

FIGURE 9–53 Although the abnormally thickened capsule in most patients with capsular contracture appears isoechoic, (**left**, *c*), in a few cases, it can be hyperechoic (**right**, *c*).

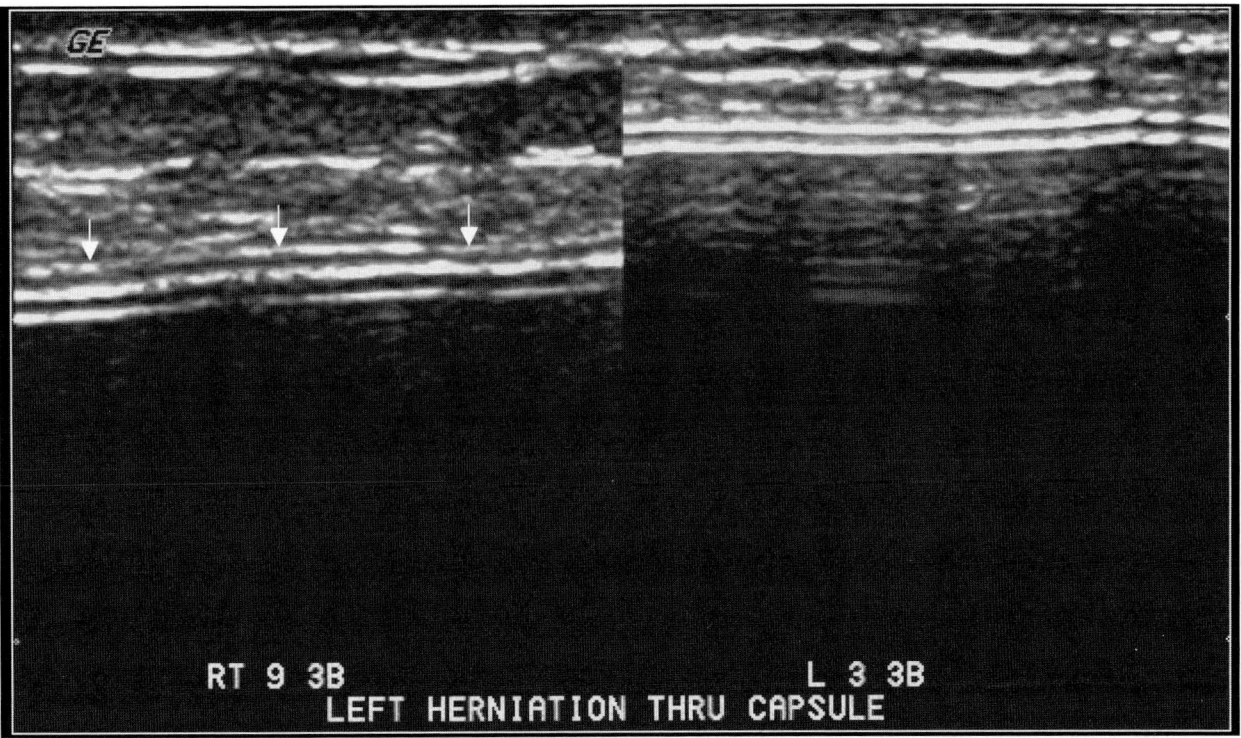

RT 9 3B   L 3 3B
LEFT HERNIATION THRU CAPSULE

FIGURE 9–54 On the side of the herniation (**right**, patient's left side), there are only two echogenic lines. The echogenic line that represents the superficial surface of the capsule is absent, the shell is focally thinned, and overlying breast tissues are thinned. On the normal contralateral side (**left**, patient's right side), there are three echogenic lines. The echogenic line that represents the outer surface of the capsule is present, the shell is thicker, and the overlying breast tissues are thicker.

are only two thin, echogenic lines instead of the three echogenic lines seen elsewhere in the ipsilateral or contralateral breast. The two lines represent the leading and trailing edges of the herniated implant shell. The capsular echoes are absent (Fig. 9–54). In bulges without herniation, the capsule and shell can be focally thinned, but the echogenic line that represents the outer surface of the capsule is not absent (Fig. 9–55).

2. Focal thinning of the implant shell in the area of herniation in comparison to other locations in the ipsilateral or contralateral breast (Fig. 9–54).

3. Abnormally superficial position of the implant shell relative to other locations in the ipsilateral or contralateral breast (Fig. 9–54). Herniation can also be manifest as a focal bulge along the edge of the shell without actually protruding closer to the skin (Fig. 9–56).

Herniations can cause palpable abnormalities and, as is the case for radial folds, can be positional. Herniations might only be present in the upright position, and in such cases, can be diagnosed only if the patient is scanned in the upright position (Fig. 9–57).

The focal thinning of the implant shell in the area of the herniation weakens the shell in that location, making

rupture more likely. Thus, it is not unusual to see intracapsular rupture (if the capsule is focally thinned but not torn) or extracapsular rupture (if there is a defect in the capsule) in association with implant herniation (Fig. 9–58).

Implant Rupture

The concept of intracapsular versus extracapsular rupture is valid in patients who have either single-lumen silicone gel implants or double-lumen implants but is not relevant in patients with saline implants. Rupture of saline implants is associated with immediate and complete collapse of the shell and its surrounding fibrous capsule that is readily apparent to the patient and her referring physician and is evident mammographically (Fig. 9–5). A completely collapsed saline implant shell may be seen as an incidental finding during targeted sonography for evaluation of a palpable or mammographic abnormality. It appears as a collection of parallel, horizontally oriented echogenic lines, very similar to the "linguini sign" described in the MRI literature. When high-frequency transducers are used, a double echogenic line represents each fold of the collapsed implant shell (Fig. 9–59). Although collapse of the ruptured

(text continued on page 240)

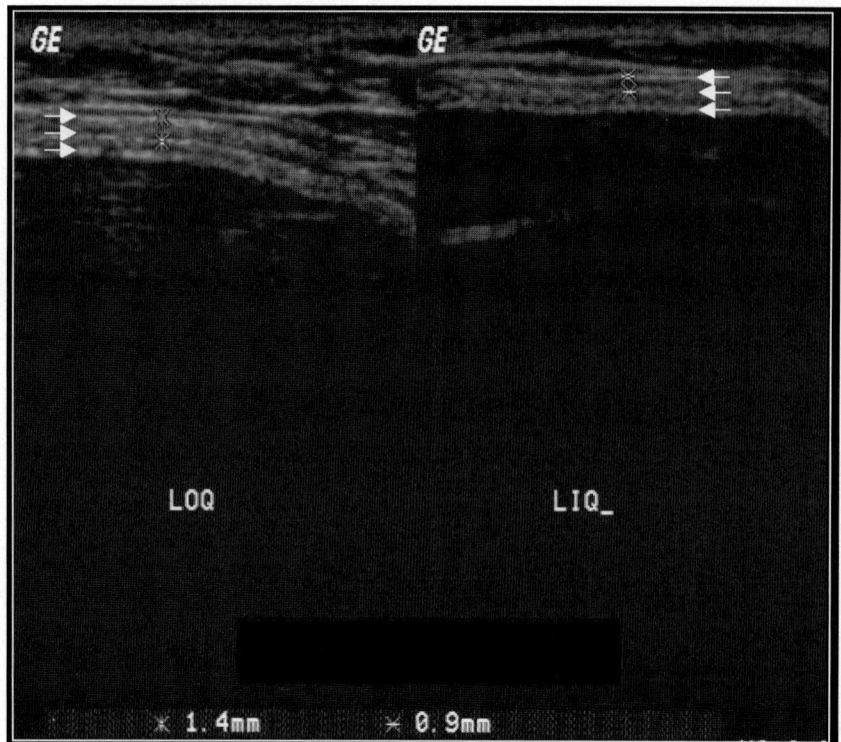

FIGURE 9–55 In a focal bulge, the capsule and the shell can be abnormally thin, but the echogenic line that represents the outer surface of the capsule is intact. There is a focal bulge in the lower inner quadrant *(LIQ)*. The lower outer quadrant *(LOQ)* of the ipsilateral breast has been used as a frame of normal reference for these split-screen images.

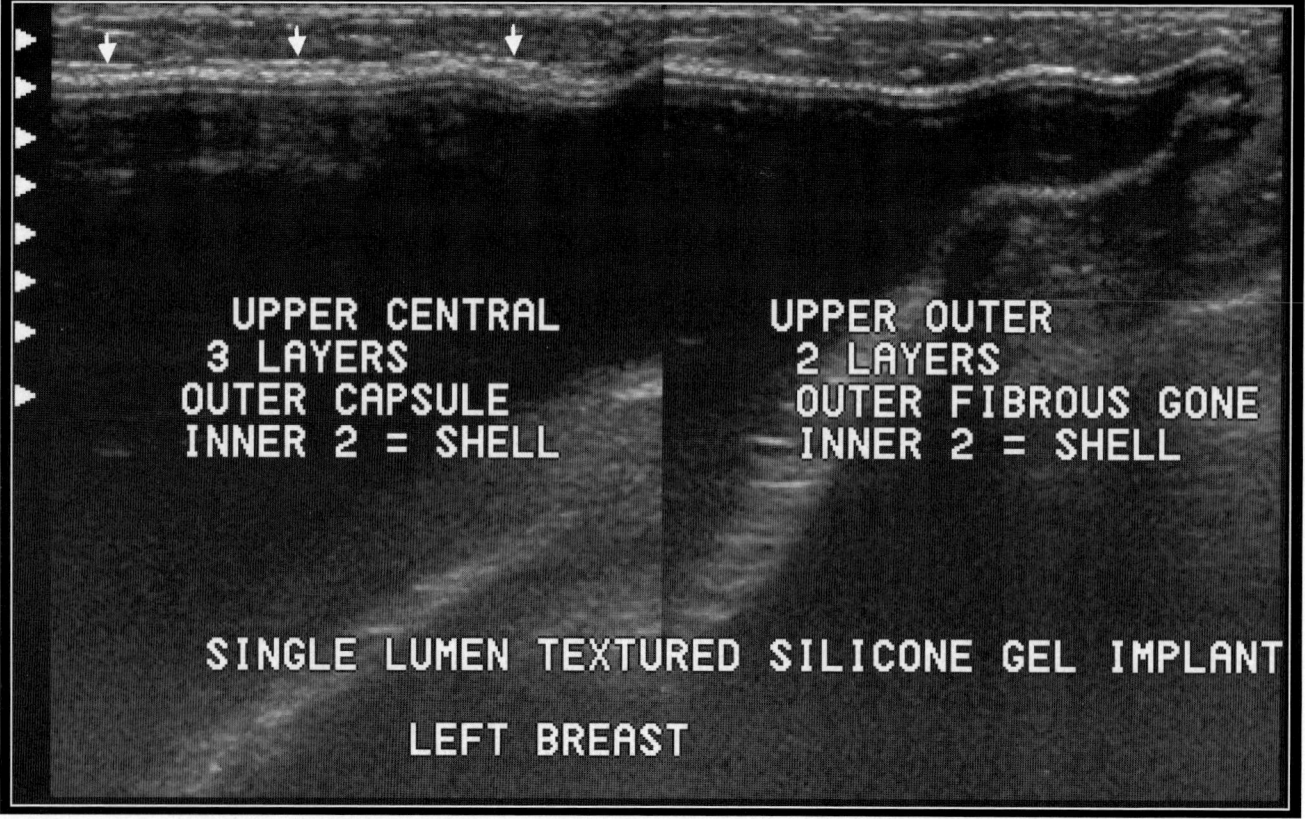

FIGURE 9–56 This case of focal herniation of the left implant bulges laterally from the edge of the implant rather than anteriorly and therefore has occurred without thinning the overlying breast tissues. Note that the echogenic line that represents the superficial surface of the capsule is present in the upper central left breast (**left** split-screen image, *arrows*) but is absent in the area of herniation in the upper outer quadrant (**right** split-screen image).

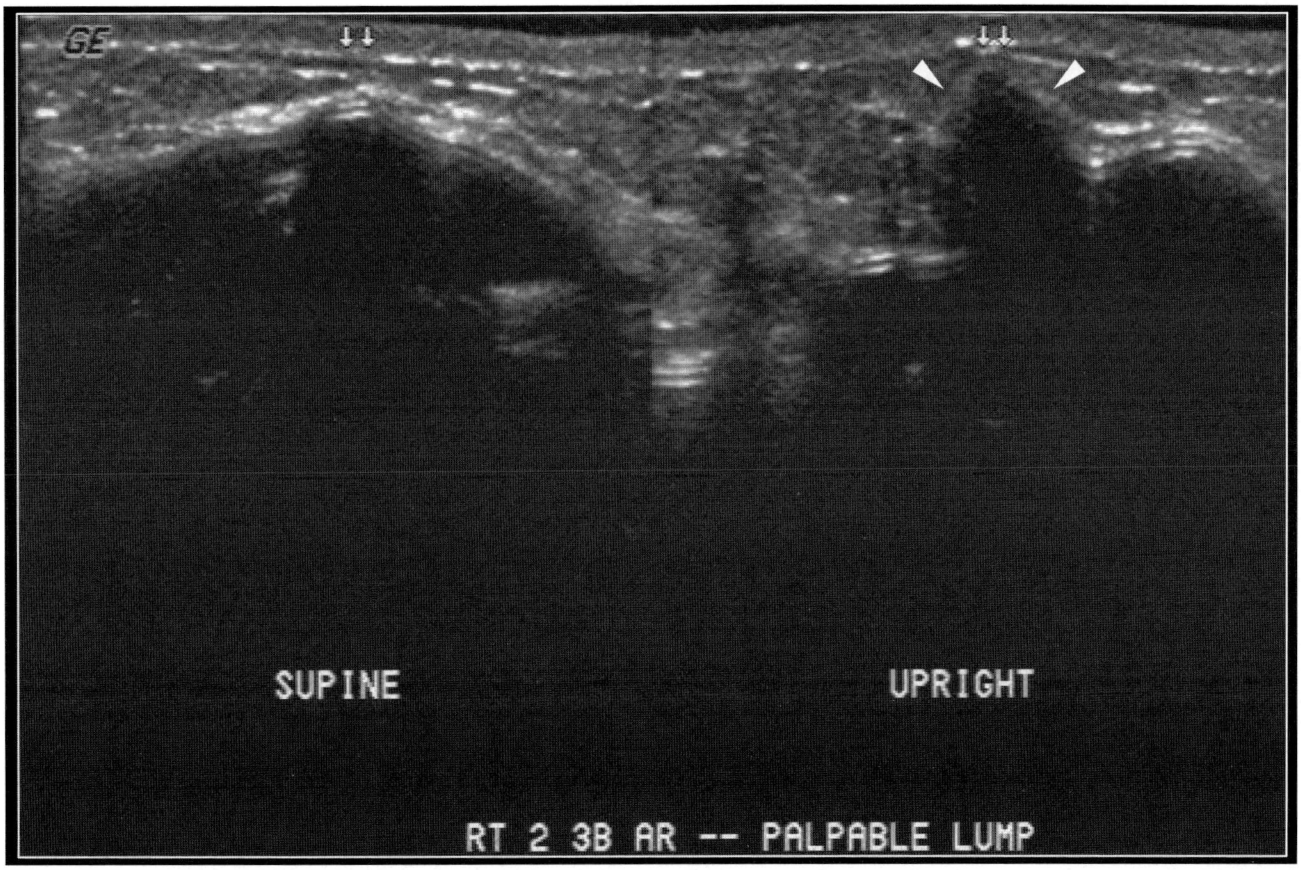

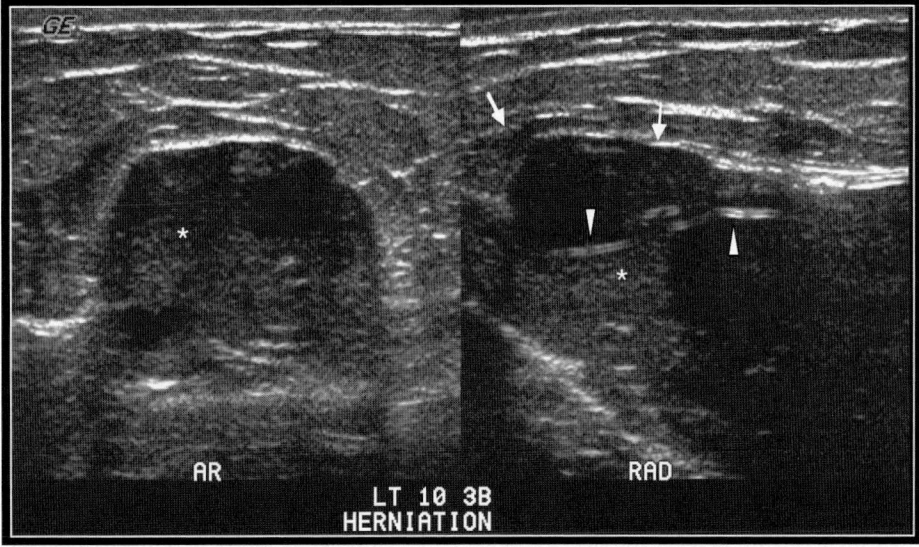

FIGURE 9–57 This palpable implant herniation is present and palpable in the upright position (**right**, *arrowheads*) but not in the supine position (**left**).

FIGURE 9–58 The thinning of the implant shell that occurs in conjunction with implant herniation weakens it and predisposes it to rupture. In this patient, there is evidence of intracapsular rupture within the implant herniation. There is abnormal separation of the shell *(arrowheads)* from the abnormally thinned capsule *(arrows)* and abnormally echogenic extravasated silicone gel *(*)* outside the shell.

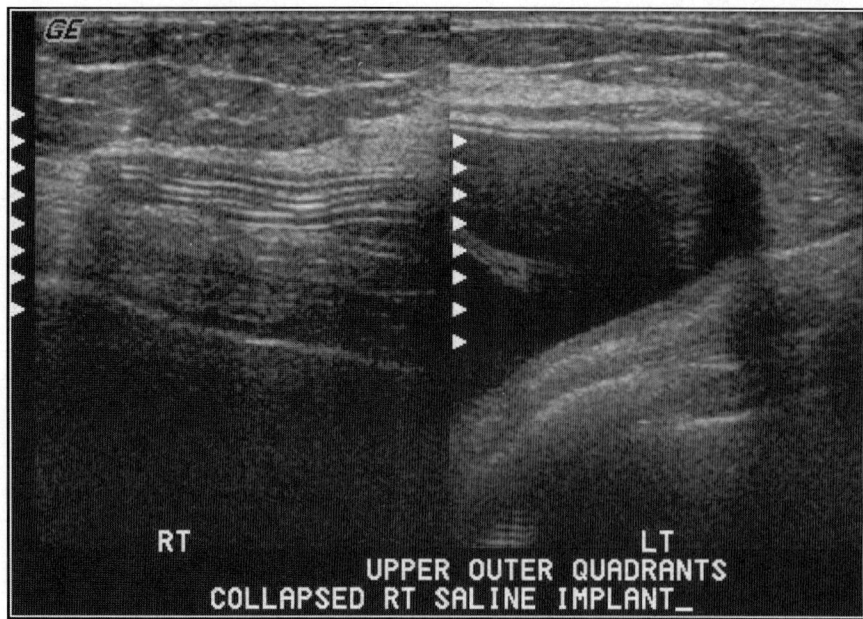

GE

RT

LT
UPPER OUTER QUADRANTS
COLLAPSED RT SALINE IMPLANT

FIGURE 9–59 Split-screen mirror-image scans of the right and left implants show an intact single-lumen saline implant on the patient's left side but a completely collapsed implant shell containing no saline on the right side. The layered folds of collapsed implant shell create an appearance similar to linguini; thus, this finding has been termed the "linguini sign" in the magnetic resonance imaging literature.

saline implant and resorption of the extravasated saline are both usually complete, in certain cases, collapse may be incomplete, and some saline that is not under pressure may remain within folds of the implant shell.

Extracapsular Rupture

The hallmark of extracapsular rupture is the presence of macroscopic amounts of silicone gel outside of both the implant shell and the periimplant capsule. The presence of extracapsular silicone gel implies that there is either simultaneous or preexisting intracapsular rupture. However, intracapsular rupture is not always sonographically demonstrable in patients who have extracapsular rupture. If the shell and capsule rupture simultaneously, the extravasated gel may move straight into the extracapsular space without ever accumulating within the intracapsular space. Therefore, extracapsular silicone may be seen without any sonographic evidence of intracapsular rupture in certain patients, whereas in others, there may be sonographic evidence of both intracapsular and extracapsular rupture.

Extracapsular extravasated silicone gel is rapidly walled off by inflammatory response that leads to formation of a silicone granuloma. Such granulomas may cause tender or nontender palpable lumps, or they may be asymptomatic and unsuspected clinically. The classic sonographic description of silicone granuloma is that of the "snowstorm" appearance—a nodule that is markedly and homogeneously hyperechoic; has a well-circumscribed, rounded anterior border; and causes "dirty" incoherent shadowing posteriorly that obscures its posterior border (Fig. 9–60A). However, not all extravasated extracapsular silicone results in the classic snowstorm appearance. In fact, there is a spectrum of sonographic appearances of silicone granulomas. Some extravasated silicone gel collections have a complex cystic appearance (Fig. 9–60B). Others can appear to be isoechoic solid nodules. Very old silicone granulomas can progress to the fibrotic phase of foreign-body reaction and can become spiculated mammographically and cause acoustic shadowing on sonography that is suspicious for malignancy. The entire spectrum may be present in a single patient who has had either extensive extracapsular rupture or injections of free silicone.

Being aware only of the snowstorm appearance of silicone granulomas will lead to disappointing sensitivity for extracapsular rupture. Being aware of and searching for the entire spectrum of appearances of extravasated silicone gel is essential to maximize the sensitivity of sonography for extracapsular rupture.

Although understanding the wide spectrum of sonographic appearances of extravasated silicone gel improves sensitivity, it does not necessarily enable us to always make a specific diagnosis without histologic proof. In cases in which the extravasated silicone has a classic snowstorm appearance, a definitive diagnosis of silicone granuloma is possible with ultrasound alone. However, in cases that have appearances other than the snowstorm appearance, findings can be nonspecific, and histologic diagnosis may be necessary.

The variation in the appearances of silicone granulomas appears to be related to several factors—the size of extravasate silicone gel droplets, the amount of fibrous and foreign-body reaction, and the age of the collection.

Complex cystic and snowstorm phases commonly coexist. Using ultrasound-guided core needle biopsy in a patient who had silicone granulomas of both snowstorm and complex cystic variety has helped to elucidate the causes of the varying sonographic appearances of silicone granulomas (Fig. 9–61). The snowstorm appearance occurs in granulomas that have smaller globules of silicone gel and more inter-

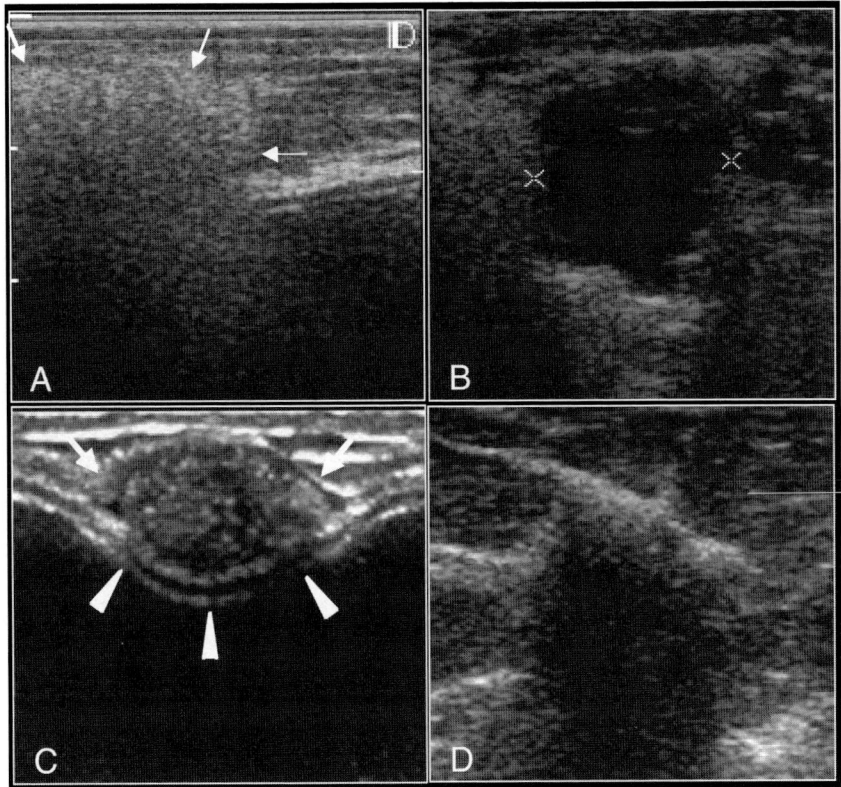

FIGURE 9–60 A: The classic sonographic appearance of silicone granulomas is the "snowstorm" appearance *(arrows)*. However, silicone granulomas have a spectrum of appearances. **B:** Large, acute extravasations of silicone gel tend to have a complex cystic appearance. **C:** Silicone granulomas of intermediate age can present as isoechoic solid nodules. **D:** In very old silicone granulomas, the foreign-body reaction to the extravasated silicone gel can become so intensely fibrotic that it creates an ill-defined acoustic shadowing that simulates malignancy. There is a general tendency for progression of silicone granulomas over time from one appearance to another.

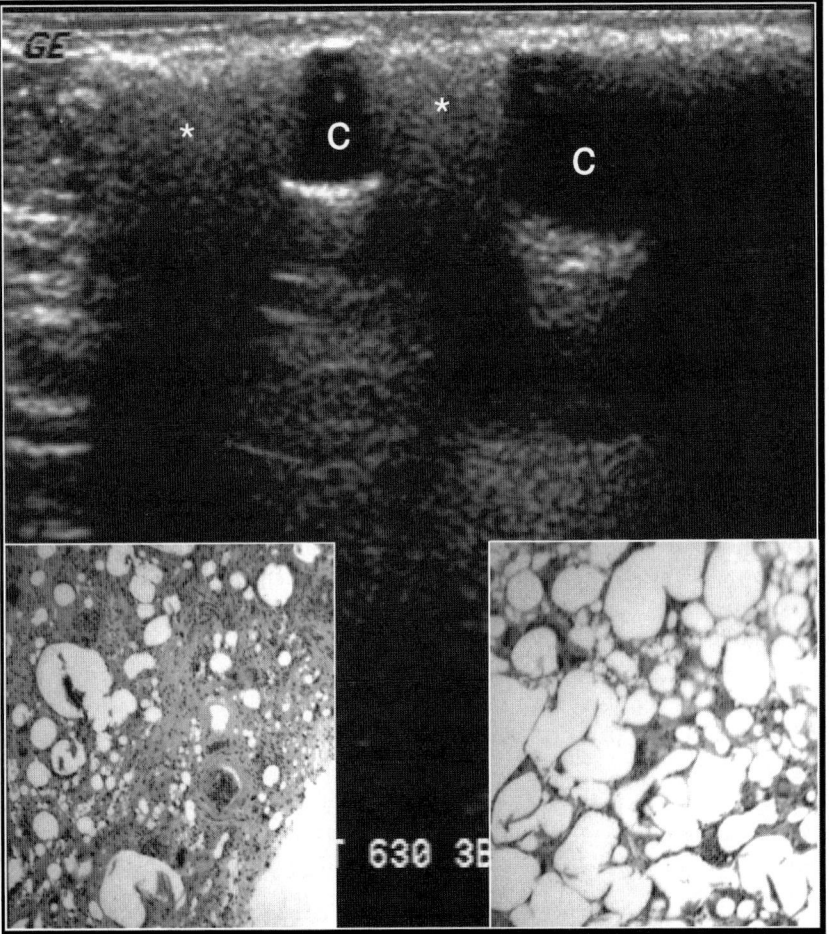

FIGURE 9–61 Snowstorm and complex cystic appearances of extravasated extracapsular silicone gel commonly coexist. Large core needle biopsies were targeted to silicone granulomas having both snowstorm and complex cystic appearances. The biopsy results of the granulomas having the snowstorm appearance *(*)* showed small silicone globules, extensive fibrosis, and foreign-body reaction between the silicone gel globules (histology, **lower left**). Biopsy results of the granulomas having a complex cystic appearance showed larger silicone gel globules and less fibrous and foreign body reaction (histology, **lower right**).

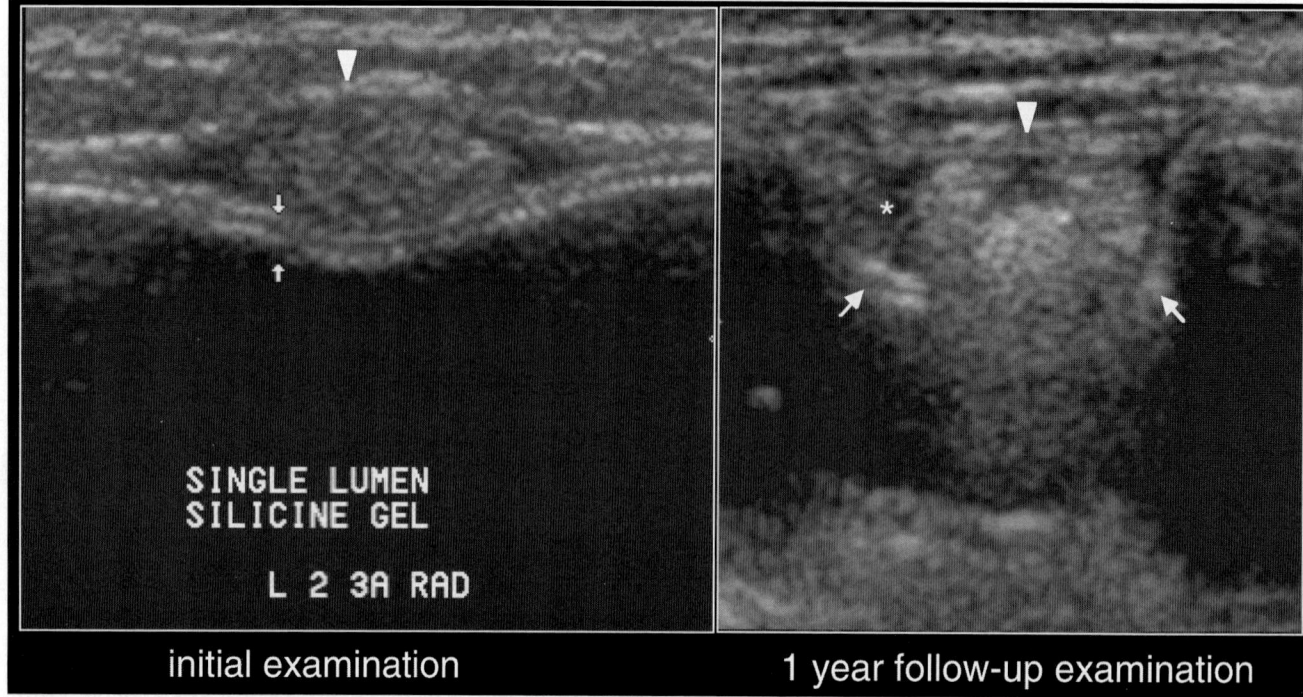

initial examination | 1 year follow-up examination

FIGURE 9–62 The sonographic appearance of silicone granulomas tends to progress over time. This granuloma had an isoechoic solid nodule appearance on the initial examination **(left)**. One year later, the granuloma had progressed to a classic snowstorm appearance **(right)**. Not all silicone granulomas are extracapsular. This granuloma was intracapsular.

vening foreign-body and fibrotic reaction (Fig. 9–61, lower left). The complex cystic appearance occurs in silicone granulomas that have larger globules of silicone gel and less fibrous and foreign-body reaction (Fig. 9–61, lower right). Larger globules of silicone gel transmit sound like fluid. Smaller globules of silicone gel interspersed with foreign-body and fibrous reaction greatly affects the ultrasound beam. The innumerable interfaces between fibrous tissue, which transmits sound at 1,540 m/s, and droplets of silicone gel, which transmits sound more slowly, leads to reflection and refraction of the beam. The reflections from these innumerable interfaces make the silicone granuloma hyperechoic and the refractions make the ultrasound beam incoherent, leading to dirty shadowing deep to the granuloma.

Silicone granulomas tend to progress from one appearance to another over time (Fig. 9–62). Large acute extravasations generally have a complex cystic appearance. The next phase is the isoechoic solid nodule appearance. The third phase is the classic snowstorm appearance. The last phase is the fibrotic phase. The snowstorm appearance is the most frequently seen, the complex cystic appearance the next most common, and the isoechoic solid nodule and fibrotic phases the least frequently seen. Multiple phases can coexist in the same patient, depending on the size and chronicity of the leakage.

It is essential to scan the entire surface area of the implant completely, especially along the entire periphery of the implant. The most common location of silicone granulomas is the periphery of the implant, where the shell is the thinnest and where the radius of curvature is smaller, predisposing this portion of the shell to fatigue fractures. In many cases of extracapsular rupture, scans obtained through the center of the implant appear completely normal, and the only evidence of extracapsular rupture is the presence of a single silicone granuloma at one point along the periphery of the implant (Fig. 9–63). Silicone granulomas that are found along the anterior aspect of the implant usually arise from fatigue fractures at the apex of radial folds (Fig. 9–62). As noted earlier, radial folds are dynamic, forming and unforming with changes of position. The radii of curvature at the apex of radial folds are the smallest that occur anywhere in the shell; thus, the apices of radial folds are especially prone to fatigue fractures. Extracapsular ruptures can occur on superficial or deep surfaces of the implant, but most are superficial. Although sonography occasionally demonstrates a silicone granuloma on the deep surface of the implant (Fig. 9–64), MRI is generally superior to ultrasound for posterior collections. At least part of the examination of implants must be performed at a depth of field that allows the posterior surface of the implant and chest wall to be seen in order to improve the chances of detecting posterior leaks sonographically.

The configuration of silicone granulomas varies greatly. In some cases, the granulomas are nodular and

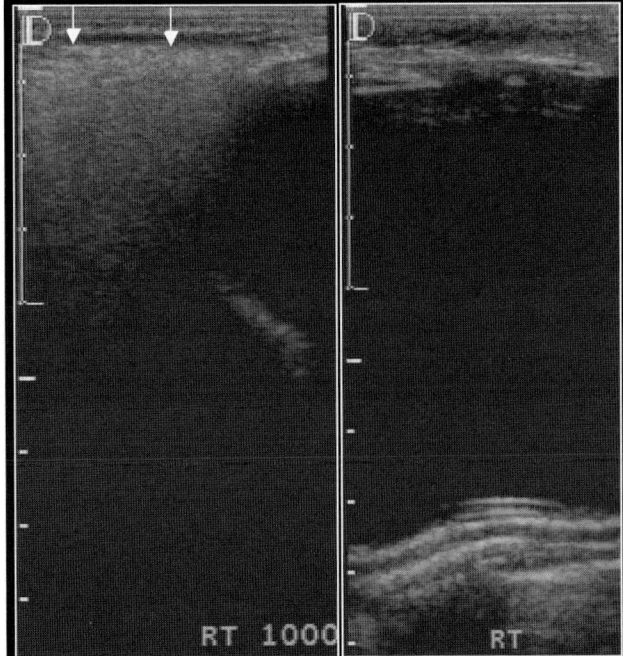

FIGURE 9–63 It is necessary to scan the entire surface of the implants before concluding that there is no extravasated extracapsular silicone gel. Scans of the central portions of the implant are frequently normal (**right**). Silicone granulomas are most frequently found along the edges of the implant, where the shell is thinner and more prone to rupture than it is along the anterior aspect of the implant (**left**).

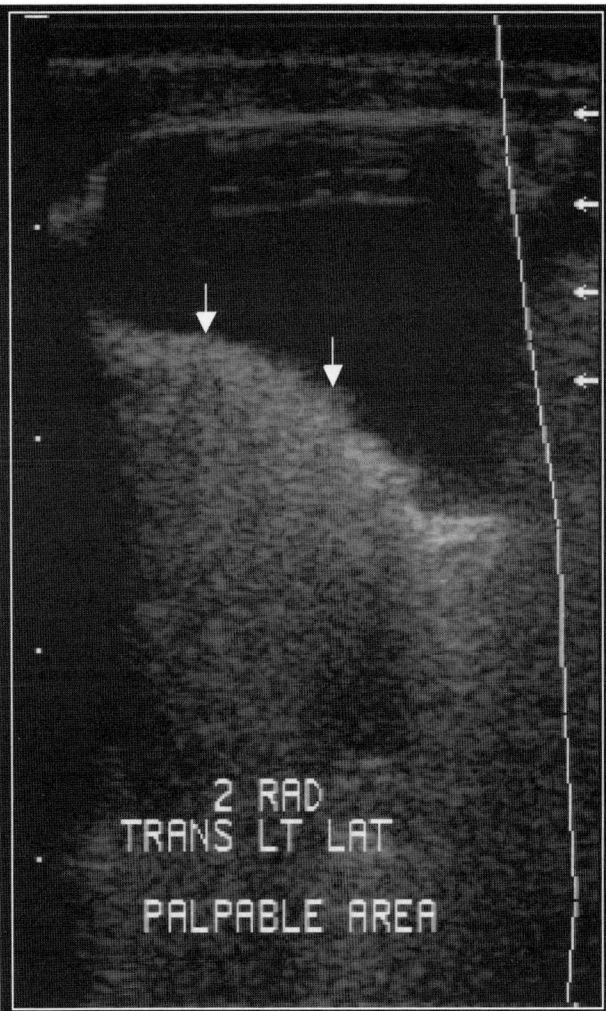

FIGURE 9–64 Sonography showed a silicone granuloma with a snowstorm appearance that lies on the posterior aspect of the implant (*arrows*) in this case. In most cases, however, magnetic resonance imaging is more sensitive for posterior ruptures.

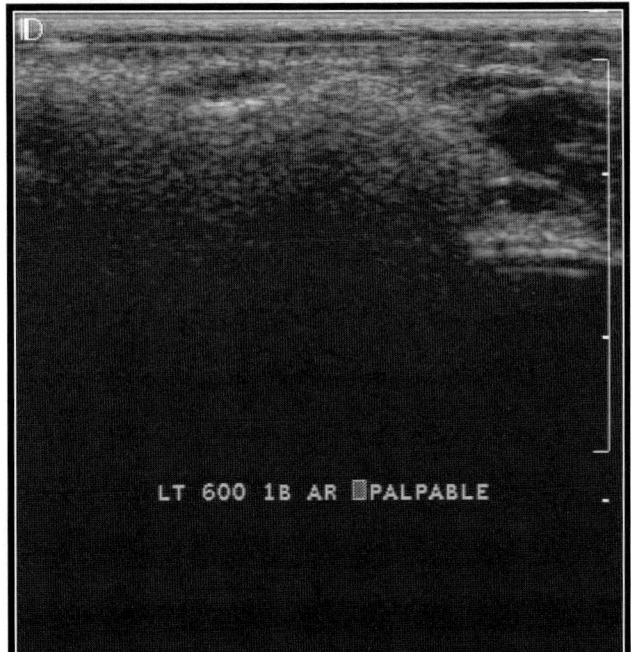

FIGURE 9–65 Silicone granulomas are frequently nodular in shape and can be palpable if located anteriorly.

cause palpable masses (Fig. 9–65). In other cases, the extravasated silicone may spread out in a thin sheet along the outer surface of the capsule that is too thin to be palpable (Fig. 9–66). At surgery, such sheetlike collections of extravasated silicone are so thin and subtle that they might be detectable only by tactile "stickiness" of the shell. Sheetlike collections of extravasated silicone gel can be difficult to distinguish from extensive capsular calcification sonographically (Fig. 9–41).

Migration of Extravasated Silicone Away from the Implant
Extravasated silicone gel can migrate away from the edges of the implant along the chest wall onto the upper abdomen, back, or axilla (Fig. 9–67). Extracapsular silicone can also dissect into tissue planes between muscles and even within muscles. We have seen silicone within pectoralis

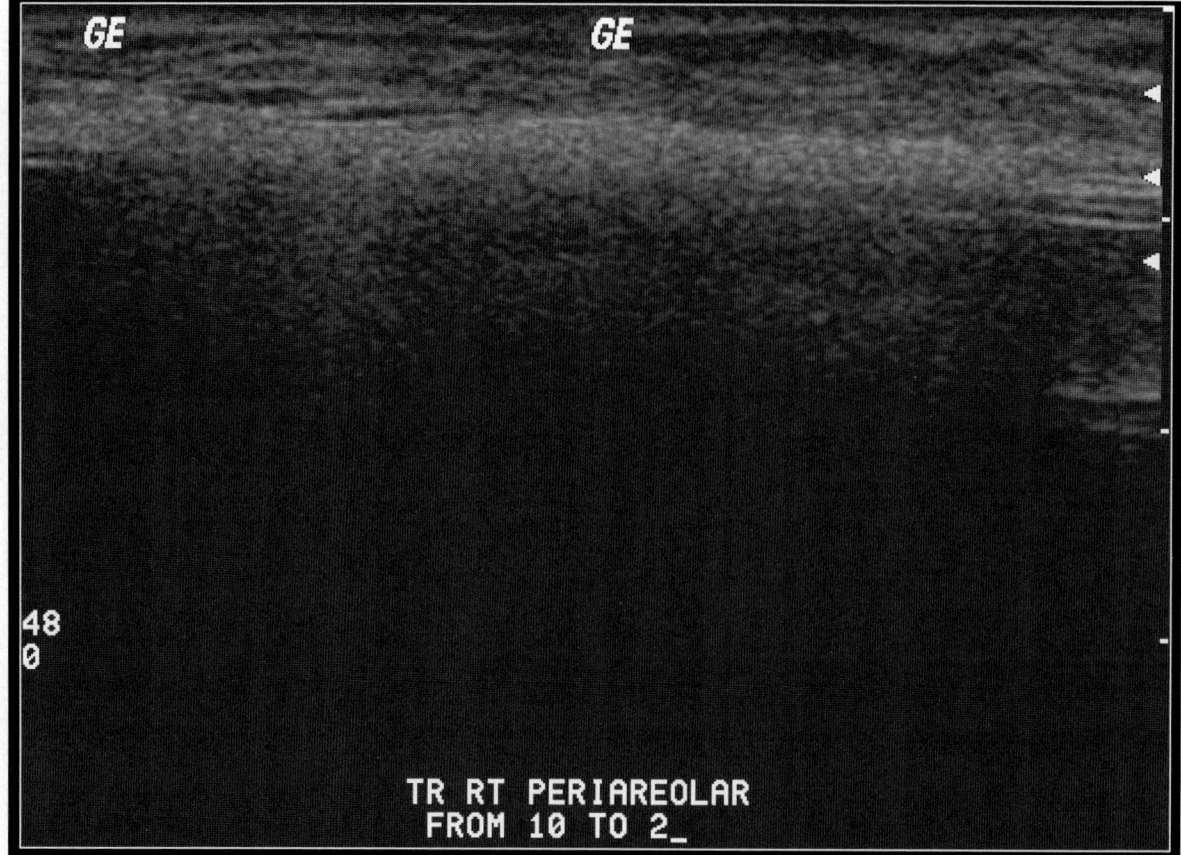

GE   GE

48
0

TR RT PERIAREOLAR
FROM 10 TO 2_

FIGURE 9–66 In other cases, the extravasated extracapsular silicone spreads out in thin, nonpalpable sheets over the anterior surface of the implant or along its edges. This appearance can be simulated by extensive capsular calcification.

and serratus muscles. The appearance of such migrated silicone collections is similar to that of hyperechoic snow-storm-type silicone granulomas within breast tissue and differs only because of location. Thus, if there is evidence of extracapsular rupture, the examination should be extended to include chest wall and axillary tissues. If the patient undergoes explantation or reimplantation, the surgeon will likely want to remove all of the extravasated silicone gel possible, especially if the patient is having any symptoms suggestive of adjuvant disease.

Silicone in Lymph Nodes

Microscopic amounts of silicone can be found within intramammary and axillary lymph nodes even in patients with intact silicone implants, presumably because of microscopic gel bleed. Such small amounts of silicone are not identifiable by imaging studies. However, in the presence of implant rupture, macroscopic amounts of silicone can be carried through lymphatic channels to axillary lymph nodes in amounts sufficient to be demonstrable on ultrasound.

At sonography, macroscopic amounts of silicone within lymph nodes appear hyperechoic, beginning in the hilum and progressing outward through the cortex with

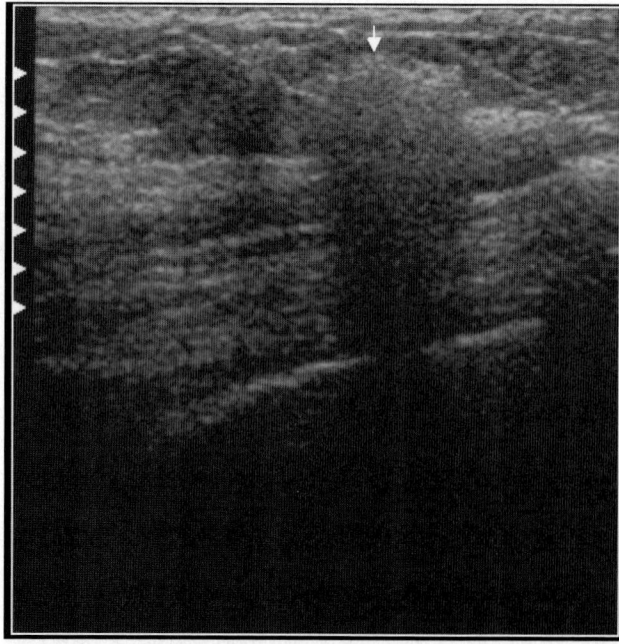

FIGURE 9–67 Extravasated extracapsular silicone gel can migrate away from the edges of the implant onto the upper abdominal wall, axilla, and back. This granuloma had migrated several centimeters away from the inferior edge of the ruptured implant onto the anterior abdominal wall.

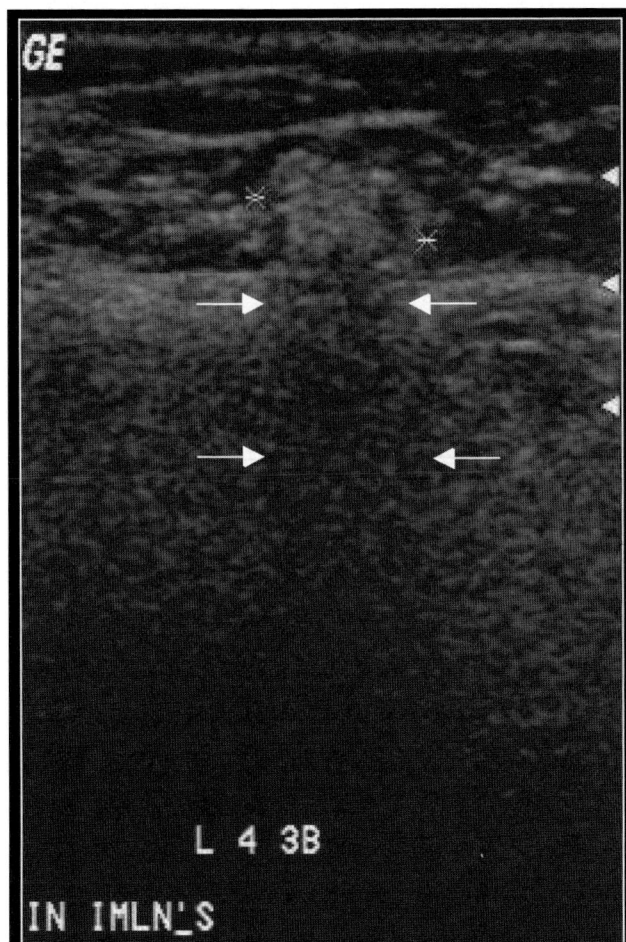

FIGURE 9–68 Extravasated silicone gel, like other foreign bodies, accumulates within the medullary sinuses of the lymph node that lie within the mediastinum of the lymph node. The silicone in the mediastinum makes it echogenic, but it is difficult to distinguish the hyperechogenicity of the silicone gel from the normal echogenicity of the mediastinum unless the silicone gel gives rise to "dirty" acoustic shadowing *(arrows)*.

time and amount of silicone. The earliest finding is increased echogenicity within the lymph node mediastinum that is difficult to distinguish from the normal echogenicity of the lymph node mediastinum unless dirty shadowing is also present (Fig. 9–68). Split-screen images of contralateral mirror-image lymph nodes for comparison is very helpful. What might represent an increase in lymph node hilar echogenicity too subtle to be diagnosed when only the abnormal node is evaluated might be obviously abnormal when compared with contralateral lymph nodes in a mirror-image location (Fig. 9–69). As the amount of silicone within lymph nodes further increases, echogenicity and snowstorm shadowing spread from the hilum side outward, decreasing the apparent thickness of the hypoechoic cortex and making it more difficult to define the structure as that of a lymph node (Fig. 9–70). When there is a snowstorm appearance, demonstration of the thin, echogenic

lymph node cortex or the lymph node capsule is critical in identifying a silicone gel–containing lymph node (Fig. 9–71, left). In very severe cases, the lymph node may have a snowstorm appearance, but the definition of the thin, echogenic cortex cannot be identified. In such cases, the abnormal silicone gel–containing lymph node cannot be distinguished from extravasated silicone that has migrated away from the implant, except by biopsy (Fig. 9–71, right).

The significance of silicone within axillary lymph to the surgeon performing explantation or reimplantation depends on whether there is suspicion of an autoimmune disturbance. If silicone truly does cause an autoimmune disorder or human adjuvant disease, and a patient with ruptured silicone implants is to undergo explantation, the surgeon might elect to remove silicone-bearing lymph nodes at the time of explanation.

Ruptured Silicone Gel Implants Reimplanted with New Single-Lumen Silicone Gel Implants

In most cases of definite extracapsular rupture, the patient will elect to undergo explantation or reimplantation. At surgery, as much extravasated silicone gel as possible is removed, but in many instances, some remains within the breast even after explantation or reimplantation.

Residual extravasated silicone gel offers no diagnostic problem if the patient has not undergone reimplantation or has elected to undergo reimplantation with single-lumen saline implants because it is clear that the silicone granuloma must have originated from the old implant (Fig. 9–72). However, residual extravasated silicone gel can create a diagnostic dilemma if the patient elects to undergo reimplantation with a silicone gel or double-lumen implant because it cannot be determined with certainty whether the silicone granuloma is a residual of the old implant or is a result of extracapsular rupture of the new silicone gel implant (Fig. 9–73). Therefore, demonstration of a silicone granuloma does not necessarily imply the presence of an extracapsular rupture of the new implant. This diagnostic dilemma arises mainly when the replacement implant was placed before 1992 and when it was another silicone gel implant. Replacement implants placed since 1992 in our area have almost all been saline implants.

Residual silicone granulomas can be seen adjacent to the periimplant capsule but are more likely to remain after explantation if the silicone has migrated along the chest wall away from the implant or has been transported to intramammary or axillary lymph nodes.

If a silicone granuloma is identified in a patient with a replacement silicone gel implant, comparison with old mammograms, sonograms, or MRI studies may reveal whether the silicone granuloma is old or new. If these old imaging studies are not available, a careful search for signs of intracapsular rupture of the current silicone implant should be undertaken. Because all extracapsular ruptures must have an associated intracapsular rupture, demonstration of intracapsular rupture of the current implant would

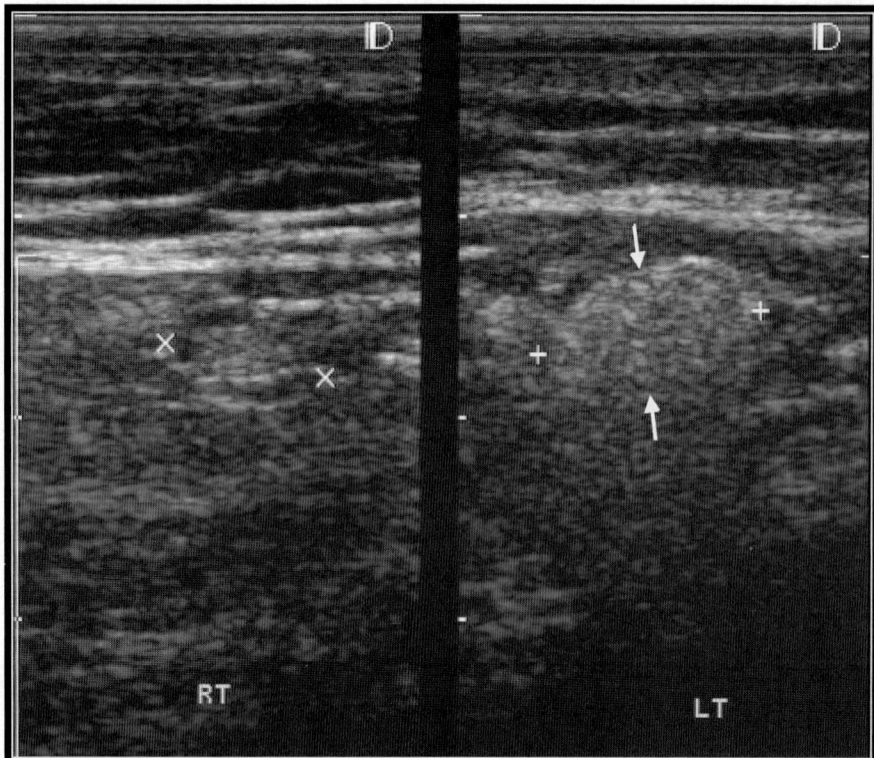

FIGURE 9–69 Split-screen images comparing right and left axillary lymph nodes facilitate sonographic assessment of the hyperechogenicity of the silicone gel–bearing left axillary lymph node (**right**, *arrows*).

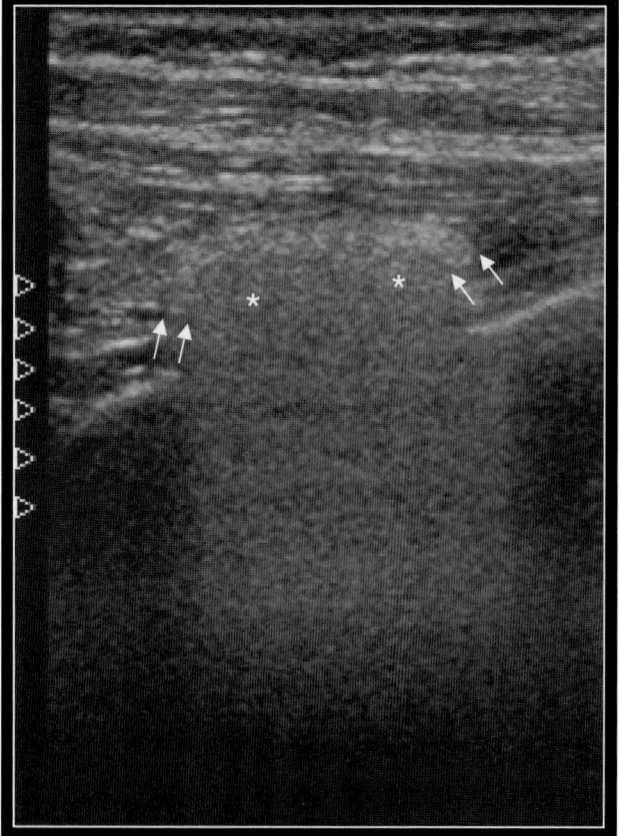

FIGURE 9–70 In severe cases of silicone gel accumulation within lymph nodes, the cortex of the node *(arrows)*, as well as the mediastinum *(*)*, can become hyperechoic and give rise to "dirty" incoherent shadowing.

imply that the granuloma is the result of rupture of the current implant. The lack of evidence of intracapsular rupture would favor the granuloma having originated from rupture of the previous implant. However, some extracapsular ruptures do not have an intracapsular rupture that can be identified by imaging studies, even when meticulously performed, so that lack of imaging evidence of intracapsular rupture does not preclude origin of a silicone granuloma from rupture of the current implant. Conversely, despite evidence of intracapsular rupture of the present implant, the extracapsular silicone granuloma may still be a residual from the old, removed ruptured implant.

Intracapsular Rupture

Intracapsular implant ruptures occur when silicone gel escapes through a rent in the shell but remains confined within the surrounding fibrous capsule. There is a continuous spectrum of intracapsular ruptures, depending on the size of the defect in the shell and degree of collapse of the implant. The spectrum ranges from tiny defects that cannot be found at surgery and are evident only because the shell has a sticky consistency to complete disintegration of the elastomer membrane with extravasation of all of the silicone gel. Small defects can be missed sonographically unless they also have extracapsular silicone granulomas or subtle sonographic counterparts to the MRI "keyhole sign." In most patients with single-lumen implants, the keyhole sign represents nothing more than a radial fold. The apices of radial folds are common places for fatigue

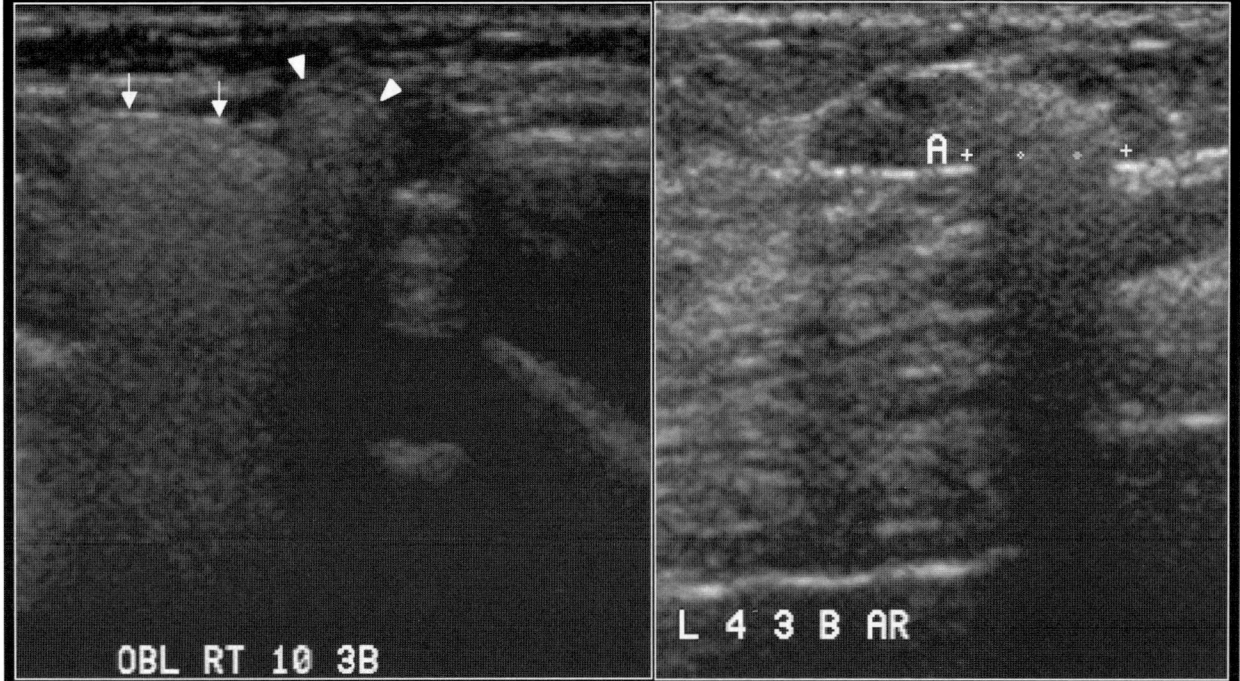

FIGURE 9–71 Identifying the thin, echogenic line that represents the lymph node capsule can be important in differentiating silicone-bearing lymph nodes (**left**, *arrows*) from extravasated free silicone gel that has migrated into the lower axilla. If the capsule is not identified, it is not possible to make the distinction. The lack of a demonstrable capsule in this biopsy-proven silicone-bearing intramammary lymph node (**right**) prevented sonographic determination that it was a lymph node.

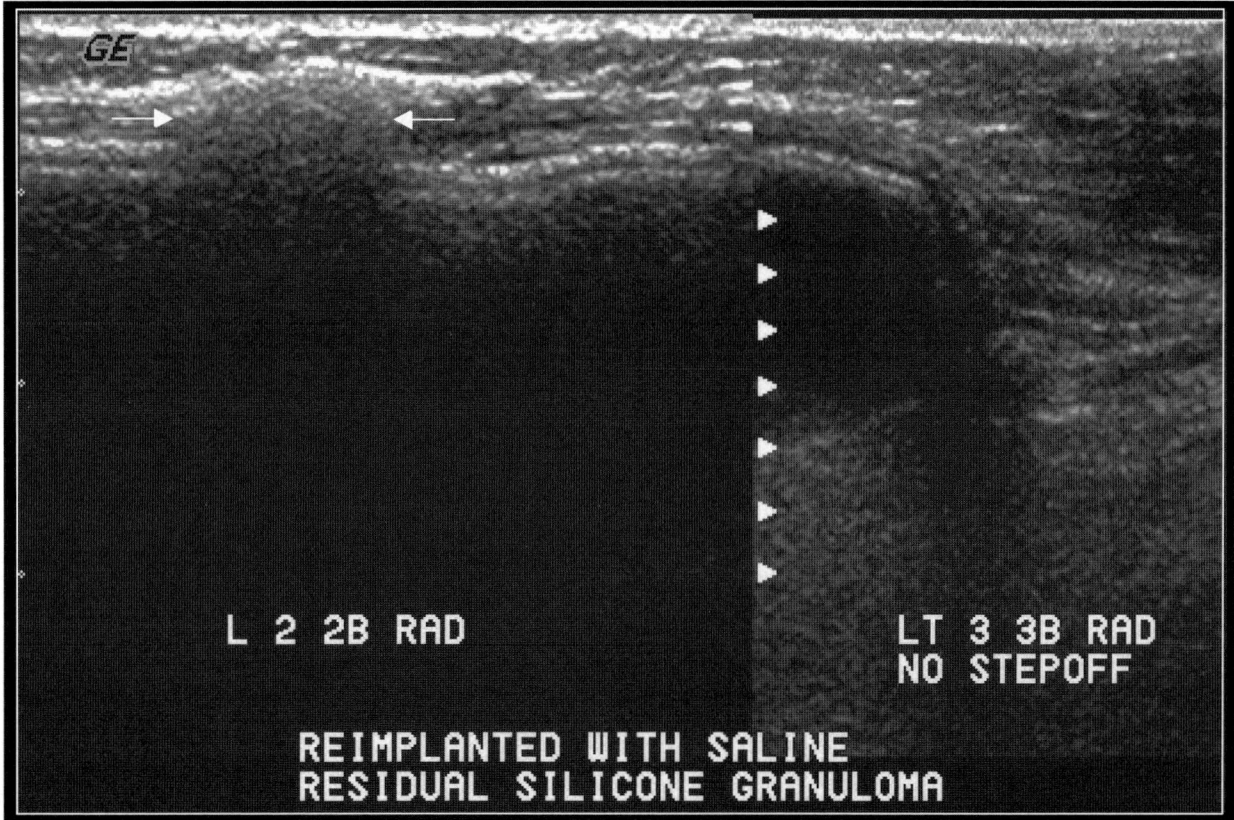

FIGURE 9–72 When a silicone granuloma that has a classic snowstorm appearance is identified in a patient who has been reimplanted with a single-lumen saline implant, it is clear that that granuloma must be a residual from the ruptured explanted silicone gel implant.

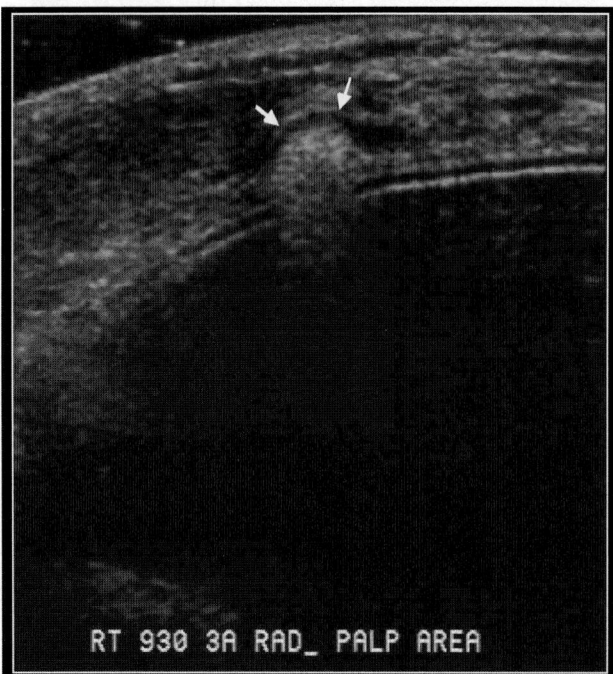

FIGURE 9–73 When there is a residual silicone granuloma or residual silicone-bearing lymph node in a patient who has been reimplanted with a single-lumen silicone gel implant, it cannot be determined with certainty whether the extravasated gel has originated in the new or old implant unless there is evidence of intracapsular rupture in the current implant.

fractures to occur and therefore are common sites for intracapsular rupture to begin. Whether the sonographic keyhole sign is merely an indication of a normal radial fold or evidence of intracapsular rupture requires evaluation of the echogenicity of the fluid within the fold and is not always certain.

The classically described sonographic findings in intracapsular rupture are (a) the presence of abnormally echogenic extravasated silicone gel that lies outside the implant shell but remains confined within the intracapsular space, and (b) the "stepladder sign" (the sonographic counterpart to the MRI linguini sign). The abnormally increased echogenicity of fluid between the capsule and shell is facilitated by comparing it to the echogenicity of the gel remaining within the implant and in split-screen imaging to the gel in the contralateral mirror image (Fig. 9–74). Additionally, folds of the collapsing elastomer membrane may be seen as a series of thin, double echogenic lines that course parallel to the probe face. This has been called the stepladder sign in the sonographic literature because the parallel lines of the membrane folds simulate the rungs on a ladder (Fig. 9–75). It is the sonographic counterpart to the MRI finding called the linguini sign. Hyperechogenicity and the stepladder sign can occur individually or together (Fig. 9–76). The silicone gel between some rungs of the ladder is nearly anechoic, indicating that it still lies within the shell, whereas the fluid between other rungs is

(text continued on page 251)

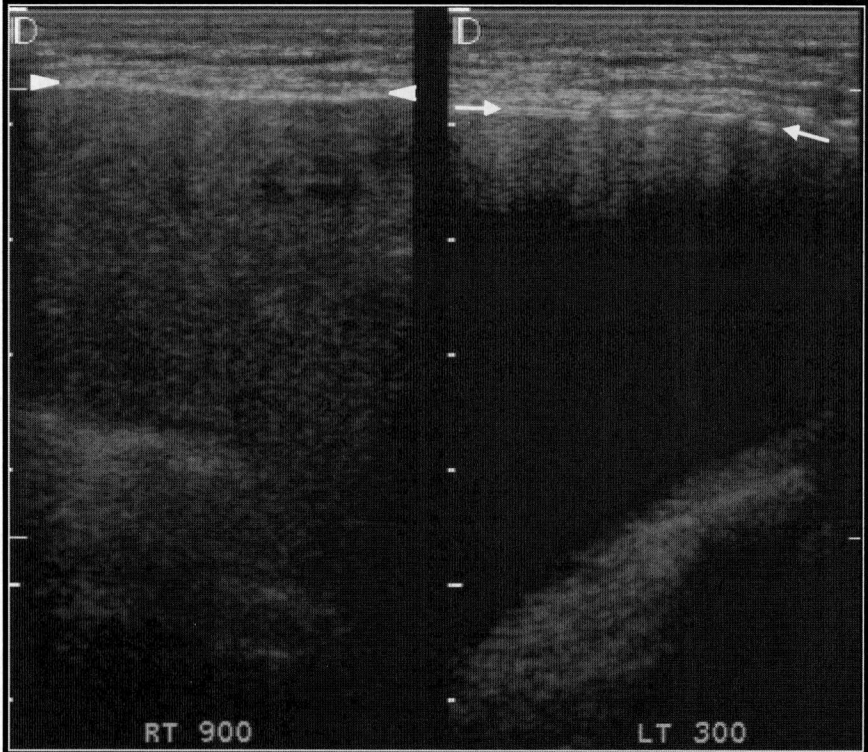

FIGURE 9–74 One of the classic signs of intracapsular rupture is hyperechoic extravasated intracapsular silicone gel (**left** split-screen image, patient's right side). Assessing echogenicity of gel is best done on split-screen mirror-image scans of the right and left sides.

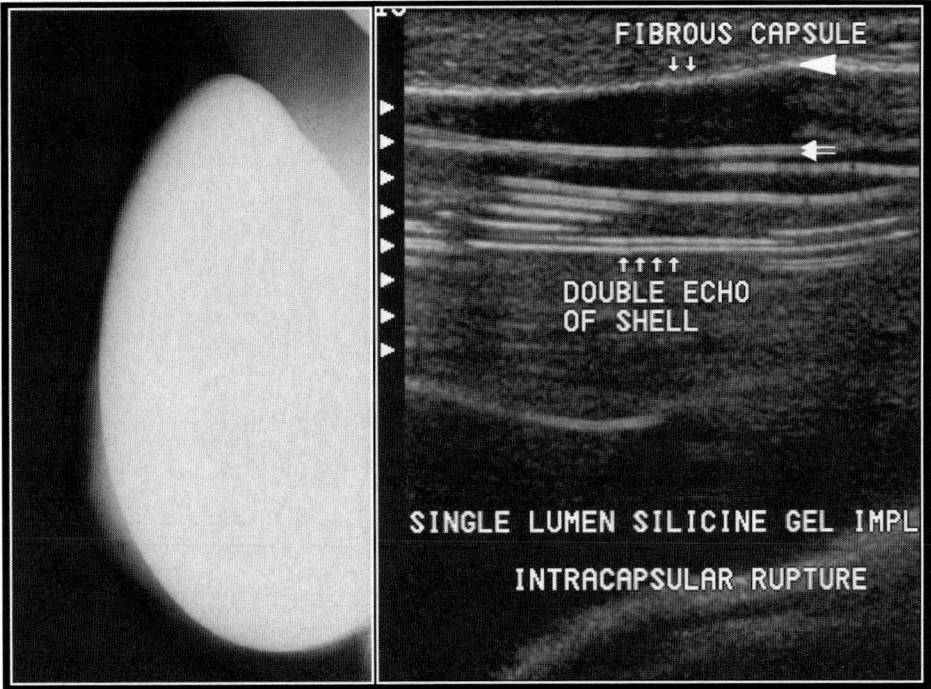

FIGURE 9–75 The other classic finding in intracapsular rupture is the "linguini sign" described in the magnetic resonance imaging literature or the "stepladder sign" described in the sonography literature. The multiple folds of the collapsed implant shell that is floating within a sea of extravasated silicone gel create horizontal echoes that are arranged parallel to each other like the rungs of a stepladder. Note that the mammogram is incapable of showing intracapsular rupture because the mammographic density of the collapsed silicone elastomer shell and the surrounding extravasated silicone gel are identical.

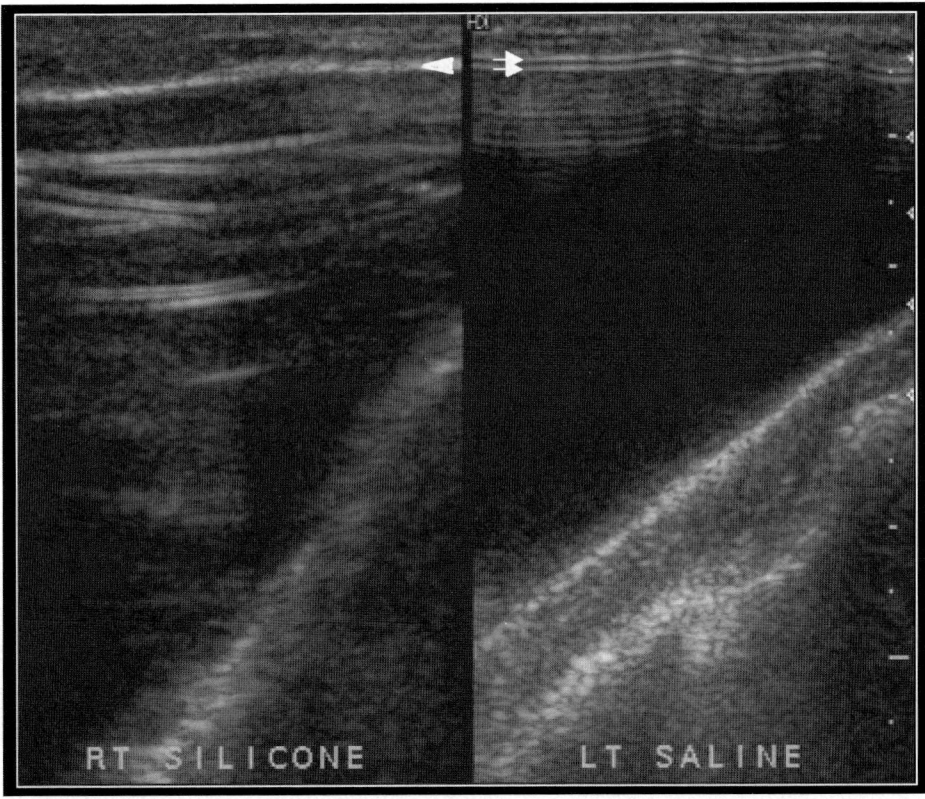

FIGURE 9–76 Hyperechoic extravasated intracapsular silicone gel and the stepladder sign often occur together (left image, patient's right side).

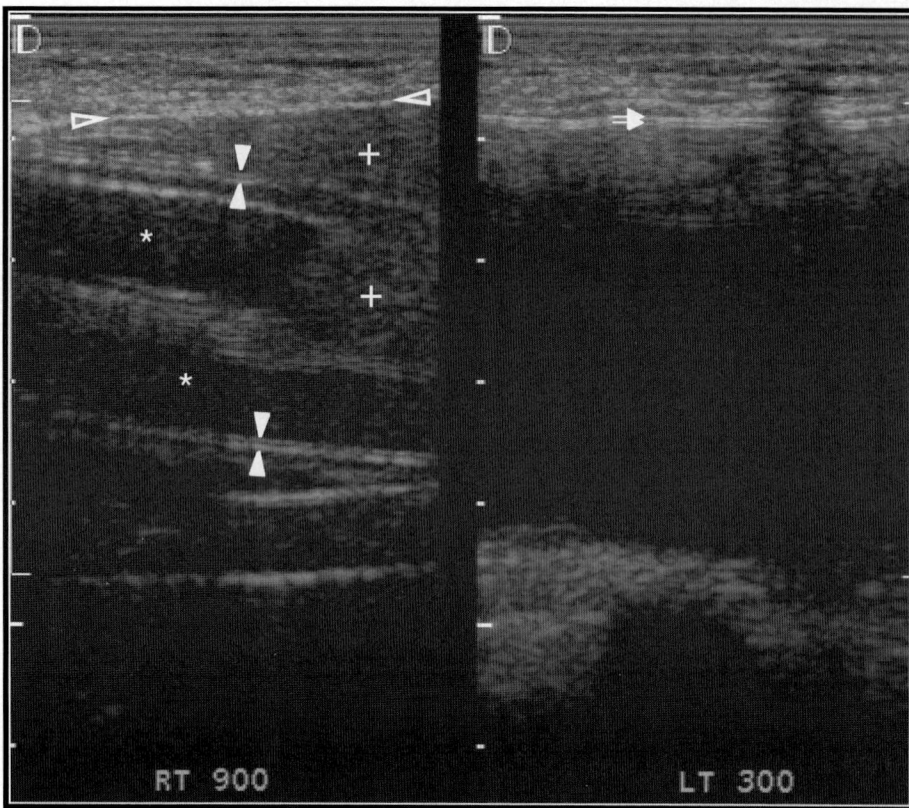

FIGURE 9–77 Split-screen images of the lateral parts of the right and left sides show the stepladder sign on the patient's right side. The double echogenic lines of the shell are part of the rungs of the stepladder *(solid arrowheads),* indicating that the shell is collapsed and folded. Some of the silicone gel on the right is anechoic, and some is hyperechoic. The anechoic gel remains within the partially collapse shell *(*),* whereas the hyperechoic gel has extravasated into the intracapsular space (+).

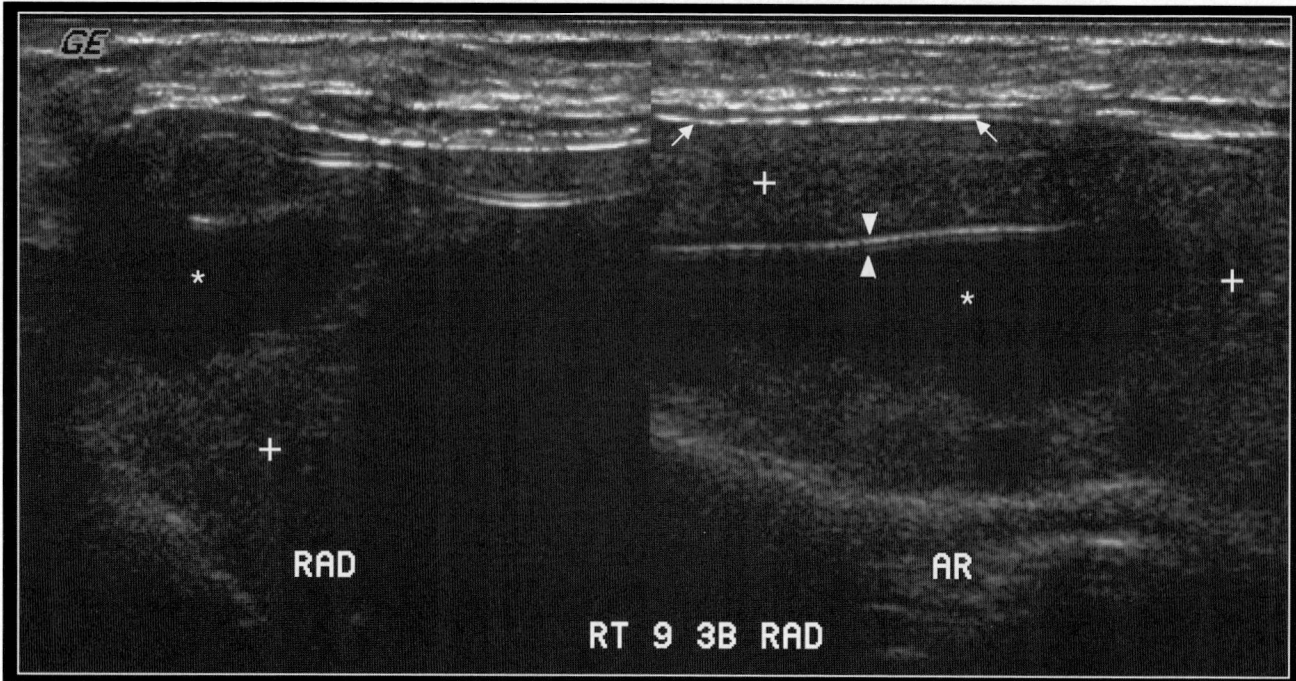

FIGURE 9–78 There is extensive intracapsular rupture with about 50% collapse of the shell. The silicone gel that has not yet extravasated from the shell remains anechoic *(*).* There is abnormal separation between the shell *(arrowheads)* and the capsule *(arrows),* and the extravasated gel that lies between the capsule and shell has become hyperechoic (+).

echogenic because it has extravasated (Fig. 9–77). It is usually easy to distinguish horizontally oriented folds of a collapsed shell from radial folds, which have a general vertical orientation perpendicular to the outer elastomer membrane and can be shown to attach to the outer membrane when viewed in short axis to the fold. A few very long radial folds, however, can curve enough that a part of them lies parallel to the anterior membrane of the implant, even when viewed in their short axis.

Completely collapsed elastomer membranes may float but more commonly fall to the posterior aspect of intracapsular gel. Therefore, their demonstration requires a depth-of-field setting that shows the posterior aspect of the implant and chest wall. If the deep surface of the implant and chest wall cannot be seen with a 7.5-MHz probe, a 5.0-MHz linear or curved linear transducer should be used. In cases in which there has been disintegration of the elastomer membrane, the extravasated intracapsular gel will be echogenic, but there will be no stepladder sign.

The classic findings of intracapsular rupture, the stepladder sign, and abnormally increased echogenicity of intracapsular extravasated gel are definitive but are insensitive because they are present only in patients in whom the rupture is large and the collapse of the implant shell is complete or nearly complete. However, not all cases of implant rupture result in complete collapse of the shell; therefore, not all cases of intracapsular rupture show the stepladder sign. There is a wide spectrum of intracapsular rupture that varies with the size of the defect in the shell and the degree of collapse. In most patients with intracapsular rupture, the shell defect is small, and the degree of collapse is much less than complete (Fig. 9–78). Traditionally, MRI has been reported to have the advantage over sonography in cases with less than complete collapse because sonographers have only looked for the classic findings, which are associated only with complete collapse of the implant. However, the sensitivity of sonography for intracapsular rupture is actually quite good and competitive with MRI, even for ruptures in which collapse is only partial, if the normal sonographic appearances of the fibrous capsule and implant shell are kept in mind.

In intracapsular rupture, gel extravasates from the shell into the space between the capsule and shell, resulting in an abnormal widening of the space between the capsule and the shell. Thus, the key finding in intracapsular rupture is the presence of an abnormal space between the capsule and the shell (of which the stepladder sign or linguini sign is only the final and most complete stage). The degree of separation between the fibrous periimplant capsule and the shell is directly proportional to the degree of extravasation of silicone from the implant and the degree of collapse of the shell (Fig. 9–79).

In complete or nearly complete collapse, the separation may be wide enough that with transducer frequencies of 10

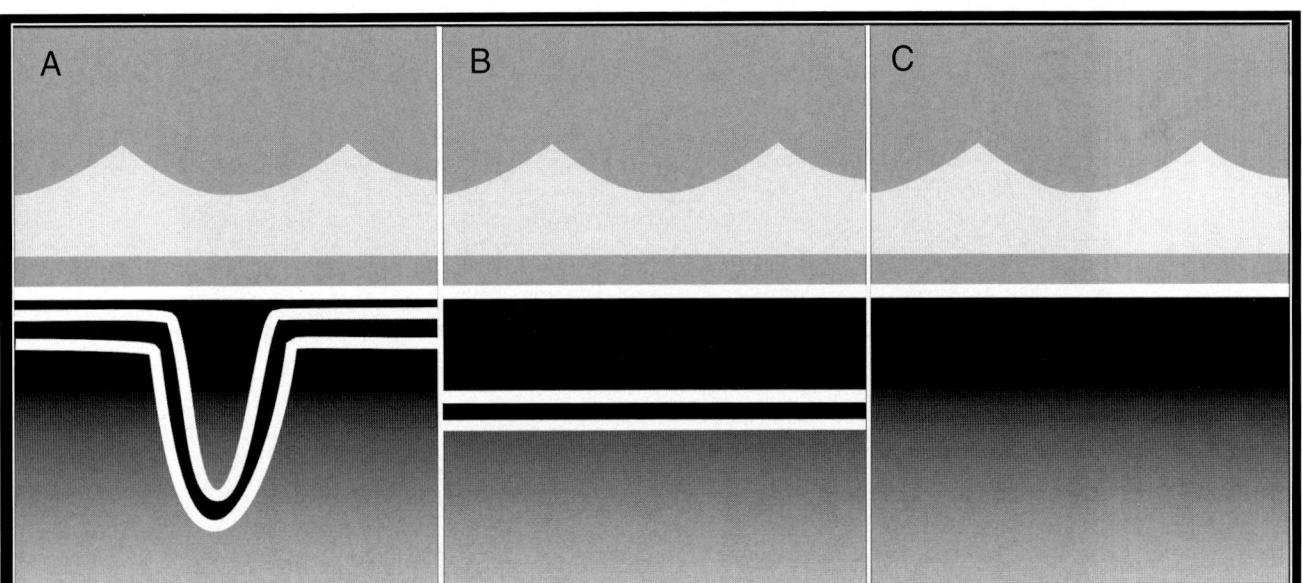

FIGURE 9–79 To maximize sensitivity, it is necessary to search for various degrees of abnormal separation of the shell from the periimplant effusion. When the degree of collapse is large, only the single echogenic line that represents the periimplant capsule may be demonstrable *(C)*. With milder degrees of collapse, the space between the shell and the capsule becomes abnormally large in two orthogonal planes *(B)*. In the earliest phases of intracapsular rupture, a stress fracture may develop within the shell at the apex of a radial fold *(A)*. There is a continuous spectrum of findings from a completely normal-appearing radial fold to definitive evidence of intracapsular rupture confined to a radial fold.

MHz or greater and standard small-parts depths of fields, the collapsed shell may lie too deeply to visualize. Only a single echogenic line representing the intact periimplant capsule will be demonstrable. The double echogenic line will be too deep to demonstrate without using a lower-frequency transducer and a greater depth of field (Figs. 9–74 and 9–80). The extravasated gel in acute ruptures is generally anechoic, whereas the extravasated gel tends to become echogenic in more long-standing ruptures. In lesser degrees of separation, the single echogenic line representing the capsule and the double echogenic line representing the shell may be closer together, but still not tightly apposed, as is normal.

The key to achieving adequate sensitivity in the sonographic diagnosis of intracapsular rupture is identifying milder degrees of capsule–shell separation (cases in which the shell defect and the degree of shell collapse is small), which is quite possible. Unfortunately, mild degrees of separation between the capsule and shell also occur in normal radial folds, so that distinguishing between radial fold and early intracapsular rupture is important but can be tricky and difficult. The key feature that distinguishes radial folds from intracapsular rupture is the shape of the separation between the capsule and the shell. In intracapsular rupture with only mild collapse of the shell, the separation between the capsule and shell is sheetlike. The capsule and shell are separated over long distances in two orthogonal planes (Figs. 9–81 and 9–82). In a radial fold, on the other hand, the capsule–shell separation appears linear or one-dimensional. The separation between the capsule and shell is long in the axis that is obtained parallel to the long axis of the fold, whereas it is short and keyhole-like when obtained perpendicular to the fold (Figs. 9–83 and 9–84).

The extravasated silicone gel that lies within the sheetlike separation between the capsule and the shell can be anechoic or nearly anechoic, like silicone gel that remains within the shell, or hyperechoic. The echogenicity of extravasated intracapsular silicone gel depends on the age of the intracapsular rupture. Newly extravasated gel tends to be anechoic or nearly anechoic, but over time, it tends to become hyperechoic (Fig. 9–85). Harmonics and real-time spatial compounding can help to demonstrate hyperechoic extravasated gel by suppressing near-field artifacts (see Chapter 2, Figs. 2–18 and 2–27).

To summarize, in evaluating a patient with silicone gel–containing implants for intracapsular rupture, three questions must be asked:

(text continued on page 255)

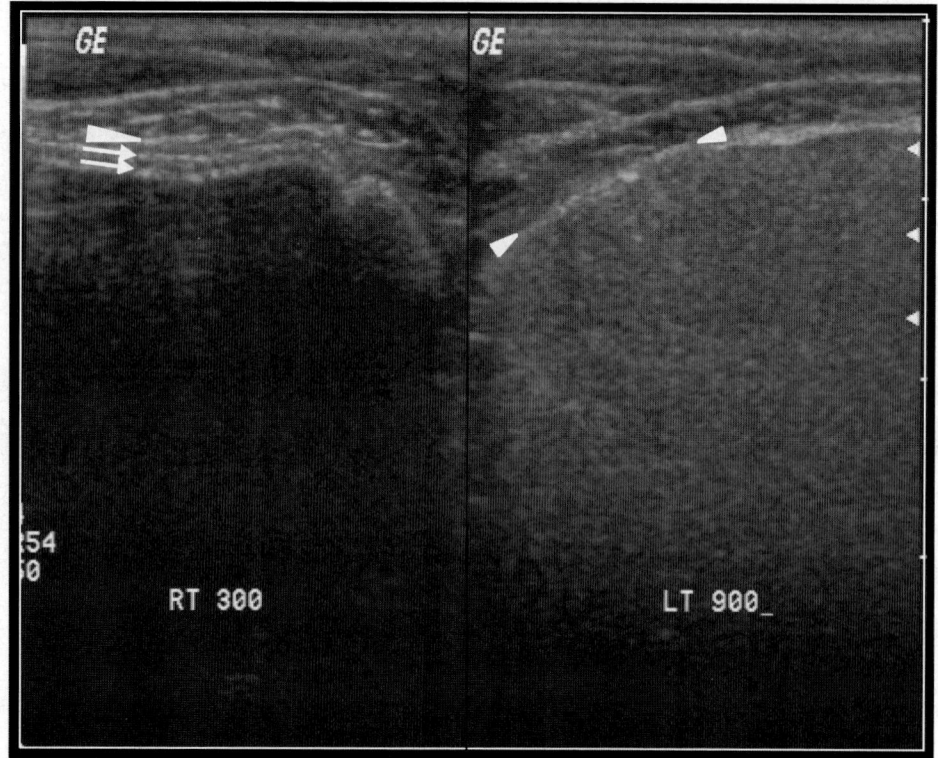

FIGURE 9–80 The normal triple echogenic line representing the intact capsule–shell complex is present on the patient's intact right implant (*arrows* indicate shell; *arrowheads* indicate superficial surface of capsule). Only a single echogenic line representing the fibrous periimplant capsule *(arrowheads)* is present on the patient's left side, where the implant is ruptured. The extravasated gel on the patient's left side is hyperechoic, and the completely collapsed shell has fallen posteriorly away from the capsule and is not visualized in these images.

long axis view
short axis view

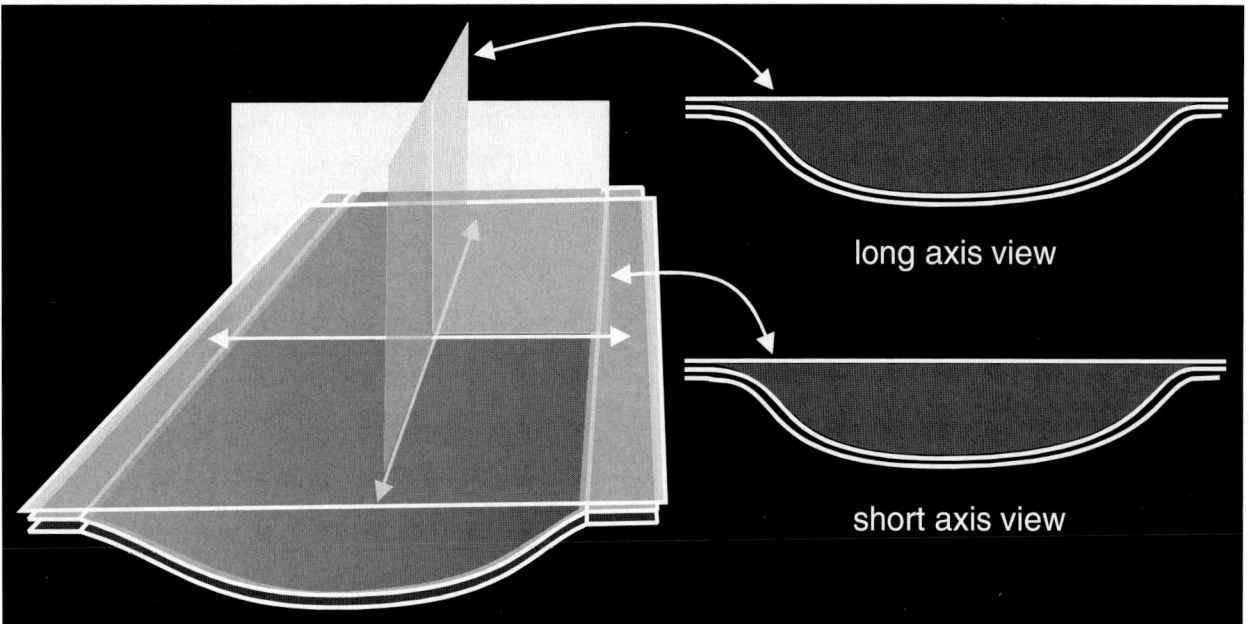

FIGURE 9–81 Definitive sonographic evidence of intracapsular rupture with partial collapse requires that the abnormal separation between the capsule and shell be sheetlike and present over long distances in two orthogonal planes.

C
S
C
S
rad
A
ar
GE
GE
rad
B
ar

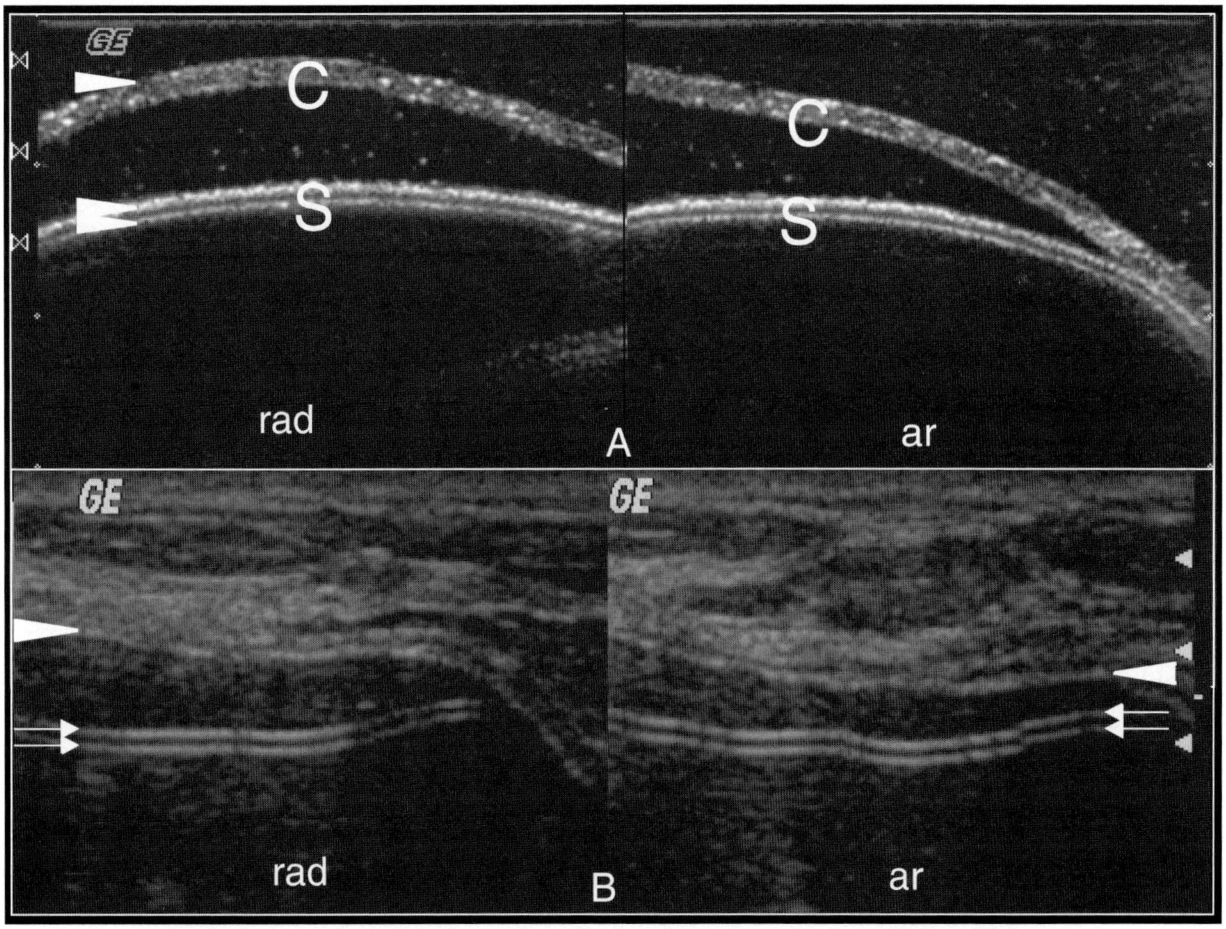

FIGURE 9–82 Intracapsular rupture with partial collapse presents as a 2-D sheetlike abnormal separation between the capsule and the shell. **A:** This is an *in vitro* model of intracapsular rupture with partial collapse in which there is abnormal separation between the slice of ham (*c*, capsule) and the shell of the implant *(s)* that is present in two orthogonal planes. **B:** This is an *in vivo* intracapsular rupture with sheetlike separation of capsule *(arrowheads)* and shell *(arrows)* that is present in two orthogonal planes.

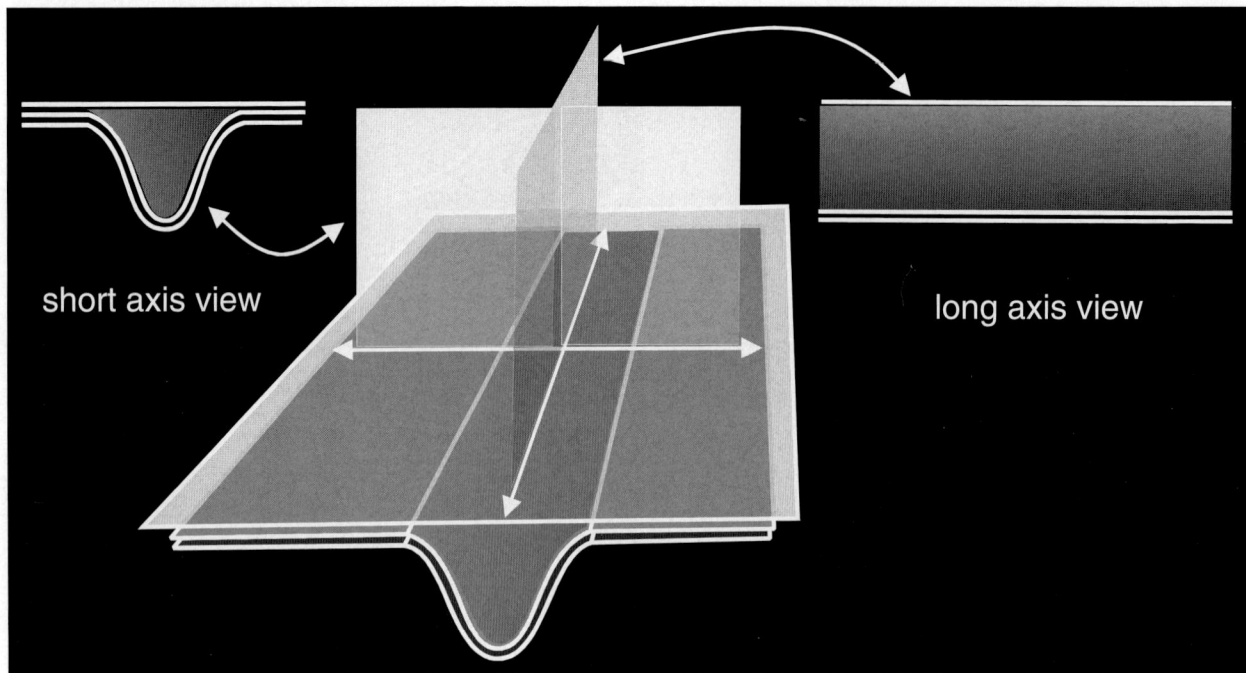

short axis view

long axis view

FIGURE 9–83 The separation between the capsule and the shell in radial folds is 1-D. The separation occurs over a long distance when obtained parallel to the long axis of the fold but is short and V shaped when obtained perpendicular to the long axis of the fold.

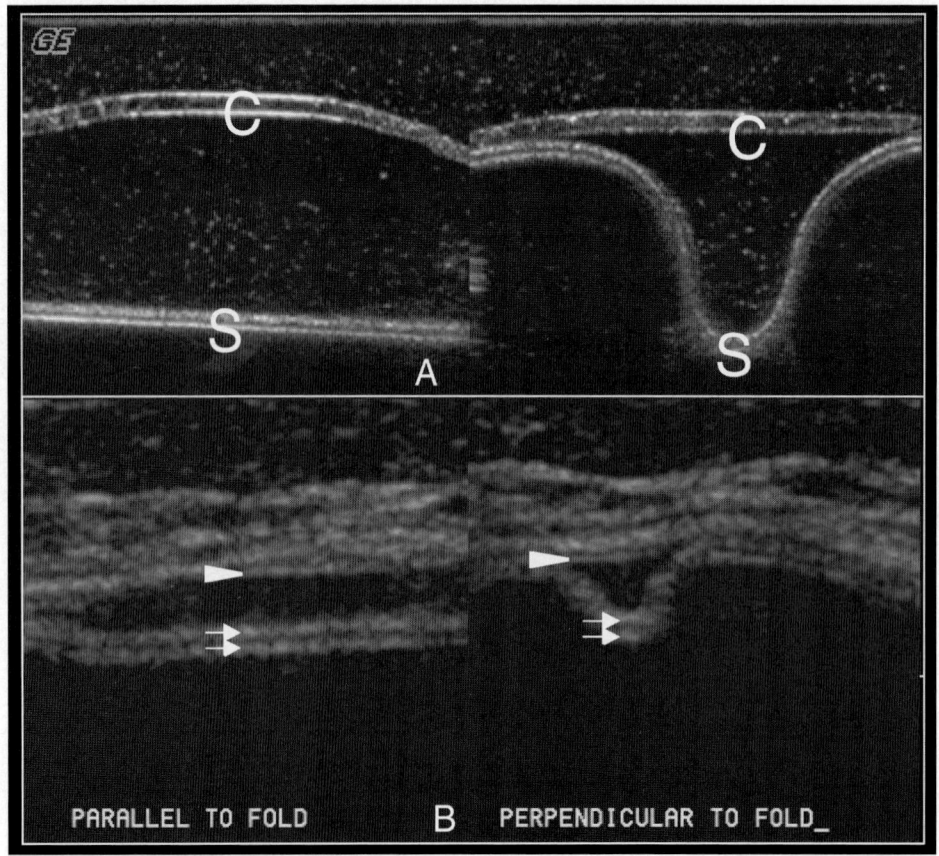

PARALLEL TO FOLD   B   PERPENDICULAR TO FOLD_

FIGURE 9–84 **A:** This *in vitro* radial fold was scanned in a water bath. The separation between the ham (c, capsule) and shell (s) extends over a long distance when obtained parallel to the long axis of the fold but is short and V shaped when obtained perpendicular to the long axis of the fold. **B:** This *in vivo* radial fold shows a long separation between the capsule *(arrowhead)* and shell *(arrows)* when obtained parallel to the long axis of the fold but a short V-shaped separation in the plane that lies perpendicular to the fold.

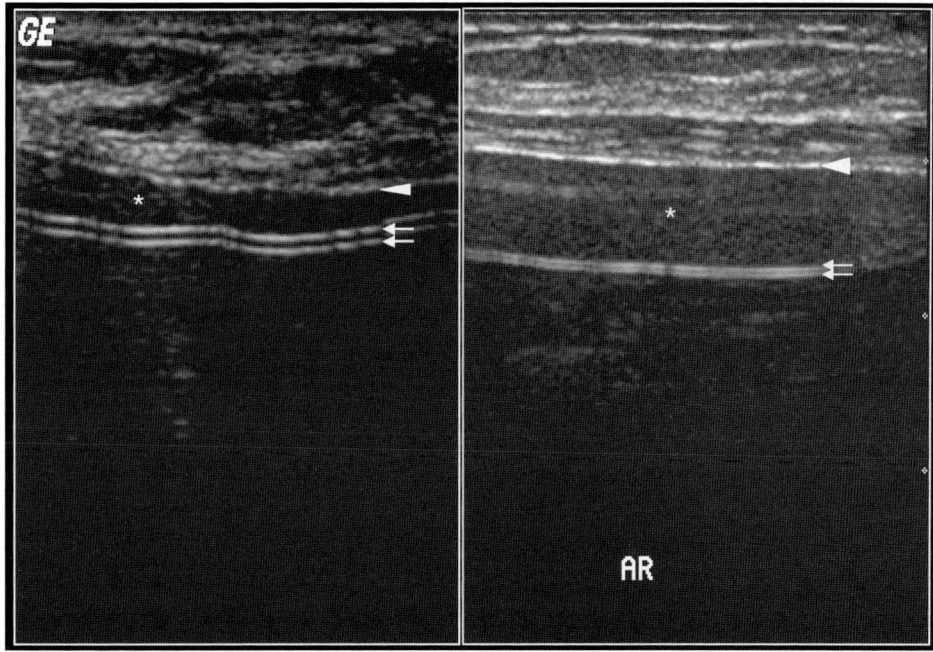

FIGURE 9–85 The extravasated silicone gel that lies in the space *(*)* between the abnormally separated capsule *(arrowhead)* and shell *(arrows)* can be anechoic or nearly anechoic in acute intracapsular ruptures **(left)** but tends to become hyperechoic over time in chronic intracapsular ruptures **(right)**.

1. Is there a separation between the capsular and shell echo complexes?
2. Is the configuration of the separation sheetlike or foldlike?
3. Is the fluid in the space between the capsule and the shell abnormally echoic?

Whether separation of the shell and capsule or echogenicity of the fluid within the space is more important in diagnosing intracapsular rupture depends on the configuration of the separation. If the separation is sheetlike, it represents a "hard finding." The presence of intracapsular rupture and the echogenicity of the fluid in the space between the capsule and shell is merely a "soft finding" that supports the diagnosis and suggests that the rupture is chronic rather than acute.

On the other hand, if the separation is foldlike, the echogenicity of the fluid is more important in determining whether the separation merely represents a radial fold or whether it represents a radial fold in which a fatigue fracture has occurred at the apex (Figs. 9–86 and 9–87). If the fluid within the fold is anechoic, it cannot be determined with certainty whether the fluid within the fold is merely the normal periimplant effusion, gel bleed without rupture, or acutely extravasated silicone gel that has not had time to become echogenic. Because radial folds are variants of normal in most patients and far more common than intracapsular rupture, it is prudent to assume

that such folds are normal. Mildly echogenic fluid within the fold can represent echogenic periimplant effusion, gel bleed, or extravasated silicone gel due to an intracapsular rupture of intermediate age. Although the risk for intracapsular rupture is slightly higher than when fluid is anechoic, in the absence of other findings that suggest intracapsular rupture, most cases of mildly echogenic fluid within radial folds should be assumed to represent echogenic periimplant effusion. This can be confirmed by scanning the effusion at the edge of the implant. Only in cases in which the fluid becomes frankly hyperechoic or assumes a classic snowstorm appearance can a diagnosis of intracapsular rupture at the apex of the fold be made with absolute certainty.

The apex of radial folds is a likely point for fatigue fractures to occur, and radial folds are thus the likely starting point for intracapsular rupture in many cases. The radial fold becomes gradually wider in its short axis as the degree of extravasation within the fold increases. Thus, there is a continuous spectrum of capsule–shell separations from foldlike radial folds to sheetlike separation that is definitive for intracapsular rupture. Patients may be seen at any point in time along this spectrum (Fig. 9–88). An important corollary is that all intracapsular ruptures that are not caused by major acute trauma are likely localized in the beginning. Thus, the abnormal separation of the shell and capsule will be found in most patients only if the entire implant surface is assessed. The

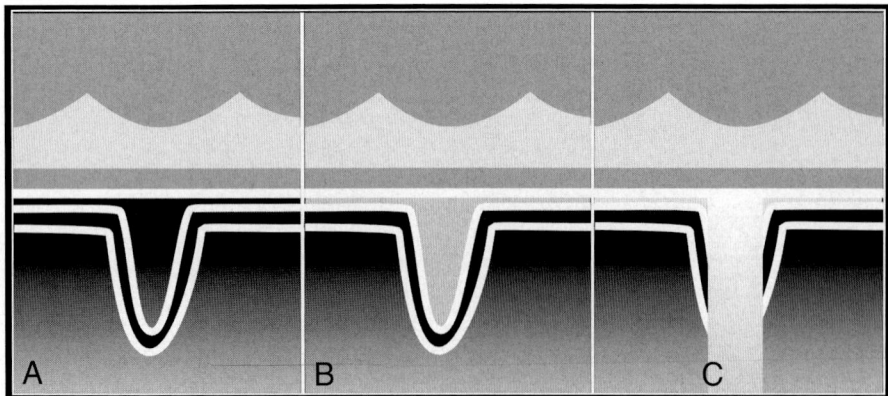

FIGURE 9–86 Radial folds are normal in most cases, but the apices of radial folds can be the sites of fatigue fractures in some. The key to making the diagnosis of intracapsular rupture that has resulted from a fatigue fracture at the apex of a radial fold is to assess the echogenicity of the substance that lies within the radial fold. Fluid that lies within the radial fold can be anechoic (**A**), mildly echogenic (**B**), or hyperechoic and snow-storm-like (**C**).

capsule will be closely apposed to the periimplant capsule over most of the implant surface. Only with time and further leakage of silicone gel from the shell will the separation between the capsule and shell become generalized and demonstrable over the entire surface of the implant.

Another site where the risk for intracapsular rupture is increased is in an area of implant herniation, where focal bulging and thinning of the implant shell weakens it and predisposes it to rupture (Fig. 9–58).

Although the intracapsular extravasated silicone gel in cases of isolated intracapsular rupture usually main-

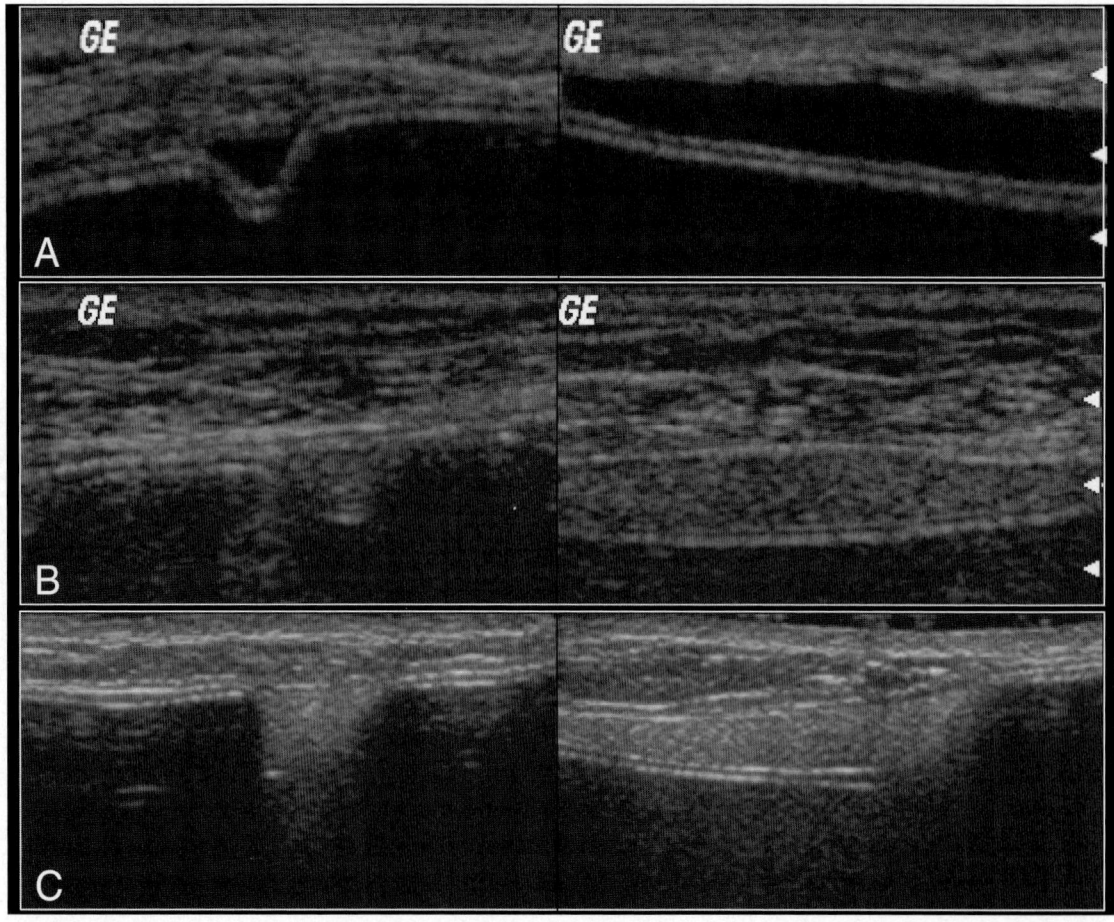

FIGURE 9–87 These split-screen images of radial folds are obtained parallel to the long axis of the fold on the **right** and perpendicular to the long axis of the fold on the **left**. **A:** Anechoic fluid within the fold can be normal periimplant effusion, gel bleed, or acutely extravasated silicone gel that has not had time to become echogenic. Because most folds with anechoic fluid are normal, in the absence of any other finding suggesting intracapsular rupture, it is prudent to assume all such folds are normal. **B:** The fluid within this fold is mildly echogenic. This can represent echogenic periimplant effusion, chronic gel bleed without rupture, or extravasated gel resulting from intracapsular rupture of intermediate age. The risks for rupture are slightly higher than if the fluid is anechoic, but in most cases, low-level echoes merely represent echogenic periimplant effusion. **C:** The contents of the fold have a hyperechoic, snowstorm appearance, which is definitive evidence that a fatigue fracture at the apex of the fold has resulted in extravasation of silicone gel into the fold. The intracapsular rupture is chronic.

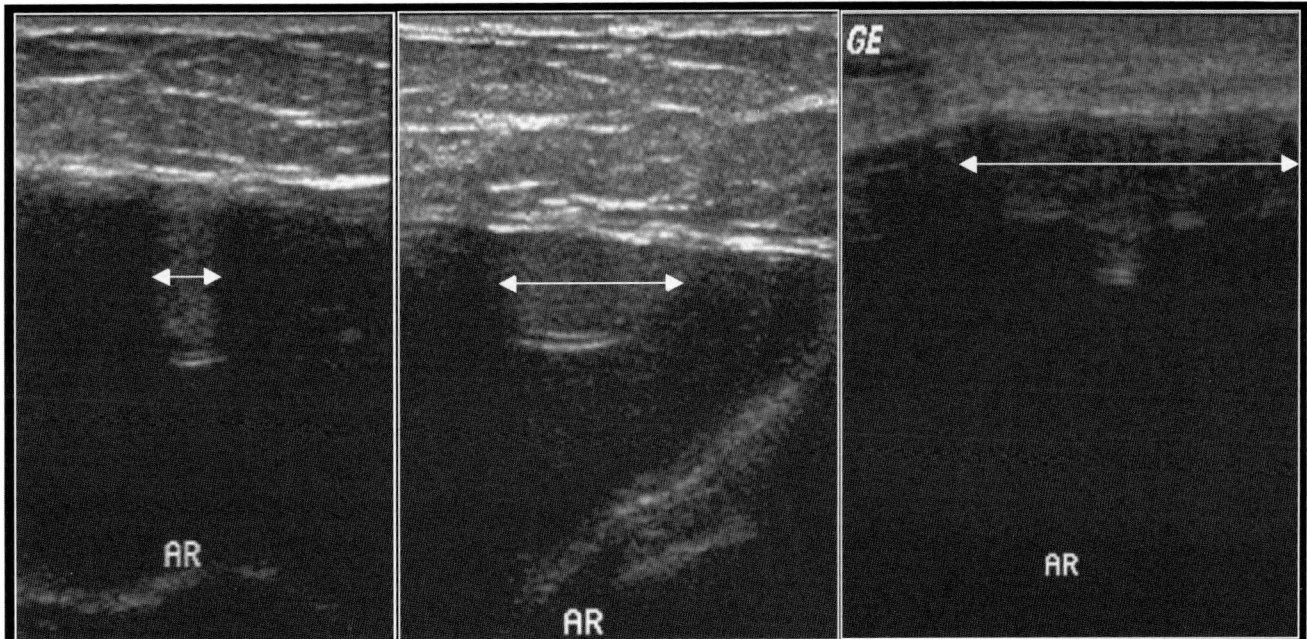

FIGURE 9–88 Many intracapsular ruptures begin as fatigue fractures at the apices of radial folds. Over time, as the amount of extravasated silicone gel within the fold increases, the fold becomes wider. Thus, there is a continuous spectrum between linear radial folds and sheetlike separations of the capsule and shell. The patient may be evaluated sonographically at any point along this spectrum.

tains a gelatinous consistency similar to that of nonextravasated gel, in some cases, the foreign-body reaction to the gel is so severe that it becomes solidified by granulomatous reaction. This process can result in formation of a silicone granuloma that is sonographically indistinguishable from an extracapsular silicone granuloma except for its intracapsular location. Thus, intracapsular collections of extravasated silicone gel can have a classic snowstorm appearance (Fig. 9–89).

Sonography can demonstrate abnormal separation between the capsule and shell best along the anterior aspect of the implant with a high degree of sensitivity but is less sensitive for abnormal separations and echogenicity on the deep surface of the implant because of limitations in beam focusing in the far field. MRI shows the anterior and posterior aspects of the shell and capsule nearly equally well and therefore has a theoretical advantage in showing isolated mild posterior intracapsular rupture. Despite this advantage of MRI, there are cases in which sonography can show a posteriorly located capsule–shell separation (Fig. 9–90). Furthermore, isolated posterior separations are less common than suggested by MRI. Patients are scanned prone in MRI and supine in ultrasound. The implant shell and the silicone gel that remains within the shell tend to fall to a dependent position within the intracapsular space. In the supine position used during sonography, the partially collapsed shell tends to fall posteriorly, and the abnormal separation between the capsule and shell tends to occur anteriorly, where the performance of sonography is strong.

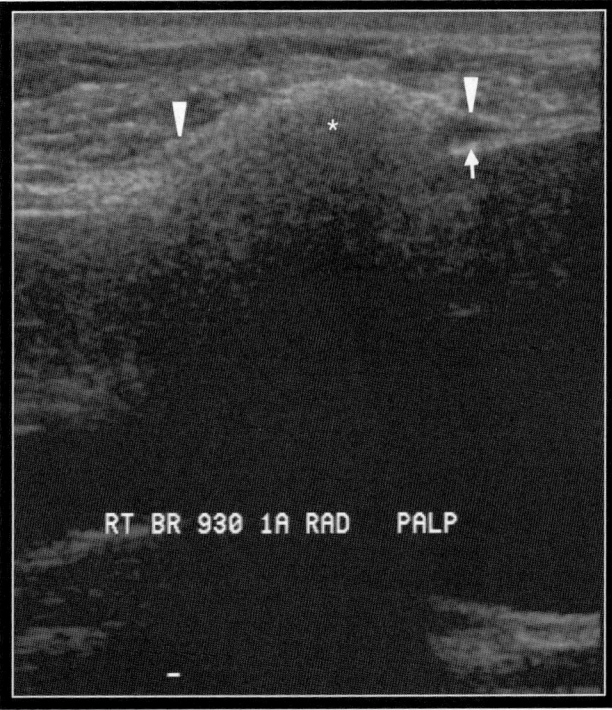

FIGURE 9–89 Most extravasated silicone gel that remains intracapsular maintains a gelatinous consistency and appears nearly anechoic or only mildly echogenic sonographically. In a few cases, foreign-body reaction to intracapsular extravasated gel may be more intense and can progress to granuloma formation with the classic snowstorm appearance. Note that this silicone granuloma lies within the capsule *(arrowheads)* but outside the shell *(arrows).*

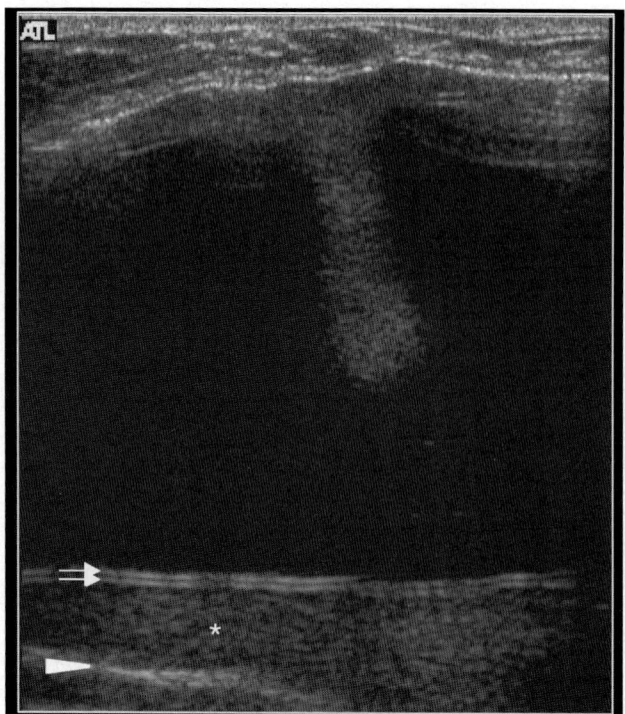

FIGURE 9–90 Magnetic resonance imaging generally is better at showing posteriorly located intracapsular rupture than is sonography. However, in certain case, we can demonstrate posterior capsule–shell separations sonographically. The double echogenic line that represents the posterior portion of the shell *(arrows)* is abnormally separated from the posterior periimplant capsule *(arrowhead)* by abnormally echogenic extravasated silicone gel *(*)*. There is also evidence of anterior intracapsular rupture in this case that appears to have originated within a radial fold.

In the prone position used for MRI, the shell tends to fall anteriorly, creating separation between the capsule and shell posteriorly, where MRI has an advantage. Cases that appear to be posterior separations on MRI can actually appear to be anterior separations on ultrasound because of different patient positioning and gravity-induced changes in position of the partially collapsed shell within the capsule. In such cases, the advantage of MRI over sonography is minimized.

Near-field reverberation echoes can simulate intracapsular rupture of a single-lumen silicone gel implant. However, counting the number of echogenic lines enables us to distinguish between intracapsular rupture and reverberation echoes (Fig. 9–91). In the case in which reverberation echoes within the implant simulate a shell that is abnormally separated from the capsule, there will be triple echogenic lines at the superficial edge of the implant–capsule complex that represent the capsule (single outer echogenic line) and the shell (inner two echogenic lines) that are closely apposed to each other. In intracapsular rupture, a single echogenic line will be present at the superficial edge of the implant–capsule complex. That single echogenic line represents the fibrous capsule.

Near-field artifacts other than reverberation echoes can obscure the true echogenicity of the fluid that lies between the capsule and the shell anteriorly. Coded harmonics can clear much of this artifact, allowing echogenicity to be more accurately assessed (see Chapter 2, Fig. 2–18).

In summary, sonographic findings of *intracapsular* rupture include:

- The specific but insensitive classic findings of abnormally echogenic extravasated silicone gel and the stepladder sign, which are present only in the small minority of patients with intracapsular rupture in whom collapse of the implant shell is complete or nearly complete
- The more sensitive but less specific sign of a two-dimensional, sheetlike, abnormal separation of the shell from the capsule
- The more sensitive but less specific radial fold that contains abnormally echogenic extravasated silicone gel, including (a) the most sensitive, least specific sign of radial fold containing anechoic fluid; (b) the less sensitive, more specific sign of radial fold containing echogenic fluid; and (c) the least sensitive, highly specific sign of radial fold containing the snowstorm appearance

Signs of intracapsular rupture may or may not be associated with signs of extracapsular rupture (Fig. 9–92). Evidence for intracapsular rupture should be sought in cases of known extracapsular rupture, especially if the patient will undergo explantation and replacement. In any case of suspected intracapsular rupture, evidence of extracapsular rupture should be sought. Many patients with isolated intracapsular rupture elect not to undergo explantation or reimplantation, but most patients with extracapsular rupture do elect to undergo explantation or reimplantation. Additionally, the type of explantation may depend on whether the rupture is extracapsular. Patients with extracapsular rupture are more likely to undergo explantation with capsulectomy, whereas patients with isolated intracapsular rupture are more likely to undergo explantation or reimplantation without capsulectomy.

Intracapsular rupture is more common than extracapsular rupture. However, historically, it has more often missed by sonography than has extracapsular rupture. Several studies have shown sonography to be less sensitive for intracapsular rupture than is MRI. Most of the published studies comparing sonography and MRI used a constellation of MRI findings to diagnose intracapsular rupture while using only the classic, but insensitive, findings of the stepladder sign with or without abnormal echogenicity to diagnose rupture. Searching for the more sensitive finding of an abnormal separation between the capsule and shell will improve sonographic sensitivity for intracapsular rupture and make sonography more competitive with MRI for detection of intracapsular rupture. The advantage of sonography for detecting intracapsular rupture is that it is much

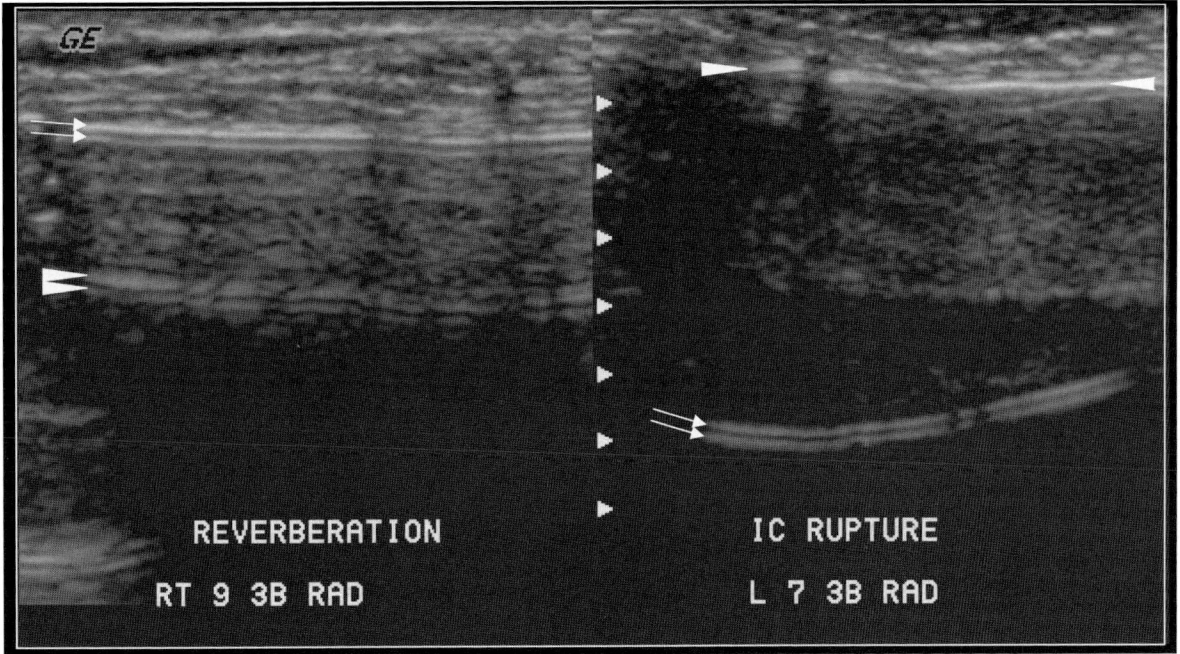

FIGURE 9–91 It is important not to mistake reverberation echoes from intracapsular rupture. The double echogenic reverberation lines **(left)** are reflected into the substance of the implant *(arrowheads)*, but the double echogenic line that represents the true shell remains at the anterior edge of the silicone *(arrows)*. In intracapsular rupture **(right)**, the double echogenic line that represents the true shell *(arrows)* is present within the substance of the implant, but only a single echogenic line that represents the periimplant capsule *(arrowheads)* is present at the anterior margin of the silicone.

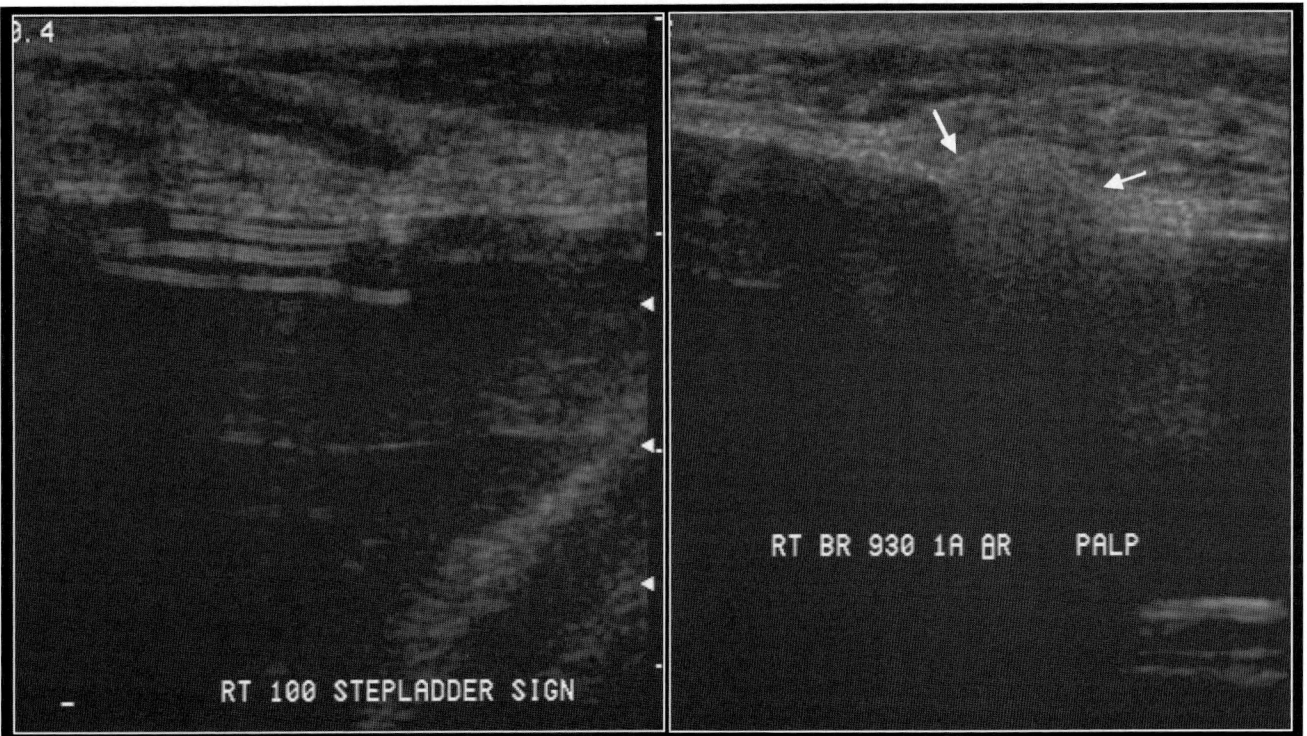

FIGURE 9–92 Many patients show findings of both extracapsular and intracapsular rupture. In most cases, extracapsular rupture **(right)** is preceded by intracapsular rupture **(left)**. On the other hand, many cases of intracapsular rupture do not have associated extracapsular rupture.

less expensive than MRI and more widely available. Its disadvantage, as always, is that it is very operator dependent.

Sonographic Evaluation of Double-Lumen Implants

Sonographic evaluation of double-lumen implants is more difficult than evaluating single-lumen implants and offers several special challenges:

1. Periimplant effusion can simulate the outer saline compartment of double-lumen implants.
2. Double-lumen implants in which the outer saline shell has collapsed may simulate single-lumen silicone gel implants.
3. Mixing of saline and silicone gel components due to loss of integrity of the inner shell, although probably not clinically significant, can cause a mottling of echogenicity within the implant, simulating intracapsular rupture with partial collapse of the shell that occurs in patients who have single-lumen silicone gel implants.

These problems are the result of not knowing with certainty the type of implant present. Obviously, every effort should be made to obtain either the surgical report or recent mammograms to help determine the type of implant and minimize the sonographic diagnostic dilemmas. However, in cases in which surgical history and mammograms are not immediately available, sonography can be used to solve the problems. The use of speed-of-sound phenomena to identify the presence of double-lumen implants was discussed earlier and is illustrated in Fig. 9–14. A useful finding is the shape of the outer water-containing structure. Most periimplant effusions are not under pressure. Therefore, the peripheral aspect of the effusion forms an acute angle. The outer saline-containing compartment of a double-lumen implant, on the other hand, usually has a rounded, peripheral margin. These differences are imperfect in distinguishing a periimplant effusion from the outer saline compartment of a double-lumen implant, however (Fig. 9–93). A more definitive method of making the distinction is to count the number of echogenic lines. A double echogenic line represents each shell. Double-

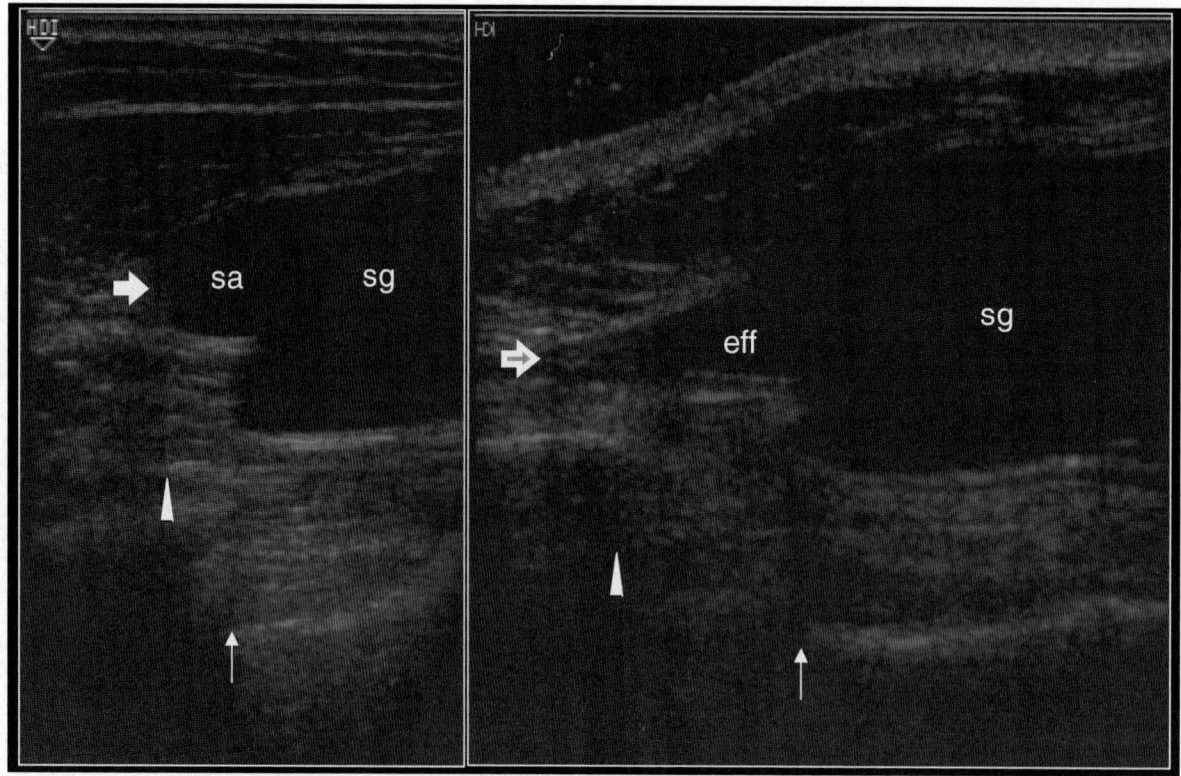

FIGURE 9–93 Speed of sound changes in the chest wall at the edges implants are not helpful in distinguishing periimplant effusions **(right)** from the outer saline-filled compartment of double-lumen implants **(left)**. In both cases, there is a step-off at the edge of the silicone gel–containing compartment *(arrows)*. Neither the periimplant effusion nor the saline-filled outer compartment of a double-lumen implant causes a step-off at its edge *(arrowhead)*. However, the peripheral edge of the effusion makes an acute angle *(large gray arrow)*, whereas the peripheral edge of the outer saline-filled compartment of a double-lumen implant is convex outward *(large white arrow)*. sg, silicone gel; sa, saline compartment of double-lumen implant; eff, periimplant effusion.

lumen implants have two shells and one capsule and thus should be represented by five echogenic lines. The most superficial line represents the superficial surface of the capsule, the middle two lines represent the surfaces of the outer shell, and the inner two lines represent the surfaces of the inner shell (Fig. 9–94, left). Single-lumen implants with periimplant effusions have one capsule and one shell and thus generally demonstrate only three echogenic lines. The most superficial line represents the outer surface of the capsule, and the two deeper lines represent the surfaces of the inner shell (Fig. 9–94, right). Thus, counting the number of echogenic lines should enable definitive distinction between double-lumen implants and various different conditions affecting single-lumen implants. This can be accomplished along the anterior aspect of the implant, where the shells and capsule are parallel to the transducer face and perpendicular to the beam. However, near-field artifacts sometimes interfere with the assessment of the number of echogenic lines along the anterior aspect of the implant.

The saline compartment of normal double-lumen implants is usually not very distended, and the saline within it

is not under pressure. In most cases, there is so little saline present and it is under so little pressure that the normal compression forces all the saline in the outer compartment to the periphery of the implant. Anteriorly, directly under the transducer, the inner and outer shells will appear to be directly in contact with each other, even when the outer shell is intact. In such cases, only by scanning the periphery of the implant can we demonstrate that the outer compartment contains saline and that it has not ruptured (Fig. 9–95). It can also be useful to count the number of echogenic lines along the anterior and posterior borders of the outer water-containing compartment. Only a single echogenic line, the capsule surrounds a periimplant effusion, whereas a double or triple echogenic line surrounds the outer saline compartment of a double-lumen implant (Fig. 9–96).

Unfortunately, it can be technically difficult to count the number of echogenic lines along the anterior edge of the outer water-containing compartment because the shell and capsule are obliquely oriented with respect to the beam. It can be easier to evaluate the posterior surface of the outer water-containing compartment because it lies

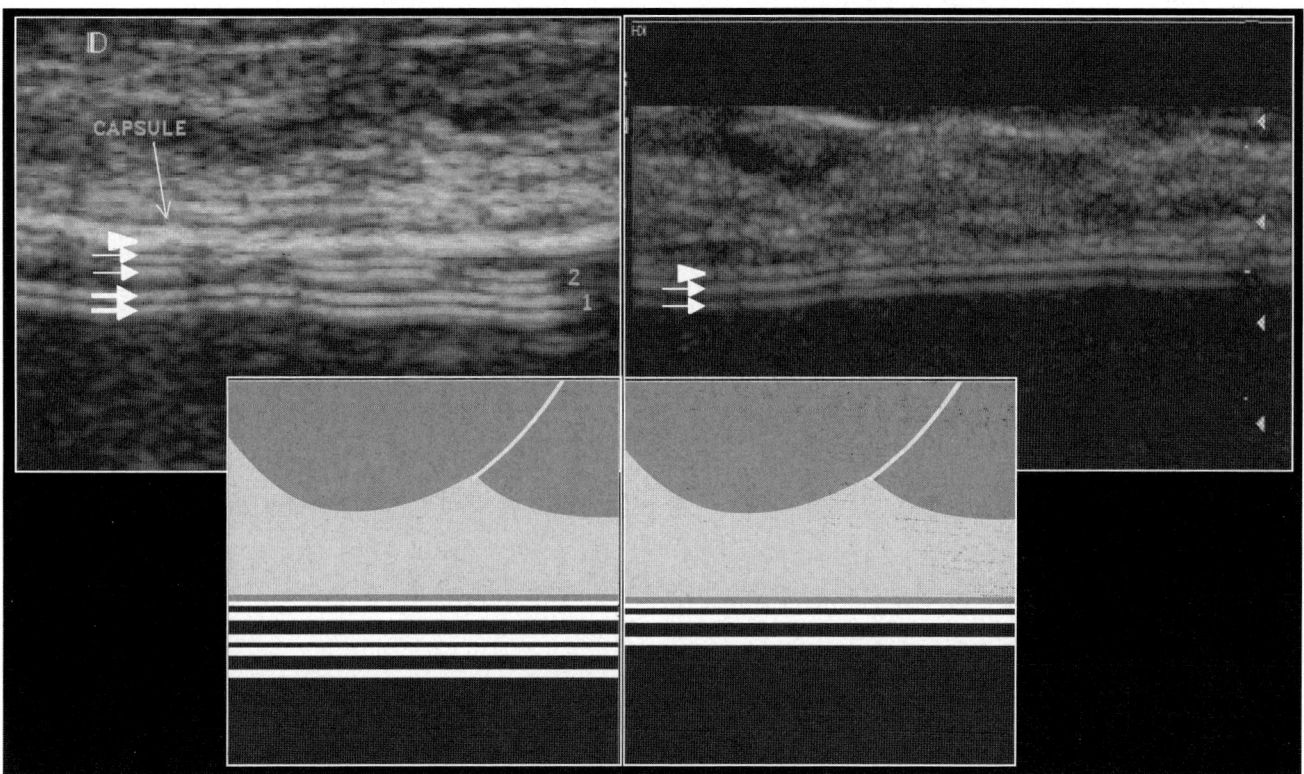

FIGURE 9–94 The **left** image shows the anterior capsule–shell echo complex of a double-lumen implant, and the **right** image shows the anterior capsule–shell echo complex of a nontextured single-lumen implant. The double-lumen complex consists of five echogenic lines. The anterior line represents the capsule *(arrowhead)*, and each of the two shells is represented by a double echogenic line *(arrows)*. The single-lumen complex consists of three echogenic lines: the anterior capsular echogenic line *(arrowhead)* and the double echogenic line that represents the shell *(arrows)*.

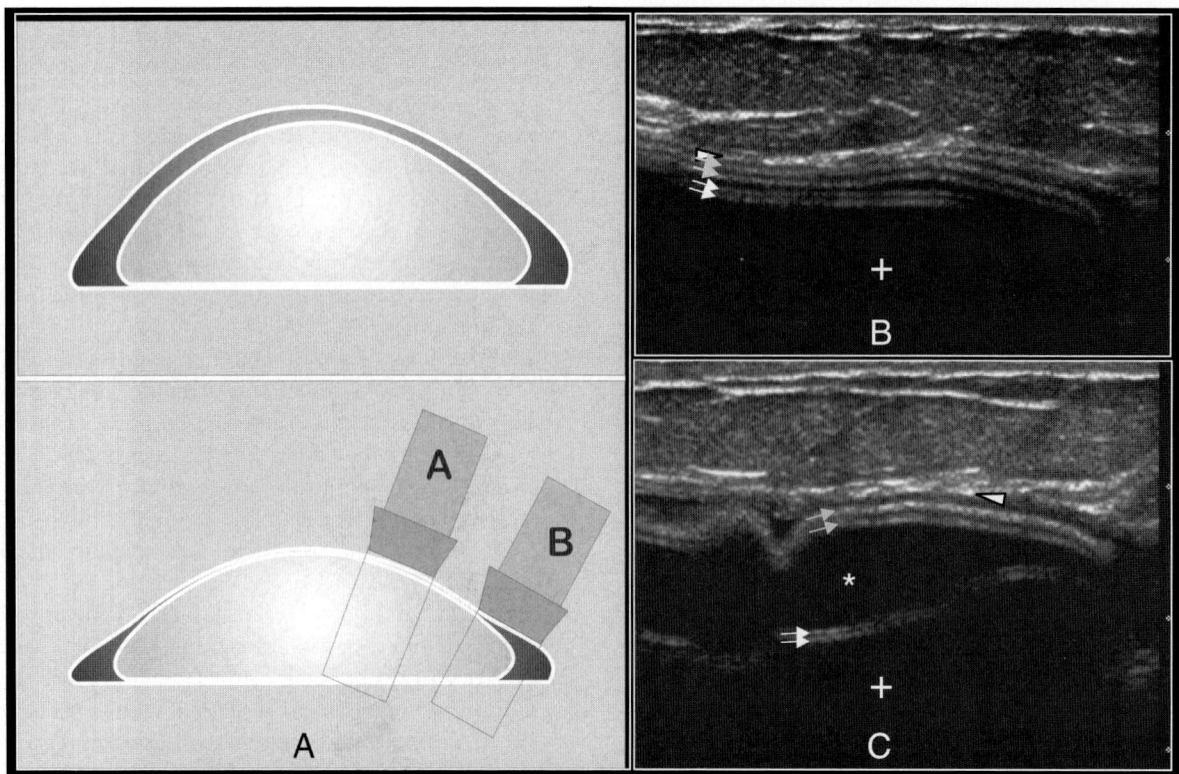

FIGURE 9–95 A: Because there is usually relatively little saline within the outer compartment of a double-lumen implant and because the saline is under very little pressure, when the outer shell is being compressed by the transducer, all of the saline can be displaced from the anterior part of the outer shell toward its periphery (**bottom**). Scans obtained on the anterior aspect of the implant (position **A**) usually show the inner and outer shells in direct contact with each other and no saline between the two shells, whereas scans obtained at the periphery of the implant (position **B**) will show saline between the inner and outer shells. This image was obtained over the anterior aspect of the implant, similar to position **A**. The saline has been displaced to the periphery, and the inner and outer shells are in direct contact with each other. **C:** This image was obtained at the periphery of the implant, similar to position **B**. Saline separates the inner and outer shells in this location. (*Arrowhead* indicates capsule, *gray arrows* indicate outer shell; *white arrows* indicate inner shell.) *, saline within outer compartment; +, silicone gel in inner compartment.

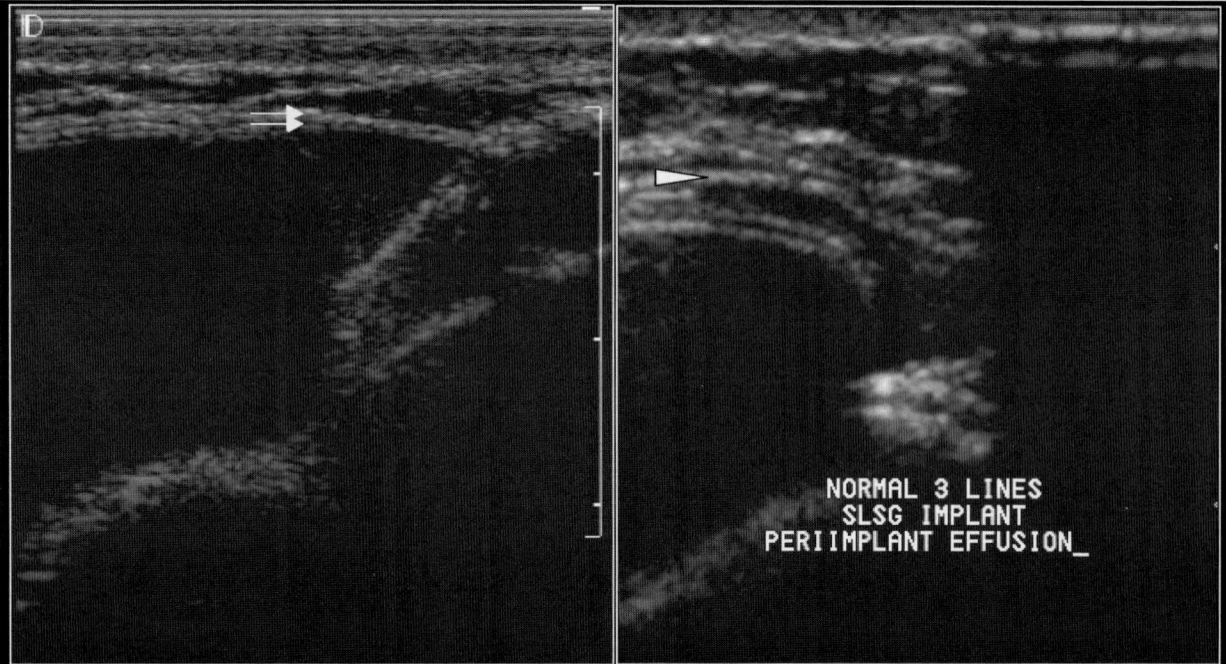

FIGURE 9–96 Assessing the anterior aspect of the periimplant effusion or outer compartment of a double-lumen implant can be helpful in distinguishing between the two. The presence of a double echogenic line *(arrows)* indicates that the fluid collection of interest is the outer compartment of a double-lumen implant (**left**). The presence of only a single echogenic line *(arrowhead)* representing the periimplant capsule indicates that the fluid collection of interest is a periimplant effusion (**right**). In patients with contracted thickened capsules, this finding can be misleading.

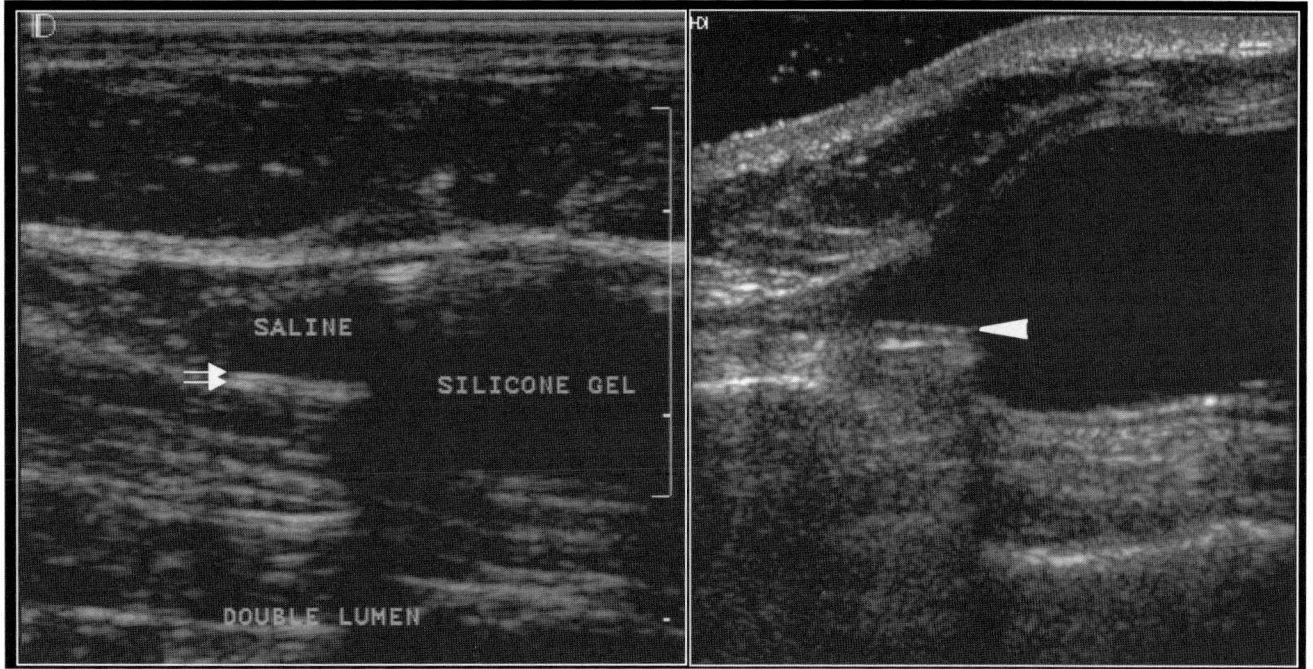

FIGURE 9–97 Assessing the posterior aspect of the periimplant effusion or outer compartment of a double-lumen implant can also be helpful in distinguishing between the two. The presence of a double echogenic line *(arrows)* indicates that the fluid collection of interest is the outer compartment of a double-lumen implant **(left)**. The presence of only a single echogenic line *(arrowhead)* representing the periimplant effusion indicates that the fluid collection of interest is a periimplant effusion **(right)**. Assessing the posterior wall is sometimes easier because it is more nearly perpendicular to the ultrasound beam.

more nearly perpendicular to the beam, than it is to evaluate the anterior margin, which is usually angled and sloping (Fig. 9–97). Unfortunately, in patients with capsular contracture, the capsule may be thickened enough to present as a double echogenic line rather than as the single echogenic line typically seen with a normal thin, fibrous periimplant capsule. The echogenicity of the fluid in the outer compartment is not helpful in distinguishing between single-lumen implants surrounded by effusion and double-lumen implants. Both periimplant effusions and saline within the outer compartment of double-lumen implants tend to be anechoic when new but become more echogenic with age (Fig. 9–98). In the double-lumen implants, the increased echogenicity that occurs over time is likely the result of long-term microscopic gel bleed, whereas in the periimplant effusions, the temporal increase in echogenicity is probably the result of chronic inflammation. Reverberation echoes that arise from the shell of a single-lumen implant can simulate echoes that arise from the inner shell of a double-lumen implant (Fig. 9–99).

Distinguishing a double-lumen implant in which the outer saline compartment has ruptured and decompressed from a single-lumen implant can be very difficult. Rupture of the outer saline compartment is common and is demonstrable both mammographically (Fig. 9–100) and sonographically. Split-screen mirror-image scans showing absence of saline-type sound transmission, with its lack of step-off at the edge of the implant on one side, are the best way to document rupture of the outer compartment (Fig. 9–101). Counting the number of echogenic lines (determining the number shells) and identifying a lack of saline between the inner and outer shells is a better way to diagnose rupture of the outer saline compartment. Scanning along the anterior aspect of the implant is not helpful in determining whether the outer saline compartment has ruptured because there is normally so little saline within the outer compartment that the inner and outer shell are directly in contact with each other along the anterior aspect of the implant. However, along the edges, there usually is enough saline to separate the inner and outer shells from each other. If the two shells are in direct contact with each other at the periphery of the implant, it indicates that the outer compartment has ruptured and that there is no saline within the outer compartment (Fig. 9–102).

Rupture of the inner silicone gel–containing compartment of double-lumen implants is much less common and more difficult to evaluate unless the inner compartment collapses completely. Because the outer shell is usually in-

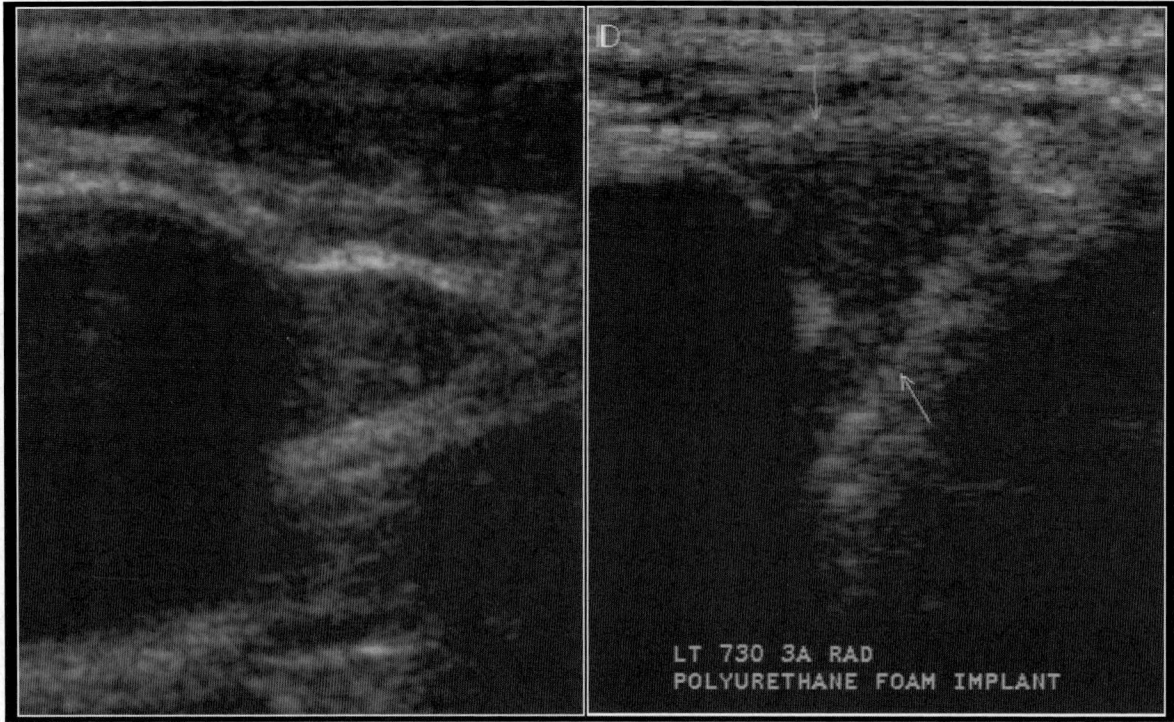

FIGURE 9–98 The echogenicity of fluid is not helpful in distinguishing periimplant effusion from the outer saline-containing shell of a double-lumen implant. Chronic effusions occasionally become more echogenic over time, especially in association with polyurethane-coated implants (**right**). Likewise, the outer saline compartment of double-lumen implants may become echogenic with time because of gel bleed through the inner shell into the outer compartment (**left**).

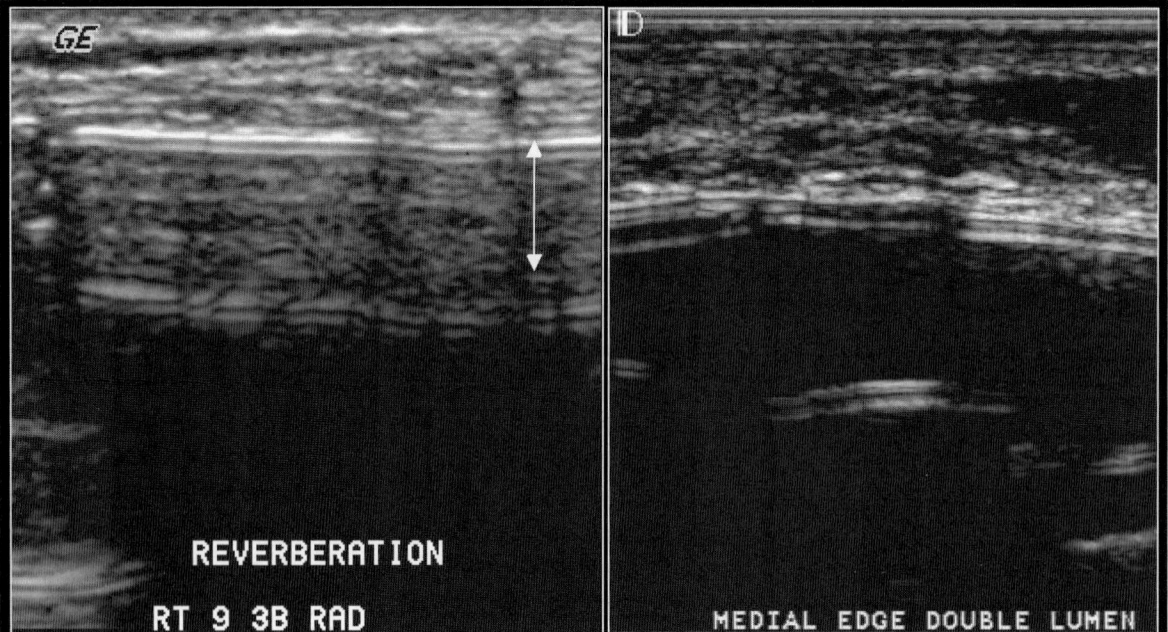

FIGURE 9–99 Reverberation echoes that lie within a single-lumen implant may mimic the double echogenic line of the inner shell of a double-lumen implant. Reverberations echoes (**left**) will remain parallel to the anterior shell of a single-lumen implant and will occur at a distance about 1.5 times the distance between the skin and the shell of the implant. Because of the slower speed of sound in silicone gel, the reverberation echoes artifactually appear deeper than they would in saline implants (the *double-headed arrow* represents the distance from the skin to the leading edge of the shell). The inner shell of a double-lumen implant that lies along the anterior aspect of the implant will usually be in direct contact with the outer shell because there is too little saline anteriorly to separate the two shells. At the edges of the implant, where there is enough saline to separate the shells, the inner shell of a double-lumen implant (**right**) will not be parallel to the outer shell and will be more variable in depth than will reverberation echoes.

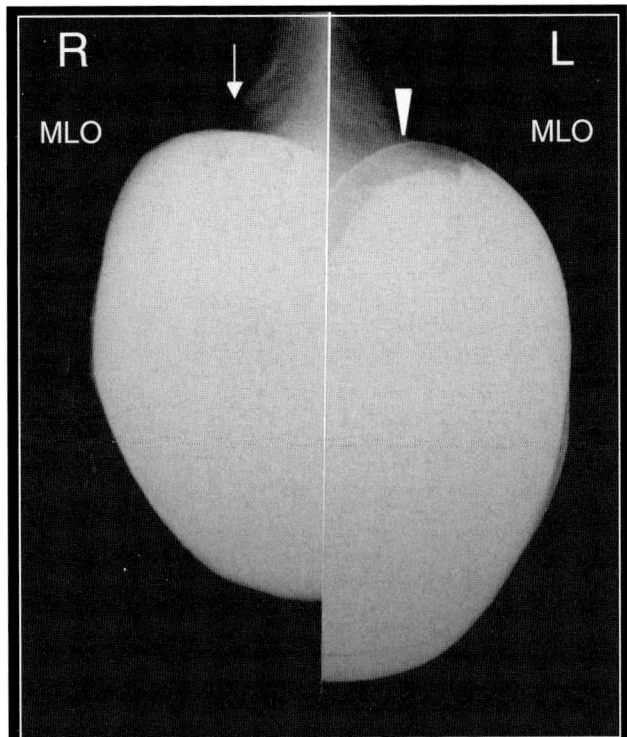

FIGURE 9–100 Mediolateral oblique mammograms of double-lumen implants show a visible outer saline-filled compartment on the left *(arrowhead)*, but no visible outer saline-filled compartment *(arrow)* on the right. This could represent a double-lumen implant on the right, where the outer shell has ruptured and the saline has leaked out, or it could represent a single-lumen silicone gel implant on the right.

tact, the outer contour of the implant in such cases usually remains normal. In acute cases of inner compartment rupture, the diagnosis may be missed because both the saline and extravasated silicone gel are anechoic. In more chronic cases, the mixing of silicone gel from the inner compartment with saline in the outer compartment can result in mottled or mixed echogenicity of the fluid within the outer compartment (Fig. 9–103). This can be difficult to distinguish from intracapsular rupture of a single-lumen silicone gel implant. However, the anechoic spaces are not surrounded by shell, as they are in intracapsular rupture of a single-lumen silicone gel implant. The significance of diagnosing rupture of the inner compartment is questionable because the usually intact outer compartment will contain the silicone gel that extravasates from the inner compartment.

Becker Expanders and Single-Lumen Saline Expanders
Becker expanders are temporary double-lumen implants that have a saline inner compartment and a silicone gel outer compartment. They are used almost exclusively in the process of breast reconstruction after mastectomy for breast cancer treatment. The inner compartment is gradually expanded by small serial injections through a valve over a period of time in order to create a space large enough to place a permanent implant. The inner saline compartment is anechoic and the outer silicone gel compartment is usually mildly echogenic. At the edge of the implant, where the silicone gel is thickest, the implant appears to be slightly

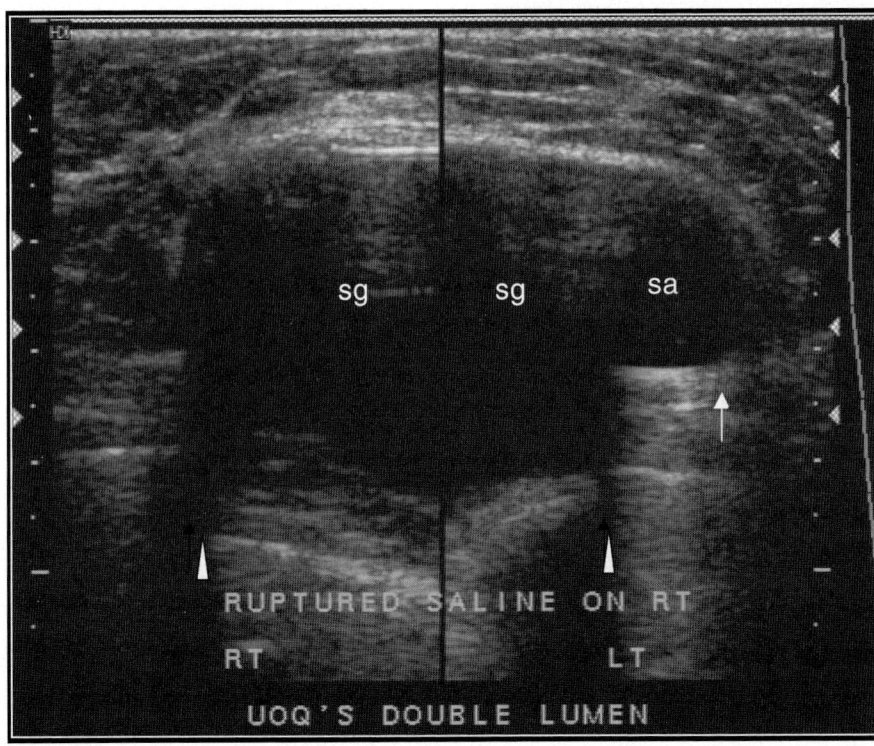

FIGURE 9–101 Split-screen mirror-image sonograms of the upper outer quadrants performed on the same patient shown in Figure 9–100 show findings similar to the mammographic findings. The patient's left side shows typical findings along the edge of a double-lumen implant. There is no step-off at the edge of the outer saline-containing compartment *(arrow)*, but there is a step-off at the edge of the inner silicone gel–containing compartment *(arrowhead)*. On the patient's right side, the outer compartment cannot be identified. This indicates either that the outer compartment has ruptured and lost all of its saline or that the patient has a single-lumen silicone gel implant on the right side.

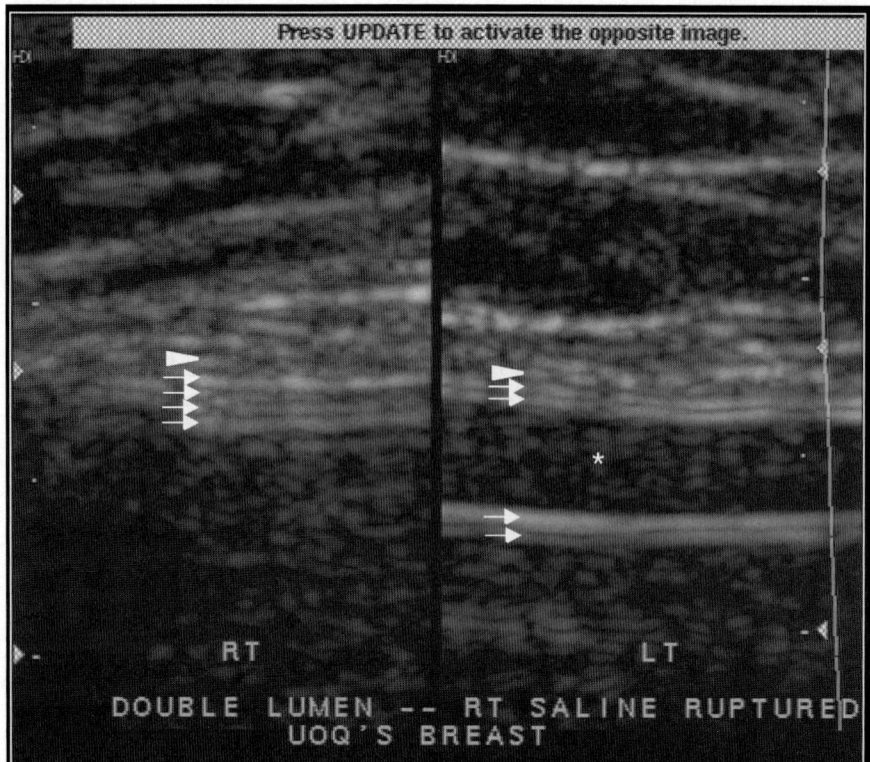

FIGURE 9–102 Magnified scans along the periphery of the implant in the patient shown in Figs. 9–100 and 9–101 indicated that there is a double-lumen implant on the right in which the outer compartment has ruptured. Split-screen mirror-image scans along the edge of the implants show saline between the two shells on the patient's left (*), but no saline between the two shells on the patient's right.

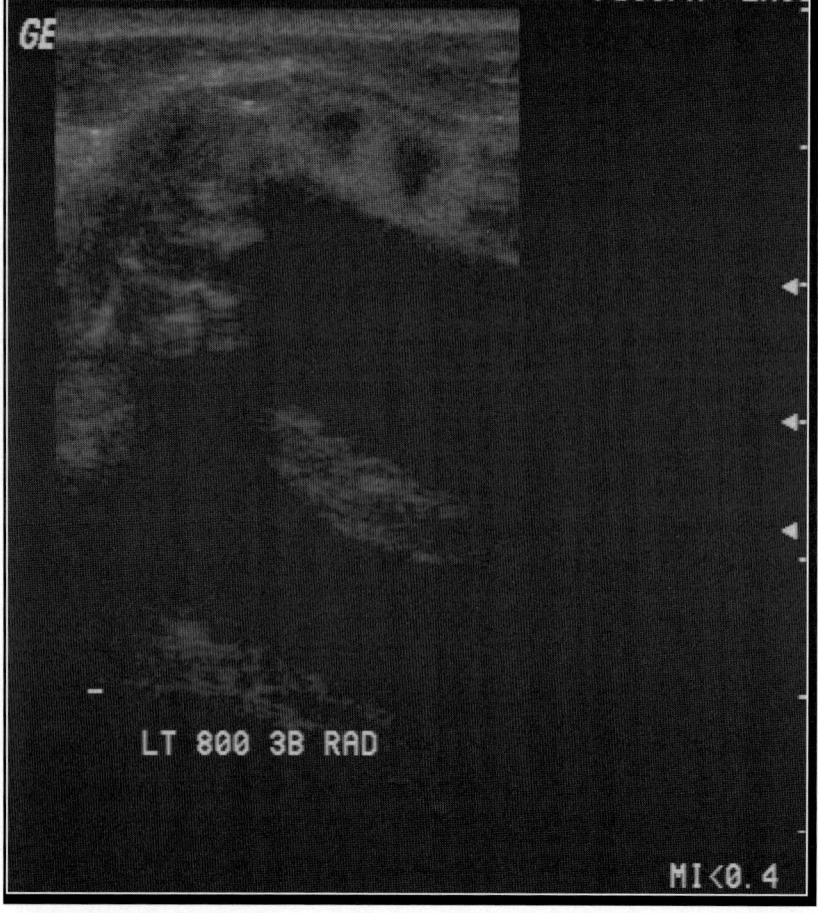

FIGURE 9–103 When the inner silicone gel–containing compartment of a double-lumen implant ruptures and releases silicone gel into an intact outer saline-containing compartment, the mixture of saline and silicone gel may result in a heterogenous texture within the outer compartment that has a spotted appearance. This is much less common than rupture of the outer saline-containing compartment and can be difficult to distinguish from intracapsular rupture of a single-lumen implant with a mixture of effusion and extravasated silicone gel within the capsule.

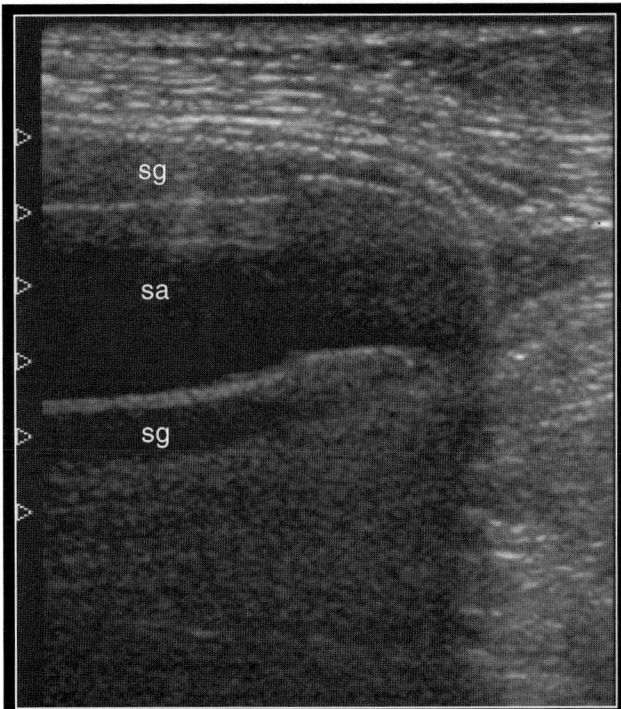

FIGURE 9–104 This partially filled Becker expander contains a central compartment filled with saline and an outer compartment filled with silicone gel. The inner compartment is filled incrementally over time with repeated small injections of saline in order to expand the tissue space gradually enough to accept a permanent implant. It is used almost exclusively for reconstructive surgery after mastectomy.

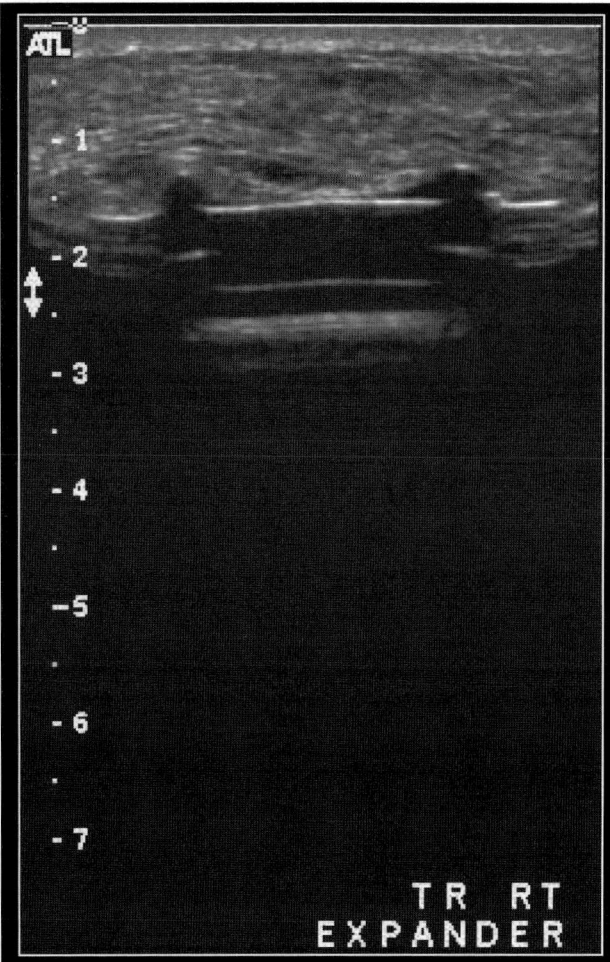

FIGURE 9–105 The fill valve for this single-lumen saline tissue expander is larger than that of single-lumen implants because it must be used repeatedly after implantation, not just a single time at implantation. Sonography can help locate the valve for sequential expanding injections of saline in some cases.

thicker than over the rest of the implant because of the slower speed of sound through silicone gel (Fig. 9–104).

Single-lumen saline expanders have been used. The fill valve of these expanders is larger than the fill valves of single-lumen saline implants (Fig. 9–105). Sonography can be helpful in guiding sequential expanding injections through the valve.

COMPLICATIONS OTHER THAN IMPLANT RUPTURE

Sonography is valuable in identifying both acute and chronic complications of implants other than implant rupture. These include hematomas, seromas, abscesses, and fat necrosis.

Hematomas and Seromas

Acute hematomas and seromas are relatively common immediately after implantation, especially in association with expanders and reconstructive surgery, but are usually not diagnostic dilemmas. Likewise, most implant infections occur in the immediate postoperative period.

Acute hematomas have a range of sonographic appearances, depending on the proportion of blood that is liquid and clotted, and the sonographic appearance typically evolves over time (Fig. 9–106). Acute hematomas are hypoechoic and largely cystic. Quickly, fluid–debris levels form and the blood begins to clot and become hyperechoic. Eventually, as the entire hematoma becomes clot, the mass becomes solid. Finally, in chronic stages, the clot can either organize and become more solid in appearance or completely liquefy.

Acute seromas may be simple cystic or may have thin septations that represent fibrinous adhesions. Like hematomas, they are most commonly associated with reconstructive surgery and expanders (Fig. 9–106).

Chronic hematomas are less common and are nonspecific in their sonographic appearance in most cases. They may appear cystic, solid, or mixed.

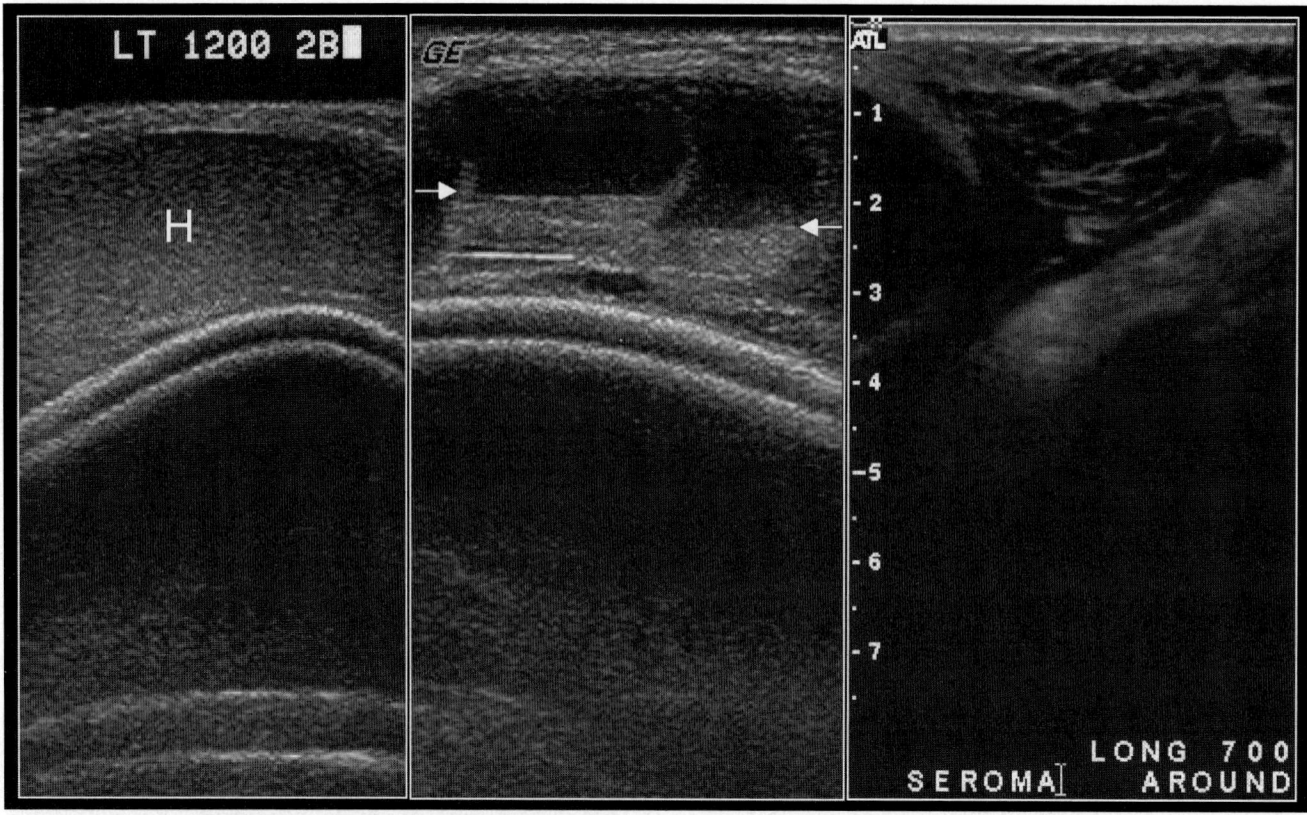

FIGURE 9–106 Most hematomas and seromas occur acutely after implantation. The echogenicity varies, depending on the amount of clot and liquid blood and the age of the hematoma. Hyperacute hematomas appear uniformly echogenic (**left**). In acute and subacute hematomas, clots and debris levels that appear hyperechoic form while other blood components liquefy and appear hypoechoic (**middle**). Acute seromas usually contain multiple fibrinous adhesions (**right**).

Occasionally, the pectoralis muscle that overlies large implants will be so thinned and stretched that it is prone to muscle tear and hematoma formation. The history and sonographic findings confirming the origin of the complex mass from the overlying muscle rather than breast tissue will help make the diagnosis. Seat-belt injuries are particularly prone to tearing the pectoralis muscle (Fig. 9–107). The long-term sequela of pectoralis tear and hematoma may be coarse dystrophic calcifications that simulate those of fat necrosis.

Implant Infection and Abscesses

Most implant infections occur immediately after implantation or in the postoperative period after explantation. Occasionally, however, an implant will become infected years after implantation. In most cases, the etiology of such infections is uncertain but is likely to be hematogenous in origin. The patient with an infected periimplant effusion and acute capsulitis will present with acute swelling and tenderness of the breast, but will usually not show outward signs of inflammation. The earliest sonographic finding is that the effusion is under tension rather than soft and compressible. This may be the only finding for 5 to 7 days. Within a few days, the capsule will begin to thicken, and fibrinous adhesions will appear within the

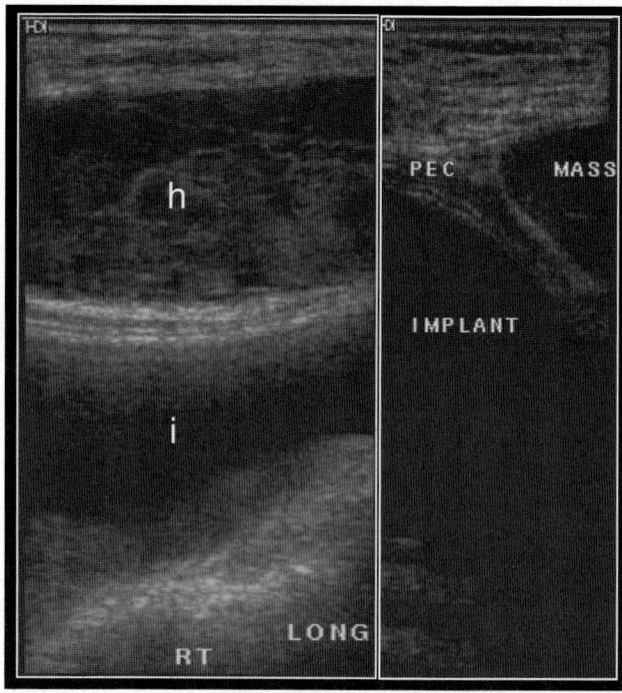

FIGURE 9–107 This hematoma developed because of a seat-belt injury sustained in a motor vehicle crash in a patient with retropectoral implants. There is an acute hematoma (*h*) anterior to the implant (*i*) on the patient's right side (**left**). A scan obtained radially in the axillary segment shows that the hematoma has arisen from a pectoralis major tear (**right**).

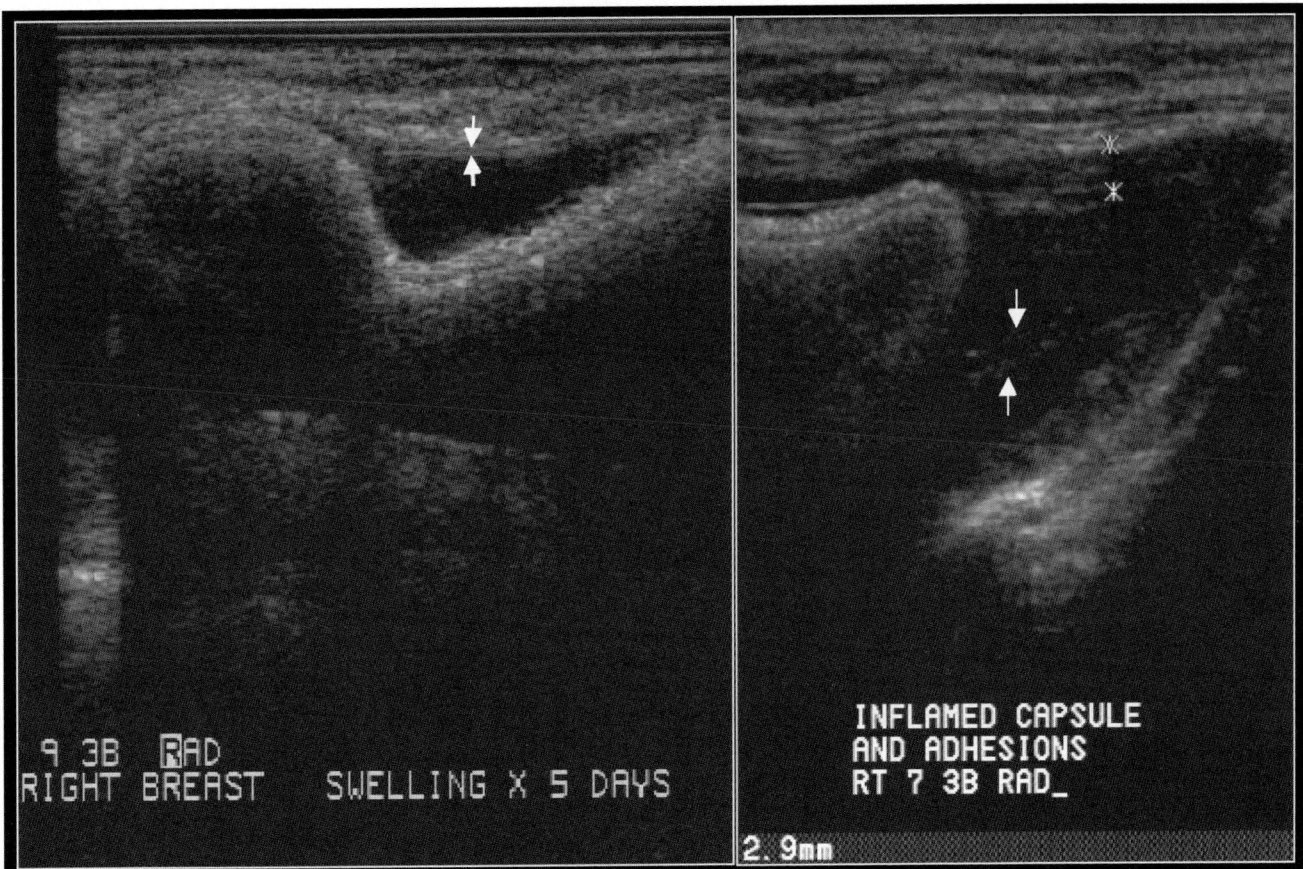

FIGURE 9–108 This patient presented with sudden onset of acute pain and swelling in her right breast years after implantation. Sonography showed a heavily textured single-lumen saline implant with a periimplant effusion, which was unusual in that it was markedly asymmetric with the patient's left side, which had no effusion. The capsule is only minimally thickened *(arrows)* 5 days after the onset of symptoms **(left)**. Because of concern about infection of the capsule, the patient was placed on antibiotics and asked to return in 10 days for reevaluation with sonography **(right)**. The follow-up exam showed evidence of acute inflammation or infection despite treatment with antibiotics. The capsule had become abnormally thickened *(calipers)*, the effusion had enlarged, and fibrinous adhesions had appeared within the effusion *(arrows)*.

effusion (Fig. 9–108). At this stage, color Doppler usually shows marked hyperemia of the thickened capsule (see Chapter 20, Fig. 20–60). Imaging-guided aspiration can be done for diagnosis, but neither ultrasound-guided repeated aspirations or placement of a drain will lead to cure of the infection because of the presence of an infected foreign body, the implant. Explantation and antibiotic treatment for several months are usually necessary to completely sterilize the implant site before reimplantation can be performed.

Explantation-related Complications

Patients who have undergone explantation occasionally require sonographic evaluation. The imaging findings after explantation vary, depending on whether the patient underwent explantation through a capsulotomy or had capsulectomy in addition to explantation.

When implants are removed through a capsulotomy, but the capsule is not removed, the capsule can undergo dense calcification, or serous fluid can accumulate within the fibrous capsule, resulting in an acute or chronic intracapsular seroma. This is more likely to occur if the removed implant was a textured polyurethane implant because polyurethane stimulates a chronic inflammatory periimplant effusion and because flecks of polyurethane are likely to remain within the capsule and intracapsular space after explantation, perpetuating the inflammatory effusion even after the implant is removed. In fact, polyurethane implants may stimulate synovial metaplasia in the cells surrounding the periimplant effusion, resulting in formation of an actively secreting bursa similar to those seen around joints. It is not surprising that once synovial metaplasia has occurred, the bursa may be maintained even after removal of the foreign-body implant that stimulated its development. Seroma formation within the capsule is also more common when the capsule around

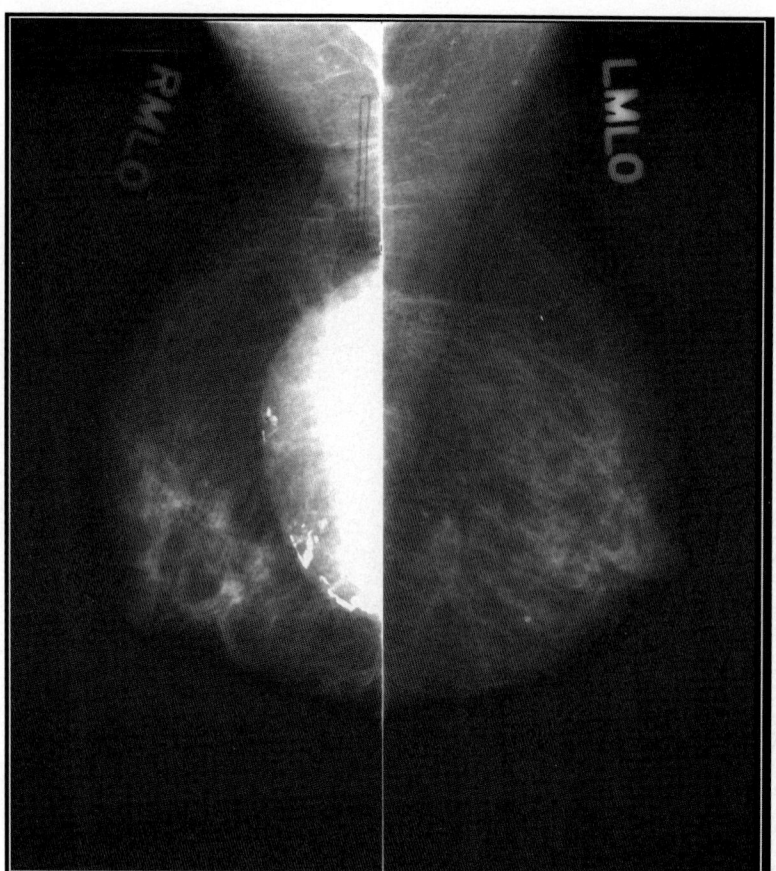

FIGURE 9–109 This patient had undergone bilateral explantation without capsulectomy because of signs and symptoms of human adjuvant disease. Attempted capsulectomy had to be abandoned because of excessive bleeding. A few weeks after explantation, the patient developed pain and tenderness in the right breast and felt as though she still had an implant. Mammograms show a mass on her right that represents a seroma-hematoma within the residual calcified right periimplant fibrous capsule that simulates the presence of an implant mammographically.

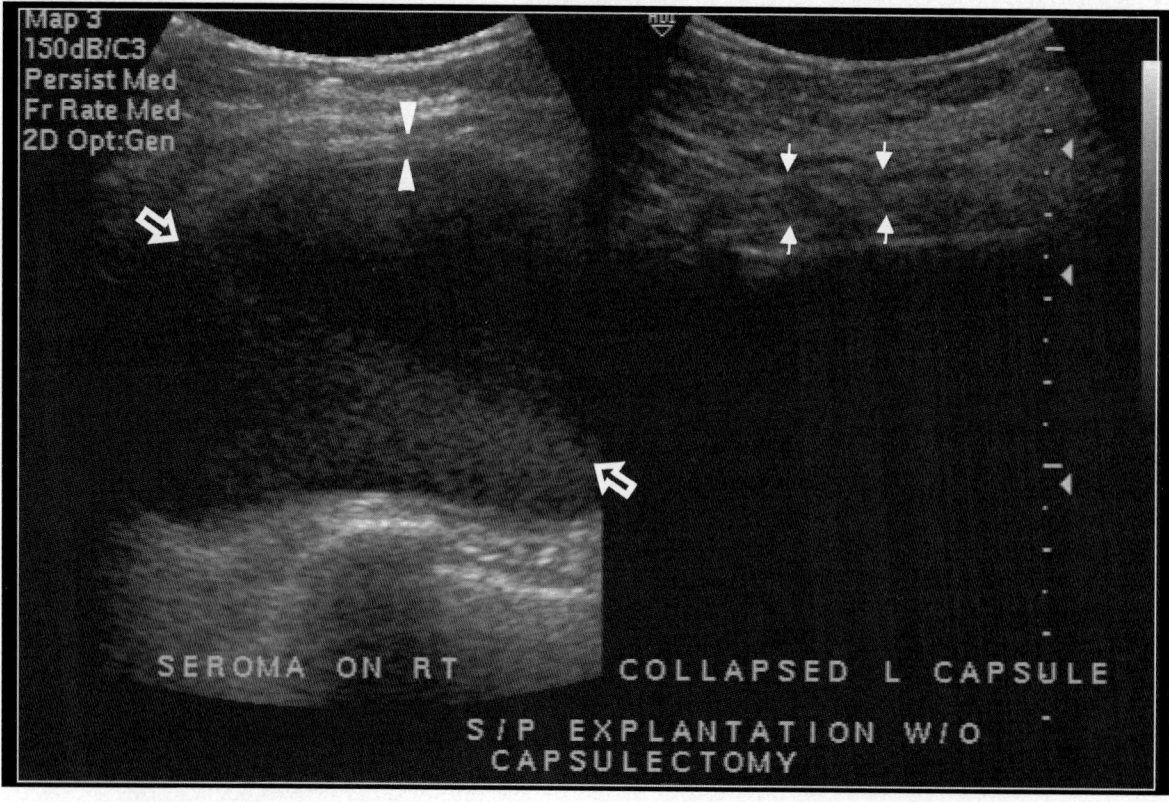

FIGURE 9–110 Split-screen mirror-image scans of the right and left sides of the patient whose mammograms are shown in Fig. 9–109 show a large, thick-walled *(arrowheads)* complex cystic structure that contains a fluid–debris level *(hollow arrows)* on the patient's right. This represents a seroma-hematoma that has accumulated within the capsule after explantation. On the patient's left side, the capsule is completely collapsed and lies directly on the chest wall *(arrows).*

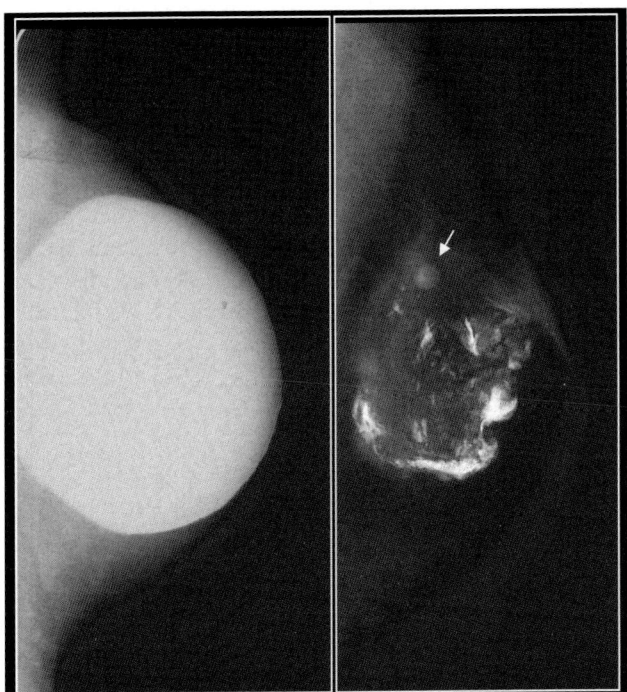

FIGURE 9–111 This patient illustrates the more typical course after explantation without associated capsulectomy. The **left** image represents the preexplantation appearance of this single-lumen silicone gel implant. The **right** image shows the residual calcified capsule after explantation. The calcifications are large and coarse and have an appearance similar to that of fat necrosis. A small droplet of intracapsular silicone gel remains *(arrow)*, indicating that either there had been intracapsular rupture before explantation or the implant had been ruptured during explantation.

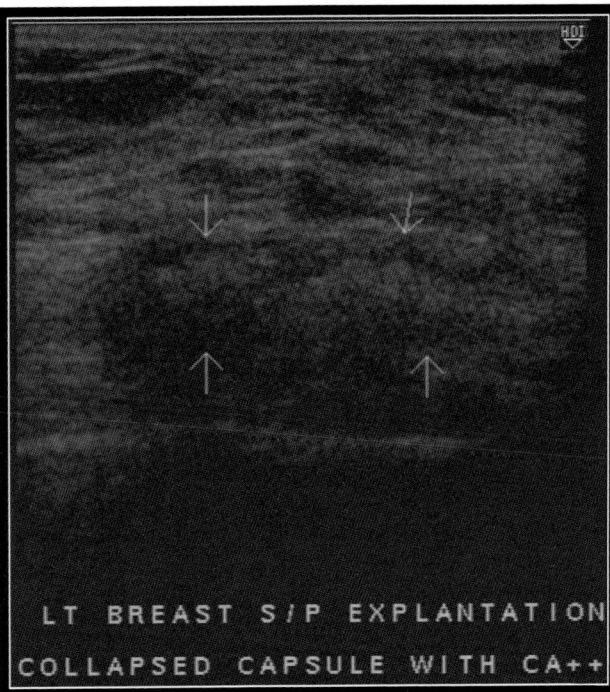

FIGURE 9–112 Sonography of the collapsed calcified capsule shown in Fig. 9–111 could potentially be worrisome if interpreted in the absence of the mammogram. It is ill-defined, mildly hypoechoic, and contains foci of hyperechogenicity that cause acoustic shadowing.

the implant was abnormally thick and contracted, even if the implant was not polyurethane coated. Finally, seroma formation after explantation is also more common when the removed implant was subglandular in location rather than retropectoral. Large intracapsular postexplantation seromas can simulate the presence of an intact implant on mammograms (Fig. 9–109). Sonographically, they appear to be complex cysts with thick echogenic walls, variable amounts of calcification within the walls or internally, and variable amounts of echogenic material within the cyst (Fig. 9–110). These complex cysts are usually very deep, lying along the chest wall within the retromammary zone. The deep location is not surprising because most implants are placed subglandular, deep to the mammary zone.

In other cases, after explantation without capsulectomy, the residual capsule may collapse and progress through the fibrotic scarring phases identical to those of fat necrosis, forming cicatrizing scars or dense calcifications (Figs. 9–111 and 9–112).

When complete capsulectomy has been performed at the time of explantation, intracapsular seromas do not form, and the sonographic findings are usually similar to lumpectomy: highly variable amounts of hematoma, scar tissue, and fat necrosis (Fig. 9–113).

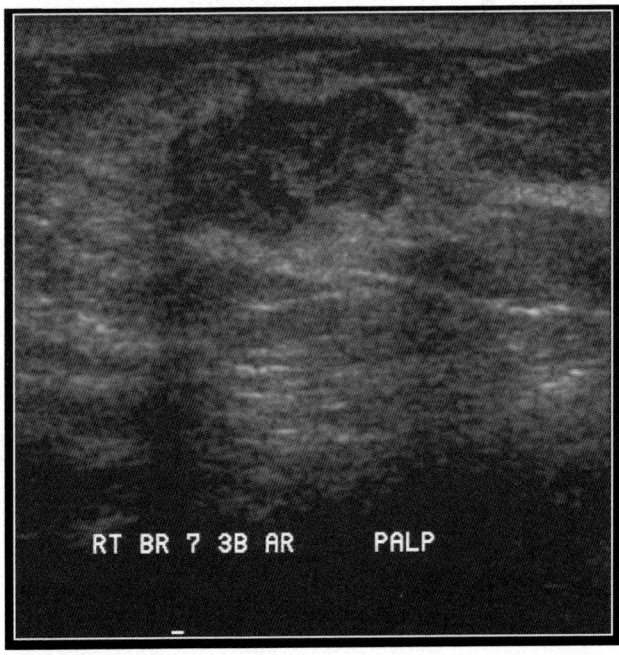

FIGURE 9–113 This small hematoma complicated explantation with capsulectomy. Its appearance is similar to that of breast hematomas that arise from any other surgical procedure.

SUMMARY

Patients with implants may undergo targeted sonography for evaluation of clinical or mammographic abnormalities or nontargeted sonography for evaluation of implant complications. The clinical or mammographic abnormality for which the study is being performed might either be related to implant abnormalities or breast pathology unrelated to the implant. Whether or not the targeted portion of the examination identifies an implant problem as the cause of clinical or mammographic findings, we evaluate the implants bilaterally for additional unsuspected complications.

In patients in whom sonography is being performed for evaluation of a palpable or mammographic abnor-mality, the sonographer or sonologist must solve the chief complaint before beginning the nontargeted evaluation of the implants. One must not be distracted from the primary goal by the presence of implants. Remember that, in addition to the potential complications associated with implants, patients with implants suffer from the same spectrum of benign breast disorders and malignant lesions as do patients without implants. Such patients have simple and complex breast cysts, fibroadenomas, and carcinomas (Fig. 9–114). It would be a tragedy to become so engrossed in incidental evaluation of the implant for complications that a palpable or mammographically visible carcinoma is not identified and evaluated sonographically.

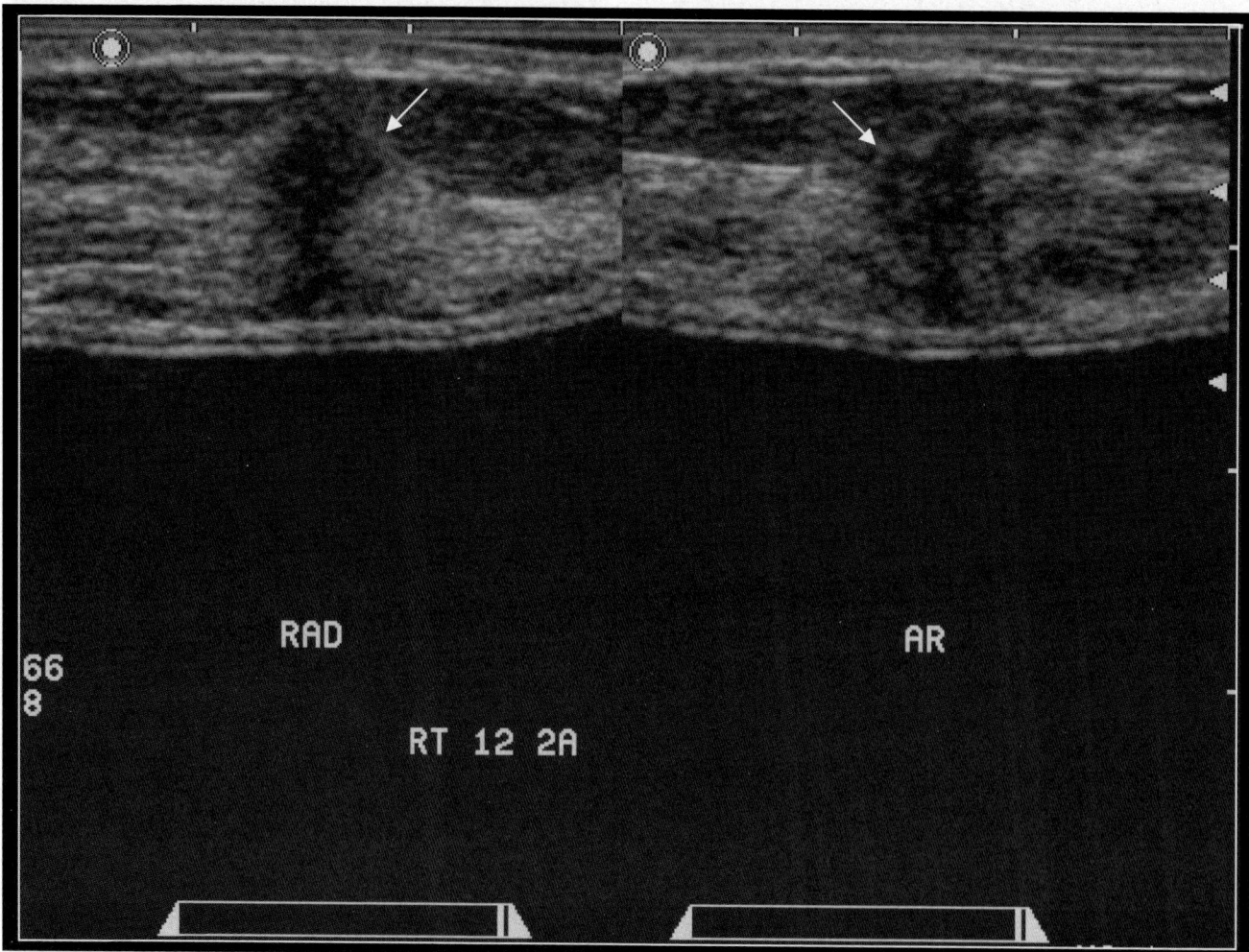

FIGURE 9–114 Most patients with breast implants who undergo sonography have either palpable lumps or a mammographic abnormality that is their chief concern. They are usually not concerned about their implants. Evaluating the implants first in such patients could be fascinating, but distracting, and could prevent accurately diagnosing the real reason for presentation. Primary attention should be directly to the chief complaint, not the implants. Only after the chief complaint is thoroughly evaluated should any attempt be made to evaluate the implants. This patient presented with a palpable lump that sonography showed to be a small, taller-than-wide BIRADS 5 solid nodule that proved to be intermediate-grade invasive ductal carcinoma. The implants were assessed only after thorough evaluation of the patient's palpable abnormality.

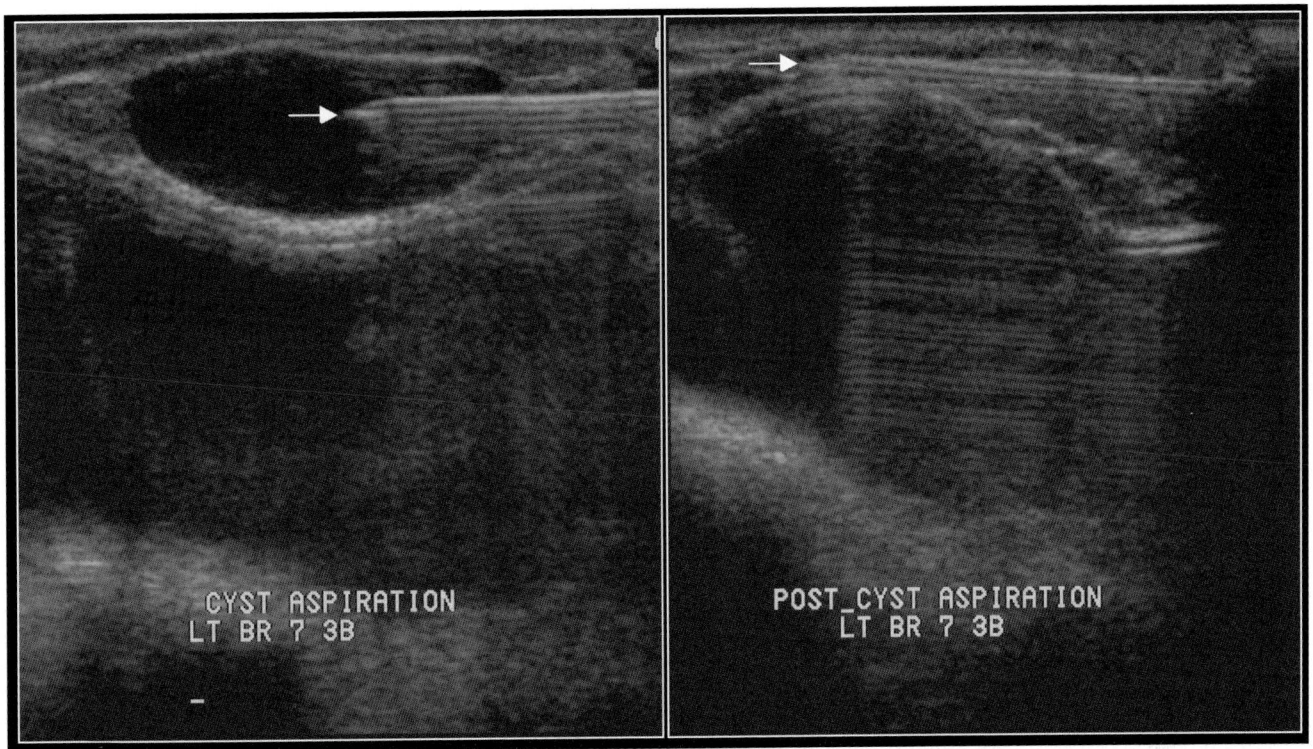

FIGURE 9–115 The presence of implants should not dissuade one from performing interventional procedures of any type. With ultrasound guidance, precise control of the needle tip *(arrow)* and bevel position can be maintained throughout the procedure with virtually no risk for puncturing the implant.

The presence of mammary implants should not dissuade one from performing necessary interventional procedures under ultrasound guidance. Cyst aspiration, needle localization, core needle biopsy, vacuum-assisted large core needle biopsy, and sentinel node injections and procedures are all quite possible and safe with real-time guidance (Fig. 9–115).

High-frequency, broad-bandwidth transducers, shallow depths of field, and magnification are necessary to demonstrate the thin, echogenic lines that represent the implant shell and its surrounding fibrous capsule. Special techniques and occasionally lower-frequency transducers are necessary for optimal evaluation of implant type and complications. Split-screen mirror-image scans of the right and left sides can be helpful. In many instances, the most valuable information about the type of implant and implant complications is found along the periphery of the implant rather than on its anterior surface.

Sonography can help determine the implant type and site of implantation. Variations are myriad, and they must be fully understood before implant abnormalities can be reliably detected.

Sonography can identify both intracapsular and extracapsular ruptures of single-lumen silicone gel implants. Sonographic diagnosis is more accurate for extracapsular ruptures than for intracapsular ruptures. There is a spectrum of findings for both intracapsular and extracapsular rupture, just as there is a spectrum in the severity of rupture and collapse of the implant shell. Better results will be obtained with sonography if the entire spectrum of findings is understood and sought in all patients than if only one or two findings are used. Sonography can detect silicone granulomas that lie within intramammary and axillary lymph nodes and within muscles as well as those within breast tissues. Complications of saline implants are usually obvious clinically and mammographically and seldom require sonographic evaluation. The role of sonography in patients with saline implants is similar to its role in patients without implants.

In patients who have had ruptured silicone implants replaced with new silicone implants, extracapsular silicone granulomas may be unrelated to rupture of the new implant. Instead, such silicone granulomas may be residuals of the old ruptured implant that were not removed at the time of reimplantation.

Sonography is valuable for assessing acute and chronic implant complications other than rupture. Abscess and hematoma, which may occur acutely or chronically, are readily identified by sonography.

Patients who have undergone explantation without complete capsulectomy can develop seromas within the residual capsule that can simulate more serious conditions sonographically and may suggest that the patient still has an implant on mammograms.

SUGGESTED READINGS

Ahn CY, Shaw WW. Regional silicone-gel migration in patients with ruptured implants. *Ann Plast Surg* 1994;33(2):201–208.

Ahn CY, et al. Comparative silicone breast implant evaluation using mammography, sonography, and magnetic resonance imaging: experience with 59 implants. *Plast Reconstr Surg* 1994;94(5):620–627.

Andersen B, et al. The diagnosis of ruptured breast implants. *Plast Reconstr Surg* 1989;84(6):903–907.

Baker JL, Bartels RJ, Douglas WM. Closed compression technique for rupturing a contracted capsule around a breast implant. *Plast Reconstr Surg* 1976;58:137–141.

Berg WA, et al. Diagnosing breast implant rupture with MR imaging, US, and mammography. *Radiographics* 1993;13(6):1323–1336.

Berg WA, et al. MR imaging of the breast in patients with silicone breast implants: normal postoperative variants and diagnostic pitfalls. *AJR Am J Roentgenol* 1994;163(9):575–578.

Berg WA, et al. Single- and double-lumen silicone breast implant integrity: prospective evaluation of MR and US criteria. *Radiology* 1995;197(10):45–52.

Berger B, Wimbish KJ. Diagnostic imaging of breast implants. *Appl Radiol* 1995;Jan:25–28.

Brumbaugh JM, Ikeda DM, Waters LM. The augmented breast and its evolution. *Appl Radiol* 1994;9:11–17.

Busch H. Silicone toxicology. *Semin Arthritis Rheum* 1994;24[1 Suppl 1]:s11–17.

Caskey CI, et al. Breast implant rupture: diagnosis with US. *Radiology* 1994;190(3):819–823.

Chung KC, et al. Diagnosis of silicone gel breast implant rupture by ultrasonography. *Plast Reconstr Surg* 1996;97(1):104–109.

Conant EF, et al. Surgical removal of ruptured breast implants: the use of intraoperative sonography in localizing free silicone. *AJR Am J Roentgenol* 1995;165(6):1378–1379.

Darnell EK, Demars RV. Ultrasonographic localization of breast tissue expander valves. *J Ultrasound Med* 1987;6:531–534.

De Bruhl ND, et al. Silicone breast implants: US evaluation. *Radiology* 1993;189(1):95–98.

DeAngelis GA, et al. MR imaging of breast implants. *Radiographics* 1994;14(4):783–794.

Destouet JM, et al. Screening mammography in 350 women with breast implants: prevalence and findings of implant complications. *AJR Am J Roentgenol* 1992;159(5):973–978.

Everson LI, et al. Diagnosis of breast implant rupture: imaging findings and relative efficacies of imaging techniques. *AJR Am J Roentgenol* 1994;163(1):57–60.

Fenske TK, Davis P, Aaron SL. Human adjuvant disease revisited: a review of eleven post-augmentation mammoplasty patients. *Clin Exp Rheumatol* 1994;12(5):477–481.

Fornage BD, Sneige N, Singletary SE. Masses in breasts with implants: diagnosis with US-guided fine-needle aspiration biopsy. *Radiology* 1994;191(2):339–342.

Friedman RJ. Silicone breast prostheses implantation and explanation. *Semin Arthritis Rheum* 1994;24[1 Suppl 1]:8–10.

Gabriel SE, et al. Risk of connective-tissue diseases and other disorders after breast implantation. *N Engl J Med* 1994;330(24):1697–702.

Ganott MA, et al. Augmentation mammoplasty: normal and abnormal findings with mammography and US. *Radiographics* 1992;12(2):281–295.

Gorczyca DP, et al. Silicone breast implants in vivo: MR imaging. *Radiology* 1992;185(11):407–410.

Gorczyca DP, et al. Silicone breast implant ruptures in an animal model: comparison of mammography, MR imaging, US, and CT. *Radiology* 1994;190(1):227–232.

Granchi D, et al. Silicone breast implants: the role of immune system on capsular contracture formation. *J Biomed Mater Res* 1995;29(2):197–202.

Hameed MR, Erlandson R, Rosen PP. Capsular synovial-like hyperplasia around mammary implants similar to detritic synovitis: a morphologic and immunohistochemical study of 15 cases. *Am J Surg Pathol* 1995;19(4):433–438.

Handel N, Silverstein MJ, Gamagomi P, et al. Factors affecting mammographic visualization of the breast after augmentation mammoplasty. *JAMA* 1992;268:1913–1917.

Hang-Fu L, Snyderman RK. State-of-the-art breast reconstruction. *Cancer* 1991;68[5 Suppl]:1148–1156.

Harris KM, et al. Silicone implant rupture: detection with US. *Radiology* 1993;187(3):761–768.

Hayes MK, Gold RH, Bassett LW. Mammographic findings after the removal of breast implants. *AJR Am J Roentgenol* 1993;160(3):487–490.

Leibman AJ, Kruse B. Breast cancer: mammographic and sonographic findings after augmentation mammoplasty. *Radiology* 1990;174(1):195–198.

Leibman AJ, Kruse BD. Imaging of breast cancer after augmentation mammoplasty. *Ann Plast Surg* 1993;30(2):111–115.

Leibman AJ. Imaging of complications of augmentation mammaplasty. *Plast Reconstr Surg* 1994;93(6):1134–1140.

Leibman AJ, Sybers R. Mammographic and sonographic findings after silicone injection. *Ann Plast Surg* 1994;33(4):412–414.

Levine RA, Collins TL. Definitive *diagnosis* of breast implant rupture by ultrasonography [Comments]. *Plast Reconstr Surg* 1991;87(6):1126–1128.

Mendelson EB. Silicone implants present mammographic challenge. *Diagn Imaging* 1992;9:70–76.

Mund DF, et al. MR imaging of the breast in patients with silicone-gel implants: spectrum of findings. *AJR Am J Roentgenol* 1993;161(4):773–778.

Noda S, Eberlein TJ, Eriksson E. Breast reconstruction. *Cancer* 1994;74[1 Suppl]:376–380.

Peters W, Pugash R. Ultrasound analysis of 150 patients with silicone gel breast implants. *Ann Plast Surg* 1993;31(1):7–9.

Peters W, Smith D. Calcification of breast implant capsules: incidence, diagnosis, and contributing factors. *Ann Plast Surg* 1995;34(1):8–11.

Petro JA, et al. Evaluation of ultrasound as a tool in the follow-up of patients with breast implants: a preliminary, prospective study. *Ann Plast Surg* 1994;32(6):580–587.

Reynolds HE, et al. Comparison of mammography, sonography, and magnetic resonance imaging in the detection of silicone-gel breast implant rupture. *Ann Plast Surg* 1994;33(3):247–255.

Reynolds HE. Evaluation of the augmented breast. *Radiol Clin North Am* 1995;33(6):1131–1145.

Rivero MA, Schwartz DS, Mies C. *Silicone* lymphadenopathy involving intramammary lymph nodes: a new complication of silicone mammaplasty. *AJR Am J Roentgenol* 1994;162(5):1089–1090.

Robinson OG Jr, Bradley EL, Wilson DS. Analysis of explanted silicone implants: a report of 300 patients. *Ann Plast Surg* 1995;34(1):1–6.

Rosculet KA, et al. Ruptured gel-filled silicone breast implants: sonographic findings in 19 cases. *AJR Am J Roentgenol* 1992;159(4):711–716.

Samuels JB, et al. Radiographic diagnosis of breast implant rupture: current status and comparison of techniques. *Plast Reconstr Surg* 1995;96(4):865–877.

Shestak KC, et al. Breast masses in the augmentation mammaplasty patient: the role of ultrasound. *Plast Reconstr Surg* 1993;92(2):209–216.

Sinclair TM, Kerrigan CL, Buntic R. Biodegradation of the polyurethane foam covering of breast implants. *Plast Reconstr Surg* 1993;92(6):1003–1013.

Skene AI, et al. Technical note: appearances on ultrasound of impalpable injection port in a double chamber breast prosthesis. *Br J Radiol* 1993;66(791):1050–1051.

Slavin SA, Goldwyn RM. Silicone gel implant explantation: reasons, results, and admonitions. *Plast Reconstr Surg* 1995;95(1):63–69.

Soo MS, et al. Seromas in residual fibrous capsules after explantation: mammographic and sonographic appearances. *Radiology* 1995;194(3):863–866.

Steinbach BG, Hardt NS, Abbitt PL. Mammography: breast implants—types, complications, and adjacent breast pathology. *Curr Probl Diagn Radiol* 1993;22(2):39–86.

Steinbach BG, et al. Breast implants, common complications, and concurrent breast disease. *Radiographics* 1993;13(1):95–118.

Stewart NR, et al. Mammographic appearance following implant removal. *Radiology* 1992;185(10):83–85.

Su CW, et al. Silicone implants and the inhibition of cancer. *Plast Reconstr Surg* 1995;96(3):513–520.

Theophelis LG, Stevenson TR. Radiographic evidence of breast implant rupture. *Plast Reconstr Surg* 1986;78(5):673–675.

Thuesen B, et al. Capsular contracture after breast reconstruction with the tissue expansion technique: a comparison of smooth and textured silicone breast prostheses. *Scand J Plast Reconstr Surg Hand Surg* 1995;29(1):9–13.

van Wingerden JJ, van Staden MM. Ultrasound mammography in prosthesis-related breast augmentation complications. *Ann Plast Surg* 1989;22(1):32–35.

Varga J, Schumacher HR, Jimenez SA. Systemic sclerosis after augmentation mammoplasty with silicone implants. *Ann Intern Med* 1989;111(5):377–383.

Weizer G, et al. Utility of magnetic resonance imaging and ultrasonography in diagnosing breast implant rupture. *Ann Plast Surg* 1995;34(4):352–361.

10

SONOGRAPHIC EVALUATION OF BREAST CYSTS

As in other organs, breast cysts can be classified as either simple or complex. Cysts arising from any organ that meet strict criteria for being simple cysts are benign with almost absolute certainty. However, complex breast cysts are generally less worrisome than complex cysts arising from other organs. For example, complex renal or hepatic cysts are relatively uncommon and are considered to carry a relatively high risk for being malignant or infected, but complex breast cysts are far more frequent and are at much lower risk for being malignant or infected. Despite the relatively low risk for malignancy or infection associated with complex breast cysts as a group, the sonographer must have a systematic method of assessing the risk for malignancy or infection within any individual complex breast cyst. This chapter describes the algorithm that we have developed for assessing complex breast cysts. This algorithm has been adapted from previously developed algorithms that are used in mammography and for sonographic assessment of solid breast nodules.

A *complex cyst* can be defined as any cyst that does not meet strict criteria for a simple cyst. Simple cysts must be anechoic and well circumscribed; have a thin, echogenic outer wall or capsule; and have enhanced through-transmission and thin edge shadows. All five of these criteria must be met to classify the cyst as simple. Absence of any of these criteria excludes a cyst from being characterized as simple and requires characterization of the cyst as complex or complicated.

Complex breast cysts are common, and unfortunately, the percentage of all breast cysts that appear to be complex is increasing. The use of higher-resolution equipment contributes to this increasing prevalence of complex breast in two ways: (a) better demonstration of real particulate matter that exists within cyst fluid, and (b) introduction of more artifactual echoes within cysts.

There are real structures that lie within benign breast cysts that can give rise to worrisome internal echoes at sonography that all histopathologists would merely classify as part of the spectrum of benign fibrocystic change (FCC). Table 10–1 lists internal structures other than papilloma or carcinoma that cause internal echoes that require a cyst to be characterized as complex rather than simple. Most of this particulate matter was too small to be resolved by older, lower-resolution ultrasound equipment. Thus, the cysts that contained them were inaccurately characterized as simple rather than complex. However, newer, higher-resolution equipment can show these particles in a much larger percentage of cases, increasing the percentage of all breast cysts that must be correctly characterized as complex or complicated.

Unfortunately, in addition to showing real particulate matter within cysts better, newer transducers that operate at the absolute limits of frequency, bandwidth, and dynamic range have a tendency to create more artifactual echoes within cysts, causing simple cysts to be falsely characterized as complex. By pushing frequency, bandwidth, and dynamic range to their absolute limits, we can minimize volume-averaging artifact and maximize spatial resolution, but this compromises contrast resolution. Table 10–2 lists various artifactual echoes that can be increased when transducer frequency, bandwidth, and dynamic range are pushed to, and sometimes, beyond their limits.

The reassuring *general rules* about complex breast cysts are that (a) malignant complex breast cysts are usually obviously suspicious, and (b) most complex cysts fall within the broad spectrum of FCC. Most malignant cystic lesions are solid suspicious nodules that have either undergone cystic or hemorrhagic degeneration or have secondarily involved a preexisting adjacent cyst. Only rarely will a malignant complex breast cyst be difficult to characterize as suspicious. However, general rules apply to populations, not individuals. Individuals are seldom reassured by general rules. Each individual patient is always sure that she is the exception to the general rule.

TABLE 10–1. CAUSES OF INTERNAL ECHOES WITHIN COMPLEX BREAST CYSTS OTHER THAN PAPILLOMA OR CARCINOMA

Cell debris

Protein globules

Cholesterol crystals

Red blood cells

Polymorphonuclear leukocytes

Lymphocytes

Plasma cells

Macrophages (histiocytes)

Foamy macrophages

Epithelial cells—floating

Epithelial cells—papillary

Apocrine cells—floating

Apocrine cells—papillary

Unlike malignant complex cystic lesions, whose appearance accurately reflects their nature, benign complex cysts caused by FCC frequently have suspicious sonographic appearances. Suspicious-appearing benign complex cysts are common. Many patients have numerous complex cysts in each breast. Such lesions are simply too numerous to be biopsied, aspirated, or even followed. In order to both avoid mischaracterizing malignant complex cysts as benign and minimize biopsies on the far more numerous suspicious-appearing benign complex cysts, the sonographer or sonologist must develop a systematic approach for evaluating the risk associated with individual complex breast cysts. Each complex breast cyst must be characterized into a Breast Imaging Reporting and Data System (BIRADS) category to assess the relative values of aspiration, biopsy, follow-up, or return to routine screening. Furthermore, most complex breast cysts must be sonographically characterized as benign (BIRADS 2) and the

TABLE 10–2. ARTIFACTUAL INTERNAL ECHOES WITHIN CYSTS[a]

Reverberations

Ring-down

Clutter

Triangulation

Side-lobe

Speckle

[a]Increased when transducer frequency, bandwidth, and dynamic range are pushed to limits.

patient returned to routine screening pool so as not to exhaust all of the funds available for breast cancer screening on unnecessary histologic or cytologic evaluation or short-interval follow-up of benign complex breast cysts.

The efficacy of any imaging algorithm must be judged by a gold standard. Developing an algorithm for characterizing complex breast cysts has been more difficult than was developing the algorithm for sonographic characterization of solid breast nodules because the gold standard for complex cysts is less certain than that for solid nodules. The gold standard for solid breast nodules is histology, whereas the gold standard for complex breast cysts has generally been either cyst fluid cytology or long-term follow-up with clinical and imaging examinations. Histology, although not perfect, is far more reliable and reproducible than is cytology of cyst fluid, which has unacceptably high false-negative and false-positive rates. Follow-up is also beset by problems, including poor patient compliance and the need to follow for up to 2 to 3 years, not just 6 months. Even surgical excision of complex breast cysts can be difficult and inaccurate. Pathologists have a tendency to underinterpret the cystic components of the biopsy. A complex cyst that is quite dominant clinically and sonographically is likely to be ruptured at surgery or in the process of histologic preparation and therefore may be completely unimpressive to the pathologist. A dominant complex cyst that has been ruptured at surgery or in the process of fixation may be misinterpreted as merely being part of the background fibrocystic process if an area of incidental atypia or ductal carcinoma *in situ* (DCIS) is discovered in the specimen. All of this makes obtaining objective feedback on an imaging algorithm for evaluation of complex breast cysts difficult and fraught with uncertainty. A busy breast imaging department can obtain reliable histology on 100 solid breast nodules in order to assess the efficacy of its imaging algorithm within a few months. However, to obtain equally reliable gold standard histologic or long-term follow-up data on 100 complex breast cysts might require an initial patient population of thousands of patients and many years.

Sonographic characterization of complex breast cysts can be divided into two levels. In level one, we simply characterize cysts into one of three categories: simple, complex, or indeterminate cystic versus solid. (Unfortunately, even with the best available equipment and a very experienced sonologist, there is still a small percentage of lesions that cannot be accurately classified as cystic or solid.) Level 1 characterization represents the traditional role of breast ultrasound. In level 2, the characterization process is taken one step further. Each breast cyst is assigned a BIRADS category. There is little controversy about level 1 characterization. It is quite similar everywhere and has not changed in decades. However, there is more controversy about level two characterizations. This controversy exists largely be-

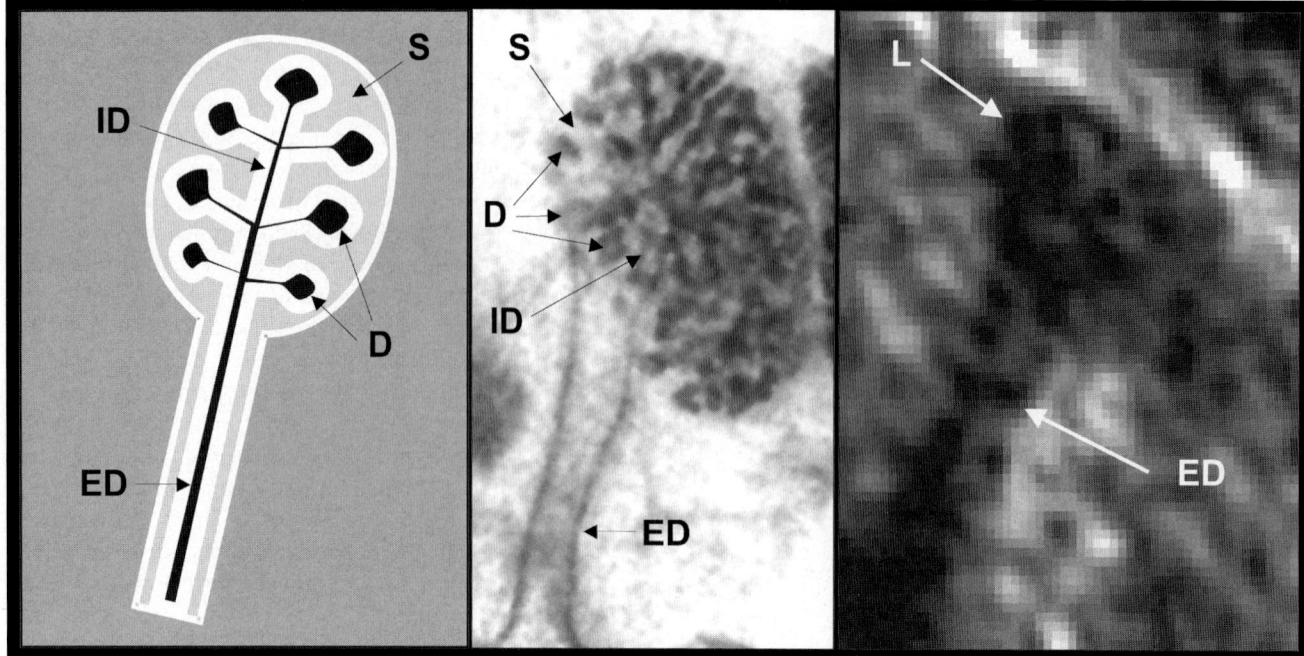

FIGURE 10–1 The individual components of the functional unit of the breast, the terminal ductolobular unit *(TDLU)*, the extralobular terminal duct *(ED)*, intralobular terminal duct *(ID)*, intralobular ductules *(D)*, and intralobular stroma *(S)*, are all equally isoechoic and indistinguishable from each other sonographically. Therefore, the normal sonographic appearance is similar to that of a tennis racket, with the racket head representing the lobule *(L)* and the handle representing the extralobular terminal duct *(ED)*.

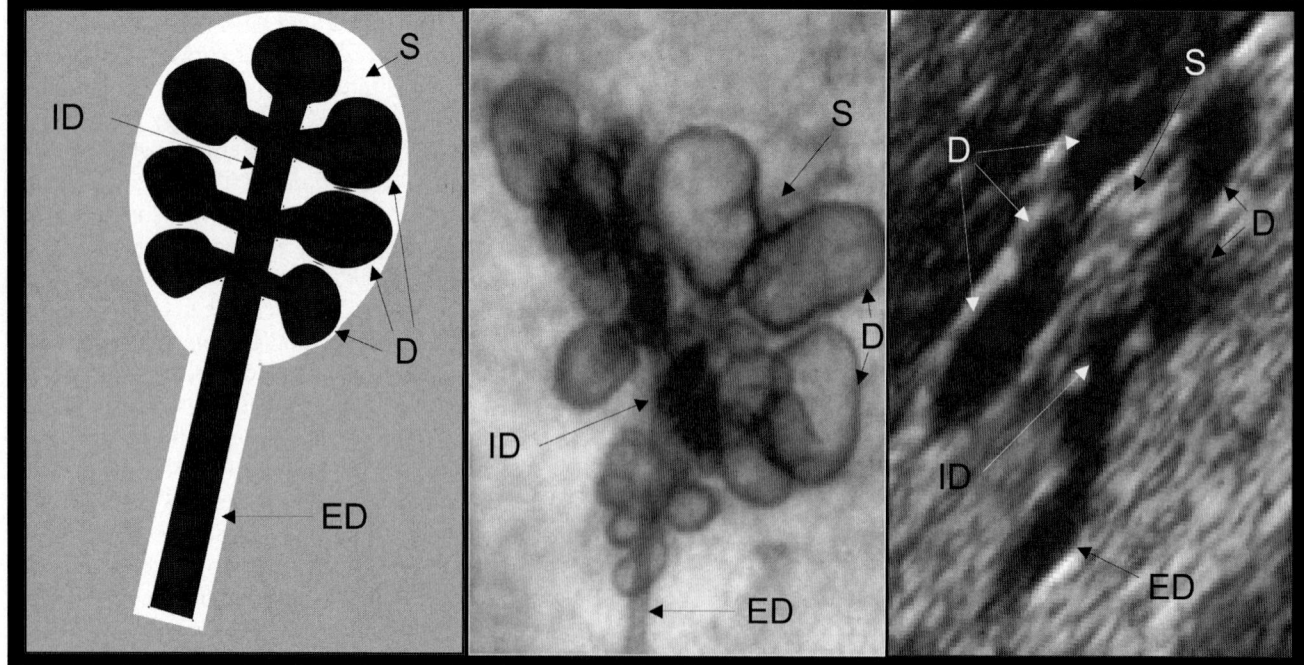

FIGURE 10–2 In early fibrocystic change, the extralobular *(ED)* and intralobular *(ID)* portions of the terminal duct and the intralobular ductules *(D)* become dilated and filled with fluid, and the normally isoechoic loose intralobular stromal tissue *(S)* becomes fibrosclerotic and appears hyperechoic. (Subgross 3-D histology courtesy of Hanne M. Jensen, MD, University of California at Davis.)

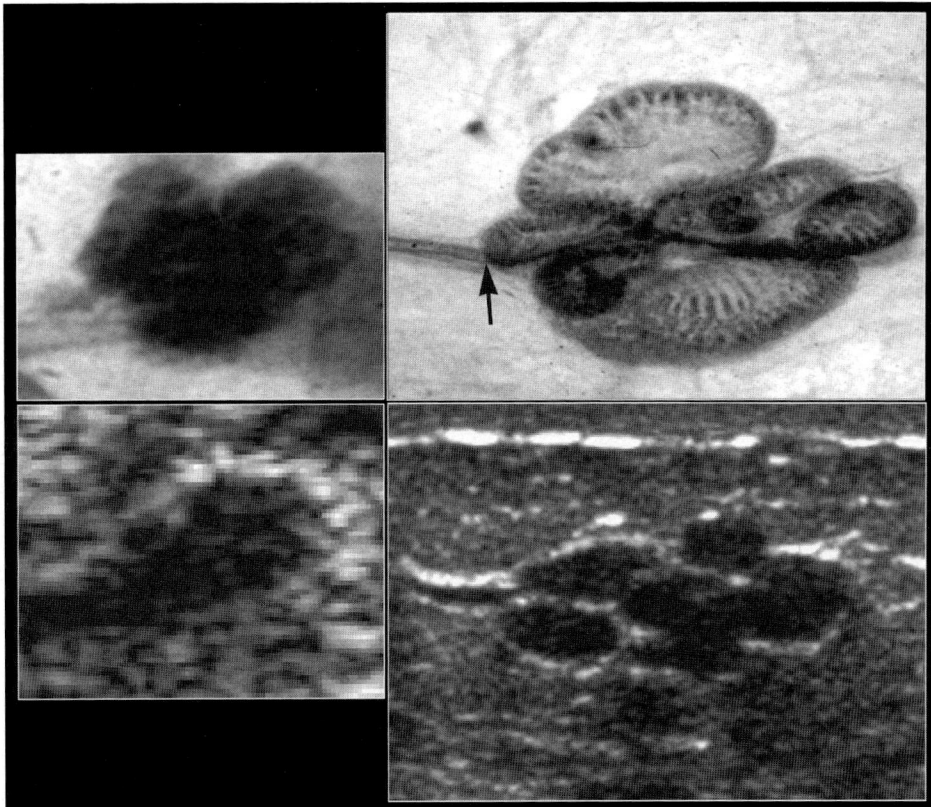

FIGURE 10–3 Comparison of normal terminal ductolobular unit (TDLU) histologically and sonographically **(left)** to moderate fibrocystic change **(right)**. Note that echoes present in the TDLU affected by fibrocystic change **(lower right)** reflect the presence of papillary apocrine metaplasia **(upper right)** within the cystically dilated ductules. (Subgross 3-D histology courtesy of Hanne M. Jensen, MD, University of California at Davis.)

cause of the difficulties with the gold standard that were discussed previously and because of a highly variable, and often unjustified, reliance on and faith in cyst aspiration and cytologic evaluation of cyst fluid.

Before defining the algorithm for level 2 characterizations of complex breast cysts, it is necessary to review the histology of FCC and its relationship to the underlying breast anatomy. Most FCC arises within the functional unit of the breast, the terminal ductolobular unit (TDLU). Cysts evolve from severe ectasia of larger, more centrally located ducts much less commonly. The TDLU consists of the intralobular and extralobular portions of the terminal duct, ductules, and intralobular stroma. The terminal duct, ductules, and intralobular stroma, all the components of the TDLU, are all isoechoic and indistinguishable from each other in lobules that are unaffected by FCC. Such lobules appear as a homogeneously isoechoic bulbous cul-de-sacs on the end of isoechoic extralobular terminal ducts (Fig. 10–1). FCC originating in the TDLU begins as dilation and effacement of intralobular ductules and of the intralobular terminal duct. The normally loose and elastic isoechoic intralobular stromal tissues that surround the

ductules undergo hyalinization and sclerosis and become hyperechoic (Fig. 10–2). The combination of cystic dilation of the ductules and fibrosclerosis of the intralobular stroma enlarges the TDLU (Fig. 10–3). The relative degree of cystic change and sclerosis varies greatly from lobule to lobule, and TDLUs unaffected by FCC can lie immediately adjacent to cystic TDLUs (Fig. 10–4). Cystic changes may predominate in one TDLU, whereas fibrosclerotic intralobular stromal changes may predominate in the adjacent lobule. Cystic changes may predominate in one part of the lobule, whereas fibrosis, sclerosis, and hyalinization may predominate in other parts of the same lobule (Fig. 10–5). This tremendous variability in lobular involvement contributes to the broad spectrum of appearances of FCC.

As the degree of cystic dilation of the ductules progresses, some of the ductules become effaced and incorporated into adjacent cystically dilated ductules, and the intralobular stromal tissue becomes compressed. Thus, the number of residual ductules within each lobule decreases as the degree of dilation increases. Ultimately, all ductules may be completely effaced and incorporated into the wall of a tension cyst, the structure we recognize as a simple

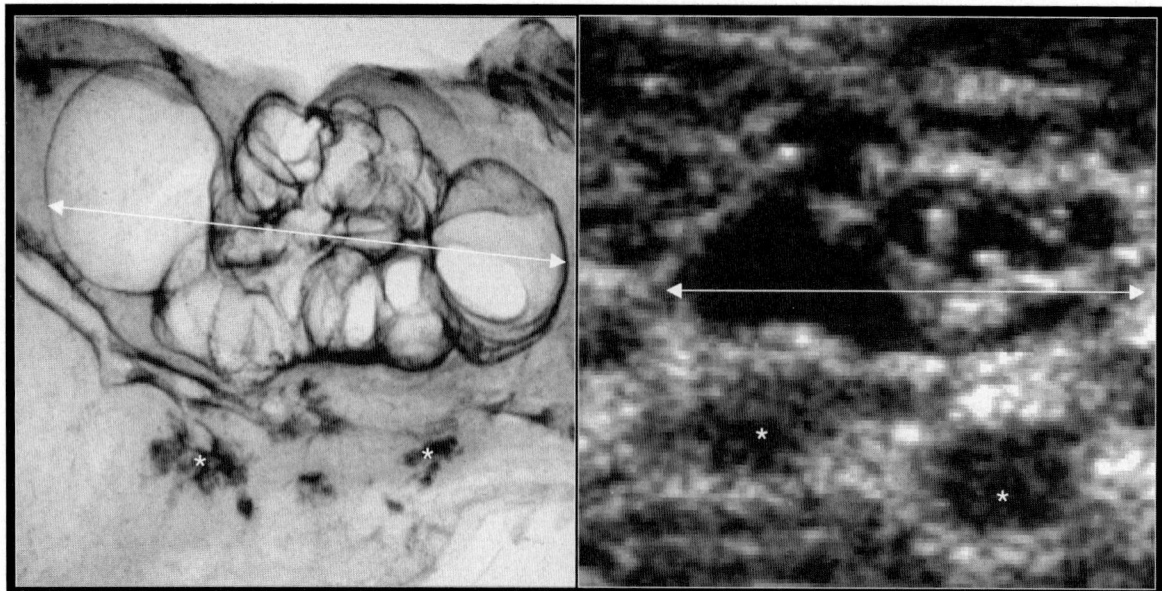

FIGURE 10–4 The anterior terminal ductolobular unit (TDLU) is moderately to severely cystically dilated *(double-headed arrow)*. The posterior TDLUs *(*)* are normal in size and appearance. (**Left,** courtesy of Hanne M. Jensen, MD, University of California at Davis.)

cyst. When the affected TDLU is imaged parallel to its long axis, FCC changes can be shown in their entirety and recognized as FCC. However, in most cases, imaging planes and histologic slices randomly cut through the TDLU in axes other than the long axis show only some of the lobular FCC changes (Fig. 10–6).

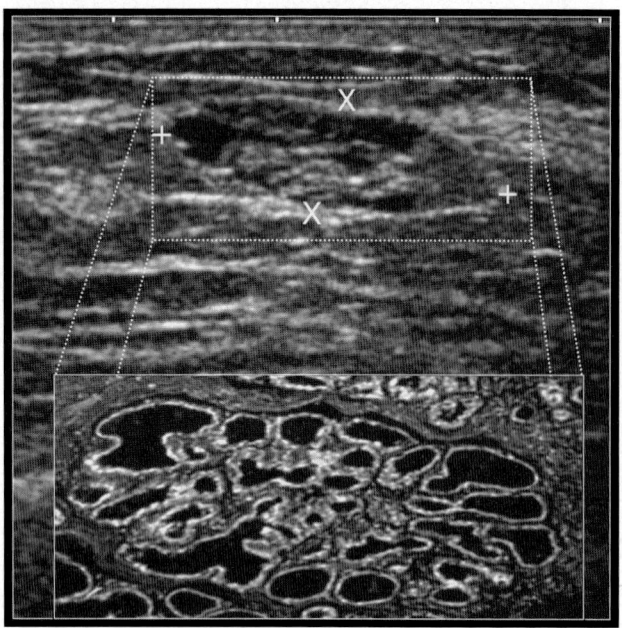

FIGURE 10–5 This terminal ductolobular unit is moderately affected by fibrocystic change, but about half the lobule is composed of microcysts and fibrosclerosis that are volume averaged to appear isoechoic. (Subgross 3-D histology courtesy of Hanne M. Jensen, MD, University of California at Davis; histology is video-inverted to make cystic areas appear black.)

The spectrum of sonographic appearances of FCC varies with the stage of development and the relative degrees of cystic dilation and sclerosis. In later stages of FCC, when cystic change predominates, sonographic diagnosis may be straightforward. However, in earlier stages, when cystic dilations are very small (microcysts), or when hyalinization, sclerosis, and papillary apocrine metaplasia predominate, FCC can cause a worrisome complex cystic appearance, or may even cause a solid, microlobulated appearance (Figs. 10–7 and 10–8). In certain cases, clustered microcysts caused by FCC can be indistinguishable from DCIS, and biopsy may be necessary (Fig. 10–9).

The algorithm that has been developed for evaluating breast cysts has been derived directly from the algorithms used to evaluate mammograms and solid breast nodules. The general algorithm for mammographic and sonographic evaluation of solid breast nodules is designed to err on the side of caution and can be summarized as follows:

1. Eliminate as many artifactual echoes as possible in pseudo complex cysts.
2. Look for suspicious findings in real complex cysts.
3. If there are no suspicious findings, look for definitively benign findings.
4. If there are no definitively benign findings, characterize the lesion into an intermediate-risk category.

A more detailed explanation of the imaging algorithm used for evaluation of complex breast cysts follows. Complex cysts differ from solid nodules in that complex cysts may be worrisome for either neoplasm or infection. First, an attempt is made to exclude simple cysts that appear complex because of artifactual internal echoes. Then, the algo-

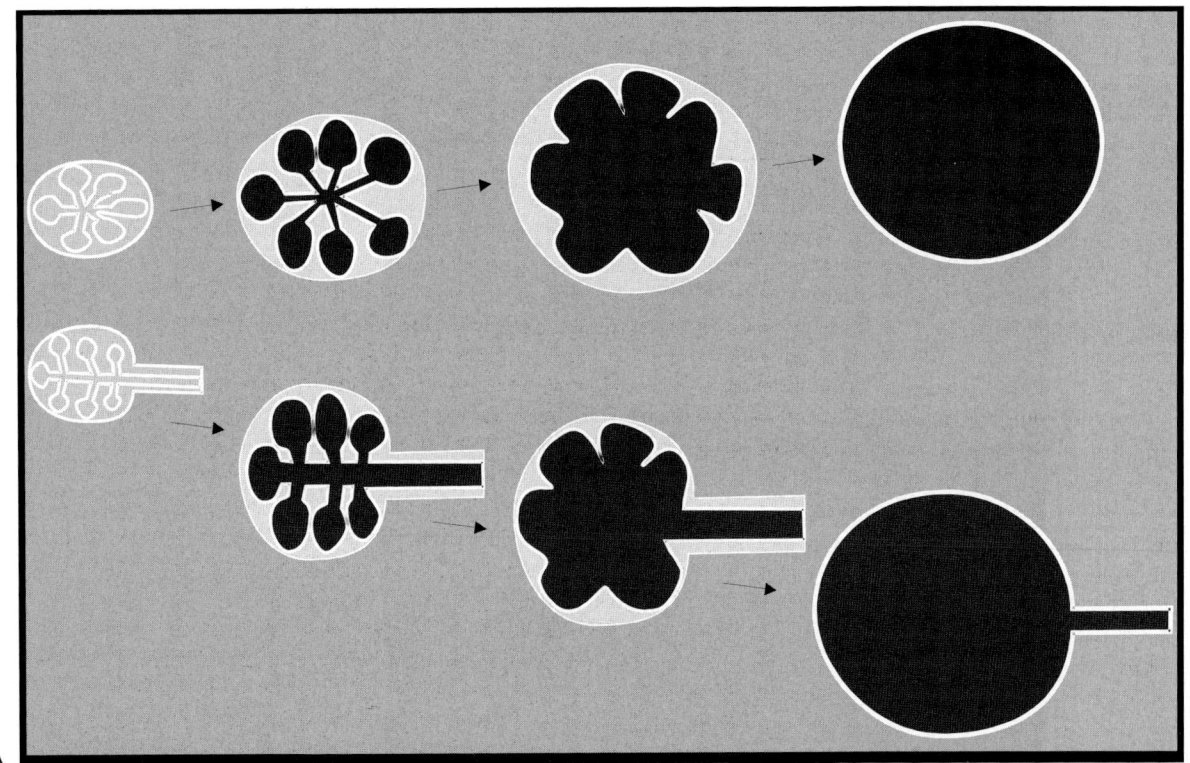

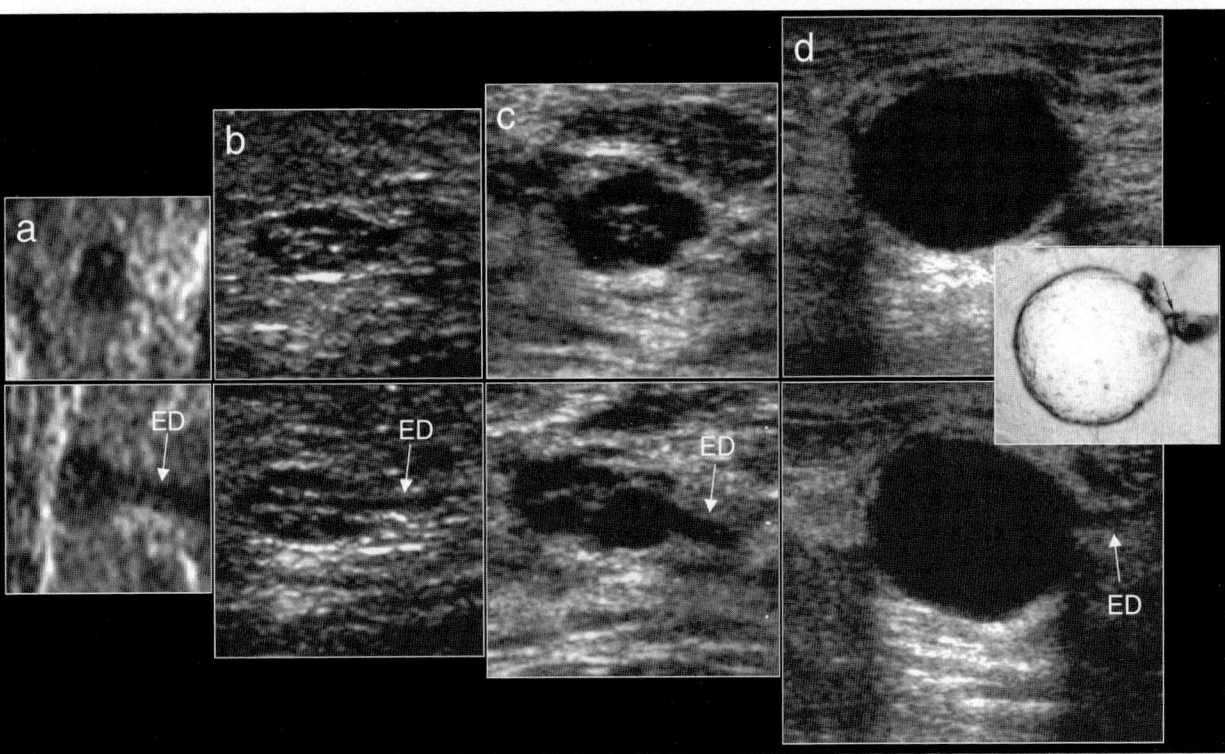

FIGURE 10–6 A: This figure illustrates the progression from a normal terminal ductolobular unit (TDLU) to severe fibrocystic change and tension cyst formation in long axis (**lower row**) and short or random axes (**top row**). Most examples of microcysts seen in real life, both sonographically and histologically, are obtained at random planes through the TDLU, much like the appearance in the **top row**. During ultrasound, however, there is an opportunity to reorient the transducer in a plane more nearly parallel to the long axis of the TDLU. **B:** This figure shows the progression from a normal TDLU *(a)*, to mild cystic dilation of the TDLU *(b)*, to moderate cystic distention of the TDLU *(c)*, to full-tension cyst formation *(d)*. The **bottom row** of images is obtained parallel to the long axis of the TDLU, and the **top row** of images is obtained perpendicular to the short axis of the TDLU. ED, extralobular terminal duct. (Subgross 3-D histology courtesy of Hanne M. Jensen, MD, University of California at Davis.)

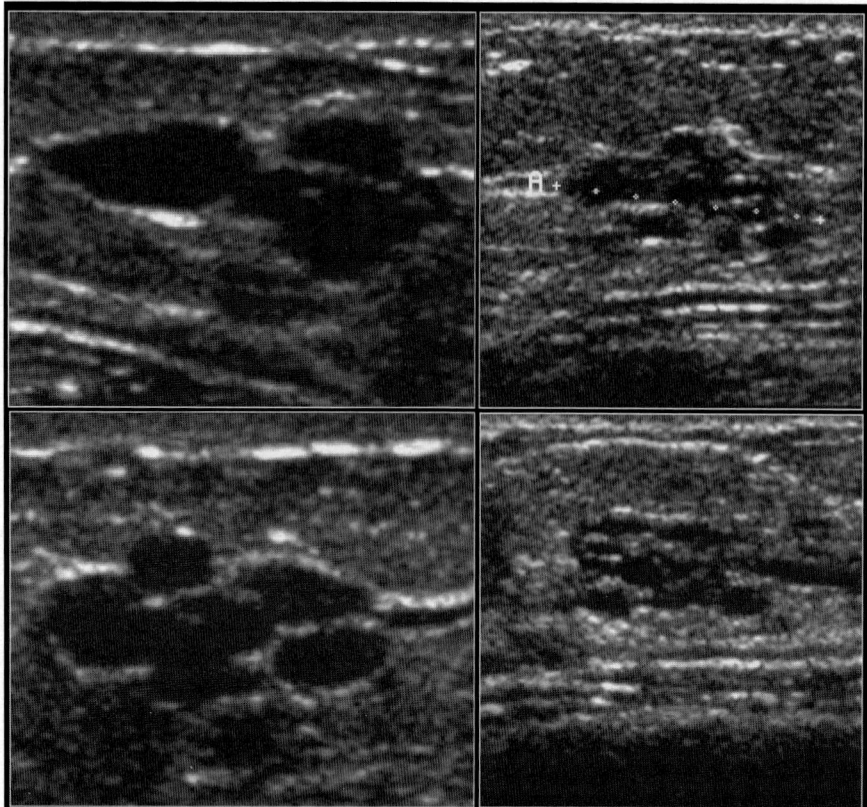

FIGURE 10–7 When cystic dilation of the terminal ductolobular unit (TDLU) is moderate or greater, few interpretive difficulties are encountered (**left**). The structure is easily identified as a cystically dilated TDLU and can be classified as either a thinly septated cyst or cluster of simple cysts. However, when dilation is minimal, microcysts may become volume averaged with the echogenic surrounding sclerotic intralobular stroma. The resulting appearance is isoechoic and microlobulated (**right**), an appearance that can be seen in ductal carcinoma *in situ* and in some cases of invasive ductal carcinoma. The **bottom row** shows the TDLU parallel to its long axis and the **top row** shows the TDLU perpendicular to its long axis.

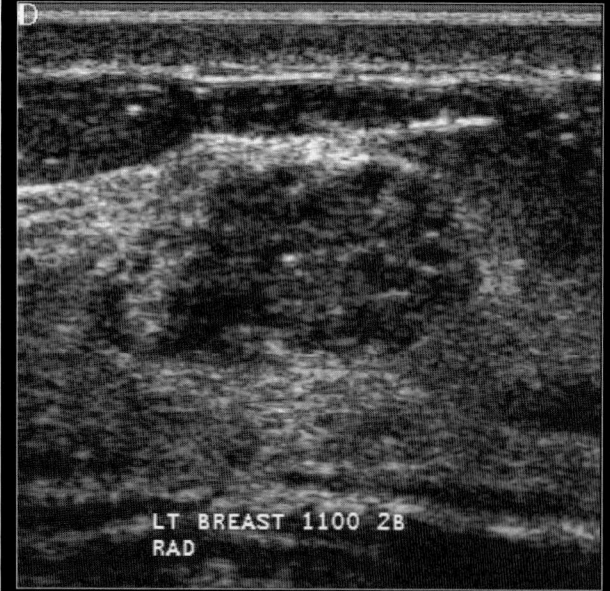

FIGURE 10–8 In some cases of fibrocystic change, the terminal ductolobular unit can become greatly expanded, but the individual cysts are either so small that they are volume averaged with surrounding fibrosclerotic stroma or are filled with echogenic secretions or papillary apocrine metaplasia. Such lesions are indistinguishable from solid microlobulated lesions. This appearance explains many cases in which histologic results are discordant with imaging findings. In most cases like this case, when a nonspecific benign diagnosis of fibrocystic change is obtained, but a specific benign or malignant diagnosis was expected, the patient may undergo repeat core needle biopsy or excisional biopsy.

rithm requires a search for findings that are worrisome for malignancy—findings that would be classified as BIRADS categories 4a, 4b, or 5. If any of these findings are detected, the cyst should be evaluated histologically. If there are no findings suspicious for malignancy (BIRADS 4a, 4b, or 5 findings), findings that are suspicious for infection are sought. Findings that are suggestive of inflammation or infection, when identified, are generally characterized as probably benign (BIRADS 3) and require aspiration, Gram stain, and culture. Cytologic evaluation of fluid is unnecessary because the sonographic and clinical concern is infection, not neoplasm. Only if there are no findings that are suspicious for either malignancy or infection are specific benign findings sought. If benign findings are identified, the cystic lesion can be characterized as benign (BIRADS 2 category), and no interventional procedure or special follow-up is necessary. If the lesion cannot be characterized as BIRADS 2, then probably benign (BIRADS 3) findings are sought. Complex cysts characterized as BIRADS 3 can be managed with attempted aspiration or short-interval follow-up. If there are no specific malignant findings, but the cystic lesion cannot strictly be classified as BIRADS 2 or 3, by default, the lesion must be characterized as BIRADS 4a and histologically evaluated with either open surgical biopsy or ultrasound-guided vacuum-assisted needle biopsy.

Table 10–3 compares the mammographic algorithm and the sonographic algorithms for characterizing solid nodules and complex cysts. Employing an algorithm for

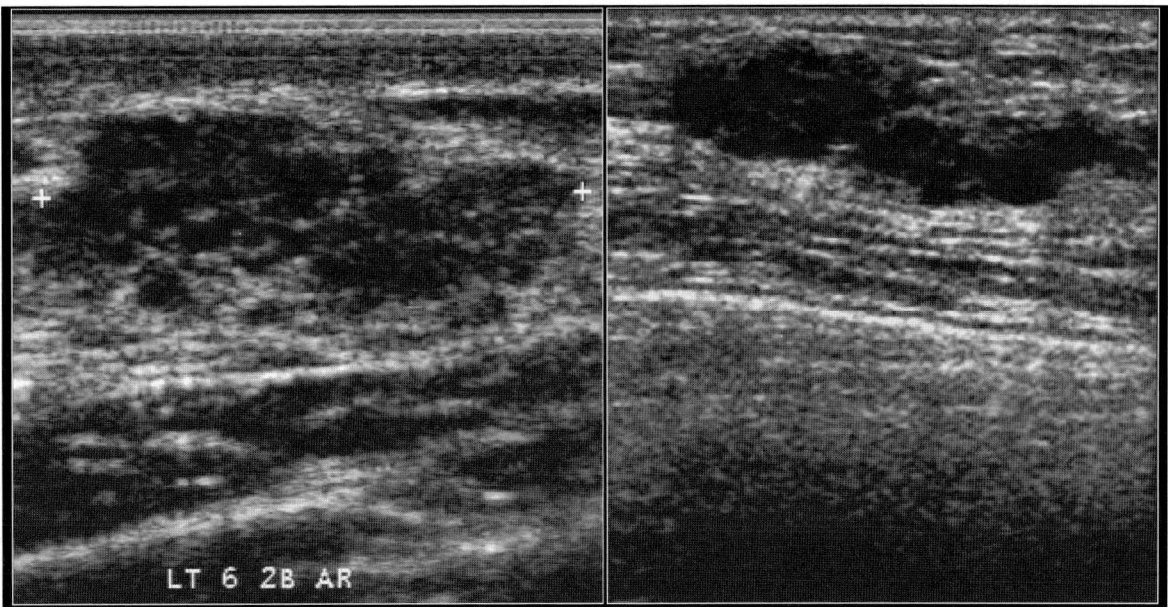

FIGURE 10–9 This illustrates the difficulties in distinguishing microlobulated fibrocystic change, with volume averaging of microcysts and fibrosclerosis causing much of the lesion to appear isoechoic and solid (**left**) from a microlobulated, markedly hypoechoic, high-nuclear-grade ductal carcinoma *in situ* (**right**). For this reason, the microcystic appearance is considered suspicious and excludes a complex cyst from benign (BIRADS 2) and probably benign (BIRADS 3) categories.

TABLE 10–3. COMPARISON OF ALGORITHMS USED FOR EVALUATING MAMMOGRAMS AND SONOGRAMS OF SOLID AND COMPLEX CYSTIC BREAST LESIONS

Mammographic Nodule Algorithm	Ultrasound Algorithm for Solid Nodules[a]	Ultrasound Algorithm for Complex Breast Cysts[b]
1. Look for BIRADS 3, 4a, 4b, and 5 findings	1. Exclude pseudo solid lesion caused by artifactual internal echoes	1. Exclude pseudo complex cystic lesion caused by artifactual internal echoes
2. If BIRADS 4a, 4b, or 5 finding: diagnostic mammograms, ultrasound, biopsy	2. Look for BIRADS 4a, 4b, and 5 findings	2. Look for BIRADS 4a, 4b, and 5 findings
3. For BIRADS 3: ultrasound	3. If found, characterize as BIRADS 4a, 4b, or 5 and biopsy	3. If found, characterize as BIRADS 4a, 4b, or 5 and biopsy
4. If no BIRADS 3, 4a, 4b, or 5 finding: look for BIRADS 2 findings	4. If no BI-RADS 4a, 4b, or 5 findings: look for strict BIRADS 2 findings	4. If not BIRADS 4a, 4b, or 5: look for BIRADS 3 inflammatory findings
5. If BIRADS 2 finding: characterize as BIRADS 2 and return to routine screening pool	5. If BIRADS 2 finding: characterize as BIRADS 2 and return to routine screening pool	5. If no BIRADS 4a, 4b, or 5 findings: look for strict BIRADS 2 findings
6. If no BIRADS 2 finding: characterize as BIRADS 1 and return to routine screening pool	6. If no BIRADS 2 finding: look for BIRADS 3[c]	6. If BIRADS 2 finding: characterize as BIRADS 2 and return to routine screening pool
	7. If strict BIRADS 3 finding: characterize as BIRADS 3 and offer options of biopsy or follow-up	7. If no BIRADS 2 findings: look for BIRADS 3 findings
		8. If BIRADS 3 finding: characterize as BIRADS 3 and offer options of attempted aspiration and short-interval follow-up
		9. If no BIRADS 3 finding: by default, characterize as BIRADS 4a and biopsy

[a]Solid nodules should never be characterized as BIRADS 1.
[b]Breast cysts should never be characterized as BIRADS 1.
[c]The only BIRADS 2 solid nodules are normal-appearing intramammary lymph nodes, lipomas, and purely hyperechoic fibrous lesions.

characterizing complex breast cysts that is very similar to the existing mammographic algorithm and the sonographic algorithm for solid breast nodules helps reduce operator dependence and promises to make mammographers more comfortable in using sonography for more than level 1 characterization—"cystic versus solid."

STEP 1: EXCLUDE PSEUDO COMPLEX CYSTS AND PSEUDO INDETERMINATE LESIONS DUE TO ARTIFACT AND SOLID LESIONS MASQUERADING AS CYSTS

The first step in characterization of cystic lesions of the breast is to exclude the presence of artifactual echoes within simple cysts than can falsely make them appear to be either solid or complex cystic. Reverberation echoes, side-lobe artifacts, clutter, volume averaging, and speckle artifact can fill all or part of cysts.

Avoiding excessive gain and power settings is important in minimizing artifactual echoes. However, care must be taken not to reduce gain so much that true internal echoes are suppressed. Gain should never be reduced enough that surrounding breast fat appears severely hypoechoic or anechoic. Demonstrating surrounding breast fat as an isoechoic structure prevents suppression of true internal echoes within complex cysts (Fig. 10–10).

Volume averaging or beam width artifact significantly degrades spatial and contrast resolution and can result in artifactual echoes within simple cysts. Volume averaging is especially troublesome in cases in which anechoic microcysts are averaged with the intervening hyalinized, hyperechoic intralobular stroma because it can result in the tissue appearing to be isoechoic and solid rather than cystic. Volume averaging has generally decreased with newer, higher-resolution transducers (Fig. 10–11) but can still be a problem in the near field and in the far field within the breast. Volume averaging, particularly in the near field, can be minimized with an acoustic standoff (see Chapter 2, Figs. 2–5 and 2–6).

Reverberation echoes usually do not result in mischaracterization of a simple cyst as complex because of their characteristic appearance. Reverberation echoes are parallel to the anterior wall of the cyst and tend to occur at intervals equal to the distance between the skin and anterior wall of the cyst or the distance between a major tissue interface and the anterior cyst wall (Fig. 10–12). They are worse for near-field cysts than for far-field cysts and are worse for nontense, flattened cysts (Fig. 10–13) that have anterior walls that are parallel to the skin. Using lesser degrees of compression pressure will minimize reverberation echoes by increasing the depth of the cyst and also by minimizing flattening of the anterior wall. Angulating the transducer slightly so that the beam does not intersect the

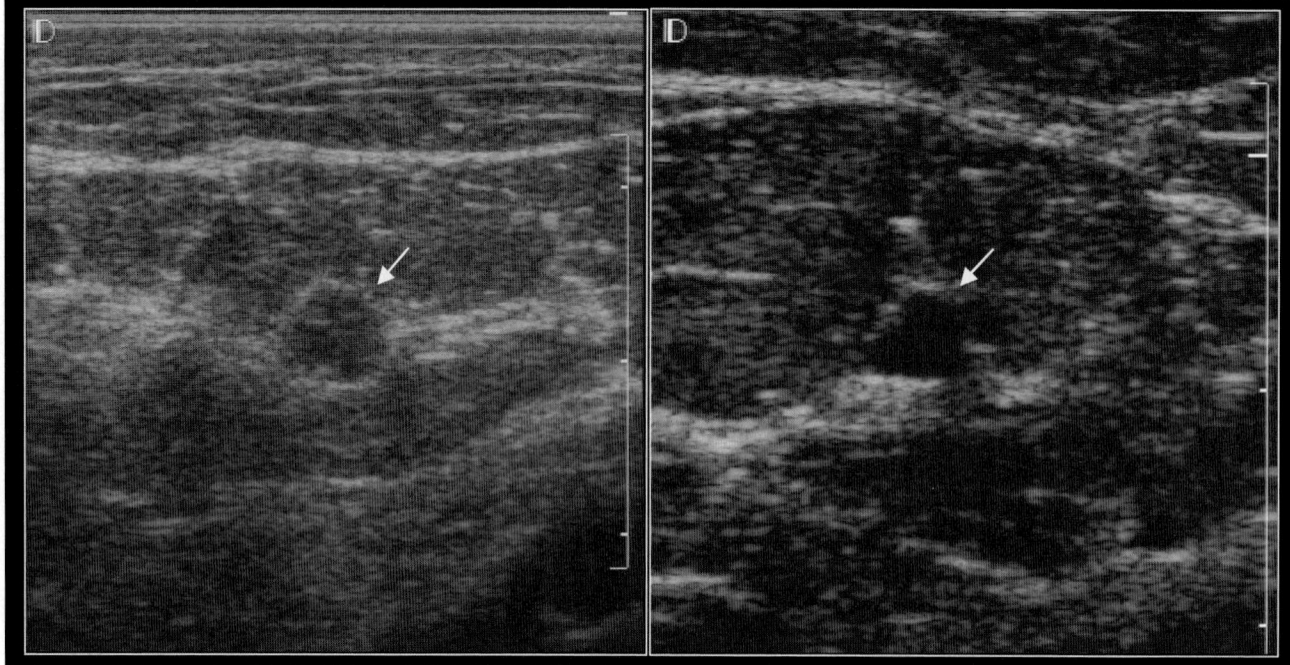

FIGURE 10–10 There is a delicate balance among using too much gain and filling simple cysts with artifact, using appropriate gain (**left**), and using too little gain and making a solid lesion falsely hypoechoic and pseudocystic in appearance (**right**). The fat should be displayed as a mid-level gray to avoid creating the pseudocystic appearance. Additionally, the heterogeneity of echoes within the lesion in the **left** image is a clue that it is solid rather than a cyst with artifact.

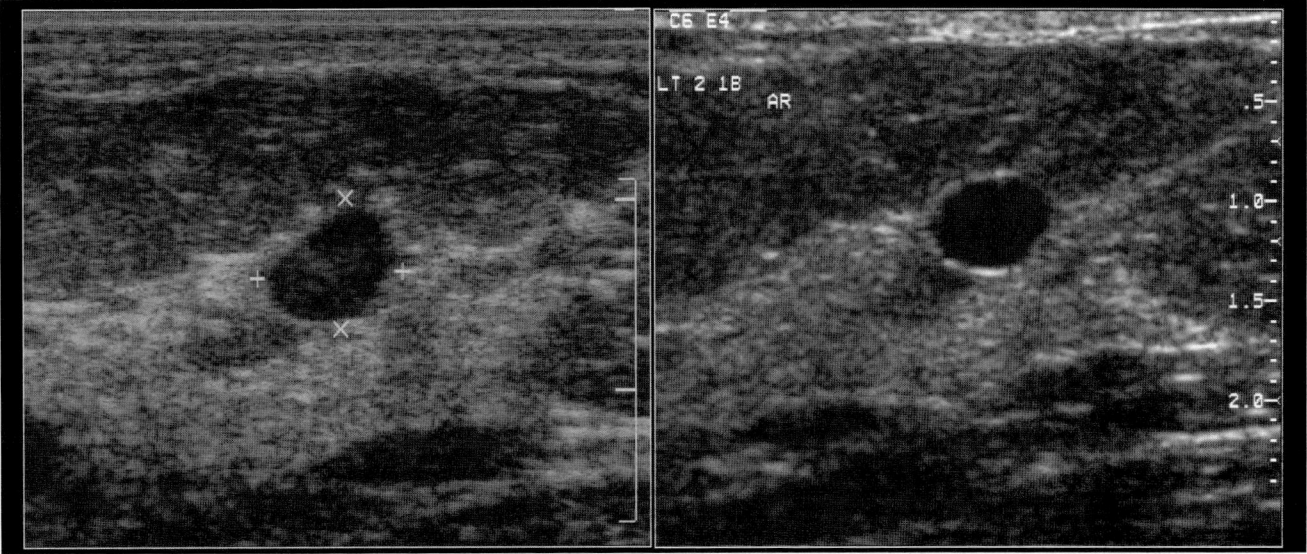

FIGURE 10–11 Older analogue equipment with lesser resolution can result in more volume averaging and other artifact **(left)** than does newer digital equipment with better resolution **(right)**. This is the same cyst scanned on two different machines the same day.

anterior cyst wall perpendicularly will also help minimize reverberation echoes (see Chapter 3, Fig. 3–7).

There have been three improvements in ultrasound equipment in recent years that can aid greatly in ridding cysts of artifactual echoes. All of these developments are discussed and illustrated in detail in Chapter 2.).

1. Electronic focusing in the short axis [1.5-dimensional (1.5-D) arrays] can reduce volume averaging in the near field. This decreases beam width and minimizes volume averaging, especially in the near field (between the skin and 1 cm). This effect is most pronounced for sebaceous cysts (see Chapter 2, Fig. 2–10).

2. High-frequency coded harmonics has reduced clutter, reverberation, and speckle artifacts within cysts, allow-

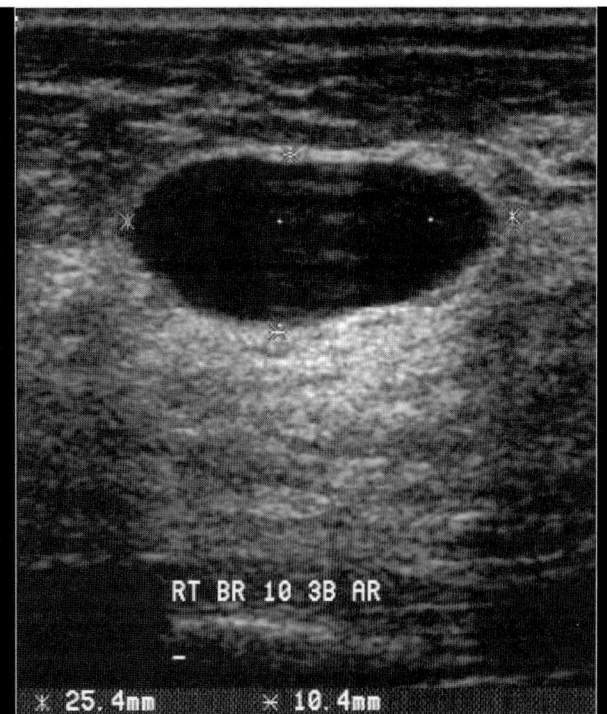

FIGURE 10–12 This is an example of multiple reverberation echoes within a cyst. The spacing between them is the same as the distance between the fat and fibrous interface that lies just superficial to the anterior wall of the cyst.

FIGURE 10–13 In a larger, less tense, flatter cyst, the reverberation echoes are longer and involve a greater percentage of the cyst volume because a longer segment of the anterior cyst wall is perpendicular to the ultrasound beam.

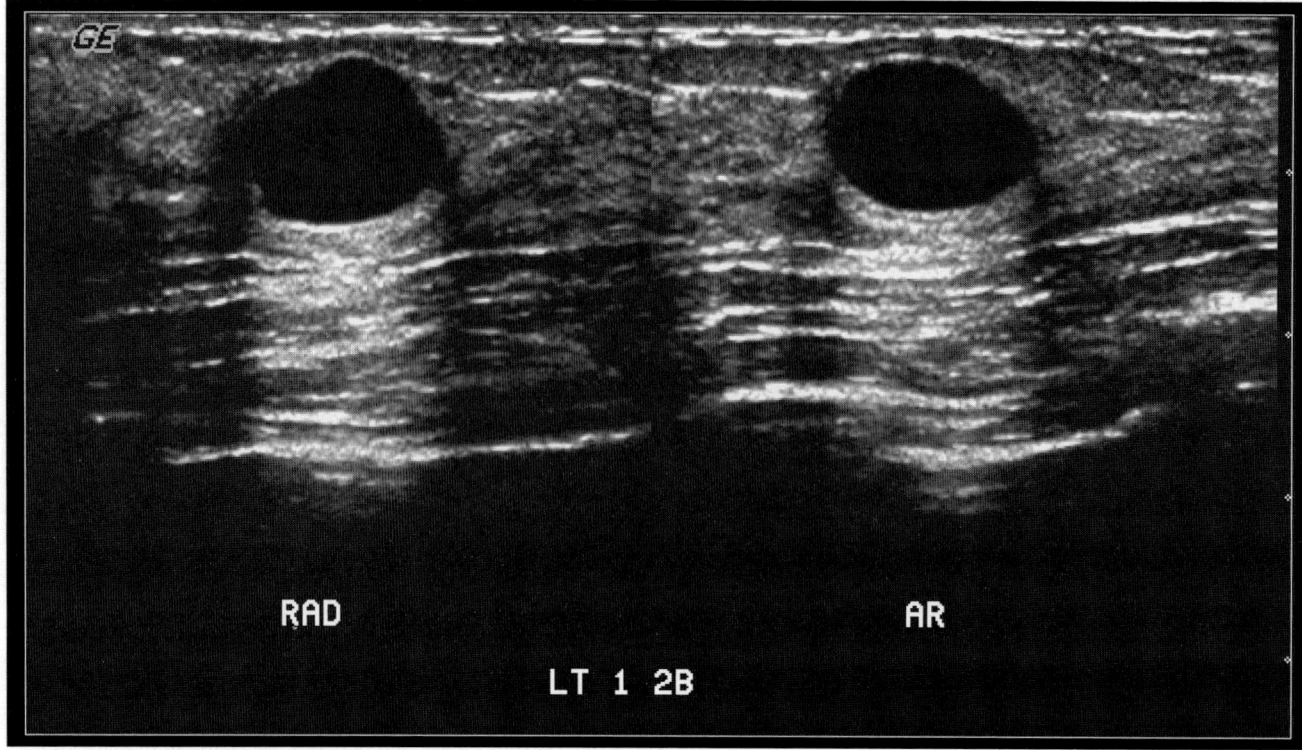

FIGURE 10–14 This cyst meets strict criteria for being a simple cyst. It is shown in radial *(rad)* and antiradial *(AR)* planes. It is anechoic, well circumscribed, and completely encompassed within a thin, echogenic wall; has enhanced through-transmission deep to it; and produces thin edge shadows.

ing some cysts that would have been classified as complex to be reclassified as simple (see Chapter 2, Figs. 2–14 and 2–15). There are even cases of indeterminate cystic or solid lesions that can be reclassified as simple cystic when evaluated with digitally encoded harmonics (see Chapter 2, Fig. 2–16). Interestingly, in the complex cysts that have real internal echoes, the echogenicity is increased with coded harmonics (see Chapter 2, Fig. 2–17). Thus, coded harmonics appears to allow us to better distinguish real internal echoes that exist within some cysts from the artifactual echoes that exist within others, even though they may appear identical to each other with fundamental imaging.

3. Helping to evaluate breast cysts better is spatial compounding of the image. The compounding builds up and accentuates real internal echoes and tends to average artifactual echoes temporally and, like high-frequency coded harmonics, helps us to distinguish complex cysts with real internal echoes from simple cysts that merely appear complex because of artifactual internal echoes (see Chapter 2, Fig. 2–26). The physics, engineering, and principles of electronic focusing in the short axis, high-frequency coded harmonics, and real-time compounding are all discussed in detail in Chapter 2.

After all available methods are employed to ensure that simple cysts containing artifactual echoes are not incorrectly classified as complex or indeterminate cystic versus solid, three groups of lesions remain: simple cysts, complex cysts, and indeterminate. Complex cysts and indeterminate lesions must undergo level 2 characterization. Cysts meeting strict criteria for a simple cyst may be classified as simple and can be characterized as BIRADS 2, benign with virtual 100% certainty (Fig. 10–14). The strict criteria that must be met for a cyst to be classified as simple are as follows:

- Central anechogenicity
- Well-circumscribed margins
- Completely encompassed by a thin, echogenic capsule
- Enhanced through-transmission
- Thin edge shadows

Simple cysts do not need to undergo biopsy, be aspirated, or be even followed for diagnostic purposes. In general, we aspirate simple cysts only for symptomatic relief when they are exquisitely tender or when they prevent adequate compression to be applied during mammography. Simple cysts are so common that they are virtually variants of normal between 35 and 50 years of age. Simply showing that a simple cyst exists in the same quadrant as either a

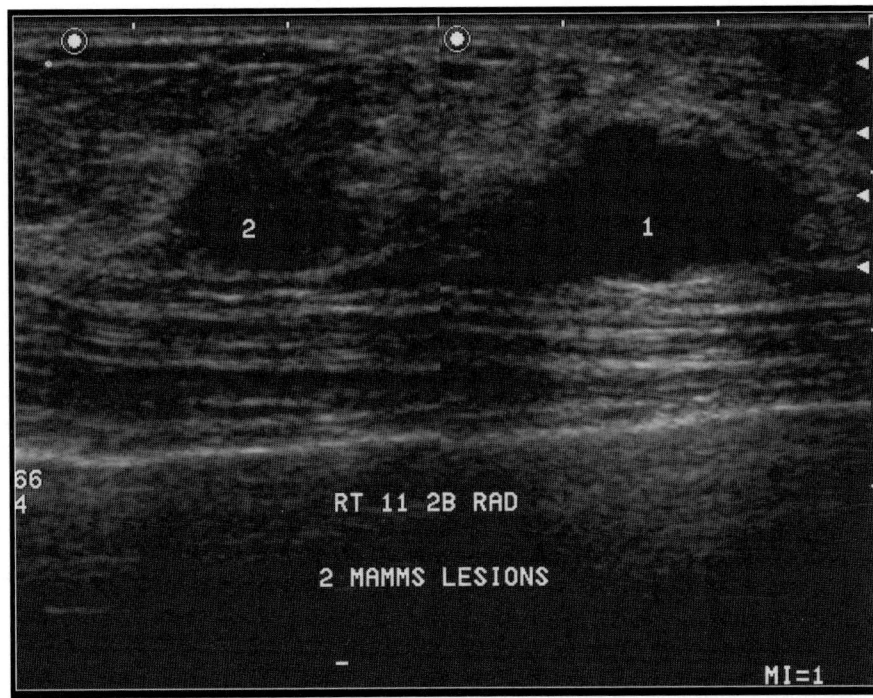

FIGURE 10–15 In patients who present with palpable lumps, it is important to palpate the lump while scanning it. Showing that a simple cyst exists in the same quadrant of the breast as a palpable lump does not prove that the cyst causes the lump. Simultaneous scanning and palpation in this patient showed the cyst to be soft, compressible, and nonpalpable *(1)*. The palpable lump was caused by the malignant solid nodule *(2)* was in the vicinity of the cyst.

palpable lump or mammographic abnormality does not by itself prove that the cyst is the cause of the lump or mammographic nodule. Although simple cysts are always benign, they can occur in the same vicinity as breast carcinomas (Fig. 10–15). The lump or mammographic abnormality in such cases may be caused by the malignancy, with the cyst being an incidental finding. It is necessary to palpate and scan the cyst simultaneously to be sure it is the cause of the lump and to correlate size, shape, location, and surrounding tissue density on mammography and sonography to be sure the cyst is the cause of the mammographic abnormality (see Chapter 5, Fig. 5–5). Correlating clinical and mammographic findings with sonographic findings is discussed in detail in Chapters 5 and 6, respectively.).

Cystic malignancies are rare, are usually obviously malignant sonographically, and rarely cause a diagnostic dilemma. In our experience, most cystic malignancies occur when a cancer arises next to a cyst rather than within it and secondarily involves the cyst (Fig. 10–16). Others represent nodules that would be better classified as solid with central cystic or hemorrhagic degeneration (Fig. 10–17). However, an occasional cyst with very subtle malignant findings can occur and cause diagnostic dilemmas (Fig. 10–18). The level 2 characterization of complex breast cysts is designed to detect and appropriately characterize such subtle malignant cysts as BIRADS category 4a or higher.

Some solid nodules can simulate cysts, especially if an incorrect technique is used. This is especially true of high-grade invasive ductal carcinomas that are typically markedly hypoechoic and have enhanced through-transmission (Fig.

10–19). Scanning with gain settings too low may artifactually make such lesions appear anechoic rather than hypoechoic. The false anechogenicity together with the enhanced through-transmission may make them appear to be cysts. However, even with too low a gain setting, such lesions should not be mistaken for cysts because they usually do not have a complete thin, echogenic capsule and often have

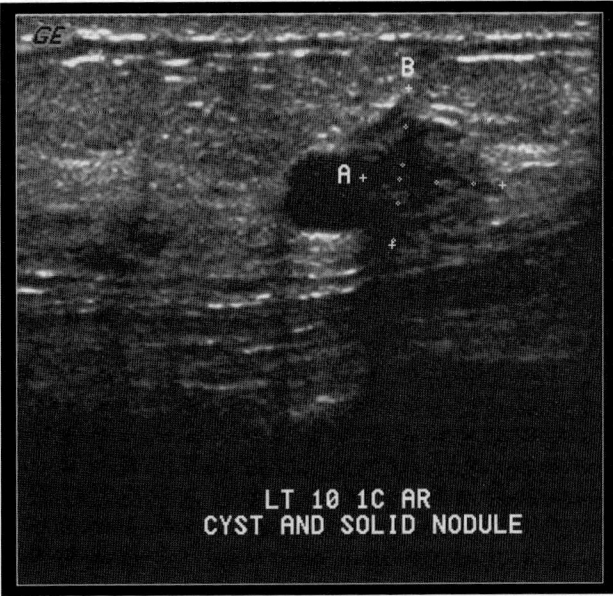

FIGURE 10–16 In most of the "malignant cysts" that we have seen, a solid malignant nodule has secondarily involved the cyst, as in this case.

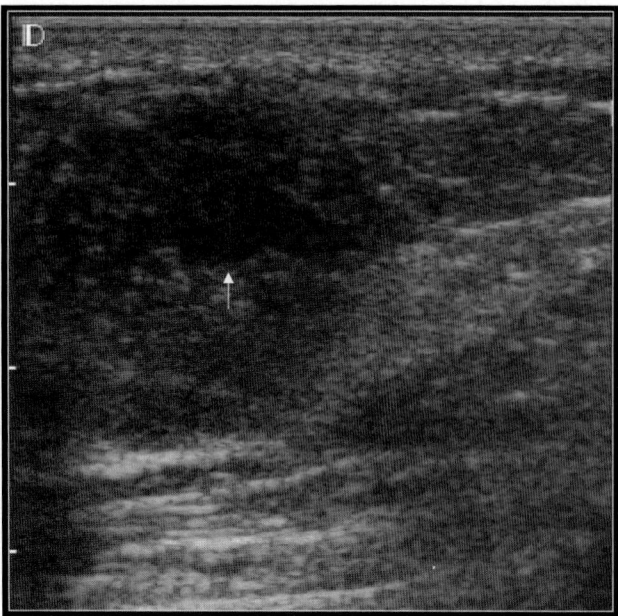

FIGURE 10–17 Other "malignant cysts" represent solid nodules that have undergone cystic or hemorrhagic degeneration centrally. This is an example of a high-grade invasive ductal carcinoma that has undergone hemorrhagic degeneration centrally *(arrow)*.

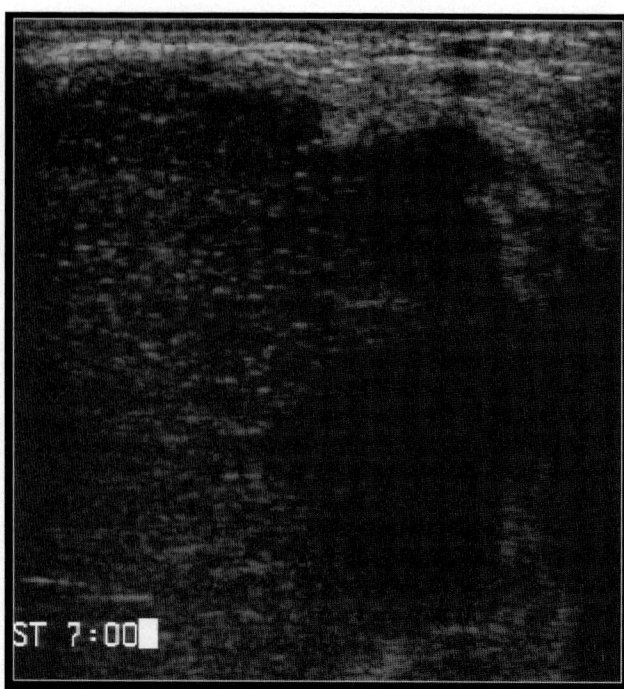

FIGURE 10–18 Only rarely will one see a primary cystic carcinoma that is subtle and difficult to distinguish from cysts that are part of the fibrocystic spectrum. This cyst was initially misinterpreted as a complex benign cyst and aspirated, but immediately recurred. Note the irregular isoechoic nodularity of the anterior wall of the cystic lesion.

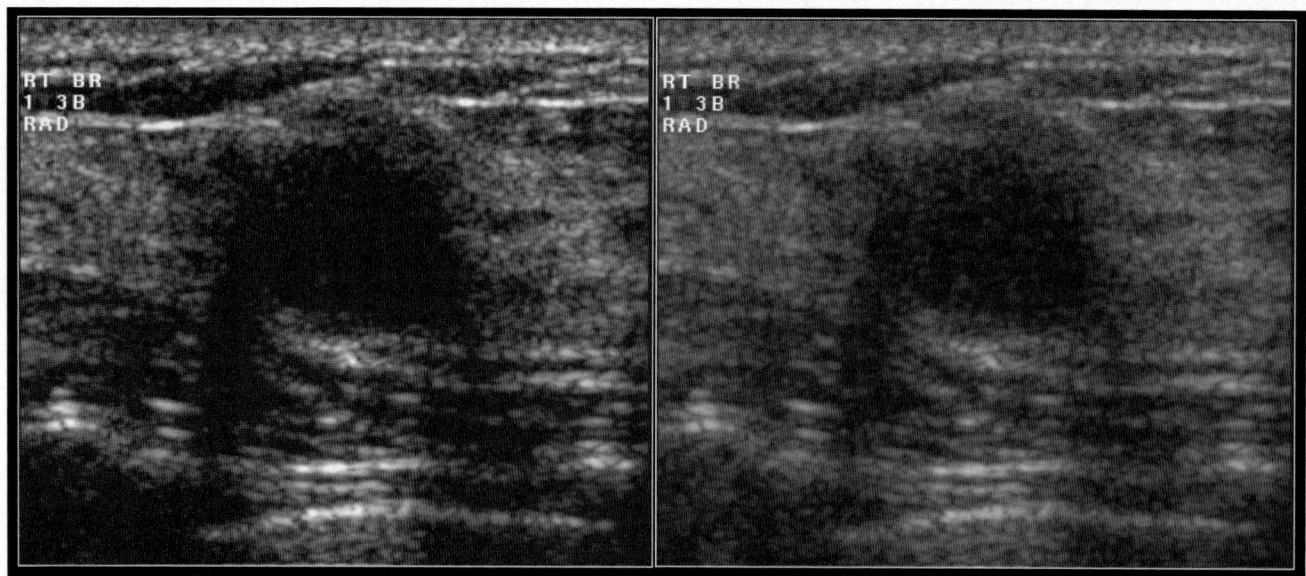

FIGURE 10–19 Some malignant solid nodules may be misinterpreted as cysts if poor imaging parameters are used. This is particular likely with lesions that are hypoechoic, are homogeneous, and have enhanced through-transmission, including high-grade invasive ductal carcinomas, medullary carcinomas, and lymphomas of the breast. These lesions appear falsely to be anechoic if gain settings that are used are too low (**left**). Together with the enhanced through-transmission, this can result in misclassification as a cyst. Even then, however, the lesion does not meet strict criteria for a simple cyst. It is not well circumscribed, does not have a thin, echogenic outer capsule, and does not have thin edge shadows. Note that the subcutaneous fat in the **left** image is inappropriately displayed as nearly anechoic. More appropriate gain settings in the **right** image display fat as gray and reduce the chances of misclassifying the lesion as cystic.

shapes and surface characteristics that suggest their true nature. Additionally, the fat within the breast may appear to be more hypoechoic than normal, offering a clue that gain is too low. Adequate gain settings should result in isoechoic fat, not markedly hypoechoic or anechoic fat. A few solid malignant nodules will appear anechoic and pseudocystic even when gain and power settings are appropriate. This most commonly occurs in medullary carcinomas (Fig. 10–20), lymphomas, and high-grade invasive ductal carcinomas. Metastases to intramammary lymph nodes or axillary lymph nodes (Fig. 10–21) can also appear anechoic. Such lesions may be misclassified as cysts but often have angular margins, taller-than-wide shape, microlobulation, partial lack of a thin capsule, or other findings that should prevent them from being misclassified as cysts. Additionally, color Doppler will often show a vessel within such anechoic-appearing solid nodules, whether primary or lymph node metastases (Fig. 10–22).

STEP 2: LOOK FOR BIRADS 4A, 4B, OR 5 FINDINGS

After artifactual internal echoes and solid nodules simulating cysts have been excluded, the true complex cysts can undergo level 2 characterization into BIRADS categories. As noted earlier, the fist step is to look for findings suspi-

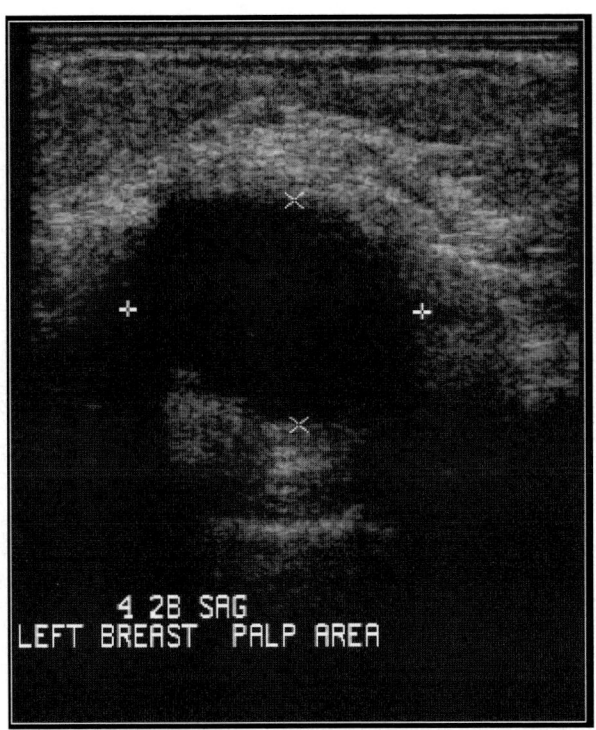

FIGURE 10–20 A few malignant solid nodules may appear anechoic or nearly anechoic even when gain settings appropriately display fat as isoechoic and midlevel gray rather than black. This is most likely to occur in medullary carcinomas, such as this case, and a few high-grade invasive ductal carcinomas.

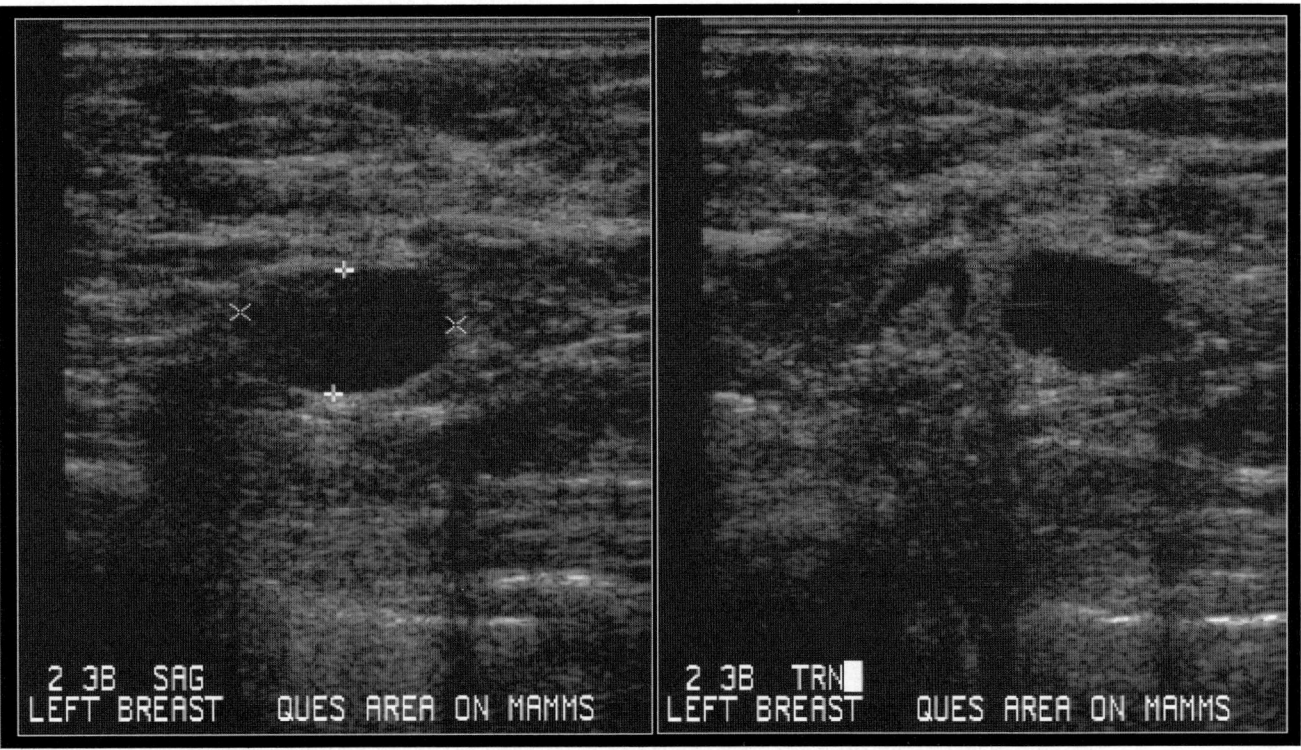

FIGURE 10–21 Metastases to axillary lymph nodes are also prone to appear anechoic or nearly anechoic, despite adequate gain settings. Note that there is a grossly abnormal axillary lymph node immediately adjacent to a sonographically normal-appearing lymph node. This is typical of malignant involvement and very unlikely to occur in inflammatory lymphadenopathy.

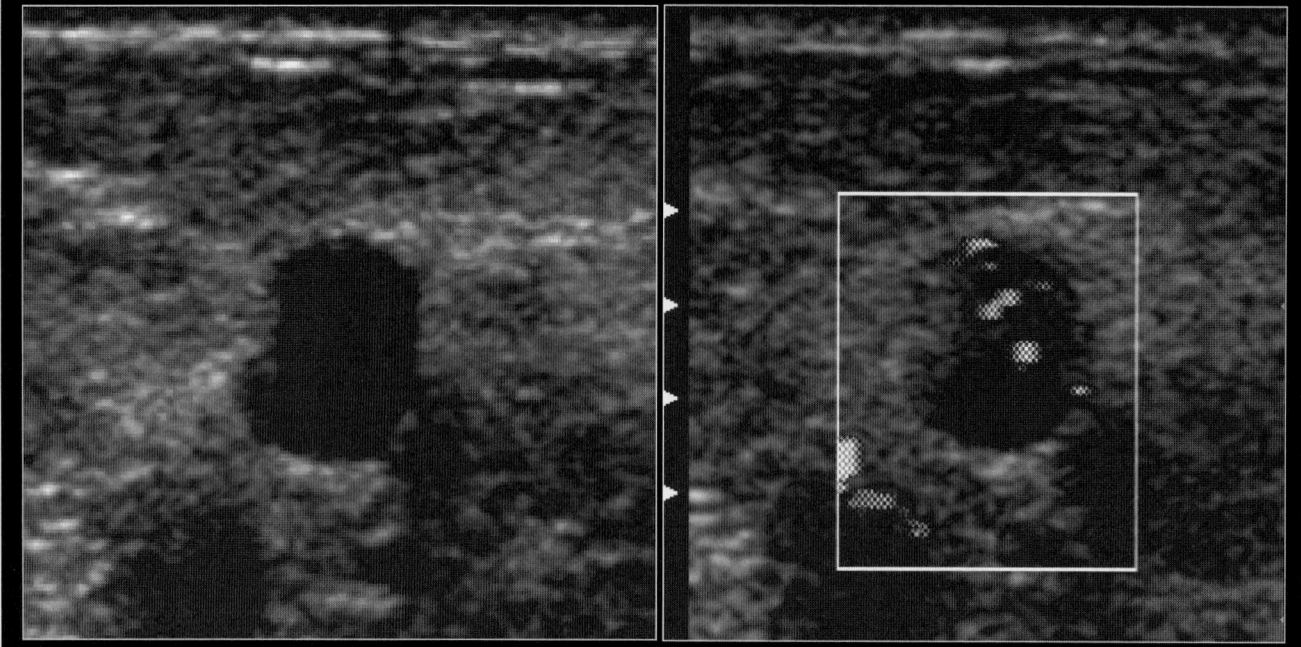

FIGURE 10–22 Color or power Doppler can be invaluable in distinguishing anechoic or nearly anechoic solid primary malignant nodules with a pseudocystic appearance from true cysts. Most anechoic-appearing malignancies are highly cellular and highly vascular. Demonstration of an internal blood vessel with color or power Doppler indicates that the lesion is solid and only pseudocystic, not truly cystic.

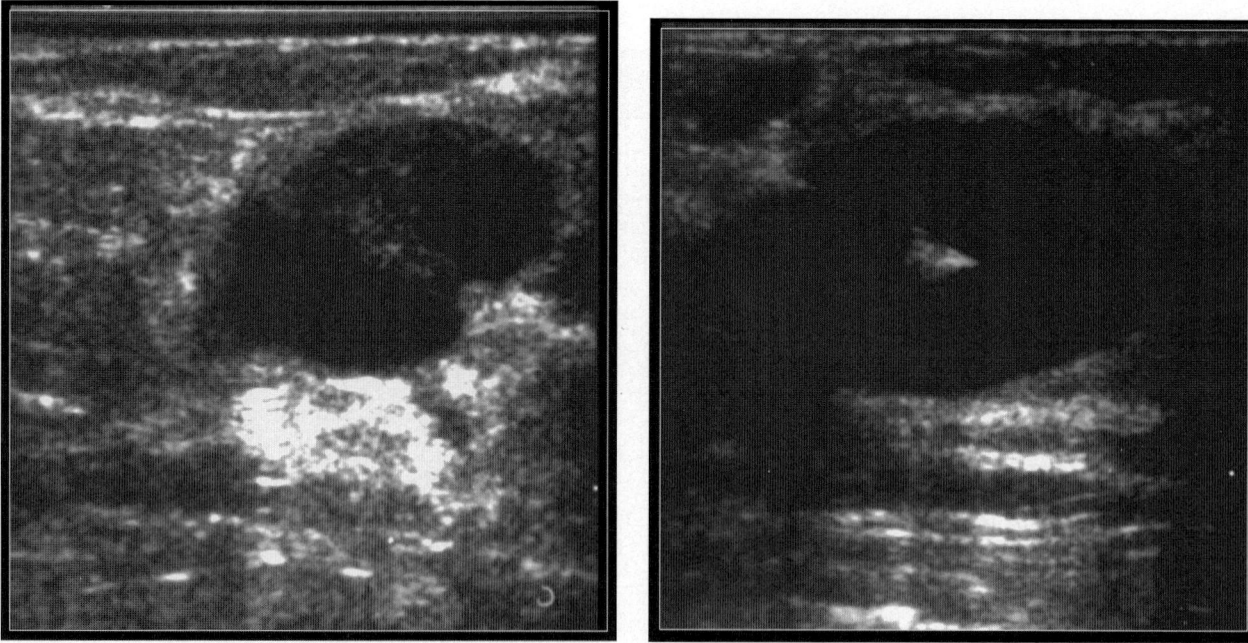

A   B

FIGURE 10–23 A: This complex cyst contains an isoechoic, thick septation, a suspicious finding that requires histologic assessment. Fluid cytology alone is unreliable in such cases. Because the septation is nearly isoechoic with surrounding tissues, it might be difficult to find and localize for surgical excision if the fluid cytology results were malignant or atypical. **B:** Aspiration of the cyst may be performed before biopsy of the thick septation in order to stabilize it for needle biopsy, but should be done under real-time guidance, so that the sonographic appearance of the residual thick septation without the surrounding fluid is known. Fluid cytology was falsely negative in this case.

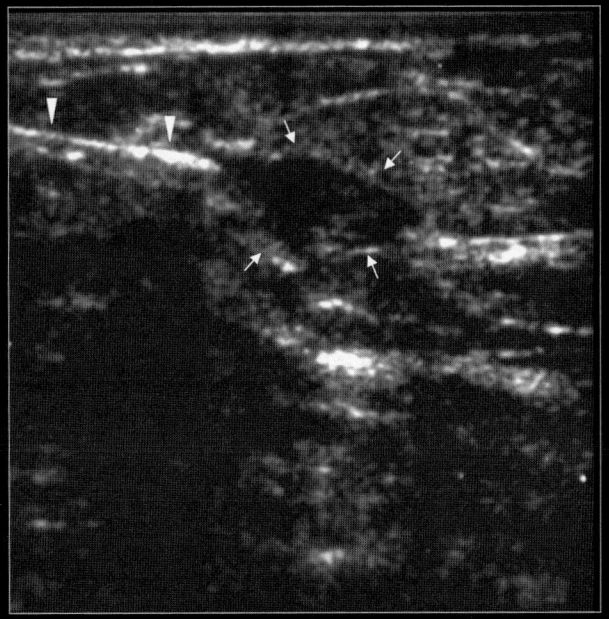 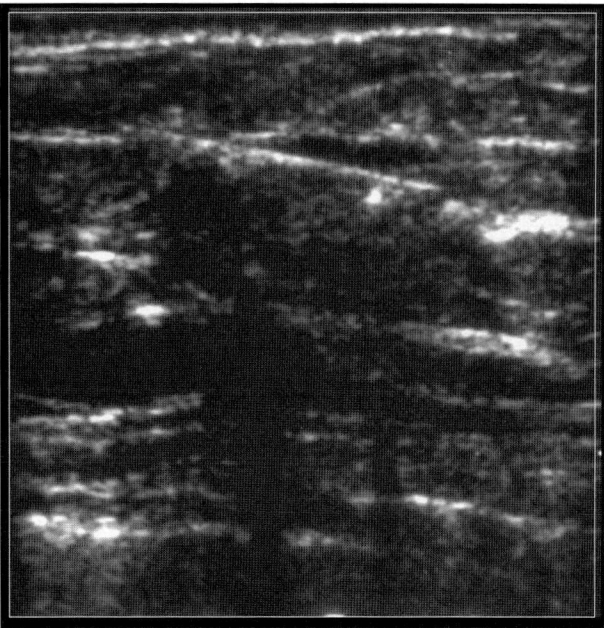

C

D

FIGURE 10–23 *(continued)* **C:** After real time US-guided aspiration of fluid, the residual thick septation is visible as a fusiform mildly hypoechoic structure *(arrows)* that is surrounded by iso-echoic fat. The large core needle *(arrowheads)* is in its prefire position immediately before core needle biopsy. **D:** The large core needle has passed through the lesion and is in its postfire position. The lesion was marked with medicinal charcoal to facilitate excisional biopsy should the results of histology be malignant or atypical. Today, ultrasound-guided vacuum-assisted biopsy would be performed rather than core biopsy, and the site would be marked with a mammotomy clip rather than charcoal. The biopsy revealed invasive ductal carcinoma, and the patient was treated with lumpectomy and radiation.

cious for intracystic malignancy. If even one suspicious finding is identified, the lesion is characterized as BIRADS 4a or higher and undergoes biopsy. We do not aspirate cysts with findings worrisome for malignancy, and we do not rely on cyst fluid cytology in such cases. Only if there are no suspicious findings for malignancy or infection does the algorithm progress to looking for benign findings that would allow the cyst to be characterized as benign, BI-RADS category 2.

The major sonographic findings in complex cysts that are worrisome for intracystic neoplasm are as follows:

• Thick, isoechoic septations
• Certain mural nodules
• Presence of a fibrovascular stalk
• Microcystic microlobulated appearance

As is the case for solid nodules or for mammographic interpretation, if even a single one of these suspicious findings is present, the lesion must be excluded from BIRADS 2 or 3 categories and must be classified a minimum of BI-RADS 4a and undergo biopsy.

Intracystic neoplasm includes both benign and malignant intracystic papillary lesions (ICPLs); benign papillomas constitute about 85% to 90% of such lesions, whereas intracystic papillary carcinomas constitute about another 6% to 7%. Benign papillomas in which atypical ductal

hyperplasia has developed within the surface epithelium account for another 6% to 7%. Other types of breast malignancies that have undergone cystic or hemorrhagic degeneration or that have secondarily involved adjacent simple cysts constitute less than 1%.

Complex cysts that have one or more findings that are suspicious for a true intraductal papillary lesion are classified as BIRADS 4a or higher and should not be aspirated and evaluated with cytology alone. Such lesions require histologic, not cytologic, evaluation. The risk for falsely negative cyst fluid cytology is far too high. In fact, aspiration alone is risky because removal of the fluid may make it difficult to find the residual thickened septation or mural nodule for surgical excision at a later time if the fluid cytology is malignant or atypical. If aspiration is performed, it should be done under continuous real-time guidance and monitoring, so that the appearance of the residual solid components is known, as a prelude to ultrasound-guided biopsy (Fig. 10–23). Our initial approach to worrisome complex cystic lesions was to aspirate, then perform ultrasound-guided large core needle biopsy, leaving medicinal charcoal to stain the area for later excision should the histology be malignant. However, with the advent of 11-gauge directional vacuum-assisted biopsy (DVAB), we now perform ultrasound-guided DVAB of such lesions and always deploy a marker clip to facilitate later identification and localization of the area for excision should the histology be malignant.

Findings Worrisome for Intracystic Malignancy

Thick, Isoechoic Internal Septations

Internal septations within complex cysts may be thick and isoechoic or thin and hyperechoic. Thick, isoechoic septations are worrisome for intracystic papilloma or carcinoma (Fig. 10–24, right). On the other hand, thin, echogenic septations merely represent the residual normal walls of the cystically intralobular dilated ductules (Fig. 10–24, left). It is far more reassuring and teleologically more correct to think of a complex cyst with thin, echogenic septations as a cluster of simple cysts rather than as a single complex cyst. Clusters of simple cysts, like individual simple cysts, can be characterized as BIRADS category 2, and aspiration, biopsy, and short-interval follow-up can all be obviated in most cases.

Certain Mural Nodules

Intracystic mural nodules are common, but intracystic papillomas and intracystic carcinomas cause only a small minority of them. Most mural nodules are caused by a benign proliferative disorder that is part of the fibrocystic spectrum: papillary apocrine metaplasia (PAM). Additionally, an echogenic lipid layer floating on cyst fluid can simulate an ICPL in certain situations. Isolated fat–fluid levels unaccompanied by other worrisome findings are definitively benign and can be classified as BIRADS 2. Fat–fluid levels are discussed in detail later in this chapter under BIRADS 2 findings.

Because intracystic mural nodules are so often merely manifestations of FCC with PAM, not indicators of intracystic papillomas or carcinomas, it is useful to try to characterize mural nodules sonographically. Biopsy of all mural nodules would have an unacceptably low biopsy rate for malignancy. Avoiding biopsies of mural nodules caused by FCC and PAM would be preferable. Fortunately, there are subtle differences between the appearances of mural nodules caused by intracystic papillomas and carcinomas and those caused by papillary apocrine metaplasia that aid us in distinguishing between them. (*Although PAM is a benign proliferative disorder that can indicate a slightly increased risk for later development of malignancy, the risk is generalized, and removal of the lesion does not alter this underlying risk. Thus, removal of all lesions containing PAM is not warranted.*)

The differences in the sonographic appearances between mural nodules caused by intracystic papillomas or

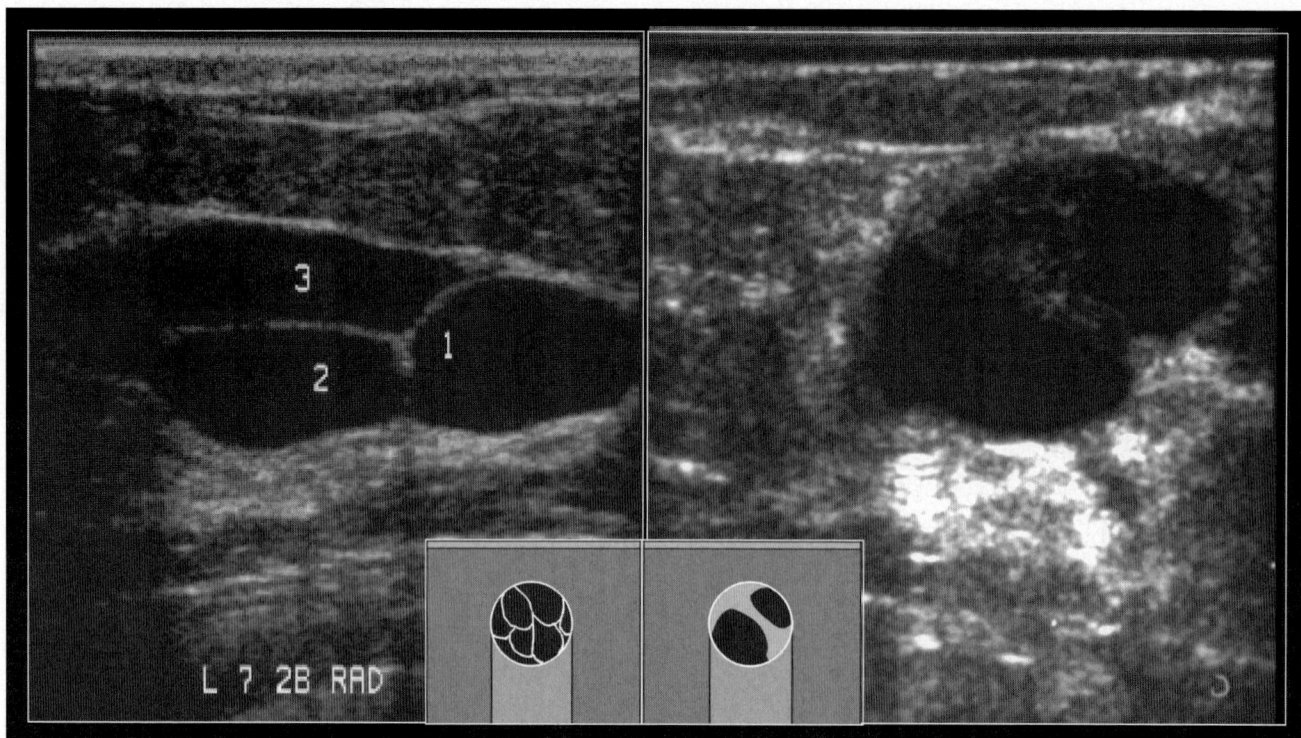

FIGURE 10–24 The thinly septated cyst shown on the **left** is a cluster of three simple cysts. At biopsy, the thick isoechoic septation (**right**) was shown to be an intracystic invasive ductal carcinoma.

growth of ICP
mural nodules

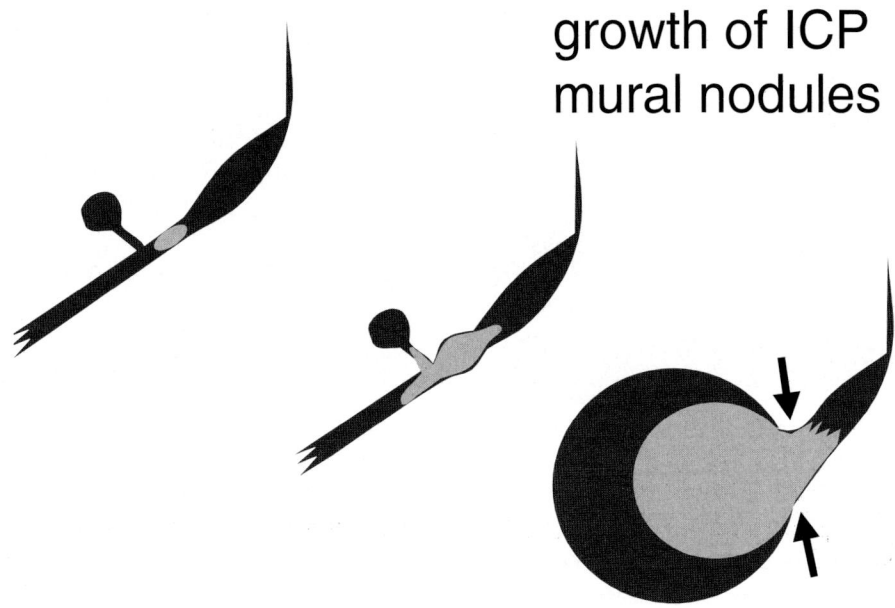

FIGURE 10–25 A key feature of mural nodules caused by papillomas and papillary carcinomas is the sonographic appearance at the point of attachment to the cyst wall. The appearance is affected by the order in which the nodule and cyst develop. The lesion begins as an intraductal papillary lesion that, by a combination of fluid secretion and obstruction of the duct, secondarily creates the cyst. Thus, there is absence of the thin, echogenic line at the point at which the mural nodule is attached to the wall and often a projection of the nodule into the duct that courses away from the cyst, usually toward the nipple.

carcinomas and those caused by FCC with PAM are influenced by the sequence in which the cyst and nodule arise, differences in blood supply, and to a much lesser extent, texture and internal surface characteristics. An intraductal papillary lesion usually precedes the development of the cyst that contains a true ICPL, such as intracystic papilloma or intracystic carcinoma. By a combination of secretion of fluids and obstruction of a duct, the underlying papillary lesion causes a cyst to form secondarily, usually distal to the underlying lesion (Figs. 10–25 and 10–26).

Intracystic papillomas and intracystic carcinomas, because they exist in the ducts before the formation of the cyst, often extend into the surrounding ducts that lead from the cyst to the nipple. On the other hand, in FCC with PAM, formation of a primary cyst with a single layer of apocrine cells usually precedes formation of the mural nodule caused by secondary focal papillary growth of metaplastic apocrine cells. The shape of the lesion and the sonographic appearance of the wall to which the mural nodule is attached are directly affected by whether the cyst or papillary

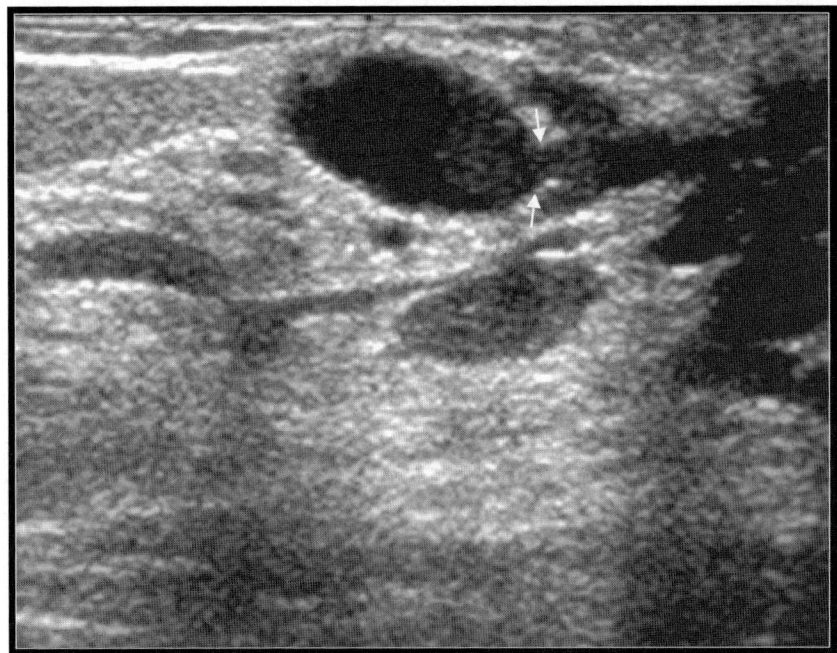

FIGURE 10–26 This small papilloma has formed within a branch duct and secondarily created a distal cyst that represents an obstructed terminal ductolobular unit (TDLU). Note that the papilloma protrudes beyond the point at which the wall of an oval cyst would be interpolated into the duct that courses toward the nipple, as illustrated in the bottom drawing in Fig. 10–25 *(arrows).*

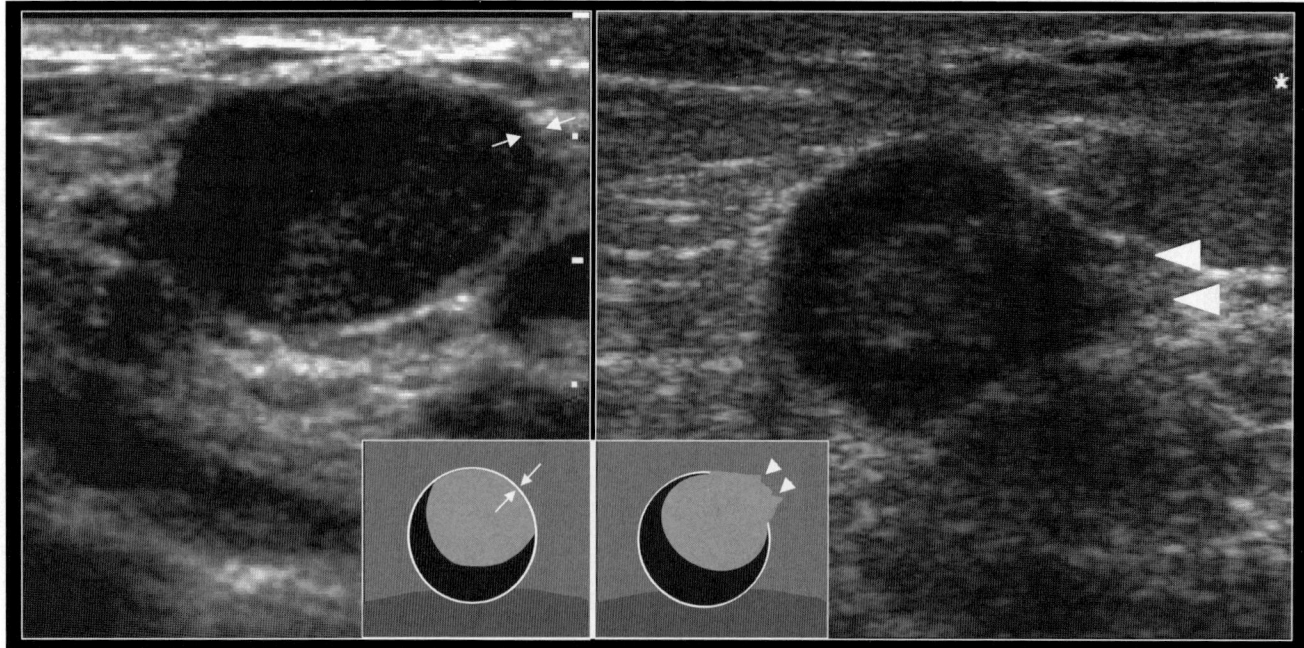

FIGURE 10–27 The mural nodule caused by papillary apocrine metaplasia shown in the **left** image has a smooth attachment to the cyst wall, and the thin, echogenic capsule all along the points of attachment to the cyst wall is preserved *(arrows)*. The intracystic papilloma shown in the **right** image, on the other hand, has an angular and irregular point of attachment to the cyst wall and lacks a thin, echogenic capsule *(arrowheads)*.

growth formed first. Scanning complex cysts in a radial plane and specifically searching for the relationship of nearby mammary ducts to the mural nodule can offer the best clues to the order in which the cyst and mural nodule were formed. This finding cannot be evaluated in the antiradial plane in most cases.

The growth of true intracystic papillomas and carcinomas into surrounding draining ducts results in two sonographic findings. First, the wall to which the mural nodule attaches may be angular or irregular and may not have a thin, echogenic capsule. This differs from the appearance of mural nodules caused by PAM, which

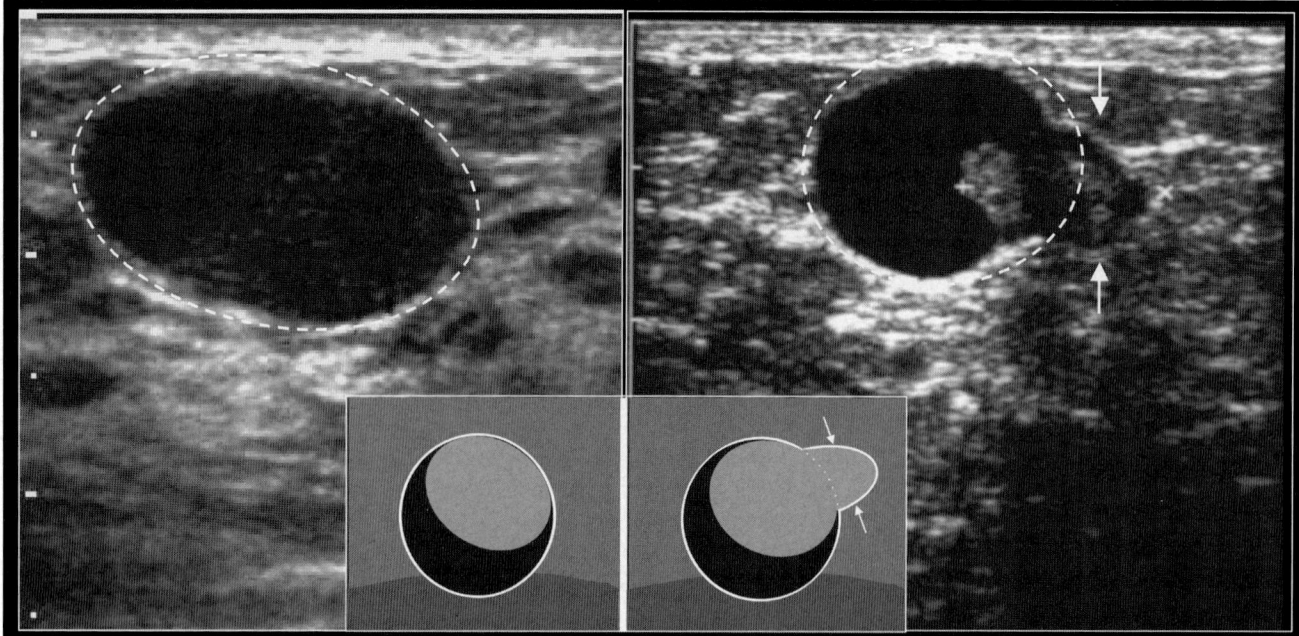

FIGURE 10–28 The mural nodule caused by papillary apocrine metaplasia shown in the **left** image remains confined within the oval shape of the cyst *(dotted line)* in which it developed. The intracystic papilloma shown in the **right** image, on the other hand, grows into a duct coursing away from the cyst toward the nipple *(arrows)*, causing the mural nodule to protrude beyond the oval shape of the cyst *(dotted line)* that it has secondarily created.

formed inside a preexisting cyst, where the attachment of the mural nodule is smooth and where the thin, echogenic outer cyst wall is intact (Fig. 10–27). Second, the papillomas or carcinomas that extend into the draining ducts beyond cyst may grossly distend the duct that changes the shape of a normally spherical or oval cyst to a keyhole shape. The projection of papillary growth from the cyst into a grossly distended duct yields a configuration we have termed *duct extension* that can also be seen in association with purely solid nodules and that is discussed in detail in Chapter 12. The duct extension seen with papillomas and carcinomas differs from the sonographic shape of cysts containing mural nodules caused by PAM. Even the most florid cases of PAM tend to occur in cysts that have a circular or oval shape. Mural nodules caused by PAM do not distend draining ducts enough to alter the shape of the cyst containing the mural nodule from its normal circular or oval shape (Fig. 10–28).

The absence of capsule and presence of duct extension are both considered hard imaging findings that strongly suggest that the cyst contains a true papilloma or carcinoma rather than PAM. Presence of one or both of these two hard findings excludes a lesion from BIRADS 2 or 3 categories, requires BIRADS 4a classification or higher, and requires that biopsy be performed.

Internal Echotexture

The underlying histologic differences between ICPLs and papillary apocrine metaplasia also cause differences in their internal echotexture. Intracystic papillomas and carcinomas are usually multifrondular. Each frond contains two layers of epithelium, two variable layers of myoepithelium, two basement membranes, a loose fibrous core, and a vascular stalk. Between each frond is a layer of fluid. All of these layers and the interfaces between fronds tend to make most intracystic papillary lesions appear echogenic and coarse in echotexture. PAM, on the other hand, tends to grow across the cyst lumen in thin, gracile bridges that are only one or two cells wide. The fluid spaces between the papillae are larger. This makes PAM appear less echogenic and less heterogeneous in echotexture than are intracystic papillomas and carcinomas. Additionally, intracystic papillomas and carcinomas more frequently have associated hemorrhage within them that contributes to their echogenic, coarse texture. Thus, the texture of intracystic papillomas and carcinomas can usually be described as echogenic and coarse, whereas the texture of PAM can usually be described as hypoechoic and lacy (Fig. 10–29).

Additionally, although both true ICPLs and PAM may be multifrondular, the tips of the fronds of PAM lack the multiple layers of papilloma fronds and are more difficult

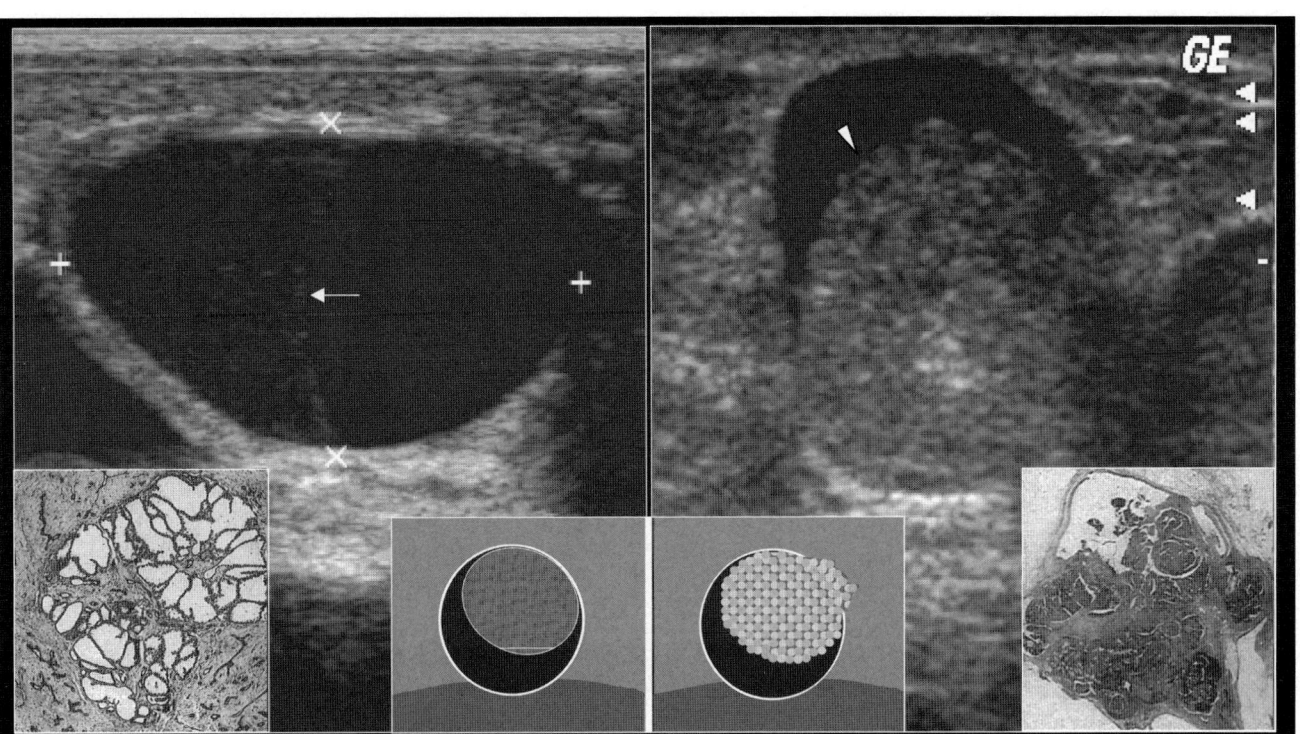

FIGURE 10–29 The mural nodule caused by papillary apocrine metaplasia shown in the **left** image has an echotexture that is hypoechoic, uniform, and lacy. Its inner margin is a thin, echogenic line *(arrow)*. The mural nodule caused by intracystic papilloma shown in the **right** image, on the other hand, has an echotexture that is coarse, heterogeneous, and echogenic. The surface of the papilloma is heavily microlobulated *(arrowhead)*. (Histopathologic images courtesy of Laszlo Tabar.)

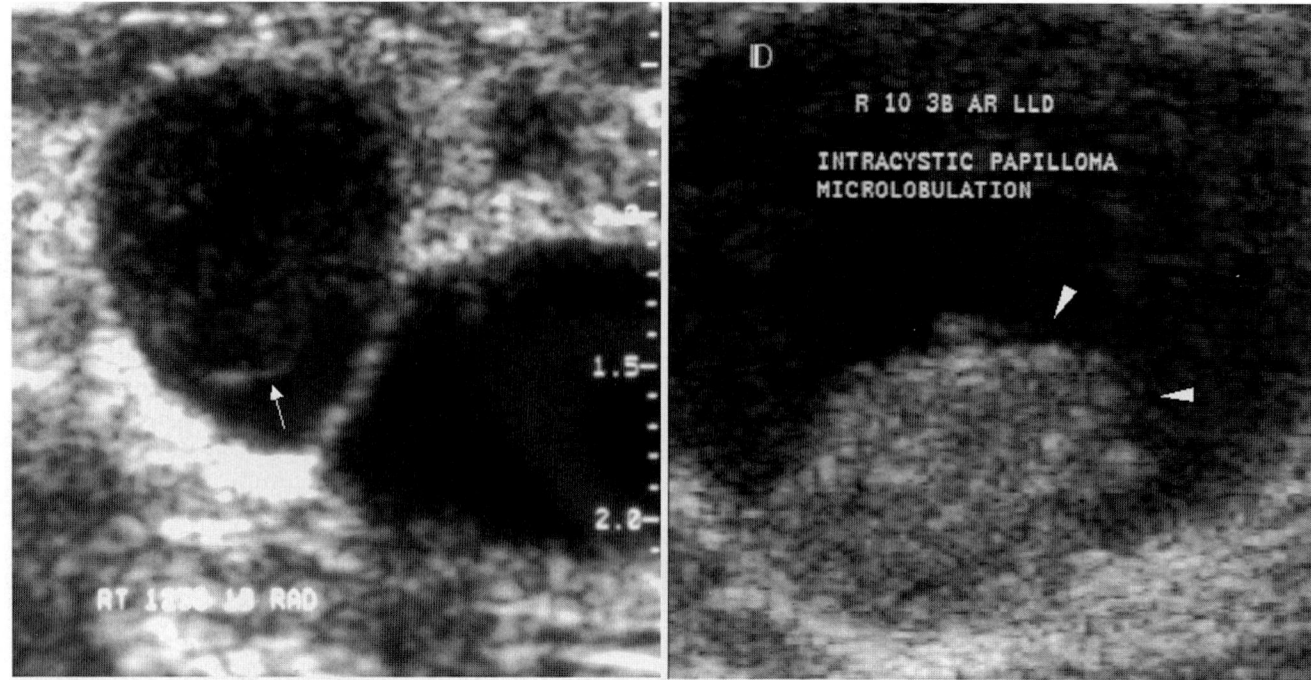

FIGURE 10–30 The mural nodule caused by papillary apocrine metaplasia shown in the **left** image has an echotexture that is hypoechoic, uniform, and lacy. Its inner margin is a thin, echogenic line *(arrow)*. The mural nodule caused by intracystic papilloma shown in the **right** image, on the other hand, has an echotexture that is coarse, heterogeneous, and echogenic. The surface of the papilloma is heavily microlobulated *(arrowheads)*.

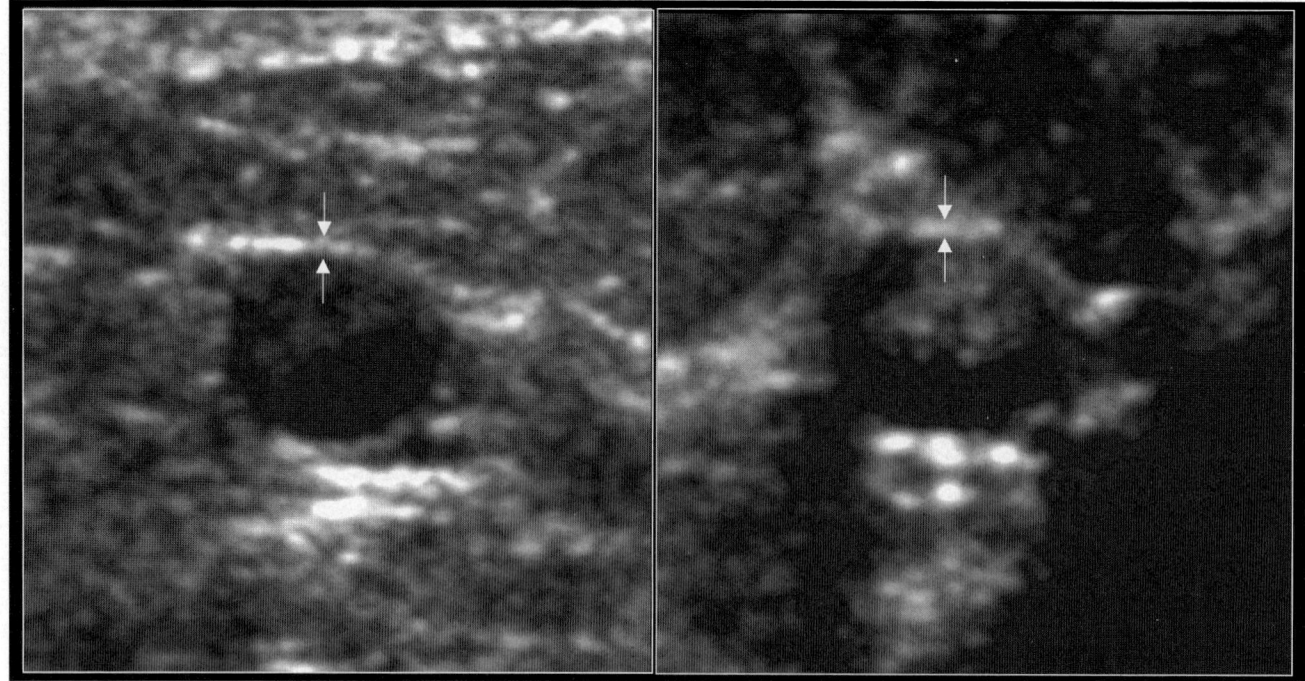

FIGURE 10–31 Although most eccentric cyst wall thickenings caused by papillary apocrine metaplasia (PAM) are concave inward and have an inner surface parallel to the outer wall **(left)**, a significant minority have a convex inner border in the configuration of a mural nodule **(right)**. Even though only a small fraction of PAM is convex inward, PAM so greatly outnumbers intracystic papillomas (ICPs) and carcinomas that most convex inward mural nodules are caused by PAM, not ICPs. Thus, the shape of the inner margin is not very useful. More useful is whether the thin outer capsule is intact all along the attachment of the eccentric thickening to the outer cyst wall. Cases of PAM have an intact thin, echogenic capsule *(arrows)* along their entire lengths of attachment.

to see. The coarser fronds of ICPLs can result in a heavily microlobulated appearance to the inner surface of the mural nodule, whereas the thin, gracile inner surface of the fronds in PAM is relatively inapparent, often leading the appearance of a smooth inner margin (Fig. 10–30).

The echotexture and inner surface characteristics of mural nodules caused by PAM and true ICPLs vary and overlap more than do the outer surface characteristics. A small percentage of cases of PAM may be echogenic and have a coarse echotexture. Conversely, the hemorrhagic infarction that occurs relatively frequently in papillomas and papillary carcinomas can make them appear more hypoechoic and lacy in texture than usual. Because of the greater variability and lower reliability of the echotexture and inner surface characteristics of mural nodules, these findings are considered too soft to be used alone and are used only in conjunction with hard findings discussed earlier.

Whether the inner surface of the mural nodule is convex or concave in shape is not very helpful in distinguishing a mural nodule caused by FCC with PAM from one caused by a papilloma or carcinoma. Most eccentric wall thickenings caused by papillomas have convex inner margins, whereas only a small percentage of mural nodules caused by PAM are inwardly convex (Fig. 10–31). Most eccentric wall thickenings caused by PAM have a concave inner margin that parallels the outer wall. However, because complex cysts containing PAM so greatly outnumber complex cysts containing papillomas or carcinomas, most complex cysts that present with convex mural nodules are caused by FCC with PAM, not papillomas or carcinoma. Furthermore, many apparent mural nodules represent mobile fat–fluid levels that change configuration when the patient position changes. Thus, whether the shape of the inner margin is concave or convex has been of little help, is the softest of all of the sonographic findings, and is no longer used as to differentiate FCC with PAM from papilloma or carcinoma. Fat–fluid levels that simulate mural nodules are discussed later in this chapter.

Mobility of an Apparent Mural Nodule

Tumefactive sludge, pus, or clot can simulate a mural nodule. The apparent nodule should be viewed with the patient in different positions to assess its mobility and to distinguish an attached mural nodule from dependent debris, pus, or clot. True papillary nodules are attached to the wall and do not move when the patient is changed from a supine position to either left lateral decubitus or upright positions (Fig. 10–32). Tumefactive sludge, on the other hand, will shift to the dependent portion of the cyst if enough time is allowed (Fig. 10–33). Intracystic clot can become adherent to the wall and fail to shift; hence, lack of a shift does not indicate with absolute certainty the presence of a papillary nodule. However, no papillary lesions will move with changes in patient position. Therefore, demonstration of movement is more valuable than demonstration of lack of motion.

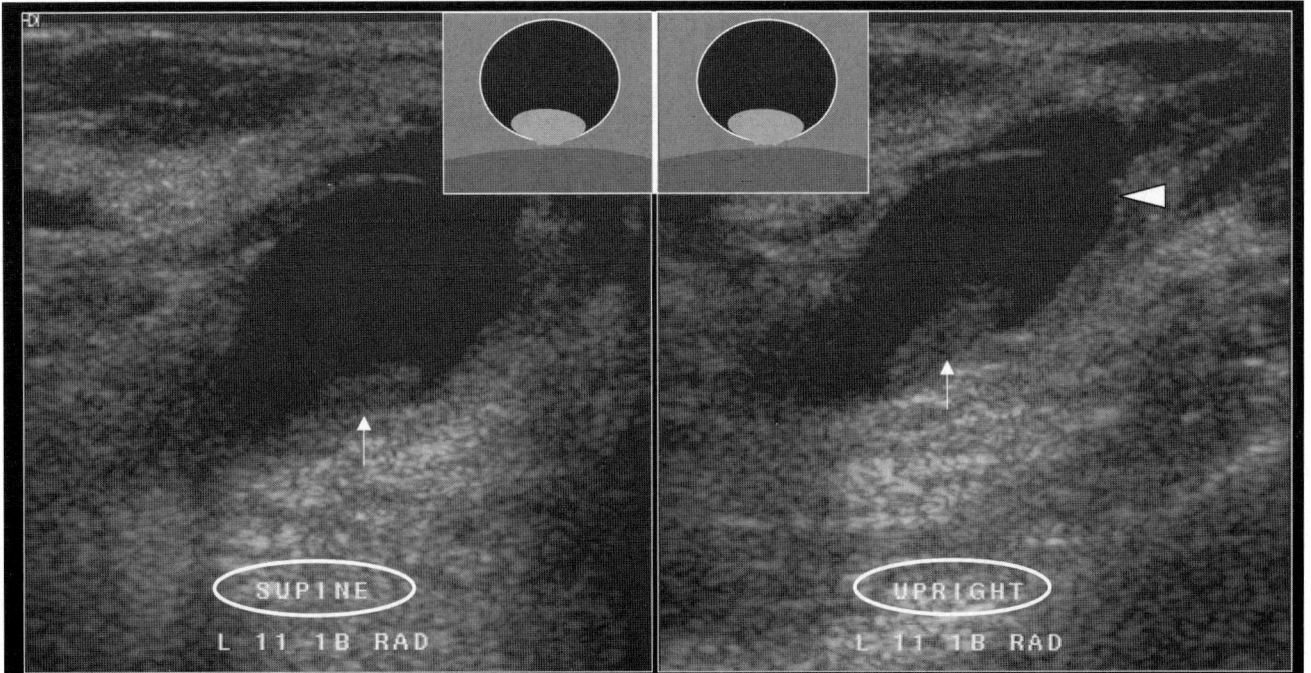

FIGURE 10–32 This mural nodule *(arrows),* caused by an intracystic papilloma, does not fall to the dependent portion of the cyst *(arrowhead)* in the upright position because it is firmly attached to the cyst wall.

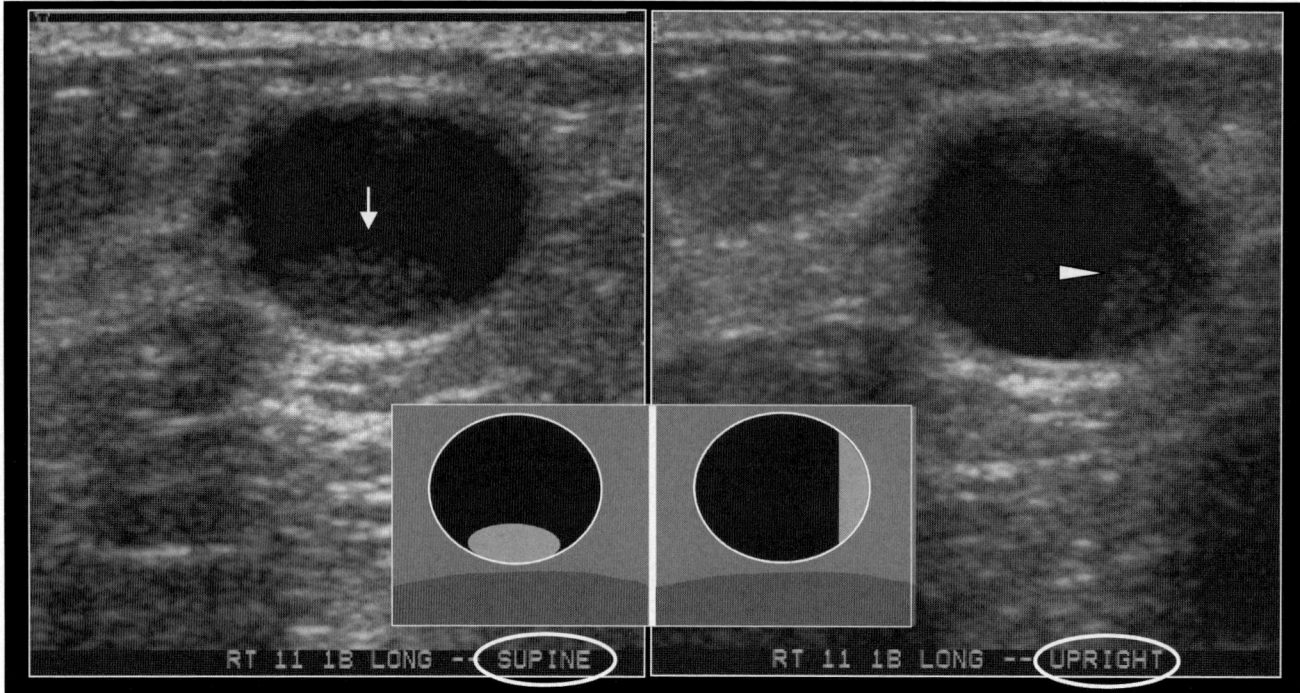

FIGURE 10–33 This inflamed cyst has tumefactive sludge or pus *(arrow)* that simulates a mural nodule when the patient is supine **(left)**. In the upright position **(right)**, the pus redistributes to the dependent inferior wall of the cyst *(arrowhead).*

Power Doppler Vocal Fremitus Transmission

The ability of an apparent mural nodule to transmit vocal vibrations can also help distinguish a mural nodule from nonattached echogenic debris within the cyst, regardless of whether the debris is largely lipid in content and floats or whether it is heavier than cyst fluid and sinks to the bottom of the cyst. The information obtained on transmission of vibrations will be similar to that obtained by assessing mobility. The only advantage of power Doppler is that it may save a few minutes because both fluid–debris levels and fat–fluid levels may take 5 or 10 minutes to show definitive evidence of relocation within the cyst after changing the patient's position. The use of power Doppler fremitus is discussed in detail and illustrated in the color panels in Chapter 20. True papillary nodules and septations will transmit vibrations from the surrounding tissues into the cyst regardless of whether the nodule is attached to the dependent or nondependent wall of the cyst (see Chapter 20, Figs. 20–93, 20–94 and 20–95). On the other hand, tumefactive sludge and floating lipid debris will not transmit vibrations into the cyst (see Chapter 20, Figs. 20–96 and 20–97). Although transmission of vibrations is reliable, we have seen a few papillary lesions that did not transmit fremitus. On a theoretical basis, adherent clot could transmit vibrations, but we have never observed it.

Fibrovascular Stalk

There are differences in the blood supply to mural nodules caused by papillomas and carcinomas and PAM. Papillomas and the atypical and malignant lesions that arise from them are among the most vascular lesions in the breast. The use of color and power Doppler in assessment of complex breast lesions is discussed and illustrated in the color plates of Chapter 20. Even small intraductal or intracystic papillary lesions only a few millimeters in diameter usually have blood flow within their fibrovascular stalks that is demonstrable by color or power Doppler (see Chapter 20, Fig. 20–29). On the other hand, PAM, no matter how florid, seldom develops a fibrovascular core that can be demonstrated by Doppler (see Chapter 20, Fig. 20–28). We have seen thousands of cases of PAM florid enough to cause mural nodules, but only two cases in which there was a Doppler-demonstrable fibrovascular core. Pulsed Doppler spectral analysis is useful in showing arterial waveforms when there is a question of whether a color signal within the mural nodule is real or artifactual (Fig. 10–34). Thus, like angular attachment margins and duct extension, the presence of demonstrable arterial flow within a mural nodule is considered a hard finding for an intracystic neoplasm and requires BIRADS 4a or higher classification and biopsy. In cases in which a true ICPL has undergone hemor-

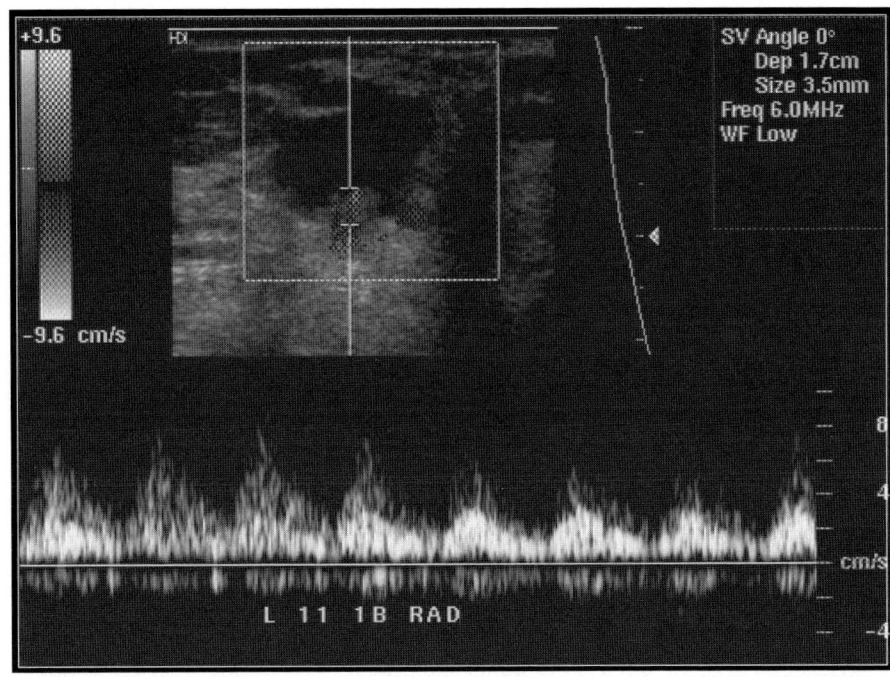

FIGURE 10–34 Pulsed Doppler spectral analysis that shows arterial waveforms can be helpful when there is question about whether the color signal within a mural nodule is real or an artifact.

rhagic infarction and the cyst is filled with blood, color Doppler can help to distinguish the papillary lesion from the blood and clot (see Chapter 20, Fig. 20–32).

It must be emphasized, however, how soft and sensitive to pressure the flow within the fibrovascular stalk of papillomas and papillary carcinomas is. Papillomas and papillary carcinomas not only are among the most vascular lesions in the breast but also are among the softest and most compressible lesions in the breast. The blood flow within the stalk is extremely sensitive to transducer pressure and can be completely eradicated with only slightly too much scan pressure. Thus, when interrogating a mural nodule for blood flow with color or power Doppler, it is imperative that a large amount of acoustic gel be used and that scan pressure be very light to avoid false-negative findings (see Chapter 20, Fig. 20–14).

The color or power Doppler appearance of the fibrovascular core of a mural nodule has been helpful in predicting whether the mural nodule is benign or malignant. Even large mural nodules caused by benign intracystic papillomas tend to be fed by a single vessel (see Chapter 20, Fig. 20–31, left). Malignant intracystic mural nodules, on the other hand, tend to generate multiple feeding vessels (see Chapter 20, Fig. 20–31, right). Thus, the presence of more than one vessel feeding an intracystic mural nodule predicts that it is malignant.

As is always the case with color or power Doppler, the value of a positive finding is greater than that of a negative finding. Thus, the presence of a fibrovascular core that is demonstrable with color or power Doppler is a better indicator of the presence of an intracystic papilloma or carcinoma than is absence of blood flow an indicator of FCC with PAM. Papillomas and carcinomas undergo hemorrhagic infarction often enough that a lack of demonstrable flow does not exclude their presence. Likewise, the presence of multiple feeding vessels is a stronger predictor of malignancy than is a single vessel a predictor of benignity.

Microcystic Complex Appearance, Microlobulated Outer Contour

Microlobulated outer contour has just recently added to the list of complex cystic worrisome findings. In the earlier discussion of how cysts form within TDLUs, it should be clear that many cases of early FCC could have a microlobulated appearance. When the cystically dilated ductules are large enough to resolve individually, there is no diagnostic dilemma. However, when the cystically dilated ductules are too small to resolve and are volume averaged with the fibrosclerotic echogenic component of FCC, the averaged echotexture may appear to be isoechoic, the same as for many solid nodules. Additionally, many clusters of cysts contain PAM, which creates enough internal echogenicity to make such lesions appear to be solid. Thus, in certain cases, TDLUs with microcysts are characterized as solid rather than cystic. Multiple enlarged ductules filled with high-nuclear-grade DCIS can appear nearly anechoic and microlobulated and can simulate the appearance of clusters of microcysts. We have seen high nuclear grade DCIS that simulated clustered microcysts triple in size in a matter of months (Fig. 10–35).

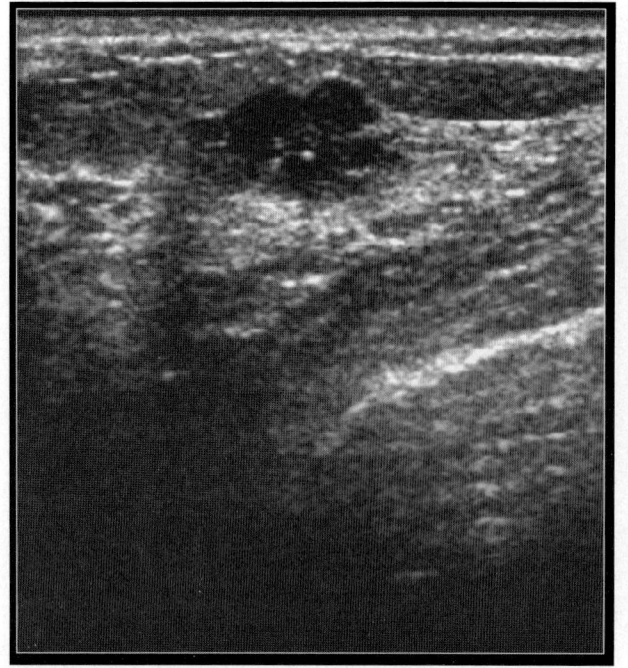

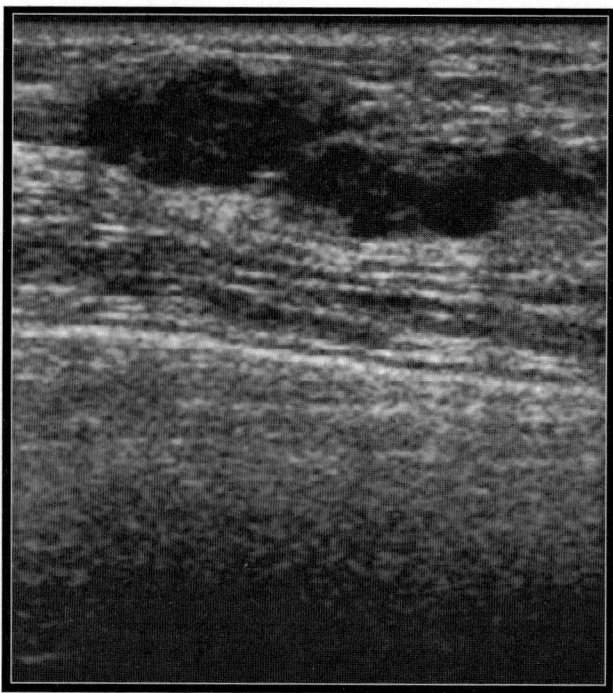

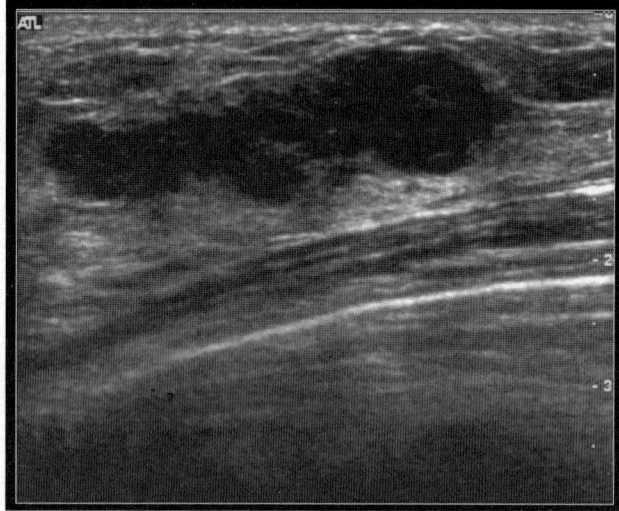

FIGURE 10–35 A: Microlobulated clusters of complex cysts should be viewed as worrisome. Most represent fibrocystic change, with volume averaging or apocrine metaplasia causing the echoes within the microcysts. However, ductal carcinoma *in situ* (DCIS), particular high-nuclear-grade DCIS, can have a similar appearance. This palpable microlobulated lesion was misinterpreted as a cluster of cysts and characterized as probably benign with a recommendation for 6-month follow-up. **B:** The palpable abnormality had enlarged in 5 weeks; hence, the patient returned for follow-up. The lesion had enlarged from a diameter of 14 mm on the first examination to a maximum diameter of 31 mm on the second examination. Biopsy the same day showed high-nuclear-grade DCIS. Each apparent microcyst is actually a duct distended with DCIS and necrotic debris. **C:** At the time of mastectomy 8 weeks after the initial examination and 3 weeks after the second examination, the lesion had enlarged to a maximum diameter of 50 mm. The microlobulated complex cyst, although usually a manifestation of fibrocystic change, can represent very aggressive high-nuclear-grade DCIS.

Table 10–4 summarizes the differences between low-risk mural nodules caused by PAM and high-risk mural nodules caused by true intracystic papillary neoplasia.

STEP 3: LOOK FOR BIRADS 3 FINDINGS OF INFLAMMATION OR INFECTION

The algorithm for evaluation of complex cysts differs from that of solid nodules in that it must take into account the possibility of infection as well as neoplasm. Although complex cysts that are worrisome for neoplasm should undergo biopsy and histologic evaluation, those that are worrisome for inflammation require only aspi-

ration, Gram stain, and culture. When the concern is infection rather than neoplasm, cytologic evaluation of cyst fluid adds little but expense. The clinical findings of pain, tenderness, erythema, and fever and the clinical laboratory findings of leukocytosis and elevated sedimentation rate are usually present in addition to the sonographic findings.

The sonographic findings that are worrisome for inflammation and infection are as follows:

- Uniform, isoechoic thickening of the cyst wall
- Hyperemia of the cyst wall
- Fluid–debris level

Frequently, all three findings coexist.

TABLE 10–4. FINDINGS THAT HELP DISTINGUISH PAPILLOMA OR CARCINOMA FROM FIBROCYSTIC CHANGE (FCC) WITH PAPILLARY APOCRINE METAPLASIA (PAM)

	High-Risk Findings: Intracystic Papillary Lesions	Low-Risk Findings: PAM
Hard finding	Angular attachment margins, no capsule	Thin, echogenic capsule preserved at attachment point
Hard finding	Duct extension into surrounding tissue	No duct extension, circular or oval shape maintained
Hard finding	Fibrovascular stalk	No fibrovascular stalk
Hard finding	Microlobulated outer surface	Smooth, gently curved outer surface
Soft finding	Echogenic	Hypoechoic
Soft finding	Coarse texture	Lacy texture
Soft finding	Microlobulated inner surface	Smooth inner surface
Soft finding	Convex inner margin	Concave inner margin

Circumferential, Uniform, Isoechoic Wall Thickening

The outer wall or capsule around simple cysts and most noninflamed complex cysts is thin (1 mm or less) and echogenic. In inflamed cysts, the normally thin, echogenic wall becomes edematous, thicker, and less echogenic (isoechoic with fat) (Fig. 10–36). The involvement tends to be circumferential and uniform, unlike the thickening in papilloma or carcinoma, which is eccentric. Additionally, the isoechoic circumferential thickening is concave inwardly,

and inner and outer surfaces of the thickened wall parallel each other. The uniform, circumferential wall thickening of inflamed cysts is usually seen in association with the second and third findings of inflammation, hyperemia, and fluid–debris levels. Occasionally the inflammation is more asymmetric. In other patients, the degree of wall thickening may be so severe that it virtually fills the cyst (Fig. 10–37).

There are causes of uniform wall thickening other than inflammation that must be taken into account when evaluating such cysts, including PAM and fibrosis. The sonographic appearance of PAM that involves a cyst

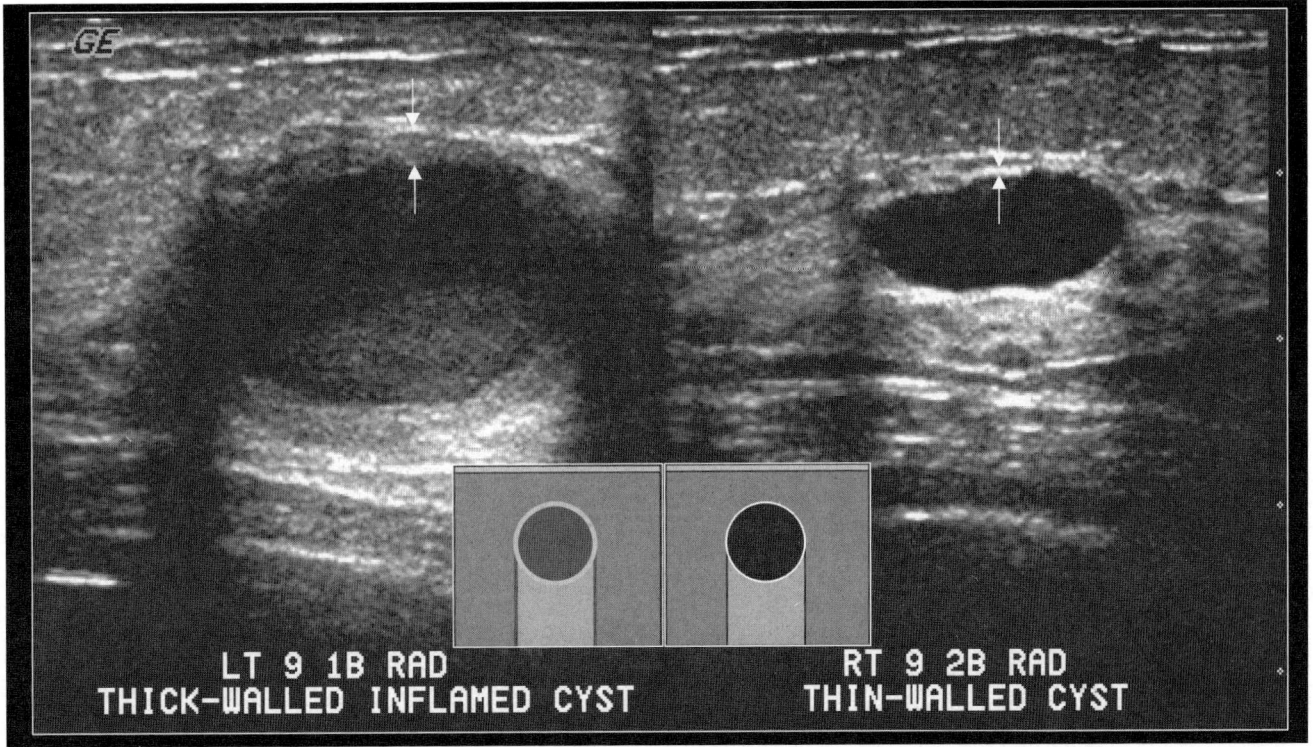

LT 9 1B RAD
THICK-WALLED INFLAMED CYST

RT 9 2B RAD
THIN-WALLED CYST

FIGURE 10–36 This figure illustrates two cysts in the same patient. The inflamed cyst in the left breast has a uniformly thickened and isoechoic wall (**left**). The noninflamed cyst in the right breast has the usual thin, echogenic wall (**right**).

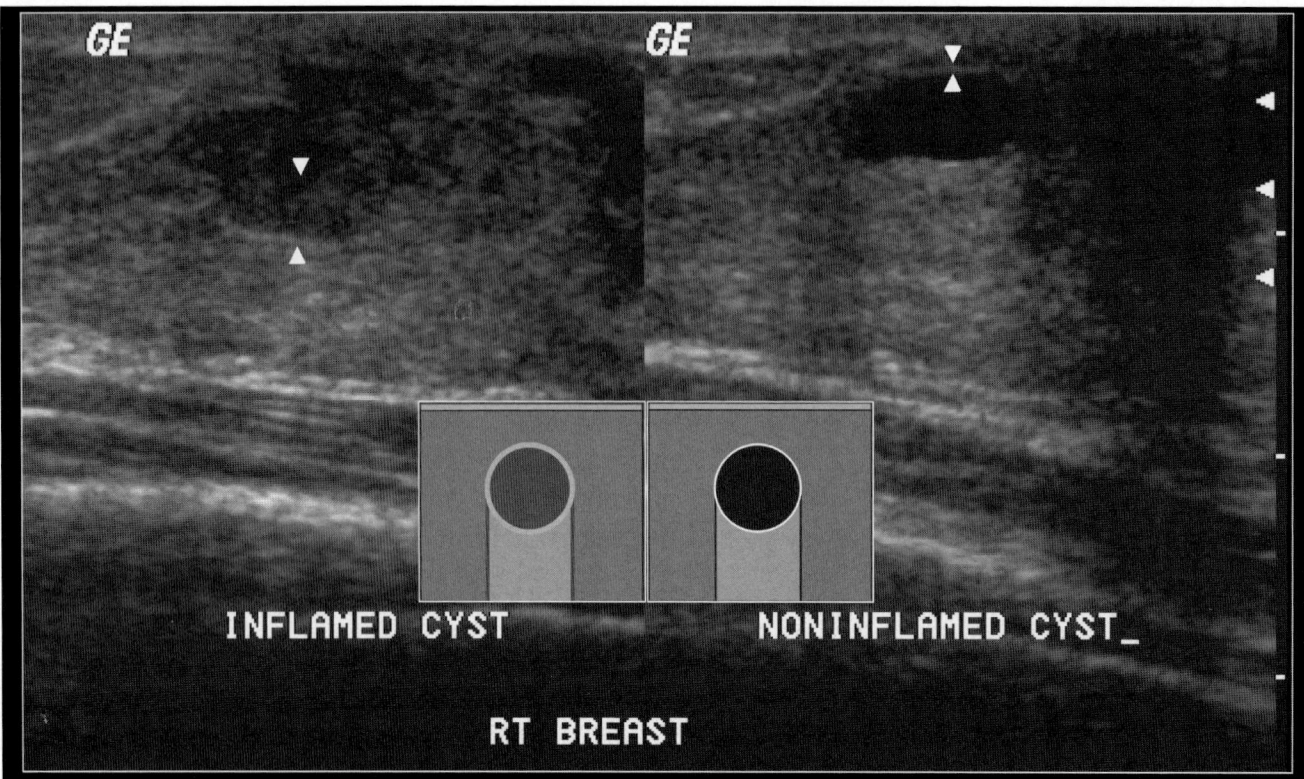

FIGURE 10–37 This figure shows two cysts in the same breast, one inflamed (**left**) and one non-inflamed (**right**). The inflamed cyst has a markedly thickened wall of uniform thickness. The non-inflamed cyst, on the other hand, has a normally thin and echogenic wall.

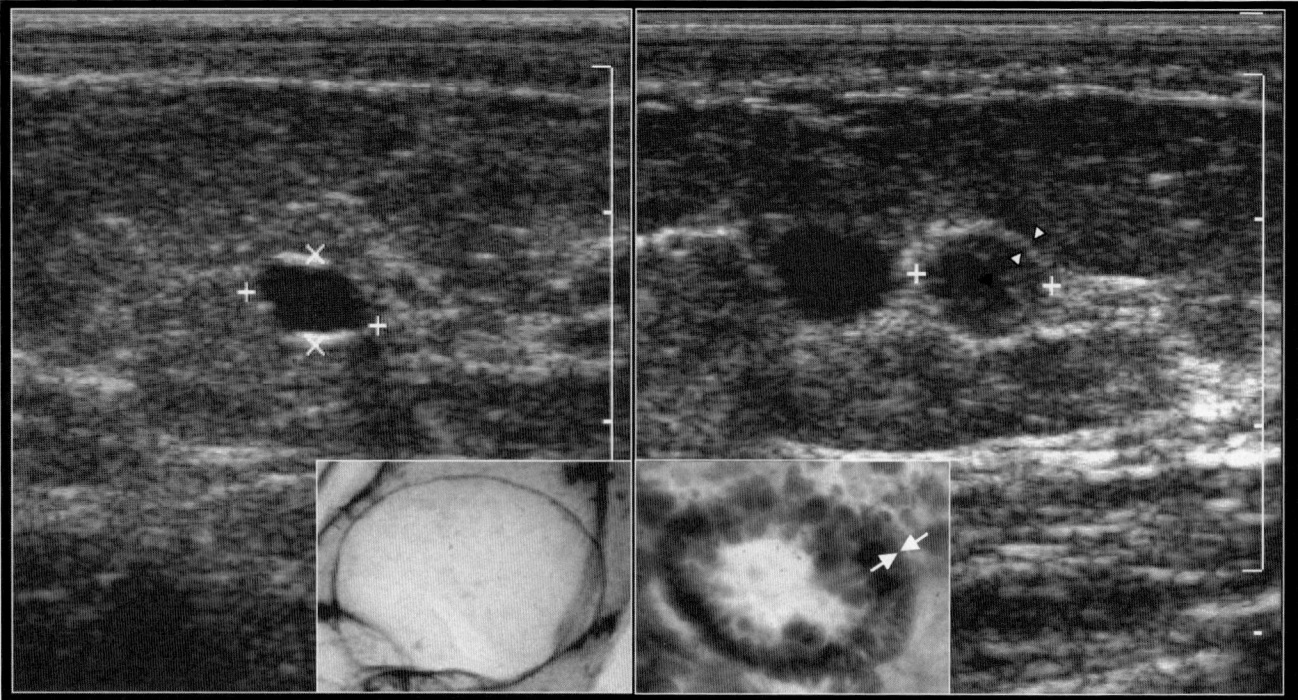

FIGURE 10–38 Papillary apocrine metaplasia can cause circumferential wall thickening as well as mural nodules. It differs from inflammation in that the outer echogenic capsule is preserved (*arrowheads*) and the inner border is irregular because of the multiple papillary projections of apocrine cells. (Subgross 3-D histology courtesy of Hanne M. Jensen, MD, University of California at Davis.)

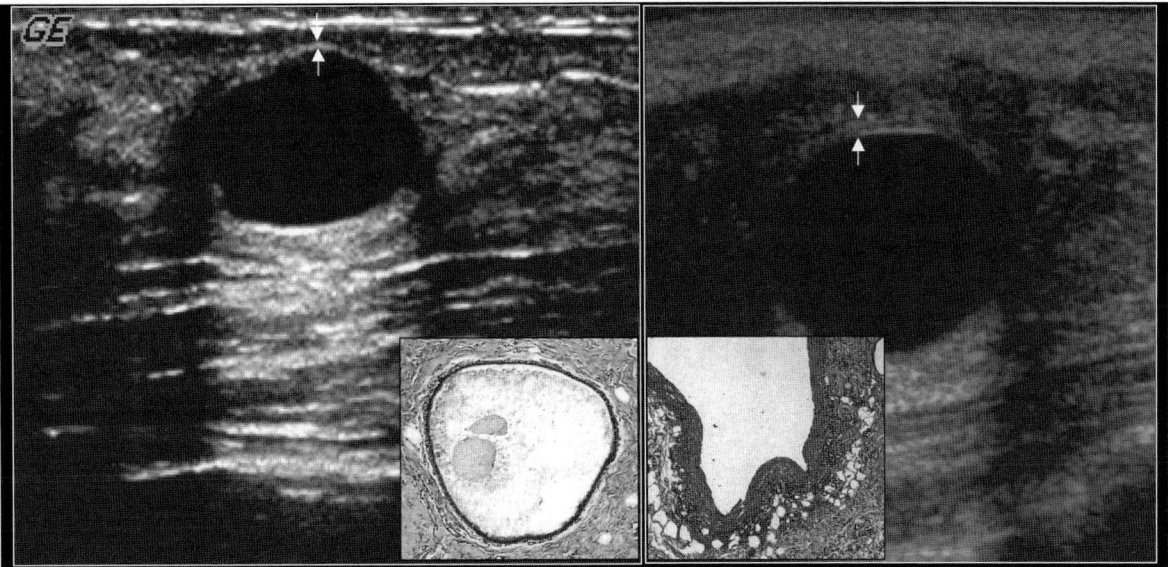

FIGURE 10–39 Uniform wall thickening can also be caused by fibrosis (**right**). The thickened wall in fibrosis is similar to that seen in acute inflammation because fibrosis is usually the end stage of inflammation. The thickened wall seen in fibrosis differs slightly from that in acute inflammation in that in fibrosis, the degree of wall thickening is usually slightly less, the echogenicity is slightly greater, and inflammatory hyperemia is absent. Although the echogenicity of the mildly thickened wall in fibrosis is slightly greater than that of fat and acute inflammation, it is less echogenic than the normal thin cyst wall (**right**).

circumferentially may have a sonographic appearance that is similar, but not identical, to that of an inflamed cyst. PAM usually causes slightly more eccentric and less uniform wall thickening; has a preserved thin, echogenic outer capsule; and in inner border, is usually microlobulated because of the papillary nature of the apocrine metaplasia (Fig. 10–38). That fibrosis may cause wall thickening similar to that of an inflamed cyst should not be surprising because fibrosis is thought to be a long-term sequela of epithelial rupture and inflammation of the cyst wall. Cyst wall fibrosis results in uniform wall thickening that differs from that of an acutely inflamed cyst wall in two ways: (a) it is mildly hyperechoic rather than isoechoic, and (b) it is not hyperemic (Fig. 10–39).

Hyperemia of the Cyst Wall

The normal thin, echogenic capsule around noninflamed breast cysts has so little blood flow that it is not demonstrable with color or power Doppler. The presence of blood flow within a cyst wall is abnormal, and the presence of blood flow within a uniformly thickened, isoechoic cyst wall strongly suggests acute inflammatory hyperemia (see the color images in Chapter 20, Fig. 20–40). The simple presence or absence of flow on color or power Doppler is all that is necessary to make the diagnosis of inflammation. Pulsed Doppler spectral analysis is not necessary unless there is a question of the color signal being artifactual. Demonstration of hyperemia within the thickened portion of the cyst wall is especially helpful in confirming the sus-

picion of inflammation in cases in which the inflammatory thickening of the wall is not uniform (Fig. 10–40). Doppler-demonstrable blood flow is almost never present in the other two entities that can cause uniform cyst wall thickening, fibrosis (see Chapter 20, Fig. 20–41), and PAM; thus, the presence of blood flow in a thickened cyst wall virtually excludes them. Interestingly, the direction in which the vessel courses differs in inflamed cysts from the direction of the fibrovascular stalk in ICPLs that cause eccentric wall thickening. The vessels in inflamed cysts lie parallel to the thickened wall of the cyst. The vessels within the fibrovascular stalk of intrapapillary lesions course perpendicular to the wall because they are feeding structures inside the wall rather than the wall itself (see Chapter 20, Fig. 20–42).

Fluid–Debris Levels

The presence of fluid–debris levels implies dependent particles that are large and heavy, that is, cellular in size: white or red blood cells. Cysts that have fluid–debris levels usually, but not always, also demonstrate uniform, isoechoic wall thickening. The coexistence of uniform wall thickening and fluid–debris levels strongly suggests that the debris is pus, especially if there are clinical findings of inflammation and demonstrable inflammatory hyperemia in the cyst wall. A fluid–debris level that contains surface tension may cause the sludge to assume a shape that simulates a mural nodule (i.e., tumefactive sludge, as discussed earlier). Changing the patient's position and watching for a shift of the sludge to the dependent wall of the cyst will prevent misinterpretation

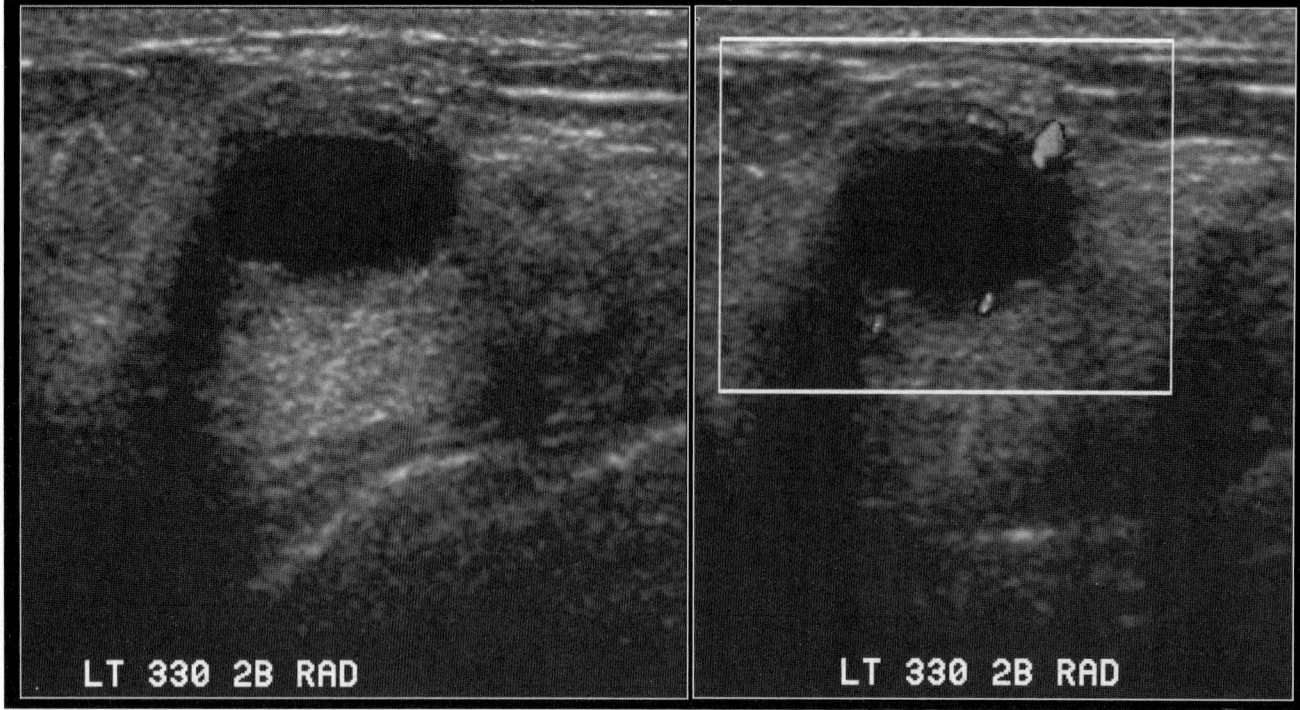

FIGURE 10–40 Occasionally, acute inflammatory changes in cyst walls are eccentric and not uniform (**left**). Demonstration of inflammatory hyperemia in the eccentrically thickened portion of the wall is helpful in confirming the suspicion of inflammation. The course of vessels in inflammatory hyperemia is parallel to the outer cyst wall, unlike those feeding intracystic papillary lesions, which course perpendicular to the cyst wall.

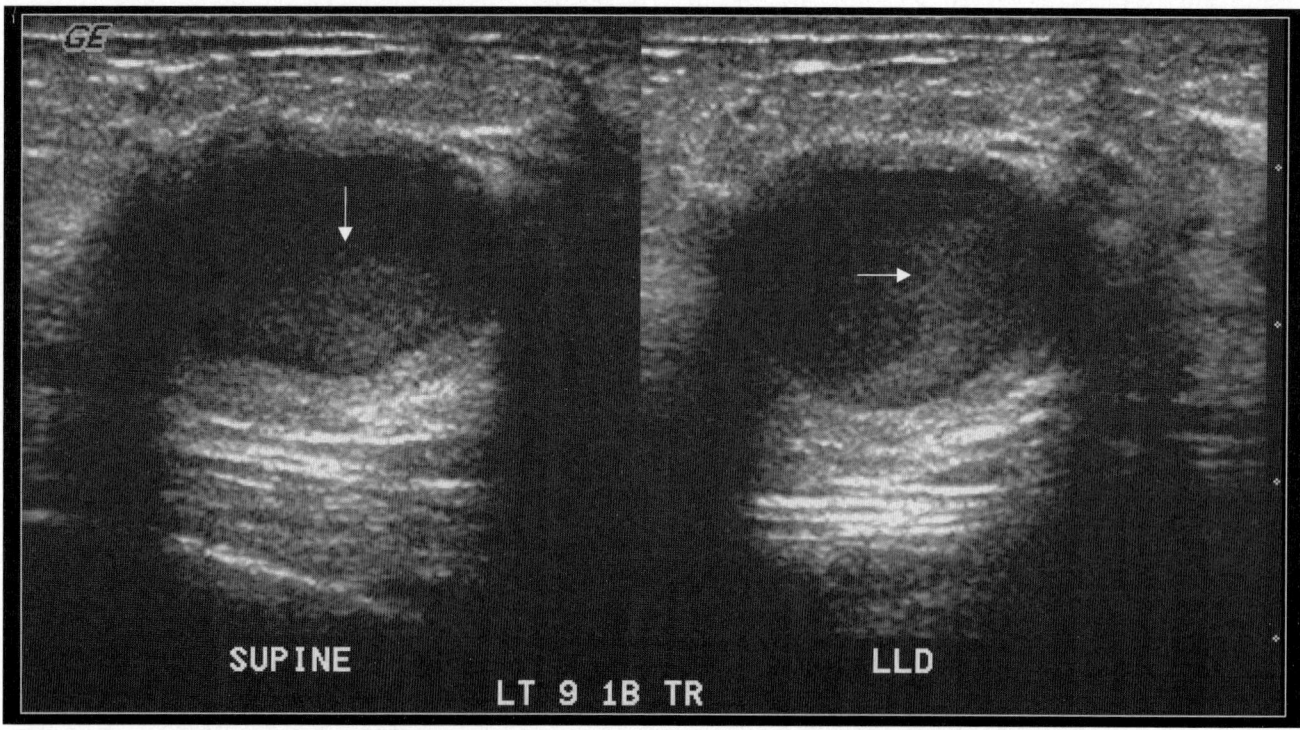

FIGURE 10–41 This acutely inflamed or infected cyst has a fluid–debris level as well as uniform isoechoic wall thickening. There was also hyperemia of the cyst wall on color Doppler. Acutely inflamed cysts usually, but not always, show all three findings. Note the shift in the fluid–debris level when the patient is changed from a supine to left lateral decubitus position *(arrows)*. Demonstrating the shift in position of the debris is necessary to help distinguish it from an intracystic mural nodule.

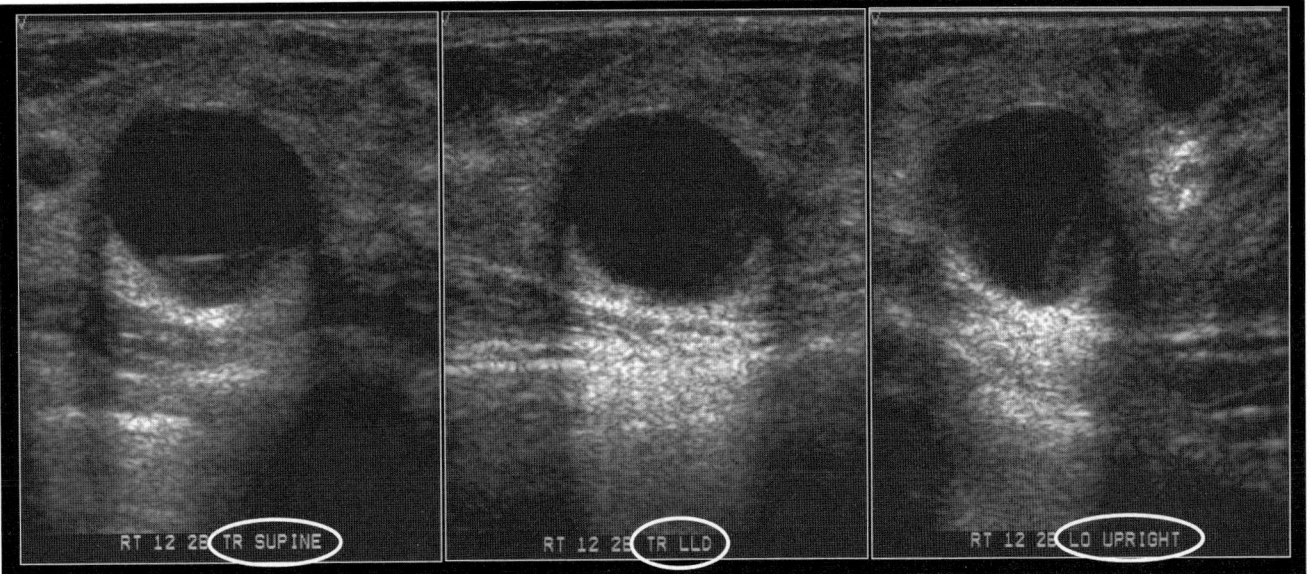

FIGURE 10–42 Either upright or left lateral decubitus (LLD) positioning can be used to show redistribution of debris to a newly dependent position within the cyst. When LLD positioning is used, the cyst is evaluated in the transverse plane. When upright positioning is used, the cyst is evaluated in the longitudinal plane.

of sludge as a mural nodule (Figs. 10–32, 10–33 and 10–41). Turning the patient from the supine to the left lateral decubitus position while viewing transversely, or scanning supine and upright while viewing longitudinally, is necessary to demonstrate the shift in position of the debris level (Fig. 10–42). This is analogous to demonstrating the shift of sludge within the gallbladder. The contents of an inflamed cyst with a fluid–debris level may be very viscous and therefore slow moving. It may take 5 or even 10 minutes to show a complete shift of a debris level to the dependent part of the cyst (Fig. 10–43). Waiting an insufficient time for the shift to the dependent wall of the cyst to occur can make a debris level falsely appear to not shift and may result in the transactive sludge being misdiagnosed as a mural nodule.

It is common to have bland inflammation in the spectrum of FCC. This is likely the result of chemical mastitis resulting from a breach in the epithelium of the cyst wall and leakage of irritating lipid-laden fluid into surrounding tissues. The presence of one or more of the three findings discussed earlier is a strong indicator of inflammation but not necessarily of infection. In fact, most cysts with these findings are affected with bland inflammation, but not infected. Unfortunately, however, in symptomatic patients, there is no way to distinguish a blandly inflamed cyst from an infected cyst with absolute certainty sonographically, clinically, or even after inspection of the aspirate. The clinical findings and sonographic appearances of bland inflammation and infection are identical. Both bland inflammation and infection can lead to pain, tenderness, erythema, and even fever. In most cases, after the fluid is

completely aspirated from the inflamed or infected cyst, the residual thick wall of the collapsed cyst will persist (Fig. 10–44). The aspirates obtained from both blandly inflamed cysts and infected cysts are identical: grossly purulent or bloody and purulent (Fig. 10–45). Only Gram stain and culture of the aspirate can distinguish between the two.

Not all complex cysts showing evidence of inflammation need to be aspirated. If the patient is asymptomatic and not in a high-risk group for infection, the presence of bland inflammation rather than infection can usually be assumed. On the other hand, if the patient is symptomatic, aspiration, Gram stain, and culture are always performed.

Because even after aspiration and visual inspection of the aspirate, there is uncertainty about whether the cyst is infected or merely inflamed, the approach we have chosen is to place the patient on a 3-day prescription of dicloxacillin (*Staphylococcus* species is the most likely organism) while we await Gram stain and the 72-hour culture results. If the Gram stain and 72-hour culture are negative, no further treatment or follow-up is necessary. The aspiration alone usually relieves symptoms in most cases. However, if the Gram stain and culture are positive, the antibiotic prescription is extended 7 days or changed to a different antibiotic based on the organism grown and its antibiotic sensitivity.

The terms *inflamed* or *infected cyst* and *breast abscess* should not be used interchangeably. Inflammation or infection of a cyst must be distinguished from a classic breast abscess in patients at high risk for abscess formation. Inflammation or infection of cysts represents a secondary process involving a preexisting noninflamed cyst and are thus well circumscribed, unilocular, and easily drained

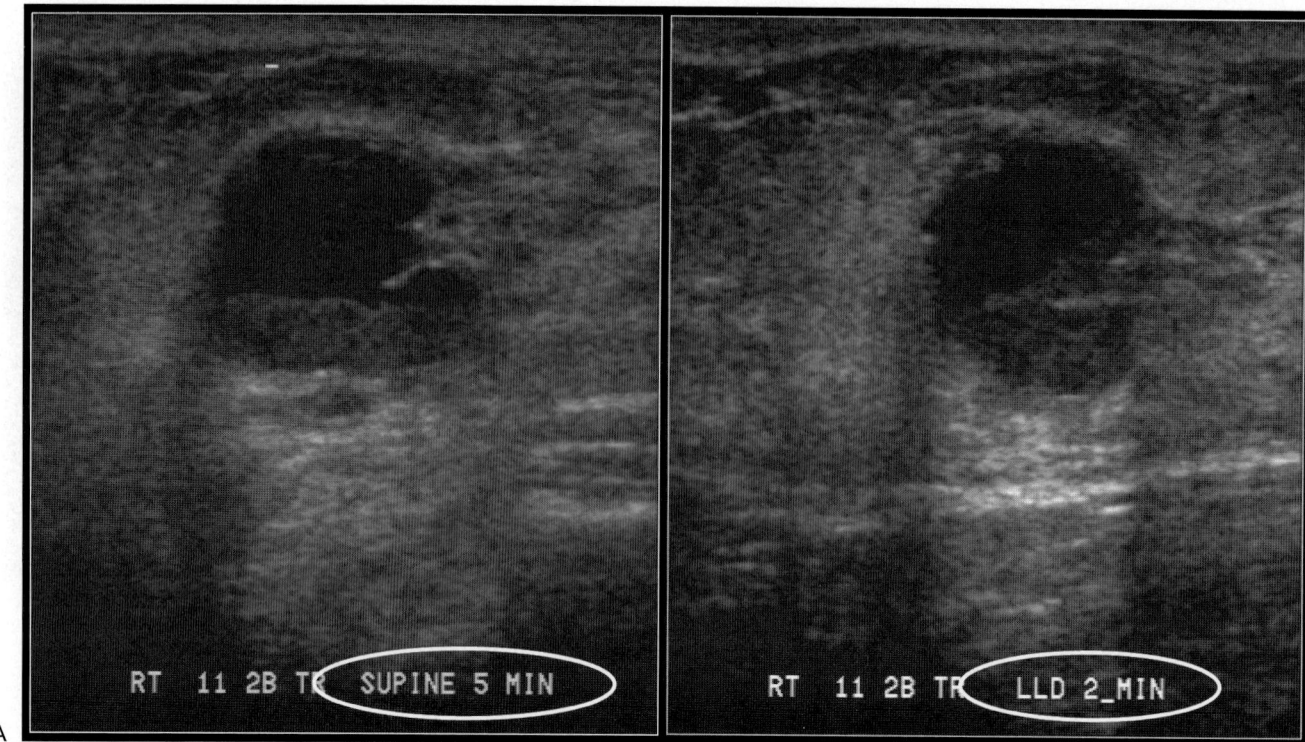

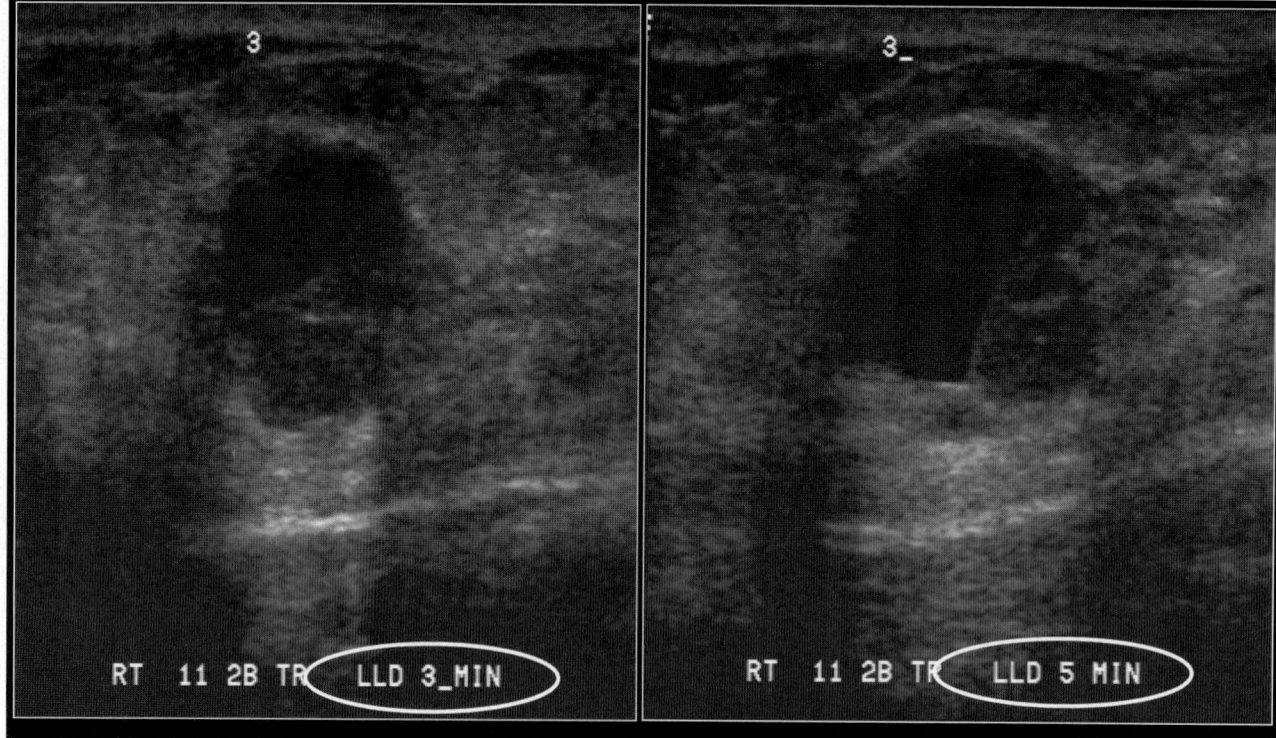

FIGURE 10–43 A: The fluid and debris within acutely inflamed cysts is often very viscous and moves very slowly. It is not possible to turn the patient into a left lateral decubitus position or place the patient in an upright position and see an immediate shift in the position of the debris. A period of 5 to 10 minutes is often necessary for the debris to equilibrate completely to the new dependent position within the cyst after a change in patient position. Waiting an insufficient time may lead to the false impression that the debris is attached to the wall and represents a mural nodule. In this case, the debris has only begun to shift at 2 minutes. **B:** At 3 minutes, the debris has still not moved completely to the dependent portion of the cyst. Not until 5 minutes has passed has it completely redistributed to the newly dependent left side of the cyst.

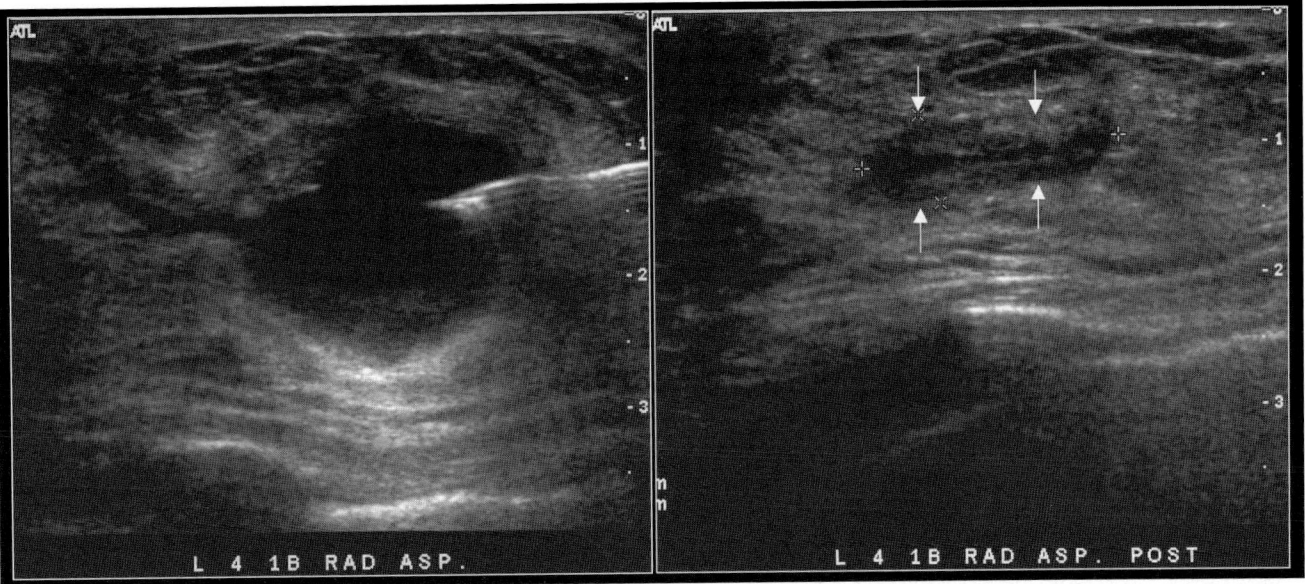

FIGURE 10–44 Although most acutely inflamed cysts can be completely aspirated of fluid and debris, the residually thickened wall remains after aspiration *(arrows)*. This is not a concern because the sonographic findings before aspiration clearly indicate inflammation or infection and not neoplasm. For this reason, the fluid from acutely inflamed cysts is evaluated with Gram stain and culture, but not cytology.

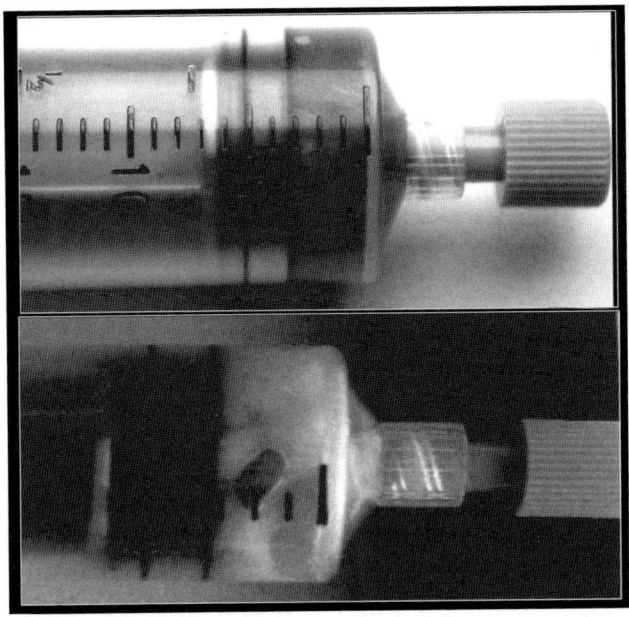

FIGURE 10–45 The fluid from acutely inflamed cysts is frankly purulent, regardless of whether the inflammation is caused by infection or is bland (**bottom**). Because of the high degree of hyperemia present, it is common to get bleeding into the purulent fluid (**top**).

percutaneously with a needle. On the other hand, a puerperal abscess that forms in a lactating patient represents an area of liquefactive necrosis of breast tissue caused by severe infection and does not involve a preexisting cyst. Puerperal and nonpuerperal periareolar abscesses are much less well defined than inflamed or infected cysts and more likely to be multilocular (Fig. 10–46). The contents of abscesses are much thicker, more viscous, and more heterogeneous—usually a mixture of liquefied and nonliquefied necrotic breast tissue. In a patient with postpartum mastitis or in a patient with typical periareolar inflammation and a history of nipple discharge of plucking or areolar hairs, a straightforward diagnosis of abscess, not inflamed cyst, should be made. The diagnosis and treatment of breast abscess may vary greatly from the diagnosis and treatment of an inflamed or infected cyst. For an inflamed cyst, aspiration is usually all that is necessary for both diagnosis and treatment. For breast abscess, aspiration alone is often inadequate, and placement of drain tubes or catheters is more likely to be necessary. In the worst abscess cases, surgical incision, drainage, lysis of adhesions, or even excision may be necessary. Puerperal and nonpuerperal abscesses are discussed in greater detail in Chapter 11.

Fluid–debris levels that are not associated with isoechoic thickening or hyperemia of the cyst wall are usually not of significance. Some patients with FCC can develop enough heavy cell debris to create a fluid–debris level. If the cyst is not tender and is completely surrounded by a

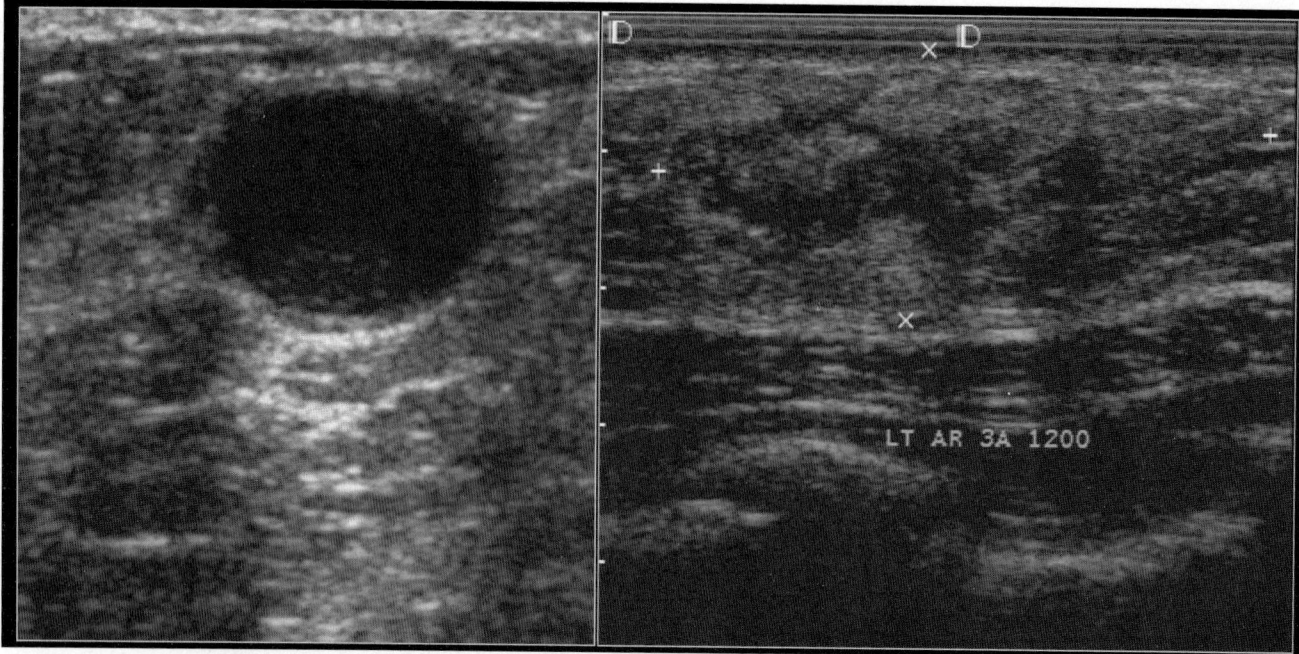

FIGURE 10–46 It is important to realize that both infected and noninfected acutely inflamed cysts have a markedly different appearance from abscesses that develop within patients with puerperal mastitis. In the former, the inflammation or infection involves a previously well-defined structure, a cyst (**left**). In the latter, severe infection leads to irregular liquefactive necrosis, which can be ill defined early. Only later will a defined cavity develop (**right**). Do not look for a structure that has the appearance of an acutely inflamed cyst in puerperal mastitis patients.

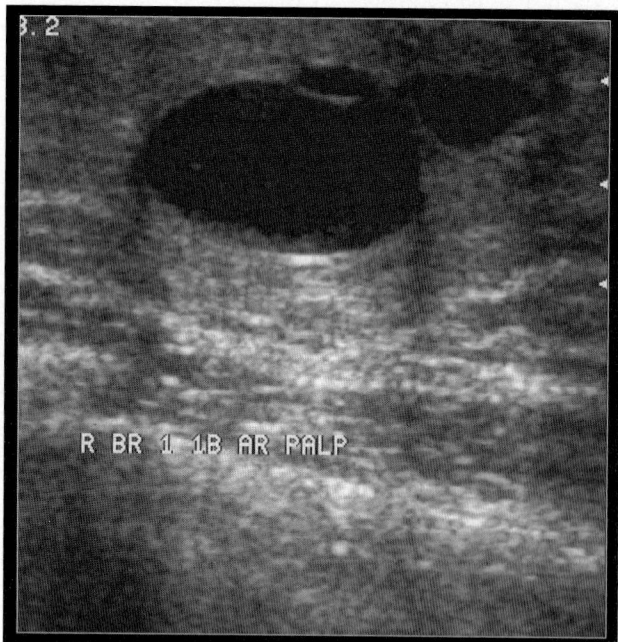

FIGURE 10–47 Occasionally, fluid–debris levels will be seen in asymptomatic cysts that are noninflamed. These have thin, echogenic and avascular walls and are not tender during scanning. Such cysts are usually of little concern and yield typical greenish black or greenish brown cyst fluid when aspirated. Cytology and culture are invariably negative. The debris represents the residual fragments of cells that inhabit the cyst in fibrocystic change, protein globules, and cholesterol crystals.

normal-appearing thin echogenic wall, it usually merely represents FCC (Fig. 10–47).

STEP 4: IF THERE ARE NO BIRADS 4A, 4B, OR 5 FINDINGS AND NO BIRADS 3 FINDINGS OF INFLAMMATION, LOOK FOR BIRADS 2 FINDINGS

Benign findings can be sought only after searches for BIRADS 4a, 4b, and 5 findings suspicious for true intraductal papillary lesions, and BIRADS 3 findings of inflammation failed to disclose any suspicious findings. In addition to simple cysts, many other types of complex cysts can be characterized as definitively benign, BIRADS 2. Several of these BIRADS 2 findings are simply mammographic findings that have been applied directly to ultrasound. BIRADS 2 types of complex cysts include the following:

- Clusters of simple cysts
- Thin, echogenic septations
- Milk of calcium[a]
- Circumferential calcification of cyst walls[a]—eggshell calcifications
- Punctate calcifications in cyst walls
- Lipid cysts[a]
- Fat—fluid levels[a]

- Mobile cholesterol crystals
- Cysts of skin origin

a Mammographic BIRADS 2 findings applied to ultrasound.

Clusters of Simple Cysts

Clusters of individual simple cysts that meet criteria for BI-RADS 2 are assigned to the same risk category as the individual simple cysts, i.e., BIRADS 2. Clustered cysts are virtually always peripheral in origin and arise at the level of the TDLU, and each of the cysts in the cluster represents a cystically dilated ductule. The cysts must be large enough that there is no volume averaging with surrounding intralobular stroma, and there should be no PAM within each cyst (Fig. 10–48). With higher-resolution transducers, smaller individual cysts can be characterized as clustered cysts. Regardless of the transducer resolution, some clustered cysts are either too small to rid of volume averaging or contain enough papillary epithelial growth that they must be considered clusters of complex microcysts (Fig. 10–49). As noted earlier, these clustered complex microcysts can be difficult to differentiate from DCIS distended ductules, should be excluded from the category of clustered simple cysts, and should be characterized as BIRADS 4a or higher.

Cysts Containing Thin, Echogenic Septations

Cysts containing thin, echogenic septations may be thought of as clusters of simple cysts, each representing BI-

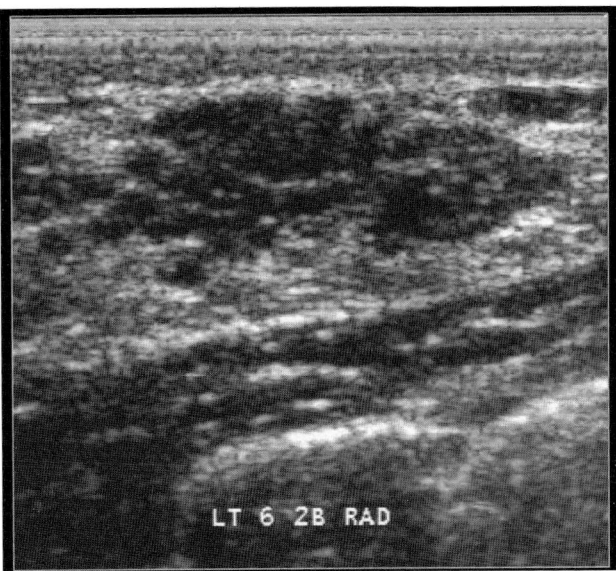

FIGURE 10–49 Even with the highest-resolution equipment, some microcysts are either too small to resolve completely without volume averaging or contain enough papillary apocrine metaplasia to cause difficulties in diagnosis. These should be viewed with suspicion, classified as microcysts, characterized as mildly suspicious (BIRADS 4a), and undergo biopsy. They can easily be confused with high-nuclear-grade ductal carcinoma *in situ* sonographically (Figs. 10–9 and 10–35). Biopsy of this lesion revealed only fibrocystic change.

RADS category 2 risks. Thinly septated cysts, like clustered cysts, virtually always arise at the level of the TDLU, and each of the cystic components represents a dilated intralobular tubule (Fig. 10–50). Thinly septated cysts differ from clustered cysts discussed earlier only in the size of the individual cysts.

Milk of Calcium

Milk of calcium is a definitively mammographic benign finding that can be directly applied to ultrasound (Fig. 10–51). The milk of calcium appears sonographically as tiny stones in the dependent portion of the cyst. Like gallstones, the tiny calculi within breast cysts can be made to shift to different parts of the cyst by changing the patient's position. In the supine position, they lie along the posterior wall of the cyst; in the left lateral decubitus position, they lie along the left wall of the cyst; and in the upright position, they lie along the inferior wall of the cyst (Fig. 10–52). Changes in position between the supine position and left lateral decubitus position need to be viewed in the transverse plane. Changes in the position between the supine and upright position need to be viewed in the longitudinal plane. The calcifications seen in milk of calcium do differ from gallstones in one important way: milk of calcium calculi are too small to shadow. To shadow, a calcification must be as wide as the ultrasound beam. The

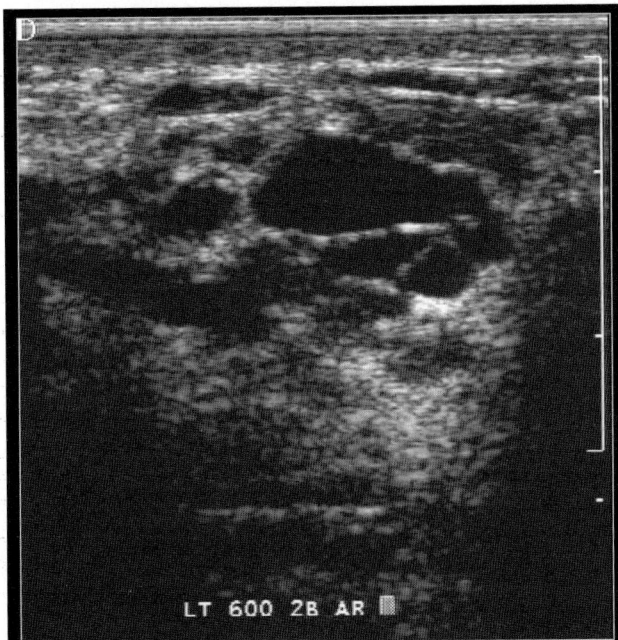

FIGURE 10–48 Clusters of simple cysts are benign (BIRADS 2) and have the same significance as thinly septated cysts and individual simple cysts.

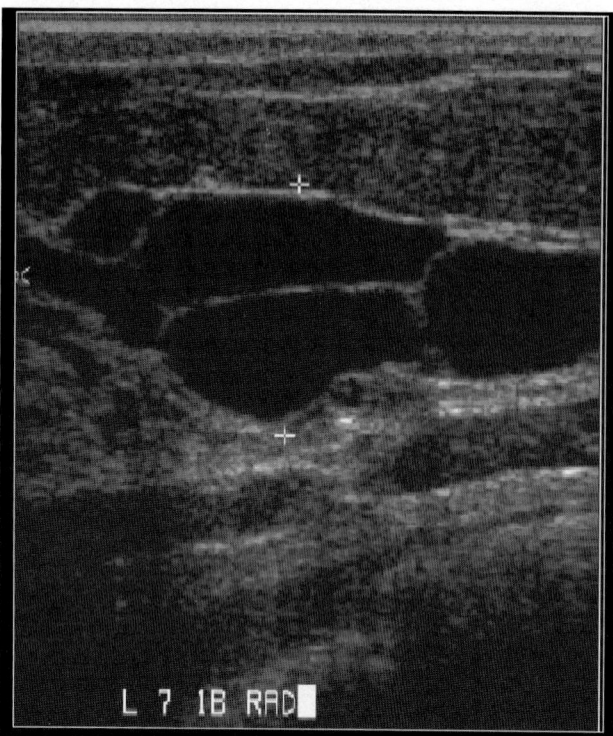

FIGURE 10–50 Thinly septated cysts are benign (BIRADS 2) and can be thought of as clusters of simple cysts with implications identical to that of a single simple cyst. Essentially, there is no distinction between thinly septated cysts and clusters of simple cysts.

individual calculi in milk of calcium are large enough to reflect sound and to appear as bright echoes, but generally are not large enough individually to result in acoustic shadowing. However, a layer of numerous tiny calculi may be large enough to occlude the ultrasound beam and cause acoustic shadowing, even though the individual calculi are too small to cause such shadowing (Fig. 10–53).

Although mammography is generally more sensitive for calcifications than sonography, sonography is actually more sensitive at demonstrating milk of calcium because it can show a single intracystic stone changing position, whereas mammography needs enough stones (dozens) to form a classic "tea cup" appearance on the horizontal beam film. Thus, sonography routinely demonstrates milk of calcium in cases in which mammography is unable to do so. Sonography is so sensitive for milk of calcium in comparison to mammography that it may have a role in evaluating clustered calcifications seen at mammography.

In certain cases of clustered nonspecific or probably benign calcifications seen on mammography, sonography may show definitive evidence of milk of calcium when only a single calcification is present within each of several small cysts (Fig. 10–54). In such cases, using sonography changes the mammographic BIRADS category from 4a or 3 to sonographic BIRADS 2, and either biopsy or follow-up can potentially be avoided. Such a change in management of clustered calcifications by sonography is only theoretical

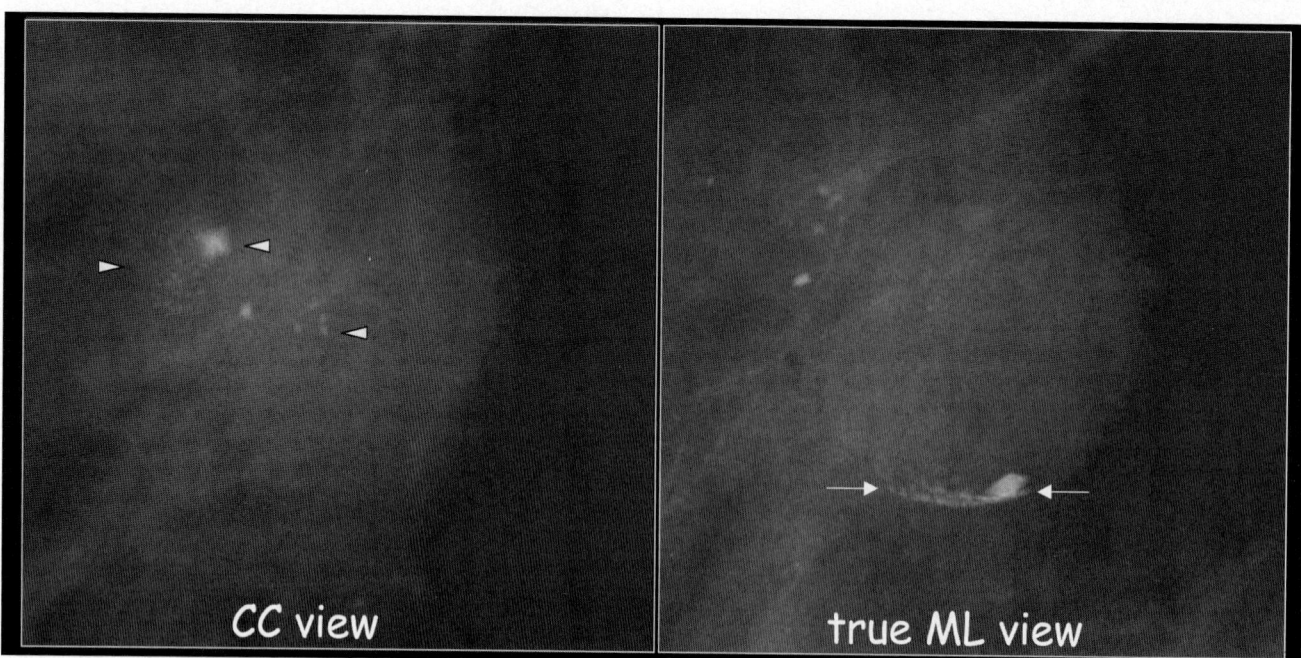

FIGURE 10–51 Milk of calcium is a previously described, definitively benign (BIRADS 2) mammographic finding that can be used in sonography. On the craniocaudal (CC) view, taken with a vertical beam, the calcifications are punctate or granular, variable in size, and nonspecific *(arrowheads)*. On the true mediolateral (MLO) view, however, taken with a horizontal beam, the calculi layer is in the dependent portion of the cyst. The appearance has been likened to milk in the bottom of a tea cup.

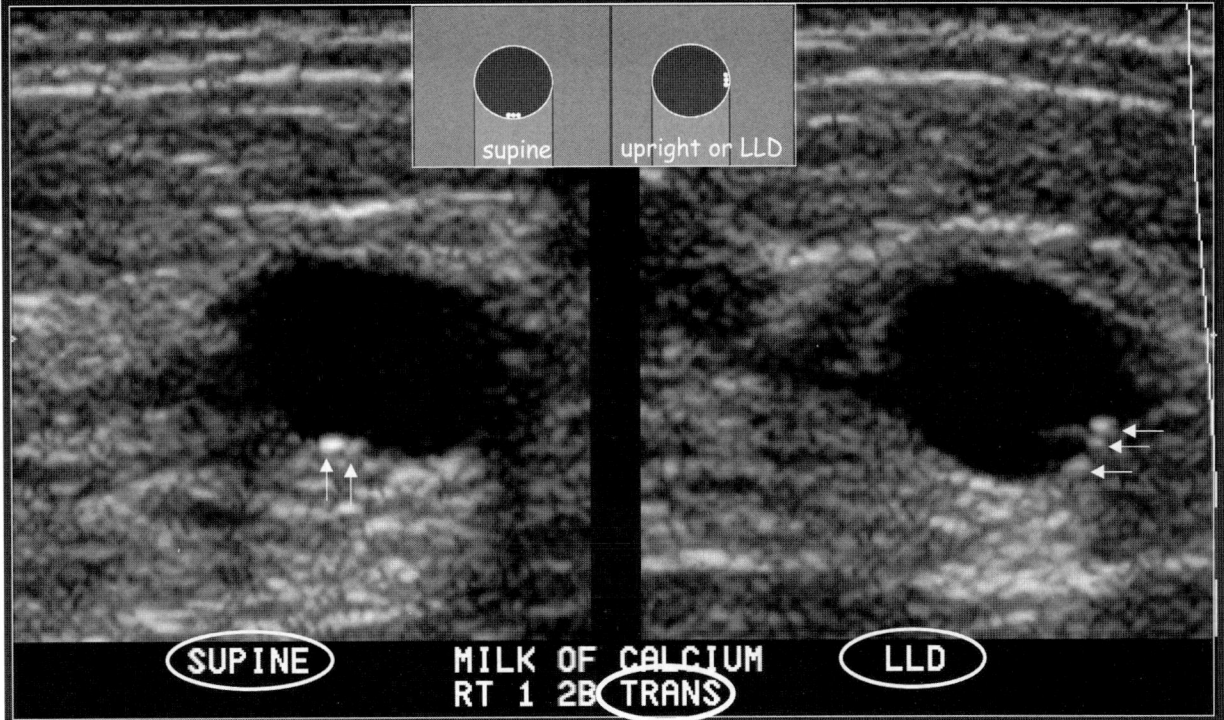

FIGURE 10–52 Milk of calcium is not milk at all, but tiny intracystic calculi of variable size and number. The individual calculi are too small to cause acoustic shadowing but are large enough to create a bright echo within the cyst. In the supine position, they lie along the posterior wall of the cyst. In the left lateral decubitus position, they move to the left lateral wall of the cyst. Although mammography is capable of showing smaller calcifications than can ultrasound, sonography can actually show milk of calcium when there are fewer calculi present. Sonography can show a single stone moving within a cyst, whereas mammography may require dozens of calculi within an individual cyst before a classic tea cup configuration is visible.

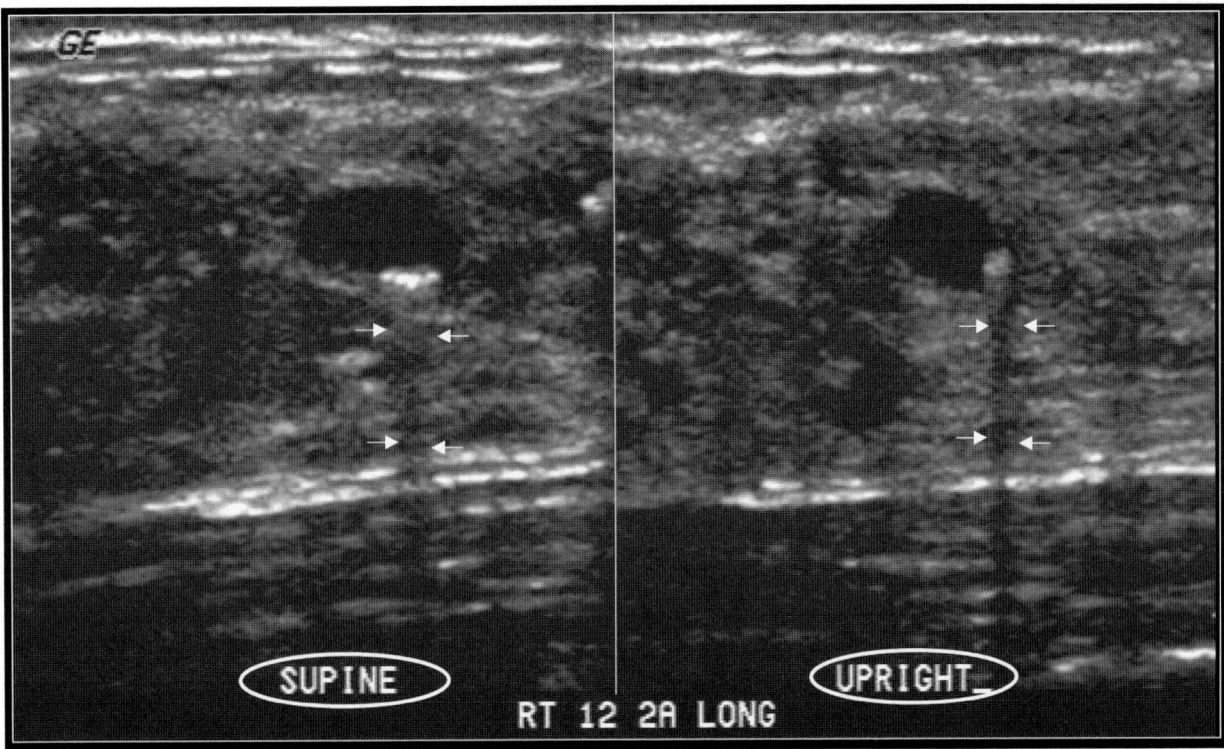

FIGURE 10–53 Although individual calculi in cysts with milk of calcium are too small to shadow, a clump of numerous calculi together may create acoustic shadowing *(arrows)*, as in this case.

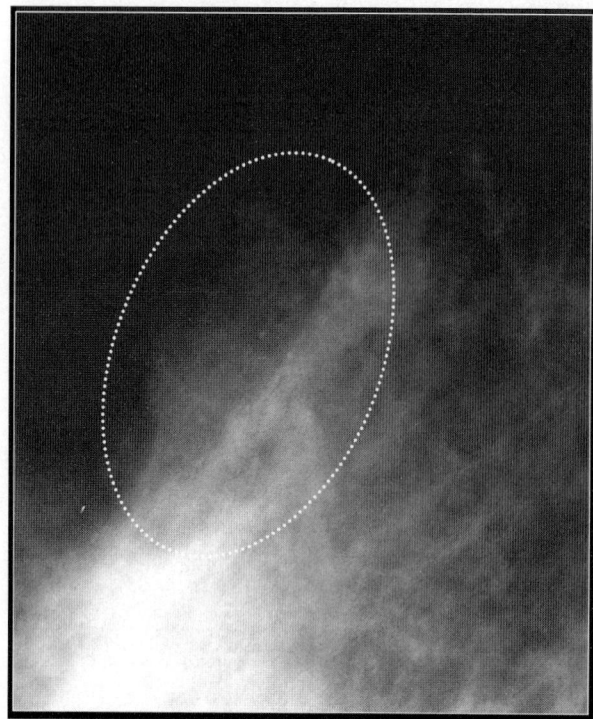

A

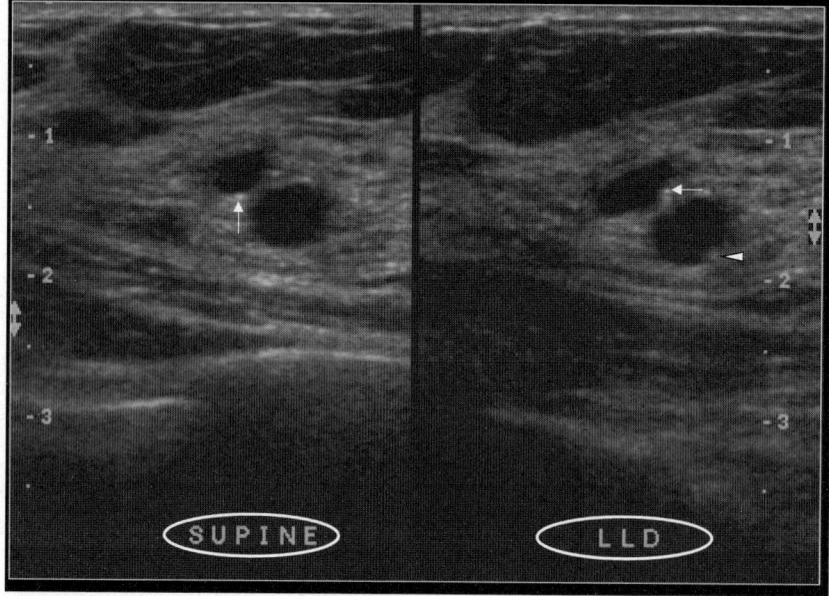

B

FIGURE 10–54 A: The true mediolateral view of the axillary segment of the right breast showed nonspecific punctate calcifications because none of the cysts that contained calculi had enough calculi to form recognizable tea cup configurations. **B:** Sonography of the axillary segment showed several cysts that each contained one or two calculi *(arrows and arrowhead).* This case illustrates the ability of ultrasound to document definitive evidence of milk of calcium when mammography cannot. It suggests that high-quality sonography in experienced hands could have a role in assessment of nonspecific punctate calcifications. The role of sonography in management of mammographic calcifications, however, remains theoretical because there are no published studies documenting the ability of sonography to minimize benign biopsies in patients with clustered calcifications to date.

at this point because there is to date no definitive published evidence of the efficacy of sonography for such purposes. However, our preliminary findings are that sonographic accurately shows strong evidence of benign FCC in at least some patients with mammographically nonspecific or worrisome calcifications.

Punctate Calcifications in the Thin, Echogenic Cyst Wall

Punctate calcifications that lie entirely within the thin, echogenic cyst capsule are benign and, in essence, represent incomplete circumferential or "eggshell" calcifications. Like milk of calcium, the punctate calcifications within the wall of cysts may be too small to cause acoustic shadowing but large enough to cause a bright echo within the wall of a cyst (Fig. 10–55). When the punctate calcification lies within the dependent wall of the cyst, it may be indistinguishable from milk of calcium calculus without turning the patient to see if the calcification is mobile. Coded harmonics and real-time compounding improve sonographic demonstration of punctate calcifications within cyst walls by suppressing speckle artifact (Figs. 10–56 and 10–57).

(text continued on page 315)

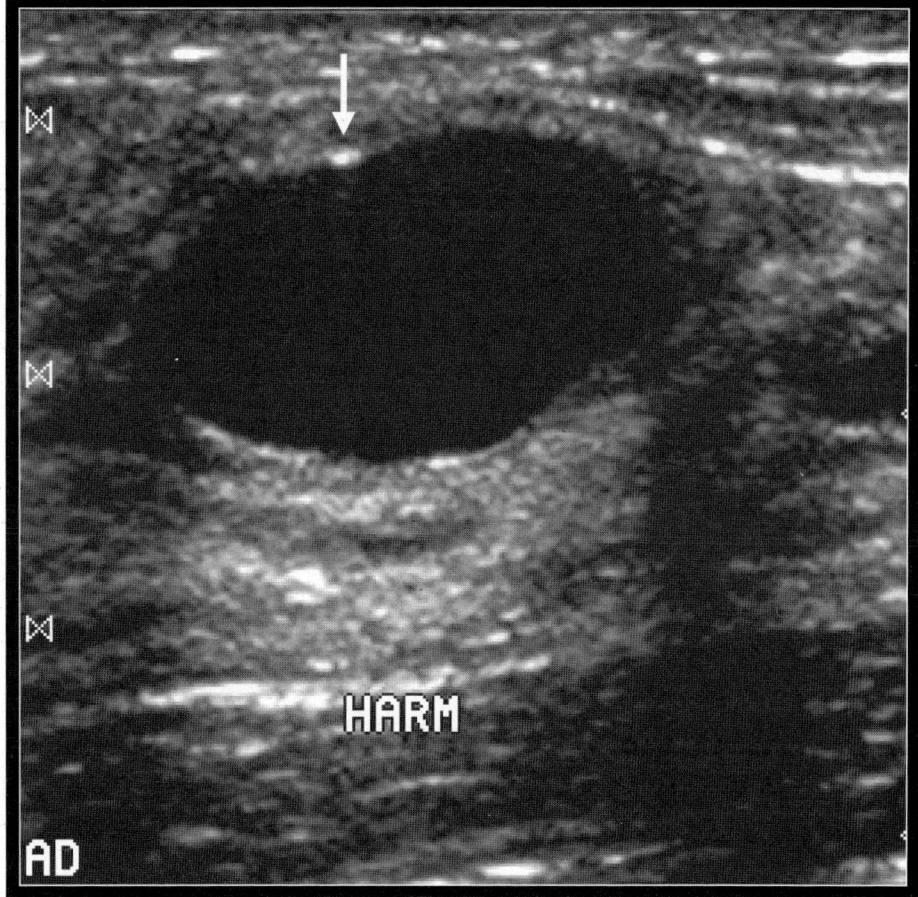

FIGURE 10–55 Punctate calcifications in the cyst wall *(arrow)* are benign (BIRADS 2). This punctate calcification occurred in a fibrotic cyst wall that had caused mild uniform isoechoic thickening of the wall and is likely a long-term sequela of inflammation or hemorrhage into the cyst.

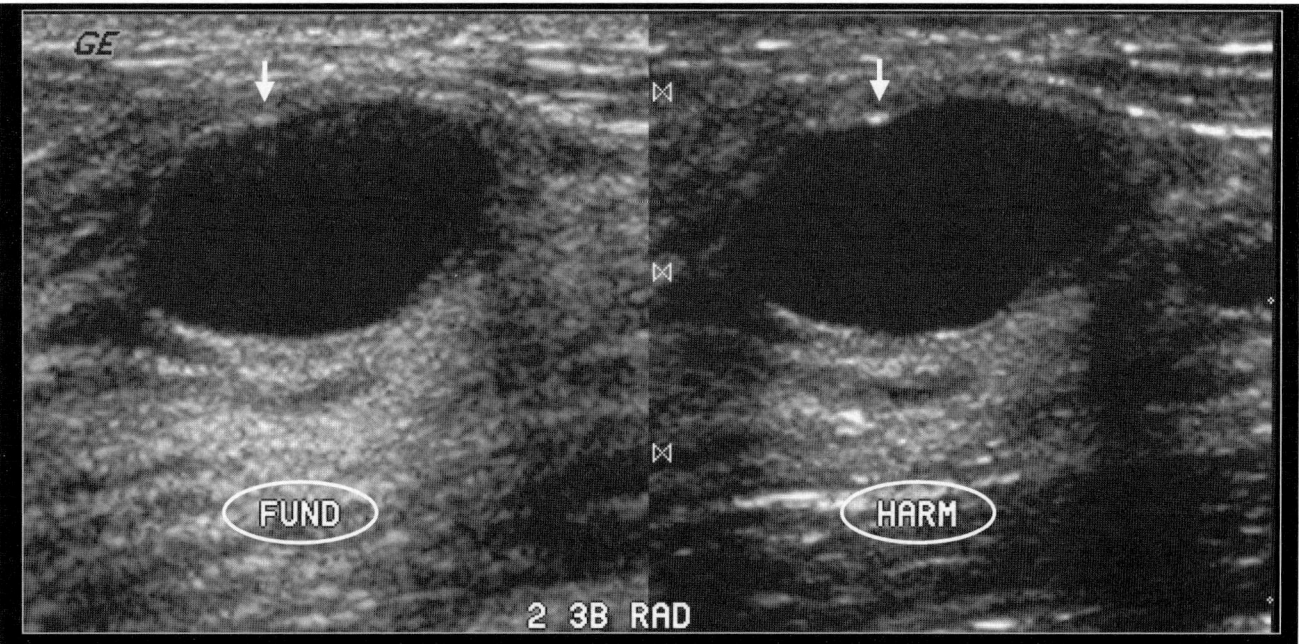

FIGURE 10–56 Punctate wall calcifications are better shown with coded harmonics (**right**) than with fundamental imaging (**left**). This is likely due to suppression of speckle artifact with coded harmonics. Speckle creates artifactual little white dots that tend to obscure punctate calcifications, which are real little white dots.

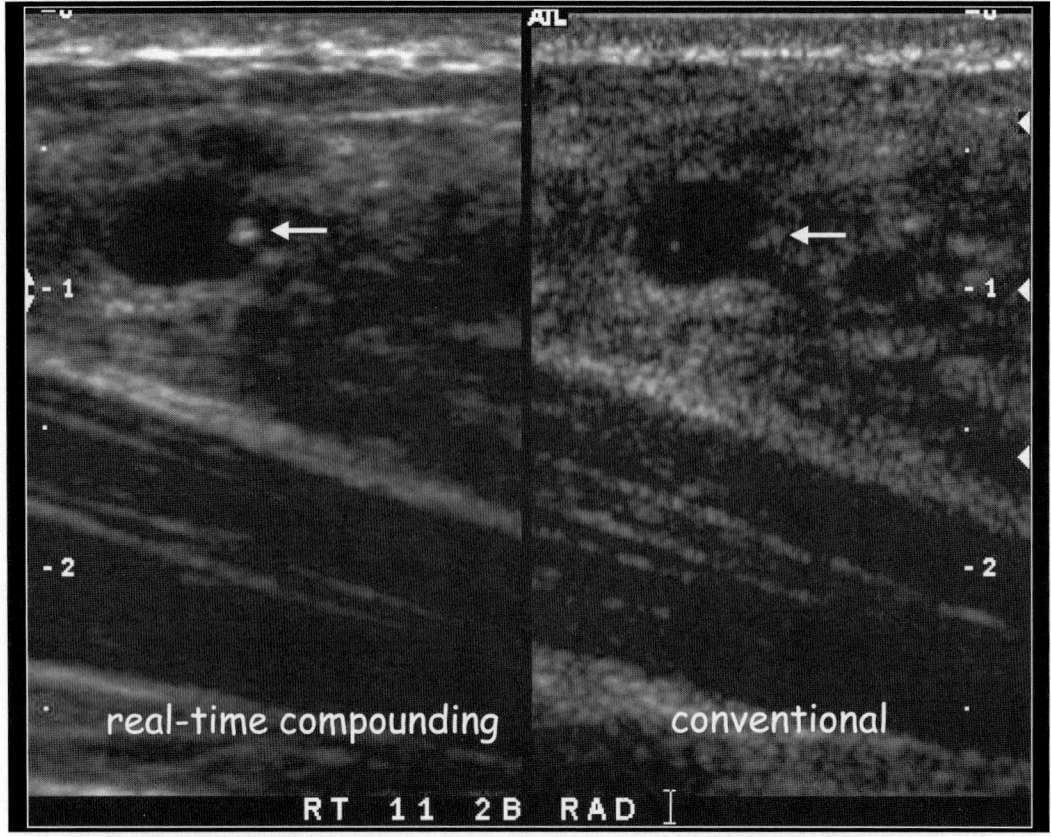

FIGURE 10–57 Real-time compounding also suppresses speckle artifact. This enables punctate wall calcifications to be better demonstrated with real-time compounding (**left**) than with conventional imaging (**right**).

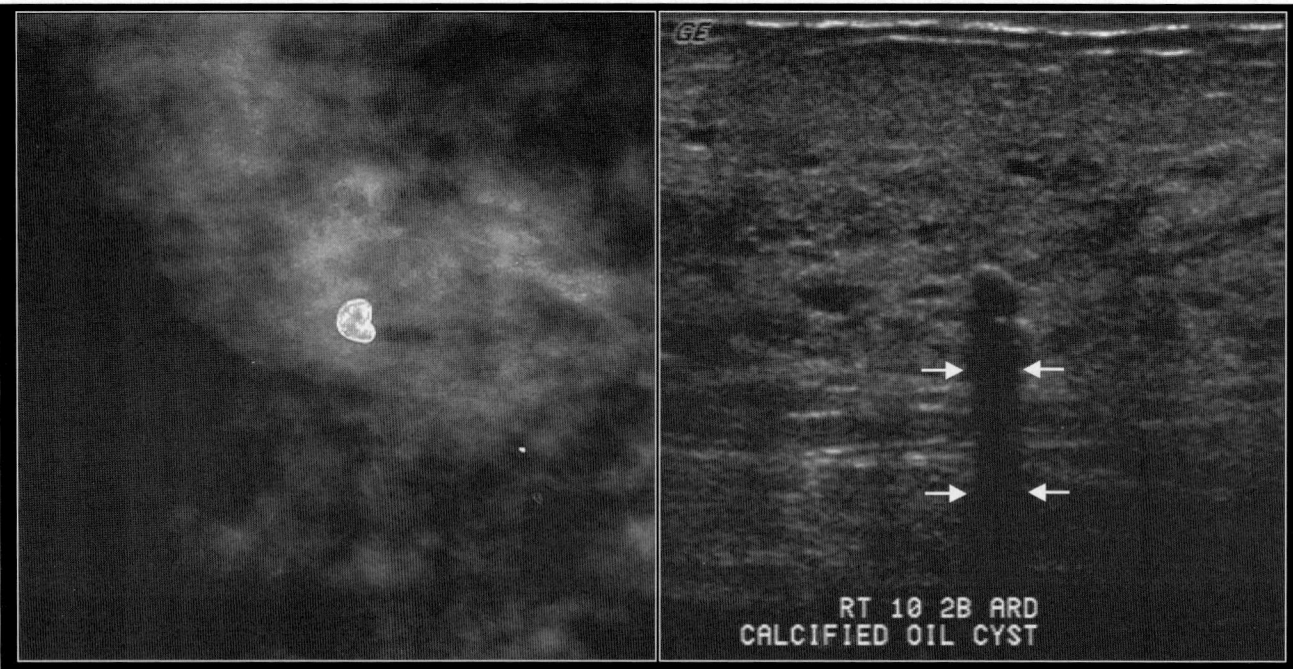

FIGURE 10–58 Circumferential wall calcifications are simply more extensive wall calcifications than punctate wall calcifications (**left**). They have been termed "eggshell calcifications" in the mammography literature and are benign (BIRADS 2). Sonography can also show eggshell calcifications that can also be characterized as BIRADS 2 (**right**). Dense calcification of the cyst wall causes acoustic shadowing *(arrows)* that may be so dense it obscures the posterior wall of the cyst. Most eggshell calcifications are thought to arise within lipid-filled cysts, but calcification may also result from inflammation of the cyst wall or hemorrhage into a cyst.

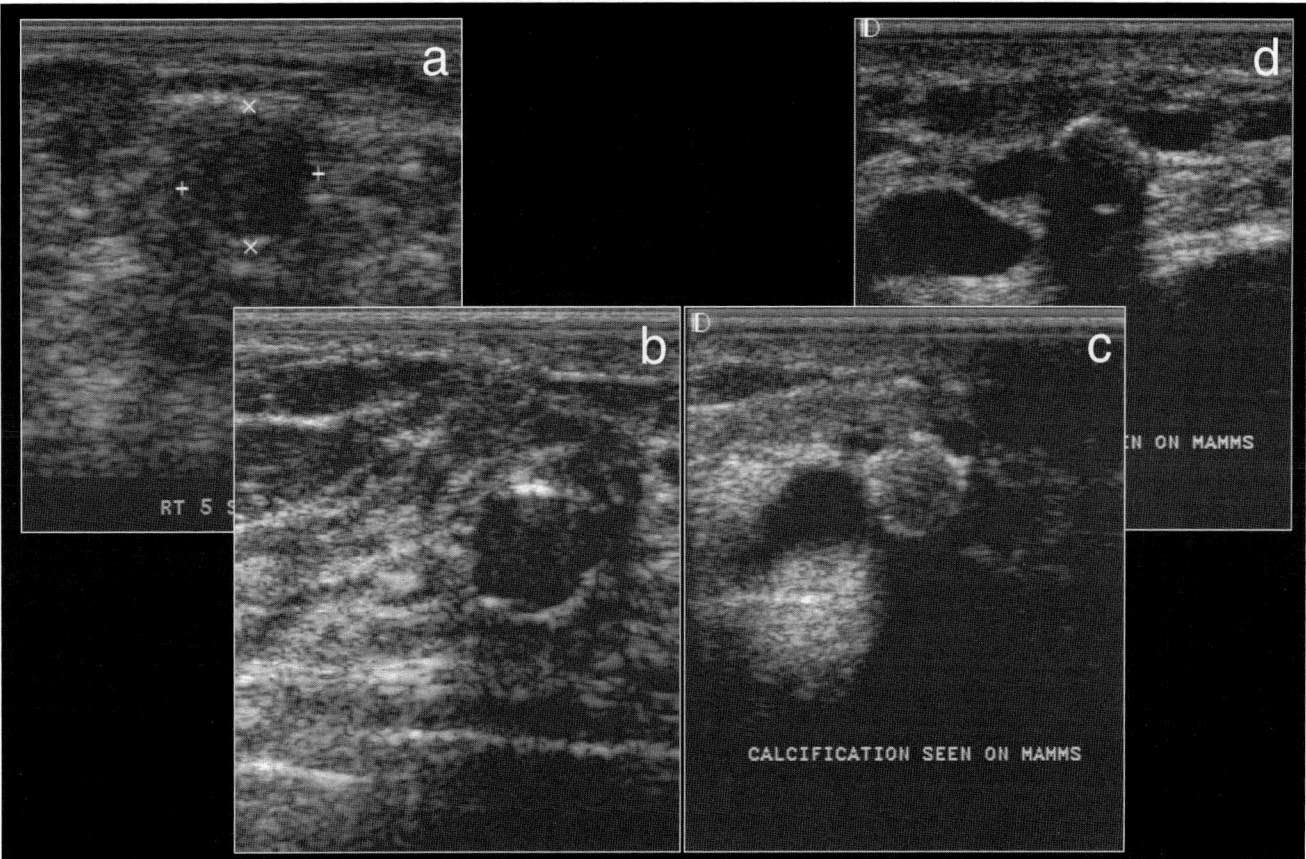

FIGURE 10–59 The appearance of eggshell calcifications varies greatly on ultrasound, depending on the thickness, density, and distribution of calcification within the cyst wall. When calcification is early or light, the wall may merely create artifact that makes the cyst appear echogenic *(a)*. The lipid contents of such cysts also likely contribute to the echogenicity of the cyst fluid. As calcification becomes thicker and denser, the wall of the cyst becomes hyperechoic, but only begins to shadow *(b)*. As the calcification becomes even thicker and denser, the cyst contents, as well as the wall, may appear hyperechoic *(c)*. In the end stage, when calcification is very thick and dense, it may give rise to intense acoustic shadowing that obscures the posterior wall of the cyst *(d)*.

Circumferential or Eggshell Calcifications in the Cyst Wall

Eggshell calcifications are definitively benign mammographic findings that are directly applicable to ultrasound (Fig. 10–58). The sonographic appearance is surprisingly variable, depending on the extent and thickness of calcifications and whether they are tangential to the beam. Eggshell calcifications progress through a series of stages. In the earliest stage, the cyst appears filled with echoes, but the wall has normal echogenicity (Fig. 10–59A). This occurs because most cysts that develop eggshell calcifications are lipid filled, and the lipid contents are echogenic. In the next stage, the wall becomes abnormally thick and echogenic, but does not cause shadowing (Fig. 10–59B). In later stages, the cyst wall contents and the cyst wall become echogenic and cause shadowing (Fig. 10–59C). In the last stage, the cyst wall becomes so calcified that only the ante-

rior wall is visible and the deeper portions of the cyst are completely obscured by intense shadowing (Fig. 10–59D).

The wall calcifications are not always uniform and symmetric and may involve primarily cyst walls that are either perpendicular or parallel to the x-ray or mammographic beam, thus affecting the imaging appearances greatly. In general, the mammographic finding of eggshell calcification is so definitively benign that sonographic evaluation is not warranted. However, and somewhat surprisingly, in some cases, sonography may be more sensitive to eggshell calcifications than mammography because the mammographic appearance also depends on whether the calcifications project *en face* or in tangent to the mammographic beam. Calcifications in the cyst wall that lie tangential to the beam appear bright white mammographically, whereas thin calcifications that lie along the walls perpendicular to the x-ray beam and that are projected *en face* may be mammographically inapparent. In certain

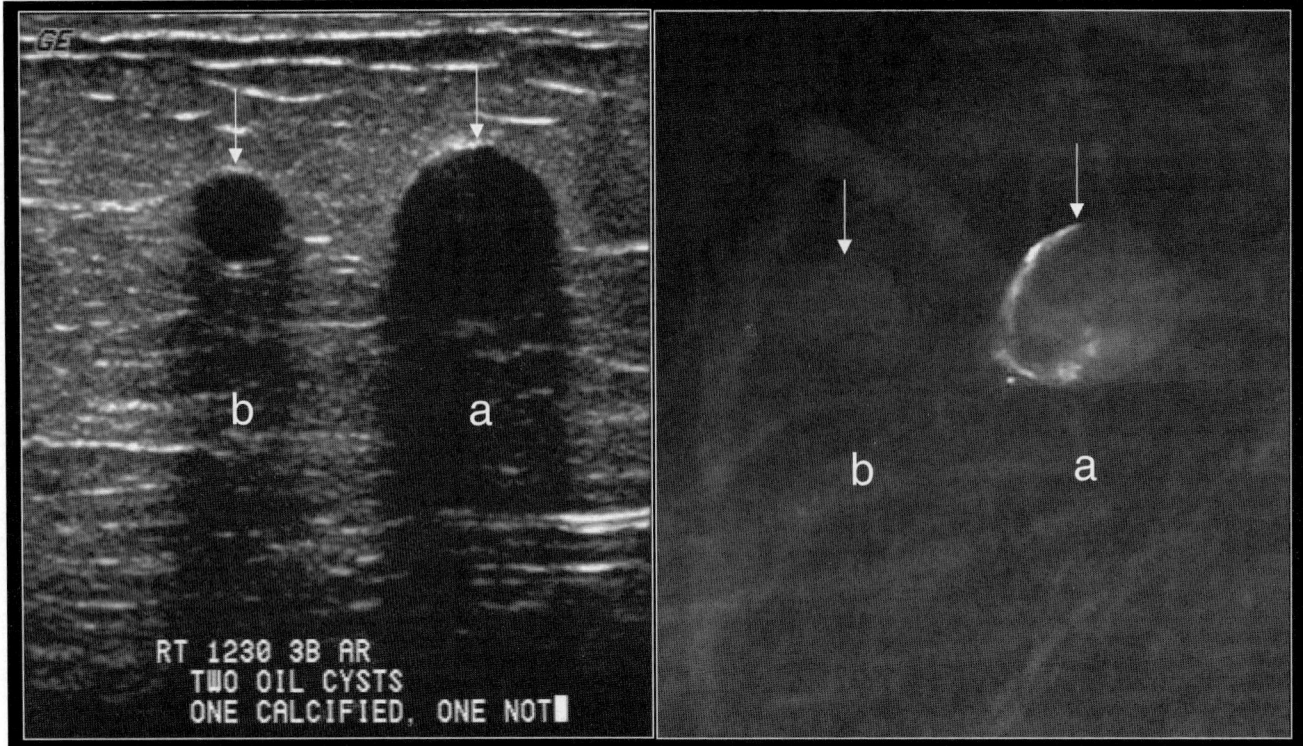

FIGURE 10–60 In general, mammography has the advantage over sonography in demonstrating eggshell calcifications. There is no need to evaluate such calcifications on ultrasound because they are definitively benign mammographically. However, there are times when sonography actually shows eggshell calcifications better than mammography. This occurs when the calcifications do not lie tangentially to the x-ray beam. Mammography shows eggshell calcification of cyst *a* well because the calcifications lie tangential to the beam. However, mammography fails to show the calcified wall of cyst *b* well because the calcifications lie *en face*, not tangential to the beam. Sonography shows both well.

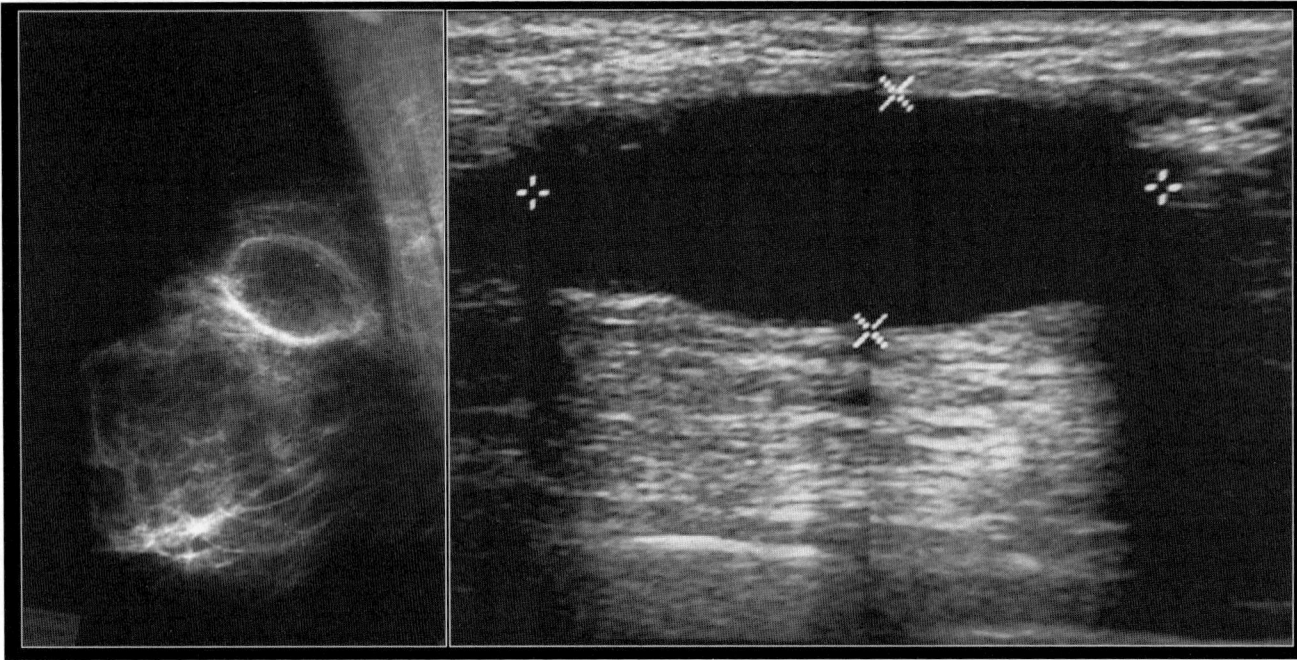

FIGURE 10–61 Lipid or oil cysts are definitively benign (BIRADS 2) mammographically. They can be definitively benign sonographically also, if they appear as simple cysts, as in this case. However, most lipid cysts do not appear to be simple cysts on sonography.

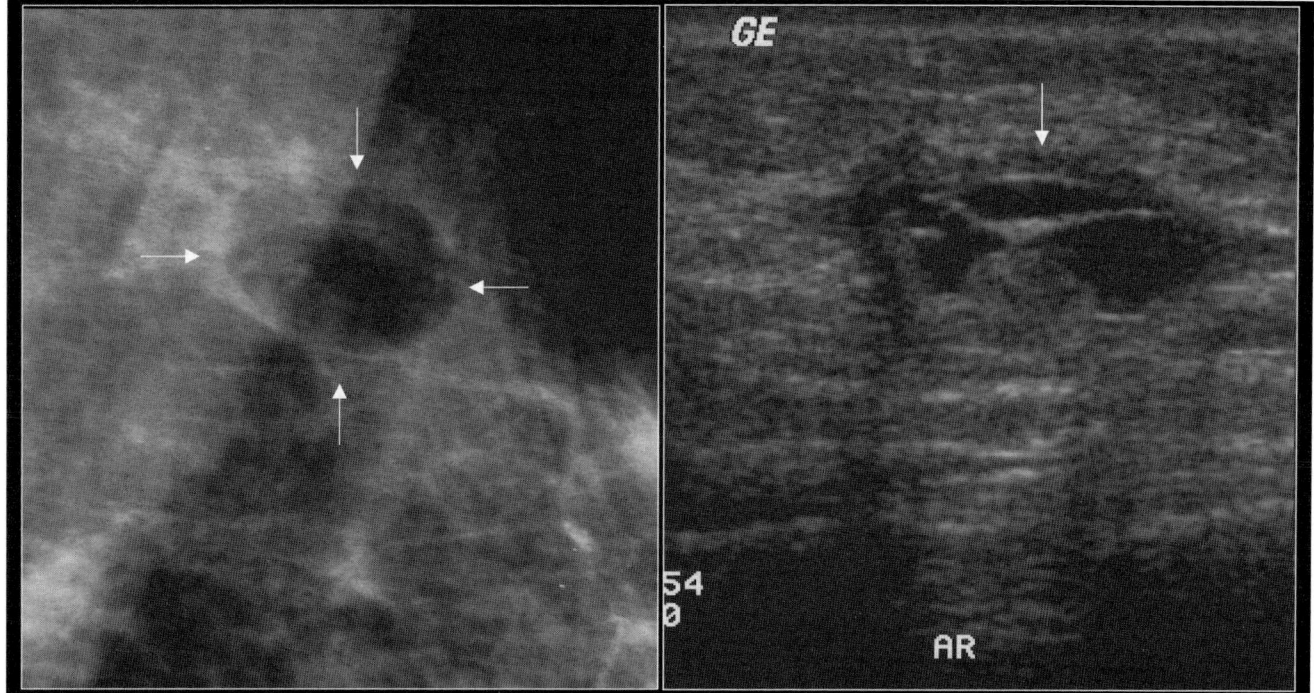

FIGURE 10–62 This definitively benign (BIRADS 2) oil cyst at mammography appears more worrisome sonographically. It has a thick wall and a mural nodule (BIRADS 4a). This discrepancy in the sonographic and mammographic BIRADS categories is, unfortunately, common. Because of this, when mammography shows an oil cyst, but sonography shows a worrisome-appearing complex cyst, the sonographic findings should be ignored, and the mammographic findings should be relied on.

cases, such calcifications will be shown well sonographically, regardless of which wall they involve (Fig. 10–60).

Lipid Cysts

Lipid cysts or oil cysts are definitively benign mammographically, but unfortunately, frequently appear more worrisome sonographically than they do mammographically. The appearance of lipid cysts varies much more sonographically than it does mammographically. Most mammographically benign lipid cysts have to be classified as suspicious sonographically. The thickness of the lipid cyst walls often appears irregular sonographically (Fig. 10–61). Sonography also frequently shows findings worrisome for neoplasm such as mural nodules or thick, isoechoic septations (Fig. 10–62). Certain lipid cysts appear at sonography to be solid because the inspissated fatty material within them is so echogenic. Based on sonography alone, most lipid cysts would have to undergo biopsy unnecessarily.

The complex and somewhat worrisome sonographic appearances of lipid cysts should not be surprising because they are nearly identical to those of the hematomas, seromas, and biopsy or lumpectomy cavities in which lipid cysts frequently arise. Partial compressibility and lack of Doppler-demonstrable blood flow within thickened walls, septations, and mural nodules are all sonographic findings that can be reassuring in postsurgical patients but that are less reassuring in patients who have never had breast surgery or trauma. In general, when there is any possibility that a complex cyst could be a lipid cyst (posttrauma or postsurgical), spot compression mammograms are likely to yield more definitively benign (BIRADS 2) characteristics than is ultrasound. In this setting, spot compression mammography should be obtained before deciding to biopsy such a lesion. Because of the propensity of sonography to produce false-positive findings, when mammography shows a definitively benign lipid cyst and sonography shows a complex cyst with one or more worrisome findings, more reliance should be place on the benign mammographic finding. Using such an approach, unnecessary biopsy can be avoided in most cases.

The sonographic evaluation of hematomas, seromas, and lumpectomy cavities are discussed in greater detail in Chapter 18.

Fat–Fluid Levels

A fat–fluid level within a cyst is another definitively benign mammographic finding that can be directly applied to

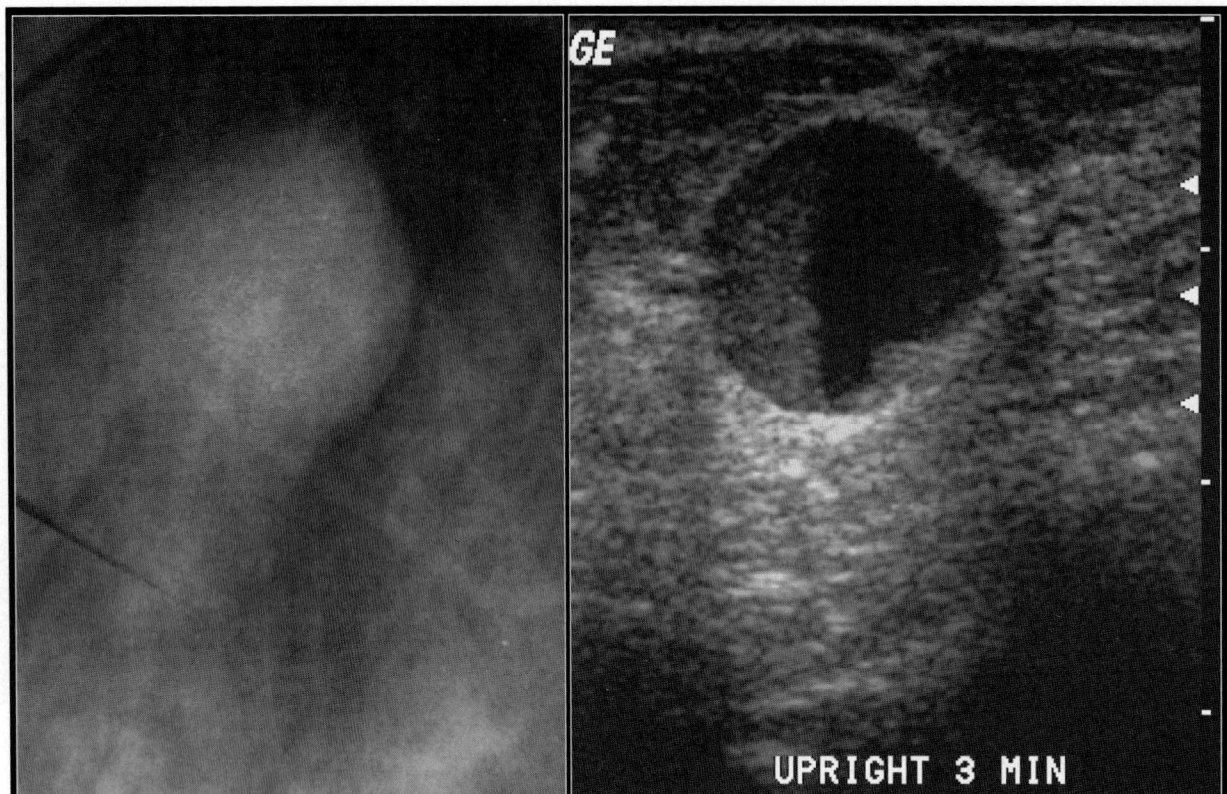

FIGURE 10–63 Fat–fluid levels are benign (BIRADS 2) mammographic findings that can also be identified and characterized as BIRADS 2 by sonography. Fat–fluid levels are typically only seen in galactoceles on mammography but are very frequently seen in routine fibrocystic change sonographically and are thus far more commonly seen sonographically than mammographically. In many cysts that have classic fat–fluid levels on sonography (**right**), the lipid layer cannot be identified mammographically (**left**).

sonography. However, fat–fluid levels are rarely demonstrated mammographically and are usually associated with classic galactoceles. On the other hand, the fat–fluid levels are far more frequently demonstrated sonographically and are usually part of the fibrocystic spectrum and not associated with galactoceles. Sonography is more sensitive than mammography for the detection of fat–fluid levels, probably because the mediolateral oblique view is not truly a horizontal beam and because mammographic compression temporarily disrupts the fat–fluid interface and mixes lipid and water components of cyst contents (Fig. 10–63). The lipid layer within cysts containing fat–fluid levels is composed of phospholipid cell membrane debris from the various cells that inhabit the cyst and from the internal contents of foamy macrophages. Why the lipid layer in cysts that contain fat–fluid levels is echogenic while the fat in pure lipid cysts is often nearly anechoic is uncertain. The lipid layer in FCC also tends to be more echogenic than the lipid layer within the less common galactocele (Fig. 10–64). The relative proportions of water and fat within cysts can vary greatly. The fat layer may be smaller than, the same size as, or larger than the fluid layer (Fig. 10–65). When the lipid

layer fills most of the cyst, leaving only a thin layer of fluid along one edge of the lesion, care must be taken not to mistake the cyst for a solid nodule (Fig. 10–66).

The shape and orientation of the echogenic lipid layer can also vary in appearance from patient to patient. The interface may be straight, convex away from the echogenic fat, concave toward the fat, or sigmoid in shape and may be oriented horizontally, obliquely, or vertically (Fig. 10–67). The shape and orientation of the fat–fluid interface may also vary in an individual patient from radial to antiradial view and over time with changes in patient position (Fig. 10–68). In certain cases, the echogenic lipid layer may be indistinguishable from the eccentric wall thickenings and mural nodules caused by papillary apocrine metaplasia or other papillary neoplastic lesions. Only a change in alignment of the fat–fluid interface that occurs when the patient position is changed enables us to distinguish a lipid layer from a mural nodule (Fig. 10–69). As is the case with fluid–debris levels, enough time must be allowed for gravity to move the water layer to the dependent portion of the cyst and to enable the lipid layer to float to the nondependent part of the cyst. The contents of cysts

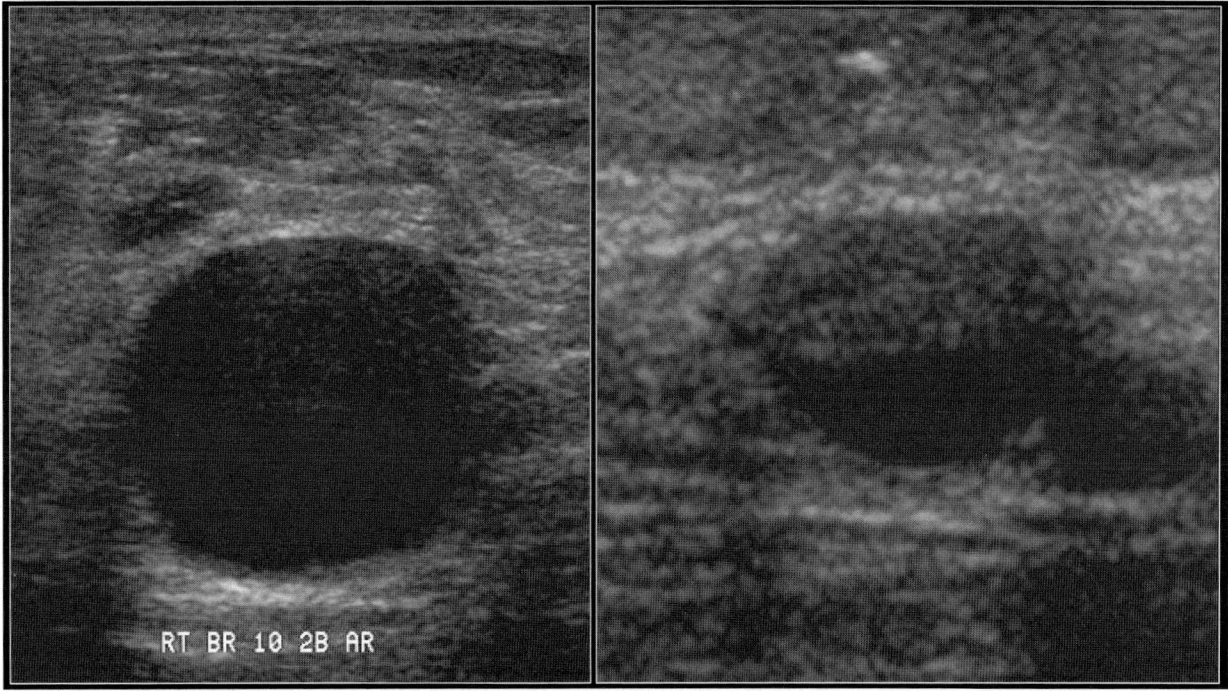

FIGURE 10–64 The lipid layer in cysts that contain fat–fluid levels varies from markedly hypoechoic to isoechoic. The hypoechoic lipid layer on the **left** lies in the nondependent portion of a galactocele. The isoechoic lipid layer in the cyst on the **right** lies in the nondependent portion of a typical cyst of fibrocystic change.

with fat–fluid levels are frequently thick and viscous, and it may take as long as 10 minutes for a complete shift of the fat–fluid level to occur (Fig. 10–70). If insufficient time is allowed for the change in position to occur, the echogenic lipid layer can falsely appear immobile and can then be mistaken for a mural nodule. With changes in patient position, both the shape and the alignment of the

fat–fluid interface change. However, while in the process of equilibrating to its new position, the fat–fluid interface is sigmoid in shape and obliquely oriented. This obliquely oriented and sigmoid interface shape is so reliably present during patient position changes that we believe it may be definitive evidence of the presence of a fat–fluid level in transition even without changing the patient position

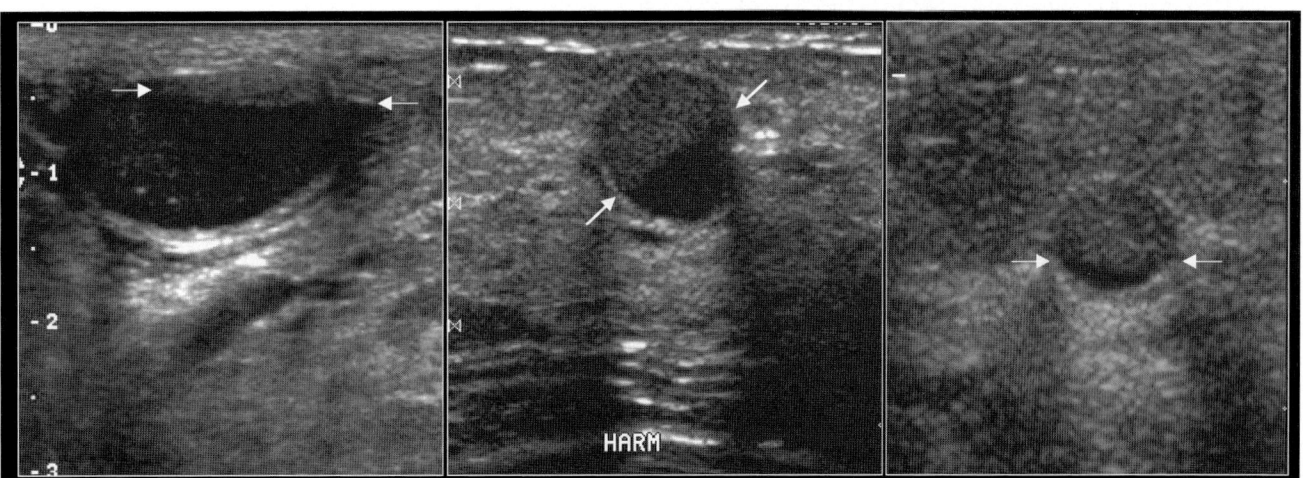

FIGURE 10–65 The echogenic lipid layer in cysts that contain fat–fluid levels varies in size. The lipid layer may fill a minority of the cyst (**left**), half the cyst (**middle**), or nearly all the cyst (**right**). Lipids completely fill some cysts.

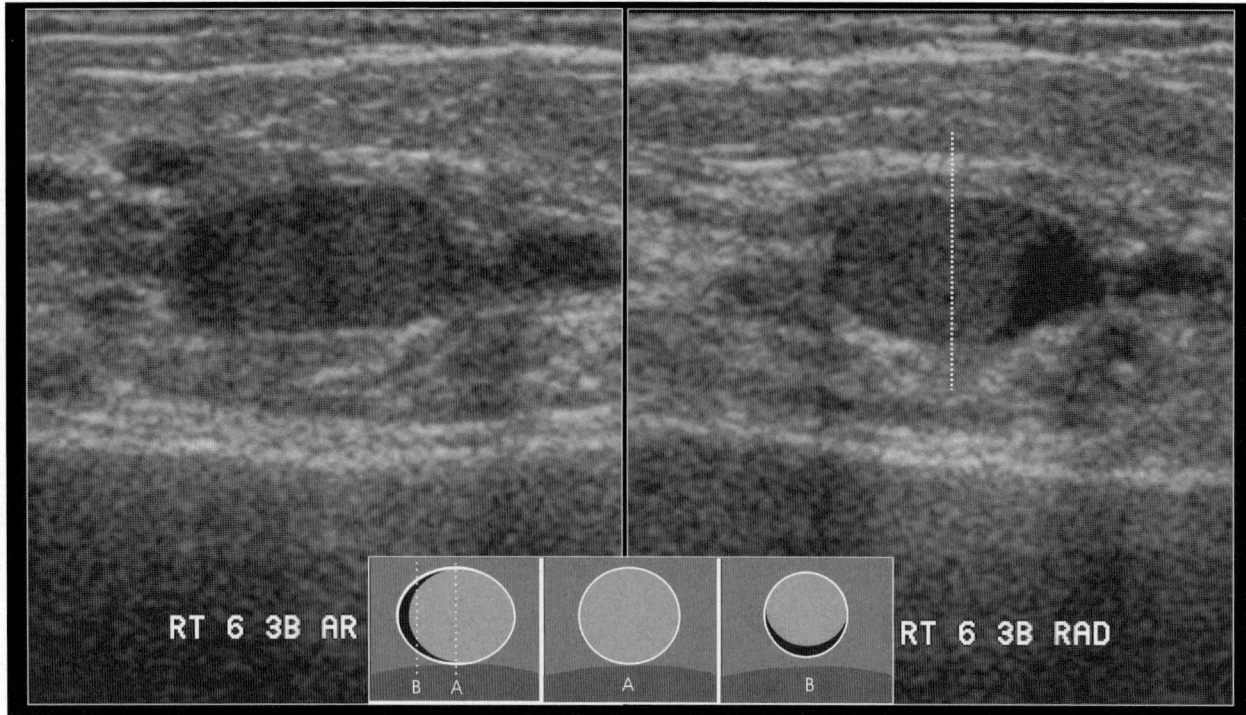

FIGURE 10–66 In cases in which the lipid layer nearly fills the cyst, scanning through the cyst in certain planes may make the cyst appear to be a solid nodule. The radial plane through the cyst *(RAD)* shows a small crescent of fluid at one end of the cyst. An orthogonal antiradial plane through the white line shows what appears to be a solid nodule. It is important to identify cysts with fat–fluid levels correctly because they can be characterized as BIRADS 2 and require neither aspiration nor additional evaluation. On the other hand, solid nodules with such an appearance must be characterized as BRIADS 3 and require at least short-interval follow-up.

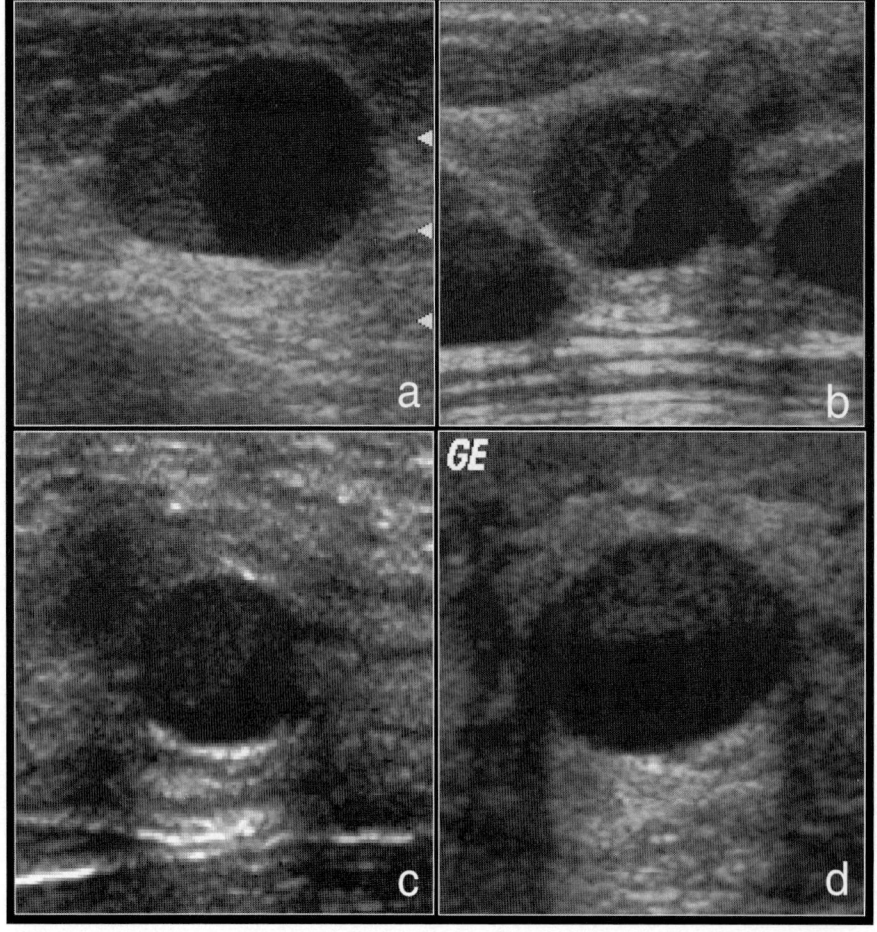

FIGURE 10–67 The shape of the fat–fluid interface varies. It may be concave *(a)*, sigmoid shaped *(b)*, convex *(c)*, or straight *(d)*. The shape in individual cysts also varies with time and position.

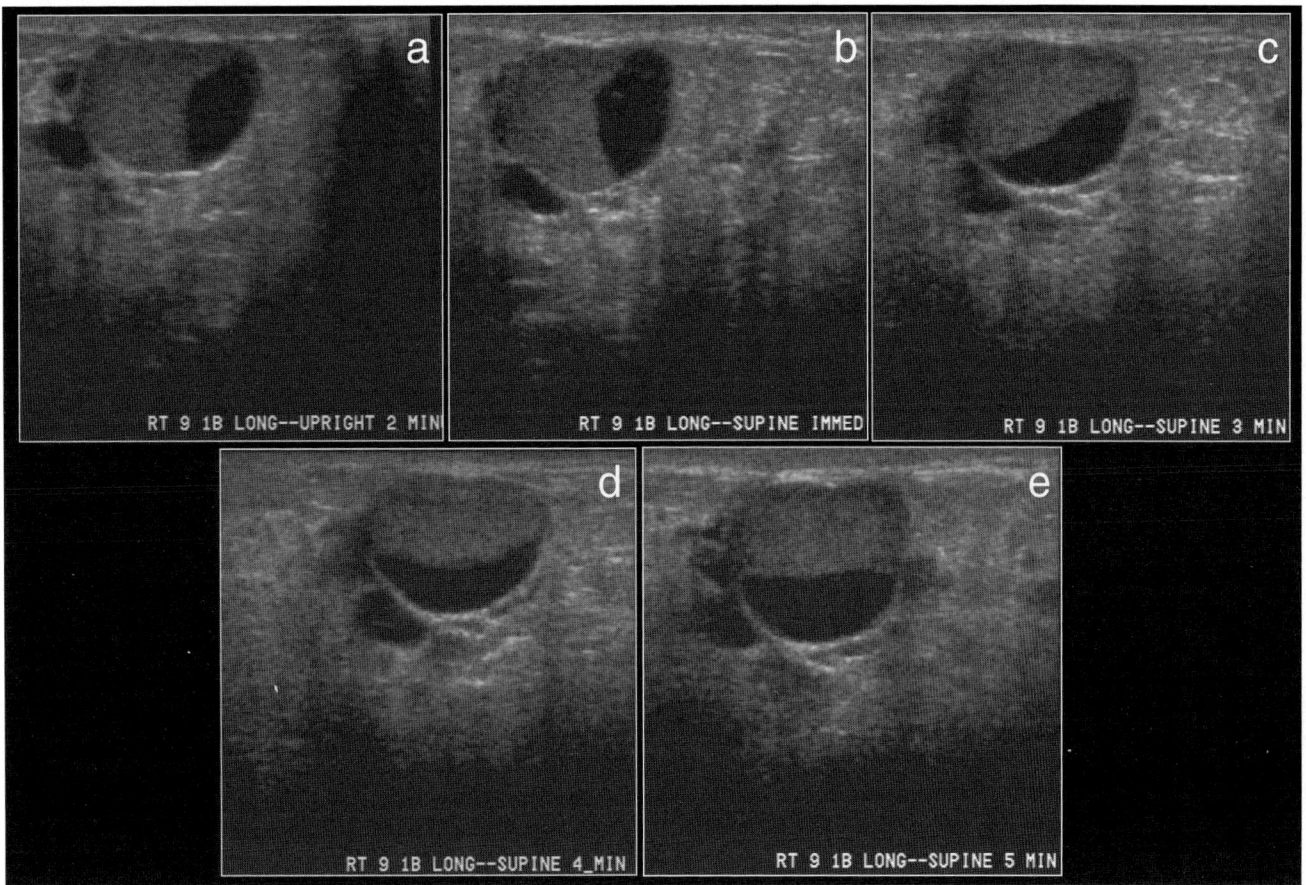

FIGURE 10–68 The shape of the fat–fluid interface changes with patient position. When fully equilibrated and in relatively large cysts, the interface may be concave, convex, or straight. In this case, in the upright position, it was concave and vertically oriented *(a)*. In the longitudinal plane, immediately after placing the patient supine, there was no change in the fat–fluid interface position or configuration *(b)*. After 3 minutes, the interface is obliquely oriented and has a sigmoid configuration *(c)*. After 4 minutes, the fat–fluid interface had become horizontally oriented and convex in shape *(d)*. After 5 minutes, it had fully equilibrated and become straight as well as horizontal *(e)*. The sigmoid shape and oblique orientation are so typical of a fat–fluid level in transition from one position within the cyst to another that the orientation and shape alone suggest the presence of a fat–fluid level.

(Fig. 10–71). The obliquely oriented and sigmoid-shaped fat–fluid interface is frequently seen during routine scanning because scans are begun immediately after the patient has lain down, before the fat–fluid level has equilibrated to the new nondependent position it must assume when the patient is supine. Thus, most fat–fluid levels are naturally scanned in a state of transition from the upright to the supine position. In the longitudinal plane, after the patient lies down, as the lipid level shifts from the craniad to the anterior portion of the cyst, and as the fat–fluid interface approaches a 45-degree angle, the posterior part of the lipid layer assumes a convex shape, and the anterior portion assumes a concave shape.

Because cysts with fat–fluid levels are definitively benign, there is seldom need to aspirate for diagnostic pur-

poses. However, when aspiration is deemed necessary, such cysts can be completely aspirated (Fig. 10–72). Interestingly, when cysts with fat–fluid levels are aspirated through a small needle, the fat becomes completely emulsified within the cyst fluid. Because the fat is emulsified within the fluid, a lipid layer is not immediately visible within the aspirated fluid (Fig. 10–72). The test tube may need to be left undisturbed in an upright position for a few hours before the lipid layer separates out again. Cytology of such cysts typically shows benign FCC. Although epithelial cells, foamy macrophages (histiocytes), metaplastic apocrine cells, red blood cells, and various white blood cells can sometimes be seen, the aspirates from most cysts with fat–fluid levels are acellular or paucicellular, with large amounts of cellular debris and lipids (Fig. 10–72).

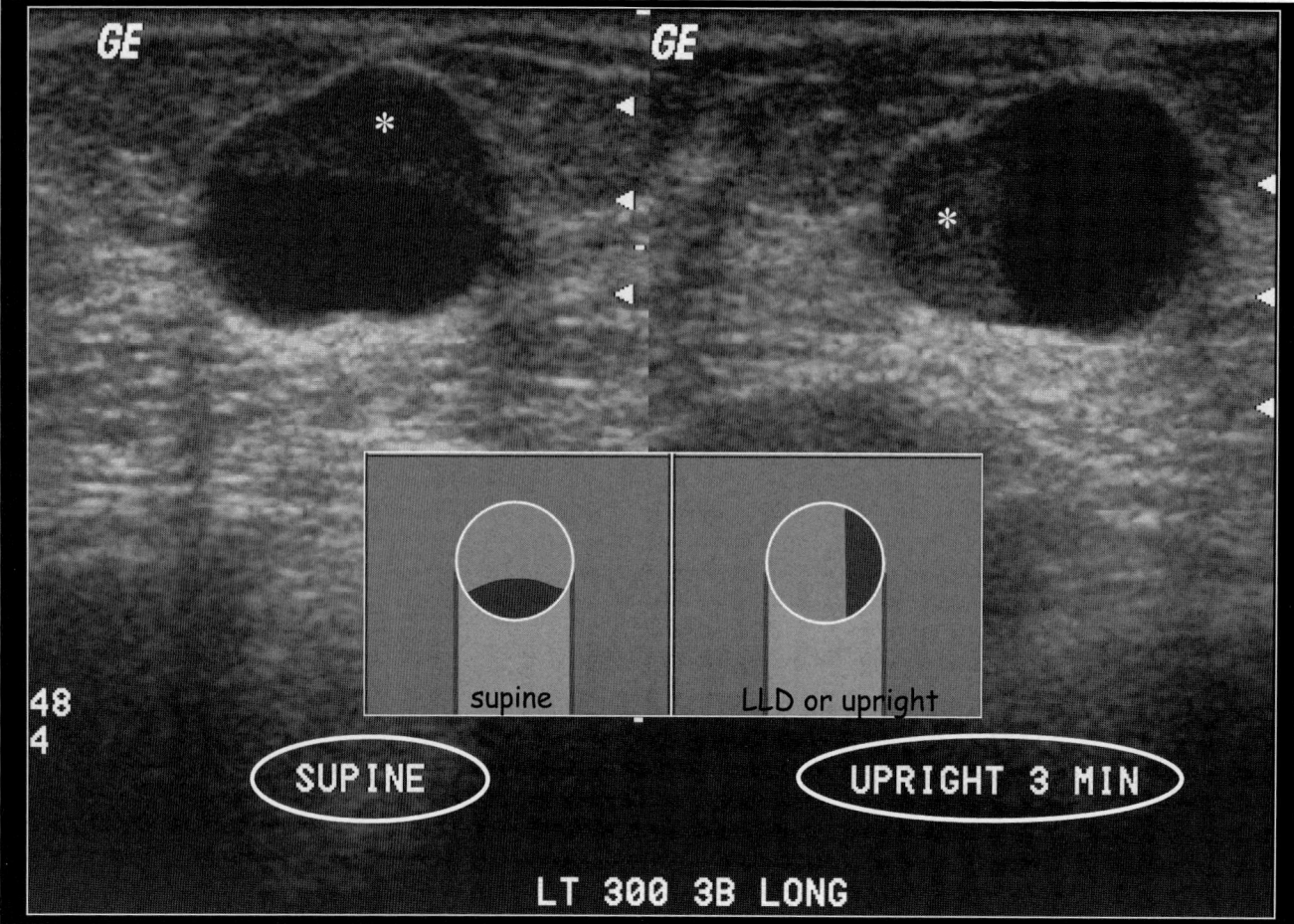

FIGURE 10–69 The echogenic lipid layer *(*)* lies in the nondependent part of the cyst in the supine position. When viewed in the longitudinal plane, the lipid layer redistributes to the new nondependent portion of the cyst along the superior wall.

Mobile Internal Particles

In some cysts, the diffuse low-level internal echoes can be moved solely by the energy of the ultrasound beam (not by percussing or deforming the cyst or changing the patient's position). To demonstrate motion of particles, it may be necessary to override the default low-transmit power setting at which most ultrasound machine boot up. (Low-power settings are used by default in order to minimize potential hazardous effects of ultrasound.) The higher the transmission power used, the faster the particles can be made to move. This movement is best demonstrated by capturing a video loop on a picture archiving and communications system (PACS) but can also be documented on split-screen images, with the low-power image demonstrated on one side and the high-power image demonstrated on the other side. The stationary internal echoes

appear punctate with low power but appear smeared in the anteroposterior dimension on freeze-frame images obtained with high power (Fig. 10–73). Motion of particles can more easily be demonstrated by use of color or power Doppler, which requires higher power and supplies more energy than does the B-mode ultrasound beam. As the particles are displaced posteriorly within the center of the cyst by the color or power Doppler beam, vertically oriented trails of color are created within the cyst that have been termed "color streaking." Color and power Doppler–induced movement can also be captured on cine loops or freeze-frame images (see the color images in Chapter 20, Fig. 20–33). That such particles can be moved by the very-low-energy levels of the ultrasound beam implies that these particles are extremely small, light, and subcellular in size. Red or white blood cells, epithelial cells, apocrine cells, and tumor cells are all too large and heavy to be moved by the

(text continued on page 325)

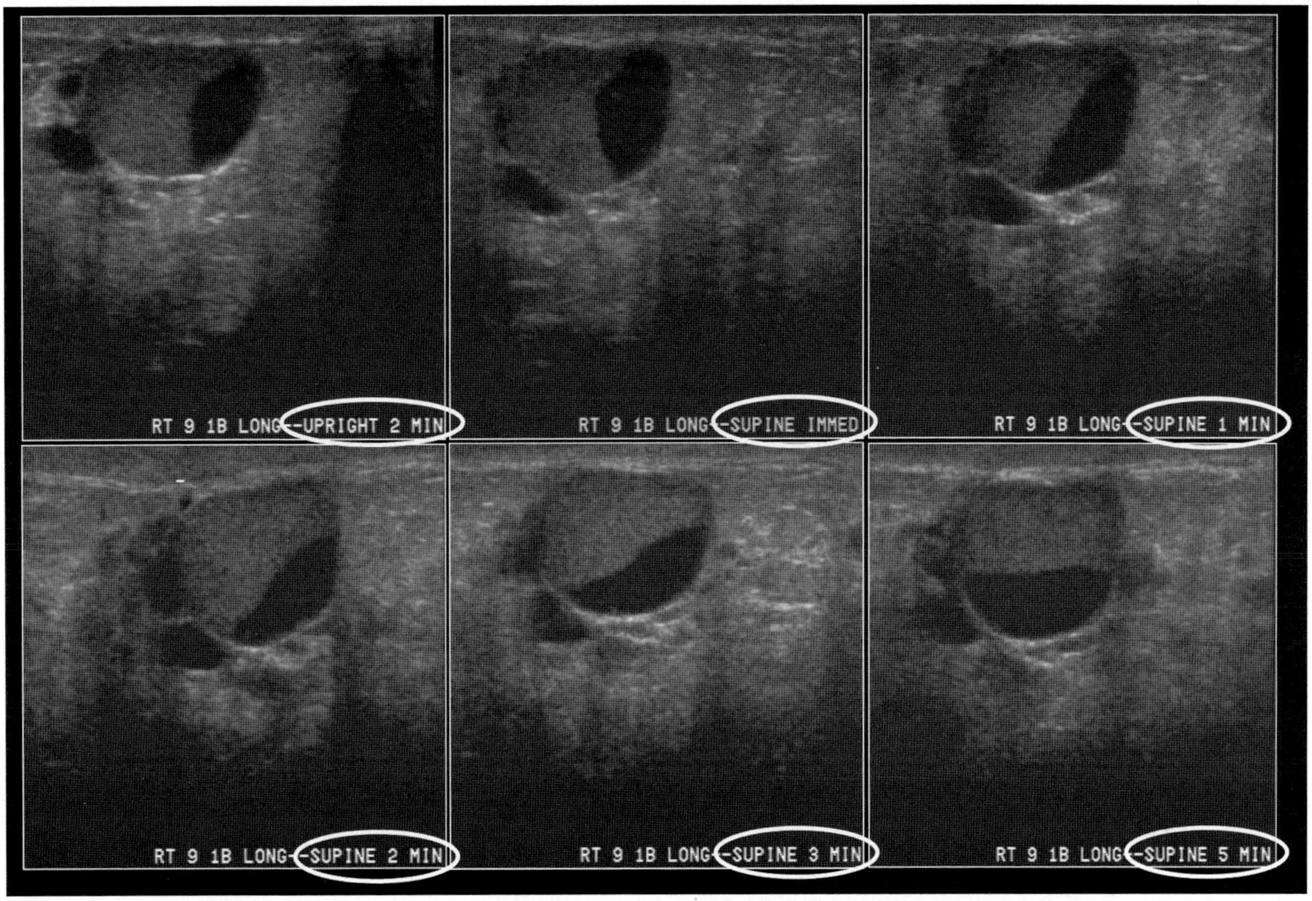

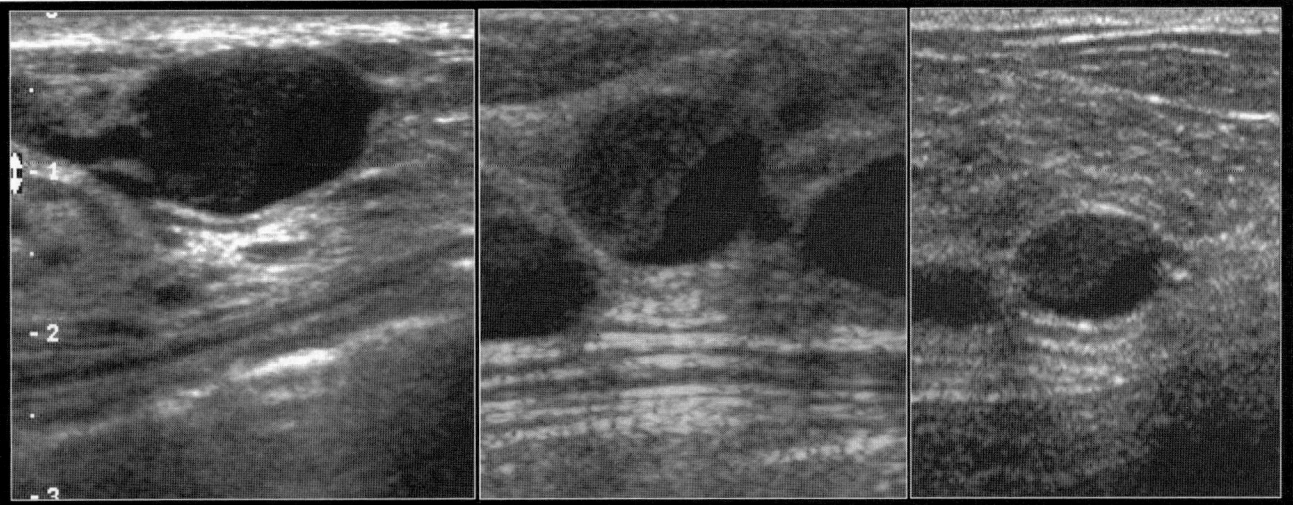

RT 9 1B LONG—UPRIGHT 2 MIN   RT 9 1B LONG—SUPINE IMMED   RT 9 1B LONG—SUPINE 1 MIN

RT 9 1B LONG—SUPINE 2 MIN   RT 9 1B LONG—SUPINE 3 MIN   RT 9 1B LONG—SUPINE 5 MIN

FIGURE 10–70 The fluid and lipid layer in cysts that contain fat–fluid levels tends to be very viscous and slowly moving. It may take 5 or 10 minutes for the lipid layer to equilibrate in its new nondependent position. If enough time is not allowed for this to occur, it may falsely appear that the lipid layer represents a mural nodule and is attached to the wall.

FIGURE 10–71 The typical configuration and alignment of a fat–fluid level in transition from one part of a cyst to another is a sigmoid shape and an oblique orientation. The sigmoid shape and oblique orientation are so typical of fat–fluid levels in transition that they may allow definitive diagnosis of a fat–fluid level without waiting for full equilibration in the new patient position to occur. Because scanning is frequently commenced immediately after the patient walks into the room and lies down in the supine position, before the shift is complete, the sonographer frequently sees obliquely oriented sigmoid-shaped fat–fluid interfaces early in the ultrasound examination.

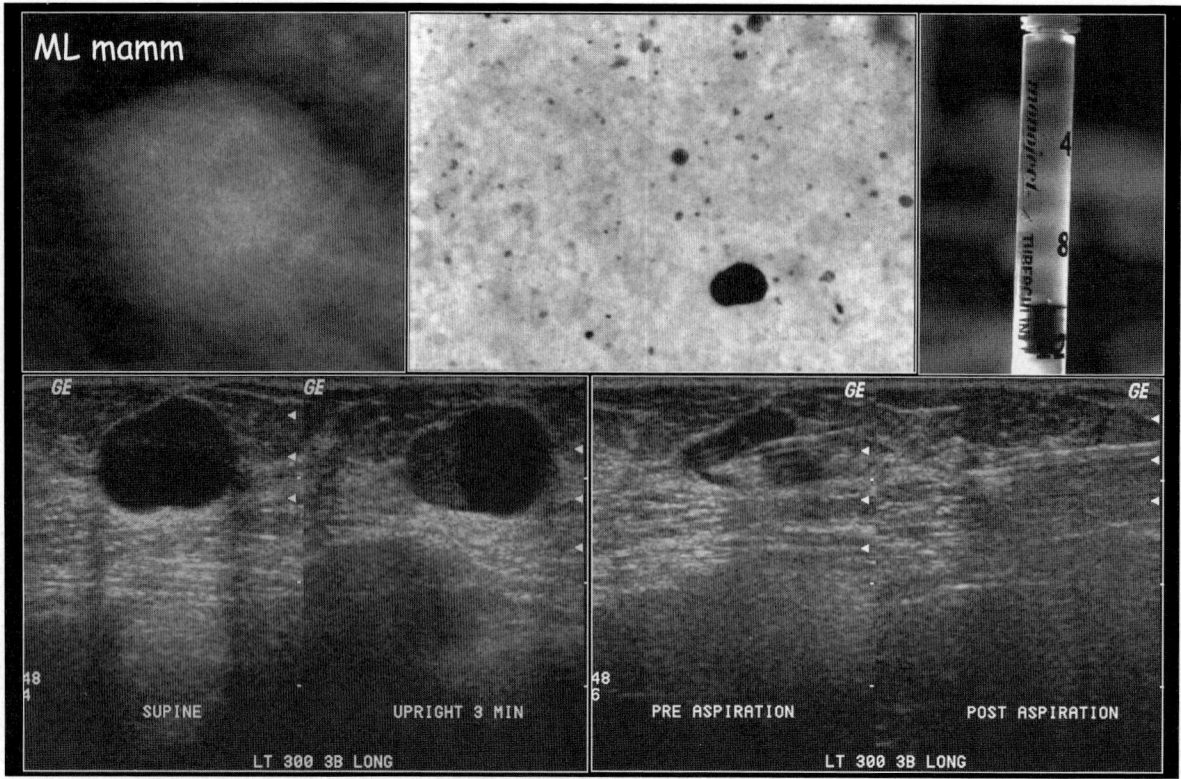

FIGURE 10–72 Cysts that contain fat–fluid levels can be completely aspirated. In the process of passing through the needle and into a vacuum, the lipid layer becomes completely emulsified within the cyst fluid. Thus, the aspirated fluid appears homogeneous and does not show a lipid level immediately after aspiration. After a few hours to a few days, a white lipid layer separates out. Cytology of the lipid layer is usually acellular.

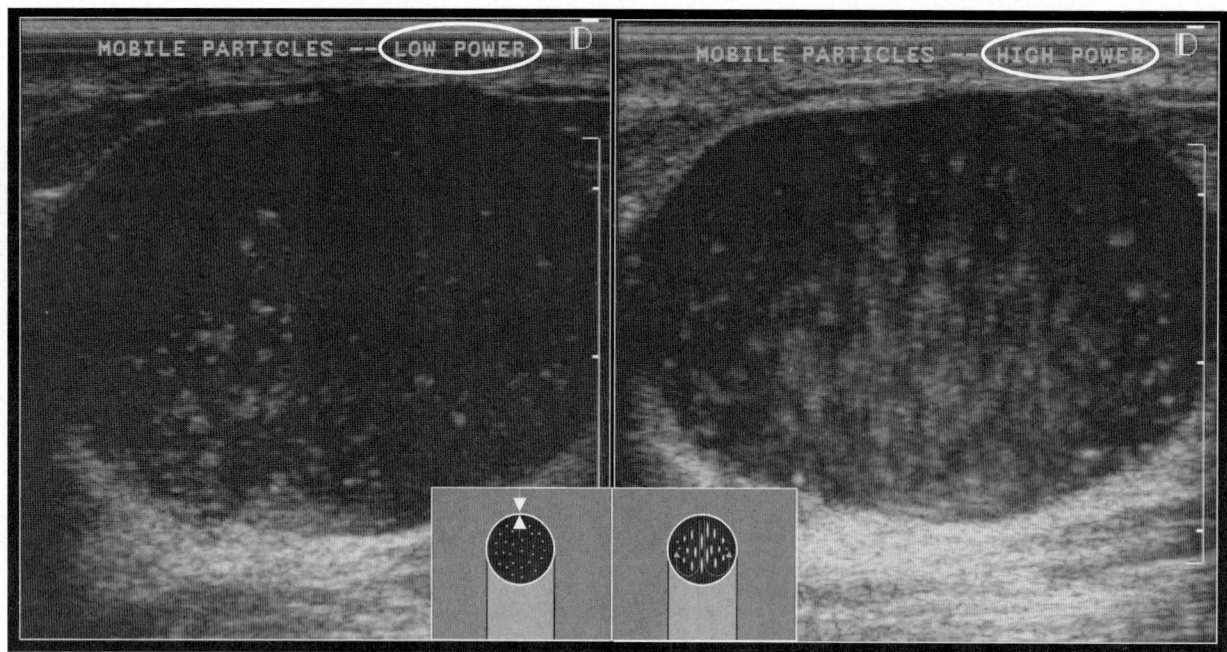

FIGURE 10–73 This cyst contains mobile echoes that can be moved solely by the energy of the ultrasound beam. The low power at which most ultrasound machines boot up in order to minimize possible harmful effects to the patient may be inadequate to move the particles within the cyst. Thus, it is necessary to turn the transmit power higher to demonstrate the motion. The **left** images show the internal echoes within the cyst at low power. They appear punctate and well defined because they are not moving. However, at high transmit power, they appear elongated in the anteroposterior direction and ill defined because they are being pushed posteriorly by the energy of the ultrasound beam.

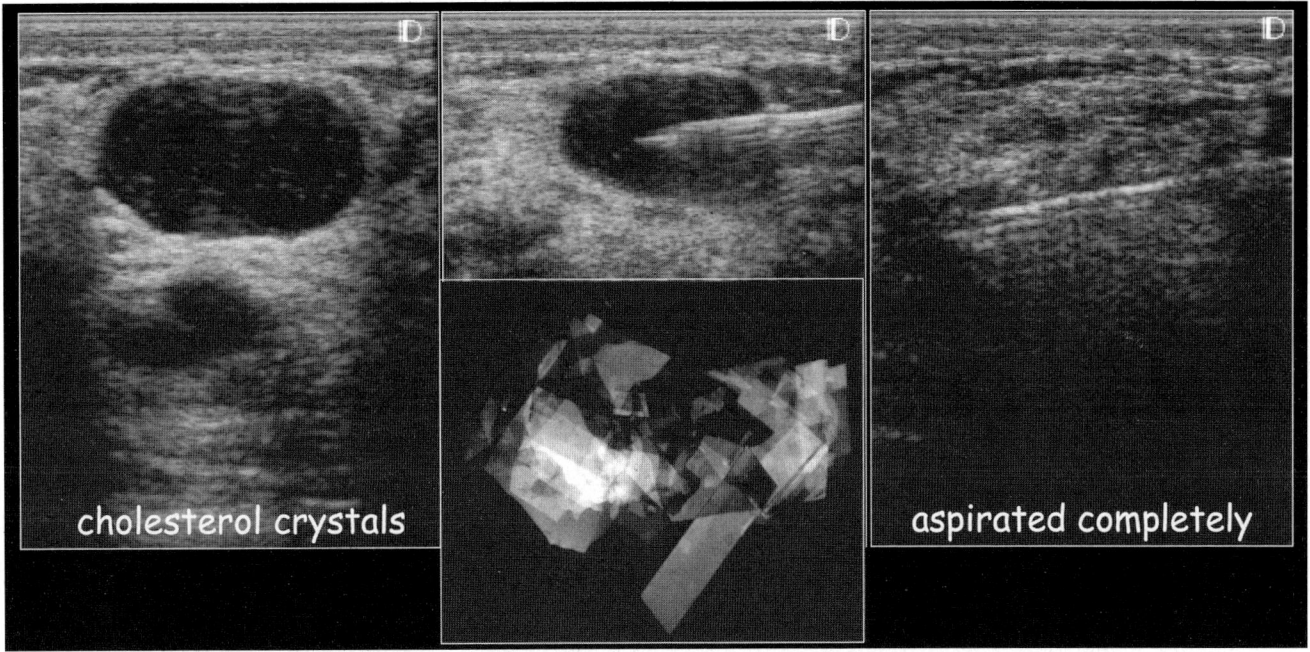

FIGURE 10–74 Cysts with mobile particles or color streaking can be completely aspirated. In dozens of cases, the cytology has been benign and typical of fibrocystic change. When the fluid is viewed with polarized light, cholesterol crystals can be identified. Cholesterol crystals are thought to be the particles that are being moved by the ultrasound and Doppler beams.

energy of the ultrasound beam. Cysts containing mobile particles can usually be completely aspirated (Fig. 10–74). The fluid within such cysts is typically greenish brown or greenish gray and has cytology typical of FCC. When the fluid from such cysts is examined with polarized light, an unusually large number of cholesterol crystals are present, suggesting that the mobile particles are cholesterol crystals (Fig. 10–74).

Cysts of Skin Origin

Cysts of skin origin include sebaceous cysts, Montgomery gland cysts, and epidermal inclusion cysts. Three sonographic findings can confirm origin in the skin (Fig. 10–75):

1. The lesion lies entirely within the skin. Most of the lesions that lie entirely within the skin are small and do not offer diagnostic difficulty if they are appropriately scanned with an acoustic standoff (Fig. 10–76). However, without an acoustic standoff, it may be difficult to appreciate that the lesion lies within the skin.

2. Most of the lesion lies within the subcutaneous tissues, but a "claw sign" of hyperechoic skin can be shown around that edge of the lesion. With use of an appropriate acoustic standoff, it is easy to demonstrate the hyperechoic skin enveloping the edges of the lesion. However, as sebaceous cysts become larger, they protrude farther into the subcutaneous fat, and it becomes more difficult to demonstrate the

claw sign. The claw sign may not be equally well seen around all the edge of the lesion, and a specific effort must be made to demonstrate origin from the skin (Fig. 10–77).

3. The lesion lies entirely within the subcutaneous fat, but the gland neck or hair follicle within which the lesion arose can be shown coursing through the skin. In sebaceous cysts with visible gland necks, there are two sonographic appearances. In the first case, the neck of the obstructed gland becomes dilated and funnel shaped. The narrow part of the funnel lies superficially, and the wide part is contiguous with the rounded fundus of the gland that lies within the subcutaneous fat. The overall shape is similar to that of a spindle top. The spindle top shape will only be seen in the tissue plane that is in the long axis to the obstructed sebaceous gland. However, in the short axis, enough of the gland lies within the skin that the claw sign is demonstrable (Fig. 10–78). The second appearance is subtle and far more difficult to appreciate. The gland neck or the hair follicle into which the gland drains is only minimally dilated and tubular in shape, and the fundus of the gland appears to lie entirely within the subcutaneous fat (Fig. 10–79). As is the case with the spindle-top shape, the tubular gland neck is visible only when the scan plane is parallel to the long axis of the obstructed sebaceous gland. In other planes, it is not demonstrable. In sebaceous cysts with narrow gland necks, the obstructed fundus of the gland lies

(text continued on page 329)

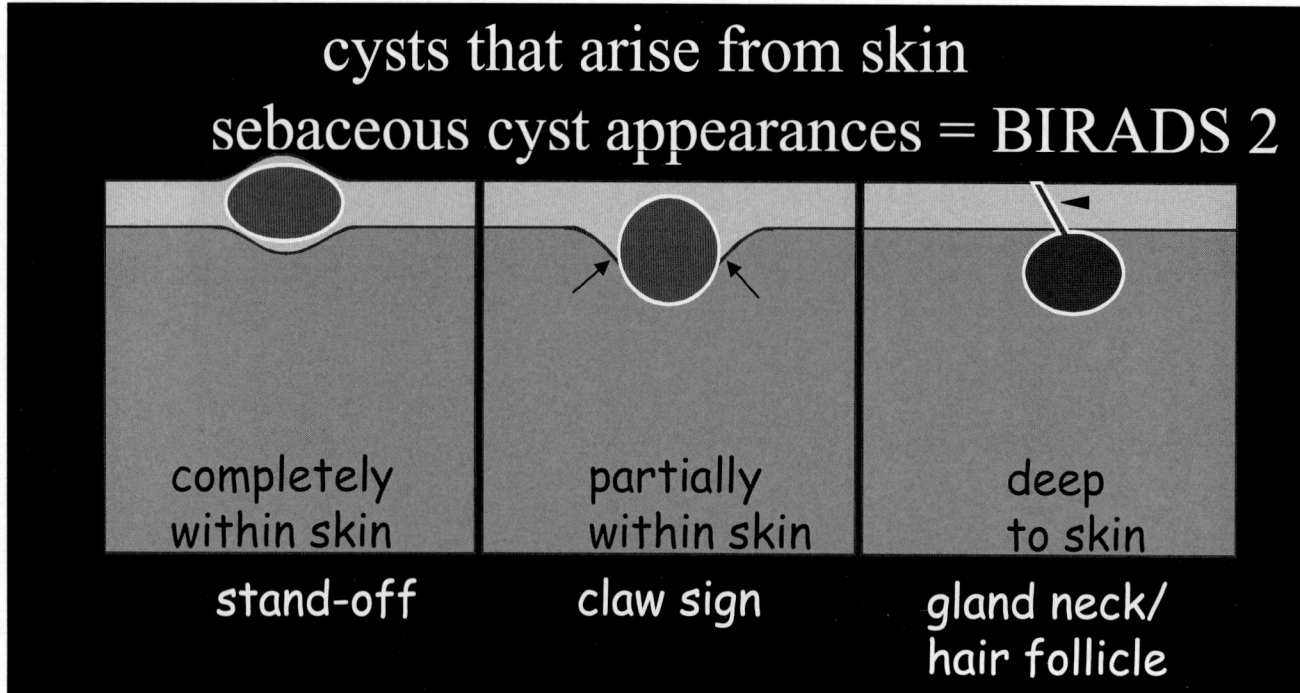

cysts that arise from skin
sebaceous cyst appearances = BIRADS 2

completely within skin	partially within skin	deep to skin
stand-off	claw sign	gland neck/ hair follicle

FIGURE 10–75 Complex cysts of skin origin are benign (BIRADS 2). Complex cysts of skin origin (mostly sebaceous cysts) can have three different sonographic appearances. The lesion may lie entirely within the skin (**left**). The cyst may lie mainly within the subcutaneous fat, but careful evaluation of the edges of the cyst may show skin wrapping around the lesion in the configuration of a claw (**middle**). Finally, the entire lesion may appear to lie in the subcutaneous fat deep to the skin, but careful scanning with very-high-resolution equipment may show the hair follicle into which the gland drains *(arrowhead)*.

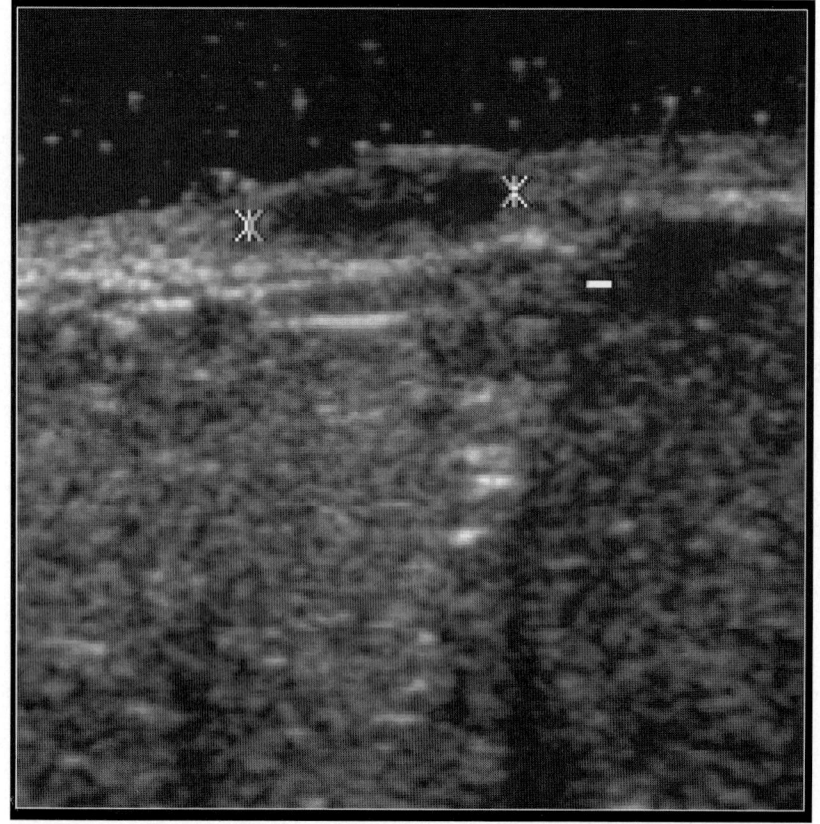

FIGURE 10–76 This complex sebaceous cyst lies entirely within the skin and is benign (BIRADS 2). As in this case, an acoustic standoff of gel is usually necessary.

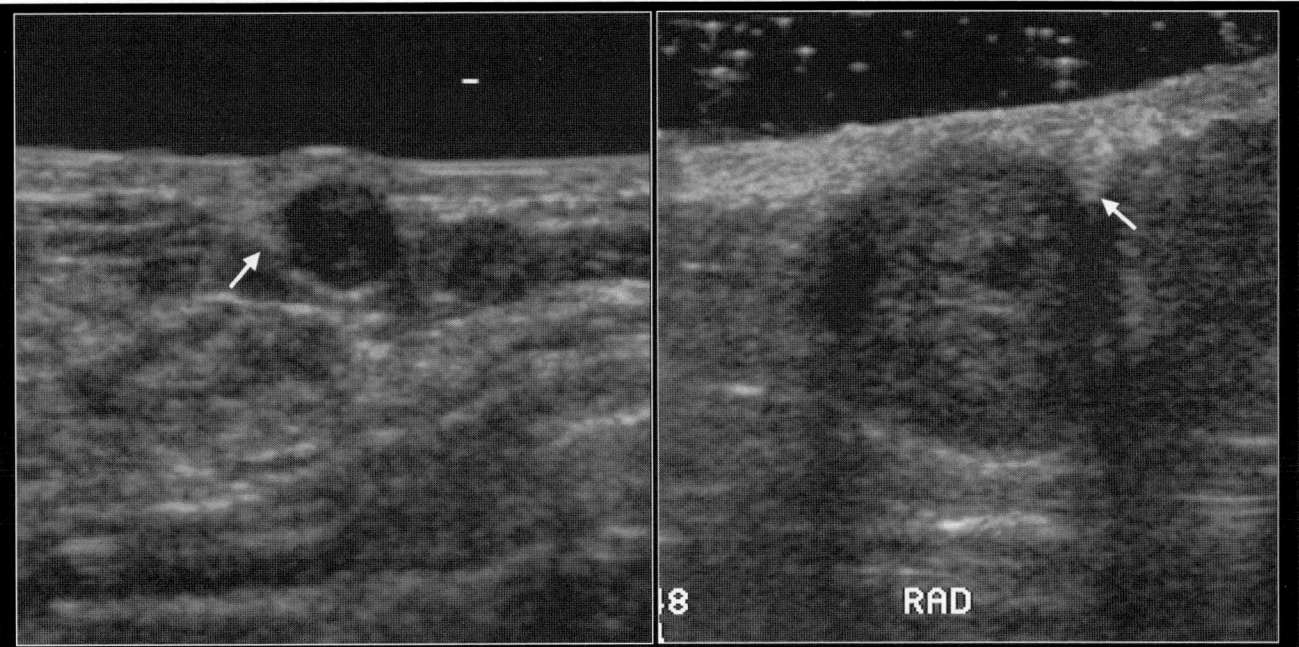

FIGURE 10–77 Both the large complex sebaceous cyst shown on the **right** and the smaller complex sebaceous cyst shown on the **left** lie within the subcutaneous fat. In each case, however, a "claw" of hyperechoic skin *(arrows)* wraps around the edge of the lesion. Note that a standoff pad was used for the **left** image, and a standoff of acoustic gel was used to obtain the **right** image. Without a standoff or a 1.5-D array transducer, the claw sign is difficult to demonstrate.

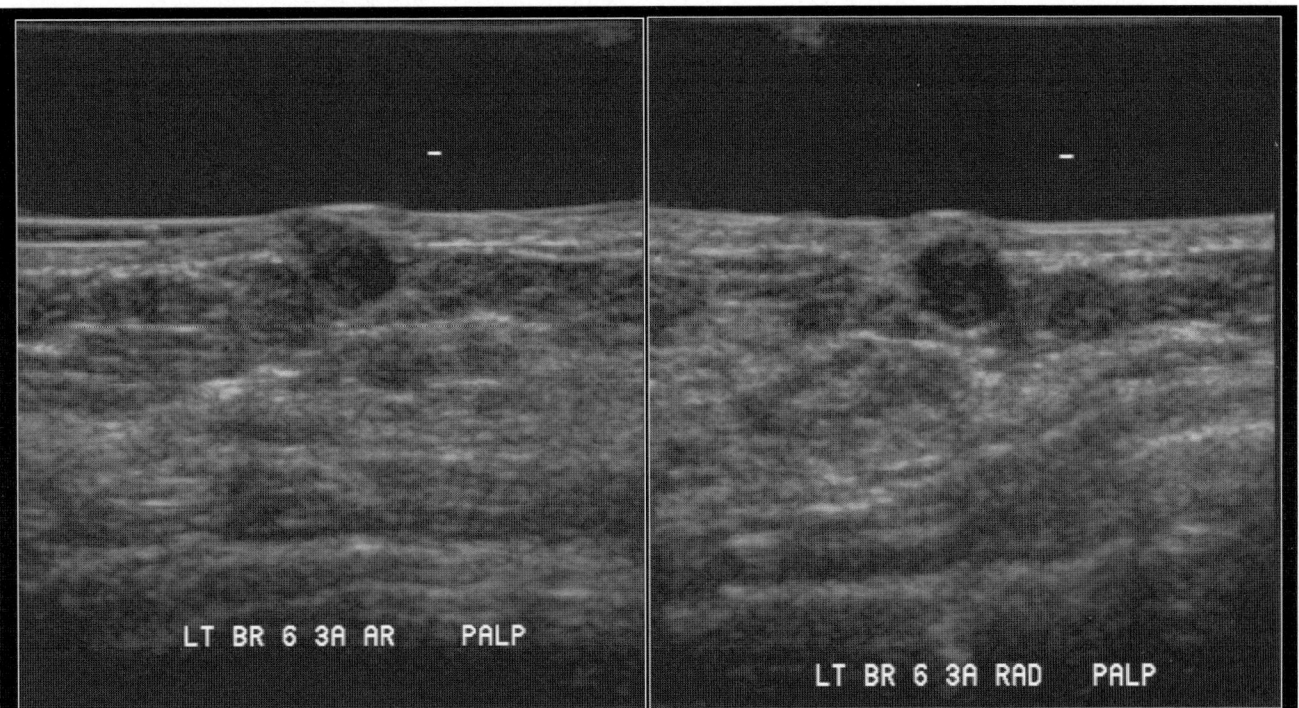

FIGURE 10–78 This complex sebaceous cyst lies in the subcutaneous fat, but the dilated gland neck that has a funnel shape protrudes through the hyperechoic skin. The extension of the gland neck or hair follicle through the skin is seen only in the antiradial view.

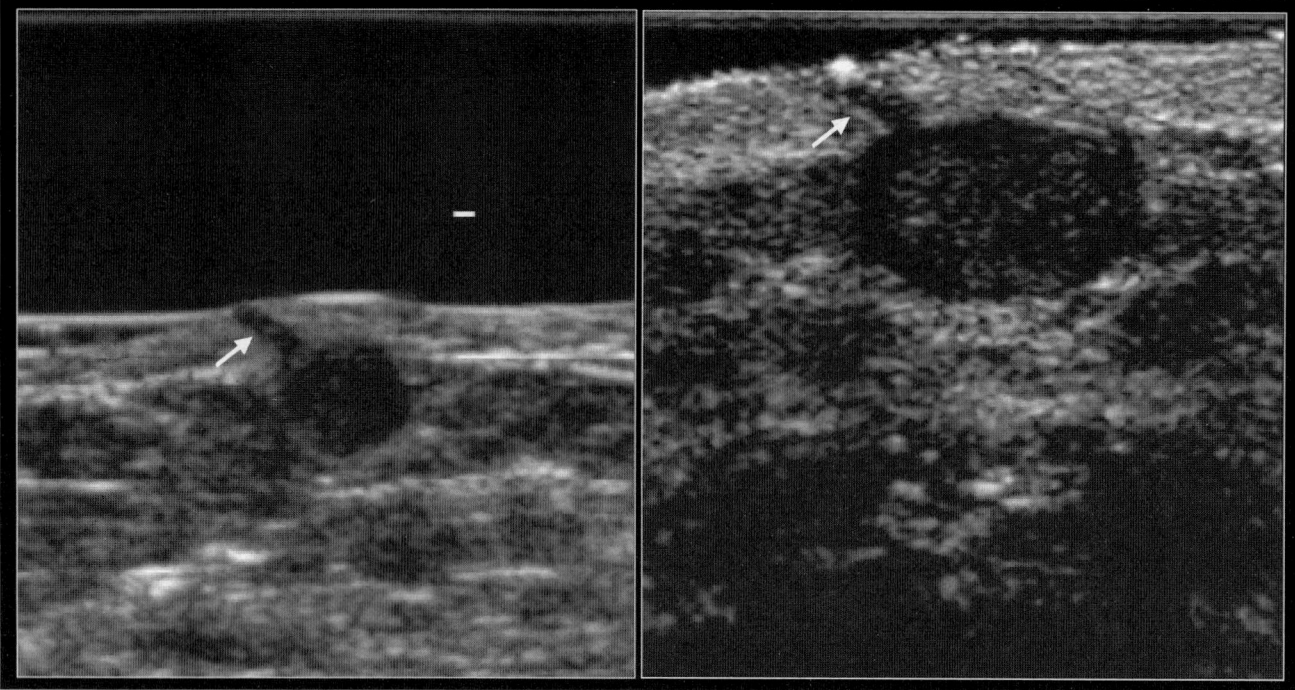

FIGURE 10–79 These sebaceous cysts lie within the subcutaneous fat rather than within the skin. However, the gland neck or hair follicle into which the sebaceous gland drains is seen as a hypoechoic tubular structure *(arrows)* passing through the hyperechoic skin. The **left** image was obtained with an 8-mm acoustic standoff pad. The **right** image was obtained with a thin layer of gel and a 1.5-D array transducer.

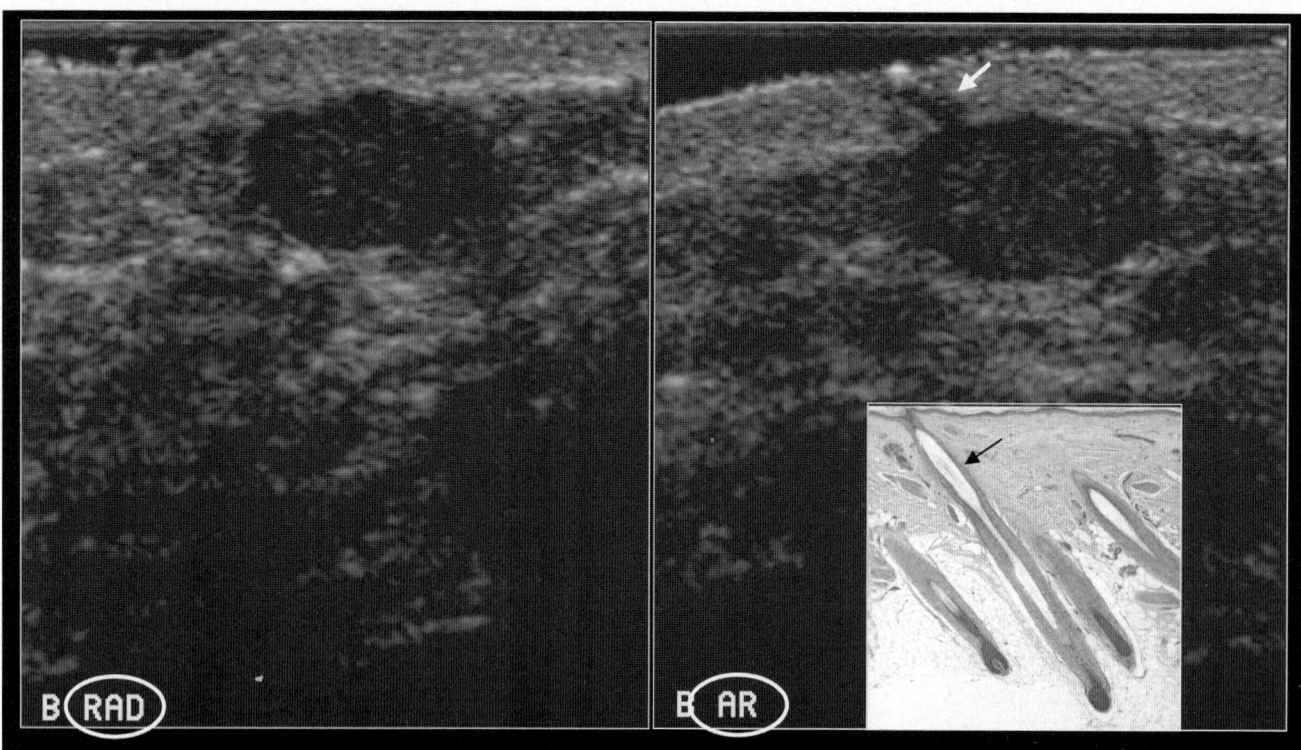

FIGURE 10–80 The gland neck or hair follicle that passes through the skin *(arrow)* is seen only in one view of this complex sebaceous cyst. This structure must be specifically sought in any superficially located lesion, or it will not be identified. Because the hair follicle into which the sebaceous cyst drains is obliquely oriented, "heeling or toeing" of the transducer may be necessary to improve the angle of incidence. In the left image, obtained with a straight anterior approach the hair follicle cannot be seen. In the antiradial view (**right**), the left end of the transducer was place closer to the skin (heeled) in order to better demonstrate the hair follicle.

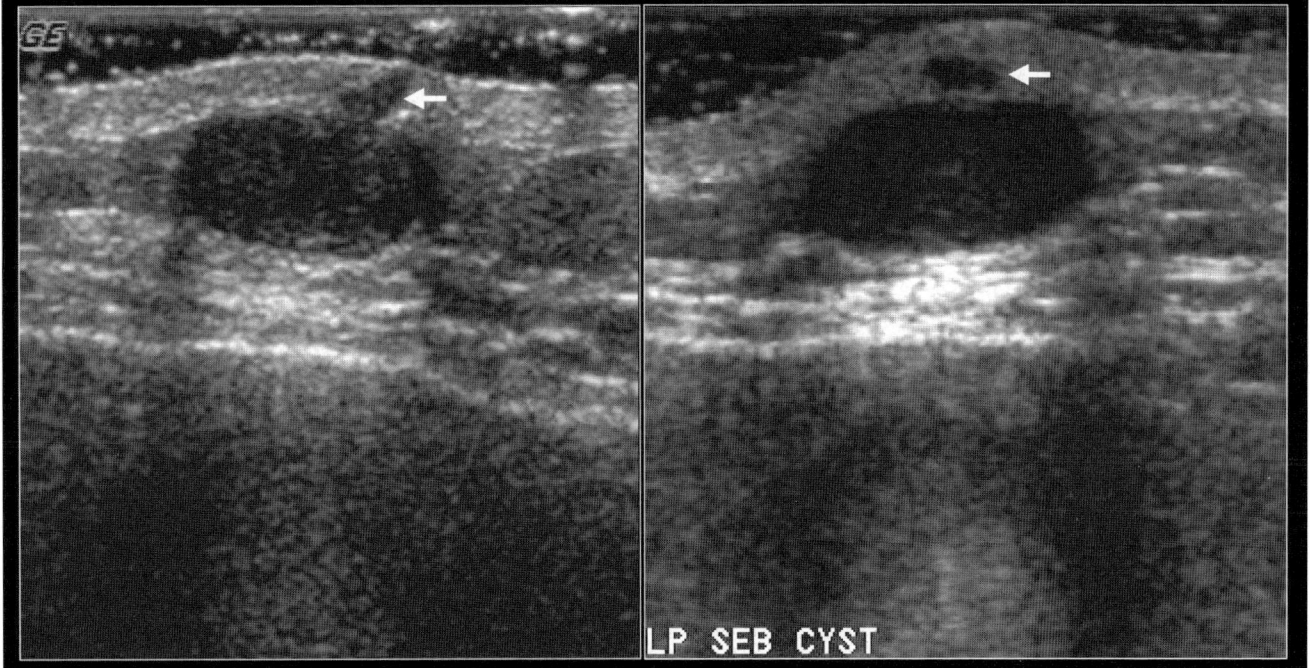

FIGURE 10–81 The gland neck appearance changes with time, and in chronic sebaceous cysts, it may become smaller or even disappear. The image on the **left** was obtained on the initial examination. The image on the **right** was obtained 1 year later. Note that most of the gland neck is no longer visible.

entirely within the subcutaneous fat deep to the skin; hence, there is no demonstrable claw sign (Fig. 10–80). The tubular gland neck is so superficial (less than 2 mm deep) that even with an acoustic standoff, it is better demonstrated with a 1.5-D array transducer (see Chapter 2, Fig. 2–10). The presence of a demonstrable swollen hair follicle is associated with sebaceous cysts of recent onset. Over time, the hair follicle can become less inflamed and less apparent (Fig. 10–81).

Regardless of the shape and depth of the sebaceous cyst, the internal echogenicity varies tremendously, from anechoic to hyperechoic, depending on the duration of obstruction and relative amounts of fluid and keratin (Fig. 10–82). The more fluid and the more acute the obstruction, the more likely a sebaceous cyst is to appear anechoic or nearly anechoic. The more chronic the obstruction and the more lipid and keratinaceous material within the cyst, the more likely it is to become hyperechoic.

Sebaceous cysts frequently become inflamed. The sonographic findings are similar to those of inflammation elsewhere in the body. In sebaceous cysts that lie within the skin completely, the inflammation caused the skin around the lesion to become thicker, less echogenic, and hyperemic (Fig. 10–83). Noninflamed sebaceous cysts have no demonstrable blood flow. Inflamed sebaceous cysts that lie within the subcutaneous tissue become more hypoechoic,

develop thickened walls, and cause the surrounding fat to become hyperechoic and hyperemic.

Although demonstrating origin within the skin is extremely strong evidence of benignity, remember than cancer can secondarily involve the skin. Large cancers that involve the skin will not be confused with sebaceous cysts and do not cause diagnostic difficulties. However, a small percentage of TDLUs are "ectopic" and lie within the subcutaneous zone near the skin. Small malignancies that arise within these ectopic TDLUs may involve the skin at a very early stage. In such cases, the sonographic findings may appear at first glance similar to those of certain sebaceous cysts (Fig. 10–84). Usually one or more suspicious findings are present and prevent misdiagnosis as a sebaceous cyst.

Epidermal inclusion cysts are similar to sebaceous cysts but have features that help distinguish them from sebaceous cysts sonographically. Epidermal inclusion cysts can be caused by surgery, needle biopsy, or penetrating trauma but can also arise in preexisting sebaceous cysts when squamous epithelium grows down into the fundus of the gland. The squamous epithelium continuously forms layers of keratin that slough into the cavity of the cyst, resulting in characteristic sonographic appearances. The sloughed keratin may form multiple, loosely adherent layers that appear echogenic on sonograms. The multilaminar echogenic

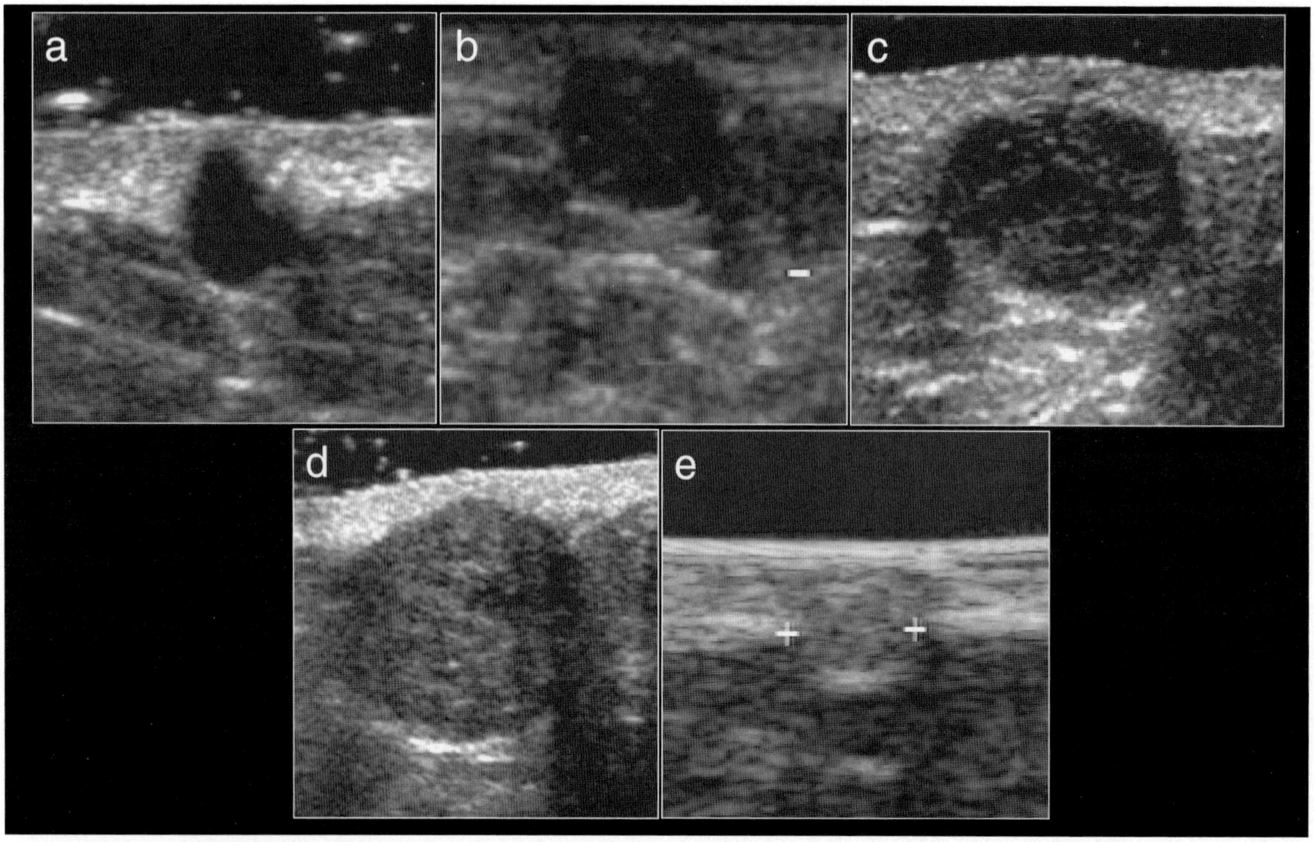

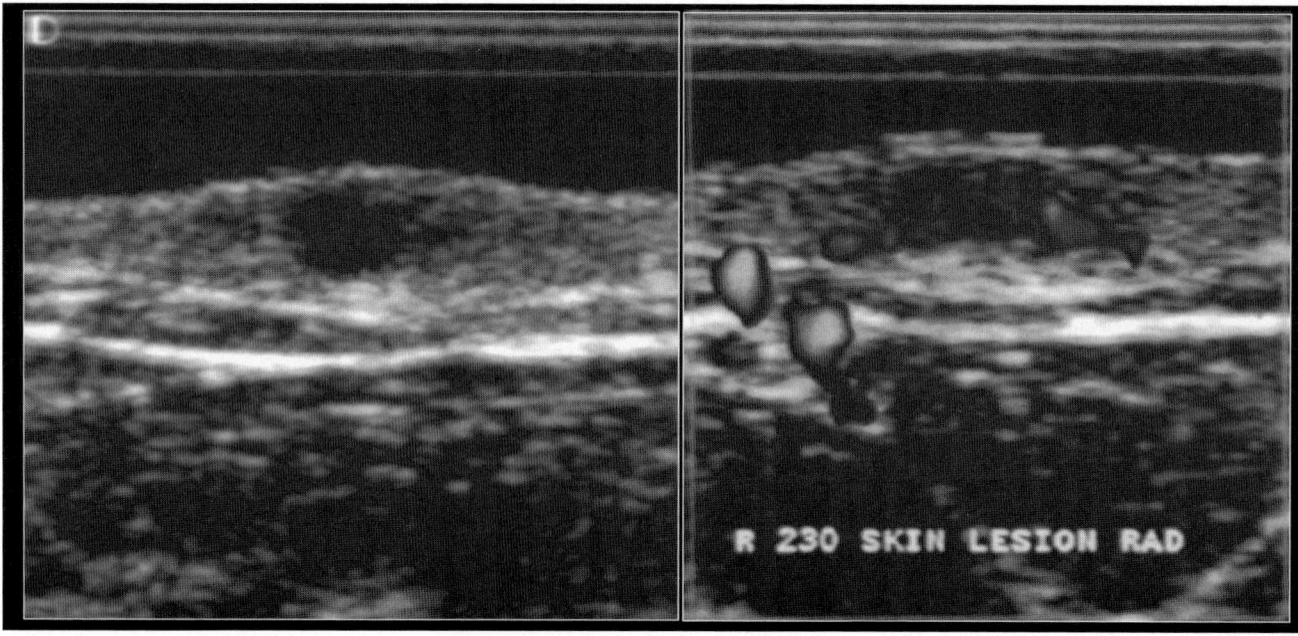

FIGURE 10–82 The echogenicity of sebaceous cysts varies tremendously. They can appear anechoic *(a)*, severely hypoechoic *(b)*, mildly hypoechoic *(c)*, isoechoic *(d)*, or even hyperechoic *(e)*.

FIGURE 10–83 When sebaceous cysts become inflamed, the skin around them becomes thickened, less echogenic, and hyperemic.

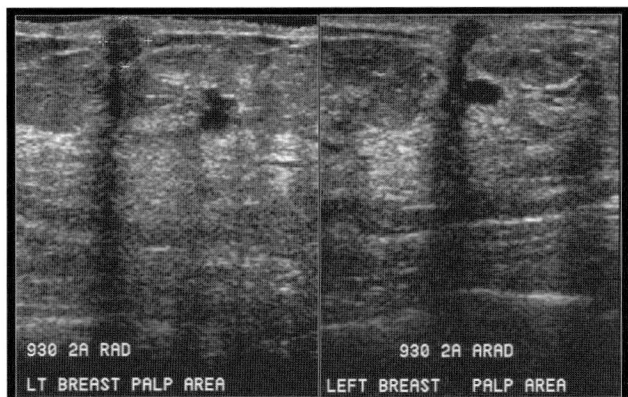

FIGURE 10–84 Occasionally, a small malignancy arising within an ectopic terminal ductolobular unit that lies within a Cooper's ligament may involve the skin at an early stage and simulate a sebaceous cyst.

appearance can be described as onion-skin–like (Fig. 10–85). When the sloughed keratin is more disorganized, it may form a central nodule surrounded by fluid that has strands of keratin adhering to its surface, causing a "stringy" appearance (Fig. 10–86). When the sloughed keratin forms a denser nodule within the cyst, it may have a pearl-like appearance similar to the appearance of sebum within an ovarian dermoid that may cause acoustic shad-

owing, even when not calcified. The keratin nodule may also calcify (Fig. 10–87).

Any complex cyst can have a mixture of benign BI-RADS 2 findings and suspicious BIRADS 4a findings. As is always the case with any lesion having multiple different findings in different BIRADS categories, the entire lesion should be assigned to highest BIRADS category finding present. The finding with the lower BIRADS risk category is always ignored because we must assign risk in such a fashion to take into account that breast cancer is heterogeneous, not only from lesion to lesion, but sometimes even within an individual lesion. Thus, a malignant breast lesion may have a mixture of benign and worrisome findings. The only way to avoid false-negative findings in such cases is to ignore the more benign findings and assign the characteristics of the higher-risk findings to the lesion as a whole. For example, milk of calcium and cholesterol crystals can sometimes be associated with higher-risk findings such as eccentric wall thickening or fluid–debris levels. When milk of calcium (BIRADS 2) is associated with eccentric wall thickening (BIRADS 4a), the milk of calcium is ignored, and the overall characterization of the complex cysts is that of the eccentric wall thickening (Fig. 10–88). Similarly, when mobile internal echoes (BIRADS 2) are associated with an isoechoic thickened cyst wall (BIRADS 3), the mobile echoes are ignored, and the complex cyst is assigned to the category of the fluid–debris level.

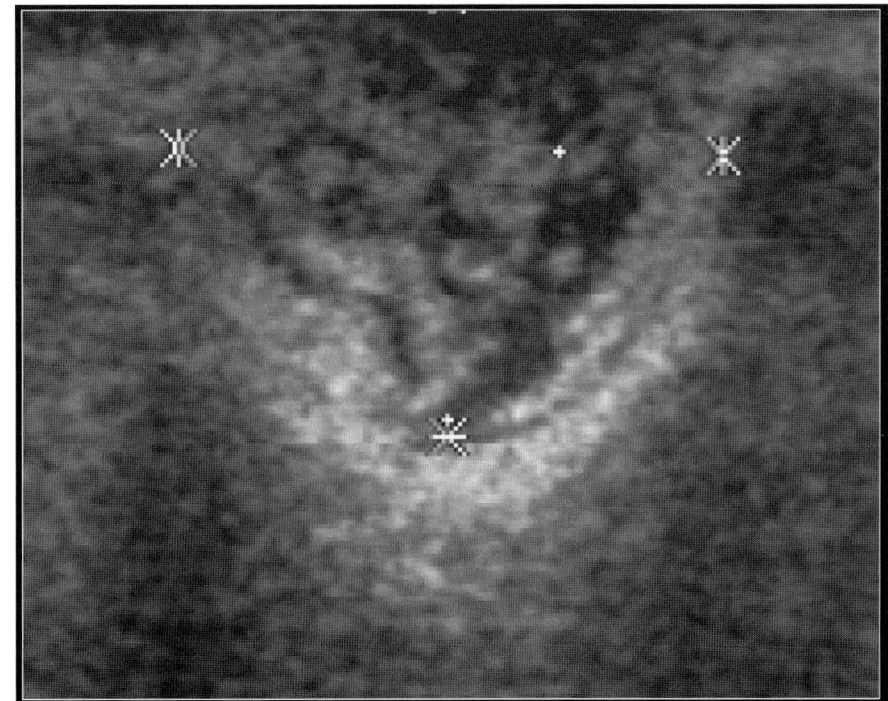

FIGURE 10–85 Epidermal inclusion cysts differ from sebaceous cysts in that squamous cells within the cyst produce keratin that can have one of several different appearances. Epidermal inclusion cysts may result from surgery, needle procedures, or penetrating trauma, but they can also arise from squamous metaplasia within sebaceous cysts. One of the sonographic appearances typical of epidermal inclusion cysts is a hyperechoic, multilaminar appearance, like an onion skin. The multiple layers represent layers of sloughed keratin within the cyst.

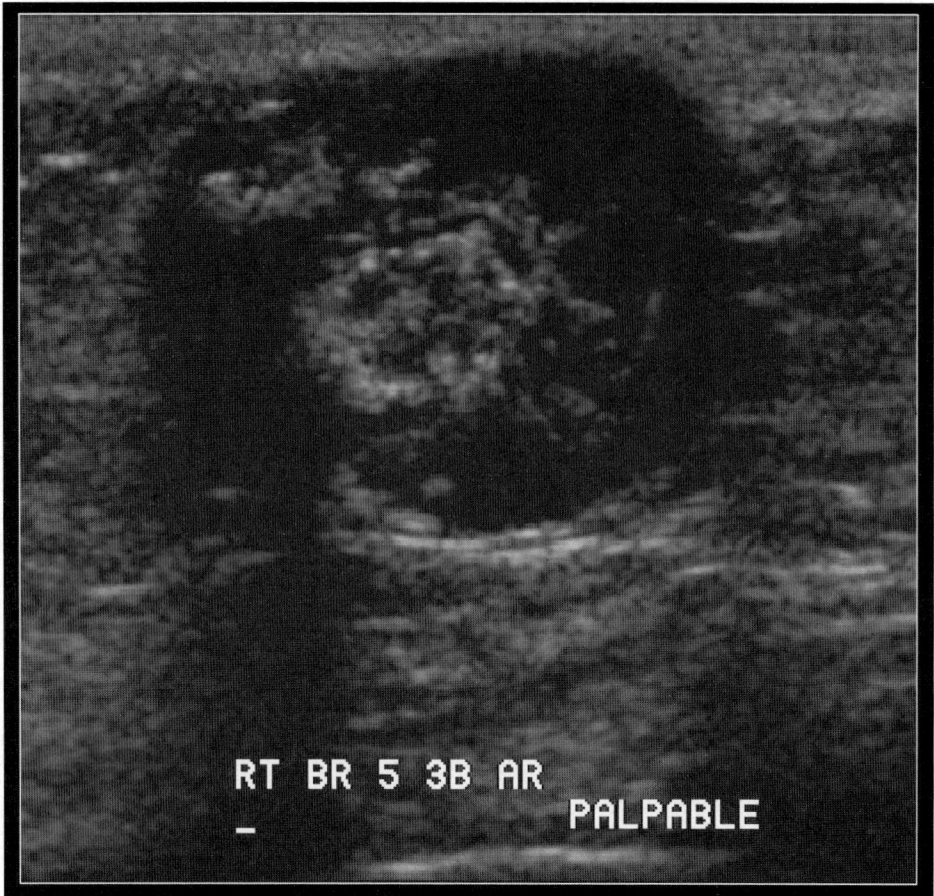

FIGURE 10–86 The keratin produced within an epidermal inclusion cyst can give rise to a central nodule that has strands of keratin attached to its surface, producing a stringy appearance.

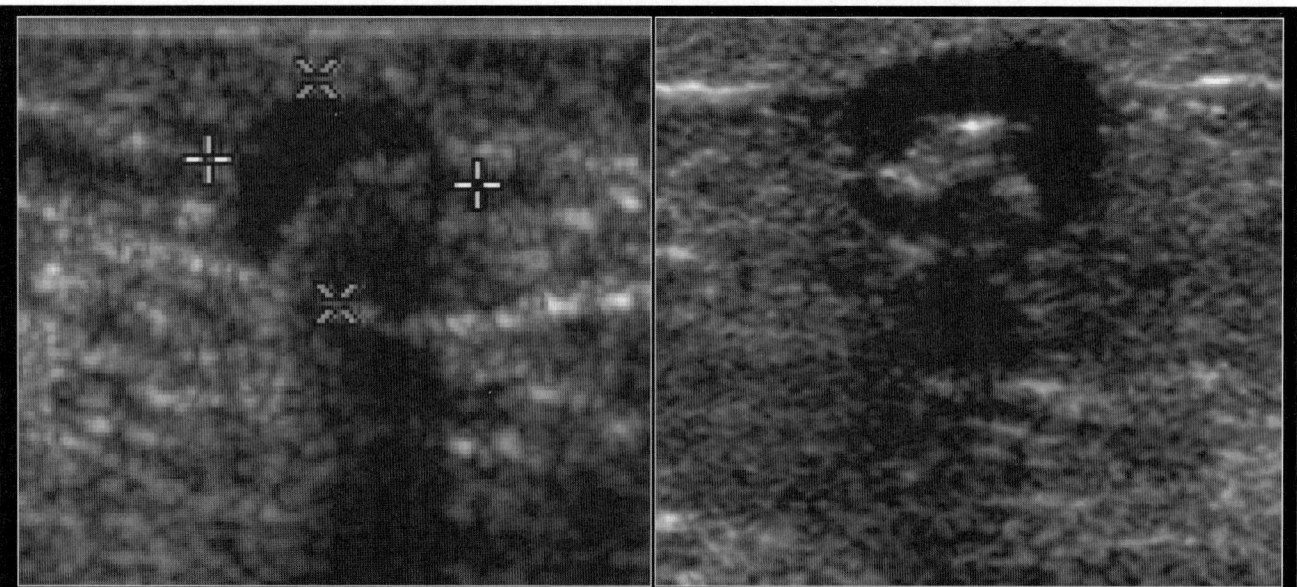

FIGURE 10–87 The keratin within the epidermal inclusion cyst can form a dense central nodule that may give rise to acoustic shadowing, even without being calcified. This appearance is similar to that of sebum within an ovarian dermoid **(left)**. The dense nodule of keratin that lies within an epidermal inclusion cyst may calcify, as in this case.

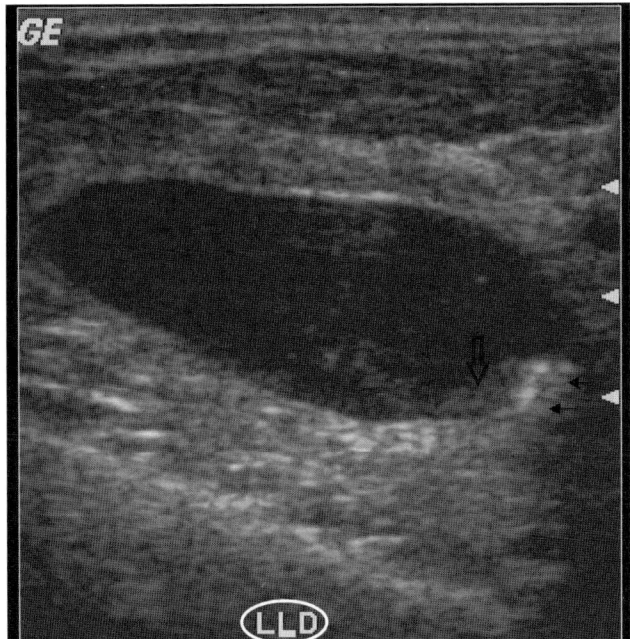

FIGURE 10–88 Some cysts have a combination of findings that must be assigned to different BIRADS categories. In this case, definitively benign milk of calcium (BIRADS 2) coexists with a fluid–debris level (BIRADS 3). Whenever a mixture of findings is present, the overall lesion characterization is that of the highest BIRADS finding. Thus, the milk of calcium is ignored, and the cyst is assigned to the BIRADS category of the fluid–debris level. This must be done because of the heterogeneity of breast cancer. Many cancers have mixtures of benign and suspicious findings that require us to err on the side of caution.

STEP 5: IF BIRADS 2 FINDINGS CANNOT BE IDENTIFIED, SEARCH FOR BIRADS 3 FINDINGS

BIRADS 3 findings include the following:

- Eccentric, nonmobile concave wall thickening (acorn cyst)
- Diffuse, low-level echoes filling entire cyst
- Indeterminate cystic versus solid lesions

Eccentric Concave Wall Thickening

The typical appearance of PAM is as an eccentric wall thickening that has a concave inner margin that parallels its intact thin, echogenic outer capsule. Only a small minority of cases of PAM present as mural nodules with convex inner margins. The key sonographic findings supporting the diagnosis of PAM are preservation of the thin echogenic capsule, lack of a fibrovascular stalk, as discussed earlier in the section on Certain Mural Nodules, and a slightly stringy internal margin because of the papillary nature of the apocrine metaplasia (Fig. 10–89). The risk for malignancy in such lesions is less than 2%, and the lesions, therefore, can be classified as BIRADS category 3, probably benign. Because the concave thickening has a configuration similar to the cap on an acorn, we have termed such complex cysts acorn cysts. Options for acorn cysts are like those for any BIRADS 3 category lesions and include attempted aspiration and short-interval follow-up.

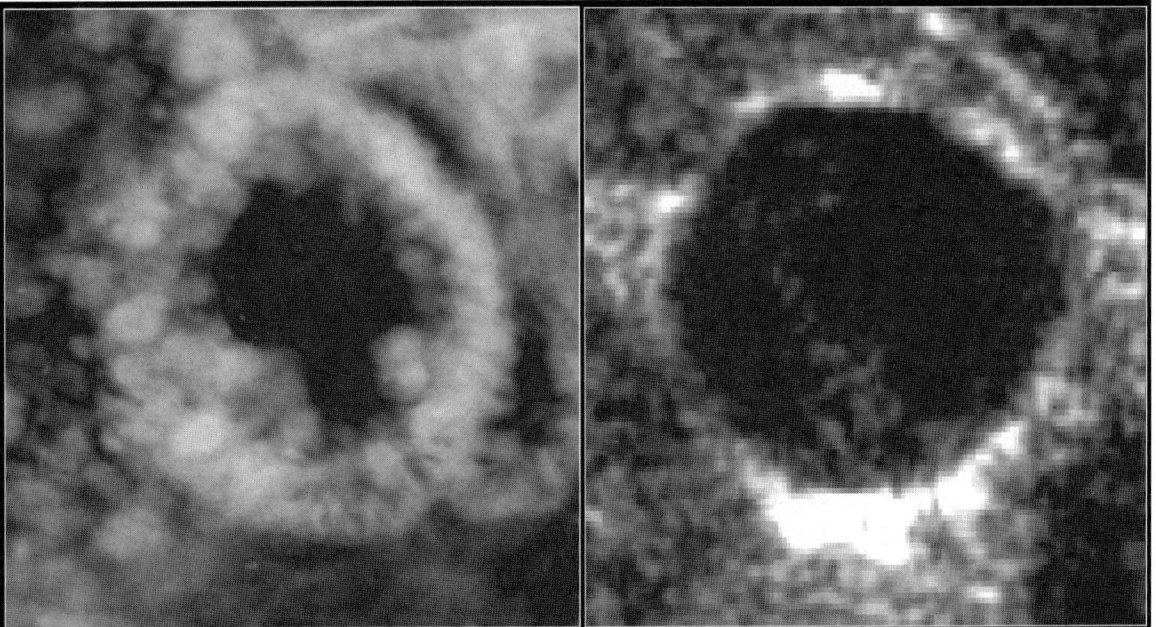

FIGURE 10–89 Although mural nodules caused by papillary apocrine metaplasia (PAM) have been discussed earlier, the most common sonographic appearance of PAM is that of an eccentric wall thickening that is concave inward and parallel to the thin, echogenic cyst wall. The inner margin is irregular because of the papillary nature of the apocrine growth. The texture is hypoechoic and lacy. Because the apocrine growth within the cyst has an appearance similar to the cap on an acorn, such cysts have been termed "acorn cysts." (Gross 3-D histology, video inverted, courtesy of Hanne M. Jensen, MD, University of California at Davis.)

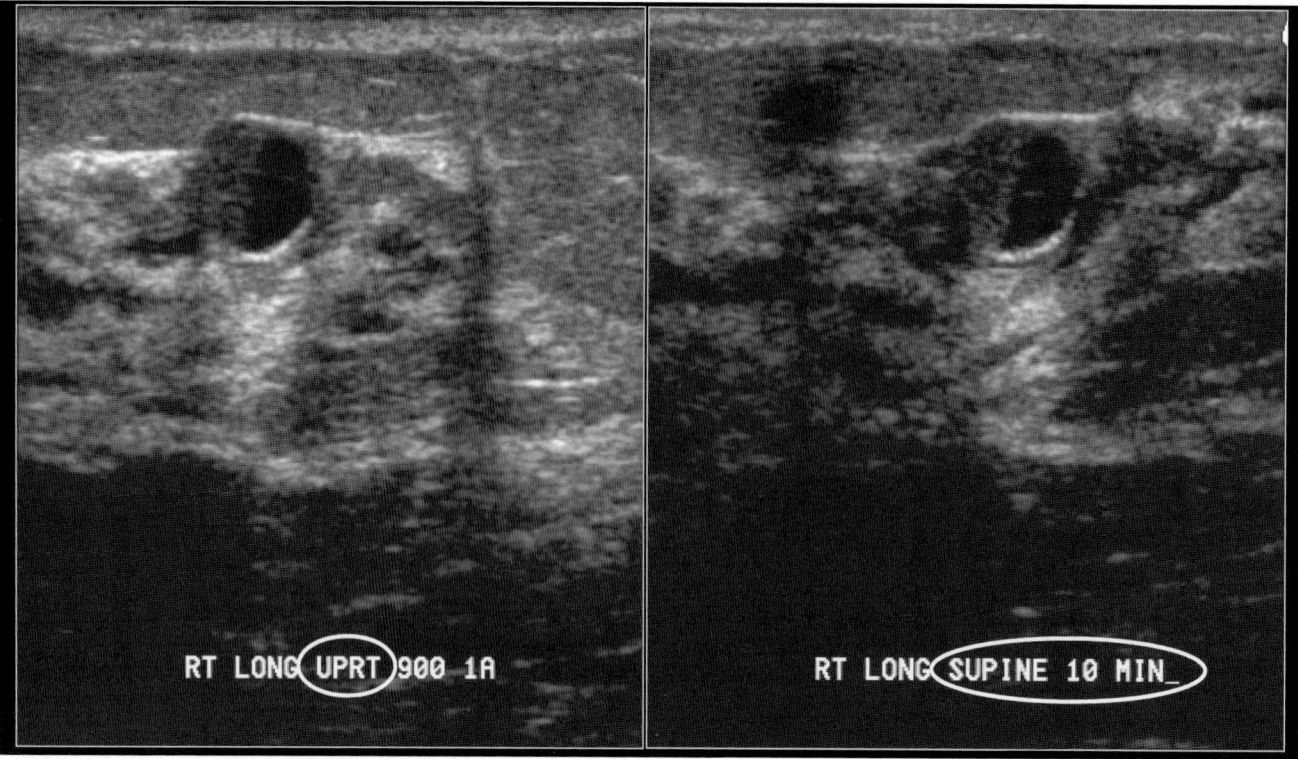

FIGURE 10–90 The sonographic appearance of papillary apocrine metaplasia (PAM) is very similar to that of the lipid layer in cysts that contain fat–fluid levels. However, the position of the PAM is fixed. It does not shift within the cyst when the patient position is changed, and there is no fixed relationship to either the dependent or nondependent position within the cyst. The shape of the interface also differs somewhat from that of a fat–fluid interface.

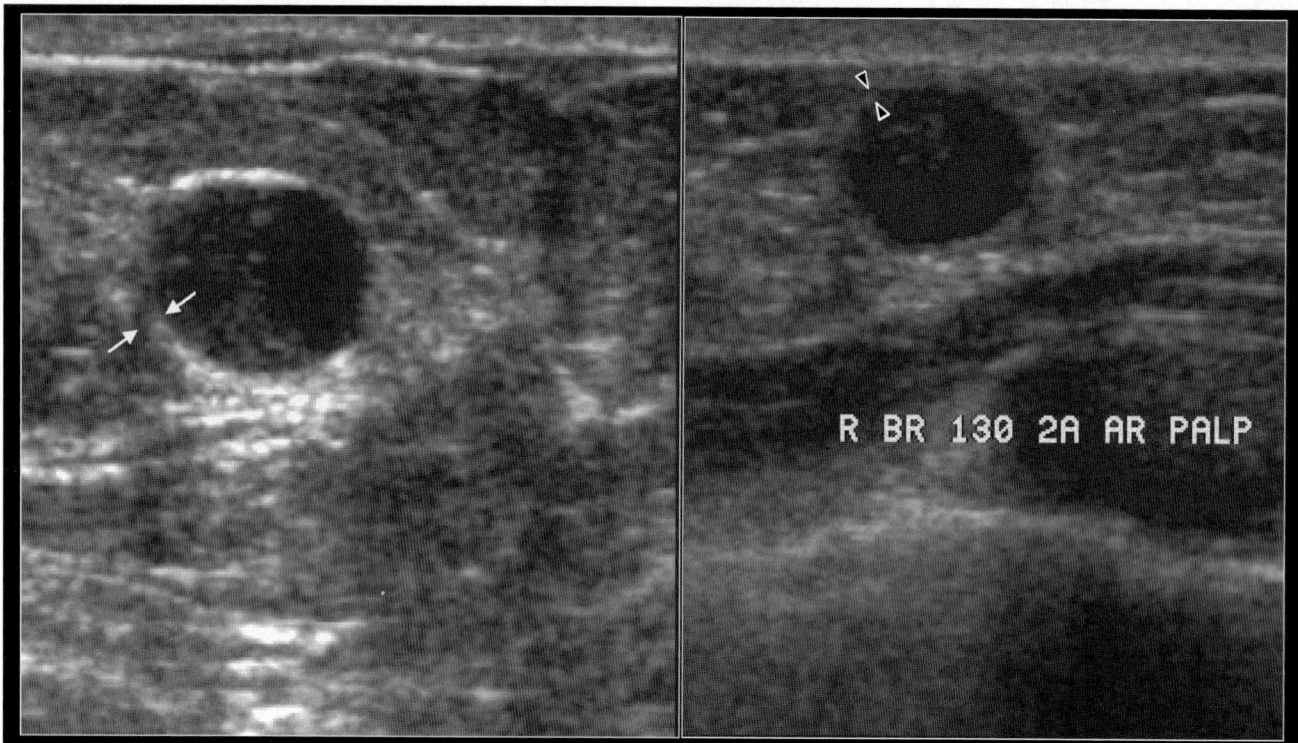

FIGURE 10–91 The shape of the interface between the papillary apocrine metaplasia and the cyst fluid is usually concave (**left**) but is convex inward in a significant minority of cases (**right**). Regardless of the shape of the papillary growth, the thin, echogenic capsule all along the point of attachment of the papillary growth is preserved *(arrows and arrowheads)*. Differences between the appearance of mural nodules caused by papillary apocrine metaplasia, intracystic papilloma, and intracystic carcinoma are discussed in greater detail earlier in the chapter text and illustrated in Figs. 10–25 through 10–31 and 10–34.

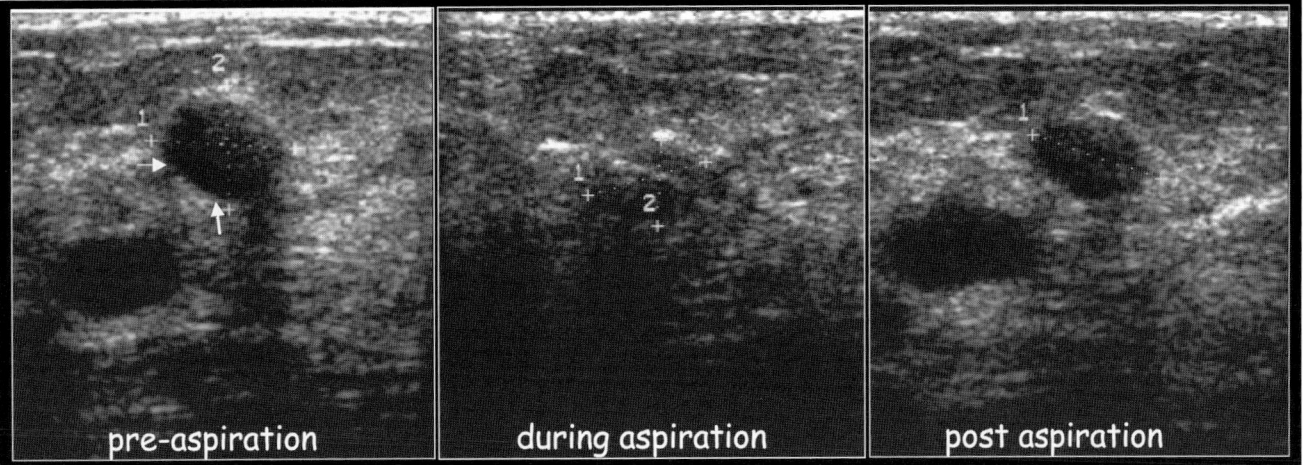

FIGURE 10–92 Acorn cysts caused by papillary apocrine metaplasia (PAM) can only be partially aspirated. The fluid contents *(arrows)* can be aspirated, but the papillary apocrine growth is firmly attached to the cyst wall and cannot be aspirated. The residual lesion (**right**) is the size of the PAM component before aspiration (**left**).

A cyst with a fat–fluid level in which the fatty layer is concave can simulate an acorn cyst. However, changing the patient's position should always enable us to distinguish between PAM and a fat–fluid level if adequate time is allowed for the change in the position of the fat–fluid level. Fat–fluid levels will eventually change to a new nondependent position in the upright or left lateral decubitus position (Figs. 10–68 to 10–70), but PAM remains fixed in position that is unrelated to the nondependent wall of the cyst (Fig. 10–90).

Although the shape of the inner surface of papillary apocrine metaplasia is concave and parallel to the outer cyst wall in most cases, the shape is convex in a significant minority of patients (Fig. 10–91). The convex configuration of PAM is more difficult to distinguish from papillomas or carcinoma. In such cases, it is important to assess the capsule along the point of attachment, to determine its shape (Figs. 10–27 and 10–28), and to assess for the presence of a fibrovascular stalk with color or power Doppler as discussed in the section above on assessment of mural nodules and illustrated in the color prints in Chapter 20 (see Figs. 20–28 to 20–32).

Conversely, although papillomas and carcinomas usually have a convex inner border, a minority will have a concave inner margin that can simulate the usual case of PAM. The papillomas or carcinoma will more often show evidence of loss of the outer thin, echogenic capsule and duct extension (Figs. 10–27 to 10–28) and will be far more likely to have a Doppler demonstrable fibrovascular stalk.

Acorn cysts caused by PAM can also be differentiated from similar-appearing cysts that contain fat–fluid levels by attempting to aspirate them. As noted earlier, cysts with fat–fluid levels can be completely aspirated. On the other

hand, cysts containing PAM filling a significant portion of the cyst can only be partially aspirated—the fluid contents can be aspirated, but the papillary apocrine growth is attached firmly enough to the wall that it will remain at the end of the procedure and will require biopsy for confirmation of diagnosis (Fig. 10–92).

Complex Cysts Filled with Diffuse, Low-Level Echoes and Indeterminate Cystic Versus Solid Lesions

The discussions of complex cysts filled with diffuse, low-level internal echoes and indeterminate cystic versus solid lesions must be undertaken together. There is so much overlap in the sonographic findings that, in most cases, it cannot be determined with certainty whether a lesion is a cyst filled with diffuse low-level echoes or a solid nodule. To shorten the description of such lesions, they will be termed indeterminate cystic versus solid (ICS) lesions for the remainder of this section.

There are several different histologic entities that can give rise to the ICS lesion appearance:

- Solid lesions such as fibroadenoma
- Encysted papillomas that completely fill a cyst
- Papillary apocrine completely filling a cyst
- Cysts that contain echogenic fluid (such cysts have been called inspissated cysts, gel cysts, foam cysts, and muco-celes in the literature):
- Lipid-laden fluid similar in echogenicity to the lipid layer in cysts that contain fat–fluid levels (the fluid aspirated from such cysts appears to be white and foamy; thus, such cysts have been termed foam cysts)

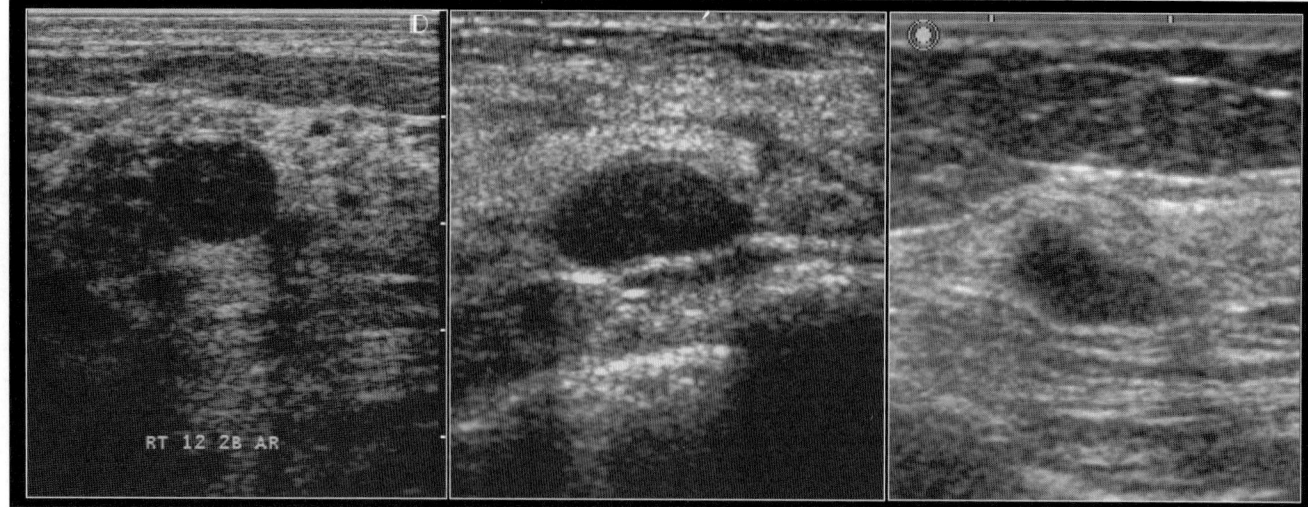

FIGURE 10–93 The shape of cysts that contain diffuse low-level internal echogenicity ("foam cysts" or "gel cysts") or indeterminate cystic versus solid lesions varies. The shape may be spherical (**left**), elliptical, wider than tall (**middle**), or gently lobulated and wider than tall (**right**).

• Inspissated proteinaceous debris that has become gelatinized (the fluid from such cysts appears greenish or yellowish and gelatinous in consistency; thus, such cysts have been termed gel cysts)

Sonographically, these entities usually appear identical to each other; therefore, it is not possible to distinguish between these entities with sonography alone in most cases.

Thus, options for evaluation in most cases include the following:

• Doppler to determine whether the lesion is solid
• Assuming the lesion is solid and characterizing it into a BIRADS category
• Short-interval follow-up
• Attempting to aspirate the lesion

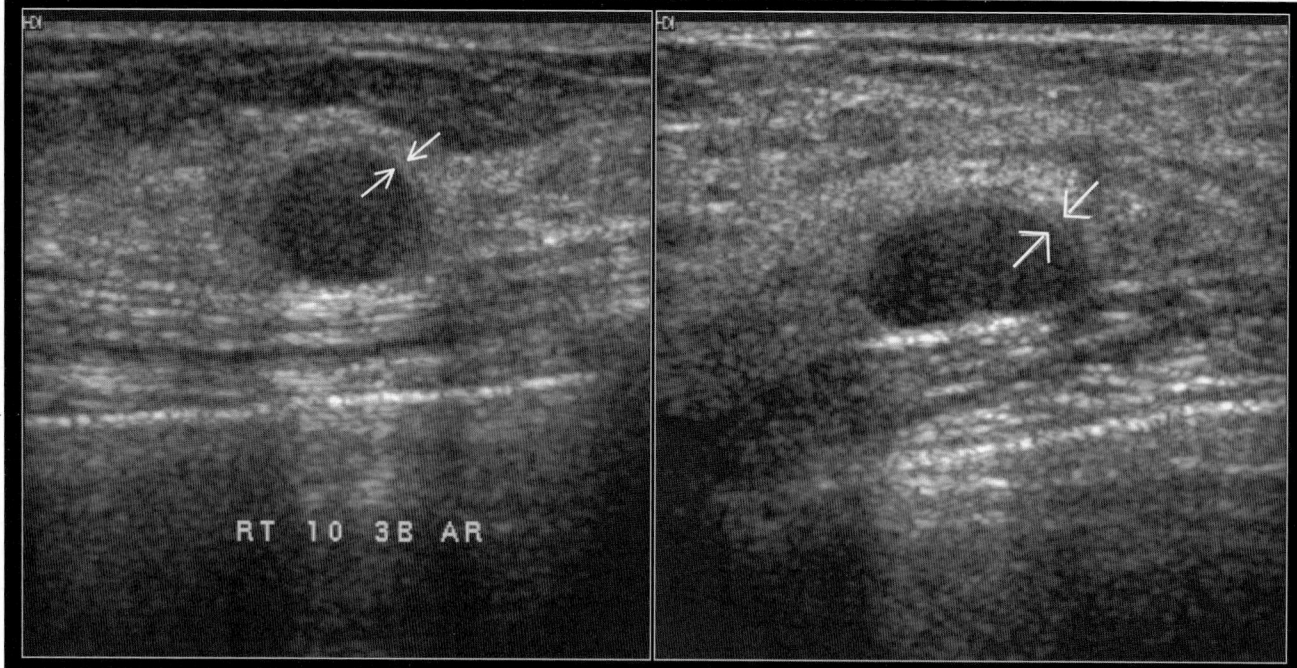

FIGURE 10–94 Most foam or gel cysts or indeterminate cystic versus solid lesions are encompassed in a thin, echogenic capsule (*between arrows*), regardless of shape.

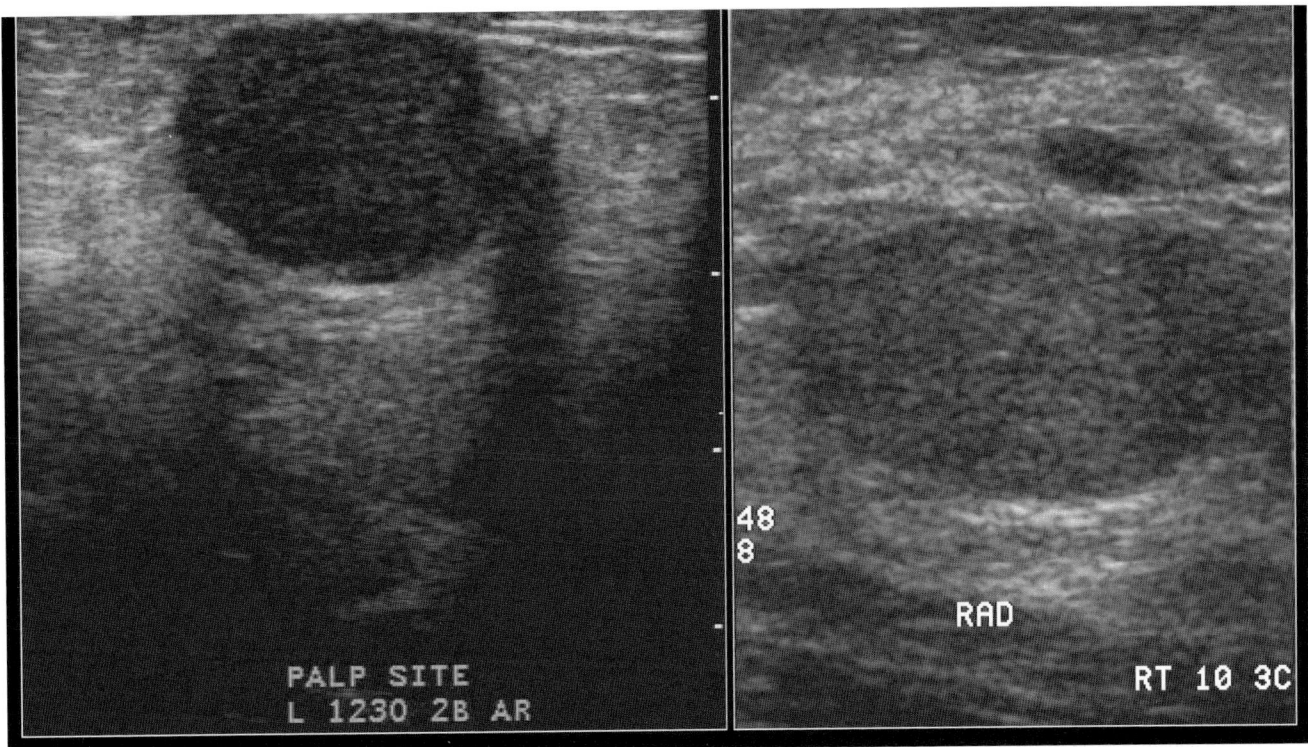

FIGURE 10–95 The echogenicity of foam or gel cysts or indeterminate cystic versus solid lesions varies from hypoechoic (**left**) to isoechoic (**right**).

- Large core needle or vacuum-assisted needle biopsy, depending on the BIRADS category

Most ICS lesions are spherical in shape, but some are oval or gently lobulated (Fig. 10–93). All ICS lesions are encompassed completely by a thin, echogenic capsule (Fig. 10–94). Most ICS lesions are mildly hypoechoic, but some are isoechoic with fat (Fig. 10–95). Most ICS lesions have through-transmission, but a few have normal sound transmission (Fig. 10–96).

In most cases, sonography alone cannot determine the histologic basis for ICS lesions, but an effort should be made to do so because in a minority of cases, differentiation is possible.

First, color Doppler should be used to determine whether there is internal flow. Solid lesions, such as fibroadenomas (see the color images in Chapter 20, Figs. 20–5 and 20–23) and encysted papillomas that completely fill cysts (see the color images in Chapter 20, Fig. 20–24), often have Doppler-demonstrable internal flow. PAM, no matter how florid, virtually never develops a fibrovascular stalk, and foam and gel cysts never have internal flow (Fig. 10–97). Care must be taken not to mistake internal color streaking in a cyst that contains cholesterol crystals for flow within a blood vessel (see the color images in Chapter 20, Fig. 20–33). Pulsed Doppler spectral analysis that shows an

arterial waveform will be found in fibroadenomas but cannot be obtained from the color signal in cysts with cholesterol crystals (Fig. 10–98).

Second, the entire volume of the ICS lesion should be assessed carefully for the presence of a thin, peripheral crescent of fluid that indicates the presence of a mural nodule or lipid layer nearly completely filling the cyst (Fig. 10–99). It is important to scan the whole volume of the cyst in two planes to look for subtle collections of fluid in the periphery. Views taken in one plane, through either the lipid layer or mural nodule, may falsely make the lesion appear to be solid, whereas orthogonal views show it to definitely be a complex cyst (Figs. 10–66 and 10–92).

Once it has been established that the lesion does not have a central vessel or a peripheral crescent of fluid, cysts with mural nodules or fat–fluid levels and definitely solid nodules are excluded, and true ICS lesions remain. General rules can be used to try to distinguish between complex cysts and solid nodules, but as is usually the case, general rules do necessarily reassure individual patients. The general rules that help distinguish complex cysts filled with low-level internal echoes from solid nodules are that the classic complex cysts with diffuse low-level echoes are more typically spherical and hypoechoic and have more through-transmission than do solid nodules. The classic fibroadenoma is elliptical in shape and isoechoic with fat and shows

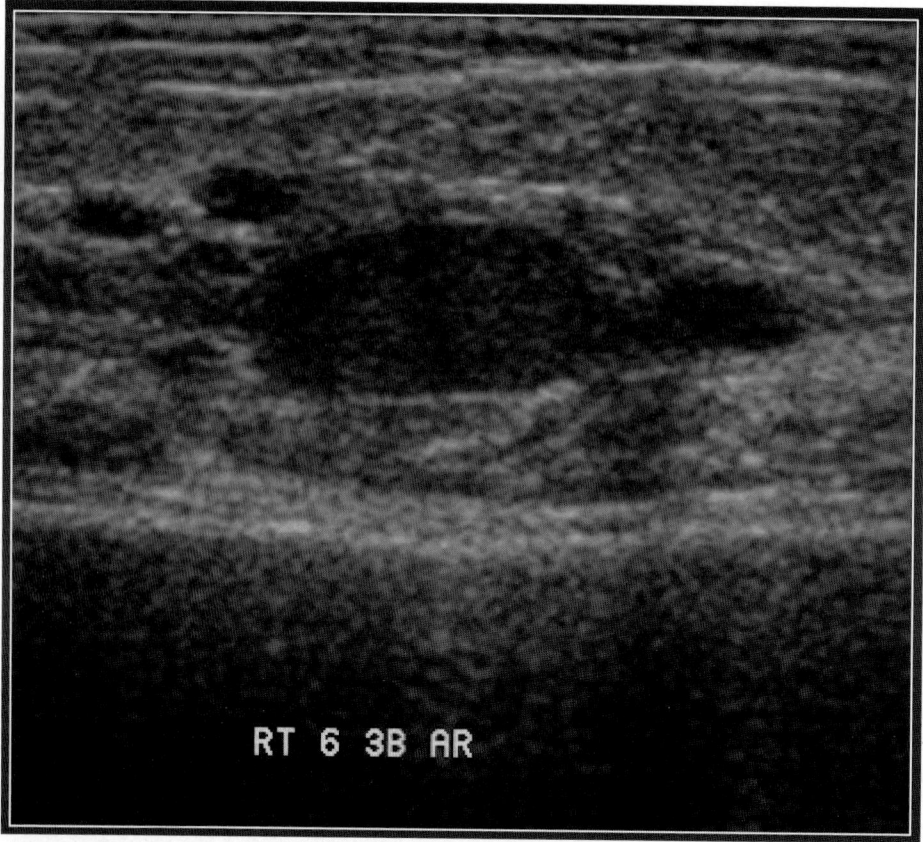

FIGURE 10–96 The sound transmission through foam or gel cysts or indeterminate cystic versus solid lesions varies from normal (**left**) to enhanced (**right**).

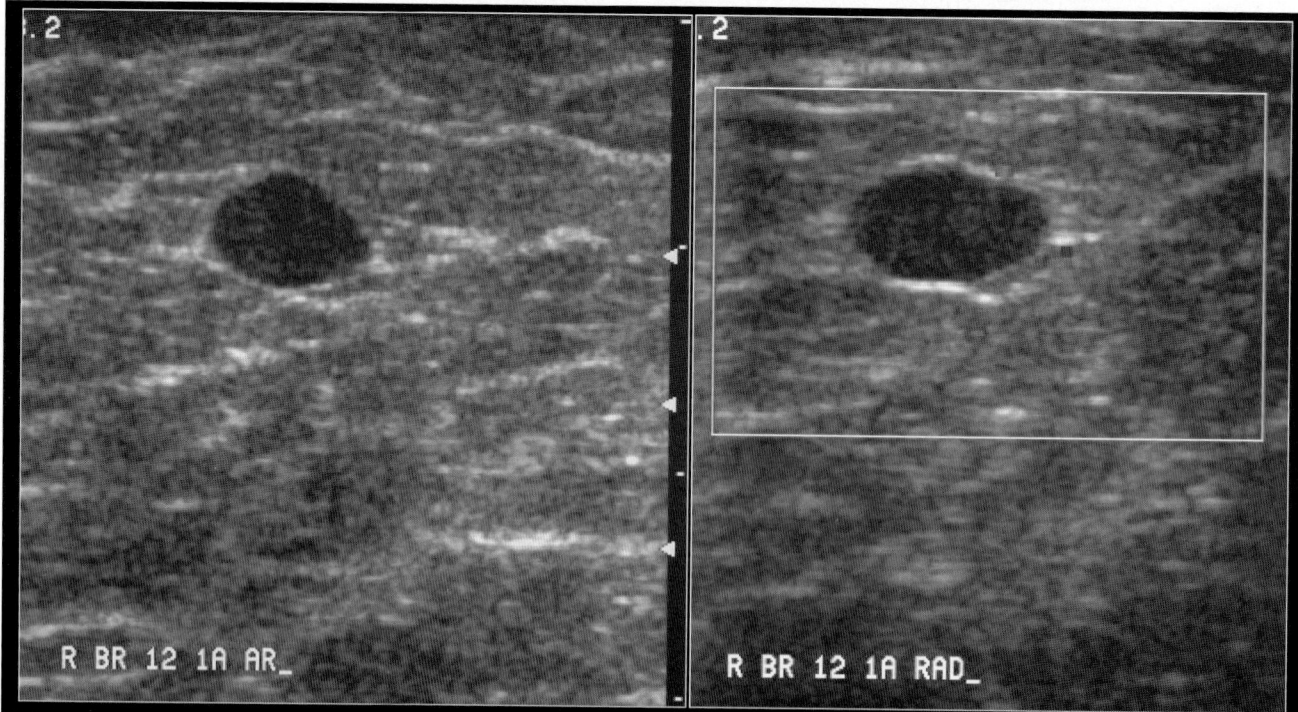

FIGURE 10–97 This indeterminate cystic versus solid lesion has no demonstrable internal flow on color Doppler, indicating that it is more likely to be cystic. It proved to be a foam cyst that could be completely aspirated. The aspirated fluid had a white, foamy appearance typical of a foam cyst.

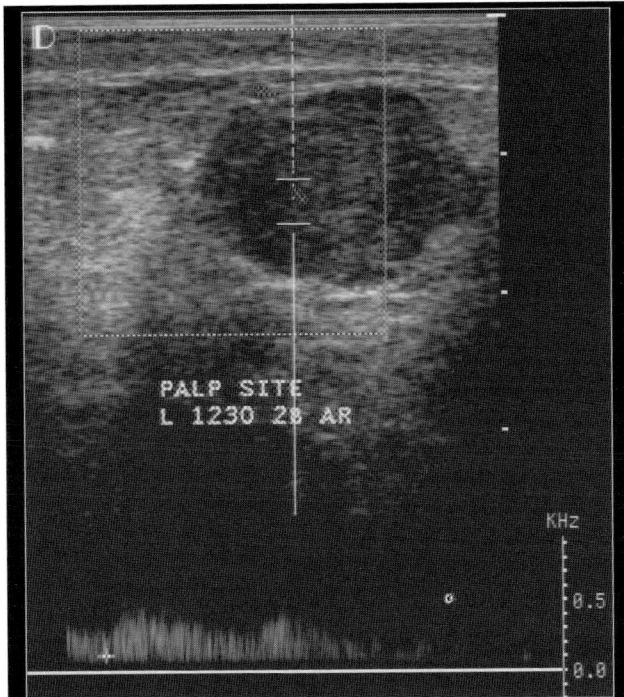

FIGURE 10–98 Pulsed Doppler spectral analysis is helpful in distinguishing blood flow within an indeterminate cystic versus solid lesion from artifact or color streaking. An arterial waveform is more helpful than a venous waveform because it can more easily be distinguished from the random noise created by color streaking. An arterial waveform indicates a solid nodule or encysted papillary lesion with certainty.

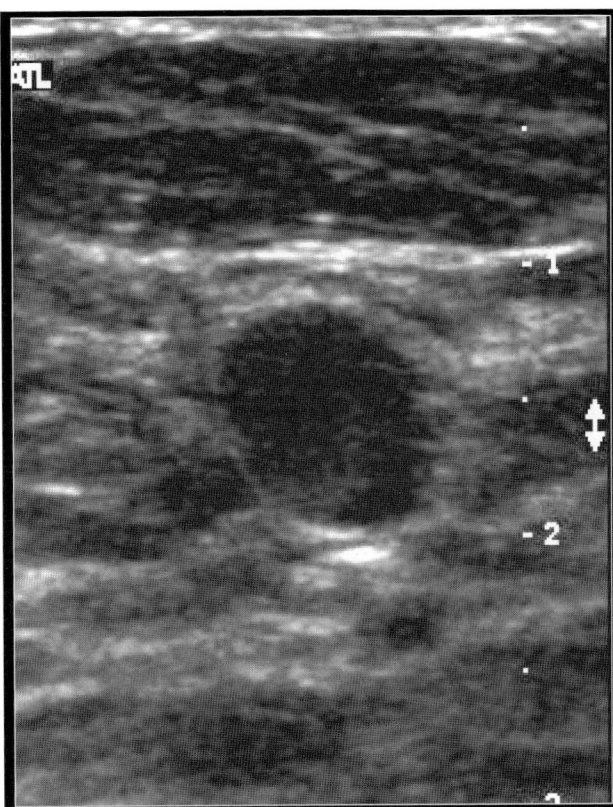

FIGURE 10–99 Demonstration of a thin crescent of fluid indicates the presence of a complex cyst rather than a solid nodule. Such fluid collections can be very subtle.

normal through-transmission (Fig. 10–100). Another general rule is that the echotexture of fibroadenomas is coarse and heterogeneous, whereas that of foam and gel cysts is finer and uniform (Fig. 10–101). The problem with the general rules is that many complex cysts and fibroadenomas are not classic in appearance. Thus, some complex cysts have one or more features typical of solid nodules. A complex cyst may be elliptical rather than spherical in shape, may be isoechoic rather than hypoechoic, and may have normal rather than enhanced through-transmission (Fig. 10–102). Similarly, certain fibroadenomas have one or more features typical of the classic complex cyst. Thus, fibroadenomas may be nearly spherical rather than elliptical in shape, may be hypoechoic rather than isoechoic, and may have enhanced rather than normal through-transmission (Fig. 10–103). Although heterogeneity is probably more reliable for diagnosing solid nodules in comparison to the other general rules listed previously, occasionally, the echotexture of complex cysts may be more heterogeneous than that of fibroadenomas (Fig. 10–104). This is particularly true of fibroadenomas with myxoid or highly cellular stroma. The bottom line is that for any individual nodule, if the overlap in sonographic features is taken into account, an absolute distinction cannot be made between a complex

cyst with low-level internal echoes and a fibroadenoma (Fig. 10–105).

Once all noninvasive sonographic methods of distinguishing cystic from solid have been exhausted, three choices remain:

1. The ICS lesion can be assumed to be solid and characterized as such into a BIRADS category. Using this approach, most ICS lesions are characterized as probably benign (BIRADS 3), and the patient can be offered the options of follow-up, attempted aspiration, or biopsy. Most patients will choose short-interval follow-up. ICS lesions that can be characterized as BIRADS 3 are common, so common that it would be impractical to biopsy or even aspirate them all. It is not unusual for a patient who has numerous cysts in each breast to have five or more ICS lesions in each breast. ICS lesions that do not meet strict criteria for BIRADS 3 category will have to undergo biopsy. Characterization of solid breast nodules is discussed in detail in Chapter 12.
2. The ICS lesion can undergo direct excisional or image-guided needle biopsy. This is generally not the best choice because ICS lesions are so common. The yield

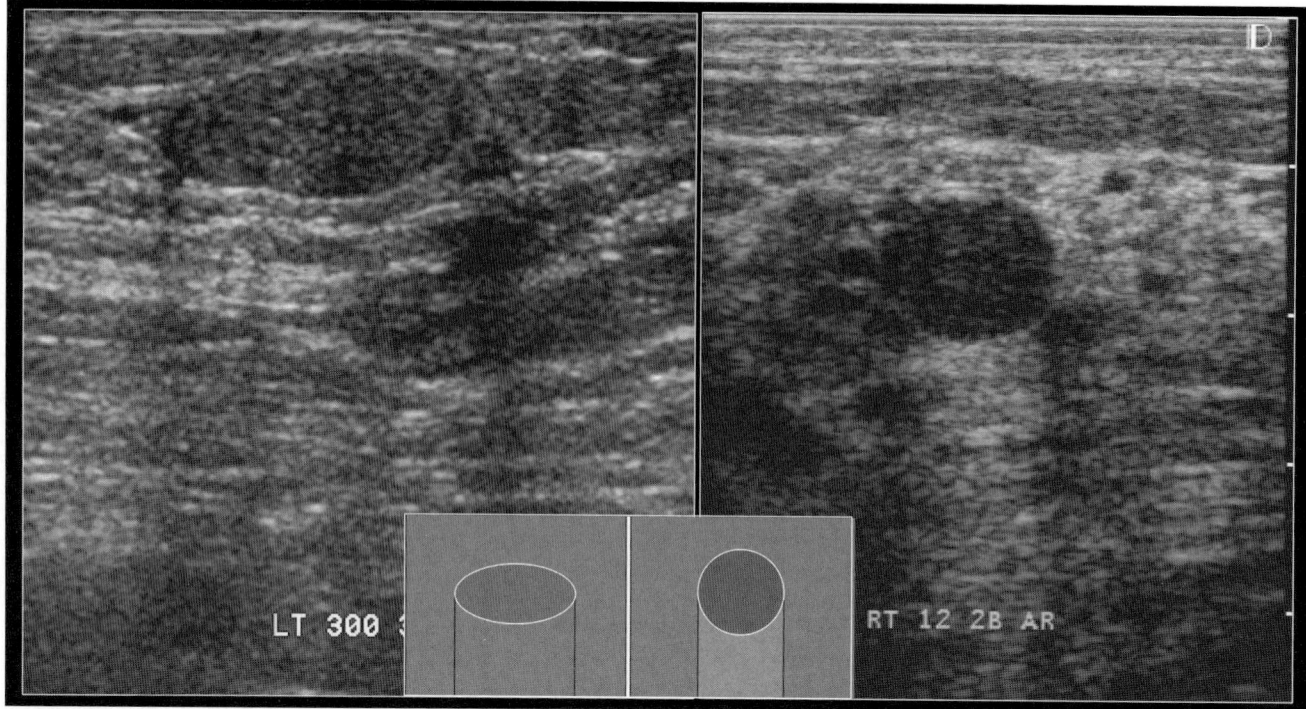

FIGURE 10–100 The typical fibroadenoma (**left**) is elliptical in shape, wider than tall, and iso-echoic with fat and has normal through-transmission. The typical foam or gel cyst (**right**), on the other hand, is spherical in shape and mildly to moderately hypoechoic and has enhanced through-transmission. Unfortunately, exceptions to the typical appearances are common.

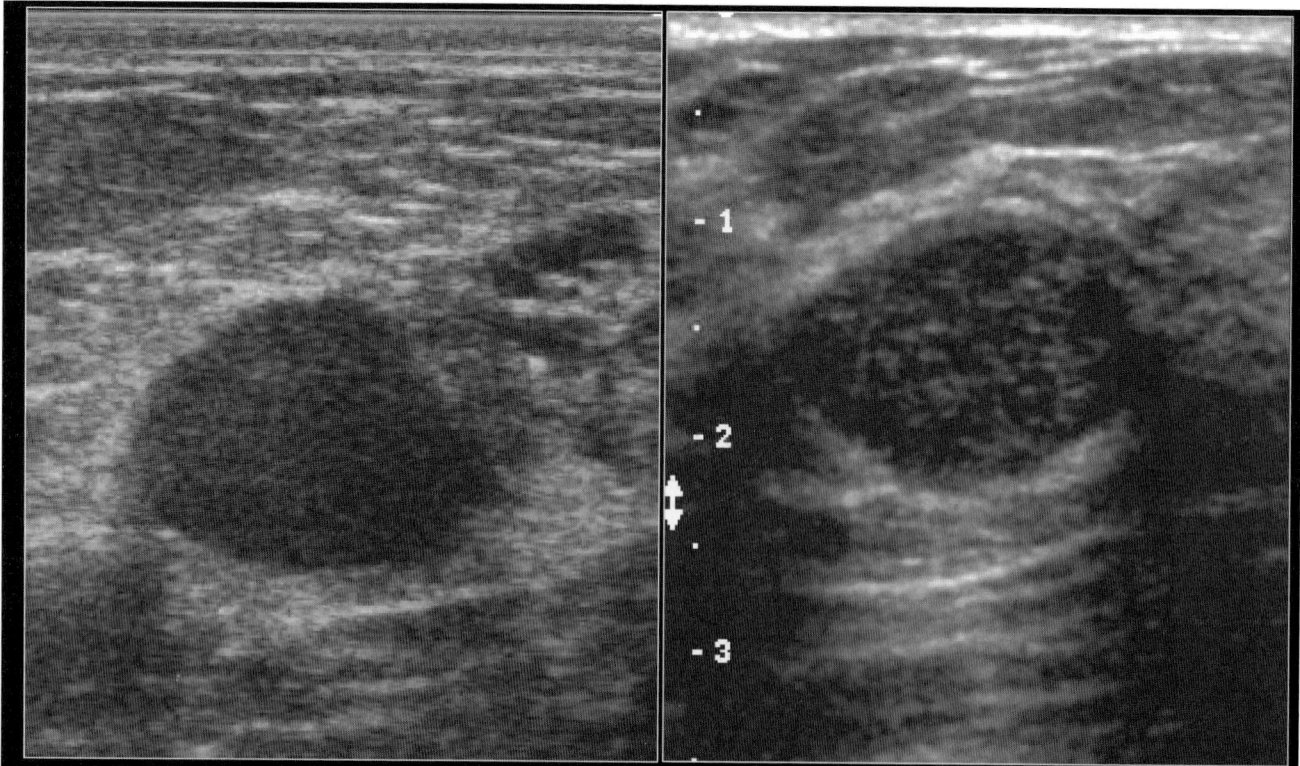

FIGURE 10–101 The echotexture of foam or gel cysts and fibroadenomas generally differs. The echotexture of foam or gel cysts is likely to be fine and relatively uniform (**left**). The echotexture of solid nodules, on the other hand, is more likely to be coarse and heterogeneous (**right**).

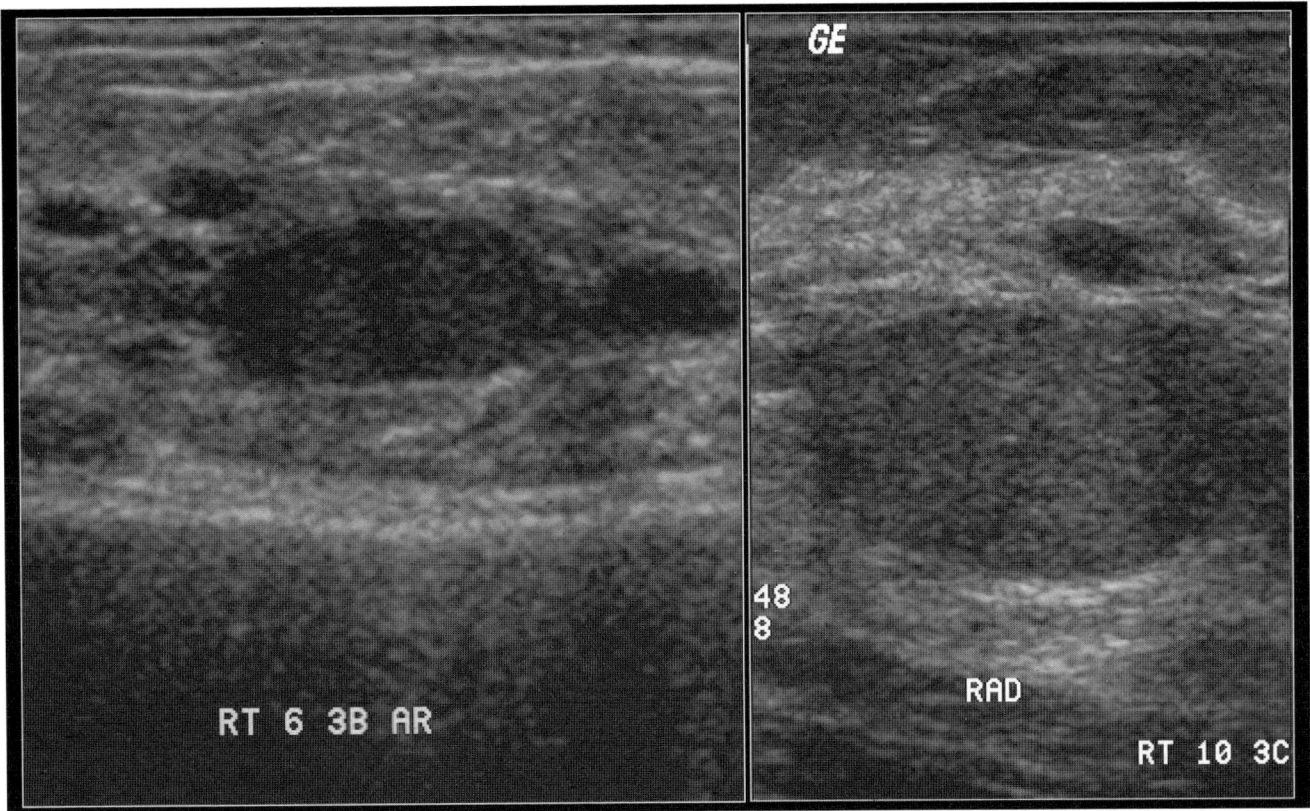

FIGURE 10–102 Foam or gel cysts may not be typical in appearance. Foam cysts may be elliptical rather than spherical in shape (**left**), have normal rather than enhanced through-transmission (**left**), and may be isoechoic rather than hypoechoic (**right**).

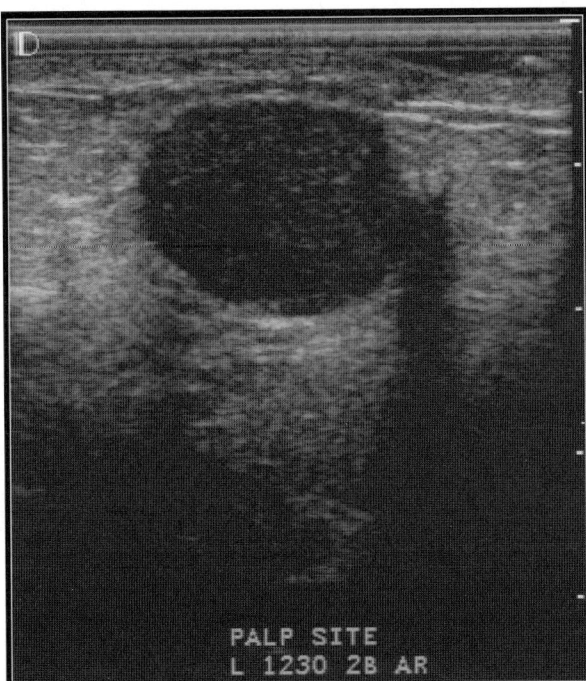

FIGURE 10–103 Solid nodules such as this fibroadenoma may have sonographic appearances that are not typical. The shape may be spherical rather than elliptical, the lesion may be hypoechoic rather than isoechoic, and there may be enhanced rather than normal through-transmission.

of positive biopsies would be very low. Sonographic characterization is a better approach, reserving biopsy for lesions that cannot be characterized as BIRADS 3 and for those patients who choose biopsy despite a BIRADS 3 characterization.

3. Aspiration of the ICS lesion can be attempted. The results of attempted aspiration will, of course, depend on the underling histologic basis for the sonographic finding of the ICS lesion. If the lesion is actually solid, aspiration will not be possible at all (Fig. 10–106). If the lesion contains echoes by virtue of being completely filled with PAM, aspiration will not be possible. If the lesion contains diffuse, low-level echoes caused by gelatinized proteinaceous debris or is completely filled with lipid, the cyst can be completely aspirated if a large enough needle and enough vacuum are used (Fig. 10–107). ICS lesions whose internal echoes are caused by a mixture of PAM and echogenic fluid can be only partially aspirated (Fig. 10–92). Because sonography alone cannot determine the precise cause of the internal echoes in most cases, sonography alone cannot predict the success of aspiration (Fig. 10–108). Only after attempting aspiration can it be determined whether aspiration has succeeded. Two adjacent cysts may have identical sonographic features, and one may be

(text continued on page 344)

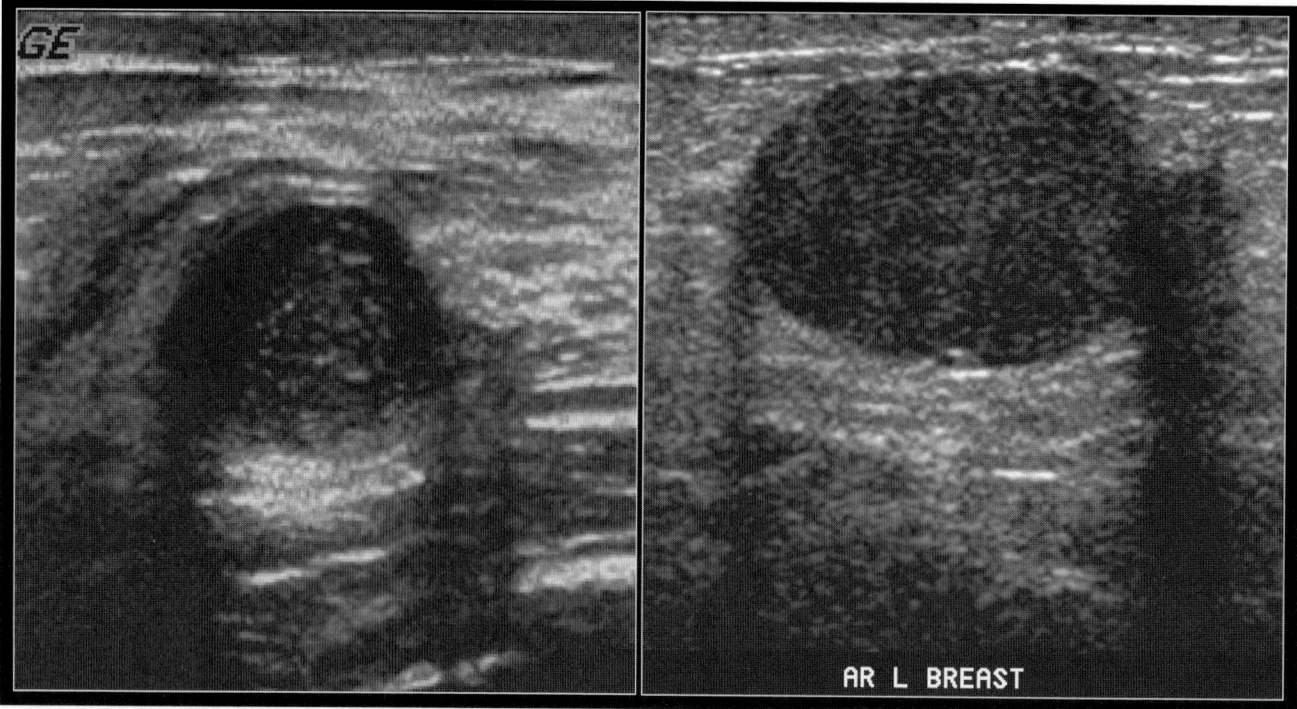

FIGURE 10–104 There are also exceptions to the general rule about the echotexture of complex cysts and solid nodules. Certain complex cysts may have a texture that is coarse and heterogeneous (**left**), and certain solid nodules may have a texture that is fine and homogeneous (**right**).

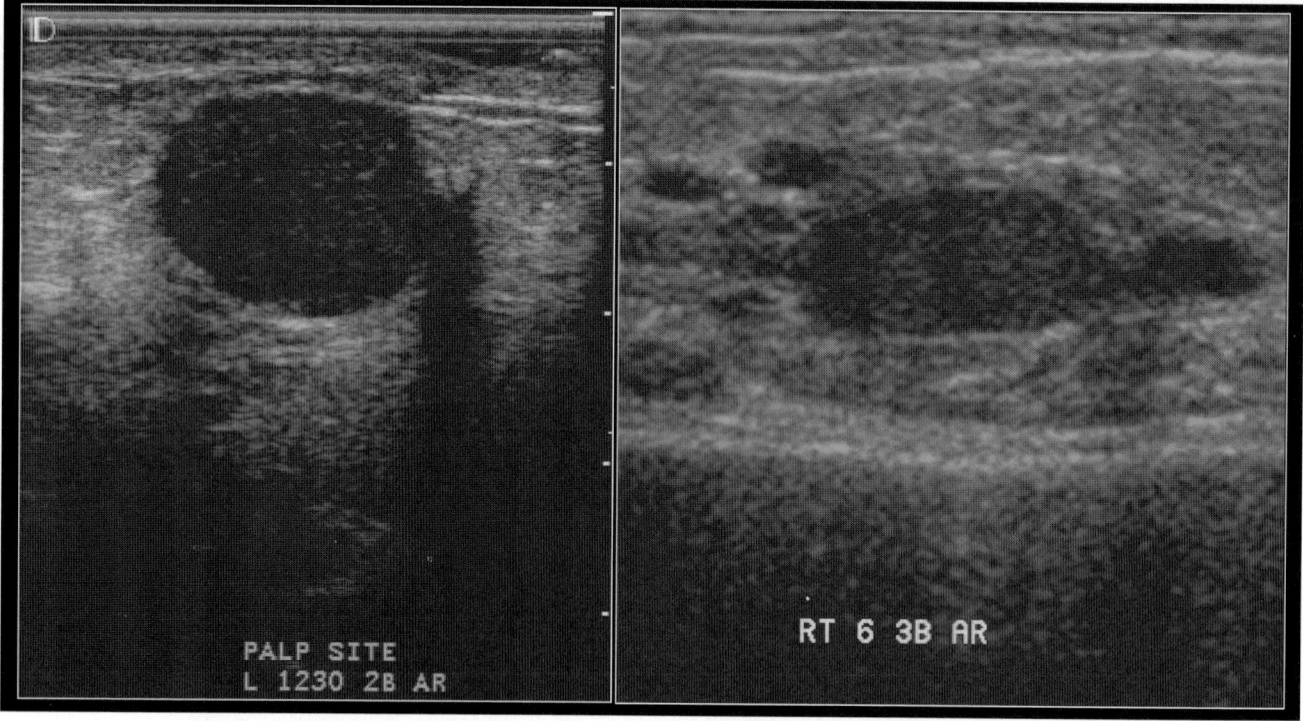

FIGURE 10–105 The exceptions to the general rules are so prevalent that for any individual lesion, it may be impossible to determine with certainty from sonography alone whether the lesion is complex cystic or solid. The fibroadenoma shown in the **left** image has sonographic features that are typical of complex cysts. It is spherical in shape, is hypoechoic, and has enhanced through-transmission. The foam cyst shown in the **right** image has sonographic features that are typical of a fibroadenoma. It is elliptical in shape, wider than tall, and only mildly hypoechoic and has normal through-transmission. Because of this overlap in sonographic features, it is prudent to assume the worst, that the lesion is solid, and then either characterize it or attempt to aspirate it.

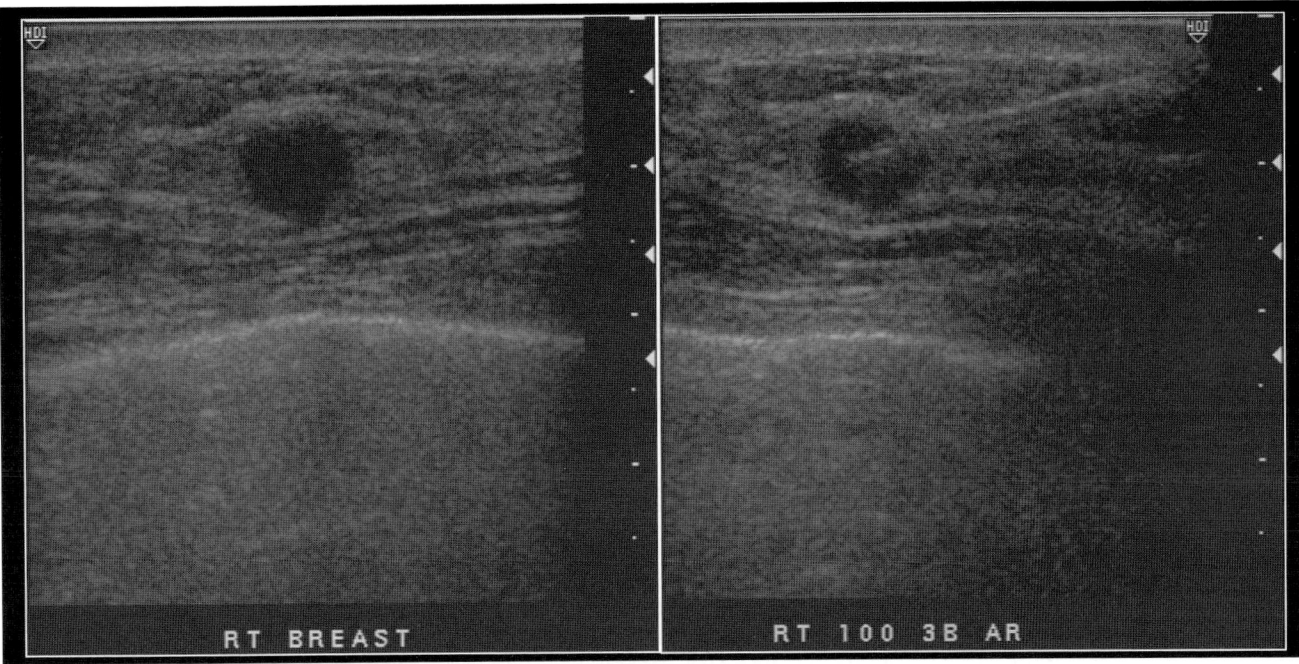

FIGURE 10–106 This indeterminate cystic versus solid lesion could not be aspirated at all because it was a solid nodule. Biopsy that followed showed it to be a fibroadenoma. **Left:** Before aspiration. **Right:** During attempted aspiration.

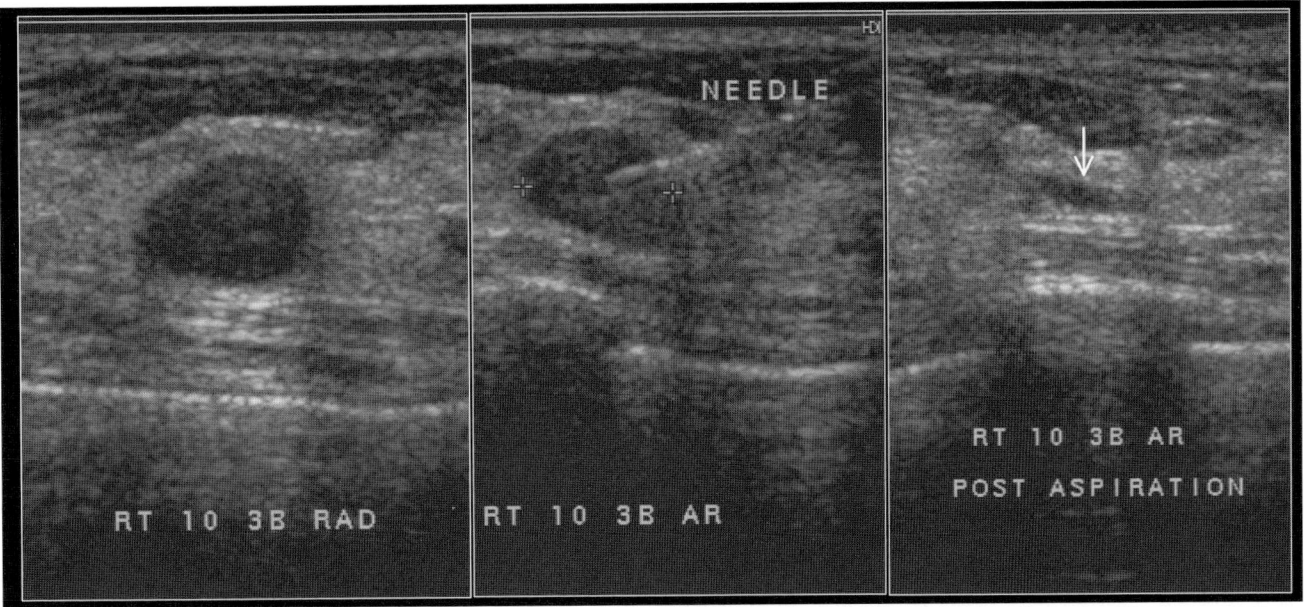

FIGURE 10–107 This indeterminate cystic versus solid lesion had more sonographic features suggesting that it was solid than features suggesting that it was cystic. It did have enhanced through-transmission but was elliptical in shape rather than spherical and was isoechoic with fat rather than hypoechoic. However, the lesion could be completely aspirated. **Left:** The lesion pre-aspiration. **Middle:** during aspiration. **Right:** After aspiration. *Arrow* indicates collapsed cyst after aspiration.

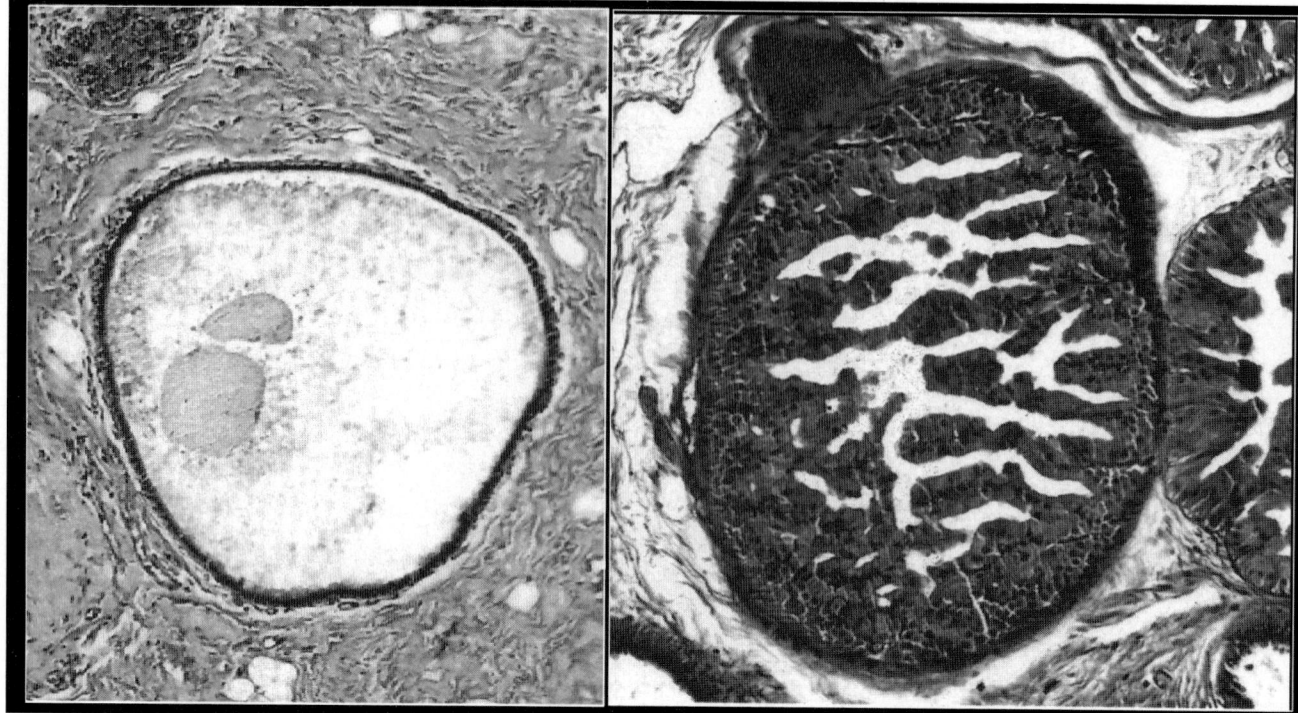

FIGURE 10–108 Sonography alone cannot predict the success of attempted aspiration because the complex cysts shown above appear identical sonographically. The cyst on the **left** will have diffuse, low-level echogenicity because of the thick proteinaceous and gelatinous fluid that it contains, but it will be possible to aspirate it completely. The cyst on the **right** will have diffuse, low-level internal echoes because of the papillary apocrine metaplasia that fills it. It will not be possible to aspirate it at all. Some cysts may have a mixture of papillary apocrine metaplasia and equally echogenic proteinaceous or lipid-laden fluid that is indistinguishable from the apocrine metaplasia. It will be possible to partially, but not completely, aspirate such cysts.

completely drained and the other completely nonaspiratable (Fig. 10–109).

Even in cases in which the ICS lesion cannot be aspirated at all, some useful information about whether the lesion is cystic can be gleaned from attempting to move the needle tip within the lesion. In a solid lesion, the tip of the needle is fixed within the lesion. Attempting to rock the needle tip anteriorly and posteriorly within the solid nodule will not change its position relative to the anterior and posterior margins of the lesion (Fig. 10–110). However, nonaspiratable cysts filled with apocrine metaplasia differ from solid nodules. The strands of apocrine metaplasia that fill the cyst are thin and gracile, usually only one or two cells thick, and easily disrupted. Thus, even though the papillary apocrine growth within the cyst is attached to the wall and cannot be aspirated, it offers little resistance to the rocking motion of the needle. Thus, the needle tip can be rocked from the anterior wall of the lesion to the posterior wall without difficulty (Fig. 10–111). In the process of rocking the needle, "snouts" of papillary apocrine cells can be broken loose and aspirated. The cyst will not be drained completely, but even the tiny amount of aspirate that is possible after rocking the needle may be enough to evaluate

(text continued on page 347)

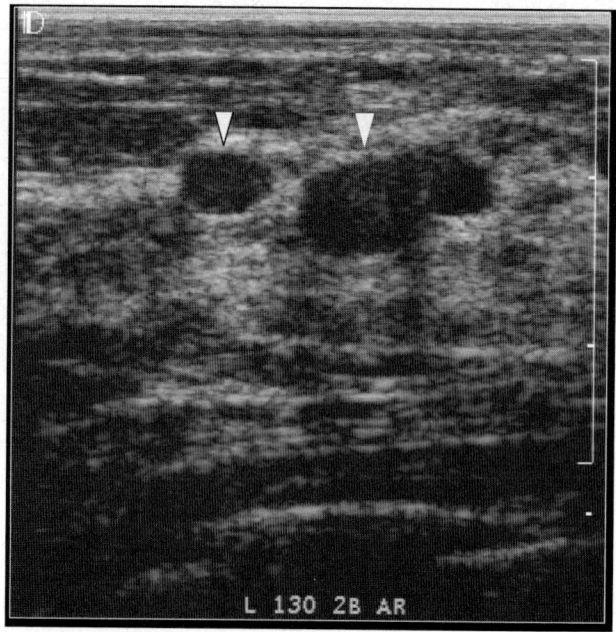

A

FIGURE 10–109 A: It is not possible to determine with sonography alone whether it will be possible to aspirate a foam or gel cyst or indeterminate cystic versus solid lesion. Their sonographic appearances are identical. Except for size, these two complex cysts *(arrowheads)* are sonographically identical in appearance, and aspiration of both was attempted.

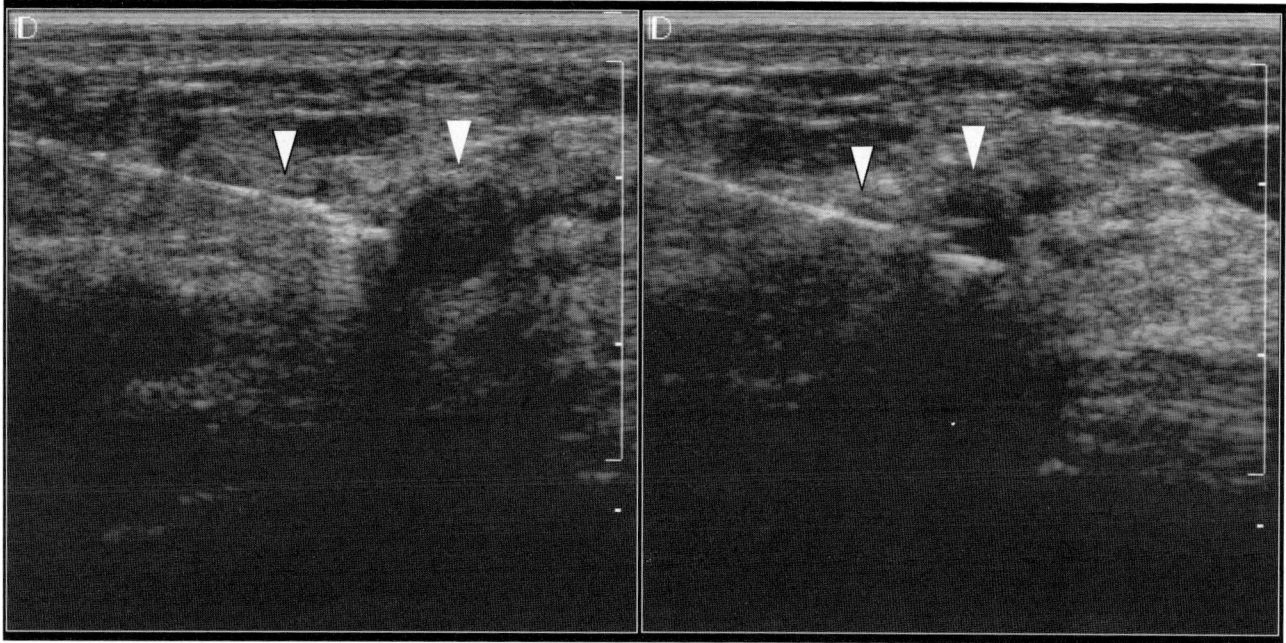

B

FIGURE 10–109 *(continued)* **B:** During aspiration, a needle path was chosen that would allow aspiration of both cysts. The smaller of the two lesions could be completely aspirated *(solid arrowhead)*. The large and deeper of the two lesions could not be aspirated at all.

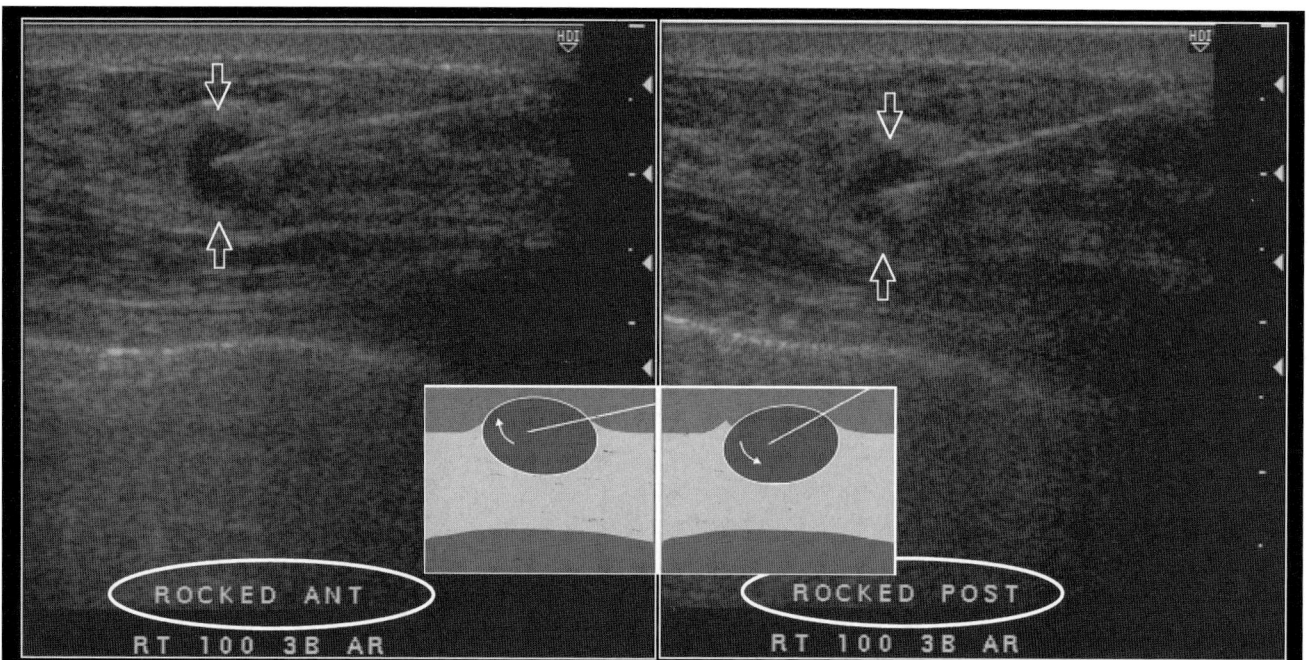

FIGURE 10–110 This is the lesion that could not be aspirated shown in Fig. 10.106. An attempt was made to rock the needle tip within the lesion. Note that the position of the needle tip relative to the anterior and posterior capsules of the lesion *(arrows)* did not change during the maneuver, indicating that the aspiration failed because the lesion was solid. Biopsy that followed showed the lesion to represent a fibroadenoma.

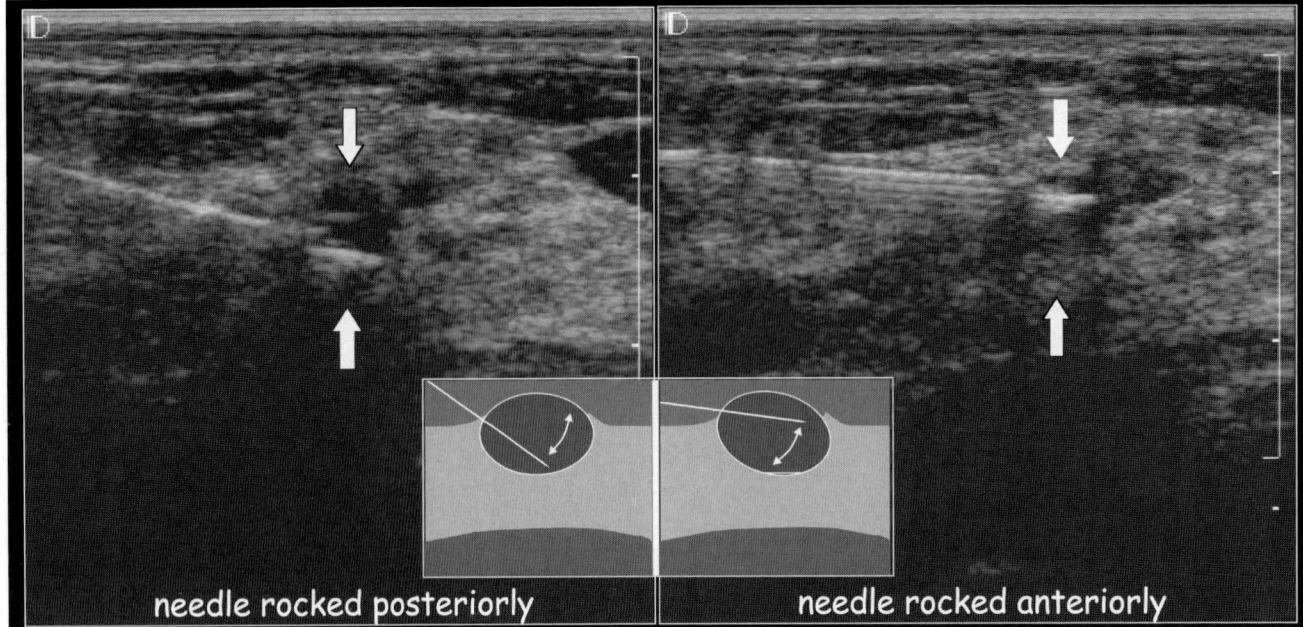

FIGURE 10–111 This is the larger, deeper indeterminate cystic versus solid lesion that could not be aspirated shown in Fig. 10.109. When the needle was rocked in the anteroposterior plane, the needle tip could be moved within the lesion from the anterior capsule (**left**, *hollow arrow*) to the posterior capsule (**right**, *hollow arrow*). The movement of the needle tip within the lesion indicated that the lesion was a complex cyst rather than a solid nodule. The movement of the needle within the lesion also facilitated aspiration of a droplet of fluid that revealed clumps of papillary apocrine cysts on cytologic evaluation.

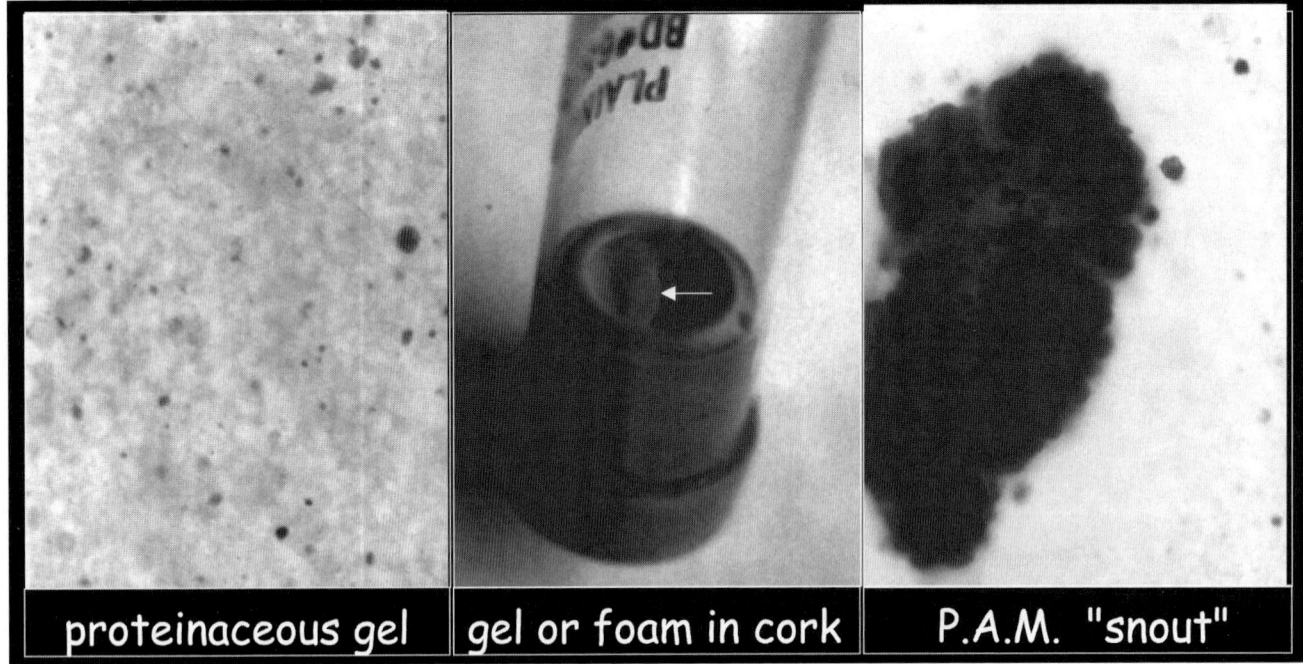

FIGURE 10–112 When the rocking maneuver causes the needle tip to move within the indeterminate cystic versus solid lesion, it tends to facilitate aspiration of small amounts of fluid from the cyst. The amount may be so small that if a Vacutainer system is used, there may be only a droplet or two within the red cork (**middle**, *arrow*) and no fluid visible within the glass part of the tube. Cytologic evaluation of these small aspirates may yield definitive findings of fibrocystic change, such as clumps of apocrine cells (**right**) or acellular proteinaceous or lipid material (**left**). In such cases, a failed aspiration becomes a fine-needle aspiration biopsy.

cytologically (Fig. 10–112). The appearance of clumps of pink-staining apocrine cells is characteristic enough to make a definitive diagnosis of benign FCC in most cases. Thus, a failed aspiration can become a fine-needle aspiration biopsy (FNAB).

STEP 6: IF BIRADS 3 FINDINGS CANNOT BE IDENTIFIED, THE LESION MUST BE CHARACTERIZED AS BIRADS 4A OR HIGHER AND UNDERGO BIOPSY

Any sonographic algorithm for characterizing cystic or solid lesion must err on the side of caution. The goal is to prevent biopsy, when possible, by identifying findings that have a 98% or greater chance of being benign (BIRADS 3 or lower category). However, if there is even a single suspicious finding or if strict criteria for BIRADS 2 or BIRADS 3 categories are not met, the lesion must be characterized as BIRADS 4a or higher and must undergo biopsy.

It should also be remembered that not all lesions diagnosed histologically as FCC will appear to be cystic sonographically. In FCC, there is a mixture of fibrosclerotic, benign proliferative, and cystic change. Cystic changes may predominate in some cases, but in others, the fibrosclerotic or benign proliferative changes (such as PAM) may predominate. When noncystic changes predominate, the lesion tends to have a solid and microlobulated appearance that is worrisome (Fig. 10–113). Such lesions account for most cases in which the histology obtained from core needle biopsy is considered nonconcordant with the sonographic finding. In such cases, the imaging findings suggest a specific malignant diagnosis such as high-nuclear-grade DCIS or a specific benign diagnosis such as papilloma, but the histologic findings yield the unexpected nonspecific benign diagnosis of FCC. When the histologic results are nonconcordant with the imaging findings, there is always concern that the random sampling pattern of spring-loaded large core needle biopsy has yielded a false-negative diagnosis, and repeat large core needle biopsy or surgical

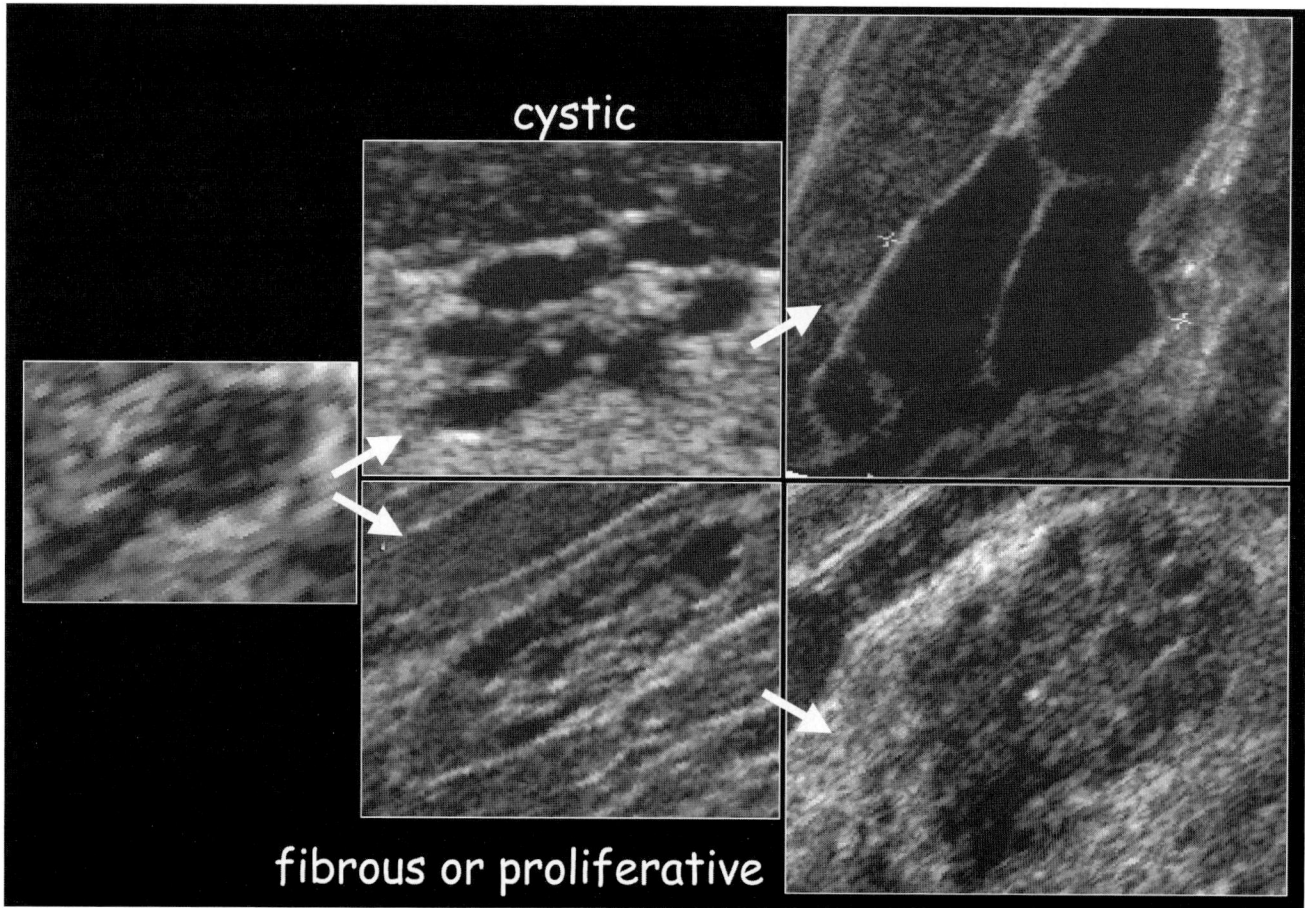

FIGURE 10–113 In the lesions shown in the **top row**, cystic change predominates, and the diagnosis of fibrocystic change is obvious sonographically. However, in the **bottom row**, fibrosclerotic and proliferative changes predominate, which in combination with volume averaging of microcysts, make the lesions appear solid, microlobulated, and worrisome. Such lesions should be characterized as BIRADS 4a or higher and are better evaluated with 11-gauge directional vacuum-assisted biopsy rather than spring-loaded core needle biopsy.

excisional biopsy is considered. Nonconcordant imaging and histologic findings are the main reason that 11-gauge vacuum-assisted biopsy is favored over large core needle biopsy for small lesions. As a practical matter, lesions less than 1.3 cm in maximum diameter can be completely removed with vacuum-assisted 11-gauge needle biopsy. If the entire lesion is removed by vacuum-assisted biopsy and completely evaluated histologically, there is no chance of false-negative biopsy. Thus, the nonspecific benign histologic diagnosis of FCC can be believed without resorting to repeat needle biopsy or excision. For this reason, when a lesion is solid and microlobulated and might represent FCC simulating a more worrisome condition, we feel that the more complete sampling technique of vacuum-assisted 11-gauge needle biopsy, rather than the random sampling technique of large core needle biopsy, should be employed instead of spring-loaded core needle biopsy.

SUMMARY

Most complex breast cysts are benign and part of the fibrocystic spectrum. Most malignant breast cysts are obviously cystically or hemorrhagically degenerated solid nodules or solid nodules that have secondarily involved a cyst. However, although these general rules are reassuring in studies of populations of patients, they are frequently not reassuring enough to either the patient or referring physician in individual cases. Therefore, the sonographer or sonologist must have a systematic method of assessing the risk of each complex cyst for neoplasm and infection. Complex cysts are too common to assume that all are worrisome. In women who have multiple cysts, it is common to see many different complex cysts of different types in each breast (Fig. 10–114).

The algorithm for evaluating complex breast cysts is similar to that used for mammographic evaluation and for

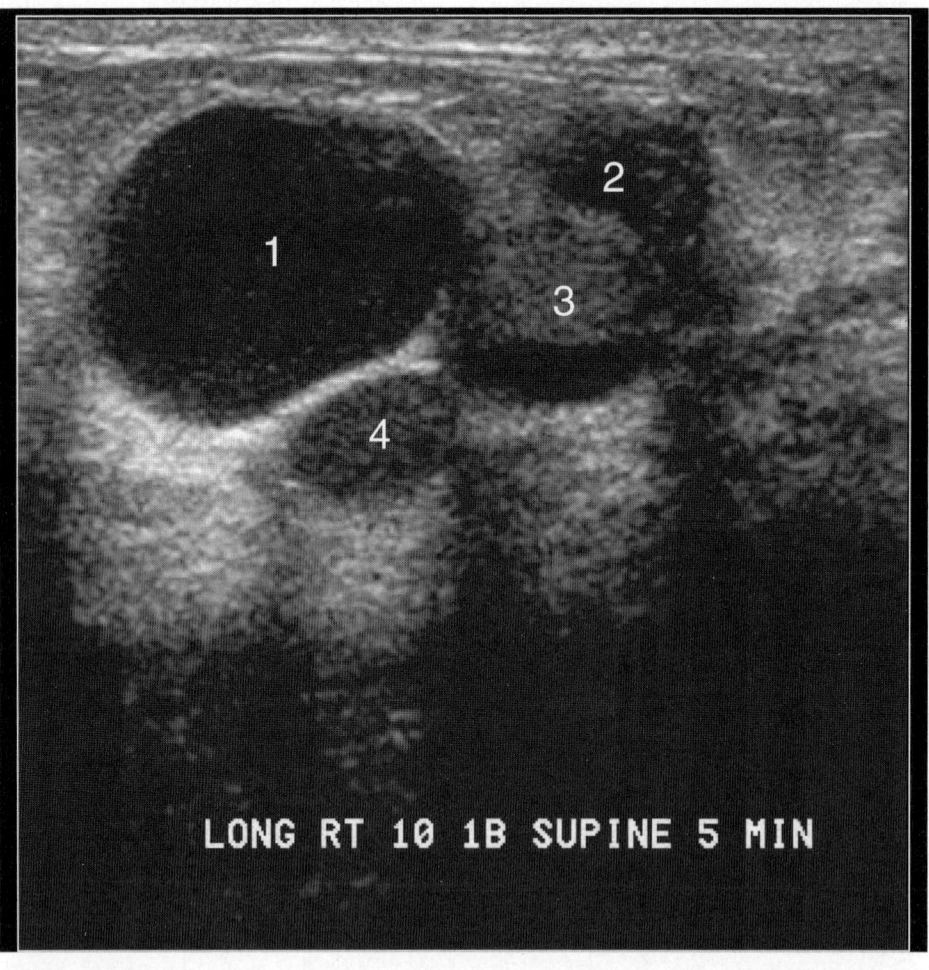

LONG RT 10 1B SUPINE 5 MIN

FIGURE 10–114 This patient illustrates the importance of characterizing complex breast cysts. Complex cysts are simply too frequently seen to biopsy, aspirate, or even follow all of them. In women with multiple cysts, it is common to find multiple complex cysts of varying types in each breast. In one field of view in this patient, there are four different types of complex cysts. Cyst 1 has diffuse low-level echoes, a fluid–debris level, and mobile echoes caused by cholesterol crystals. Cyst 2 has an isoechoic, thickened wall caused by papillary apocrine metaplasia. Cyst 3 contains a fat–fluid level. Cyst 4 is an indeterminate cystic versus solid lesion and is most likely a complex cyst completely filled with either viscous lipid or proteinaceous debris.

sonographic evaluation of solid breast nodules. The algorithm for complex cysts differs only in that it contains an extra step for assessing the risk for infection. Generally, the mammographic algorithm and sonographic algorithm for evaluation of solid breast nodules are concerned only with neoplasm.

First, artifactual echoes are excluded to the extent possible in order to maximize the percentage of cysts characterized as simple and to minimize the percentage characterized as complex cystic. This currently is best accomplished using coded harmonics and spatial compounding.

Second, worrisome features for intracystic neoplasm or inflammation are sought. If even a single feature worrisome for neoplasm is present, the nodule must be characterized as BIRADS 4a or greater and subjected to histologic evaluation. Currently, ultrasound-guided vacuum-assisted large core needle biopsy with clip deployment is the method of choice. If no features worrisome for neoplasm are found, sonographic features indicating inflammation are sought. If features of inflammation are found, aspiration for Gram stain and culture is performed.

Third, if no findings suspicious for a true ICPL of acute inflammation are found, benign features are sought. If BIRADS 2 features are found, the lesion can be characterized as BIRADS 2, and no further evaluation is necessary.

If BIRADS 2 features cannot be found, BIRADS 3 features are sought. If BIRADS 3 features are found, the lesion is characterized as BIRADS 3, and either attempted aspiration or short-interval follow-up is performed. The algorithm, like that for mammography and sonography of solid breast nodules, is designed to err on the side of caution but also to minimize the percentage of cases in which biopsy, aspiration, or short-interval follow-up are necessary. If strict criteria for BIRADS 3 cannot be met, the lesion can undergo attempted aspiration or biopsy.

The small percentage of lesions that cannot be determined with certainty to be either cystic or solid either can be assumed to be solid and characterized as such or can be assessed with attempted aspiration. If assumed to be solid, most have BIRADS 3 characteristics and therefore can be followed. Even failed aspirations may yield enough aspirate for cytologic evaluation, which often shows clumps of apocrine cells indicating that the complex cyst is filled with papillary apocrine metaplasia as a part of the benign fibrocystic spectrum.

There are almost certainly many different algorithms that could be developed to deal successfully with complex cysts. This algorithm has been patterned after the algorithms used for mammography and sonographic evaluation of solid breast nodules, to minimize the need to "reinvent the wheel." We have found the algorithm described previously to be useful in assessing the risk for malignancy and infection in complex cysts. However, judging the success of any algorithm for evaluation of complex breast cysts is and will be more difficult than assessing the efficacy of mammography for calcifications or sonography for solid nodules because the old gold standards for complex breast cysts are less satisfactory than those for mammography and sonographic evaluation of solid breast nodules in most cases—fluid cytology or follow-up rather than the histology.

SUGGESTED READINGS

Bardales RH, Suhrland MJ, Stanley MW. Papillary neoplasms of the breast: fine-needle aspiration findings in cystic and solid cases. *Diagn Cytopathol* 1994;10(4):336–341.

Barki Y, et al. Infarcted cystadenofibroma of the breast. *J Ultrasound Med* 1987;6:213–215.

Bargum K, Nielsen SM. Case report: fat necrosis of the breast appearing as oil cysts with fat-fluid levels. *Br J Radiol* 1993; 66(788): 718–720.

Bassett LW, Kimme-Smith C. Breast sonography: technique, equipment, and normal anatomy. *Semin Ultrasound CT MR* 1989; 10(2):82–89.

Bassett LW, Kimme-Smith C. Breast sonography. *AJR Am J Roentgenol* 1991;156(3):449–455.

Brenner RJ, et al. Spontaneous regression of interval benign cysts of the breast. *Radiology* 1994;193(2):365–368.

Ciatto S, Morrone D, Bravetti P. Differential diagnosis of intracystic breast lesions in hemorrhagic cysts. *Radiol Med* (Torino) 1991; 81(5):592–596.

Cilotti A, et al. The diagnostic imaging of complex breast nodules. *Radiol Med* (Torino) 1992;84(3):198–203.

Cooke CG, Grant EG, Cigtay OS. Ultrasound demonstration of giant malignant breast cyst undetected by xeromammography. *J Clin Ultrasound* 1981;9(10):461–462.

Crowe DJ, Helvie MA, Wilson TE. Breast infection. Mammographic and sonographic findings with clinical correlation. *Invest Radiol* 1995;30(10):582–587.

Drukker BH. Breast cysts and solid lesions: the role of fine-needle aspiration. *Curr Opin Obstet Gynecol* 1994;6(6):492–494.

Dyreborg U, et al. Needle puncture followed by pneumocystography of palpable breast cysts. A controlled clinical trial. *Acta Radiol* 1985;26(3):277–281.

Fajardo LL, Bessen SC. Epidermal inclusion cyst after reduction mammoplasty. *Radiology* 1993;186(1):103–1066.

Fallentin E, Rothman L. Intracystic carcinoma of the male breast. *J Clin Ultrasound* 1994;22(2):118–120.

Fitzal P, Wolf G. Comparison of the diagnostic value of the individual examination steps (triple diagnosis) in breast cysts. *Ultraschall Med* 1990;11(4):202–205.

Franquet T, Cozcolluela R, De Miguel C. Stereotaxic fine-needle aspiration of low-suspicion, nonpalpable breast nodules: valid alternative to follow-up mammography. *Radiology* 1992;183(3): 635–637.

Gorins A, et al. Breast cysts. *Verh K Acad Geneeskd Belg* 1991; 53(2):101–120.

Hayes R, Michell M, Nunnerley HB. Acute inflammation of the breast—the role of breast ultrasound in diagnosis and management. *Clin Radiol* 1991;44(4):253–256.

Hilton SV, et al. Real-time breast sonography: application in 300 consecutive patients. *AJR Am J Roentgenol* 1986;147(3): 479–486.

Hogg JP, Harris KM, Skolnick ML. The role of ultrasound-guided needle aspiration of breast masses. *Ultrasound Med Biol* 1988;1: 13–21.

Ikeda DM, et al. The role of fine-needle aspiration and pneumocystography in the treatment of impalpable breast cysts. *AJR Am J Roentgenol* 1992;158(6):1239–1241.

Jackson VP. The current role of ultrasonography in breast imaging. *Radiol Clin North Am* 1995;33(6):1161–1170.

Jackson VP, The role of ultrasound in breast imaging. *Radiology* 1990;177:305–311.

Jellins JE, et al. Detection and classification of liquid-filled masses in the breast by gray scale echography. *Radiology* 125;(10):205–212.

Kenlson MH, el Yousef SJ, Goldberg RE, et al. Intracystic papillary carcinoma of the breast: mammographic, sonographic, and MR appearance with pathologic correlation. *J Comput Assist Tomogr* 1987;11:1074–1076.

Khaleghian R. Breast cysts: pitfalls in sonographic diagnosis. *Australas Radiol* 1993;37(2):192–194.

Lee ME, Hashimoto B, Carter L. Role of direct contact, real-time breast ultrasound: one year's experience. *Ultrasound Med Biol* 1988;1:109–112.

Leucht WJ, Rabe DR, Humbert KD. Diagnostic value of different interpretative criteria in real-time sonography of the breast. *Ultrasound Med Biol* 1988;1:59–73.

Liberman L, Feng T, Susnik B. Case 35: intracystic papillary carcinoma with invasion. *Radiology* 2001;219:781–784.

McCulloch GL, Evans AJ, Yeoman L, et al. Radiological features of papillary carcinoma of the breast. *Clin Radiol* 1997;52(11):865–868.

Mercado CL, Hamele-Bena D, Singer C, et al. Papillary lesions of the breast: evaluation with stereotactic directional vacuum-assisted biopsy. *Radiology* 2001;221:650–655.

Meyer JE, et al. Image-guided aspiration of solitary occult breast 'cysts.' *Arch Surg* 1992;127(4):433–435.

Mitnick JS, Vazquez MF, Harris MN, et al. Invasive papillary carcinoma of the breast: mammographic appearance. *Radiology* 1990;177:803–806.

Muller JW. Diagnosis of breast cysts with mammography, ultrasound and puncture. A review. *Diagn Imaging Clin Med* 1985;54(3–4):170–177.

Navas MDM, et al. Intracystic papilloma in male breast: ultrasonography and pneumocystography diagnosis. *J Clin Ultrasound* 1993;21(1):38–40.

Nightingale KR, et al. A novel ultrasonic technique for differentiating cysts from solid lesions: preliminary results in the breast. *Ultrasound Med Biol* 1995;21(6):745–751.

Nyirjesy I, Billingsley FS. Management of breast problems in gynecologic office practice using sonography and fine-needle aspiration. *Obstet Gynecol* 1992;79(5 Pt 1)):699–702.

Omori LM, et al. Breast masses with mixed cystic-solid sonographic appearance. *J Clin Ultrasound* 1993;21(8):489–495.

Piccoli CW. Current utilization and future techniques of breast ultrasound. *Curr Opin Radiol* 1992;4(5):139–145.

Ravichandran D, et al. Cystic carcinoma of the breast: a trap for the unwary. *Ann R Coll Surg Engl* 1995;77(2):123–126.

Reuter K, D'Orsi CJ, Reale F. Intracystic carcinoma of the breast: the role of ultrasonography. *Radiology* 1984;153(10):233–234.

Rosner D, Blaird D. What ultrasonography can tell in breast masses that mammography and physical examination cannot. *J Surg Oncol* 1985;28(4):308–313.

Rotili G, et al. The percutaneous treatment of breast cysts. A proposed new method. *Radiol Med* (Torino) 1994;88(3):225–227.

Roy M, et al. Study of benign superficial cysts by fine needle aspiration cytology. *J Indian Med Assoc* 1995;93(1):8–9, 13.

Savjak D, Pikula B. Relation of epithelial metaplasia and calcification with epithelial proliferation in fibrocystic breast disease. *Med Arh* 1991;45(1–2):59–62.

Schepps B, Scola FH, Frates RE. Benign circumscribed breast masses. Mammographic and sonographic appearance. *Obstet Gynecol Clin North Am* 1994;21(3):519–537.

Schneider JA. Invasive papillary breast carcinoma: mammographic and sonographic appearance. *Radiology* 1989;171(5):377–379.

Schwarz E, Kiesler J. Diagnosis of (intra)-cystic breast cancer. *Rontgenblatter* 1986;39(8):216–219.

Sneige N, Fornage BD, Saleh G. Ultrasound-guided fine-needle aspiration of nonpalpable breast lesions. Cytologic and histologic findings. *Am J Clin Pathol* 1994;102(1):98–101.

Soo MS, Williford ME, Walsh R, et al. Papillary carcinoma of the breast: imaging findings. *AJR Am J Roentgenol* 1995;164(2):321–326.

Sterns EE. The natural history of macroscopic cysts in the breast. *Surg Gynecol Obstet* 1992;174(1):36–40.

Tobin CE, Hendrix TM, Resnikoff LB, et al. Breast imaging case of the day. *Radiographics* 1996;16:720–722.

Urbanowicz Z, et al. Comparison of mammography and sonography in diagnosis of breast cysts. *Ginekol Pol* 1992;63(2):82–83.

Venta LA, et al. Sonographic evaluation of the breast. *Radiographics* 1994;14(1):29–50.

Weiss H, et al. Sonographic detection of intracystic breast tumors. *Ultraschall Med* 1985;6(4):233–236.

11

NONMALIGNANT BREAST DISORDERS THAT HAVE COMPLEX CYSTIC PHASES

Several conditions of the breast in their classic phases are complex cystic but in other phases may appear solid sonographically. These conditions include the following:

1. Galactocele
2. Mastitis and abscess
   a. Puerperal mastitis and abscess
   b. Duct ectasia–periductal mastitis complex (nonpuerperal abscess)
3. Seroma, hematoma, and lymphocele
4. Fat necrosis
5. Mondor's disease—superficial thrombosis of breast veins
6. Hemangioma, venous malformation, and lymphangioma

The histologic and imaging findings of these various conditions overlap because most have inflammatory or granulomatous components. The histologic and imaging findings of inflammation are similar, regardless of the etiology. In some cases, it is not possible to distinguish one of these conditions from another. Two or more of these entities may coexist, and one condition may, over time, evolve into another. For instance, patients who have undergone lumpectomy may have postoperative seroma and hematoma that become secondarily infected, becoming abscesses, and that finally may evolve into various forms of fat necrosis. A chronic or recurrent galactocele may become secondarily infected and evolve into an abscess. Fat necrosis may evolve from a hematoma. Thus, clinical findings and the timing of events must be taken into account when interpreting imaging or histologic findings in such patients.

GALACTOCELE

General Pathologic Classification, Epidemiology, and Clinical Findings

Galactoceles have been described as cystically dilated terminal ducts and terminal ductules that are filled with milk and lined by the normal double layer of breast epithelium and myoepithelium.

The classic clinical history of galactocele is a painless lump that appears a few weeks to a few months after cessation of breast-feeding. However, galactoceles can be seen during breast-feeding and even during the third trimester of pregnancy as well as after cessation of breast-feeding. In our experience, most patients who have developed galactoceles while still breast-feeding have recently decreased the frequency of feedings after returning to work. Galactoceles have been reported in infants in whom they form in response to maternal hormones in breast milk. Rare cases of galactocele have been reported after reduction mammoplasty or in association with birth control pills.

Enzymes can denature the breast milk protein over time, essentially curdling the milk. Lipids that are initially suspended in a uniform emulsion of tiny droplets within the milk may separate into larger globules or even fat–fluid layers.

Mammographic Findings

Mammography may be the initial imaging procedure in patients who have stopped breast-feeding for a few weeks, but sonography typically is performed in place of mammography in patients who are still lactating.

In the unusual case in which mammography is performed first, sonography may be unnecessary if mammography shows classic galactocele findings of a lipid cyst, a lesion with fat–fluid levels on horizontal beam films, or a lesion containing randomly distributed mixtures of water and fat density.

The mammographic appearance of the galactocele depends on its stage. An acute galactocele is a suspension of emulsified tiny fat globules in a watery base that usually appears to be a nonspecific water-density mass mammographically. In a subacute galactocele, the tiny fat globules within milk coalesce into large fat globules that remain suspended within a watery base. Because the larger fat globules remain suspended in water, the subacute galactocele, like the acute galactocele, appears to be a nodule of water density mammographically. More mature galactoceles, in which the fat globules may become even larger and more unevenly distributed, result in a heterogeneous, mixed fat and water-density mammographic mass. At this stage, if the patient does not change position for a while, fat may rise through the water portion of the galactocele to its nondependent part, creating a fat–fluid level. Finally, a chronic galactocele, if not secondarily infected, may appear as a pure lipid cyst due to complete resorption of the water component.

The mammographic appearance of early galactoceles as water-density masses is completely nonspecific. The mammographic differential for mixed fat and water-density lesions is narrower, however, and includes benign entities: (a) galactocele; (b) hematoma, which usually is associated with a history of trauma or attempted aspiration or biopsy; (c) intramammary lymph node, in which the fatty density is central and represents the hilum or mediastinum of the lymph node; and (d) fibroadenolipoma (hamartoma), which is frequently large, often nonpalpable, and unrelated to breast-feeding.

Sonographic Findings

The sonographic appearance of a galactocele, like the mammographic appearance, varies with the stage of development of the galactocele and with the location. Fresh milk is nearly anechoic, which can be seen by examining the lactiferous sinuses during the letdown phase of breast-feeding. This nearly anechoic appearance corresponds to the acute phase of galactocele formation, in which tiny globules of fat are emulsified and homogenously suspended throughout a water base. Thus, new or fresh galactoceles that represent acutely obstructed, milk-filled, dilated terminal ductolobular units (TDLUs), usually appear to be anechoic or nearly anechoic. They present as either unilocular simple cysts (Fig. 11–1) or thinly septated multiloculated cysts (Fig. 11–2). However, in certain cases, acute galactoceles may have diffuse low-level internal echoes because of the innumerable interfaces that exist between the lipid globules and water components of the galactocele (Fig. 11–3). The location of galactoceles can also affect the appearance. Peripheral galactoceles are often multilocular (Fig. 11–2) or have the appearance of dilated distal ducts and lobules (Fig. 11–4). Centrally located

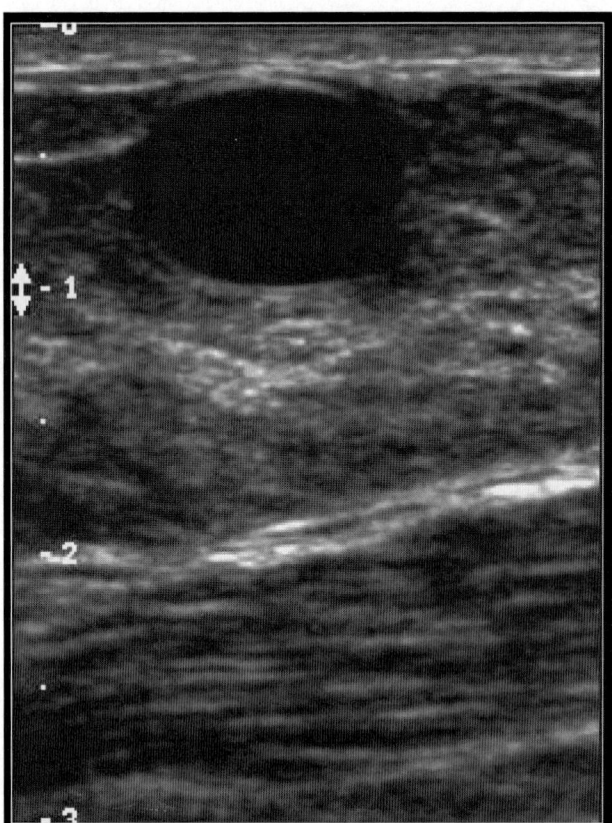

FIGURE 11–1 Acute galactoceles can be anechoic and simple cystic.

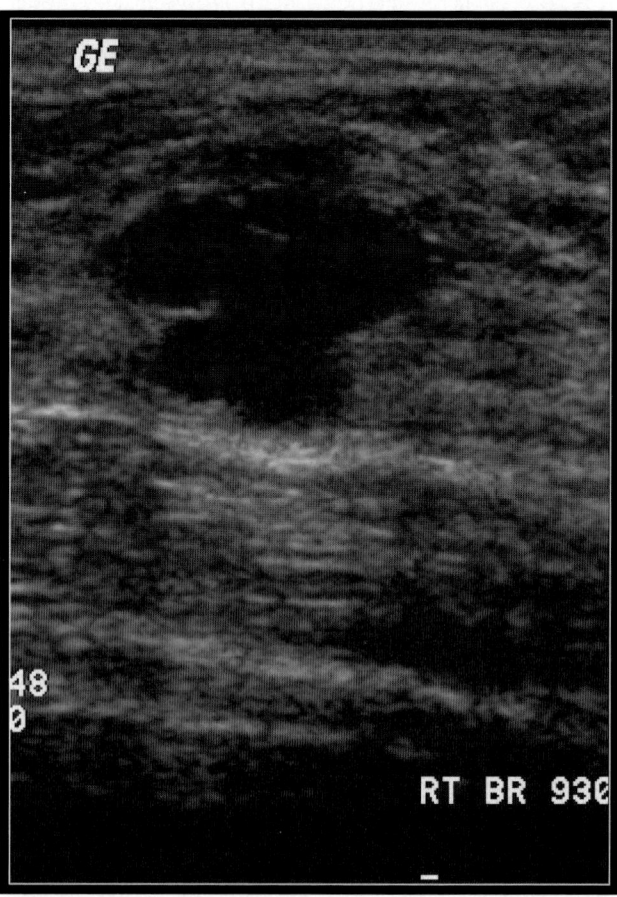

FIGURE 11–2 Acute galactoceles can be nearly anechoic and multiloculated.

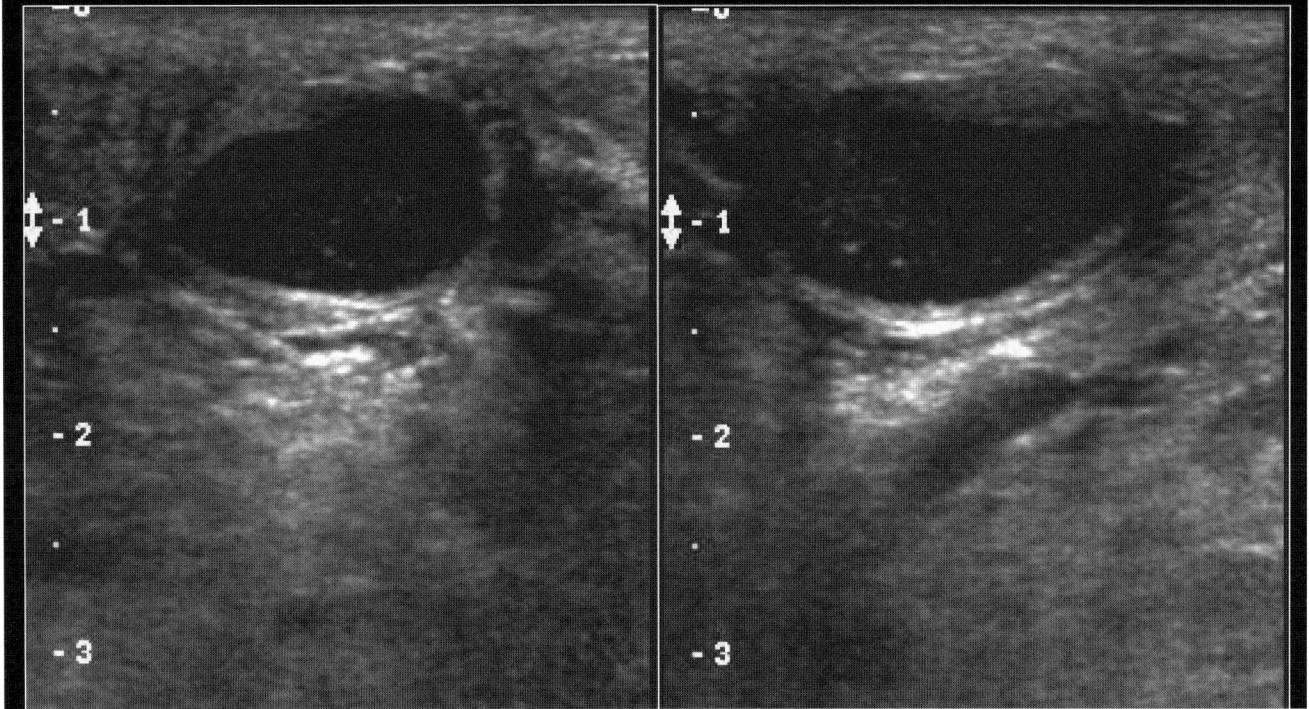

FIGURE 11–3 The milk within galactoceles can have a diffuse, low-level echogenicity because of the innumerable interfaces between incompletely emulsified fat globules and water.

galactoceles are more likely to be unilocular or bilocular and involve only the lactiferous sinus portion of a single duct and one or two central branches (Fig. 11–5). The peripheral variety is more common. An especially common place for galactoceles to form is in accessory breast tissue within the axillary segment of the breast. The peripheral glands and ducts within accessory breast tissue are frequently able to function and produce milk under the influence of the hormones of pregnancy, but the milk is unable to drain from the accessory breast because there are

no major ducts connecting the accessory tissue to the nipple. Thus, the lobules and peripheral ducts within the accessory breast tissue become engorged with milk (Fig. 11–6).

Galactoceles tend to become mildly to moderately echogenic as they age. The lipid components in older galactoceles become less well emulsified and coalesce into larger fat globules that have more prominent and echogenic interfaces with the water component of milk in which they are suspended. Such galactoceles either appear to have

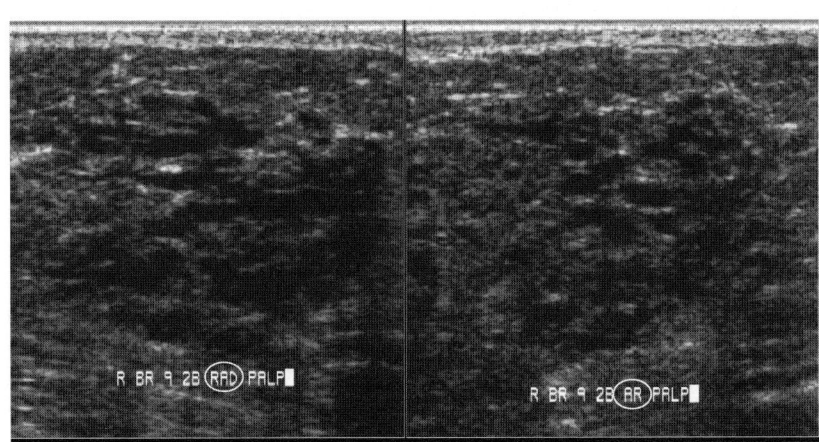

FIGURE 11–4 In peripheral galactoceles that are less dilated than the one shown in Fig. 11–2, the shape and configuration of obstructed distal ducts and lobules is easier to appreciate. Radial scans *(rad)* show the distal ducts and lobules in their long axes, and antiradial *(ar)* views show the distal ducts and lobules in their short axes.

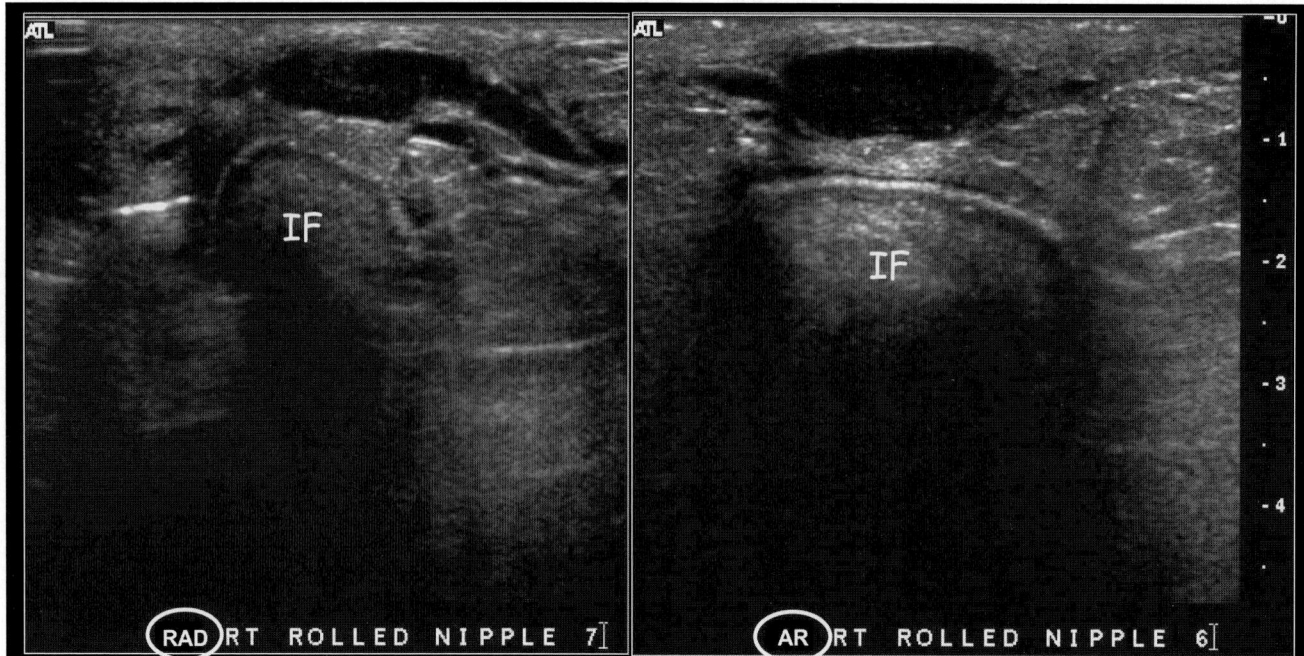

FIGURE 11–5 Occasionally, a central galactocele will involve the lactiferous sinus and even extend into the base of the nipple. RAD, radial plane; AR, antiradial plane; IF, index finger of nonscanning hand.

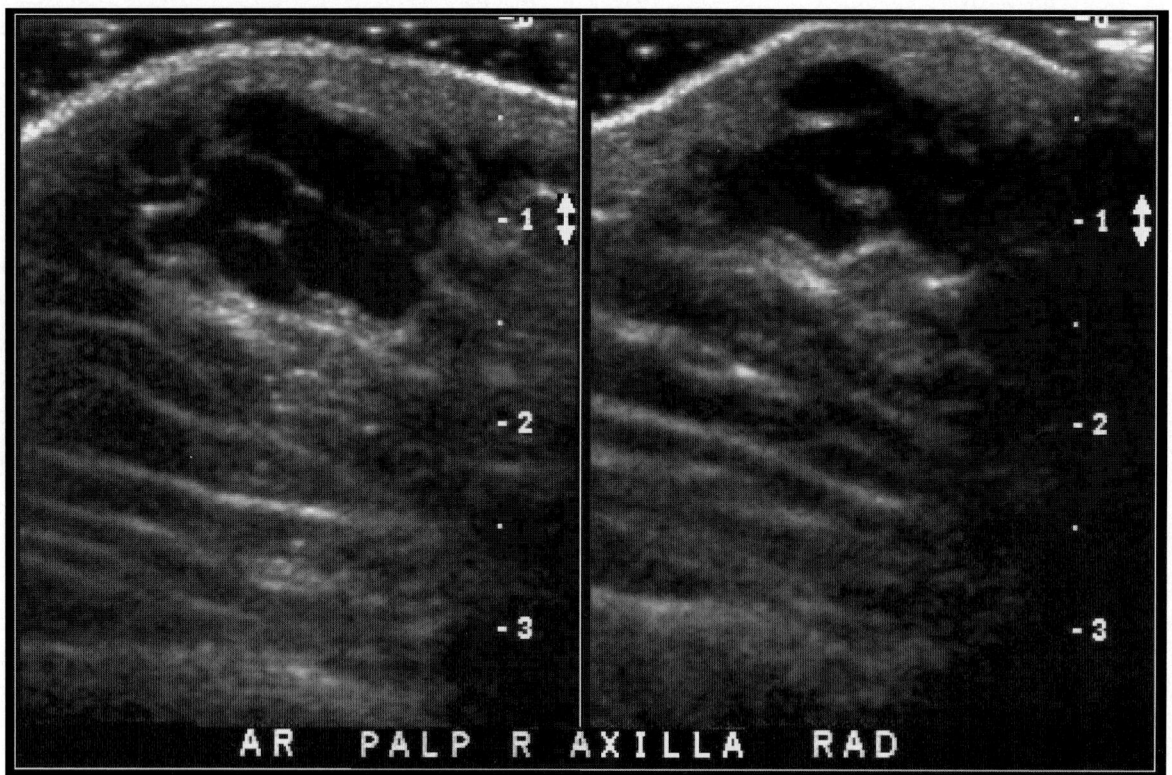

FIGURE 11–6 Galactoceles commonly develop within accessory breast tissue in the axillary segment or axilla. The tissue there is hormonally sensitive and capable of secreting milk, but the accessory breast tissue usually does not have a duct that drains it to the nipple. Thus, milk produced in the accessory breast tissue is trapped within, causing dilation of the rudimentary ducts and lobules within it. Galactoceles that develop within accessory breast tissue tend to present earlier than galactoceles in other parts of the breast—often during the third trimester of pregnancy.

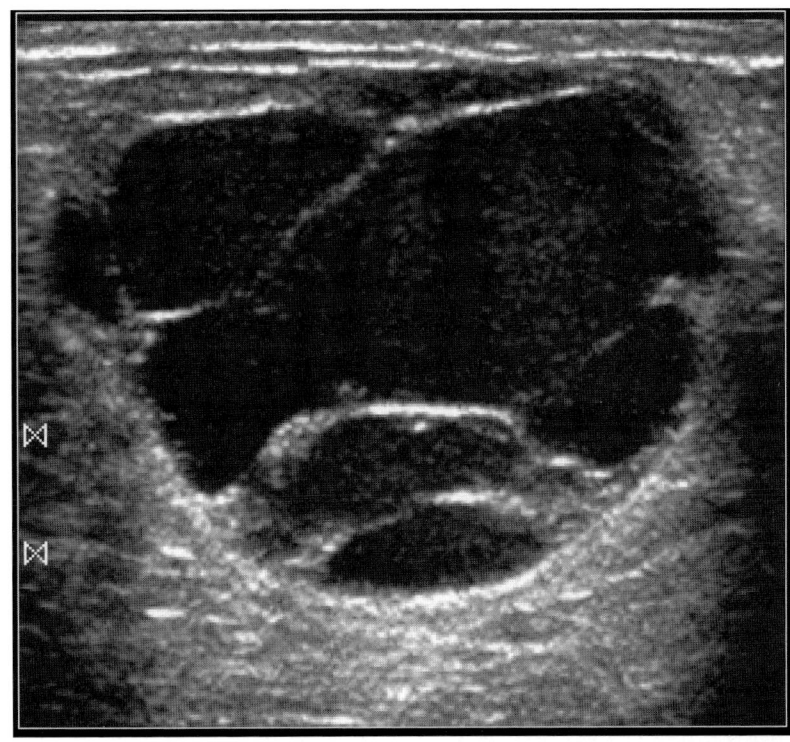

FIGURE 11–7 As galactoceles age, the trapped milk tends to become more echogenic because the lipid contents become less well emulsified, forming larger droplets of suspended lipids. The larger droplets form larger interfaces with the water components in which they are suspended, creating innumerable tiny fat–fluid interfaces that increase echogenicity.

homogeneous diffuse, low-level internal echoes when the lipid and water components are uniformly mixed (Fig. 11–7) or may have heterogenous echogenicity when the lipid components are not uniformly mixed (Fig. 11–8). Galactoceles in which protein has been extensively denatured and in which the milk has curdled may even appear sonographically solid and hyperechoic to varying degrees (Fig. 11–9). Despite the underlying obstructive process from which galactoceles arise, and despite their solid appearance on sonography, hyperechoic galactoceles may still be fairly soft and compressible (Fig. 11–10).

The acute, nearly anechoic phase of the galactocele corresponds to a water-density mass phase mammographically. The hyperechoic, solid-appearing galactocele phase can correspond to either water-density or mixed fat and water-density mammographic lesions.

Distinguishing a galactocele that has a solid hyperechoic appearance from a true solid mass, such as a fibroadenoma or breast cancer, is important. Mammographic demonstration of a pure fatty density or a mixed fat and water-density mass may be the most definitive way to make this distinction in cases in which there is enough fat within the galactocele to be mammographically visible. However, in cases in which the classic mammographic appearance is not present, color Doppler may be helpful.

There are two methods of distinguishing solid-appearing complex cysts such as galactoceles from true solid lesions, and Doppler can be helpful in both:

1. Demonstrate blood vessels in the center of the lesion.
2. Create a "color swoosh" by ballottement of the lesion with the transducer.

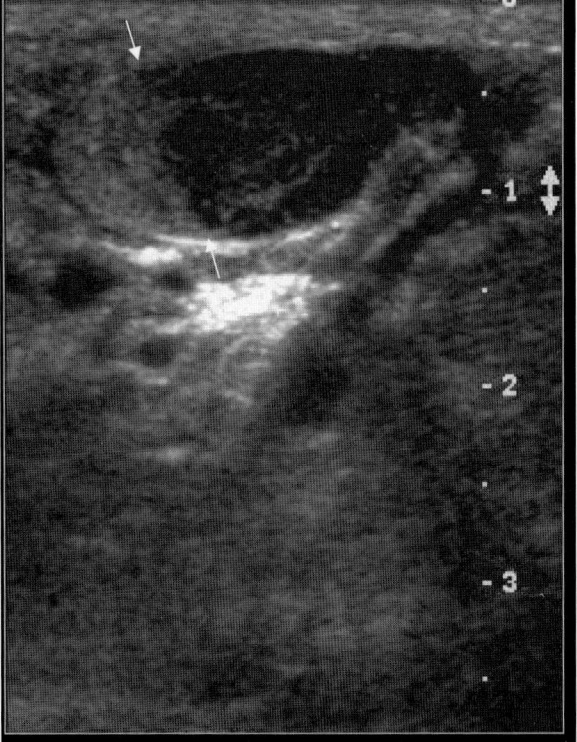

FIGURE 11–8 With prolonged stasis in subacute or chronic galactoceles, lipid droplets become larger. When lipid droplets become very large, they tend to mix less evenly with the water components of the trapped milk, causing heterogeneous texture within the galactocele. In this case, the echogenic lipid components could be seen streaming to the nondependent portion of the galactocele after the patient changed position. Eventually, the echogenic contents formed the fatty layer of a fat–fluid level *(arrows)*.

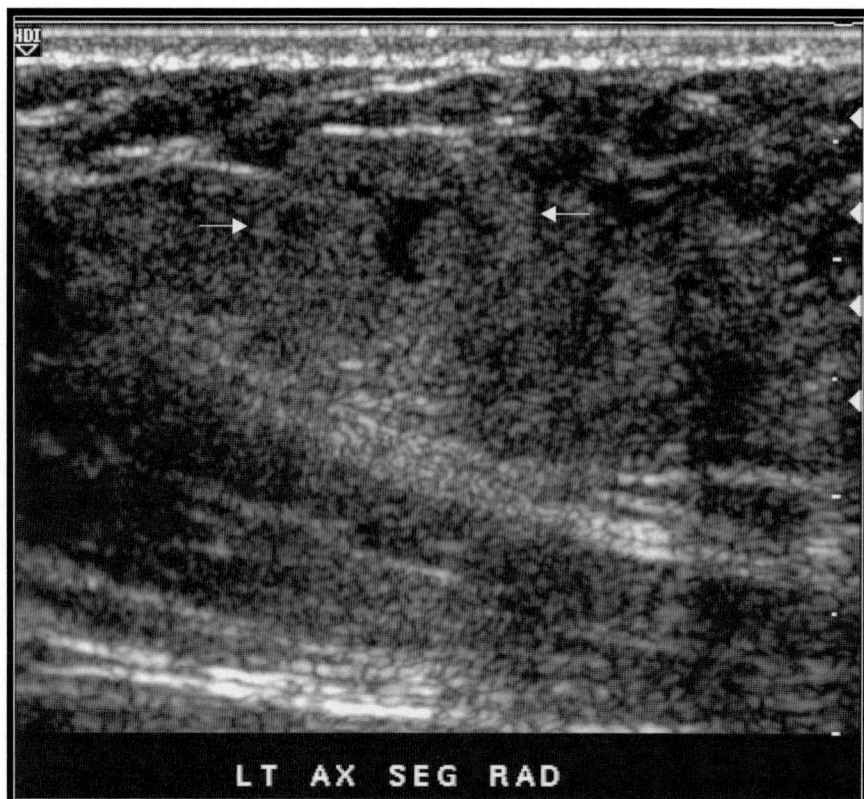

FIGURE 11–9 In chronic galactoceles, enzymatic action denatures the protein components of milk, causing the milk to become mildly hyperechoic *(arrows)*. In such cases, the galactocele can appear to be solid and hyperechoic and may be difficult to distinguish from surrounding glandular tissue.

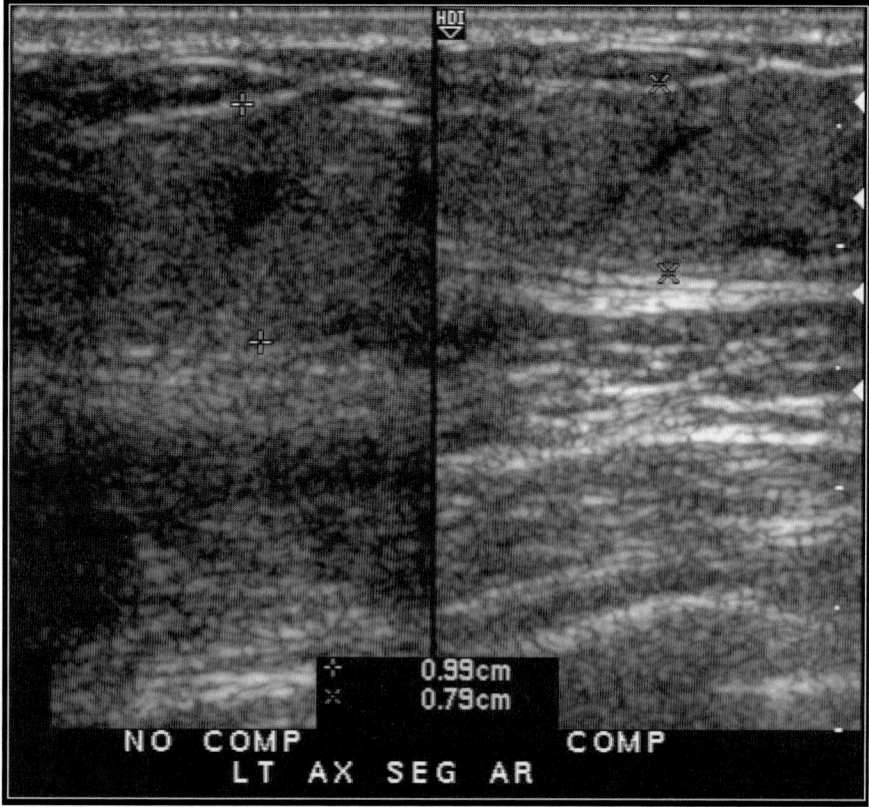

FIGURE 11–10 Despite the underlying obstructive process that gives rise to galactoceles, many galactoceles are soft and compressible.

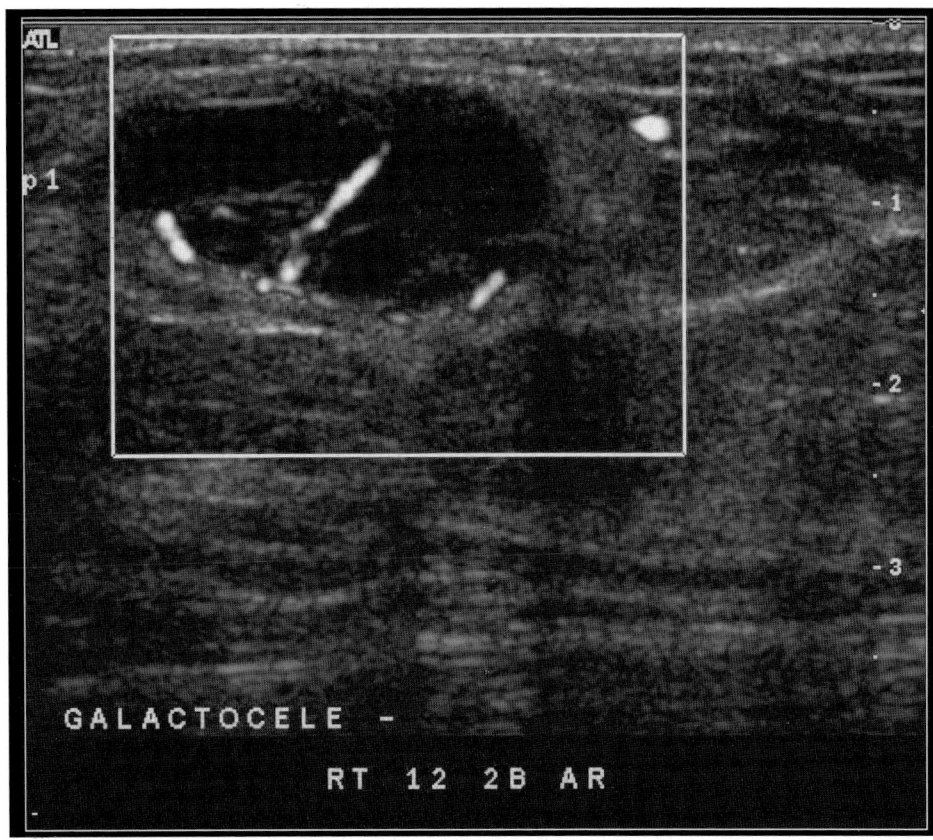

FIGURE 11–11 Galactoceles may have flow in their walls, but not centrally. There is almost invariably demonstrable flow in the hormonally stimulated surrounding glandular breast tissues. However, flow may be demonstrable with color or power Doppler within the thin, echogenic septations that bridge certain galactoceles.

Regarding the first method, galactoceles have no internal blood flow that is demonstrable by color Doppler, but flow may be demonstrable in the hyperemic outer wall and in the surrounding breast tissue. Septated galactoceles may also have blood vessels within the thin, echogenic internal septations (Fig. 11–11). Although cancers and fibroadenomas do not always have central color Doppler–demonstrable blood flow during the nonlactating state, most are so hormonally stimulated during lactation that internal vascularity can easily be demonstrated with Doppler (see Chapter 20, Figs. 20–5, 20–7, 20–16). The presence of vascularity within an echogenic mass, therefore, indicates that the mass is solid.

Regarding the second method, duplex sonography of solid nodules is discussed in more detail in Chapter 20. Ballottement of a hyperechoic galactocele with the transducer can demonstrate movement of particles that can be important in confirming that the mass is actually complex cystic rather than solid. The movement of echogenic milk induced by ballottement shows a to-and-fro pattern, with echogenic milk moving in one direction during compres-sion with the transducer and sloshing back in the opposite direction during release of compression. The moving echogenic structures are fat globules or denatured milk proteins rather than blood because there is no blood flow within the lumen of a galactocele. The ballottement-induced particle motion can be demonstrated with either real-time B-mode imaging or color or power Doppler imaging. Although there is no blood flow within the lumen of a galactocele, the hyperemic surrounding lactating glandular tissue usually has readily demonstrable blood flow. It is important to distinguish between color Doppler signals caused by blood flow in surrounding glandular tissue and the color swoosh of echogenic milk within the lumen of a galactocele. Pulsed Doppler spectral analysis can be helpful, showing arterial waveforms within glandular tissue and random noise within sloshing echogenic milk. Similar to-and-fro flow of debris can be shown within early puerperal abscesses before they become well circumscribed. This should not be surprising because it is likely that many puerperal abscesses arise within preexisting galactoceles. Flow of debris within an infected galactocele is shown in

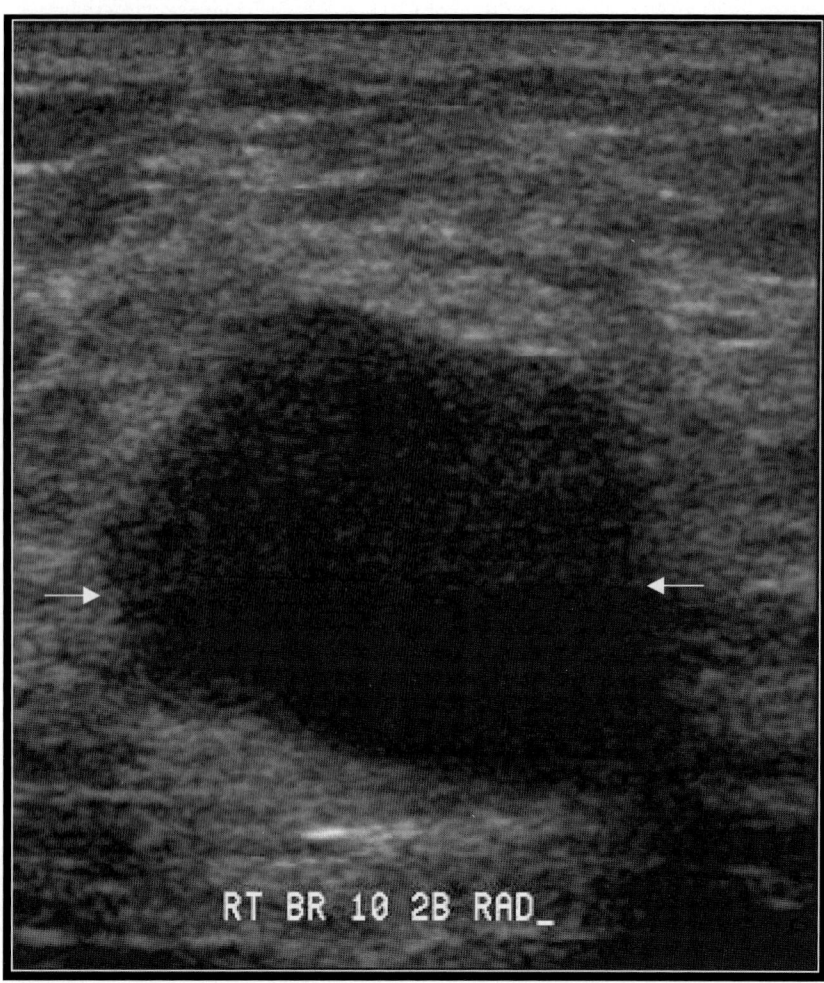

FIGURE 11–12 When fat globules become too large to remain emulsified, they eventually separate into a lipid layer that floats on the denser water components of the galactocele, forming a fat–fluid level (*arrows* indicate fat–fluid interface). Fat–fluid levels are definitively benign findings (BIRADS 2) but can be seen in fibrocystic change as well as within galactoceles. In fact, most cysts that contain fat–fluid levels do not occur during lactation or immediately after cessation of breast-feeding and are asymptomatic incidental findings during ultrasound (see Chapter 10).

the section on puerperal abscesses later in this chapter (see also Chapter 20, Fig. 20–35).

As galactoceles continue to age, the milk curdles and fat and water elements separate to a greater degree, becoming more heterogeneously distributed. Galactoceles then appear to have a mixed cystic and solid texture, corresponding to the mixed fat and water-density mammographic phase. In certain cases, a fat–fluid level may be apparent sonographically, comparable to the mammographic appearance (Fig. 11–12). The mildly echogenic fat floats on the gravity-dependent water-density component of the galactocele. In cases in which the lipid layer is only minimally echogenic or is very small, showing movement of the lipid layer to the newly nondependent portion of the cyst when the patient's position is changed from supine to upright or left lateral decubitus is helpful (Fig. 11–13). The appearance is similar to the fat–fluid levels seen in fibrocystic change (discussed in Chapter 10). Chronic galactoceles in which water components have been completely resorbed may become pure lipid cysts. Such galactoceles have either a simple cystic appearance or a complex cystic appearance similar to that of foam or gel cysts that are characterized by

low-level internal echoes and are discussed in Chapter 10. Mammographically, these lesions may be indistinguishable from lipid cysts associated with fat necrosis, especially if eggshell calcifications develop within the cyst wall. Examples of a lipid cyst are shown in Chapter 10 and later on in this chapter in the section on fat necrosis.

The natural history of most galactoceles is spontaneous resolution. The palpable lump and tenderness may resolve fairly quickly with conservative treatment—over a few days to a few weeks. In many patients, the lesions regress rapidly on follow-up sonograms (Fig. 11–14). However, in some patients, the lesion remains visible at sonography for much longer than they are symptomatic. We have seen galactoceles that are no longer symptomatic persist for years (Fig. 11–15).

In cases in which mammographic, sonographic, and Doppler findings are not definitive, ultrasound-guided aspiration is usually diagnostic and is often curative (Fig. 11–16). Successful aspiration may cause the palpable abnormality to disappear and confirms the suspicion of galactocele by yielding milky fluid. Occasionally, a successfully aspirated galactocele will recur. A recurrent galactocele, like

(text continued on page 361)

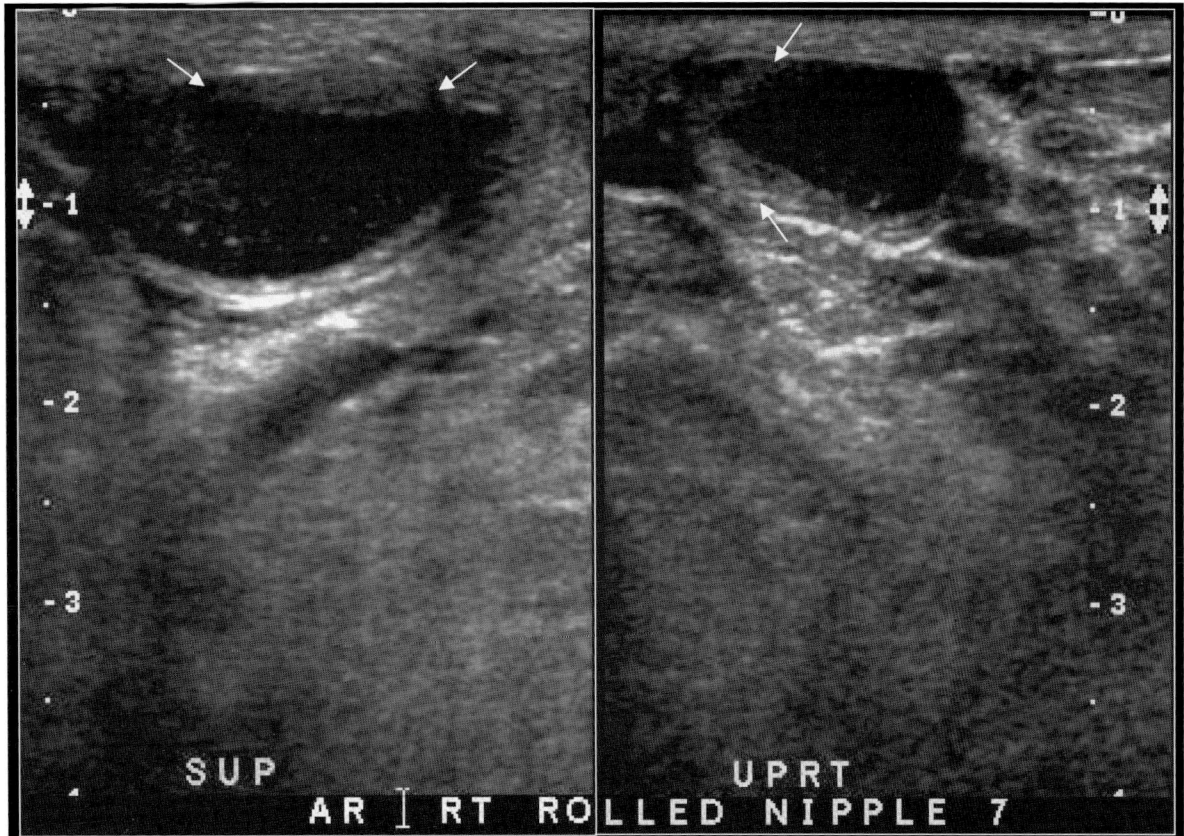

FIGURE 11–13 Echogenic lipid layers may simulate abnormal thickening of the galactocele wall or mural nodules. Therefore, it is essential to demonstrate that fat–fluid levels move and reorient themselves when the patient changes position in order to distinguish them from mural nodules that are immobile because they are attached to the wall of the lesion. The echogenic lipid layer floats anteriorly when the patient is supine but moves to the cranial portion of the galactocele when the patient is upright or to the right side of the lesion when the patient is placed into a left lateral decubitus position.

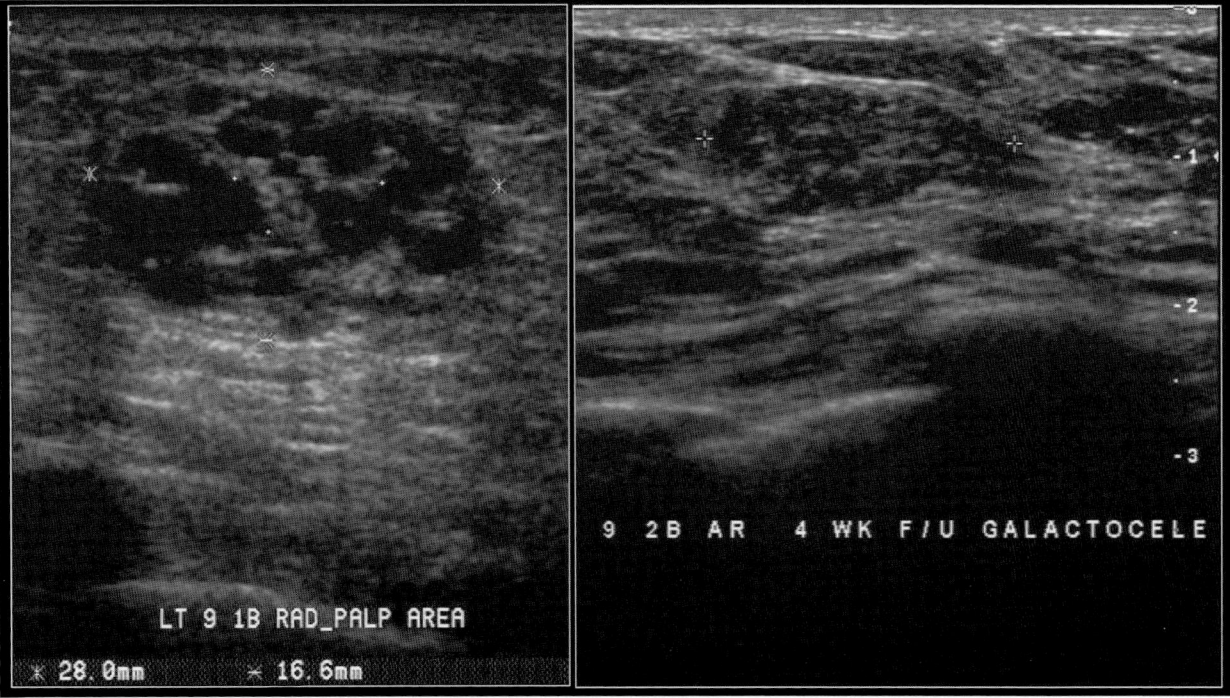

FIGURE 11–14 Most galactoceles eventually regress spontaneously over a few days to weeks. This galactocele gradually regressed over 4 weeks.

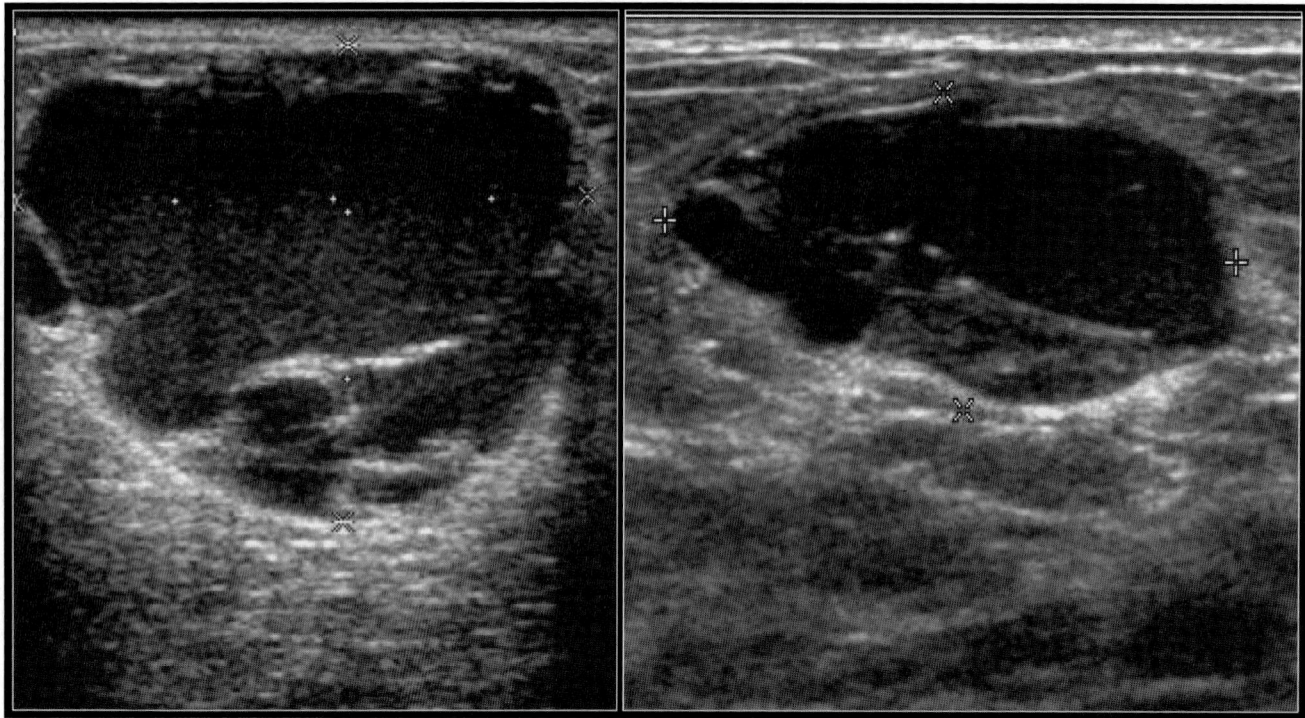

FIGURE 11–15 The resolution of certain galactoceles is protracted and may take months. In others, the lesion becomes chronic and never completely regresses. This lesion became gradually smaller over a period of years but never completely disappeared.

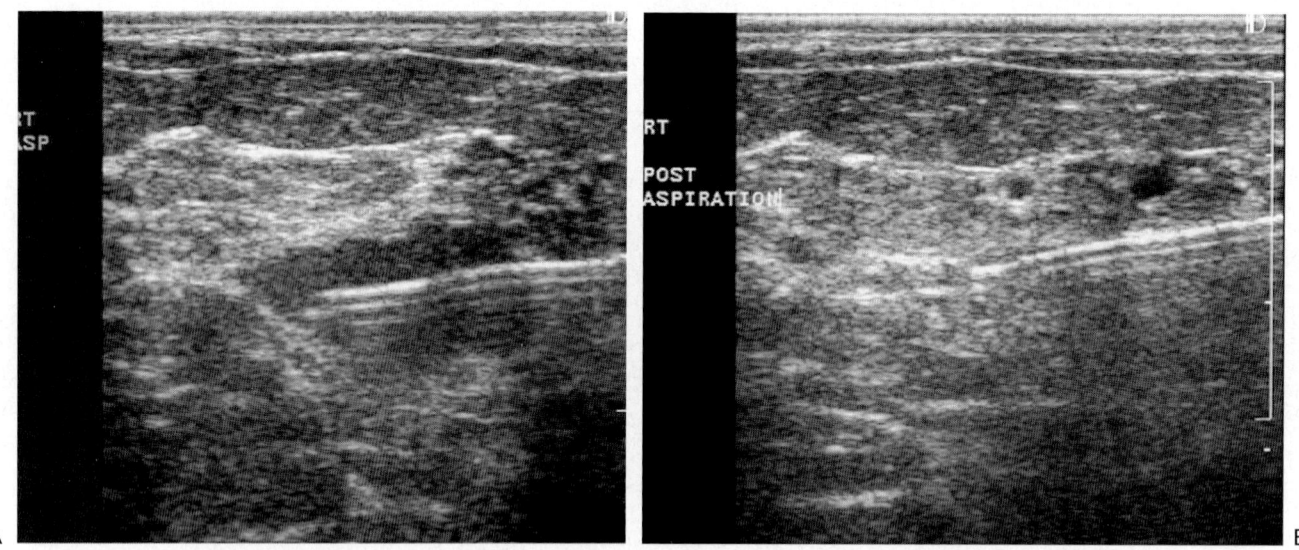

FIGURE 11–16 A: The tender galactocele was aspirated under ultrasound guidance, the fluid was sent for Gram stain and culture, and the patient was placed on antibiotics. **B:** At the completion of aspiration, there was no residual fluid left within the tender galactocele. The Gram stain and culture were negative, and the pain and tenderness resolved immediately after aspiration. The antibiotics were discontinued immediately after the negative 72-hour culture results were obtained.

any static fluid collection, is prone to secondary infection and may progress to mastitis and abscess formation. Therefore, if there is any tenderness or erythema or if the aspirate appears purulent, evaluation of the aspirate with Gram stain and culture and sensitivity will be necessary.

PUERPERAL ABSCESS FORMATION AND MASTITIS (LACTATIONAL MASTITIS)

General Pathologic Classification, Epidemiology, and Clinical Findings

Mastitis is inflammation of the breast that may be either infectious or noninfectious in origin.

Infectious mastitis most commonly is acute, occurs during lactation (*puerperal mastitis*), and may progress to tissue necrosis and abscess formation. Nipple fissure is an important underlying condition, allowing skin bacteria, usually *Staphylococcus aureus,* to penetrate through the skin into the ducts and deeper parts of the breast. Obstruction and stasis are also contributing factors. The subareolar inflammation caused by nipple fissures may lead to obstruction of the mammary ducts. Stasis of the milk lying within ectatic and obstructed ducts or within persistent or recurrent galactoceles ultimately predisposes to puerperal or lactational mastitis. The milk within obstructed ducts or lobules is an excellent culture medium for bacterial growth. Persistent untreated infection can then progress to abscess formation.

Patients with acute puerperal mastitis have localized or generalized edema and erythema of the breast, along with pain, tenderness, warmth, fever, and leukocytosis. If there is a mature abscess or underlying infected galactocele, there may be a tender, palpable, fluctuant lump. If the abscess is "pointing," the skin over the area of pointing will be stretched, thinned, and discolored. Additionally, some patients may have purulent nipple discharge.

Mammographic Findings

Mammography is usually not very helpful, showing only enlargement and increased density resulting from edema of the inflamed segments of the breast. If there is a well-developed abscess, an ill-defined high-density mass may be visible, but the lesion is often obscured by the surrounding inflamed and radiographically dense lactational tissue. Sonography is more useful than mammography both for identifying a drainable abscess in patients with puerperal mastitis and for following the effectiveness of treatment.

Sonographic Findings

Sonography is the examination of choice in patients with puerperal mastitis and is almost always the first imaging study performed. Early in the course of puerperal mastitis, before tissue necrosis leads to a well-defined abscess cavity, edema may be the only sonographic finding (Fig. 11–17). The edema affects all of the tissue layers in the area of inflammation. The skin and subcutaneous fat are thickened and become hyperechoic. Cooper's ligaments are also thickened. The normally hyperechoic Cooper's ligaments and interlobular stromal fibrous tissue become less echogenic, less

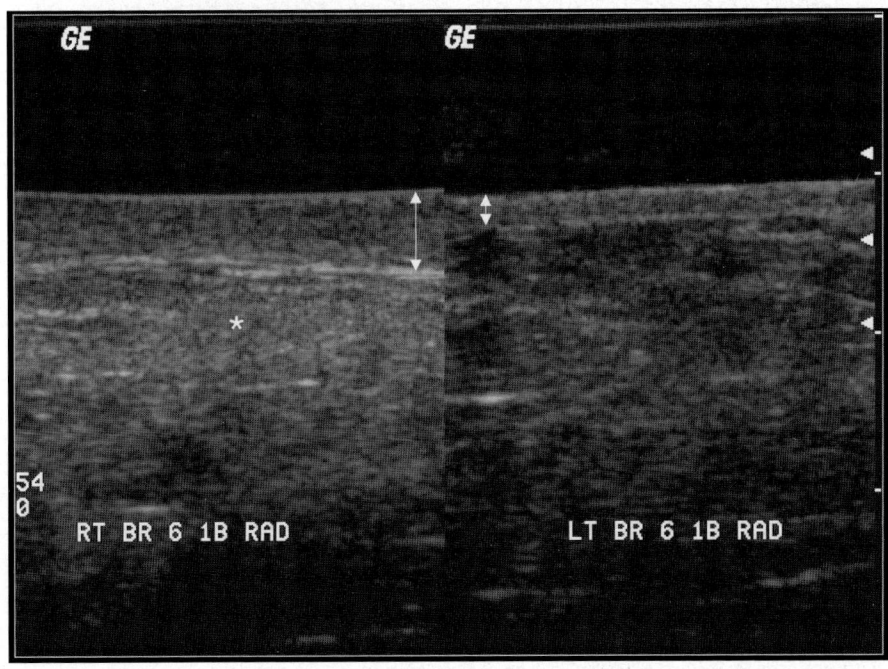

FIGURE 11–17 These split-screen mirror images of a patient with right-sided puerperal mastitis compare the affected right side with the unaffected left side. Puerperal mastitis causes edema. Edema of subcutaneous fat causes the fat to be hyperechoic *(*)* with respect to fat in uninvolved portions of the ipsilateral breast or compared with normal fat in the mirror-image location of the contralateral breast. The skin also becomes abnormally thick and usually mildly hypoechoic *(two-headed arrow)*. These changes caused by edema are most easily and accurately appreciated on split-screen images comparing the symptomatic area to uninvolved areas of the ipsilateral or contralateral breast. An acoustic standoff pad was used to demonstrate skin changes.

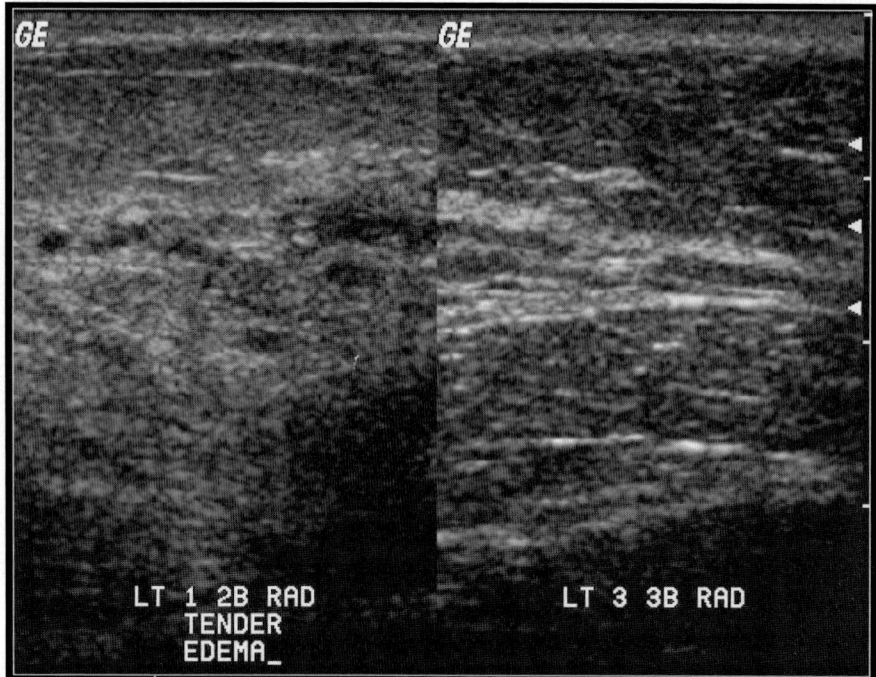

FIGURE 11–18 These split-screen images compare the infected 1:00 position of the left breast with the uninfected 3:00 position. The severe edema has made the fat at 1:00 markedly hyperechoic and the normally hyperechoic fibrous tissue less echogenic than normal. In the infected area of the breast, the distinction between fat and fibrous tissue is less clear than it is in the normal 3:00 location. The infected areas is thickened enough and penetration decreased enough that the chest wall at 1:00 is inadequately visualized.

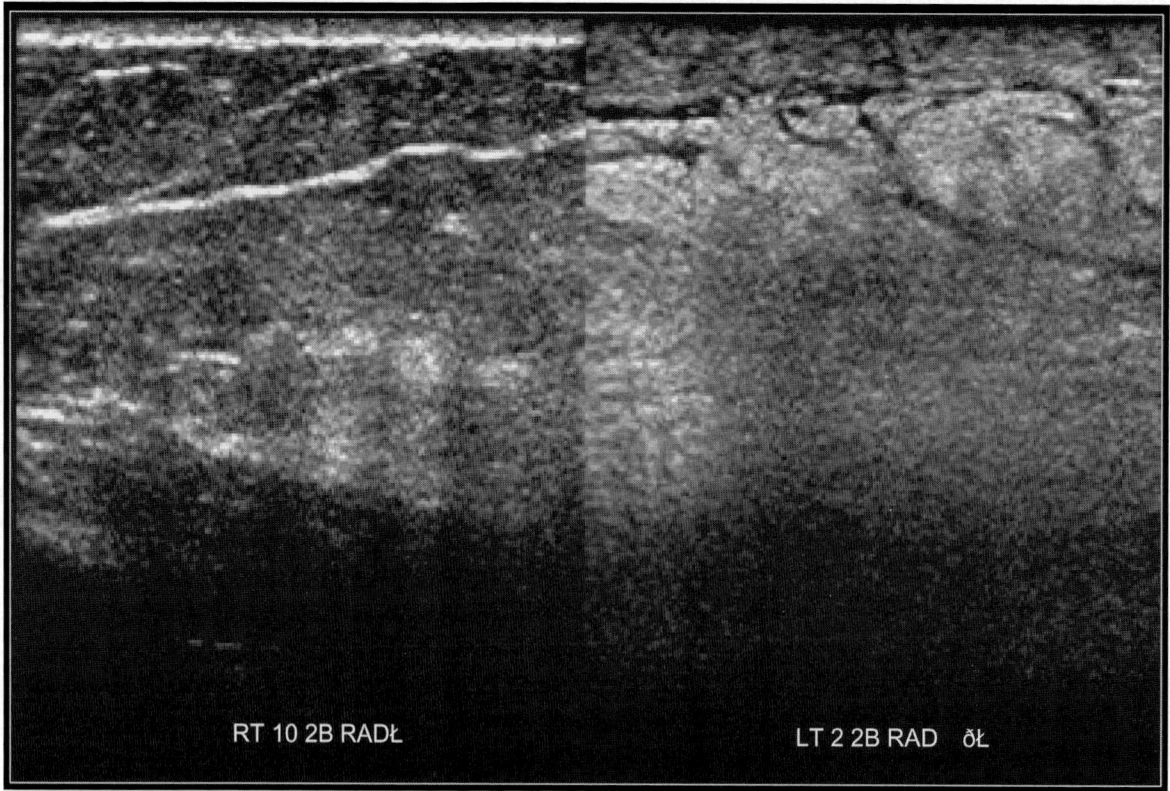

FIGURE 11–19 These split-screen images compare mirror-image locations on the right and left side in a patient who has very severe puerperal mastitis on the left. The edema in the left breast is so severe that all distinction between different types of tissue has been lost, and penetration to the chest wall is inadequate. Evaluation with a 5-MHz curved linear array transducer was necessary to exclude abscess and underlying inflammatory carcinoma. Involvement this severe usually occurs just before tissue necrosis and abscess development.

well defined, and more difficult to distinguish from the abnormally echogenic fat (Fig. 11–18). In the advanced stage, just before liquefactive necrosis, the distinction between ducts, lobules, and surrounding fibrous tissue disappears (Fig. 11–19). The entire breast thickness increases. The hyperechogenicity of fat, skin thickening, and loss of distinction between different types of breast tissues is most readily appreciated if comparison is made to the mirror-image location in the contralateral breast with documentation on split-screen images.

The engorged, edematous, and infected breast of the patient with puerperal mastitis may be difficult to penetrate with the standard high-frequency near-field 7- to 12-MHz transducers typically used for breast ultrasound. The breasts become difficult to penetrate because (a) lactating patients have thicker breasts than nonlactating patients, (b) mastitis further increases the breast thickness, and (c) edema decreases sound transmission through the breast as well as scattering sound, adversely affecting focusing characteristics. Excluding abscess formation deep within the breast is impossible if the sound beam cannot penetrate coherently to the chest wall (Fig. 11–19). Achieving adequate penetration and resolution in patients with puerperal mastitis often requires the more deeply focused and better penetrating 5-MHz linear probe, which is generally discouraged in diagnostic breast ultrasound. Puerperal mastitis represents one of the select few indications for breast ultrasound in which a 5-MHz probe may outperform 7- to 12-MHz transducers.

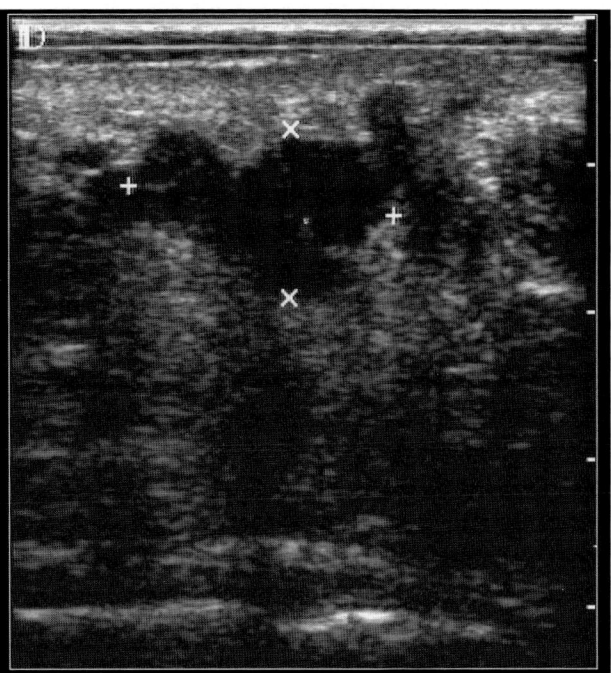

FIGURE 11–21 Abscesses that develop within peripheral galactoceles are more likely to reflect the underlying multiloculated configuration of peripheral galactoceles than are centrally located abscesses.

Although puerperal mastitis can spread to involve the entire breast, its origin is typically lobar or sublobar. The sonographic appearance of early puerperal mastitis reflects whether the central or peripheral portion of the lobe is more involved. The patterns of involvement can be peripheral, central, or nonspecific. The peripheral and central patterns have well-defined, obstructed, fluid-filled ducts or lobules early in the course that facilitate early diagnosis of abscess formation. On the other hand, the nonspecific pattern of mastitis results in formation of an abscess cavity only late in the course of infection, and early diagnosis of abscess is very difficult.

In the *peripheral pattern*, the underlying obstruction is at the level of the peripheral sublobar ducts or lobules, and the infection typically develops within a preexisting galactocele. Thus, abscess develops very early in the course of the disease and has sonographic characteristics that are similar to those of the peripheral galactocele in which it arose. The abscess is usually relatively well defined very early in its development. The wall of the abscess is thicker than the wall of an uninfected galactocele (Fig. 11–20). It is often multilobulated or multilocular or septated (Fig. 11–21). Solid necrotic tissue or denatured milk may float within the pus (Fig. 11–22).

In the *central pattern* of acute puerperal mastitis, the infection originates within the ectatic central ducts rather

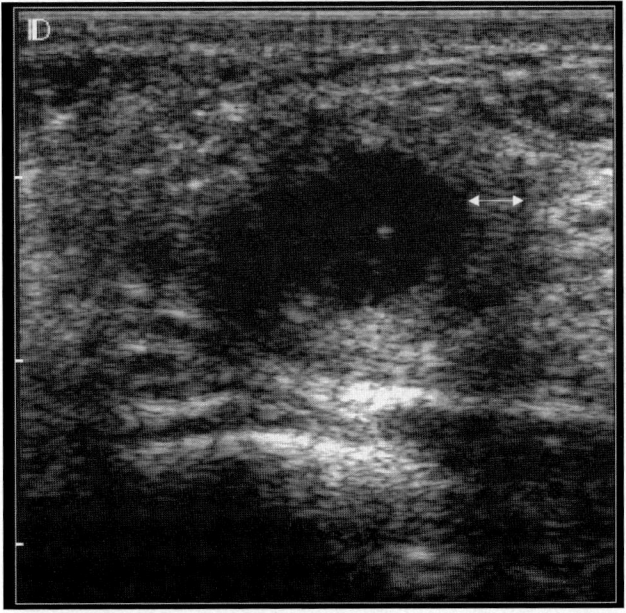

FIGURE 11–20 The wall of the abscesses that have developed from galactoceles is thicker than the wall of the galactoceles from which they arose *(two-headed arrow).*

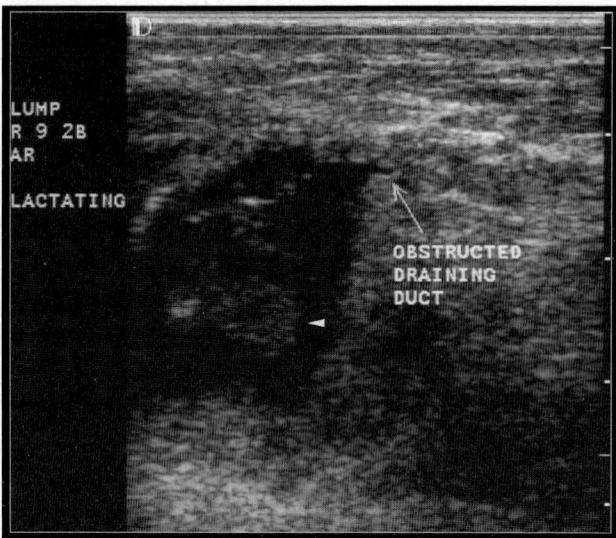

FIGURE 11–22 Echogenic necrotic debris or inspissated milk may lie within the central cavity of peripheral puerperal abscesses.

than within a preexisting galactocele. The walls of infected ducts, like the walls of inflamed cysts, are thick and isoechoic rather than thin and echogenic (Fig. 11–23). If the ducts are obstructed, they may contain denatured solid, echogenic "milk plugs" within their lumina. Split-screen image comparisons with contralateral ducts or even ipsilateral ducts from an uninfected lobe readily demonstrate the differences in the sonographic appearances between obstructed, infected ducts and normal ducts (Fig. 11–24). The findings are nonspecific indicators of stasis and inflammation. The involvement is initially lobar in distribution but may rapidly spread to involve the whole breast. Color or power Doppler may demonstrate hyperemia within the thickened, isoechoic duct walls (see Chapter 20, Figs. 20–45 and 20–46). The sonographic appearances of ducts that are acutely inflamed are identical, regardless of whether the cause of inflammation is infection (puerperal mastitis) or chemical (duct ectasia–periductal mastitis complex). Thus, the history of breast-feeding, rather than the sonographic appearance, is the key to distinguishing between inflamed ducts caused by infection and the duct ectasia–periductal mastitis complex.

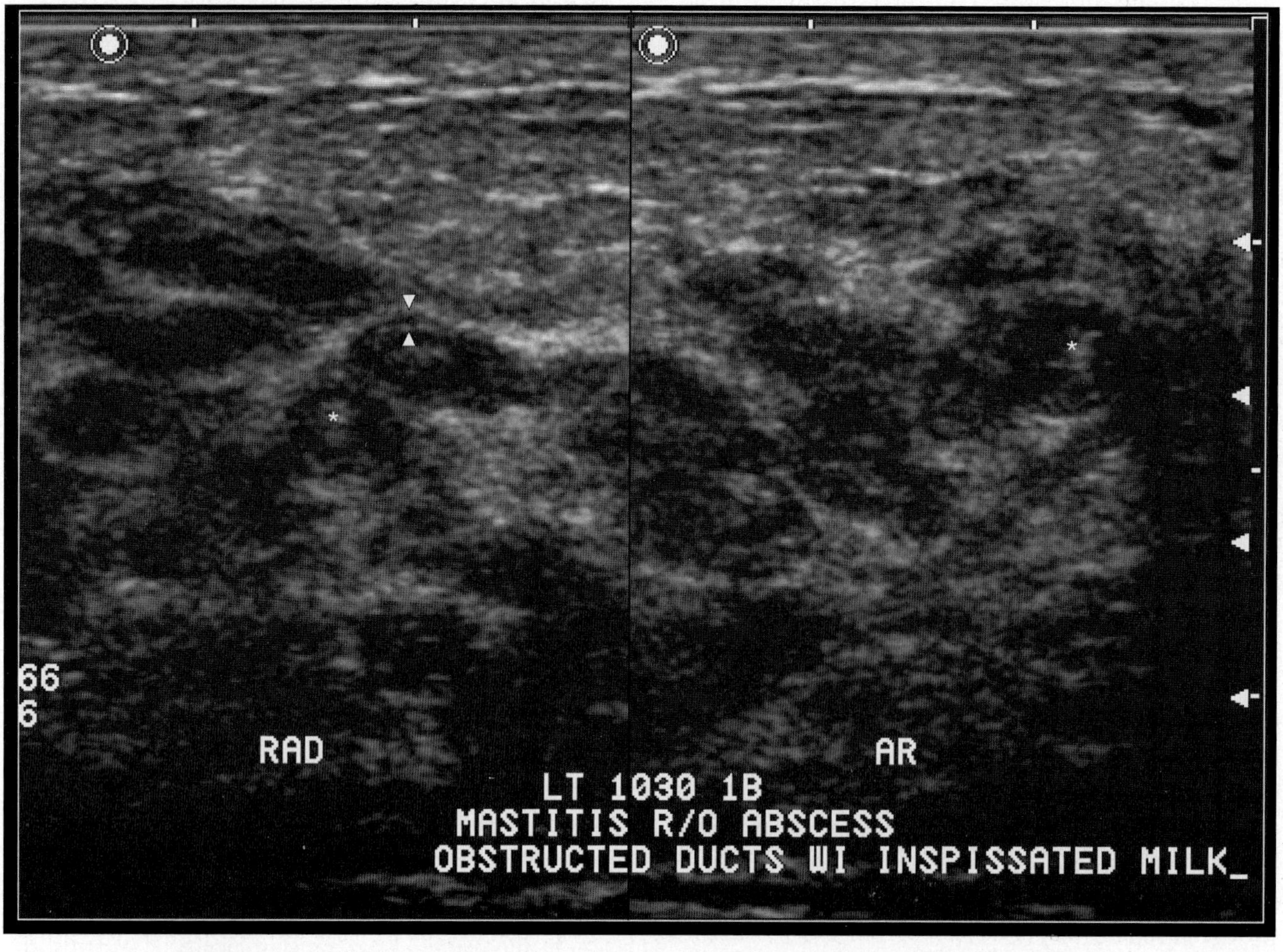

FIGURE 11–23 In the central form of acute puerperal mastitis, there is no underlying galactocele. The central ducts are infected and dilated and contain echogenic inspissated milk *(*)*. The duct walls are abnormally thickened and isoechoic *(between arrowheads)*.

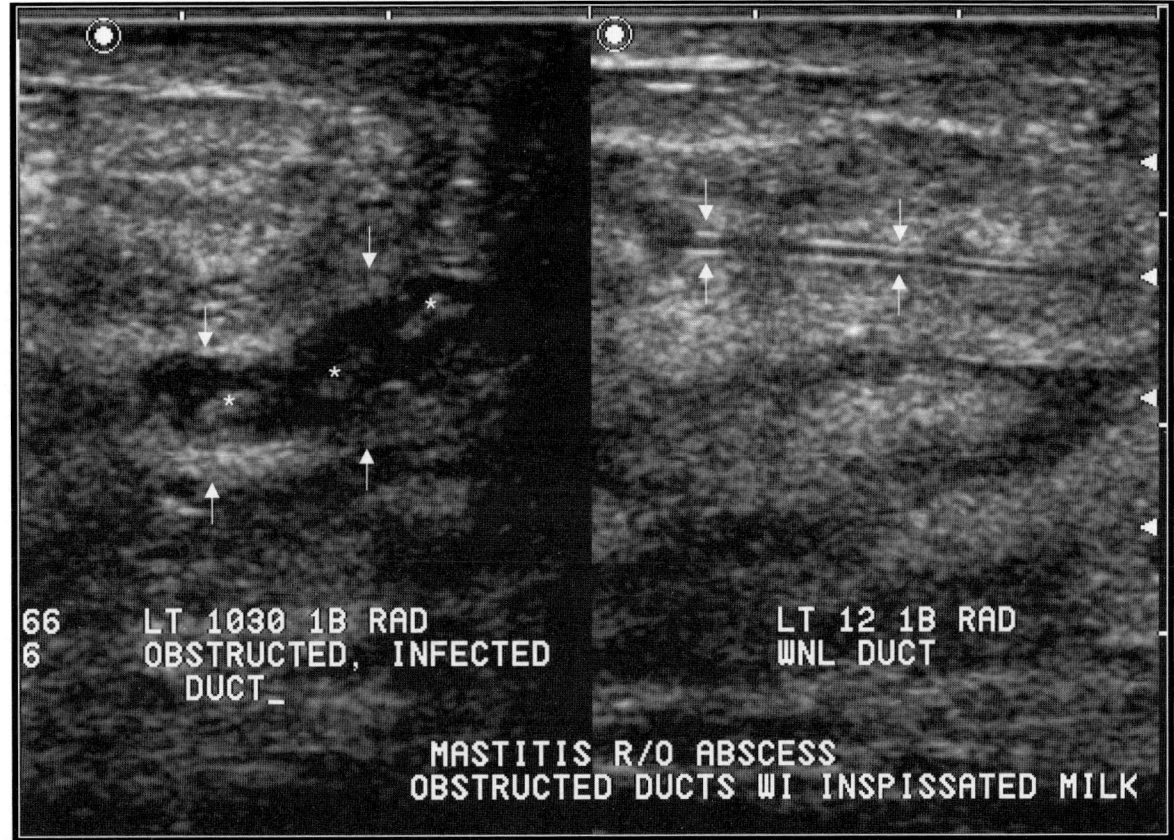

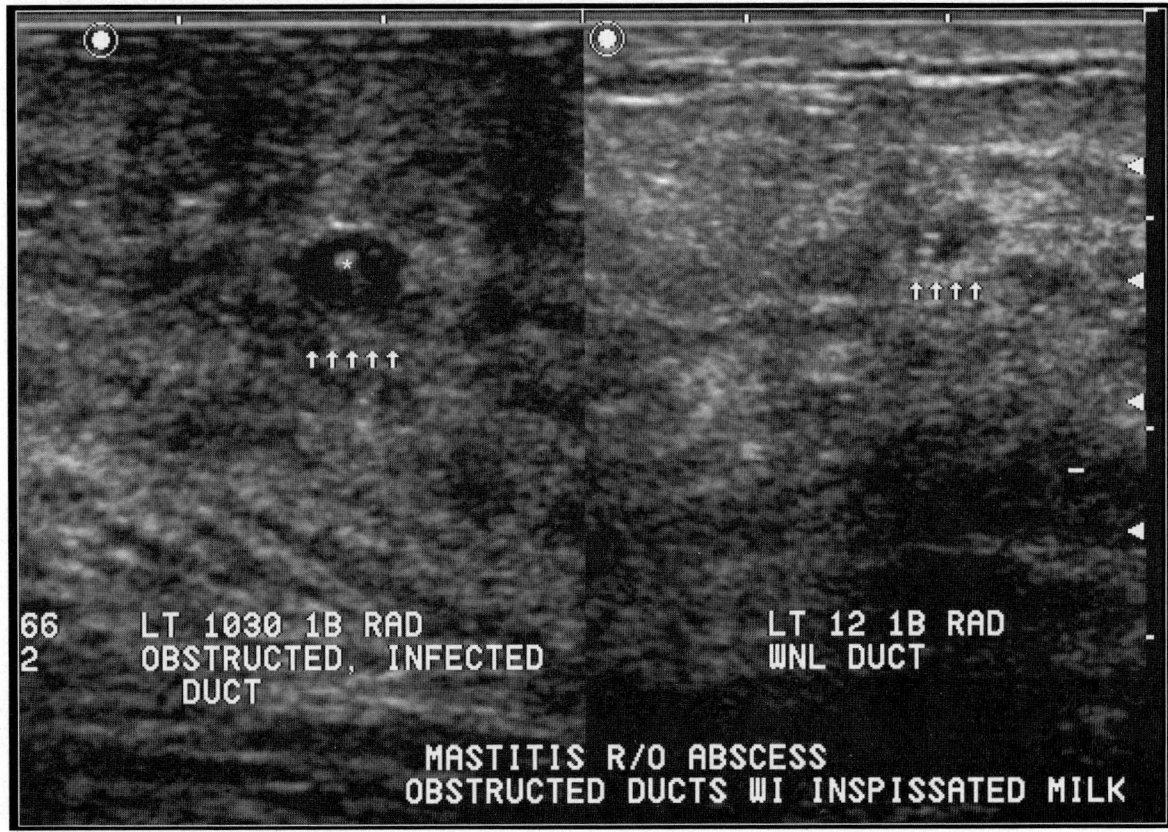

FIGURE 11–24 A: These are split-screen long-axis images of an infected duct at 10:30 (**left**) and an uninfected duct at 12:00 (**right**) in the left breast. Note that the normal duct is only minimally dilated and has thin, echogenic walls (**right**, *arrows*). The infected duct (**left**) is abnormally dilated, contains echogenic inspissated milk *(*)*, and has an abnormally thick and ill-defined wall (**left**, *arrows*) **B:** These are split-screen short-axis images of an infected duct at 10:30 (**left**) and an uninfected duct at 12:00 (**right**) in the left breast. Note that the normal duct is only minimally dilated and has thin, echogenic walls (**right**, *arrows*). The normal duct is surrounded by isoechoic loose periductal stroma fibrous tissue. The infected duct (**left**) is abnormally dilated, contains echogenic, inspissated milk (*), and has an abnormally thick and ill-defined wall (**left**, *arrows*).

If successfully treated with antibiotics before frank abscess formation, the severity of duct dilation (Fig. 11–25), thickening of the duct wall, and duct wall hyperemia all gradually improve. The inspissated milk plugs also lyse and disappear. Hyperemia regresses before imaging findings improve (see Chapter 20, Fig. 20–47).

When abscess develops from the central pattern of infection, it results from necrosis and rupture of the walls of one or more central ducts and leakage of infected milk into the surrounding tissues. Thus, the shape and location of abscesses resulting from the central pattern of mastitis differ from those with the peripheral pattern of mastitis. The underlying structure whose shape is reflected is that of a severely obstructed and dilated central duct, not that of obstructed peripheral ducts and lobules. The abscess cavity is more likely to be oval, parallel to the subareolar ducts, unilocular, thick walled, and centrally located (Fig. 11–26). When the central pattern of mastitis is inadequately treated, infection may lead to necrosis and rupture of multiple duct walls, leading to multiple abscesses whose

distribution parallels that of the underlying ducts in which they arose (Fig. 11–27). The sonographic findings in patients who have the central pattern of puerperal mastitis are indistinguishable from those of duct ectasia and acute periductal mastitis (chemical mastitis), except for the history of breast-feeding.

Because obstruction is one of the factors contributing to infection, many patients with mastitis have more dilated ducts on the infected side than on the contralateral, asymptomatic side. However, assessment of dilated ducts in lactating patients must be tempered with the knowledge that the degree of physiologic duct dilation during lactation varies greatly, depending on when the patient last breast-fed and with letdown. Physiologic letdown is associated with dilation of the lactiferous sinus portion of the ducts, and unilateral letdown might create a false impression of pathologic ectasia caused by obstruction. However, in patients with central mastitis, the degree of ductal asymmetry is more than would be expected with asymmetric letdown. Split-screen mirror images of the subareolar ducts on the

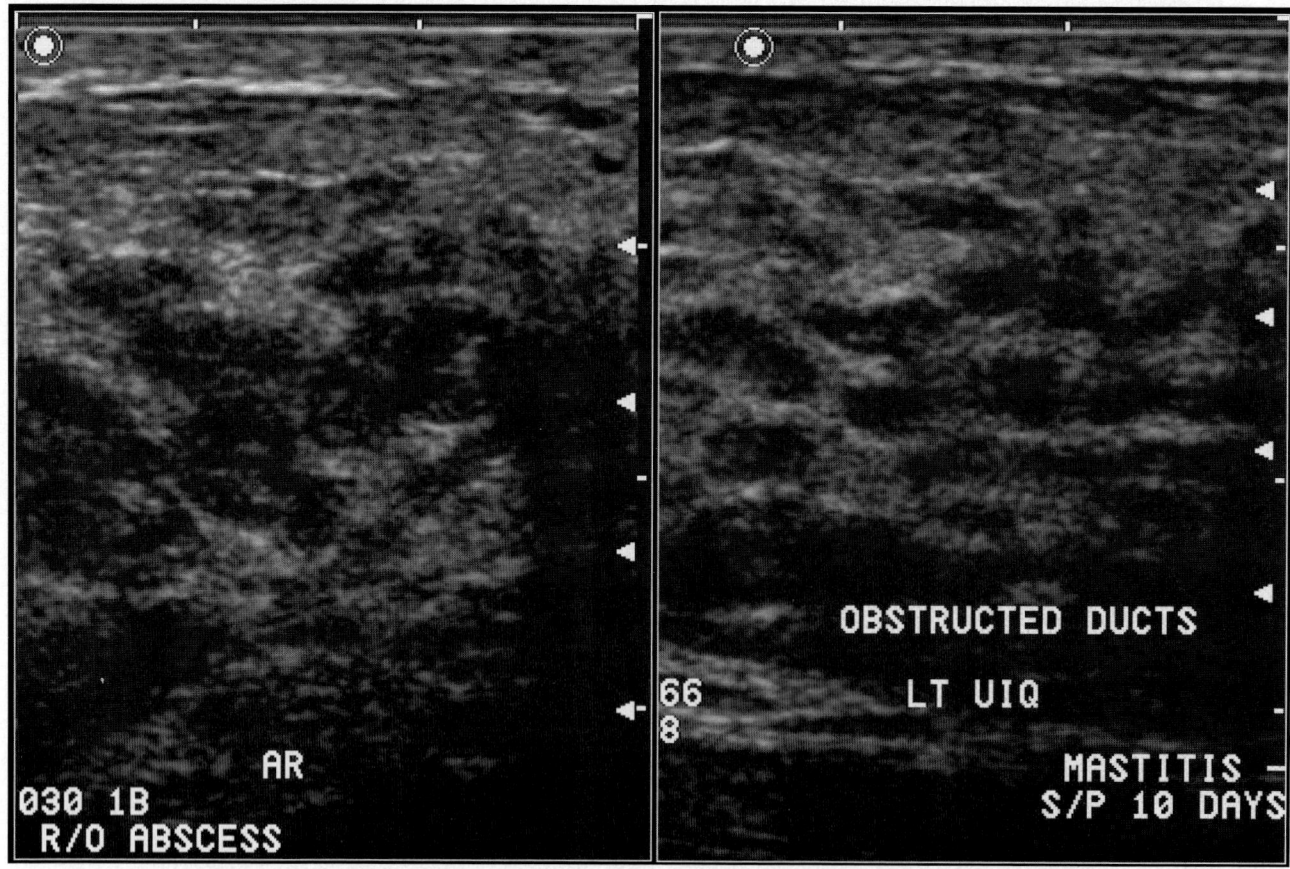

FIGURE 11–25 A: These antiradial images of the infected area of the left breast are obtained through the short axis of the infected ducts at the time of diagnosis (**left**) and after 10 days of antibiotic treatment (**right**). Note that the ducts are less dilated (less obstructed) and have slightly thinner walls on the follow-up examination. Note also that on the follow-up examination, there is less inspissated milk within the lumen to act as a nidus for continued infection.

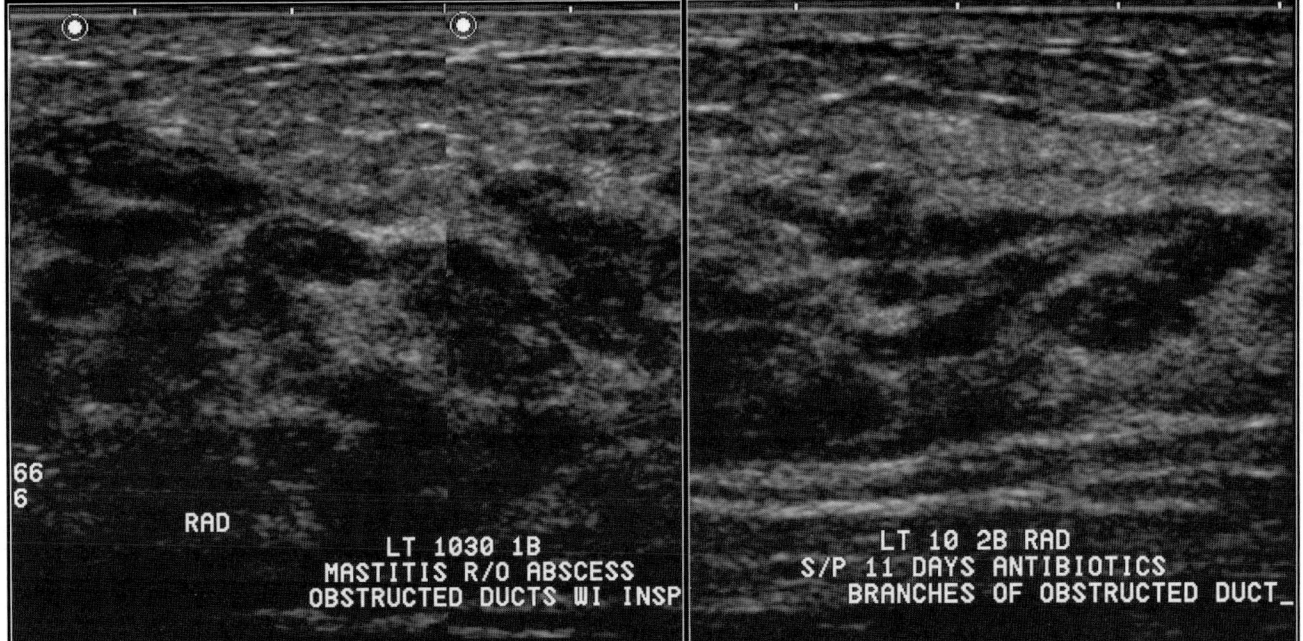

RAD

LT 1030 1B
MASTITIS R/O ABSCESS
OBSTRUCTED DUCTS WI INSP

LT 10 2B RAD
S/P 11 DAYS ANTIBIOTICS
BRANCHES OF OBSTRUCTED DUCT

66
6

B

FIGURE 11–25 *(continued)* **B:** These radial images of the infected area of the left breast are obtained through the long axis of the infected ducts at the time of diagnosis (**left**) and after 10 days of antibiotic treatment (**right**). Note that the ducts are less dilated (less obstructed) and have slightly thinner walls on the follow-up examination. Note also that on the follow-up examination, there is less inspissated milk within the lumen to act as a nidus for continued infection. Additionally, note that the infection is lobar in distribution. The ducts are so severely dilated on the initial examination that it is difficult to appreciate the lobar configuration. However, on the follow-up examination, the degree of dilation has decreased enough to show that all of the ducts are branches of a single lobar duct.

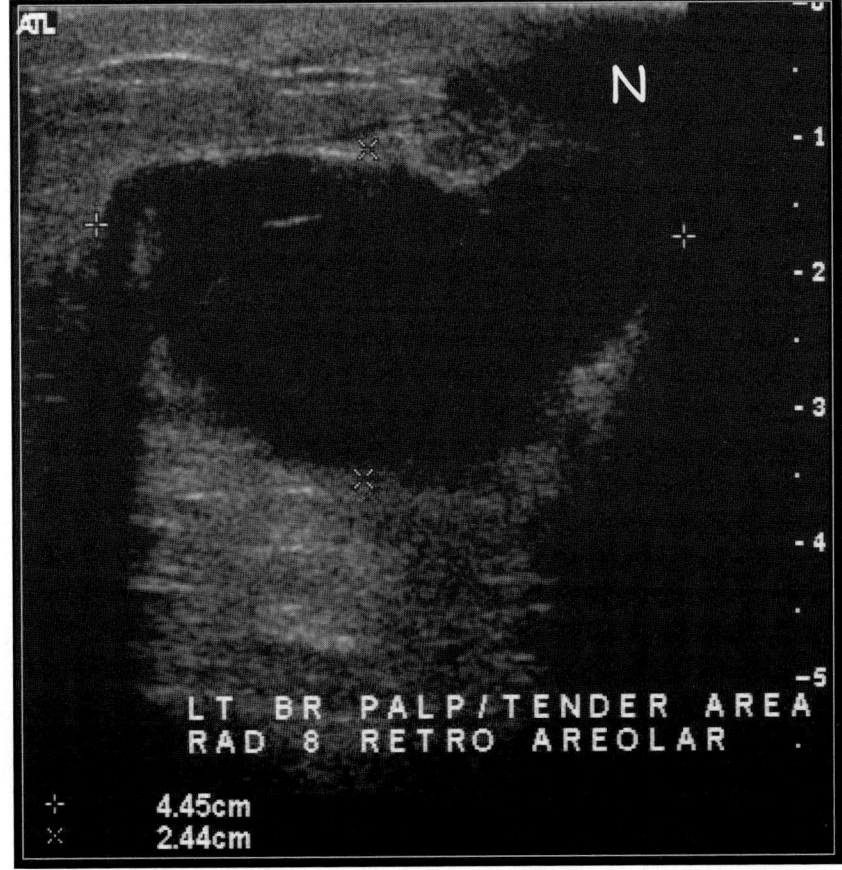

LT BR PALP/TENDER AREA
RAD 8 RETRO AREOLAR

4.45cm
2.44cm

FIGURE 11–26 Centrally located puerperal abscesses are more likely to be unilocular and elongated in an axis parallel to the central ducts than are peripheral abscesses because they originate from rupture of severely infected central ducts. N, nipple.

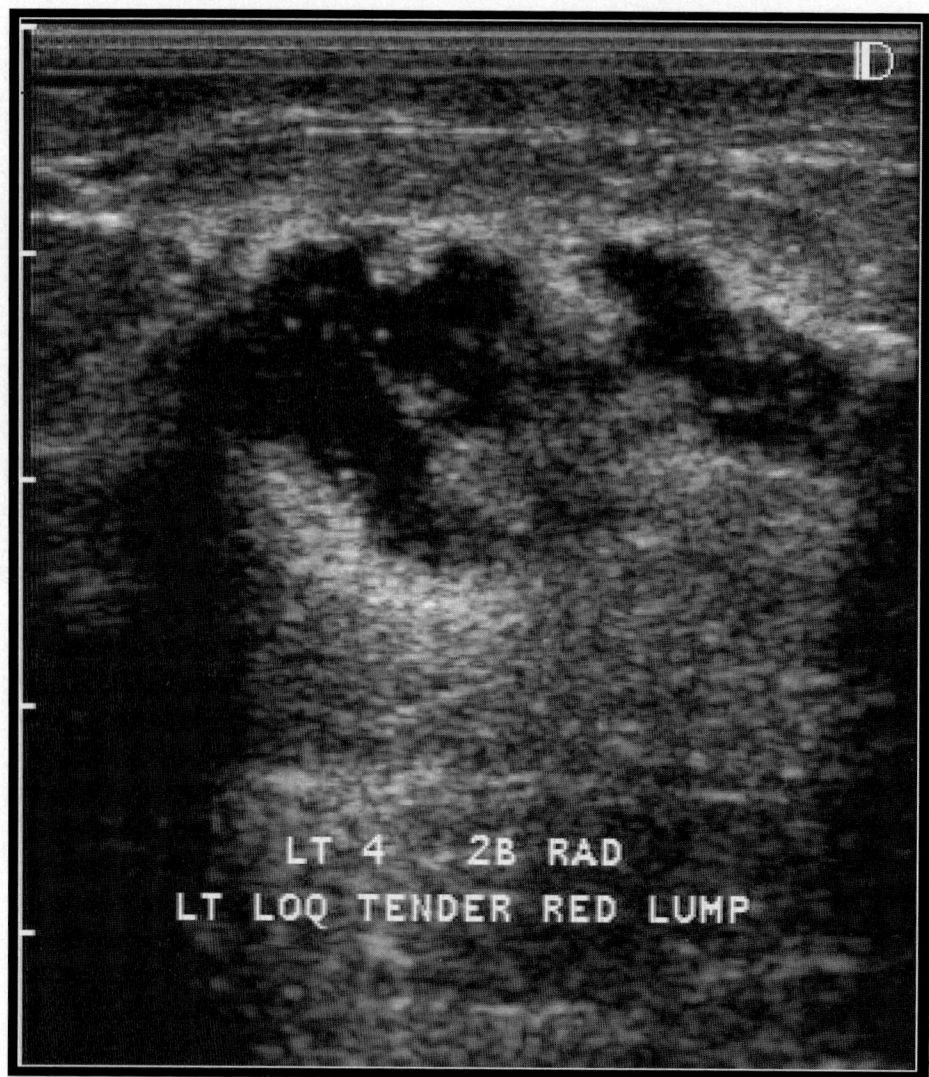

FIGURE 11–27 Occasionally, central puerperal abscesses are multiloculated because multiple central ducts have become necrotic and ruptured. The long axis of each of the loculations courses parallel to the long axis of the central ducts.

right and left sides or in different parts of the same breast not only allow comparison with the symptomatic area with other areas of the breast but also equalize stimuli that cause letdown.

In the *nonspecific pattern* of puerperal mastitis, no fluid-filled underlying obstructed peripheral or central structures can be identified. There are no identifiable galactoceles or dilated periareolar ducts, only ill-defined edema and hyperemia. There are no sonographically demonstrable dilated ducts or lobules in which the infection develops. In such cases, a well-defined abscess cavity develops only very late in the infectious process, after liquefactive necrosis has occurred. Consequently, it is difficult to diagnose abscess formation with ultrasound early in these patients.

Most important, most puerperal breast abscesses developing from the nonspecific pattern of mastitis do not have the classic, well-defined sonographic characteristics of secondarily infected or inflamed cysts described in Chapter 10. Puerperal breast abscesses vary tremendously in appearance, depending on age and maturity of the lesion. Untreated or unsuccessfully treated puerperal mastitis can cause tissue necrosis. Ultimately, this devitalized tissue undergoes liquefactive necrosis. Early in the liquefactive process, the echotexture of the devitalized tissue may be nearly identical to that of the surrounding viable breast tissues, despite the presence of necrosis. The only clues to the presence of early necrosis may be slight alterations in the echogenicity and homo-

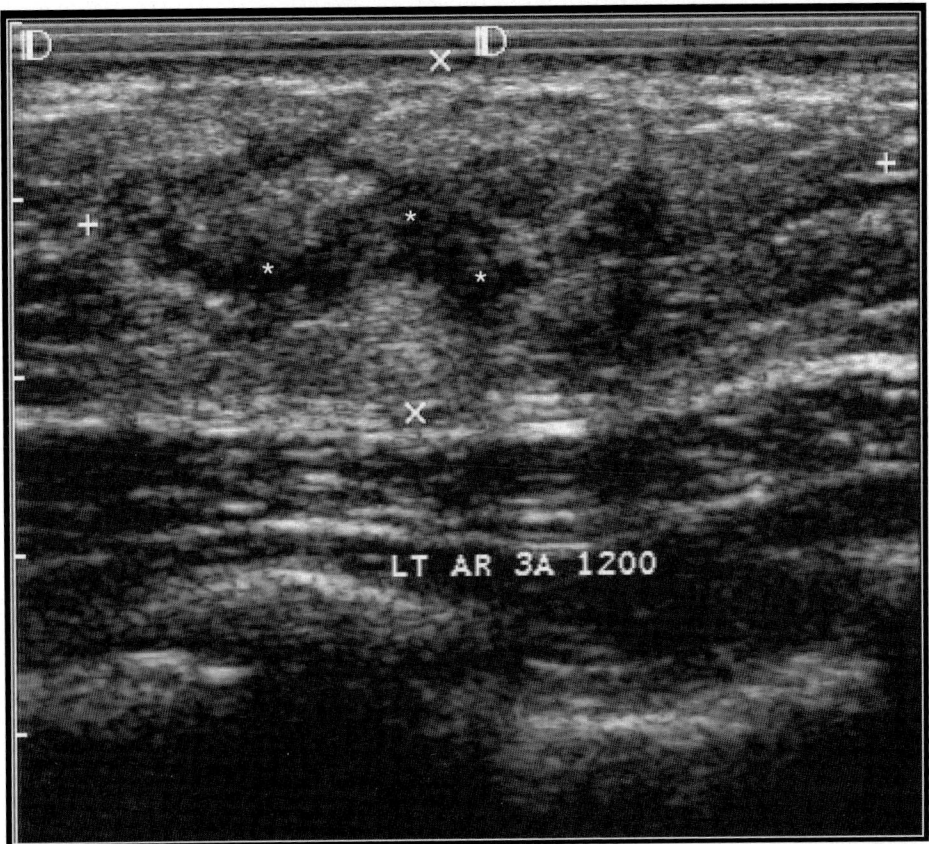

FIGURE 11–28 Abscesses that have a nonspecific pattern may be very difficult to identify early in the course of development. The area of liquefactive necrosis that will later become a well-defined abscess is usually slightly hypoechoic (*) and heterogeneous with respect to surrounding breast tissues, but the margins remain ill defined until the abscess wall matures.

geneity relative to surrounding viable lactational tissue. Tissues that have undergone liquefactive necrosis are usually minimally more hypoechoic and heterogeneous than surrounding viable tissue (Fig. 11–28). The liquefied and necrotic tissue sloughs into the central cavity of the developing abscess, whose walls remain ill defined. At this still early stage of abscess development, distinguishing devitalized necrotic from surrounding viable tissue by sonographic appearances alone may be possible only by showing that the necrotic tissue is unattached and moves during gentle ballottement of the breast. The sloshing, to-and-fro movement of the necrotic debris is readily apparent with routine B-mode real-time imaging but can be documented in a single hard-copy freeze-frame image by using color or power Doppler during ballottement. The detached necrotic debris is echogenic enough to create a color signal as it sloshes to and fro within the developing abscess cavity during ballottement. The color slosh in ill-defined and early abscesses is very similar to the color swoosh caused by ballottement

of ectatic ducts that are filled with echogenic secretions (Fig. 11–29). The color signal resulting from debris movement within the abscess cavity should be distinguished from blood flow. Of course, there will be no demonstrable blood flow within areas of liquefactive necrosis, but the surrounding viable infected tissues will usually be hyperemic.

In other cases, pointing of mildly hypoechoic tissue through the anterior mammary fascia into the subcutaneous zone will be a clue the presence of liquefactive necrosis. Because of near-field volume averaging, pointing may be better demonstrated with the use of an acoustic standoff (Fig. 11–30). Pointing is usually evident clinically as a focal erythematous bulge in which the skin is thinned and glistening.

As the liquefactive process progresses, necrotic tissues and rancid milk within the cavity may liquefy at varying rates. Thus, the abscess contents become generally more hypoechoic but also more heterogeneous. The tissues that are liquefying more slowly create solid debris of varying

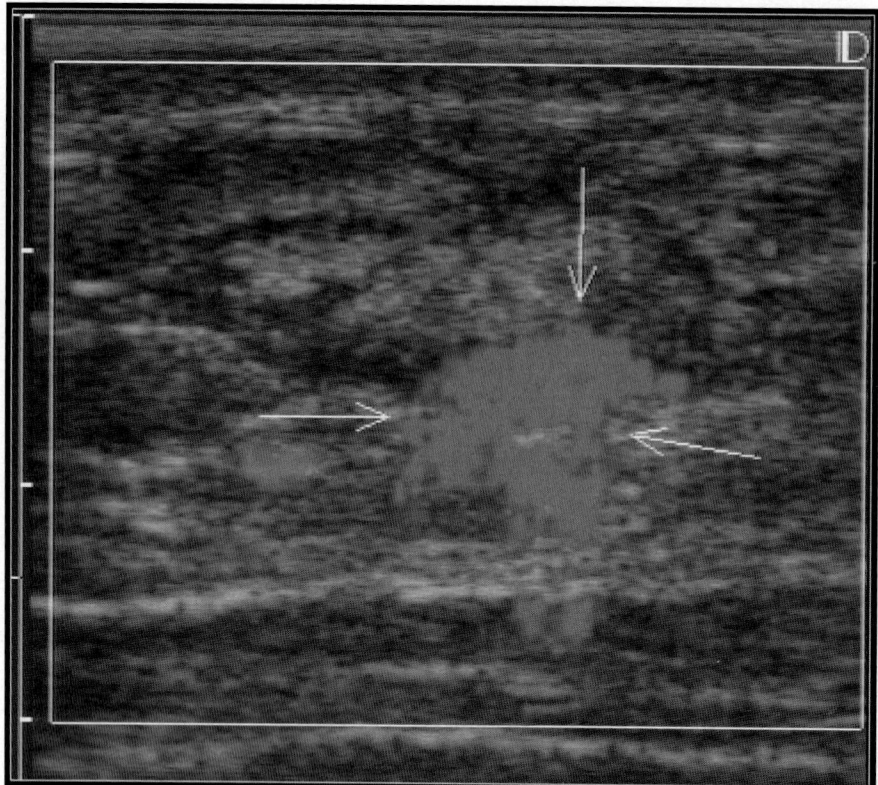

FIGURE 11–29 Gentle ballottement of the inflamed area with the transducer may cause detached necrotic debris to slosh back and forth, defining the nascent abscess cavity. The movement to and fro, the color swoosh of necrotic tissue *(arrows)* during ballottement, can be documented on a single freeze-frame image with color or power Doppler. The echogenicity of the necrotic tissue may be so close to that of surrounding viable tissue that it may not be identifiable on the image alone (same case as Fig. 11–28).

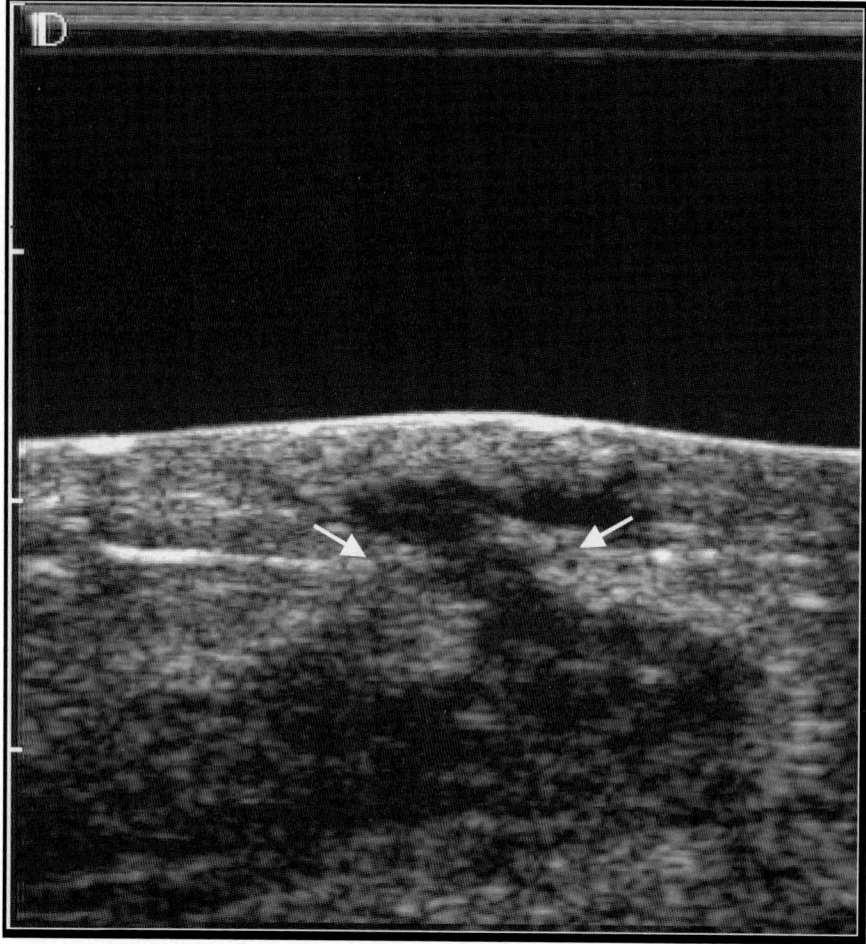

FIGURE 11–30 The spontaneous "pointing" of this solid-appearing early abscess through the anterior mammary fascia *(arrows)* and into the subcutaneous fat is best shown with an acoustic standoff pad.

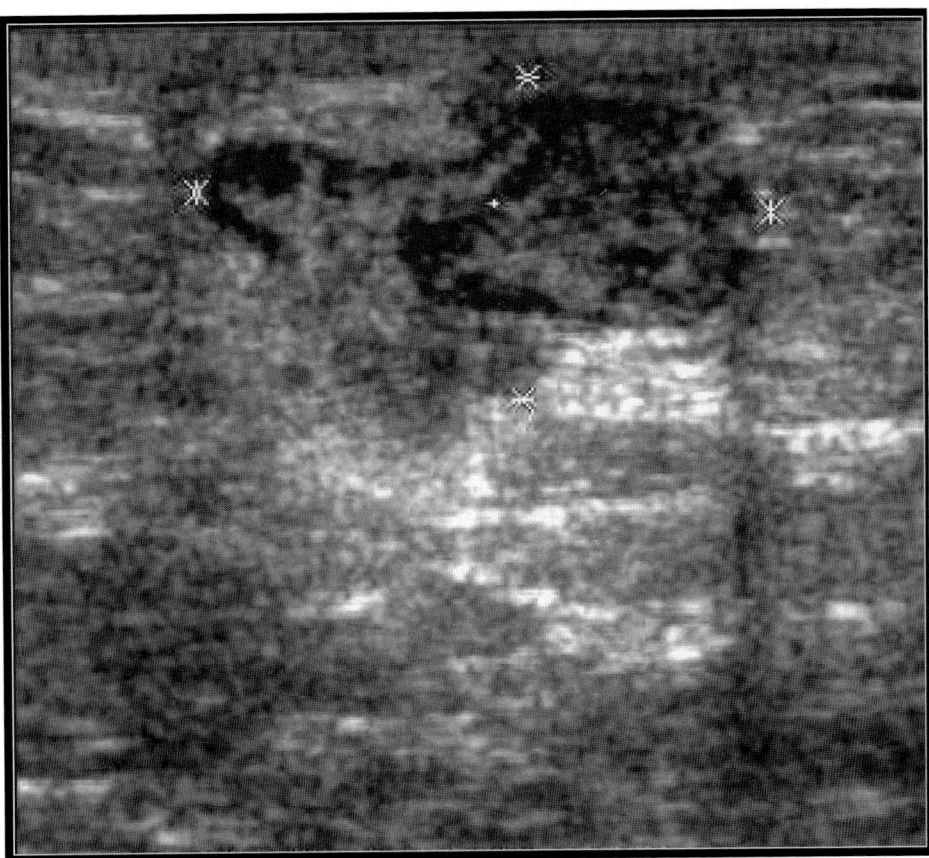

FIGURE 11–31 Chronic abscesses may have sonographic appearances that are difficult to distinguish from solid nodules.

size and echogenicity that floats within the more hypoechoic and completely liquefied tissues. Only in the latest stages of abscess formation does a mature, relatively well-defined, thick, echogenic wall form around the abscess that we recognize as the classic sonographic appearance of an abscess.

Abscesses that are not adequately treated with surgery, percutaneous drainage procedures, or antibiotics may become chronic and may develop a solid appearance that is difficult to distinguish from other worrisome solid nodules. Such lesions may require biopsy for definitive diagnosis (Fig. 11–31).

In summary, the goal of sonography in patients with puerperal mastitis is to diagnose abscess formation as early as possible, to obtain fluid for culture and sensitivity before results are confused or obscured by antibiotic treatment, and as often as possible, to drain the lesion percutaneously by either repeated ultrasound-guided aspiration or ultrasound-guided catheter drainage. To establish early diagnosis and treatment, patients with puerperal

mastitis are frequently scanned within 24 hours of the onset of symptoms. Such early diagnosis and ultrasound-guided percutaneous drainage are usually feasible and straightforward in the peripheral and central forms of puerperal mastitis and abscess, in which an underlying, obstructed, fluid-filled structure is present before it becomes infected (Fig. 11–32). However, diagnosis will frequently be delayed in the nonspecific form of mastitis because liquefactive necrosis is a late sequela of infection. In such cases, the area of developing liquefactive necrosis may be difficult or impossible to demonstrate sonographically in the first 24 to 48 hours of the onset of symptoms. If no abscess cavity is demonstrable on the first examination, a short-interval follow-up examination should be scheduled within 1 or 2 days, by which time an abscess cavity may be apparent. The abscess cavity that eventually does develop in such patients responds less well to repeated aspirations than do the abscesses in the central and peripheral forms of mastitis, and more frequently requires surgical incision and drainage.

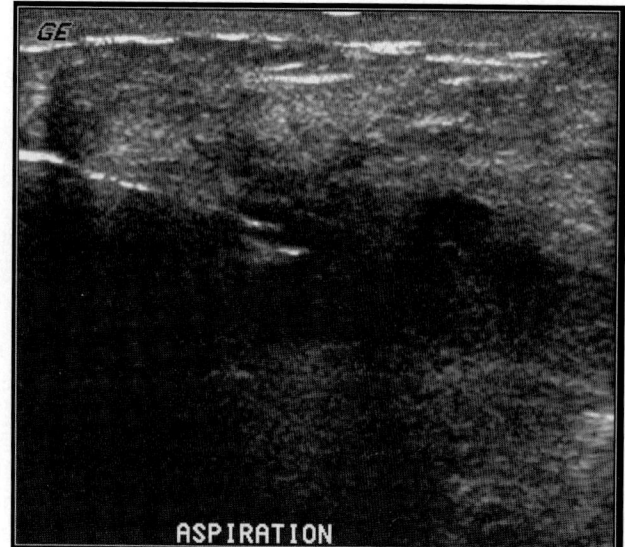
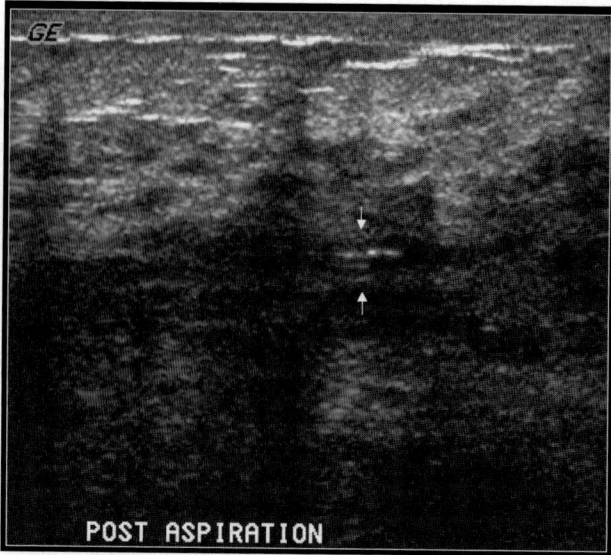

FIGURE 11-32 A: The nonspecific form of abscess responds less well to percutaneous aspiration than better defined central or peripheral abscesses because the necrotic debris is too viscous to pass through the needle in many cases. Nevertheless, attempted aspiration is worth the effort in most cases that appear to be unilocular. Certain abscesses that appear unlikely to be aspiratable can be completely drained and respond well to a single or to repeated aspirations. Additionally, even when the abscess cannot be completely drained, the aspirate can be sent for culture and sensitivity to make sure that the patient is placed on appropriate antibiotics. **B:** Despite the solid appearance shown in the image in part **A**, this abscess was virtually completely drained with ultrasound-guided aspiration. The patient was placed on antibiotics and did not require additional aspirations or drain placement.

NONPUERPERAL (PERIAREOLAR ABSCESS) AND NONPUERPERAL MASTITIS: THE DUCT ECTASIA–PERIDUCTAL MASTITIS COMPLEX (NONLACTATIONAL MASTITIS, CHEMICAL MASTITIS, PERIDUCTAL MASTITIS, PLASMA CELL MASTITIS)

General Pathologic Classification, Epidemiology, and Clinical Findings

Acute mastitis may also occur in nonlactating patients (nonpuerperal mastitis) who usually have underlying ductal ectasia, or less commonly, breast cysts. Such cases probably begin as chemical inflammation due to rupture of ectatic ducts or cysts. The inflammation in such patients is chemical rather than infectious in origin, but secondary bacterial infection may supersede. The organism causing the secondary infection is more often anaerobic and less often *Staphylococcus* species than is the case for typical puerperal mastitis. Causative bacteria usually are normal mouth or vaginal flora.

Duct ectasia is an inflammatory condition of the larger-order mammary ducts. Whether dilation occurs first, leading to stasis and secondary inflammation, or whether inflammation of the walls of the ducts leads to loss of elastic fibers in the duct wall and secondarily results in dilation or stasis is controversial. There is also some evi-

dence to suggest that hyperprolactinemia is an important factor in this process. However, only a small percentage of cases of hyperprolactinemia are caused by pituitary tumors. Duct ectasia is usually asymptomatic. Only about 30% to 40% of patients with duct ectasia complain of nipple discharge. In early duct ectasia, the discharge can be milky or greenish, but in later phases of the process that are most likely to be associated with periductal mastitis, the secretions can be thick, pasty, or cheesy and whitish to yellowish in color.

Inflammatory weakening of the duct wall accompanies stasis and luminal dilation. Lipid-rich, highly inflammatory secretions accumulate within the duct lumen. The inflamed and weakened duct wall can rupture spontaneously or from normally insignificant minor trauma, releasing fatty secretions into the periductal tissues and causing an intense periductal chemical mastitis. When periductal inflammation is complicated by necrosis and infection, abscess formation can occur. Abscesses that occur in association with duct ectasia are termed *nonpuerperal abscesses* and are most typically periareolar in location, simply reflecting the underlying location of the inflamed central ducts from which they arise. Such abscesses are prone to form periareolar skin fistulas that are very difficult to eradicate by antibiotic treatment, percutaneous aspiration, or even open incision and drainage. Even when open excision of the abscess is performed, periareolar abscesses can recur if the entire fistulous tract is not removed with the abscess. In most cases of periareolar fistulas, surgical excision of the entire fistula complex is required for effective treatment.

Chronic duct ectasia usually involves more than one lobar ductal system on each side. Thus, over time, different ducts may rupture, leading to repeated migratory episodes of focal periductal mastitis or periareolar abscesses. Acute episodes of periductal mastitis may cause transient episodes of nipple retraction that resolve as the inflammation abates. Acute periductal mastitis can also progress to chronic periductal mastitis and, ultimately, to periductal and intraductal fibrosis and permanent nipple retraction that simulates the nipple retraction caused by scirrhous breast cancer clinically, mammographically, and sonographically. Intraluminal fibrosis may obliterate the duct lumen, causing a classic garland pattern of fibrosis to develop within the ducts. The combination of periductal and intraductal fibrosis results in enlarged solid-appearing ducts that simulate high-nuclear-grade ductal carcinoma *in situ* (DCIS) sonographically. Duct ectasia is also discussed in Chapter 9 as it pertains to the sonographic evaluation of nipple discharge and in Chapter 21 as a cause of sonograms that are falsely positive for cancer.

Because the spectrum of findings in duct ectasia is so broad and changes so much over time, the recent trend has been to lump the various forms under the category of duct ectasia–periductal mastitis complex. The term *duct ectasia* literally means dilated duct but implies much more—obstruction, inflammation, occasionally superimposed infection, and fibrosis. Combining it with the term *periductal mastitis complex* more clearly connotes the presence of disease processes in addition to simple dilation of the duct lumen.

The duct ectasia–periductal mastitis complex affects two different groups of patients: women in their perimenopausal years, and women in their late teens and early 20s. The underlying histologic basis for the complex differs in the two groups. The younger group usually has underlying congenital nipple inversion that is associated with squamous metaplasia involving variable lengths of the distal ends of the ducts of one or more lobes. It is normal to have squamous metaplasia lining the distal 2 or 3 mm of the mammary ducts within the nipple. However, in the younger group prone to periareolar nonpuerperal abscess, the squamous metaplasia may extend proximally for several centimeters and even into duct branches. The squamous cells produce keratin plugs that obstruct the duct and lead eventually to duct dilation, stasis, inflammation, and infection. The duct ectasia that develops in the perimenopausal group is not associated with congenital nipple inversion or squamous metaplasia of the distal ducts in most cases. Its etiology is more difficult to define, controversial, and likely multifactorial. It may be hormonal and related to prolactin, estrogen, and progesterone. It does not, however,

appear to be related to previous breast-feeding because the incidence of duct ectasia is similar in patients who have breast-fed and those who have not. Although smoking is not likely to be an underlying cause of the duct ectasia–periductal mastitis complex, women with duct ectasia who smoke are more likely to develop the severe complications of periductal mastitis than are those who do not smoke. It is likely that products of cigarette smoke either exacerbate inflammatory changes in the duct or cause superimposed ischemic changes in the duct wall that interfere with healing.

The duct ectasia–periductal mastitis complex is a leading cause of noncyclical focal breast pain. Patients with the complex frequently have a history of repeated migratory episodes of focal breast pain that resolve either spontaneously or on antibiotic treatment over 1 or 2 weeks. Careful sonographic evaluation of the focal area of pain often shows definitive evidence of ductal and periductal inflammation. The value of antibiotics in such patients is debatable. Although acute periductal mastitis is usually chemically induced rather than infectious in origin, in some cases, there is undoubtedly secondary bacterial infection. In fact, a significant percentage of asymptomatic patients with duct ectasia have been shown to have bacteria colonizing their ducts. Rupture of ectatic ducts colonized by bacteria is likely to result in periductal abscess formation. Early antibiotic treatment may prevent formation of periductal abscess. Unfortunately, chemical periductal inflammation cannot be readily distinguished from periductal infection clinically or by imaging findings. Thus, it seems prudent to treat cases of suspected acute periductal mastitis with antibiotics, even though most patients are likely merely to have chemical mastitis.

Inflammation and rupture of inflamed cysts can also lead to focal chemical mastitis or abscess formation. The ruptured cysts that give rise to mastitis and abscess formation are of lobular origin and are more likely to be peripheral in location than are the focal areas of inflammation and abscess formation resulting from ruptured ducts. Although the locations of inflammation around ruptured ducts and cysts are different, the histology is not. In both cases, the release of lipid-rich fluid contents into surrounding tissues causes an intense focal chemical mastitis.

Mammographic Findings

The mammographic findings in nonpuerperal mastitis are nonspecific. There are two categories of findings: those related to the underlying ductal ectasia or fibrocystic change, and those related to the focal mastitis or abscess formation. The findings of ductal ectasia vary with the stage of the disease. There may be numerous prominent subareolar ducts, usually bilaterally symmetrical. Typical intraductal secretory-type calcifications or periductal calcifications may be present and are definitively benign [Breast Imaging

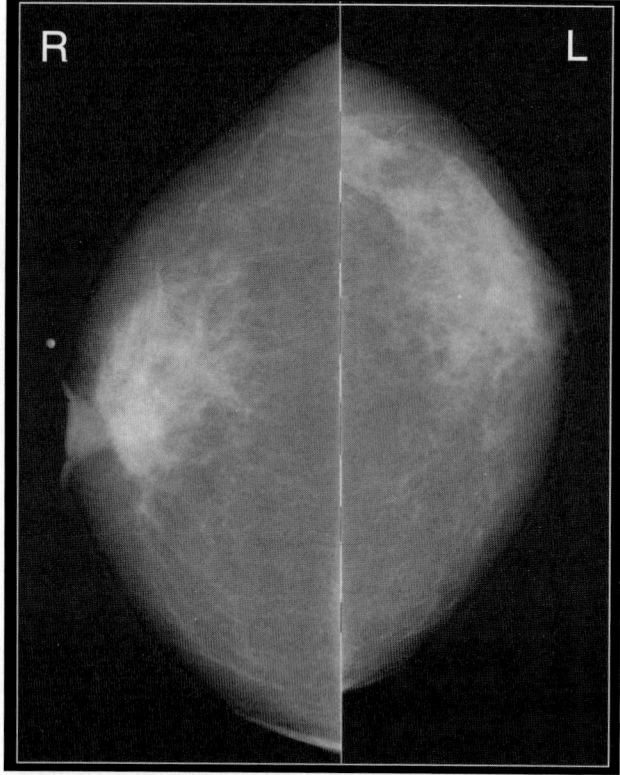

FIGURE 11–33 The nipple retraction seen on the right side is the result of end-stage duct ectasia—periductal mastitis complex that has progressed to severe periductal fibrosis. The mammographic finding simulates nipple retraction caused by malignancy.

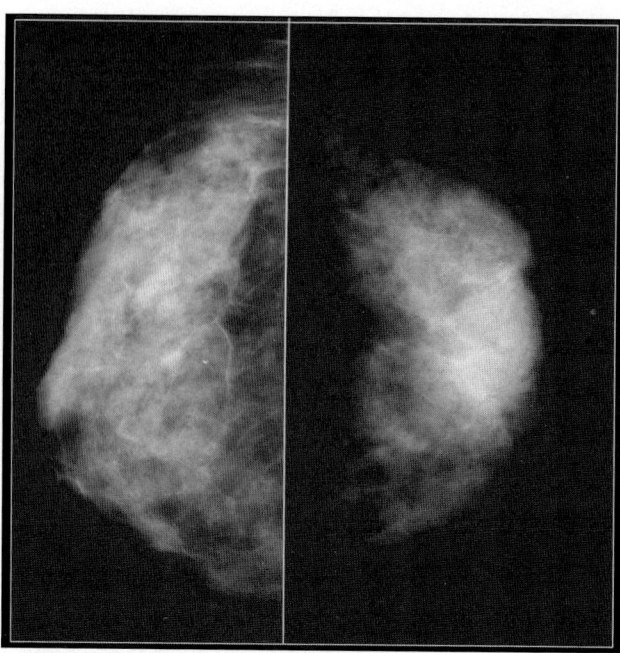

FIGURE 11–34 Nonpuerperal periareolar abscess, like puerperal abscess, causes nonspecific mammographic findings of increased density and ill-defined mass.

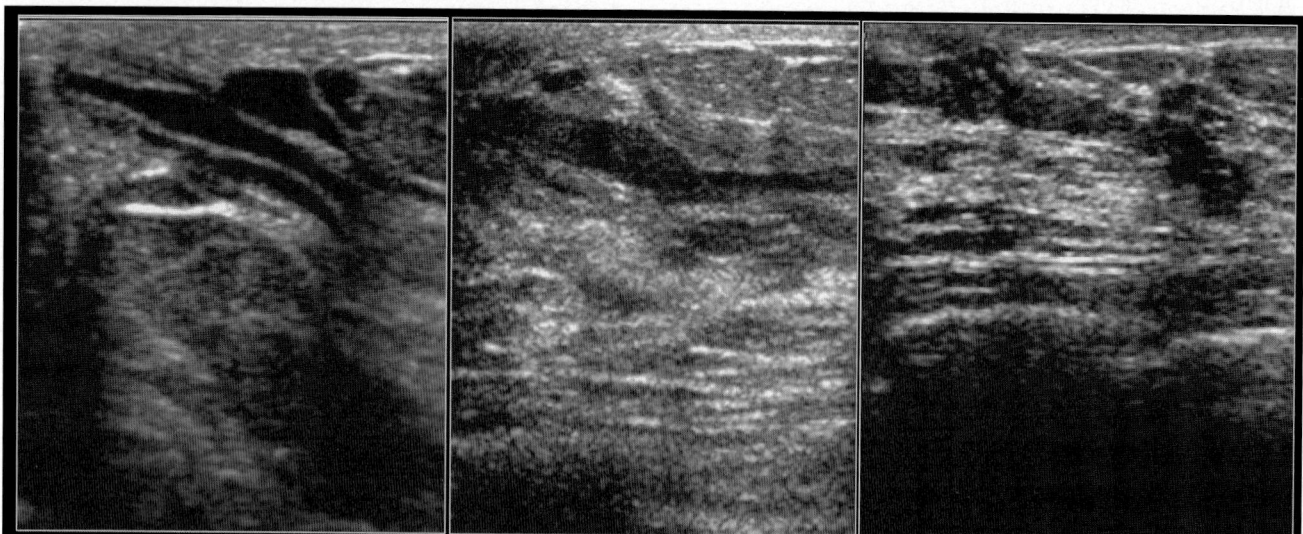

FIGURE 11–35 The secretions within the ectatic ducts may be nearly anechoic, mildly echoic, or isoechoic with periductal fat and solid appearing. The echogenicity of the secretions increases with the fat content of the secretions and the duration of stasis. The solid-appearing secretions typically represent inspissated, highly fatty secretions that have a pasty or cheesy appearance similar to that caused by comedo ductal carcinoma *in situ*.

Reporting and Data System (BIRADS) category 2]. However, earlier in the process of calcification, when calcification is incomplete, and before the appearance becomes classic, the calcifications may resemble those seen in DCIS closely enough to require biopsy. In later stages, when periductal fibrosis and scarring is the dominant feature, there may be an ill-defined or frankly spiculated subareolar mass with nipple retraction that simulates infiltrating malignancy (Fig. 11–33). Focal mastitis causes a nonspecific area of ill-defined increased density that can be difficult to distinguish from asymmetric glandular tissue, compression artifact, or even occult malignancy. A periductal abscess, if detectable, will appear as an indistinct high-density mass or nodule, usually in the subareolar area. The focal increased density caused by edema resulting from a ruptured or leaking cyst is usually located farther peripherally than that associated with the duct ectasia–periductal mastitis complex. Multiple other circumscribed or partially circumscribed isodense nodules that represent multiple other noninflamed cysts may be present. The inflamed and leaking cyst, if still present, may have more indistinct margins than the other nodules. Unfortunately, some patients with acute periductal mastitis or nonpuerperal abscess are too tender to tolerate adequate mammographic compression, making the whole ipsilateral breast appear small and dense (Fig. 11–34).

Sonographic Findings

Sonographic findings, like mammographic findings of nonpuerperal mastitis and abscess, are a reflection of the chronic underlying ectatic condition and of the superimposed acute or chronic inflammatory process. The sonographic findings of periductal mastitis associated with ductal ectasia other than abscess are discussed and illustrated in detail in Chapter 8.

The sonographic appearance of the affected duct varies depending on the stage of the disease and the contents of the dilated ducts. In the early and intermediate phases of the disease, dilated fluid-filled subareolar ducts are usually demonstrable. The fluid within such ducts may be anechoic, mildly hypoechoic, or even isoechoic with surrounding fatty tissues, depending on the composition of the fluid within the duct (Fig. 11–35). Thin secretions within the ducts appear either anechoic or markedly hypoechoic with diffuse low-level internal echogenicity. In more long-standing duct ectasia, especially after episodes of acute inflammation, the secretions have a grossly different consistency and therefore a different echotexture. The secretions grossly become more viscous and have a pasty or cheesy texture similar to the cheesy comedo paste of necrotic high-nuclear-grade DCIS. The viscous fluid contains numerous foam cells, inflammatory cells, or crystalline materials within the duct lumen that result in the fluid being more echogenic and often nearly isoechoic with normal breast fat.

The sonographic findings of focal, acute, nonpuerperal mastitis are similar to those of puerperal mastitis, except for being more localized. Sonographically recognizable changes involve both the wall of the inflamed ectatic duct and the tissues surrounding the duct.

There are changes that occur in the walls of acutely inflamed ectatic ducts that are readily demonstrable with ultrasound and Doppler. The walls of both normal ducts and ectatic noninflamed ducts are thin and echogenic and have no Doppler-demonstrable blood flow. Acutely inflamed duct walls, on the other hand, are abnormally thickened and isoechoic and hyperemic on color Doppler. The degree of wall thickening varies greatly, from mild to so severe that it virtually obliterates the lumen (Fig. 11–36). The involvement of ducts is not at all uniform. Although duct ectasia may involve several different lobar ducts, and over time

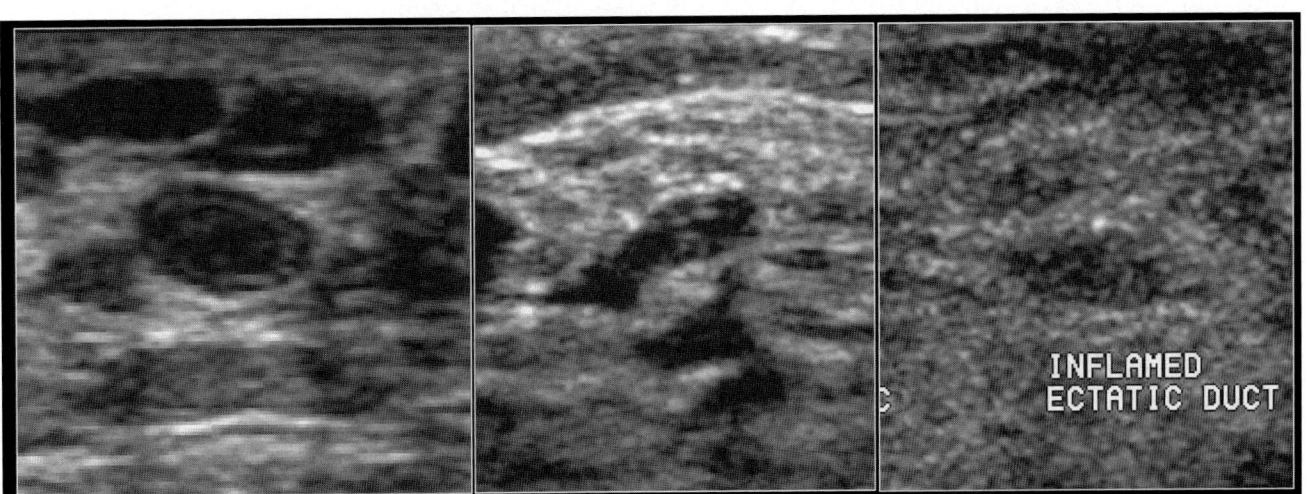

FIGURE 11–36 In the duct ectasia–periductal mastitis complex, the wall of acutely inflamed ectatic ducts becomes abnormally thick and isoechoic, much like the ducts in acute central puerperal mastitis shown in Figs. 11–23 to 11–25. The degree of thickening is proportional to the degree of acute inflammation.

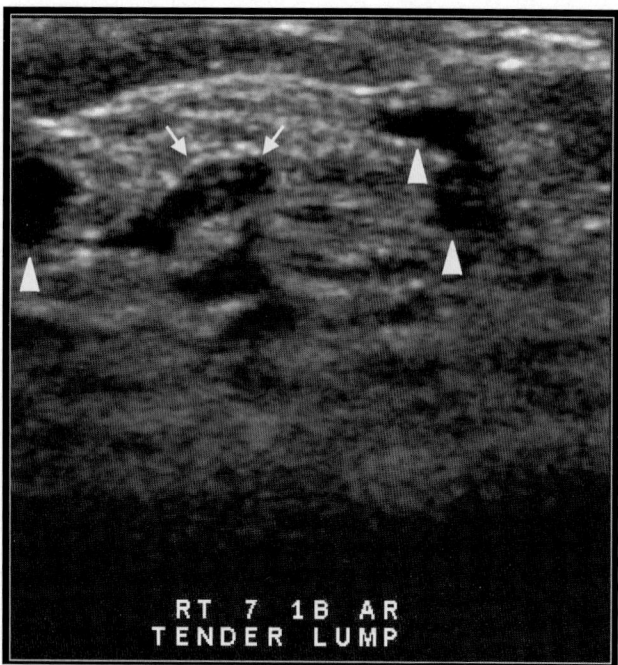

FIGURE 11–37 In patients who are evaluated with ultrasound for acute noncyclical pain, it is important to evaluate all of the ducts for wall thickening. This patient has several ectatic ducts that have thin, noninflamed walls *(arrowheads)*. Such ducts are unlikely to be the cause of pain. However, one duct does have a thick isoechoic wall *(arrows)* that indicates that it is acutely inflamed and, in the absence of solid nodules or secondary signs of malignancy, fairly strong evidence that the duct ectasia—periductal mastitis complex is the cause of this patient's pain.

inflammation may affect all of the ectatic ducts, only one lobar duct is acutely inflamed at any time. Thus, severe wall thickening and hyperemia may be seen in the acutely inflamed duct and its branches, whereas the immediately adjacent ectatic duct wall remains thin and echogenic (Fig. 11–37). When inflammation of the duct wall is severe, color or power Doppler can demonstrate inflammatory hyperemia within the isoechoic thickened duct wall (see Chapter 20, Figs. 20–45 to 20–47, 20–51, and 20–52). Inflammatory hyperemia, like wall thickening, is nonuniform. The tender, acutely inflamed and hyperemic duct may lie immediately adjacent to a thin-walled and avascular duct (see Chapter 20, Fig. 20–52). The secretions caused by duct ectasia are usually not bloody. However, the epithelium of acutely inflamed ectatic and markedly hyperemic cuts can ulcerate, leading to frankly bloody discharge (see Chapter 20, Figs. 20–50 and 20–51). Occasionally, acute episodes of duct wall and periductal inflammation will lead to transient episodes of nipple retraction that resolve completely when the inflammation abates (Fig. 11–38).

When inflammation involves the periductal tissues as well as the duct wall, it causes sonographically detectable changes in the periductal soft tissues. The changes are easiest to appreciate on split-screen images when the inflamed duct is surrounded by fat. The inflamed periductal fat becomes hyperechoic and hyperemic (Fig. 11–39). When the inflamed duct is surrounded by hyperechoic interlobular stromal fibrous tissue, inflammatory changes are much more difficult to appreciate sonographically in most cases.

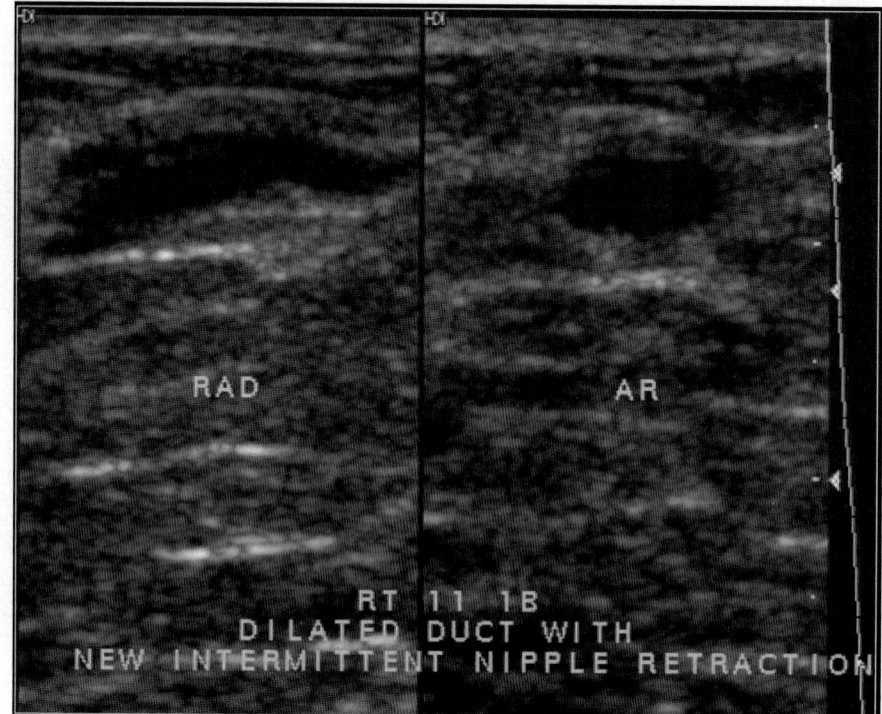

A

FIGURE 11–38 A: Acute periductal mastitis can cause temporary nipple retraction. This patient presented with acute pain in the periareolar upper outer quadrant of the right breast and acute onset nipple retraction. The ectatic duct at the 11:00 position was focally tender and had an abnormally thickened and isoechoic wall. *(Continues)*

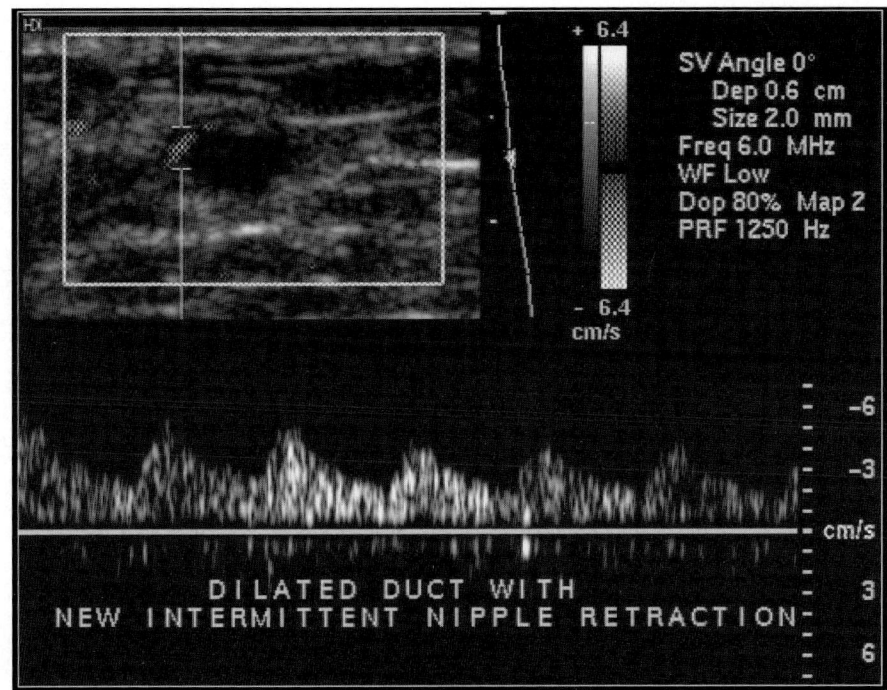

B

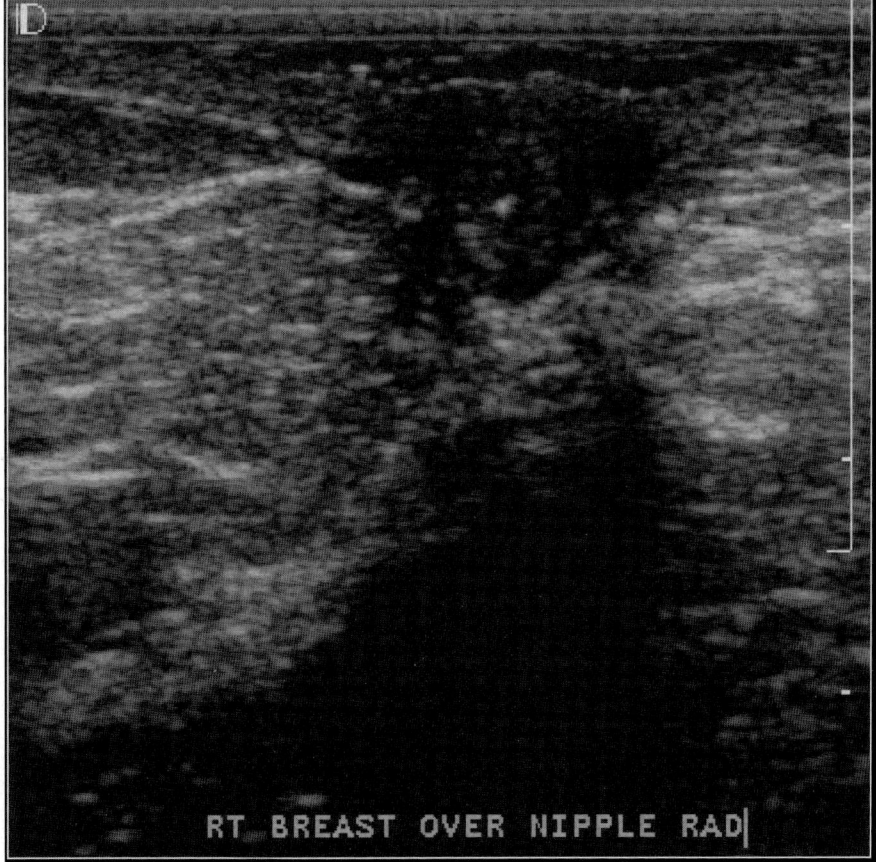

C

FIGURE 11–38 *(continued)* **B:** Color Doppler showed hyperemia within the thickened wall of the ectatic duct at 11:00 and pulsed Doppler spectral analysis confirmed the presence of hyperemia. **C:** Transverse scan over the nipple using a standoff of acoustic gel shows the acute nipple retraction. The patient was treated with broad-spectrum antibiotics, and the pain of the nipple retraction resolved over about 2 weeks. The patient had a history of at least two other episodes of transient nipple retraction associated with acute pain. It is likely that at some point in the future, fibrosis will develop around the offending duct and the nipple retraction will become permanent.

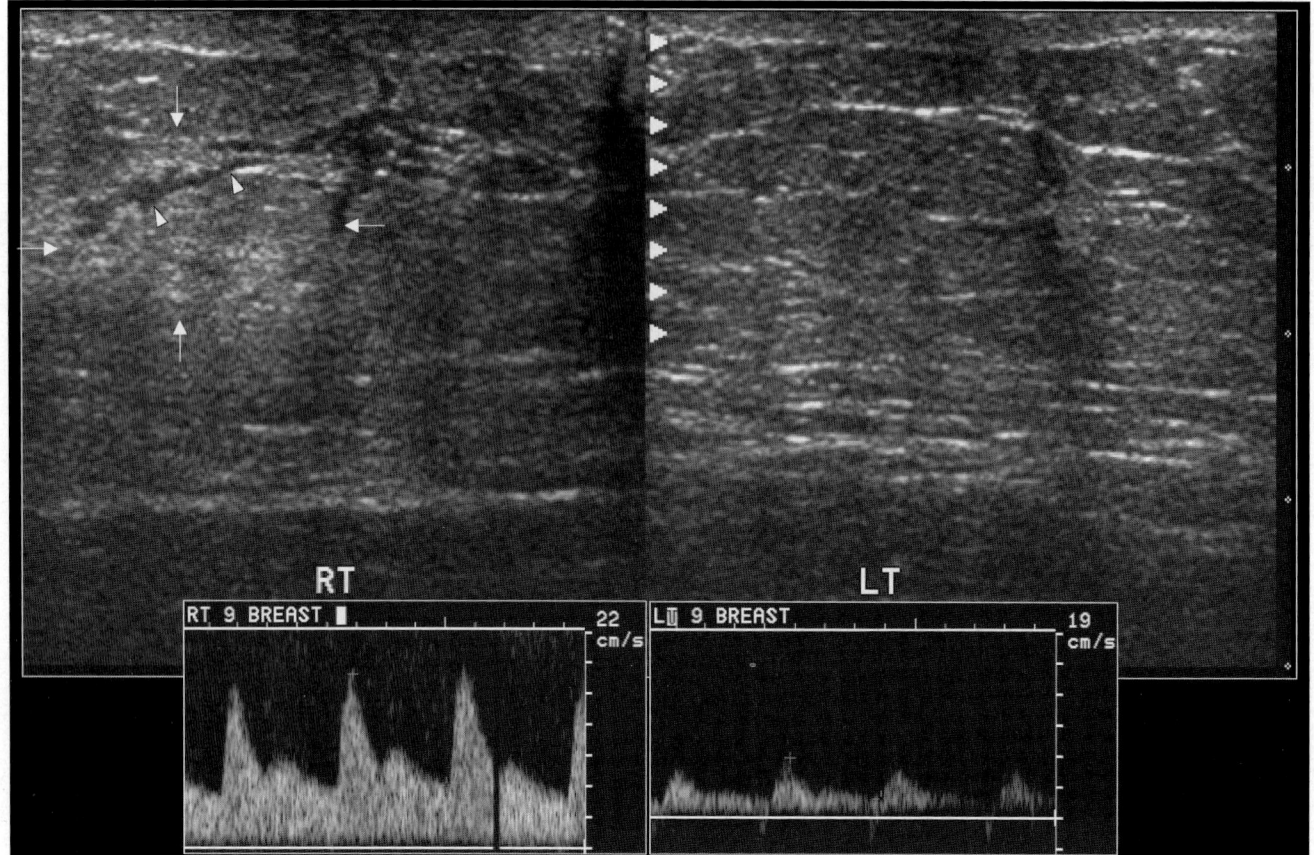

FIGURE 11–39 This figure illustrates focal acute periductal mastitis surrounding a small peripheral duct at the 9:00 position on the **right**. The patient presented with acute pain in the 9:00 position of the right breast. Split-screen mirror-image scanning of the lateral aspects of both breasts (**left** side location is mislabeled, should be 3:00) shows a focal area of hyperechoic fat *(arrows)* in the area of symptoms on the **right**, indicating acute edema. In the center of the edema is a mildly ectatic duct *(arrowheads)*. Color and power Doppler spectral analysis showed hyperemia within the edematous tissues. Note that the velocities are higher and the resistivity indices lower in hyperemic area on the **right** side than on the **left**. The presence of focal edema and hyperemia centered around an ectatic duct indicate the presence of acute periductal mastitis.

The normally hyperechoic fibrous tissue becomes slightly less echogenic. In cases of very severe periductal inflammation, the fat may become so hyperemic and the fibrous tissue echogenicity may decrease enough that the distinction between fat and fibrous tissue becomes less (Fig. 11–40).

The imaging and Doppler changes that occur in the duct wall and periductal tissues in patients with acute periductal mastitis usually cause focal pain and tenderness. In the past, it has been sufficient to evaluate focal, noncyclical pain with targeted ultrasound and be satisfied with a negative sonogram that showed neither a worrisome solid nodule nor a tender cyst. However, a negative ultrasound merely rules out a few causes of pain. It does not diagnose the cause of pain. It would be better to diagnose the cause of pain definitively. We believe that the sonographic findings of the duct ectasia and acute periductal mastitis are definitive enough to make a specific diagnosis of the cause of pain in a significant percentage of cases.

As the acute edema phase regresses and subacute periductal inflammation persists, a band of isoechoic fibrosis forms around the outside of the duct that is easy to appreciate when the duct is surrounded by hyperechoic fibrous tissue (Fig. 11–41) but more difficult to identify when the duct is surrounded by fat (Fig. 11–42). At this stage, the focal pain and tenderness of which the patient complained has already improved, usually spontaneously, and the hyperemia that was present in the acute phase has markedly decreased or disappeared.

Periductal mastitis that does not completely resolve and becomes chronic can present sonographically as a solid nodule. Periductal mastitis nodules have a propensity to form in the bases of Cooper's ligaments (Fig. 11–43). It

(text continued on page 381)

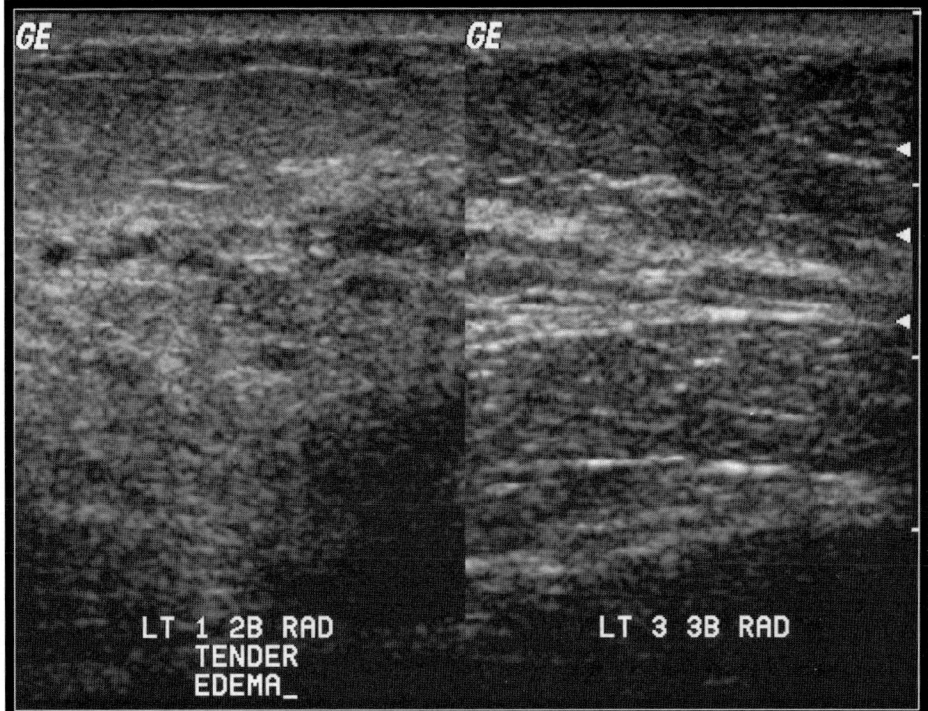

FIGURE 11–40 When acute periductal mastitis occurs around ducts that are surrounded by fibrous tissue, changes can be difficult to demonstrate unless comparison is made to uninvolved areas. The fibrous tissue becomes less echogenic, and the fat becomes more echogenic, decreasing the contrast between fat and fibrous tissue and partially obscuring tissue planes. The changes are focal and occur only around the acutely inflamed ectatic duct.

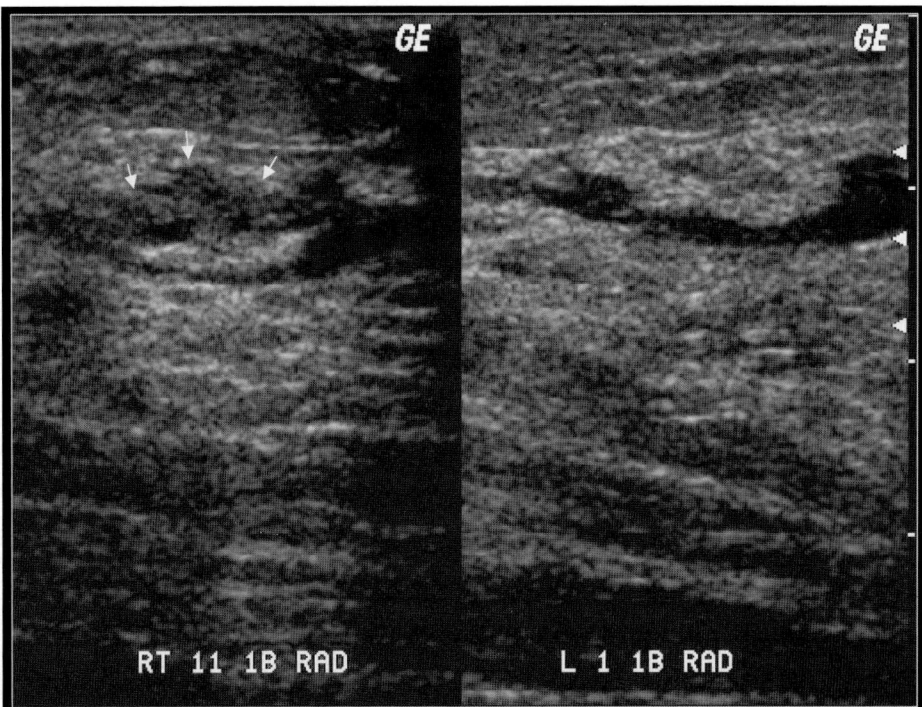

FIGURE 11–41 When periductal mastitis becomes chronic, inflammatory tissues or fibrosis may persist along the outside of the duct. The isoechoic tissues that surround the anterior aspect of the branch duct at 11:00 (**left**, *arrows*) represent chronic periductal mastitis. Note that the ectatic duct at 1:00 on the **left** has normal hyperechoic interlobular stromal fibrous tissue surrounding it. Note that the chronic periductal mastitis around the 11:00 duct on the **right** is compressing and distorting the duct lumen.

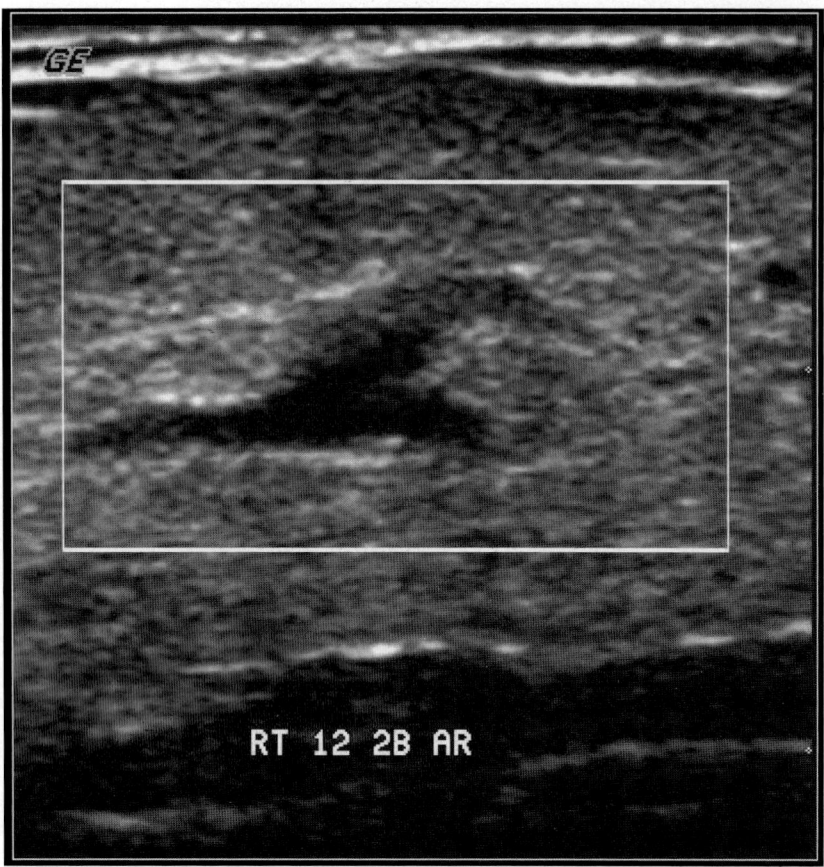

FIGURE 11–42 The isoechoic tissue along the anterior aspect of this ectatic branch duct is caused by subacute periductal mastitis. This patient had an acute episode of pain in the 12:00 position of the right breast. By the time her sonogram was performed, 2 weeks later, the pain and tenderness had almost completely spontaneously resolved. Note that despite the persistent imaging evidence of periductal inflammation, there is no demonstrable hyperemia. The presence of hyperemia is a sign of acute periductal mastitis, but will be absent in subacute and chronic phases of periductal mastitis.

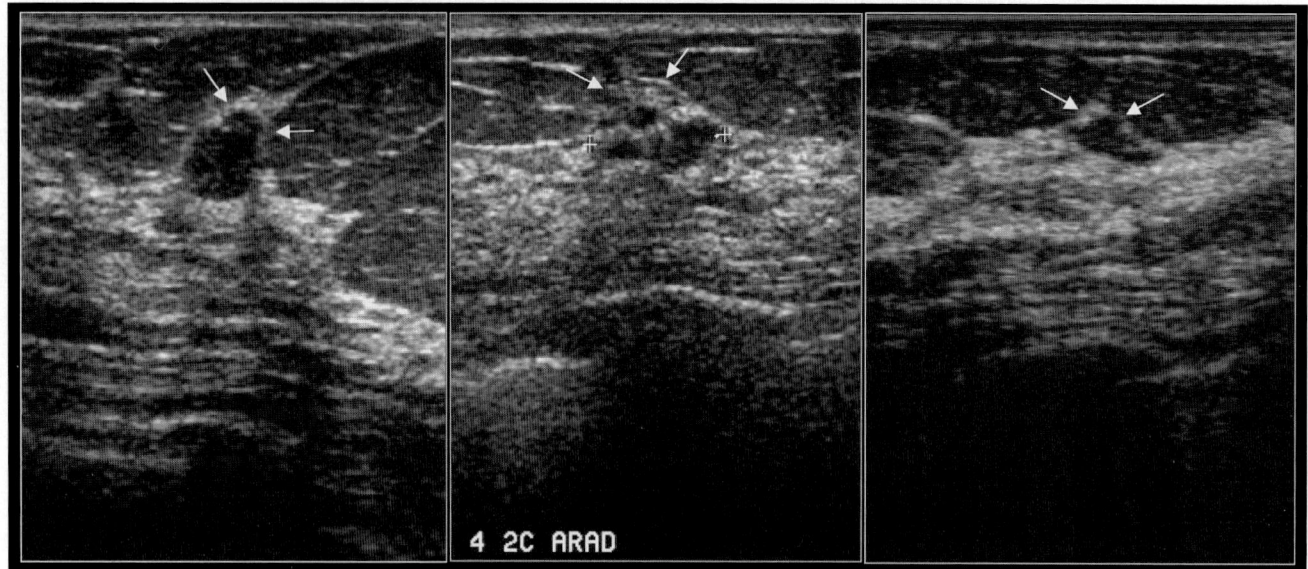

FIGURE 11–43 Occasionally, ultrasound-guided biopsy of apparent solid nodules will yield a histologic diagnosis of focal mastitis. The histologic features are identical to those of acute periductal mastitis, but there is no sonographically visible ectatic duct in the area. Such episodes of mastitis may have been related to ruptured cysts or to duct ectasia that has been obliterated by fibrosis. The typical location of focal mastitis is at the base of Cooper's ligaments *(arrows)*. This suggests that mechanical factor may be at play. The Cooper's ligaments may place traction on cysts or ectatic ducts that lie at the base the ligament, predisposing them to rupture.

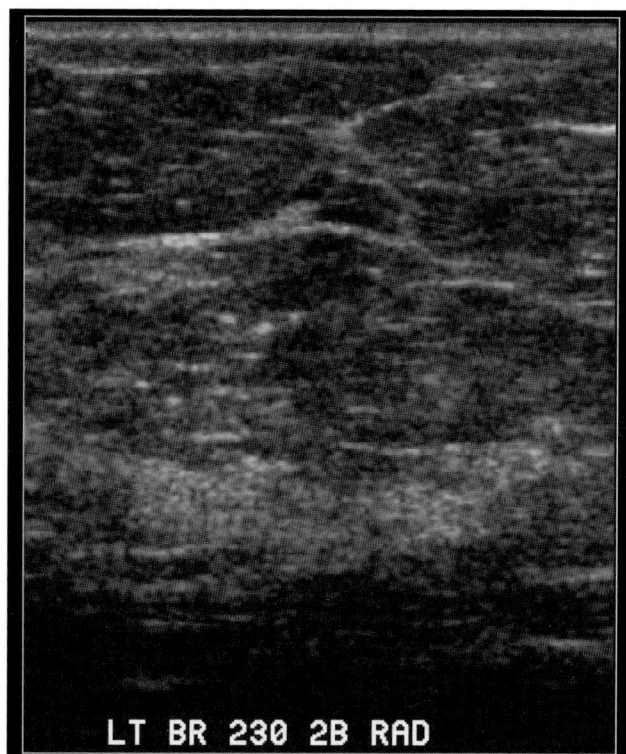

LT BR 230 2B RAD

FIGURE 11–44 Rupture of an inflamed ectatic duct or inflamed cyst releases lipid-laden fluid into the surrounding tissues and can give rise to periductal mastitis and formation of a cholesterol granuloma. The main significance of cholesterol granulomas is that they appear to be solid nodules with some atypical features that may make them difficult to distinguish from malignant nodules. This cholesterol granuloma was associated with chronic periductal mastitis and has angular margins and microlobulations, findings that are suspicious for malignancy.

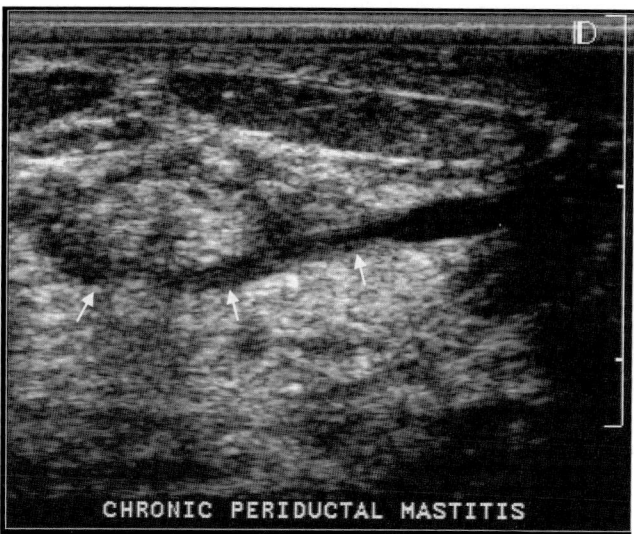

CHRONIC PERIDUCTAL MASTITIS

FIGURE 11–45 In the end stages of the duct ectasia—periductal mastitis complex, obliterative periductal fibrosis compresses the duct lumen and may completely obliterate it. In certain cases, intraductal fibrosis also contributes to obliteration of the lumen. Sonographically, we are usually not able to resolve whether the isoechoic tissue is intraductal or periductal. The duct appears to be solid and isoechoic and has a sonographic appearance that can be absolutely identical to ductal carcinoma *in situ* (DCIS) filling the lumen. There is no way to distinguish between obliterative periductal fibrosis and DCIS sonographically in such cases and biopsy is necessary. Note that the duct lumen is preserved in the lactiferous sinus portion of the duct, but that the more peripheral portions of the duct lumen are obliterated by fibrosis *(arrows).*

seems likely the ligaments place traction on the weakened and inflamed ducts, predisposing ducts that that lie deep to the ligaments to rupture. Focal mastitis nodules often develop in granulomatous foreign-body reaction to extravasated cholesterol crystals. The granulomatous reaction that envelops the extravasated lipids creates cholesterol granulomas that are significant mainly because they can be mistaken for malignant nodules (Fig. 11–44).

In the end stages of duct ectasia, obliterative periductal fibrosis envelops and compresses the duct lumen. Fibrosis may also develop intraductally, filling the residual lumen that is not compressed by periductal fibrosis, but sonographically, the duct may be so compressed that it is difficult to determine whether the fibrosis is intraductal or periductal and merely compressing the duct (Fig. 11–45). Periductal fibrosis is far more common than is intraductal fibrosis. The net result is that the duct appears solid and mildly enlarged on sonography, sometimes involving several branch ducts as well as the main duct (Fig. 11–46).

Unfortunately, end-stage periductal or intraductal fibrosis is sonographically indistinguishable from DCIS filling the duct and virtually always requires biopsy. Chronic periductal inflammation and subsequent fibrosis makes the margins of the affected ducts appear to be irregular, again simulating extensive ductal tumor involvement (Fig. 11–47). A patient with chronic duct ectasia may develop intraductal calcifications as well as periductal fibrosis. When the calcifications are fully developed, they are definitively benign in mammographic appearance (BIRADS 2) and require no further evaluation. However, the intraductal calcifications may be seen at an early stage, when they are still incomplete. Incomplete calcifications cannot be distinguished from those in DCIS. Like DCIS, periductal fibrosis and intraductal calcifications may be extensive, involving nearly an entire breast lobe (Fig. 11–48). Periductal and intraductal fibrosis can ultimately lead to permanent nipple retraction (Fig. 11–49).

The spectrum of sonographic findings for nonpuerperal abscesses is the same as for puerperal abscesses, as discussed in the preceding section. The findings that help distinguish nonpuerperal abscesses from puerperal

(text continued on page 385)

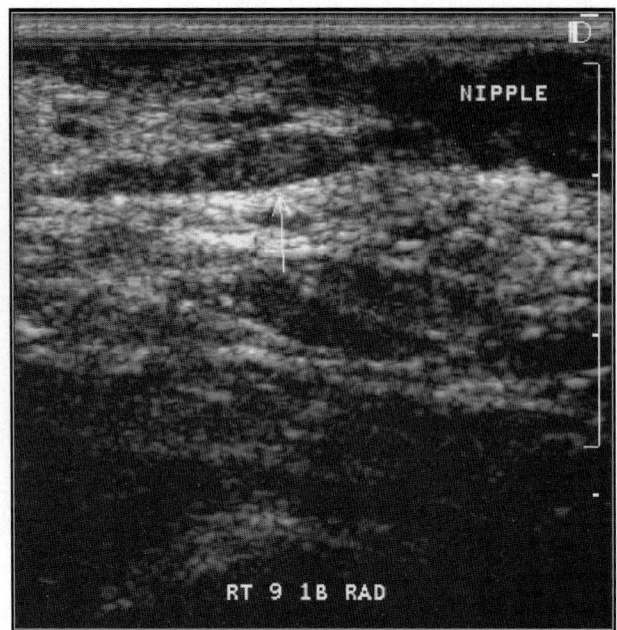

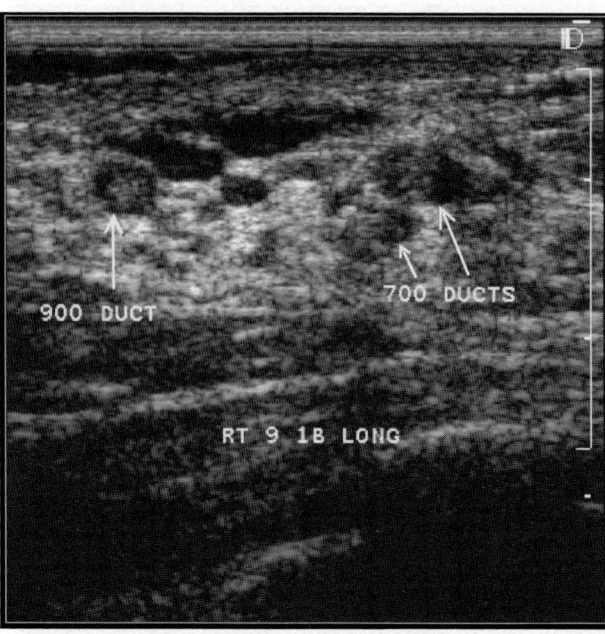

FIGURE 11–46 A: Intraductal and periductal fibrosis may involve several branches as well as the main lobar duct. This radial view of the main duct shows it to be filled with solid material that is sonographically indistinguishable from ductal carcinoma *in situ* (DCIS). **B:** Antiradial view shows several branch ducts that are enlarged and isoechoic because of intraductal and periductal fibrosis. The patient underwent biopsy because the sonographic findings so strongly suggested DCIS.

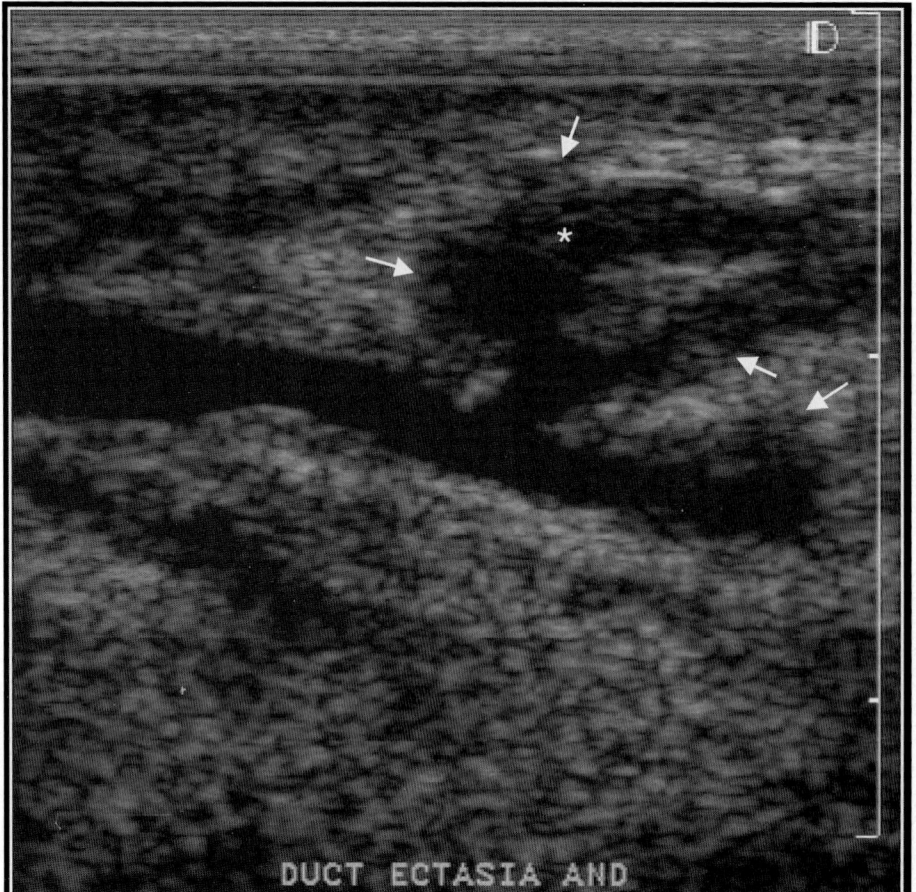

FIGURE 11–47 Radial view of a severely ectatic duct shows isoechoic intraductal fibrosis filling the lumen of the anterior-most branch *(*)* and periductal fibrosis compressing three branches *(arrows)*. The periductal fibrosis makes the margins of the duct ill defined, raising concerns about periductal tumor invasion.

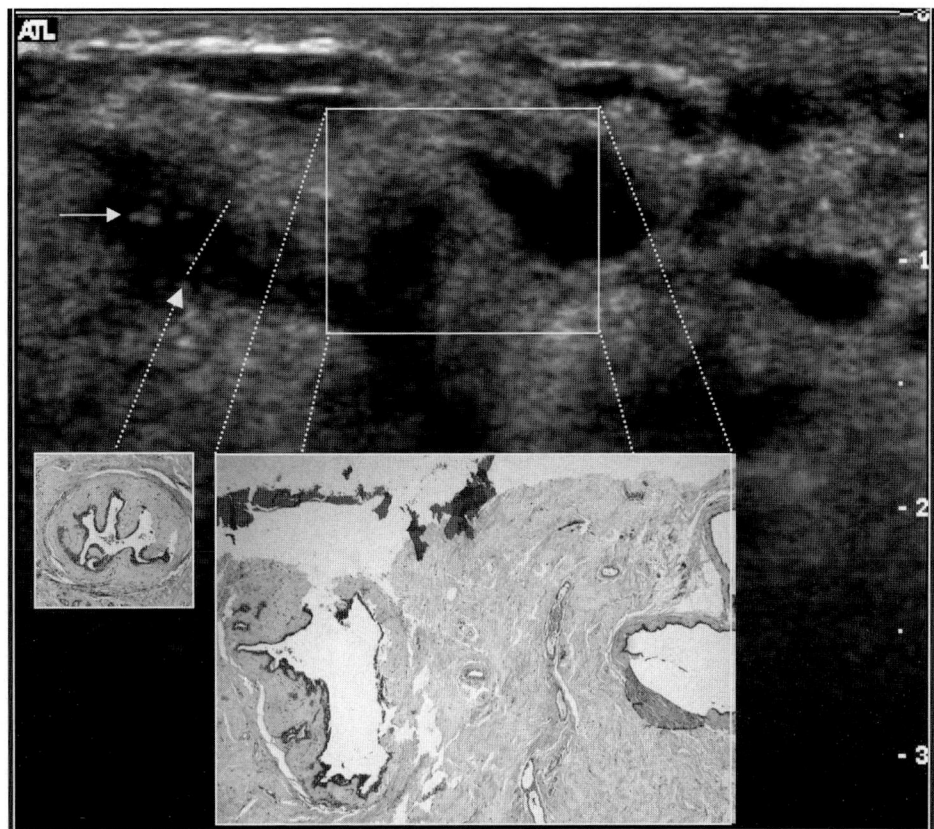

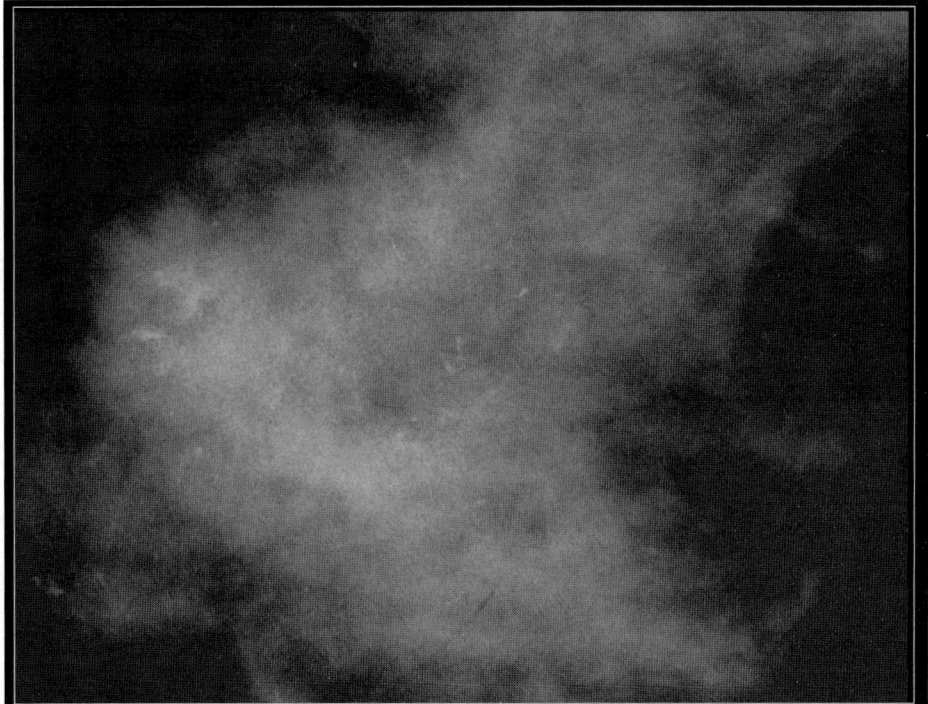

FIGURE 11–48 A: The wall of the duct in the center of the image is irregularly thickened by periductal fibrosis *(*)*. To its right is a duct that is more sonographically normal, but does have mild periductal fibrosis at biopsy *(#)*. On the left side of the image is a duct with calcifications in the lumen *(arrow)* that is more severely compressed by periductal fibrosis. The calcifications were visible mammographically and were suspicious for ductal carcinoma *in situ* (DCIS), not classic secretory calcifications. Both mammographic and sonographic findings were suspicious enough for DCIS that imaging-guided vacuum-assisted 11-gauge needle biopsy was necessary. **B:** Spot compression magnification mammogram of the calcifications shown in the image in part **A** shows that the calcifications are granular and pleomorphic and therefore suspicious for DCIS. They are not classically benign secretory calcifications, despite being the result of the duct ectasia—periductal mastitis complex. *(Continued.)*

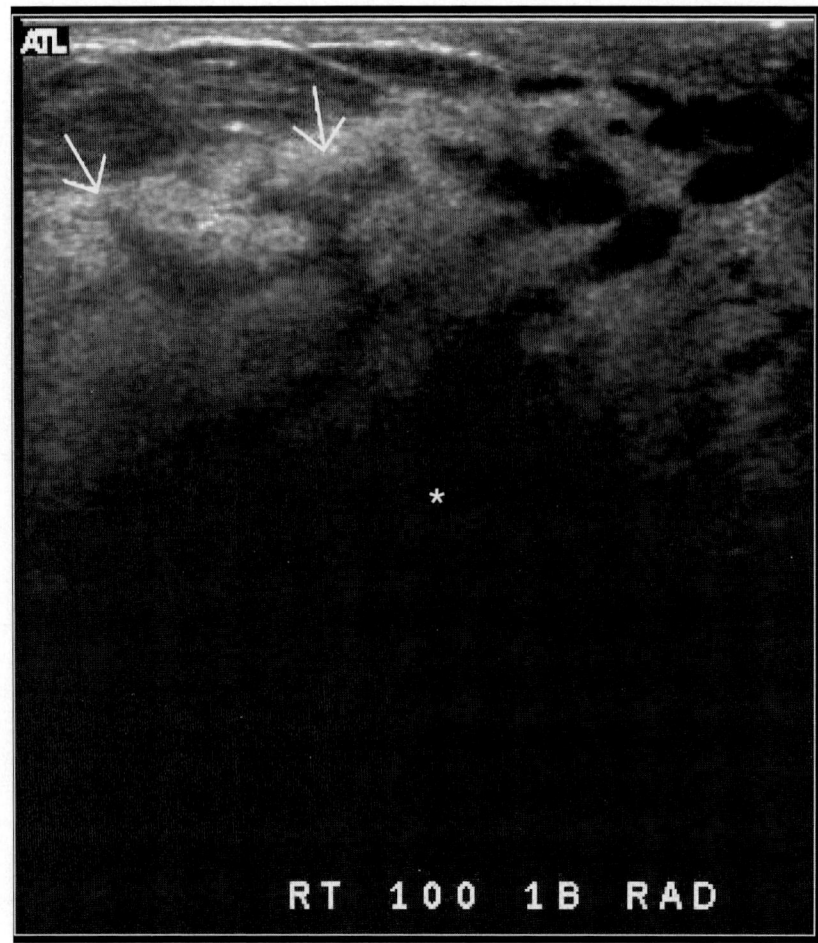

C

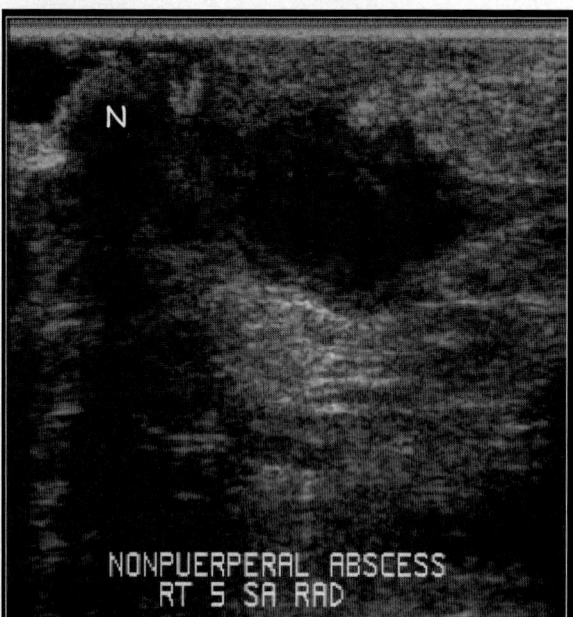

FIGURE 11–48 *(continued)* **C:** Several branches of the main lobar duct are completely obliterated by periductal fibrosis *(arrows)*. The markedly hypoechoic area deep in the breast that causes intense acoustic shadowing is suspicious for invasive carcinoma (*). The appearance is quite typical for invasive lobular carcinoma. Biopsy revealed granulomatous giant cell foreign-body reaction interpreted by the pathologist to represent fat necrosis or breast infarct. The foreign-body reaction and granulomatous mastitis are nonspecific and can result from a variety of etiologies, including trauma or surgery, hemorrhage, ruptured inflamed cysts, and periductal mastitis.

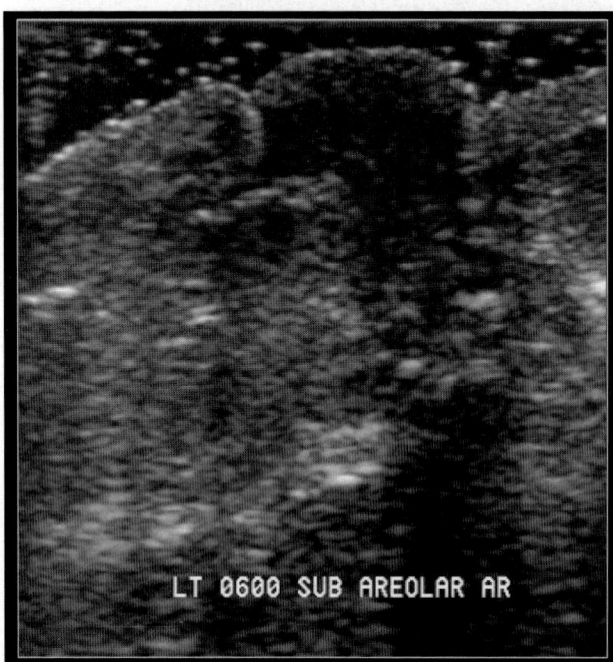

FIGURE 11–49 Periductal fibrosis resulting from the chronic duct ectasia—periductal mastitis complex can lead to permanent nipple retraction.

FIGURE 11–50 The typical nonpuerperal periareolar abscess is thick walled, is elongated in an axis parallel to the subareolar ducts, and involves the nipple or areola. The axis lies parallel to the subareolar ducts because it arises when an inflamed ectatic duct ruptures, extravasating highly inflammatory, lipid-rich secretions into the periductal soft tissues. The abscess has caused nipple retraction, which gradually resolved with aspiration and antibiotic treatment over a period of weeks. The thick-walled appearance is typical of periareolar abscesses in perimenopausal patients who have a history of chronic duct ectasia. N, nipple.

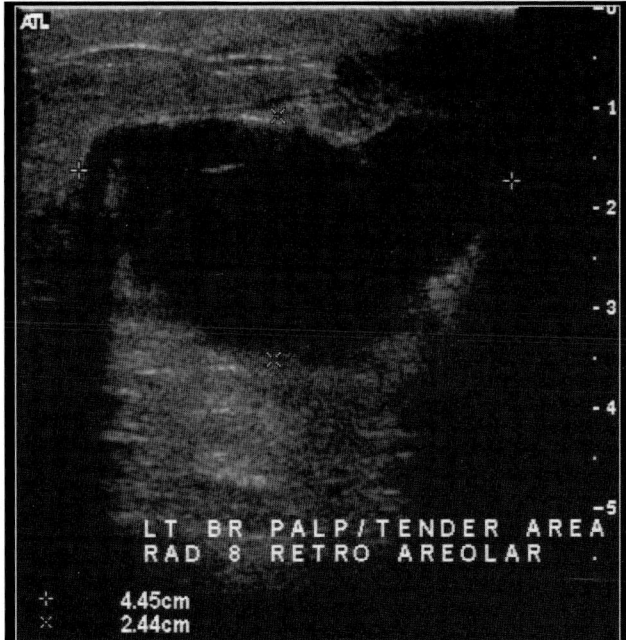

FIGURE 11–51 This periareolar abscess in a teenager is relatively thin walled but is elongated in an axis that is parallel to the major subareolar ducts and extends to the base of the nipple. The thin wall is more typical of first-time abscesses that occur in the younger age group, where congenital nipple inversion and squamous metaplasia rather than chronic duct ectasia, are the etiologies.

abscesses are the lack of relationship to lactation, the association with duct ectasia, and the typical periareolar location. The sonographic appearance does differ between the perimenopausal group, in whom the underlying etiology is chronic duct ectasia, and those in their late teens and 20s, in whom the underlying etiology is congenital nipple inversion and squamous metaplasia. The nonpuerperal periareolar abscess in perimenopausal patients is typically thick walled, angular, elongated in an axis parallel to the ducts, directly subareolar in location, and more likely to involve the areola and base of the nipple (Fig. 11–50). Peripheral compression, two-handed compression, and rolled-nipple techniques can be helpful in demonstrating these findings. The initial nonpuerperal abscess in the younger age group is more likely to be relatively thin walled, oval or lobulated, at the edge of the areola in location, and not directly involving the areola and nipple (Fig. 11–51). Particularly in the perimenopausal group, the intense inflammation associated with nonpuerperal periareolar abscesses, their tendency to recur, and the scarring associated with their healing may lead to nipple retraction that may be transient or permanent. The intense scarring that can result from a subareolar abscess can be very difficult to distinguish from a cancer that retracts the nipple (Fig. 11–52). Nonpuerperal abscesses can be aspirated once or repeatedly, treated with percutaneous catheter drainage, or treated surgically.

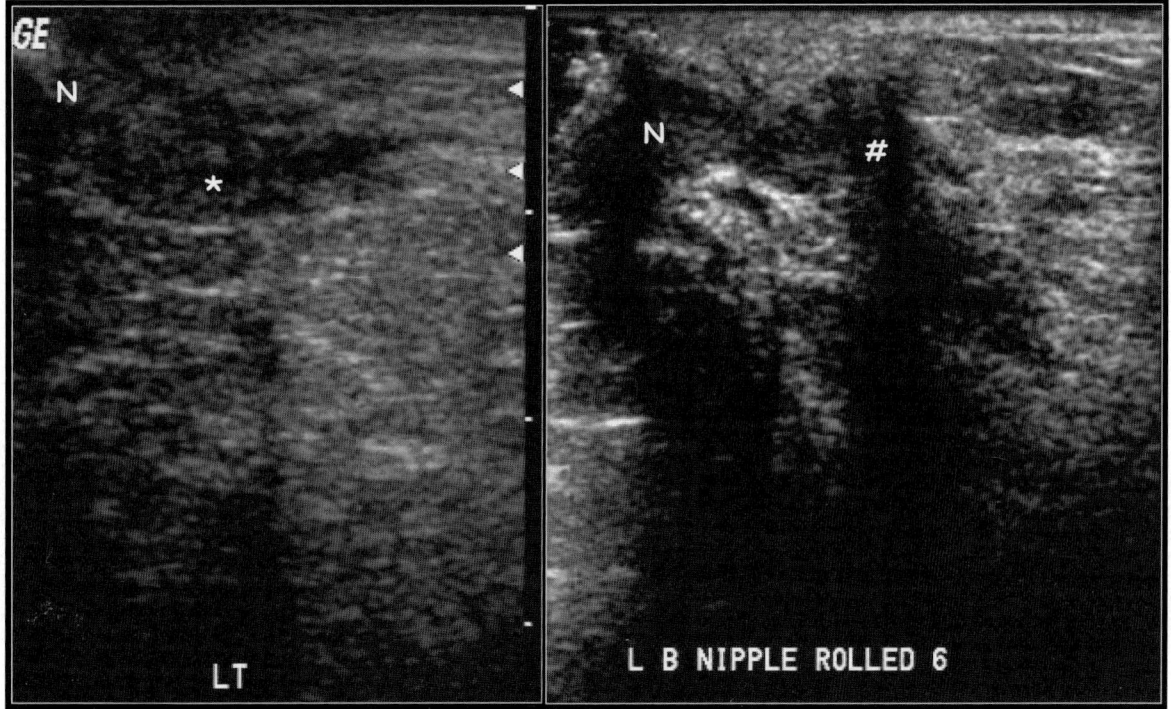

FIGURE 11–52 The chronic periareolar abscess in the image shown on the **left** (*) has become solid in appearance and caused nipple retraction. The invasive carcinoma shown in the **right** image (#) has grown within the ducts into the nipple and caused nipple retraction that is clinically indistinguishable from that caused by the chronic periareolar abscess. N, nipple.

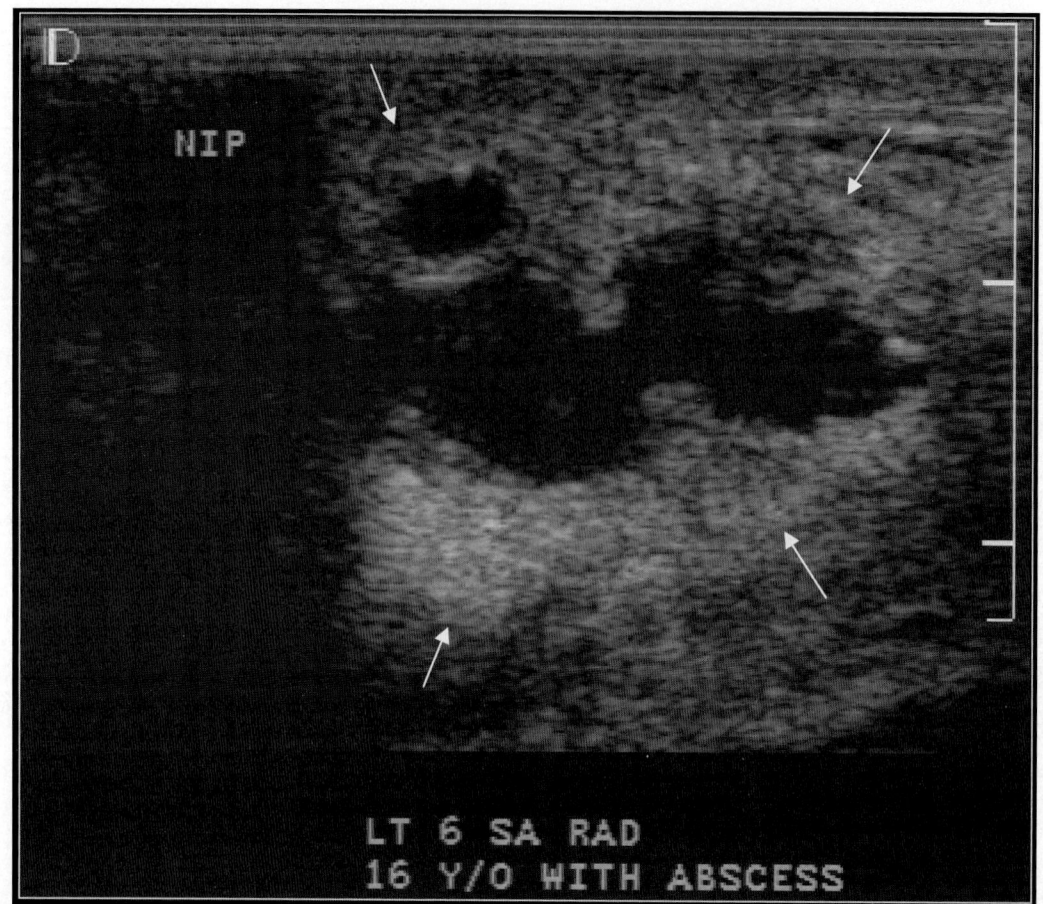

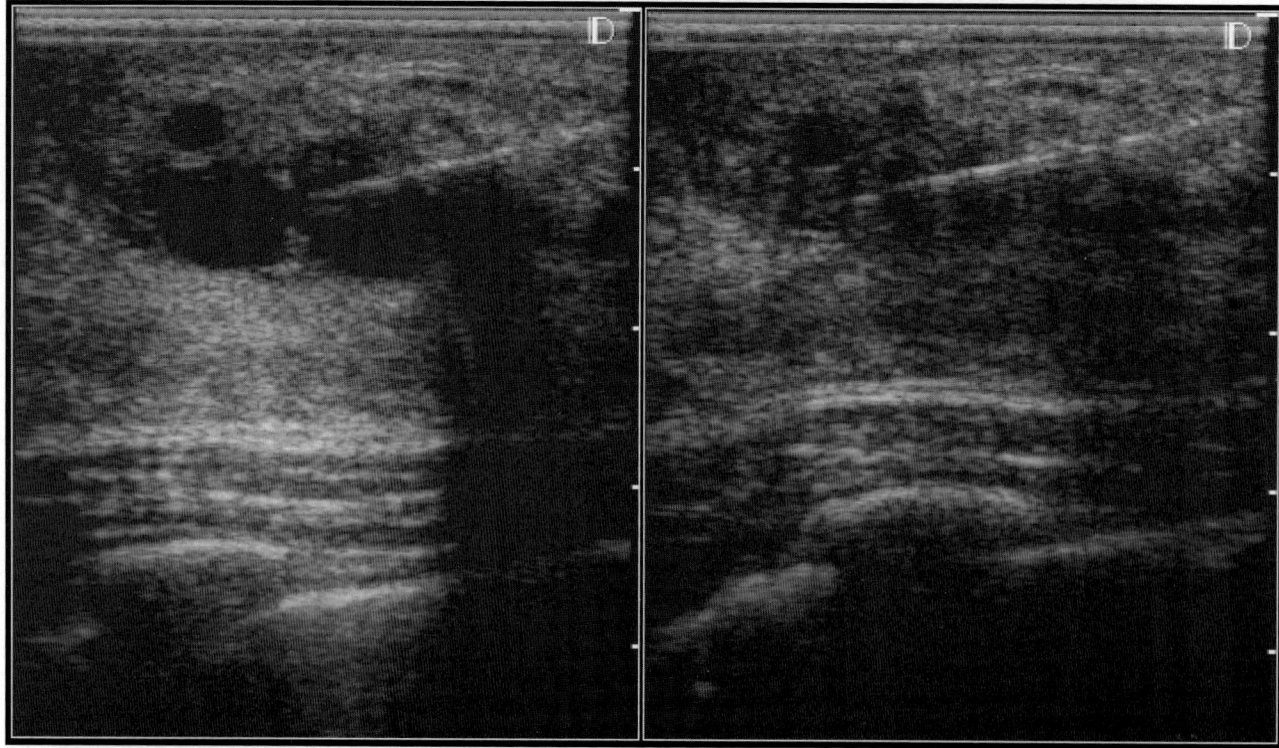

FIGURE 11–53 A: Thin-walled, periareolar abscesses in the younger age group that are the result of congenital nipple inversion and squamous metaplasia generally respond well to single ultrasound-guided aspiration and antibiotic treatment. The long axis of this lobulated abscess is parallel to the axis of the central ducts. There is edema surrounding the abscess that represents an intense periabscess focal mastitis *(arrows)*. **B:** Ultrasound-guided aspiration completely drained the pus from the abscess. Pain and tenderness were improved immediately after aspiration, and residual inflammation resolved gradually over 10 days on broad-spectrum antibiotic treatment. Culture revealed mixed flora. Despite congenital nipple inversion, there has been no recurrent abscess to date.

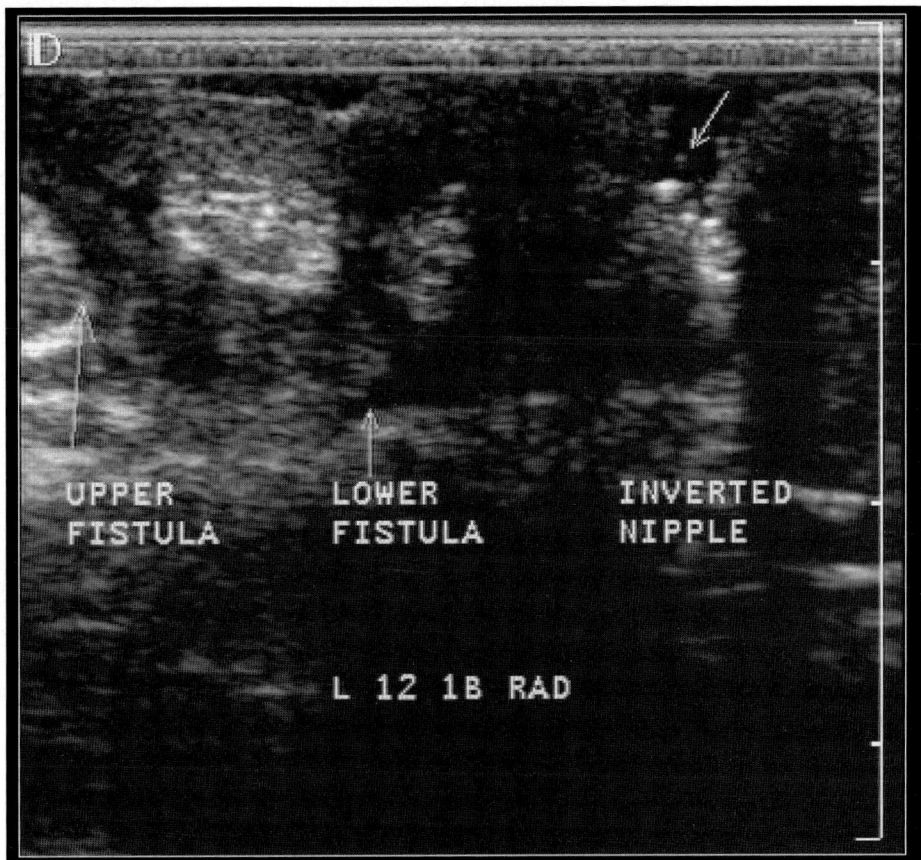

FIGURE 11–54 Periareolar nonpuerperal abscesses that are not aspirated or surgically drained may point and spontaneously drain through the skin. The fistulous tract through which the abscess drains is difficult, if not impossible, to eradicate with conservative treatment in almost all cases and thus usually must be surgically excised completely for healing to occur. This patient had developed two fistulous tracts as well as severe nipple retraction. Antibiotic treatment was successful only at stopping purulent drainage from one of the fistulous tracts or the nipple, but not from all three. The patient developed "ping-pong" drainage that moved back and forth serially from the upper fistulous tract to the lower tract, then to the nipple, and then back to the upper tract again. Several cycles of this drainage pattern occurred before the patient underwent definitive surgery.

First-time periareolar abscess in the younger group respond well to single aspirations and antibiotics (Fig. 11–53). Periareolar abscesses in the perimenopausal group can also be aspirated under ultrasound guidance but are more likely to require repeated aspirations or more definitive drainage. It is important to drain these abscesses because if they are not drained, they will eventually point and establish spontaneous drainage through the skin, which may result in chronically draining fistulous tracts that require complete surgical excision (Fig. 11–54). Antibiotics alone seldom succeed in healing fistulas or nonpuerperal abscesses. Some abscesses can require many weeks or months of oral antibiotics before completely resolving (Fig. 11–55). Even when successfully aspirated or drained completely, nonpuerperal abscesses have a tendency to recur in both the peri-

menopausal and younger groups. Abscesses recur in the perimenopausal group because of the underlying ductal ectasia and periductal mastitis, and in the younger group because of underlying nipple inversion and squamous metaplasia. Nonpuerperal periductal mastitis and subareolar abscesses have a particular propensity to involve the nipple (Fig. 11–56). Only tiny fluid collections that we have deemed too small to warrant drainage may be present within the nipple (Fig. 11–57). Such involvement seems to respond poorly to antibiotics (Fig. 11–58), but in most cases, there is too little abscess fluid to aspirate. Thus, patients usually require prolonged antibiotic treatment and follow-up sonography.

The underlying cause of peripherally located nonpuerperal abscess is more often fibrocystic change (FCC)

(text continued on page 391)

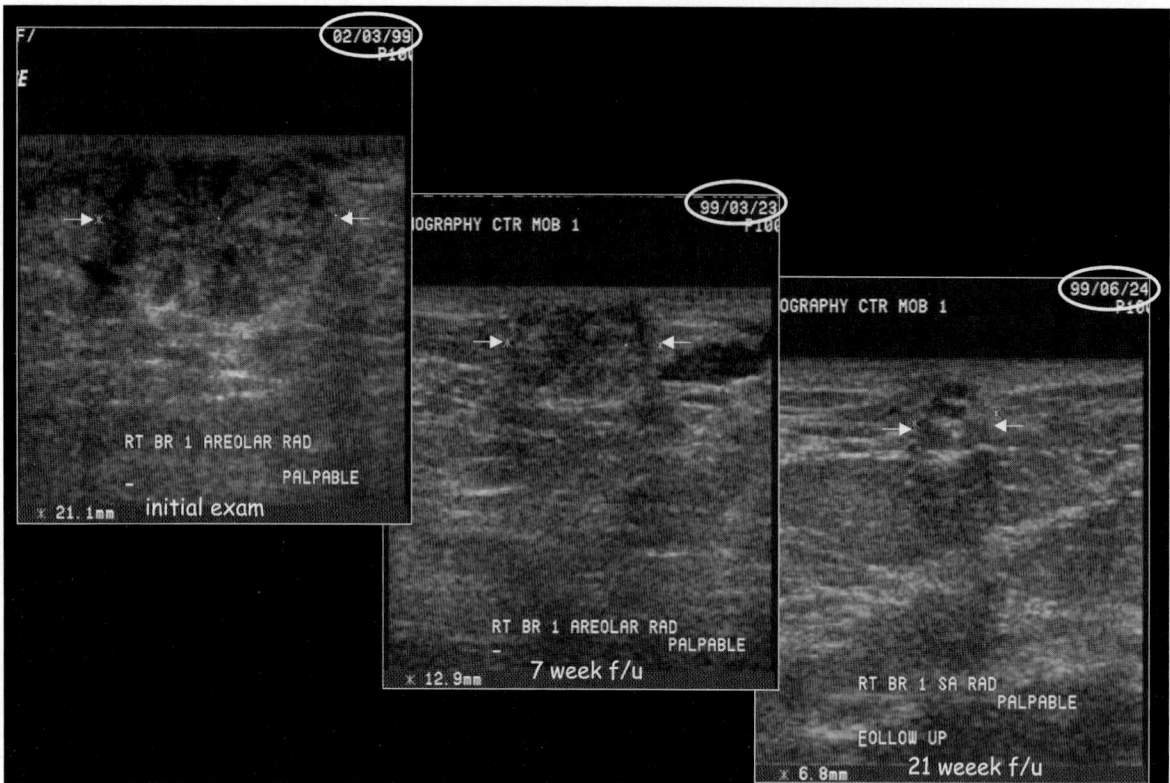

FIGURE 11–55 The resolution of periareolar nonpuerperal abscesses on antibiotic treatment alone is slow and very protracted, if it can be achieved at all. This chronic abscess had too much solid component to be drained percutaneously. Image-guided core needle biopsy revealed chronic abscess. The patient refused surgery. The patient was then placed on long-term antibiotic treatment, and the lesion gradually resolved over a period of more than 5 months.

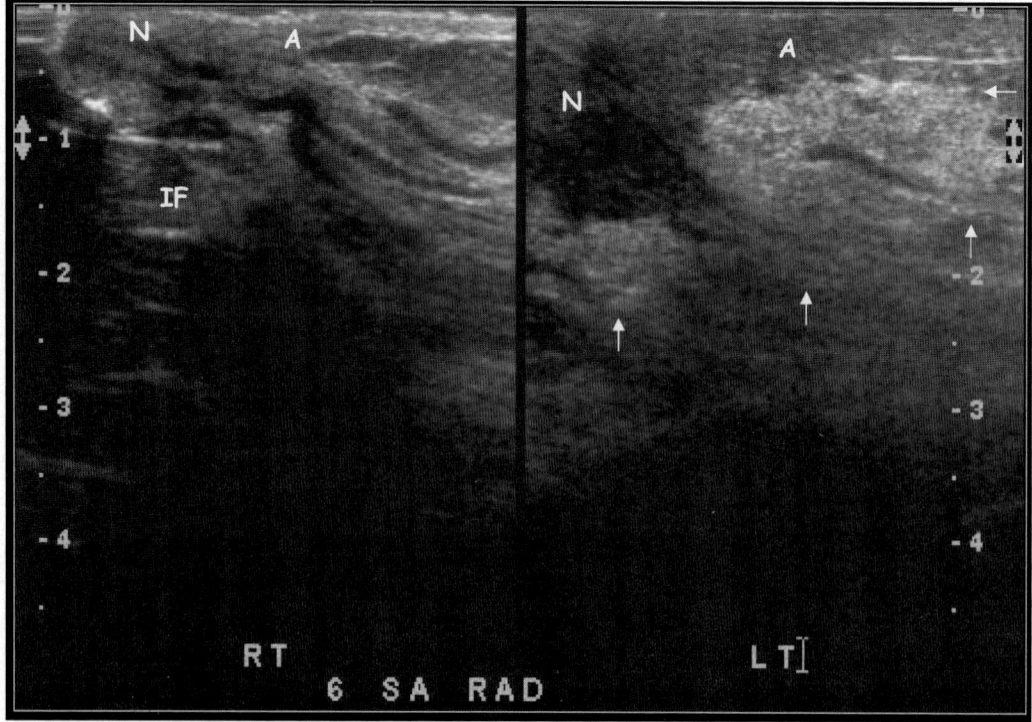

FIGURE 11–56 Acute nonpuerperal periductal mastitis resulting from either chronic duct ectasia or congenital nipple inversion and squamous metaplasia is particularly prone to involve the nipple and areola. These split-screen radial images show the normal nipple, areola, and subareolar ducts on the patient's right side (**left**) and the acutely infected nipple *(N)*, areola *(A)*, and subareolar soft tissues on the patient's asymptomatic left side (**right**). The left nipple and areolar are thickened and less echogenic than on the normal right side, whereas the subareolar fat and loose connective tissues are more echogenic than normal *(arrows)*. Note that there is mild duct ectasia present bilaterally, indicating that patient is at risk for additional episodes of acute and chronic periductal mastitis bilaterally. The rolled-nipple technique has been used to show the intranipple ducts on the patient's right side, but edema and pain prevented using the maneuver on the patients left side, where only the peripheral compression technique was possible. IF, index finger of nonscanning hand.

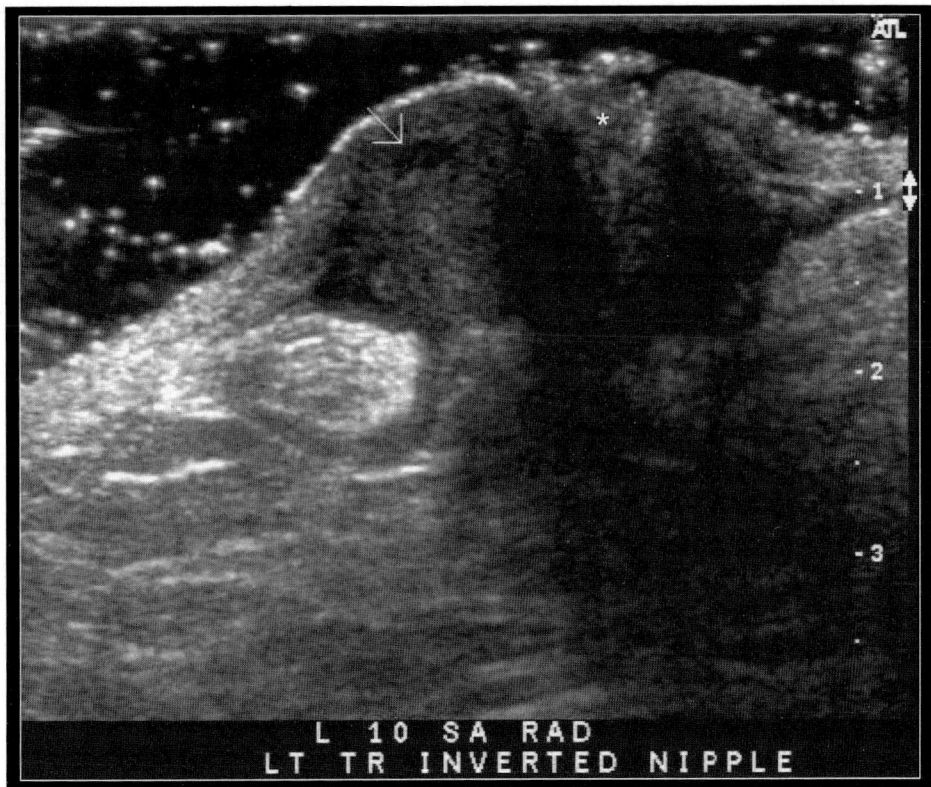

FIGURE 11–57 Involvement of the nipple and areola by acute periductal mastitis is generally not accompanied by fluid collections large enough to warrant percutaneous drainage *(arrow)*. Note the congenital nipple inversion (with associated squamous metaplasia) that predisposed this patient to infection and the crusted purulent discharge within the depressed nipple (*).

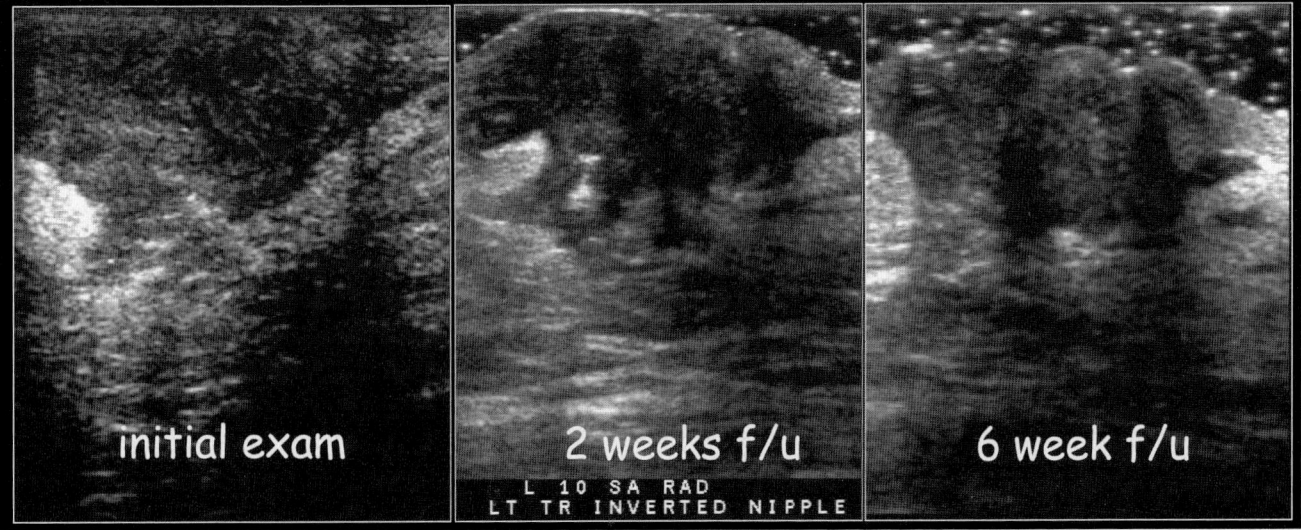

FIGURE 11–58 Involvement of the nipple and areola by acute periductal mastitis responds poorly to antibiotic treatment alone, but there seldom is much fluid to drain. In such cases, nipple resection is a poor option, and surgery is a generally a last resort. Prolonged antibiotic treatment over weeks to months should be anticipated. In this patient, little improvement was noted over a 6-week period in which the patient underwent three 14-day courses of antibiotic treatments. She was placed on long-term antibiotics and had gradual improvement over a period of several months. The lack of immediate response to antibiotics in such patients always raises concerns about an underlying inflammatory carcinoma; thus, any evidence of an associated solid nodule warrants aggressive biopsy.

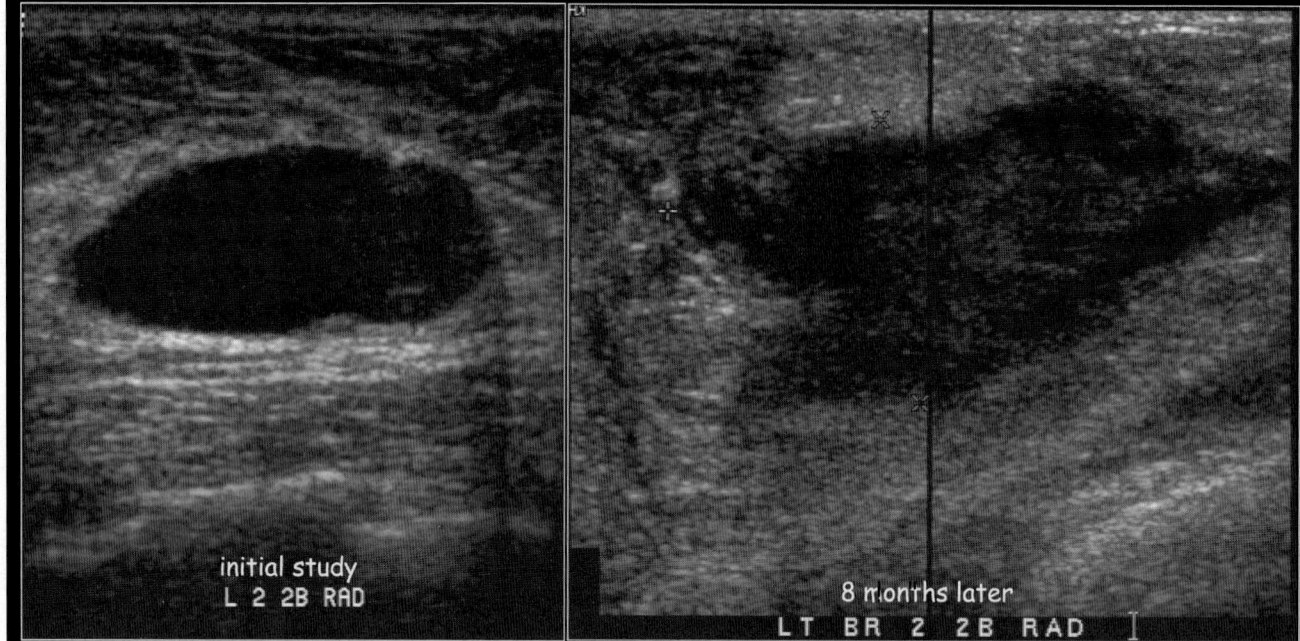

FIGURE 11–59 Not all nonpuerperal abscesses result from duct ectasia or congenital nipple inversion with squamous metaplasia. This patient had neither nipple discharge nor sonographic evidence of duct ectasia but developed a nonpuerperal abscess. The patient had a large, simple cyst from which the abscess apparently developed. Whether the abscess resulted from rupture of the cyst and release of lipid-laden contents into the surrounding tissue, communication of the cyst with a ductal system colonized by bacteria, or hematogenous seeding is uncertain.

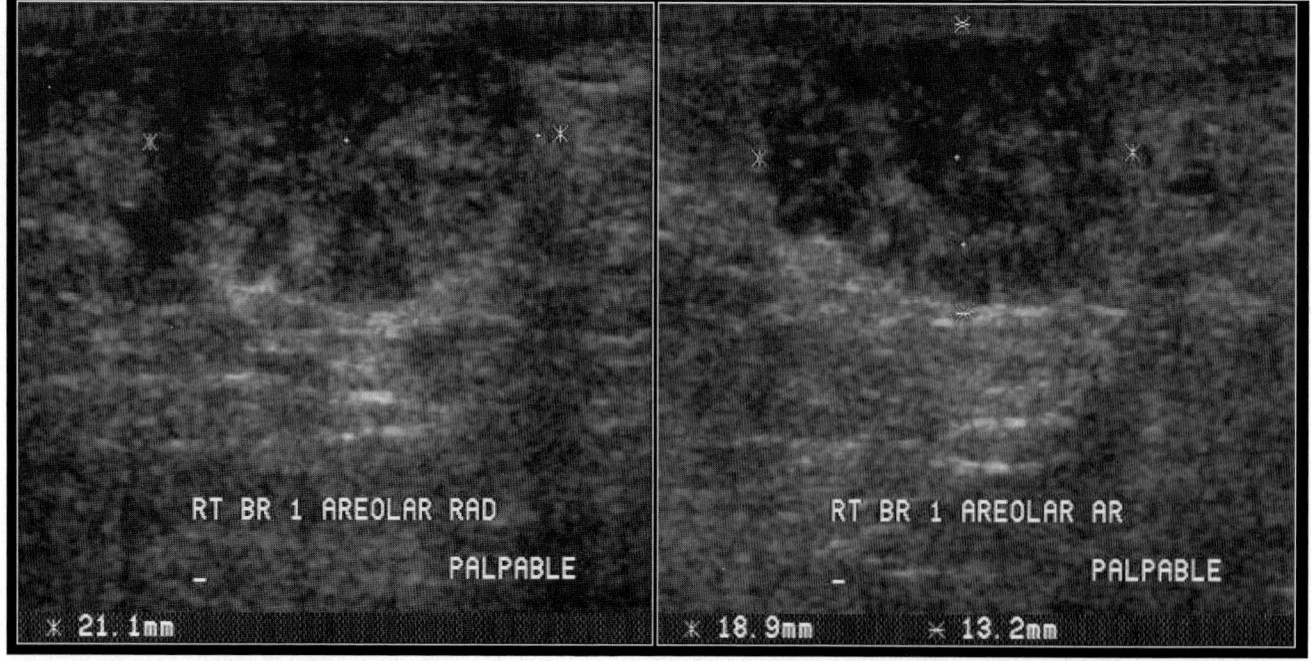

FIGURE 11–60 Like puerperal abscesses, nonpuerperal abscesses may become chronic and may appear solid sonographically.

than duct ectasia (Fig. 11–59). Secondary infection of a preexisting cyst usually requires coexisting conditions: (a) intervention (attempted aspiration), (b) hematogenous seeding, or (c) secondary inflammation and communication with a ductal system that has been colonized by bacteria. An underlying inflamed cyst may not always be demonstrable because the event causing focal mastitis and abscess formation is often spontaneous rupture of an inflamed cyst. In certain cases, however, the focal mastitis may have been caused by leakage from a cyst that has not completely ruptured. The findings in acutely inflamed cysts are discussed in detail in Chapter 10 and include (a) diffuse, isoechoic, circumferential thickening of the cyst wall (as opposed to the thin echogenic wall seen around uncomplicated breast cysts), and (b) either diffuse low-level echogenicity within the cysts lumen or the presence of a fluid–debris level within the cyst. These findings are indicative of inflammation rather than frank infection. Acutely inflamed, infected cysts that give rise to focal mastitis often have hyperemia within the wall and the immediately surrounding tissue

that can be demonstrated with color Doppler (see Chapter 20, Figs. 20–40 to 20–42). A noninfected (sterile), inflamed cyst cannot be distinguished sonographically or clinically from an acutely infected cyst. Only aspiration, Gram stain, and culture can distinguish an infected from a noninfected, inflamed cyst. However, over time, the infected cyst becomes more irregular.

Nonpuerperal abscesses are far more likely than puerperal abscesses to recur and become chronic because of the underlying chronic ductal inflammation or obstruction. Chronic or recurrent nonpuerperal abscesses associated with chronic focal mastitis may contain sufficient granulation tissue and fibrosis to simulate solid nodules (Fig. 11–60).

Mastitis with or without abscess, whether puerperal or nonpuerperal, must be distinguished from inflammatory carcinoma. Both cause severe edema and inflammation. Both can have masses that appear markedly hypoechoic and have enhanced acoustic through-transmission (Fig. 11–61).

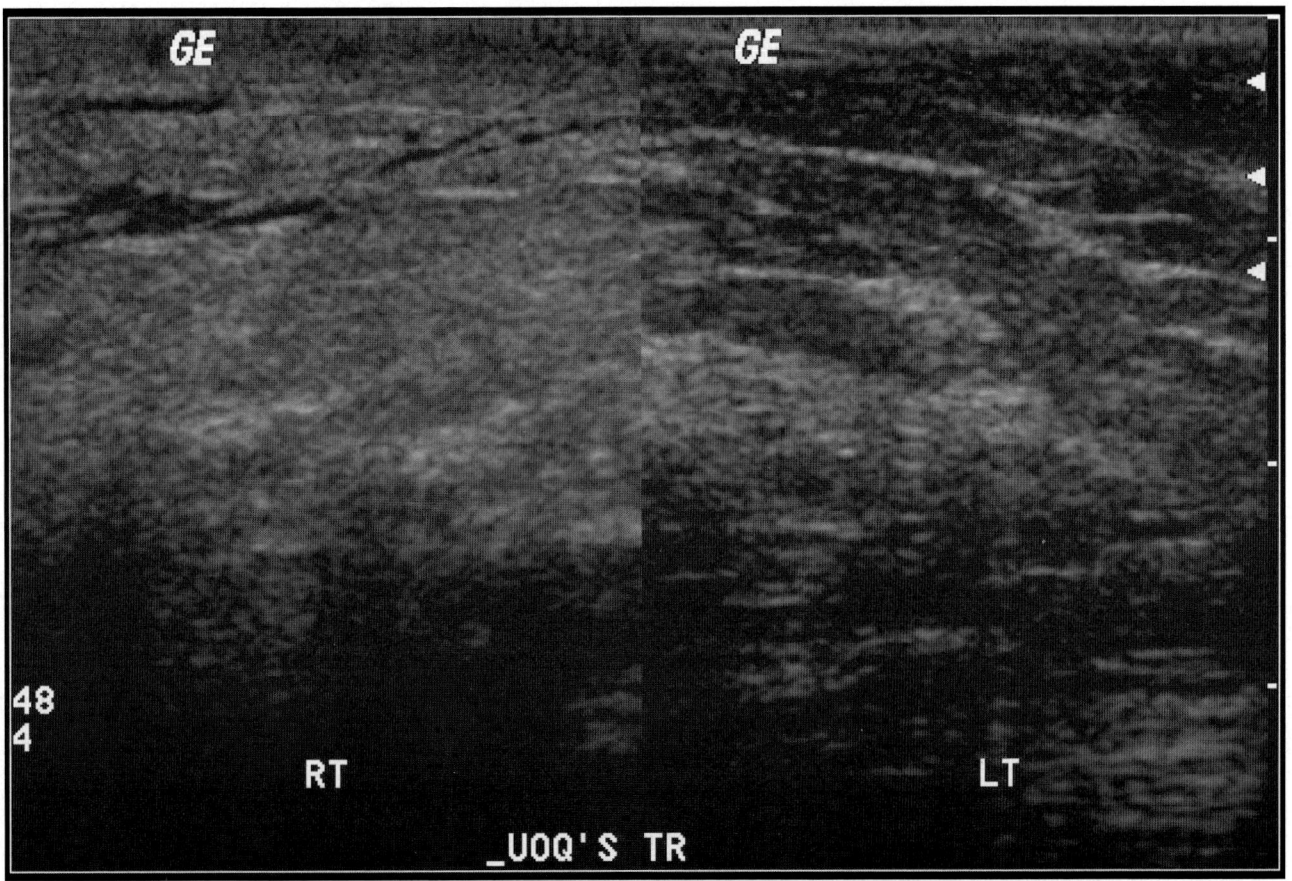

FIGURE 11–61 A: In all cases of nonpuerperal mastitis, the possibility of inflammatory carcinoma must be kept in mind. The edema caused by inflammatory carcinoma appears identical to the edema caused by mastitis clinically and sonographically. The edema adversely affects sonographic penetration; thus, lower frequency transducers (such as 5-MHz linear or curved linear array) may be necessary to exclude an underlying carcinoma in some cases. *(Continued.)*

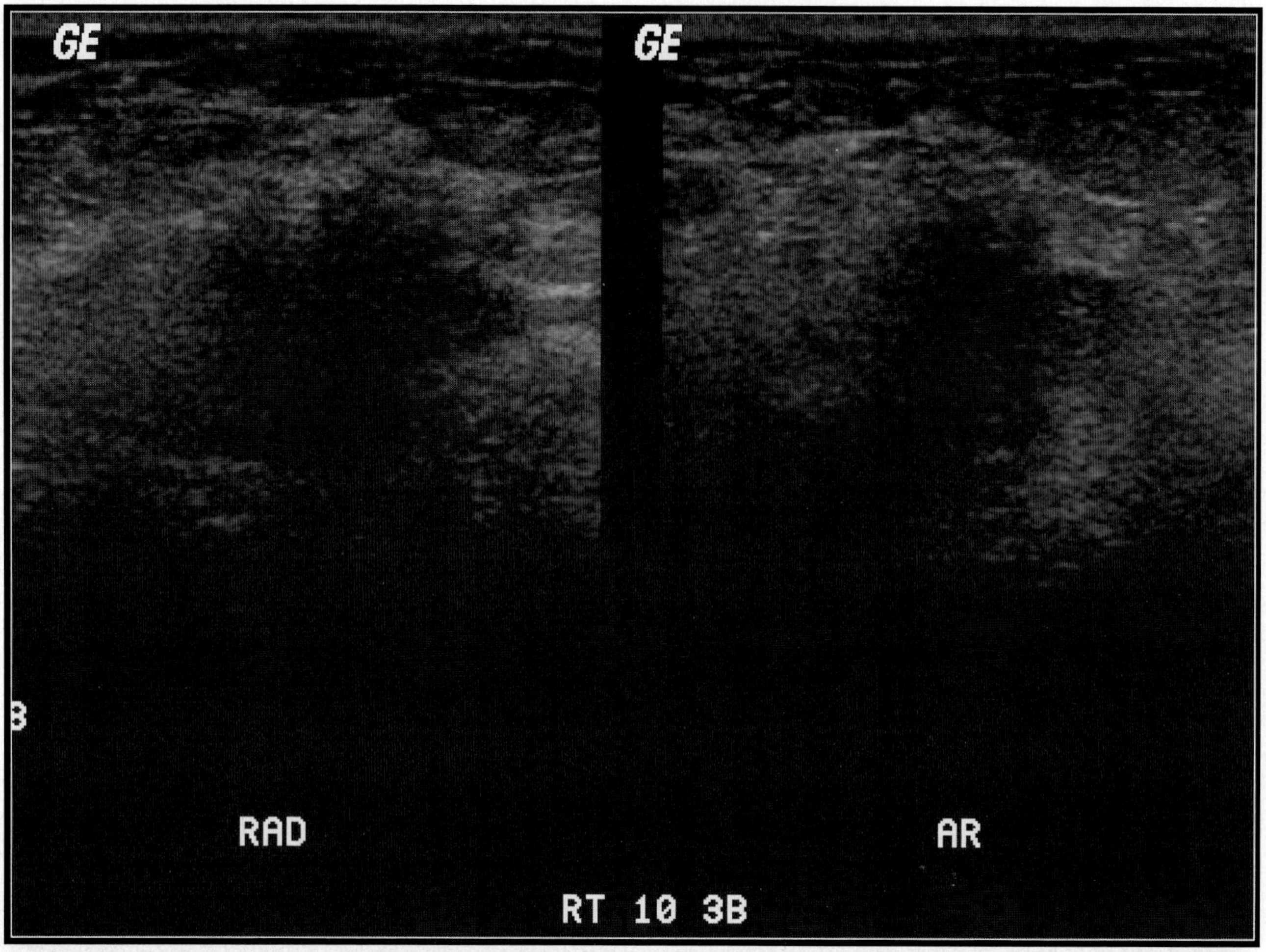
GE
GE
RAD
AR
RT 10 3B

B

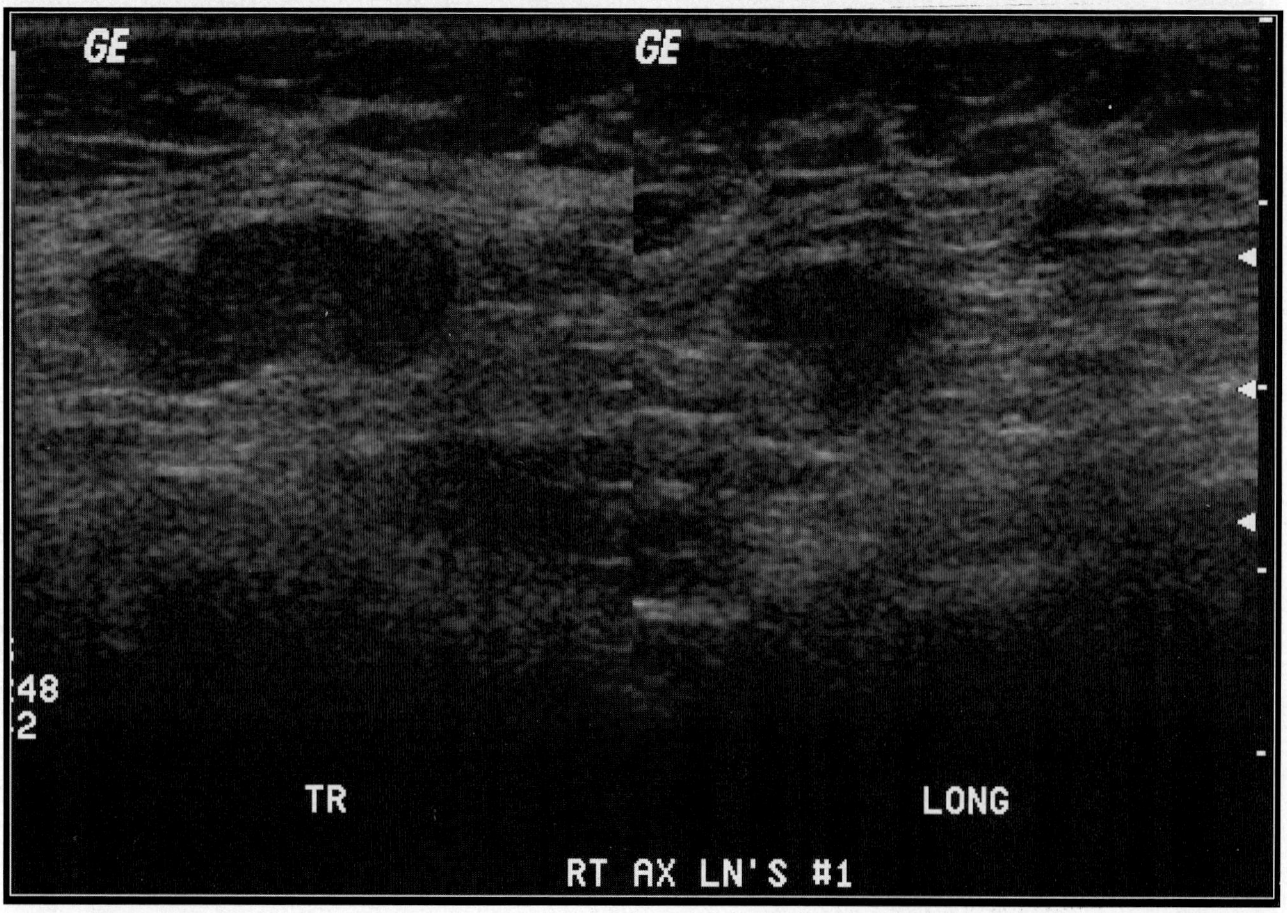
GE
GE
TR
LONG
RT AX LN'S #1

C

Ultrasound-guided Abscess Drainage of Nonpuerperal Abscesses

Sonographic guidance is important in both the diagnosis and the treatment of breast abscesses. The aspirate obtained from an ultrasound-guided aspiration can be evaluated with Gram stain and culture. Abscesses that are well defined, mature, and entirely liquefied centrally may be amenable to complete aspiration and treatment with antibiotics, potentially not requiring an indwelling drainage tube. Recurrences may be treated with repeat aspiration. On the other hand, early abscesses that contain large amounts of solid debris or several loculations generally cannot be adequately aspirated and require placement of an indwelling catheter in conjunction with antibiotic treatment. Abscesses that contain numerous loculations or that contain large amounts of solid debris are more likely to be inadequately drained by catheters and may respond better to surgical incision and drainage. However, even in these cases, a therapeutic trial with percutaneous drainage is usually warranted. Abscess drainage is discussed in greater detail in Chapter 17.

SEROMAS

A seroma is a localized collection of serous fluid within the breast. Most seromas result from minimally invasive interventional procedures or surgical procedures and are unwanted complications of the procedure. The more extensive the surgery, the more likely a seroma is to develop. The larger the seroma, the longer it will take to resolve and the more likely it is to be complicated by secondary infection. Additionally, lymphatic disruption due to axillary dissection predisposes to seroma formation.

Although seromas are generally viewed as troublesome complications to be avoided, there are three instances in which the development of a seroma may be helpful: (a) in certain cases in which lumpectomy is performed, (b) after ultrasound-guided large core vacuum-assisted needle biopsy (mammotomy), and (c) in association with augmen-

tation implant surgery. These situations are discussed later in the section about ultrasound findings of seromas.

Seroma Development in Lumpectomy Cavities

Lumpectomy cavities may be sutured closed at the time of surgery or may intentionally be left open to accumulate blood or serous fluid in hopes that the accumulated fluid will prevent indentation and deformity of the contour of the breast. The surgeon is most likely not to close the cavity in cases in which the amount of tissue excised is very large in comparison to the breast size. The strategy is fraught with potential problems, however, because the cavity is just as likely to accumulate blood as serum, and the more blood, the more likely there is to be severe fat necrosis and late scar retraction. Thus, a better early cosmetic result may, in some cases, lead to more deformity later on.

Seromas within lumpectomy cavities may also be an advantage to radiation therapists because the skin scar is not an accurate reflection of the location of the lumpectomy cavity. The seroma far more accurately shows the location of the actual lumpectomy cavity than does the skin incision, and this can be readily demonstrated in the radiation oncology suite with ultrasound guidance. Additionally, ultrasound-guided brachytherapy is more easily and more accurately performed when there is a seroma within the lumpectomy cavity than when the cavity is collapsed or closed. Saline and contrast may be injected into the cavity to facilitate stereotactic placement of brachytherapy needles.

It is common for serous fluid and blood to coexist within a surgical cavity. Thus, many postsurgical fluid collections are mixed seromas and hematomas, not pure seromas, and distinguishing between them can be difficult in certain cases.

Seromas in Mammotomy Cavities

Seromas or hematomas may develop within the cavity created by directional vacuum-assisted large core needle biopsy (DVAB, mammotomy). Although such seromas are

FIGURE 11–61 *(continued)* **B:** Radial and antiradial images show the carcinoma causing the edema and inflammatory hyperemia shown in the image in part **A. C:** The edema and inflammation caused by inflammatory carcinoma results from invasion of lymphatic channels, which, in turn, increases the likelihood of finding abnormal axillary or internal mammary lymph nodes. This patient had grossly abnormal lymph nodes sonographically, as do most patients with inflammatory carcinoma. Ultrasound-guided biopsies of the primary tumor, skin, and axillary lymph nodes showed intermediate-grade invasive ductal carcinoma, tumor within lymphatic vessels in the skin, and metastatic breast cancer in axillary lymph nodes. The primary tumor was marked with a mammotomy clip, and the patient underwent 6 weeks of induction chemotherapy before surgery that made the edema and lesion almost completely disappear and the lymph nodes shrink dramatically. At mastectomy and axillary dissection, only a small, residual primary tumor was found. The lymphatic tumor emboli and metastases to axillary lymph nodes had completely resolved. At least in some patients, and at least in the short term and for local control, the prognosis for inflammatory carcinoma is better than previously believed. The long-term prognosis is still uncertain.

complications of the procedure, they can be of great bene-fit in patients in whom all sonographic evidence of disease is removed at the time of mammotomy and in whom bi-opsy reveals malignancy. Such patients must later undergo needle localization lumpectomy. Sonographic localization of mammotomy cavity seromas are discussed and illus-trated in greater detail later in this chapter in the section about sonographic findings of seromas.

Seromas around Implants

The periimplant effusion that forms between the fibrous periimplant capsule and the implant shell is essentially a de-sired seroma. Periimplant effusion seroma most commonly occurs around textured implants and is thought to decrease the likelihood of capsular contracture. It may also provide for some freedom of movement of the implant within the capsule, minimizing the chances of the implant rupturing with minor trauma. However, the periimplant effusion or seroma may become secondarily inflamed or infected in cer-tain cases. Additionally, in cases in which explantation is per-formed without excising the periimplant capsule, seromas may reaccumulate within the capsule. Periimplant seromas are discussed and illustrated in greater detail later in this chapter in the section on sonographic findings of seromas.

Mammographic Findings of Seromas

The mammographic findings of seromas are nonspecific and depend on the etiology as well as the tension and com-pressibility of the fluid collection. The appearance is that of a water-density mass of varying size and density. A seroma that is soft and compressible has low density and ill-defined margins. A seroma that is tense and incompressible presents as a high-density, well-circumscribed mass or nodule. The shape of a seroma may be irregular because the serous fluid accumulates within an irregularly shaped surgical defect. Because soft and compressible seromas within lumpectomy cavities have a low-density mammographic appearance that is not very worrisome for recurrent tumor, the mammo-graphic findings in patients with postlumpectomy seromas are often more reassuring than are the sonographic findings.

Sonographic Findings

Most seromas present sonographically as simple cysts or complex cysts with diffuse low-level internal echoes (Figs. 11–62 and 11–63). However, fibrinous adhesions may cause multiple avascular thin, echogenic or thick, isoechoic septa-tions that bridge the fluid collection (Fig. 11–64). In cases in which the seroma was initially mixed with some blood,

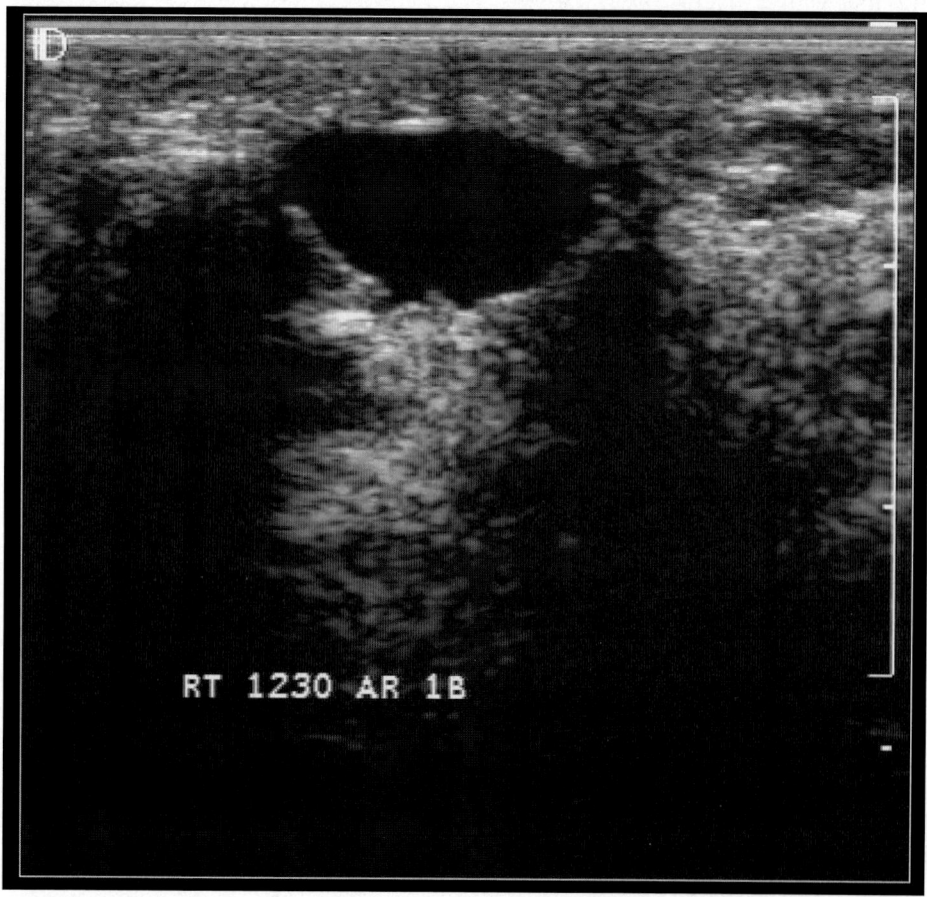

FIGURE 11–62 Some seromas are simple cystic.

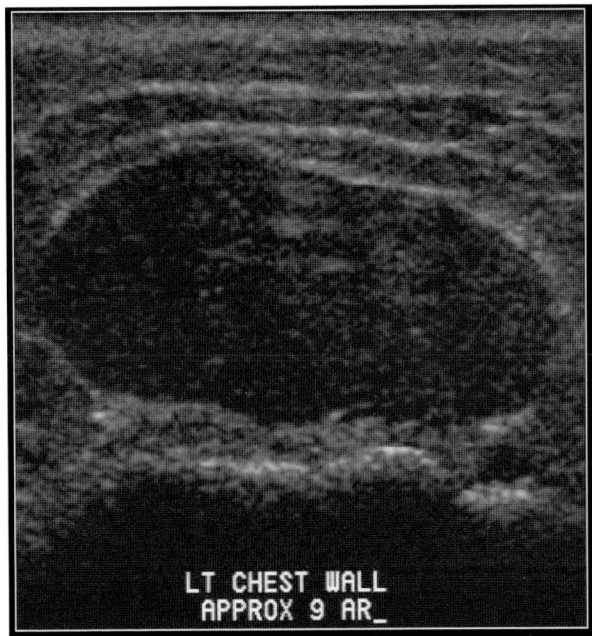

FIGURE 11–63 Other seromas may have diffuse low-level internal echogenicity.

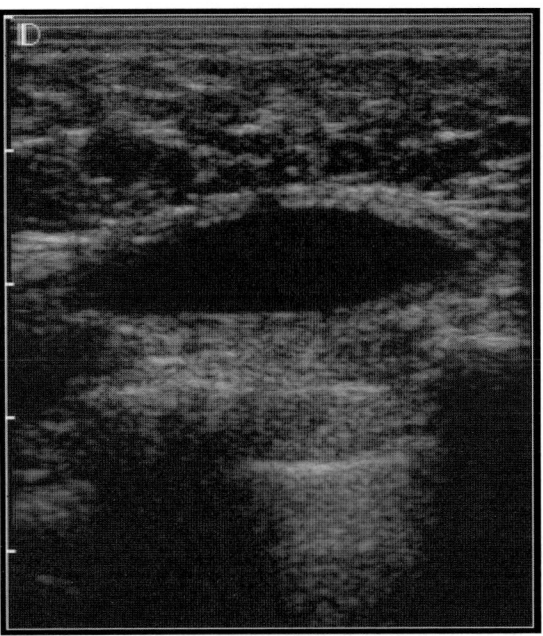

FIGURE 11–65 Many seromas arise mixed with small amounts of blood. In such seromas, the wall tends to be mildly thickened.

the wall of the seroma may be thick and isoechoic (Fig. 11–65) or echogenic, irregular, or nodular (Fig. 11–66). The wall of the seroma and the septations will remain avascular on color Doppler a few months after surgery (Fig. 11–67). Seromas conform to the size and shape of the surgical defect created. Thus, larger surgical procedures are more likely to cause seromas, the seromas are more likely to be large, and complications such as infection are more likely. The seromas associated with mastectomy (Fig. 11–68) are larger than those caused by lumpectomy (Figs. 11–62 to 11–67), which, in turn, are larger than those caused by mammotomy. When axillary dissection is performed, the disruption of lymphatic and venous drainage patterns makes development of large seromas even more likely (Fig. 11–69).

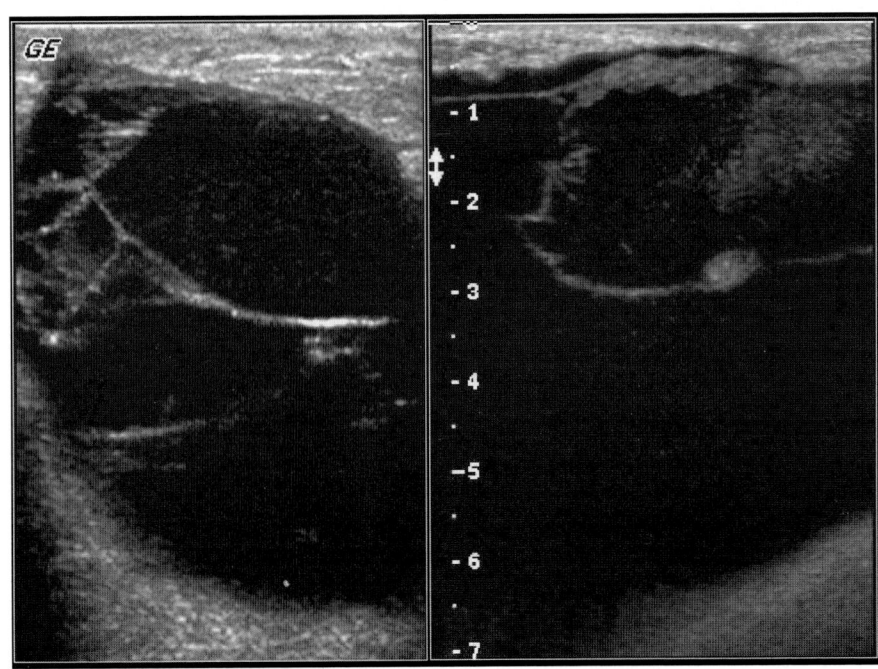

FIGURE 11–64 Fibrinous adhesions or thin, echogenic septa may bridge seromas (**left**). Seromas that initially contained some blood are more likely to have thick isoechoic internal septations (**right**).

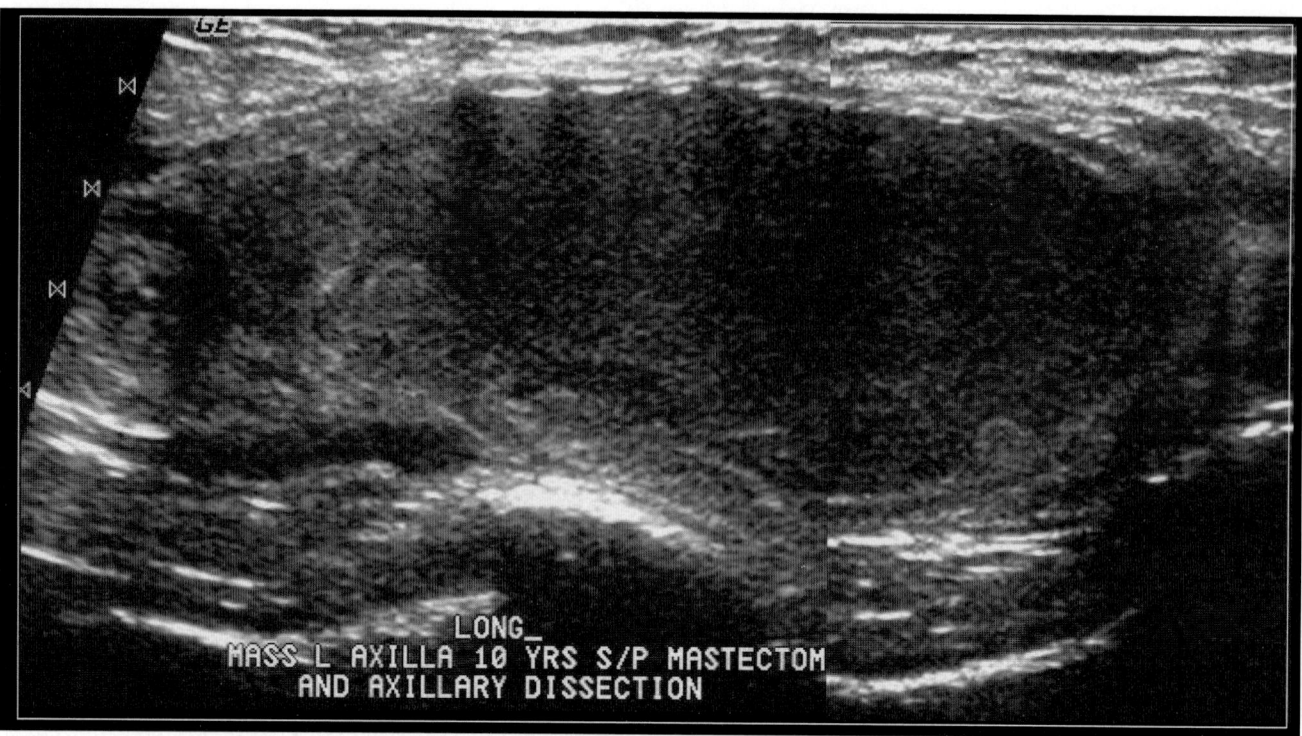

FIGURE 11–66 Seromas that initially contained some blood are more likely to have irregular wall thickening, mural nodules, and echogenic fluid.

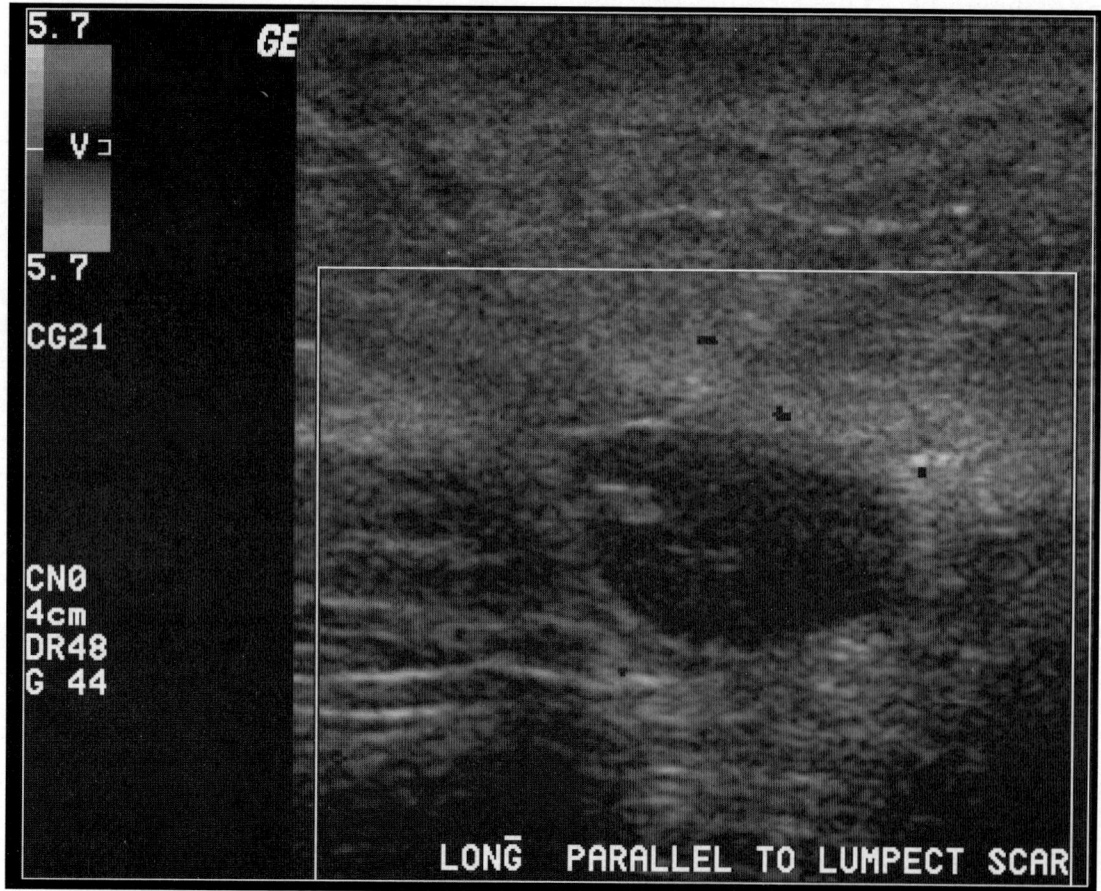

FIGURE 11–67 Unless infected, seromas will have no blood flow within the thickened walls, mural nodules, or thick septations, helping to distinguish them from intracystic papilloma or intracystic carcinoma.

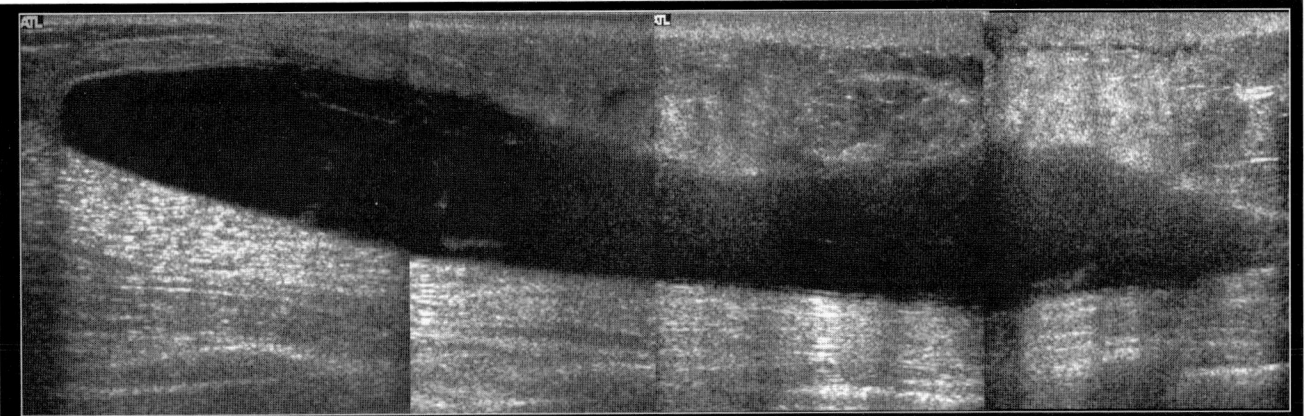

FIGURE 11–68 Postsurgical seromas conform to the size and shape of the surgical defect. Thus, more extensive surgeries lead to larger seromas. Mastectomy leads to the largest seromas. This seroma extended over the entire length of the mastectomy scar.

Because lumpectomy cavities are irregular and asymmetric in shape, the seromas that form within the cavities also are irregular and asymmetric in shape. The lumpectomy cavity seroma is usually elongated in an axis parallel to the long axis of the surgical scar but may be either flattened or circular in the plane that lies perpendicular to the scar, depending on whether the defect was sutured closed (primary closure) or not (Fig. 11–70). Lumpectomy scars can be sutured closed at the time of surgery or left open. When the lumpectomy cavity is not primarily closed, the hope is that a seroma will accumulate within the potential cavity and prevent indentation and deformity of the overlying skin. If the lumpectomy cavity is large or the underlying breast size is small, primary closure may pull the overlying skin inward toward the

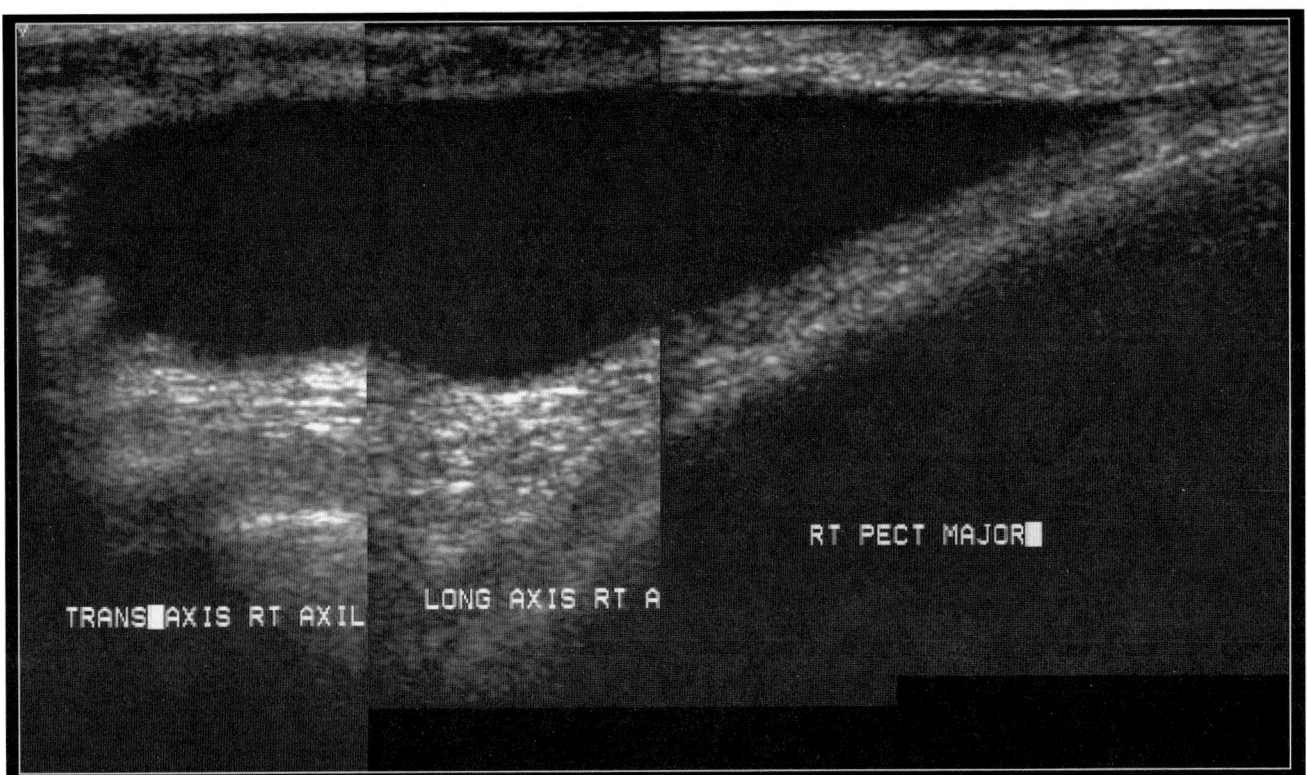

FIGURE 11–69 Axillary dissection increases the likelihood of seroma and the size of seromas that do develop because of interruption of lymphatic and venous drainage. This is just one of the reasons for the move away from full axillary dissection to more limited low axillary dissection or sentinel node procedures.

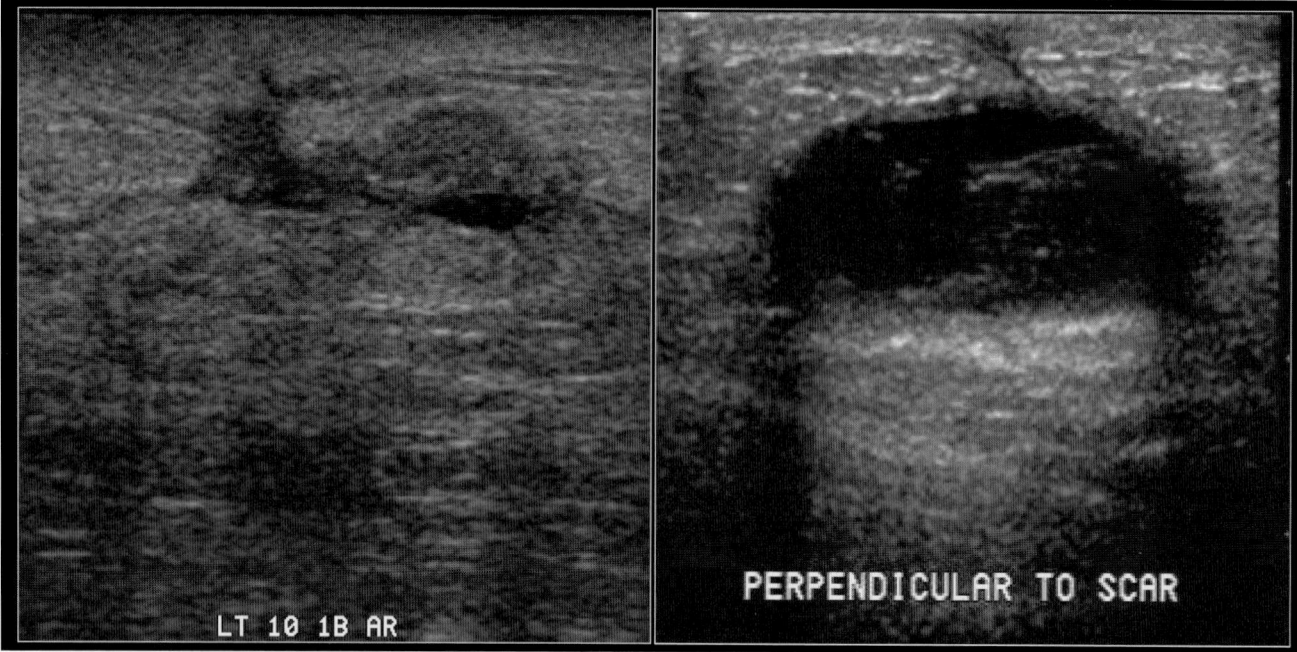

FIGURE 11–70 Surgical cavities that are sutured closed at the time of surgery have flattened, small seromas that are not worrisome in appearance **(left)**. Surgical cavities that are not sutured closed at the time of surgery accumulate large seromas or hematomas. This tends to prevent indentation and deformity of the skin line, but the seromas or hematomas that develop within the open cavity later can cause mammographic and sonographic concerns about recurrent tumor and may also increase the risk for postoperative infection **(right)**.

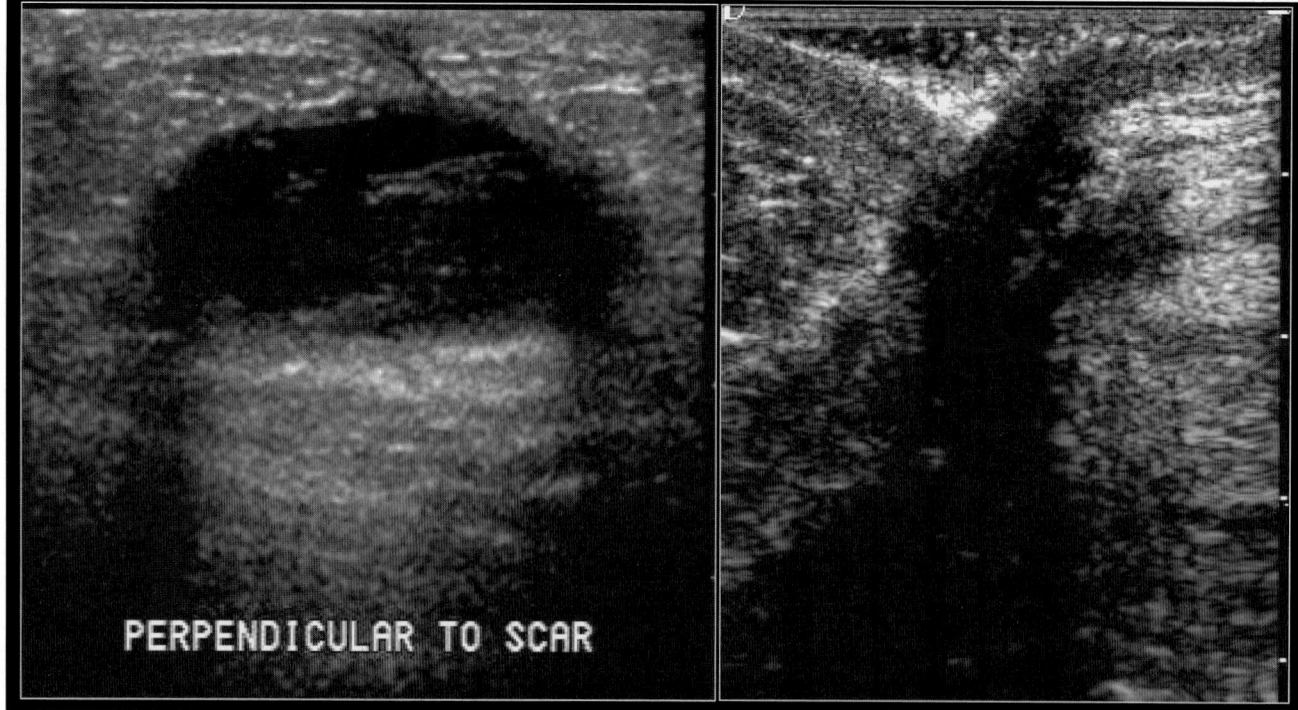

FIGURE 11–71 This figure illustrates the rationale for not primarily closing the lumpectomy cavity. When the volume of tissue removed at lumpectomy is large or when the underlying breast size is small, suturing the cavity closed is more likely to result in indentation of the overlying skin **(right)**. On the other hand, by not suturing the lumpectomy cavity closed and allowing serum or blood to accumulate within the cavity, the skin line is maintained **(left)**.

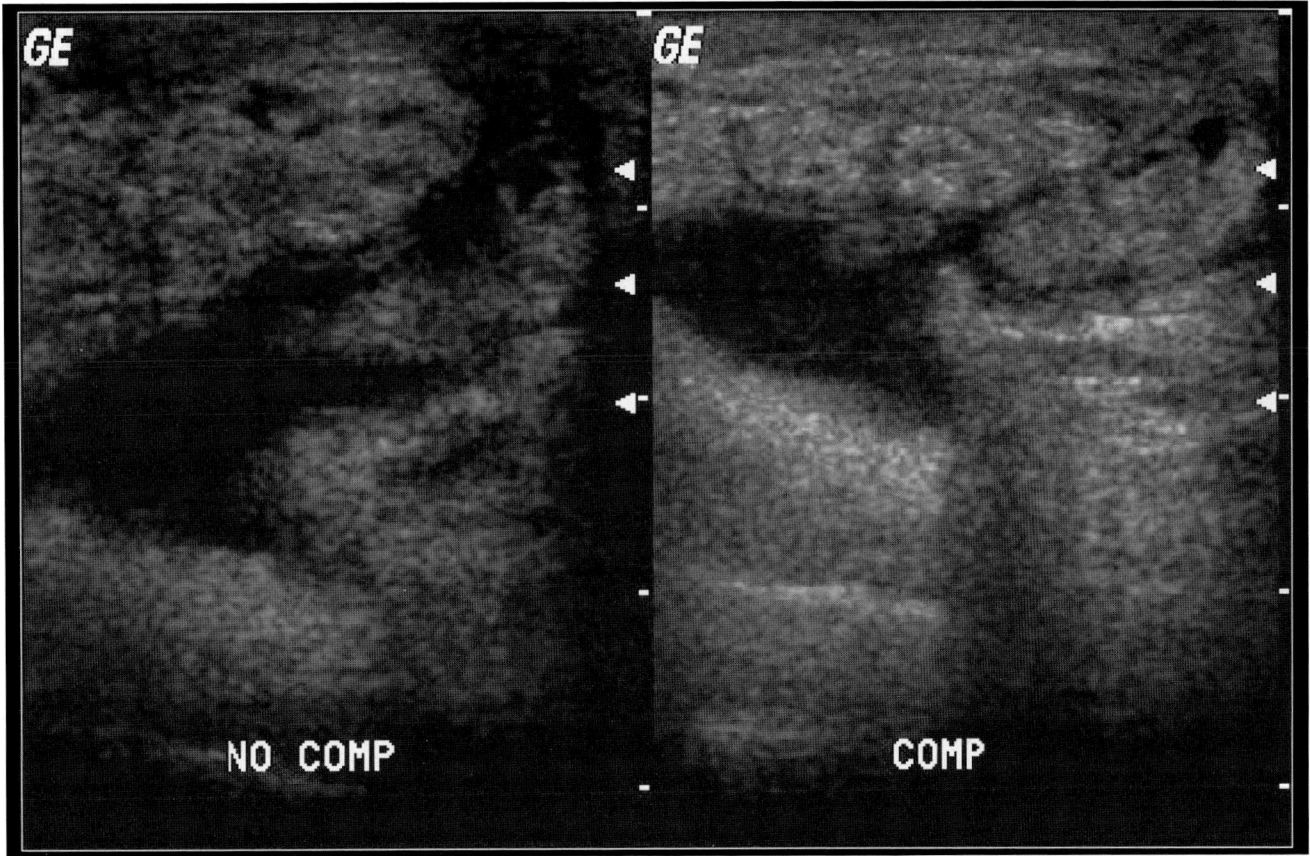

FIGURE 11–72 Many lumpectomy cavities are irregular or angular in shape. Thus, the seroma that forms within the cavity has angular margins that may raise concerns about recurrent malignancy. However, most angular seromas are not tense or under pressure (fluid collections that are tense or under pressure become rounded) and therefore are softer and more compressible than recurrent tumor. Split-screen images with and without compression can be reassuring in some cases. This angular seroma is very soft and highly compressible.

lumpectomy site (Fig. 11–71). Different methods of surgical management of the lumpectomy cavity are discussed and illustrated in more detail in Chapter 18.

Because lumpectomy cavities often have angular margins, the seromas that develop within such cavities may also have angular margins. Angular margins present difficulties in sonographically distinguishing between recurrent carcinoma and echogenic seroma. Color Doppler can be helpful in such cases because angular seromas have no demonstrable blood (Fig. 11–67) but angular recurrent neoplasms frequently do. As is always the case with Doppler, a positive finding, the presence of blood flow, is more valuable than a negative finding, absence of flow, because some recurrent tumors may not have enough blood flow to be demonstrable with color Doppler. Compressibility may also be used to distinguish between seroma and recurrent tumor. The seromas that have angular margins do so because they are not tense or under pressure. Thus, they are usually quite soft and compressible, which can be demonstrated with split-screen images obtained with and without compression (Fig.

11–72). Recurrent tumor, on the other hand, will be relatively incompressible.

As noted earlier, seromas can be beneficial under certain circumstances. Leaving the lumpectomy cavity open to accumulate serum can prevent skin deformity when excisional volume is large compared with the original presurgical volume of the breast (discussed earlier and in Chapter 18).

The serous effusion that forms between the periimplant fibrous capsule and implant shell represents a seroma that is generally desirable (Fig. 11–73). Periimplant effusion or seroma is thought to decrease the risk for capsular contracture and to enable the implant to move within the capsule, minimizing its chances of being compressed and ruptured with minor trauma. However, not all periimplant seromas are desirable. Some represent significant complications. Large postoperative seromas can be painful and deforming and also increase the risk for postoperative infection. Such periimplant seromas are more likely to demonstrate evidence of inflammation, such as capsular thickening, fibrinous adhesions, and hyperemia. Normal

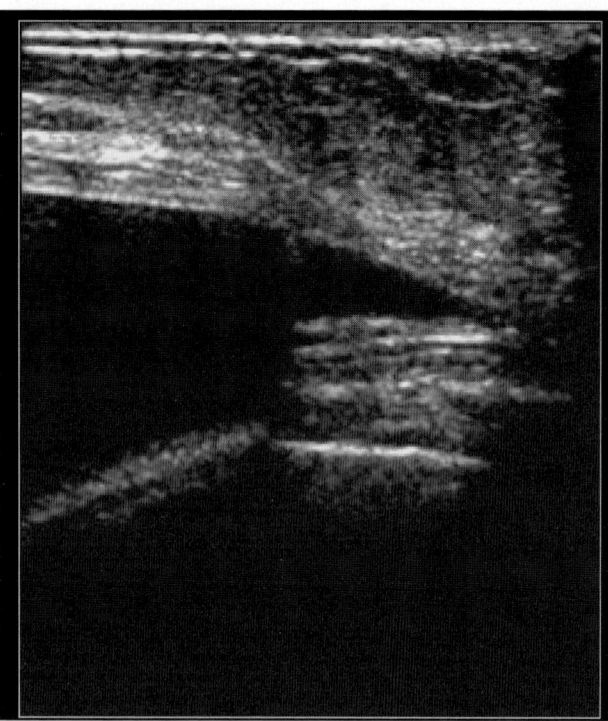

FIGURE 11–73 The periimplant effusion that develops around textured implants is essentially a seroma that is desirable and beneficial to the patient. The development of a normal, small periimplant seroma is thought to decrease the likelihood of capsular contracture and may protect the implant from traumatic rupture by allowing it to move away from compression pressure within the capsule. Normal periimplant effusions or seromas are anechoic, distributed around the periphery of the implant, and not loculated anteriorly, and they contain no fibrinous adhesions.

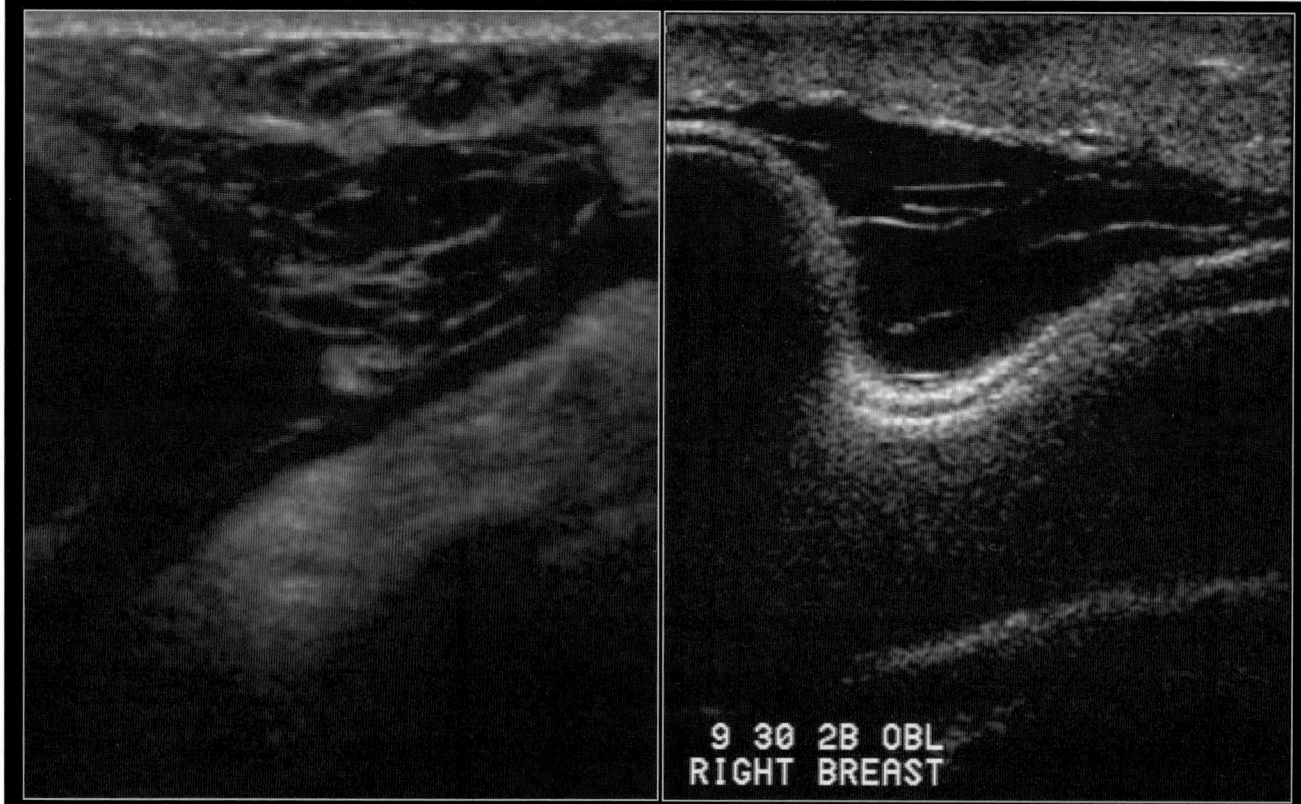

FIGURE 11–74 Large, undesired periimplant seromas with an exudative component that forms fibrinous adhesions are most likely to occur in patients who are undergoing mastectomy and immediate reconstruction. This is even more likely in patients who are also undergoing axillary dissection. These usually distribute around the periphery of the implant (**left**). Loculated effusions (seromas) along the anterior aspects of the implant do not normally occur and suggest a pathologic fluid collection (**right**).

periimplant effusions are usually distributed around the periphery of the implant, so that loculation of periimplant effusion along the anterior aspect of the implant shell also suggests the presence of a clinically significant seroma (Fig. 11–74). Occasionally, periimplant effusions can become infected years after implantation (see Chapter 20, Fig. 20–60).

A seroma may accumulate within the residual periimplant capsule after explantation without capsulectomy or reimplantation. If the fluid collection is not tense, tender, or infected, the patient is often happy with the seroma because it adds to postexplantation breast size (Fig. 11–75). However, in some patients, too much serous fluid may accumulate within the capsule, causing pain and tenderness

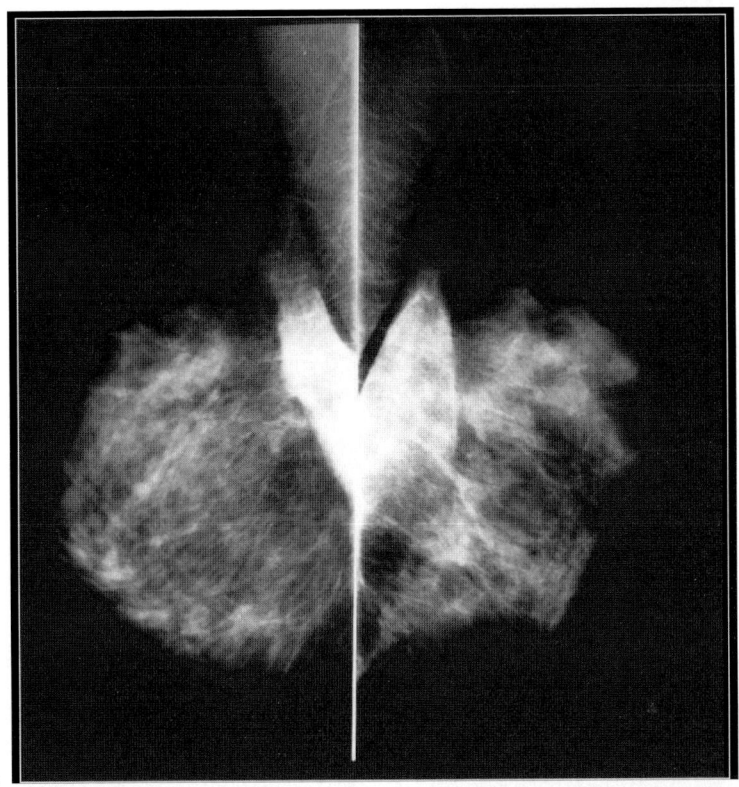

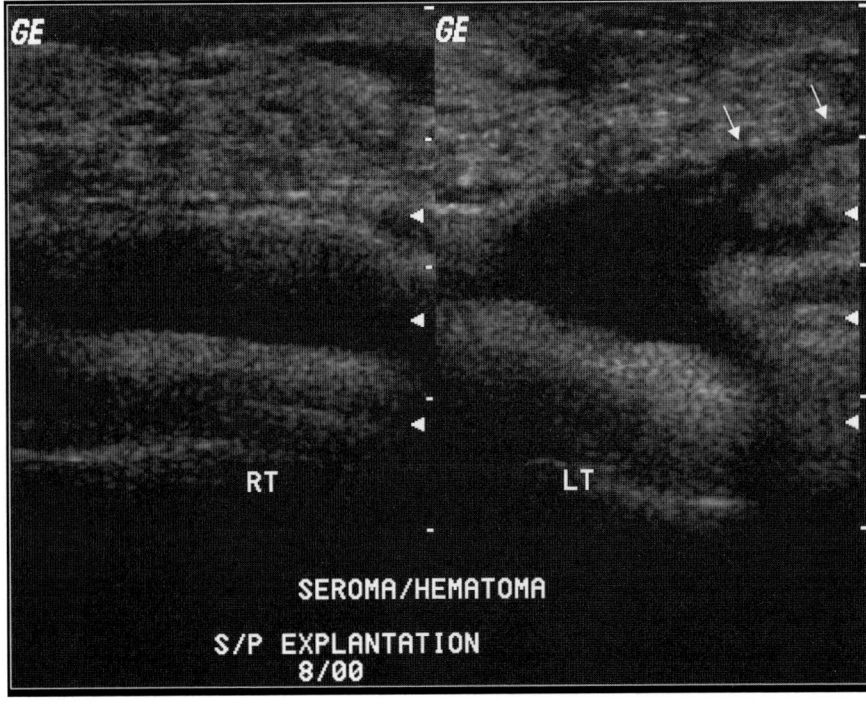

FIGURE 11–75 A: In patients who undergo explantation without capsulectomy, seromas may form within the residual periimplant fibrous capsule. As long as these seromas are relatively symmetric in size, not tense and tender, and not infected, they may be desirable to the patient. Postexplantation seromas may help maintain breast size. **B:** The patient was very happy that these seromas developed within the residual capsule after explantation because her breasts decreased in size less than she had expected them to decrease. The seromas were not tender and were roughly symmetric in size. Unfortunately, the left seroma communicated with the infraareolar scar on the left *(arrows)*, causing skin retraction.

(Fig. 11–76). Such seromas usually cannot be managed adequately with serial aspirations and must be managed by surgical capsulectomy.

Finally, the seromas that develop within mammotomy cavities may be beneficial if the biopsy reveals malignancy and if all imaging evidence of the lesion was removed at the time of mammotomy. Such patients will require needle localization lumpectomy. The seroma within the mammotomy cavity enables the mammotomy site to be localized with ultrasound rather than mammography. The seromas that fill the mammotomy cavity are frequently markedly elongated in an axis parallel to the needle tract in patients who underwent stereotactic biopsy because the tissues were compressed in an axis parallel to the needle during biopsy.

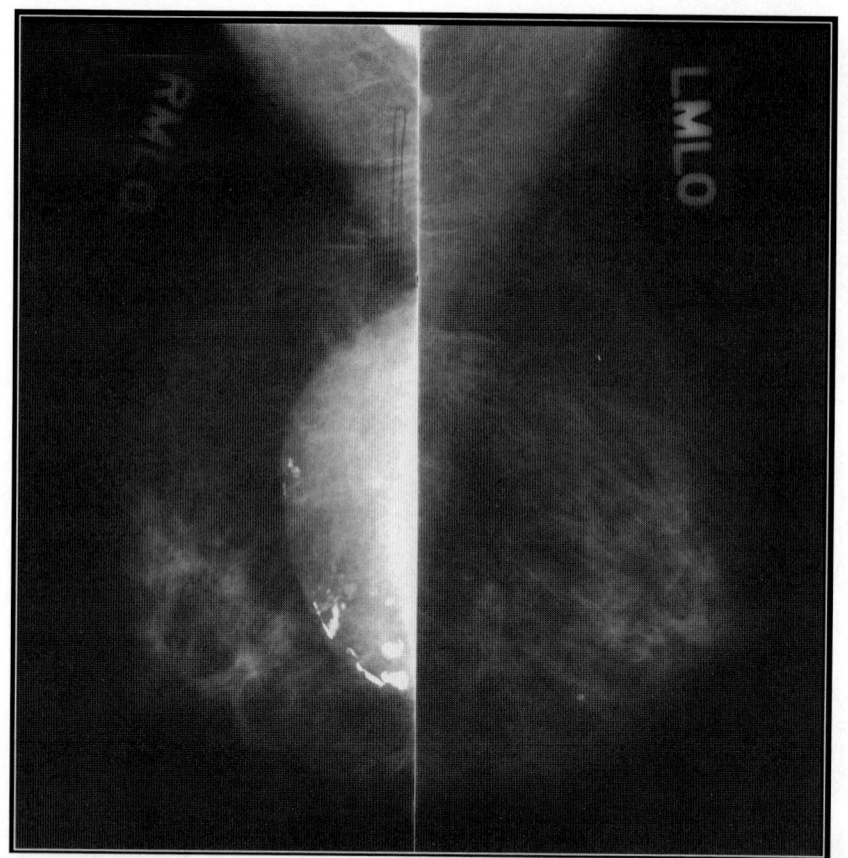

A

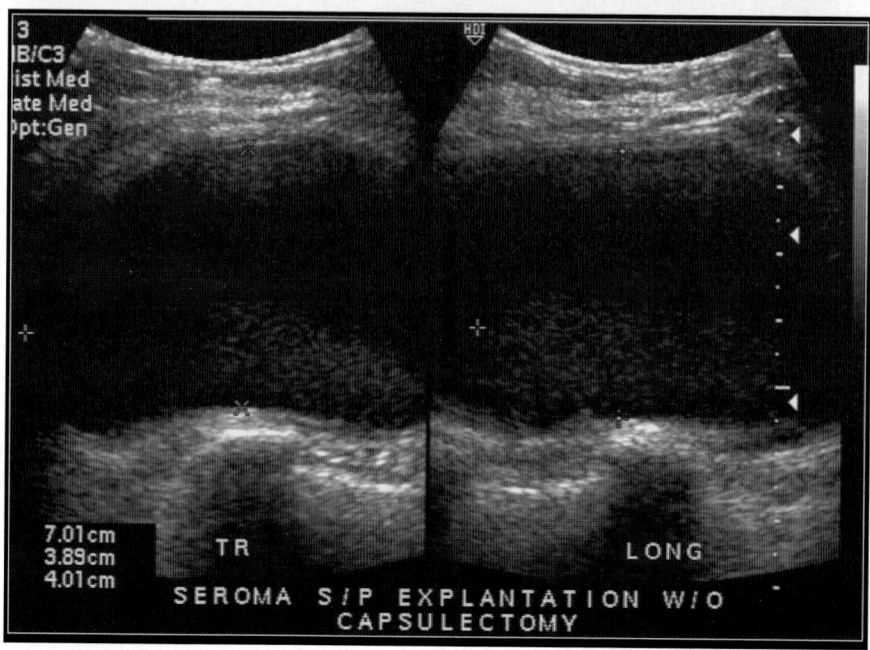

B

FIGURE 11–76 A: Although postexplantation seromas are generally viewed favorably by the patient, they can be very undesirable if they are markedly asymmetric, tender, painful, or secondarily infected. This patient developed a very tense and painful postexplantation seroma on the right, but not on the left. Explantation was performed because of intracapsular rupture bilaterally, but the patient also had severe capsular contracture on the right. The surgeon had planned to perform capsulectomy in addition to explantation. Unfortunately, the patient was being anticoagulated because of massive pulmonary embolus and it was deemed unsafe to discontinue anticoagulation. Severe bleeding problems were encountered during attempted capsulectomy on the right; thus, only explantation was accomplished. Attempts at capsulectomy were abandoned. The mammograms showed a large right postexplantation seroma that simulates a residual implant. The residual capsule on the right is heavily calcified. **B:** The postexplantation seroma on the right was so large that a 5-MHz curved linear probe was necessary to evaluate it adequately. The seroma contained a fluid—debris level that could not be appreciated with the 12-MHz linear transducer. At aspiration, the debris was old blood that presumably had accumulated at the time of the first attempted capsulectomy.

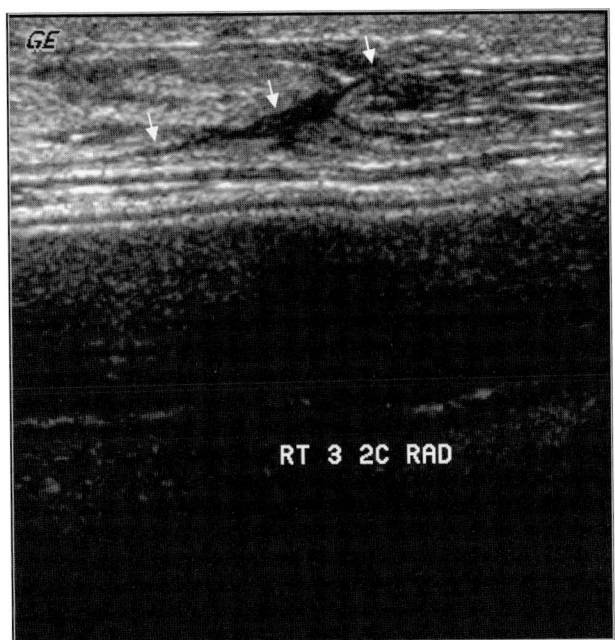

FIGURE 11–77 The seroma that develops within a mammotomy cavity and persists for 2 to 6 weeks is a minor complication that is desirable if the biopsy reveals malignancy that must be localized for lumpectomy a few days to a few weeks later. The seroma that results from stereotactic biopsy tends to be very elongated along the needle tract because the breast was compressed in that axis during the biopsy. The cavity that develops during stereotactically guided mammotomy is spherical or mildly oval while the breast is in compression but becomes markedly elongated after compression is released *(arrows).*

After stereotactic biopsy, when mammographic compression is released, the cavity elongates along the axis that was compressed during biopsy (Fig. 11–77). Mammotomy cavities created under ultrasound guidance, on the other hand, tend to be nearly spherical or only mildly elliptical in shape (Fig. 11–78). As noted earlier, the seroma is a useful target for ultrasound-guided needle localizations. If residual solid nodule can be identified along the edges of the mammotomy cavity seroma, the nodule is localized directly (Fig. 11–79). However, if there is a seroma within the mammotomy cavity and there is no visible residual lesion along the edges of the cavity, the center of the cavity rather than the mammotomy clip should be localized (Fig. 11–80). Localization of the nodule should be reserved for cases in which localization mammotomy clip must be performed under mammographic guidance because the seroma has been completely resorbed. Ultrasound-guided needle localization of the mammotomy seroma is much easier and more accurate than is mammographically guided localization of the mammotomy clip in virtually all cases in which a seroma is still present in the mammotomy site. The mammotomy marker is clipped to one of the walls of the mammotomy cavity and thus is deployed eccentrically and is not deployed within the center of the cavity. If there is residual disease along the edges of the mammotomy cavity (80% of the time there is residual disease after mammotomy), the residual tumor is equally likely to be on the wall of the cavity opposite from the clip as it is to be on the

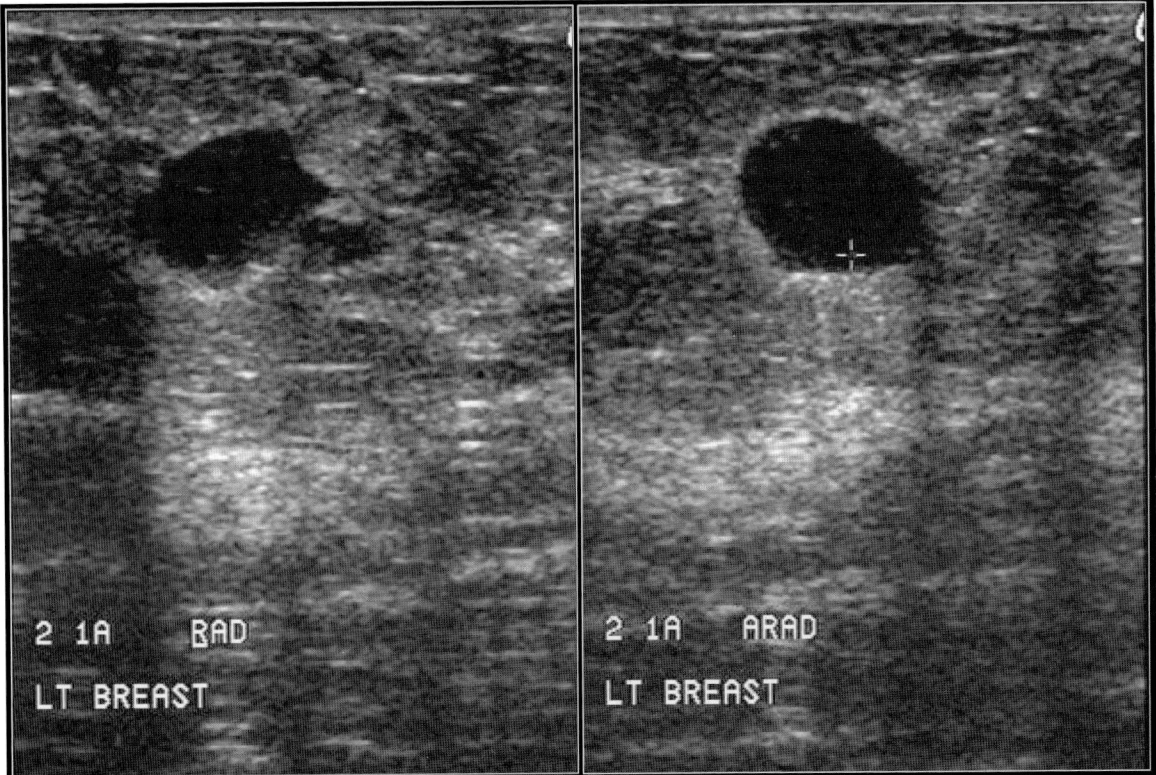

FIGURE 11–78 The cavity that develops after ultrasound-guided mammotomy is more likely to be spherical or mildly elliptical in shape and is not as elongated along the axis of the needle as is the cavity that results from stereotactically guided biopsy.

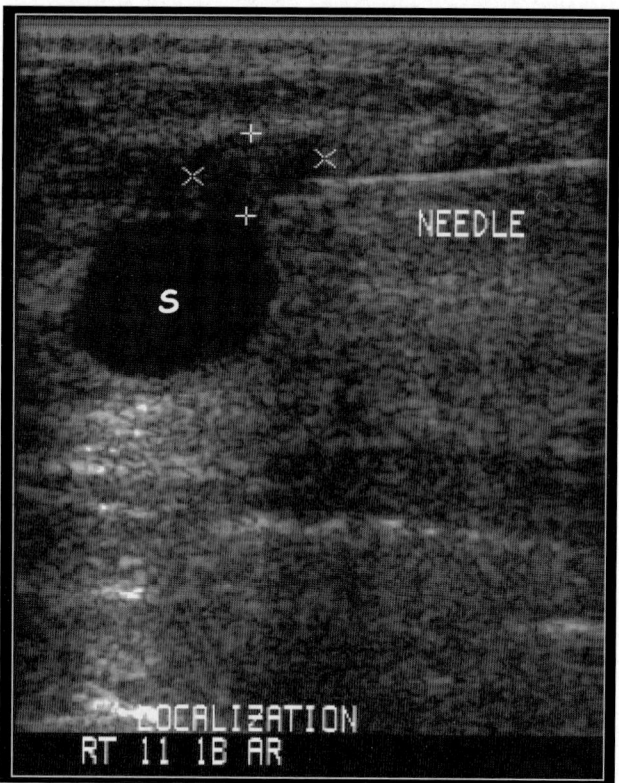

FIGURE 11–79 If there is sonographic evidence of residual tumor *(calipers)*, the residual disease, rather than the seroma within the mammotomy cavity *(S)*, should be localized.

same wall as the clip. In some cases, localizing the mammotomy clip mammographically could result in the localization wire being farther away from the residual disease than if the mammotomy cavity is localized under ultrasound guidance. This is illustrated and explained in Fig. 11–81. (Newer DVAB localizing pledgets can be deployed within the center of the mammotomy cavity and are preferable to the old clips.)

LYMPHOCELES

Lymphoceles are localized collections of lymphatic fluid. They occur in patients who have had lumpectomy or mastectomy with axillary node dissection for treatment of breast cancer. The axillary dissection disrupts lymphatics, causing leakage of lymph and blocking drainage of lymph and serum that accumulates in the surgical wound. Lymphoceles in breast cancer patients are almost always in the axillary area. Many surgeons do not distinguish between lymphoceles and seromas, considering them to be similar complications of surgery.

Mammographic Findings

Because of their location in the axilla and because they most frequently occur in patients who have had mastectomy as well as axillary dissection, lymphoceles may be too

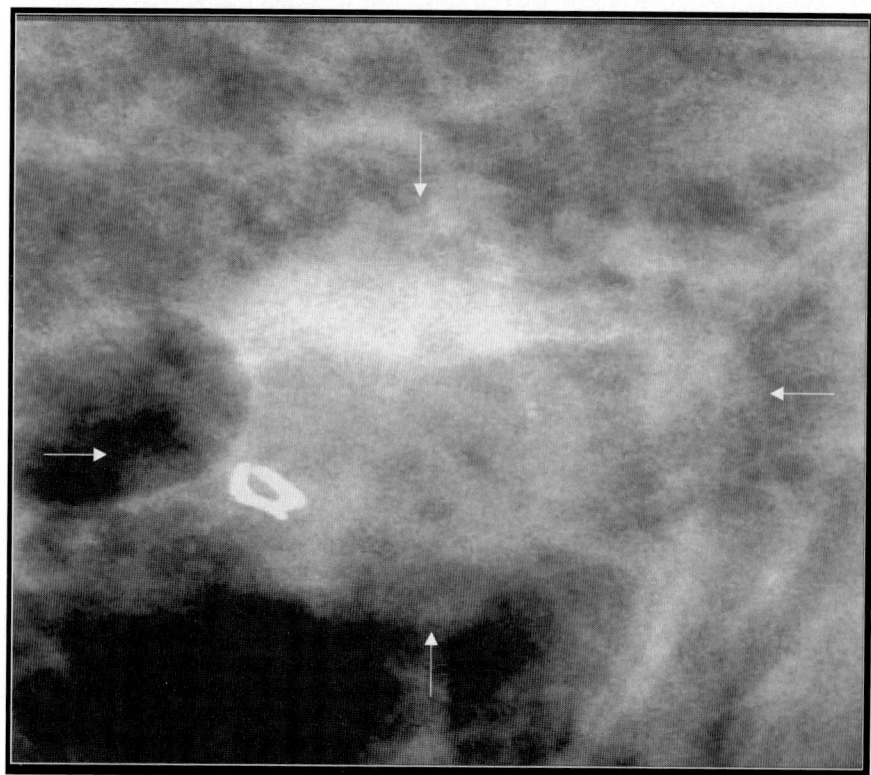

A

FIGURE 11–80 A: The mammotomy clip is deployed in one of the walls of the mammotomy cavity *(arrows)*, not in the center of the cavity. The oval mammotomy cavity is filled with serum, and the clip lies along the inferior left edge of the seroma in about the 8:00 position. *(Continued.)*

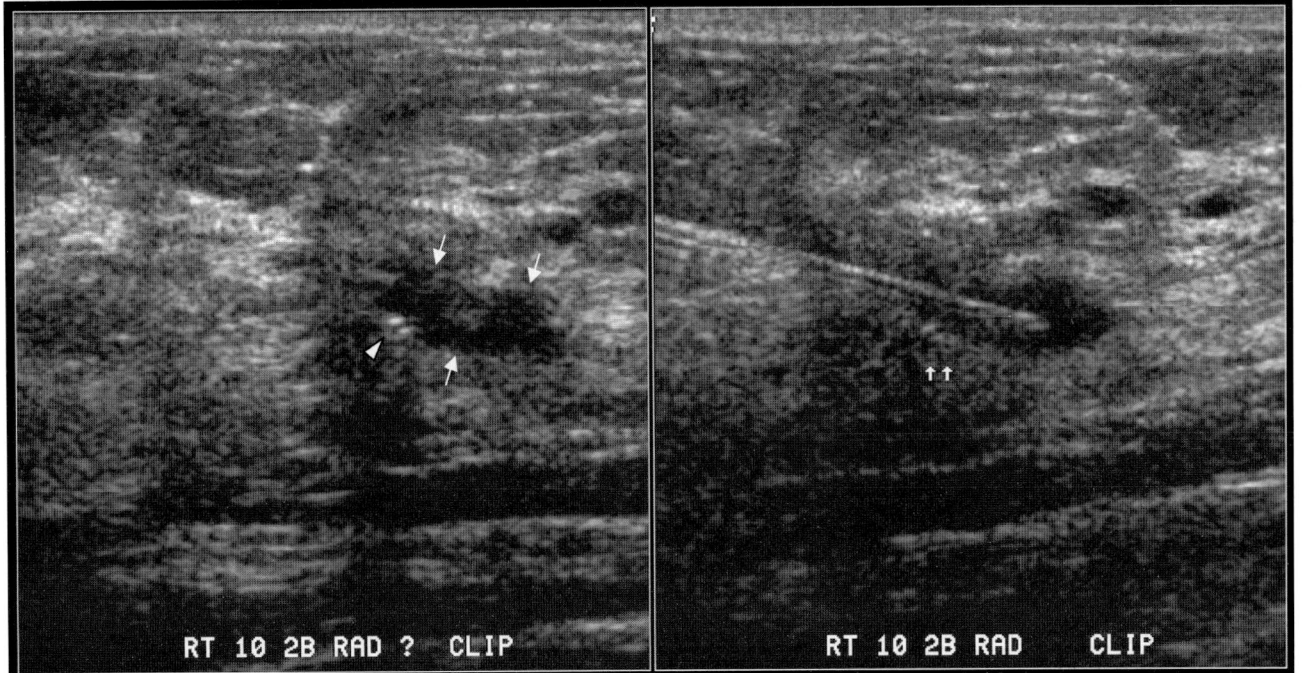

B

FIGURE 11–80 *(continued)* **B:** The seroma within the oval mammotomy cavity is readily demonstrable. In this view (**left**), the mammotomy clip (**left,** *arrowhead*) can be seen along the inferior left edge of the seroma (**left,** *arrows*), not within the center of the seroma. The ultrasound-guided needle placement is to the center of the seroma (**right**), not to the mammotomy clip (**right,** *arrows*).

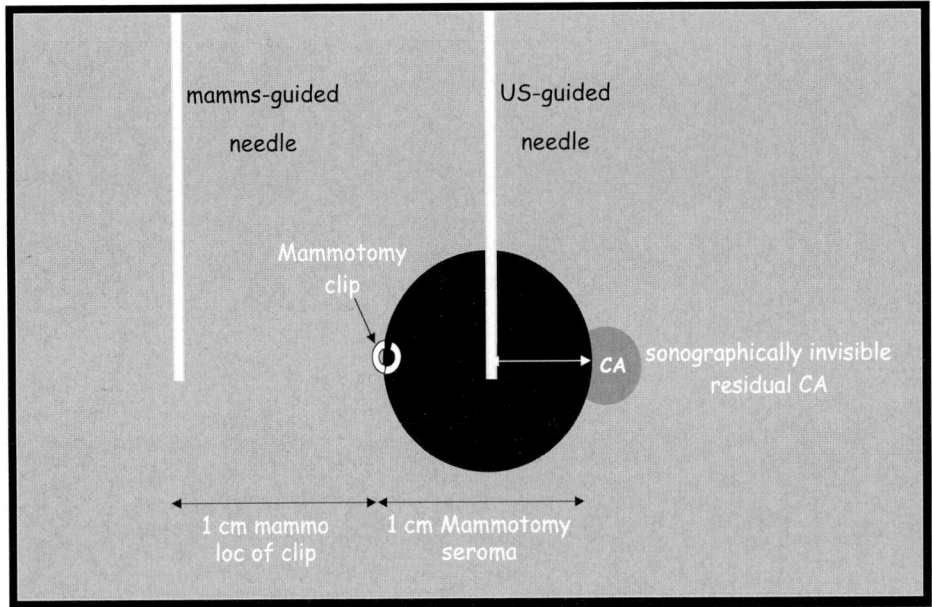

FIGURE 11–81 The theoretical advantage to localizing the center of the seroma within the mammotomy cavity rather than the mammotomy clip is shown in this illustration. If the seroma within the mammotomy cavity is 1 cm in diameter, if there is a small focus of residual carcinoma along one wall of the seroma, and if the center of the cavity is localized under ultrasound guidance, the farthest from the residual disease that the needle can be is 0.5 cm. The mammotomy clip may be on any wall of the lesion. In at least one-fourth of cases, the clip is on the opposite wall of the seroma from the residual disease. If ultrasound-guided localization of the mammotomy clip is performed, the needle will be 1 cm from the residual disease in about one-fourth of cases. If a mammographic localization of the mammotomy clip is performed and a needle position plus or minus 1 cm from the clip is accepted, the tip of the needle might be as far as 2 cm from the residual disease. Thus, not only is sonographic localization of the seroma within the mammotomy cavity much quicker and technically easier than the mammographic localization of the clip, but in a significant minority of cases, it will more accurately localize the residual disease.

high in the axilla to image mammographically. When seen, they are identical to seromas in their mammographic appearances.

Sonographic Findings

Pure lymphoceles are similar to seromas that have a simple cystic appearance. They do not have fibrinous adhesions, thickened or nodular walls, or septations and are usually anechoic or have only minimal low-level echogenicity. Lymphoceles that are mixtures of lymph and serum have the sonographic features of complex seromas—diffuse low-level internal echogenicity, thick walls, mural nodules, fibrinous adhesions, and internal septations—and should be considered seromas rather than lymphoceles (Fig. 11–82).

HEMATOMAS

General Pathologic Classification, Epidemiology, and Clinical Findings

A hematoma is a localized collection of extravasated blood within the breast. The collection may be liquid, clotted, or a mixture. The appearance, like all other cystic structures discussed in this chapter, evolves as the hematoma ages.

Hematomas usually follow a traumatic event or an interventional procedure such as cyst aspiration, needle biopsy, or excisional biopsy. However, occasionally there is spontaneous hemorrhage into a preexisting cyst. This most commonly occurs in acutely inflamed cysts, but whether the inflammation is the cause or a result of the hemorrhage cannot always be determined. When a spontaneous hemorrhage not associated with a breast cyst occurs, an underlying degenerating neoplasm should be suspended unless the patient is being anticoagulated. Warfarin sodium (Coumadin) may precipitate breast necrosis and secondary hematoma formation in some patients. A hematoma may gradually be completely resorbed and disappear or may be only partially resorbed and persist as chronic hematoma. An incompletely resorbed chronic hematoma may evolve into fat necrosis and a classic lipid cyst, but may remain water density and may have an appearance indistinguishable from a chronic seroma.

Mammographic Appearance

The mammographic appearance of an acute hematoma varies but most typically is that of a mixed fat and water-density mass (Fig. 11–83). Galactoceles, intramammary lymph nodes, and hamartomas may also have mixed fat

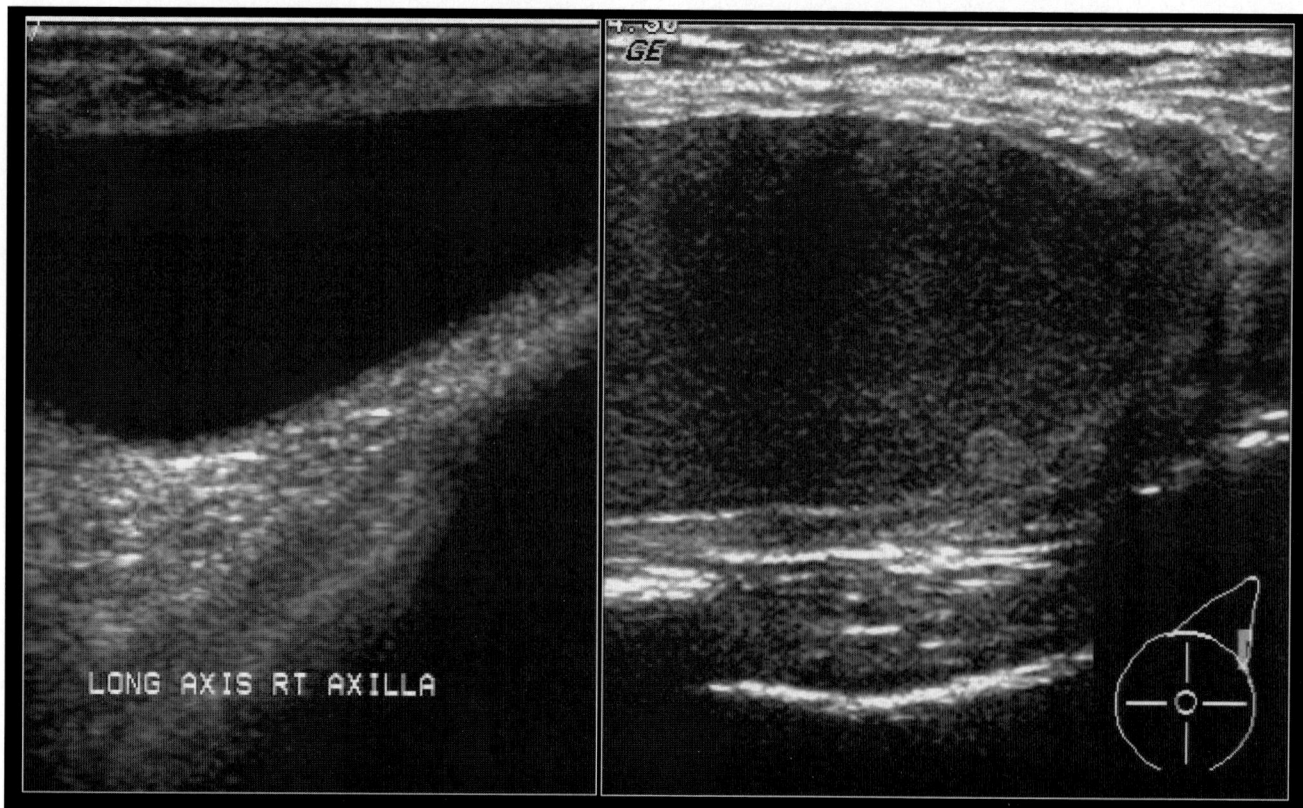

FIGURE 11–82 Lymphoceles that are composed of pure lymphatic fluid appear to be simple cysts **(left)**. Lymphoceles that are mixtures of blood or serum and lymph have sonographic features that reflect the blood or serous fluid components. Lymphoceles occur after axillary dissection.

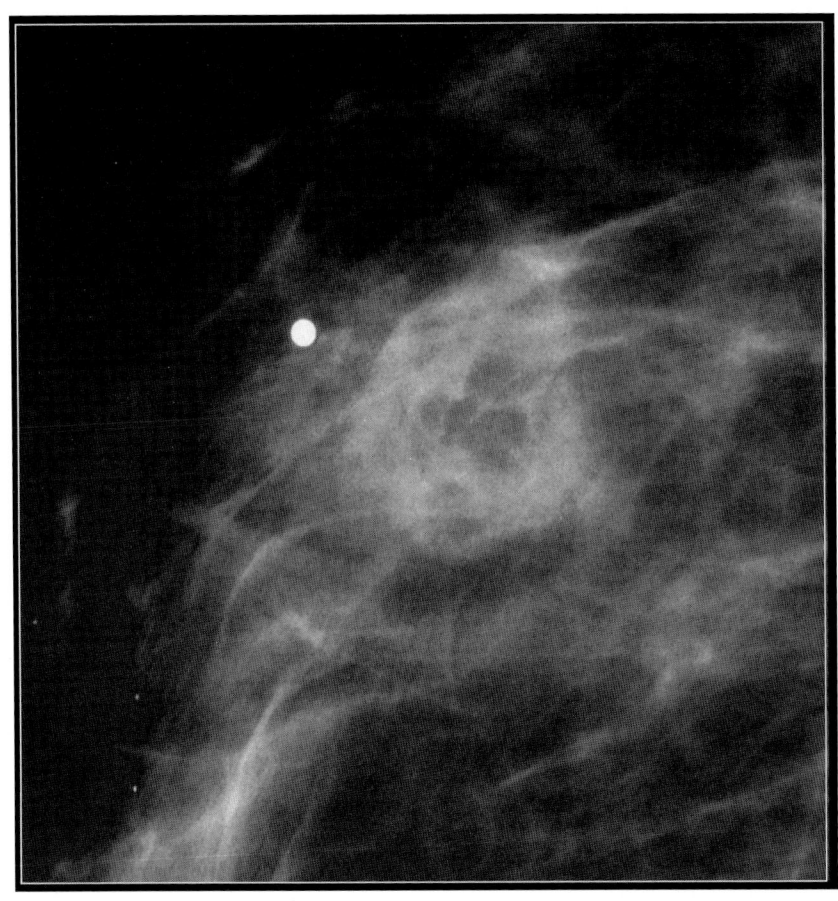

FIGURE 11–83 Most hematomas appear to be mixed water and fat density on mammography. Very large hematomas, particular those that accumulated within surgical cavities, may be nonspecific and pure water density.

and water density but usually do not have a history of trauma or surgery.

Sonographic Appearance

Hyperacute hematomas may be completely anechoic but do not remain that way for very long (Fig. 11–84). Acute hematomas are markedly *hypoechoic*, with very-low-level, but generally heterogeneous, internal echotexture, that reflects the interfaces between clots and fibrin strands (Fig. 11–85). However, as the clotting process begins, the blood within the hematoma may become diffusely hyperechoic (Fig. 11–86). The hyperechoic components of blood may also layer into an echogenic debris level (Fig. 11–87). On the other hand, subacute hematomas usually appear as irregularly marginated complex cystic masses with thickened *hyperechoic* walls, mural nodules, or irregularly thickened but avascular internal septations (Fig. 11–88). A chronic hematoma may vary greatly in echotexture. Chronic hematomas or the lipid cysts into which they evolve may be anechoic, markedly hypoechoic with diffuse homogeneous low-level internal echoes, anechoic or hypoechoic with a subtle fluid–debris level, or diffusely mildly echogenic. Most chronic hematomas are hypoechoic with internal

septations and mildly thick and irregular walls. In fact, it is actually quite difficult to classify the age of hematomas because many contain a mixture of reliquefied blood and residual clots of varying ages within the same lesion (Fig. 11–89). Regardless of the internal echotexture, chronic hematomas demonstrate enhanced through-transmission of sound unless the hematoma wall calcifies (as the hematoma evolves into fat necrosis). As the wall surrounding the lipid cyst calcifies, sound transmission diminishes, and the wall becomes brighter (more reflective). Ultimately, calcification becomes dense and thick enough to result in complete or partial acoustic shadowing (Fig. 11–90). Chronic organizing hematomas occasionally appear solid rather than cystic (Fig. 11–91). Other chronic hematomas evolve into lipid cysts, and the echogenic lipid contents make them appear hyperechoic and solid (Fig. 11–92). Spot compression mammograms are often more definitive than sonography in such cases. In acute and subacute phases of hematoma evolution, the migration of blood breakdown products into surrounding breast tissues irritates them and causes edema that is sonographically visible and ecchymosis that is visually apparent in the overlying skin (Fig. 11–93). The edema of the fat surrounding a hematoma causes the fat to become hyperechoic and the distribution of edematous

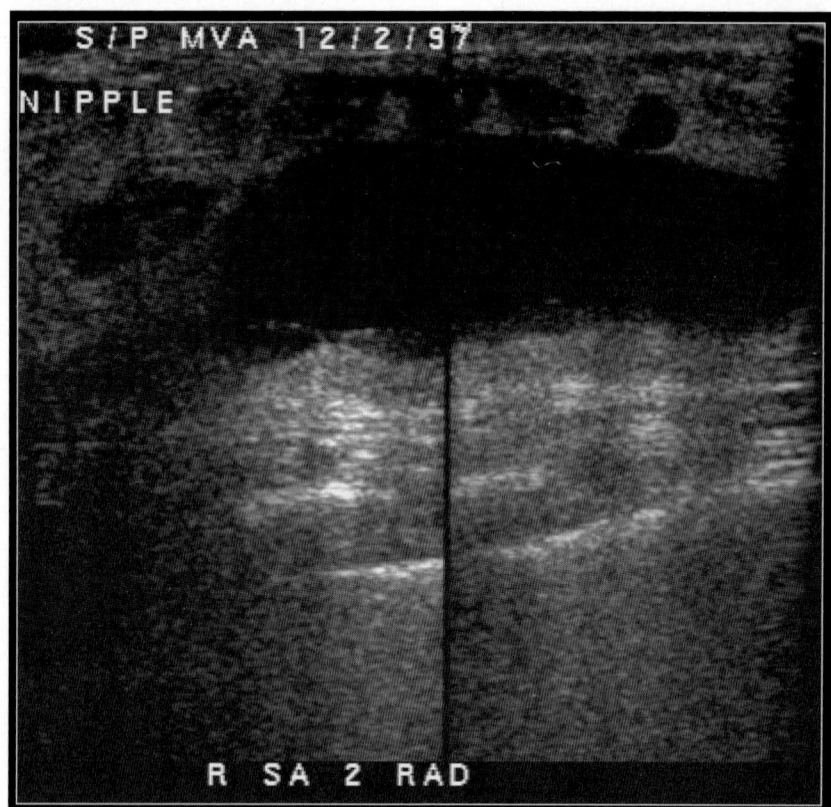

FIGURE 11–84 Hyperacute hematomas may be nearly anechoic. However, as soon as clotting begins, they become heterogeneous.

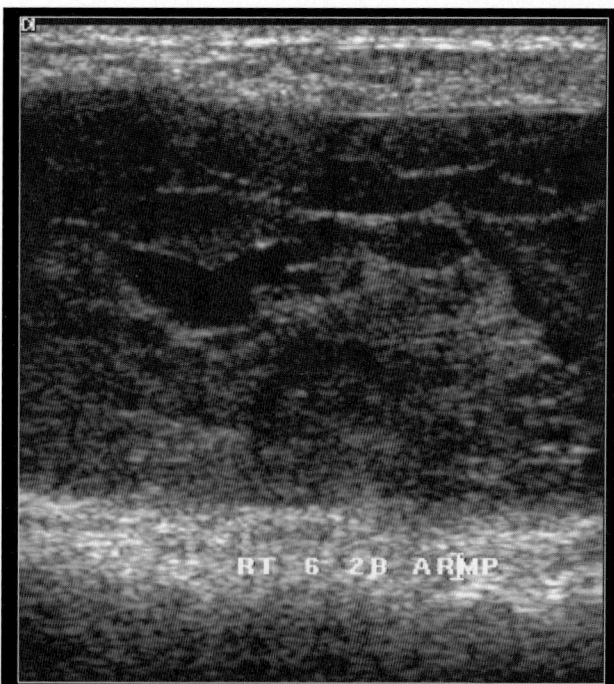

FIGURE 11–85 Acute hematomas are hypoechoic and heterogeneous. Areas of increased echogenicity represent older clots. Linear echoes represent fibrinous stands or interfaces between liquid blood and clots or between different clots.

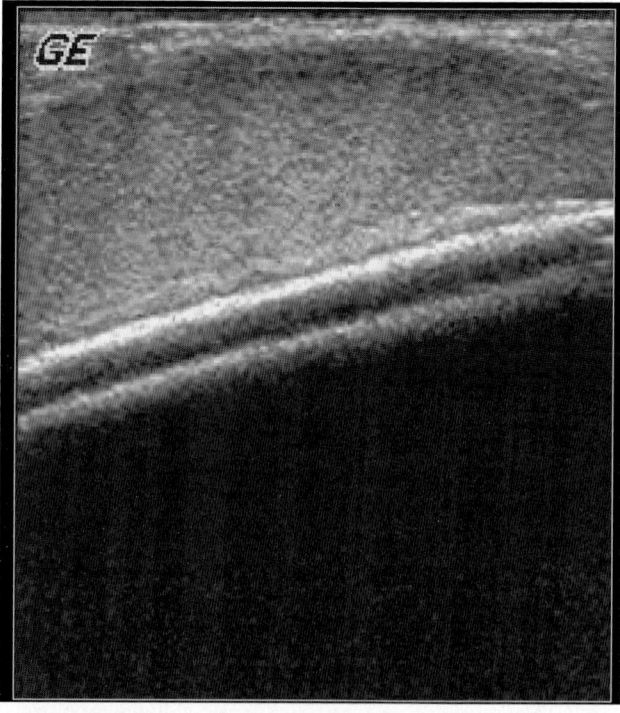

FIGURE 11–86 An acute hematoma may be purely hyperechoic as blood starts to clot diffusely.

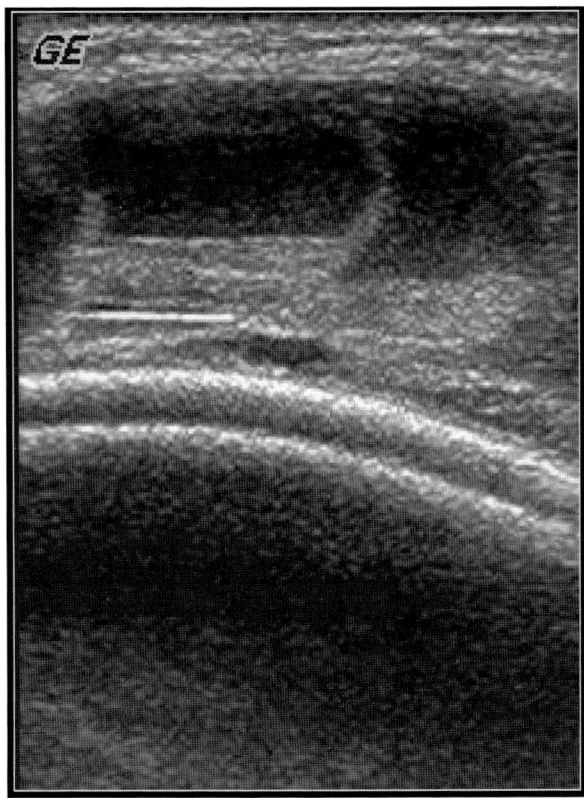

FIGURE 11–87 Acute hematomas may layer into fluid—debris levels, with serum rising to the nondependent portion of the hematoma, and clotted platelets and red blood cells falling to the dependent portion of the hematoma.

and hyperechoic fat parallels the distribution of overlying visible skin ecchymosis. In milder cases of acute trauma, when there is ecchymosis but no hematoma formation, only edema of the tissues may be apparent sonographically (Fig. 11–94).

Subacute and chronic hematomas that have thick internal septations or mural nodules can be difficult to distinguish from intracystic papilloma or carcinoma. However, there are a few subtle differences that can help distinguish hematoma from intracystic neoplasm.

First, color or power Doppler may be helpful. Papillomas and intracystic papillary malignancies have a true fibrovascular stalk. If color Doppler or power Doppler demonstrates blood flow within a thickened intracystic septation or mural nodule, it indicates that there is a fibrovascular stalk and that the complex cyst contains a true papillary neoplasm. On the other hand, an adherent clot within an acute and subacute hematoma that manifests itself as a thick internal septation or mural nodule does not have an internal blood supply. Therefore, color or power Doppler will not show internal vascularity within the thick septations or mural nodules within hematomas (see Chapter 20, Fig. 20–30). (Chronic organizing hematomas, on the other hand, may have some internal vascularity.) However, remember that whereas the presence Doppler documented flow within the solid parts of a complex cyst indicates the presence of a papillary neoplasm and rules out an acute or subacute hematoma, the lack of demonstrable flow is much less helpful. Both benign and malignant in-

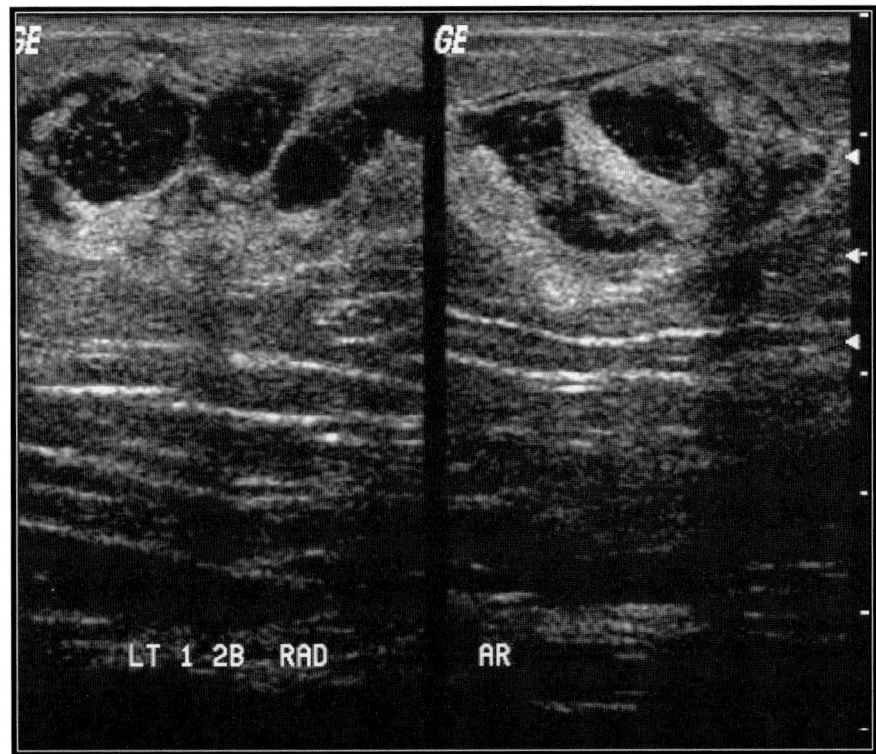

FIGURE 11–88 Subacute hematomas develop thick, echogenic walls and internal septations that are avascular on color Doppler. The echogenic part of the hematoma represents older clot, whereas the markedly hypoechoic areas represent either more acute clot or liquified clot.

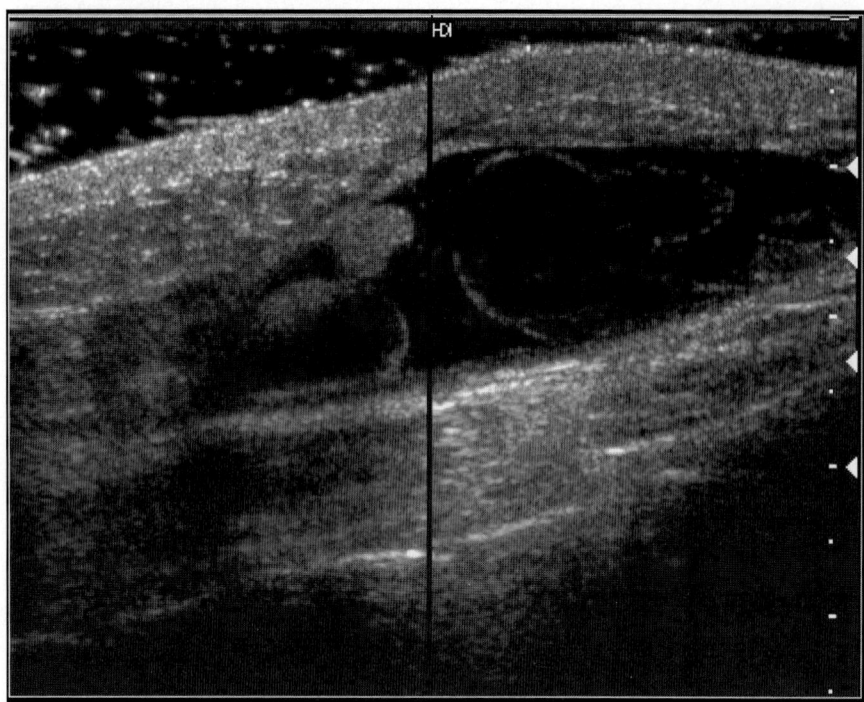

FIGURE 11–89 In most cases, it is difficult to assign a precise age to a clot because the bleeding and clotting occur over a period of time, resulting in a very heterogeneous mass with liquid and clotted components of various ages.

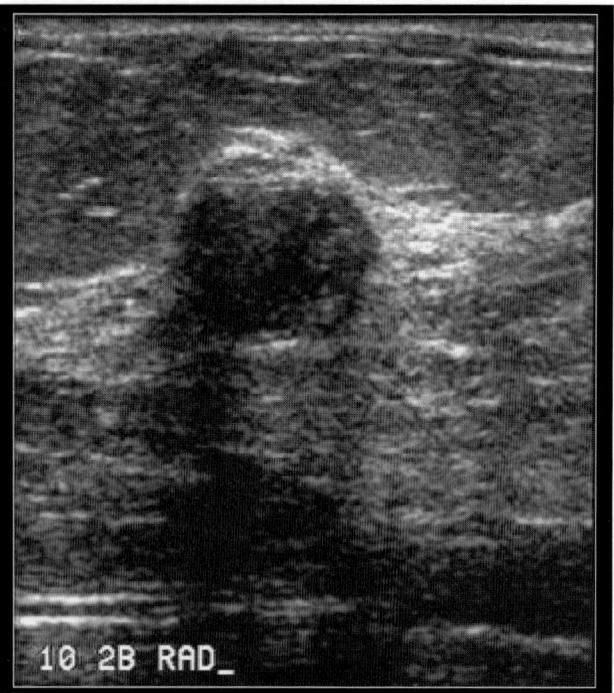

FIGURE 11–90 Chronic hematomas that have evolved to lipid cysts may develop dense enough calcification within their walls to cause acoustic shadowing.

tracystic papillary lesions may undergo hemorrhagic infarction and therefore may not have enough flow to be detectable with current Doppler equipment (see Chapter 20, Figs. 20–31 and 20–32).

Second, blood may layer in the dependent portion of the cyst, creating a sonographically demonstrable fluid–debris layer. The fluid–debris level may change with repositioning of the patient from supine to the right or left lateral decubitus or upright positions (Fig. 11–95). Intracystic neoplasms, benign and malignant, are firmly attached to the cyst wall and will not shift with changes in patient position. However, intracystic papillary neoplasms can be associated with bleeding that layers in the dependent portion of the cyst and obscures the underlying mural nodule (Fig. 11–96A). Therefore, the dependent wall of the cyst, which may be obscured by layered debris when the patient is in a supine position, should be evaluated when the debris is shifted to a different part of the cystic lesion by placing the patient in either the upright or left lateral decubitus position (Fig. 11–96B). Interpretation of findings can be further complicated by clot within an acute hematoma that adheres to the hematoma wall and therefore, like an intracystic neoplasm, does not shift when the patient position is changed. In such cases, color or power Doppler may be the only method of distinguishing between hematoma with adherent clot and intracystic neoplasm (Fig. 11–97).

(text continued on page 415)

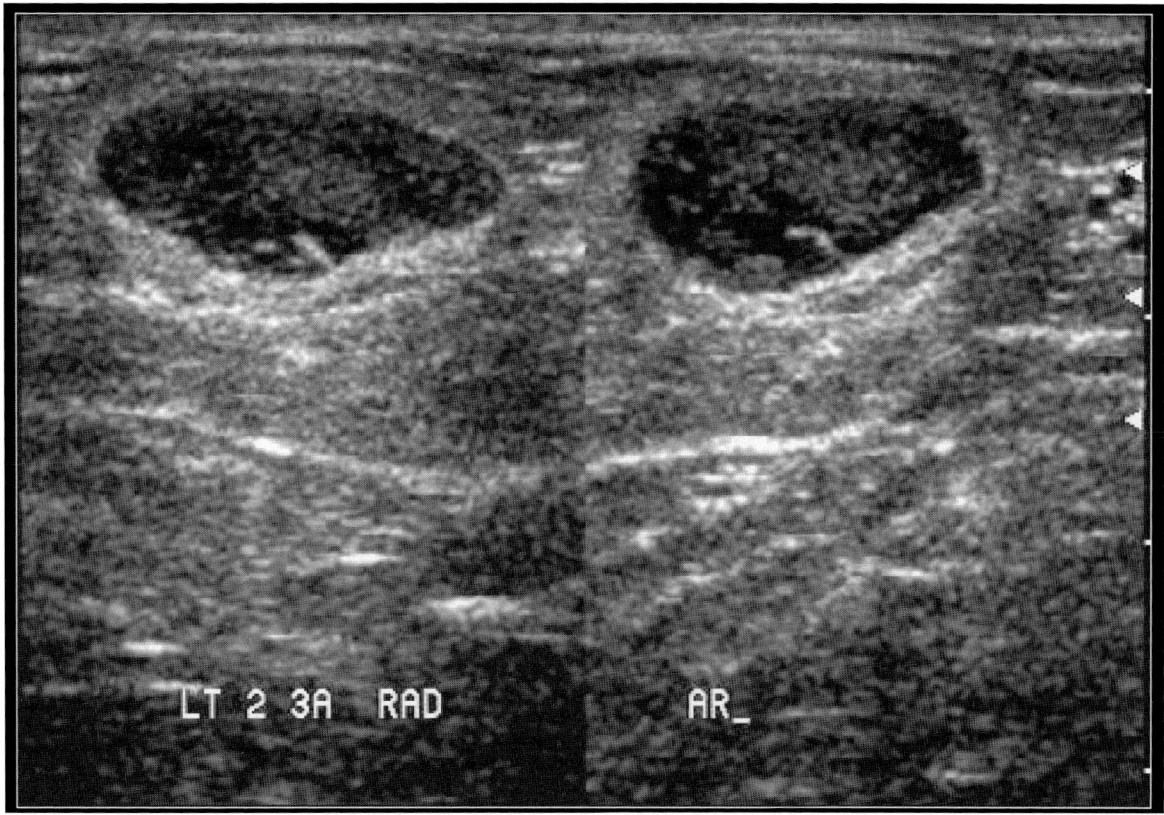

FIGURE 11–91 Chronic hematomas that organize may appear to be solid at sonography.

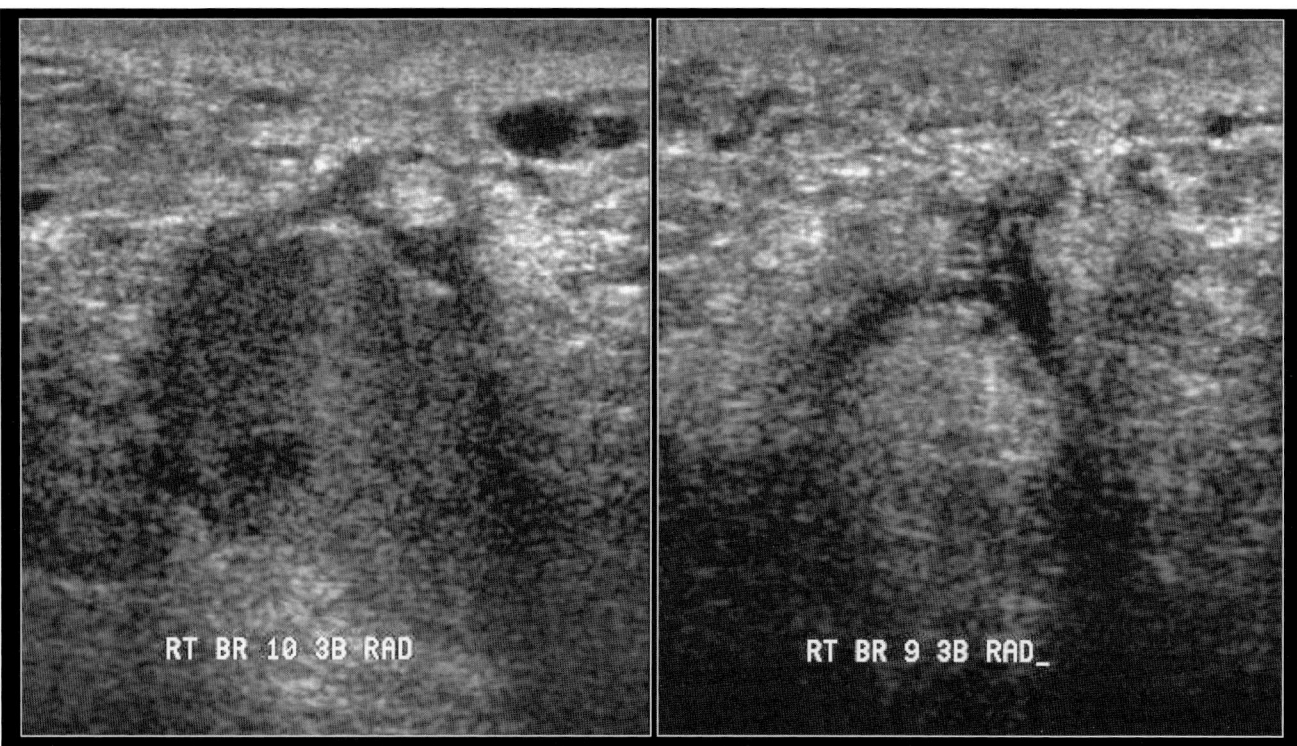

FIGURE 11–92 Some chronic hematomas that have evolved into lipid cysts become echogenic and have a solid appearance because the lipids they contain are echogenic. The echogenicity of lipid cysts is highly variable and can range from nearly anechoic to hyperechoic. This patient had a large hematoma caused by trauma more than a year earlier. The hematoma had evolved into a lipid cyst. The patient had two lipid cysts with echogenic contents. One was isoechoic (**left**), and the other contained hyperechoic lipid contents (**right**).

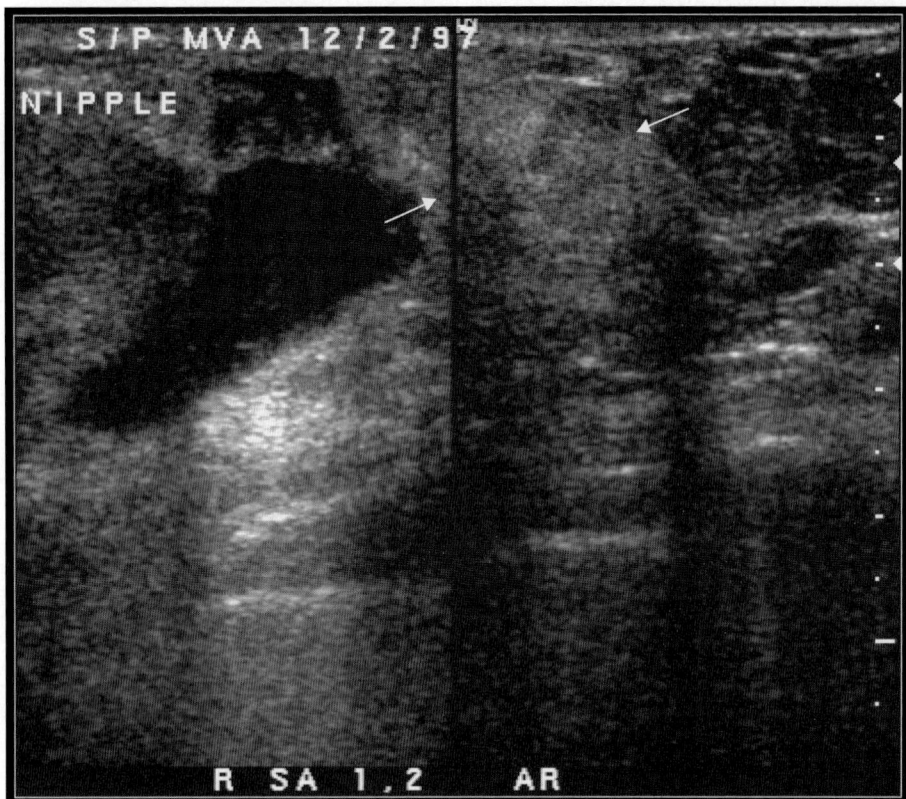

FIGURE 11–93 Edematous, hyperechoic tissues may surround hematomas of any age *(arrows)*. Acute hematomas are often surrounded by ecchymosis, whereas blood breakdown products cause a localized mastitis in the tissues surrounding subacute and chronic hematomas.

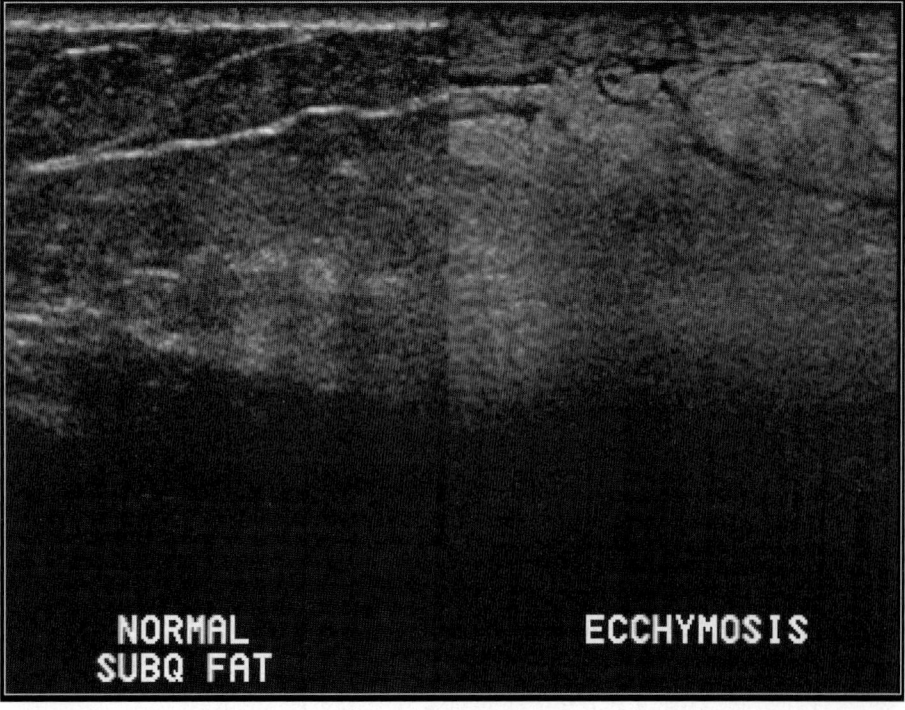

FIGURE 11–94 In some cases of trauma, there is ecchymosis and edema, but no discrete hematoma. This patient sustained a seat-belt injury in a motor vehicle accident. In the area of ecchymosis, the fat is severely hyperechoic, and small effusions bridge the fat along the normally hyperechoic Cooper's ligaments. The echotexture is nonspecific and compatible with severe edema of any etiology. Only the history of trauma and the presence of skin ecchymosis suggests that this represents subcutaneous ecchymosis rather than edema of other etiologies.

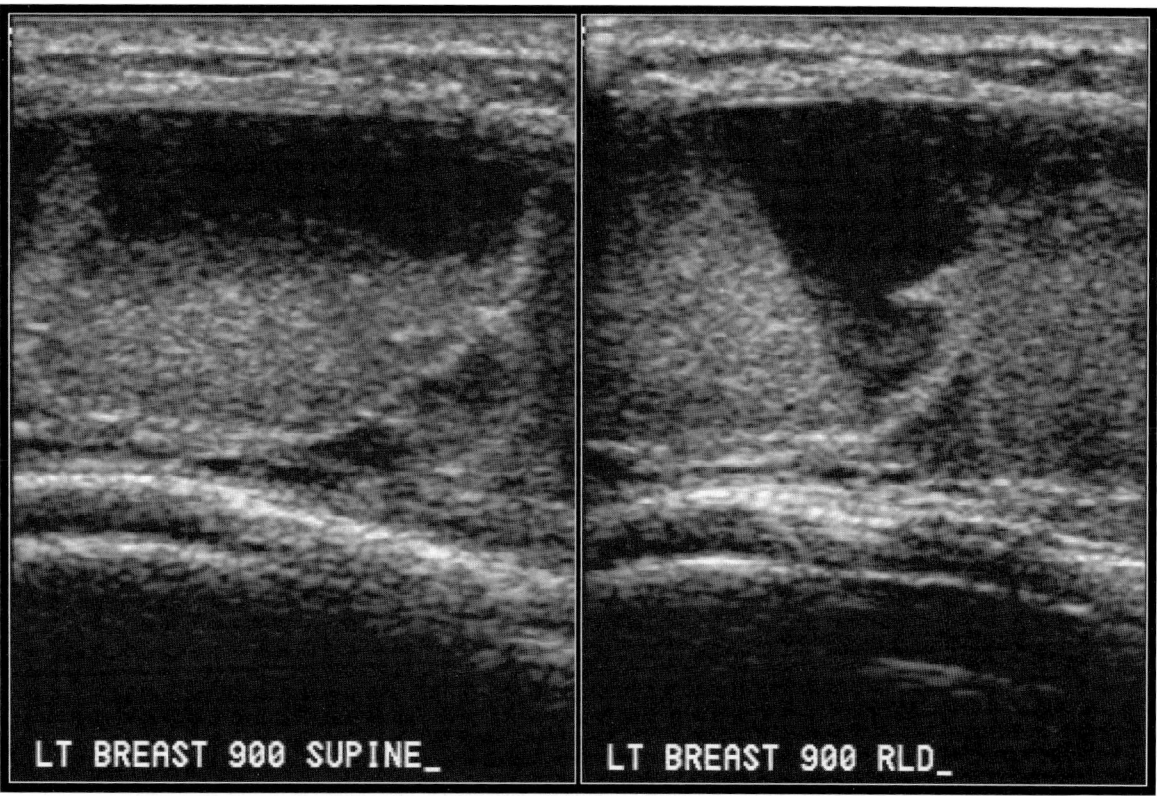

FIGURE 11–95 The debris level in hematomas that contain fluid—debris levels may simulate a mural nodule or may obscure an underlying nodule that is causing intracystic bleeding. Causing the debris to shift to a different part of the cyst by placing the patient in an upright or lateral decubitus position can prove that the debris is not a mural nodule that is attached to the wall. Once the debris moves to a different part of the cyst, the wall that was obscured by the debris in the supine position can be more accurately assessed for the presence of an underlying mural nodule.

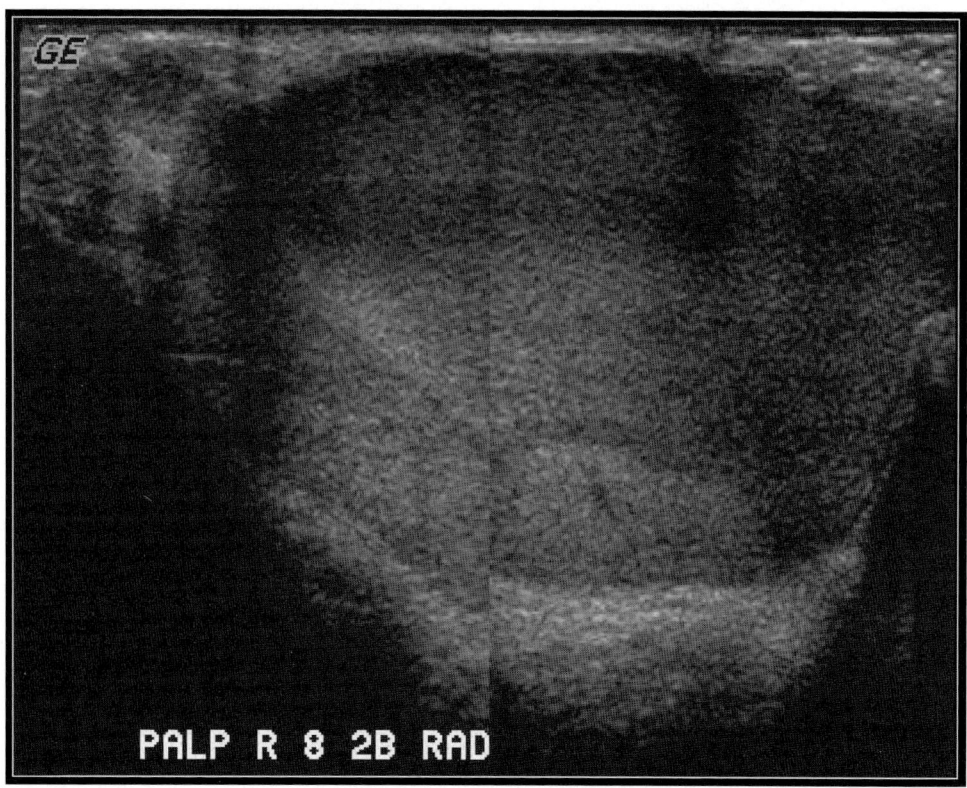

A

FIGURE 11–96 A: This large complex cyst with echogenic fluid contains what appears to be a debris level along its posterior wall. *(Continued.)*

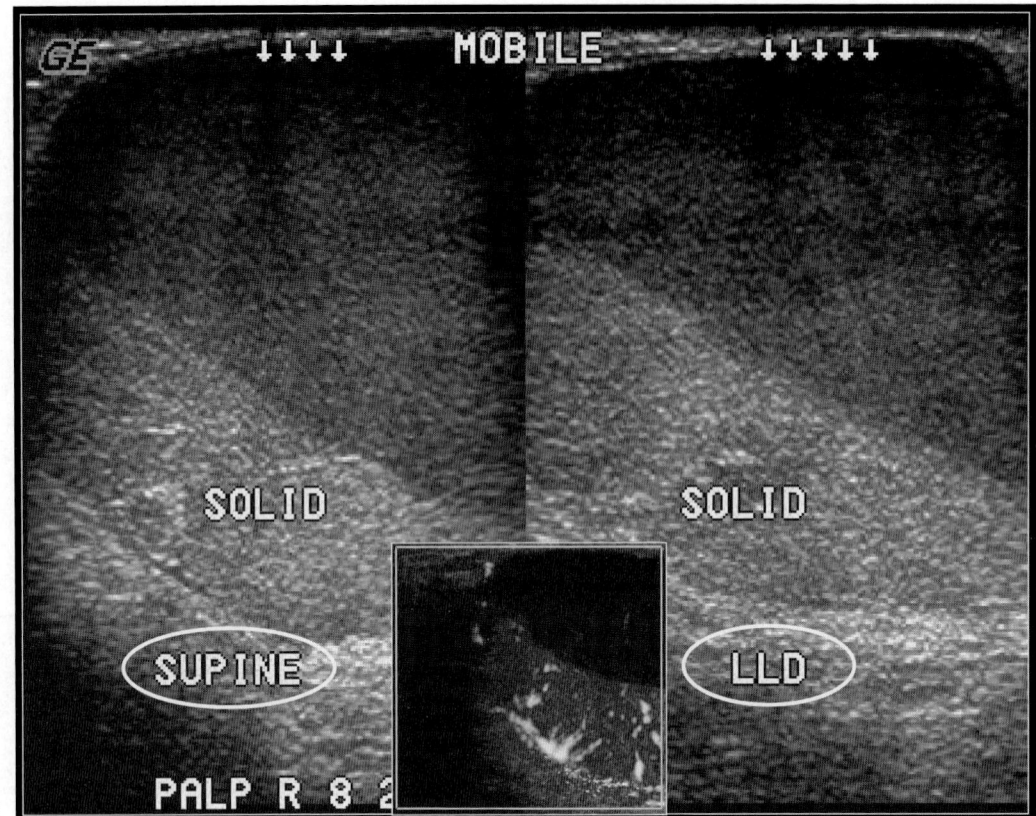

FIGURE 11–96 *(continued)* **B:** The apparent debris level is attached to the wall and does not fall to the left side of the cyst when the patient is placed in the left lateral decubitus position. The apparent debris level also has multiple fibrovascular stalks. Both the attachment to the wall and the vascularity prove that this is not simply a debris level, but an intracystic neoplasm that has caused secondary bleeding into the cysts.

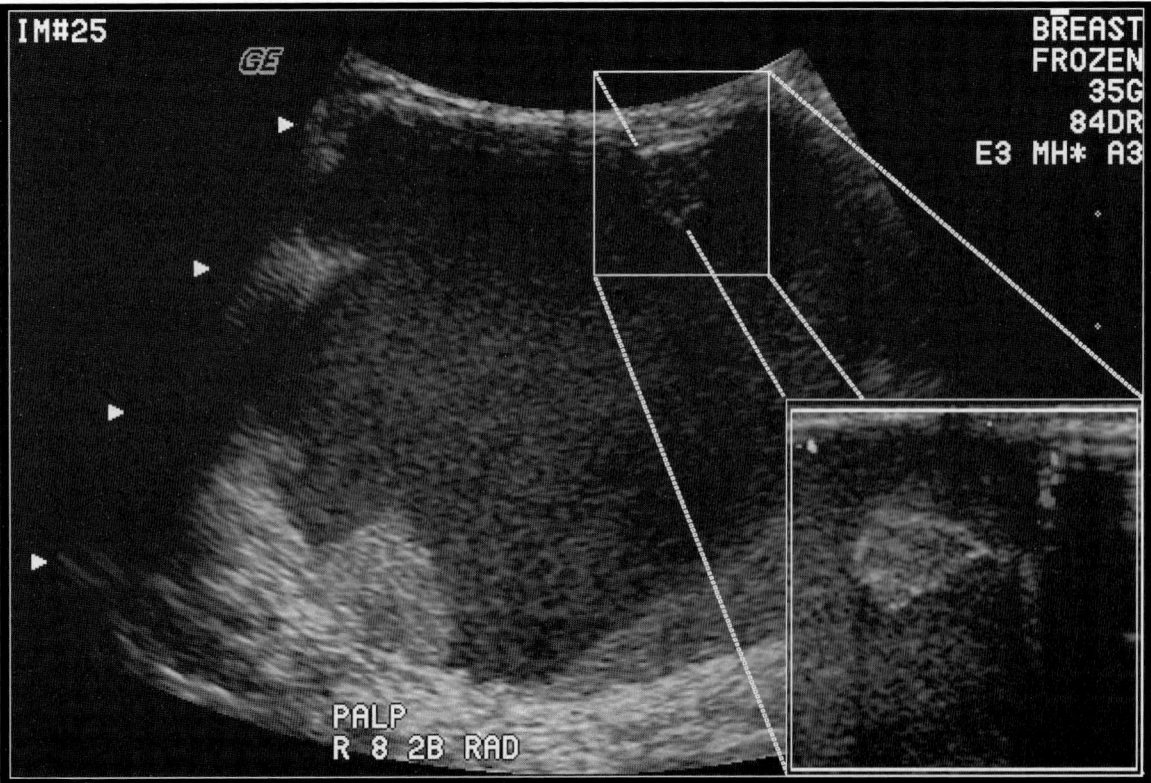

FIGURE 11–97 This mural nodule likely represents adherent clot rather than a tumor nodule because it is avascular on color Doppler evaluation. However, the findings should be interpreted with caution because a negative Doppler assessment is of less value than a positive assessment when evaluating mural nodules. Neoplastic mural nodules often undergo hemorrhagic infarction, in which case they will have no internal blood flow demonstrable by Doppler.

Hematomas are frequent minor complications of excisional biopsy and lumpectomy. As is the case for seromas, larger hematomas generally occur with wider excisions. As discussed earlier for seromas, the surgeon may encourage hematoma formation within the lumpectomy cavity in certain cases by not primarily closing the lumpectomy cavity in order to minimize deformity of the breast. In general, the smaller the breast or the larger the excision, the more likely a surgeon is to leave the cavity open. It is likely that not primarily closing the lumpectomy cavity does improve the early appearance of the surgical site. However, long-term results are less clear. The larger hematomas that accumulate within unclosed lumpectomy cavities are more likely to become chronic and to progress to the fibrotic and retracted phase of fat necrosis. Thus, in some cases, a better early cosmetic result may lead to greater deformity later. The progression to fat necrosis with cicatrix formation is exacerbated in patients who have undergone radiation therapy after lumpectomy. Furthermore, the chronic hematoma–fat necrosis complex that results from not closing the lumpectomy scar can result in more late diagnostic dilemmas because the exuberant fibrosis of end-stage florid fat necrosis can be difficult to distinguish sonographically from recurrent tumor. Spot compression magnification views and contrast-enhanced magnetic resonance imaging with the rotating delivery excitation off-resonance (RODEO) sequence help in some patients, but in many cases, biopsy is necessary to make the distinction. The appearance of chronic hematoma and fat necrosis within lumpectomy scars is discussed in the following section and also in Chapter 18.

FAT NECROSIS

General Pathologic Classification, Epidemiology, and Clinical Findings

Fat necrosis is also discussed and illustrated in Chapter 18. Because certain phases of fat necrosis are cystic and most cases of fat necrosis likely arise from cystic hematomas or seromas, it is prudent to include a discussion of the cystic phases of fat necrosis in the section on complex cysts.

Fat necrosis results from injury to breast fat. Although classic cases have a history of previous surgery or trauma at the site of development, certain cases do not have such a specific history. Causes other than direct trauma or surgery include ischemia and chemical irritation. A more complete list of contributing factors is presented in Table 11–1.

In some cases, multiple different factors contribute to the development of fat necrosis. For example, in patients undergoing reduction mammoplasty, surgical trauma, ischemia due to surgical disruption of blood supply, and chemical irritation due to bleeding into the surgical defects all contribute to the high incidence of fat necrosis. In patients undergoing lumpectomy and radiation therapy, multiple factors contribute to the development of fat necrosis: (a) hemorrhage into the lumpectomy site, (b) chronic granulomatous inflammatory changes caused by blood breakdown products, (c) early ischemia resulting from surgical disruption of blood supply to fat immediately surrounding the lumpectomy cavity, and (d) late ischemia resulting from radiation-induced arteritis and small vessel obliteration.

Fat necrosis may be asymptomatic or may cause tender or nontender palpable lumps. The clinical findings often are indistinguishable from those of the underlying contributing processes, such as surgical scarring, hematoma, or periductal mastitis. Distinguishing fat necrosis from recurrent tumor in breast cancer patients who have undergone lumpectomy and radiation is an especially troublesome clinical and imaging problem.

The earliest histologic findings of fat necrosis are inflammatory changes and hemorrhage into fat. These result in injury to adipocytes. Individual injured fat cells release their lipid contents into the interstitium of the adipose tissue. The released lipid material is broken down into liquefied fatty acids, which further chemically irritate and inflame surrounding tissues, perpetuating and extending the process. A fibrous capsule may eventually form around the oily fatty acids. Within this encapsulated collection of oily fatty acids, salts of the fatty acids may accumulate along the capsule. The fatty acids in the wall may undergo saponification, causing calcium to precipitate along the wall and ultimately forming circumferential eggshell calcifications typical of lipid cysts. In addition, the fatty acids that are not encapsulated can be viewed by the immune system as foreign bodies and result in a chronic granulomatous, giant cell, foreign-body–like reaction in the surrounding tissues. Processes other than fat necrosis can release fatty acids into surrounding tissues and incite a virtually indistinguishable histologic response. For example, the lipid contents of some cysts and inflamed ectatic ducts are virtually identical to the lipids released into the interstitium by fat necrosis. Thus,

TABLE 11–1. CAUSES OF FAT NECROSIS

Trauma

Surgical trauma, especially wide excisions, including:
    Lumpectomy for cancer
    Reduction mammoplasty

Ischemia
    Large, pendulous, fatty breasts
    Disruption of blood supply caused by extensive excision of tissue
    Arteritis as a result of radiation therapy

Chemical irritation
    Bleeding into fatty tissues
    Rupture of cysts
    Rupture of ectatic ducts, plasma cell mastitis

Hemorrhage into preexisting cyst

rupture of a lipid-containing cyst or ectatic duct results in a chemical inflammation or mastitis that is identical to that resulting from fat necrosis. Over time, the chronic granulomatous or foreign-body reaction caused by fat necrosis leads to fibrosis of varying degrees. In certain cases, the fibrotic reaction is so severe that it retracts and deforms surrounding tissues. Such exuberant fibrosis or cicatrix formation may simulate the scirrhous response elicited by some breast cancers. Similarly, the fibrotic reaction induced by cyst rupture can lead to fibrosis that simulates malignancy, and the periductal and intraductal fibrosis resulting from the chronic duct ectasia–periductal mastitis complex can lead to nipple retraction similar to that caused by malignancy.

Mammographic Findings

The mammographic findings of fat necrosis vary greatly and depend on the stage of development and the relative amounts of lipid cyst formation and fibrous scarring. Very early in the course, there may be no mammographic findings. Later, a mixed lipid and water-density lesion may be present (Fig. 11–98). Out of the mixed-density lesion, a

well-circumscribed, low-density lipid cyst that has a thin water-density capsule may develop. With time, as calcified salts of fatty acids precipitate along the capsule of the oil cyst, spherical or elliptical calcifications with low-density centers (eggshell calcifications) may form in the breast (*liponecrosis macrocystica calcificans*). These lesions are usually multiple and can be several millimeters to a few centimeters in size. (Lipid cysts are also discussed in Chapters 10 and 18.) These lipid cysts, whether they have water-density capsules or calcified capsules, have a characteristic and definitively benign (BIRADS 2) mammographic appearance (Fig. 11–99). Lesions with eggshell calcifications do not require additional mammographic or sonographic evaluation. In patients in whom the fibrotic phase of fat necrosis has become predominant, frank spiculation or less specific architectural distortion with or without a water-density mass (chronic hematoma) may predominate. Exuberant fibrotic scarring is most likely to occur in cases in which fat necrosis develops within a large hematoma, particularly a hematoma within a lumpectomy cavity that was not primarily closed, and is also usually more pronounced in patients who have also had radiation therapy. In such

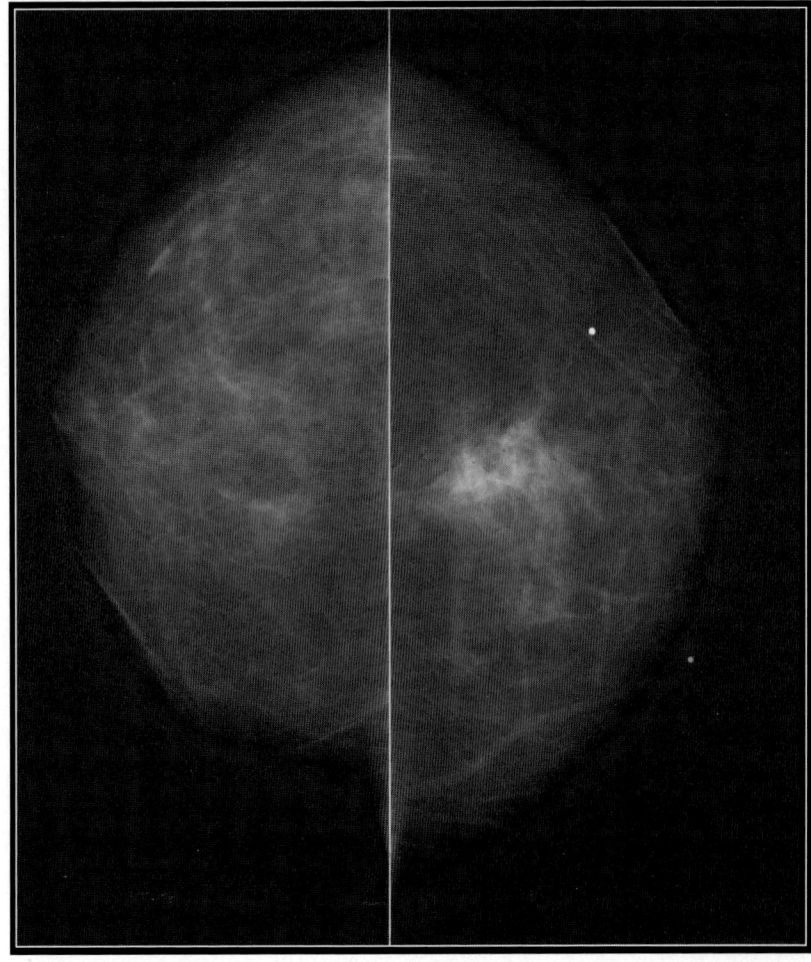

FIGURE 11–98 The earliest mammographic finding in fat necrosis is the presence of a mixed fatty and water-density mass that actually represents the hematoma from which fat necrosis will develop.

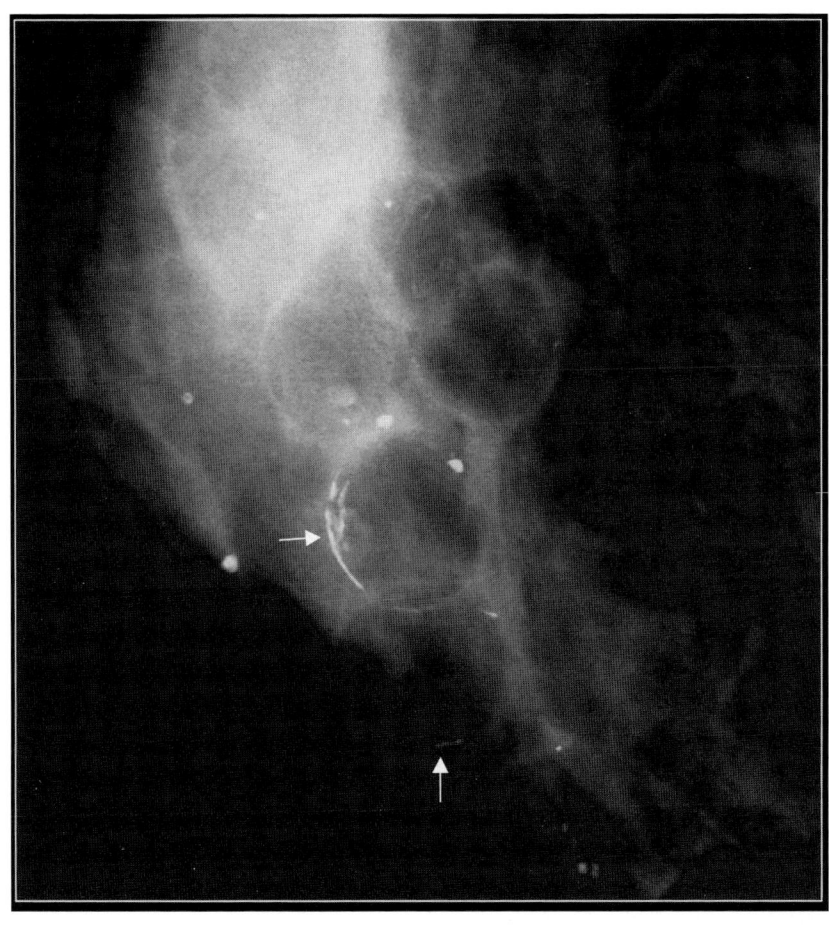

FIGURE 11–99 When multiple lipid cysts are present, they may be at different stages of development. Note that two cysts are at different stages of calcification, whereas multiple other lipid cysts have no calcification yet.

patients, the spiculated water-density mass may be difficult to distinguish from recurrent malignancy in the lumpectomy site. However, most scars related to surgery are linear in shape, at least in one view (Fig. 11–100). All phases of fat necrosis may be present simultaneously in the same breast.

Patients who have undergone reduction mammoplasty are particularly likely to have multiple areas of mammographically evident fat necrosis in various phases throughout both breasts (Fig. 11–101).

Sonographic Findings

The sonographic appearance of fat necrosis, like the mammographic appearance, varies greatly, depending on both the stage of development and the relative degrees of lipid cyst formation and fibrosis. It must be remembered that fat necrosis is a nonspecific response to the injury of fat that could be ischemic, chemical, surgical, or traumatic. Frequently, more than one etiology is operative, and one etiology may evolve into another. There are pure findings of fat necrosis, which are described later. However, in many cases, the dominant findings are those of the associated condition, that is, the surgical scar, hematoma, or seroma.

In postsurgical patients, all of the possible etiologies may be active: ischemic injury from surgical disruption of blood vessels and lymphatics, surgical scarring, hematoma, seroma, and chemical injury to fat surrounding the wound and hematoma from blood breakdown products. Thus, fat necrosis in postsurgical patients tends to have the most varied and complex of all etiologies.

In the earliest phases, only edema of one or more fat lobules is demonstrable. Edema of fat either homogeneously or heterogeneously increases its echogenicity relative to the surrounding normal fatty tissues (Fig. 11–102). If the extent of fatty edema is limited to a small area, the abnormal hyperechogenicity of the involved fat will be readily apparent and distinguishable from the normal surrounding isoechoic fat. However, if the edematous area is so extensive that the area of involvement is wider than the ultrasound transducer, it may be difficult to appreciate the hyperechogenicity without split-screen mirror-image scanning of the contralateral side enabling comparison to the echogenicity of normal breast fat (Fig. 11–103). The hyperechoic edema induced by fat necrosis is indistinguishable from edema of any other etiology. Thus, the edema resulting mastitis appears identical sonographically to the

(text continued on page 420)

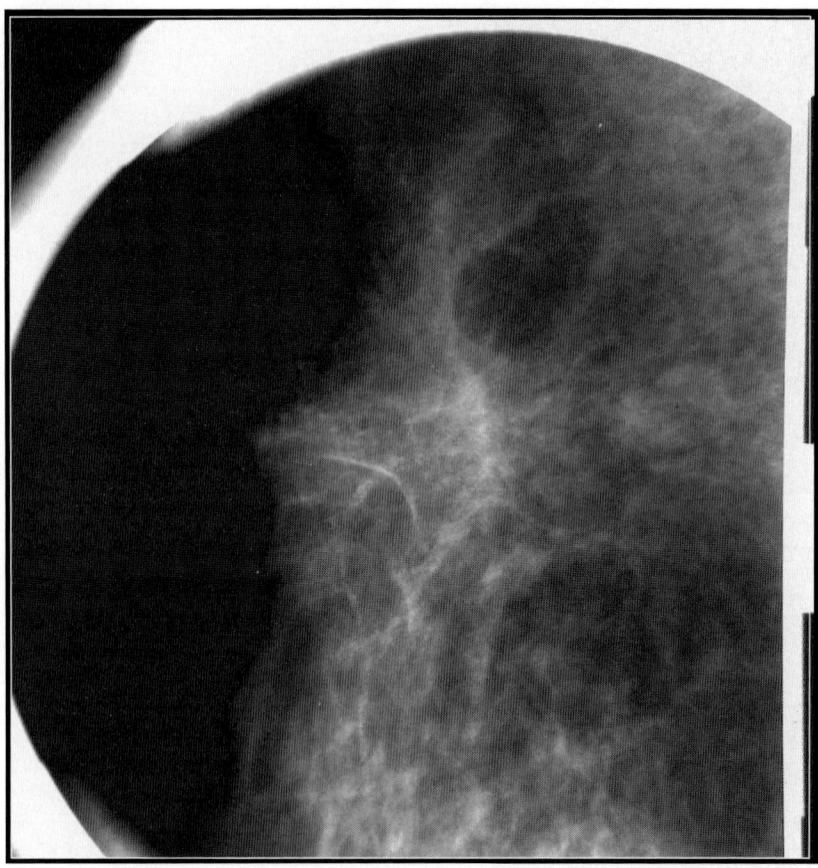

FIGURE 11–100 If fat necrosis progresses to the fibrous phase, it may cause architectural distortion and spiculation that is worrisome for malignancy. The fat necrosis associated with surgical scars is often linearly shaped.

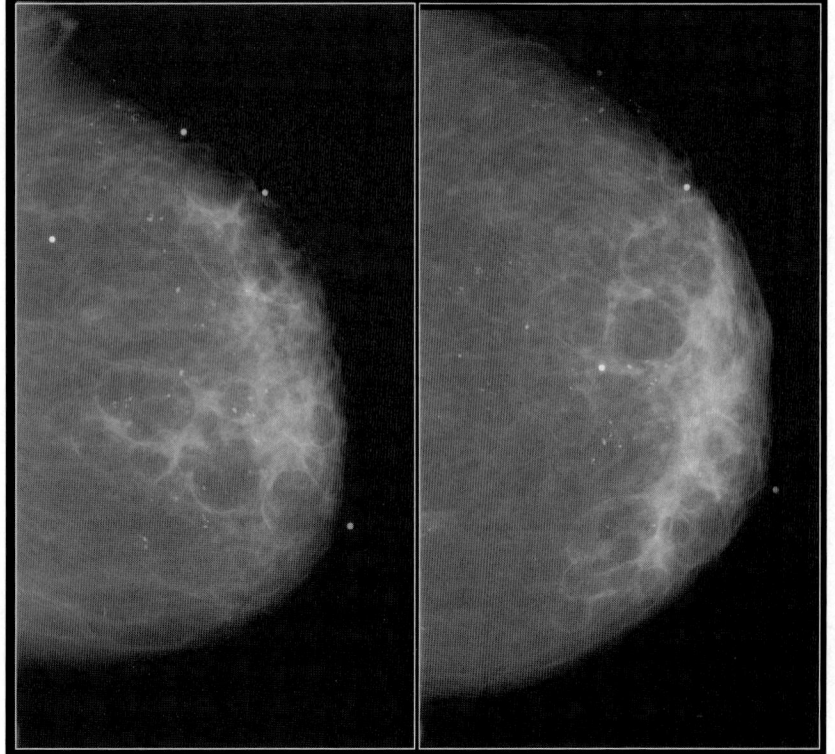

FIGURE 11–101 Reduction mammoplasty is the most common etiology for multiple lipid cysts and fat necrosis in multiple stages scattered throughout both breasts.

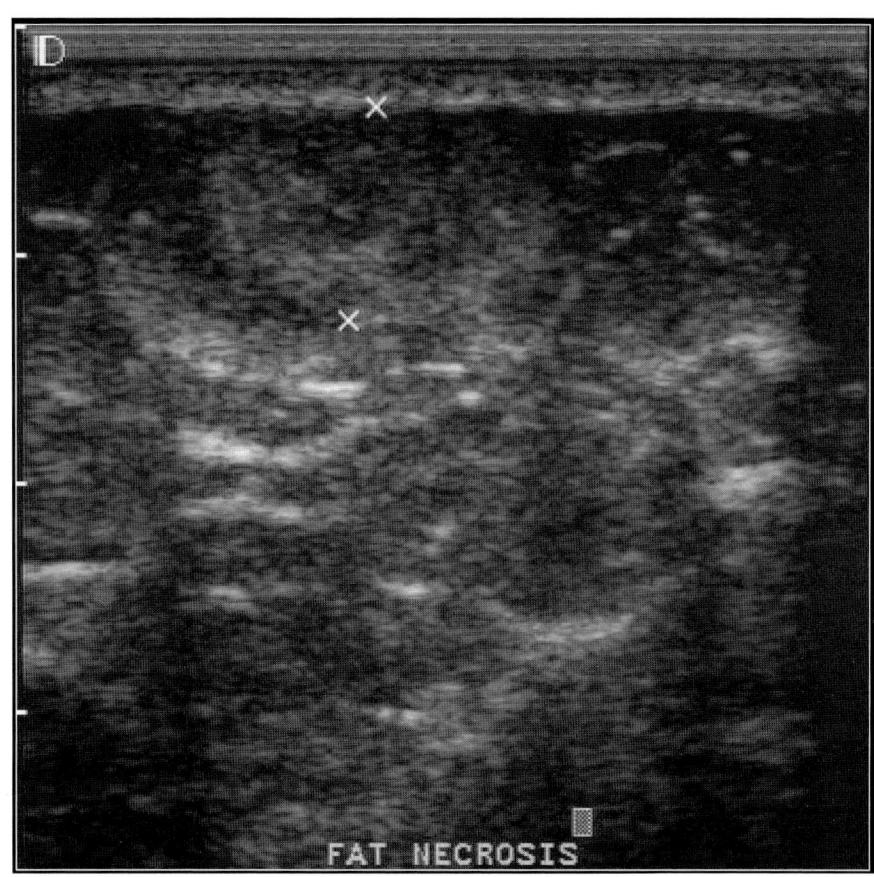

FIGURE 11–102 The earliest sign of fat necrosis is edema of fat, which makes the fat either homogeneously or heterogeneously hyperechoic. When only a single fat lobule is involved, it may be difficult to distinguish early mild fat necrosis from a subcutaneous lipoma.

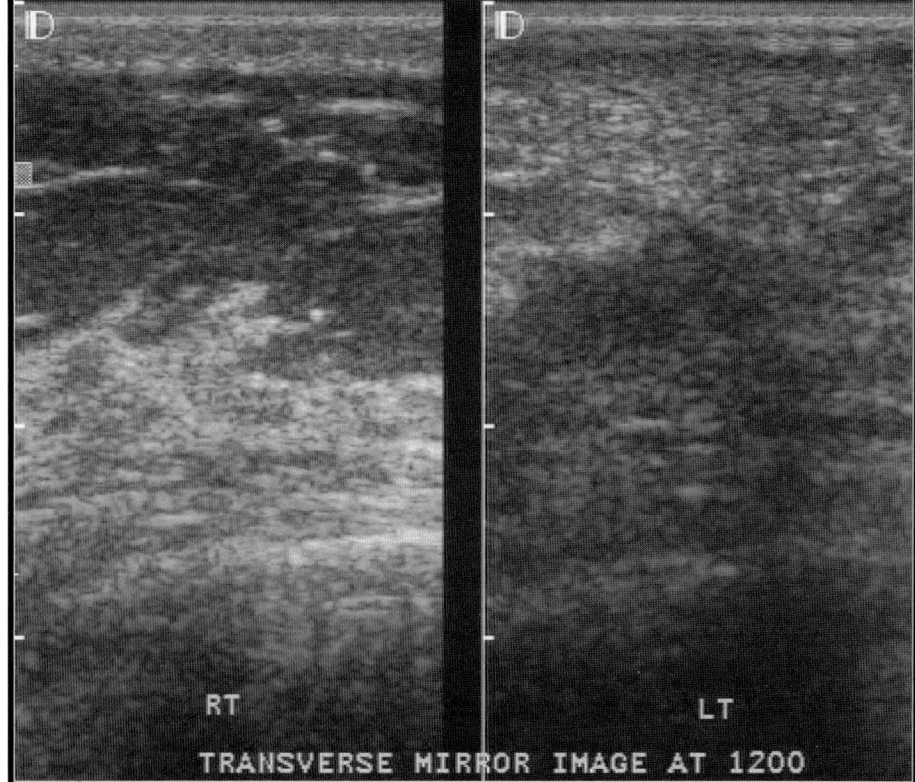

FIGURE 11–103 When early fat necrosis is severe and extensive, the pattern of edema is nonspecific and may not be sonographically distinguishable from edema of other causes such as mastitis or inflammatory carcinoma. The edema in fat necrosis is usually not associated with inflammatory hyperemia, but both mastitis and trauma with diffuse ecchymosis can be hyperemic and may progress to fat necrosis. These split-screen mirror-image scans of the 12:00 areas of right and left breasts show severe edema on the patient's left side.

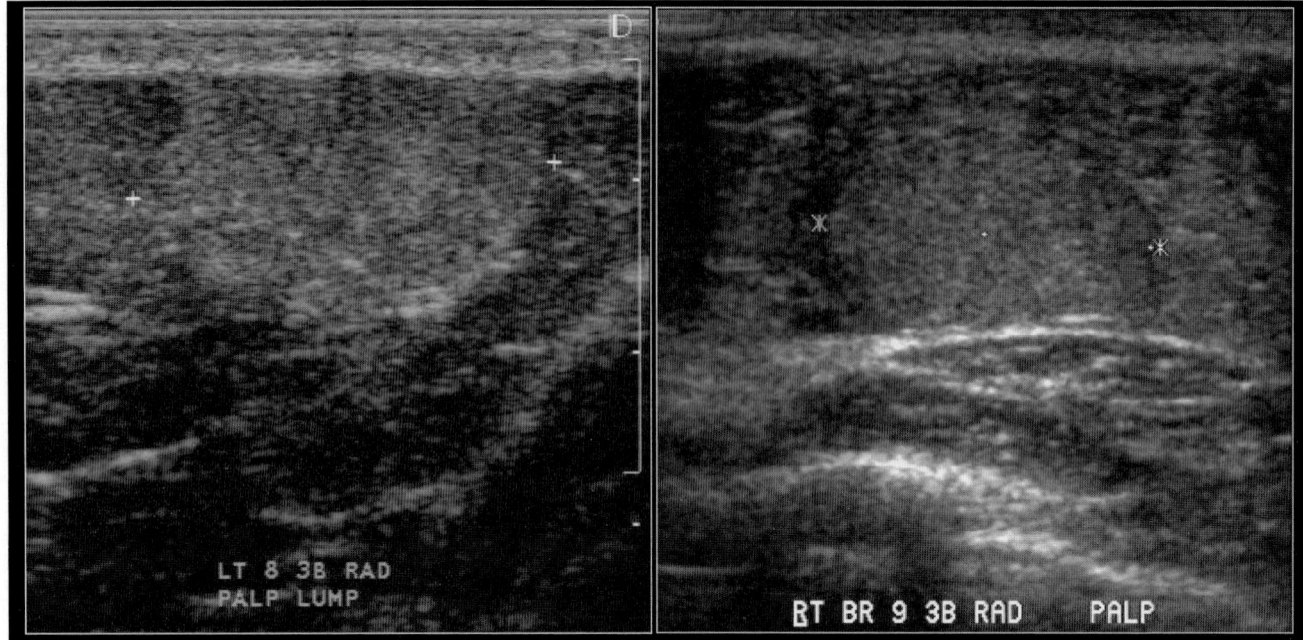

FIGURE 11–104 These figures illustrate the similarity in the appearance of early fat necrosis involving a single fat lobule (**left**) and a mildly hyperechoic lipoma (**right**).

edema of fat necrosis. It can also be difficult to distinguish fat necrosis that is limited to a single fat lobule from certain lipomas that also appear mildly echogenic because of a higher than normal fibrous content (Fig. 11–104). Obviously, the early changes of fat necrosis described previously may be isolated, but they are often associated with sonographic findings of the surgical scar, hematoma, or seroma.

The complex cystic phases of fat necrosis have multiple different origins: (a) liquefaction of fat from pure fat necrosis, (b) hematomas, and (c) seromas. In cases in which fat necrosis is an isolated process, the sonographic features of the complex cyst are typical of lipid cysts in various phases. However, in the cases in which fat necrosis is postsurgical, the early sonographic characteristics of the le-

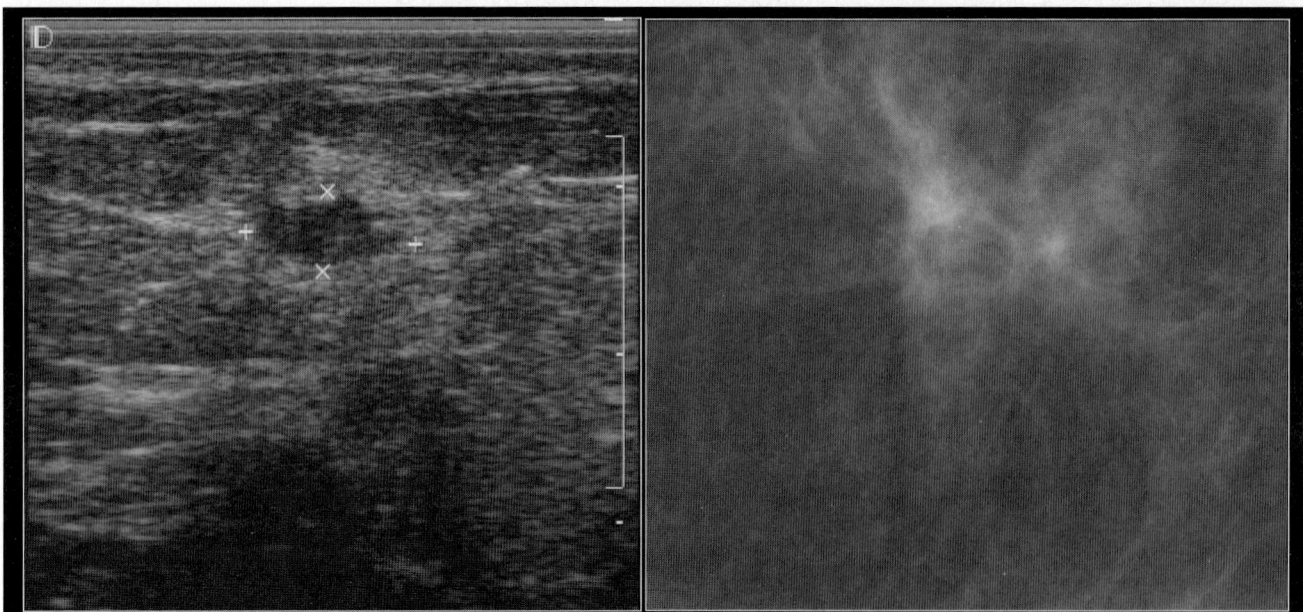

FIGURE 11–105 Necrotic fat liquefies, forming an ill-defined collection of fluid on ultrasound and a thick-walled lipid cyst on mammography.

sion are merely a reflection of the characteristics of the hematoma or seroma within the surgical site from which fat necrosis evolved. The cysts that form after surgery reflect the irregular shape of the surgical defect, not a circular or oval shape. Postsurgical hematomas and seromas can be associated with ischemia or chemical mastitis in the fat surrounding the surgical site, leading to fat necrosis in those tissues. Thus, the pattern of postsurgical fat necrosis complex cystic lesions is often mixed, reflecting the mixed etiologies—surgical scar, periscar ischemia, hematoma, and perihematoma chemical mastitis.

As isolated fat necrosis progresses beyond the edema stage, ill-defined complex cystic areas that represent fibrous encased circular or oval lipid cysts appear within the edematous fat (Fig. 11–105). With additional time, a thin, echogenic, well-defined lipid cyst wall develops (Fig. 11–106). These early lipid cysts may demonstrate diffuse low-level echogenicity; thin, echogenic capsules; and sometimes multiple loculations. However, even when pure lipid cysts are multiloculated, each loculation tends to be smooth, well defined, and either circular or oval (Fig. 11–107). In cases in which fat necrosis and lipid cyst develop from a preexisting hematoma, the sonographic appearance is merely a reflection of the sonographic appearance of the underlying hematoma. With time, as saponified calcified fatty acids form in the cyst lumen and are deposited within the lipid cyst capsule, both the cyst contents and cyst wall become more echogenic. The calcification of the lipid cyst wall progresses from mildly in-

creased echogenicity to intense hyperechogenicity, and the enhanced through-transmission that was present before calcification is gradually replaced by increasing acoustic shadowing (Fig. 11–108). The echogenicity of the lipid cyst contents also increases enough in certain cases that the lesion appears to be solid rather than cystic, including the following:

1. In cases in which fat necrosis evolves from a hematoma, the resulting complex lipid cyst is more likely to have a thick, relatively echogenic wall, mural nodules, or thick septations and to contain echogenic debris—all features that are typical of chronic hematomas (Fig. 11–109).
2. In cases in which fat necrosis evolves from a seroma, the resulting complex lipid cyst is likely to have an isoechoic wall of medium thickness, in some instances, thin, echogenic internal septations, and nearly anechoic to mildly echogenic fluid—all features that are typical of seromas (Fig. 11–110).

Because the shape of the complex lipid cysts that develop in postsurgical fat necrosis have an angular or irregular shape that reflects the irregular shape of the surgical cavity, they may simulate angular malignant lesions sonographically (Fig. 11–111). The shape depends heavily on whether the surgical cavity was sutured closed or left open to accumulate blood and serum. In cases in which the lumpectomy cavity has been sutured closed, the appearance of the lipid cyst within the surgical cavity differs de-

(text continued on page 425)

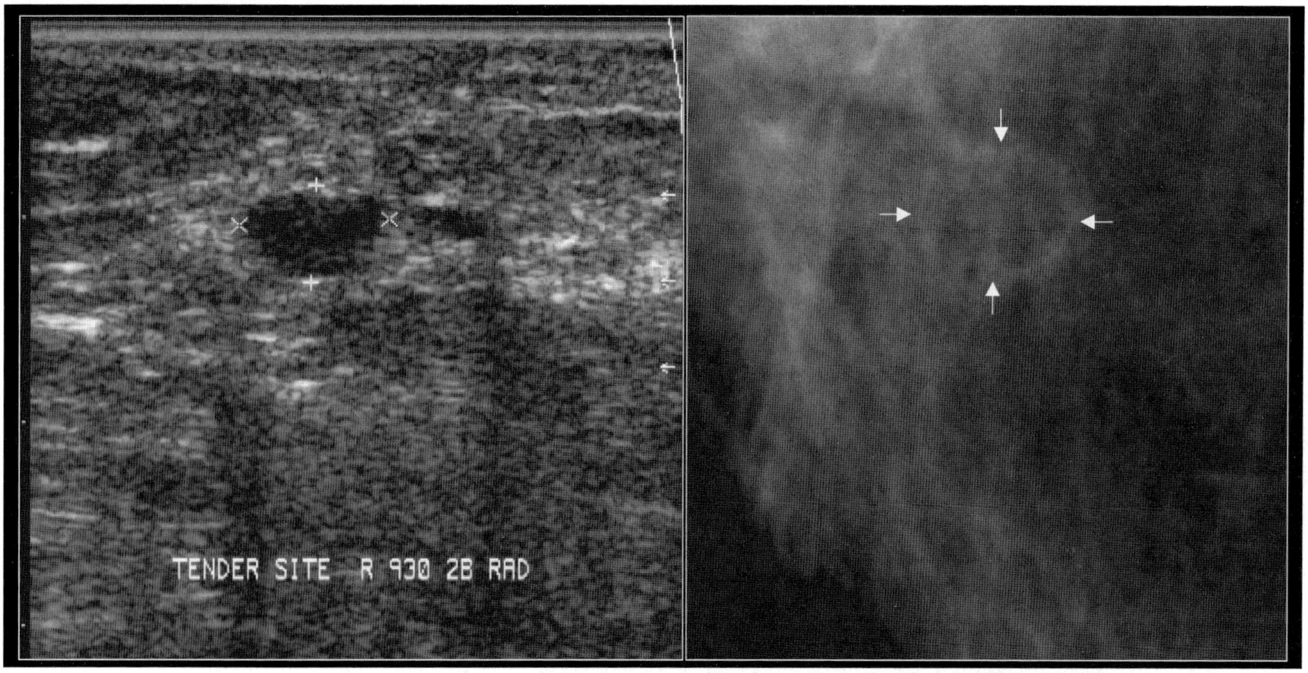

FIGURE 11–106 A wall of fibrous tissue encases the liquefied fat. The lipid cyst develops a thin, echogenic wall on ultrasound, and its wall becomes thinner and better defined on mammograms.

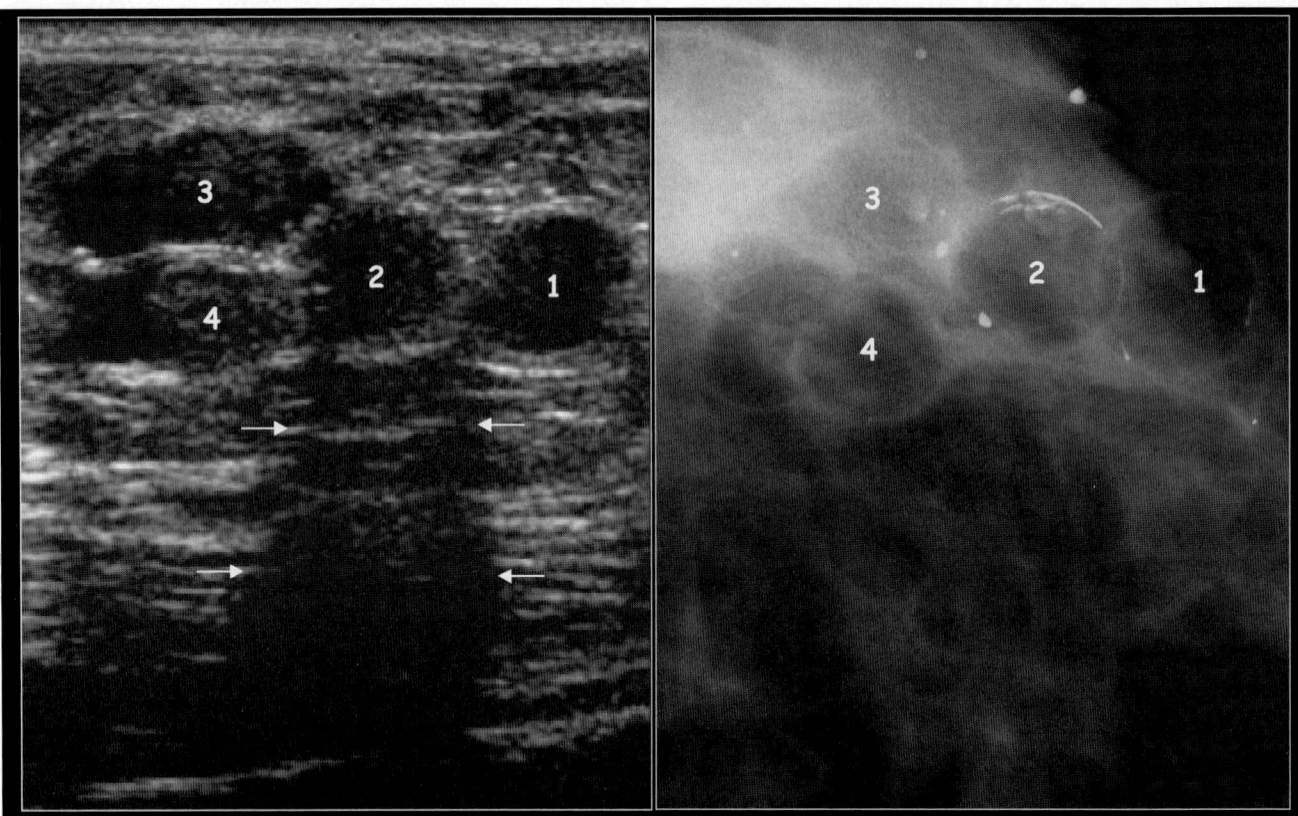

FIGURE 11–107 Even when lipid cysts are multilocular, each component appears to be a circular or oval structure with a benign mammographic appearance. On ultrasound, the appearance is less certain. The lipid contents of the multiple lipid cysts vary from cysts to cyst. The cyst that is calcifying casts an acoustic shadow *(#2, arrows)*.

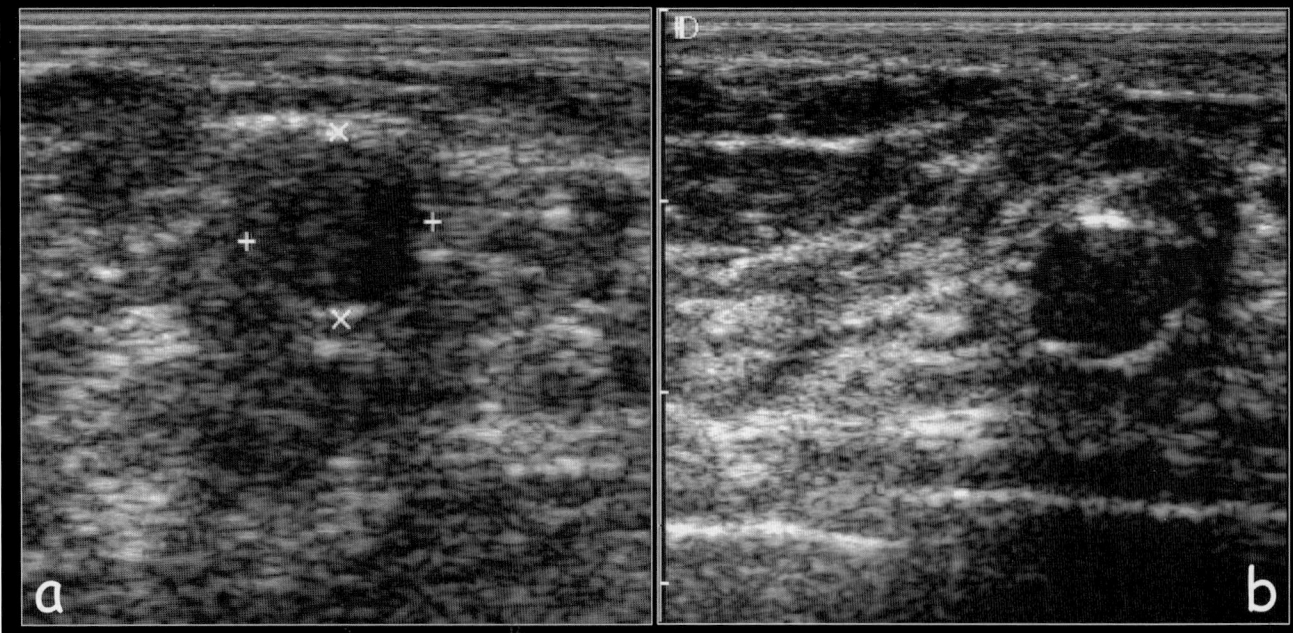

FIGURE 11–108 **A, B:** The sonographic appearance of lipid cysts changes as the degree of wall calcification increases. With early calcification (**A**), the echogenicity of the wall may not be appreciably increased, but the normally enhanced sound transmission may decrease to become similar to that of surrounding tissue. The diffuse, low-level internal echogenicity is caused by the lipid contents of the cyst, not the calcification in the wall. As wall calcification increases, the wall may become hyperechoic, but the calcium is only thick enough to cause mild shadowing (**B**). *(Continued.)*

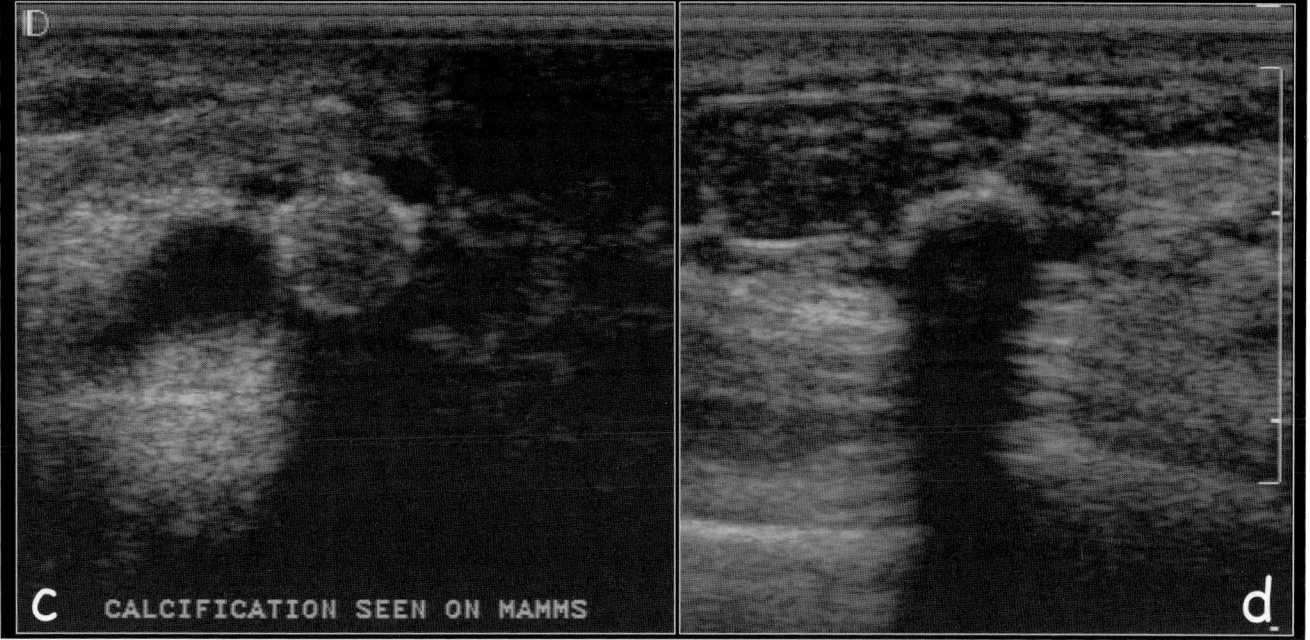

FIGURE 11–108 *(continued)* **C, D:** As calcification in the lipid cyst wall progresses, the hyperechoic wall appears thicker and brighter, and saponified calcified salts of fatty acids floating within the cyst fluid may make the cyst contents appear mildly hyperechoic (**C**). The calcification is now thick and dense enough to cause moderately severe acoustic shadowing. Finally, when calcification is dense and complete enough to cause a classic "eggshell" calcification on mammograms, the shadowing may be so intense that only the anterior wall of the calcified lipid cyst is visible. The posterior aspects of the cyst are completely obscured by acoustic shadowing.

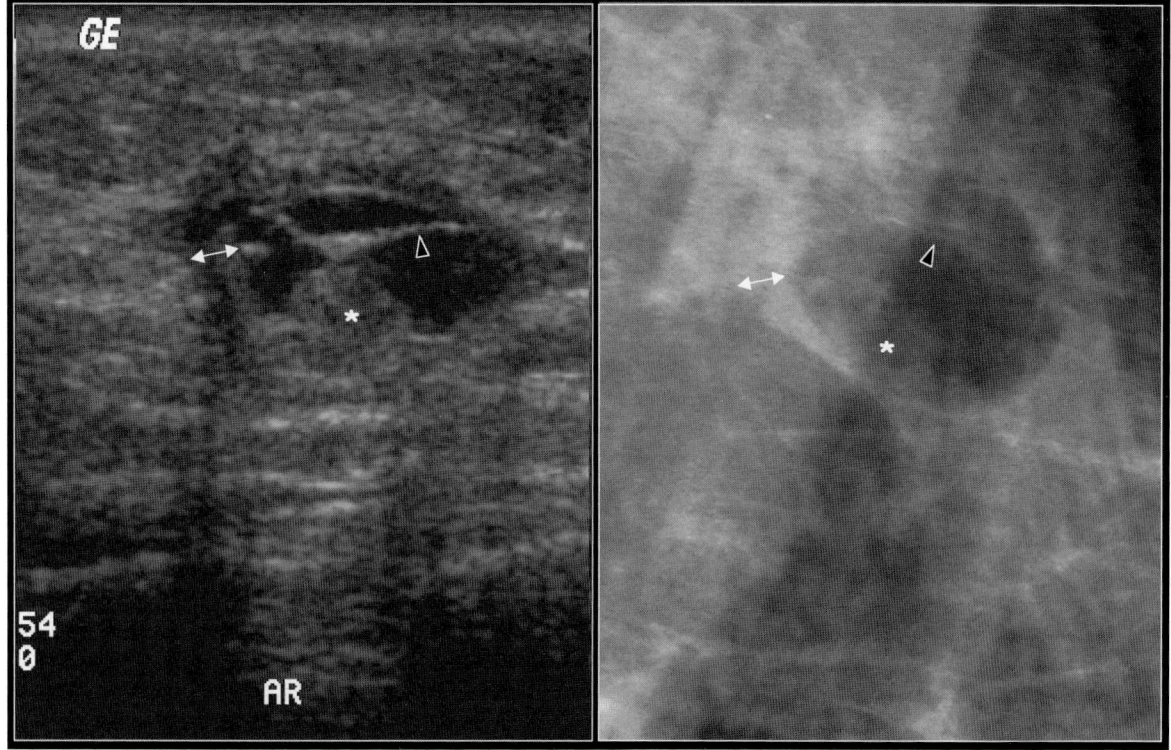

FIGURE 11–109 Lipid cysts that evolve from hematomas often have multiple mildly suspicious sonographic findings, such as thick walls, septations, and mural nodules, but appear to be classically benign lipid cysts (BIRADS 2) mammographically. When mammographic findings and sonographic findings are discordant, and when mammography shows a lipid cyst, more reliance should be placed on the mammographic findings. Note that the thick wall along the left edge of the nodule *(double-headed arrow)*, the mural nodule *(*)*, and the internal septations *(arrowheads)* are all visible mammographically but are hard to distinguish from superimposed tissues. The key to mammography being reassuring is the lipid density, which mammography can show, but sonography cannot.

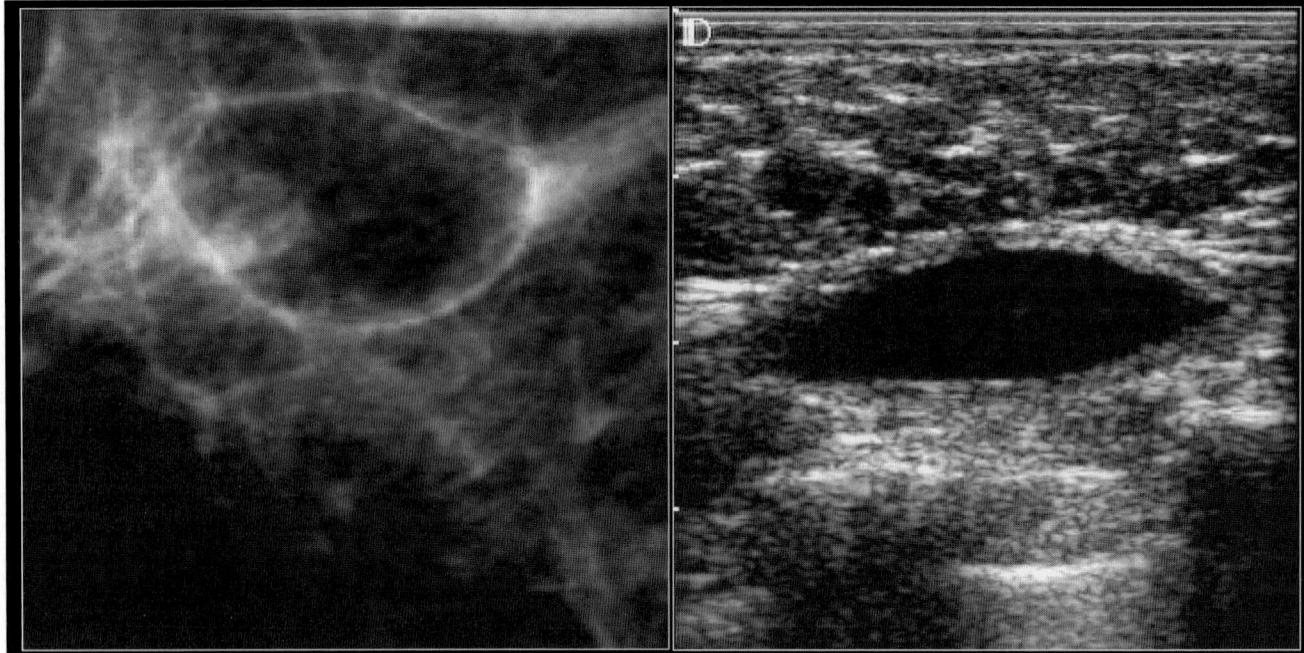

FIGURE 11–110 Lipid cysts that develop from seromas are more likely to be anechoic and less likely to have mural nodules or thick septations than those that develop from hematomas. They may, however, still have a mildly thickened wall.

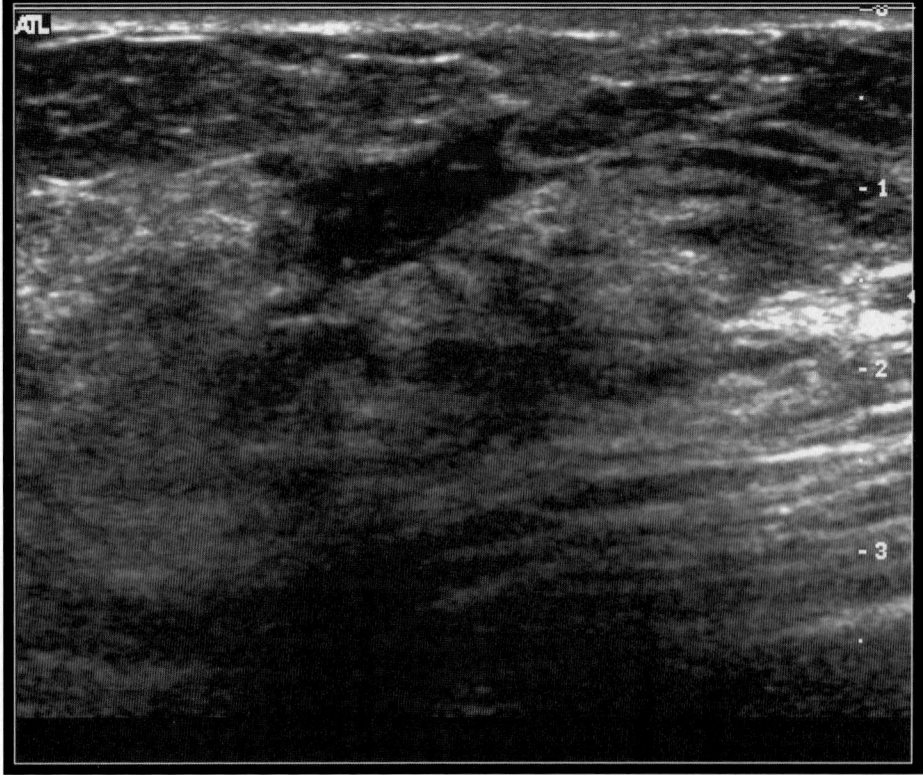

FIGURE 11–111 The shape of lipid cysts that develop within lumpectomy cavities reflects the irregular and angular shape of the lumpectomy cavity if the lipid cyst is flaccid and not under tension.

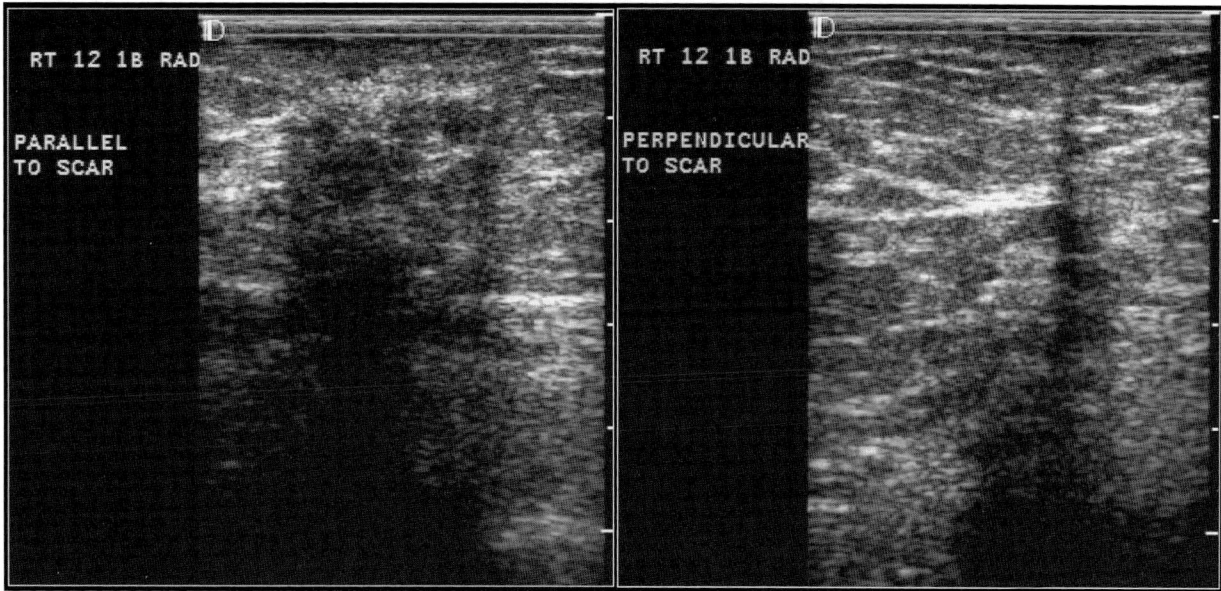

FIGURE 11–112 The shape of a lumpectomy cavity that has been sutured closed differs from a cavity that has been left open. Cavities that have been sutured closed appear linear when scanned in an axis that is perpendicular to the long axis of the scar. However, when scanned parallel to the scar, the cavity appears more worrisome and masslike.

pending on whether it is scanned parallel or perpendicular to the scar. When scanned parallel to the scar, the fat necrosis or lipid cyst may appear masslike and worrisome. However, when scanned perpendicular to the scar, the configuration of the fat necrosis is linear and reassuring (Fig. 11–112). On the other hand, when the surgical cavity is left open, the fat necrosis within it appears masslike and more worrisome for recurrent tumor, regardless of the scan plane (Fig. 11–113).

Transducer angulation, split-screen compression imaging, and Doppler may be helpful in distinguishing fat necrosis from recurrent tumor. Some of the apparent

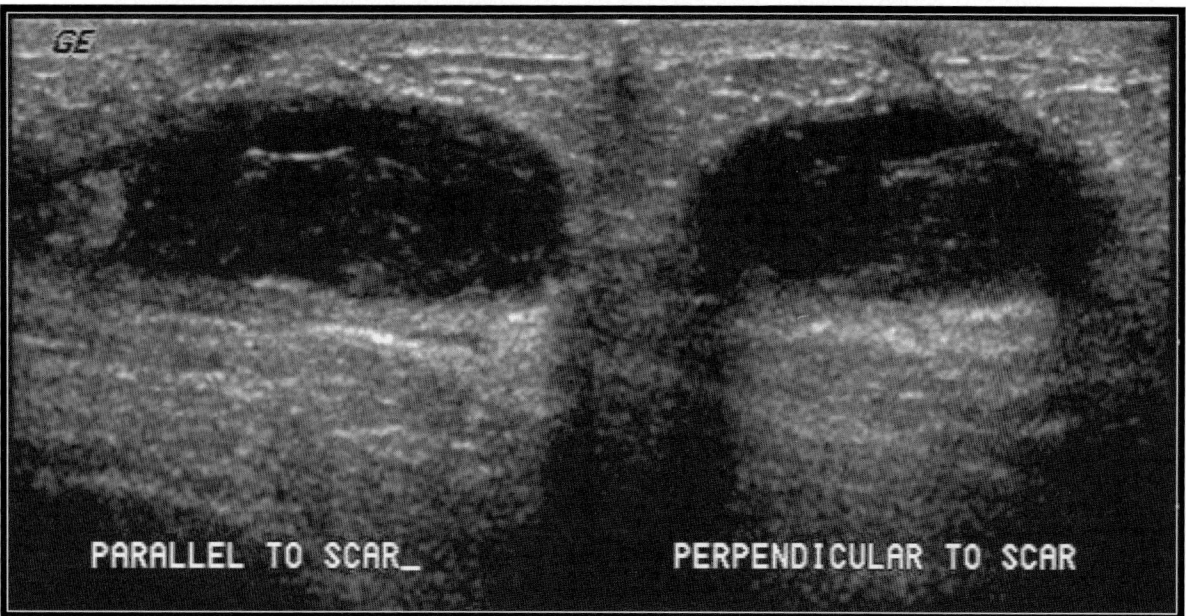

FIGURE 11–113 A lumpectomy cavity that has not been primarily closed will accumulate serum or blood that will eventually evolve into a lipid cyst. The fluid collection appears masslike in both long and short axis to the scar. This lipid cyst is under tension and therefore fairly smooth and oval shaped. However, when the lipid cyst within the open lumpectomy cavity is flaccid and the cavity is irregular in shape, distinguishing between recurrent carcinoma and fat necrosis may be more difficult than in patients who have had primary closure.

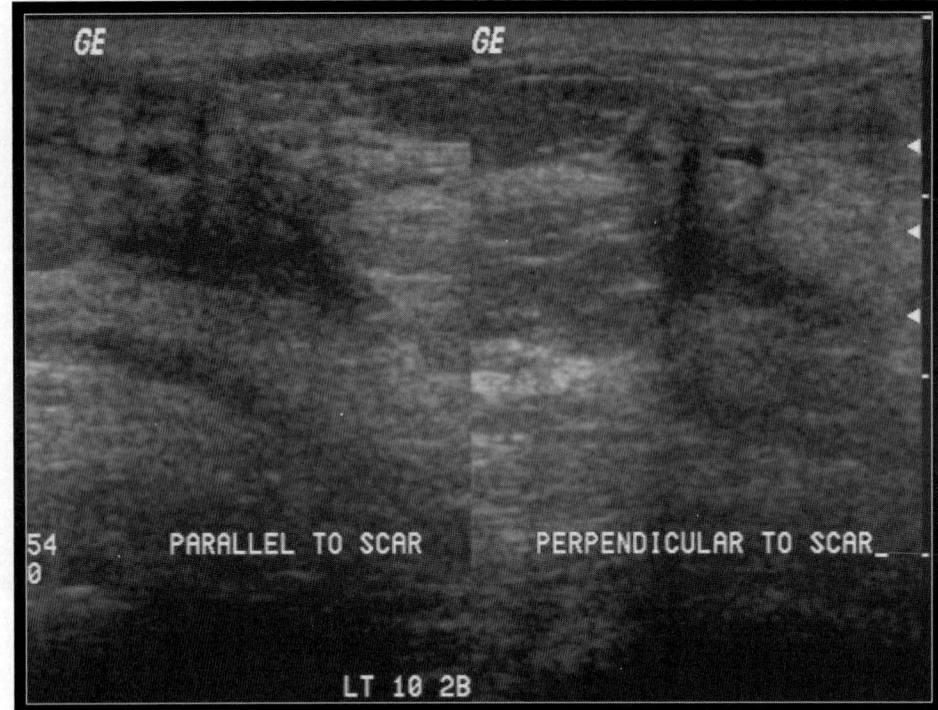

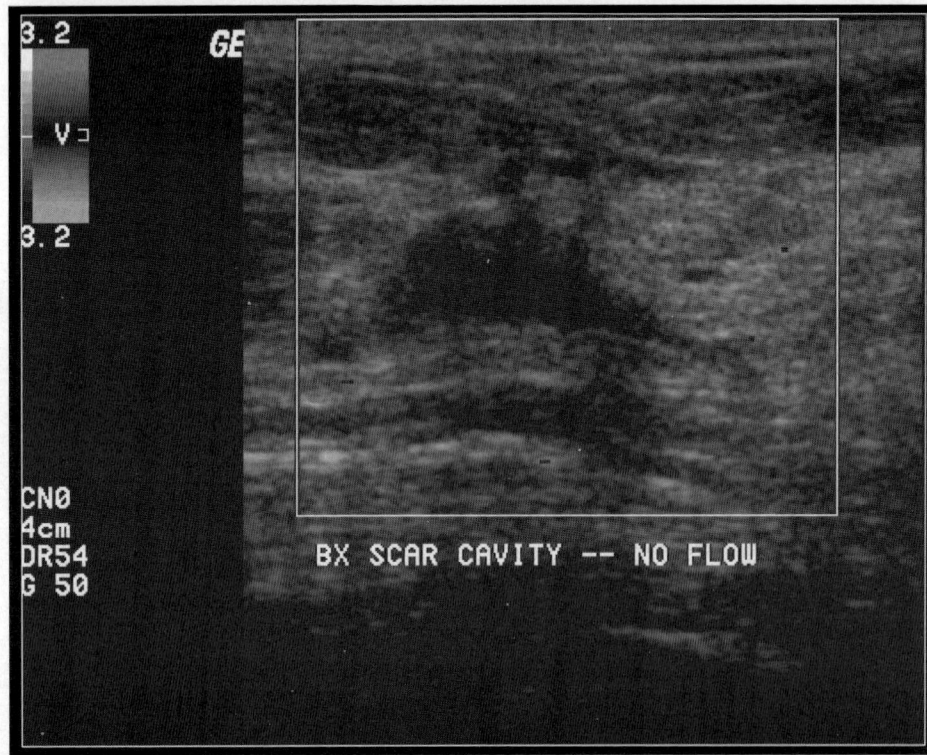

FIGURE 11–114 A: This lumpectomy cavity was not sutured closed. The seroma that collected within the cavity has evolved into a flaccid lipid cyst that is mildly echogenic and angular in shape in both the long and short axes of the scar. Recurrent carcinoma can have a similar appearance. **B:** Color Doppler assessment of fat necrosis and lipid cysts more than 6 months after surgery shows no blood flow. Fat necrosis is, by definition, avascular after granulation tissue that is present early after surgery matures to fibrous scar tissue. Recurrent tumor, on the other hand, is far more likely to have internal blood flow.

masslike effect of fat necrosis is actually caused by critical angle shadowing, not true mass effect. Angling the transducer so that an angle of incidence is more nearly perpendicular to the scar can change the configuration of the scar from worrisome and masslike to reassuring linear. Recurrent carcinoma, on the other hand, appears nodular or masslike regardless of the angle of incidence. Split-screen images performed with and without compression are also helpful because the angular lipid fluid collections that outline the surgical cavity are usually not tense. (Tense lipid cysts would compress the walls of the surgical defect into a spherical or oval shape.) Instead, they are soft and easily compressed, despite their worrisome angular shape. Irregularly shaped recurrent carcinoma, on the other hand, is not compressible. The principles are the same as for seromas and hematomas and have been discussed and illustrated earlier.

In some cases, scanning the lumpectomy site parallel and perpendicular to the scar, angling the transducer, and evaluating with compression are not definitive enough to aid in the distinction between fat necrosis and recurrent tumor (Fig. 11–114A). In such cases, color Doppler can be used to help distinguish an irregularly shaped lipid cyst that lies within a biopsy defect from recurrent tumor. Fat necrosis, by definition, is avascular and therefore has no demonstrable internal blood flow when evaluated with color or power Doppler (Fig. 11–114B). A recurrent tumor nodule, on the other hand, often has enough internal

blood flow that it can be shown by color or power Doppler (Fig. 11–115). There are two *caveats*. The first is that some recurrent tumor nodules may not have Doppler-demonstrable blood flow, so that a negative Doppler study is not as useful as a positive. The second is that a healing surgical scar may form granulation tissue that has demonstrable flow. This process is usually complete by 6 months after surgery. Additionally, radiation treatments performed in the months after surgery may temporarily cause some hyperemia-related radiation mastitis. Thus, Doppler tends to be less helpful in evaluating the wound site in the first 6 months after surgery in patients who have not had radiation therapy but for a few months longer in patients who have had radiation as well as surgery.

Very late in the fat necrosis process, fibrosis may become the dominant pathologic process. The sonographic appearance of severe fibrosis can be very worrisome on sonography. In the most severe cases, it can cause angular, markedly hyperechoic, spiculated, intensely shadowing lesions that are sonographically indistinguishable from scirrhous carcinoma (Fig. 11–116). Severe fibrotic changes are most likely to develop in patients who have had postlumpectomy radiation and are also more likely to develop in patients who had large hematomas in the immediate postoperative period. Angulation and compression are not helpful in distinguishing between the fibrous phase of fat necrosis and recurrent tumor, but as is the case for angular lipid cysts, Doppler may be of use. Additionally, spot

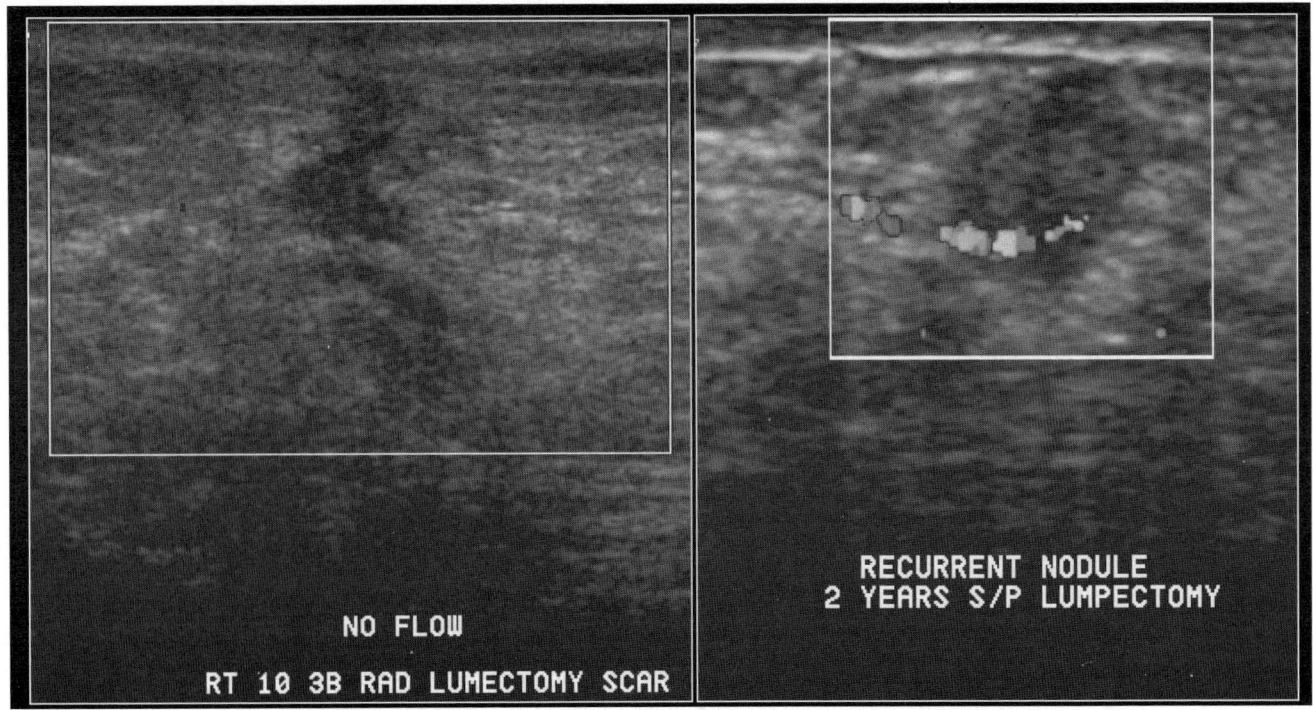

FIGURE 11–115 This figure shows a solid nodule resulting from fibrous phase of fat necrosis to be avascular (**left**), whereas a small solid nodule caused by recurrent tumor in the chest wall to have internal blood flow (**right**).

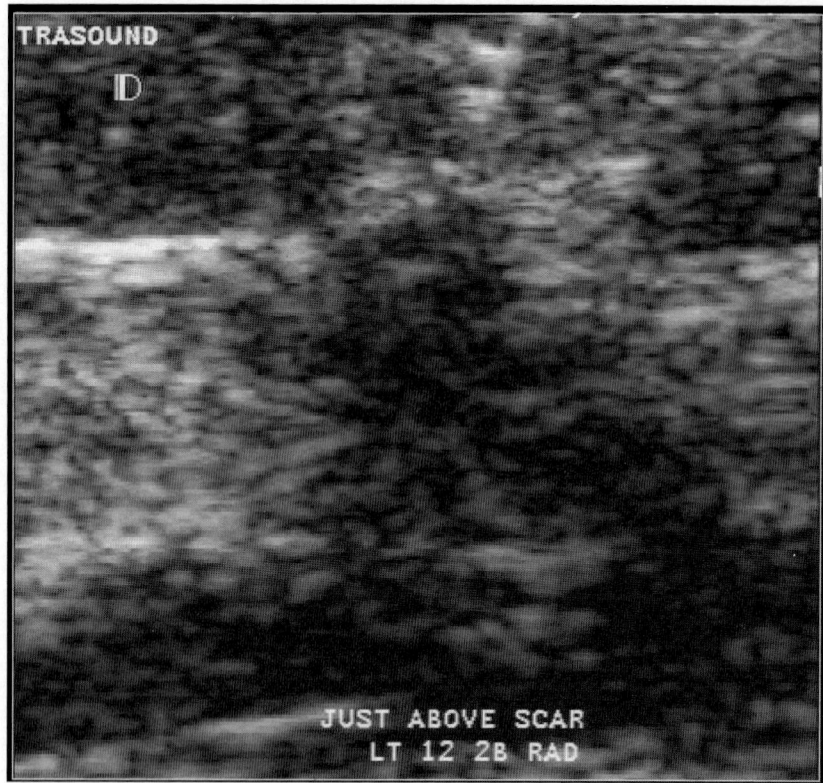

FIGURE 11–116 In the end stages of fat necrosis, fibrosis may be so severe that it causes spiculation on both mammograms and on sonograms. In such cases, spot compression mammography may be more useful than sonography because it may be capable of showing definitive evidence of associated lipid cysts that sonography cannot show.

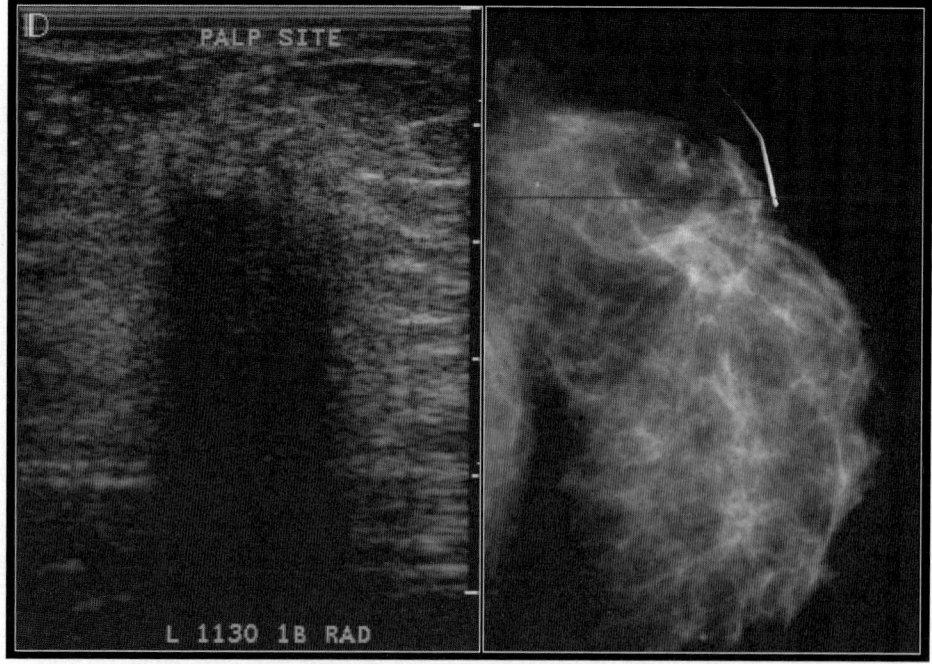

FIGURE 11–117 The intensely shadowing, markedly hypoechoic, angular lesion on ultrasound is caused by the dense fibrous phase of fat necrosis. The sonographic findings are very worrisome for recurrent tumor. The mammograms, however, show the spiculated lesion to lie along the inferior edge of a large lipid cyst. Review of serial mammograms showed slowly retracting scar over about 4 years, but no new developing density. The mammographic findings were more suggestive of fat necrosis than were the sonographic findings because serial studies were available showing no developing density and because mammography showed a lipid cyst closely associated with the spiculation.

compression mammograms may be reassuring. The severe fibrotic phase of fat necrosis often does not occur alone. It is accompanied by edema and lipid cyst formation. The lipid cysts may have an irregular shape that contributes to the worrisome findings produced by fibrosis sonographically. However, mammography will show the definitively benign lipid or oil cysts surrounding the spiculated central scar, suggesting the diagnosis of fat necrosis (Fig. 11–117).

MONDOR'S DISEASE: ACUTE SUPERFICIAL THROMBOSIS OF BREAST VEINS

Thrombosis of superficial breast veins is not truly a cystic condition of the breast, but acute thrombus may be nearly anechoic and may simulate a cystic condition of the breast. Venous thrombosis is a vascular condition that can affect vessels in any part of the body, not just the breast.

General Pathologic Classification, Epidemiology, and Clinical Findings

Mondor's disease is a rare disorder in which superficial veins within the subcutaneous breast tissues thrombose. In most cases, there is a history of breast surgery or direct trauma to the area. Seat-belt injuries to the breast are among the most common of causes. In other cases, there is a history of severe exertion and dehydration. Superficial thrombosis may occur spontaneously during pregnancy. Underlying breast cancer has been reported in up to 12% of cases, but we believe associated breast cancer is much less common. Mondor's disease has also been seen in patients with central venous pressure catheters, especially if the internal mammary vein is accidentally catheterized. We have also seen spontaneous thrombosis of venous malformations of the breast. Mondor's disease can occur in males as well as in females.

The vein most commonly thrombosed is the thoracoepigastric vein, which courses from the inferomedial aspect of the breast toward the axilla. (Interestingly, the shoulder harness component of seat belts closely parallels the course of this vein.) The vein second most commonly involved is the lateral thoracic vein, which courses from the lateral aspect of the breast to the axilla. However, in patients in whom Mondor's disease is a complication of central venous pressure lines, the veins in the medial aspect of the breast that drain into the internal mammary vein are involved.

Patients with acute Mondor's disease usually present with pain, tenderness, and a generally linear area of skin erythema. There is often a tender palpable cord rather than a palpable nodule. However, because the thrombosed vein is usually tortuous and varies in caliber and is unevenly thrombosed, the palpable abnormality may be a tortuous row of small nodules that has been described as a "string of beads." In very severe cases, the inflammatory reaction around the acutely thrombosed vein may cause retraction and dimpling that may be noticeable only in the upright position. Although the acute clinical findings would appear to be definitive enough to allow diagnosis without imaging, there are several reasons that the imaging specialist often first suggests the diagnosis. First, Mondor's disease is rare enough that most primary care clinicians will personally never have seen a case before and will not suspect the diagnosis. Second, the patient often does not present in the acute phase immediately after trauma. Instead, the patient presents a few weeks later, when the history of trauma has been forgotten, the acute signs of trauma and inflammation have resolved, and only a palpable abnormality remains. By this time, there may have been partial recanalization of the thrombosed vein so that the classic palpable cord or string of beads abnormality is no longer present. Finally, to minimize the number of physician visits, patients with breast complaints are often referred directly to a breast-imaging center before being seen by the clinician.

The natural history of Mondor's disease is for the thrombosed vein to recanalize and for the clinical findings to resolve gradually and spontaneously. Low-dose aspirin may accelerate recanalization.

Mammographic Findings

Mammograms are usually negative. In cases in which the thrombosed vein is not obscured by overlying dense tissue, an abnormally prominent vein may be visible—usually a tortuous tubular or beaded structure projecting through the subcutaneous fat. When the diagnosis of Mondor's disease is suspected clinically, the possibility of obtaining adequate demonstration mammographically is improved by performing tangential views. However, because most cases are not suspected clinically before mammography, additional diagnostic views are usually not obtained. Instead, most patients with Mondor's disease are referred to sonography for targeted evaluation of pain or a palpable abnormality.

Sonographic Findings

Although Mondor's disease does not produce either a cyst or a solid breast nodule in the strictest sense, the thrombosed breast vein can appear to be a cyst or an abnormally enlarged mammary duct to the sonographer who does not suspect the correct diagnosis.

Normal superficial breast veins course through the subcutaneous fat just deep to the skin. They can be completely collapsed with transducer pressure (Fig. 11–118). In fact, they are so soft and compressible that they often are completely collapsed during scanning with normal compression pressure. They also have spontaneous flow with

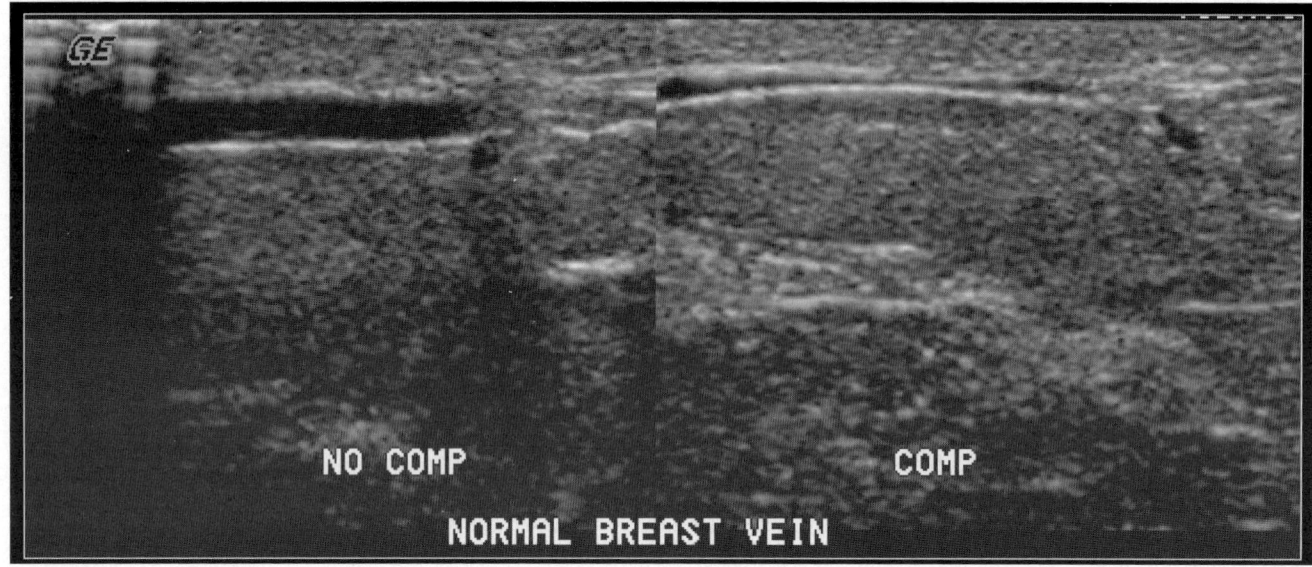

FIGURE 11–118 Normal breast veins course superficially through the subcutaneous fat, just deep to the skin, and are soft and completely collapsible with transducer compression **(right)**; the vein is open when scanned with very light scan pressure.

respiratory variation that is demonstrable on color (see Chapter 20, Fig. 20–69) or power Doppler (Fig. 11–119).

In short axis, the acutely thrombosed vein appears rounded, nearly anechoic, and cystic. It is important to scan in the long axis in order to appreciate that the structure is tubular (Fig. 11–120). Long-axis views of the thrombosed vein may show a tubular or beaded shape (Fig. 11–121). As is always the case in peripheral venous thrombosis, compression sonography and Doppler are the key to determining that the vein is clotted and not merely distended. The acute clot is incompressible (Fig. 11–122), and there is no Doppler-demonstrable flow, even with augmentation (Fig. 11–123). The beading appearance is likely due to tortuosity of the thrombosed vein and corresponds clinically to the palpable "string of pearls." The diameter of the clot frequently varies over the length of the thrombosed segment. Areas of older, retracted thrombus appear narrower, more tubular, and more echogenic, whereas areas of more acute thrombus appear wider, more beaded, and more nearly anechoic. Near-field volume averaging of perivascular tissue

(text continued on page 433)

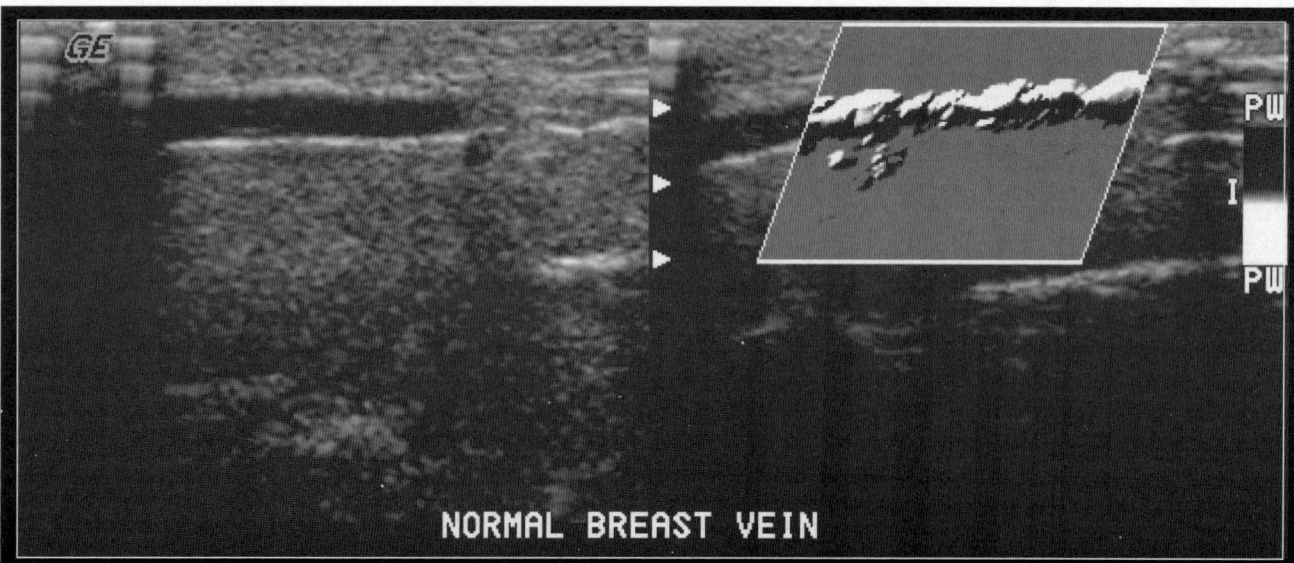

FIGURE 11–119 Blood flow is demonstrable in normal superficial breast veins with power Doppler using a variety of maps. This is a gray-scale topographic map.

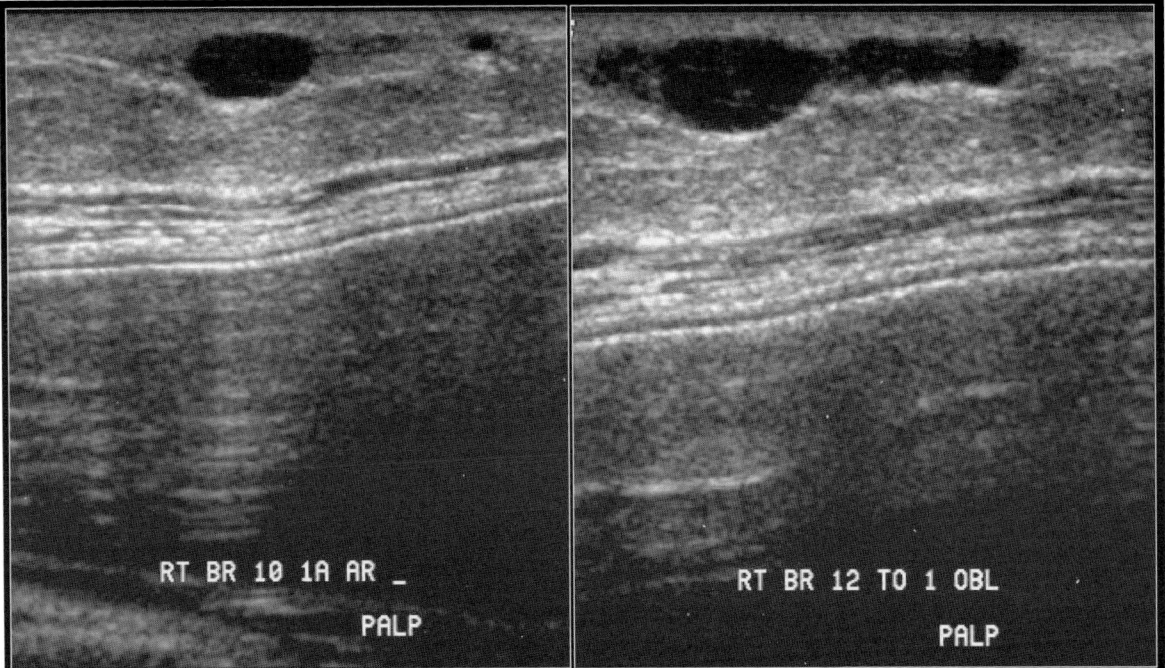

FIGURE 11–120 Acutely thrombosed superficial breast veins (Mondor's disease) are markedly hypoechoic. In short axis, an acutely thrombosed vein may simulate a breast or skin cyst (**left**). In long axis, the tubular nature of the structure is evident, but it might still be mistaken for a dilated duct (**right**). That mistake should not be made, however, because acutely thrombosed veins do not have a radial distribution relative to the nipple and almost always lie within the subcutaneous fat, rather than within the mammary zone, where the mammary ducts lie.

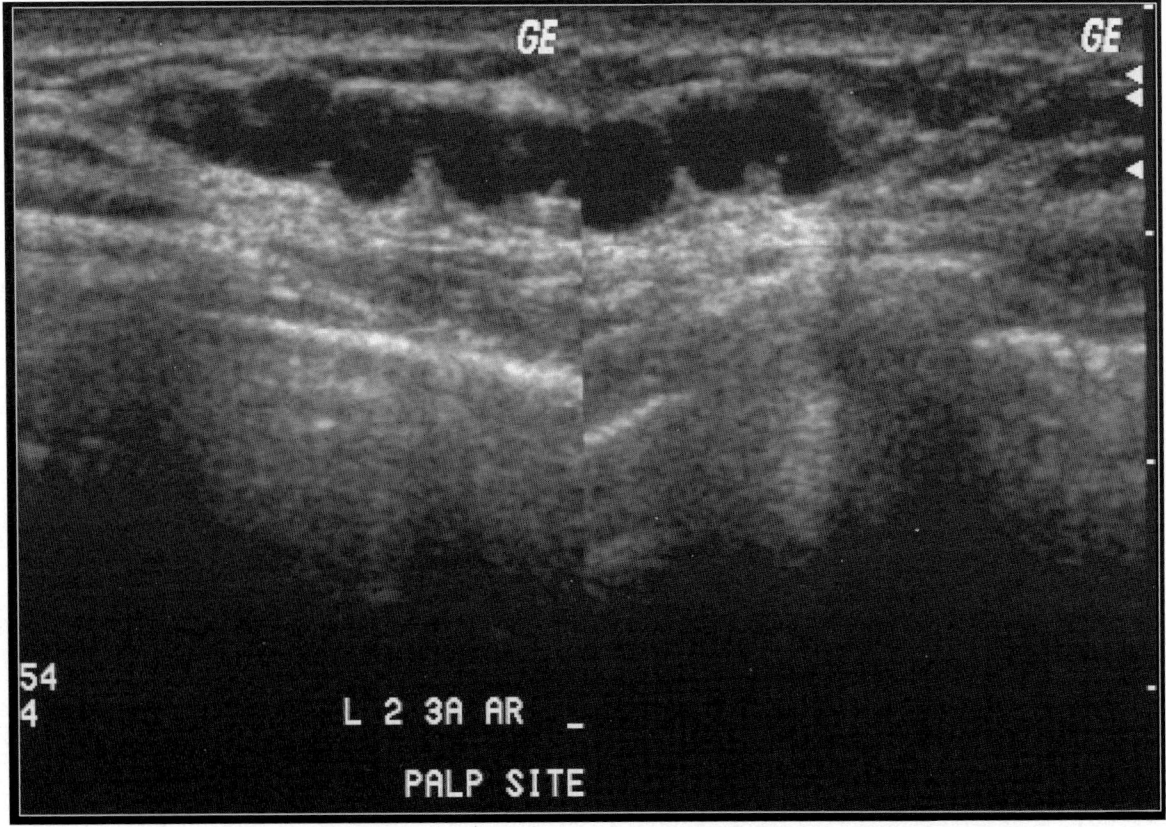

FIGURE 11–121 Acutely thrombosed superficial breast veins usually have a beaded appearance. This could be related to tortuosity; it is less likely to be associated with valves because the lobulations are too close together.

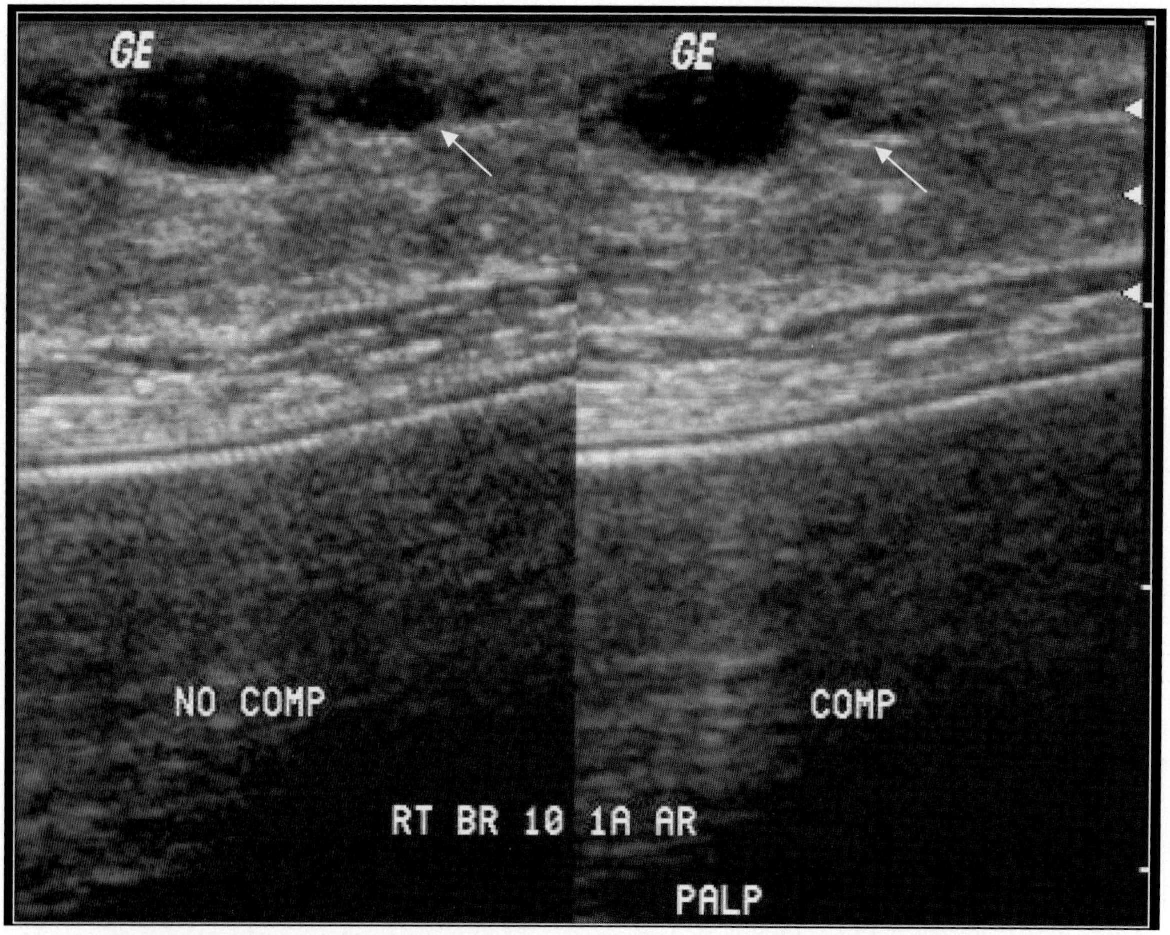

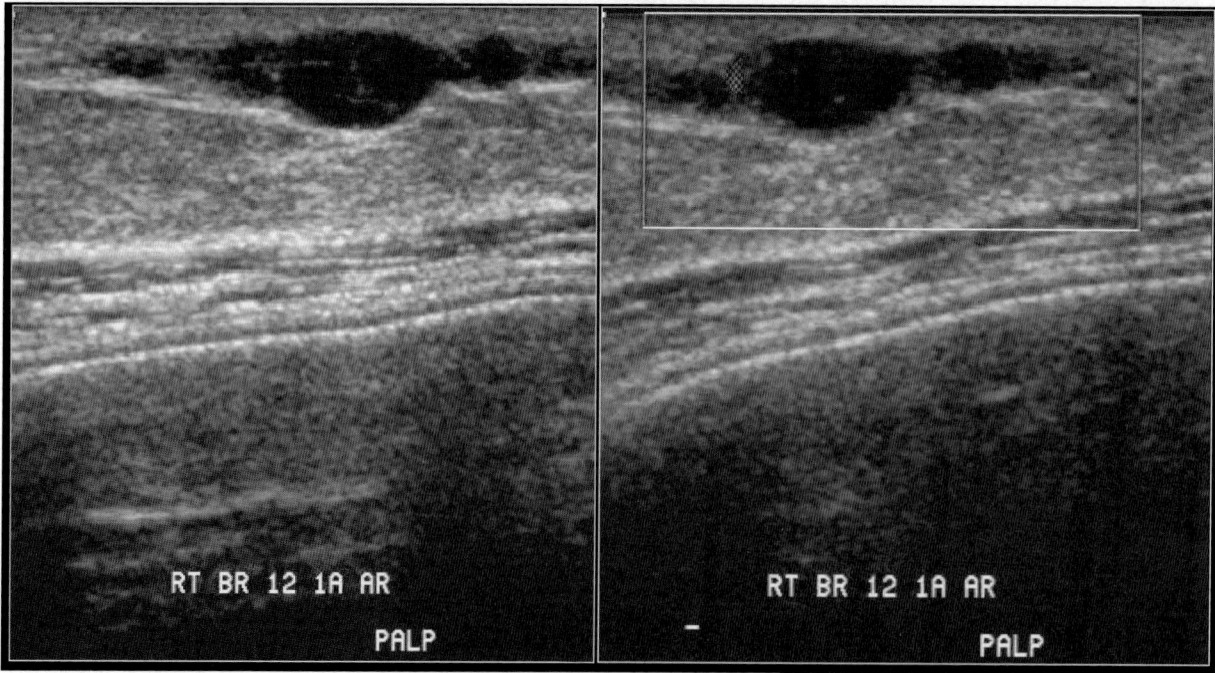

FIGURE 11–122 The two signs of acute thrombosis for veins anywhere in the body are incompressibility and lack of flow on color Doppler. This acutely thrombosed and completely occluded vein *(*)* is incompressible. The small tributary vein next to the main acutely thrombosed vein is partially compressible, indicating partial thrombosis *(arrows)*.

FIGURE 11–123 This acutely thrombosed superficial breast vein has no blood flow on color Doppler, indicating that the thrombus is completely occlusive.

with the clotted vein may contribute to the narrow segments appearing more echogenic (Fig. 11–124). In some cases, the older thrombus retracts so much and becomes so echogenic that it can no longer be distinguished from surrounding tissues, leaving a series of short segments of acutely clotted vein separated by what appears to be normal breast tissues (Fig. 11–125). The thrombus may extend into tributary veins, showing a branching pattern. The course of the thrombosed vein is variable but most often corresponds to that of the thoracoepigastric vein or lateral thoracic vein (parallel to the shoulder strap of a seat belt). The inferior mammary fold is so often involved that we question whether underwire bras might not also be a contributing factor. Mondor's disease usually involves veins that lie just deep to the skin, but it can involve more deeply lying veins (Fig. 11–126). Thrombosis of deep breast veins usually represents extension of thrombus in the axillary, subclavian, or internal mammary veins into collateral veins that have developed in the breast. Thus, thrombosis of breast veins that are more deeply located within the breast is likely to indicate a more serious underlying venous problem that is often a complication of peripherally inserted central catheter or central venous pressure lines.

Although identification of vein valves has not been reported, the widened areas should represent the thrombus with the lumen proximal to valves of origin, and the narrower areas should represent the nonthrombosed lumen distal to valves, similar to thrombosis of other peripheral veins. The hypoechoic thrombus within the vein lumen should not be mistaken for tumor or inspissated secretions within breast ducts. First, the thrombosed vein is virtually always within the subcutaneous fat, superficial to the mammary zone and therefore superficial to the location of major breast ducts. Additionally, the thrombosed veins in Mondor's disease are not radially oriented with respect to the nipple as are ectatic ducts.

Over time, the thrombosed vein becomes more difficult to identify sonographically. The hyperechoic perivenous edema associated with acute thrombosis helps make hypoechoic acute clot more conspicuous. As times passes, the edema subsides, the perivenous fat becomes less echogenic, and the clot retracts and becomes more echogenic. All of these changes make the chronically thrombosed vein much more difficult to demonstrate sonographically (Fig. 11–127). Chronic Mondor's disease that is still faintly palpable as a nontender cord may become invisible sonographically. In other cases, clot dissolves, and the vein gradually recanalizes.

Because the veins involved by Mondor's disease are typically so superficial, diagnosis presents severe near-field volume averaging problems for sonography, even with very-high-frequency transducers. Using a standoff pad or a standoff of acoustic gel or a 1.5-dimensional array transducer facilitates diagnosis in most patients.

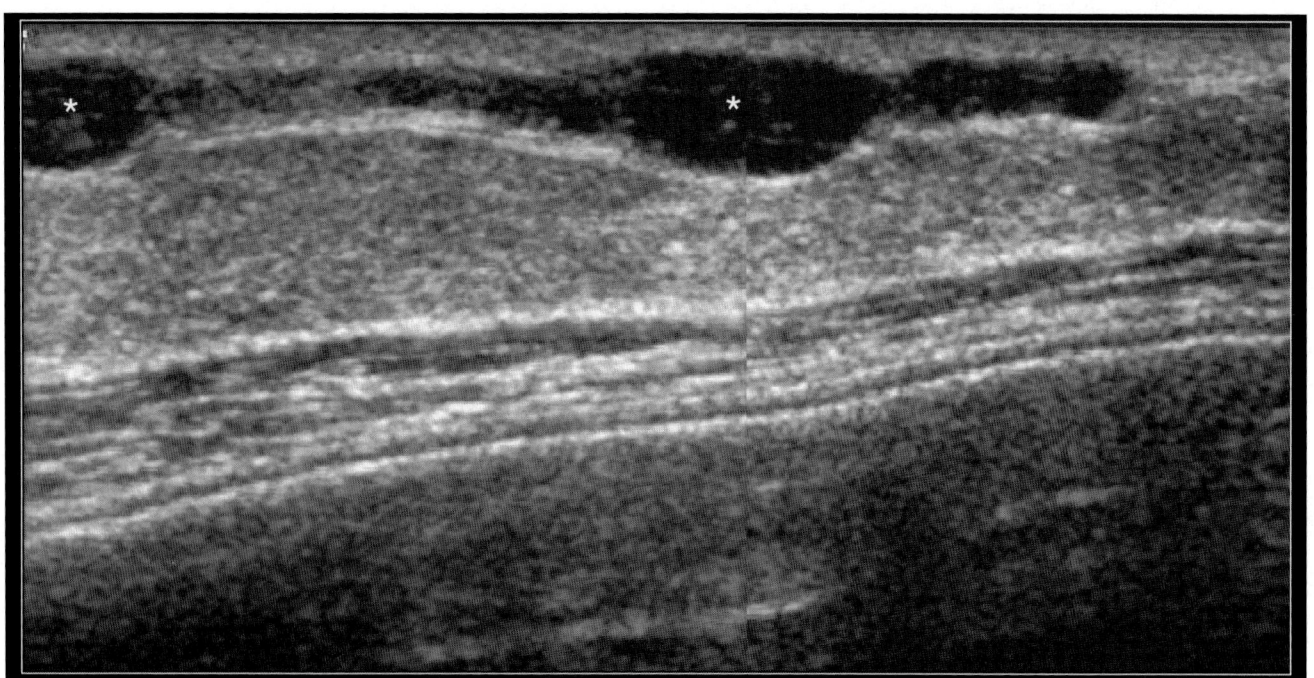

FIGURE 11–124 The degree of venous distention can vary, especially if the process of thrombosis is ongoing. In areas where clot is more acute (*), the clot is more nearly anechoic, the lumen is more distended, and the shape is more beaded. In portions of the vein where the clot is older and retracted, the vein is more echogenic, more tubular in shape, and less distended.

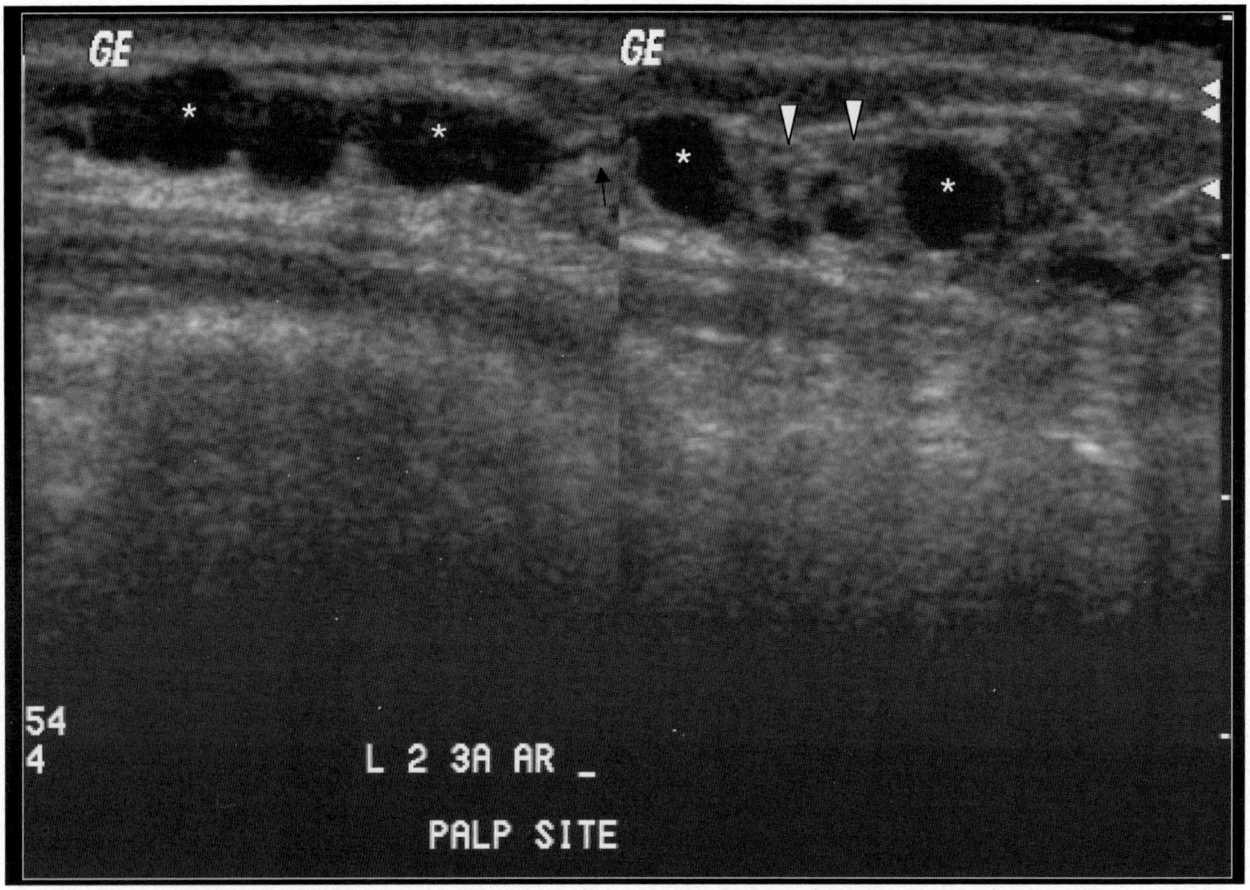

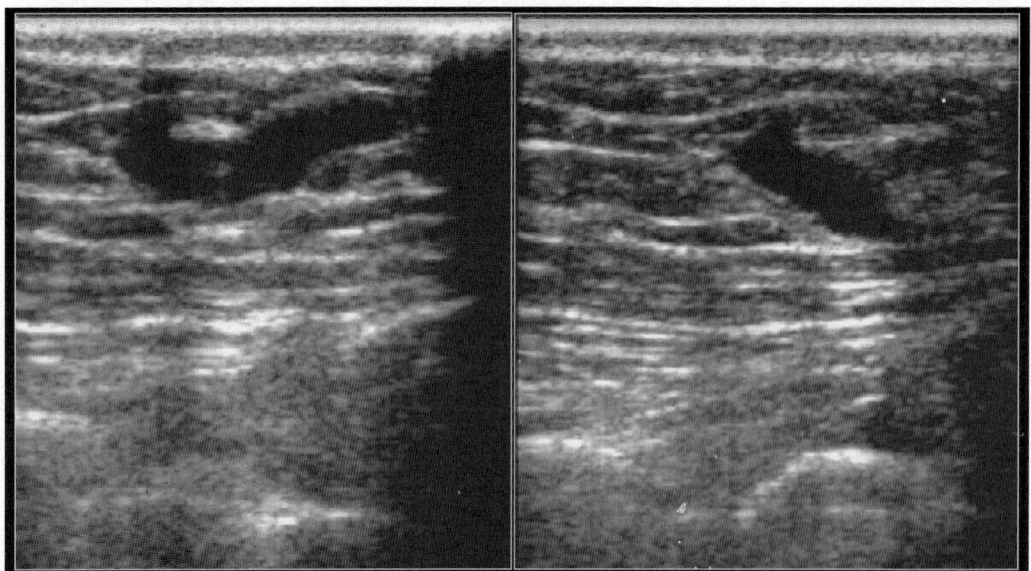

FIGURE 11–125 In certain cases of superficial venous thromboses, the acute thrombotic process (*) appears to be segmental. Generally, no flow is demonstrable between the acutely clotted and distended segments, suggesting that old clot has obliterated these segments *(arrowheads)*. In other cases, the vein is severely retracted and barely visible between the acute clots *(arrow)*. Segmental thromboses such as these are responsible for the clinical finding of a palpable "string of pearls."

FIGURE 11–126 Occasionally, acute thrombosis involves more deeply located veins within the breast. In such cases, the thrombus is usually an extension thrombosis that involves either the internal mammary vein or axillary vein. The vessels may represent collaterals that have developed in the breast in order to bypass thromboses in more central veins that have secondarily thrombosed. The thrombosed deep vein in the axillary segment of the left breast in this case was a collateral that developed around an axillary vein thrombosis. Thrombus had propagated from the axillary vein into the collateral veins passing through the breast.

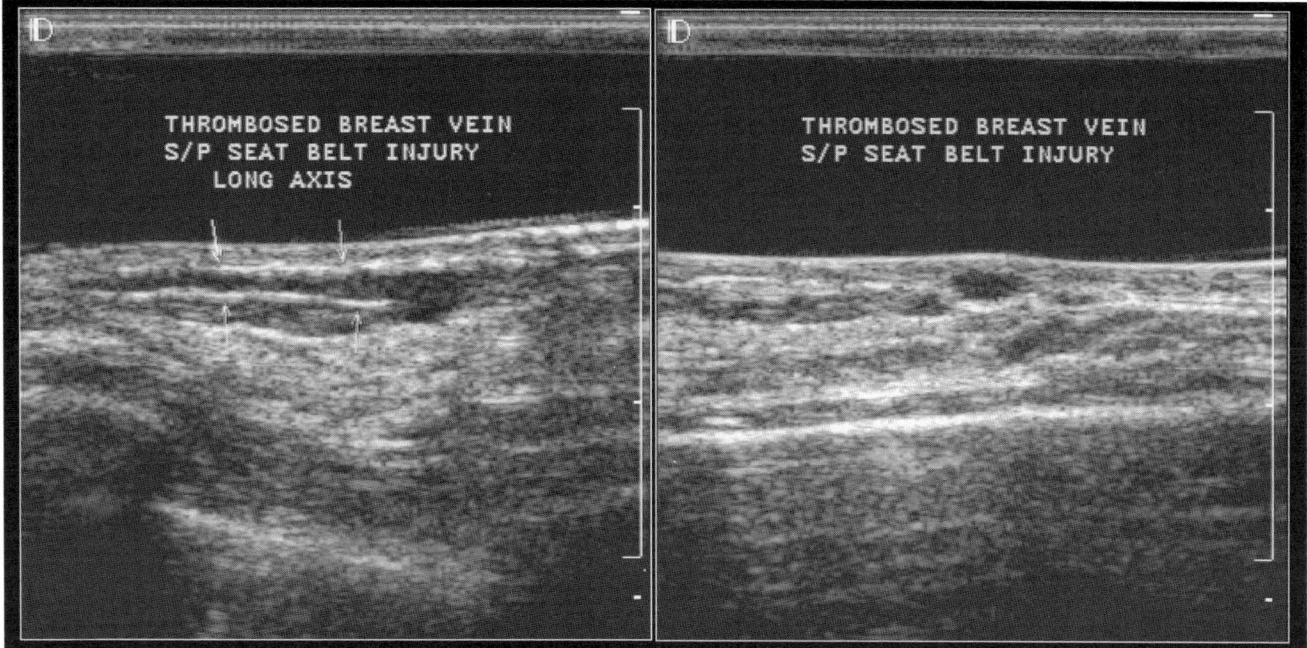

FIGURE 11–127 This chronically thrombosed, superficial breast vein is isoechoic rather than hypoechoic or nearly anechoic. As the clot retracts, it becomes more echogenic, smaller, and less beaded in appearance. Some superficial veins completely recanalize, some partially recanalize, but most remain thrombosed. Breast veins have lower flow requirements than lower extremity veins and are less likely to recanalize. This patient had suffered a seat-belt injury about 6 weeks earlier that had caused her superficial venous thrombosis.

The importance of Mondor's disease to the sonographer is that the process is usually a benign, self-limited condition that requires neither biopsy nor excision if the correct diagnosis can be suggested. On the other hand, if the diagnosis of Mondor's disease is not suspected, biopsy will likely be required. Mondor's disease may be mistaken for more suspicious superficially located pathology. However, even when the sonographic diagnosis of Mondor's disease is correctly suggested, thorough scanning of the involved areas of the breast is important because it has been reported that up to 12% of cases of Mondor's disease are associated with occult malignancy.

HEMANGIOMAS AND VENOUS MALFORMATIONS OF THE BREAST

Like Mondor's disease, breast hemangiomas and venous malformations are not truly cystic conditions of the breast. In fact, capillary hemangiomas appear solid and are usually hyperechoic with respect to fat. However, cavernous hemangiomas and venous malformations that involve the breast may be mistaken for cystic conditions that arise from breast tissue. Furthermore, venous malformations are prone to spontaneous thrombosis and, when thrombosed, are indistinguishable from Mondor's disease.

General Pathologic Classification, Epidemiology, and Clinical Findings

Hemangiomas are usually very small, clinically inapparent, and incidental findings at histology. However, larger hemangiomas may present as nonpalpable mammographic nodules. Small, microscopically detectable, perilobular hemangiomas are almost always incidental findings at histology. These lesions are relatively common, occurring in about 5% of benign biopsies and in up to 11% of autopsy studies. Perilobular hemangiomas are smaller than one low-power microscopic field and are generally imperceptible on clinical and imaging studies. Despite the name "perilobular," most of these lesions are intralobular. The major significance of perilobular hemangiomas to pathologists is that these vascular tumors may be difficult to distinguish from low-grade angiosarcomas histologically, especially if there is any endothelial atypia. Perilobular hemangiomas are usually less than 2 mm in maximum diameter, whereas clinically detected angiosarcomas are almost always larger than 3 cm in diameter.

Macroscopic hemangiomas are larger than 4 mm but usually less than 2 cm in diameter and rarely palpable. These lesions can present as mammographic masses and therefore necessitate ultrasound evaluation. The tumors can be classified as cavernous or capillary, depending on the size of vessels contained within. Cavernous hemangiomas and mixed cavernous and capillary hemangiomas are both more common than pure capillary hemangiomas. In fact, most cavernous hemangiomas of the breast also contain areas of capillary-sized vessels within them.

Unlike perilobular hemangiomas, which occur within the parenchyma (mammary zone), most macroscopic hematomas lie superficial to the mammary zone within the subcutaneous tissues. Thus, similar to hemangiomas that occur within the subcutaneous fat anywhere in the body, they can be thought of as lesions of the skin.

At gross pathology, hemangiomas are dark, reddish to brown in color, and relatively soft and spongy. These masses are usually well circumscribed, although certain lesions may have peripheral vessels that grow into surrounding normal soft tissues.

The diagnosis of hemangioma is not possible with fine-needle aspiration biopsy but can be made with large core needle biopsy or mammotomy as well as excisional biopsy.

Venous malformations are postcapillary vascular malformations that have slow flow and show no evidence of arteriovenous shunting. The slow flow makes these lesions prone to spontaneous thrombosis. Venous malformations may involve any venous system in the body and therefore may involve the veins of the breast. Most of the large breast veins course rather superficially through the subcutaneous fat. Therefore, most venous malformations of the breast, like larger hemangiomas, involve the subcutaneous fat rather than the mammary zone. Similar to lymphatic malformations (cystic hygromas, lymphangioma), venous malformations of the breast frequently involve the axillary area.

Mammographic Findings

Perilobular hemangiomas are not visible mammographically. Occasionally, a macroscopic cavernous or capillary hemangioma may cause a mammographic nodule. These lesions are low to medium density, round or lobulated in shape, with a circumscribed margin. Hemangiomas may contain calcifications that are, in essence, phleboliths. However, because the channels are irregular in shape, the calcifications usually do not have the classic rounded shapes expected with phleboliths forms in other parts of the body. Instead, the phleboliths associated with hemangiomas are usually amorphous or granular in appearance.

Venous malformations may cause findings similar to cavernous hemangiomas. However, because the venous malformations are so frequently located within the axillary area, they are difficult to demonstrate mammographically.

Sonographic Findings

Perilobular hemangiomas are not identifiable sonographically. The sonographic appearance of macroscopic heman-

giomas depends on the size of the vessels contained within and the presence or absence of fibrosis, scarring, thrombosis, or phleboliths.

Pure capillary hemangiomas do not appear to be cystic at all. In fact, pure capillary hemangiomas have a solid, hyperechoic appearance very similar to that of hemangiomas of the liver (Fig. 11–128). The margins are sharply defined and the sound transmission is normal or increased. The shape of capillary hemangiomas of the breast is more elliptical than that of liver hemangiomas, however, because soft, compressible breast hemangiomas are invariably mildly to moderately flattened in the anteroposterior dimension by transducer pressure. Split-screen images with and without compression pressure can be helpful in distinguishing soft hemangiomas from firmer focal fibrosis, which can have an identical ellipsoid uniformly hyperechoic appearance (Fig. 11–129).

Cavernous hemangiomas may be mildly hypoechoic, isoechoic, or mildly hyperechoic and are usually heterogeneous in texture. The lesion is composed of vessel lumina, which are hypoechoic, and vessel walls, which are hyperechoic. The dominant lesion echogenicity will depend on size of the vascular channels. The larger the channels, the more hypoechoic the lesion will appear. The vessel lumina

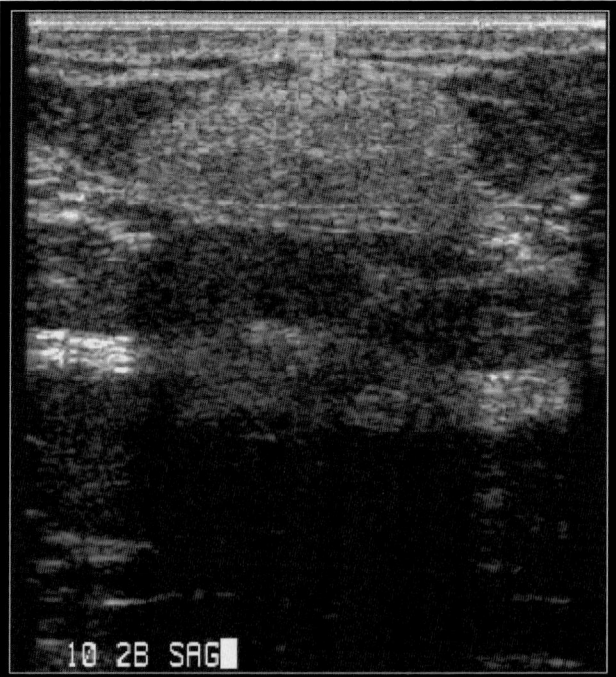

FIGURE 11–128 Capillary hemangiomas appear to be hyperechoic solid nodules rather than cysts. They usually lie within the subcutaneous fat and can be thought of as skin lesions rather than breast lesions. The appearance is similar to that of liver hemangiomas except that breast hemangiomas are typically oval because the transducer compresses them in the anteroposterior dimension.

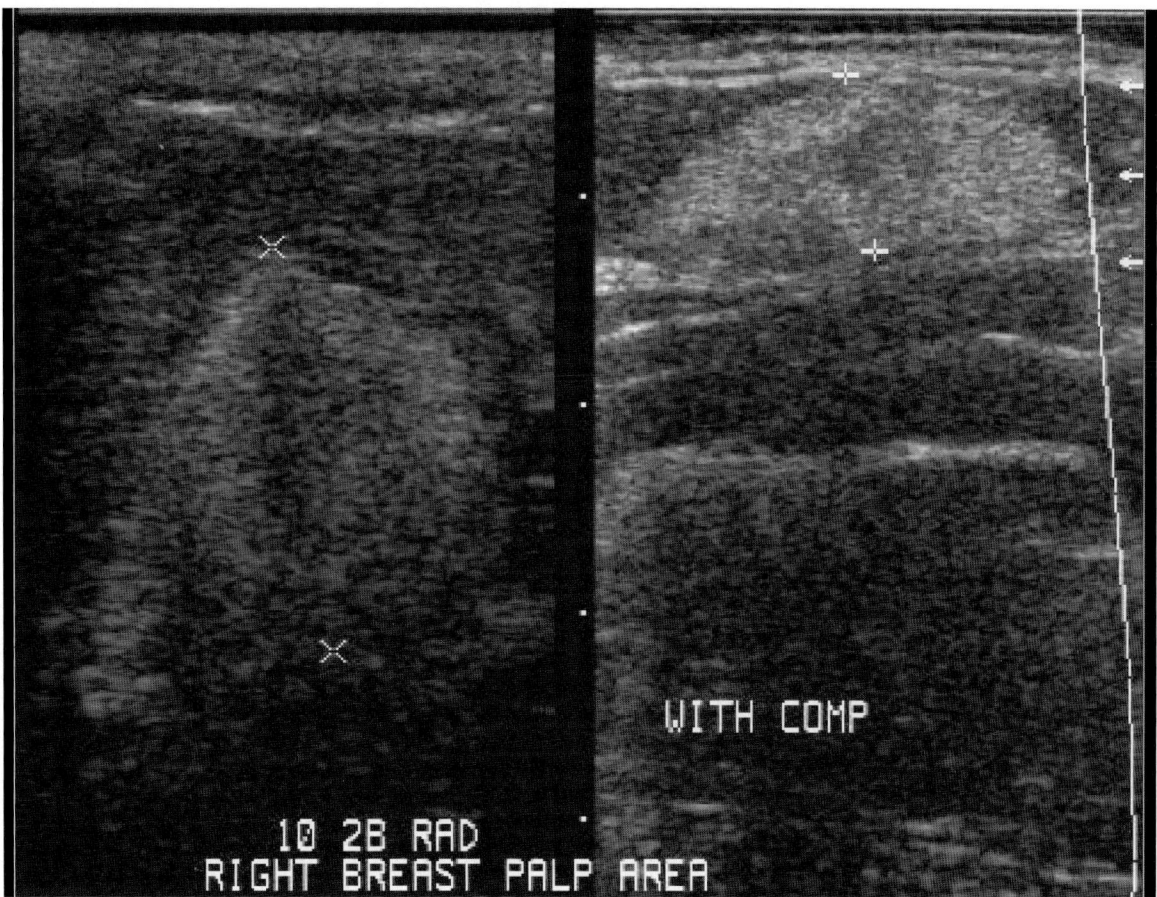

FIGURE 11–129 Despite their rigid solid appearance, capillary hemangiomas of the breast are quite soft and compressible. The more they are compressed, the more echogenic they become, and the better the sound transmission. Flow within capillary hemangiomas is too little and too slow to show with color or power Doppler.

are nearly anechoic, and the vessel walls are echogenic (Fig. 11–130). If vessel channels are large, the echogenic walls are widely spaced, and the dominant echogenicity of the lesion is that of the vessel channels—hypoechoic. On the other hand, the smaller the vascular channels, the more echogenic the lesion will be. If vessels are very small, the echogenic vessel walls will be very close together and will create the dominant echogenicity of the lesion—echogenic. The size of vascular channels is often nonuniform and may vary throughout the lesion, causing heterogeneous texture. Color or power Doppler is helpful in showing that the hypoechoic spaces within the lesion are venous channels and in excluding secondary spontaneous thrombosis of venous channels (see Chapter 20, Fig. 20–72). Flow within the lesion may be so slow that compression augmentation is necessary to demonstrate it (see Chapter 20, Fig. 20–74). Phleboliths will appear as areas of markedly increased echogenicity that may or may not shadow, depending on the diameter of the calcification relative to the beam width. Phleboliths may occur centrally within the lesion, where they are surrounded by patent vascular channels, or they may occur at the periphery of the lesion, where all of the surrounding vessels are chronically thrombosed and difficult or impossible to demonstrate sonographically (Fig. 11–131). In the latter circumstance, the phlebolith may have sonographic characteristics that are identical to those of eggshell calcifications in oil cysts.

The dilated veins within venous malformations may be quite large. Individual channels may reach 1 cm or more in size, and these vascular structures may be clustered, simulating a cluster of cysts. The veins are soft and completely compressible if not thrombosed (Fig. 11–132). Similar to the case for cavernous hemangiomas, spontaneous flow within venous malformations is usually so slow that augmentation is necessary to demonstrate it with color or power Doppler. Flow can be augmented by manually compressing portions of the malformation that do not lie directly under the transducer or by ballottement of the malformation with the transducer. The venous channels within venous malformations, like those of hemangiomas, are large enough to form sonographically visible phleboliths.

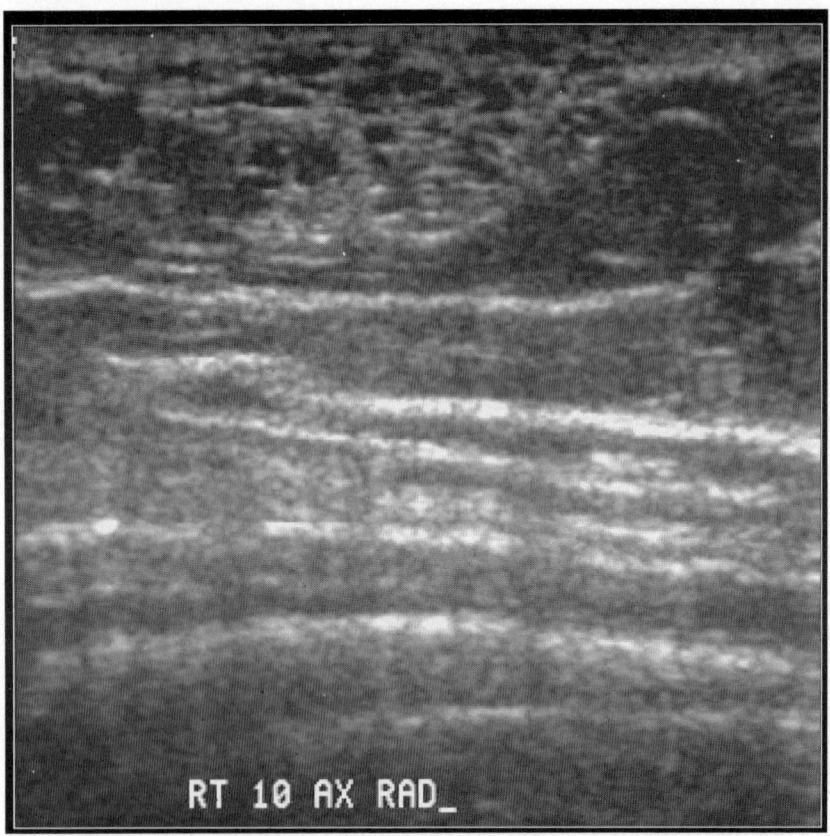

RT 10 AX RAD_

FIGURE 11–130 Cavernous hemangiomas have a complex cystic appearance. The echogenicity depends on the size of the vascular channels. The larger the channels and the farther apart the hyperechoic vessel walls, the more hypoechoic the lesion appears. On the other hand, the smaller the channels and the larger component of the lesion composed of hyperechoic vessel walls, the more echogenic the lesion. These lesions are also quite compressible. Compression of the lesion with the transducer pushes the hyperechoic vessel walls closer together and makes the whole lesion appear more echogenic. Compression may be useful for augmenting the slow flow within the lesion and assessing venous channels for spontaneous thrombosis, which is relatively common because of the slow flow within the lesion.

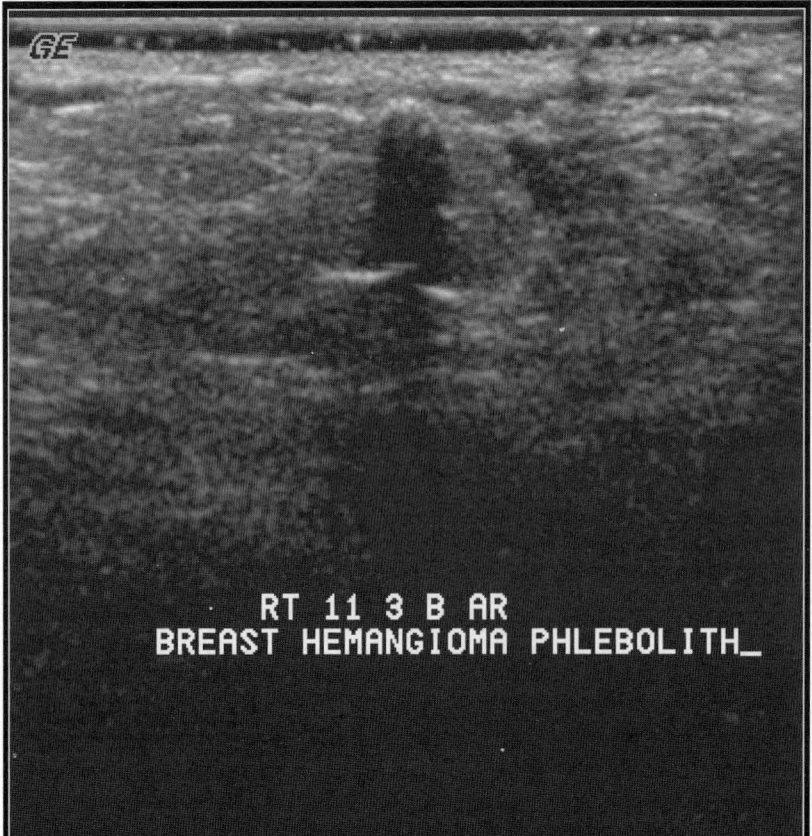

RT 11 3 B AR
BREAST HEMANGIOMA PHLEBOLITH_

FIGURE 11–131 The thrombi that result from spontaneous thrombosis within cavernous hemangiomas may calcify and form phleboliths. Sonographically, phleboliths are circular, intensely shadowing calcifications that are identical in their features to the far more commonly seen eggshell calcifications in oil cysts. Only if the calcification can be shown to be associated with a cavernous hemangioma can it be assumed to be a much less common phlebolith.

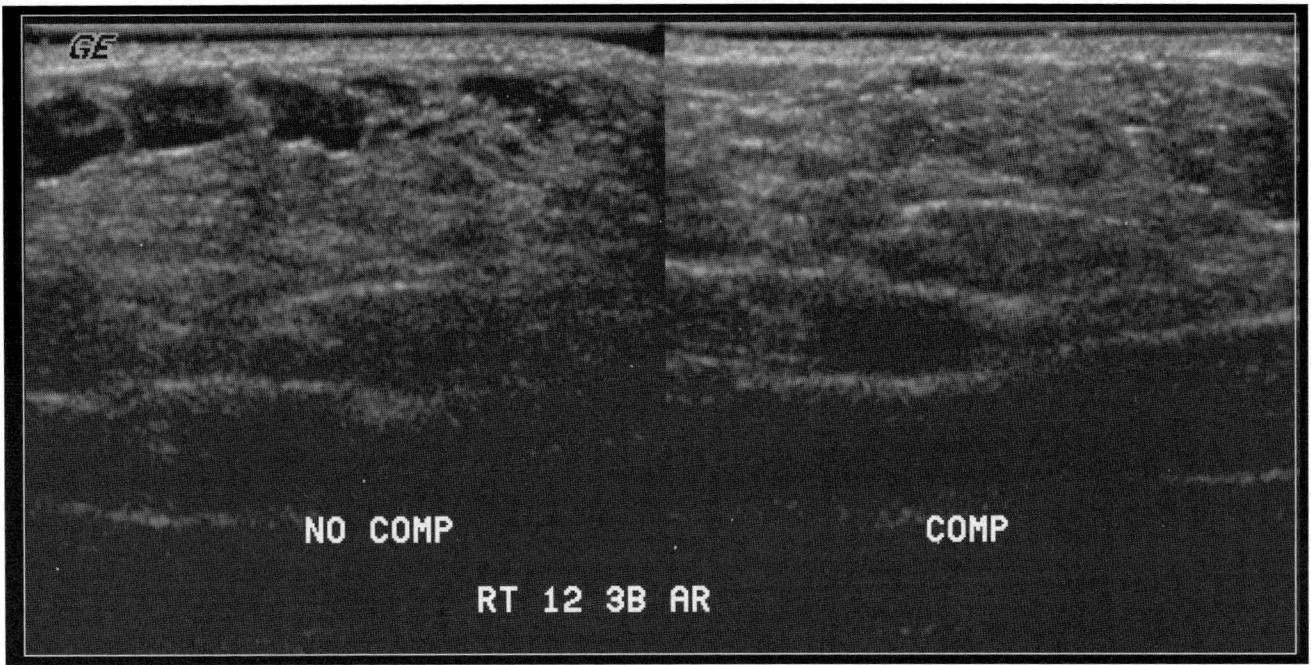

FIGURE 11–132 Venous malformations differ from hemangiomas. Hemangiomas are benign vascular tumors, whereas venous malformations are simply malformations of veins. The entire malformation is postcapillary; hence, there is no associated arteriovenous shunting, and flow is slow, not rapid. The abnormal veins in nonthrombosed venous malformations are abnormally dilated and tortuous **(left)**, are invariably incompetent, and like normal veins, can be completely collapsed with transducer pressure **(right)**. Venous malformations can occur in any venous system within the body, but in breast, like lymphatic malformations, they are most common in the axillary region. The abnormal veins in this lesion drained to the axilla.

LYMPHANGIOMAS (LYMPHATIC MALFORMATIONS, CYSTIC HYGROMA)

Like venous malformations, lymphatic malformations or lymphangiomas most commonly occur within the axillary area. Lymphangiomas are most frequent in infants but can be seen in adults. Fetal and infant cystic hygromas are lymphangiomas. The axilla is the second most likely site for development of lymphangiomas after the neck. Like hemangiomas and venous malformations, lymphangiomas are not truly breast lesions but rather are lymphatic disorders that happen to have occurred in the area of the breast. The dilated lymphatic channels within a lymphangioma may be mistaken for cysts or dilated ducts that can occur within accessory breast tissue in the axilla.

Mammographic Findings

The findings in lymphangiomas are nonspecific. Because of the frequent location high in the axilla it may not be possible to image these lesions adequately using mammography. Additionally, many occur in infants, in whom it is desirable to avoid radiation if possible. When visible, the mammographic appearance of lymphangiomas is similar to that of hemangiomas and venous malformations—usually dilated, tortuous vessels within the subcutaneous fat.

Sonographic Findings

Lymphangiomas have a sonographic appearance similar to a cluster of simple cysts or dilated ducts. However, the echogenicity, like that of hemangiomas, will depend on the size of the lymphatic channels. When the channels are large, the echogenic lymphatic vessels walls are widely displaced, and the overall echogenicity of the lesion most closely resembles that of the vessel lumina—nearly anechoic. However, when lymphatic channels are small, the echogenic vessel walls are close together, and the overall echogenicity most closely resembles that of the vessel walls—hyperechoic. When lymphatic vessel channels are prominent, the sonographic appearance can be very similar to that of duct ectasia that occurs within accessory breast tissue within the axilla (Fig. 11–133). However, the lymph-filled vessels are very soft and compressible and may be completely flattened during routine scanning. Thus, very light scan pressure must be used to demonstrate lymphangiomas adequately. The compressibility of lymphatic vessels may be used to help distinguish lymphangiomas from

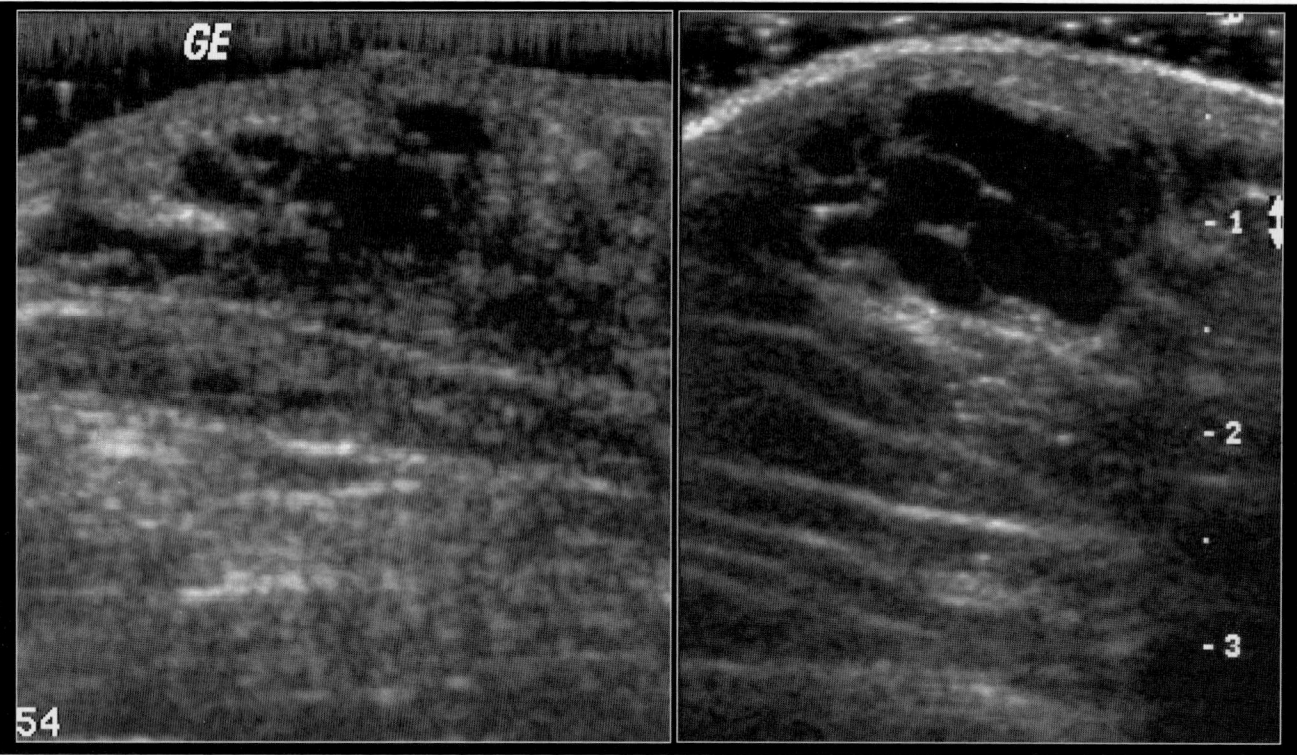

FIGURE 11–133 Lymphangiomas of the breast are most common in the axillary segment and axilla. The dilated lymphatic channels of a lymphangioma (**left**) may simulate ectatic ducts in accessory breast tissue within the axillary or axillary segment of the breast (**right**). The lymphatic vessels in a lymphangioma can be completely collapsed with transducer pressure, whereas the ectatic ducts within accessory breast tissue cannot.

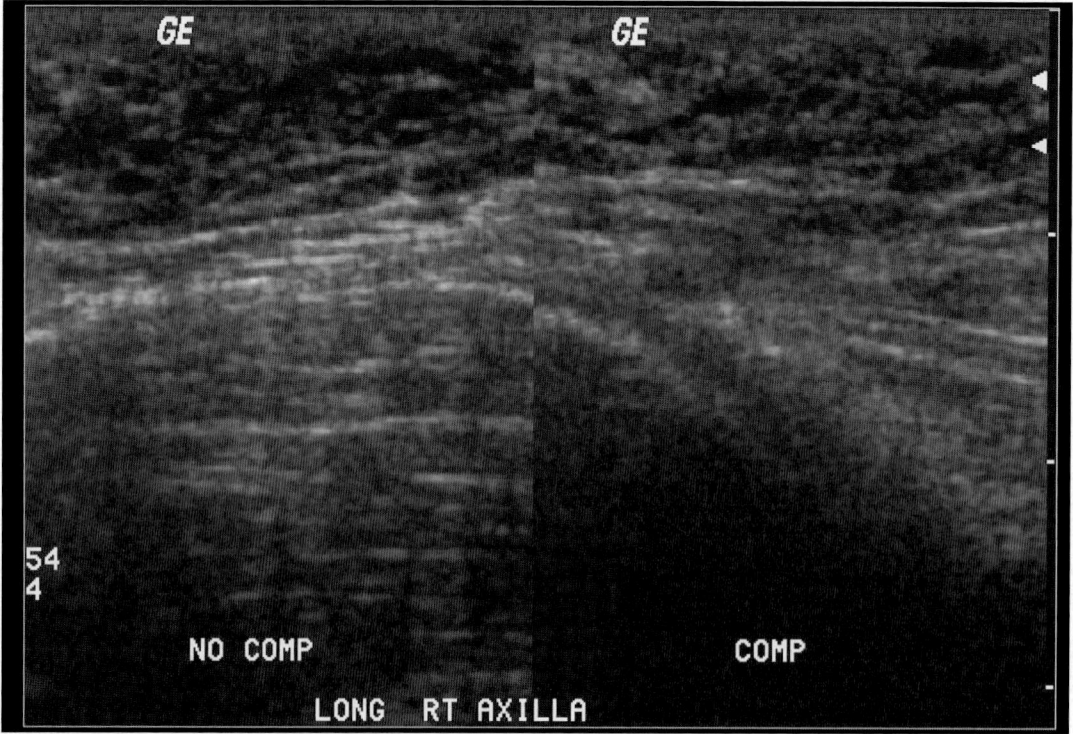

FIGURE 11–134 Most lymphangiomas are seen in newborns and infants and may be associated with cystic hygromas of the neck. However, this small lymphangioma caused focal pain in a young adult that instigated diagnostic sonography. The lesion is soft and compressible, and the lymphatic channels can be completely collapsed with transducer compression (**right**). The lymphatic channels are very small, and much of the lesion is composed of lymphatic vessel walls, accounting for the echogenic parts of the lesion.

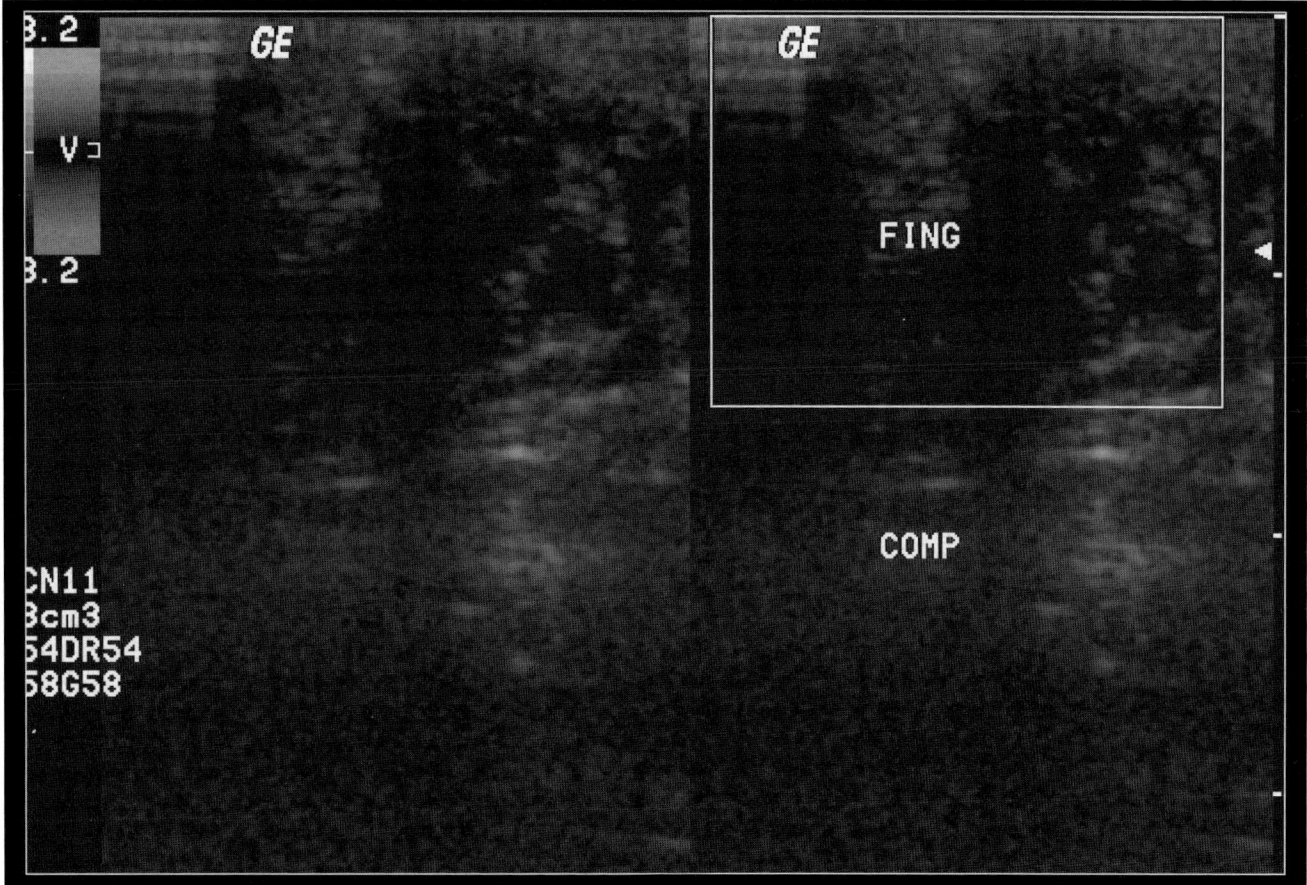

FIGURE 11–135 Unlike venous malformations or hemangiomas, lymphangiomas do not have enough spontaneous flow to be demonstrable with color Doppler. However, there are enough internal echoes within lymphatic fluid that, with augmentation, a very weak color signal can be obtained.

ectatic ducts. The lymphatic channels within lymphangiomas can be completely collapsed with transducer compression, whereas ectatic ducts are mildly compressible but cannot be completely collapsed (Fig. 11–134). Lymphangiomas do not develop internal calcifications similar to the phleboliths that develop within venous malformations. Whatever spontaneous lymph fluid flow there is within lymphangiomas is too little and too slow to be demonstrated with color or power Doppler. However, augmenting lymphatic flow within the vessel using transducer ballottement may create enough flow to create a color signal within the lesion (Fig. 11–135).

SEBACEOUS CYSTS, EPIDERMAL INCLUSION CYSTS, AND MONTGOMERY GLAND CYSTS

Sebaceous cysts, epidermal inclusion cysts, and Montgomery gland cysts are discussed in Chapter 10 in the discussion on types of BIRADS 2, definitively benign cysts.

INTRACYSTIC PAPILLOMAS AND INTRACYSTIC PAPILLARY CARCINOMAS

Intracystic papillary lesions and their distinction from fibrocystic change with papillary apocrine metaplasia are discussed in Chapter 10. Nipple discharge and papillary lesions of the breast are also discussed in Chapter 8.

SUGGESTED READINGS

General

Drukker BH. Breast disease: a primer on diagnosis and management. *Int J Fertil Womens Med* 1997;42(5):278–287.

Khaleghian R. Breast cysts: pitfalls in sonographic diagnosis. *Australas Radiol* 1993;37(2):192–194.

Galactocele

Cassier C, et al. Radiographic aspects of galactoceles. *Radiology* 1986;67(11):803–806.

Gomez A, et al. Galactocele: three distinctive radiographic appearances. *Radiology* 1986;158(1):43–44.

Hall FM. Galactocele: three distinctive radiographic appearances [Letter]. *Radiology* 1986;160(3):852–853.

Mezi S, et al. The use of mammary echotomography in the diagnosis and monitoring of the pregnant and puerperal breast: three cases of galactocele. *G Chir* 1990;11(4):238–242.

Nokes SR, Osteen PK, Fincher RL. Radiological case of the month: galactocele. *J Ark Med Soc* 1992;89(7):353–354.

Salvador R, et al. Galactocele of the breast: radiologic and ultrasonographic findings. *Br J Radiol* 1990;63(746):140–142.

Puerperal Mastitis and Abscess

Crowe DJ, et al. Breast infection: mammographic and sonographic findings with clinical correlation [non-puerperal mastitis in real time and color Doppler ultrasound]. Breast masses. Mammographic and sonographic evaluation. *Invest Radiol* 1995;30(10): 582–587.

Dixon JM. Repeated aspiration of breast abscesses in lactating women. *Br Med J* 1988;297:1517–1518.

Harris VJ, Jackson VP. Indications for breast imaging in women under age 36 years. *Radiology* 1989;172(2):445–448.

Karstrup S, et al. Ultrasonically guided percutaneous drainage of breast abscesses. *Acta Radiol* 1990;31(2):157–159.

Karstrup S, et al. Acute puerperal breast abscesses: US-guided drainage. *Radiology* 1993;188(3):807–809.

Loyer IM, Harmeet K, David CL, et al. Importance of dynamic assessment of the soft tissues in the sonographic diagnosis of echogenic superficial abscesses. *J Ultrasound Med* 1995;14:669–671.

Perlmutter S, Licht M, Gold M, Price A, et al. Ultrasound ringdown artifact in breast abscess. *J Womens Imaging* 2001;3:108–111.

Duct Ectasis, Periductal Mastitis, Nonpuerperal Abscess, and Granulomatous Mastitis

Blohmer JU, et al. Non-puerperal mastitis in real time and color Doppler ultrasound. *Geburtshilfe Frauenheilkd* 1994;54(3):161–166.

Boisserie-Lacroix M, Lafitte JJ, Sirben C, et al. Inflammatory and infectious lesions of the breast: contribution of sonography. *J Chir* 1993;130(10):408–415.

Bunddred NJ, Dover MS, Coley S, et al. Breast abscesses and cigarette smoking. *Br J Surg* 1992;79:58–59.

Chantra PK, et al. Circumscribed fibrocystic mastopathy with formation of an epidermal cyst. *AJR Am J Roentgenol* 1994;163(4):831–832.

Dixon JM, Ravisekar O, Chetty U, Anderson TJ. Periductal mastitis and duct ectasia: different conditions with different etiologies. *Br J Surg* 1996;83:820–822.

Fem. SE. Breast abscesses in Nigeria: lactational vs. non-lactational. *J R Cull Surg Edina* 1995;40(1):25–27.

Ferrara JJ, et al. Nonsurgical management of breast infections in nonlactating women: a word of caution. *Am Surg* 1990;56(11):668–671.

Furlong AJ, al-Naked L, Knox WF, et al. Periductal inflammation and cigarette smoke. *J Am Cull Surg* 1994;179:417–420.

Gilles M, Kopp W, Beaufort F. Diagnosis, incidence and course of nonpuerperal mastitis. *Radiology* 1985;25(2):87–92.

Graveled IH. The radiology of periductal mastitis. *Br J Clin Pract Symp Suppl* 1989;68:73–75, 87–89.

Grajower MM, Sas N. Danazol therapy for periareolar abscess [Letter]. *N Engl J Med* 1986;314(14):923.

Han BK, Choe YH, Park JM, et al. Granulomatous mastitis: mammographic and sonographic appearance. *AJR Am J Roentgenol* 1999;173:317–320.

Hayes R, Michell M, Nunnerley HB. Acute inflammation of the breast—the role of breast ultrasound in diagnosis and management. *Clin Radiol* 1991;44(4):253–256.

Hughes LE. The duct ectasia/periductal mastitis complex. In: *Benign disorders and diseases of the breast: concepts and clinical management*, 2nd ed. London: WB Saunders, 2000:143–165.

Khoda J, Lantsberg L, Yegev Y, et al. Management of periareolar abscess and mammilary fistula. *Surg Gynecol Obstet* 1992;175(2):306–308.

Maier WP, Au FC, Tang Ck. Nonlactational breast abscess. *Am Surg* 1994;60(4):247–250.

Mansel RE, Hughes LE. Breast pain and nodularity. In: *Benign disorders and diseases of the breast: concepts and clinical management*, 2nd ed. London: WB Saunders, 2000:95–118.

Matriacardi L, Lovati R. Ultrasonic appearance of a case of mammary duct ectasia. *J Clin Ultrasound* 1991;19(9):568–570.

Miller SD, McCollough ML, DeNapoli. Periductal mastitis: masquerading as carcinoma. *Dermatol Surg* 1998;24:383–385.

Nani NT, Bernael P, Nocentini C, et al. Mammary duct ectasia: nodologic assessment. Features and echographic incidence. *Radiol Med* (Torino) 1993;85(6):748–752.

Pahnke VG, et al. Nonpuerperal mastitis: a disease with increasing clinical relevance? *Geburtshilfe Frauenheilkd* 1985;45(1):29–35.

Paredes Lopez A, Moreno G. Non-puerperal mastitis: clinical study of 30 patients. *Ginecol Obstet Mex* 1995;63:226–230.

Peters H, Geisthovel F, Schuulze-Tollert J, et al. Non-puerperal mastitis: clinical aspects and therapy. *Dtsch Med Wochenschr* 1985;110(3):97–104.

Peters F, Schuth W. Hyperprolactinemia and nonpuerperal mastitis (duct ectasia). *JAMA* 1989;261(11):1618–1620.

Reddin A, McCrea ES, Keramati B. Inflammatory breast disease: mammographic spectrum. *South Med J* 1988;81(8):981–988.

Reynolds HE, Cramer HM. Cholesterol granuloma of the breast: a mimic or carcinoma. *Radiology* 1994;191:249–250.

Smith GL, et al. Cholesterol granuloma of the breast presenting as an intracystic papilloma. *Br J Radiol* 1997;70(839):1178–1179.

Sweeney DJ, Wylie EJ. Mammographic appearances of mammary duct ectasia that mimic carcinoma in a screening program. *Australas Radiol* 1995;39(1):18–23.

Umbach G, Mosny D, Bender HG. Nonpuerperal mastitis: three possible causes including mammography correlates. *Fortschr Med* 1989;107(2):65–66.

van Overhagen H, Zonderland HM, Lameris JS. Radiodiagnostic aspects of non-puerperal mastitis. *ROFO Fortschr Geb Rontgenstr Nuklearmed* 1988;149(3):294–297.

Watt-Boolsen S, Rassmussen NR, Blichert-Toft M. Primary periareolar abscess in the nonlactating breast: risk of recurrence. *Am J Surg* 1987;153(6):571–573.

Webster DJT. Infections of the breast. In: *Benign disorders and diseases of the breast: concepts and clinical management*, 2nd ed. London: WB Saunders, 2000:187–196.

Wilhelmus JL, Schrodt GR, Mahaffey LM. Cholesterol granulomas of the breast: a lesion which clinically mimics carcinoma. *Am J Clin Pathol* 1982;77:592–597.

Hematoma, Seroma, and Lymphocele

Burak WE, Goodman PS, Young DC, et al. Seroma formation following axillary dissection for breast cancer: risk factors and lack of influence of bovine thrombin. *J Surg Oncol* 1997;64:27–31.

Gollentz B, et al. Breast hematoma and cytosteatonecrosis: apropos of 55 cases *J Radiol* 1990;71(1):33–43.

Harlow CL, et al. Sonographic detection of hematomas and fluid after imaging guided core breast biopsy. *J Ultrasound Med* 1994; 13(11):877–882.

O'Dwyer PJ, O'Higgins NJ, James AG. Effect of closing dead space on incidence of seroma after mastectomy. *Surg Gynecol Obstet* 1991;172:55–56.

Pignatelli V, et al. Hematoma and fat necrosis of the breast: mammographic and echographic features. *Radiol Med* (Torino) 1995; 89(1–2):36–41.

Sa EJ, Choi YH. Cystic lymphangioma of the breast. *J Clin Ultrasound* 1999;27:351–352.

Tadych K, Donegan WL. Postmastecomy seromas and wound drainage. *Surg Gynecol Obstet* 1987:483–487.

Warren HW, Griffith CD, McLean L, et al. Should breast biopsy cavities be drained? *Ann R Coll Surg Engl* 1994;76(1):39–41.

Watt-Boolsen S, Nielsen VB, Jensen J, et al. Postmastectomy seroma: a study of the nature and origin of seroma after mastectomy. *Dan Med Bull* 1989;36:487–489.

Woodworth PA, McBoyle MF, Helmer SD, et al. Seroma formation after breast cancer surgery: incidence and predisposing factors. *Am Surg* 2000;66:444–450.

Fat Necrosis

Andersson I, Adler DD, Ljungberg O. Breast necrosis associated with thromboembolic disorders. *Acta Radiol* 1987;28(5):517–521.

Baker KS, Stelling CB. Mammographic appearance of Coumadin-induced fat necrosis [Letter]. *AJR Am J Roentgenol* 1992;158(3):689–690.

Balu-Maestro C, et al. Ultrasonographic surveillance of treated breast cancer. *Radiology* 1991;72(12):655–661.

Balu-Maestro C, et al. Ultrasonographic posttreatment follow-up of breast cancer patients. *J Ultrasound Med* 1991;10(1):1–7.

Beeckman P, et al. The ultrasound aspect of the skin and subcutaneous fat layer in various benign and malignant breast conditions. *J Belge Radiol* 1991;74(4):283–288.

Boyages J, et al. Fat necrosis of the breast following lumpectomy and radiation therapy for early breast cancer. *Radiother Oncol* 1988; 13(1):69–74.

Brown FE, Sargent SK, Cohen SR, et al. Mammographic changes following reduction mammoplasty. *Plast Recontstr Surg* 1987; 80(5):691–698.

Chaudary MM, et al. New lumps in the breast following conservation treatment for early breast cancer. *Breast Cancer Res Treat* 1988;11(1):51–58.

Dershaw DD, et al. Differentiation of benign and malignant local tumor recurrence after lumpectomy. *AJR Am J Roentgenol* 1990; 155(1):35–38.

Di Piro PJ, et al. Seat belt injuries of the breast: findings on mammography and sonography. *AJR Am J Roentgenol* 1995;164(2): 317–320.

el-Deeb NA. Fat necrosis of the breast: an unusual complication of lumpectomy and radiotherapy in breast cancer. Review of literature and report of four new cases. *Eur J Surg Oncol* 1990;16(3): 248–250.

Evers K, Troupin RH. Lipid cyst: classical and atypical appearances. *AJR Am J Roentgenol* 1991;157:271–273.

Fajardo LL, Bessen SC. Epidermal inclusion cyst after reduction mammoplasty. *Radiology* 1993;186(1):103–106.

Harrison RL, Birtton P, Warren R, et al. Can we be sure about a radiological diagnosis of fat necrosis of the breast? *Clin Radiol* 2000; 55:119–123.

Harvey JA, Moran RE, Maurer EJ, et al. Sonographic features of mammary oil cysts. *J Ultrasound Med* 1997;16:719–724.

Hogge JP, Robinson RE, Magnant CM, et al. The mammographic spectrum of fat necrosis of the breast. *Radiographics* 1995;15: 1347–1356.

Linden SS, Sickles EA. Sedimented calcium in benign breast cysts: the full spectrum of mammographic presentations. *AJR Am J Roentgenol* 1989;152(5):967–971.

Mendelson EB. Evaluation of the post-operative breast. *Radiol Clin North Am* 1992;30(1):107–138.

Miller JA, Festa S, Goldstein M. Benign fat necrosis simulating bilateral breast malignancy after reduction mammoplasty. *South Med J* 1998;91:765–767.

Pignatelli V, et al. Hematoma and fat necrosis of the breast: mammographic and echographic features. *Radiol Med* (Torino) 1995; 89(1–2):36–41.

Pollack AH, Kuerer HM. Steatocystoma multiplex: appearance at mammography. *Radiology* 1991;180(3):36–38.

Rostom AY, el-Sayed ME. Fat necrosis of the breast: an unusual complication of lumpectomy and radiotherapy in breast cancer. *Clin Radiol* 1987;38(1):31.

Solomon B, et al. Delayed development of enhancement in fat necrosis after breast conservation therapy: a potential pitfall of MR imaging of the breast. *AJR Am J Roentgenol* 1998;170(4): 966–968.

Soo MS, Kornguth PJ, Hertzberg BS. Fat necrosis in the breast: sonographic features. *Radiology* 1998;206(1):261–269.

Stigers KB, et al. Abnormalities of the breast caused by biopsy: spectrum of mammographic findings. *AJR Am J Roentgenol* 1991; 156(2):287–291.

Van Gelderen WF. Atypical fat necrosis of the breast: the "mycetoma" appearance. *Australas Radiol* 1994;38(1):76–77.

Mondor's Disease: Superficial Thrombosis

Camiel MR. Mondor's disease in the breast. *Am J Obstet Gynecol* 1985;152(7):879–881.

Catania S, et al. Mondor's disease and breast cancer. *Cancer* 1992; 69(9):2267–2270.

Chiedozi LC, Aghahowa JA. Mondor's disease associated with breast cancer. *Surgery* 1988;103(4):438–439.

Conant EF, et al. Superficial thrombophlebitis of the breast (Mondor's disease): mammographic findings. *AJR Am J Roentgenol* 1993;160(6):1201–1203.

Cooper RA. Mondor's disease secondary to intravenous drug abuse. *Arch Surg* 1990;125(6):807–808.

Decembrini P, et al. Mondor's disease: our experience. *G Chir* 1994;15(8–9):355–357.

Fiorica JV. Special problems: Mondor's disease, macrocysts, trauma, squamous metaplasia, miscellaneous disorders of the nipple. *Obstet Gynecol Clin North Am* 1994;21(3):479–485.

Fornero G, Rosato L, Ginardi A. Rare venous pathology: Mondor's disease. *Minerva Chir* 1994;49(11):1179–1180.

Mahesh KS, Watson AB. Mondor's disease of the breast: sonographic and mammographic findings. *AJR Am J Roentgenol* 2000;177: 893–896.

Miller DR, Cesario TC, Slater LM. Mondor's disease associated with metastatic axillary nodes. *Cancer* 1985;56(4):903–904.

Hemangioma

Carreira C, Romano C, Rodriguez R, et al. A cavernous haemangioma of breast in male: radiological-pathologic correlation. *Eur Radiol* 2001;11(2):292–294.

Courcoutsakis NA, et al. Breast hemangiomas in a patient with Kasabach-Merritt syndrome: imaging findings. *AJR Am J Roentgenol* 1997;169(5):1397–1399.

Dener C, Sengui N, Tez S, et al. Haemangiomas of the breast. *Eur J Surg* 2000;166(12):977–979.

Galindo LM, Shienbaum AJ, Dwyer-Joyce L, et al. Atypical hemangioma of the breast: a diagnostic pitfall in breast fine-needle aspiration. *Diagn Cytopathol* 2001;24(3):215–218.

Gembala RB, et al. Color Doppler detection of a breast perilobular hemangioma. *J Ultrasound Med* 1993;12(4):220–222.

Leseur GC, Brown RW, Bhathal PS. Incidence of perilobular hemangioma of the breast. *Arch Pathol Lab Med* 1983;107:308–310.

Perugini G, et al. Cavernous hemangioma of the pectoralis muscle mimicking a breast tumor. *AJR Am J Roentgenol* 1994;162(6):1321–1322.

Rosen PP. Vascular tumors of the breast. V. Nonparenchymal hemangiomas of the mammary subcutaneous tissues. *Am J Surg Pathol* 1985;9:723–729.

Webb LA, Young JR. Case report: haemangioma of the breast—appearances on mammography and ultrasound. *Clin Radiol* 1996;51(7):523–524.

12

ULTRASOUND OF SOLID BREAST NODULES: DISTINGUISHING BENIGN FROM MALIGNANT

RATIONALE FOR SONOGRAPHIC CHARACTERIZATION

General and Specific Goals of Diagnostic Breast Ultrasound

The general goal of diagnostic breast ultrasound is to make a more specific diagnosis than can be made with clinical findings and mammography alone. Important specific goals of diagnostic breast ultrasound are to prevent as many unnecessary biopsies as possible and to find cancers missed by mammography. Neither the general nor the specific goals can be achieved without sonographic characterization of solid breast nodules.

Common Wisdom

For many years, the common wisdom was that there is so much overlap between the sonographic findings of benign and malignant solid nodules that it is impossible to distinguish all benign from all malignant solid nodules and therefore that all solid nodules must undergo biopsy, regardless of the sonographic findings.

Problems with the Common Wisdom

The common wisdom was not invented out of thin air. It was based on multiple published studies from the late 1970s and early 1980s in which ultrasound was found inadequate for distinguishing solid benign from solid malignant nodules.

However, these studies were plagued by several problems. First, they were performed using old, lower-resolution ultrasound equipment. The use of lower-resolution equipment was unavoidable because that was all that was available at the time. Additionally, the attempt to automate whole breast ultrasound resolution for purposes of primary breast cancer screening further compromised resolution. Most automated whole breast scanners were designed to scan the patient in a prone position with "hanging" breasts. The thickness of the hanging breast is often 10 cm or more, requiring frequencies as low as 3 MHz to achieve adequate penetration. The need for low-frequency transducers to achieve adequate penetration to those depths severely degraded both spatial and contrast resolution. Critical angle shadowing in hanging breasts further contributed to interpretive difficulties. Improvement in the resolution of high-frequency near-field hand-held transducers since that time has been remarkable. Current high-frequency transducers can routinely resolve normal lobules and, under ideal circumstances, can demonstrate calcifications as small as 200 μm.

Second, in old studies, the ability of sonography to distinguish benign from malignant was usually assessed on the basis of single sonographic findings. Breast cancer is far too heterogeneous to be evaluated with single findings. We learned this long ago in mammography. That is why mammographers do not rely on only a single finding for detection of and characterization of breast lesions. Instead, mammographers use a battery of suspicious findings (Table 12–1). If even a single one of these suspicious findings is present, mammographers must perform additional evaluation. Only if none of these findings is present can the patient be allowed to return to routine annual screening.

Third, the goals of these studies were overly ambitious and unrealistic:

- To replace mammography as the primary breast cancer screening tool. The attempt to achieve this cannot be criticized. The goal was laudable. Unfortunately, ultrasound was less effective at primary breast cancer screening than was mammography. The problem is that early mammographers who were involved in these studies for too long inappropriately used the failure of sonography as a screening tool to condemn all breast ultrasound, regardless of whether it was used for whole breast screening or in a targeted diagnostic fashion.

TABLE 12–1. SUSPICIOUS FINDINGS IN BREAST IMAGING

Mammographic Suspicious Findings	Sonographic Solid Nodule Suspicious Findings
Mass	Shadowing
Nodule	Hypoechoic echotexture
Spiculation	Spiculation
Irregular margins	Angular margins
Indistinct margins	Thick, echogenic halo
Microlobulation	Microlobulation
Architectural distortion	Taller than wide
Asymmetric density	Duct extension
Developing density	Branch pattern
Calcifications	Calcifications

- To distinguish all benign from all malignant solid breast nodules. We agree that there is a large overlap in sonographic findings between benign and malignant solid breast nodules. We also agree that it is impossible to distinguish all benign from all malignant solid breast nodules using sonographic criteria. However, we strongly disagree with the premise that no attempt should be made to distinguish benign from malignant solid breast nodules using sonographic criteria. We believe that trying to characterize all solid breast nodules is an unreasonable goal. It is important to have realistic goals for ultrasound or any other imaging test. A reasonable and achievable goal for diagnostic breast ultrasound is to identify a subgroup of solid nodules that has such a low risk for malignancy that the option of short-interval follow-up can be offered as a viable alternative to biopsy. This subgroup is identified every day in mammography as the Breast Imaging Reporting and Data System (BI-RADS) 3 (probably benign) risk category. The BIRADS 3 subgroup can also be identified with a high degree of accuracy using multiple sonographic findings in a strict algorithmic approach. Thus, identifying a subgroup that meets criteria for BIRADS 3 classification is a reasonable goal for diagnostic breast sonography.

The Sonographic Algorithm Is the Mammographic Algorithm Directly Applied to Ultrasound—Not a Radical Departure from Current Mammographic Management Rules

It is important to realize that offering short-interval follow-up sonography, as an alternative to biopsy, does not represent a radical departure from current mammographic practice. Most who perform breast ultrasound are also involved in mammography. We do not need to "reinvent the wheel." Mammography is almost certainly the most intensely scrutinized of all the imaging modalities and perhaps is the most intensely scrutinized diagnostic or screening examination, of any type, in the history of medicine. Although far from perfect, mammography has withstood this scrutiny quite well. For this reason, as many of the principles of mammographic interpretation and patient management should be adapted by and directly applied to sonographic evaluation as is possible.

The cornerstones of the mammographic algorithm that have led to its success are the following:

- By employing multiple suspicious findings, it takes into account the heterogeneity of breast cancer—not only from nodule to nodule but also within individual nodules.
- If even a single suspicious finding is present, additional evaluation is required.
- It categorizes all lesions or structures into standardized risk categories (BIRADS categories).
- It errs on the side of caution in defining the probably benign category (BIRADS 3). Sensitivities and negative predictive values must be 98% or greater to categorize a lesion as BIRADS 3 and to offer the patient the option of follow-up instead of biopsy.
- Management algorithms have been developed and are relatively standardized for each BIRADS category.

Although the mammographic algorithm is certainly far from perfect, its success at detecting and diagnosing cancer may be rivaled only by the success of Papanicolaou smears at detecting cervical cancer. Thus, we have incorporated the mammographic cornerstones into the algorithm that we have developed for sonographic evaluation of solid breast nodules.

The first cornerstone of mammographic evaluation that can directly be applied to sonographic evaluation of solid breast nodules is the use of multiple sonographic findings to account for the heterogeneity of breast cancer. A mammographer would never rely on a single finding such as spiculation or calcification because too many cancers would be missed. Instead, mammographers rely on a battery of findings, including mass, nodule, asymmetric density, spiculation, architectural distortion, certain types of calcification, and developing density. Similarly, no sonologist should expect to be successful in identifying malignancy using a single finding. A battery of multiple sonographic findings is necessary to evaluate solid breast nodules. Table 12–1 shows lists of findings that are used in mammography and sonography to identify malignant lesions. Note that the lists are more similar than dissimilar and that several sonographic findings are simply mammographic findings that have been applied directly to ultrasound. Duct extension and branch pattern are also mammographic findings that are largely limited to calcifications, but that find broader application in ultrasound, with which noncalcified extensions of tumor into surrounding ducts can be readily identified. Only during galactography can mammography show such noncalcified ductal growth.

The second cornerstone of mammographic interpretation that can be applied directly to sonographic evaluation is that the individual findings must be used in a rigidly followed algorithm (Table 12–2). Each suspicious finding must be sought in each and every case. If even a single suspicious mammographic finding is detected, further evaluation is mandated. Because mammography is a primary screening tool as well as a diagnostic tool, additional evaluation after mammography could include one or more of many different methods. For example, a mammographic finding could be characterized as an "Aunt Minnie" benign finding; it could be compared to old films or subjected to follow-up. It might also be evaluated with additional views, spot compression and magnification, ultrasound, or biopsy. Only if there are no suspicious mammographic findings can the mammographic study be reported as negative and can the patient return to the routine screening pool.

The algorithm that we use for sonographic findings is also rigid and closely parallels the mammographic algorithm. We look for the battery of sonographic findings suspicious for malignancy shown in Table 12–1. If even a single one of those findings is present, the nodule must be excluded from benign and probably benign risk categories (BIRADS 2 and 3 categories), must be characterized as BI-RADS 4a or higher, and must be further evaluated. The list of additional evaluations for BIRADS 4 to 5 solid nodules is much shorter for sonography than for mammography because sonography is a secondary or diagnostic examination rather than a primary screening examination. In gen-

eral, additional evaluation of solid nodules with one or more sonographic suspicious findings includes only biopsy.

Not only is the sonographic algorithm for evaluation of solid breast nodules as strict as the mammographic algorithm, but also it actually includes an extra step of assurance that does not exist in mammography. Mammograms are considered negative so long as no suspicious findings are present. On the other hand, solid nodules detected at sonography are a positive finding. Thus, a simple absence of any sonographic findings that are suspicious for malignancy can never constitute a negative study. Therefore, after concluding that there are no suspicious findings, one of three strictly defined benign findings must be identified before the nodule can be characterized as benign or probably benign (BIRADS 2 or 3). Even if there are no suspicious findings, if one of three benign findings cannot be specifically identified, the nodule must by default be characterized as mildly suspicious (BIRADS 4a), and biopsy must be recommended. Furthermore, because solid nodules characterized as probably benign (BIRADS 3) are positive findings, they must undergo short-interval follow-up. Table 12–2 shows the algorithms for mammographic and sonographic evaluation, respectively.

The third cornerstone of mammographic management that can and should be directly applied to sonographic management is the use of and definition of sonographic BIRADS categories. For biopsy avoidance, the definition of the probably benign BIRADS 3 risk category is particularly important.

In 1995, we published a prospective study that demonstrated that a low-risk group of solid breast nodules could be identified by using multiple sonographic findings in a strictly followed algorithm. A total of 750 solid nodules were prospectively characterized with sonography into

TABLE 12–2. BREAST IMAGING ALGORITHMS

Mammographic Algorithm	Sonographic Solid Nodule Algorithm
1. Look for suspicious findings	1. Look for suspicious findings
2. If a single finding is present do something more:	2. If a single finding is present, do something more:
Old films, follow-up, additional views, ultrasound, biopsy	Biopsy
3. If no suspicious findings, routine screening	3. If no suspicious findings, look for benign findings[a]
4. If BIRADS 3 categories, short-interval follow-up	4. If benign findings, no biopsy, but follow-up needed
	5. If no benign findings, BIRADS 4: biopsy[a]

[a]Extra step that does not exist in the mammographic algorithm. These steps make the sonographic algorithm more conservative than the mammographic algorithm.

three risk classes: benign, indeterminate, or malignant. The entire group of 750 solid nodules had a 16.7% prevalence of cancer. The odds ratio of a benign classification was 0.029, representing a greater than 33-fold reduction in the risk for a nodule being malignant from the baseline prevalence (16.7%) in the entire group of 750 nodules. The negative predictive value and odds ratio for a benign ultrasound classification were competitive with those published for needle-localization breast biopsy and image-guided large core needle biopsy. More important, the sensitivity for cancer was 98.4% (123 of 125 of malignant nodules were correctly classified as either indeterminate or malignant). The negative predictive value was 99.5% (424 of 426 nodules classified as benign were benign). The false-negative rate was 2 of 125 (1.6%). Thus, the goal of achieving a sensitivity of 98% or greater and a false-negative rate of 2% or less was achieved in the overall group, and a subgroup of nodules was identified in which the negative predictive value is 98% or greater.

The study that was published in *Radiology* in 1995 was begun before the advent of the American College of Radiology BIRADS classification system and therefore did not utilize BIRADS classes. Furthermore, the goal that we had in mind at the beginning of that study was to identify a subgroup of nodules in which there was a 5% or less risk for malignancy. That we were able to identify a subgroup with benign sonographic appearances that had less than a 2% risk for malignancy was serendipitous. Only after the BIRADS categories were widely employed in mammographic reporting did it become apparent that our goal should be to identify a subgroup of nodules with a 2% or lower risk for malignancy, similar to the BIRADS 3 risk class in mammography. For this reason, we have performed a new study in which solid nodules are characterized into BIRADS categories. The specific goals of the new study were to identify a subgroup of nodules that met strict criteria of BIRADS 3, but also to assess the ability of sonography to stratify solid nodules into all of the BIRADS risk categories.

Both mammographic and sonographic lesions that are characterized as BIRADS 3 now must have 2% or less chance of being malignant. To prove that sonography can identify a BIRADS 3 subpopulation of nodules within a larger group of nodules, the negative predictive value of nodules in the BIRADS 3 subgroup that undergo biopsy should be 98% or greater, the sensitivity for breast carcinoma in the entire population of nodules should be 98% or greater, and the false-negative rate in the entire population of nodules should be 2% or less. Thus, to achieve the specific sonographic goal of preventing biopsy of some solid nodules, sonography need only to be able to identify a subgroup of solid nodules that can be characterized into the BIRADS 3 category. Achieving the old unrealistic goal of distinguishing all benign from all malignant solid nodules is neither possible nor necessary.

The precedent for offering the option of follow-up in patients who have lesions with less than a 2% risk for malignancy has been established in several large mammographic series. If the BIRADS 3 category established by ultrasound has the same cancer risk as does the mammographic BIRADS 3 category (it does, ≤2%), offering short-interval follow-up as an option to biopsy to patients who have solid nodules that are characterized as BIRADS 3 by sonography cannot be considered a radical departure from the mammographic standard of care.

Table 12–3 shows the BIRADS categories that we currently use, the expected risks for malignancy in each category, and the actual percentages of malignancy within each category at the time of biopsy, based on ongoing prospective sonographic BIRADS characterization of 1,211 solid nodules that have undergone biopsy to date. Note that we are able to characterize lesions into BIRADS risk categories using sonography appropriately. For each BIRADS category, the actual percentage of malignant nodules lies within the expected range of percentages predicted.

We have modified the standard BIRADS categories only in that we have divided the BIRADS 4 into two cate-

TABLE 12–3. PROSPECTIVE CHARACTERIZATION OF 1,211 SOLID NODULES INTO BIRADS CATEGORIES[a]

BIRADS Category	No. of Nodules Undergoing Biopsy	No. of Malignant Nodules	Expected Risk for Cancer (%)	Actual Risk for Cancer (%)
2	15	0	0	0
3	231	1	≤2	0.4
4a	515	52	3–49	10
4b	191	118	50–89	62
5	259	236	≥90	91
Totals	1,211	407		34

[a]All 1,211 nodules have undergone biopsy. No solid nodules can be classified as BIRADS 1. Overall negative-to-positive biopsy ratio is 2:1.

gories divided at 50%. The risk for malignancy within the BIRADS 4 category extends all the way from greater than 2% to less than 90%—a huge range. For this reason, we have subdivided the BIRADS 4 category into two subcategories: 4a and 4b. We define BIRADS 4a risk for malignancy to extend from more than 2% to less than 50%. In BIRADS category 4b, the risk for malignancy is 50% or greater, but less than 90%. Dividing the BIRADS 4 category at 50% makes some sense because 50% or greater usually defines the medical and legal concept of "probable." In this study, solid nodules can never be characterized as BIRADS 1 because solid nodules do not represent a normal sonogram. Solid nodules characterized as BIRADS 2 and BIRADS 3 are considered negative, and nodules characterized into BIRADS 4a, 4b, and 5 categories are considered positive for purposes of correlation with histology. The sensitivity in the ongoing study is presently 99.8%, the negative predictive value of BIRADS 3 characterization is 99.6%, and the false-negative rate is 0.2%—all better than in the 1995 study. Furthermore, the risk for malignancy in each of the BIRADS categories from 2 through 5 is precisely within the expected range defined by mammography (Table 12–3). Thus, sonographic characterization of solid breast nodules into BIRADS categories is quite feasible.

The final cornerstone of mammography that can be applied to sonography is management by BIRADS categories. If both ultrasound and mammography can stratify patients into BIRADS categories, and if the risk for malignancy is the same for sonography and mammography within each category, then the management of sonographic lesions within any given category should be identical to management of mammographic lesions in the same category. If a patient with a mammographic lesion that is characterized as BIRADS 3 can be offered the option of follow-up rather than biopsy, then a patient with a sonographic lesion that meets strict criteria for BIRADS 3 can also be offered the option of follow-up. If all mammographic lesions that are BIRADS 4 or 5 must undergo biopsy, then all sonographic lesions characterized as BIRADS 4 or 5 must undergo biopsy.

Gross Morphology Versus Histology

Sonography directly demonstrates the gross morphology of solid nodules, not the histology. Sonography only indirectly demonstrates findings that reflect the underlying histology. This limitation must always be kept in mind, but it does not completely preclude our ability to distinguish benign from malignant. There will always be some circumscribed malignant lesions that appear to have benign gross morphologic features (Fig. 12–1) and some benign lesions that appear to have grossly malignant morphology (Fig. 12–2). With proper choice of sonographic findings that are employed in a logical algorithm, subgroups of solid

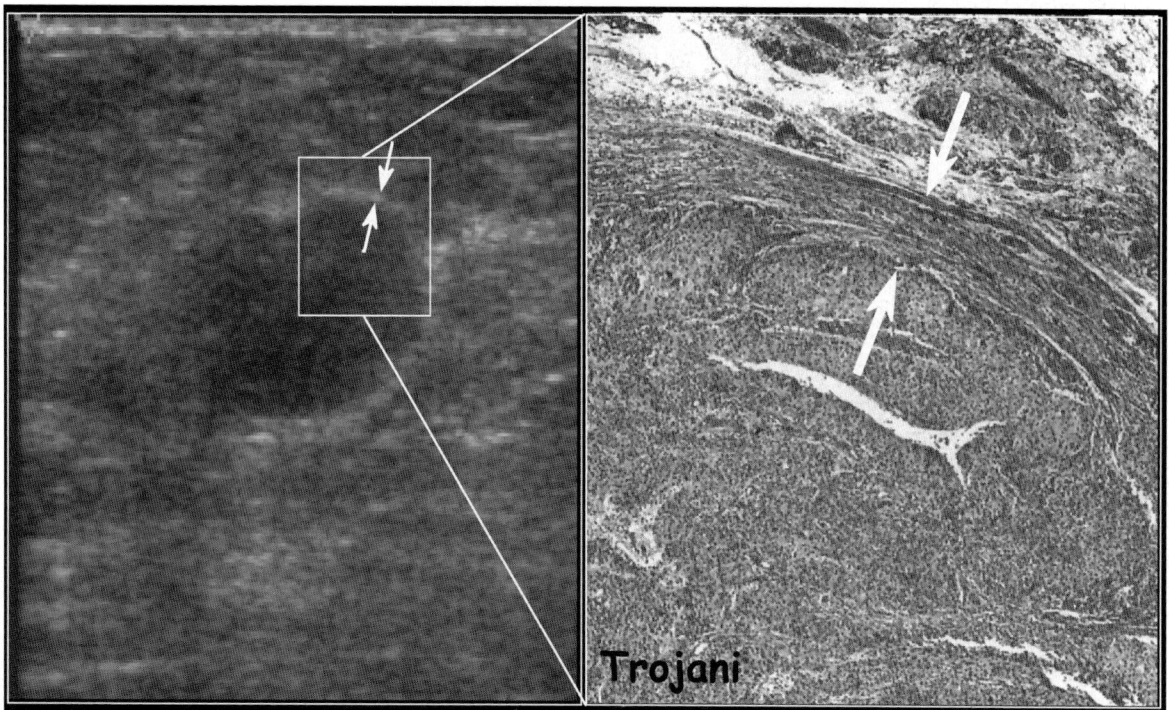

FIGURE 12–1 Sonographic features of benign and malignant solid nodules overlap. Some malignant nodules are circumscribed and at least partially encompassed by a thin capsule, findings more commonly associated with benign nodules.

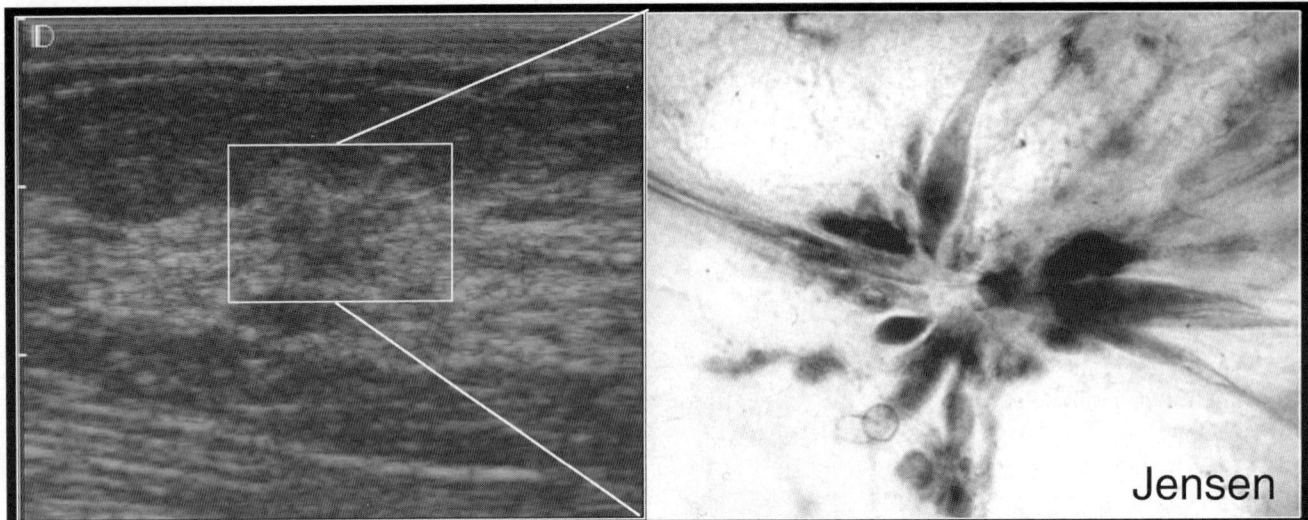

FIGURE 12–2 Sonographic features of benign and malignant solid nodules overlap. Some benign solid nodules are spiculated, a feature more commonly associated with malignant nodules. (Subgross histology courtesy of Hanna Jansen, University of California, Davis.)

nodules that have either a greater than 90% chance of being malignant (BIRADS 5) or more than a 98% chance of being benign (BIRADS 3) can be identified. Within the subpopulations that have multiple suspicious sonographic findings, the gross morphology indirectly, but accurately, indicates the invasive histology of the lesion (Fig. 12–3). Within the subgroup that completely lacks suspicious sonographic findings, the presence of characteristic sonographic shapes and margin characteristics indirectly reflects the benign histology of the nodule (Fig. 12–4).

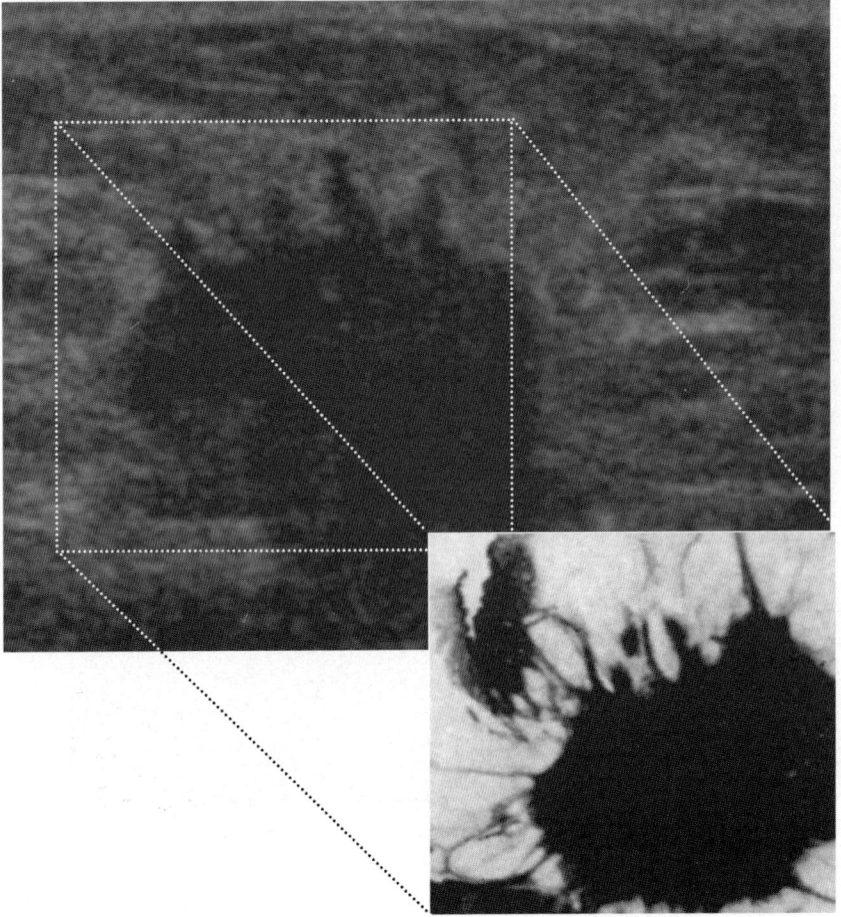

FIGURE 12–3 Sonography directly demonstrates gross morphology, not histology. However, in many cases, the gross morphologic features shown by sonography are characteristic, as in this spiculated malignant lesion.

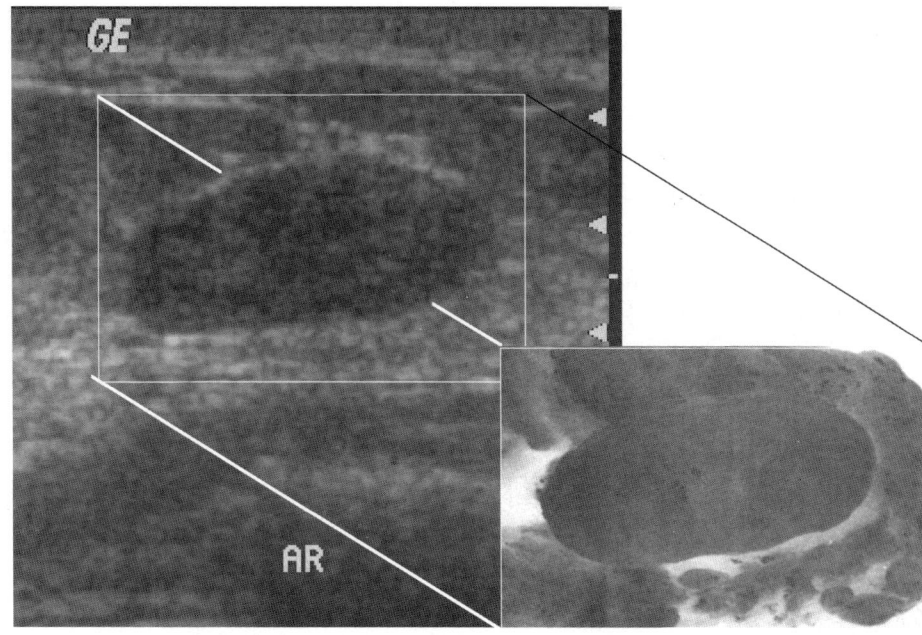

FIGURE 12–4 Sonography directly demonstrates gross morphology, not histology. However, in many cases, such as this benign nodule, the gross morphologic features shown by sonography are characteristic.

The Heterogeneity of Breast Cancer and How to Account for It

Breast cancer is not homogeneous. It varies greatly, not only from one nodule to another, but even within an individual nodule. Parts of an internally heterogeneous malignant nodule may have a gross morphology that simulates a benign lesion, whereas other parts of the same lesion may have malignant characteristics. Any imaging algorithm designed to characterize solid nodules must take into account the heterogeneity of breast cancer from nodule to nodule and within individual nodules if it is to achieve adequate sensitivity.

We can illustrate the heterogeneity of malignant breast nodules from nodule to nodule in a simplified fashion with a spectrum that ranges from circumscribed nodules at one end of the spectrum to spiculated lesions at the other end of the spectrum (Fig. 12–5). The middle peak of the spectrum represents an internally heterogeneous group of mixed lesions that are partially circumscribed and partially spiculated. Unfortunately, the histology and gross morphology of spiculated and circumscribed malignant solid nodules, and thus the sonographic features, differ greatly from each other and in many cases are opposites. Internally heterogeneous lesions that lie within the middle peak demonstrate some histologic, morphologic, and sonographic features from each end of the spectrum.

From the imager's point of view, the lesions that lie on the spiculated end of the spectrum are classic "crablike" malignant nodules. Detection of spiculated lesions sonographically can cause problems, but correctly characterizing the lesion as suspicious by sonography rarely does. On the other hand, circumscribed malignant solid nodules are usually easy to detect but have gross morphologic features that overlap those of benign lesions such as fibroadenomas,

making sonographic characterization more difficult. The gross morphologic and sonographic features of spiculated and circumscribed malignant solid nodules are often opposite from each other.

Let us compare some of the histologic and morphologic features of circumscribed and spiculated malignant solid nodules and how this affects their sonographic appearances. Desmoplasia, cellularity, and vascularity are all histologic, morphologic, and sonographic features that are nearly opposite from each other in circumscribed and spiculated malignant solid nodules.

Host Response to the Neoplasm—Desmoplasia Versus Inflammation

There is a misconception that all malignant breast lesions are abundantly desmoplastic. Desmoplasia constitutes a much larger percentage of the volume of spiculated than of circumscribed malignant solid nodules. Desmoplasia can be thought of as a host response to the tumor—an attempt to wall it off from the surrounding tissues with fibrosis and elastosis in order to keep it from spreading. Desmoplasia, like sclerosis in a bone lesion, is a slowly developing response to tumor and can fully manifest itself only when the tumor grows slowly enough to allow its gradual development. Thus, spiculated lesions that are abundantly desmoplastic are usually low- to intermediate-grade malignancies that grow slowly enough for desmoplasia to develop.

On the other hand, most circumscribed carcinomas are high-grade invasive ductal carcinomas that grow so rapidly that desmoplasia does not have time to develop. Instead, these more rapidly growing carcinomas incite a more rapidly developing inflammatory response. Thus, circum-

breast cancer is <u>heterogeneous</u>

<u>circumscribed</u>
- cellular
- high grade
- inflammatory hr
- enhanced transmission
- Doppler +
- elastography -

... and mixed circumscribed
and spiculated ...

<u>spiculated</u>
- paucicellular
- low grade
- desmoplastic
- shadowing
- Doppler -
- elastography +

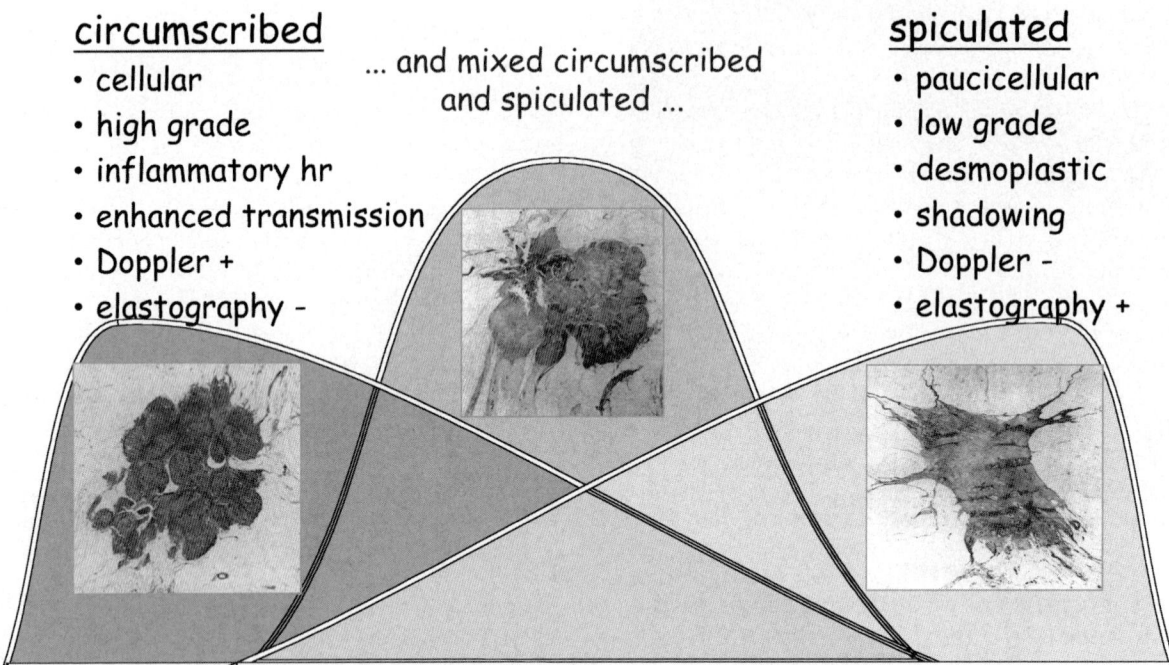

FIGURE 12–5 The gross morphologic features of malignant nodules span a spectrum from circumscribed to spiculated. Additionally, there are heterogeneous lesions in the middle of the spectrum that have mixed features. The gross morphology at one end of the spectrum is the opposite from that at the other end, and thus, the sonographic features that represent the morphology are also opposite. As a result, individual sonographic features can identify nodules at one end of the spectrum and some of the mixed lesions in the center, but not at the opposite end of the spectrum. No single finding can identify nodules at both ends of the spectrum. Thus, any sonographic algorithm designed to achieve high sensitivity for malignant nodules must employ multiple findings, some of which identify nodules at one end of the spectrum, and others that identify nodules at the other end of the spectrum.

scribed malignant nodules tend to have smaller components of desmoplasia and larger components of inflammation (lymphocytes, plasma cells, or both).

Whether a tumor incites a desmoplastic or inflammatory response is not all or nothing. It is merely a matter of degree. Spiculated lesions contain relatively larger amounts of desmoplasia and relatively smaller amounts of inflammatory response, whereas circumscribed lesions are more likely to have large inflammatory and small desmoplastic components. Mixed spiculated and circumscribed malignant nodules may contain nearly equal components of inflammation and desmoplasia.

Tumor Cellularity

Circumscribed lesions are much more cellular than spiculated lesions. Spiculated malignant solid nodules contain relatively few tumor cells surrounded by abundant hypocellular desmoplasia. Circumscribed carcinomas, on the other hand, contain both large numbers of tumor cells and large numbers of lymphocytes, plasma cells, or both.

Effects of Desmoplasia and Cellularity on Sonographic Features

The relative amounts of desmoplasia and cellularity in malignant solid nodules greatly affect their sonographic appearance. The acoustic shadowing deep to some malignant tumors is actually caused by desmoplasia, not the tumor cells. Thus, lower-grade spiculated lesions that contain abundant desmoplasia tend to cause complete or partial acoustic shadowing. On the other hand, tumor cells and inflammatory cells both transmit sound better than normal breast tissues. Thus, high-grade, highly cellular circumscribed carcinomas tend to have enhanced through-transmission rather than acoustic shadowing.

The difference in sound transmission between the circumscribed and spiculated ends of the malignant solid nodule spectrum creates a diagnostic dilemma for those who wrongly believe that desmoplasia is a dominant feature of all breast carcinomas. If solid nodules are evaluated with only a single finding, such as acoustic shadowing, virtually all high-grade invasive carcinomas and many special-type tumors that lie within the circumscribed end of the spectrum and have enhanced acoustic through-transmission will be missed. A single sonographic finding such as acoustic shadowing can identify lesions at the spiculated end of the spectrum and some of the internally heterogeneous nodules that lie in the middle of the spectrum but cannot identify nodules at the circumscribed end of the spectrum.

A similar problem exists when other single parameters, such as stiffness, are evaluated by a modality such as elastography. Desmoplasia causes malignant nodules to be stiff. Thus, spiculated nodules that contain abundant desmoplasia are stiff and positive on elastography. On the other hand, circumscribed lesions that contain very little desmoplasia are not stiff and therefore are likely to be missed by elastography.

Vascularity of Neoplasm—Angiogenesis Factors, Inflammatory Hyperemia, and Doppler

Circumscribed lesions tend to be far more vascular than are spiculated lesions. All living tissues—malignant nodules, benign nodules, and normal tissues—have blood flow. However, spiculated lesions do not necessarily have perceptibly more blood flow than do benign lesions or normal tissues. The reason for this is that spiculated tumors are paucicellular. The relatively few tumor cells within spiculated lesions generate relatively small amounts of angiogenesis factors; thus, there is relatively little tumor neovascularity. Additionally, desmoplasia requires little blood flow. On the other hand, most circumscribed malignant nodules are markedly more vascular than normal tissues or benign nodules. The much larger numbers of tumor cells generate abundant angiogenesis factors. Furthermore, the extensive inflammatory infiltrates incite a hyperemic response. The combination of extensive tumor neovascularity and inflammatory hyperemia causes these tumors to be obviously hypervascular in comparison to normal tissue and benign lesions.

The differences in blood flow to spiculated and circumscribed lesions affects the sensitivity of Doppler for detecting breast cancer. Doppler will inherently be less sensitive for spiculated lesions that have relatively little tumor neovascularity and virtually no inflammatory hyperemia than it will for circumscribed lesions that have both abundant tumor neovascularity and intense inflammatory hyperemia. Once again, we can see that a single parameter, such as Doppler-detectable blood flow, will detect virtually all high-grade circumscribed lesions that lie at one end of the spectrum but may miss a significant per-

centage of spiculated lesions that lie at the spiculated end of the spectrum.

Spectrum from Spiculated to Circumscribed Benign Solid Nodules

Complicating matters further is that there is a spectrum of benign nodules that also ranges from spiculated to circumscribed (although the percentage of benign lesions that fall in the spiculated end of the spectrum is much smaller than for the malignant spectrum). There may actually be more overlap in gross morphologic findings between circumscribed benign and circumscribed malignant lesions than there is between the circumscribed and spiculated ends of the benign or malignant spectrum. Similarly, there may be more overlap between the gross morphologic features of spiculated benign and spiculated malignant lesions than there is the between circumscribed and spiculated ends of either the benign or malignant spectrum. This complex overlap can be illustrated as a Venn diagram (Fig. 12–6). A single finding, such as shadowing, which detects the presence of desmoplasia, may reliably distinguish spiculated from nonspiculated lesions, but not necessarily benign from malignant lesions (Fig. 12–7). Using shadowing as the only finding, and assuming that absence of shadowing is a definitively benign finding, biopsy could be avoided in most fibroadenomas because very few fibroadenomas cause acoustic shadowing. However, there would be an unacceptably high number of false-negative findings because many circumscribed malignancies do not cause acoustic shadowing and therefore would be missed.

However, if progressively more sonographic findings are employed, and the complex Venn diagram is divided from different angles, the number of benign biopsies of fibroadenomas that can be prevented is decreased, but the number of false-negative findings is also decreased. Eventually, if enough findings are used, we can reduce the false-negative rate of 2% or less, while still classifying a significant percentage of nodules as probably benign, enabling us to offer short-interval follow-up as an alternative to biopsy (Fig. 12–8). The rationale behind multiple sonographic findings is that certain findings are more sensitive for one end of the malignant spectrum, whereas other findings are more sensitive for the other end of the spectrum. Only by using more than one finding can we expect to detect lesions at both circumscribed and spiculated ends of the spectrum. Of course, by using multiple findings, we are able to characterize fewer fibroadenomas as probably benign, BI-RADS 3, and therefore are able to prevent fewer biopsies. Preventing fewer biopsies is the price that must be paid to keep the false-negative rate below 2%. The goal of future studies is to fine-tune the findings used in order to achieve the largest possible BIRADS 3 group while maintaining sensitivity and negative predictive value of 98% or greater.

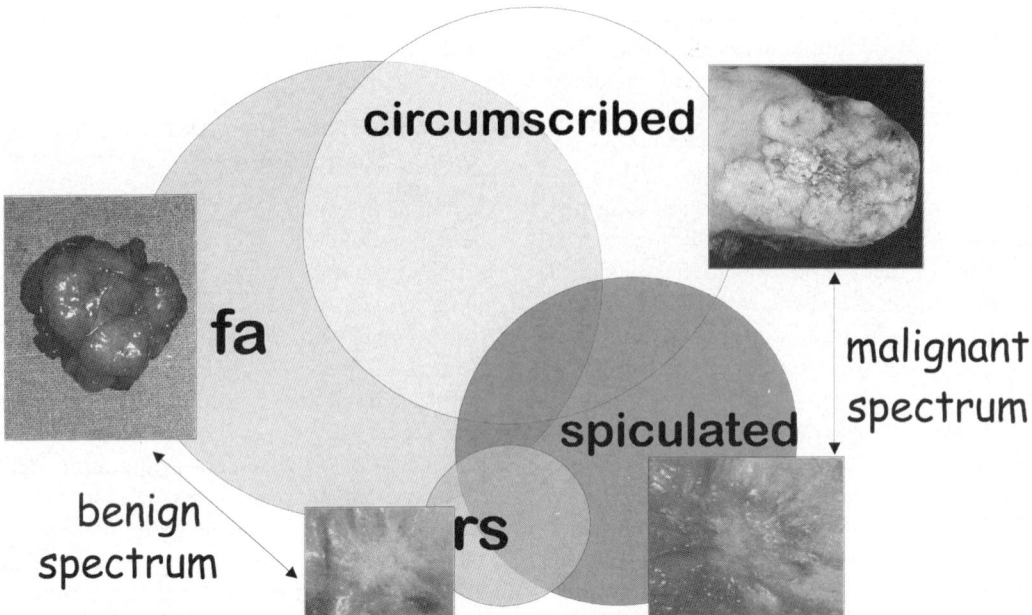

FIGURE 12–6 Complicating the evaluation of solid nodules further, there is a parallel spectrum of benign nodules spanning from circumscribed to malignant. There is complex overlap among all four types of lesions. Fa = fibroadenoma. Solid breast nodules—complex spectrum of gross morphology for both benign and malignant nodules that overlap extensively.

Because of the heterogeneity of breast carcinoma, individual findings can only identify nodules at one end of the spectrum and some of the internally heterogeneous cases in the middle of the spectrum. Any algorithm that can identify malignant nodules with 98% or greater certainty must use multiple findings.

In an ideal world, two perfect findings—one perfect for detection of speculated lesions and one perfect for circumscribed lesions—would be all that was necessary to characterize solid breast nodules. Unfortunately, none of the findings we use has 99% or greater sensitivity for either end of the spectrum, so we have had to develop an algo-

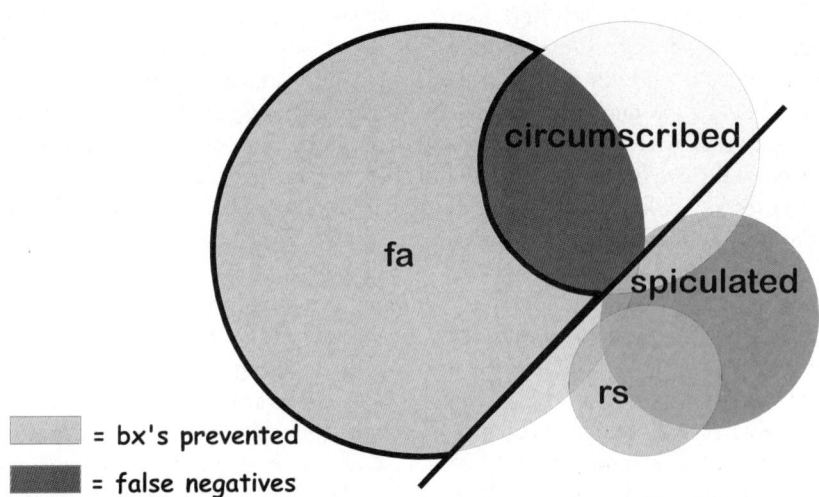

FIGURE 12–7 Single suspicious features cannot identify a benign population with 98% or greater certainty without missing an unacceptably high percentage of malignant nodules. A single morphologic and sonographic feature such as acoustic shadowing does an excellent job of discriminating spiculated from circumscribed lesions, but does not necessarily do an adequate job of distinguishing benign from malignant nodules. Using only the lack of acoustic shadowing to identify benign nodules could help prevent biopsy on most fibroadenomas *(black part of Venn diagram)* because very few fibroadenomas cause shadowing. However, an unacceptably high percentage of circumscribed carcinomas would be misclassified as benign *(light gray part of Venn diagram)* because they do not cause shadowing. Fa = fibroadenoma. Single criterion—high true negatives, high false negatives a single finding cannot identify a group of benign nodules with an acceptable false negative rate.

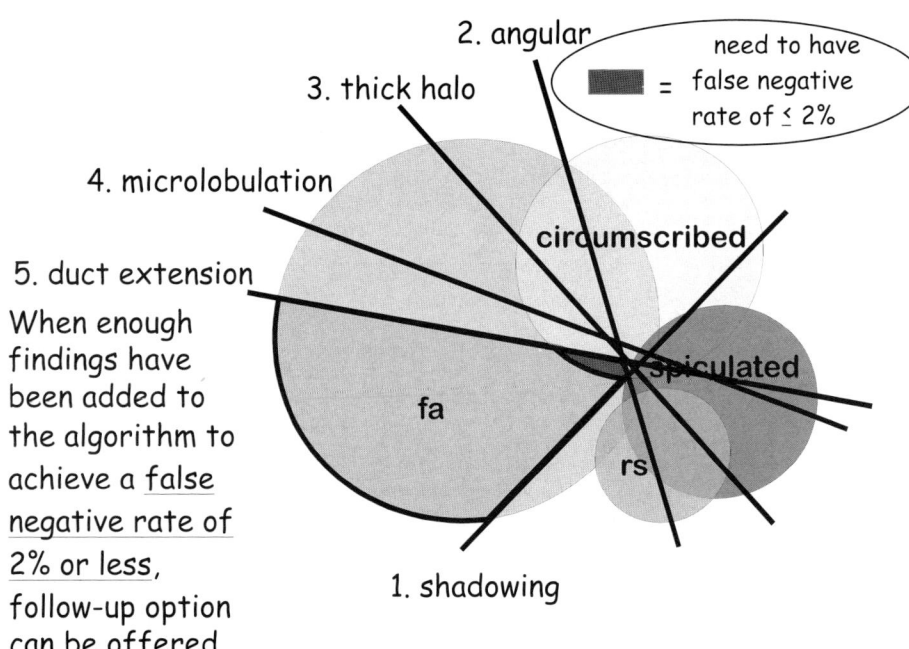

2. angular

3. thick halo

4. microlobulation

5. duct extension

When enough findings have been added to the algorithm to achieve a <u>false negative rate of 2% or less</u>, follow-up option can be offered.

need to have false negative rate of ≤ 2%

circumscribed

spiculated

fa

rs

1. shadowing

FIGURE 12–8 If enough sonographic features are employed, both spiculated and circumscribed ends of the malignant spectrum can be identified with a 98% or greater sensitivity. The cost of using multiple suspicious findings is that the percentage of the benign nodules that lack all of the suspicious sonographic features is reduced. fa = fibroadenoma.

rithm with more than two findings in order to achieve our stated goals of 98% or greater sensitivity and negative predictive value and 2% or lower false-negative rate.

Mammography Has an Established Standard of Care to which Sonographic Practice Must Adhere

The use of multiple sonographic findings in a complex and rigid algorithm is based on the premise that a subgroup of probably benign (BIRADS 3) solid breast nodules can be identified that is benign with 98% or greater certainty (less than 2% false-negative rate). Patients with lesions characterized as BIRADS 3, whether by sonography or mammography, can be offered three options: (a) short-interval follow-up, (b) image-guided large core needle biopsy or mammotomy, or (c) excisional biopsy (with image-guided needle localization for nonpalpable lesions). Later in this chapter, the actual results of the patients' decisions are presented.

There are several large published mammographic series on which adding short-interval follow-up to the list of options for patients with probably benign lesions is based. Therefore, the conclusions of our sonographic study published in 1995 and of our current ongoing study should not be considered unduly risky or out of the mainstream. The standard of care for mammographic management of probably benign lesions has already been established and implemented by mammographers and is logically based on a solid foundation of gross morphologic and histopathologic correlation. The methods we are employing in sonographic evaluation of solid breast nodules are also solidly based on the gross morphology and histopathology of breast cancer and adhere strictly to the standard of care already established by

mammographers. It is perplexing that some mammographers have been hesitant to accept and employ a sonographic algorithm that is so completely based on the mammographic algorithm that they use every day. The sonographic algorithm has directly evolved from the mammographic algorithm. In effect, mammography has established the rules by which breast lesion characterization must be undertaken. To practice the standard of care, sonographers must accept those rules and follow them. Sonography, like mammography, can identify a subpopulation of BIRADS 3 nodules that has less than a 2% chance of being malignant. Like patients who have BIRADS 3 lesions identified mammographically, patients who have BIRADS 3 lesions identified by sonography should be offered the option of short-interval follow-up in addition to the various options for biopsy. To treat sonographically characterized solid breast nodules that have less than a 2% risk for malignancy differently from mammographic lesions that have less than a 2% risk for malignancy is illogical. A lesion that has a 1% risk for malignancy has the same risk, regardless of whether that risk is defined by mammography or sonography. The resistance to the acceptance of sonographic identification of a BIRADS 3 subgroup of solid nodules is based on emotion, not science, and is certainly not in the best interest of the patient.

THE IMAGING FINDINGS, THEIR HISTOLOGIC AND MORPHOLOGIC BASIS, AND THE IMAGING ALGORITHM IN WHICH THEY ARE USED

Table 12–4 lists the nine suspicious findings used in the sonographic algorithm for evaluation of solid breast nod-

TABLE 12–4. SONOGRAPHIC FINDINGS SUSPICIOUS FOR MALIGNANCY

Characteristic	Finding
Surface	Spiculation; thick, echogenic halo
	Angular margins
	Microlobulation[a]
Shape	Taller than wide
	Duct extension[a]
	Branch pattern[a]
Internal	Sound transmission
	Echogenicity
	Calcifications

[a]Soft finding.

ules. The suspicious findings are the same findings for both the study that was published in *Radiology* in 1995 and the ongoing study. Three of the findings represent surface characteristics, three represent shapes, and three represent internal characteristics. Each of the findings has a solid basis in the gross morphology and histopathology of breast cancer. The algorithm in which these findings are used is detailed later in Table 12–7.

Each suspicious finding can also be thought of as being hard, soft, or mixed. Hard findings are more likely to be associated with invasive malignancy and have higher positive predictive values. Hard findings include spiculation, angular margins, and acoustic shadowing. Soft findings are more likely to be associated with ductal carcinoma *in situ* (DCIS)—either in pure DCIS or as intraductal components in lesions that have both invasive and DCIS components. Soft findings include duct extension, branch pattern, and calcifications. Using soft findings in addition to hard findings increases the sensitivity of the algorithm, especially for DCIS, but reduces the positive predictive value for breast cancer. A relatively large percentage of lesions that contain only soft findings are caused by nonmalignant entities, but a significant minority of such case will represent DCIS. The use of soft findings also helps assess the true extent of disease in patients who have invasive duct carcinomas with extensive intraductal components. Mixed findings such as microlobulations, taller-than-wide shape, and hypoechogenicity can be seen with both inva-

TABLE 12–5. INDIVIDUAL BENIGN SOLID NODULE FINDINGS

Pure and intensely hyperechoic texture

Elliptical shape (wider than tall)

Gently lobulated shape (three or fewer lobulations and wider than tall)

Complete thin capsule

TABLE 12–6. GROUPED BENIGN SOLID NODULE FINDINGS

Pure and intensely hyperechoic texture

Elliptical shape, wider than tall, complete thin, echogenic capsule

Gently lobulated (less than four) shape (wider than tall); complete thin capsule

sive carcinoma and DCIS and have positive predictive values intermediate between those of hard and soft findings.

Table 12–5 lists the individual benign findings used in the sonographic algorithm for evaluation of solid breast nodules. There are four individual findings, but the elliptical and gently lobulated shapes cannot stand alone and must be completely encompassed by a thin, echogenic capsule, resulting in three total benign categories that are shown in Table 12–6. Benign findings can only be sought after suspicious findings are sought and not found. If there is even a single suspicious finding, the lesion must be excluded from the probably benign (BIRADS 3) category, and benign findings should be sought.

The malignant and benign findings must be used within the context of a rigidly followed algorithm. The algorithms used for the 1995 study and the current ongoing study are listed in Table 12–7.

It can be seen in Table 12–7 that the algorithm for sonographic evaluation of solid nodules has not changed much since the 1995 study. One key difference between the 1995 study and the current study is that the 1995 study assigned lesions to one of three risk categories—benign, indeterminate, or malignant—whereas the current study uses modified BIRADS categories—BIRADS 2,3, 4a, 4b, and 5. The second key difference is that the definition of benign has changed. In 1995, lesions that had 5% or lower risk for malignancy were considered benign. In the current study, 2% or less risk for malignancy is required for inclusion in the BIRADS 3, probably benign category. The change in the risk for malignancy from 5% to 2% or less has been based on the results of several large mammographic studies in which it was proposed that lesion with 2% or lower risk could be followed rather than undergo biopsy.

Sonographic Findings Suspicious for Malignancy in Solid Nodules

Spiculation and Thick, Echogenic Halo

Spiculation is a gross morphologic finding that has been borrowed from mammography and directly applied to the sonographic evaluation of solid breast nodules. It is also a hard finding, indicating the presence of invasion of the lesion into the surrounding tissues. Spiculation consists of alternating hypoechoic and relatively hyperechoic straight

TABLE 12–7. ALGORITHMS FOR SONOGRAPHIC EVALUATION OF SOLID BREAST NODULES

1995 Study	Current Ongoing Study
1. Look for malignant findings	1. Look for malignant findings
2. If malignant findings, classify as malignant, biopsy	2. If malignant findings, classify as BIRADS 4a, 4b, or 5 and biopsy
3. If no malignant findings, look for benign findings	3. If no malignant findings, look for benign findings
4. If benign findings (≤5% risk for cancer), classify as benign; offer three options— needle biopsy, surgical biopsy, follow-up	4. If benign findings (<2% risk for cancer), classify as BIRADS 2 or 3; for BIRADS 3, offer three options—needle biopsy, surgical biopsy, follow-up
5. If benign findings not found, classify indeterminate and biopsy	5. If benign findings not found, classify as BIRADS 4a and biopsy

lines radiating out perpendicularly from the surface of the nodule (Fig. 12–9). However, it is relatively rare to see both hypoechoic and hyperechoic spiculations in an individual nodule. In general, only spiculations of one echogenicity are visible, depending on the echogenicity of the background tissues in which the lesion develops (Fig. 12–10). Thus, in invasive nodules that are surrounded by fat, only hyperechoic spiculations are visible, whereas in lesions surrounded by hyperechoic fibrous tissues, only hypoechoic spiculations are seen. Sonography does not play much of a diagnostic role in fat-surrounded spiculated lesions because they are readily visible on the mammograms that have usually been performed before sonography. The roles of sonography in most fat-surrounded spiculated lesions are localizing the lesion for ultrasound-guided biopsy and determining extent of disease. However, sonography does play a valuable diagnostic role in lesions that have hypoe-

choic spiculations because the dense, hyperechoic fibrous tissue that surrounds the spiculated lesions often obscures them on mammograms.

Because breast cancer may be heterogeneous not only from nodule to nodule, but also within the same nodule, spiculations may be present only on part of the surface of the nodule (Fig. 12–11). Recognizing that spiculations may be present only on part of the surface is important for two reasons. First, unless the entire surface of the nodule has been scanned in two orthogonal planes, it cannot be determined whether the lesion is spiculated. Accepting two images obtained in longitudinal and transverse planes through the widest part of the lesion is inadequate for purposes of evaluating surface characteristics. Second, even if most of the nodule is well circumscribed and thinly encapsulated, the presence of spiculation over only part of the surface of a nodule excludes the nodule from the BIRADS

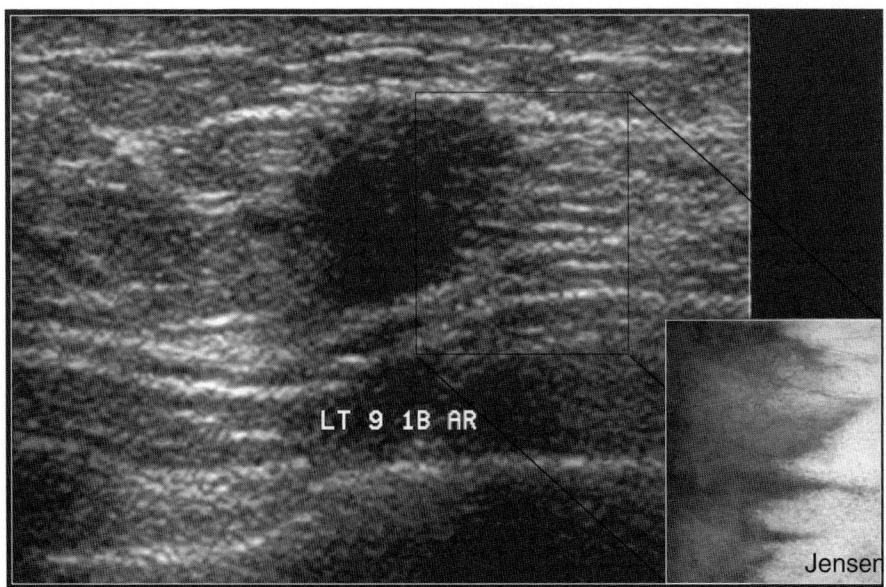

LT 9 1B AR

Jensen

FIGURE 12–9 In some malignant nodules, spiculations appear as alternating hypoechoic and hyperechoic lines radiating out perpendicularly from the surface of the nodule. The hypoechoic components represent either fingers of invasive tumor or intraductal components of tumor growing into the surrounding tissue. The hyperechoic components represent the interfaces between tumor and the surrounding breast tissues.

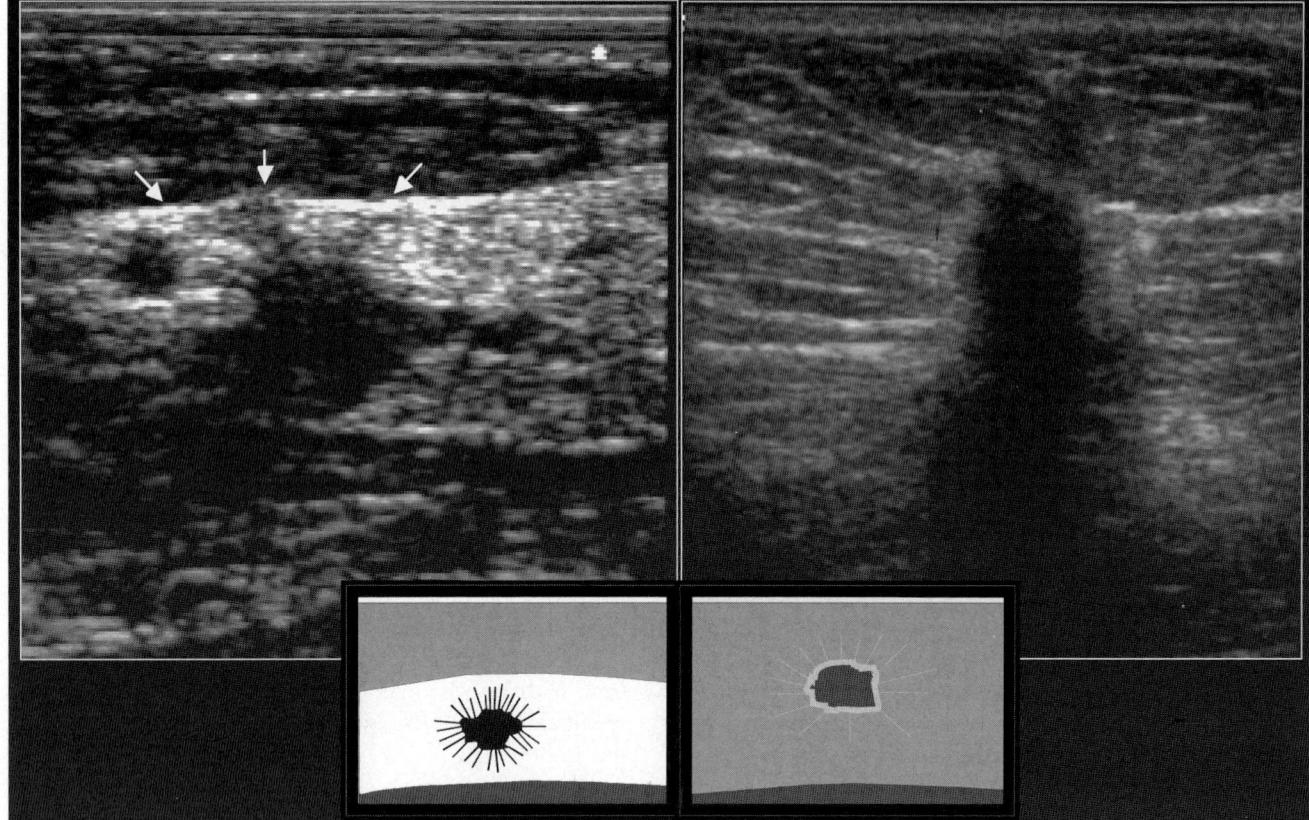

FIGURE 12–10 The malignant nodule on the **left** has visible hypoechoic spiculations that are highlighted by the hyperechoic surrounding fibrous tissue. It was neither palpable nor mammographically visible, but did cause focal pain. The malignant nodule on the **right** has hyperechoic spiculations that are contrasted by the isoechoic fat that surrounds the lesion. The lesion was visible as a spiculated nodule on mammography. Sonography was performed to localize the lesion for excision.

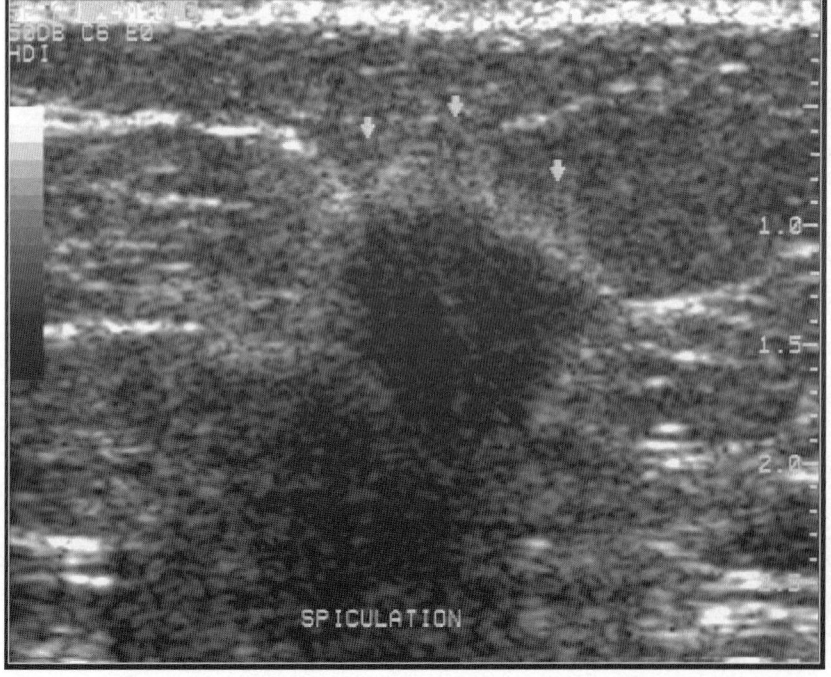

FIGURE 12–11 Breast cancer can be heterogeneous not only from nodule to nodule but also within an individual nodule. Thus, spiculations may only involve part of the nodule's surface (*arrows*). For this reason, (1) the entire nodule surface must be assessed in two planes before concluding that there are no spiculations, and (2) if part of the nodule surface is smooth and part is spiculated, the smooth surface should be ignored, and the nodule should be classified as spiculated.

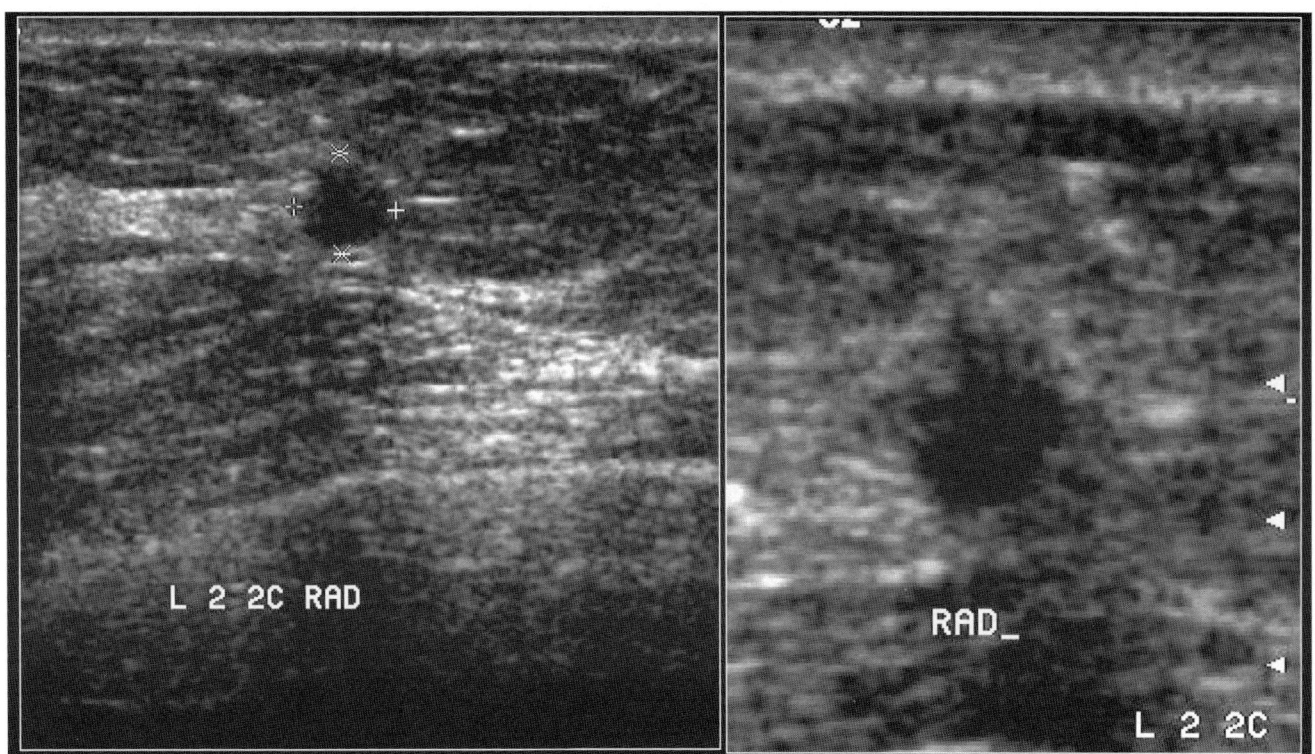

FIGURE 12–12 Write magnification can facilitate demonstration of surface characteristics such as spiculations. Note that the hypoechoic spiculations are better seen on the magnified view (**right**) than on the nonmagnified view (**left**).

3, probably benign category. The nodule must be characterized as BIRADS 4a or higher. Whenever there is a mixture of suspicious and benign findings within an individual nodule, the benign findings must be ignored, and the characteristics of the suspicious lesion must be applied to the overall BIRADS category of the nodule.

Magnification views of the nodule may aid in evaluating its surface characteristics such as spiculation, just as it does for mammography (Fig. 12–12). "Write magnification," rather than "read magnification," should be employed to best assess surface characteristics. In write magnification modes, scan lines are rewritten in order to maintain or even increase line density and spatial resolution. In read magnification mode, each pixel is merely magnified, making all nodules look more jagged. Under ideal circumstances, when the magnification box uses less than half of the elements and channels, half-line scanning modes may double the line density within the magnification box.

Real-time compounding is a recent technical development that helps identify spiculations by better demonstrating spicules that are not precisely perpendicular to the ultrasound beam (Fig. 12–13).

Spiculation has a very good positive predictive value but a low sensitivity (Table 12–8). To improve the sensitivity of spiculations, we now consider the presence of a thick, echogenic halo around the nodule to be a variant of spicu-

lations. Thus, in the current study, the presence of either a thick, echogenic halo or frank spiculations is considered positive for spiculations. We believe that the thick, echogenic halo represents hyperechoic spicules that are too small to resolve sonographically. The sonographic demonstration of frank spiculations depends on the echogenicity of surrounding tissues, the size of the spiculations, and the spatial resolution of the ultrasound equipment. In at least some cases, it is possible to demonstrate frank spiculations with high-end equipment when low-end equipment shows only a thick, echogenic halo (Fig. 12–14). Such cases have convinced us that the presence of a thick, echogenic halo should be considered to represent unresolved spiculations.

Typical thick, echogenic halos caused by unresolved spiculations are thicker along the lateral edges of the lesion and either thinner or less apparent along the anterior and posterior aspects of the lesion (Fig. 12–15). The reason for the halo appearing thicker along the lateral edges of the lesion is that the spicules are nearly perpendicular to the ultrasound beam along the sides of the lesion and therefore make strong spicular reflectors. The spicules that lie along the anterior and posterior edges of the lesion are nearly parallel to the ultrasound beam, make poor spicular reflectors, and thus are poorly shown sonographically.

Some very small malignant nodules may have a very small hypoechoic central nidus and a very thick halo (Fig.

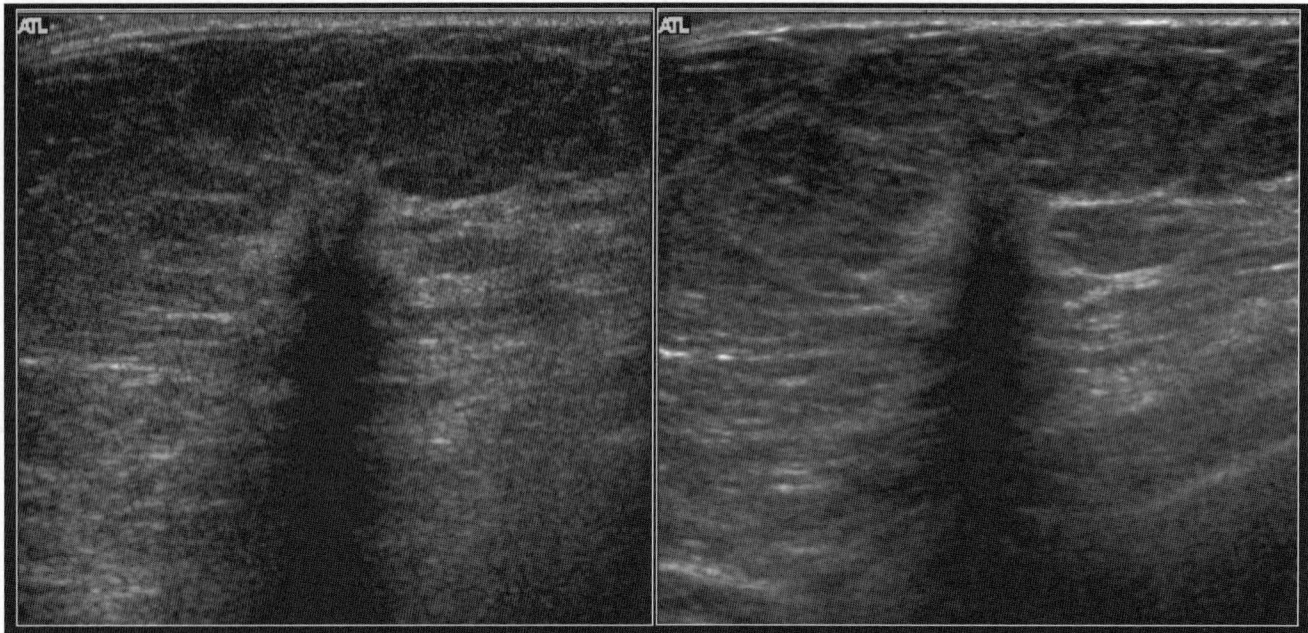

FIGURE 12–13 Real-time spatial compounding can improve our ability to demonstrate spicula-tions. The alternating hypoechoic and hyperechoic spiculations seen along the lateral edges of the nodule are better seen with spatial compounding (**right**) than with conventional imaging (**left**).

12–16). If the lesion is not scanned carefully, it can be mis-taken for a purely hyperechoic benign lesion. This is partic-ularly true if the lesion lies in the near field and is subject to volume-averaging artifact or if the entire lesion is not scanned carefully and tangential images through the halo are obtained without obtaining any images through the hy-poechoic central nidus. These technical errors resulting in false-negative benign characterizations are discussed and il-lustrated later in this chapter in the section on benign find-ings in purely hyperechoic lesions and in Chapter 21 in the discussion of false-negative findings and technical errors. We have never seen and do not believe that there are purely hyperechoic malignant lesions. Either equipment resolu-tion must be inadequate or technical errors must be made

to create the appearance of a purely hyperechoic malignant solid nodule.

Occasionally, a thick, ill-defined, echogenic halo is the result of peritumoral edema rather than unresolved spicu-lations (Fig. 12–17). The halo resulting from peritumoral edema has a more uniform echotexture than that of spiculations and does not become linear in texture, regard-less of the spatial resolution of the ultrasound equipment. Peritumoral edema can be caused by either intense peritu-moral inflammation (typical in high-grade invasive and medullary carcinomas) or from lymphatic obstruction due to lymphatic invasion. Inflammatory peritumoral edema randomly occurs along any and all surfaces of the tumor that have an intense inflammatory host response. Peritu-

(text continued on page 463)

TABLE 12–8. SENSITIVITY AND POSITIVE PREDICTIVE VALUES (PPV) FOR SPICULATION AND THICK, ECHOGENIC HALO

	1995 Study (750 Nodules)[a]		Current Study (1,211 Nodules)[b]	
		PPV		PPV
	Sensitivity	Odds Ratio	Sensitivity	Odds Ratio
Spiculations	36%	92% (5.5)	36%	87% (2.7)
Thick halo	—	—	35%	74% (1.9)
Spiculation or halo	—	—	71%	80% (2.4)

[a]Prevalence, 16.7%.
[b]Prevalence, 32.8%.

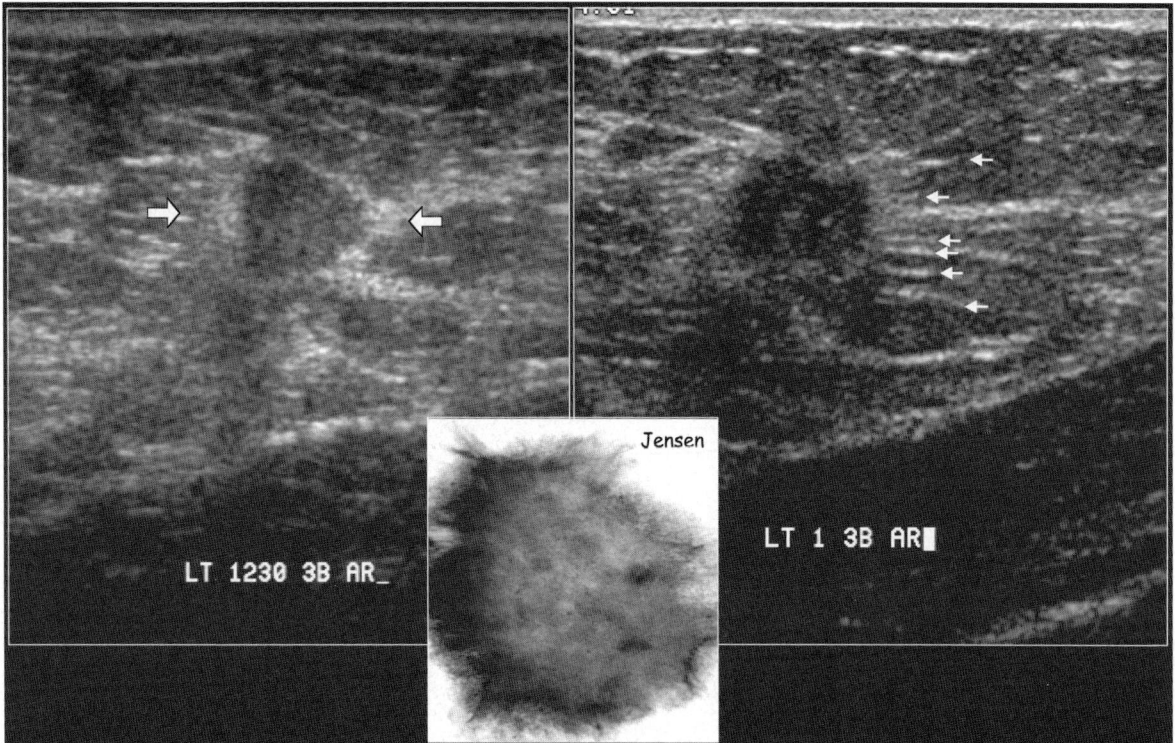

FIGURE 12–14 Whether sonography is able to show frank spiculations or a thick echogenic halo depends on the size of the spiculations and the spatial resolution of the ultrasound equipment being used. What appears to be a thick, echogenic halo (unresolved spiculations) with a cheaper machine (with inherently lower spatial resolution) may appear as frank spiculations when scanned with a machine that has higher spatial resolution. These images show the same nodule scanned on the same day with machines of different spatial resolution. The image on the **left,** which was obtained with a lower-resolution machine, shows an ill-defined thick, echogenic halo *(block arrows)*, whereas the image on the **right,** which was obtained with a higher-resolution machine with a 1.5-D array, shows frank echogenic spiculations along the lateral edges of the nodule where the spicules are perpendicular to the beam *(arrows)*. Note that some spiculations on gross morphologic specimens are so tiny that they appear hairlike. (Subgross histology courtesy of Hanna Jansen, MD, University of California, Davis.)

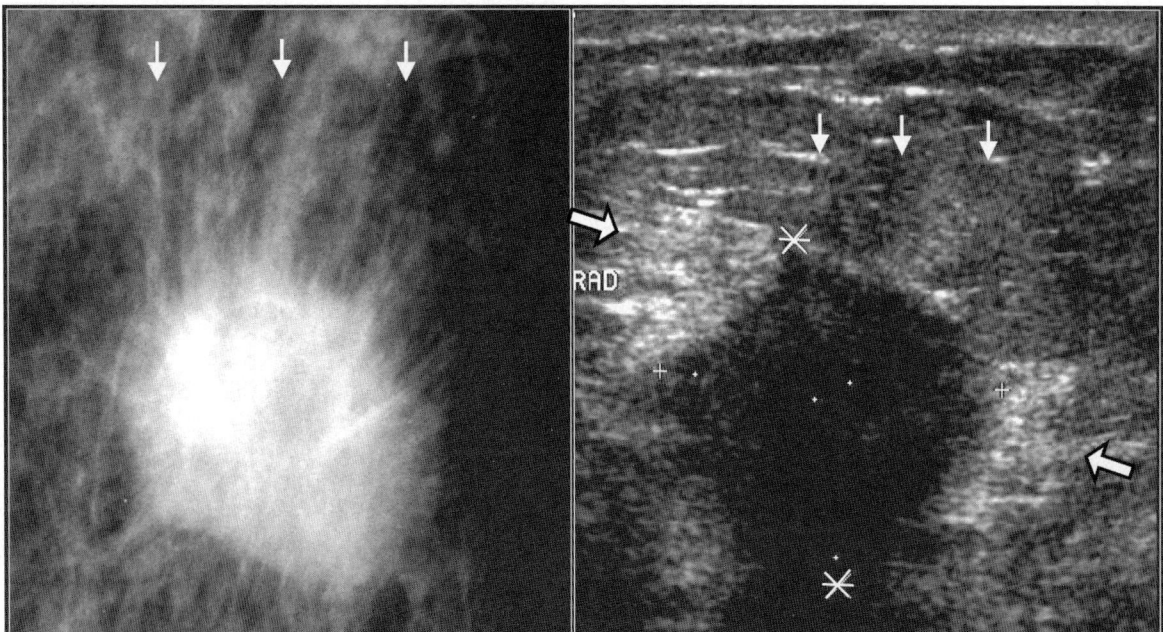

FIGURE 12–15 Note that even though the superficially located spiculations are the most prominent spiculations mammographically, they are poorly shown sonographically *(arrows)*. Typically, the thick, echogenic halo is thicker and brighter along the lateral edges of the nodule *(block arrows)* because that is where the spicules are perpendicular to the ultrasound beam and make bright specular reflectors. Typically, the halo is thinner and less bright anteriorly and posteriorly because that is where the spicules are parallel to the ultrasound beam and make poor specular reflectors. Acoustic shadowing that typically occurs with spiculated lesions also tends to obscure spiculations that lie along the deep surface of the nodule, as they do in this case *(*)*.

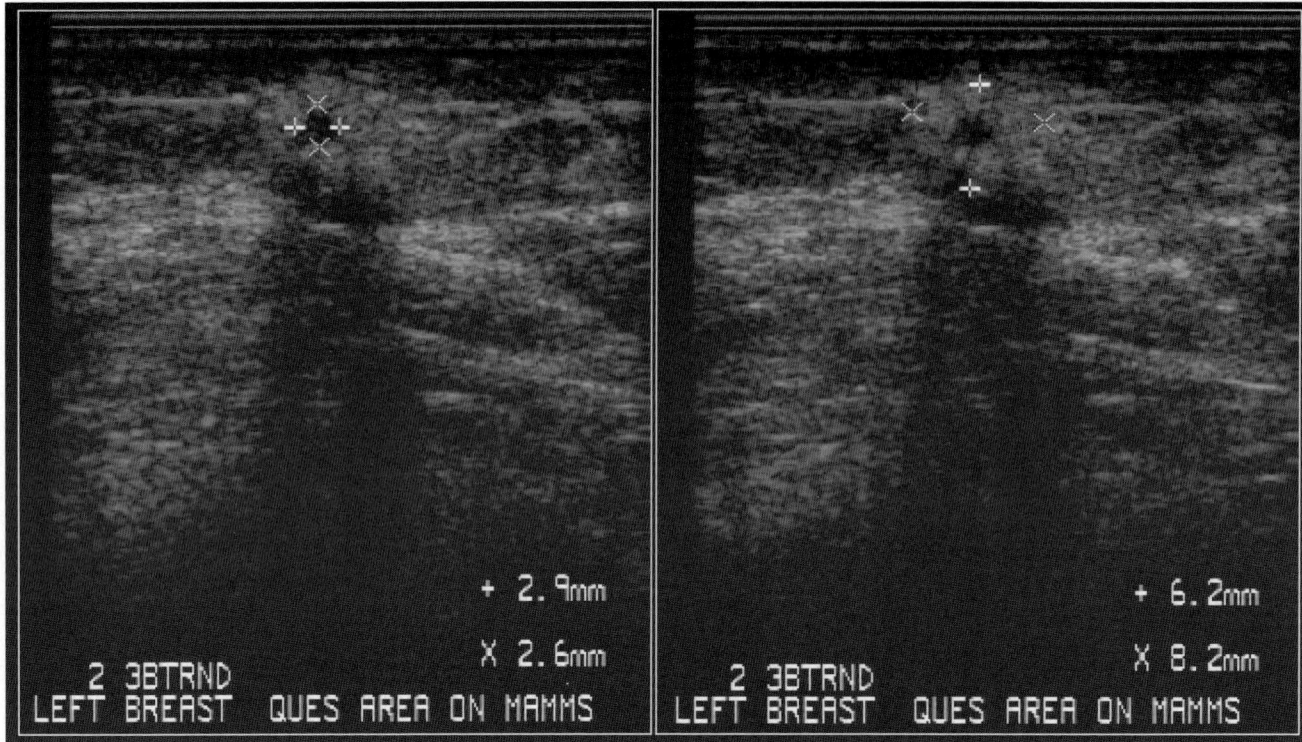

FIGURE 12–16 We have never seen a purely hyperechoic, malignant solid nodule. However, in some cases, the central hypoechoic tumor nodule may be very small (less than 3 mm in **left** image), and the thick echogenic halo can be much larger (8 mm maximum diameter, **right**). Near-field volume averaging or tangential images obtained through the edges of the thick, echogenic halo could lead to a false impression that the lesion is purely hyperechoic.

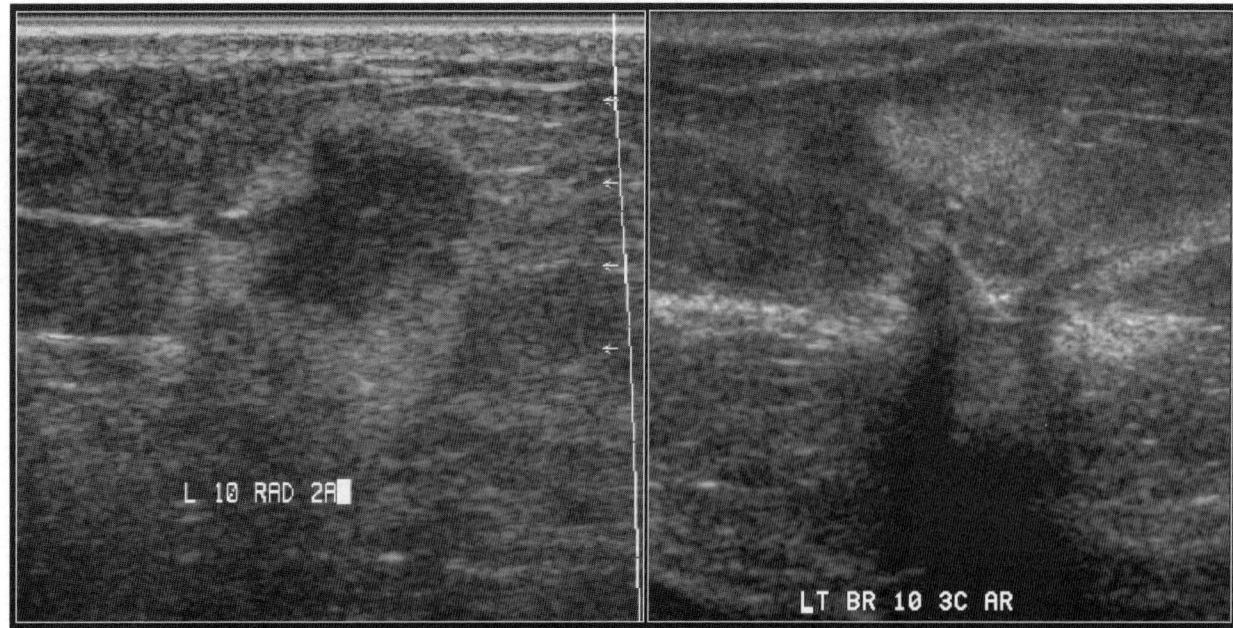

FIGURE 12–17 Not all thick, echogenic halos arise from unresolved spiculations. Edema in peritumoral fat may make the fat appear hyperechoic instead of its usual isoechoic appearance. Peritumoral edema may result from an intense peritumoral inflammatory response that occurs in high-grade invasive ductal carcinomas and medullary carcinomas. Inflammatory peritumoral edema occurs randomly along any inflamed surface of the tumor (**left**). Lymphedema due to lymphatic invasion and obstruction can also cause an ill-defined thick, echogenic halo. The halo caused by lymphedema typically occurs superficial to the nodule (**right**) because the usual pattern of lymphatic drainage from the mammary zone is superficially toward the subdermal network, to the periareolar area, and finally to the regional (usually axillary) lymph nodes.

moral lymphedema typically occurs superficially, between the solid nodule and the skin, because lymphatic drainage from malignant tumors typically is in a superficial direction, toward the subdermal lymphatic network. Peritumoral edema that occurs only superficial to a suspicious solid nodule indicates a higher than normal likelihood of lymph node metastasis.

Of course, there are benign entities that can be spiculated and simulate malignancy. Radial scar is the most common. Sclerosing adenosis, fat necrosis, and biopsy scar are other histologic entities that can be spiculated mammographically and sonographically. The sonographic features of such entities are discussed and illustrated in Chapters 13, 15, and 18.

Table 12–8 shows the sensitivities and positive predictive values for frank spiculations in the 1995 study and the sensitivities and positive predictive values for frank spiculations; thick, echogenic halo; and either spiculations or halo in the current ongoing study. Note that by combining thick halo with spiculations, the positive predictive value has been reduced mildly, bur the sensitivity of spiculation has been more than doubled, and the overall accuracy has also been improved.

Angular Margins

The presence of angular margins is the most accurate of all sonographic findings suspicious for malignancy. Angular margins are the same as the irregular or jagged margins that have been the most commonly reported suspicious finding in the literature during the past 20 years. Angularity of the nodule margin is a mammographic finding that has been applied to sonography. The presence of angular margins is a hard finding, indicative of invasive malignancy in most instances.

The presence of angular margins is especially valuable because it can occur in both spiculated and circumscribed malignant nodules. In some circumscribed malignant nodules, angular margins are the only hard suspicious findings present.

The angles on the surface of the solid nodule may be very acute, 90 degrees, or even obtuse. Some angles are so acute that they may be difficult to distinguish from thick spiculations (Fig. 12–18). As is always the case, the heterogeneity of breast cancer must be kept in mind when evaluating the nodule surface for angular margins. Breast cancer may have mixed characteristics. Thus, angular margins may be very localized and may be present only on one sur-

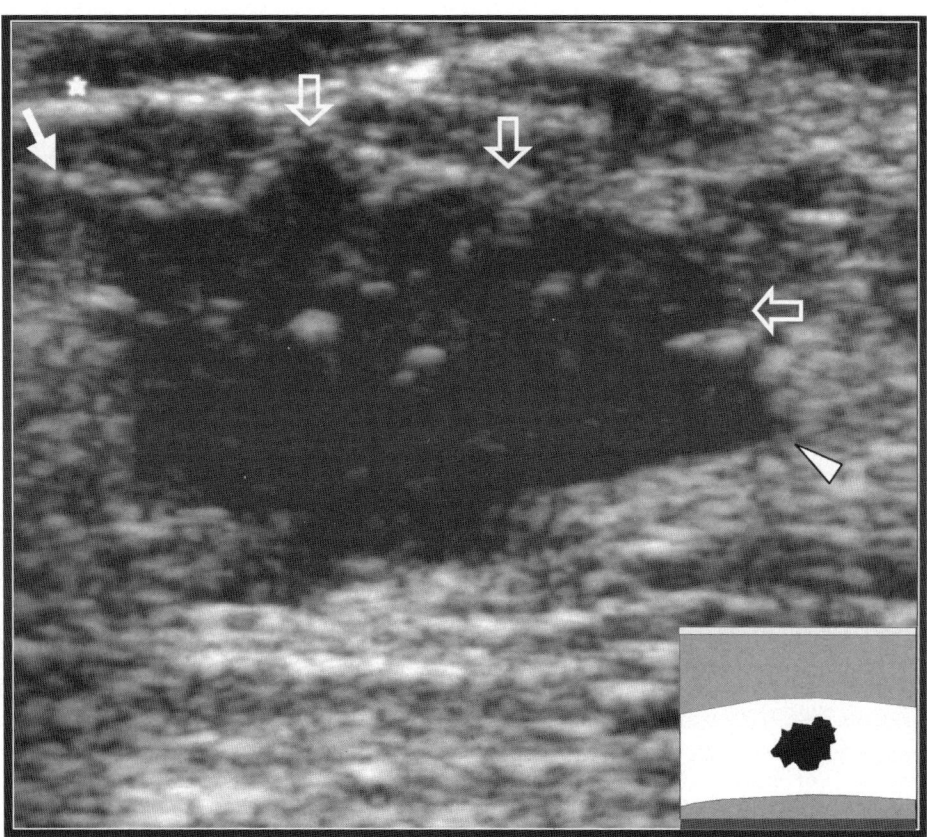

FIGURE 12–18 The angles formed along the surface of the nodule may be very acute, like a large spiculation *(arrow)*, acute *(hollow arrow)*, 90 degrees *(arrowhead)*, or obtuse. The presence of a single angle on any surface of the nodule must exclude the nodule from the BIRADS 3 category.

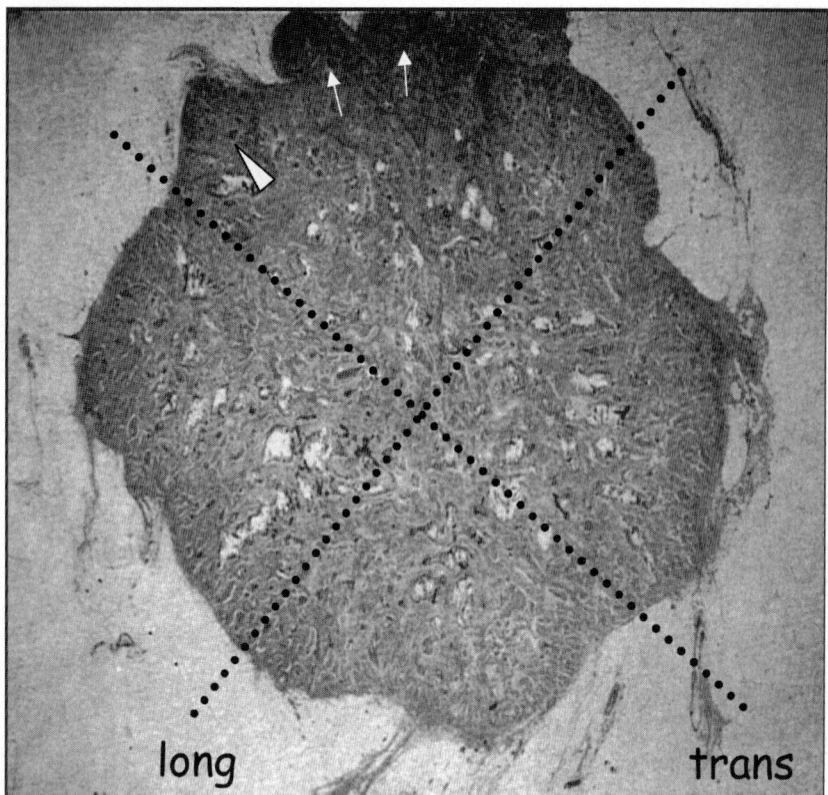

long   trans

FIGURE 12–19 Because of the internal heterogeneity of breast cancer, angular margins may involve only one surface of the nodule. Note that in this circumscribed carcinoma, the angular margin *(arrowhead)* and microlobulations *(arrows)* that involve only one surface of the nodule would have been missed by traditional longitudinal and transverse planes through the widest part of the nodule *(dotted black lines)*. Thus, to exclude the presence of angular margins, the entire nodule must be scanned in two planes, preferably radial and antiradial planes. Furthermore, even if only one angular margin is identified, the lesion must be excluded from the BIRADS 3 category.

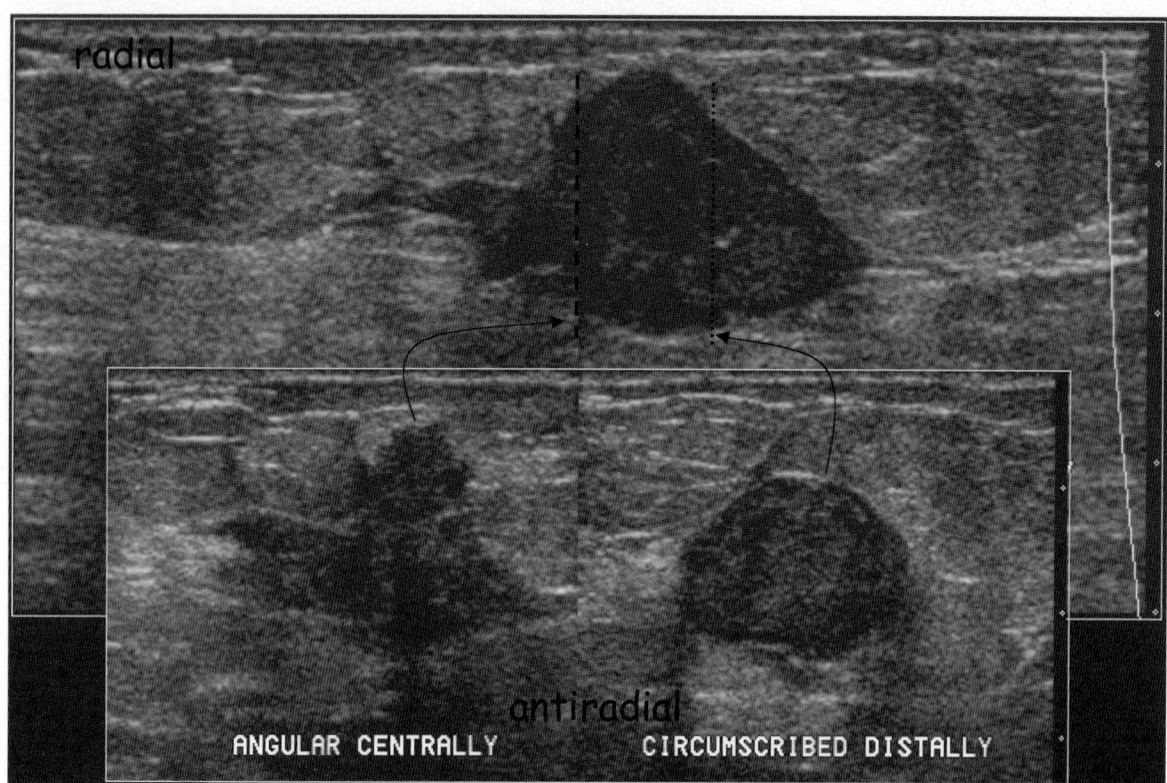

radial

antiradial

ANGULAR CENTRALLY   CIRCUMSCRIBED DISTALLY

FIGURE 12–20 This large, intermediate-grade invasive ductal carcinoma demonstrates the heterogeneity of breast cancer within a single nodule. The **upper** image shows a radial view through the nodule. The **lower** split-screen images show two antiradial planes through the lesion. The **right lower** image was obtained at the level of the *dotted black line* and shows a portion of the tumor that has a wider-than-tall, gently lobulated shape that we typically associate with benign lesions. The **lower left** image was obtained at the level of the *dashed black line* and has numerous angular margins and microlobulations that clearly indicate the true nature of the lesion. Internal heterogeneity of lesions is the reason that suspicious findings cannot be excluded unless the entire surface area and substance of the nodule are assessed.

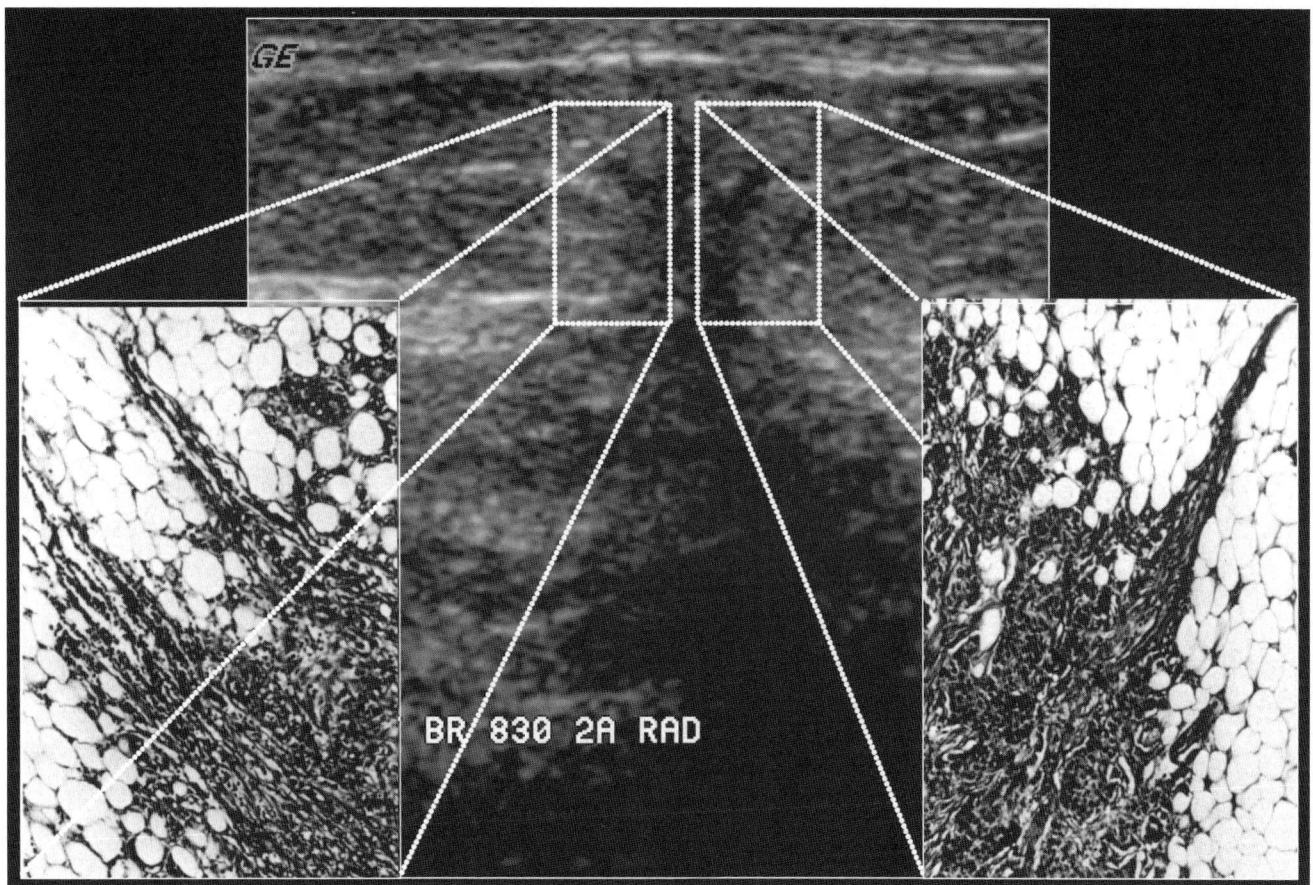

FIGURE 12–21 Angular margins occur along surfaces of the nodule that offer the lowest resistance to invasion. In malignant nodules that are surrounded by fat, there is little resistance of invasion in any direction. Therefore, angular margins and spiculations can be found along any surface of a spiculated nodule that is surrounded by fat.

face of a nodule. The entire surface of the nodule must be evaluated in two orthogonal planes before it is concluded that there are no angular margins present. Even if most of the nodule surface of the nodule is smooth, rounded, and thinly encapsulated, but there is an angular margin along one surface, the nodule must excluded from the BIRADS 3 or probably benign category (Figs. 12–19 and 12–20). Even a single angle on any surface of the nodule should exclude the nodule from the BIRADS 3 class and requires characterization into BIRADS 4a category or higher. It is important to understand that the presence of angular margins and a thin, echogenic capsule are not mutually exclusive findings. It is possible to have a thinly encapsulated angular margin. In such cases, the benign finding, the thin, echogenic capsule, is ignored, and the nodule is assigned the more suspicious risk category of the angular margin.

Invasion into surrounding tissues follows the paths of least resistance. Fat offers little resistance to invasion in any direction (Fig. 12–21). Thus, fat-surrounded lesions tend to have angles randomly distributed along all surfaces. However, denser fibrous tissues and the anterior mammary fascia offer higher resistance to direct invasion and tend to

force tumor growth into predictable patterns. Fibrous tissue presents intermediate resistance, depending on whether the lesion grows parallel or perpendicular to the collagen fibers. Angular margins in fibrous-surrounded lesions tend to occur along the lateral edges of the lesion and resemble thick, hypoechoic spiculations (Fig. 12–22). Densely fibrotic support ligaments and the anterior and posterior mammary fascia offer even higher resistance to direct invasion than do hyperechoic fibrous elements.

Angular margins are most frequently and easily demonstrated at the point at which Cooper's ligaments intersect the surface of the malignant nodule. The higher relative resistance of the anterior mammary fascia to invasion by malignancy explains this. The anterior mammary fascia is not an absolute barrier to invasion because cancer may invade through it, but it offers enough resistance that in most cases malignancy will grow along the undersurface of the fascia until it reaches a point of lower resistance to invasion. The anterior mammary fascia is not a completely intact envelope in which ducts and lobules are contained. Rather, it is discontinuous at each point at which Cooper's ligament attaches (Fig. 12–23A). At each ligament, the an-

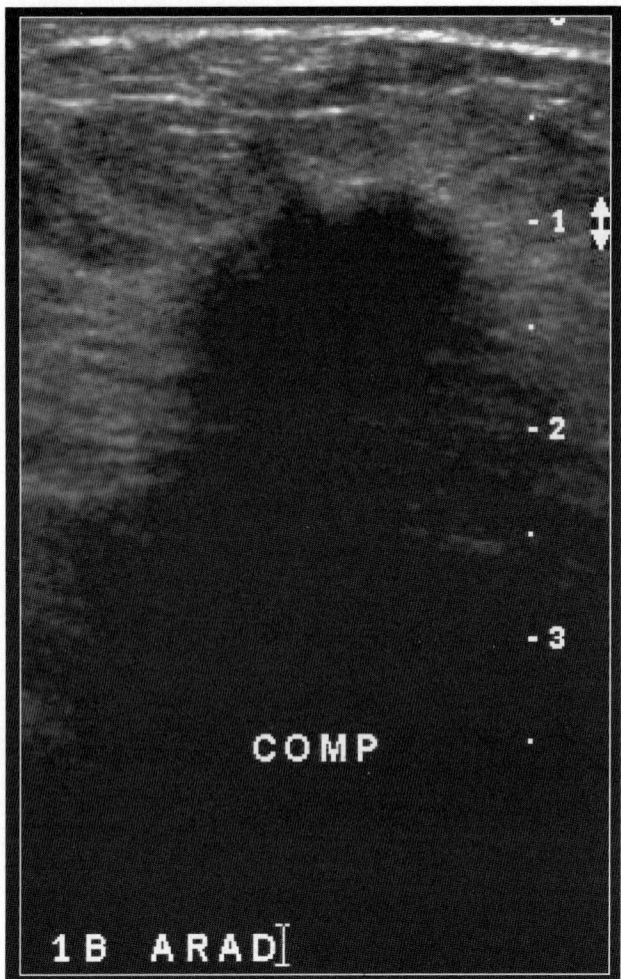

FIGURE 12–22 In malignant nodules that are surrounded by fibrous tissue, the paths of low resistance tend to be between collagen fibers that are horizontally oriented. Thus, the angular margins tend to lie along the lateral edges of the nodule and to resemble thick spiculations.

terior mammary fascia continues up to the skin along one surface of Cooper's ligament, attaches to the skin, and then courses back down along the other side of the ligament, eventually continuing horizontally as the anterior mammary fascia. Thus, each Cooper's ligament is composed of two layers of fascia that are closely opposed to each other except at its deep end, where the two layers of fascia separate from each other to continue as the anterior mammary fascia. The shape of the space between the leaves of fascia as they separate is triangular. The potential space between the leaves of fascia that form the base of each Cooper's ligament, unlike the anterior mammary fascia, presents a path of low resistance for the growth of invasive malignancy. If we think of the anterior mammary fascia as a fence, the base of each Cooper's ligament represents a potential gate in the fence. The invasive malignancy that grows through the fence conforms to the triangular space between the two leaves of fascia that form Cooper's ligaments, forming points or angles at the base of each ligament that intersects the surface of the invasive malignant nodule (Fig. 12–23B). Thus, the key to identifying angular margins with the highest sensitivity possible is to follow hyperechoic Cooper's ligaments posteriorly through the subcutaneous fat until they intersect the surface of the nodule. If the lesion is an invasive malignancy, angles will be formed at the points at which Cooper's ligaments touch the surface of the nodule (Fig. 12–24). It is not at all unusual to see invasive malignant nodules that have numerous angles at points along the surface that are intersected by Cooper's ligaments (Fig. 12–25). Angular margins can occur along paths of low resistance of invasion other than the bases of Cooper's ligaments. Some angles can occur when tumor invades loose periductal stromal tissue, and

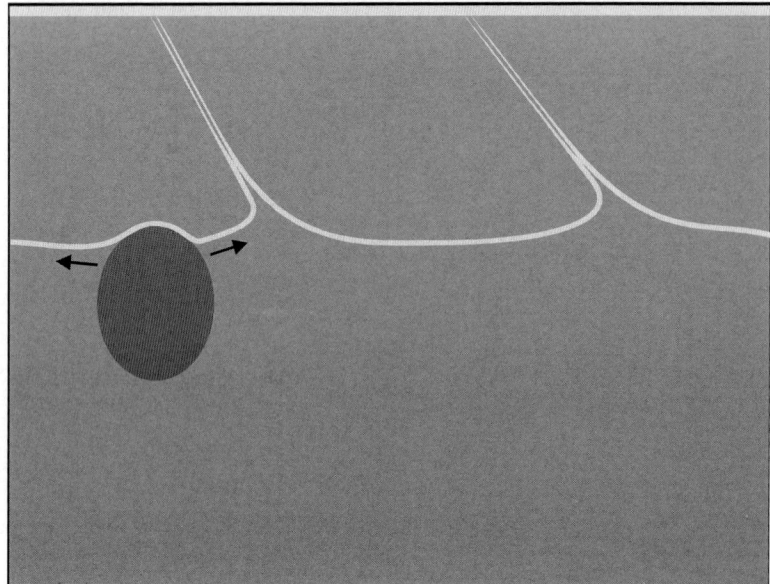

A

FIGURE 12–23 A: The anterior mammary fascia has a relatively high resistance to direct invasion by carcinomas. Thus, cancers that lie adjacent the fascia tend to be forced into a horizontal growth pattern along the undersurface of the fascia until they encounter a point of low resistance to invasion. The points of low resistance are at the intersection of Cooper's ligaments with the anterior mammary fascia. Each ligament is composed of two layers of fascia that are continuous with the anterior mammary fascia. *Continued.*

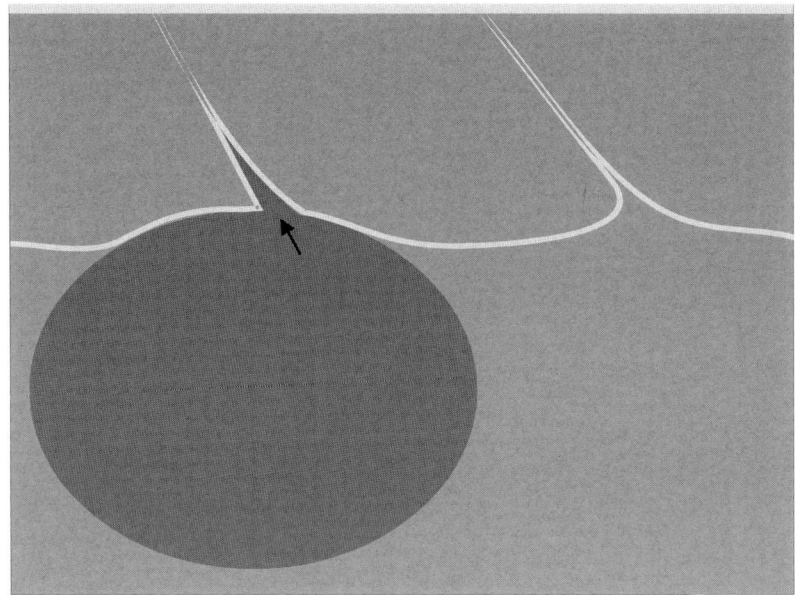

B

FIGURE 12–23 *(continued)* B: As the nodule enlarges horizontally along the undersurface of the anterior mammary fascia, it encounters the base of a Cooper's ligament, where the anterior mammary fascia is absent and where the resistance to invasion is low. Tumor grows into the base of Cooper's ligament, assuming the angular shape of the base of the ligament. Thus, one of the keys to identifying angular margins is to identify the echogenic Cooper's ligaments and follow them down to their interfaces with the nodule's surface.

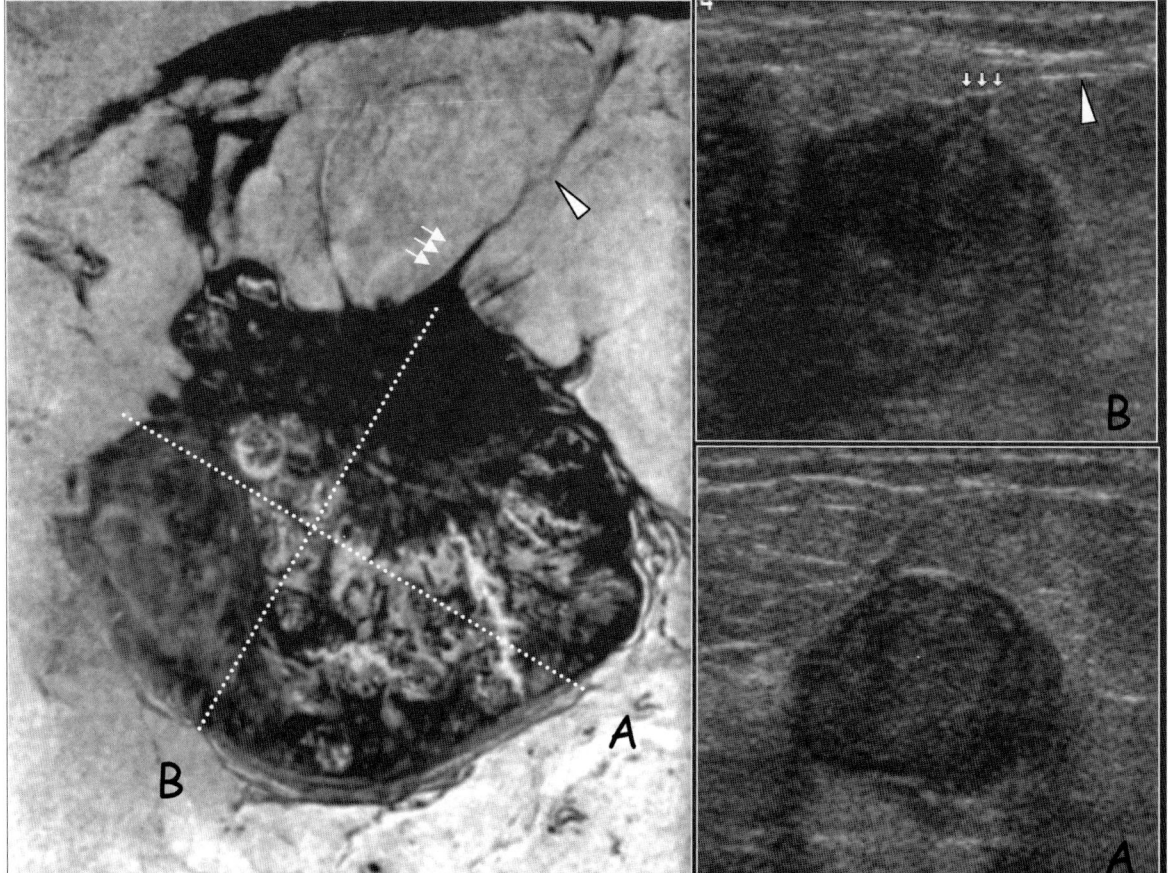

FIGURE 12–24 This circumscribed malignant nodule illustrates how to maximize the sensitivity of angular margins. Note that the plane through this nodule shows only one angular margin. The remainder of the nodule is only gently lobulated. If an image were obtained through plane *A*, sonography would only show a gently lobulated nodule with features that suggest benignity. However, if the *echogenic Cooper's ligament is identified* (white arrowhead) and followed deeply to its intersection with the surface of the nodule, the angular margin that represents invasion into the space at the base of Cooper's ligament *(three arrows)* is readily demonstrable.

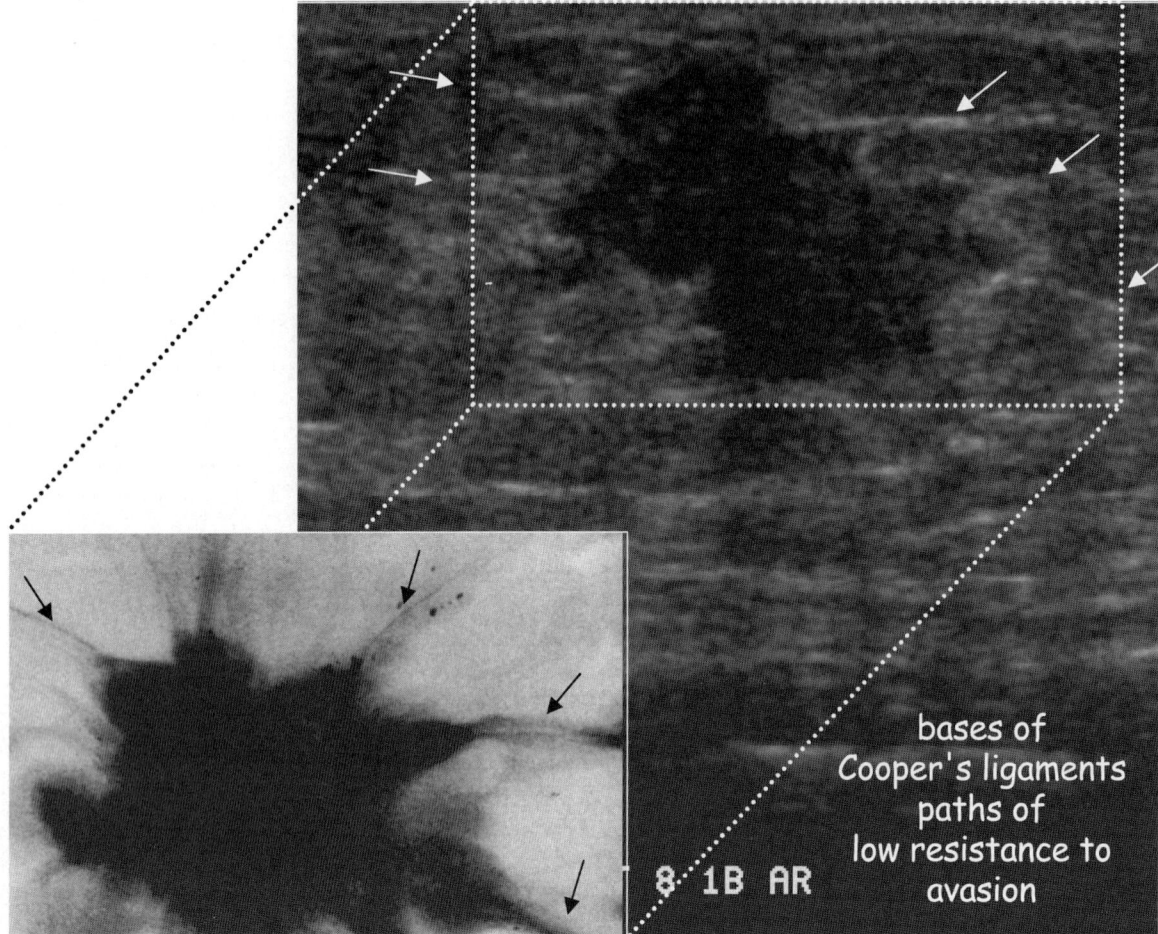

bases of
Cooper's ligaments
paths of
low resistance to
avasion

8 1B AR

FIGURE 12–25 Note that angular margins associated with invasion of the bases of Cooper's ligaments are common and often multiple.

others can occur as tumor grows horizontally along the undersurface of Cooper's ligaments. However, careful attention to the intersection of Cooper's ligaments with the surface of solid nodules is the most useful way to improve detection of angular margins in solid nodules that are malignant and invasive.

Table 12–9 shows the sensitivities and positive predictive values for angular margins in the 1995 study and in the current ongoing study. The improvement in sensitivity between the 1995 study and the current study is the result of careful examination of the intersection of Cooper's ligament with the surface of the malignant solid nodules. The overall accuracy of angular margins is 75% in the current study.

Microlobulation

Microlobulation is a surface characteristic and a mammographic finding that has been applied to sonography. It is a

**TABLE 12–9. SENSITIVITY AND POSITIVE PREDICTIVE VALUES (PPV)
FOR ANGULAR MARGINS**

	1995 Study (750 Nodules)[a]		Current Study (1,211 Nodules)[b]	
		PPV		PPV
	Sensitivity	Odds Ratio	Sensitivity	Odds Ratio
Angular margins	83%	68% (4.0)	90%	59% (1.8)

[a]Prevalence, 16.7%.
[b]Prevalence, 32.8%.

mixed finding that can be seen with both invasive carcinoma and pure DCIS. Microlobulations should be distinguished from large gentle lobulations that are several millimeters in size and few in number. In fact, three or fewer gentle large lobulations are considered to be a benign finding. Microlobulations are much smaller (1 or 2 mm), more numerous, and closer together. Because breast cancer is heterogeneous not only from nodule to nodule, but also within an individual nodule, only part of a malignant nodule may be microlobulated. Thus, as is always the case, the entire surface of the nodule must be scanned in two orthogonal planes before it is concluded that there are no microlobulations. If part of the nodule is smooth and part is microlobulated, the smooth part must be ignored, and the entire nodule must be assigned to the higher risk category of the microlobulations.

As is true for any surface characteristic, write magnification may improve the scan resolution and the definition of surface characteristics such as microlobulations (Fig. 12–26). Additionally, real-time compounding may help to better define microlobulations (Fig. 12–27).

There are three possible histologic explanations for microlobulation that include both invasive and intraductal features: (a) micronodular invasive tumor, (b) intraductal components of tumor, and (c) cancerized lobules. It is not always possible to determine whether microlobulations reflect the presence of a micronodular pattern of invasive malignancy or the presence of DCIS in either pure form or in combination with invasive components of tumor. However, there are clues that suggest the etiology in certain cases:

1. Microlobulations that have angular configurations or are associated with a thick, echogenic lesion suggest the presence of a micronodular invasive tumor (Fig. 12–28).
2. Microlobulations that are rounded and thinly encapsulated suggest the presence DCIS. If all of the other suspicious findings that are associated with microlobulation are soft (calcifications, duct extension, and branch pattern), the lesion is more likely to represent pure DCIS or DCIS with microinvasion. On the other hand, if microlobulations coexist with hard findings (spiculations, thick halo, angular margins), the lesion is likely to

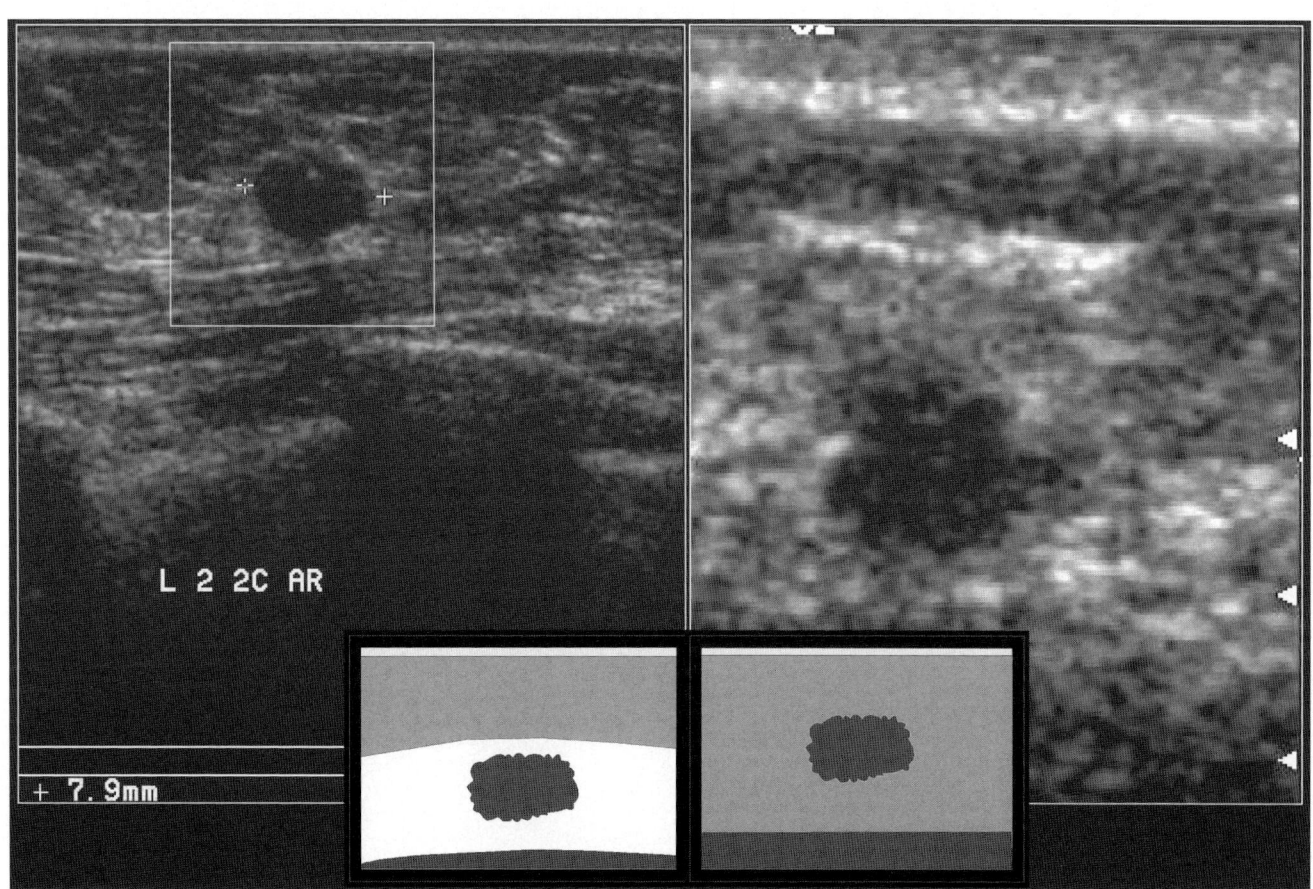

FIGURE 12–26 Like spiculations and other surface characteristics, microlobulations are frequently better demonstrated when viewed with write magnification. Note that when magnified **(right)**, the microlobulations in this circumscribed malignant nodule are much better demonstrated than they are without magnification **(left)**.

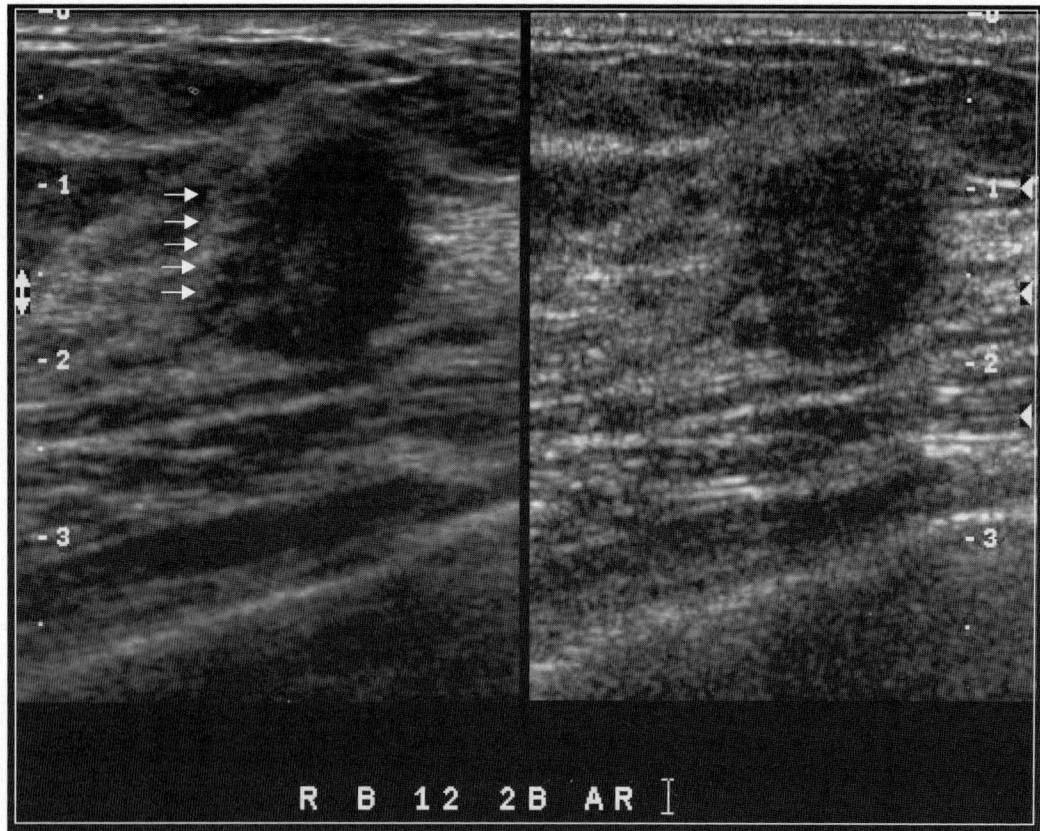

FIGURE 12–27 Microlobulations *(arrows)*, like other surface characteristics, are frequently better demonstrated with real-time spatial compounding (**left**) than they are with conventional imaging (**right**).

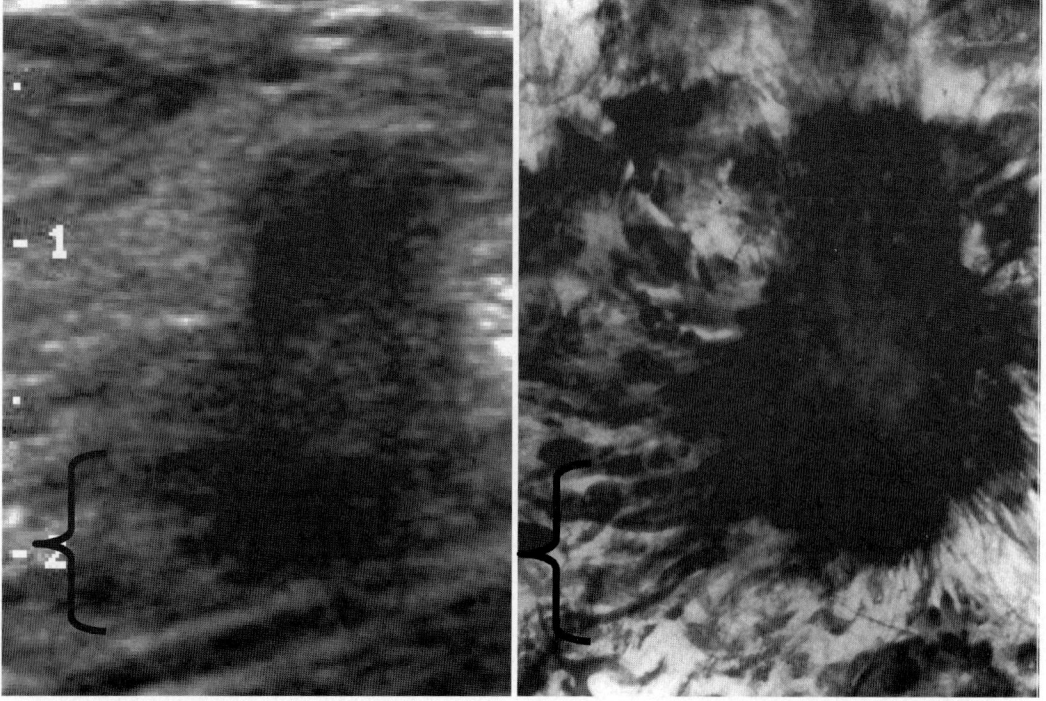

FIGURE 12–28 Microlobulations that are angular and that are associated with a thick, echogenic halo most commonly represent fingers of tumor invading the surrounding tissues. There is a continuous spectrum from microlobulations to spiculations. (Subgross histology image courtesy of Laszio Takar, MD.)

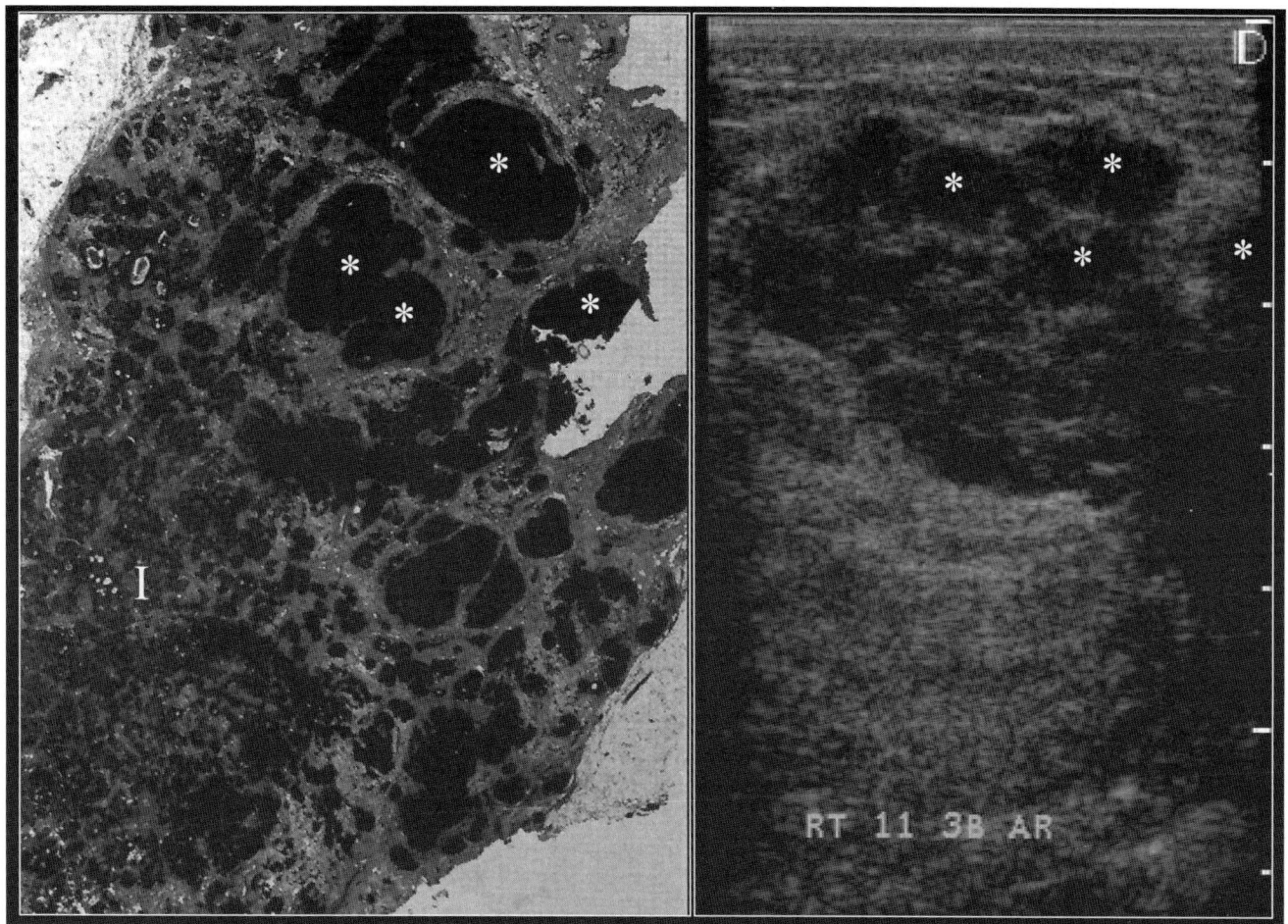

FIGURE 12–29 About 85% of invasive ductal carcinomas have ductal carcinoma *in situ* (DCIS) components. In such cases, the cords of invasive tumor *(I)* are most typically centrally located, and the DCIS components of tumor are located in the periphery. The microlobulated surface of such lesions is the result of the intraductal (DCIS) components of tumor *(*)* rather than the centrally located invasive components.

contain both invasive and intraductal (DCIS) components. More than 80% of invasive ductal carcinomas have components of DCIS within them. In most such cases, the cords of invasive tumor lie centrally within the nodule, and the DCIS distended ducts are in the periphery of the nodule. Thus, the surface characteristics in such lesions result from DCIS components of the tumor rather than the invasive components (Fig. 12–29).

3. Breast cancer can grow inside the breast through the ductal system. Cancer may grow within the ducts centrally toward the nipple or peripherally into lobules, "cancerizing" them. Cancerized lobules can become abnormally enlarged (Fig. 12–30), and the presence of multiple enlarged cancerized lobules may contribute to microlobulation. In malignant solid nodules that contain extensive intraductal components of tumor, both intraductal components of tumor and cancerized lobules can cause microlobulations (Fig. 12–31).

Interestingly, in malignant nodules that are composed of both invasive and intraductal components of tumor, the size of microlobulations correlates with the histologic grade of carcinoma (Fig. 12–32). High-grade invasive ductal carcinomas tend to have high-nuclear-grade DCIS components of tumor. High-nuclear-grade DCIS is more likely to have grossly distend ducts, creating relatively large microlobulations. Low-grade invasive ductal carcinoma is most likely to have low-nuclear-grade DCIS components. Ducts that contain low-nuclear-grade DCIS are less likely to be distended and thus are more likely to cause small microlobulations. Intermediate-grade invasive ductal carcinoma is most likely to have medium-sized microlobulations. Thus, the larger the microlobulations, the more likely the lesion is to be high grade.

Microlobulation is a mixed finding that most frequently results from DCIS components of tumor rather than fingers of invasive tumor. Microlobulation is especially helpful in avoiding false-negative findings in circum-

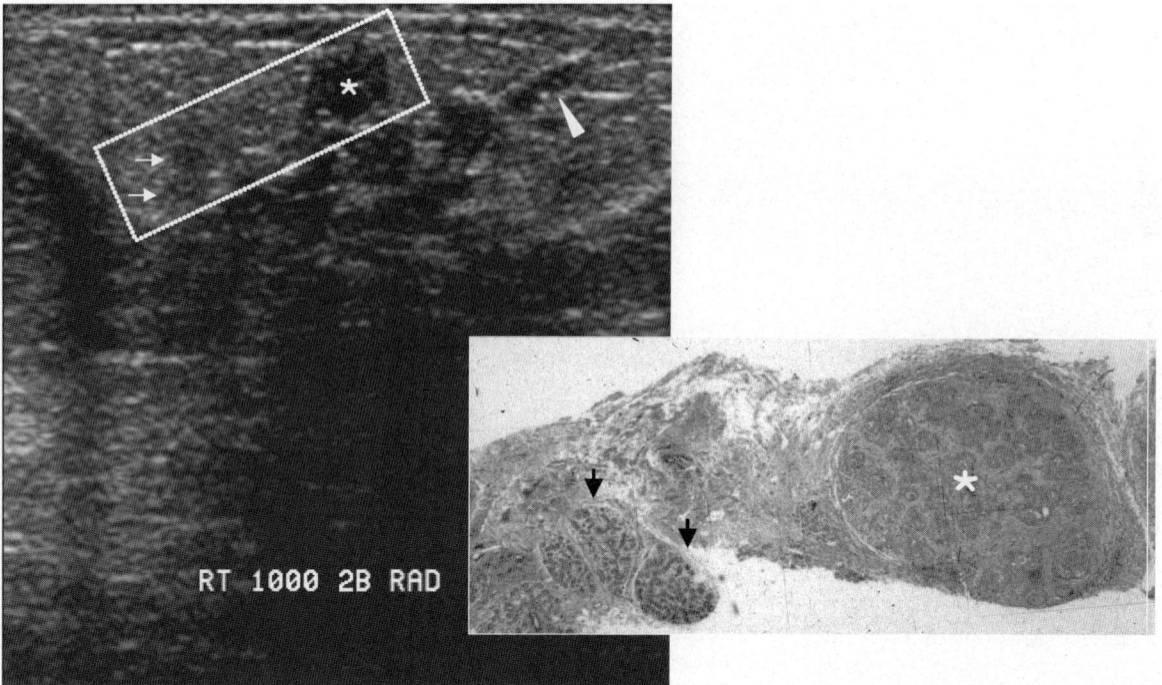

FIGURE 12–30 This heavily microlobulated lesion is caused by high-nuclear-grade ductal carcinoma *in situ* (DCIS) with microscopic invasion. An ultrasound-guided core biopsy was obtained along the course of the *dotted box*. The large microlobulation *(*)* represents a lobule that has been "cancerized." The smaller lobules *(arrows)* are sonographically and histologically normal. The core biopsy and excisional biopsy revealed high-nuclear-grade DCIS with no evidence of invasion. Note the hypoechoic linear structure *(arrowhead)* that extends beyond a cancerized lobule *(+)*. This represents microscopic invasion sonographically. The lobule is the end of the ductal system, a cul-de-sac, beyond which there are no ducts. Any evidence of tumor located more peripherally than the lobule indicates the presence of invasion. Based on this finding, the axillary nodes were evaluated, an abnormal-appearing node was identified and underwent biopsy, revealing invasive carcinoma that had been missed by the random sectioning technique employed by the pathologists. Repeat serial sectioning of the lumpectomy specimen revealed microscopic invasion that had been missed by random sectioning technique. Even though sonography shows gross morphology rather than histology, a thorough understanding of how breast cancer grows and spreads within the breast and of the underlying breast anatomy can reveal tremendous amounts of information that helps manage patients.

scribed lesions. In some circumscribed malignant nodules, microlobulation may be the only suspicious finding present. However, the improved sensitivity of soft findings for DCIS comes with a price—more false-positive sonograms and a lower positive predictive value. Microlobulation is not unique to DCIS. It is frequently seen in fibrocystic change, particularly in the microcystic variety. It is also frequently seen in benign proliferative disorders such as sclerosing adenosis. Many benign intraductal papillomas are also microlobulated. Even some hyalinized or complex fibroadenomas may be microlobulated. The net result is that the sensitivity of microlobulations is the highest of all findings, but its positive predictive value is the lowest of any of the suspicious findings.

The sensitivities and positive predictive values of microlobulation for breast carcinoma in the 1995 study and the current ongoing study are shown in Table 12–10.

The overall accuracy of microlobulations in the current study is 67%.

Taller-than-Wide Shape

Taller-than-wide shape is unique to sonography. It is a mixed finding that can occur with either invasive malignancy or pure DCIS, but has its origin in the shape of the DCIS from which invasion arose. Taller-than-wide indicates that the lesion's anteroposterior (AP) dimension is larger than either of its horizontal dimensions (Fig. 12–33) The finding was first described in the Japanese literature, but later Fornage et al. (1989) showed that having a larger AP dimension was primarily a feature of small malignant nodules that had a volume of less than 1 mL. Our data supports that of Fornage. Taller-than-wide carcinomas are primarily small lesions with maximum diameters less than 1.5 cm.

Because breast cancer is heterogeneous not only from nodule to nodule, but also within an individual nodule, it is possible for an image obtained through one part of a malignant nodule to be taller than wide and an image obtained though another part of the same malignant nodule to be

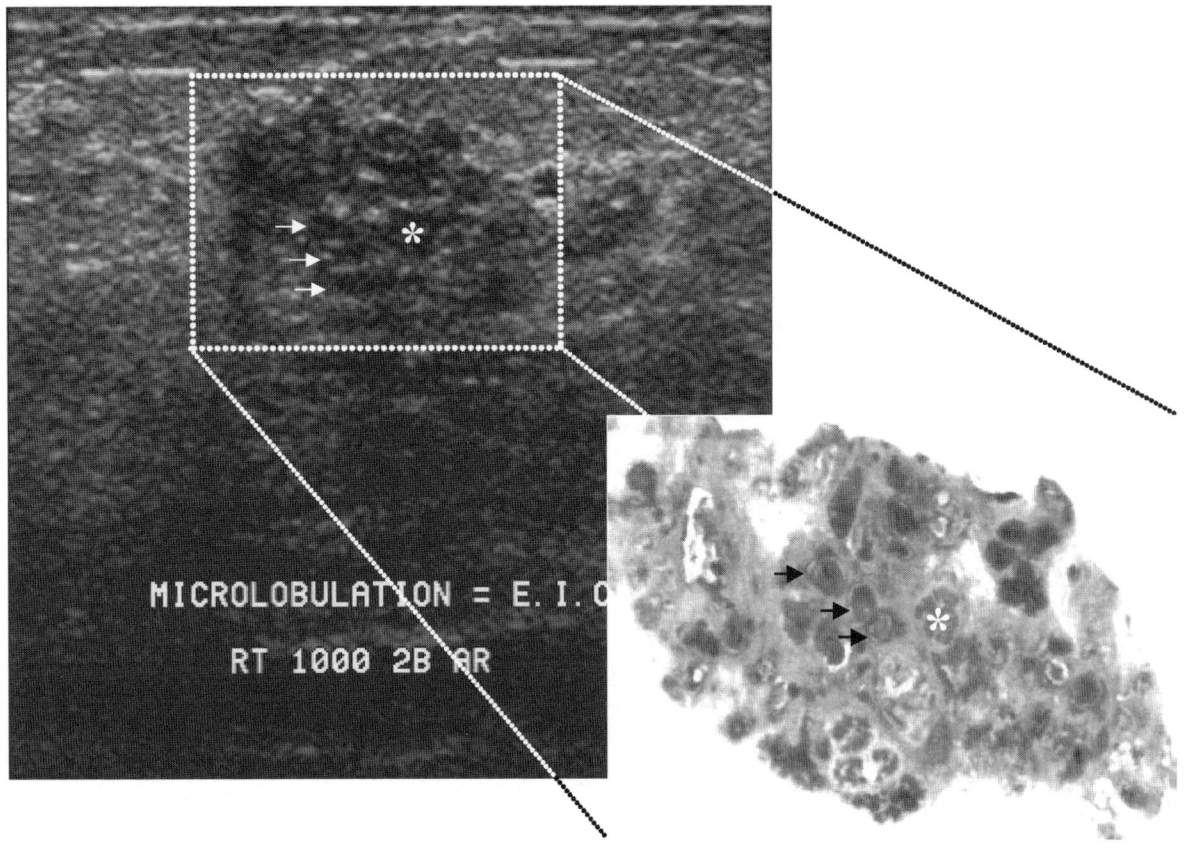

FIGURE 12–31 The numerous microlobulations throughout this nodule are the result of a combination of intraductal components of tumor *(arrows)* and cancerized lobules *(*)*.

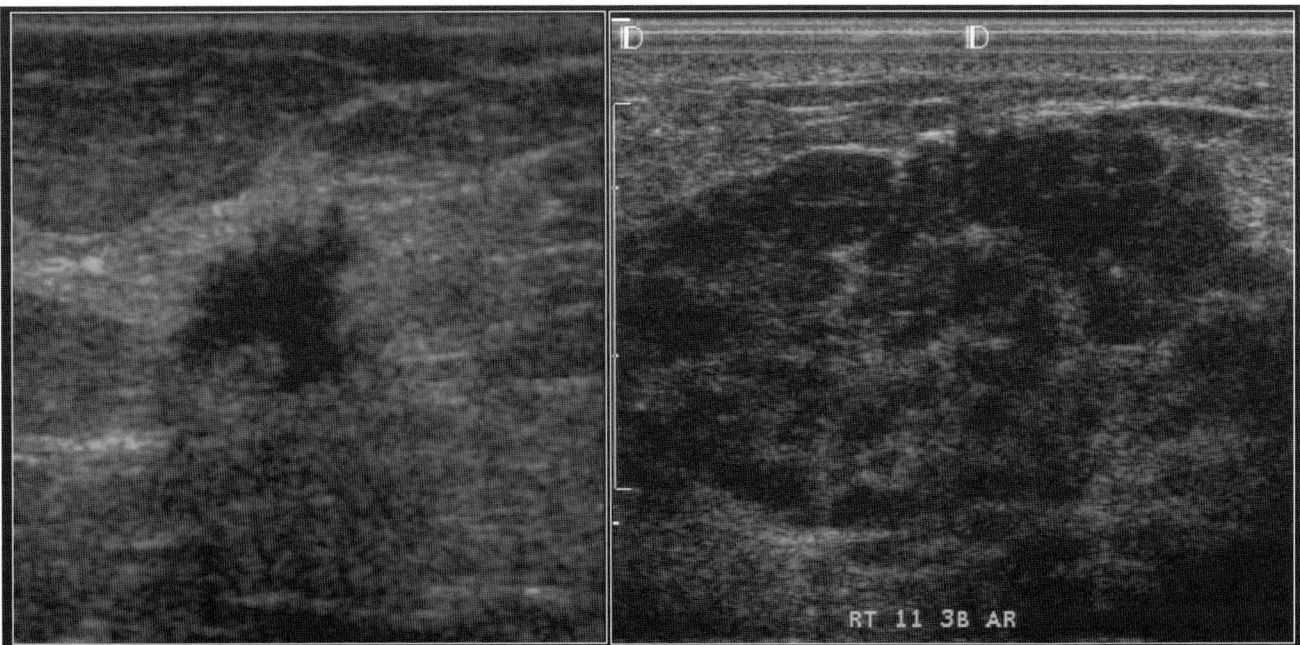

FIGURE 12–32 The size of microlobulations is frequently related the nuclear grade of ductal carcinoma *in situ* (DCIS) components and the histologic grade of the invasive components of the tumor. High-grade invasive carcinomas tend to have high-nuclear-grade DCIS components, and low-grade invasive ductal carcinomas tend to have low-nuclear-grade DCIS components of tumor. For reasons that will be explained in detail in Chapter 14, high-nuclear-grade DCIS tends to enlarge the ducts more grossly than does low-nuclear-grade DCIS. Thus, large microlobulations suggest the presence of a high-grade lesion, and small microlobulations suggest the presence of a low-grade lesion. Intermediate-sized microlobulations tend to correspond to intermediate-grade lesions.

TABLE 12–10. SENSITIVITY AND POSITIVE PREDICTIVE VALUES (PPV) FOR MICROLOBULATIONS

	1995 Study (750 Nodules)[a]		Current Study (1,211 Nodules)[b]	
		PPV		PPV
	Sensitivity	Odds Ratio	Sensitivity	Odds Ratio
Microlobulations	75%	48% (2.9)	92%	50% (1.5)

[a]Prevalence, 16.7%.
[b]Prevalence, 32.8%.

wider than tall (Fig. 12–34). Thus, the entire volume of a nodule must be scanned in two orthogonal planes before it can be concluded that no part of the nodule has a taller-than-wide configuration; even if only a part of the nodule is taller than wide, the nodule must be excluded from the BI-RADS 3 category, and biopsy must be recommended.

There are several theories about why small malignant solid nodules are larger in the AP dimension than in any of the horizontal dimensions. One is that only the central hypoechoic nidus of the nodule is being measured. If the thick, echogenic halo or spiculations that surround the nodule were to be included in the measurement, the nodule would not be taller than wide. Another theory is that the tissue planes in the breast of a patient who is being scanned in the supine position are horizontally oriented.

Benign lesions remain confined within and grow parallel to the tissue planes and therefore are wider than tall. Malignant lesions, on the other hand, can invade across normal tissue planes and grow in an axis that lies perpendicular to the axis of the tissue planes. Another theory is that malignant lesions are stiff and not compressible in the AP dimension because of associated desmoplasia, whereas many benign lesions are soft enough to be compressible in the AP dimension (see Chapter 3, Figs. 3–13, 3–14 and 3–15). Finally, some steeply obliquely oriented benign lesions can be rotated into a wider-than-tall configuration with transducer compression because they are not fixed to surrounding tissues. Invasive malignant lesions, on the other hand, are fixed to surrounding tissues and cannot be rotated flat in the AP plane (see Chapter 3, Fig. 3–17).

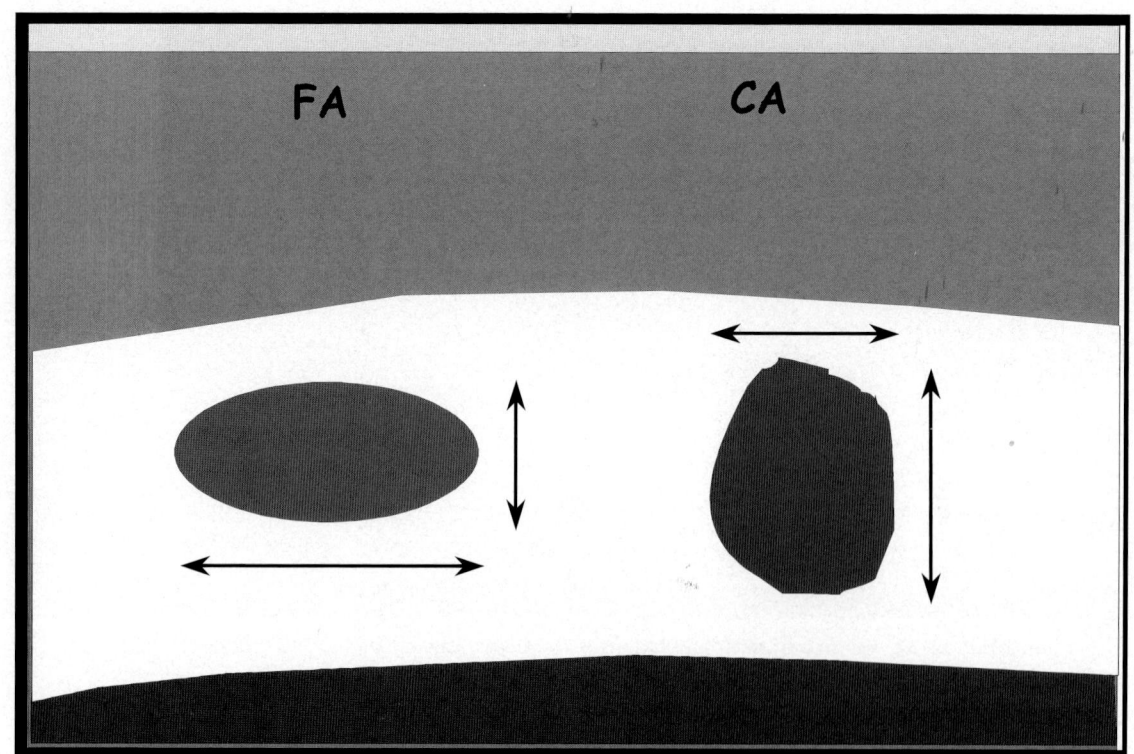

A

FIGURE 12–33 A: "Taller than wide" indicates that a nodule is larger in the anteroposterior dimension than it is in any horizontal plane. Taller than wide is a feature of small malignant nodules. Benign lesions are typically wide than tall. *(Continued.)*

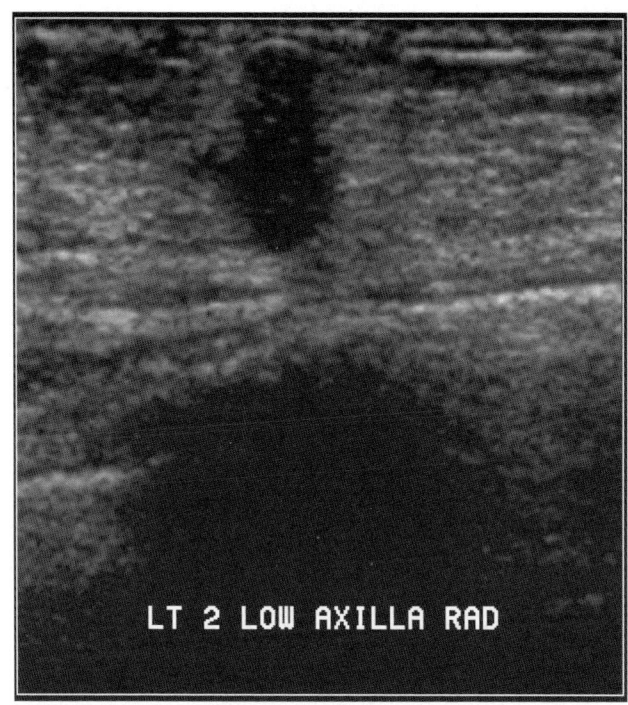

B

FIGURE 12–33 *(continued)* **B:** This small invasive ductal carcinoma is taller than wide.

All of the possible explanations discussed previously have some merit, but we believe that there is a better explanation for small malignant solid nodules being taller than wide. We believe that the taller-than wide shape in small, but not large, cancers reflects the shape of the underlying lobule in which the carcinoma arose. Most cancers are thought to arise at the level of the terminal ductolobular unit (TDLU), at the junction of the extralobular terminal duct with the lobule. The DCIS then grows proximally in the terminal duct toward the large ducts and peripherally into the lobule, cancerizing the intralobular ductules. The net result of this growth pattern is an axis of growth that is parallel to the long axis of the lobule in which it arose. The taller-than-wide shape of small malignancies that involve primarily a single lobule progresses from racket shaped to spindle-top shaped (Fig. 12–35). Fibroadenomas also arise within the lobule but cannot grow down the terminal duct into the main ductal system and therefore are forced into a growth axis that is perpendicular to the long axis of the underlying lobule (Fig. 12–36).

From Teboul, we learned that the average mammary lobar duct has several rows of vertically oriented TDLUs arising from it: more rows growing anteriorly that have long extralobular terminal ducts and fewer rows growing posteriorly that have short extralobular terminal ducts (Fig.

(text continued on page 479)

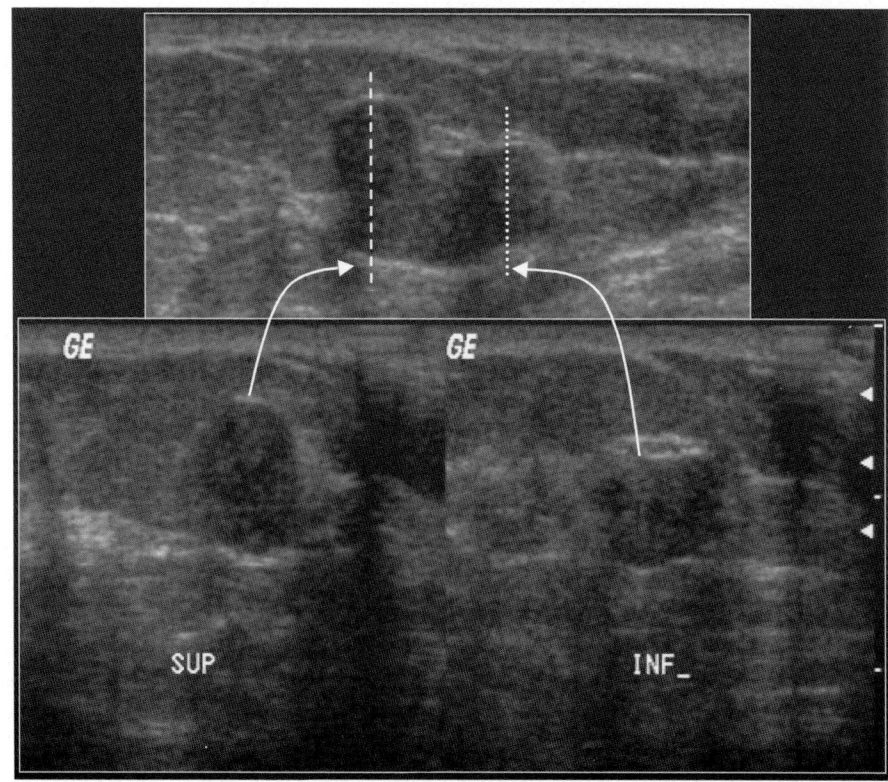

FIGURE 12–34 Because breast cancer may be heterogeneous within an individual nodule, if any part of the nodule is taller than wide, the entire lesion must be considered taller than wide and excluded from the BIRADS 3 category. The **upper** image shows a lobulated nodule in the radial plane. The **lower right** image shows antiradial views of the nodule through the level shown by the *dotted white line*, while the **lower left** image shows the antiradial view through the plane of the *dashed white line*. Note that the lesion is wider than tall through the plane of the *dotted white line* but taller than wide through the plane of the *dashed line*. The lesion must be considered taller than wide and excluded from BIRADS 3 classification. (Histology revealed fibroadenoma.)

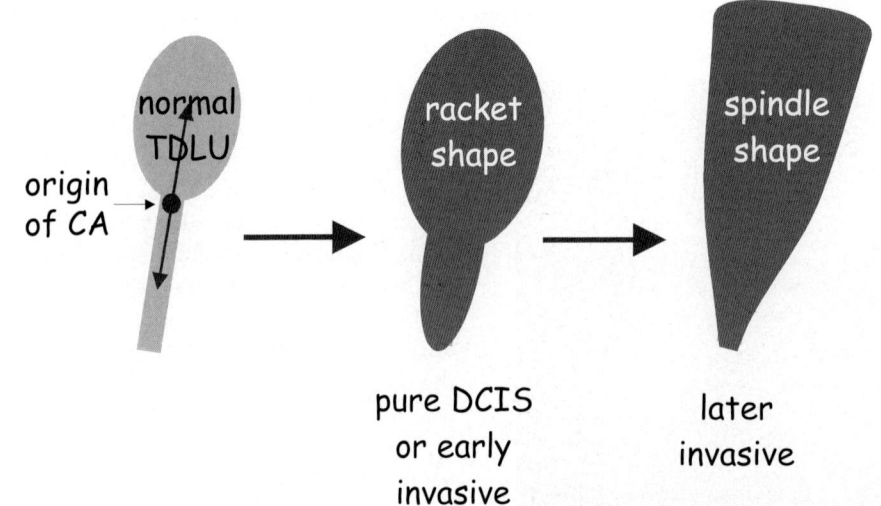

A

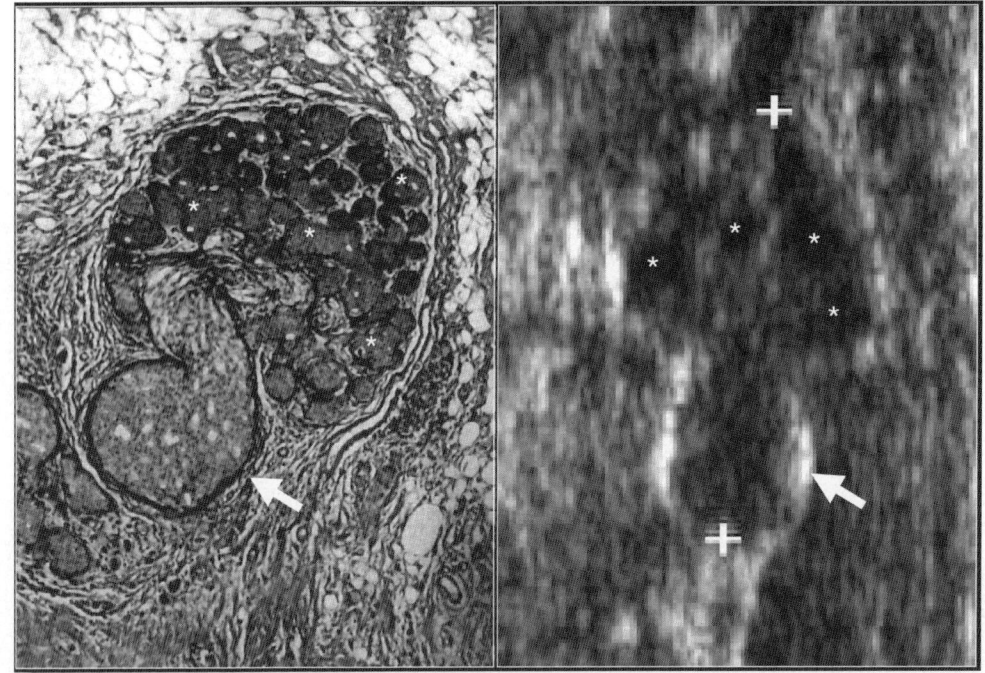

B

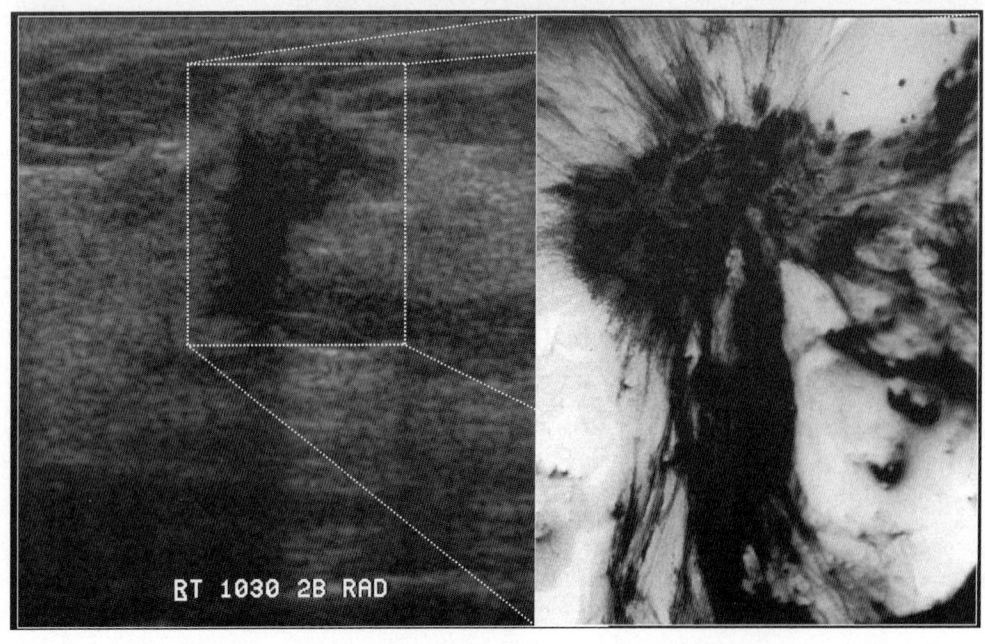

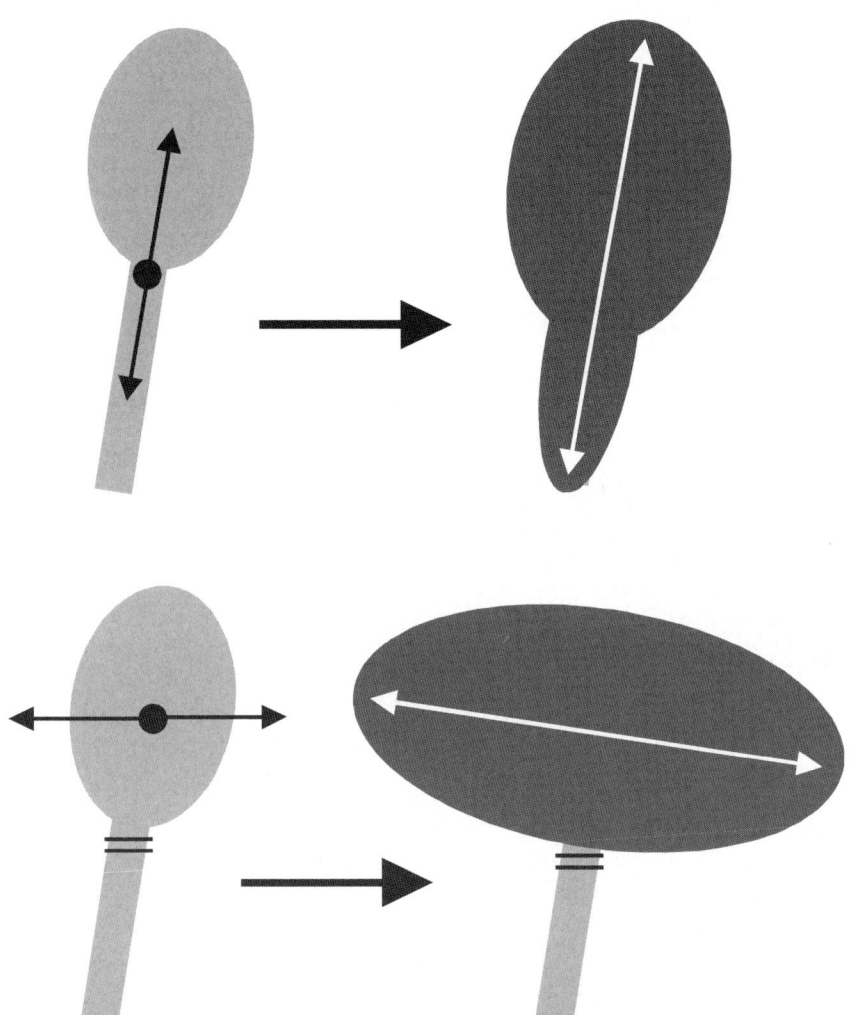

FIGURE 12–36 Fibroadenomas also arise within the lobule but cannot grow down the extralobular terminal duct and are forced to grow in a plane that is perpendicular to the long axis of the terminal ductolobular unit. **Top row:** Growth pattern of carcinomas. **Bottom row:** growth pattern of fibroadenomas.

FIGURE 12–35 A: The **left** image shows a normal terminal ductolobular unit (TDLU). Most breast carcinomas are thought to arise within the TDLU at the level of the junction of the extralobular terminal duct and the lobule. Growth of the tumor is then peripherally into the lobule (cancerization of the lobule) and centrally down the extralobular terminal duct into the main ductal system. The net result of this pattern of growth is that small malignant lesions have a long axis that is parallel to the long axis of the lobule in which they arose. The shape of small cancers that involve primarily a single lobule (and surrounding tissues in the case of invasive lesions) is racket shaped (**middle**) or spindle shaped (**right**). Pure ductal carcinoma *in situ* (DCIS) tends to demonstrate the racket shape. The shape tends to progress from racket-like to spindle-like as invasion develops and progresses. **B:** These images illustrate DCIS involving a single TDLU. The TDLU has a racket-like shape. Note the grossly distended extralobular terminal duct (*arrows*, the racket handle) and the distended ductules (***) within the enlarged lobule (the racket head). Note that the long axis of the small malignant lesion is parallel to the long axis of the TDLU in which it arose. The enlarged ductules within the TDLU can be very difficult to distinguish from microcysts in fibrocystic change. **C:** This small invasive not otherwise specified carcinoma retains the shape of the anterior lobule in which it arose. Invasion from the lobule into surrounding tissues has changed the shape from racket-like to that of an asymmetric spindle. (Subgross histology image courtesy of Laszlo Tabar, MD.)

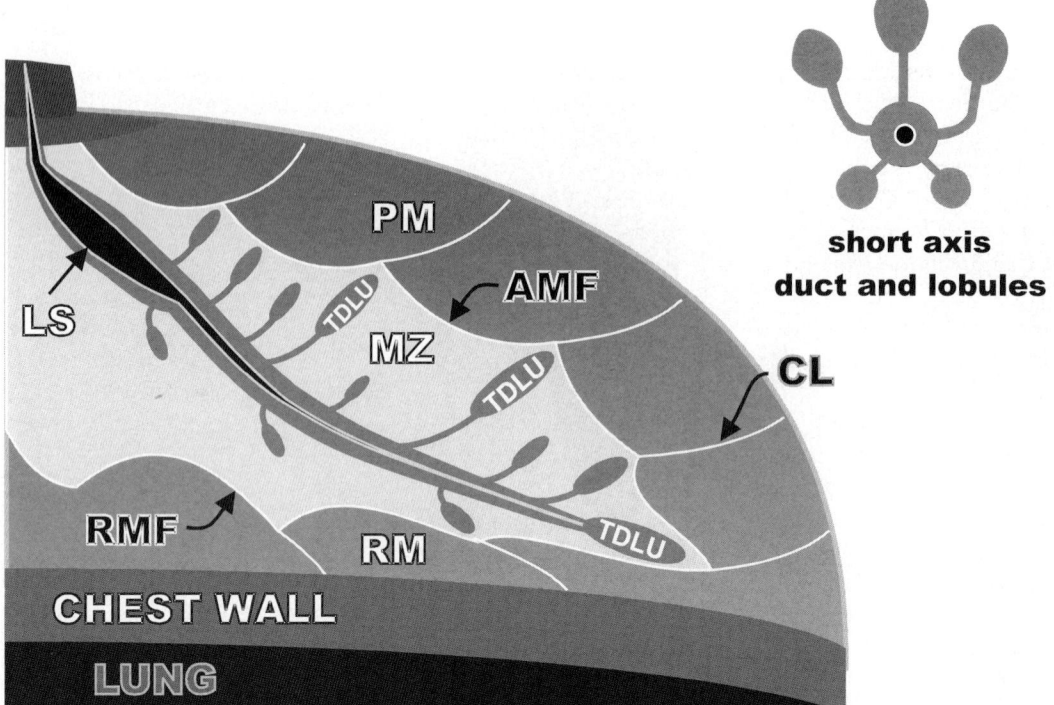

**short axis
duct and lobules**

FIGURE 12–37 The shape of a small carcinoma will reflect the shape of the terminal ductolobular unit (TDLU) in which it arose. From Teboul, we have learned that the typical lobar duct has several rows of vertically oriented TDLUs arising from it: more anteriorly and fewer posteriorly. Additionally, some TDLUs are on the terminal ends of ducts and are horizontally oriented. The anterior three rows of lobules tend to have long extralobular terminal ducts, and the posterior rows of lobules tend to have short extralobular terminal ducts. Small carcinomas arising from anterior and posteriorly located TDLUs will be taller than wide for a period of time. On the other hand, small cancers arising from terminal lobules will never be taller-than-wide at any point in time.

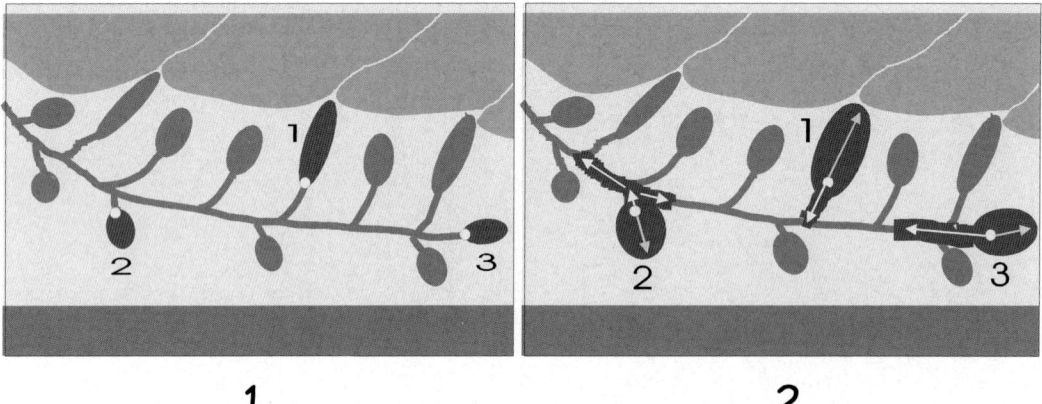

1   2

FIGURE 12–38 The **left** image shows the three types of lobules in the breast. The terminal lobule is horizontally oriented *(#3)*, whereas the posterior and anterior lobules are vertically oriented. The anterior lobules have long extralobular terminal ducts, whereas the posterior lobules have short extralobular terminal ducts. The **right** image shows that the orientation of small carcinomas reflects the orientation of the terminal ductolobular units (TDLUs) in which they arise. Small carcinomas that arise and grow parallel to the long axis of terminal lobules will always be wider than tall. Thus, the suspicious finding of taller than wide can never have a sensitivity of 100%. Small carcinomas arising within and growing parallel to the long axis of posterior lobules will be taller than wide for a very short period of time. However, because the extralobular terminal ducts of posterior lobules are so short, the carcinoma reaches the horizontally oriented main ducts system and assumes a horizontal growth pattern relatively early in its life, quickly becoming wider than tall. Small carcinomas arising within and growing parallel to the long axis of anterior lobules will remain within the lobule and reflect the shape of the TDLU for a much longer time because the extralobular terminal ducts of anterior lobules are long and it will take a longer period of time for the carcinoma to reach the main ductal system and to begin growing horizontally. Because TDLUs are more numerous and because the dwell time of small carcinomas within anterior lobules is longer, most small taller-than-wide carcinomas that we see arise from anterior lobules.

12–37). There are also terminal lobules that lie at the peripheral end of the lobar ductal system and are horizontally rather than vertically oriented. The shape of a small malignant nodule will reflect the underlying shape of the lobule in which it arose (Fig. 12–38). Malignancies that arise in the terminal TDLUs will grow parallel to the horizontally oriented TDLU and will never (at any point in their development) be taller than wide. Thus, taller than wide can never be expected to have 100% sensitivity. Malignancies that arise in the posterior lobules will be taller than wide for a short while, but because the extralobular terminal duct is short, they will gain access to the main lobar duct relatively early in their lives. Once the lesion has gained access to the horizontally oriented lobar ducts, the lesion rapidly grows in a horizontal axis and becomes wider than tall. Malignancies that arise from the anterior lobules will remain taller than wide for a longer time than will posterior lobules because it takes longer for the tumor to grow down the extralobular terminal duct and reach the main lobar ducts. We do see a few taller-than-wide lesions that have arisen in posterior lobules. However, because the dwell time within anterior lobules is longer than it is within posterior lobules and because there are more anterior lobules than posterior lobules, most of the small taller-than-wide lesions we see in ultrasound arise from anterior lobules.

The shape of small taller-than-wide carcinomas that arise from anterior lobules is very characteristic. In early phases, the small taller-than-wide cancer has an appearance of a tennis or badminton racket (Fig. 12–39). In small cancers arising from anterior lobules, the racket-shaped lesion lies in the superficial half of the breast with the handle oriented posteriorly. Small cancers arising from posterior lobules will lie in the deep half of the breast and will have the racket handle oriented anteriorly. Small cancers arising from terminal lobules will lie at mid-breast depths and will have the appearance of a racket lying on its side. In later phases, the appearance is more like that of a spindle top, in which the depth and orientation of the pointed end of the spindle indicate the type of lobule from which the lesion arose. In some cases, the extension of tumor into the main duct is visible (Fig. 12–40).

As the tumor enlarges and grows into the main ductal system, both its growth pattern and long axis have a tendency to become horizontally oriented. The sensitivity of the taller-than-wide shape is inversely proportional to the

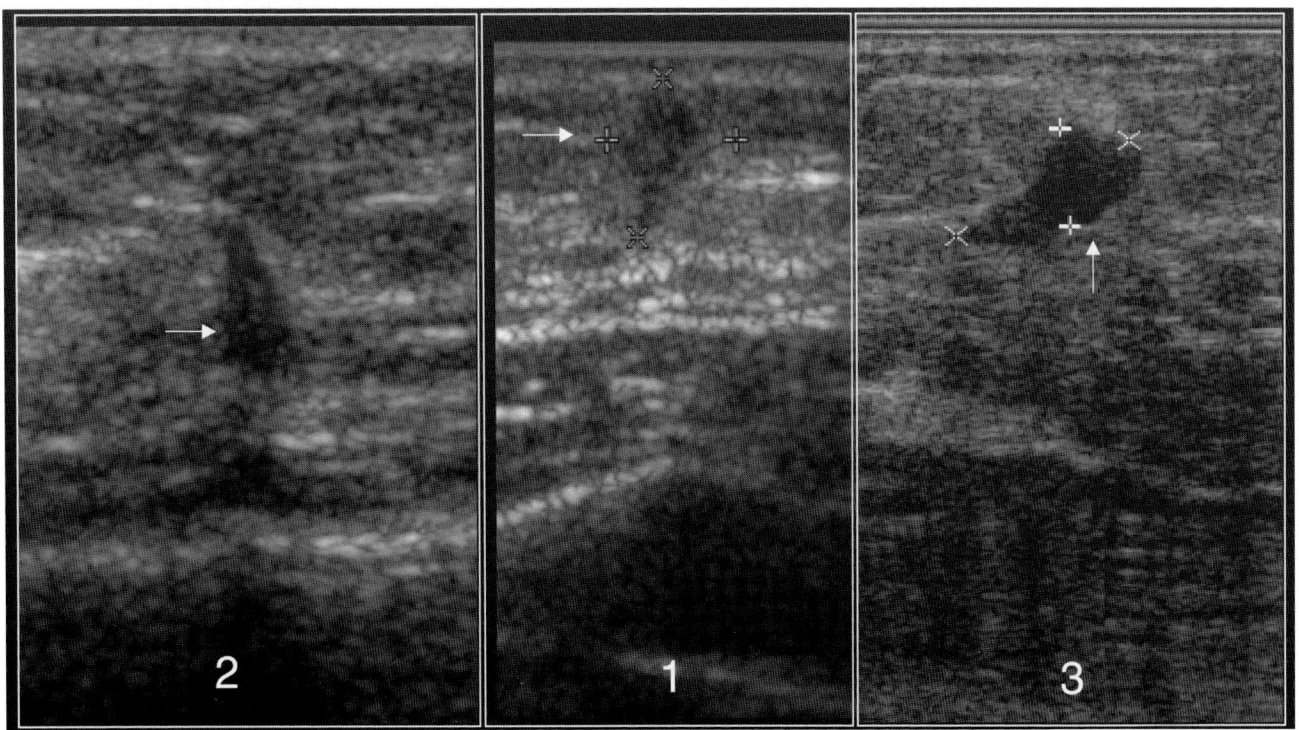

FIGURE 12–39 The **left** image shows a small taller-than-wide carcinoma arising from a posterior lobule. It has the shape of a racket with the handle pointed anteriorly and lies within the deep half of the breast. The **middle** image shows a typical small taller-than-wide carcinoma arising from an anterior lobule. It is racket shaped with the handle pointed posteriorly and lies within the superficial half of the breast. The **right** image shows a typical small racket-shaped carcinoma that is wider than tall and arose within a terminal lobule. The handle of the racket points centrally, and the lesion lies within the middle third of the breast. From its very inception, it has been wider than tall because the terminal ductolobular unit in which it arose is horizontally oriented.

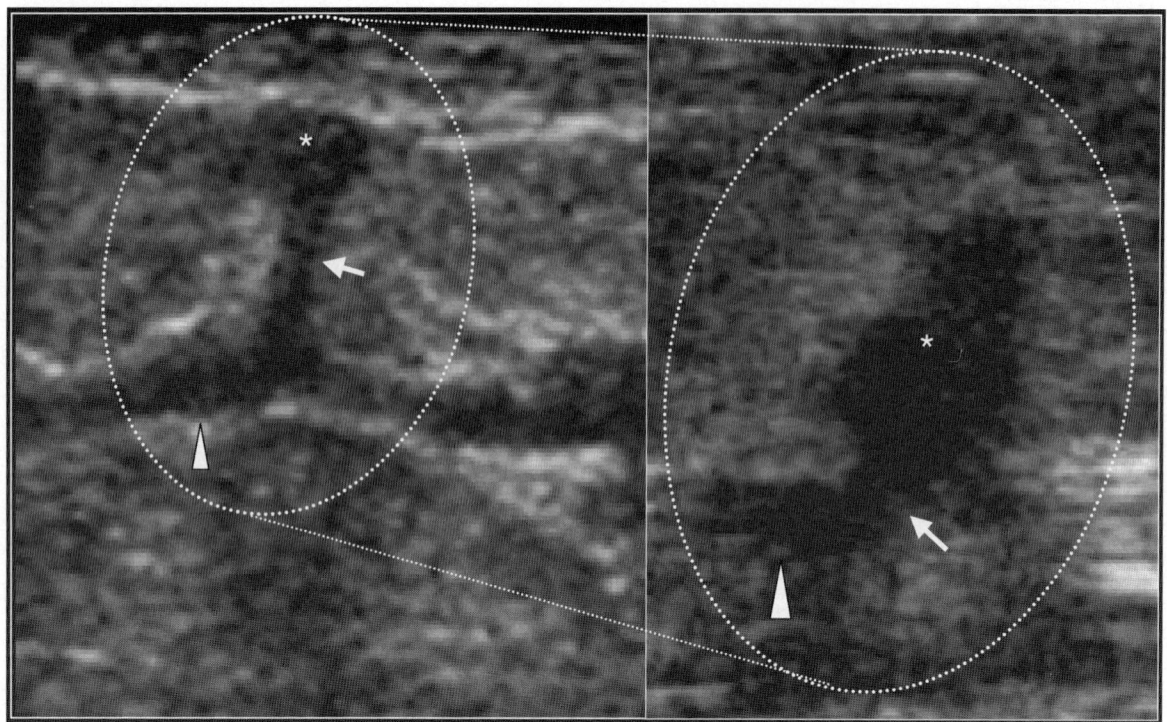

FIGURE 12–40 Within the *oval line* lies a typical anterior lobule and a short segment of the main ductal system (**left**). A small invasive ductal carcinoma (**right**) involves the lobule *(*)*, the extralobular terminal duct *(arrow)*, and a short segment of the extralobular terminal duct *(arrowhead)*.

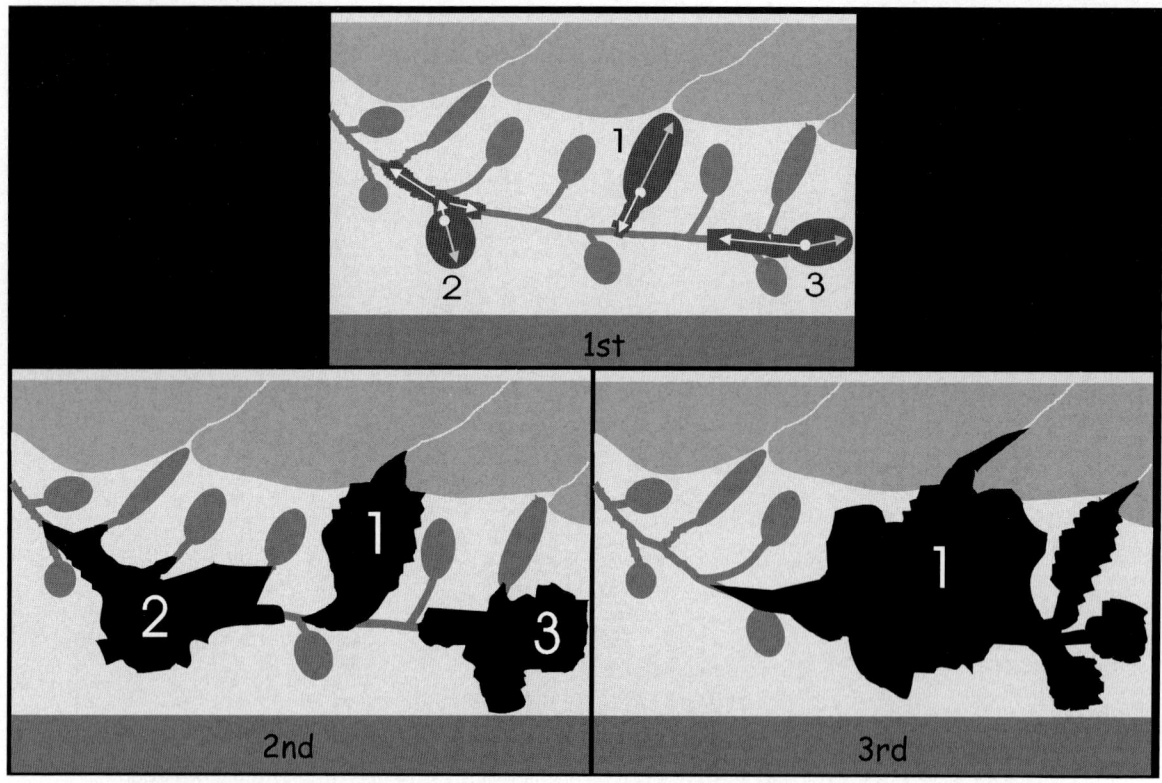

A

FIGURE 12–41 A: Once a carcinoma has begun growing within the main ductal system, its growth pattern becomes horizontal, and the lesion rapidly becomes wider than tall. The larger the maximum diameter of a malignant solid nodule, the more likely it is to have become wider than tall and the less likely it is to remain taller than wide. Carcinomas arising within terminal lobules are wider than tall from inception *(lobule 3)*. Carcinomas arising from posterior lobules become wider than tall relatively early in their development *(lobule two,* **lower left***)*. Carcinomas arising from anterior lobules must become larger before they can reach the lobar duct and assume a horizontal growth pattern *(lobule 1,* **lower right***)*. *(Continued.)*

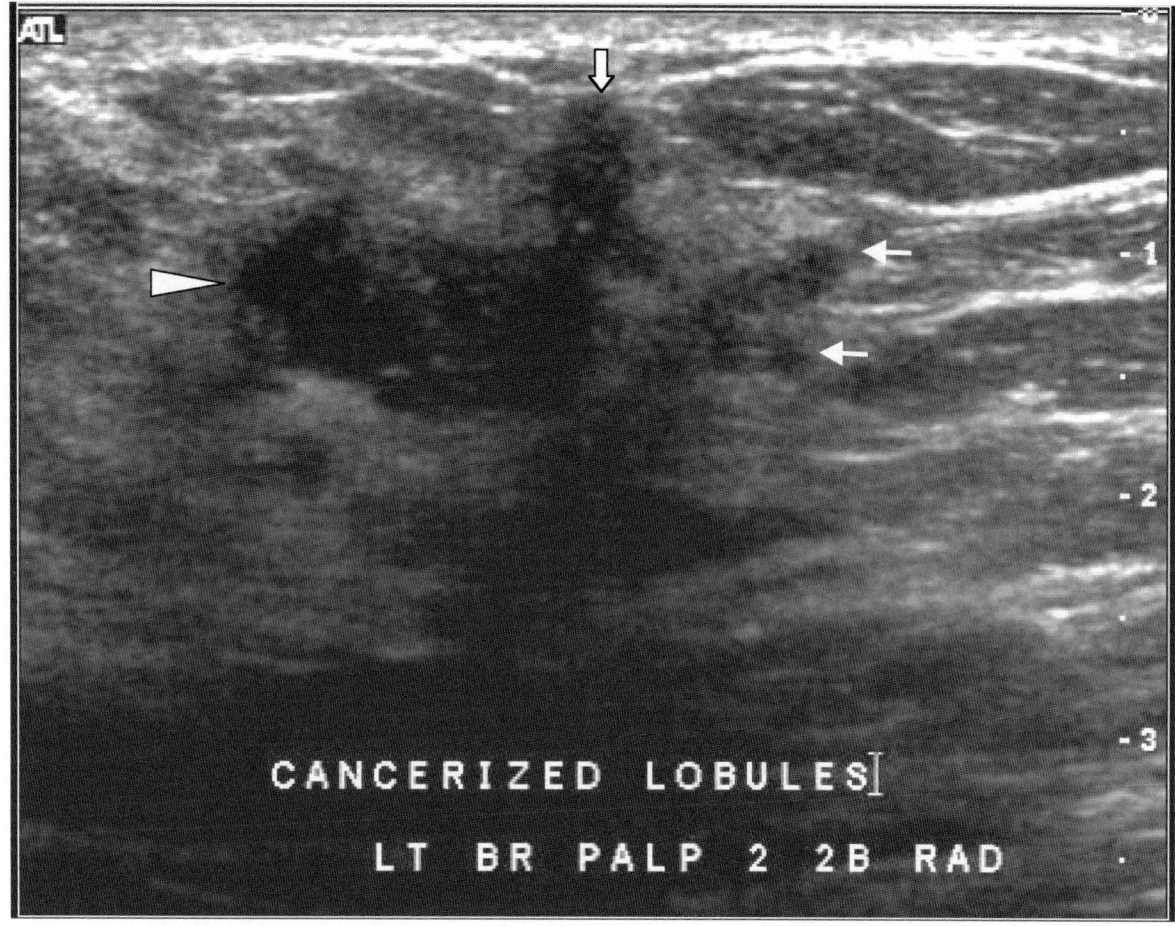

FIGURE 12–41 *(continued)* **B:** This large mixed invasive and intraductal carcinoma has become wider than tall. It likely arose within an anterior lobule *(block arrow)*, but now has grown horizontally within a grossly distended lobar duct *(arrowhead)* and has cancerized two horizontally oriented terminal lobules *(arrows)*.

size of the nodule. The larger the nodule, the more likely the tumor is to have grown into the main ductal system and assumed a horizontal growth pattern. Thus, the larger the size, the less likely a malignant neoplasm is to be taller than wide, and the lower the sensitivity of taller than wide as a sonographic finding (Fig. 12–41). In the entire series of 1,211 solid nodules, the sensitivity is less than 50%.

However, for lesions less than 1.5 cm in maximum diameter, the sensitivity is 63%, whereas for lesions larger than 15 mm, the sensitivity is only 35%. Table 12–11 shows the sensitivity and positive predictive values for taller-than-wide shape.

Note that although the sensitivity of the taller-than-wide shape decreases as maximum diameter of the lesion in-

TABLE 12–11. SENSITIVITY AND POSITIVE PREDICTIVE VALUES (PPV) FOR TALLER-THAN-WIDE SHAPE

| Taller than Wide | 1995 Study (750 Nodules)[a] | | Current Study (1,211 Nodules)[b] | |
	Sensitivity	PPV Odds Ratio	Sensitivity	PPV Odds Ratio
All sizes	42%	81% (4.9)	48%	74% (2.2)
≤15 mm	—	—	63%	82% (2.5)
>15 mm	—	—	35%	88% (2.7)

[a]Prevalence, 16.7%.
[b]Prevalence, 32.8%.

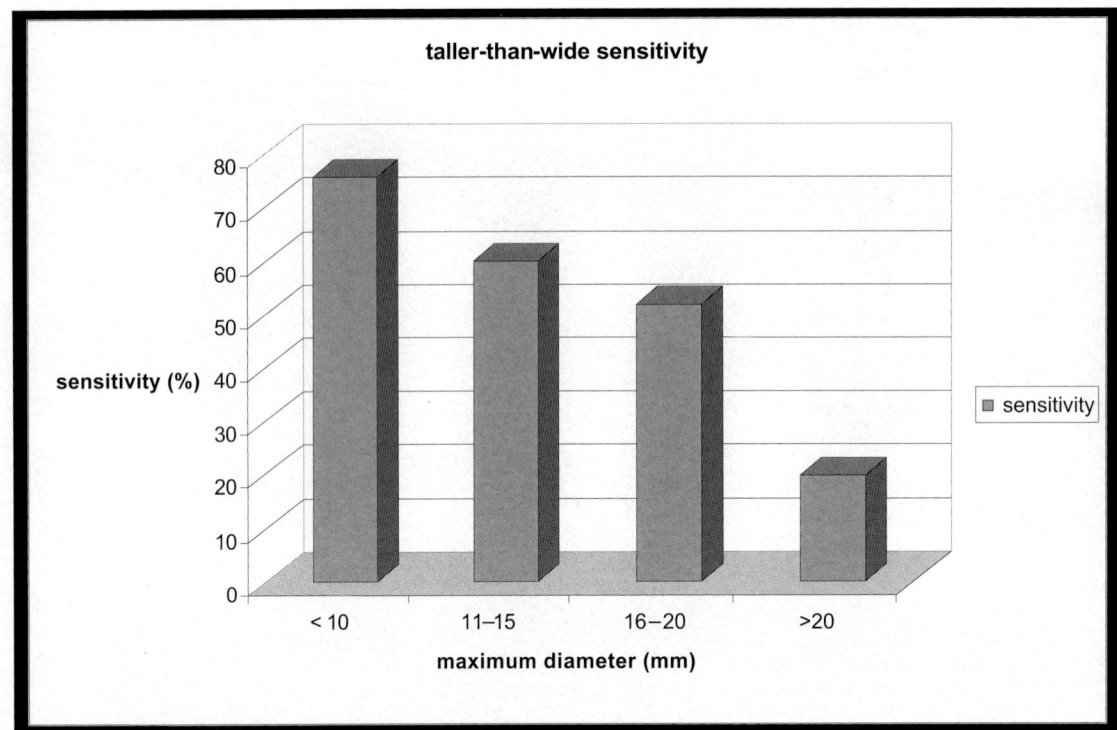

FIGURE 12–42 The sensitivity of taller-than-wide shape falls as size increases.

creases, the positive predictive value actually increases. Thus, large lesions that have a taller-than-wide shape are more likely to be malignant than are small taller-than-wide lesions.

Figure 12–42 shows graphically how the sensitivity of the taller-than-wide shape decreases as maximum diameter of the lesion increases.

Duct Extension and Branch Pattern

Duct extension and branch pattern are shape findings that are used in mammography when evaluating calcifications that we have applied to sonographic assessment of solid breast nodules. Duct extension and branch pattern are soft findings typically associated with either pure DCIS or DCIS components in lesions that are mixtures of invasive and intraductal tumor. Like all soft findings, they improve the sensitivity of sonography for DCIS but reduce positive predictive value because duct extension and branch pattern can also be seen in benign lesions such as intraductal papillomas.

Duct extension and branch pattern are generally not identified unless specifically sought. These findings usually are missed if a solid nodule is scanned only in longitudinal and transverse planes through the widest part of the lesion. Detecting duct extension and branch pattern requires interrogating the lesion in the radial plane. The external radial plane, as discussed in earlier chapters, is a plane similar to that of the spoke of a wheel relative to the hub of the wheel. It is very important to recognize that the external radial plane is merely a starting point for evaluating the nodule. The key to detecting duct extension and branch pattern is to assess the ducts in the region of the nodule and how the lesion interacts with the ducts. This requires scan planes that are parallel to the long axis of the ducts in the region of the nodule—the internal radial plane. Mammary ducts may be oriented exactly parallel to the external radial plane, but tortuosity of central ducts and more peripherally located branch ducts may not lie in the external radial plane. Thus, the scan of the nodule should be begun in a true external radial plane, but then must be adjusted by variable amounts to identify the internal radial plane that is parallel to the long axis of the ducts that lie in the vicinity of the nodule.

Duct extension is usually a single large projection of tumor within a relatively centrally located duct that extends away from the primary lesion toward the nipple. Because the duct extension may involve the large and very distensible lactiferous sinus portion of the central duct, it may be several millimeters in size. Duct extensions can be up to 5 mm in diameter. Branch pattern involves smaller peripheral ducts that lie away from the nipple. Some of the ducts involved with branch pattern are so small that they are difficult to distinguish from spiculations (Figs. 12–43 and 12–44).

There are two reasons for evaluating the ducts adjacent to solid nodules. Both reasons are based on the tendency of

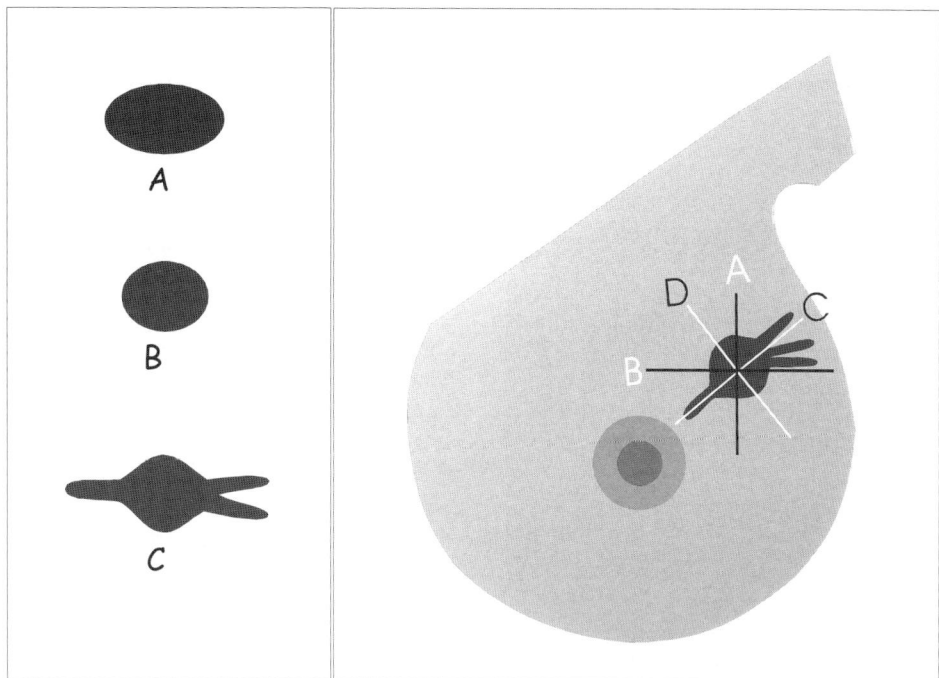

FIGURE 12–43 Solid nodules should be scanned in axes that are parallel and perpendicular to the ducts that lie in the vicinity of the nodule. This generally involves starting with a scan plane that is truly radially oriented with respect to the nipple. However, because lobar ducts can be tortuous and because lesions have arisen within tributaries of the lobar duct that are not truly radially oriented with respect to the nipple, the scan plane may have to be adjusted slightly off the true radial plane. What is really important is scanning parallel to the long axis of the local duct system to determine whether the duct is involved with tumor. Scanning solid nodules in random longitudinal or transverse planes or in planes that are unrelated to the long axis of the local ductal system may make the nodules appear to have circular or oval shapes that we typically associate with benign lesions, potentially leading to false-negative characterization of the lesion as BIRADS 3. On the other hand, scanning parallel to the long axis of the local ductal system may show projections of intraductal tumor or periductal invasion that project toward the nipple from the lesion (duct extension) or multiple smaller projections away from the nipple (branch pattern) that suggest to us that there is intraductal growth of the lesion, findings that are suspicious for neoplasm and exclude a lesion from BIRADS 3 classification.

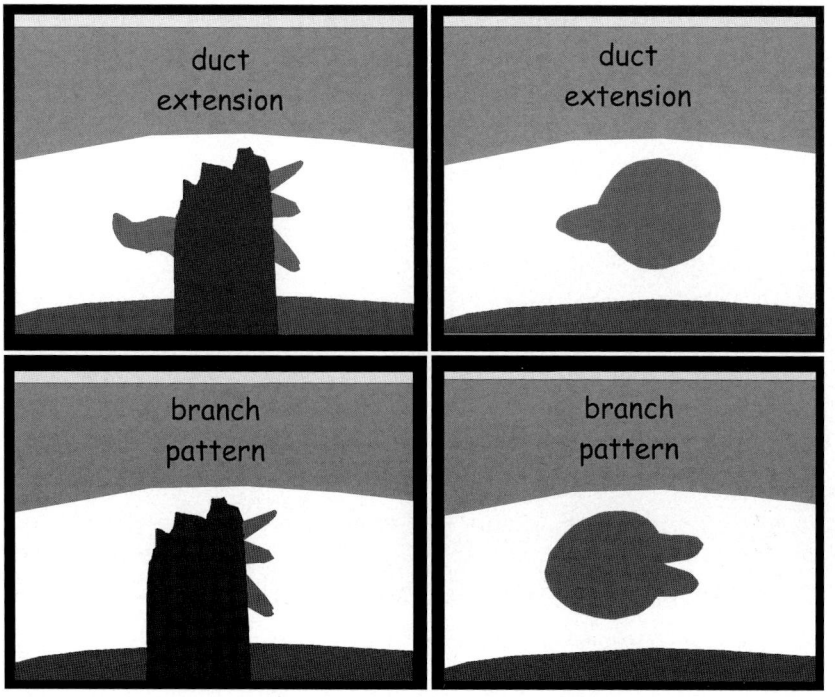

FIGURE 12–44 Duct extension and branch pattern can be associated with other hard, suspicious sonographic findings (**left**) or unassociated with any other suspicious findings (**right**). Duct extension is usually a single, relatively large projection toward the nipple. It may achieve a diameter of several millimeters if it involves the capacious and highly distensible lactiferous sinus portion of the lobar duct. Duct extensions that are associated with other hard suspicious findings usually represent intraductal [ductal carcinoma *in situ* (DCIS)] components of tumor in lesions that are mixed invasive and intraductal. Duct extensions and branch patterns that are unassociated with any other suspicious findings (**right**) usually represent benign papillomas, but about 13% of these lesions represent either DCIS or atypical ductal hyperplasia (ADH). Because such lesions are not benign with the 98% or greater certainty required for BIRADS 3 characterization, such lesions must be considered BIRADS 4a and excluded from the BIRADS 3 category.

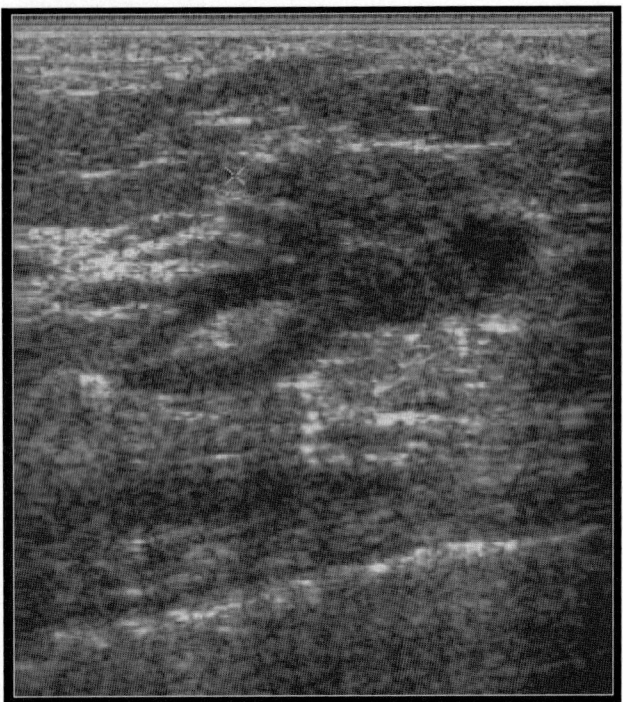

FIGURE 12–45 This internal radial view of a palpable mass shows branch pattern *(arrows)* that represent ductal carcinoma *in situ* (DCIS) components of the carcinoma. The branch pattern is a soft finding that helps avoid false-negative findings in cases of pure DCIS.

breast cancer to grow and spread within the ductal system of the breast. By detecting abnormally enlarged ducts that pass from the lesion into surrounding tissues we hope to accomplish the following: First, we hope to reduce false-negative findings by detecting a shape that suggests intraductal growth and therefore is suspicious for malignancy (Fig. 12–45).

Second, we hope to detect extensive intraductal components of tumor in lesions that are mixtures of invasive and intraductal tumor, leading to more complete diagnosis and treatment of the lesion with a single surgical procedure (Fig. 12–46). When a nodule that has duct extension or branch pattern has other findings that are suspicious for malignancy, especially hard findings that are more suspicious for invasion (spiculation; thick, echogenic halo; angular margins; acoustic shadowing), the lesion likely contains mixed invasive and DCIS components. The duct extension and branch pattern, if prominent, may represent extensive intraductal components of tumor that extend several centimeters away from the main lesion and that affect the chances of local control and reoccurrence (Fig. 12–47). Postoperative radiation therapy has been used in an attempt to eradicate residual intraductal components of tumor, but the latest data suggest that radiation does not kill the intraductal components but instead merely delays their growth and development into invasive lesions. Thus,

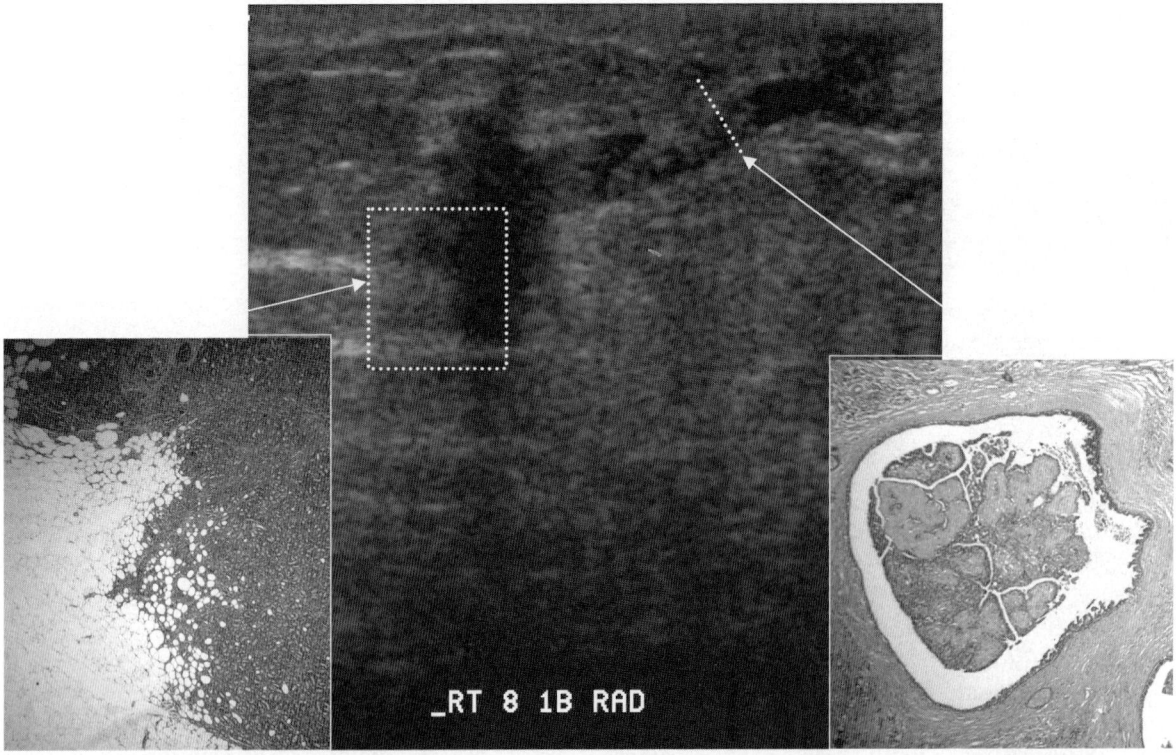

FIGURE 12–46 The internal radial view of this mixed invasive and intraductal carcinoma shows a prominent duct extension (soft finding) that represents the ductal carcinoma *in situ* component of the tumor *(dotted line)* and an angular mass with a thick, ill-defined echogenic halo (hard findings) that represents the invasive portion of the carcinoma *(dotted box)*.

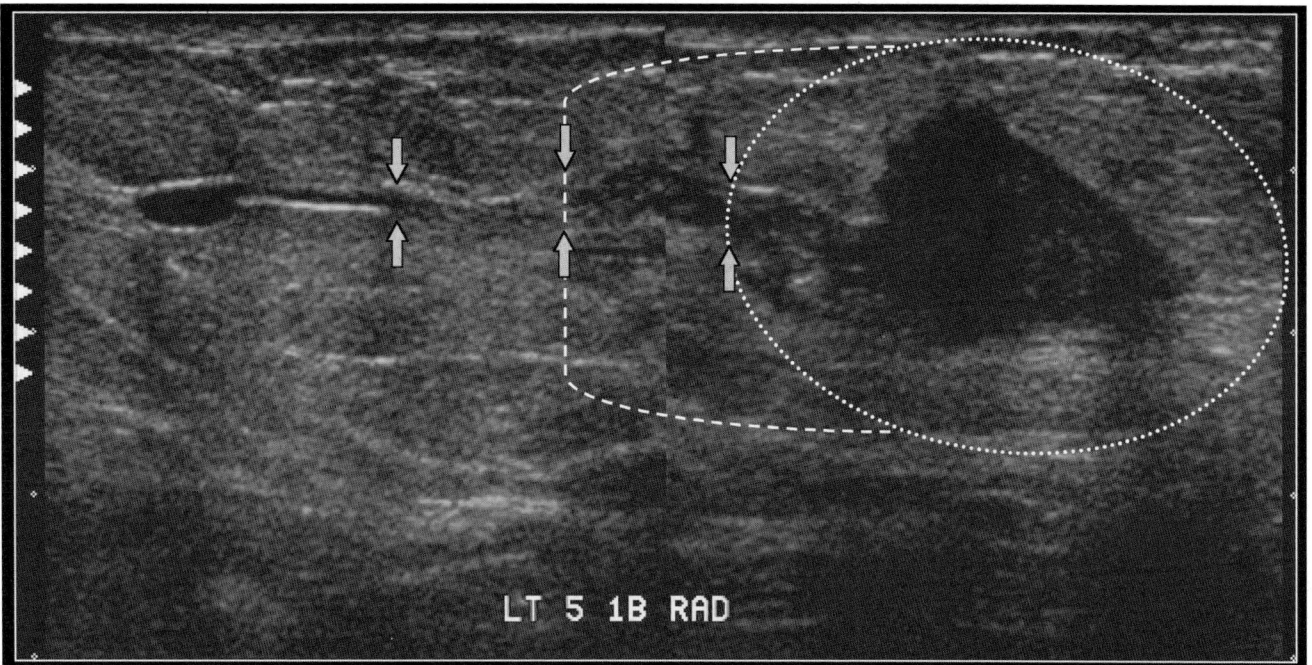

LT 5 1B RAD

FIGURE 12–47 This internal radial view of an intermediate-grade invasive ductal carcinoma shows a long duct extension *(arrows)* that can only be shown by interrogating the lesion in a plane that is parallel to the long axis of the regional ducts. If the surgeon is not informed of the presence of the duct extension, he or she will likely perform a wide excision (1-cm margins within the *dotted oval*). If the surgeon orients the specimen, and the pathologist carefully inspects the inked margins, they will likely find positive margins at the arrows at the left edge of the oval. The surgeon will need to reexcise the positive margin to the middle set of arrows *(dashed line)*, but will still have positive margins. The surgeon will then need to inform the patient that the disease can be removed only by mastectomy, but it will have taken three surgeries to arrive at the appropriate treatment. Even worse, there is a chance that the positive margin will be missed at the time of lumpectomy and that the patient will return later with recurrent carcinoma arising from the unresected ductal carcinoma *in situ* components of the lesion. If the radiologist performs ultrasound-guided core needle biopsy on the main mass and ultrasound-guided vacuum-assisted needle biopsy of the intraductal component of the tumor away from the main mass, the diagnosis of invasive carcinoma with extensive intraductal components can be established before lumpectomy, and the patient can appropriately be offered mastectomy or a trial of induction chemotherapy before inappropriate performance of lumpectomy. The chances of needing multiple surgeries and incomplete resection resulting in early recurrence can be minimized.

it is as important as ever to gain complete local control of malignancies. In other cases, radial scans may show the overall size of the combined invasive and intraductal components of the tumor to be too large to be cured by lumpectomy or to involve structures such as the nipple that require more extensive surgical procedures than just lumpectomy (Fig. 12–48). Patients with such involvement may be better treated with skin-sparing mastectomy and reconstruction than with lumpectomy or segmentectomy. Alternatively, such patients may undergo a trial of induction chemotherapy before surgery in an attempt to shrink the lesion enough to enable it to be removed with lumpectomy.

Third, we hope to detect multifocal disease. Careful serial section studies have shown that multifocal disease usually represents multiple separate foci of invasion that are connected by DCIS-filled ducts and which lie within a single mammary lobe. Scanning the primary lesion in a ra-

dial plane and identifying the lobar ductal system with which it is associated makes it more likely that the additional foci of invasion will be sonographically identified (Fig. 12–49). The likely sites for invasion to occur within the lobar ductal system are at branch points of the duct and in cancerized lobules.

The negative predictive values of lack of duct extension and branch pattern for excluding the presence of intraductal components of tumor are highly variable and depend on the grade of the lesion. As noted in the section on microlobulation, invasive ductal carcinomas have intraductal components in more than 80% of cases. High-grade invasive ductal carcinomas tend to have high-nuclear-grade DCIS components that grossly distend the ducts. The gross distention of the ducts caused by high-nuclear-grade DCIS components is readily detectable both as duct extension and branch pattern on ultrasound. However, low-grade invasive ductal carci-

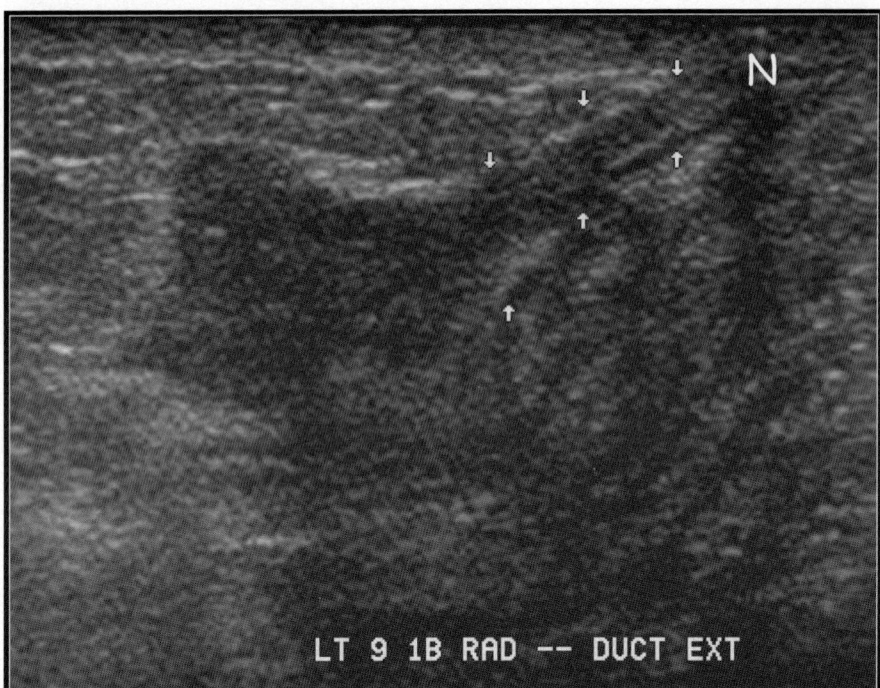

FIGURE 12–48 Demonstration of the extent of duct extension can affect treatment and diagnostic decisions. In this case, the radial scans suggested duct extension to at least the base of the nipple *(N)*, a contraindication to simple lumpectomy. Based on the sonographic findings of duct extension, biopsy proved involvement of the nipple and indicated the need for skin-sparing mastectomy rather than simple lumpectomy.

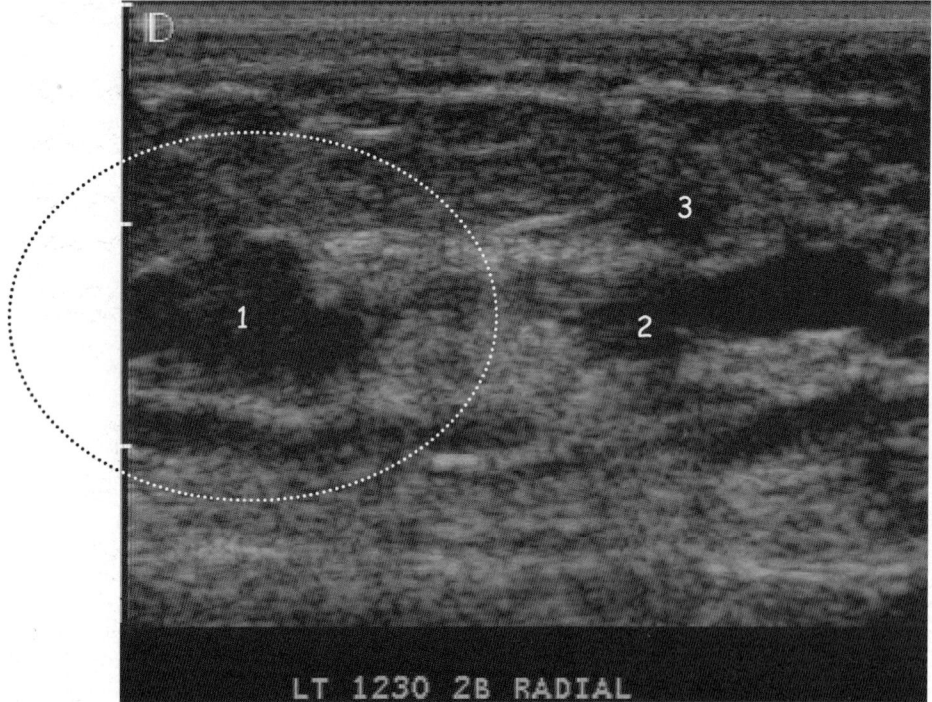

FIGURE 12–49 Scanning in the internal radial plane can also improve our ability to detect multifocal invasive carcinoma, which serial section studies have been shown to represent multiple individual foci of invasion in a single lobar ductal system connected by ductal carcinoma *in situ*. Points of low resistance to invasion are at duct branch points *(#2)* and within cancerized lobules *(#3)*. As was the case with extensive intraductal components, the surgeon cannot appropriately treat what he or she does not know exists. Routine longitudinal and transverse scans through the widest point of the main lesion *(#1)* would miss the multifocal disease and lead to inappropriate wide excision (1-cm margins within the *dotted oval*). If positive margins were detected, the patient would need reexcision. If not detected, the patient would likely have recurrent disease within a relatively short period of time.

noma usually has low-nuclear-grade DCIS components that are far less likely to distend the involved ducts enough for them to be detected by ultrasound. Intermediate-grade lesions cause intermediate degrees of ductal distention. Thus, the sensitivity of the sonographic findings of duct extension and branch pattern depends on the grade of the lesion. The sensitivity is good for high-grade lesions, poor for low-grade lesions, and intermediate for intermediate-grade lesions. The presence of duct extension and branch pattern has a fairly high positive predictive value, but the absence of duct extension and branch pattern does not exclude the presence of DCIS components. Additionally, the sensitivity of sonography cannot be viewed in a vacuum. Contrast-enhanced magnetic resonance imaging (MRI) with the rotating delivery excitation off-resonance (RODEO) sequence is likely more sensitive for intraductal components in low-grade lesions. However, even with the apparent superiority of MRI for detection of low-nuclear-grade components of tumor, second-look ultrasound may be necessary for biopsy guidance. Thus, even when high-resolution MRI is available, it is important for the sonography to be able to recognize and demonstrate intraductal components of tumor.

The size of branch patterns can be of use in predicting the histologic grade of a lesion. Branch pattern is more predictive of grade than is duct extension because the ducts involved by branch pattern are normally small enough that only high-nuclear-grade DCIS can grossly distend them. Large branch patterns correspond to high-nuclear-grade DCIS malignant components or to preexisting papillomas. Medium-sized branch pattern tends to correspond to inter-

mediate-grade lesions, and very small branch patterns that are difficult to distinguish from prominent spiculations usually correspond to low-grade lesions (Fig. 12–50). Duct extension is not a reliable predictor of histologic grade because the central portions of the ductal system (especially the lactiferous sinuses) that are involved by duct extension are so easily distensible that even low-nuclear-grade DCIS and benign papillomas can grossly distend them.

Duct extension and branch pattern are soft suspicious findings that may either be associated with other, harder suspicious findings or that may occur alone. When duct extension or branch pattern occurs in the absence of any other suspicious findings, the lesion is a benign intraductal papilloma in about 90% of cases (Fig. 12–51). However, biopsy of many of these lesions has revealed a 7% risk for DCIS, and an additional 6% of lesions have atypical ductal hyperplasia (ADH) involving the surface epithelium of a papilloma. Thus, even isolated duct extension or isolated branch pattern carries a 13% risk for either DCIS or ADH—far too high for the lesion to be characterized as BIRADS 3.

The sensitivities and positive predictive values for duct extension and branch pattern in the 1995 and current ongoing studies are shown in Table 12–12. Note that the sensitivity has increased, especially for duct extension, in the current study. However, the positive predictive value has decreased. This is a reflection of the expanding role of ultrasound in the evaluation of nipple discharge. A large percentage of all lesions that have duct extension represent benign intraductal papillomas that are found when evaluating patients with nipple discharge. The overall accuracy for duct extension in

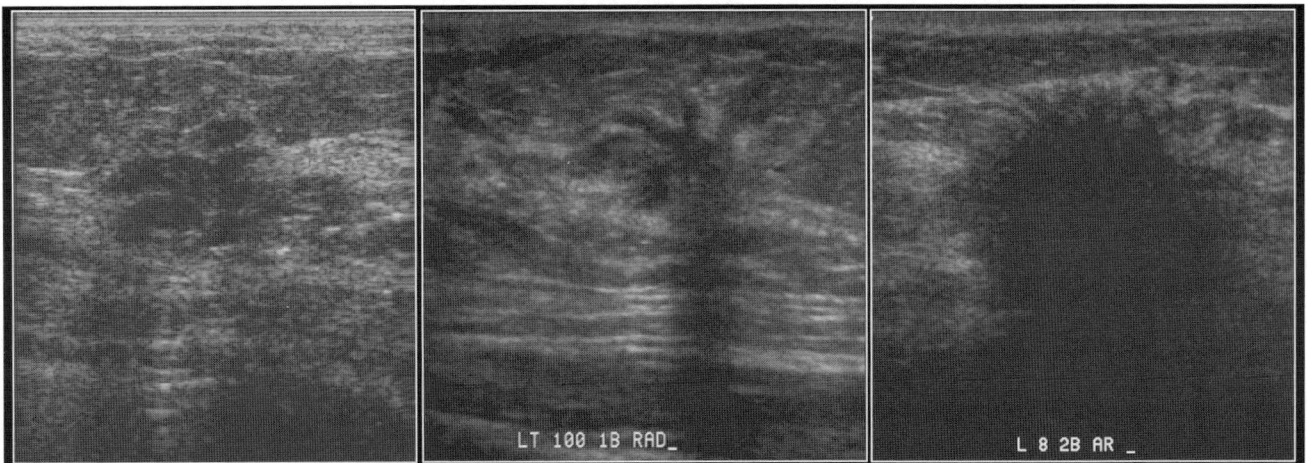

FIGURE 12–50 Like microlobulations, the size of branch pattern reflects that grade of the carcinoma. Large branch patterns (**left**) tend to be the result of high-grade invasive ductal carcinomas with high-nuclear-grade ductal carcinoma *in situ* (DCIS) components or papilloma. Small branch pattern (**right**) tends to reflect low-grade invasive ductal carcinoma with low-nuclear-grade DCIS components. Small branch pattern may be difficult to distinguish from thick spiculations. Intermediate-sized branch pattern (**middle**) tends to be associated with intermediate-grade invasive ductal carcinoma and intermediate-nuclear-grade DCIS. Unlike branch pattern, duct extension appears to be unrelated to the grade of the lesion. The lactiferous sinus portion of the duct that is frequently involved by duct extension is so distensible that even low-grade lesions and benign papillomas can grossly distend the duct.

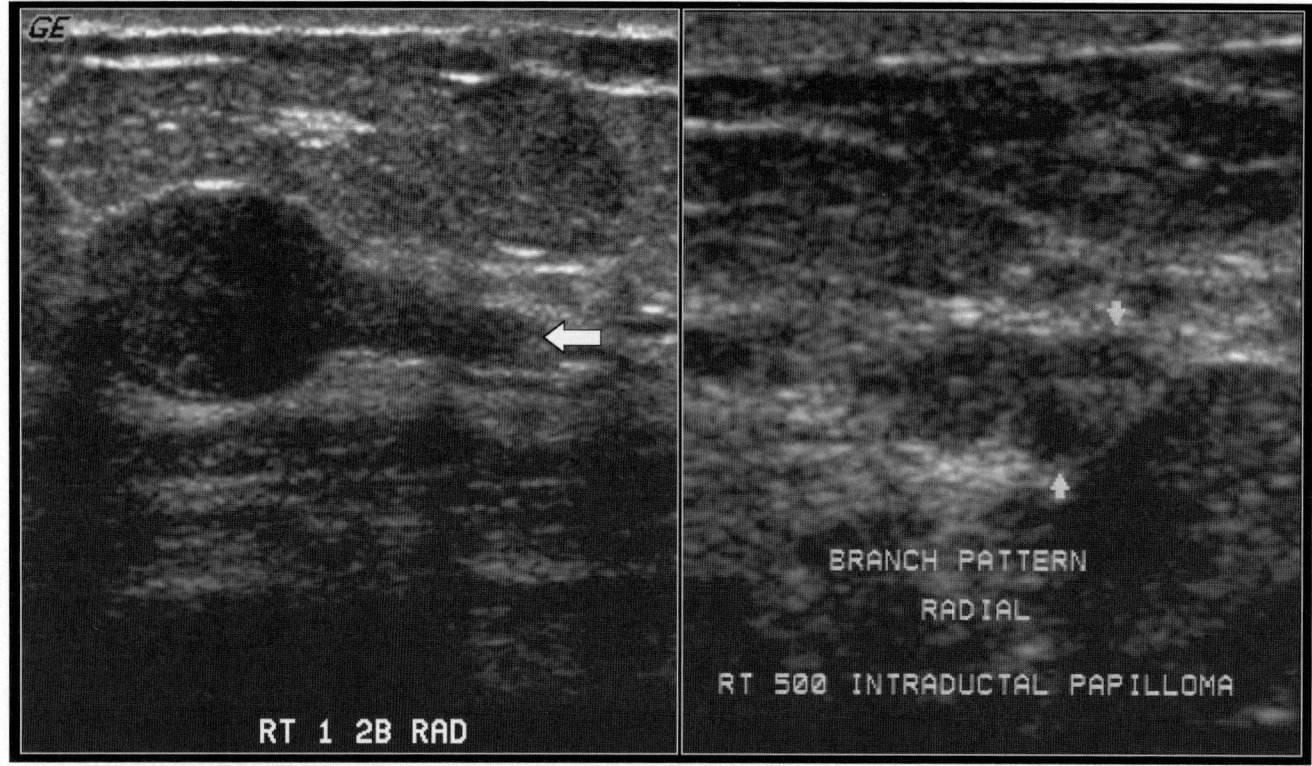

FIGURE 12–51 Solid nodules that have only a single soft finding, such as duct extension (**left**) or branch pattern (**right**), are benign papillomas in nearly 90% of cases. However, the risk for ductal carcinoma *in situ* (DCIS) is 6%, and the risk for atypical ductal hyperplasia (ADH) is 7%. Thus, the risk for DCIS or ADH is 13%, more than the less than 2% risk necessary for BIRADS 3 characterization. Such lesions must be excluded from the BIRADS 3 category and must be classified as BIRADS 4a and should undergo biopsy.

distinguishing benign from malignant solid nodules is 63%. The overall accuracy of branch pattern is 70%.

Acoustic Shadowing

Acoustic shadowing is an internal characteristic that is unique to sonographic evaluation of solid breast nodules and has no mammographic counterpart. Shadowing was one of the first findings ever detected and described on the older whole breast water-path scanners. Acoustic shadowing is a hard finding that reflects the desmoplasia induced by malignant nodules that lie primarily at the spiculated end of the spectrum. Many circumscribed breast carcinomas contain relatively little or even no desmoplasia. Thus, the sensitivity of acoustic shadowing can never be 100%.

The degree of acoustic shadowing caused by a malignant nodule depends on the frequency of the ultrasound beam with which it is scanned. Thus, lesions scanned at 12

TABLE 12–12. SENSITIVITY AND POSITIVE PREDICTIVE VALUE (PPV) FOR DUCT EXTENSION

Taller than Wide	1995 Study (750 Nodules)[a]		Current Study (1,211 Nodules)[b]	
	Sensitivity	PPV Odds Ratio	Sensitivity	PPV Odds Ratio
Duct extension	25%	51% (3.0)	49%	46% (1.4)
Branch pattern	30%	64% (3.8)	44%	60% (1.8)

[a]Prevalence, 16.7%.
[b]Prevalence, 32.8%.

MHz will cause more acoustic shadowing than those scanned with a 7-MHz beam.

Because breast cancer is heterogenous not only from nodule to nodule, but also within an individual nodule, part of a malignant lesion may be desmoplastic and cause acoustic shadowing, whereas other parts of the same lesion may contain relatively little desmoplasia and not cause shadowing (Fig. 12–52). The entire substance of a solid nodule should be scanned in two orthogonal planes before it can be concluded that there is no acoustic shadowing. If acoustic shadowing occurs in only a portion of the lesion, the entire nodule should be considered positive for acoustic shadowing, the nodule cannot be characterized as BIRADS 3, and biopsy should be recommended. Internal heterogeneity and partial shadowing are manifestations of the polyclonal nature of many malignant nodules.

Although acoustic shadowing is a hard suspicious finding, the presence of normal or enhanced through-transmission should not be considered at all reassuring in nodules that have any other suspicious findings. In fact, the sound transmission of malignant solid nodules is almost evenly distributed between those that cause acoustic shadowing, those with normal through-transmission, and those that demonstrate enhanced acoustic through-transmission. Circumscribed malignant nodules that represent high-grade invasive ductal cancers nearly always have enhanced through-transmission, whereas intermediate-grade lesions frequently demonstrate normal through-transmission or mixed areas of shadowing and enhancement (Fig. 12–53).

Enhanced through-transmission predicts a highly cellular lesion at the circumscribed end of the malignant spectrum that has grown too rapidly for desmoplasia to have developed. As noted earlier, such circumscribed lesions are also more likely to be hypervascular on color Doppler. Thus, one might expect that the presence of enhanced through-transmission in a nodule with other suspicious characteristics would predict the presence of abundant internal blood flow on color Doppler. In fact, this is true with such reliability that we consider enhanced through-transmission in suspicious solid nodules to repre-

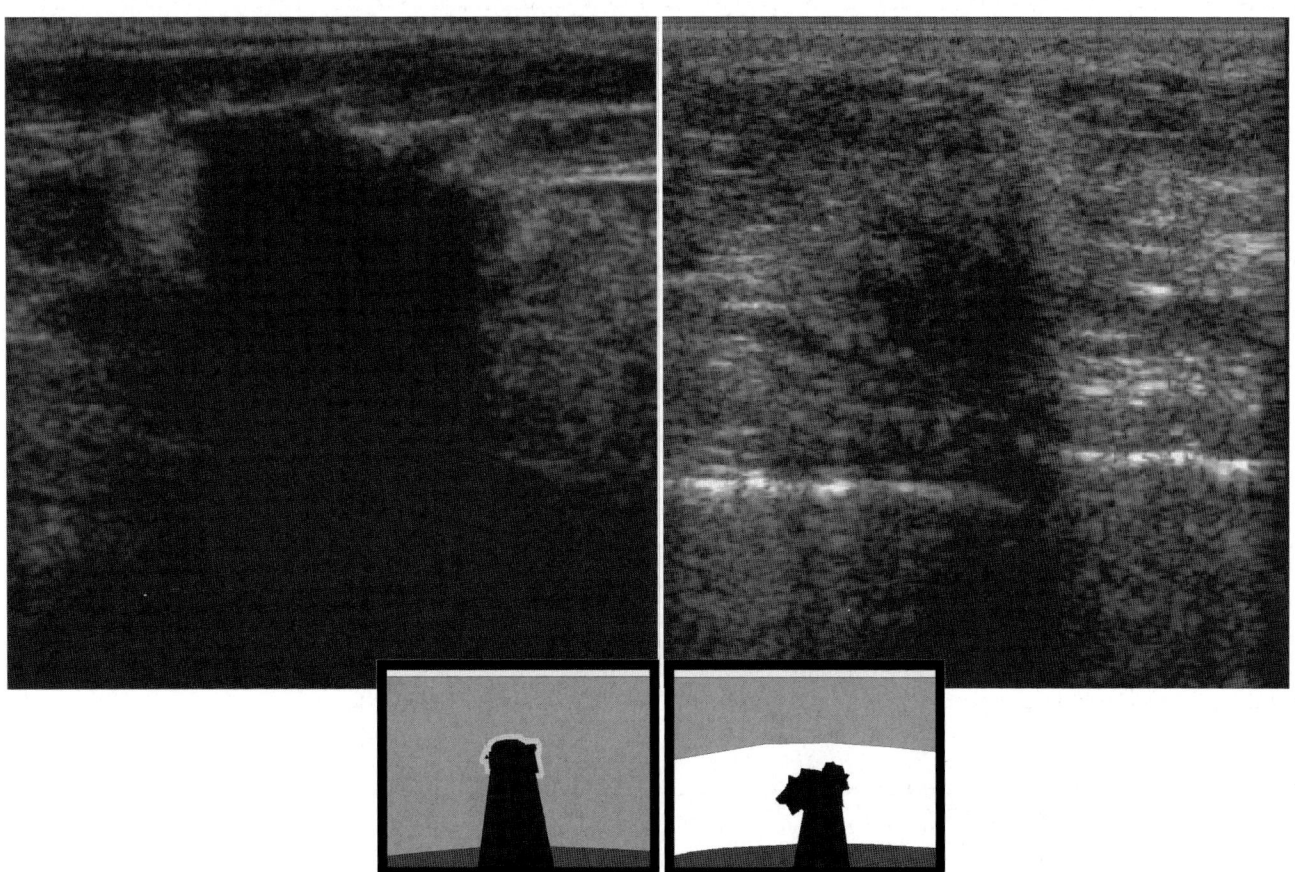

FIGURE 12–52 Acoustic shadowing is a hard suspicious finding suggesting the presence of a spiculated invasive malignancy with significant amounts of desmoplastic response. Because breast cancer can be heterogeneous within an individual nodule, only part of the nodule may incite the desmoplastic response. Thus, the shadowing can be intense and complete, even obscuring the posterior margin of the lesion when desmoplasia is extensive throughout the lesion, or the shadowing may be partial and faint when desmoplasia is less extensive and involves only part of the lesion.

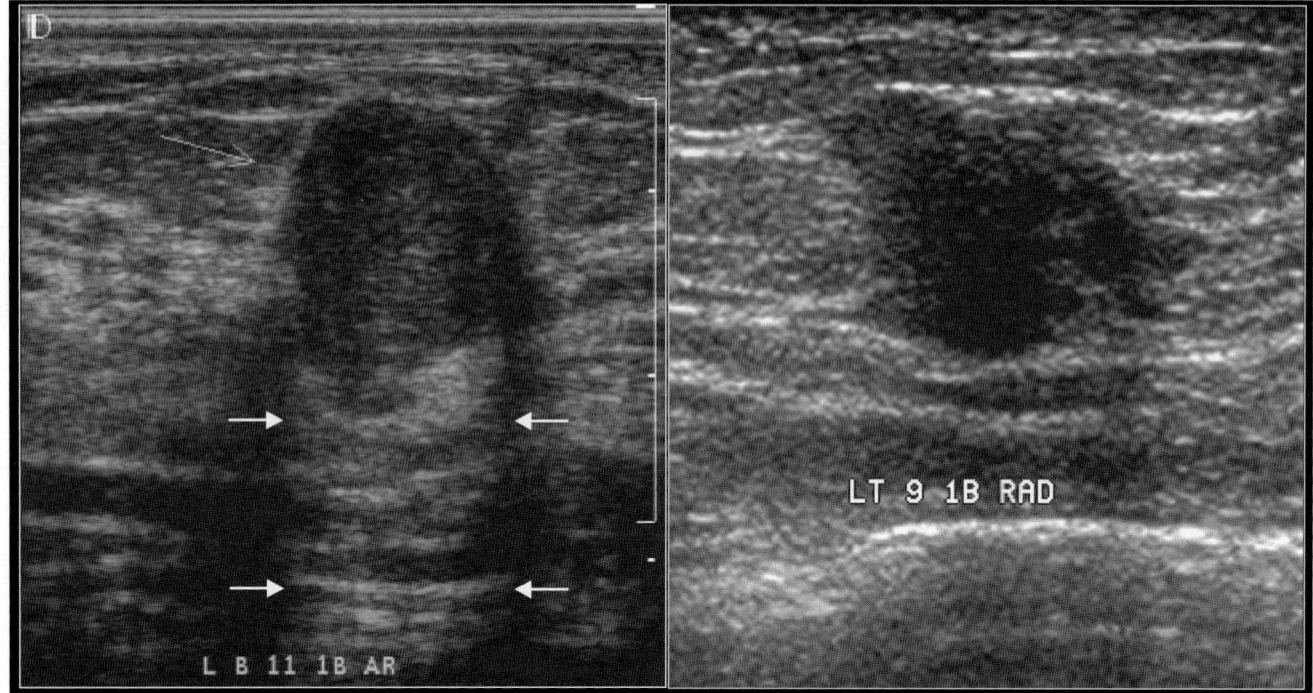

FIGURE 12–53 All malignant nodules do not cause acoustic shadowing. In fact, most malignant nodules have either enhanced or normal through-transmission of sound. This high-grade invasive ductal carcinoma has incited an intense inflammatory response and has incited virtually no desmoplastic response. It not only does not cast an acoustic shadow but also shows intense acoustic enhancement deep to the lesion (**left**). Intermediate-grade invasive lesions tend to have normal through-transmission of sound (**right**) or mixtures of small areas of shadowing and enhancement.

sent "poor man's color Doppler". However, such lesions are soft and compressible enough that internal blood flow can be obliterated if too much compression pressure is used (see Chapter 20, Fig. 20–12B). Thus, if color Doppler is to be used in evaluation of solid breast nodules, it must be performed with very little compression pressure.

Table 12–13 shows the percentage of all solid malignant nodules that show each type of sound transmission.

The sound transmission associated with malignant nodules can be used to determine their histologic grades with some limitations. Most lesions that have intense acoustic shadowing are low- to intermediate-grade lesions. On the other hand, high-grade invasive ductal carcinomas usually demonstrate enhanced acoustic through-transmission. Intermediate-grade lesions tend to have either normal

TABLE 12–13. SOUND TRANSMISSION IN 369 SOLID MALIGNANT NODULES

Acoustic shadowing (complete or partial)	35%
Normal through-transmission	32%
Enhanced though-transmission	28%
Mixed sound transmission	5%
Total	100%

through-transmission or mixed patterns, in which most of the transmission is normal, but there are small foci of either enhanced or diminished through-transmission. The histologic grading of malignant solid nodules is far from perfect. Sound transmission is more effective at distinguishing high-grade from low- and intermediate-grade lesions than it is for distinguishing low-grade from intermediate-grade lesions because there is a lot of overlap in the sound transmission characteristics of low- and intermediate-grade invasive ductal carcinomas. Enhanced through-transmission doubles the odds ratio of a lesion being high grade and almost halves its odds ratio of being low or intermediate grade. Acoustic shadowing or normal sound transmission halves the odds ratio of a lesion being high grade (Table 12–14).

Grading based on acoustic through-transmission is confounded by the size of the lesion. Larger lesions are more likely to have enhanced through-transmission, but larger lesions are also likely to be more dedifferentiated and of higher grade. The natural progression of untreated malignant nodules is for the grade of the lesion to increase as the size of the lesion increases. Very small lesions, those with diameters of less than 5 mm, are most likely to have normal through-transmission, regardless of their histologic grade. Apparently, a threshold or critical mass of either inflammatory cells or desmoplasia is necessary in order to af-

TABLE 12–14. SOUND TRANSMISSION VERSUS HISTOLOGIC GRADE OF INVASIVE DUCT CARCINOMA (202 NODULES)

Sound Transmission	Low Grade		Intermediate Grade		High Grade	
	Percentage of Cases	Odds Ratio	Percentage of Cases	Odds Ratio	Percentage of Cases	Odds Ratio
All nodules	37	1.0	37	1.0	26	1.0
Enhanced	23	0.6	26	0.7	51	2.0
Shadowing	45	1.2	42	1.1	13	0.5
Normal	42	1.1	40	1.0	13	0.5

fect sound transmission. Small lesions are less likely than large lesions to have developed a threshold amount of either desmoplasia or inflammatory response.

Despite the obvious limitations of sound transmission in predicting the histologic grade of solid malignant nodules, it is remarkable that a single sonographic finding can predict grade as well as it does. It seems likely that a multifactorial assessment that uses the presence of spiculation; thick, echogenic halo; size of microlobulations; and size of branch pattern together with sound transmission will achieve much better results.

Unfortunately, sound transmission may be affected by technical factors. Artifactual acoustic shadowing that simulates malignant shadowing can result from critical angle phenomena created by steeply obliquely oriented tissue planes such as Cooper's ligaments (Fig. 12–54). Such artifactual shadowing can usually be eradicated with firmer compression (Fig. 12–55). Acoustic shadowing that results from malignancy, however, may be decreased but generally cannot be completely eradicated with higher degrees of transducer compression. Enhanced through-transmission deep to high-grade invasive ductal carcinomas or special-type tumors may

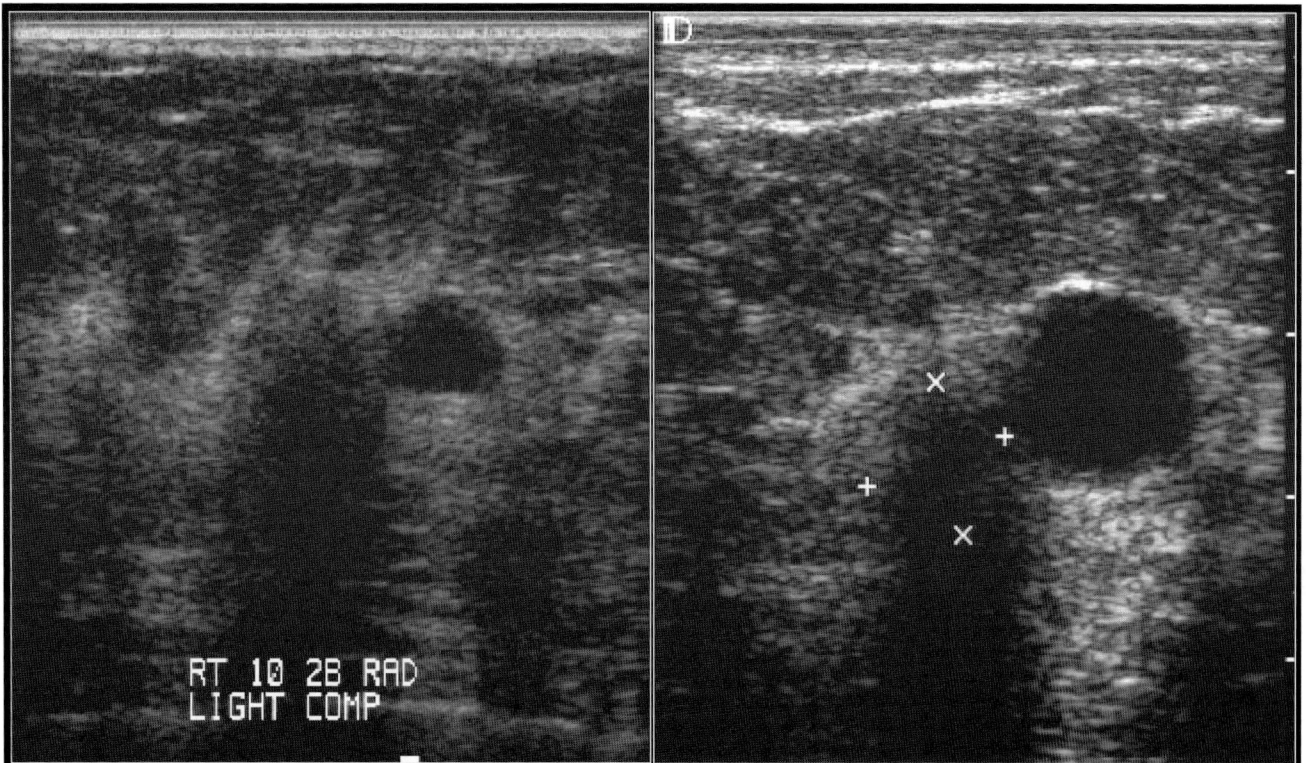

FIGURE 12–54 Artifactual acoustic shadowing caused by critical angle phenomena can simulate a malignant nodule that causes acoustic shadowing. The **left** image shows artifactual shadowing caused by critical angle shadowing arising in steeply obliquely oriented Cooper's ligaments that are coursing through the subcutaneous fat. The **right** image shows a shadowing tubular carcinoma next to a simple cyst.

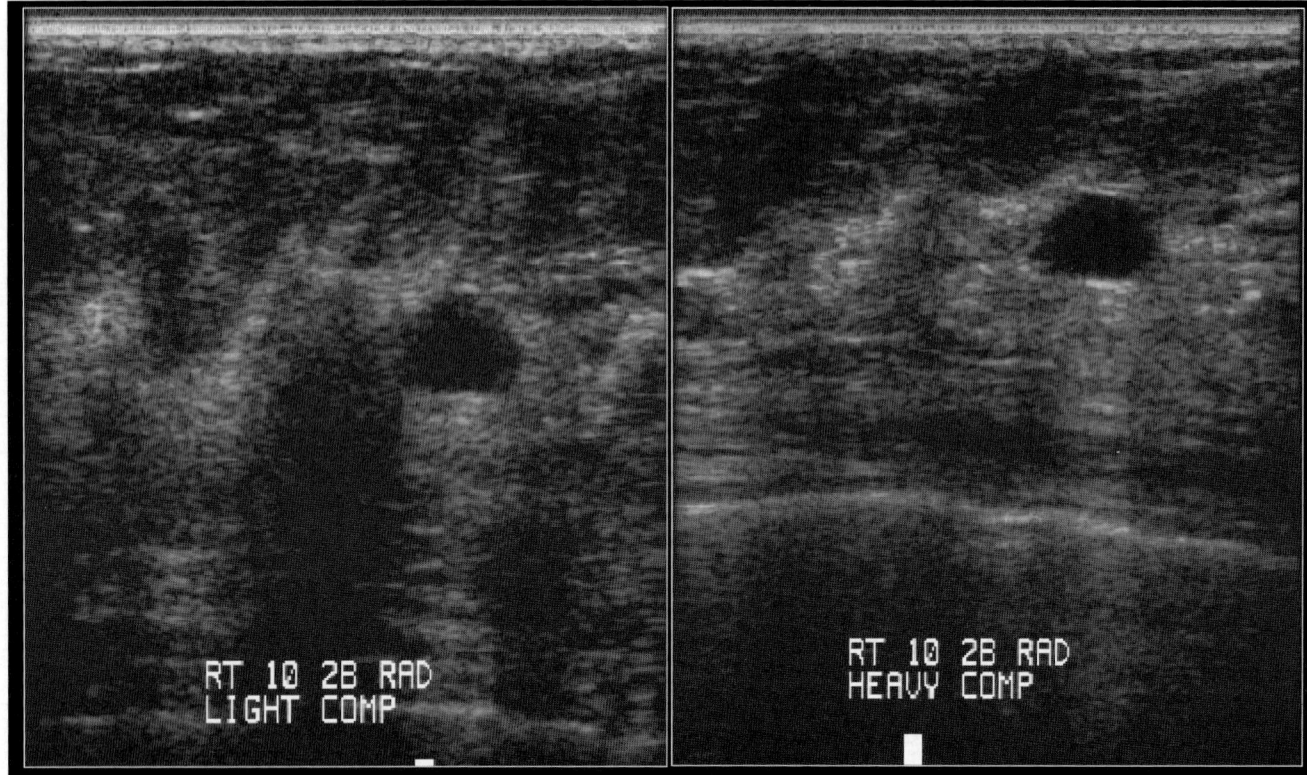

FIGURE 12–55 Artifactual acoustic shadowing resulting from obliquely oriented tissue planes, such as Cooper's ligaments **(left)**, can be reduced or obliterated by using heavier scan pressure that forces the shadowing tissue planes into a more horizontal orientation **(right)**. Increasing scan pressure may reduce, but will not completely obliterate, acoustic shadowing caused by malignant nodules.

be better demonstrated with higher degrees of compression pressure (Fig. 12–56). Another technical factor than can affect both acoustic shadowing and enhanced through-transmission is spatial compounding. By steering the beam from multiple angles of incidence per frame, the degree of both acoustic shadowing and enhanced through-transmission can be reduced (Fig. 12–57).

Remember that not all spiculated lesions that cause acoustic shadowing are low-grade invasive ductal carcinomas and that not all lesions associated with enhanced through-transmission are high-grade invasive ductal carcinomas. There is a differential diagnosis for malignant-appearing solid nodules that have enhanced through-transmission that includes the rare special-type tumors in addition to high-grade invasive ductal carcinomas. Thus, the differential diagnosis for malignant-appearing nodules that demonstrate enhanced through-transmission, in order of prevalence, includes: high-grade invasive ductal carcinoma, colloid (mucinous) carcinoma larger than 1.5 cm, medullary carcinoma, metaplastic carcinoma, and invasive papillary carcinoma. Likewise, some special-type tumors and lobular carcinoma must be considered in the differential of malignant-appearing nodules that cause acoustic shadowing. The differential

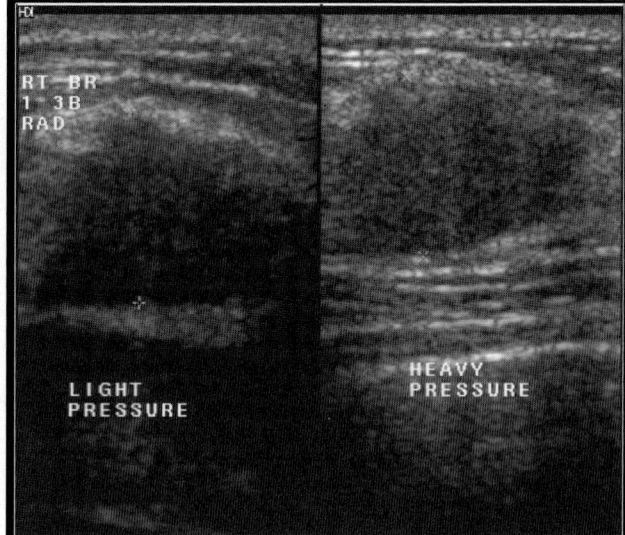

FIGURE 12–56 The degree of compression pressure used during scanning can also affect the appearance of enhanced through-transmission. Nodules that appear to have normal through-transmission with relatively light degrees of scan pressure **(left)** can show markedly enhanced through-transmission when scanned with a higher degree of compression pressure **(right)**.

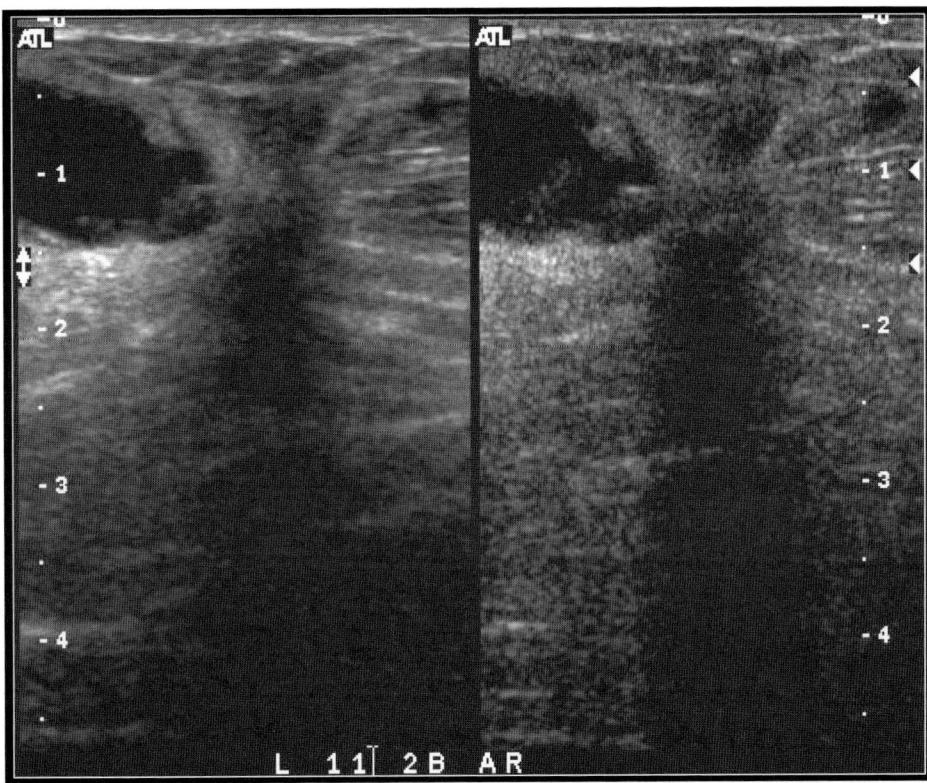

FIGURE 12–57 Real-time compounding diminishes acoustic shadowing by steering the beam in at multiple different angles. This can decrease intense acoustic shadowing (**left**) in comparison to conventional imaging (**right**), but more important, can completely eradicate mild or partial shadowing in other cases.

diagnosis for lesions that cause acoustic shadowing, in order of prevalence, includes: low-grade invasive ductal carcinoma, invasive lobular carcinoma, tubular carcinomas 1.5 cm or larger, and tubulolobular carcinoma. The differential diagnosis for lesions with normal through-transmission, in order of prevalence, includes: intermediate-grade invasive ductal carcinoma, small tubular carcinomas less than 1.5 cm, small colloid carcinomas less than 1.5 cm, and small tubulolobular

carcinomas less than 1.5 cm in maximum diameter. Table 12–15 shows the sound transmission characteristics of breast malignancies other than invasive ductal carcinoma. The sound transmission characteristics of special-type tumors are illustrated in Chapter 14.

Entities other than malignant nodules can also cause acoustic shadowing. Biopsy scar and fat necrosis can cause shadowing. This is illustrated and discussed in greater de-

TABLE 12–15. SOUND TRANSMISSION CHARACTERISTICS OF BREAST MALIGNANCIES OTHER THAN DUCTAL CARCINOMA

	Shadowing	Normal	Enhanced
Medullary carcinoma	0%	0%	100%
Colloid carcinoma	0%	29%	71%
Colloid carcinoma > 1.5 cm	0%	0%	100%
Tubular carcinoma	57%	43%	0%
Tubular carcinoma > 1.5 cm	67%	33%	0%
Tubulolobular carcinoma	100%	0%	0%
Invasive lobular carcinoma	59%	36%	5%

TABLE 12–16. SENSITIVITY AND POSITIVE PREDICTIVE VALUE (PPV) FOR ACOUSTIC SHADOWING

| | 1995 Study (750 Nodules)[a] | | Current Study (1,211 Nodules)[b] | |
| | | PPV | | PPV |
	Sensitivity	Odds Ratio	Sensitivity	Odds Ratio
Complete shadow	42%	81% (4.9)	16%	69% (2.1)
Partial shadow	—	—	19%	57% (1.7)
Any shadow	—	—	35%	62% (1.9)

[a]Prevalence, 16.7%.
[b]Prevalence, 32.8%.

tail in Chapter 18. Radial scar can be associated with acoustic shadowing and is discussed and illustrated in Chapter 15. Densely calcified fibroadenomas may result in acoustic shadowing and are discussed and illustrated in Chapter 13. Calcified lipid cysts can cast acoustic shadows and are discussed and illustrated in Chapters 11 and 18.

Table 12–16 shows the sensitivities and positive predictive values of acoustic shadowing in the 1995 study and in the current ongoing study. The overall accuracy is 69% for complete shadowing, 68% for partial shadowing, and 71% for either partial or complete shadowing.

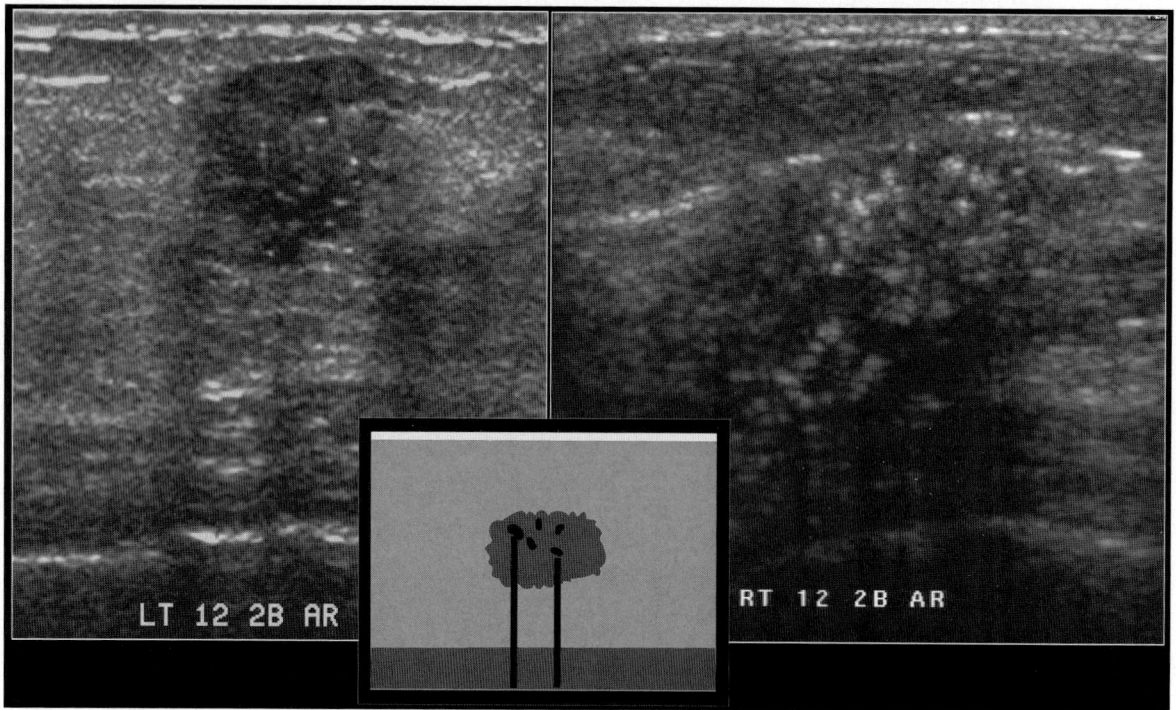

FIGURE 12–58 Most calcifications within malignant nodules lie within ductal carcinoma *in situ* (DCIS) components of the tumor. The **left** image shows microcalcifications in pure DCIS. Each hypoechoic microlobulation within the lesion represents a duct filled with necrosis, and in the center of each microlobulation is a punctate bright echo that represents calcifications within the area of central necrosis. The **right** image shows calcifications in an invasive ductal carcinoma that, like 80% of invasive ductal carcinomas, had intraductal components. Even in invasive ductal carcinomas, the calcifications usually lie within the DCIS (intraductal) components of the tumor. The calcifications within malignant nodules are often large enough to create bright echoes, despite being volume averaged with surrounding tumor substance, but are too small to create acoustic shadows in most cases. Malignant calcifications cast acoustic shadows only when so numerous that they are clumped or when the calcifications are relatively coarse, such as in cases of high-nuclear-grade DCIS *(drawing)*.

Calcifications

The presence of punctate calcifications within solid nodules is a mammographic finding applied to sonography. The presence of calcifications represents a soft sonographic finding more typically associated with DCIS or intraductal components of tumor than with invasive components (Fig. 12–58). Sonography is only 80% as sensitive as mammography for detection of calcifications within malignant nodules. Thus, it generally should be expected that mammography will show all calcifications seen sonographically, but that sonography may fail to show some calcifications that are mammographically visible. However, in occasional cases, sonography may show calcifications that are not prospectively seen on routine mammograms. Such calcifications are usually seen in retrospect on the original films or are demonstrable on spot compression magnification views (Fig. 12–59).

The width of the ultrasound beam in typical high-resolution near-field imaging equipment is 1 to 1.5 mm at the elevation plane focal depth. However, with very-large-aperture, 1.5-dimensional (1.5-D) array transducers operated at 12 MHz, beam widths of less than 1 mm can be obtained. Most of the calcifications that occur in malignant nodules have diameters much smaller than the width of the beam and therefore are subject to volume averaging. Whether volume averaging prevents demonstration of the calcifications depends heavily on the echogenicity and heterogeneity of the background tissue in which the calcifications lie. Most benign calcifications that occur as a result of fibrocystic change or benign proliferative disorders lie within a background of heterogeneous hyperechoic tissues. The volume averaging of the echogenic calcifications with the echogenic background tissues obscures the calcifications. However, most calcifications that occur within malignant nodules lie within a background of relatively homogeneous hypoechoic to isoechoic tissue. Even when volume averaging of bright calcifications with the dark-background tumor matrix occurs, the calcifications are still visible as bright echoes within the solid nodule. Thus, because of the more homogeneous and hypoechoic background tumor substance, sonography has a propensity to show malignant calcifications better than it does benign calcifications. Of course, if benign calcifications occur within the lumen or wall of a cyst or dilated duct filled with anechoic fluid, they will be more likely to be sonographically demonstrable (Fig. 12–60). Similarly, punctate calcifications that occur in homogeneously isoechoic areas of adenosis may be sonographically demonstrable (Fig. 12–61).

Although individual calcifications that are much smaller in diameter than the width of the ultrasound beam may remain visible despite volume averaging, they will not cast acoustic shadows (Fig. 12–62). The calcification must be wide enough to completely occlude the ultrasound

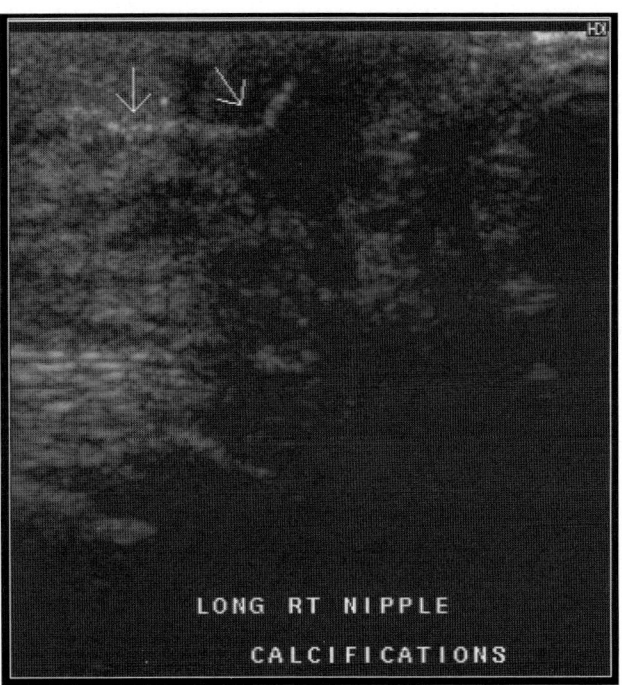

FIGURE 12–59 In general, mammography is more sensitive for calcifications than sonography. However, in some cases, sonography can show calcifications that are not readily visible on routine mammograms but that may be well shown on spot compression magnification views. In this case, calcifications within ductal carcinoma *in situ* (DCIS) could be seen coursing into the nipple on ultrasound but could not be seen on the routine mammogram, owing to overpenetration of the skin line on the routine mammogram. After sonography, spot compression magnification mammograms confirmed the presence of DCIS calcifications within the nipple.

beam in order to cast an acoustic shadow. The calcifications that occur within malignant tumors are too small to occlude the beam. Thus, malignant calcifications appear sonographically as small, bright echoes that do not cast acoustic shadows. Only if calcifications are the coarse type seen in high-nuclear-grade DCIS, or are so numerous and tightly clustered that they are nearly in direct contact with each other or stacked on one another, do they cause acoustic shadowing (Fig. 12–63).

Calcifications can occur in the invasive parts of malignant tumors but more commonly occur within the DCIS components. They are the result of necrosis and occur within the lumen of DCIS-containing ducts. Under ideal circumstances, sonography has the ability to show individual calcium-containing ducts distended with tumor. Thus, calcifications are most often seen within duct extensions (Fig. 12–64), branch patterns (Fig. 12–65), and microlobulations that represent individual tumor-distended ducts (Fig. 12–66). Individual ducts that become distended enough to be visible sonographically are more likely to occur with high-nuclear-grade DCIS components.

(text continued on page 499)

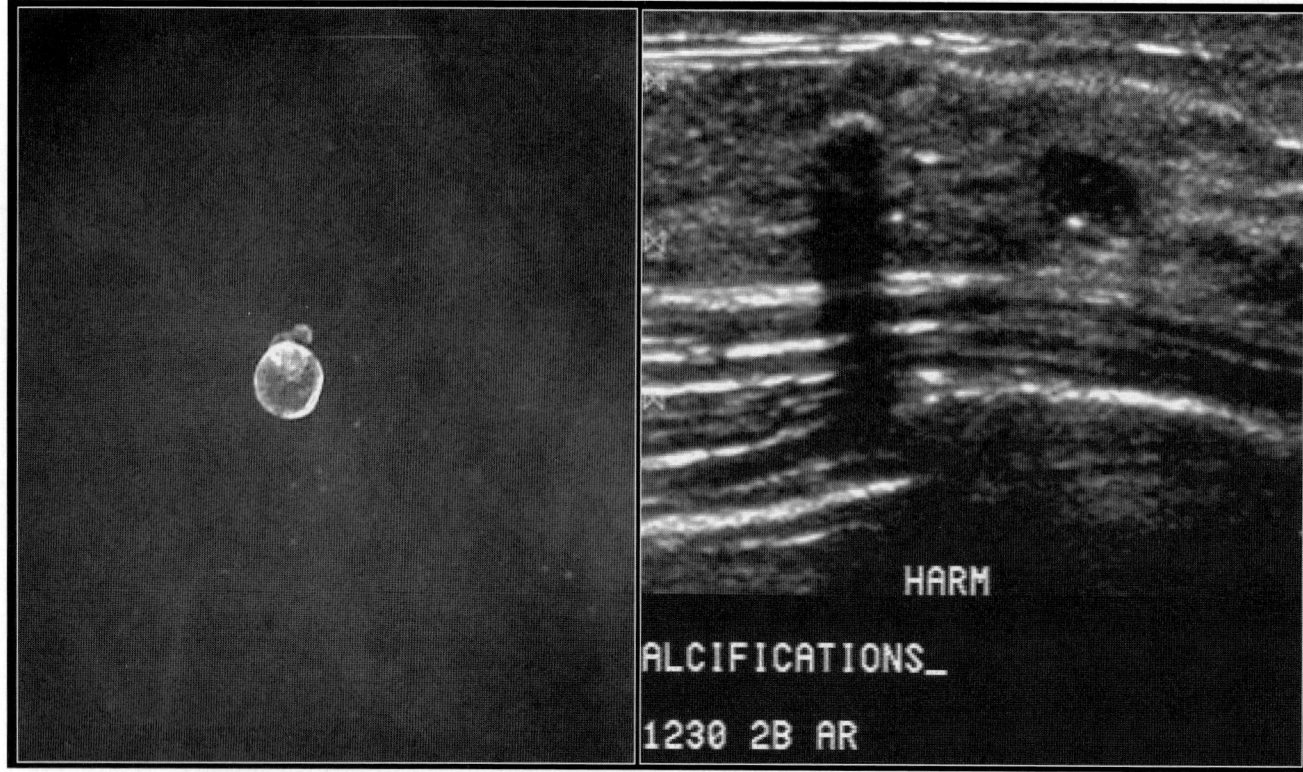

FIGURE 12–60 Sonography shows malignant calcifications more routinely than it shows benign calcifications because the malignant calcifications that are volume averaged with the uniformly isoechoic or hypoechoic tumor substance are still visible as bright echoes, whereas benign calcifications that are volume averaged with hyperechoic fibroglandular elements generally become indistinguishable from the background hyperechogenicity. However, when benign calcifications occur within the wall or lumen of cysts, within ducts, or within a background of uniformly isoechoic adenosis, they may remain visible as bright echoes despite volume averaging. In this case, benign calcifications that are visible include milk of calcium, intraductal calcifications, and oil cyst calcifications.

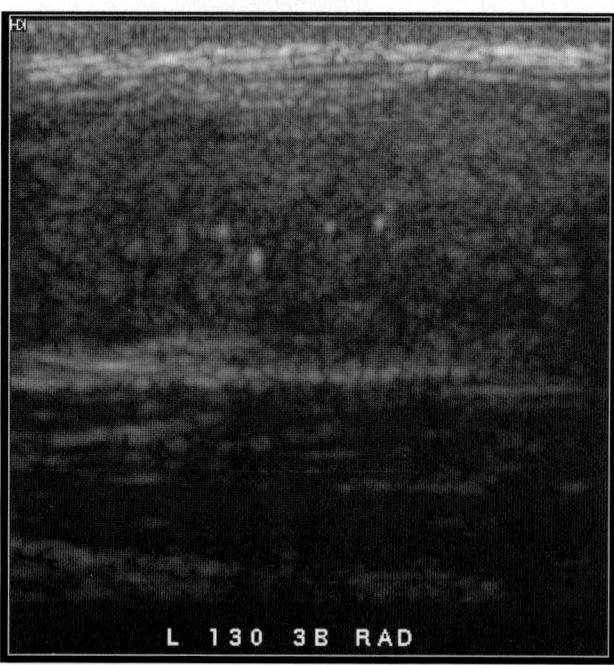

FIGURE 12–61 The small punctate calcifications within adenosis are visible in this patient because they occur in a background of homogeneous isoechoic glandular tissue. Despite volume averaging, the tiny calcifications are visible as punctate, bright echoes.

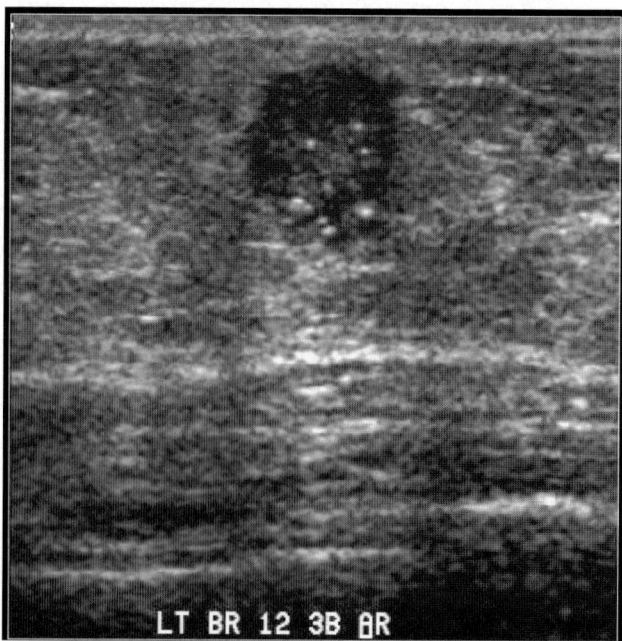

FIGURE 12–62 Although most calcifications within malignant nodules are visible as small, punctate, bright echoes despite volume averaging, they do not cast acoustic shadows because they are too narrow to occlude the beam. To cast an acoustic shadow, a calcification must be wide enough to occlude the ultrasound beam.

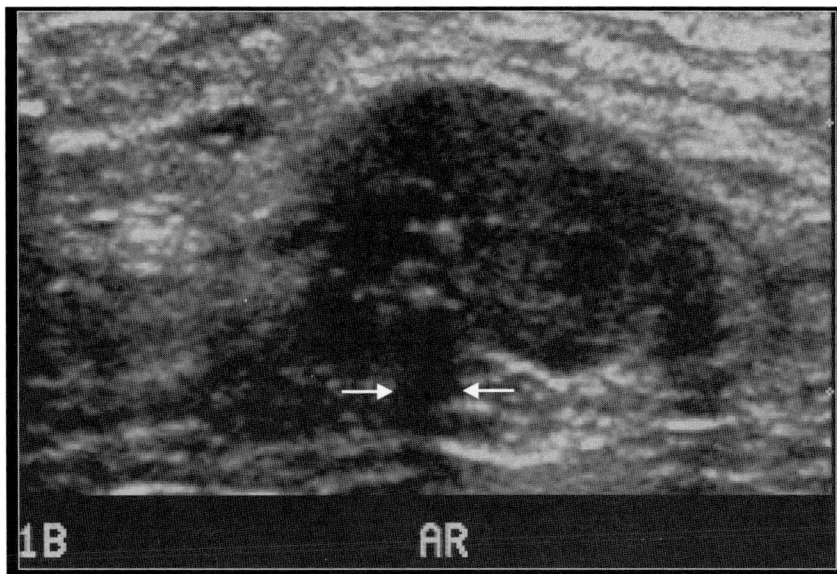

FIGURE 12–63 Occasionally, calcifications may be close enough together to be clumped. A clump of calcifications can be wide enough to occlude the ultrasound beam and cast an acoustic shadow even though the individual calcifications do not cast shadows. Large and coarse calcifications that occur in high-nuclear-grade ductal carcinoma *in situ* can also cast acoustic shadows.

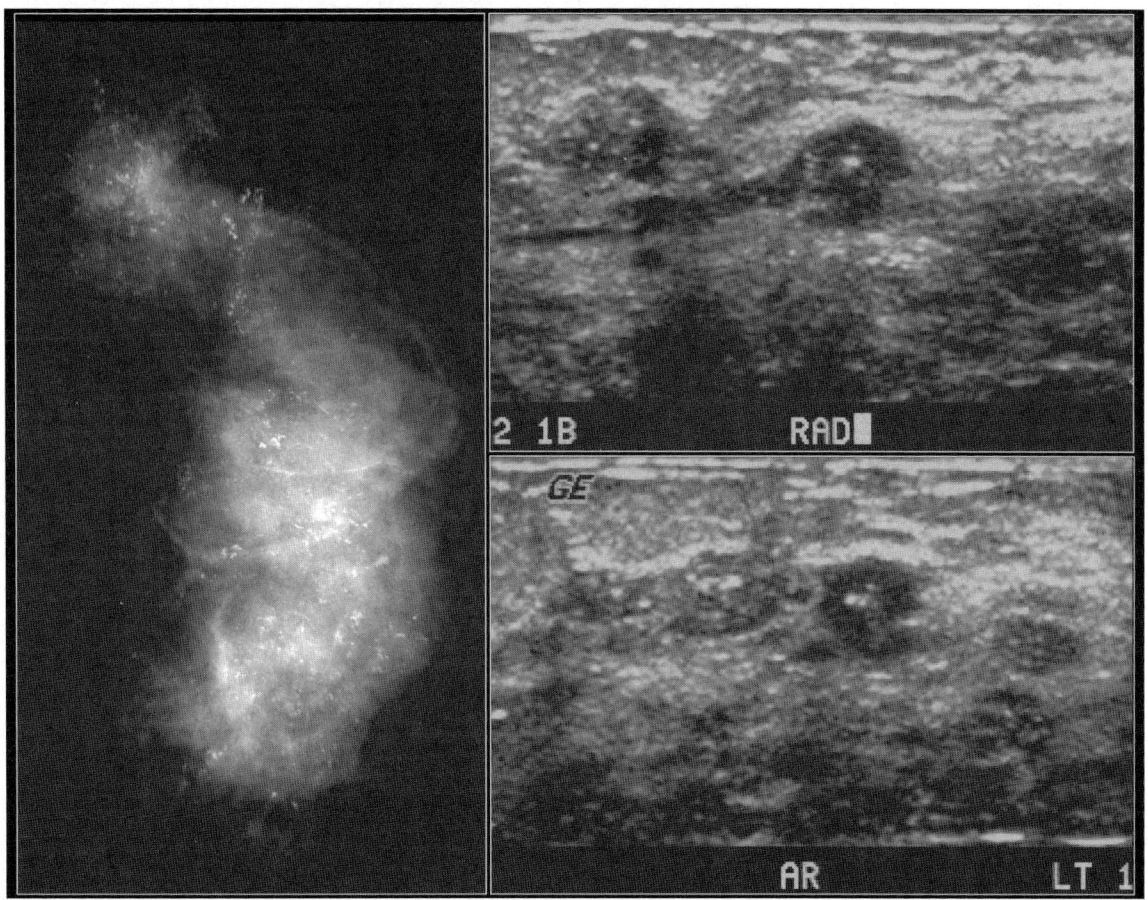

FIGURE 12–64 Coarse linear and branching calcifications involve almost the entire breast in this patient. Such calcifications lie within the necrosis in the center of the lumen of ducts distended with high-nuclear-grade ductal carcinoma *in situ* (DCIS). These calcifications are BIRADS 5 category by mammography alone, so that sonography is not necessary for diagnosis. However, if sonography shows a solid mass in this breast, the mass is most likely to represent the invasive parts of this tumor. Biopsy of calcifications under stereotactic guidance will appropriately yield a diagnosis of high-nuclear-grade DCIS, but will likely underdiagnose the presence of invasion. Biopsy of the solid nodule within this breast under ultrasound guidance will be more likely to diagnose the invasive component of the lesion. The calcifications that lie within the high-nuclear-grade components of the lesion shown in the mammogram lie within enlarged ducts and lobules. Internal radial (**upper right**) and antiradial (**lower right**) views show a grossly distended duct containing central necrosis and calcification.

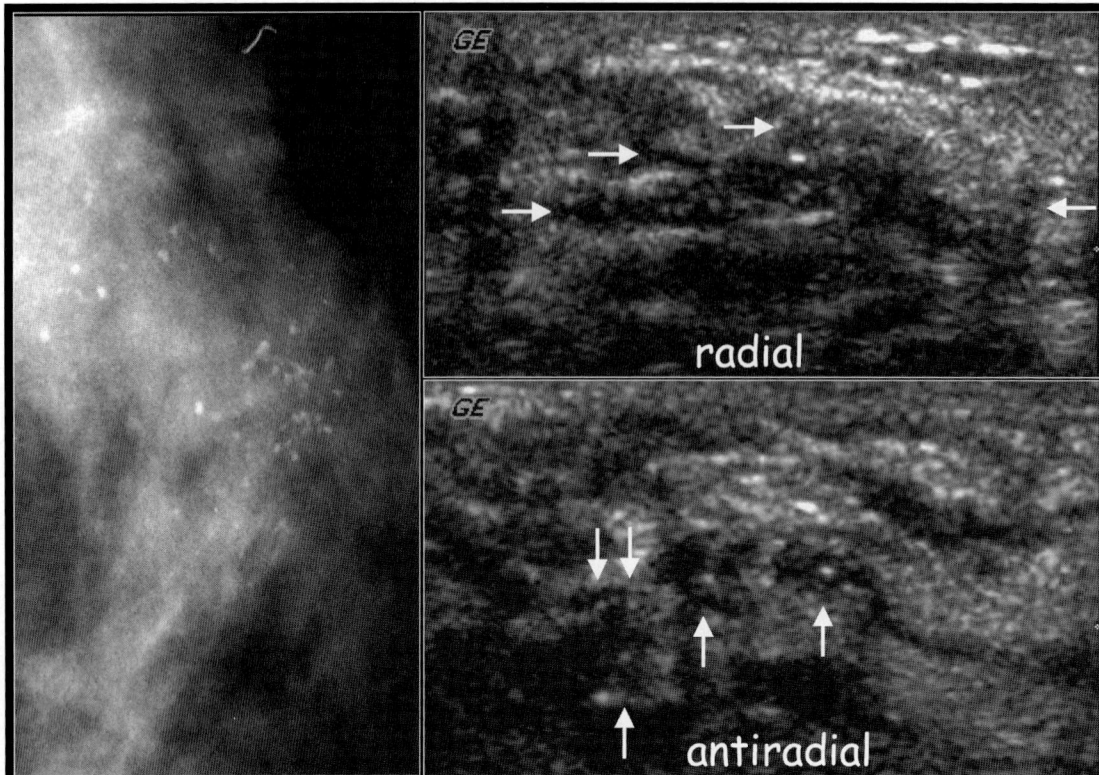

FIGURE 12–65 Calcifications can be associated with branch pattern. Internal radial (**upper right**) and antiradial (**lower right**) views demonstrate multiple branch ducts that are distended with tumor and necrosis and contain central calcifications *(arrows)*.

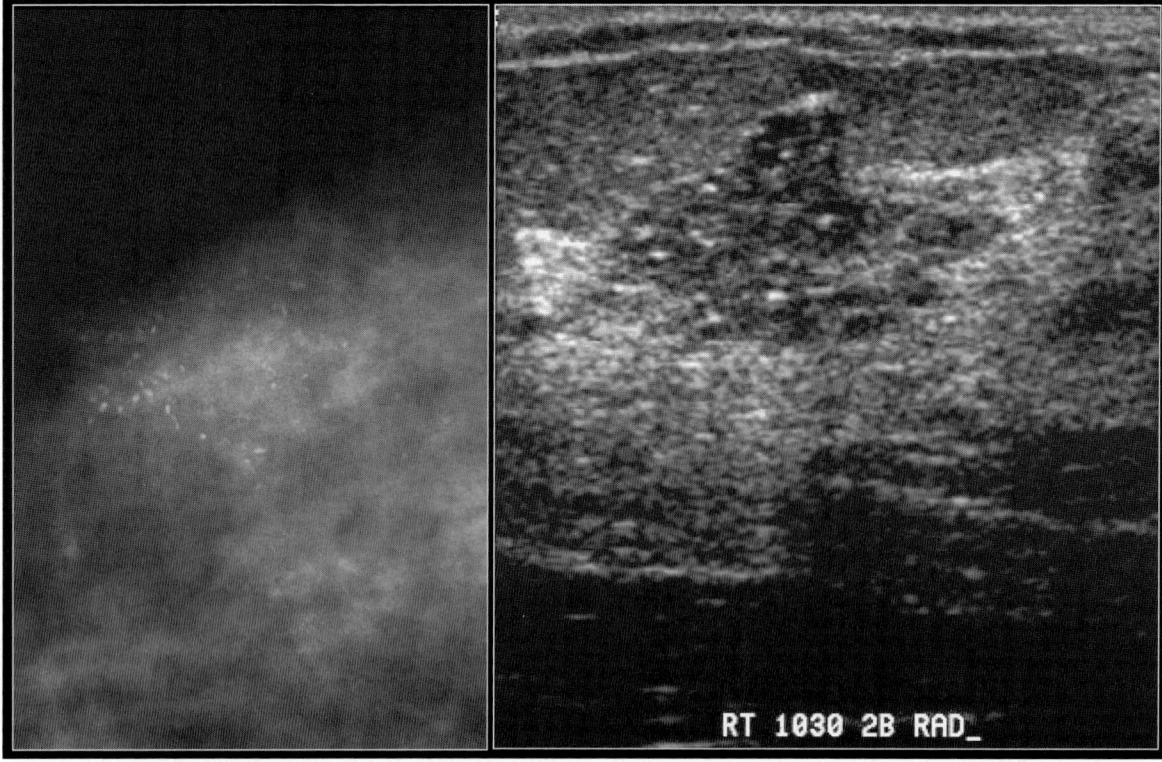

FIGURE 12–66 These segmentally distributed clustered pleomorphic calcifications are suspicious for ductal carcinoma *in situ* by mammography alone. Each calcification lies within the center of a microlobulation that represents a duct distended with tumor and necrosis.

Because the sensitivity of sonography is less than that of mammography for calcifications, the value of positive ultrasound findings is greater than the value of negative ultrasound findings. Thus, seeing calcifications within a solid nodule excludes the nodule from being characterized as BI-RADS 3. However, calcifications that are not seen sonographically but are mammographically visible are not necessarily reassuring.

The greater sensitivity of mammography and the limitations of a completely negative ultrasound do not mean that sonography has absolutely no role in evaluation of clustered calcifications. In fact, ultrasound may play a very important role when it shows positive findings.

For example, if a mammogram shows extensive calcifications in an area of water density, the dense tissues could obscure a mass that may be associated with the calcifications. The calcifications are most likely to be associated with the DCIS components of a tumor that tend to lie in the periphery of the lesion. The DCIS diagnosed may be pure DCIS, but may be part of a mixed invasive and intraductal lesion. If the calcifications undergo stereotactically

guided vacuum-assisted large core needle biopsy, the diagnosis of pure DCIS is likely to be obtained, but the presence of invasive malignancy is like to be underdiagnosed. The degree of underdiagnosis of invasive malignancy is even greater for core biopsy than for mammotomy. However, if instead, sonography is first used to evaluate the area of calcifications and shows a BIRADS 4a or higher category solid nodule, and if the nodule undergoes biopsy with ultrasound guidance, an accurate diagnosis of invasive malignancy is more likely to be made than if only stereotactic biopsy of the calcifications is performed (Fig. 12–67). Thus, identifying a solid nodule associated with calcifications can lead to more rapid and accurate diagnosis of invasive malignancy. Early diagnosis of invasion is more likely to lead to appropriate surgical management with the fewest number of surgical procedures.

In certain situations, sonography may show definitively benign forms of calcifications when mammography cannot. One example of this is milk of calcium. Although mammography may show more calcifications than sonography, numerous calcifications must be present within an

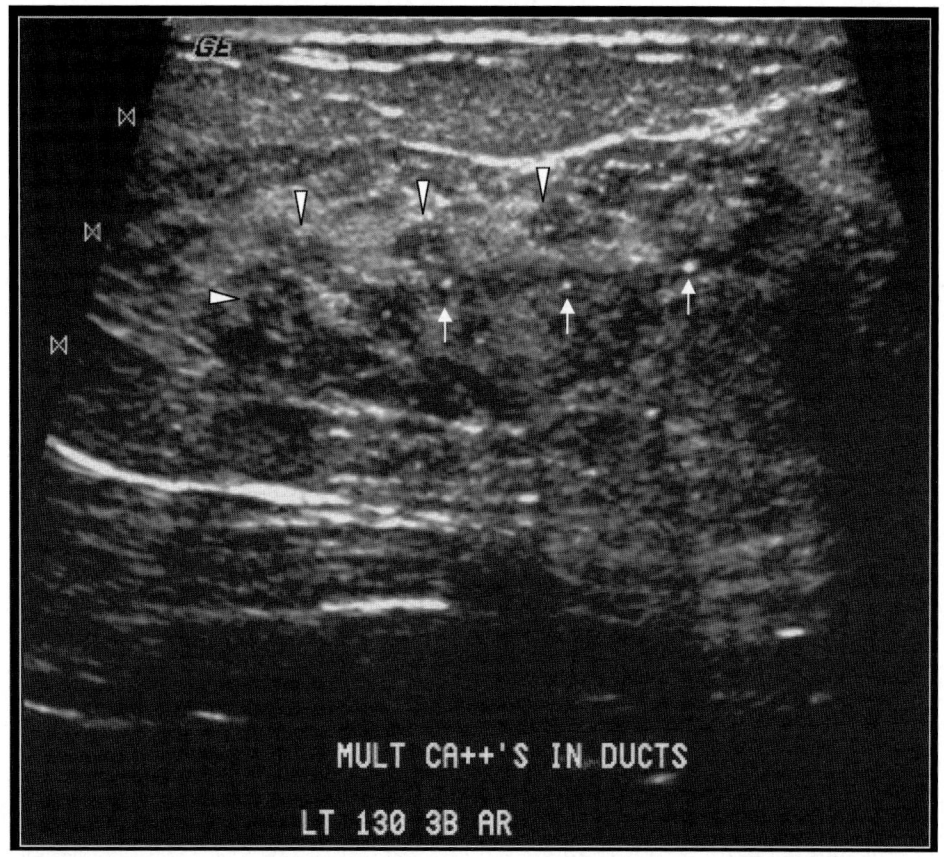

FIGURE 12–67 A: Most of the calcifications seen within malignancies lies within necrotic ductal carcinoma *in situ* (DCIS) components that distend ducts and lobules. This case of extensive high-nuclear-grade DCIS shows calcifications within enlarged ducts *(arrows)* and within cancerized lobules *(arrowheads)* that are involved with DCIS and necrosis. This patient's mammogram is shown in Fig. 12–65. *(Continued.)*

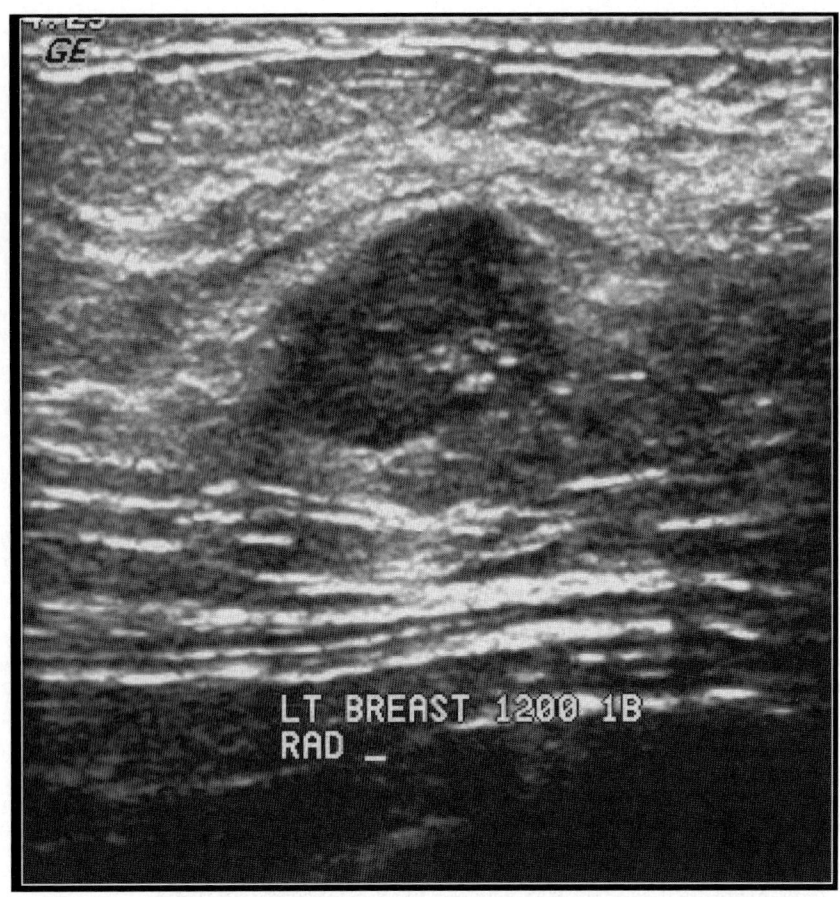

B

FIGURE 12–67 *(continued)* **B:** This solid mass in the patient with the mammogram shown in Fig. 12–65 contained invasive components of the neoplasm not shown on the mammogram that were confirmed by ultrasound-guided large core needle biopsy.

individual cyst to form a classic "tea cup" configuration of true mediolateral mammograms. Sonography, on the other hand, can show milk of calcium within a cyst that contains only a single calcification. If sonography shows a cluster of cysts, each with only one or two mobile internal calcifications, the diagnosis of fibrocystic change can be made with confidence (Fig. 12–68A, B).

The role of sonography in evaluation of calcifications has not been developed to as great a degree possible because of the misconception that sonography is not capable of showing calcifications very often. This is not at all true. Calcifications in the 500-μm size range are routinely shown by sonography, and with 1.5-D array 12-MHz transducers, calcifications in the 200 to 300 μm size range can be demonstrated. The key point that must be remembered by all who would evaluate calcifications sonographically, however, is that the value of a negative ultrasound in patients with mammographically suspicious calcifications is virtually nil. Only positive sonograms that show either solid nodules or milk of calcium are of value. Biopsy of isolated calcifications has the lowest yield of all indications for biopsy. Despite the limitations of sonography in evaluation of calcifications, we have found that sonography shows either solid nodules or milk of calcium often enough that it has the potential to improve the positive biopsy yield in patients with calcifica-

tions and to decrease the underdiagnosis of invasion without missing the diagnosis of malignancy. A prospective study of the role of sonography in management of mammographically suspicious calcifications would be warranted.

Table 12–17 shows the sensitivities and positive predictive values of sonographically detected calcifications within solid nodules. Note that since the 1995 study, the sensitivity of sonography for calcifications has increased from 27% to 40%. Mammography detects calcifications in about 50% of all malignancies and in a greater percentage of pure DCIS lesions. Thus, the sensitivity of ultrasound has increased from about one-half as sensitive as mammography to about 80% as sensitive (40%/50%) as mammography. Note also that the positive predictive value of sonographically demonstrable calcifications is decreasing. This is largely because better-resolution ultrasound equipment results in less volume averaging, which, in turn, reduces the dependence of demonstration of calcifications on background echogenicity. The better the resolution of the ultrasound equipment, the less propensity sonography has to show only the malignant calcifications.

The improvement in the sensitivity of sonography for calcifications is related to improvements in equipment as well as greater awareness of the potential role of sonography in evaluation of calcifications in recent years. Most of

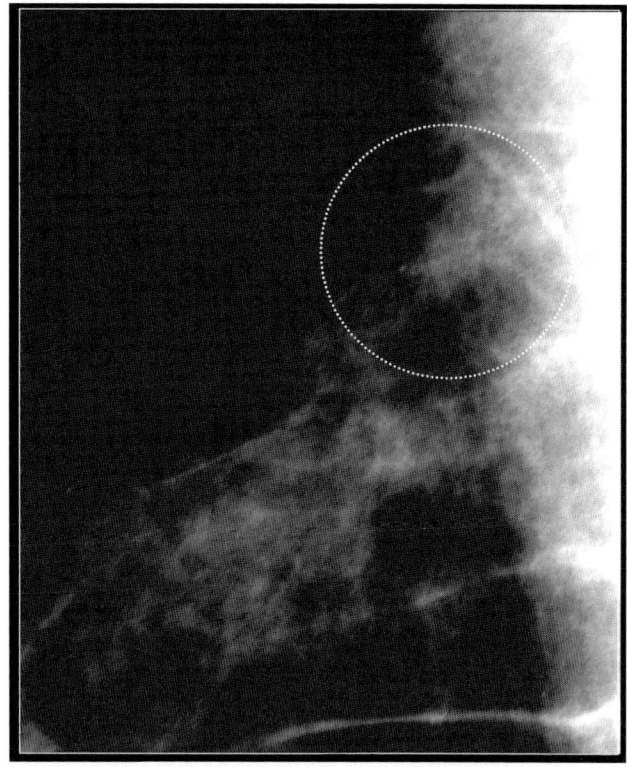

A

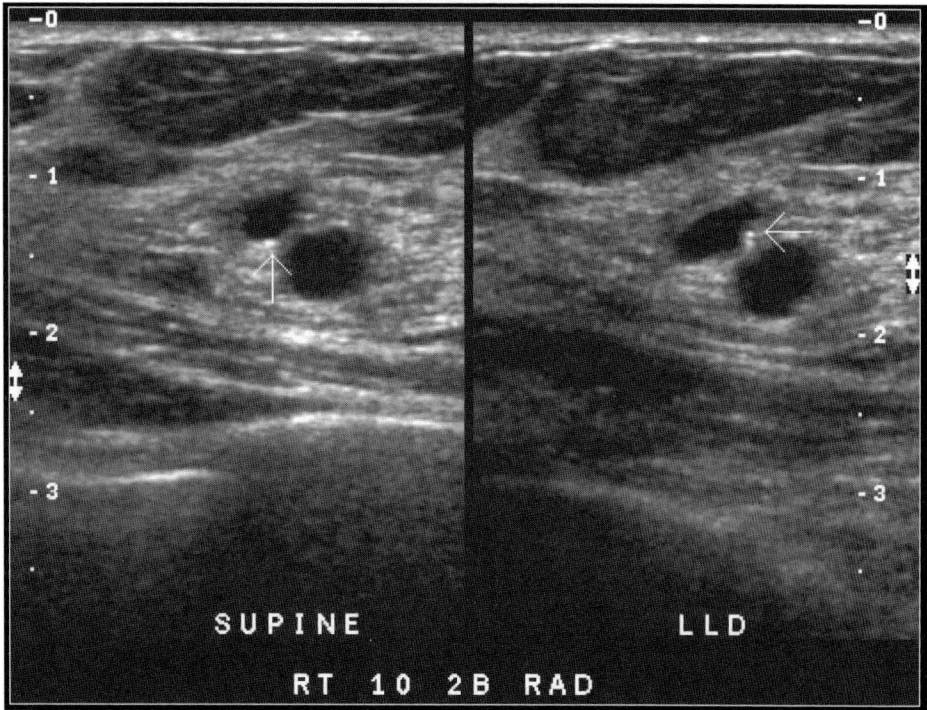

B

FIGURE 12–68 A: Although mammography is more sensitive than sonography for calcifications and can show more calcifications than sonography, sonography sometimes is more definitive than mammography. This cluster of punctate calcifications within an asymmetric density in the upper outer quadrant of the right breast is mammographically nonspecific, but suspicious enough to warrant biopsy. There is no evidence of a benign pattern, such as milk of calcium, that would allow us to avoid biopsy. **B:** Sonographic evaluation of the asymmetric density and clustered calcifications shown in this figure showed a cluster of tiny cysts, each containing only a single calcification of the milk of calcium type. Together, the individual milk of calcium calcifications created the clustered appearance seen mammographically. Mammography requires numerous calcifications within each cyst to demonstrate the classic "tea cup" configuration indicating the presence of milk of calcium. Sonography, on the other hand, can make the diagnosis of milk of calcium even with single calcifications within cysts; thus, in this case, sonography provided more specific information about the nature of the calcifications.

TABLE 12–17. SENSITIVITY AND POSITIVE PREDICTIVE VALUE (PPV) FOR CALCIFICATIONS WITHIN SOLID NODULES

	1995 Study (750 Nodules)[a]		Current Study (1,211 Nodules)[b]	
	Sensitivity	PPV Odds Ratio	Sensitivity	PPV Odds Ratio
Calcifications	27%	60% (2.9)	40%	53% (1.6)

[a]Prevalence, 16.7%.
[b]Prevalence, 32.8%.

the data in the new study was accumulated without the aid of two of the best recent developments for detecting calcifications: high-frequency coded harmonics and real-time spatial compounding. Both techniques markedly improve the ability of sonography to show calcifications and should improve the sensitivity of sonography for calcifications even more.

Hypoechogenicity

Marked hypoechogenicity is a finding unique to sonography. It is a mixed finding that can be seen in both invasive carcinomas (Fig. 12–69) and pure DCIS lesions (Fig. 12–70). It has a propensity to occur in high-grade invasive ductal carcinomas and high-nuclear-grade DCIS lesions, but some low- to intermediate-grade lesions also appear to be hypoechoic, especially lesions that cast dense acoustic

shadows (Fig. 12–71). The acoustic shadowing in such cases accentuates the apparent hypoechogenicity of the lesion. Some malignant solid nodules are so hypoechoic that they can have a pseudocystic appearance. This is most typical with high-grade DCIS, medullary carcinoma, lymphoma of the breast, and metastases to intramammary lymph nodes. Such lesions are usually markedly hypervascular, so that demonstration of internal vascularity on color Doppler can help avoid mischaracterizing such lesions as clustered cysts (Fig. 12–72).

The echogenicity of solid nodules must be compared with the echogenicity of fat, not with that of hyperechoic fibrous tissues. All lesions except isolated calcifications are hypoechoic compared with interlobular stromal fibrous tissue.

The sensitivity of hypoechogenicity has decreased over the past few years. To achieve better spatial and contrast resolution, transducer frequencies and bandwidths have been increased, and routine scanning has been performed

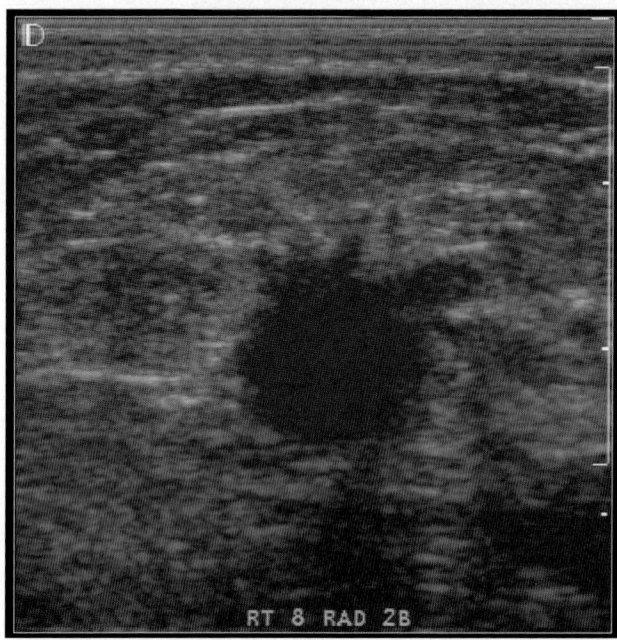

FIGURE 12–69 In most cases, such as this intermediate-grade invasive ductal carcinoma, marked hypoechogenicity indicates the presence of invasive malignancy.

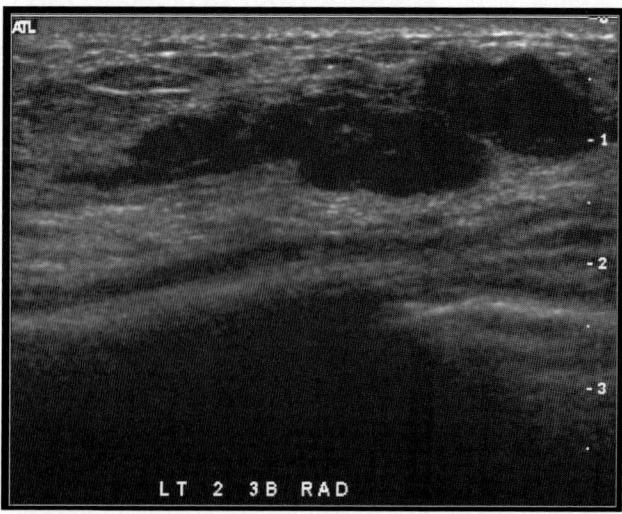

FIGURE 12–70 In some cases, such as this case, the presence of markedly hypoechogenicity indicates the presence of high-nuclear-grade ductal carcinoma *in situ* with extensive necrosis. Such lesions are usually heavily microlobulated and have demonstrable duct extensions and branch patterns.

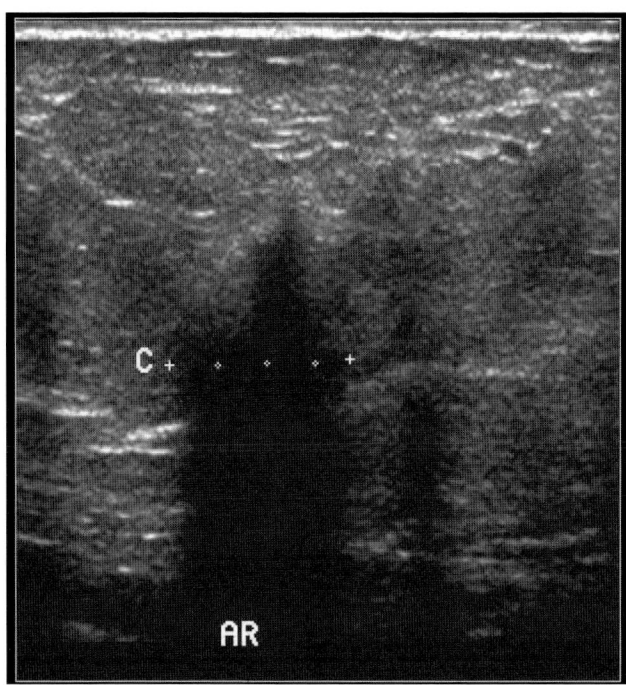

FIGURE 12–71 Some markedly hypoechoic malignant lesions, such as this lesion, are markedly hypoechoic by virtue of dense acoustic shadowing that prevents proper demonstration of the true internal echotexture. Such lesions are usually large low-grade invasive ductal, invasive lobular, or large tubular carcinomas.

at higher dynamic ranges. However, as frequency, bandwidth, and dynamic ranges have been pushed to their absolute limits, more speckle artifact and "haze" have been introduced into the image, offsetting and sometimes degrading contrast resolution. Thus, some lesions that appeared to be markedly hypoechoic on older equipment now appear only mildly hypoechoic or even isoechoic with newer equipment (Fig. 12–73). In fact, during the past 10 years, the percentage of malignant solid nodules that appear markedly hypoechoic has decreased from two-thirds to slightly less than one-half.

Two recent equipment developments that reduce speckle and other artifacts greatly have reversed the trend toward reduced sensitivity of marked hypoechogenicity: high-frequency coded harmonics and real-time compounding. Thus, lesions that appear to be isoechoic or only mildly hypoechoic with conventional imaging often appear to be much more hypoechoic when scanned with either coded harmonics or real-time compounding (Fig. 12–74).

Table 12–18 shows the sensitivity and positive predictive value of marked hypoechogenicity when sonographically evaluating solid breast nodules. Note that the sensitivity in the current ongoing study is significantly less than it was in the 1995 study. The overall accuracy in the current study is 73%.

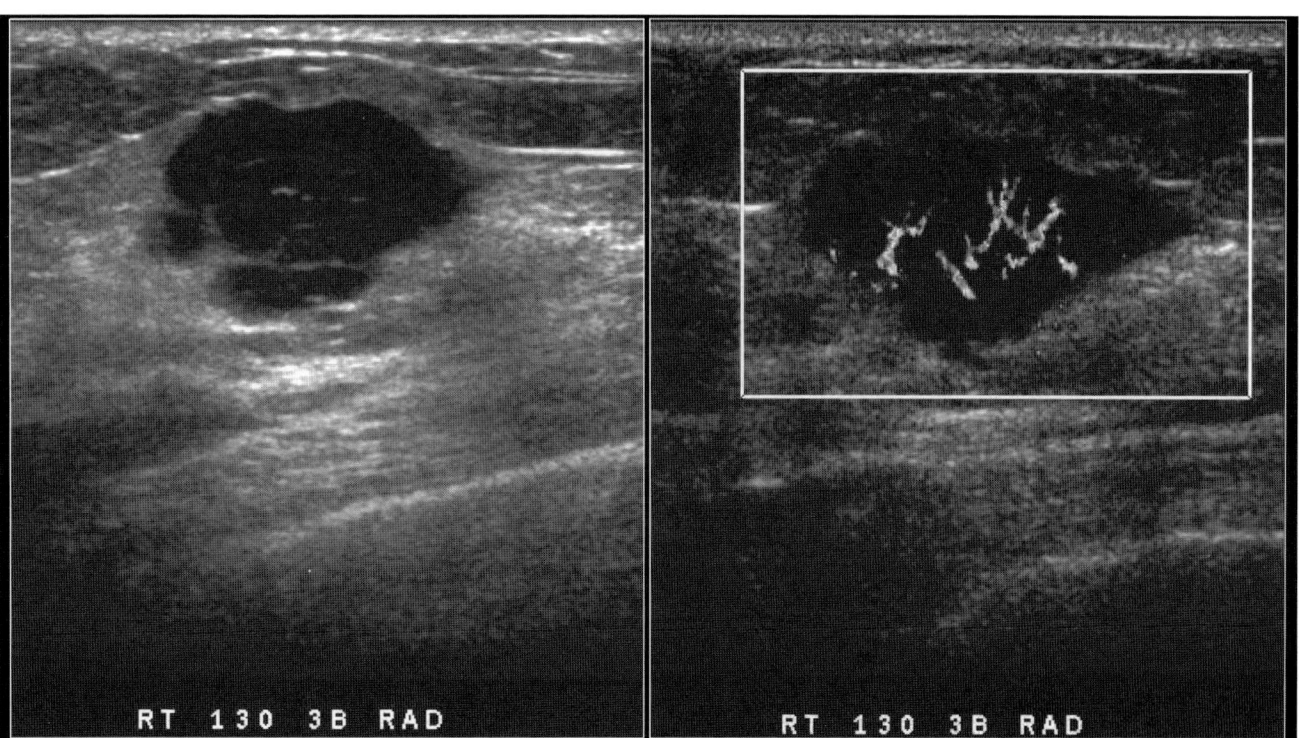

FIGURE 12–72 Certain special-type tumors, such as this medullary carcinoma, are so hypoechoic that they are nearly anechoic and have a pseudocystic appearance. Color Doppler can be helpful in avoiding misdiagnosis of such lesions as clusters of cysts. Lymphoma of the breast, metaplastic carcinoma, and some high-grade invasive ductal carcinomas may also have a pseudocystic appearance. Color Doppler shows the lesion to be markedly hypervascular internally. This helps avoid falsely characterizing the lesion as cystic and represents one of the most useful niche applications of color Doppler in evaluation of breast lesions.

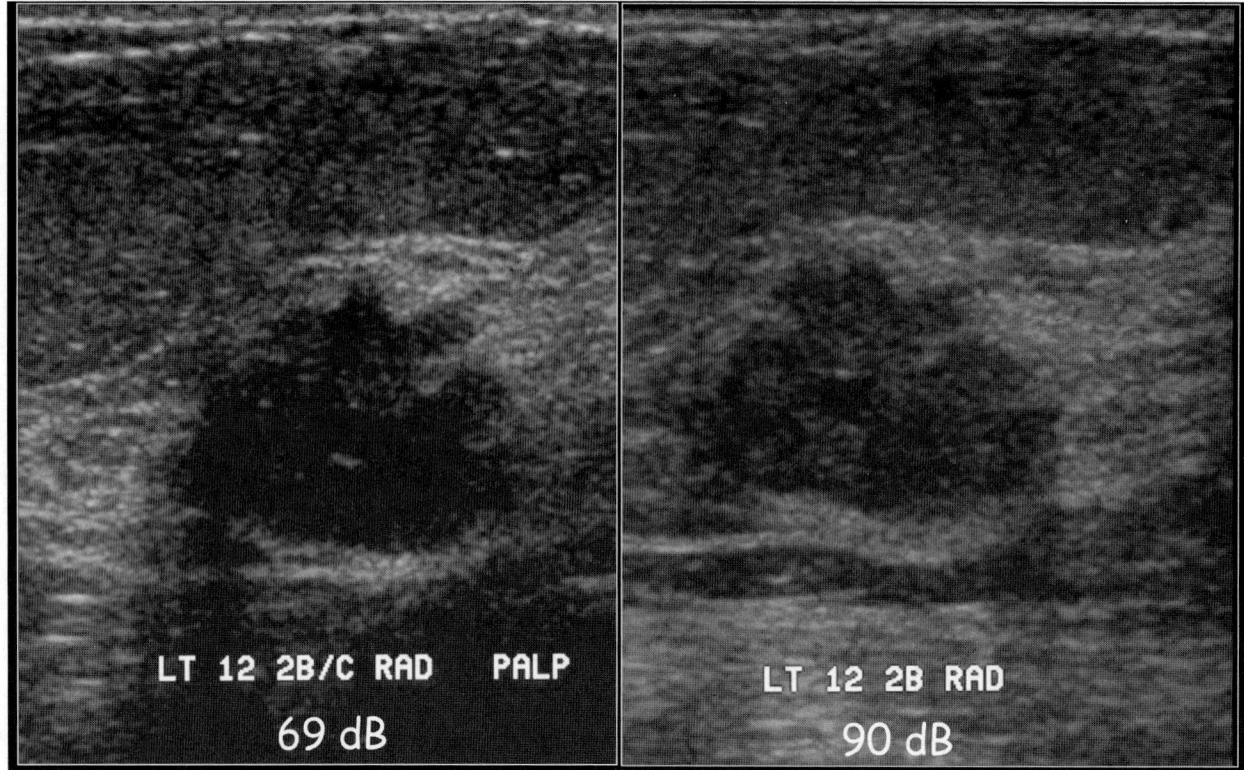

FIGURE 12–73 During the past 10 years, the portion of all malignant solid nodules that can be characterized as markedly hypoechoic has decreased from about two-thirds to one-half. This case illustrates the dependency of internal echogenicity to dynamic range. This malignant intermediate-grade invasive ductal carcinoma appears to be hypoechoic to fat when scanned with a dynamic range of 69 dB, but appears isoechoic with fat when scanned with the same transducer at a dynamic range of 90 dB.

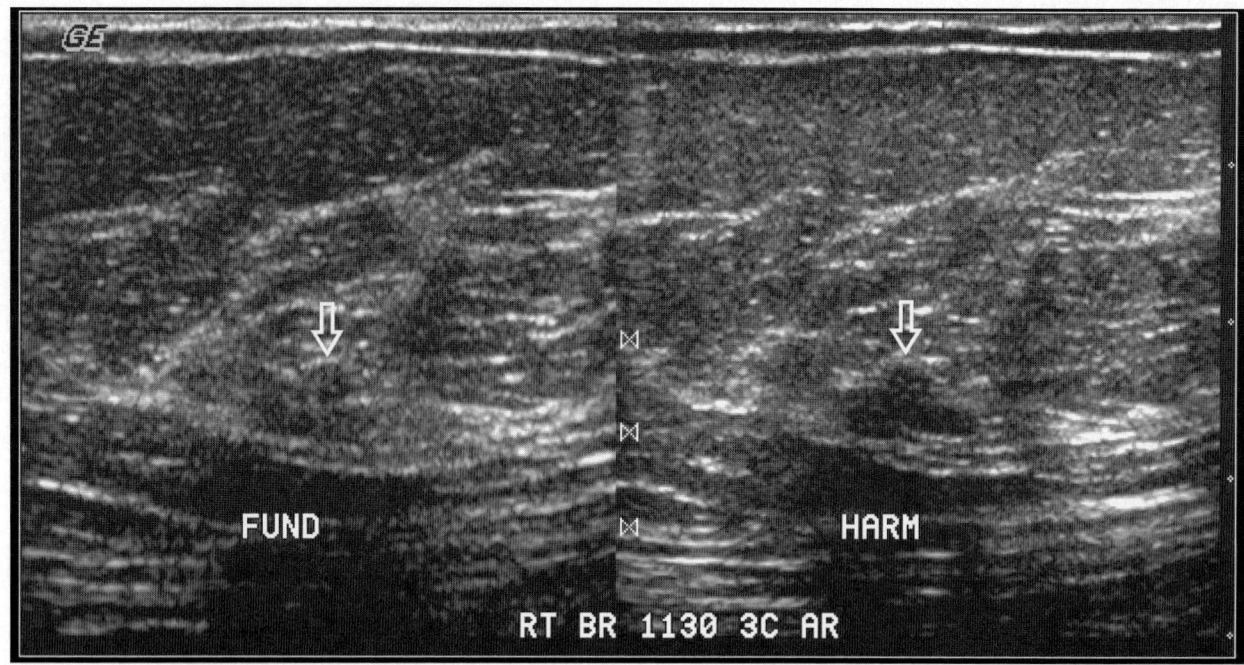

FIGURE 12–74 Coded harmonics is restoring the usefulness of hypoechogenicity as a suspicious sonographic finding. This nodule appears isoechoic and is barely visible when scanned with fundamental imaging (**left**, *arrow*). However, when the same nodule is evaluated with coded harmonics, it now appears hypoechoic with respect to surrounding fat and is readily identified (**right**, *arrow*). The transducer was not moved between the **left** and **right** images, and all scan parameters except coded harmonics were identical.

TABLE 12–18. SENSITIVITY AND POSITIVE PREDICTIVE VALUE (PPV) FOR MARKED HYPOECHOGENICITY ON SONOGRAPHIC EVALUATION OF SOLID NODULES

	1995 Study (750 Nodules)[a]		Current Study (1,211 Nodules)[b]	
	Sensitivity	PPV Odds Ratio	Sensitivity	PPV Odds Ratio
Hypoechogenicity	69%	60% (3.6)	49%	64% (1.9)

[a]Prevalence, 16.7%.
[b]Prevalence, 32.8%.

Summary of Sonographic Findings Suspicious for Malignancy

The sensitivities of the individual sonographic findings in the 1995 study and the current study are shown in Table 12–19. Note that none of the individual findings achieves the stated goal of 98% or greater sensitivity because breast cancer is too heterogeneous to be diagnosed by a single finding with high sensitivity. However, we did achieve our goal of 98% or greater sensitivity in both the 1995 study and the current study by using all of the findings in a strict algorithmic approach. The sensitivity of combined findings was 98.4% in the 1995 study and is 99.6% in the current ongoing study. The algorithm works, despite the lower sensitivities of individual findings, because the average malignant nodule has five or six positive findings. Thus, even if several of the suspicious findings are missed, it is likely that one or two of the findings will be detected, preventing the lesion from being mischaracterized as BIRADS 3.

Note that the sensitivities of most of the findings have increased since the 1995 study. The addition of thick, echogenic halo as a variant of spiculation has especially increased the sensitivity of spiculation. The routine evaluation of nipple discharge with sonography has led to the marked increase in the sensitivity of duct extension. Advances in imaging technology and increased awareness have led to other improvements. Of the findings, only acoustic shadowing and hypoechogenicity have decreased in sensitivity. Coded harmonics and real-time compounding are likely to increase the sensitivity of hypoechogenicity in the future.

Table 12–20 shows the positive predictive values and odds ratios of the individual suspicious sonographic findings. Note that all are good positive predictors of malignancy. The odds ratios are lower in the current study

TABLE 12–19. SUMMARY OF SENSITIVITIES OF INDIVIDUAL AND COMBINED FINDINGS

Sonographic Findings	1995 Study (750 Nodules)[a]	Current Study (1,211 Nodules)[b]
Microlobulations	75%	92%
Angular margins	83%	90%
Marked hypoechogenicity	69%	49%
Duct extension	25%	49%
Taller than wide	42%	48%
Branch pattern	30%	44%
Calcifications	25%	40%
Spiculations	36%	36%
Thick, echogenic halo	—	35%
Spiculations or thick halo	—	71%
Acoustic shadowing	49%	35%
Combined sensitivity	98.4%	99.6%

[a]Prevalence, 16.7%.
[b]Prevalence, 32.8%.

TABLE 12–20. SUMMARY OF POSITIVE PREDICTIVE VALUES AND ODDS RATIOS OF INDIVIDUAL FINDINGS

Sonographic Findings	1995 Study (750 Nodules)[a]	Current Study (1,211 Nodules)[b]
Microlobulations	48% (2.9)	50% (1.5)
Angular margins	68% (4.0)	59% (1.8)
Marked hypoechogenicity	60% (3.6)	64% (1.9)
Duct extension	51% (3.0)	46% (1.4)
Taller than wide	81% (4.9)	74% (2.5)
Branch pattern	64% (3.8)	60% (1.8)
Calcifications	60% (3.6)	53% (1.6)
Spiculations	92% (5.5)	87% (2.7)
Thick, echogenic halo	—	74% (1.9)
Spiculations or thick halo	—	80% (2.4)
Acoustic shadowing	65% (3.9)	62% (1.9)

[a]Prevalence, 16.7%.
[b]Prevalence, 32.8%.

because the prevalence of malignancy in nodules that undergo biopsy is higher. The reason for this is that most BIRADS 3 nodules now undergo short-interval follow-up rather than biopsy. In the 1995 study, all BIRADS 3 nodules underwent biopsy.

Sonographic Findings with Poor Predictive Values for Malignancy

Several sonographic features were not particularly helpful as findings that are suspicious for malignancy. First, maximum diameter was not helpful. Figure 12–75 shows the percentage of each 5-mm size range that is malignant. It is true that the larger the maximum diameter, the greater the risk that it is malignant, but there is no point at which the risk for malignancy is so high that a solid nodule must be considered suspicious based solely on diameter. Additionally, the presence of suspicious features is related to and dependent on the size of the lesion. The larger the lesion, the more likely it is to have one or more suspicious sonographic features and therefore to be excluded from characterization as BIRADS 3.

There is no diameter above which a solid nodule cannot be characterized as BIRADS 3 category as long as it has no suspicious features and also meets criteria for one of the benign findings discussed later. Of 37 nodules larger than 20 mm and 44 nodules between 16 and 20 mm in maximum diameter that were characterized as BIRADS 3 in the current study, none were malignant. The risk for a false-negative diagnosis is actually greater for very small lesions than for large lesions—the group in which the risk for malignancy is the lowest. Between the current study and the 1995 study, only 3 of 672 solid nodules that were characterized as BIRADS 3 were malignant. All three were less than 10 mm in maximum diameter. The only false-negative lesion characterized as BIRADS 3 in the current study was 3 mm in maximum diameter.

If 20 mm is used as a cutoff point, with lesions 20 mm or larger being considered suspicious for malignancy, the sensitivity is 22%, the positive predictive value only 44%, and the odds ratio only 1.3. Odds ratios that are near 1.0 are not very predictive. If 16 mm were used as the cutoff point, the sensitivity would improve to 40%, but the positive predictive value would decrease to 40%, and the odds ratio would decrease to 1.2.

Heterogeneous texture is worthy of comment. A review of the literature on sonographic evaluation of solid breast nodules would show that heterogeneous internal

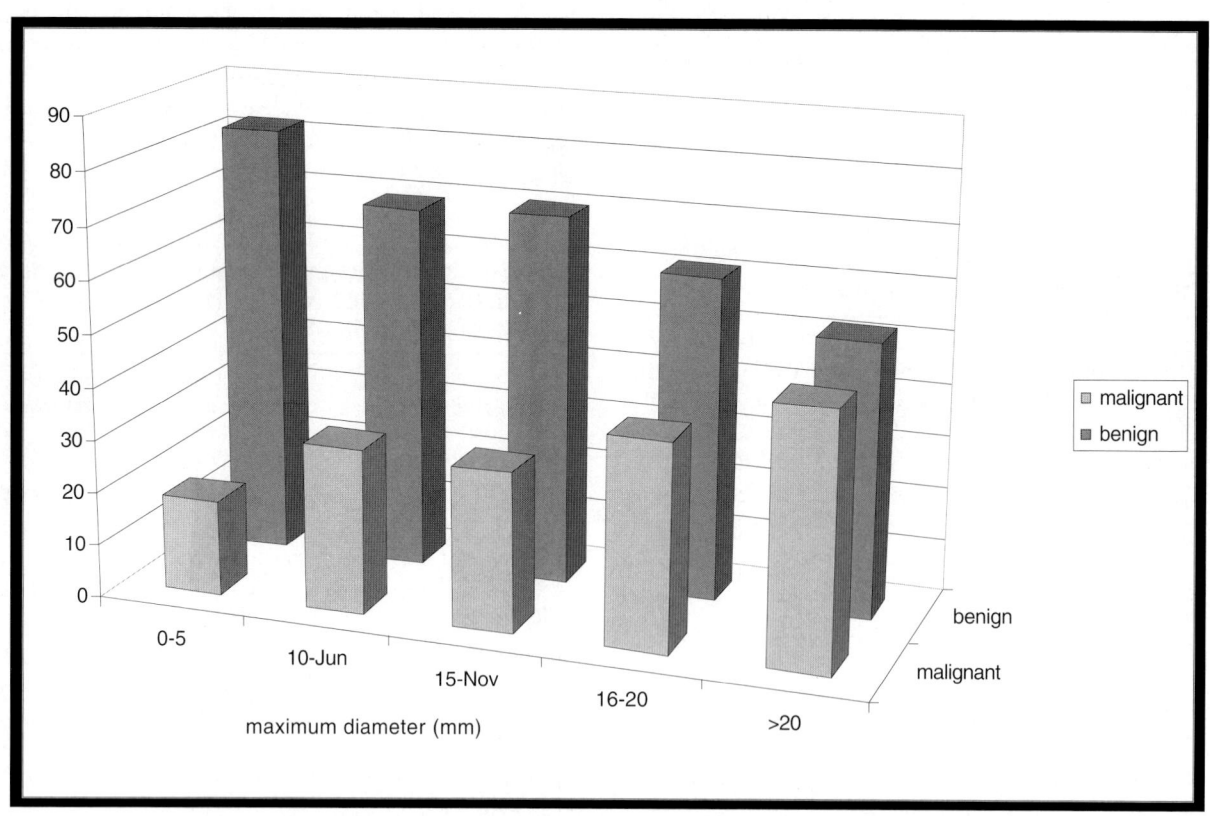

FIGURE 12–75 Although larger lesions have more risk of being malignant, there is no clear-cut diameter above which a lesion cannot be characterized as BIRADS 3. In addition, as lesions become larger, they tend to develop suspicious findings that exclude them from BIRADS 3 characterization. The malignant lesions that were falsely characterized as BIRADS 3 over the past decade were all small lesions with maximum diameters less than 10 mm rather than large lesions.

echotexture is the second most common feature of malignant nodules, trailing only angular (jagged or irregular) margins. However, in our 1995 study, we found that heterogeneous texture was present in about 20% of both benign and malignant nodules and that the odds ratio was only 1.2 for malignancy. The odds ratio of 1.2 was so close to 1.0 that heterogeneous texture was of no predictive value in characterizing solid nodules. The discrepancy between our findings and the literature can be explained by our use of calcifications as a separate finding. We believe that calcifications are the primary cause of heterogeneous texture. By creating a separate finding of calcifications, we nullified the value of heterogeneous texture. If the category of calcifications is removed and all malignant solid nodules that contain calcifications are reclassified as heterogeneous, the positive predictive value of heterogeneous texture improves to 45%, and the odds ratio increases to 2.7, restoring its value.

As noted earlier, although acoustic shadowing remains a suspicious finding for malignancy, one should not be reassured by normal or enhanced through-transmission. The rationale for this is discussed in the previous section on evaluation of sound transmission through solid nodules.

Although marked hypoechogenicity is a suspicious finding for malignancy, one should not be reassured by isoechogenicity or mild hypoechogenicity. Although 49% of malignant nodules are markedly hypoechoic with respect to fat, 51% of all malignant nodules are either isoechoic or only minimally hypoechoic.

Is the Sensitivity of 98% or Better for Malignancy Simply because the Malignant Nodules Were All Large End-stage Lesions with Poor Prognosis?

The excellent sensitivity of sonography for detecting malignant breast nodules would be of little use if all of the malignant lesions detected were so large that the patient's ultimate prognosis would be unaffected by correct sonographic characterization. Thus, it is valuable to look at two diagnostic parameters that can be gleaned from the surgical pathology: the maximum diameter of the lesion and the lymph node status in patients who underwent axillary dissection or sentinel node procedures.

The two-county data of Tabar and colleagues (1993) from Sweden show that for diameters of 15 mm or less, the 10-year survival rate is 90%, regardless of the tumor grade. Additionally, for low- and intermediate-grade lesions, the 15-year survival rate is 90%. To prove that correct characterization of malignant lesions is not simply a factor of large size and end-stage lesions, we would like to see most malignant nodules in our series have maximum diameters of 15 mm or less. In the 1995 study, 68% of nodules were 15 mm or smaller in maximum diameter. In the current study, 70% of the malignant nodules had maximum diameters of 15 mm or less. Thus, in both the 1995 study and the current study, the excellent sensitivity achieved was not simply a factor of large size and late stage, and more than two-thirds of the patients with malignant nodules were potential long-term survivors.

The two-county data from Sweden of Tabar and colleagues (1993) showed prognosis for long-term survival in patients with tumor-negative axillary lymph nodes similar to that for lesions with maximum diameters of less than 15 mm. In fact, survival is almost as good for patients with only one or two positive lymph nodes as it is when nodes are negative. In the 1995 study, 67% of patients who underwent axillary dissection had negative nodes, 6% had a single positive node, and 2% had two positive lymph nodes. Seventy-five percent had either negative nodes or one or two positive lymph nodes. In the current study, some patients underwent sentinel node procedure instead of full axillary dissection. In many, if the sentinel lymph nodes were negative, full axillary dissection was deferred. However, if any sentinel lymph node was positive, a full axillary dissection was performed. In the current study of patients who underwent either axillary dissection or sentinel node procedure, 73% had negative lymph nodes, 12% had a single positive lymph node, and 6% had two positive lymph nodes. Ninety-one percent of patients had either negative axillary lymph nodes or one or two positive lymph nodes. Therefore, based on lymph node status and analogous to the case for maximum diameter, the excellent sensitivity achieved in these two studies was not simply a factor of advanced stage. Based on lymph node status, more than 90% of these patients had negative or one or two positive lymph nodes and, thus, were potential long-term survivors.

Benign and Probably Benign Findings

Only if no findings suspicious for malignancy are found can benign findings be sought. The following sections cover the benign findings, their histologic and morphologic basis, and techniques necessary to identify the benign findings and avoid false-negative diagnosis. Tables 12–5 and 12–6 list the individual and combined benign findings. The individual benign findings are purely and markedly hyperechoic tissue, elliptical and wider-than-tall shape, gently lobulated and wider-than-tall shape, and finally, a thin, echogenic capsule that completely encompasses the nodule. Combining the elliptical or gently lobulated shapes with the presence of a complete thin, echogenic capsule is necessary because many circumscribed invasive carcinomas and most pure DCIS nodules are encompassed in a thin, echogenic capsule. However, the shape of circumscribed invasive carcinoma or pure DCIS is rarely elliptical or gently lobulated.

Hyperechogenicity

Well-circumscribed nodules that are intensely and uniformly hyperechoic are composed entirely of normal interlobular stromal fibrous tissue and are definitively benign. Such hyperechoic lesions are water density and therefore can cause mammographic masses or asymmetric densities, and because such lesions are quite firm to palpation, they can cause palpable abnormalities (Fig. 12–76).

Most women (even after menopause) have at least some hyperechoic stromal fibrous tissue within their breasts, and for this reason, its presence should not be assumed to be the cause of the mammographic or palpable abnormality. Mammographic–sonographic or clinical–sonographic correlation definitively proves it to be the cause.

For hyperechoic tissue to have 100% negative predictive value, it must be purely and intensely hyperechoic, as hyperechoic as normal interlobular stromal fibrous tissue. It must contain no isoechoic or hypoechoic tissue larger than normal ducts and lobules (Fig. 12–77). Although most isoechoic tissue larger than normal lobules merely represents TDLUs that are enlarged by benign fibrocystic change or benign proliferative disorders, certain isoechoic malignant lesions may present as enlarged lobules or isoechoic glandular tissue. Sonography can identify isoechoic lobular enlargement but cannot determine the histologic entity causing lobular enlargement. The significance of lobular prominence must be viewed in the context of the

sonographic appearances of the surrounding lobules. In general, focally enlarged TDLUs are of greater concern than generalized enlargement of TDLUs. The important thing to remember, however, is that purely hyperechoic tissue is normal tissue with virtual 100% certainty. We have never seen a purely hyperechoic carcinoma of the breast. Any hyperechoic tissue that contains isoechoic areas larger than normal ducts or lobules, however, should be viewed with more caution because the isoechoic area could contain an occult isoechoic carcinoma (Fig. 12–78). However, this does not mean that the negative predictive value of mixed hyperechoic and isoechoic tissue is poor, merely that it is not the 100% that it is for pure hyperechoic fibrous tissue. In fact, the situation is quite analogous to breast density that is routinely included in mammography reports. The sensitivity of mammography decreases as the percentage of dense tissue within the breast increases. Similarly, the negative predictive value of sonographically demonstrated normal breast tissues decreases as the relative amount of isoechoic tissue increases. It is critical to understand that the negative predictive value of any type of normal tissue is very high. It is simply slightly less than 100% when the normal tissue contains isoechoic elements that are larger than normal ducts or lobules.

We believe that power Doppler vocal fremitus can be a helpful ancillary test to help distinguish normal isoechoic glandular elements from occult isoechoic malignant nodules. Isoechoic glandular tissue tends to vibrate similarly to

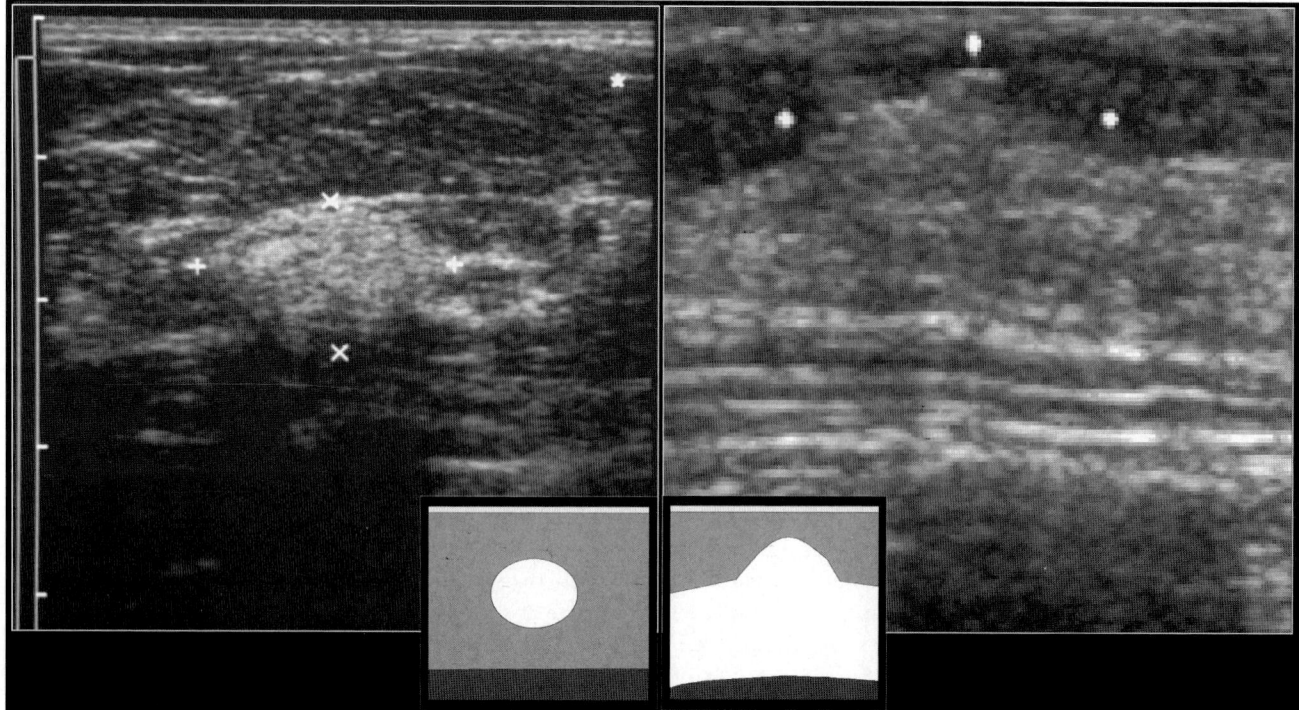

FIGURE 12–76 Purely and intensely hyperechoic breast tissues represent interlobular stromal fibrous tissue, whether it causes palpable ridges (**right**) or mammographic masses (**left**).

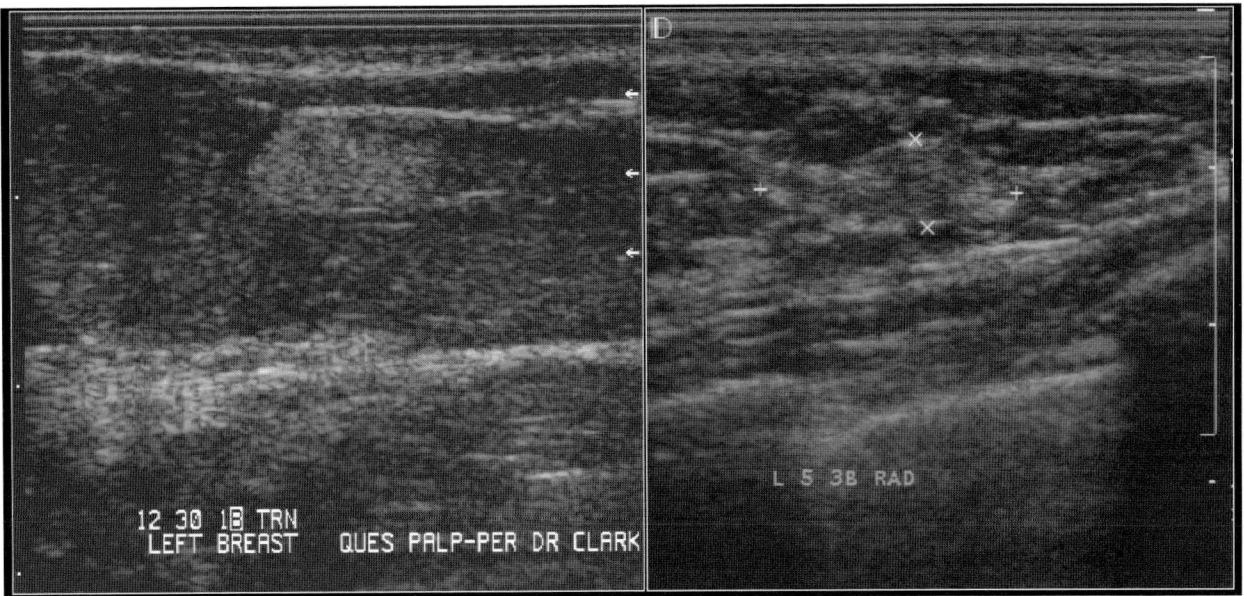

FIGURE 12-77 To be considered benign fibrous tissue with virtually 100% certainty, there should be no areas of isoechoic or hyperechoic tissue larger than normal ducts or lobules. The cause of the palpable lump or mammographic density must be purely hyperechoic. The nodule on the **left** is purely hyperechoic and therefore benign with virtually 100% certainty. The lesion on the **right**, however, includes isoechoic elements larger than normal ducts or lobules. Although such tissue is likely glandular, there is a chance that the isoechoic elements represent either isoechoic invasive malignancy or ductal carcinoma *in situ* (DCIS). Remember that one-half of all invasive malignancies are isoechoic or only mildly hypoechoic with respect to fat and that a large percentage of DCIS lesions that are sonographically visible are nearly isoechoic with fat. The risk for malignancy in the lesion on the **right** is not high (probably about 5%) but is higher than the 2% or less required for the finding to be considered probably benign (BIRAD 3).

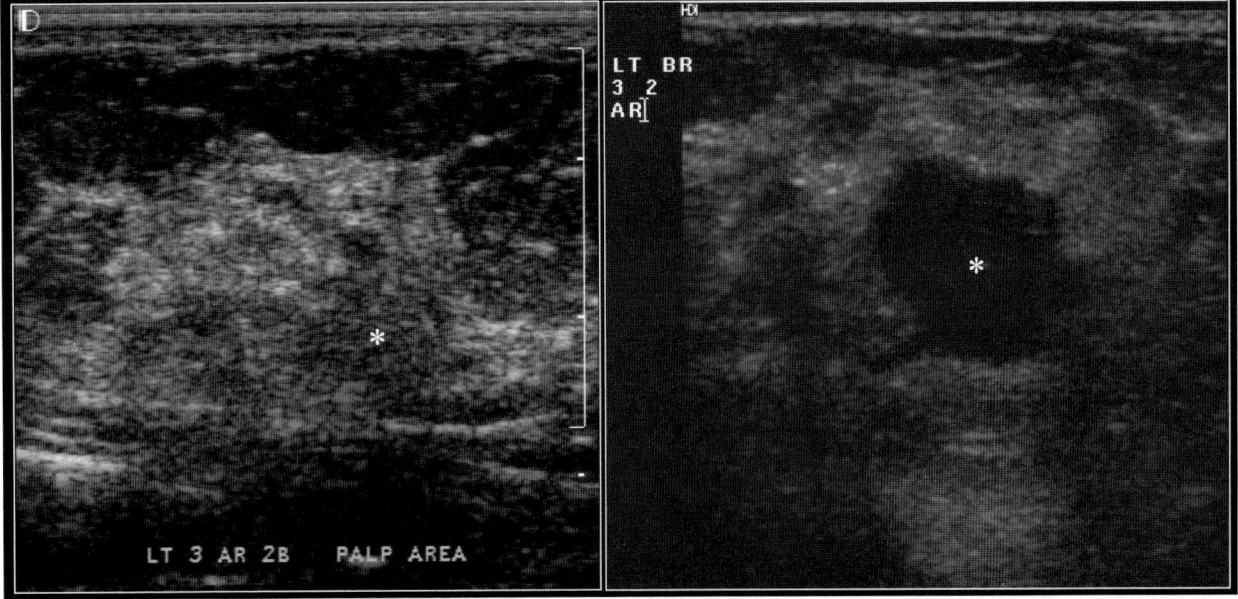

FIGURE 12-78 This case illustrates why one should not necessarily be reassured by the presence of isoechoic tissue within the tissue responsible for a palpable or mammographic abnormality. The **left** image shows the cause of a palpable abnormality to be a ridge of mixed hyperechoic and isoechoic fibroglandular tissues. A discrete nodule could not be identified. The patient was advised to return for sonographic follow-up in 6 months, but also to examine herself monthly and return earlier if there was any change in the lump. The patient detected change in the lump at 4 months and returned for follow-up sonography early. The 4-month follow-up sonogram (**right**) shows a markedly hypoechoic mass (*) that had arisen from the isoechoic tissue (*) noted on the first exam. The presence of isoechoic tissue, larger than normal ducts, or terminal ductolobular units is usually caused by fibrocystic or benign proliferative changes, but can represent malignant neoplasm in a small minority of cases.

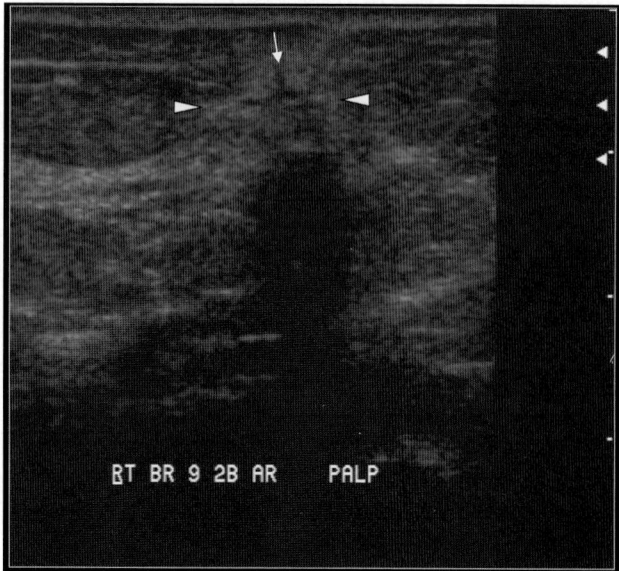

FIGURE 12–79 We have not seen a purely hyperechoic malignant neoplasm, but we have seen several malignant nodules that have a very small hypoechoic angular central nidus *(arrowheads and arrows)* surrounded by a very thick echogenic halo. Technical errors could obscure the small "dark star" that represents the central tumor nidus and falsely make the lesion appear to be purely hyperechoic.

surrounded hyperechoic fibrous tissue, creating a fairly uniform color artifact (see Chapter 20, Fig. 20–86A, B). Isoechoic neoplasms, on the other hand, tend to vibrate less, creating a defect in the color artifact induced by vibration (see Chapter 20, Fig. 20–87A, B). Thus, when a mammographic abnormality appears to be caused by fibroglandular or glandular tissues, but vocal fremitus is normal, the negative predictive value of ultrasound is increased from the 96% to 98% range to near 100%. However, when there is a fremitus defect within the isoechoic tissue, the risk for an occult isoechoic malignant nodule increases greatly. A complete discussion of power Doppler vocal fremitus is beyond the scope of this chapter, but it is presented in detail in Chapter 20.

We have never seen a purely hyperechoic malignant solid nodule and do not believe that they exist. However, certain malignant nodules may have a very tiny and subtle hypoechoic central nidus and a very thick, echogenic halo. In rare cases, the thickness of the echogenic halo may be much greater than the diameter of the central hypoechoic nidus (Fig. 12–79). There are two technical errors that the sonographer or sonologist can make that could obscure the tiny hypoechoic central nidus and falsely make the lesion appear purely hyperechoic.

The first technical error is caused by near-field volume averaging that can occur within lesions that lie within 1 cm

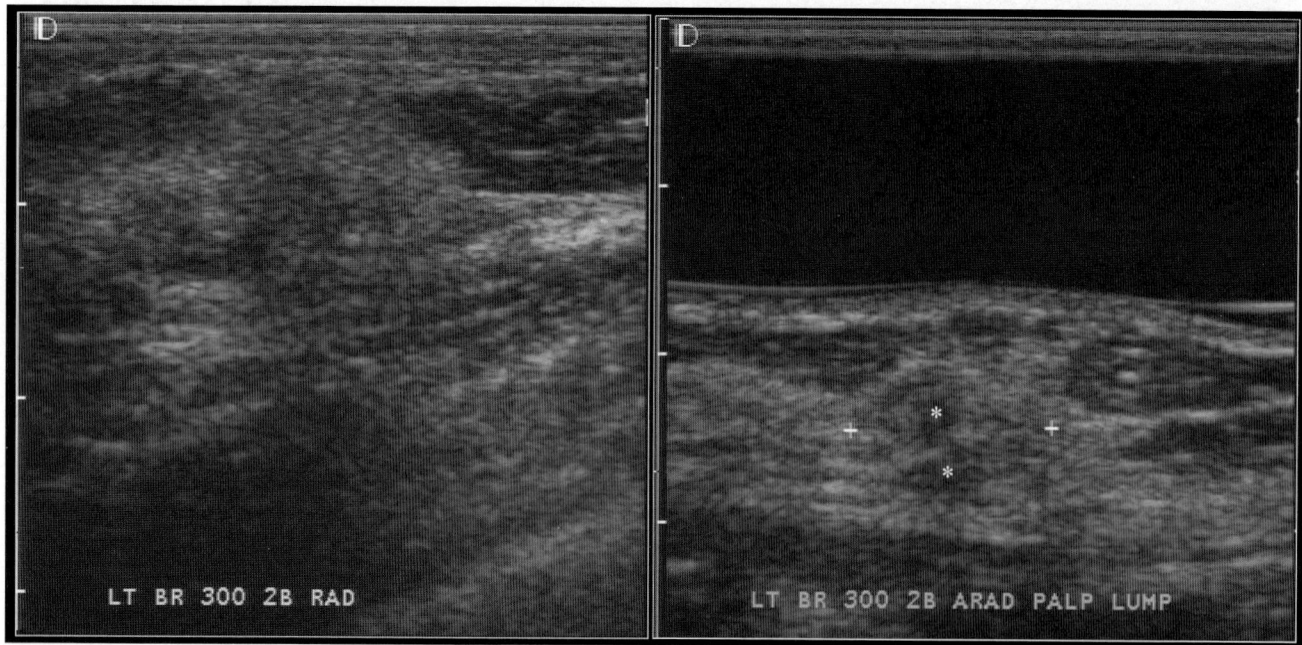

FIGURE 12–80 Near-field volume averaging can obscure a small, hypoechoic central nidus. The **left** image shows the sonogram of a pea-sized palpable lump that appears to be purely hyperechoic that was obtained without an acoustic standoff. Note that the lesion is within a centimeter of the skin, the zone where near-field volume averaging can be a problem. The **right** image was obtained with an 8-mm acoustic standoff pad and shows that what appeared to be purely hyperechoic when scanned without a standoff actually contains two hypoechoic central nidi *(*)* that represent two foci of invasive carcinoma.

of the skin. With conventional high-frequency near-field imaging transducers, the short-axis focal zone, in which the beam is only 1 to 1.5 mm wide, is located at 1.5 to 2.0 cm of depth. However, near the skin, the beam is as wide as the short axis of the transducer. The beam tapers from the width of the transducer face to 1 mm at 1.5 cm. Thus, at a depth of 5 or 6 mm, the beam may still be 4 or 5 mm wide. The small central nidus of a small and very superficially located malignant nodule with a thick, echogenic halo can be narrower than the width of the ultrasound beam and may thus be subject to volume averaging with the much more extensive surrounding hyperechoic halo. This will obscure the central nidus, making the whole lesion falsely appear hyperechoic. Volume-averaging error can and should be avoided by use of 1.5-D array transducers (an expensive solution) or an acoustic standoff (inexpensive solution) for any lesion that lies within 1 cm of the skin (Fig. 12–80).

The second technical error that can be made is to image tangentially the thick, echogenic halo and to mistakenly not identify the hypoechoic central nidus (Fig. 12–81). This mistake can be avoided by remembering that breast cancer can be heterogeneous not only from nodule to nodule, but also within individual nodules. Thus, no examination is complete without scanning the entire surface area and volume of the nodule in two orthogonal planes. Obviously, if some portion of the nodule contains hypoechoic or isoechoic tissue, the nodule cannot be considered purely hyperechoic, and the negative predictive value will be less than 100%. Careful correlation of mammographic and sonographic diameters can also help avoid this mistake for mammographically visible lesions. Tangential images obtained through the thick halo at the edges of the lesion will usually have a maximum diameter that differs from the mammographic maximum diameter by more than 10%, whereas the sonographic diameter through the portion of the lesion that contains the central nidus will be within 10% of the mammographic diameter.

The negative predictive value of pure hyperechoic fibrous tissue is 100% in both the 1995 study and in the current ongoing study. However, the prevalence of purely hyperechoic lesions within the population of nodules undergoing biopsy has dropped dramatically as referring physicians, who previously demanded biopsy proof, have now accepted purely hyperechoic tissue as normal fibrous tissue. Table 12–21 shows the negative predictive values, the odds ratios. It also shows the number of hyperechoic nodules that underwent biopsy and the prevalence of hyperechoic nodules among benign nodules that underwent biopsy.

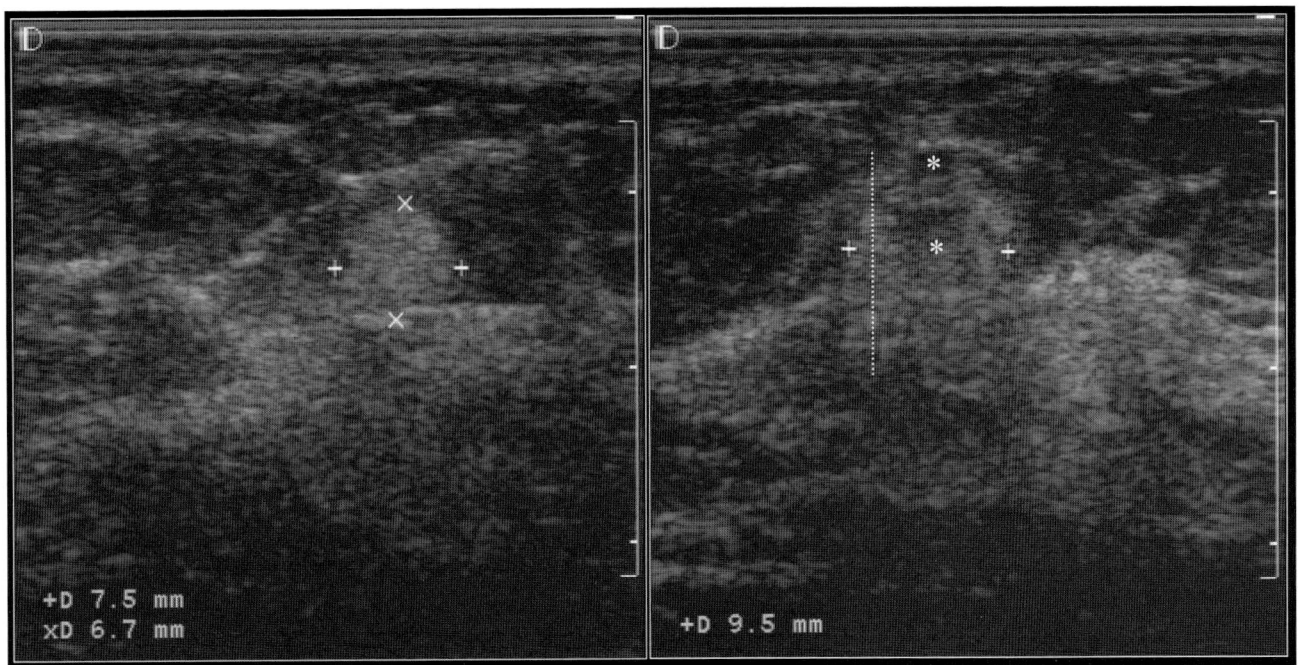

FIGURE 12–81 Tangential images obtained through the edges of a thick, echogenic halo can falsely give the impression that a malignant nodule is purely hyperechoic. The **left** image shows a 7.5-mm solid nodule that appears to be purely hyperechoic and that was thought by the sonographer to be the cause of a 13-mm mammographic nodule. However, the discrepancy in size between the sonographic structure and the mammographic structure was more than expected by measurement error alone. The **right** image shows that the lesion actually contains two angular isoechoic central nidi (*). The sonographer had falsely made the lesion appear to be purely hyperechoic by obtaining a tangential image through the thick, echogenic halo (*dotted white line*).

TABLE 12–21. NEGATIVE PREDICATIVE VALUE (NPV) AND PREVALENCE AMONG BENIGN NODULES OF PURE HYPERECHOGENICITY ON SONOGRAPHIC EVALUATION OF SOLID NODULES

	1995 Study (750 Nodules)[a]		Current Study (1,211 Nodules)[b]	
	No. of Cases (Prevalence)	NPV (Odds Ratio)	No. of Cases (Prevalence)	NVP (Odds Ratio)
Hypoechogenicity	42 (9.9%)	0% (0)	4 (1.6%)	100% (0)

[a]Prevalence, 16.7%.
[b]Prevalence, 32.8%.

Elliptical Shape

An elliptical and wider-than-tall shape is the classic shape of fibroadenomas (Fig. 12–82). The elliptical shape had a negative predictive value of 99% in the 1995 study, and 51% of all benign nodules that underwent biopsy were elliptical in shape. In the current ongoing study, a smaller percentage of all benign nodules were characterized as elliptical in shape (16%). However, the percentage of all BI-RADS 3 solid nodules that are elliptical in shape has actually increased to 57%. Thus, the prevalence of the elliptical shape among all benign nodules is not decreasing, but the percentage of elliptical nodules among all benign nodules that undergo biopsy is. The reason for this is simply that in the current environment, most classically benign elliptically shaped solid nodules undergo short-interval follow-up rather than biopsy. In fact, currently, only 19% of solid nodules that are characterized as BI-RADS 3 undergo biopsy. However, even a smaller percentage of elliptical nodules undergo biopsy (14%). Thus, it is the larger, more lobulated and more atypically appearing BIRADS 3 nodules that undergo biopsy. The situation was much different in the 1995 study, when the standard of care was to biopsy all solid nodules, regardless of sono-

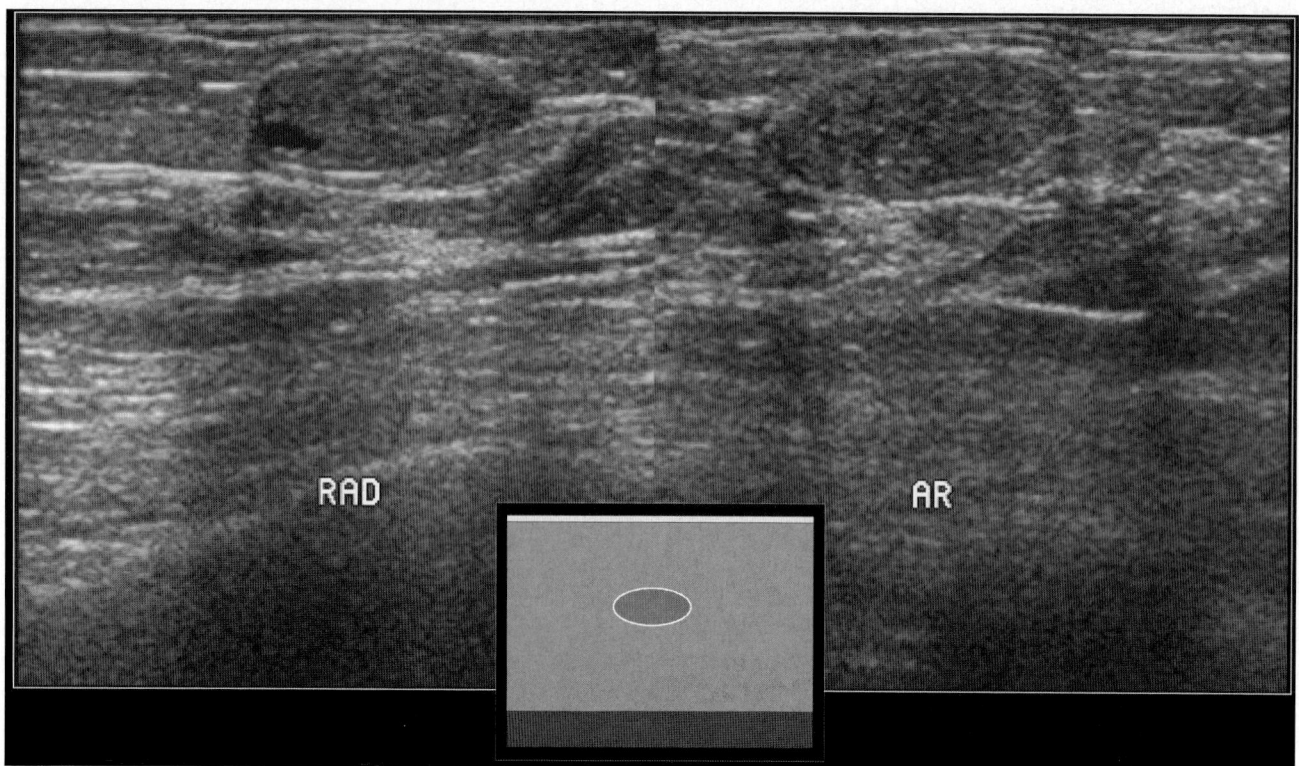

FIGURE 12–82 This benign fibroadenoma has the classically smooth, well-circumscribed, elliptical, wider-than-tall configuration.

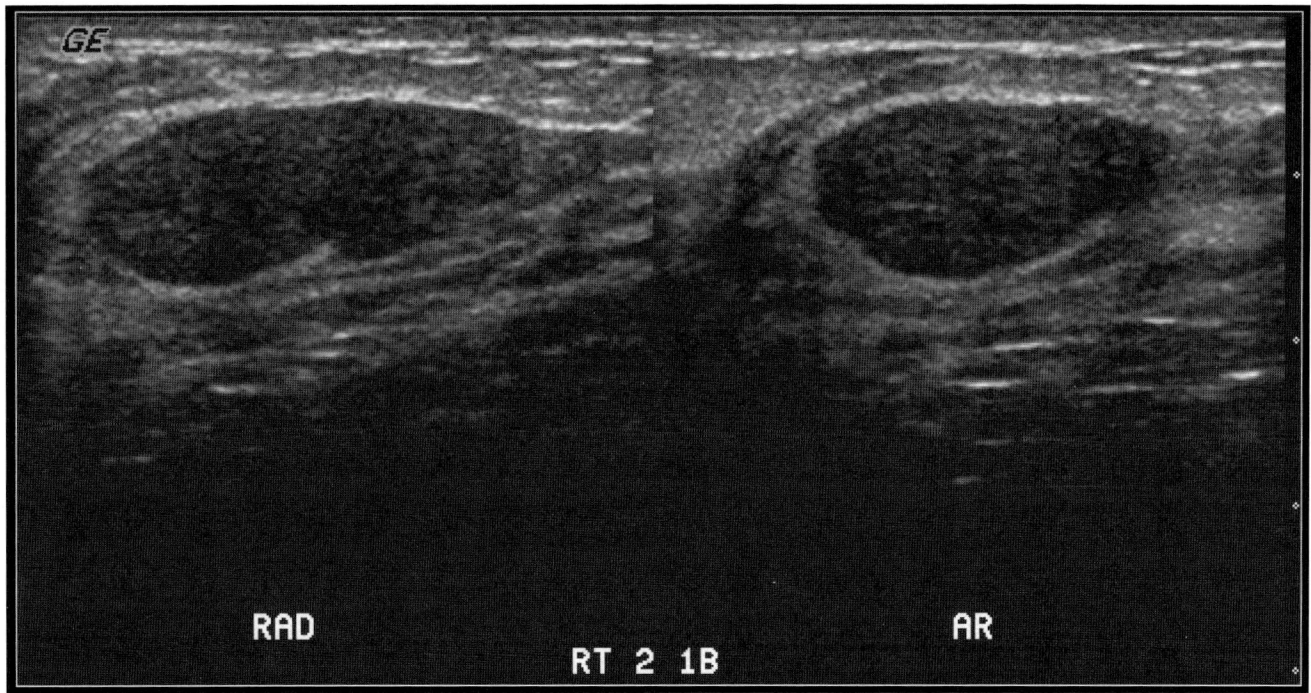

FIGURE 12–83 Many solid nodules that appear to be elliptical in shape in one plane appear to be gently lobulated in the orthogonal plane.

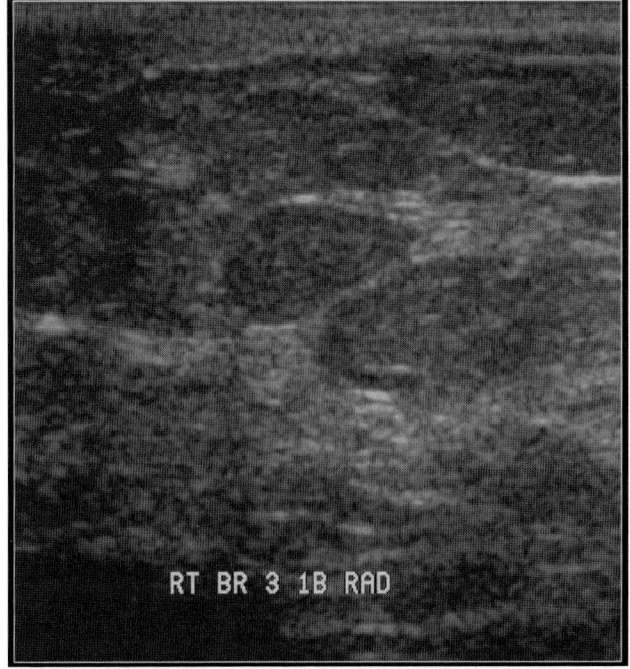

FIGURE 12–84 A teardrop shape is also a characteristic shape seen in a small minority of solid benign nodules. It is rounded on one end and pointed on the other. The pointed end actually represents an angular margin and is the only exception to the rule that even a single angle on any surface of the nodule excludes it from the BIRADS 3 category. To date, all teardrop-shaped solid nodules that have undergone biopsy have been benign fibroadenomas.

graphic appearance. The negative predictive value of the elliptical shape is lower in the current study than in the 1995 study: 97.6% versus 99.1%. Because the negative predictive value of the elliptical shape alone is less than 98%, elliptical shape must be combined with the presence of a complete thin, echogenic capsule in order to achieve the desired result of 98% or greater negative predictive value. Some lesions that appear to be elliptical in one axis appear to be gently lobulated in the orthogonal axis (Fig. 12–83).

A variant shape of the elliptical nodule is the teardrop-shaped or comma-shaped lesion (Fig. 12–84). A small percentage (2.5%) of benign solid nodules have this shape in the current study. The negative predictive value for the small number of teardrop-shaped BIRADS 3 lesions that have undergone biopsy is 100% in the current study. This shape was not recognized as a separate shape in the 1995 study. The teardrop-shaped nodule is the sole exception to the rule that a single angle on any surface of a nodule excludes it from categorization as BIRADS 3. The pointed end of a teardrop is angular.

The prevalence and negative predictive values of the combined elliptical and teardrop shapes are shown in Table 12–22.

Special mention must be made of a spherical shape, which must be distinguished from elliptical. Only seven spherical shaped nodules underwent biopsy in the current ongoing study, but two were malignant. Thus, there was a 22% chance of malignancy, and the negative predictive

TABLE 12–22. NEGATIVE PREDICATIVE VALUE (NPV) AND PREVALENCE AMONG BENIGN NODULES OF ELLIPTICAL AND TEARDROP SHAPES ON SONOGRAPHIC EVALUATION OF SOLID NODULES

	1995 Study (750 Nodules)[a]		Current Study (1,211 Nodules)[b]	
	Prevalence	NPV (Odds Ratio)	Prevalence	NPV (Odds Ratio)
Elliptical shape	51%	99.1% (0.05)	16%	97.6% (0.05)
Teardrop shape	—	—	2.5%	100% (0.00)
Elliptical or teardrop shape	—	—	18%	98% (0.06)
Spherical	—	—	1.3%	78% (0.66)

[a]Prevalence, 16.7%.
[b]Prevalence, 32.8%.

value of 78% was inadequate for classifications as BIRADS 3. The odds ratio of 0.66 is too near 1.0 for spherical shape to be predictive of benignity.

Three or Fewer Gentle Lobulations and Wider-Than-Tall-Shape

Three or fewer lobulations is a mammographic finding that we have directly applied to sonographic evaluation of solid breast nodules. These lobulations should be smooth, well circumscribed, and gently curving. For lobulation to be an effective negative predictor in ultrasound, the gently lobulated nodule must also be wider than tall (Fig. 12–85). As fibroadenomas enlarge, they tend to become more lobulated (Fig. 12–86), and as the number of lobulations increases and they become smaller, it becomes more difficult to distinguish between the gentle lobulation of a fibroadenoma and the microlobulations that can be associ-

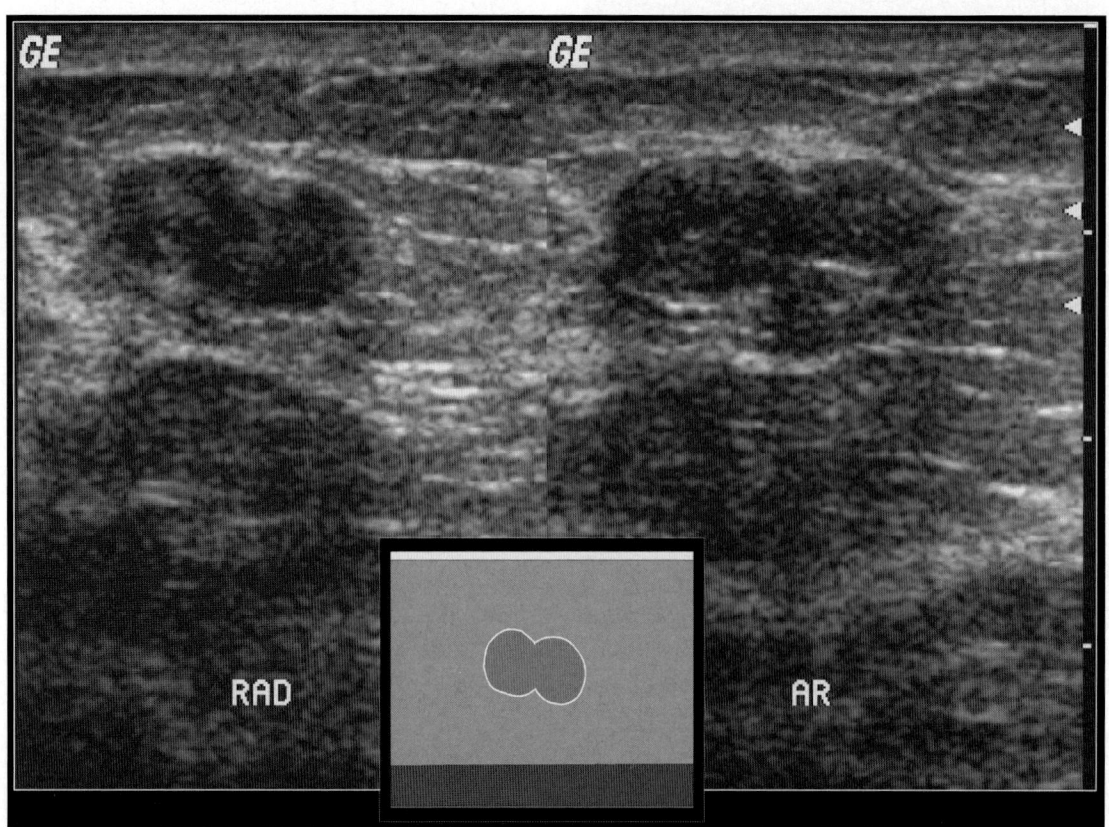

FIGURE 12–85 This benign fibroadenoma has two gentle lobulations and is wider than tall.

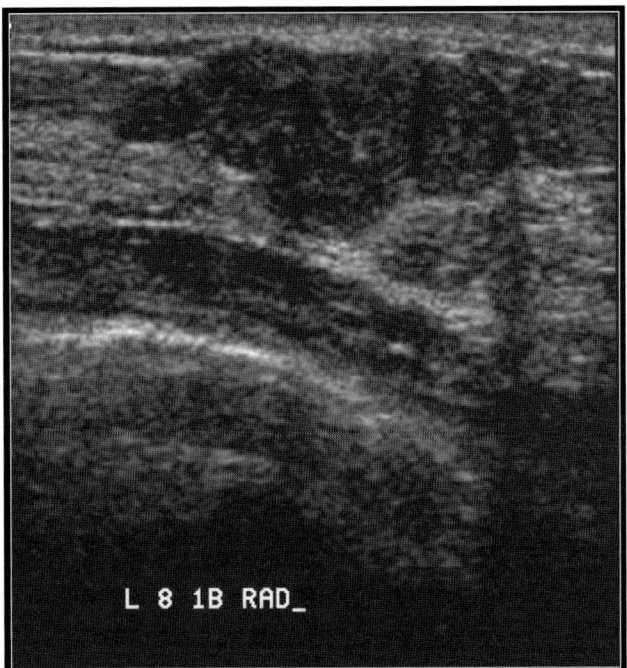

FIGURE 12–86 As benign solid nodules enlarge, they tend to become more lobulated as well as assuming other suspicious sonographic findings and thus are likely to be excluded from the BIRADS 3 category. This 3-cm fibroadenoma has too many lobulations to be classified as BIRADS 3.

the chance of malignancy increases slightly. To improve the positive biopsy rate in the BIRADS 4a group, however, it may be possible to allow a larger number of gentle lobulations. This would result in reclassification of some BIRADS 4a nodules into the BIRADS 3 group.

In the 1995 study, the negative predictive value of three or fewer gentle lobulations was 99.2%, and of all benign nodules, 19% were gently lobulated. In the current ongoing study, the negative predictive value of three or fewer gentle lobulations is 99%, and of all benign solid nodules that have undergone biopsy, 19% have been gently lobulated. Of all nodules characterized as BIRAD 3 (including the 80% that did not undergo biopsy), 31% had three or fewer lobulations. Only about one of three gently lobulated BIRADS 3 nodules currently undergoes biopsy.

The presence of more than three gentle lobulations has a significantly lower negative predictive value of 87%. Twelve percent of the benign solid nodules that underwent biopsy had more than three gentle lobulations. The odds ratio was 0.39. In the current study, the reduction of risk from the cancer prevalence of 33% to 13% was inadequate for three or more gentle lobulations to be considered BIRADS 3. Table 12–23 shows the negative predictive values, odds ratios, and prevalence of gently lobulated lesions among benign solid nodules that have undergone biopsy.

ated with malignant nodules. The three or fewer lobulations criterion was directly adopted from mammographic interpretation but may be overly strict. Mammography only shows the lobulations that are in tangent to the ultrasound beam along the edge of the nodule. Thus, a mammographic nodule that has three or fewer lobulations along one of its margins may actually have six or more total lobulations. Nevertheless, when initially applying this mammographic finding to sonography during the study published in 1995, it seemed best to be cautious. Thus, it was decided to allow no more than three lobulations for this to be a benign sonographic finding. When more than three lobulations are present, fibroadenoma is the likeliest cause, but

Thin, Echogenic Capsule Completely Encompassing the Lesion

The presence of a thin, well-circumscribed, echogenic capsule around a solid nodule indicates a slowly growing and noninfiltrating leading edge of the lesion. Such growth is typical of fibroadenomas and other benign processes. However, some circumscribed invasive malignancies and most DCIS lesions also can have a thin, echogenic capsule. Circumscribed invasive malignancies may have a thin capsule that surrounds most of the lesion, but careful interrogation of the entire surface will usually reveal areas of the surface where a thin capsule is absent and the margins are angular or ill defined. Pure DCIS is usually completely en-

TABLE 12–23. NEGATIVE PREDICTIVE VALUE (NPV) AND PREVALENCE AMONG BENIGN NODULES OF GENTLE LOBULATIONS ON SONOGRAPHIC EVALUATION OF SOLID NODULES

	1995 Study (750 Nodules)[a]		Current Study (1,211 Nodules)[b]	
	Prevalence	NPV (Odds Ratio)	Prevalence	NPV (Odds Ratio)
Less than three lobulations	19%	99% (0.05)	19%	99% (0.03)
More than three lobulations	—	—	12%	87% (0.39)

[a]Prevalence, 16.7%.
[b]Prevalence, 32.8%.

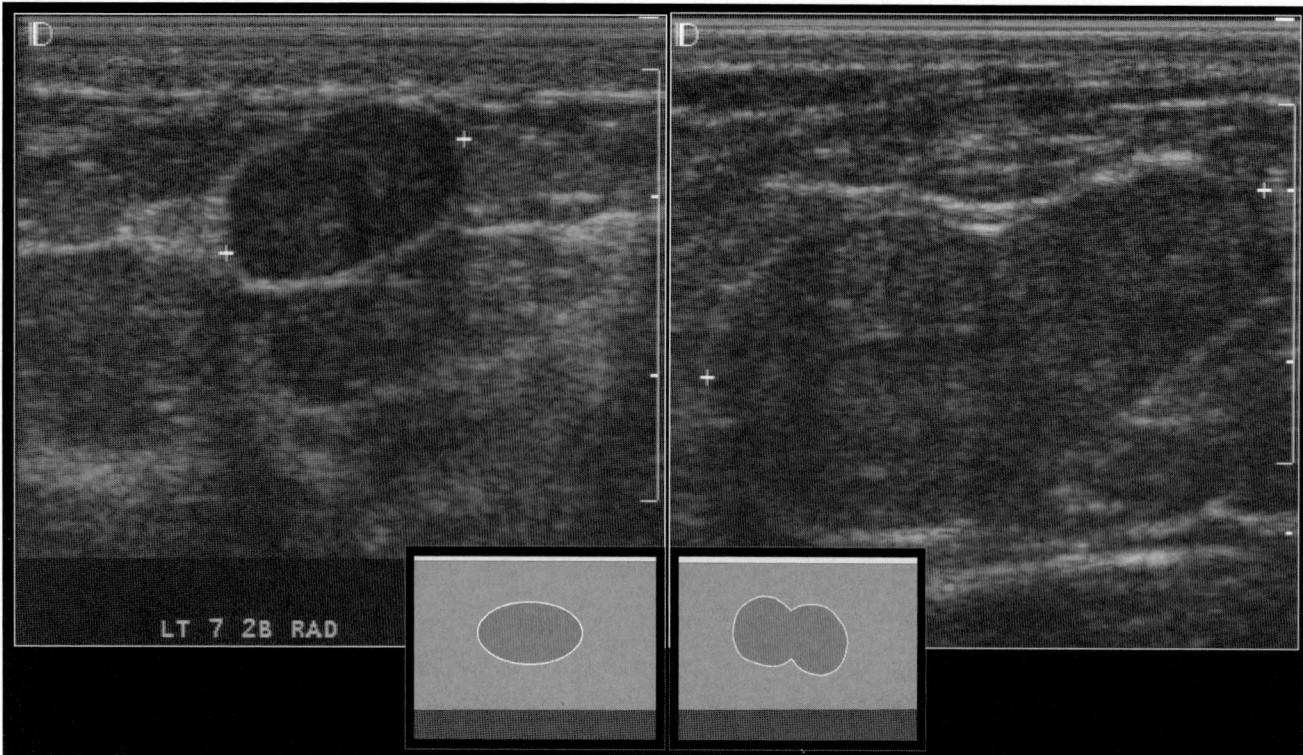

FIGURE 12–87 Benign solid nodules other than purely hyperechoic nodules must be completely encapsulated with a thin, echogenic capsule, a sign that the margins of the lesion are not infiltrating, but pushing. The problem is that circumscribed carcinomas and pure ductal carcinoma *in situ* (DCIS) nodules also have thin, echogenic outer capsules. However, neither circumscribed invasive carcinomas nor pure DCIS are elliptical or gently lobulated in shape. Instead, they are usually microlobulated and often have duct extension or branch pattern. Thus, it is necessary to combine the presence of a thin, echogenic capsule with the elliptical or gently lobulated, wider-than-tall shapes in order not to mischaracterize circumscribed invasive carcinomas and DCIS as probably benign.

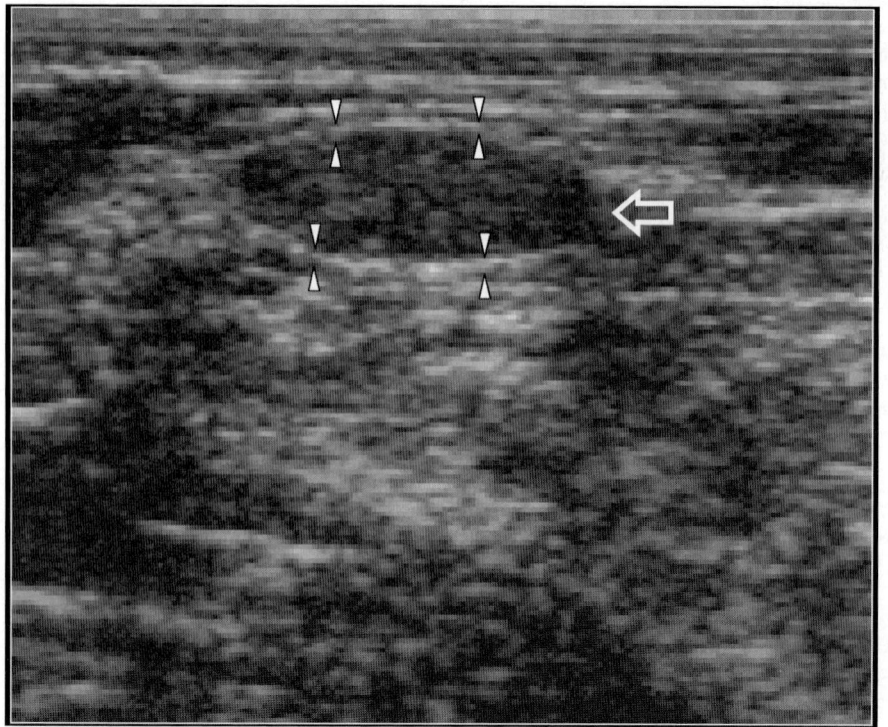

FIGURE 12–88 It is absolutely essential that the thin, echogenic capsule surrounding lesions classified as BIRADS 3 be complete. Because breast cancer can be heterogeneous within an individual nodule, it is not unusual for circumscribed invasive carcinomas to be thinly encapsulated over part, but not all, of their surfaces. This nodule has a thin, echogenic capsule that is well demonstrated along its anterior and posterior surfaces *(arrowheads)*, where the capsule is nearly perpendicular to the ultrasound beam. However, the capsule on the ends of the nodule *(arrows)* is poorly seen because of critical angle phenomena. Special maneuvers are necessary to demonstrate the thin, echogenic capsule on the ends of the nodule.

compassed by a thin, echogenic capsule that represents the intact duct wall. However, pure DCIS is almost never elliptical or gently lobulated in shape. Instead, it is usually microlobulated and frequently also shows duct extension and branch pattern shapes. Likewise, circumscribed invasive malignant nodules are rarely elliptical or gently lobulated in shape. Thus, the presence of a thin, echogenic capsule cannot stand alone as a benign finding. Instead, we must combine it with the elliptical or gently lobulated shape in order to achieve a negative predictive value of 98% or greater (Fig. 12–87).

Demonstration of a thin, echogenic capsule that only partially surrounds the lesion is insufficient evidence that the nodule is benign. Remember that breast cancer can be heterogeneous within an individual nodule. Thus, some circumscribed malignancies can have a thin, echogenic capsule that surrounds part of the lesion, but not all of it. It is absolutely essential that the thin, echogenic capsule completely surround the entire surface of the lesion in all planes evaluated. Demonstrating a complete capsule can be technically difficult because of critical angle phenomena. The capsule is usually well seen along the anterior and pos-

terior surfaces of the lesion, where it is nearly perpendicular to the beam and makes a strong specular reflector. However, the capsule on the ends of the nodule are not well shown from an anterior approach because the capsule is nearly parallel to the beam on the ends of the nodules and makes a poor specular reflector (Fig. 12–88). Some manipulation of the transducer in real time is necessary to demonstrate the thin, echogenic capsule on the ends of the nodule. This can be accomplished by rocking the transducer in its short axis and "heeling and toeing" the transducer in its long axis (Figs. 12–89 and 12–90).

Demonstrating the capsule can also be difficult in solid nodules that are surrounded by equally hyperechoic fibrous tissue (Fig. 12–91). Using lighter than normal compression can help demonstrate the capsule in such lesions. The compression normally used to maintain good skin contact and to minimize critical angle shadowing from Cooper's ligaments compresses normal fibrous tissue, making it appear more hyperechoic. Furthermore, normal compression also pushes fibrous tissue tightly against the equally echogenic capsule, helping to obscure the capsule. By scanning with lighter than normal scan pressure, the fi-

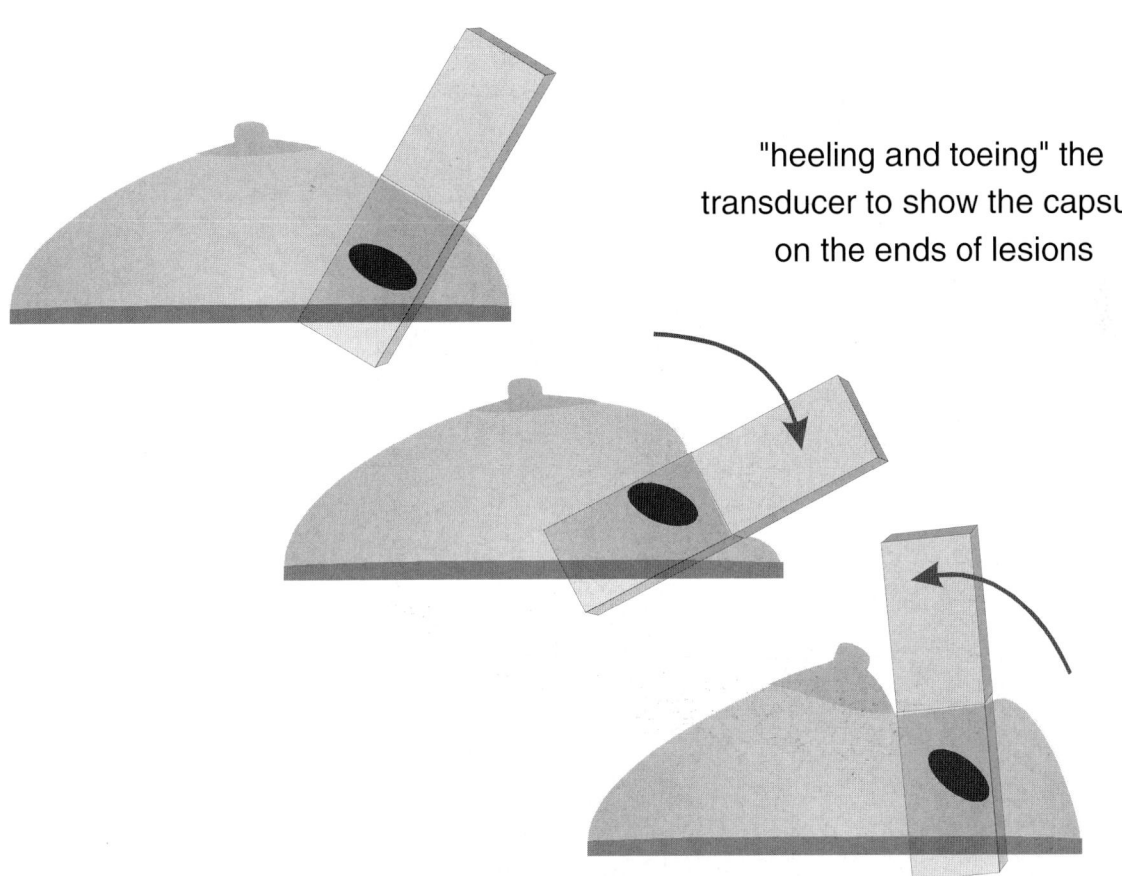

"heeling and toeing" the transducer to show the capsule on the ends of lesions

FIGURE 12–89 Rocking the transducer along its short axis and "heeling and toeing" the transducer along its long axis change the angle of incidence of the ultrasound beam with the various surfaces of the nodule and can help to demonstrate the completeness of the thin, echogenic capsule, especially on the ends of the nodule (can be converted to gray scale).

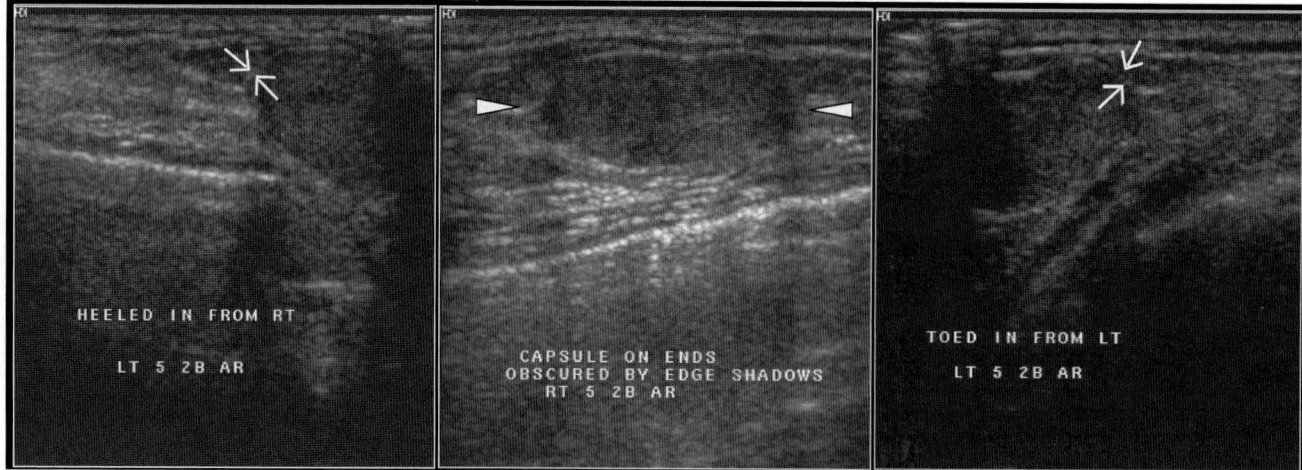

FIGURE 12–90 The **middle** image shows the appearance of a gently lobulated fibroadenoma when scanned from straight anteriorly. The thin, echogenic capsule is well demonstrated on the anterior and posterior surfaces of the nodule, where it is nearly perpendicular to the ultrasound beam, but is poorly seen along the edges of the nodule, where it is nearly parallel to the beam *(arrowheads)*. When the transducer is "heeled," the capsule along the left edge of the nodule is well-demonstrated **(left)**. When the transducer is "toed," the capsule along the right edge of the nodule is well demonstrated. It is difficult for a sonographer or mammography technologist to show the entire capsule on a few hard-copy images but relatively easy to see the whole capsule in real time.

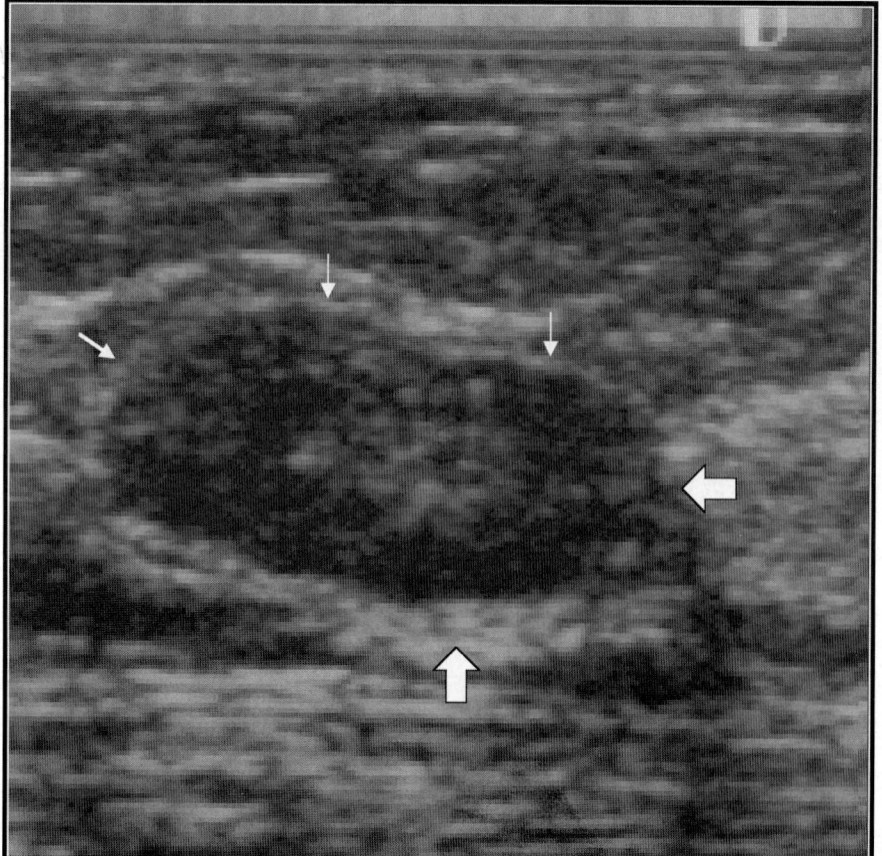

FIGURE 12–91 This gently lobulated, wider-than-tall solid nodule has a thin, echogenic capsule that is well demonstrated along the anterior aspect of the nodule where it is bordered by isoechoic fat *(small arrows)*. However, the hyperechoic fibrous tissue along the deep and right margins of the nodule obscures its capsule *(block arrows)*. Because the capsule is not complete, the lesion cannot be characterized as BIRADS category 3 from this image along. Maneuvers must be used to try to better demonstrate the thin, echogenic capsule along the margins of the lesion that are bordered by fibrous tissue that is equal in echogenicity to the capsule.

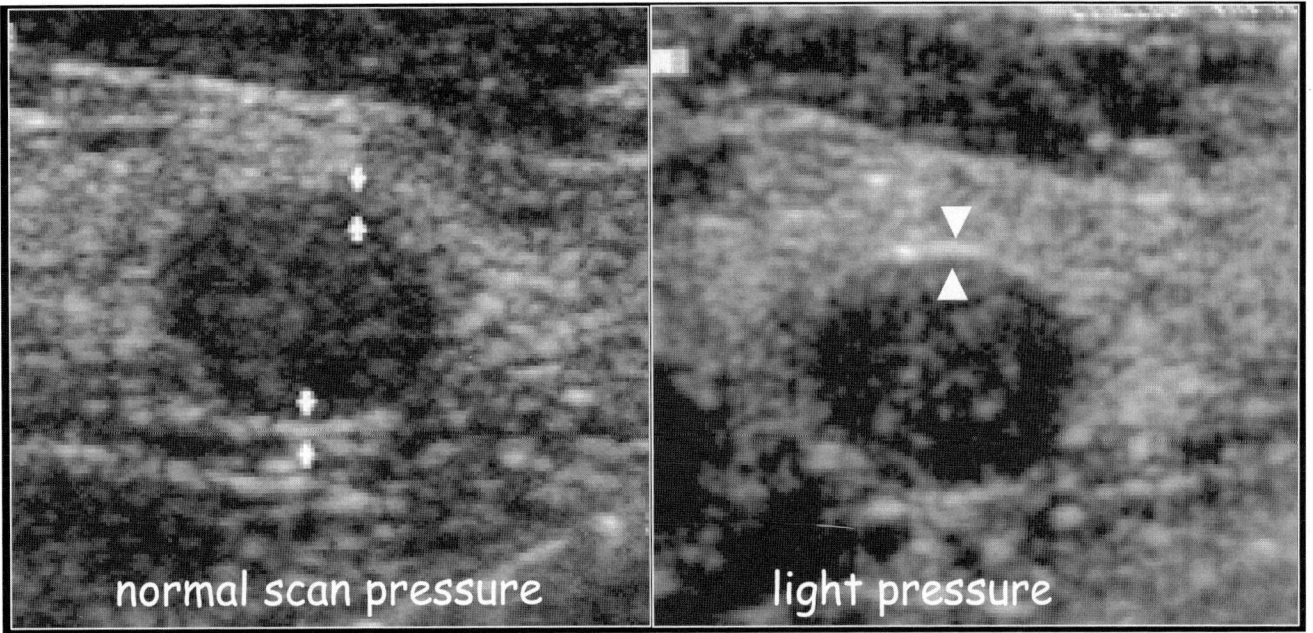

FIGURE 12–92 When scanned with normal or heavy compression pressure, the well-circumscribed, oval nodule shown in the **left** image cannot be characterized as probably benign because its thin, echogenic capsule is obscured by the equally echogenic surrounding fibrous tissue. However, when the same nodule is scanned with lighter compression pressure (**right**), the fibrous tissue expands, becomes less echogenic, and separates enough from the capsule to allow the capsule to be demonstrable. Thus, scanning with lighter scan pressure can help demonstrate the thin, echogenic capsule in benign lesions that are surrounded by echogenic fibrous tissues.

brous tissue is allowed to expand and become less echogenic and to separate away from the thin, echogenic capsule, facilitating its demonstration. Using lighter than normal compression is useful for identifying a thin, echogenic capsule that surrounds benign solid nodules regardless of whether they are surrounded by hyperechoic fibrous tissue (Fig. 12–92) or by isoechoic fat (Fig. 12–93) but is most useful in fibrous-surrounded lesions.

The problem with the very light compression that we need to use to better demonstrate the thin, echogenic capsule around solid nodules is that it tends to result in acoustic shadowing that normally does not occur when normal compression is used. Such technique-induced acoustic shadowing could prevent a benign lesion from appropriately being characterized as BIRADS 3. Therefore, the shadowing that results with very light scan pressure should not be viewed as suspicious. In certain cases, demonstrating both the presence of a thin, echogenic capsule and normal sound transmission may require variable compression—light compression to best demonstrate the thin, echogenic capsule and normal compression to demonstrate normal or enhanced sound transmission (Fig. 12–94).

In the 1995 study, 75% of all benign nodules that underwent biopsy were completely encompassed by a thin,

echogenic capsule, and the negative predictive value of a complete thin, echogenic capsule was 98%. However, in the current ongoing study, the negative predictive value of a complete thin, echogenic capsule alone is only 86%. Thus, the presence of a thin, echogenic capsule by itself is inadequate evidence of a BIRADS 3 lesion. The real value of the thin, echogenic capsule is its use in conjunction with the elliptical or gently lobulated shape. The negative predictive value of a thin, echogenic capsule together with the elliptical shape is 99.1%. Solid nodules were elliptical in shape and thinly encapsulated in 14% of all benign lesions that underwent biopsy and in 47% of all BIRADS 3 benign lesions that underwent biopsy. The negative predictive value of a thin, echogenic capsule, together with three or fewer gentle lobulations, was 100%. Solid nodules were gently lobulated and thinly encapsulated in 9% of all nodules that underwent biopsy and in 30% of all BIRADS 3 benign lesions that underwent biopsy.

Table 12–24 shows the negative predictive values and odds ratios for the presence of thin, echogenic capsule alone and in combination with the elliptical and gently lobulated shape.

There are reasons that combining the presence of a complete thin, echogenic capsule and either an elliptical,

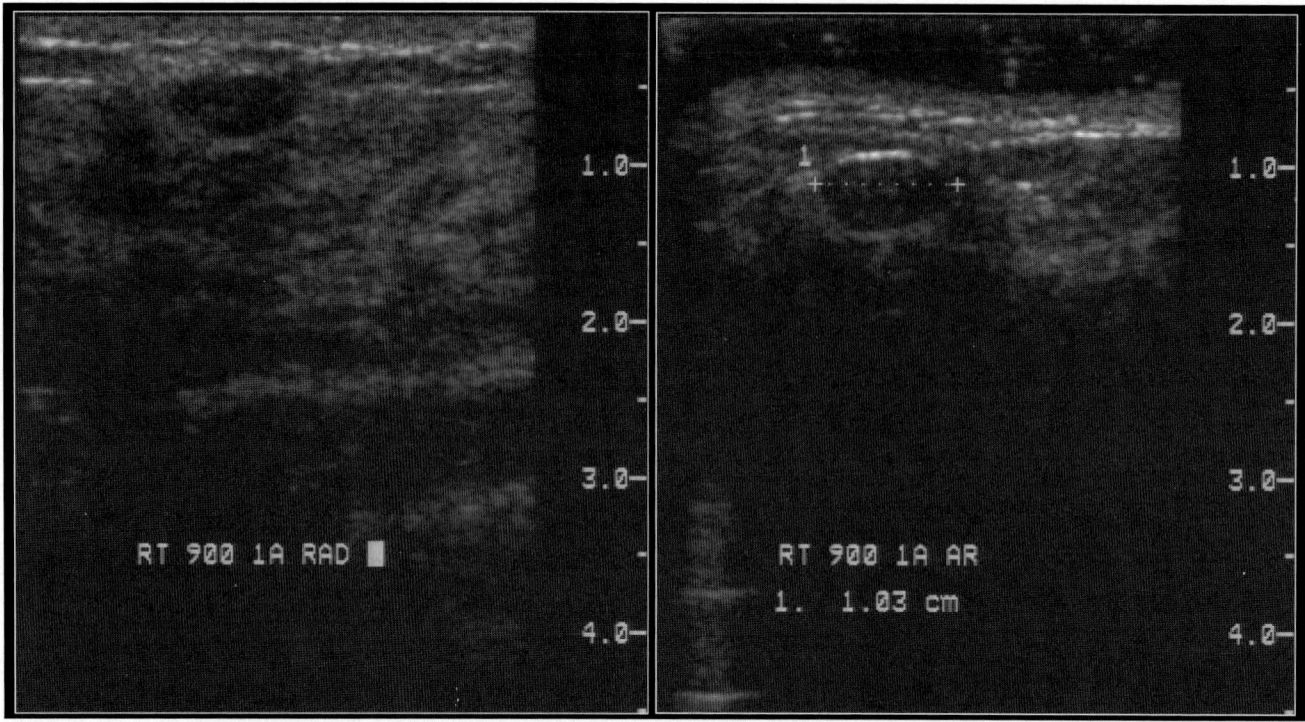

FIGURE 12–93 Even in lesions that are not completely surrounded by fibrous tissue, the capsule may be better shown with light scan pressure (**right**) than with heavy scan pressure (**left**).

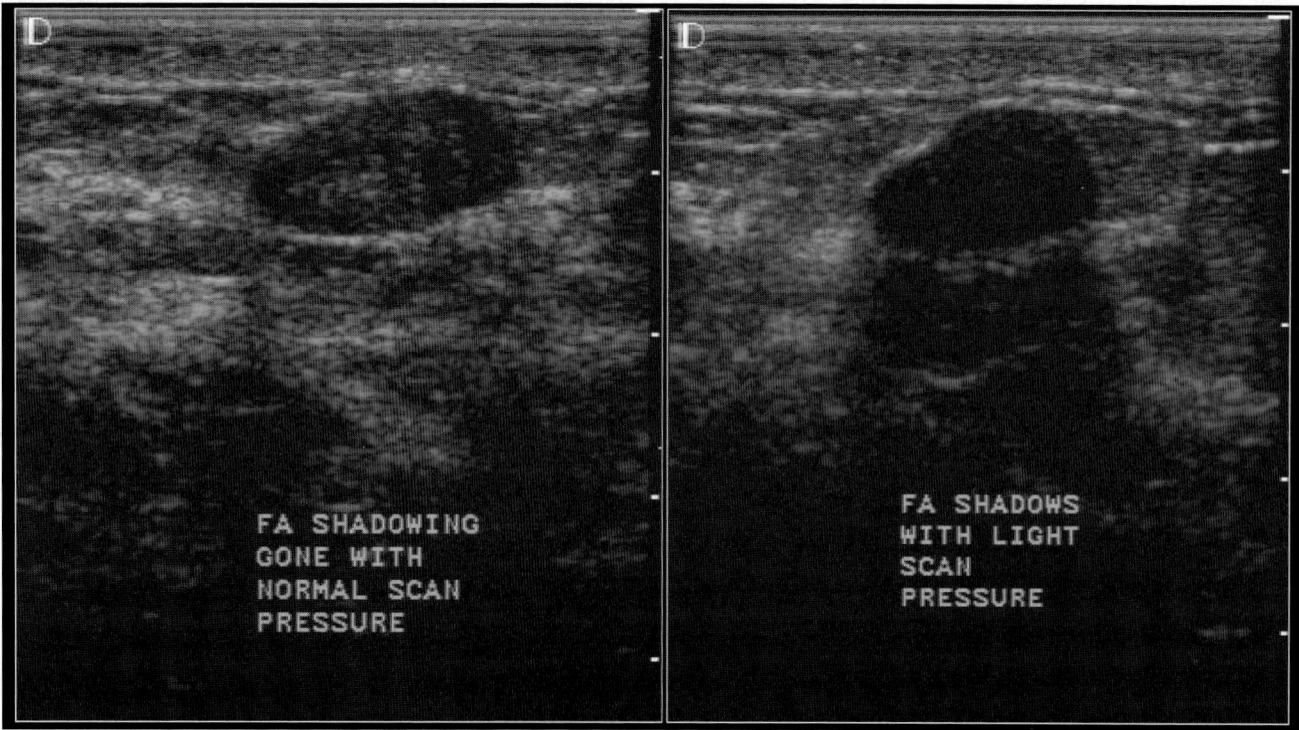

FIGURE 12–94 The problem with using light scan pressures that better demonstrates the thin, echogenic capsule that surrounds most benign solid nodules is that it can lead to artifactual acoustic shadowing deep to the lesion (**right**). Thus, a combination of normal or heavy scan pressure to show normal through-transmission (**left** image) and light scan pressure to show the capsule better (**right** image) may be necessary for complete evaluation of solid breast nodules.

TABLE 12–24. NEGATIVE PREDICTIVE VALUE (NPV) AND PREVALENCE AMONG BENIGN NODULES OF THIN ECHOGENIC CAPSULE ALONG AND WITH SHAPES

	1995 Study (750 Nodules)[a]		Current Study (1,211 Nodules)[b]	
		PPV		PPV
	Prevalence	Odds Ratio	Prevalence	Odds Ratio
Thin capsule	76%	98.8% (0.07)	61%	86% (0.42)
Capsule and elliptical	—	—	12%	99% (0.03)
Capsule and lobulated	—	—	9%	100% (0.00)

[a]Prevalence, 16.7%.
[b]Prevalence, 32.8%.

wider-than-tall shape or gently lobulated wider-than-tall shape succeeds, when shape or the presence of a capsule alone fails. First, DCIS is purely intraductal. The duct wall that contains the intraductal tumor is represented sonographically as a thin, echogenic line. However, the shape of DCIS is virtually never elliptical or solely gently lobulated. Careful interrogation almost always reveals microlobulation, duct extension, or branch pattern. Calcifications are also frequently present within the individual microlobulations, duct extensions, or branches. Furthermore, high-grade invasive ductal carcinomas and special-type tumors such as medullary carcinoma are often well circumscribed and appear generally rounded. However, they frequently have a taller-than-wide shape and usually have some surfaces that are microlobulated or angular. Even when a thin, echogenic capsule surrounds most of the circumference of a high-grade malignant lesion, it is usually missing or is thick and ill defined over part of the surface of the lesion. The presence of partial thin, echogenic capsules is merely a manifestation of the internal heterogeneity within certain malignant nodules. Thus, by combining the elliptical or gently lobulated shape with the presence of a complete thin, echogenic capsule, the chances of misdiagnosing both circumscribed invasive malignancies and pure DCIS as benign are minimized.

One special type of benign solid nodule is the intramammary lymph node. The intramammary lymph node is elliptical or gently lobulated in shape, has a hilum of variable echogenicity, and has a thin capsule surrounding it except at the hilar opening (Fig. 12–95). The sonographic appearance is similar to that of a miniature normal kidney, and the relative thickness of the cortex and hilum are proportional to that of a kidney with central atrophy and renal sinus lipomatosis. The shortest diameter is generally less than 1 cm in length, but the longest diameter may well be more than 1 cm. Lymph nodes that appear sonographically normal can be categorized as BIRADS 2 and do not require short-interval follow-up. Of 383 solid nodules characterized as lymph nodes and BIRADS category 2, 8 have been benign at biopsy, and 375 have been smaller or unchanged on follow-up. Thus, sonography is as definitive as mammography in identifying normal intramammary lymph nodes. Intramammary lymph nodes are discussed in Chapters 4 and 19.

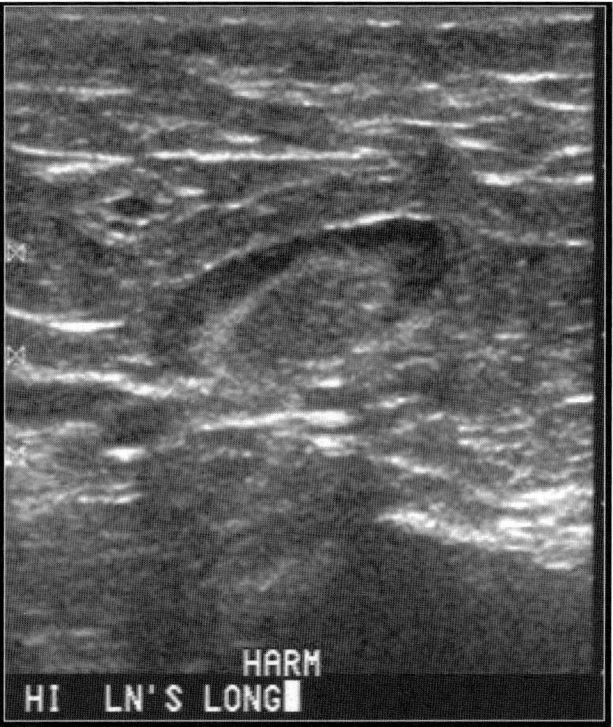

FIGURE 12–95 Lymph nodes are solid nodules with a sonographic appearance that is so typically benign that a lesion with this appearance can be classified as BIRADS category 2, definitively benign. Normal lymph nodes are elliptical or gently lobulated in shape, are wider than tall, have a hilum of variable size and echogenicity, and are encompassed within a thin, echogenic capsule (except at the opening of the hilum). The appearance is similar to that of a miniature kidney.

TABLE 12–25. SOLID NODULE FINDINGS SUSPICIOUS FOR MALIGNANCY

Soft Finding	Hard Finding	Intermediate Finding
Duct extension	Spiculations; thick halo	Hypoechoic
Branch pattern	Angular margins	Microlobulation
Calcifications	Acoustic shadowing	Taller than wide

The method of selecting BIRADS categories requires some explanation. In the 1995 study, there were only three categories: benign, indeterminate, and malignant. Any nodule with even a single malignant finding was characterized as malignant. Nodules that did not have any malignant features and had one of the three combined benign findings were characterized as benign. Nodules that had no malignant findings, but did not have specific benign findings were characterized as indeterminate. In the current ongoing study, the characterization into the BIRADS 2 and 3 categories is just as rigid, but characterization into BIRADS subcategories 4a and 4b and higher is a bit more subjective. First any lesion that is thought to be a fibroadenoma or benign intraductal papilloma, but that does not meet strict criteria for benignity, is characterized into the BIRADS 4a category. Further stratification depends on whether the suspicious findings present are soft or hard, and on how many are present. Table 12–25 lists the 9 suspicious findings into soft, hard, and intermediate categories.

As noted earlier, hard findings suggest the presence of invasive malignancy and have higher positive predictive values but, in many instances, lower sensitivity. Soft findings, on the other hand, are more frequently associated with pure DCIS or DCIS components of mixed invasive and intraductal lesions. Their sensitivities tend to be higher, but there are more false-positive findings because there is more overlap with benign processes such as papillomas, papillary duct hyperplasia, and papillary apocrine metaplasia. Because hard findings have better positive pre-

dictive values, lesions that contain them deserve higher BIRADS categories: BIRADS 4b or 5. The more hard findings present, the more likely the lesion is to be characterized as BIRADS 5. Conversely, because soft findings have lower positive predictive values, the nodules that contain only soft findings are assigned to the lowest suspicious category: mildly suspicious, BIRADS 4a.

By combining the suspicious and benign findings in the strict algorithm described earlier, the goals of 98% or greater sensitivity, 98% or greater negative predictive value, and 2% or fewer false-negative findings were achieved in both studies. Table 12–26 shows the results of findings and algorithm in the 1995 study. All nodules in all classes underwent biopsy.

The negative-to-positive biopsy ratio was 5:1. Had the 426 nodules classified as benign not undergone biopsy, the negative-to-positive biopsy ratio could have been reduced to 1.6:1. Of course, 1.6:1 is only an ideal target ratio that could never really be achieved because some patients and referring physicians are uncomfortable with follow-up rather than biopsy even when the risk for malignancy is less than 2%.

The current ongoing study differs from the 1995 study in three ways. First, even though the 1995 study achieved a negative predictive value and a sensitivity of 98% or greater, our original goal was only to achieve sensitivity and negative predictive value of 95% or greater. Second, there were only three classes in the 1995 study, whereas we have used five BIRADS categories in the current study. The third and most important way that the two studies differ is in the management of risk categories. In the 1995 study, all patients underwent biopsy regardless of their risk category. In the current study, the patient with a BIRADS 3 lesion is given three options and allowed to make the decision that is most appropriate for her. It is explained to her that the lesion is likely to be benign with greater than 98% certainty. (Even though our data would justify conveyance of a 99.5% negative predictive value, we have adhered to the BIRADS 3 definition of 98% or greater negative predictive value in order to be prudent and cautious.) She is given the options of (a) excisional biopsy,

TABLE 12–26. 1995 STUDY: CHARACTERIZATION OF SOLID BREAST NODULES

	Benign Histology	Malignant Histology	Totals
Negative ultrasound (benign)	424 (TN)	2 (FN)	426
Positive ultrasound (malignant and indeterminate)	201 (FP)	123 (TP)	324
	625	125	750

Sensitivity, 123/125 = 98.4%; negative predictive value, 424/426 = 99.5%; specificity, 424/625 = 67.8%; positive predictive value, 123/324 = 38.0%; accuracy, (424 + 123)/750 = 72.9%.
TN = true negative; FN = false negative; FP = false positive; TP = true positive.

TABLE 12–27. CURRENT STUDY: CHARACTERIZATION OF SOLID BREAST NODULES

	Benign Histology	Malignant Histology	Totals
Negative ultrasound (BIRADS 2, 3)	245 (TN)	1 (FN)	246
Positive ultrasound (BIRADS 4a, 4b, 5)	559 (FP)	406 (TP)	965
Totals	804	407	1,211

Sensitivity, 406/407 = 99.8%; negative predictive value, 245/246 = 99.6%; specificity, 245/804 = 30.5%; positive predictive value, 406/965 = 42.1%; accuracy, (245 + 406)/1,211 = 53.8%.
TN = true negative; FN = false negative; FP = false positive; TP = true positive.

(b) ultrasound-guided large core needle or vacuum-assisted needle biopsy, or (c) short-interval follow-up. She is informed that if she chooses follow-up, we are comfortable with that choice, and that the follow-up will be for 2 years, not just 6 months.

For purposes of calculating efficacy, BIRADS 2 and 3 categories are considered negative sonograms, and BIRADS 4a, 4b, and 5 are considered positive sonograms. In the current study, 1,211 nodules have undergone biopsy. Biopsy methods include surgical excision by lumpectomy or mastectomy, 14-gauge large core needle biopsy, or 14-gauge or 11-gauge vacuum-assisted needle biopsy. None of the biopsies were obtained with fine-needle aspiration. Table 12–27 shows the efficacy of the current study.

Note that the negative predictive value and sensitivity remain well over 98%. Additionally, the percentage of all biopsies that revealed malignancy is much higher in the current study. The negative-to-positive biopsy rate has decreased from 5:1 in the 1995 study to slightly less than 2:1 in the current study. Many patients with BIRADS 3 lesions (80%) in the current study have chosen to be followed rather than to undergo biopsy. Thus, we have come close the ideal goal from the 1995 study of achieving a 1.6:1 negative-to-positive biopsy ratio while not only maintaining sensitivity and negative predictive value but also improving them.

Even though the risk for malignancy in nodules meeting strict criteria for BIRADS 3 are exceedingly low, we have not felt it our position to deny biopsy to patients who are uncomfortable with the option of follow-up. It is as important that they have a healthy psyche as a healthy body. If patients feel that not undergoing biopsy or lesion removal will adversely affect their emotional status, we feel that biopsy is warranted. Thus, patients who desire biopsy are usually scheduled for biopsy before leaving the department, even when their lesion is characterized as BIRADS 3.

In patients with nodules that meet strict criteria for BIRADS 3 classification whose lesions are less that 14 mm, there is a high probability that all imaging evidence of the lesion can be removed using only the 11-gauge directional

vacuum-assisted biopsy (DVAB). Thus, not only can a definitive diagnosis can be obtained, but also any palpable and or imaging evidence of the lesion can be eradicated. This is generally reassuring to patients who elect to have biopsy. Keep in mind that removal of imaging evidence of residual disease is not at all the same as complete removal of histologic evidence disease and that DVAB is approved for diagnosis, but not treatment. Removal of imaging evidence of residual disease should be comforting to the patient and to the radiologist only if the histology is unequivocally benign. If histologic evaluation of tissue obtained at DVAB shows malignancy, atypia, or a high-risk lesion, follow-up surgical excision is required.

The predicted and actual risks for malignancy in solid nodules in each of the BIRADS categories from 2 through 5 are shown in Table 12–28. Note that in all BIRADS categories, the actual risk is within the expected risk range.

Table 12–28 gives valuable information concerning where ancillary imaging and diagnostic procedures may be helpful. Mammography has preceded ultrasound in most cases. In solid nodules that meet strict criteria for BIRADS 2 and 3, there is no need for ancillary imaging. The results are as certain as any in medical imaging. In categories 4b and 5, there is no need for additional diagnostic imaging. When the risk for cancer is greater than 50%, biopsy is required. In BIRADS category 4a, however, the chance of malignancy is only 10%. This is the category in which there is the most room for improvement in our characterization algorithm. Most BIRADS 4a lesions only have one or two soft findings. These soft findings increase sensitivity but also increase the false-positive rate. That is the price we have paid for very low false-negative rates. Only in category 4a might ancillary imaging procedures such a radionuclide sestamibi studies be helpful, and then, this is likely only in lesions 2 cm or larger.

There is also almost certainly some fine-tuning that can be done to improve the yield in the BIRADS 4a group. For instance, the cutoff in the number of lobulations allowed for BIRADS 3 classifications is probably artificially low. It is likely that 6 or even 10 lobulations do not in-

TABLE 12–28. PROSPECTIVE CHARACTERIZATION OF 1,211 SOLID NODULES INTO BIRADS CATEGORIES[a]

BIRADS Category	No. of Nodules Undergoing Biopsy	No. of Malignant Nodules	Expected Risk for Cancer (%)	Actual Risk for Cancer (%)
2	15	0	0	0
3	231	1	≤2	0.4
4a	515	52	3–49	10
4b	191	118	50–89	62
5	259	236	≥90	91
Totals	1,211	407		34

[a]All 1,211 nodules have undergone biopsy.

crease the risk for cancer as long as they are not microlobulations. Furthermore, we have always considered any intraductal lesion to be a variant of the suspicious finding of duct extension. However, in a recent study of small intraductal nodules that were removed at mammotomy at our institution, 74 of 75 lesions were benign. The risk for malignancy was less than 2%. Therefore, it is likely that small and short intraductal nodules that do not expand the duct or extend for great distances and into branch ducts can be downgraded to BIRADS 3 from the BIRADS 4a class we currently use. Finally, epithelial calcifications in complex fibroadenomas are another relatively frequent cause of false-positive findings. Perhaps, calcifications that occur in elliptical and thinly encapsulated nodules should be considered to be BIRADS 3 rather than BIRADS 4a. Each of these changes will likely improve the yield in the BIRADS 4a category without causing false-negative findings. The important thing is that by using the categories, we are able not only to assess our efficacy but also to see where there might be room for fine-tuning and improvement and where ancillary testing may be helpful.

The follow-up interval for mammographic lesions that are characterized as BIRADS 3 has been controversial. Some mammographers believe that yearly follow-up is adequate and that the first follow-up at 6 months is too soon. Malignant lesions for which mammography is falsely benign in appearance tend are said to be slowly growing lesions. However, in our experience, abandoning the 6-month follow-up sonogram for solid nodules that are characterized as BIRADS 3 would be a mistake. The malignant nodules most likely to be falsely characterized as BIRADS 3 are circumscribed carcinomas that are usually fast growing and are highly likely to show detectable changes in size or characteristics within 6 months. The more slowly growing lesions at the spiculated end of the sonographic spectrum that may not show much detectable change in 6 months are unlikely to be mischaracterized as benign. Our protocol for solid nodules that are characterized as BIRADS 3 is to perform follow-up

at 6 months, 1 year, and 2 years. If the lesion is mammographically well visualized, only a single extra sonogram at 6 months may be necessary because the 1 and 2 year follow-ups can be performed with routine annual screening mammography. However, three additional sonograms are needed only if the lesion is not visible on mammography.

Finally, when one becomes comfortable with sonographic evaluation of solid breast nodules, there is a danger of becoming too complacent. When complacency sets in, one might try to use looser rules and characterize the lesion by gut feelings rather than by the strict algorithmic approach. To analyze the danger in not adhering to a strict algorithmic approach, in the current ongoing study, we have characterized solid nodules in two ways: by the strict algorithmic approach and by subjective, gut-feeling evaluation. All decisions on biopsy were based on the strict algorithmic approach. The gut-feeling BIRADS classification was never used to make decisions about biopsy. The purpose of the gut-feeling BIRADS category was simply to determine whether the strict algorithmic approach was too strict. However, despite our considerable knowledge of and experienced in characterizing solid breast nodules sonographically, we were unable to achieve sensitivity or negative predictive value of 98% or greater with the subjective gut-feeling approach. Thus, although we were close, we could not quite identify a BIRADS 3 group of nodules that had a 2% or less chance of being malignant by gut feeling. Table 12–29

TABLE 12–29. SENSITIVITY AND NEGATIVE PREDICTIVE VALUE OF GUT FEELING VERSUS STRICT ALGORITHM

	Gut Feeling Characterization	Strict Algorithm Characterization
Sensitivity	97.2%	99.8%
Negative predictive value	97.4%	99.6%

shows the comparison of sensitivity and negative predictive values for the gut-feeling approach and the strict algorithmic approach.

SUMMARY

Because of the heterogeneity of breast cancer from nodule to nodule, single findings cannot achieve the sensitivity or the negative predictive value necessary to identify a low-risk group that can be offered the option of follow-up (BI-RADS 3 group). However, by using multiple findings in a strict algorithm, such a group can be identified. In addition, breast cancer can be heterogeneous within an individual nodule. Part of the nodule may have circumscribed features that simulate a benign lesion, whereas another part may be spiculated and obviously malignant. Only by scanning the whole surface and substance of the nodule in two orthogonal planes (radial and antiradial) can the presence of suspicious findings be excluded. If there is a mixture of benign and suspicious findings, the benign findings should be ignored.

These studies show that sonography is useful in the characterization of solid breast masses. Characterizing solid breast nodules into BIRADS categories defines carcinomas that might have been missed clinically or mammographically. It identifies a BIRADS 3 group that has far less than a 2% risk for malignancy and can offer the patient the option of follow-up rather than biopsy. Many patients with BIRADS 3 solid nodules are electing to be followed rather than to undergo biopsy, which improves the accuracy of the diagnosis of malignant breast lesions. More important, it also accurately defines a population of benign solid breast lesions that do not require biopsy when strict sonographic criteria of benignity are present.

To identify a BIRADS 3 subgroup with the desired sensitivity and negative predictive values of 98% or greater, strict adherence to the algorithm is essential. Subjective gut feelings are inadequate. When patients with BIRADS 3 nodules elect to be followed rather than undergo biopsy, follow-up should be performed in 6 months, not 1 year. The malignant lesions most at risk for being mischaracterized as BIRADS 3 tend to be high-grade invasive ductal carcinomas that grow rapidly enough for change to be readily detected at 6 months.

SUGGESTED READINGS

Adler DD, Hyde DL, Ikeda DM. Quantitative sonographic parameters as a means of distinguishing breast cancers from benign solid breast masses. *J Ultrasound Med* 1991;10(9):505–508.

Baker JA, Kornguth PJ, Soo MS, et al. Sonography of solid breast lesions: observer variability of lesion description and assessment. *AJR Am J Roentgenol* 1999;172:1621–1625.

Bamber JC, De Gonzalez L, Cosgrove DO, et al. Quantitative evaluation of real-time ultrasound features of the breast. *Ultrasound Med Biol* 1988;14[Suppl 1]:s81–s87.

Chang RF, Kuo WJ, Chen DR, et al. Computer-aided diagnosis for surgical office-based breast ultrasound. *Arch Surg* 2000;135(6):696–699.

Chao TC, Lo YF, Chen SC, et al. Prospective sonographic study of 3093 breast tumors. *J Ultrasound Med* 1999;18:363–370.

Chen DR, Chang RF, Huang YL. Computer-aided diagnosis applied to US of solid breast nodules by using neural networks. *Radiology* 1999;21(2):407–412.

Chopier J, Amram S, Maurin N, et al. Solid breast nodules: reliability of ultrasonographic and cytological studies. *J Radiol* 1995;76(5):263–266.

Cole-Beuglet C, Soriano RZ, Kurtz AB, et al. Ultrasound analysis of 104 primary breast carcinomas classified according to histopathologic type. *Radiology* 1983;147:191–196.

D'Astous FT, Foster FS. Frequency dependence of ultrasound attenuation and backscatter in breast tissue. *Ultrasound Med Biol* 1986;12(10):795–808.

Ellis RL. Differentiation of benign versus malignant breast disease. *Radiology* 1999;210:878–880.

Euno E, Tohno E, Itoh K. Classification and diagnostic criteria in breast echography. *Jpn J Med Ultrasonics* 1986;13(1):19–31.

Euno E, Tohno E, Soeda S, et al. Dynamic tests in real-time sonography. *Ultrasound Med Biol* 1988;14[Suppl 1]:53–57.

Fornage BD, Lorigan JB, Andry E. Fibroadenoma of the breast: sonographic appearance. *Radiology* 1989;172:671–675.

Fornage BD, Sneige N, Faroux MJ, et al. Sonographic appearance and ultrasound-guided fine-needle aspiration biopsy of breast carcinomas smaller than 1 cm³. *J Ultrasound Med* 1990;9:559–568.

Franquet T, De Miguel C, Cozculluela R, et al. Spiculated lesions of the breast: mammographic-pathologic correlations. *Radiographics* 1993;13(4):841–852.

Garra BS, Krasner BH, Horii SC, et al. Improving the distinction between benign and malignant breast lesions: the value of sonographic texture analysis. *Ultrason Imaging* 1993;15(4):267–285.

Garra BS, Cespedes EI, Ophir J, et al. Elastography of breast lesions: initial clinical results. *Radiology* 1997;202(1):79–86.

Golub, RM, Parsons RE, Sigel B. Differentiation of breast tumors by ultrasonic tissue characterization. *J Ultrasound Med* 1993;12:601–608.

Guyer PB, Dewbury DC, Warwick D, et al. Direct contact B-scan ultrasound in the diagnosis of solid breast masses. *Clin Radiol* 1986;37(5):451–458.

Guyer PB, Dewbury KC. Sonomammography in benign breast disease. *Br J Radiol* 1988;61(725):374–378.

Hackloer BJ, Duda V, Lauth G. Ultrasound mammography. Hamburg: Springer-Verlag, 1989.

Hall FM. Sonography of the breast: controversies and opinions. *AJR Am J Roentgenol* 1997;169(6):1635–1636.

Harper AP, Kelly-Fry E, Noe JS, et al. Ultrasound in the evaluation of solid breast masses. *Radiology* 1983;146:731–736.

Hashimoto BE, Kramer KJ, Picozzi VJ. High detection rate of breast ductal carcinoma in situ calcifications on mammographically directed high-resolution sonography. *J Ultrasound Med* 2001;20:501–508.

Heywang SH, Dunner PS, Lipsit ER, et al. Advantages and pitfalls of ultrasound in the diagnosis of breast cancer. *J Clin Ultrasound* 1985;13(8):525–532.

Hilton SW, Leopold GR, Olson LK, et al. Real-time breast sonography: application in 300 consecutive patients. *AJR Am J Roentgenol* 1986;147:479.

Huber S, Danes J, Zuna I, et al. Relevance of sonographic B-mode criteria and computer-aided ultrasonic tissue characterization in differential-diagnosis of solid breast masses. *Ultrasound Med Biol* 2000;26(8):1243–1252.

Jackson VP, Rothschild PA, Kreipke DL, et al. The spectrum of sonographic findings of fibroadenoma of the breast. *Invest Radiol* 1986;21(1):34–40.

Jackson VP. Sonography of malignant breast disease. *Semin Ultrasound CT MR* 1989;10:119–131.

Jackson VP. Management of solid breast nodules: what is the role of sonography? *Radiology* 1995;196(1):14–15.

Jokich PM, Monticciolo DL, Adler YT. Breast sonography. *Radiol Clin North Am* 1992;30(5):993–1009.

Kamio T, Hamano K, Kameoka S, et al. Ultrasonographic diagnosis of breast cancer with intraductal spreading of cancer cells. *Nippon Geka Gakkai Zasshi* 1996;97(5):338–342.

Kasumi F. Can microcalcifications located within breast carcinomas be detected by ultrasound imaging? *Ultrasound Med Biol* 1988; 14[Suppl 1]:175–182.

Kimme-Smith C. Can quantitative ultrasound measurements help avoid breast biopsy? *AJR Am J Roentgenol* 1995;165(4):825–831.

Kobayashi T. Review: ultrasonic diagnosis of breast cancer. *Ultrasound Med Biol* 1975;1(1):383–391.

Kobayashi T. Gray-scale echography for breast cancer. *Radiology* 1977;122(1):207–214.

Kobayashi T. Diagnostic ultrasound in breast cancer: analysis of retrotumorous echo patterns correlated with sonic attenuation by cancerous connective tissues. *J Clin Ultrasound* 1979;7(6):471–479.

Kobayashi T. Ultrasonic detection of breast cancer. *Clin Obstet Gynecol* 1982;25(2):409–423.

Kobayashi T, Hayashi M, Arai M. Current status of ultrasonic tissue characterization in breast cancer. *J UOEH* 1984;6(4):397–410.

Kobayashi T. Hayashi M, Arai M. Echographic characteristics and ultrasonic tissue characterization in breast tumor. *J UOEH* 1985; 7(4):419–434.

Kobayashi T, Shinozaki H, Yomon M, et al. Hyperechoic pattern in breast cancer: its bio-acoustic genesis and tissue characterization. *J UOEH* 1989;11(2):181–187.

Kopans DB. More on sonographic features in the differentiation of fibroadenoma and invasive ductal carcinoma. *AJR Am J Roentgenol* 1998;171(4):109–114.

Kossoff G. Causes of shadowing in breast ultrasound. *Ultrasound Med Biol* 1988;14[Suppl 1]:s211–215.

Lambi RW, Hodgden D, Herma EM, et al. Sonomammographic manifestations of mammographically detectable breast microcalcifications. *J Ultrasound Med* 1983;2:509–514.

LeFebvre F, Meunier M, Thibault F, et al. Computerized ultrasound B-scan characterization of breast nodules. *Ultrasound Med Biol* 2000;26(9):1421–1428.

Leucht WJ, Rabe DR, Humbert KD. Diagnostic value of different interpretive criteria in real-time sonography of the breast. *Ultrasound Med Biol Suppl* 1988;1:59–73.

Leucht WJ, ed. *Teaching atlas of breast ultrasound*. New York: Thieme Medical, 1992.

Lister D, Evans AJ, Burrell HC, et al. The accuracy of breast ultrasound in the evaluation of clinically benign discrete, symptomatic breast lumps. *Clin Radiol* 1998;53(7):490–492.

Ludwig D, Trotshel H, Gmelin E. The value of sonography in the pathologic evaluation solid breast tumors. *Rofo Fortschr Geb Rontgenstr Neuen Bildgeb Verfahr* 1989;151(6):681–687.

Marquet KL, Funk A, Fendel H, et al. The echo-dense edge and hyper-reflective spikes: sensitive criteria for malignant processes in breast ultrasound. *Beburtshilfe Frauenheilkd* 1993;53(1):20–23.

Majewski A, Rosenthal H, Wagner HH. Results of real-time sonography and raster mammography of 200 breast cancers. *Rofo Forschr Geb Rontenstr Nukear Med* 1986;144(3):343–350.

Merritt CRB. Breast nodules: sonographic characterization. *RSNA Special Course in Ultrasound*, 1996:331–337.

Michaelson J, Staija S, Moore R, et al. Observations on invasive breast cancer diagnosed in a service screening and diagnostic breast imaging program. *J Womens Imaging* 2001;3:99–104.

Moon WK, Im JG, Koh YH, et al. US of mammographically detected clustered calcifications. *Radiology* 2000;217(3):849–854.

Moss HA, Britton PD, Flower CD, et al. How reliable is modern breast imaging in differentiating benign from malignant breast lesions in the symptomatic population? *Clin Radiol* 1999;54(1):676–682.

Nightingale KR, Kornguth PJ, Trahey GE. The use of acoustic streaming in breast lesion diagnosis: a clinical study. *Ultrasound Med Biol* 1999;25:75–87

Pisano ED. Breast. In: Mittelstadt CA, ed. *General ultrasound*. New York: Churchill Livingstone, 1992:59–103.

Rahbar G, Sie AC, Hansen G, et al. Benign versus malignant solid breast masses: differentiation. *Radiology* 1999;213:889–894.

Reeve TS, Jellins J, Kossoff G, et al. Ultrasonic visualization of breast cancer. *Aust N Z J Surg* 1978;48(3):278–281.

Richter K, Willrodt RG, Opri F, et al. Differentiation of breast lesions by measurements under craniocaudal and lateromedial compression using a new sonographic method. *Invest Radiol* 1996:401–414.

Rizzato G, Chersevani R, Abbona M, et al. High-resolution sonography of breast carcinoma. *Eur J Radiol* 1997;24(1):11–19.

Rosenberg AL, Schwartz GF, Feig SA, et al. Clinically occult breast lesions: localization and significance. *Radiology* 1987;162:167–170.

Rubin E. Cutting-edge sonography obviates breast biopsy. *Diagn Imaging* 1996:Sep[Suppl]:AU14–16, 32.

Sailer M, Schuster J, Mohr W. Sonographic findings in 133 breast tumors in relation to their connective tissue content. *Rontgenblatter* 1987;40(9):302–309.

Schepps B, Scola FH, Frates RE. Benign circumscribed breast masses. Mammographic and sonographic appearance. *Obstet Gynecol Clin North Am* 1994;21(3):519–537.

Scherziner AL, Belgam RA, Carson PL, et al. Assessment of ultrasonic computed tomography in symptomatic breast patients by discriminant analysis. *Ultrasound Med Biol* 1989;15(1):21–28.

Schutze B, Marx C, Fleck M, et al. Diagnostic evaluation of sonographically visualized breast lesions by using a new clinical amplitude/velocity reference imaging technique (CARI sonography). *Invest Radiol* 1998;33:341–347.

Shimato SH, Sawaki A, Niimi R, et al. Role of ultrasonography in the detection of intraductal spread of breast cancer: correlation with pathologic findings, mammography, and MR imaging. *Eur Radiol* 2000;10(11):1726–1732.

Sickles EA. Periodic mammographic follow-up of probably benign lesions: results in 3184 consecutive cases. *Radiology* 1991;179:463–468.

Skaane P, Sauer T. Ultrasonography of malignant breast neoplasms: analysis of carcinomas missed as tumor. *Acta Radiol* 1999;40:376–382.

Stavros AT, Thickman D, Rapp CL, et al. Solid breast nodules: use of sonography to distinguish between benign and malignant nodules. *Radiology* 1995;196:123–134.

Tabar L, Duffy SW, Burhenne LW. New Swedish breast cancer detection results for women aged 40–49. *Cancer* 1993;72:1437–1448.

Teboul M. A new concept in breast investigation: echo-histological acino-ductal analysis or analytic echography. *Biomed Pharmacother* 1988:42(4):289–295.

Teboul M. Echo-histological "acino-ductal analysis." Preliminary results. *Ultrasound Med Biol* 1988;14[Suppl 1]:s89–95.

Teboul M, Halliwell M. *Atlas of ultrasound and ductal echography of the breast: the introduction of anatomic intelligence into breast imaging.* London: Blackwell Scientific, 1995.

Teboul M. Anatomy of the breast. In: *Atlas of the ultrasound and ductal echography of the breast.* Teboul M, Halliwell M, eds. Cambridge, MA: Blackwell Science, 1995:49–82.

Ueno E, Tohno E, Soeda S. Dynamic tests in real-time breast echography. *Ultrasound Med Biol* 1988;14[Suppl 1]:s53–s57.

Wilkinson EJ, Bland KI. Techniques and results of aspiration cytology for diagnosis of benign and malignant diseases of the breast. *Surg Clin North Am* 1990;70:801–813.

Williams JC. US of solid breast nodules. *Radiology* 1996;198(2): 123–134.

13

BENIGN SOLID NODULES: SPECIFIC PATHOLOGIC DIAGNOSES

FIBROADENOMAS (ADENOFIBROMAS)

Pathology

Fibroadenomas are benign tumors that arise from the terminal ductolobular unit (TDLU) and that contain variable amounts of both stromal and epithelial elements. They have been described as giant lobules with uncoordinated growth of stromal and epithelial elements.

Grossly, fibroadenomas are firm, rubbery, and elliptical or gently lobulated in shape. However, some fibroadenomas are multilobulated or even microlobulated. A rim of compressed breast tissue usually encapsulates these benign tumors, meaning that the surgeon can easily "shell" them out of surrounding breast tissues at surgery.

Fibroadenomas can be divided into two main types histologically—intracanalicular and pericanalicular—that cannot be distinguished from each other morphologically or by mammography or sonography, which only show gross morphology. Fortunately, the clinical and radiographic inability to distinguish between pericanalicular and intracanalicular fibroadenomas is not significant because their natural history and outcome are identical. In fact, many fibroadenomas contain both intracanalicular and pericanalicular elements. The only significance is for the pathologist, who must occasionally distinguish between intracanalicular fibroadenoma and phyllodes tumor.

The histology of fibroadenomas varies from one lesion to another and can even vary from one part to another within a single fibroadenoma. The amounts of stromal and epithelial elements can be equal in some lesions, but in others, either stromal or epithelial elements can predominate (fibroadenoma or adenofibroma). Nodules composed almost entirely of stromal elements may be called fibromas and those composed primarily of epithelial elements may be called adenomas. The stroma can be highly cellular or paucicellular and can also undergo myxoid change, sclero-

sis, hyalinization, and calcification. It may be difficult to distinguish fibrosclerosis from a fibroadenoma whose stroma has become hyalinized or sclerotic. The composition of the stroma can affect the palpable characteristics of fibroadenoma. Myxoid degeneration makes lesions softer, whereas sclerosis, hyalinization, and calcification increase firmness. The composition of fibroadenomas also affects the sonographic appearance—primarily influencing their echogenicity, sound transmission characteristics, and compressibility.

Fibroadenomas are thought to arise in a single TDLU and grow by incorporation of the surrounding breast tissue. These tumors may, therefore, incorporate fat and other TDLUs, primarily in the periphery of the lesion. The surrounding TDLUs that are incorporated into fibroadenomas are subject to the same proliferative and fibrocystic changes as any other TDLUs—apocrine metaplasia, ductal hyperplasia, blunt duct adenosis, and sclerosing adenosis. Thus, fibroadenomas may contain the entire spectrum of fibrocystic and benign proliferative changes. Such changes occur in up to 50% of all fibroadenomas. TDLUs that have been incorporated into fibroadenomas can also undergo secretory change during pregnancy or lactation as well as in patients taking birth control pills. Fibroadenomas that contain apocrine metaplasia, cysts, epithelial calcifications, or sclerosing adenosis have been classified as complex fibroadenomas.

Fibroadenomas are usually encapsulated by a pseudo-capsule of compressed breast tissue, indicating that the growth of the leading edge of the nodule is noninvasive or pushing rather than infiltrating.

Fibroadenomas can grow rapidly but usually do not become larger than 2 to 3 cm. Giant fibroadenomas and juvenile fibroadenomas are the exceptions, often growing rapidly larger than 3 cm, up to 6 to 10 cm. In recent years, giant and juvenile fibroadenomas are more usually termed *fibroadenomas with highly cellular stroma*. The histologic distinction of fibroadenomas with cellular stroma from benign phyllodes tumor can be difficult. These variant lesions are discussed in greater detail in the next section.

Fibroadenomas can rarely undergo total or partial infarction. This phenomenon is most common during pregnancy or lactation. Infarcted fibroadenomas tend to become irregular in shape and adherent to adjacent breast tissues, making distinction from malignant nodules on gross and sonographic examination more difficult.

Fibroadenomas rarely undergo malignant change (about 1 in 1,000). In about half of these cases, the malignancy associated with fibroadenomas is lobular carcinoma *in situ* (LCIS). About 15% of malignant degeneration is ductal carcinoma *in situ* (DCIS), and about 35% degeneration results in an infiltrating malignancy, either infiltrating ductal or lobular carcinoma. In addition, it is likely that certain phyllodes tumors evolve from preexisting cellular fibroadenomas rather than *de novo*.

Epidemiology

Overall, fibroadenomas are the third most common cause of biopsy for benign breast conditions but are the most common cause precipitating biopsy in adolescents and young adults (younger than 30 years of age). Fibroadenomas are much more common than cysts in this young age group. The peak incidence occurs during the third decade, with a second peak in the fifth decade. Estrogen stimulation is thought to be important in the formation and growth of fibroadenomas. Not surprisingly, these lesions most commonly occur during periods when anovulatory cycles (unopposed estrogen) are most frequent—adolescence and the perimenopausal years. They also tend to enlarge rapidly during the first trimester of pregnancy, when estrogen levels are very high. Although fibroadenomas are more common in younger patients, these lesions can be seen in patients in their 80s. Most postmenopausal fibroadenomas were probably present before menopause, but occasionally, *de novo* postmenopausal development can occur, usually, but not always, induced by hormone replacement therapy (HRT).

That the incidence of fibroadenomas tends to diminish with age suggests that the lesions spontaneously regress with age. The histologic composition of the stroma supports this hypothesis. Younger patients generally have more cellular stroma, whereas the stroma of fibroadenomas in postmenopausal patients is more likely to be hyalinized or calcified. Nevertheless, hyalinization and calcification may occasionally be seen in younger patients, and cellular stroma may occasionally be seen in older patients.

Multiple fibroadenomas occur in about 20% to 25% of patients. These lesions may be bilateral. A small group of patients tends to develop multiple, bilateral fibroadenomas, which recur in cycles. Fibroadenomas are more common and more often multiple, bilateral, and larger in the black population.

Not all fibroadenomas that occur in adolescents are classified as juvenile fibroadenomas. In fact, only about 5% to 10% of the fibroadenomas in adolescents meet the definition of a juvenile fibroadenoma. The diagnosis of juvenile fibroadenoma implies the presence of highly cellular stroma. Juvenile fibroadenomas are discussed in greater detail in the following section on fibroadenoma variants.

Clinical Findings

Fibroadenomas that are detected sonographically may come to ultrasound because of a palpable abnormality or a mammographic abnormality, or they may simply be incidental sonographic findings. Palpable fibroadenomas are usually firm, rubbery, mobile and not associated with pain or tenderness. The clinical findings, however, can vary with the pathology. Fibroadenomas that are undergoing infarction (usually during pregnancy or lactation) may cause pain and tenderness. When the stroma is myxomatous or cellular, the fibroadenoma is usually softer. On the other hand, fibroadenomas in which the stroma has become sclerotic or hyalinized, or in which dense calcification has occurred, are very firm to palpation. Previously infarcted fibroadenomas may become fixed to surrounding tissues and therefore nonmobile.

Mammographic Findings

Fibroadenomas that are surrounded by dense breast tissue may not be mammographically visible. Those that are visible are classically well circumscribed; round, ovoid, or gently lobulated in shape; and isodense with an equal volume of surrounding fibroglandular elements. These lesions may also be partially obscured on routine two-view mammograms. Degenerated fibroadenomas may have characteristically benign internal calcifications that show one of two patterns: dense, central calcifications having a popcorn appearance, or peripheral rimlike calcification (Fig. 13–1, left). Circular rimlike calcifications may be difficult to distinguish from calcification within a cyst wall (Fig. 13–1, middle). Calcified cysts are more likely to appear circular in shape, whereas fibroadenomas are more likely appear to be elliptical in shape.

Of course, not all fibroadenomas are mammographically classic. Some are more lobulated or even microlobulated. In general, the more numerous and smaller the lobulations, the more suspicious the findings are for malignancy. Previously infarcted fibroadenomas can have angular, jagged, or irregular margins. Hyalinized fibroadenomas can appear to be hyperdense rather than isodense. Early in the course of dystrophic calcification, before one of the two classically benign patterns has become fully developed, calcifications within a degenerating fibroadenoma can be difficult to distinguish from the granular and pleomorphic calcifications associated with malignancy (Fig. 13–1, right).

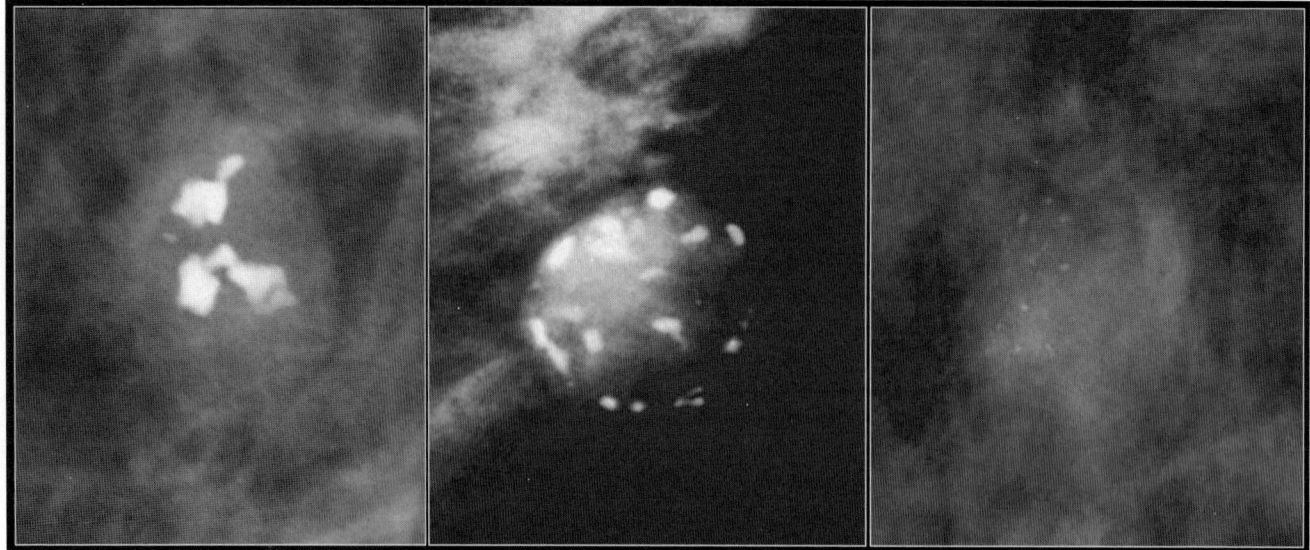

FIGURE 13–1 Coarse and dense popcorn-like calcifications are so typical of degenerated fibroadenomas that they are considered BIRADS 2, definitively benign, mammographically. Nodules that contain such calcifications do not require additional evaluation with sonography (**left**). This calcifying fibroadenoma has rimlike calcifications as well as central calcifications. Although the rim is not completely calcified yet, the pattern of peripheral rimlike calcification is also a BIRADS 2 mammographic finding that obviates further imaging evaluation and biopsy (**middle**). These clustered granular calcifications lie within a fibroadenoma. At some point, they will likely coalesce to form coarse and dense popcorn-like calcifications that are typically benign. At the present time, however, they must be considered mildly suspicious (mainly for intermediate-nuclear-grade ductal carcinoma *in situ*), must be characterized as BIRADS 4a or higher, and must undergo biopsy (**right**).

Spot compression films can better define the borders of fibroadenomas that are partially obscured on standard mammographic views. However, because ultrasound would be performed in such patients anyway to determine whether the lesion is cystic or solid, ultrasound can be employed first and will be the only examination necessary in most patients.

A round, oval, or gently curved and lobulated, well-circumscribed nodule has a 2% or less chance of being malignant based on mammographic characteristics alone. For this reason, many radiologists recommend spot compression films to confirm the presence of probably benign mammographic characteristics. The patient can then be offered short-interval mammographic follow-up. However, we believe that mammographic lesions should be as completely characterized as possible before recommending short-interval follow-up mammograms. Sonography shows whether a lesion is cystic or solid. Mammography does not. Short-interval follow-up on mammographic Breast Imaging Reporting and Data System (BIRADS) category 3 lesions would include many cysts that do not require short-interval follow-up. (Simple cysts and most complicated cysts do not require short interval follow-up. Only solid nodules that meet strict criteria for probably benign, BIRADS 3 classification and some complicated cysts require short-interval follow-up.) Thus, sonography is better for determining the management of mammographic nodules than is diagnostic mammography, and we do not see the need for spot compression mammograms in mammographic nodules that do not contain calcifications.

Sonographic Findings

The benign findings discussed in Chapter 12 correspond to classic sonographic findings. The sonographic findings for fibroadenomas may not always be classic. Nonclassic findings tend to require exclusion of the lesion from BIRADS 3 classification and characterization of the lesion as mildly suspicious, BIRADS 4a (characterization is discussed in Chapter 12).

The classic fibroadenoma displays the following sonographic findings:

- Elliptical or gently lobulated *shape*
- Larger in the transverse and craniocaudal dimensions than in the anteroposterior (AP) dimension (wider-than-tall *orientation*)
- Isoechoic or mildly hypoechoic *echotexture* with respect to fat
- Encompassed completely by a thin echogenic *capsule*
- *Sound transmission* that is either normal or increased in comparison to the transmission of the surrounding tissues

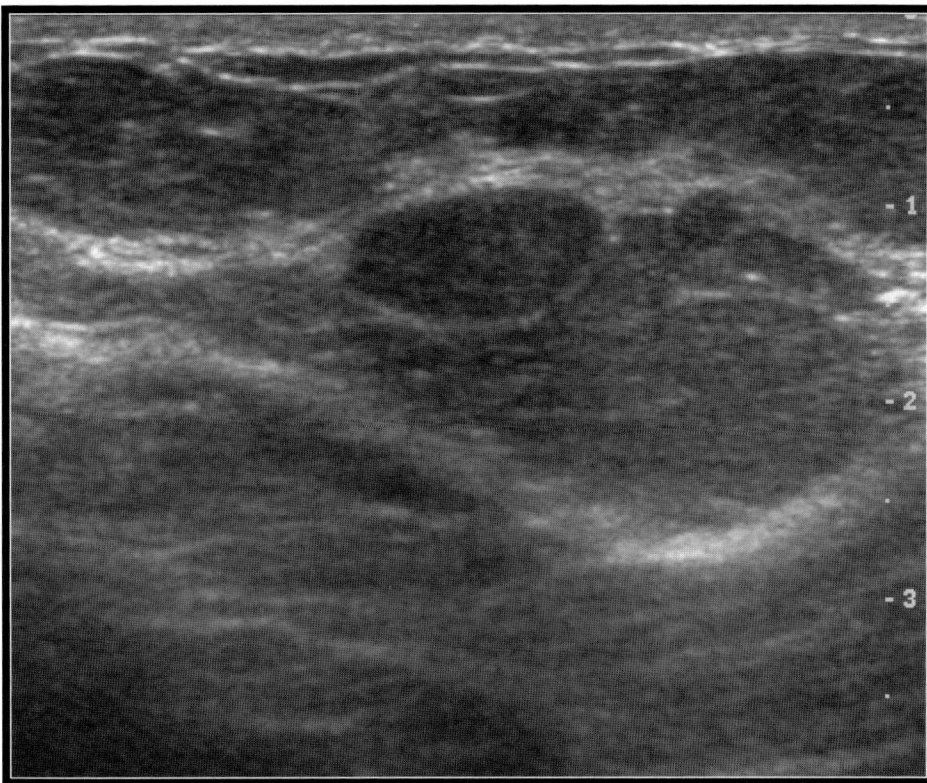

FIGURE 13–2 An elliptical, wider-than-tall shape is the most commonly seen shape of fibroadenomas, occurring in about one-half of cases.

- *Thin edge shadows*
- Mobile during palpation, not fixed to surrounding tissues
- Slightly compressible

These findings vary from nodule to nodule, reflecting the underlying histology of each fibroadenoma. Certain findings require special techniques for adequate demonstration.

Shape

The classic fibroadenoma is elliptical in shape (Fig. 13–2), possibly being gently lobulated with just two or three lobulations (Fig. 13–3). In our 1995 study, about 75% of benign solid breast nodules had either an ellipsoid or gently lobulated shape with three or fewer smoothly curving lobulations. Recent data show the percentage of lobulated fibroadenomas to be larger than the percentage of elliptically shaped fibroadenomas. Some fibroadenomas that appear to be elliptically shaped in one plane appear to be lobulated in other planes (Fig. 13–4). As fibroadenomas enlarge, they are less likely to remain elliptically shaped (Fig. 13–5). Furthermore, as fibroadenomas enlarge, they are more likely to develop more than three lobulations or microlobulations,

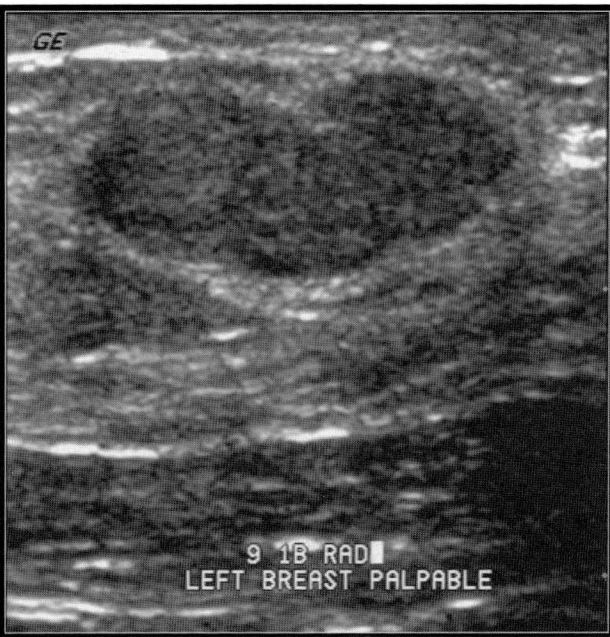

FIGURE 13–3 A wider-than-tall shape with three or fewer lobulations is the second most common shape of fibroadenomas, occurring in about one-fourth of cases.

532   *Breast Ultrasound*

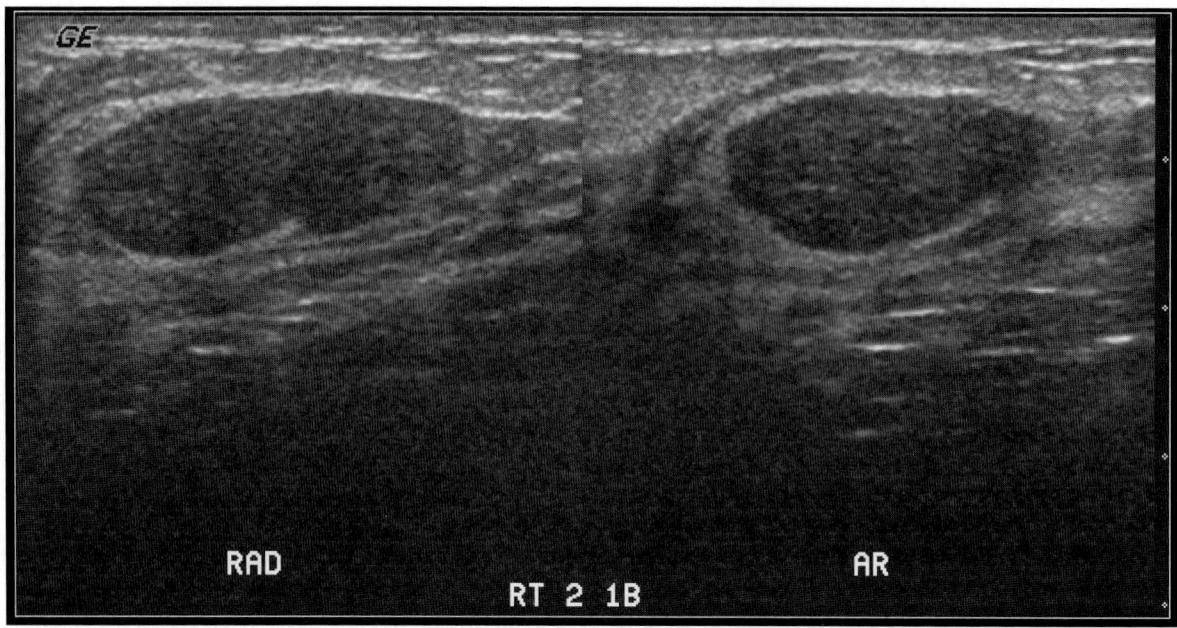

FIGURE 13–4 Whether a fibroadenoma appears elliptical in shape or gently lobulated depends on the plane in which it is examined. Many lesions may appear elliptical in one plane (**right**) but gently lobulated in the orthogonal plane (**left**). AR, antiradial, RAD, radial.

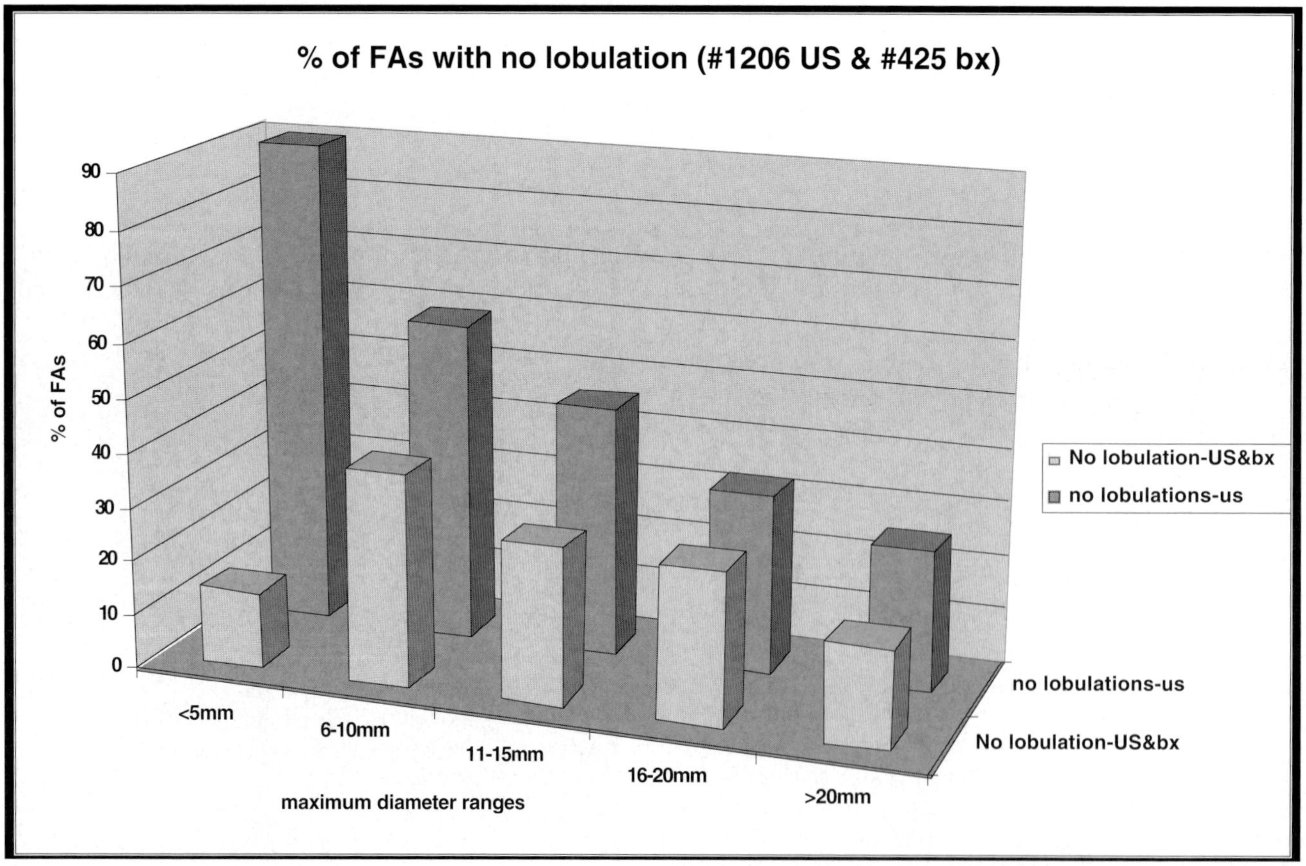

% of FAs with no lobulation (#1206 US & #425 bx)

FIGURE 13–5 As fibroadenomas enlarge, the odds of their remaining elliptical decrease. The subgroup of fibroadenomas that undergo biopsy is less likely to be elliptical than are those in the population in general.

features that currently still require BIRADS 4a classification (Figs. 13–6 to 13–8). Within the group of fibroadenomas that undergo biopsy, the percentage of fibroadenomas with more than three lobulation or microlobulations is higher than in the nonbiopsy populations, in many cases because the presence of the lobulations leads to BIRADS 4a or higher classification that mandates biopsy.

Table 13–1 shows the distribution of fibroadenomas by lobulations in the 1995 study. In this population, all solid nodules underwent biopsy, regardless of sonographic classification. Thus, this population should be representative of the entire group of fibroadenomas.

Table 13–2 shows the distribution of fibroadenomas by lobulations in the current ongoing study. This group includes the 425 fibroadenomas that underwent biopsy as well as the 871 nodules that did not undergo biopsy. The nodules that did not undergo biopsy were followed with ultrasound. On subsequent follow-up studies, none of the lesions that were sonographically classified as fibroadenomas have been shown to be malignant. In the current group that has undergone biopsy, the percentage of fibroadenomas with an elliptical shape or three or fewer lobulations is smaller than in the overall group, and the percentage of nodules with four or more lobulations or microlobulations is higher than in 1995.

Mammographic studies have shown that the more numerous and smaller the lobulations on the surface of a nodule, the greater its likelihood of being malignant. Our study confirms this hypothesis. Table 13–3 shows the risk of cancer versus the shape of the nodule. Note that solid nodules with three or fewer lobulations must also be completely encompassed within a thin, echogenic capsule for the risk for malignancy to be less than 2%. Clearly, based on these data, there is an increased risk for malignant degeneration as the number of lobulations increases and the size of the lobulations decreases. There is no certainty as to how many lobulations may be present before the risk for malignancy is increased enough that biopsy becomes essential. Possibly, the presence of three or fewer lobulations is an excessively strict criterion for benignity, and four or five lobulations would make a better cutoff point. However, study was not performed to assess what number of lobulations would make the best cutoff. Our study did show significantly increased risk for cancer in nodules that had more than three lobulations but that were not microlobulated (12.1% regardless of capsule and 5.5% when associated with a thin, echogenic capsule). This is more than the 2% or less risk required for BIRADS 3 classification, even when there is a thin, echogenic capsule. On the other hand, the risk for malignancy in elliptical or gently lobulated nodules with three or fewer lobulations was much lower (<2%), low enough for BIRADS 3 classification in the absence of other suspicious findings.

Occasionally, fibroadenomas may be spherical in shape, usually when they are less than 1 cm in size (Fig. 13–9). Such lesions may be difficult or even impossible to distinguish from complex cysts associated with fibrocystic change. Spherical shape is generally more suggestive of a fluid-containing structure under pressure, a common situation in cysts that contain actively secreting metaplastic

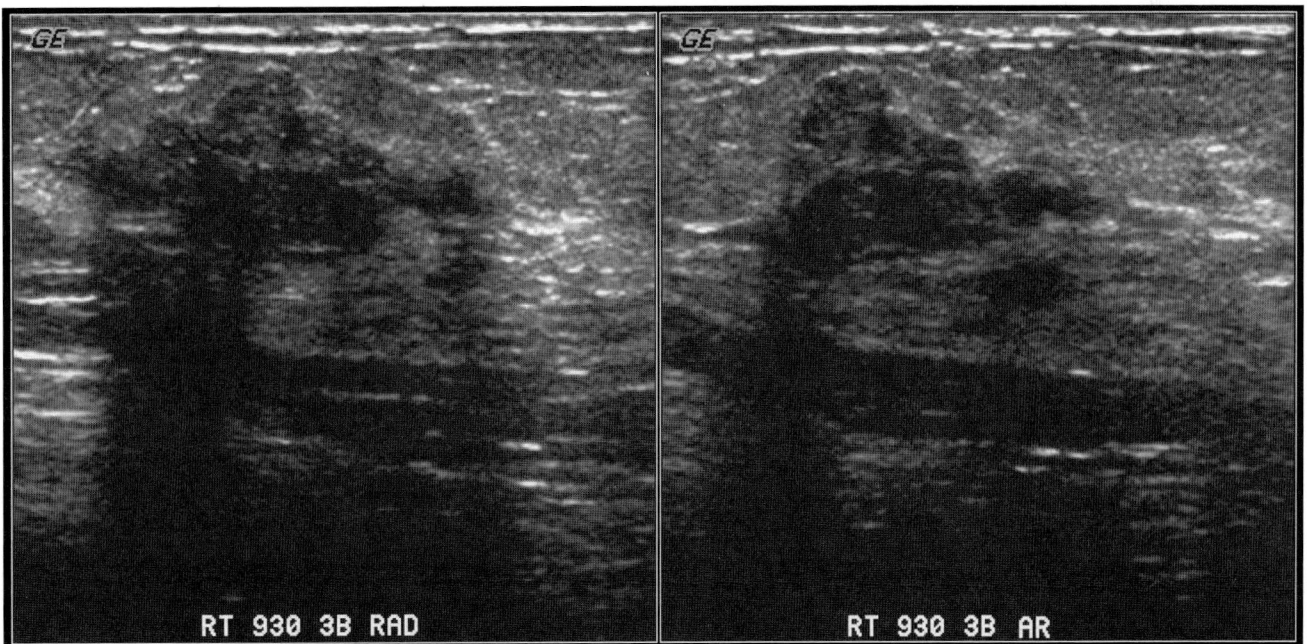

FIGURE 13–6 The larger a fibroadenoma becomes, the more likely it is to develop findings that require BIRADS 4a classification—more than three lobulations or microlobulations.

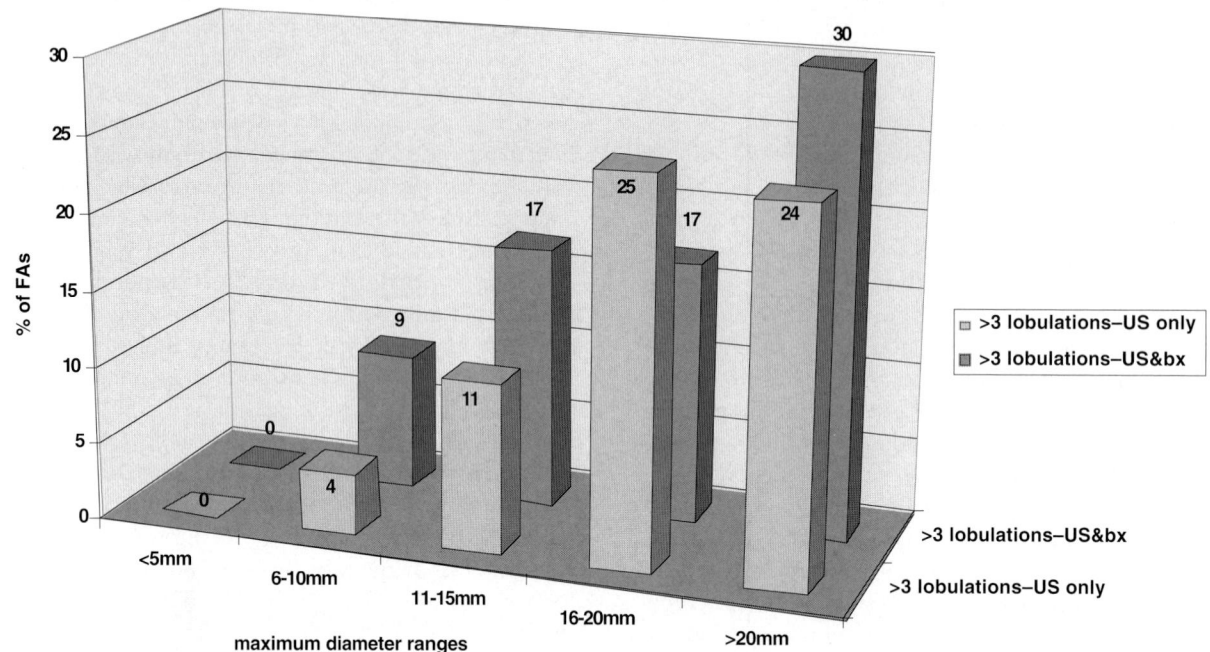

FIGURE 13–7 The larger the maximum diameter of a fibroadenoma, the more likely it is to develop more than three lobulations. This is true for both the subgroup of fibroadenomas that undergo biopsy as well as for the entire group.

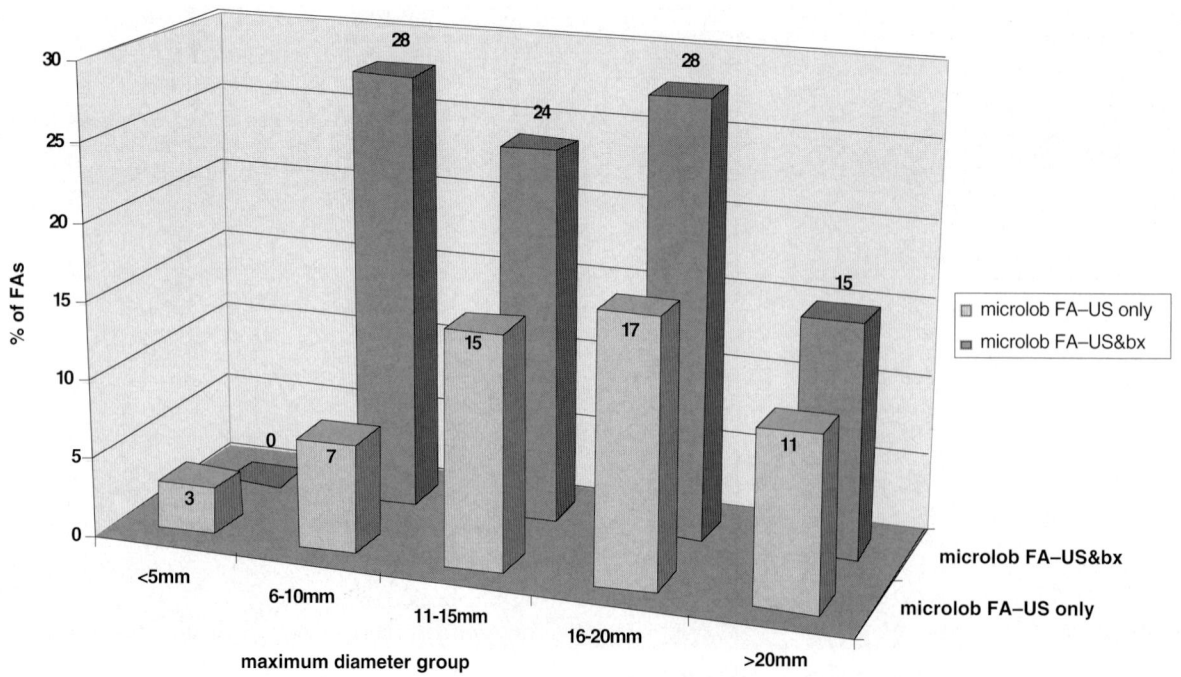

FIGURE 13–8 Microlobulation is more common in larger fibroadenomas than in smaller lesions. This is especially true for fibroadenomas that undergo biopsy.

TABLE 13–1. 1995 STUDY: ALL BIOPSY

Lobulation Pattern	No. of Fibroadenomas	Percentage of Fibroadenomas
Elliptical	173	53
Three or fewer lobulations	77	24
Four or more lobulations, but not microlobulated	31	9
Microlobulated	46	14
Total	327	100

TABLE 13–3. CURRENT STUDY: RISK FOR MALIGNANCY VERSUS LOBULATIONS (1,352 SOLID NODULES)

Nodule Shape	Percentage Malignant : Any Capsule	Percentage Malignant : Thin Capsule
Elliptical	1.9	1.7
Three or fewer lobulations	2.5	1.0
More than three lobulations, but not microlobulated	12.1	5.5
Microlobulated	51.3	21.1

apocrine cells, foam cells, macrophages, white blood cells, red blood cells, proteinaceous and cellular debris, or cholesterol crystals that give rise to internal echogenicity. In certain cases, it is impossible to distinguish between fibroadenoma and complex cysts containing diffuse, low-level, internal echogenicity (discussed in greater detail in Chapter 10).

Regardless of the lobulation pattern, there are some fibroadenomas that show angular margins along all or part of their surfaces (Fig. 13–10). Fortunately, this finding, which is worrisome for malignancy, is uncommon, occurring in only 5% of fibroadenomas. There are several possible causes for this finding in fibroadenomas: a few cases have demonstrated evidence of old infarction; others are markedly hyalinized; and still others represent complex fibroadenomas that contain florid sclerosing adenosis. (Complex fibroadenomas are discussed in greater detail later in this chapter.) Pathologists have hypothesized that the reaction of the fibroadenoma and surrounding tissue to infarction can cause the fibroadenoma to become fixed to surrounding tissues and therefore make the borders indistinct or the shape irregular.

Fibroadenomas may also assume shapes that simulate or represent duct extension and branch pattern (Figs. 13–11 and 13–12). Both of these findings are even more unusual in fibroadenomas than angular margins, each being found in only 2% of fibroadenomas. Most fibroadenomas arise within the lobule (TDLU) and grow by peripheral expansion, rather than by spreading throughout the ductal system. Fibroadenoma shapes, therefore, represent expansile, nonductal, growth patterns. However, some fibroadenomas immediately adjacent to large ducts may grow in a manner that causes indentation and invagination into the duct. Volume averaging of the duct with the invaginating portion of the fibroadenoma may simulate duct extension or branching growth patterns. Rarely, a subtype of fibroadenoma, a ductal adenoma, may arise within a duct and may manifest a ductal shape (Fig. 13–13).

Spiculation of fibroadenomas is extremely rare. Only one fibroadenoma in this series was spiculated, representing only 0.3% of all fibroadenomas. The lesion was a complex fibroadenoma in which florid sclerosing adenosis in its periphery caused spiculation.

Orientation

Most fibroadenomas, regardless of their pattern of lobulations, angular margins, duct extension, or branch pattern, grow with major axes aligned parallel to the skin (craniocaudal, transverse, radial, and antiradial directions) and the minor axes oriented in the AP dimension. The shape is, therefore, perceived as wider than tall when the patient is scanned in the supine position. There are several reasons for this orientation. First, normal tissue planes in the breast are horizontally arranged. Noninfiltrating, expansile growth shown by fibroadenomas tends to proceed within existing tissue planes along the path of least resistance. Second, most fibroadenomas are mildly to moderately compressible in the AP dimension. Third, because fibroadenomas are normally mobile, steeply or obliquely oriented fibroadenomas in the

TABLE 13–2. CURRENT STUDY: ULTRASOUND-ONLY AND ULTRASOUND AND BIOPSY GROUPS

Lobulation Pattern	No. of Fibroadenomas (%): Ultrasound-only Group	No. of Fibroadenomas (%): Ultrasound Group at Biopsy
Elliptical	644 (50)	119 (28)
Three or fewer lobulations	405 (31)	73 (17)
Four or more lobulations, but not microlobulated	120 (9)	123 (29)
Microlobulated	129 (10)	108 (26)
Total	1,296 (100)	425 (100)

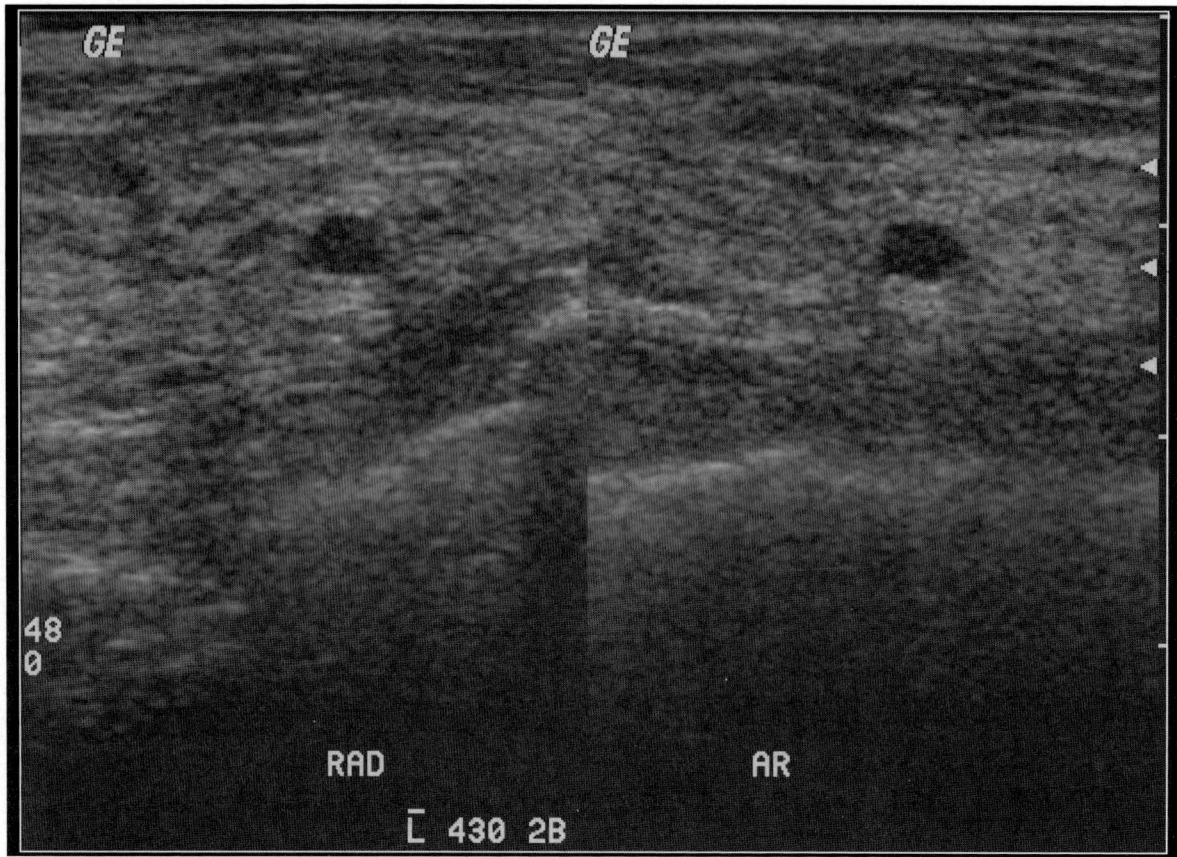

FIGURE 13–9 A small fraction of fibroadenomas are nearly spherical in shape. Such lesions can be very difficult to distinguish from complex cysts with echogenic, inspissated fluid.

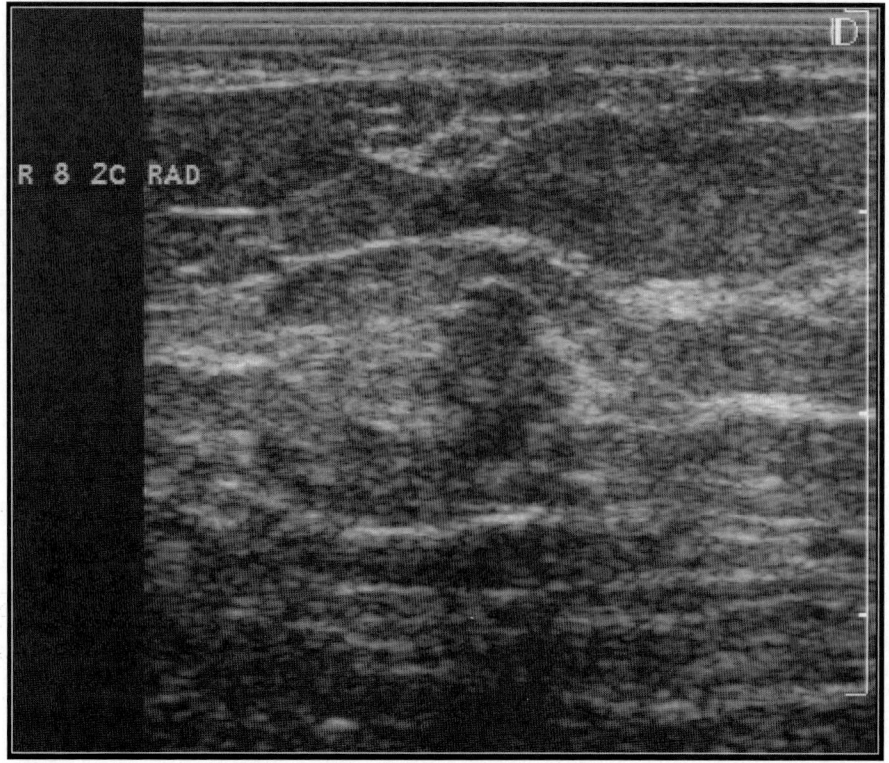

FIGURE 13–10 A small percentage of fibroadenomas develop angular margins because of previous infarction and adherence to surrounding tissues, because of intense hyalinization, or because the lesion is a complex fibroadenoma with exuberant sclerosing adenosis affecting its margins. This lesion had previously undergone infarction and was adherent to surrounding tissues.

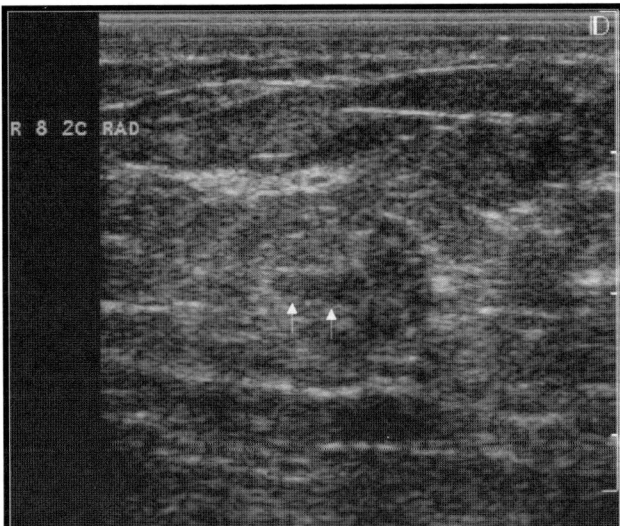

FIGURE 13–11 Duct extension *(arrows)* is a finding far more typical of malignant lesions with intraductal components than of fibroadenomas. However, occasional fibroadenomas such as this one can develop duct extensions.

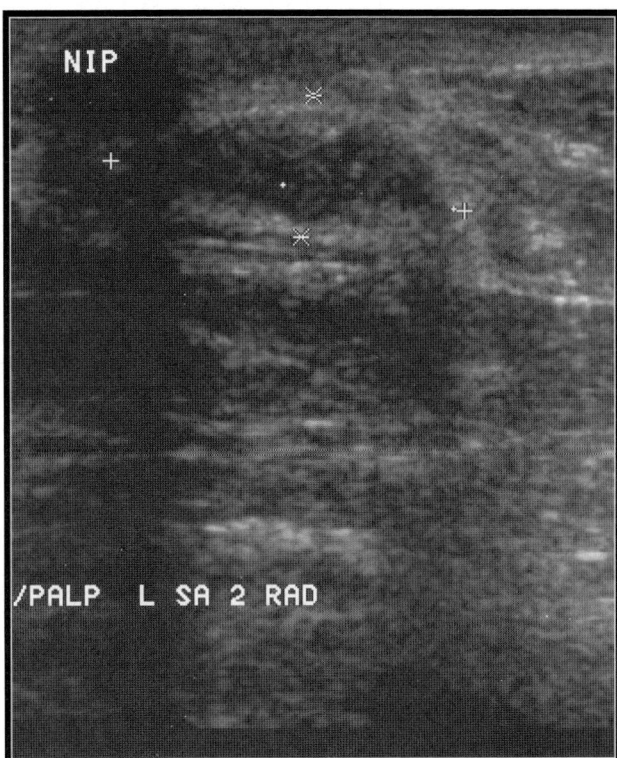

FIGURE 13–13 Rarely, a fibroadenoma may form within the periareolar ducts and give rise to what is termed a *ductal adenoma.*

absence of compression will usually rotate horizontally once the probe pressure is applied during scanning (see Chapter 3, Figs. 3–17). Although many carcinomas, especially large ones, are similar to fibroadenomas (i.e., wider than tall), only rarely are fibroadenomas likely to be taller than wide (Fig. 13–14). In this series, only 3 of 327 biopsied fibroadenomas (0.9%) were taller than wide.

Echotexture

Most fibroadenomas are isoechoic to mildly hypoechoic with respect to breast fat. In fact, in the series presented in the previous chapter, 95.4% of fibroadenomas had a background (internal) echogenicity that was either isoechoic or very mildly hypoechoic with respect to fat. Additionally, 3.1% of fibroadenomas were markedly hypoechoic, and 0.9% were completely or partially hyperechoic. Keep in mind that although marked hypoechogenicity is worrisome for carcinoma, isoechogenicity or mild hypoechogenicity is not necessarily reassuring. About 50% of carcinomas are markedly hypoechoic, but about half are nearly isoechoic and similar in echogenicity to fibroadenomas. For this reason, despite the overwhelming tendency for fibroadenomas to be isoechoic to mildly hypoechoic, this finding was not very helpful in distinguishing fibroadenomas from carcinoma.

The echogenicity of fibroadenomas tends to parallel its histologic makeup. Fibroadenomas are composed of a variable mixture of stromal and epithelial elements. In general, a higher degree of epithelial elements tend to produce a mildly hypoechoic appearance (Fig. 13–15), whereas a greater stromal composition results in an increased, more isoechoic appearance (Fig. 13–16). Homogeneous distribution of epithelial and stromal elements tends to contribute

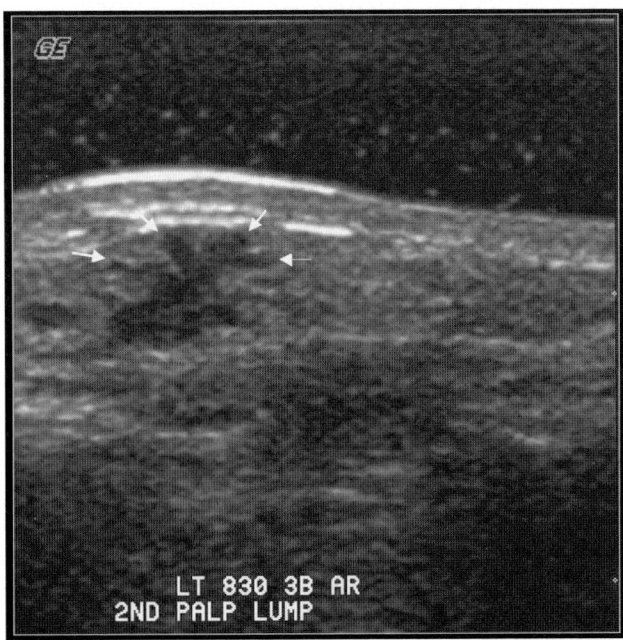

FIGURE 13–12 Findings such as duct extension and branch pattern *(arrows)* that occur far more frequently in malignant lesions can occasionally also be seen in fibroadenomas such as this previously infarcted one.

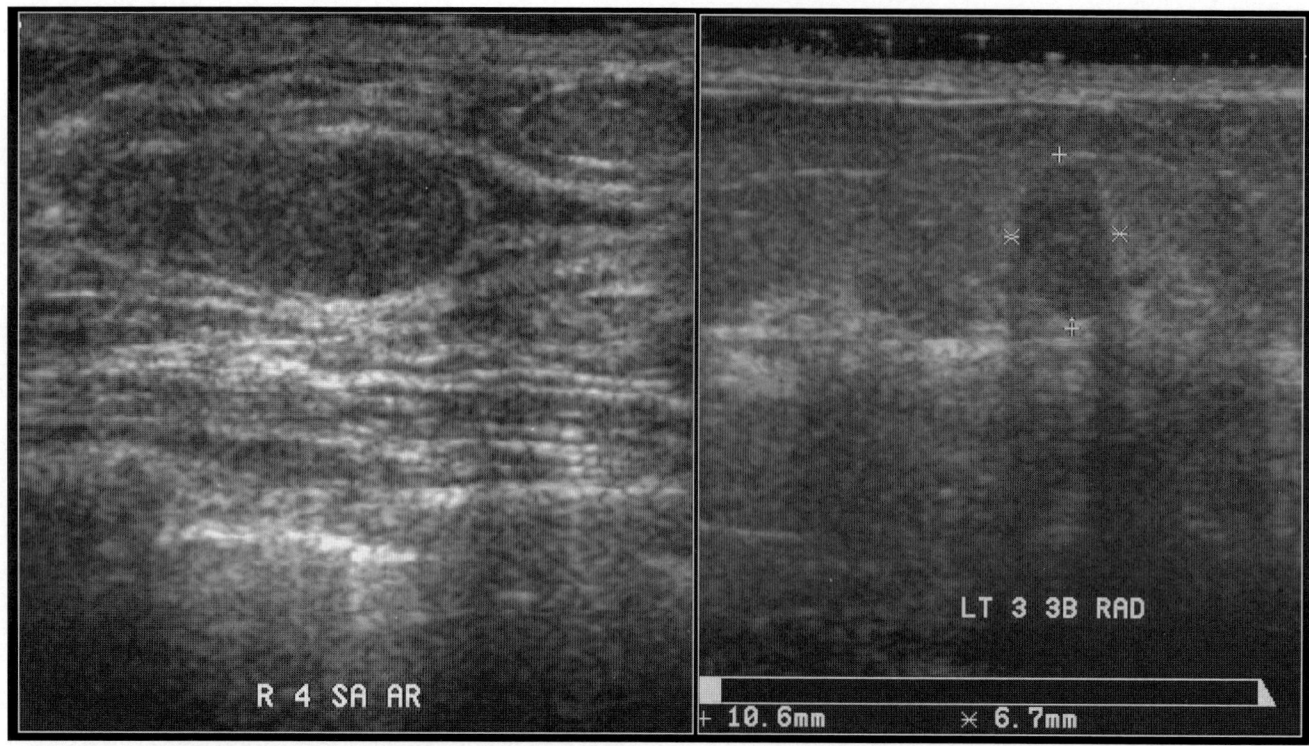

FIGURE 13–14 Most fibroadenomas are wider than tall (**left**), but a rare fibroadenoma may have a suspicious taller-than-wide shape (**right**) that excludes it from BIRADS 3 characterization and indicates the need for biopsy.

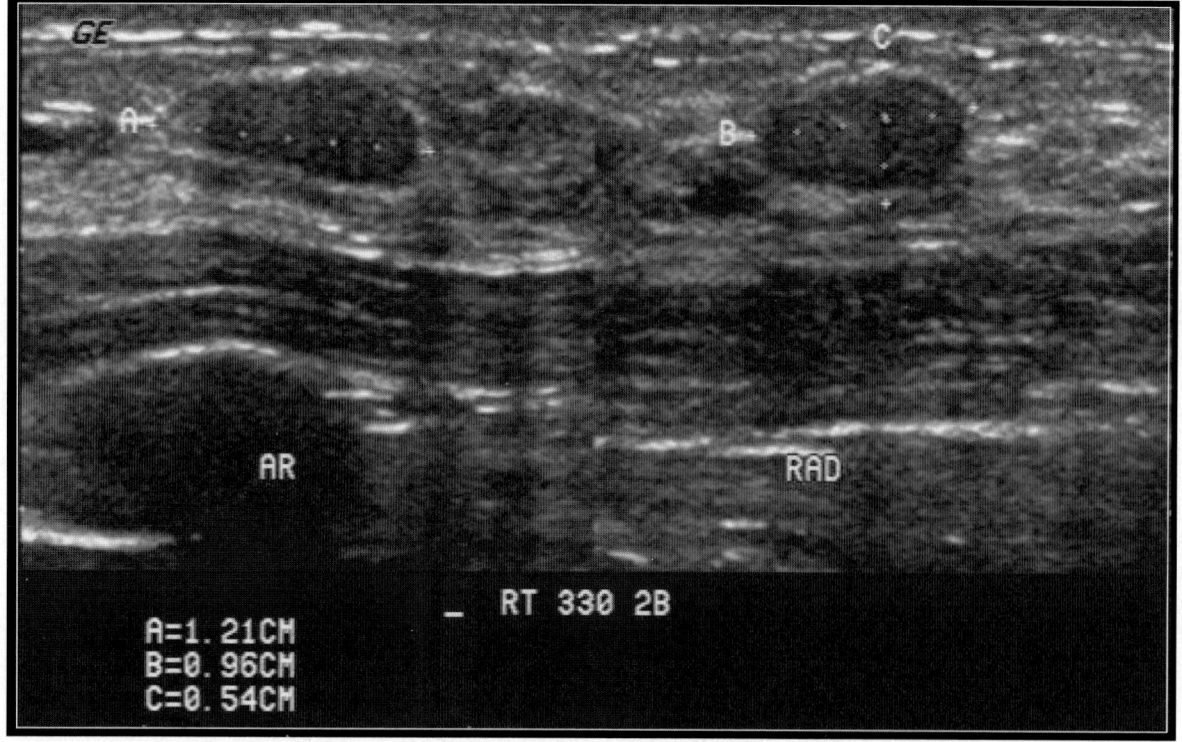

FIGURE 13–15 Most fibroadenomas are either mildly hypoechoic (such as this lesion) or iso-echoic. Histologic features contributing to hypoechogenicity are large epithelial components, homogeneous distribution of epithelial and stromal elements, and the presence of cellular stroma.

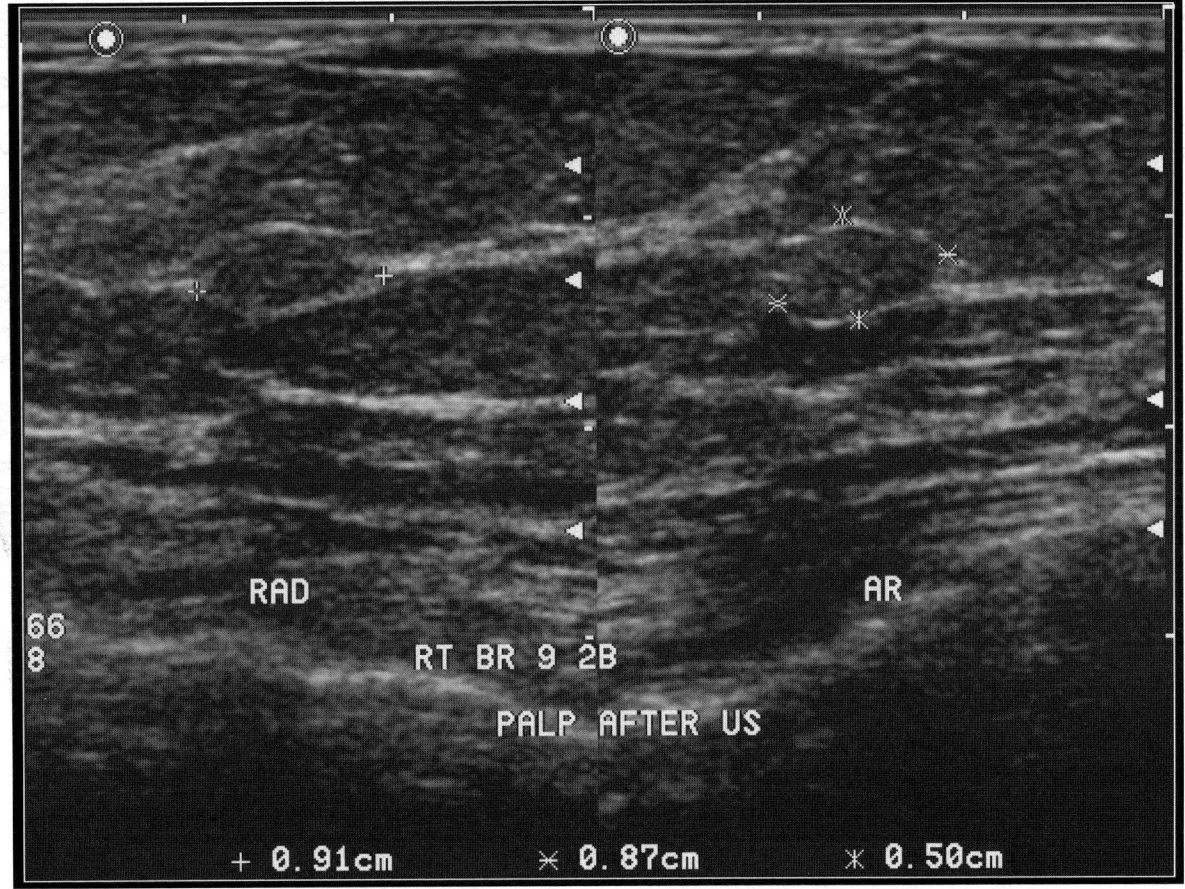

FIGURE 13–16 Fibroadenomas with relatively larger stromal components and smaller epithelial components and those that have paucicellular stroma are more likely to be isoechoic.

to hypoechogenicity, whereas heterogeneous involvement tends to increase echogenicity. In addition to variations in the relative proportions of epithelium and stroma, the composition of the stromal component varies from nodule to nodule and even within an individual nodule. The stroma may be highly cellular (fibroblasts), paucicellular (most common situation), or acellular. Fibroadenomas with cellular stroma tend to be more hypoechoic than those with paucicellular stroma (Fig. 13–17). Fibroadenomas with acellular stroma tend to be more isoechoic and can even be mildly hyperechoic if there is associated sclerosis, hyalinization, or calcification of the stroma (Fig. 13–18). Finally, the stroma may be myxomatous. In past experience, this tissue composition generally corresponds to mild hypoechogenicity. Heterogeneous areas of increased or decreased echogenicity may be present within complex fibroadenomas (those associated with apocrine metaplasia or sclerosing adenosis), which is discussed later in this chapter.

The displayed and perceived echogenicity of solid breast nodules will vary with transducer frequency and bandwidth. This concept is important to remember because nodules that are displayed as relatively hypoechoic with respect to fat or glandular tissue are more conspicuous and more easily perceived. Those nodules that are displayed as completely isoechoic are less conspicuous and more easily overlooked. Nodules that appear completely isoechoic and difficult to perceive with a 5-MHz probe have been shown often to appear mildly hypoechoic and thus are more easily perceived with a 7.5-MHz, broadbandwidth probe. Therefore, using higher-frequency and broader-bandwidth transducers minimizes the risk for overlooking certain fibroadenomas. However, even with optimal transducer frequency and bandwidth, there are fibroadenomas that will be completely isoechoic with fat.

Isoechogenicity of fibroadenomas decreases their conspicuity in patients whose breasts are completely fatty or composed of isoechoic glandular tissue (e.g., adenosis of pregnancy). A circumscribed, isodense nodule that is completely surrounded by fat on mammograms but is not readily detectable on ultrasound must be assumed to be solid and isoechoic because all simple and complex cysts would be hypoechoic compared with fat and should be easily detected sonographically. Rocking the probe on the area of interest will often be helpful because a fibroadenoma will

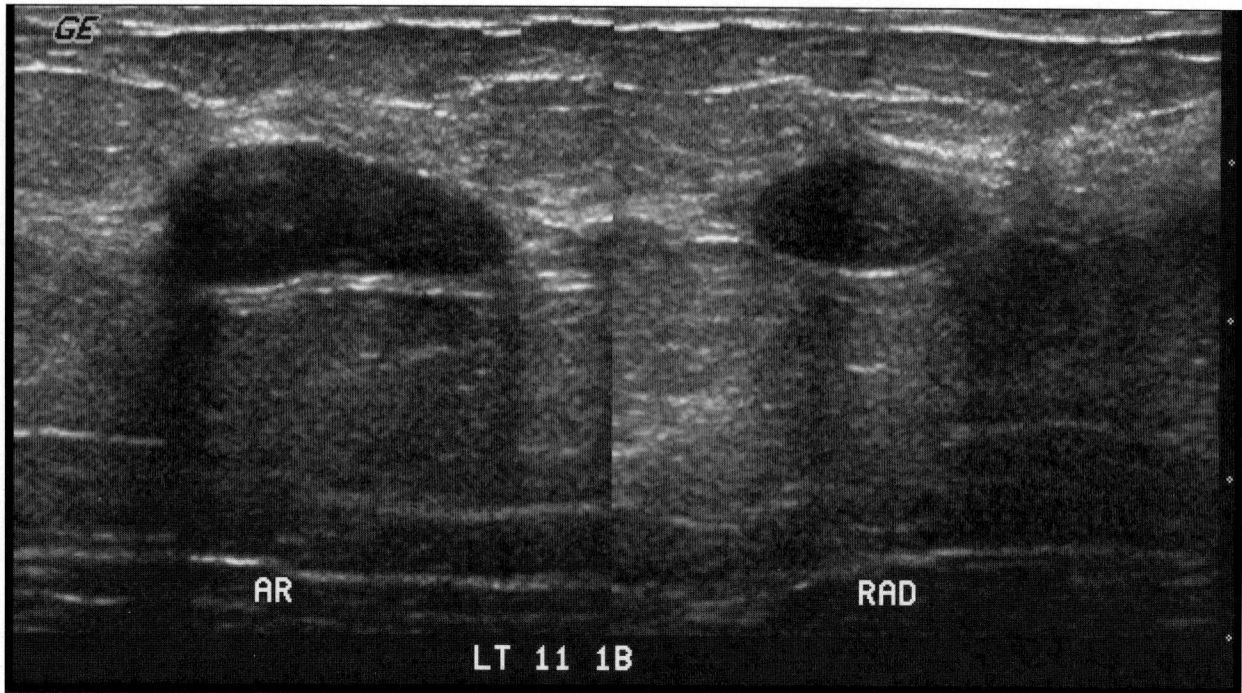

FIGURE 13–17 Fibroadenomas that have highly cellular stroma tend to be more hypoechoic than those with paucicellular stroma and tend to have enhanced through-transmission.

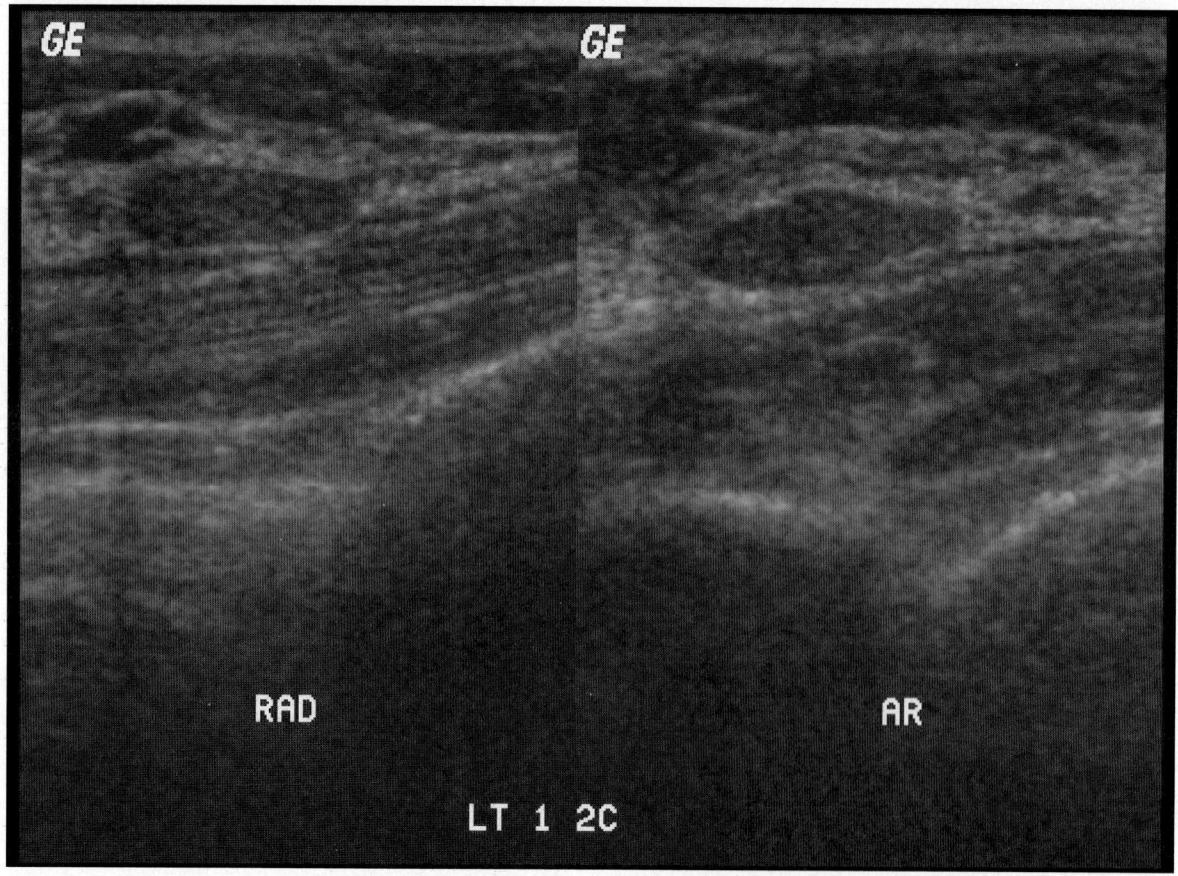

FIGURE 13–18 Fibroadenomas with paucicellular or acellular stroma tend to be isoechoic.

be completely surrounded by an echogenic capsule, appearing to flash in and out of view as the probe is rocked back and forth. Most fat lobules will not be completely circumscribed by an echogenic capsule and, with rotation of the ultrasound probe, will open into adjacent fat lobules.

In certain cases, despite all efforts, determining whether a structure is a fat lobule or the nodule is not possible. In such cases, one can attempt an ultrasound-guided aspiration or needle localization with a retractable hookwire to verify that the sonographic lesion and mammographic lesion are, indeed, the same. If the lesion can be aspirated, the mammogram is then repeated after aspiration to confirm that the lesion has disappeared. If the lesion cannot be aspirated, a retractable hookwire is placed under ultrasound guidance and a mammogram taken with the wire in place to confirm that the suspected sonographic lesion is the mammographic nodule. (This is discussed and illustrated in greater detail in Chapter 6.)

Technical developments that decrease superimposed speckle artifact make fibroadenomas and other solid nodules appear more hypoechoic and conspicuous. Coded harmonics decreases speckle artifact and in most cases makes fibroadenomas appear relatively more hypoechoic (see Chapter 2, Fig. 2–19). Because our knowledge of echogenicity and its relationship to the histology of the fibroadenoma is based on echogenicities obtained with fun-

damental imaging, the alteration induced by harmonics decreases our ability to predict histology from the echogenicity. However, the improved conspicuity of fibroadenomas with coded harmonics far outweighs the decrease in ability to predict fibroadenoma histology. Real-time compounding can also alter fibroadenoma echogenicity, primarily by decreasing speckle artifact. By decreasing superimposed artifactual echoes, real-time compounding tends to accentuate the true underlying echogenicity of hypoechoic and hyperechoic fibroadenomas, but does not alter the relative echogenicity of isoechoic fibroadenomas. Thus, hypoechoic fibroadenomas tend to become more hypoechoic (Fig. 13–19) and hyperechoic fibroadenomas tend to become more hyperechoic with real-time compounding (Fig. 13–20), but isoechoic fibroadenomas remain isoechoic.

Heterogeneity and Homogeneity of Fibroadenomas Substance

Most fibroadenomas (79%) are homogeneous in echotexture. Unfortunately, in our series, a similar percentage of carcinomas (73.6%) are also homogeneous. Similarly, there is little difference in the percentage of fibroadenomas and carcinomas that are heterogeneous in texture. Twenty-one percent of fibroadenomas and 26% of carcinomas are heterogeneous

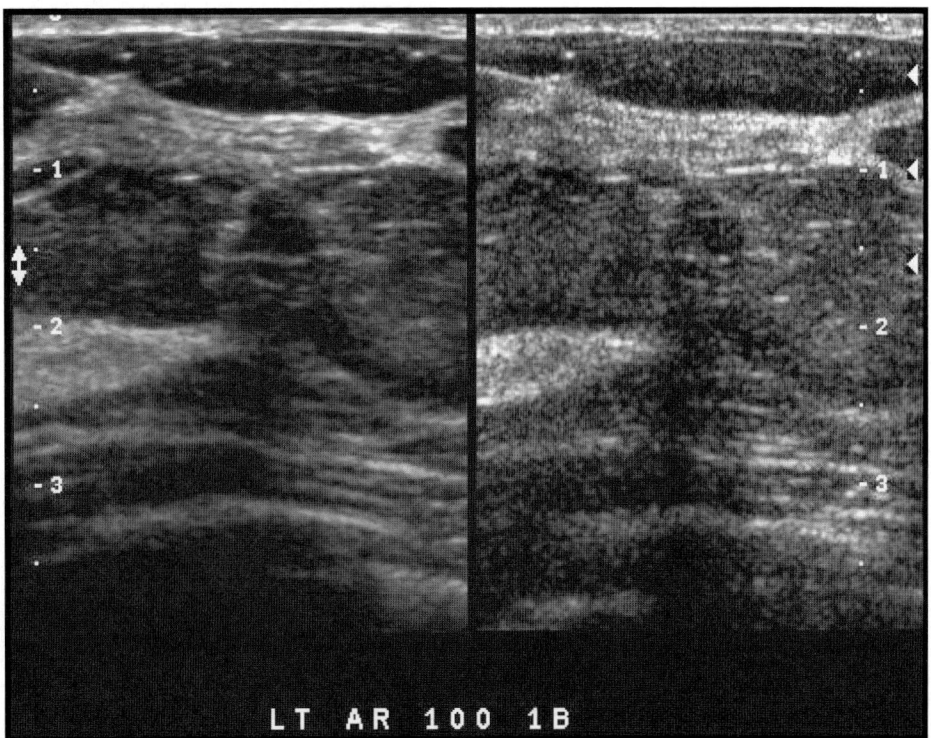

FIGURE 13–19 Spatial compounding, by reducing artifact, particularly speckle artifact, tends to exaggerate the true echogenicity of the nodule. Thus, this mildly hypoechoic fibroadenoma with conventional imaging (**right**) becomes more hypoechoic compared to surrounding fat when speckle artifact is suppressed by real-time spatial compounding (**left**).

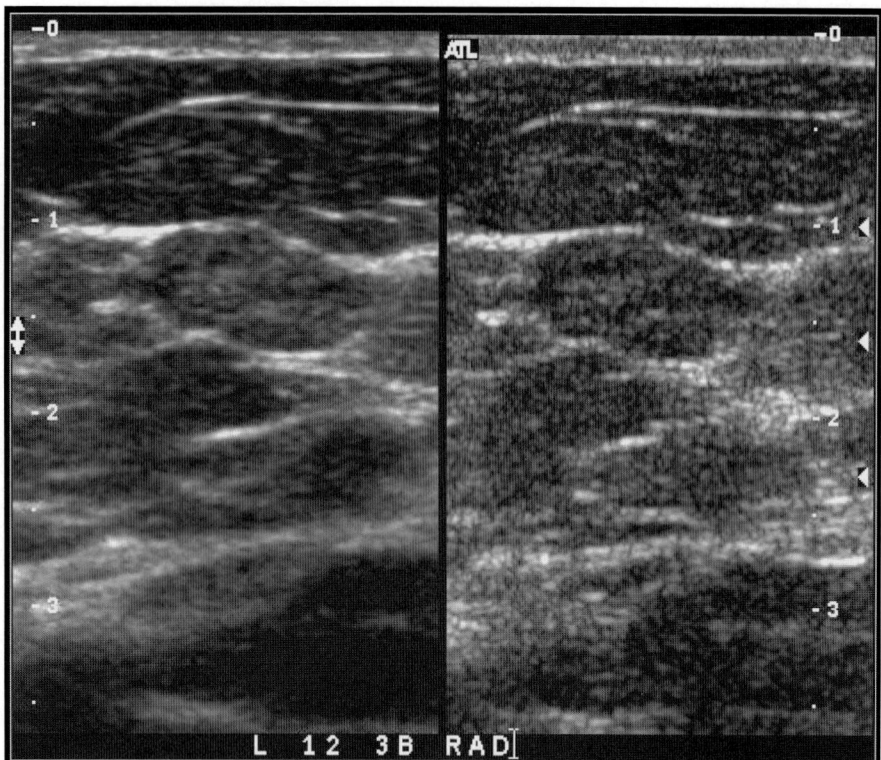

FIGURE 13–20 Just as mildly hypo-echoic fibroadenomas tend to become more hypoechoic with real-time compounding than with conventional imaging, mildly hyperechoic lesions tend to become relatively more echogenic than surrounding fat when superimposed speckle artifact is reduced by real-time compounding (**left**). The fat actually becomes more hypoechoic, making the fibroadenoma appear more echogenic. With conventional imaging (**right**) the speckle artifact superimposed over both the lesion and the surrounding fat make the lesion appear isoechoic.

in texture. Thus, whether the echotexture of a solid nodule is heterogeneous or homogeneous is of little help in distinguishing benign from malignant. This observation is in contradistinction to most of the published literature on characterizing solid breast nodules. A portion of this discrepancy is probably related to calcifications within the nodule that make it appear to have heterogeneous echotexture. Heterogeneous echotexture has predictive value only when all nodules that contain calcifications are classified as heterogeneous and calcifications are not used as a separate finding. Using calcifications as a separate finding removed heterogeneity as a useful finding in our studies.

One internal finding that is rather typical of fibroadenoma is the nonenhancing internal fibrous septation that has been described in the magnetic resonance imaging (MRI) literature. Such septa may be seen as thin, nearly straight, echogenic lines traversing the interior of otherwise probably benign-appearing nodules (Fig. 13–21). These usually extend out to the capsule on one surface of the fibroadenoma.

Thin, Echogenic Capsule

The presence of a thin, echogenic capsule, in combination with three-dimensional nodule shapes in radial and antiradial planes, is an important indicator of benignity (Fig. 13–22). In simple and complex cysts, the capsule actually represents duct or lobule walls along with various other cellular and fibrous constituents. In benign solid nodules such as fibroadenomas, however, the structure actually represents a pseudocapsule of compressed normal breast tissue.

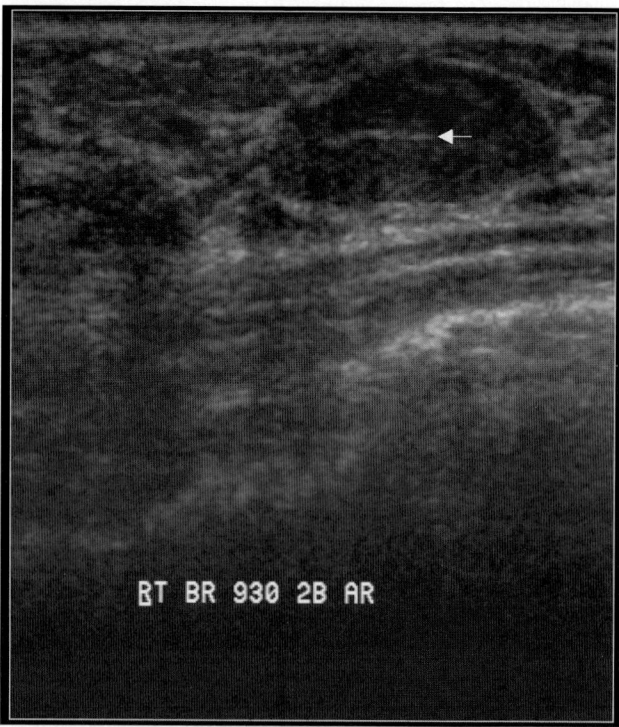

FIGURE 13–21 A minority of fibroadenomas may have a nearly straight, thin, echogenic line traversing their interior *(arrow)*. This is what has been termed the *nonenhancing fibrous septation* in the magnetic resonance imaging literature. Malignant nodules do not have straight internal septations such as these, but fat lobules frequently are subdivided into smaller fat lobules by fibrous septa. Compressibility is the best way to distinguish the nonenhancing fibrous septation within a fibroadenoma from the normal septum within a fat lobule.

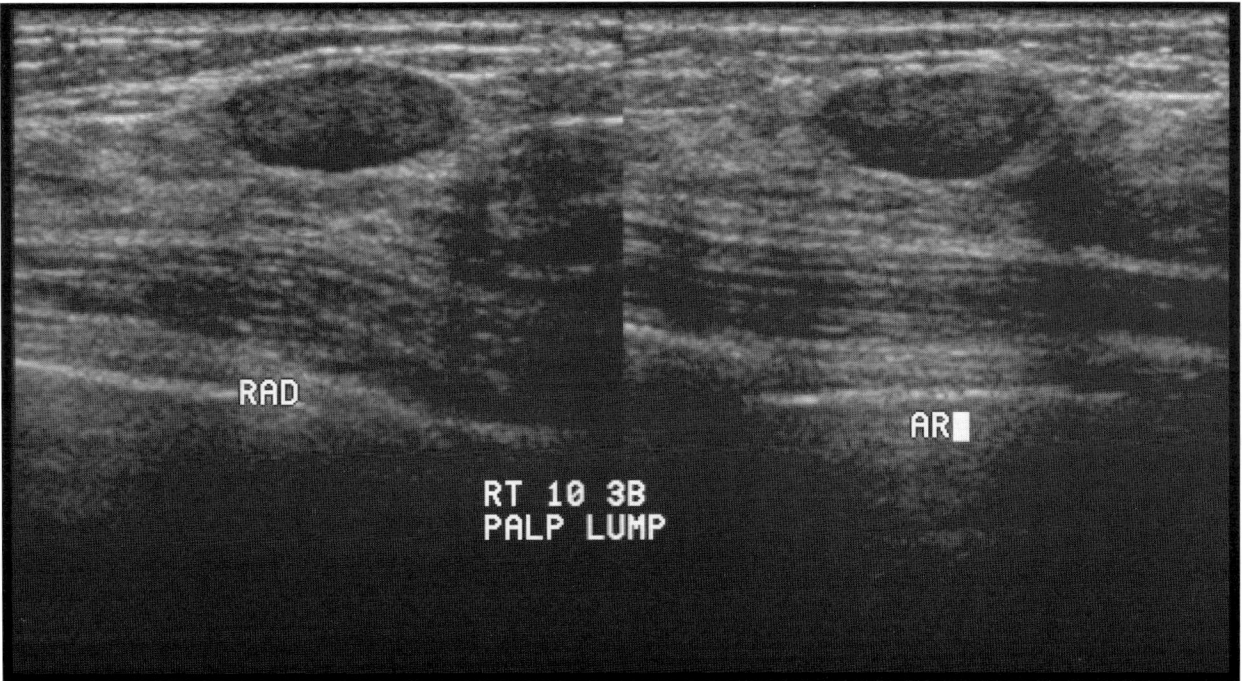

FIGURE 13–22 Fibroadenomas are completely encompassed in a thin, echogenic pseudocapsule of compressed surrounding breast tissue. The thin, echogenic capsule can usually be best shown on the anterior and posterior surfaces of the nodule and is less well shown on the ends of the nodule, where it is nearly parallel to the beam and makes a weak specular reflector. Techniques for demonstrating the entire capsule are discussed in Chapter 12.

Such a capsule indicates that the leading edge of the nodule is pushing rather than infiltrating the surrounding tissues. An indistinct margin or capsule suggests the presence of an infiltrative growth pattern, which is a strong, but not infallible, indicator of malignancy.

Showing a completely intact thin, echogenic capsule surrounding the entire periphery of the nodule is important. Partial demonstration of a thin capsule is inadequate evidence of benignity because occasional circumscribed malignant nodules may show a thin capsule around a portion of the lesion. Such circumscribed malignancies often have a capsule around a portion of the lesion, but other portions can be spiculated or encompassed in a thick, echogenic halo. Additionally, one or more of the thinly encapsulated surfaces of the nodule almost always display a worrisome sonographic shape or surface characteristic such as angularity, microlobulation, duct extension, or branch pattern. Simply obtaining two images of the nodule in the largest dimensions in longitudinal and transverse planes is inadequate because these two images may not show the suspicious features of the lesion. Thorough imaging of the entire nodule in appropriate fashion can avoid falsely classifying these special type tumors as benign.

In addition to making sure that the thin capsule is intact around the entire surface of the nodule, it is also important to make sure that the capsule is associated with either an elliptical or gently lobulated, wider-than-tall shape. Pure DCIS that has not yet invaded through the duct wall into surrounding tissues will be completely encompassed by a thin, echogenic capsule that represents the intact duct wall. However, DCIS is rarely elliptical or gently lobulated in shape. Instead, because it is growing and spreading inside the ductal system and within TDLUs, it will appear to be microlobulated and show evidence of duct extension or branch pattern. Therefore, even demonstration of a thin, echogenic capsule around a nodule that shows duct shapes should not necessarily be reassuring, and, in fact, indicates an intraductal growth pattern suspicious for DCIS. In reality, many of these lesions are merely benign intraductal papillomas, but up to 13% of such lesions represent DCIS or atypical ductal hyperplasia (ADH).

As described in Chapter 2, demonstration of the capsule around benign breast nodules is dependent on axial resolution. The higher the transducer frequency, the broader its bandwidth, and the shorter its pulse length, the better the axial resolution and the better the capsule will be demonstrated.

Equipment that improves the demonstration of the thin, echogenic capsule are also shown and illustrated in Chapter 2. Coded harmonics demonstrates the capsule to be thinner and brighter than fundamental imaging (see Chapter 2, Fig. 2–21). Real-time compounding shows the capsule on the edges of the nodule better than conventional imaging (see Chapter 2, Fig. 2–31).

Because the thin, echogenic capsule is seen as a spicular reflector, the best demonstration will be of the anterior and posterior surfaces of an ellipsoid or gently lobulated, wider-than-tall nodule, in which the capsule is parallel to the surface of the probe and perpendicular to the ultrasound beam. Additionally, the echogenic capsule may be "silhouetted" by equally echogenic interlobular stromal fibrous tissues. Sonographic techniques for best demonstrating the capsule, such as "heeling and toeing" the transducer and scanning with lighter compression, are discussed and illustrated in Chapter 12 (see Figs. 12–89 to 12–94).

Thin, echogenic capsules are most readily demonstrated around nodules that are elliptical or gently lobulated and wider than tall because more of the capsule is perpendicular to the beam when a straight anterior approach is used. As a nodule becomes more spherical, less of the surface is perpendicular to the beam and more of the capsule is steeply angled or parallel to the beam and thus more difficult to demonstrate. Additionally, the more lobulated a nodule becomes, the more the surfaces are not perpendicular to the beam and the more difficult it becomes to show an intact capsule. Finally, lesions that are taller than wide have very little capsule that is oriented perpendicular to the beam, which makes demonstration of a complete capsule exceedingly difficult in such lesions. Thus, shapes that tend to be more frequently associated with malignancy are less likely to have a demonstrable thin capsule even if one is present, helping us avoid false-negative benign classifications in such lesions.

Despite use of special sonographic maneuvers, separating the capsule from surrounding breast tissue in certain cases may still be impossible. Additionally, certain fibroadenomas will not have demonstrable capsules because of technical factors. Small, deeply located nodules in large-breasted women, especially if distal to echogenic fibrous tissue, often do not have a demonstrable capsule. This problem is most likely due to refraction and scattering of the ultrasound beam because of overlying breast tissue. Additionally, fibroadenomas that have undergone infarction often do not have a demonstrable capsule owing to adherence of the nodule to surrounding breast tissue. Any solid nodule around which a complete thin, echogenic capsule cannot be demonstrated must be characterized as at least mildly suspicious (BIRADS 4a) and must undergo biopsy.

Sound Transmission

The classic fibroadenoma has normal or increased sound transmission with respect to surrounding breast tissue, depending on its histology, the type of ultrasound equipment, and sonographic technique. Fifty-six percent of all fibroadenomas had normal through-transmission, 42% had enhanced through-transmission, and 2% had decreased through-transmission.

Fibroadenomas that have greater epithelial components and those with more cellular stroma tend to be associated with enhanced through-transmission (Fig. 13–23).

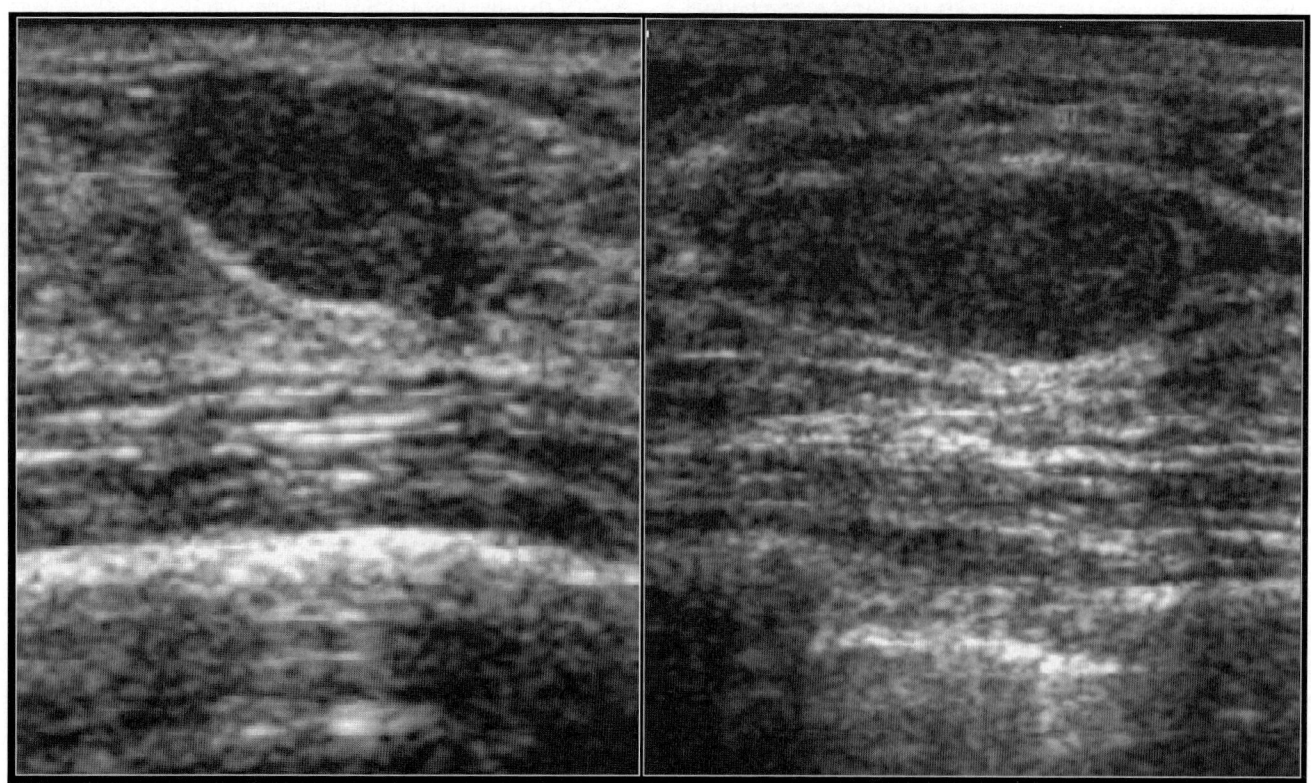

FIGURE 13–23 The sound transmission through fibroadenomas is enhanced in lesions that have large epithelial components (**left**) or highly cellular stroma (**right**), such as this lesion.

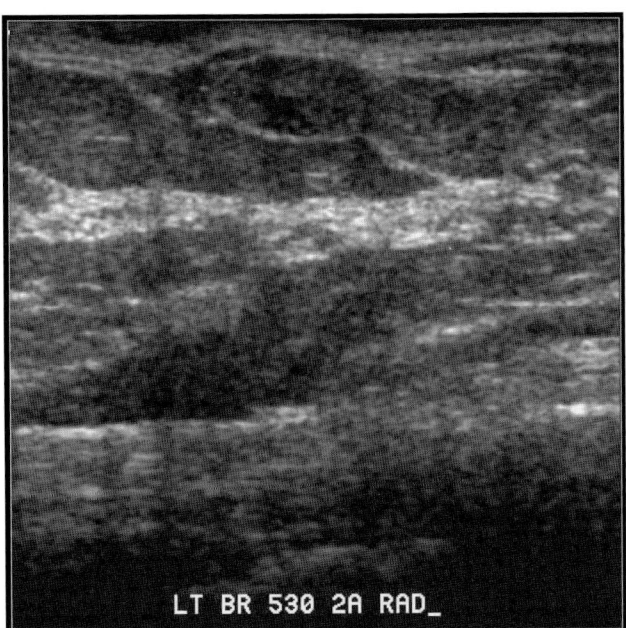

FIGURE 13–24 Fibroadenomas with small epithelial components and paucicellular stroma tend to have normal through-transmission.

The typical fibroadenoma has a small epithelial component and a paucicellular stroma and has normal sound transmission (Fig. 13–24). Fibroadenomas with secretory change due to pregnancy, lactation, birth control pills, or replacement hormone therapy and complex fibroadenomas containing areas of apocrine metaplasia or sclerosing adenosis also frequently demonstrate uniformly or heterogeneously enhanced through-transmission (discussed later). Fibroadenomas in which the stroma has become sclerotic or hyalinized can demonstrate acoustic shadowing (Fig. 13–25). Ultimately, such fibroadenomas may undergo calcification. The dystrophic calcification is usually rather coarse and dense, occurring in one of two classic patterns: dense central popcorn calcifications or peripheral circumlinear calcifications. Both types of calcifications result in decreased sound transmission and may eventually progress to produce marked shadowing (Fig. 13–26). Such fibroadenomas are usually clearly benign by mammographic criteria, however, and do not require sonographic evaluation if the mammogram is performed as the initial exam. Because fibroadenomas are most likely to be active in young patients and quiescent in older patients, enhanced sound transmission is more common in younger patients, whereas normal to decreased sound transmission is more likely to be seen in older patients. However, the relationship of sound transmission to age is variable. Young patients may have sclerosed or hyalinized fibroadenomas with decreased sound transmission, and older patients may have active fibroadenomas with enhanced sound transmission, even if not taking hormone replacement therapy.

Interestingly, fibroadenomas that have enhanced through-transmission are also more likely to show internal

flow on color Doppler evaluation (see Chapter 20, Fig. 20–5). The presence of internal flow indicates a more metabolically active lesion (regardless of whether the lesion is benign or malignant) that is more likely to grow between short-interval examinations.

The sound transmission deep to fibroadenomas will vary with the frequency of the probe. Lower-frequency probes will generally show more through-transmission than higher-frequency probes. Therefore, a nodule that has normal sound transmission with a 7.5-MHz probe may show enhanced through-transmission with a 5-MHz probe. Similarly, a nodule that shows decreased through-transmission or more worrisome frank shadowing with a 10-MHz probe may demonstrate normal through-transmission with a 7.5-MHz probe. The bandwidth of the transducer may also affect sound transmission. Broad-bandwidth probes contain low-frequency components that may enhance sound transmission. The sound transmission seen with narrower-bandwidth probes will vary with the portion of the bandwidth that is being used. With use of swept wall filters, the capability exists to select a narrow part of the transducer bandwidth at either the higher or lower end of the total transducer bandwidth. If only the upper end (higher frequency) of the spectrum is used, sound transmission will be less. If the lower end of the bandwidth is used, through-transmission will be enhanced.

Additionally, the sound transmission characteristics of a nodule can be changed by alterations in technique. In almost all cases, greater compression with the ultrasound probe will increase through-transmission. Nodules that appear to have normal or decreased sound transmission when scanned with light compression pressure frequently

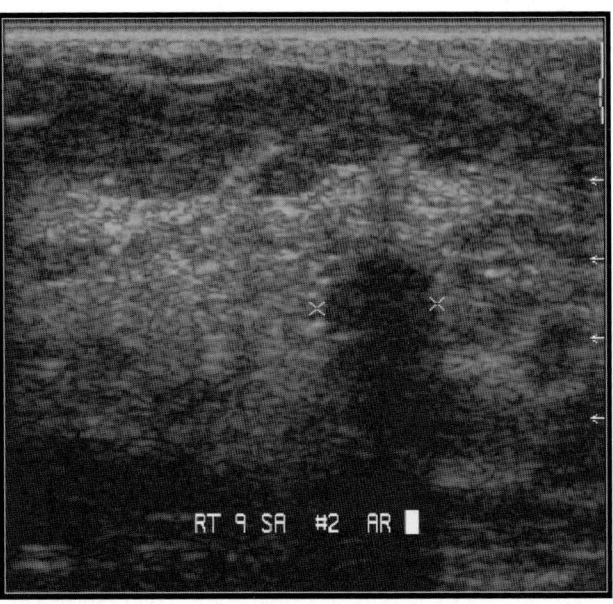

FIGURE 13–25 Fibroadenomas that have degenerated and have severely sclerotic or hyalinized stroma may demonstrate acoustic shadowing.

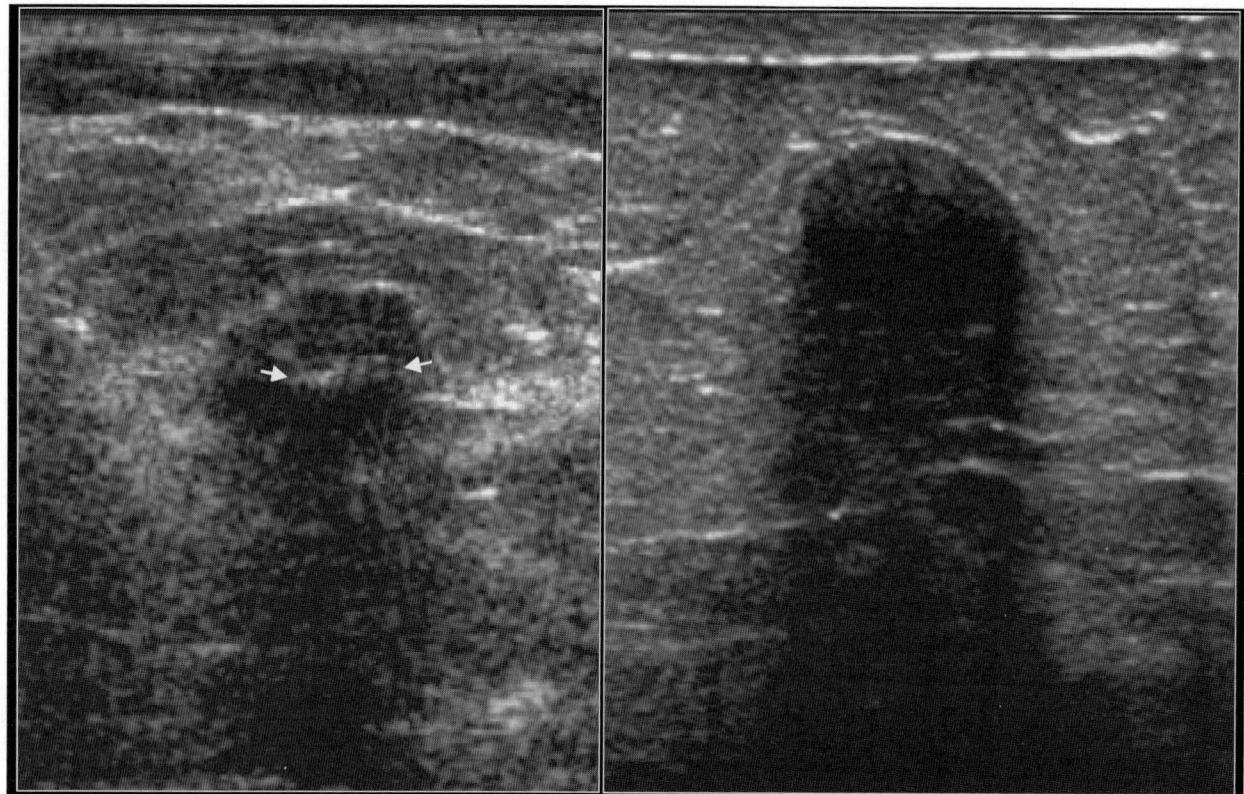

FIGURE 13–26 Fibroadenomas with dense central popcorn-like calcifications (**left**, *arrow*) or peripheral rimlike calcifications (**right**) can cause acoustic shadowing. Such lesions are definitively benign mammographically, but occasionally may be encountered unexpectedly during sonography. The mammographic image of the popcorn calcification is shown in Fig. 13–1, left and the peripheral calcification pattern is shown in Fig. 13–1, middle.

demonstrate enhanced through-transmission when vigorously compressed (Fig. 13–27). There are several reasons for this phenomenon. First, compression reduces the depth of the lesion as well as the deeper tissues. Because the penetration of the beam decreases with the square of the depth, and depth is decreased with compression, more sound will pass through the nodule into the deeper tissues in the presence of compression. Second, compression pushes tissue planes more parallel to the probe and perpendicular to the beam, decreasing refraction of the beam. This is true in the tissues surrounding the lesions but also within the lesion. Third, compression can somewhat flatten some fibroadenomas, increasing their width relative to their AP dimension. This maneuver places more of the anterior and posterior surfaces of the nodule parallel to the probe face and perpendicular to the beam, again decreasing refraction of the beam. Finally, sound transmits faster through more homogeneous compact tissue with fewer spicular interfaces than through heterogeneous loose tissue with many widely spaced spicular reflectors. Compression compacts tissue; forces spicular interfaces together, decreasing the number of major interfaces; and results in a more homogeneous texture, thus improving sound penetration and enhancing through-

transmission. For these reasons, sound transmission is generally evaluated when normal to slightly increased compression is used. Therefore, the sound transmission cannot be evaluated when the no-compression technique is being employed to better evaluate for the presence of a thin, echogenic capsule. There is usually meaningless shadowing under such circumstances.

The angle at which the ultrasound beam strikes the anterior surface of the nodule is also important in regard to sound transmission. Shadowing is more likely to occur when the beam angle is steeply oblique to the anterior surface of the nodule. Evaluating the angles of the anterior surface of the nodule in orthogonal planes permits angling of the probe in a direction that will result in a perpendicular angle of incidence. This technique results in better sound penetration and minimizes the chances of creating a false impression of tumor attenuation in an otherwise benign-appearing nodule.

Thin Edge Shadows

Thin edge shadows represent only an indirect sign of the presence of a thin, echogenic capsule along the lateral edge of the nodule (Fig. 13–28). This portion of the capsule is

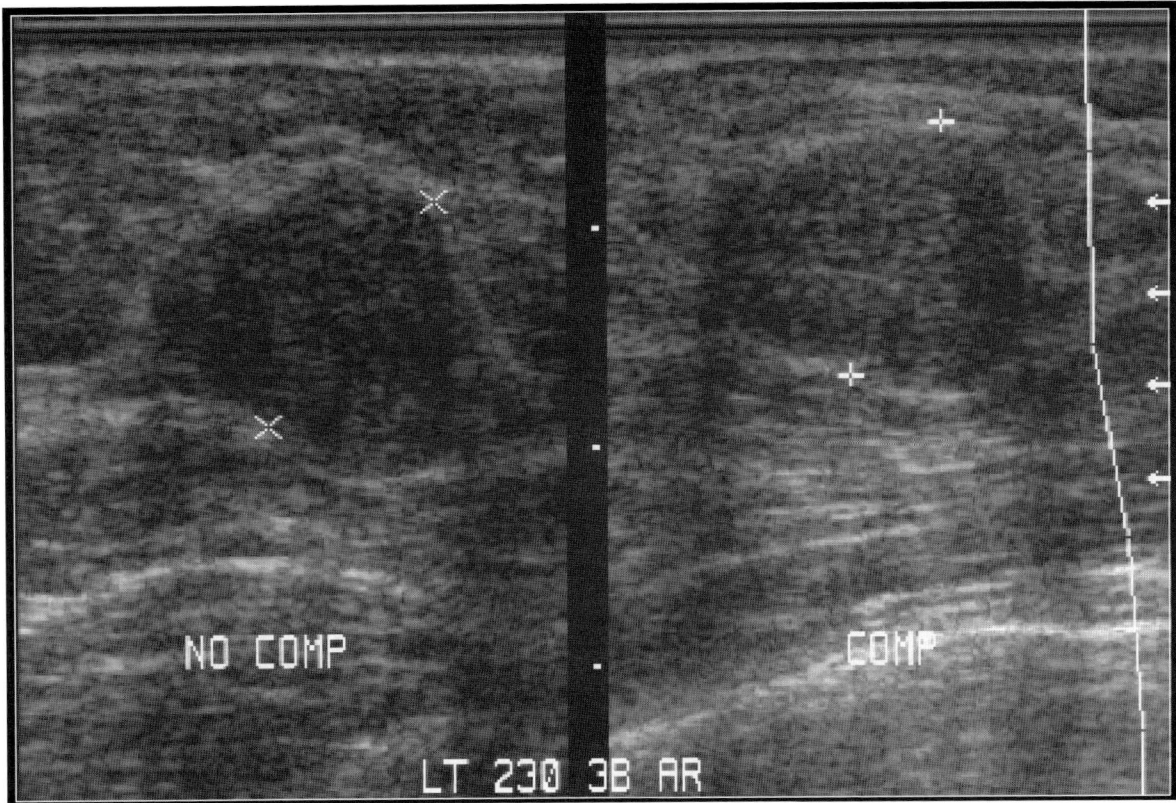

FIGURE 13–27 The degree of compression pressure affects sound transmission. In general, the more compression pressure used, the better the sound transmission and the more likely the lesion is to demonstrate enhanced through-transmission.

generally poorly demonstrated on straight anterior scans owing to refraction of the ultrasound beam by the steeply angled or parallel surfaces of the capsule on the lateral edges. Generally, direct evidence of the presence of the capsule is preferred and was discussed earlier and in Chapters 2 and 12. In cases in which heeling and toeing does not succeed and for which real-time compounding is not available, the indirect sign of the presence of thin edge shadows can be reassuring. However, thin edge shadows are considered to be a minor confirmatory finding of benignity, not a major criterion in the solid nodule characterization algorithm.

Mobility

Most fibroadenomas are not attached to surrounding breast tissues and therefore should be mobile relative to the adjacent breast parenchyma. The one exception to this rule would be fibroadenomas that have undergone infarction, become adherent to adjacent tissues, and therefore lost mobility. Mobility of a palpable nodule is usually quite apparent on the clinical exam even in the absence of imaging studies. Mobility can be confirmed during the real-time sonographic examination when the nodule moves relative to surrounding tissues during simultaneous scanning and palpation. Mobility may also be demonstrated by showing

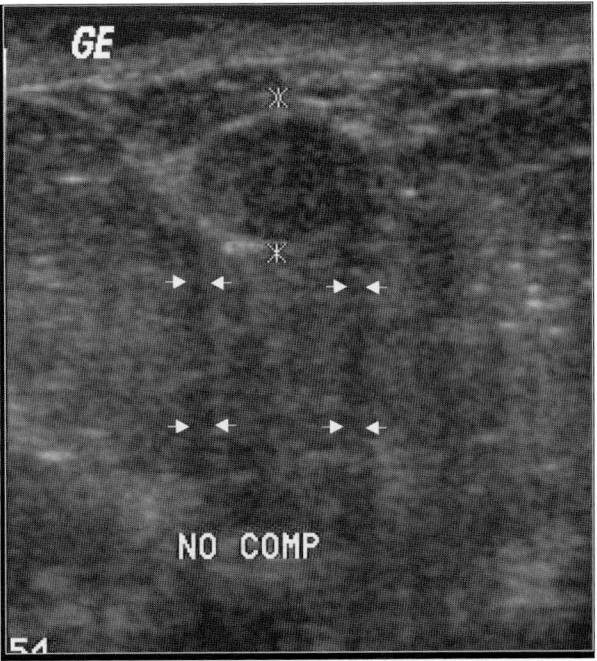

FIGURE 13–28 The presence of thin edge shadows *(arrows)* is a minor finding suggesting the presence of a thin, echogenic capsule on the ends of the lesion. However, we view such a finding as a weak indirect indicator of the presence of a thin capsule. It is far more valuable to use "heeling and toeing" or real-time compounding maneuvers to demonstrate the capsule.

that the nodule freely rotates with the surrounding soft tissue as compression is changed. This characteristic is most easily demonstrated in obliquely oriented fibroadenomas that rotate into a horizontal axis when probe pressure is applied and can be best demonstrated on split-screen images obtained with and without compression (see Chapter 3, Fig. 3–17). Mobility is viewed as a minor confirmatory finding that is helpful in a small percentage of cases. As is the case for thin edge shadows, mobility is not used as one of the major criteria for characterizing a nodule as probably benign.

Compressibility

Fibroadenomas are mildly compressible in many cases, depending on the histology. Generally, the greater the epithelial component, the softer and more compressible the nodule is. The greater the stromal component, the firmer and less compressible the nodule is. However, the histologic makeup of the stroma also affects compressibility, just as it affects sound transmission. Fibroadenomas with highly cellular or myxoid stroma usually are softer and more compressible than those with sparse cellular or acellular stroma. Fibroadenomas that have undergone secretory change due to pregnancy, lactation, birth control pills, or HRT are also softer and more compressible than the nonstimulated fibroadenomas. Complex fibroadenomas that contain extensive apocrine metaplasia and cystic change may also be unusually soft. On the other hand, fibroadenomas that contain sclerosing adenosis are often firmer than usual. With

advancing age, there is generally a tendency for the stroma to become less cellular and to undergo sclerosis, hyalinization, or calcification. Fibroadenomas that have undergone these chronic changes may become very hard and completely incompressible. Generally, fibroadenomas in young patients have histology that makes them relatively more compressible, whereas fibroadenomas in older patients have histology that makes them less compressible. However, occasionally fibroadenomas in older patients are soft and compressible, whereas fibroadenomas in younger patients may have already become sclerotic, hard, and incompressible.

Compressibility can be documented with split-screen images of the fibroadenoma: noncompressed on the left half of the image and compressed on the right. The AP dimension of the fibroadenoma is measured (outside capsule to outside capsule) in the two views, and the difference in AP dimension between the two views is divided by the AP dimension of the fibroadenoma in the noncompressed view to determine the percentage of compressibility (Fig. 13–29).

Our experience has been that many fibroadenomas compress by about 10% to 15%. However, a few fibroadenomas that have highly cellular stroma, myxoid stroma, a preponderance of epithelial elements, or epithelial secretory or apocrine changes are more compressible and may compress up to 25%. Sclerosed, hyalinized, and calcified inactive fibroadenomas may not compress at all. Most carcinomas are completely incompressible, but special-type tumors that are highly cellular and have little desmoplastic reaction, such as papillary carcinoma, mucinous carci-

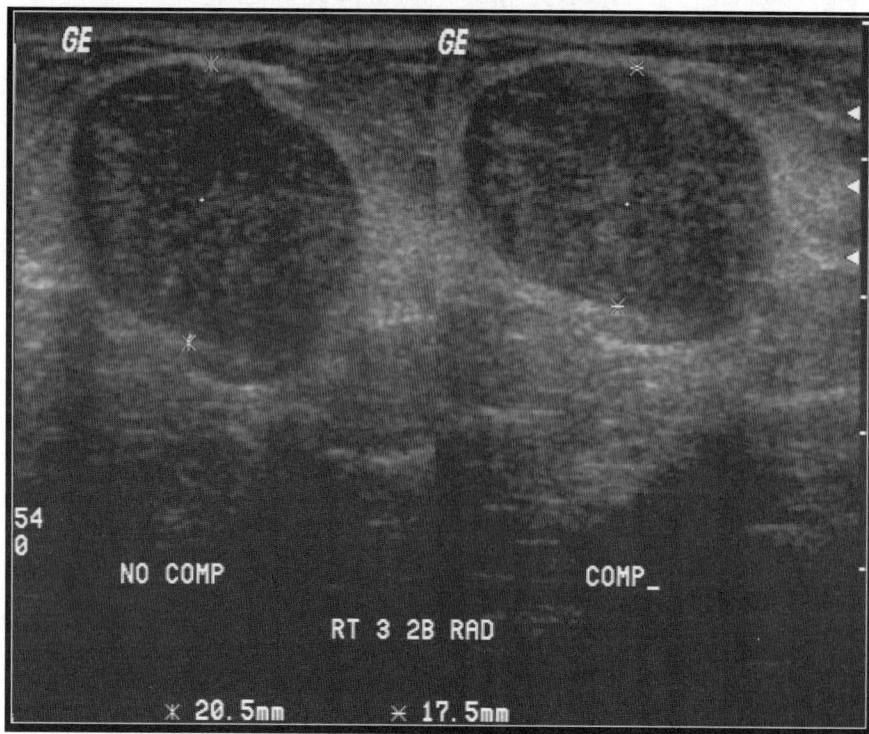

FIGURE 13–29 Fibroadenomas that have cellular (such as this fibroadenoma) or myxoid stroma or high epithelial components tend to be 10% to 25% compressible.

noma, and medullary carcinoma, may be mildly compressible. The degree of compressibility in such tumors may be similar to that of most fibroadenomas, about 10% to 15%. Unfortunately, our experience has also been that high-grade infiltrating ductal cancers, which are also highly cellular, have little desmoplastic reaction and abundant lymphocyte infiltrate, and are more likely to contain areas of frank cystic necrosis, often are mildly compressible (Fig. 13–30). Because of the large variability in compressibility of both fibroadenomas and carcinomas due to underlying variations in histology, there is considerable overlap in compressibility between benign and malignant nodules. For this reason, our algorithm for characterizing solid nodules does not use compressibility as a major criterion.

Management of Fibroadenomas

Because of the wide variation in the histologic composition of fibroadenomas, there should be surprise that the sonographic appearance of fibroadenomas varies equally widely. Only a fraction of all fibroadenomas have gross and histologic characteristics that result in a classically benign fibroadenomatous sonographic appearance, as described in

Chapter 12, that enables them to be characterized as BI-RADS 3. Those appearances include the following:

- Elliptical shape, wider-than-tall, and completely encompassed in a thin, echogenic capsule
- Gently lobulated (three or fewer), wider than tall, and completely encompassed in a thin, echogenic capsule

The fraction of fibroadenomas that meet classic criteria for benignity varies with patient population, quality of equipment, and experience of the sonographer or sonologist. Our experience is that 40% to 50% of fibroadenomas have classically benign appearances that enable us to characterize them as BIRADS 3. The other 50% to 60% of fibroadenomas have one or more suspicious characteristics that exclude them from the BIRADS 3 category, requiring characterization of BIRADS 4a or higher and biopsy. Recommending biopsy of these mildly suspicious nodules should not engender a feeling of guilt or frustration because these lesions have always undergone biopsy in the past, and the risk for malignancy is high enough to warrant biopsy in their current environment.

Nodules that meet strict criteria for benign BIRADS 3 classification have less than a 2% chance of being malignant.

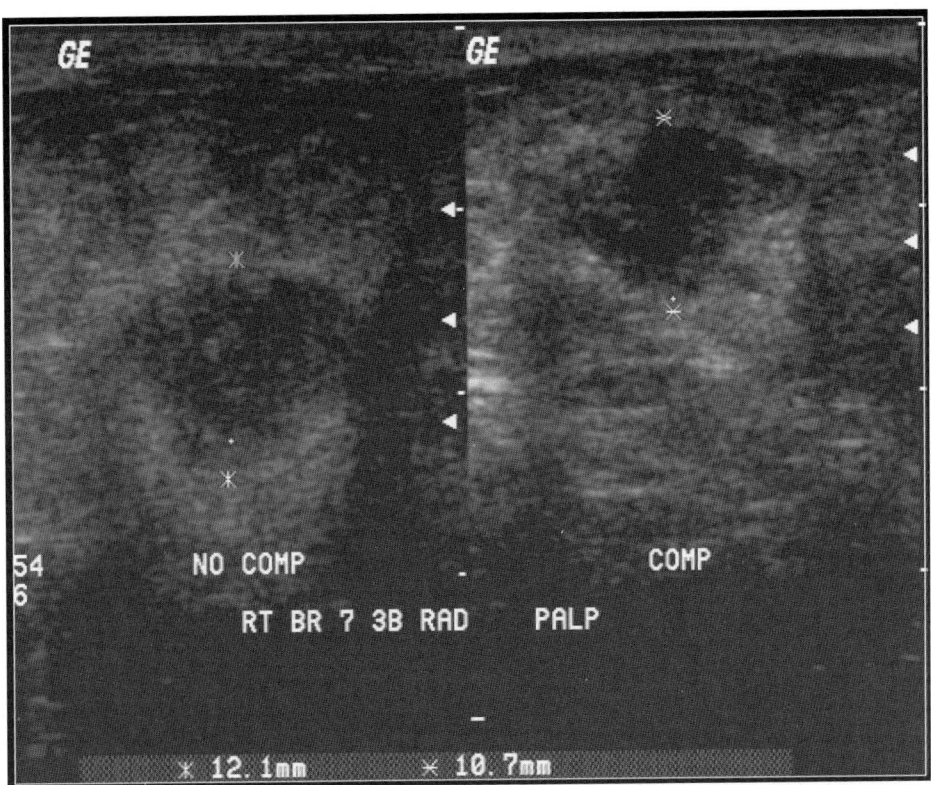

FIGURE 13–30 Some carcinomas may be mildly compressible (10% to 15%), usually lesions that lie at the circumscribed end of the spectrum and that have relatively little desmoplasia. Such lesions include high-grade invasive ductal carcinomas, colloid carcinomas, medullary carcinomas, invasive papillary carcinomas, and some metaplastic carcinomas. It is especially true of malignant lesions that have central hemorrhage or necrosis. This compressible malignant nodule is a medullary carcinoma with some central hemorrhagic necrosis.

The patient and her physician are advised of the degree of certainty and presented with three options: (a) short-interval sonographic follow-up (6 months), (b) large core needle biopsy with ultrasound guidance, or (c) excisional biopsy with or without ultrasound-guided needle localization. The patient and her referring physician use the degree of certainty based on sonographic criteria along with the knowledge of the patient's personality to choose one of these options. There are patients and referring physicians who will be uncomfortable with follow-up alone for solid nodules, regardless of the degree of certainty of benignity, and those individuals will demand biopsy. Even with less than a 1% chance of malignancy, there will be patients who prefer excisional biopsy to core needle biopsy.

Of course, nodules that have not met strict criteria for benignity, that have not been excised, and that have undergone needle biopsy proving that they are fibroadenomas must still undergo follow-up sonography.

The reasons for following lesions classified as probably benign, BIRADS 3 are (a) to detect the small percentage of malignancies that have simulated benign fibroadenoma appearance, (b) to detect rapid growth in a juvenile or giant fibroadenoma and precipitate to a smaller excision before a larger lumpectomy is required, (c) to detect benign phyllodes tumors that are usually sonographically (and sometimes histologically) indistinguishable from fibroadenomas with cellular stroma when still small but that invariably grow rapidly, and (d) to detect the extremely rare (1 in 1,000) fibroadenomas that undergo malignant degeneration.

Patients who have multiple solid nodules bilaterally are probably within the group that forms multiple bilateral fibroadenomas in cycles. The management of these lesions is much more difficult. Such patients may have as many as 8 or 10 solid nodules in each breast. Excising all of these nodules is virtually never a reasonable option because (a) many more nodules will develop in the future, (b) the extensive surgery will be disfiguring, and (c) the chances of any of these nodules being malignant is low.

Core biopsy of every single nodule is also not usually performed when there are more than three nodules on each side. In most cases in which there are multiple solid nodules bilaterally, several of the smaller lesions on each side meet the criteria for a BIRADS 3, probably benign classification. One or two on each side may be larger or have one or more suspicious findings. In such cases, we perform biopsy on the one or two largest BIRADS 3 nodules and any nodules that have suspicious criteria requiring a BIRADS 4a or higher classification to confirm that the lesions are merely fibroadenomas. We then assume the smaller more classic BIRADS 3 lesions are also fibroadenomas. This group always requires 6-month follow-up. This uncommon circumstance is one in which follow-up requires bilateral whole breast sonography because new nodules will almost certainly form in the intervals between examinations.

Histologic evidence for malignancy developing within a preexisting fibroadenoma is said to occur in 1 in 1,000 cases.

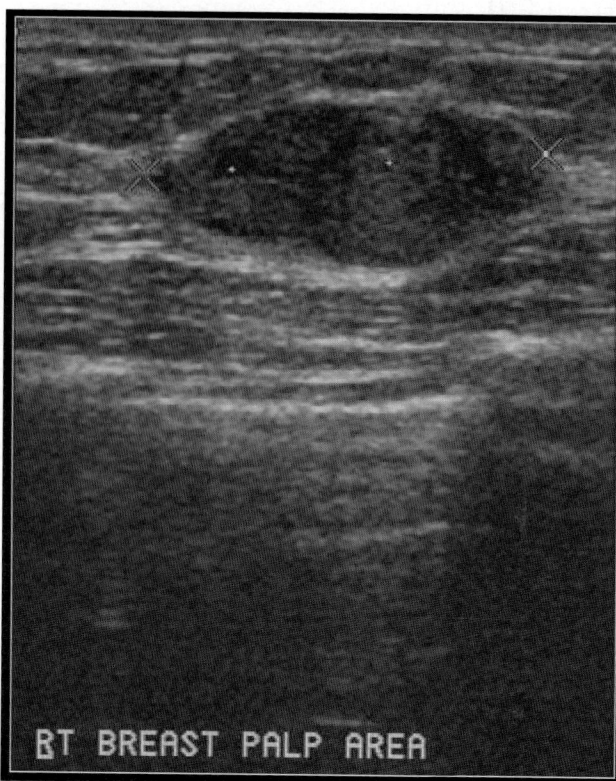

FIGURE 13–31 Malignancy rarely develops within fibroadenomas. The most frequent atypical lesion within fibroadenomas is lobular carcinoma *in situ* (LCIS), which does not have any specific findings and may be apparent only because of internal heterogeneity. This fibroadenoma unexpectedly showed LCIS at biopsy.

However, most of these are merely lobular carcinoma *in situ* (LCIS), which is really considered to be a premalignant lesion rather than a true malignancy. Sonographically, such fibroadenomas appear similar to and indistinguishable from complex fibroadenomas, having heterogeneous texture, cysts, and areas of increased echogenicity (Fig. 13–31). Ductal carcinoma *in situ* (DCIS), invasive lobular carcinoma, and invasive ductal carcinoma each develop much less commonly within the epithelium of a preexisting fibroadenoma than does LCIS, and we have not seen any cases.

It is not entirely certain whether phyllodes tumors develop *de novo* or from preexisting fibroadenomas or by both means. The overlap in sonographic and histologic features can make it difficult to distinguish between fibroadenomas with cellular stroma and benign phyllodes tumors.

Fibroadenoma Summary

Fibroadenomas have a broad spectrum of histologic findings and therefore a wide array of sonographic appearances. Only 40% to 50% of fibroadenomas have the classic findings of an elliptical or gently lobulated shape, wider-than-tall dimensions, and a complete thin, echogenic, delimiting capsule. This group of lesions can be predicted to be benign with great enough certainty (>98%) that they may be characterized as BIRADS 3 and that follow-up may be offered as an acceptable alternative to biopsy. The remainder of fibroadenomas fail to meet the strict sonographic requirements for classification as BIRADS 3, have to be characterized as BIRADS 4a or higher, and require either excisional or needle biopsy.

Of the many sonographic findings that have been reported for fibroadenomas, most have been found to be too variable and have too much overlap with malignant findings to be used as major criteria in classifying solid nodules. The criteria that are considered to be major findings and help reliably identify benign nodules with a high degree of certainty are a wider-that-tall ellipsoid shape together with a complete thin, echogenic capsule, or a wider-than-tall, gently lobulated shape (three or fewer lobulations), together with a complete thin, echogenic capsule.

The other findings discussed previously (e.g., homogeneity, mobility, compressibility, echogenicity) represent only minor or secondary or minor criteria. These less reliable criteria should not be used for determination of benignity versus malignancy. However, certain findings, such as enhanced through-transmission and compressibility, appear to reflect the presence of the histologic makeup that is likely to be associated with active growth, indicating the need for short-interval follow-up.

FIBROADENOMA VARIANTS—COMPLEX FIBROADENOMAS

Pathology

Generally, the presence of a fibroadenoma is thought to minimally increase the relative risk for subsequent breast malignancy (about twofold). However, a recent study published by Dupont, Page, Parl and associates (1994) found that fibroadenomas classified as complex are associated with a 3.10- to 3.88-fold increase in relative risk. As noted previously, fibroadenomas are composed of a variable mixture of stromal and epithelial elements. The epithelial elements within the fibroadenoma may undergo proliferative change. These changes include cyst formation, apocrine metaplasia, epithelial hyperplasia with epithelial-type calcifications, and sclerosing adenosis (Table 13–4). Fibroadenomas that contain these epithelial changes are classified as complex lesions.

TABLE 13–4. EPITHELIAL PROLIFERATIVE CHANGES WITHIN COMPLEX FIBROADENOMAS

Cyst formation

Apocrine metaplasia

Epithelial hyperplasia with calcifications

Sclerosing adenosis

About 23% of fibroadenomas in DuPont's large series were complex, and 77% were classified as simple. Patients with simple fibroadenomas had no first-degree family history of breast cancer and no increase in the relative risk for breast cancer development. On the other hand, those patients with complex fibroadenomas and a negative first-degree family history had an increase in relative risk for breast cancer development of 3.1. Those patients with complex fibroadenomas and a positive first-degree family history of breast cancer had a relative risk of about 3.9 (a 20% risk for developing breast cancer within 25 years of the initial diagnosis of complex fibroadenoma formation). The increase in relative risk is generalized—not specific for the site of fibroadenoma removal, but rather for the entirety of both breasts. Furthermore, unlike other disorders associated with increased relative risk, such as LCIS and ADH, the increased relative risk associated with complex fibroadenomas does not decrease with time and persists indefinitely. Because the average age at first diagnosis in the reported population was less than 25 years, there is a 20% chance that these patients will develop a breast cancer before 50 years of age. Based on the increased risk for developing breast cancer at an early age, suggestion has been made that these patients should undergo annual screening mammograms beginning at 35 years of age. Although there is no definitive evidence presently to support this approach, there may be a connection between the development of complex fibroadenomas and genetic predisposition to the development of carcinoma. The presence of *BRCA1* gene as well as a complex fibroadenoma, especially in patients who have positive first-degree family histories, may be such a connection.

Clinical Findings

The clinical findings of complex lesions do not differ from those of simple fibroadenomas, except for the increased relative risk for subsequent breast cancer development.

Mammographic Findings

Specific mammographic findings for complex fibroadenomas have not been reported in the literature. A reasonable assumption would be that a larger percentage of complex fibroadenoma nodules that are visible mammographically would be irregular in shape or have ill-defined contours. Additionally, one might expect that certain complex fibroadenomas would have small, punctate, lobular-type calcifications rather than the typical coarse, central, popcorn-type calcifications or the rimlike peripheral calcification associated with simple fibroadenomas.

Sonographic Findings

Although the diagnosis of complex fibroadenoma requires histologic confirmation, either by core needle or excisional biopsy, sonography may suggest the diagnosis. This assumption is important for two reasons:

1. Many benign-appearing solid nodules are now followed rather than undergoing biopsy. The presence of changes suggesting the presence of a complex rather than a simple fibroadenoma might precipitate biopsy rather than follow-up. Histologic verification of the presence of a complex fibroadenoma would lead to yearly mammographic surveillance at an earlier age and might some day lead to testing for genes associated with an increase risk for breast cancer.

2. For adjudication of core needle biopsy results. When sonographic findings are suspicious for complex fibroadenoma, the pathologist may specifically be requested to render an opinion as to whether the fibroadenoma is complex or simple. It is not necessarily standard operating procedure in all pathology departments to distinguish between complex and all other fibroadenomas.

Specific sonographic findings that are present in complex fibroadenomas absolutely exclude the lesion from being classified as probably benign. Epithelial calcifications, which may be seen within complex fibroadenomas as small, punctate echodensities, usually too small to cause

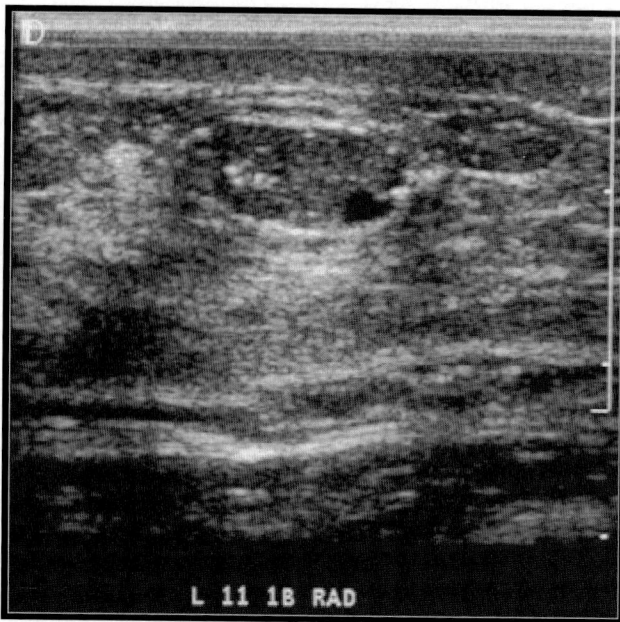

FIGURE 13–32 Punctate echoes within this fibroadenoma represent epithelial calcifications that place it in the category of complex fibroadenomas. Many epithelial calcifications in complex fibroadenomas are too small to recognize sonographically and are manifest only as heterogeneous texture.

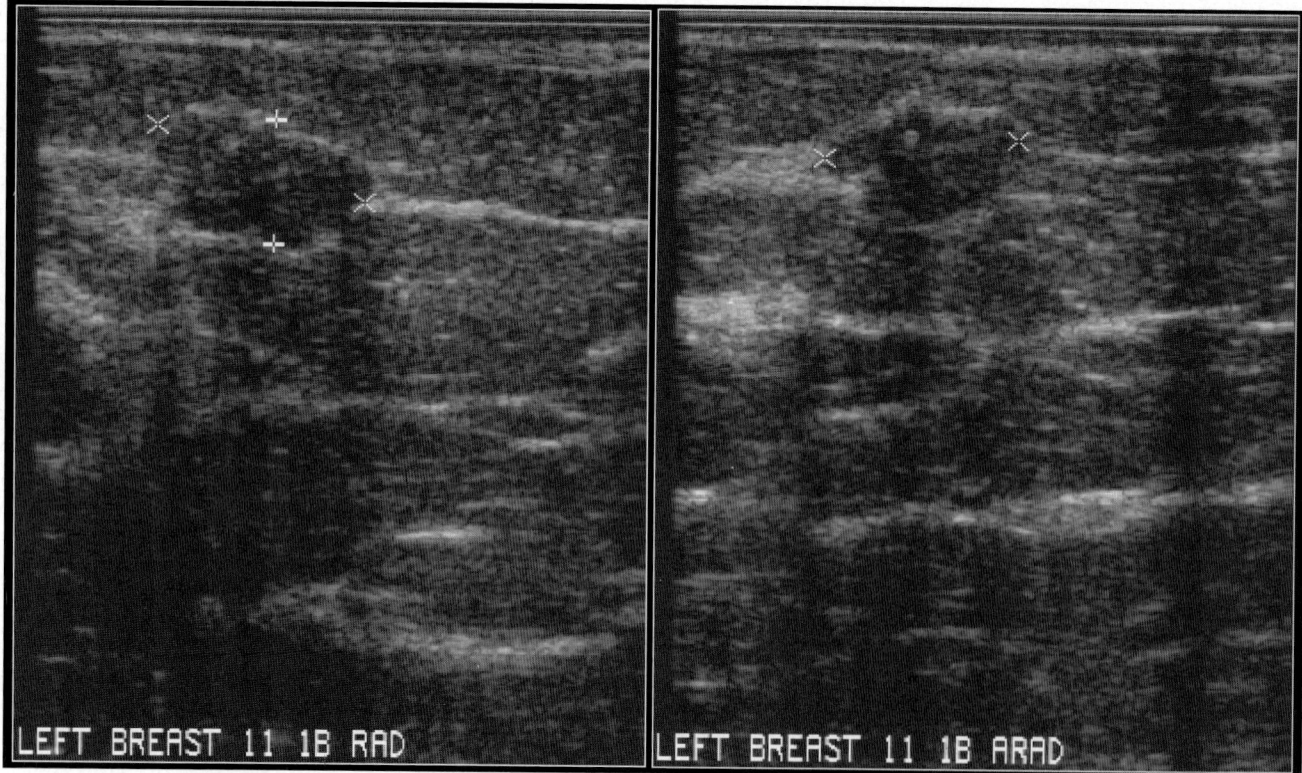

FIGURE 13–33 The presence of sclerosing adenosis within a fibroadenoma places the lesion in the category of complex fibroadenomas. Centrally located sclerosing adenosis creates heterogeneous echotexture with variable ill-defined areas of increased echogenicity, and peripherally located sclerosing adenosis may cause the margins of the lesion to become angular and irregular, as it has in this lesion.

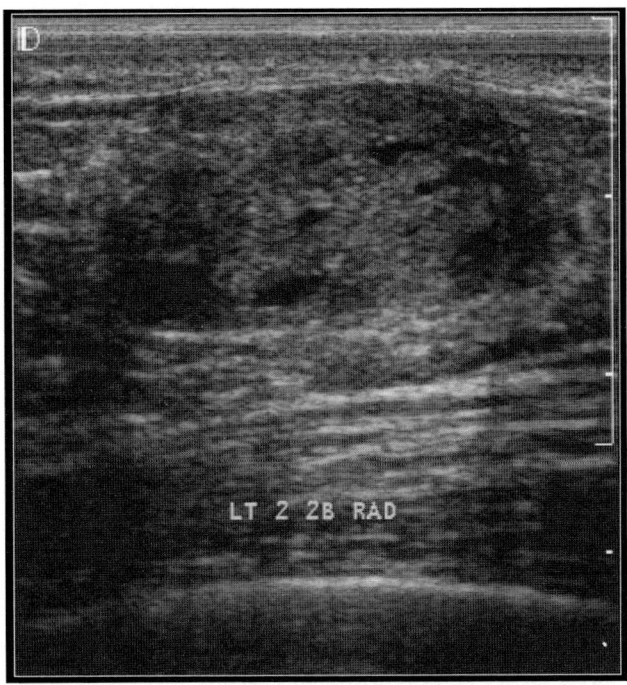

FIGURE 13–34 The presence of apocrine metaplasia within a fibroadenoma places it into the complex fibroadenoma category. However, apocrine metaplasia is not directly distinguishable from the normal epithelial or stromal interior of a fibroadenoma. The apocrine metaplasia frequently leads to internal cyst formation, however. Thus, the presence of a thin-walled, well-circumscribed cyst within a solid nodule that is thought to represent a fibroadenoma suggests that the lesion is a complex fibroadenoma that contains apocrine metaplasia.

acoustic shadowing, automatically exclude a solid nodule from classification as benign (Fig. 13–32; see also Chapter 12). These punctate calcifications differ from the dense, popcorn-like central calcifications or the rimlike peripheral calcifications that are mammographically benign and have been illustrated previously. Additionally, the presence of sclerosing adenosis within a complex fibroadenoma (typically occurring in the periphery of the nodule) often results in angular margins and excludes such a nodule from benign classification (Fig. 13–33; see also Chapter 12).

There are other sonographic findings within solid nodules, however, that may suggest the presence of a complex fibroadenoma without excluding the nodule from benign classification; these include heterogeneous internal texture, internal cysts, and internal foci of hyperechogenicity. Although the presence of apocrine metaplasia within complex fibroadenomas is not directly sonographically detectable, apocrine metaplasia frequently causes sonographically detectable small cysts to form within the nodule (Fig. 13–34). In other cases, there are ill-defined areas of increased internal echogenicity that correspond histologically to areas of sclerosing adenosis within the nodule (Fig. 13–35). In most cases, the foci of hyperechogenicity are small and ill defined, but in a few cases, large central foci of hyperechogenicity are present (Fig. 13–36). In cases in which discrete cysts or foci of hyperechogenicity are not identifiable, the texture may merely be more heterogeneous than usual (Fig. 13–37).

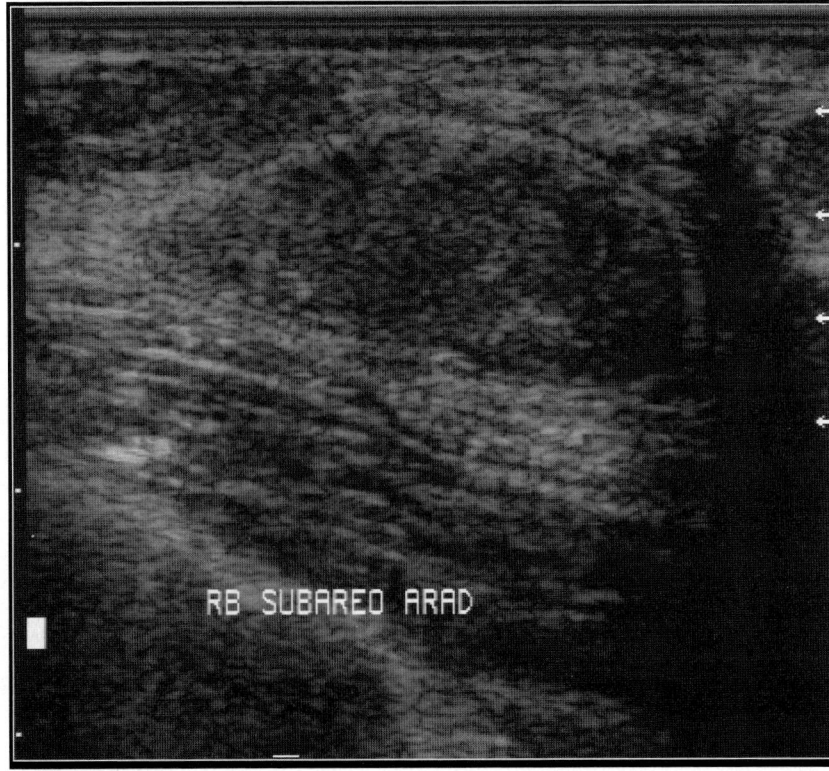

FIGURE 13–35 This heterogeneous complex fibroadenoma contains ill-defined echogenic areas that represent foci of sclerosing adenosis.

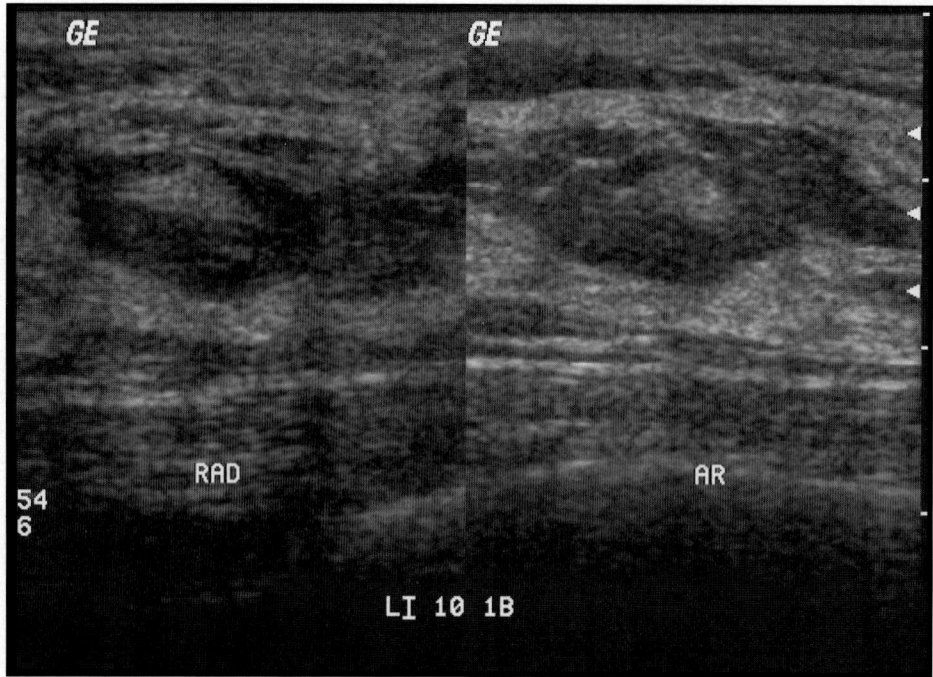

FIGURE 13–36 The large focus of hyperechogenicity within this complex fibroadenoma represents an area of sclerosing adenosis.

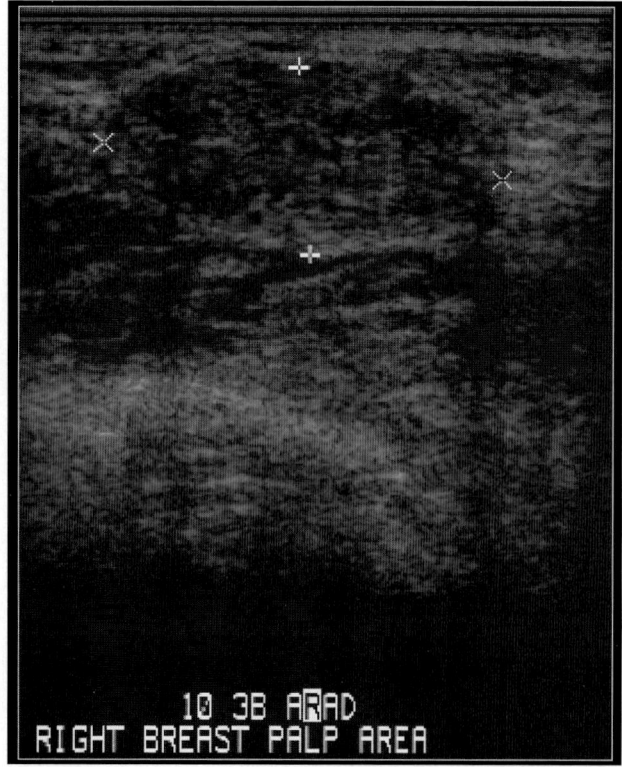

FIGURE 13–37 Discrete calcifications, cysts, or foci of hyperechogenicity cannot be identified sonographically in most complex fibroadenomas. Instead, the echotexture is merely diffusely heterogeneous.

In solid nodules that show minor findings such as internal cysts, internal foci of hyperechogenicity, or unusual heterogeneity, but have other characteristics that would allow them to be characterized as BIRADS 3, the possibility of complex fibroadenoma should be raised. This could affect the patient's decision to undergo biopsy because it might affect the frequency and timing of routine mammography and the aggressiveness in use of additional screening diagnostic imaging in the future. It is important to remember that the increased risk for future development of cancer is generalized and bilateral, not within the complex fibroadenoma.

FIBROADENOMA VARIANTS—TUBULAR ADENOMAS AND LACTATING ADENOMAS

General Pathologic Classification and Epidemiology

Tubular adenoma and lactating adenoma are terms that most likely represent a single pathologic lesion seen in different phases of physiologic activity. These lesions are related to, but not identical to, fibroadenomas. Fibroadenomas may contain foci identical to tubular adenoma and may also show foci with lactational change identical to the histology seen within lactating adenomas. Fibroadenomas represent a mixture of stromal and epithelial elements in varying amounts. Tubular and lactating adenomas, however, represent an almost pure form of epithelial growth, having very little stromal component and little cellularity of the sparse stromal elements that are present. In fact, tubular adenomas have also been called "pure" adenomas. Tubular adenomas are very rare in comparison to the incident of fibroadenomas. Many adenomas that have been reported in the past were probably fibroadenomas with a large epithelial component rather than true tubular adenomas. Lactating adenomas, are more commonly identified both clinically and pathologically. These lesions are most commonly seen during lactation or the third trimester of pregnancy, but can also present during the first and second trimesters of pregnancy. Although the time of presentation indicates a hormonal etiology, there is no reported correlation with the development of these lesions and birth control pills or HRT. Lactating adenomas may undergo infarction during lactation or the third trimester of pregnancy.

Tubular adenomas probably arise *de novo*, but there is a school of thought that lactating adenomas are the progenitor lesion. The evidence for this potential relationship is that certain lactating adenomas that developed during pregnancy or lactation, but that were not resected until after terminating breast-feeding, have shown classic histologic changes of tubular adenoma. However, an equally plausible explanation is that the tubular adenoma existed before pregnancy and merely became clinically evident after having undergone lactational change.

There are several different proposed origins for lactating adenomas. Certain lactating adenomas undoubtedly arise from preexisting fibroadenomas. More frequently, however, lactating adenomas probably arise from tubular adenomas. Other lactating adenomas may arise *de novo*. Finally, there is the belief that lactating adenomas are not all true neoplasms. Rather, some lactating adenomas represent focal areas of premature lobular proliferation and lactational activity out of phase with the surrounding breast tissue. In our experience, this explanation is especially true of areas of lactational change seen in the first two trimesters of pregnancy. Many of these "lactational adenomas" have been followed through the pregnancy and seem to disappear into a background of surrounding lactational lobular change later in the pregnancy and during lactation. In reality, lactating adenomas probably develop by all four of the proposed mechanisms, with tubular adenomas and focal lactational change out of proportion to surrounding breast tissue being most common, and fibroadenomas and *de novo* origins being less common.

Clinical Findings

Tubular adenomas can occur throughout the reproductive years, becoming uncommon after menopause. Lactating adenomas occur during the reproductive years but mainly are seen during lactation or the third trimester of pregnancy. These lesions are less commonly seen during the

first two trimesters of pregnancy. Both lesions present clinically as palpable masses or nodules. Tubular adenomas are mobile, firm, and rubbery, very similar to fibroadenomas. Lactating adenomas are also mobile, but usually are softer to palpation, unless they have undergone infarction. Lactating adenomas may enlarge rapidly during the first two trimesters of pregnancy. Infarction of lactating adenomas occurs most commonly during lactation or the third trimester of pregnancy. Infarction of a lactating adenoma is usually associated with pain and presents as a firm, tender, palpable nodule or mass. After complete resection of these lesions, there is little chance of recurrence. Neither tubular adenoma nor lactating adenoma is associated with an increase in relative risk for breast cancer development.

Gross Pathologic Findings

Both tubular and lactating adenomas are usually 4 cm or less in diameter, although occasionally these lactating adenomas may be much larger. Tubular adenomas are firm, rubbery, and circumscribed. Lactating adenomas are much softer in comparison. The surface of both lesions is smooth to finely nodular. Tubular adenomas are more typically smooth, and lactating adenomas are usually microlobulated. Although these lesions are well circumscribed, there may not be a well-defined fibrous pseudocapsule, as is usually seen with classic fibroadenomas. Lactating adenomas contain a milky substance that can be expressed during surgical excision.

Histologic Findings

Tubular adenomas are composed of noncompressed tubules made up of normal epithelial and myoepithelial elements. These tubules are indistinguishable from the tubules found within normal lobules. There is little stromal tissue surrounding the tubules, and the stroma that is present shows very little cellularity. Lactating adenomas are composed of tubules that have matured into true acini. These tubules contain actively secreting cells, and the lumina of the acini are filled with the secretions. The large fluid content within the acini accounts for the sound transmission characteristics and the softness to palpation and compressibility that produce the sonographic characteristics of lactating adenomas.

When infarction is present, it may destroy the evidence of its site of origin. It may be impossible to determine whether it has occurred within a preexisting lactating adenoma or whether it merely occurred within stimulated breast lobules.

Mammographic Findings

The mammographic findings, when present, are not specific for tubular adenoma and are indistinguishable from those of fibroadenoma. Additionally, because most lactating adenomas occur during pregnancy and lactation, when avoidance of radiation is a priority and when breast tissue is most radiographically dense and relatively incompressible, mammographic sensitivity for lactating adenomas is low. Sonography is often the first diagnostic imaging test requested in patients with lactating adenoma.

Sonographic Findings

Most of the sonographic findings that have been reported are for lactating adenomas, not tubular adenomas. However, lactating adenomas are commonly called tubular adenomas in parts of the world other than the United States. For this reason, some reports on the sonographic appearance of tubular adenomas that can be found actually describe the findings of lactating adenomas.

The sonographic appearance of a tubular adenoma is similar to that of a fibroadenoma. Tubular adenomas tend to be elliptical or gently lobulated and wider than tall (Fig. 13–38). There is a greater tendency for the lesions to appear fusiform in shape and pointed on the ends (Fig. 13–39). A minority of tubular adenomas have a microlobulated surface (Fig. 13–40). The sound transmission through tubular adenomas can be either normal or en-

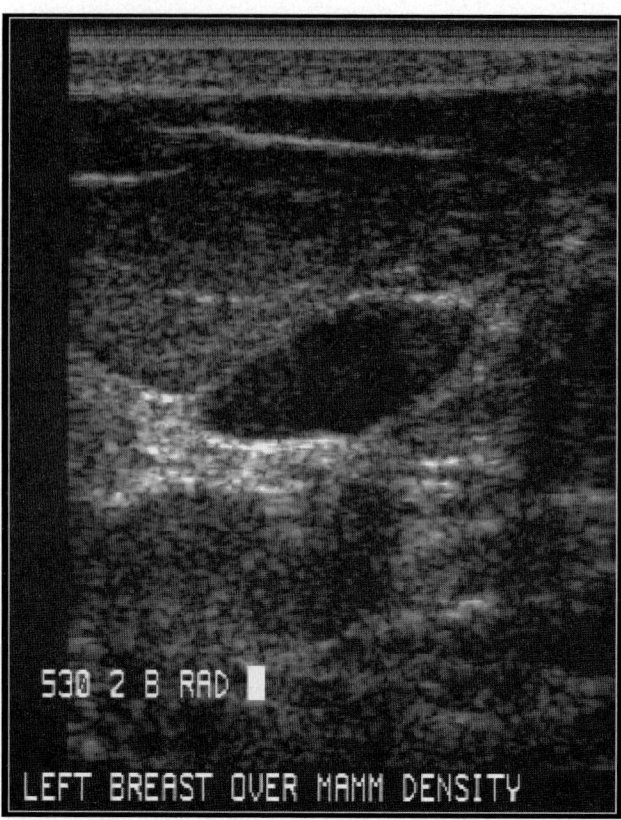

FIGURE 13–39 For reasons that are unclear, tubular adenomas are more frequently fusiform or spindle shaped than are fibroadenomas.

hanced. Enhanced through-transmission is more common because of the predominance of epithelial elements. Tubular adenomas that have undergone infarction (likely during a previous pregnancy) can demonstrate acoustic shadowing (Fig. 13–41).

Lactating adenomas are wider than tall, mildly hypoechoic, and almost invariably microlobulated and demonstrate enhanced through-transmission. The presence of microlobulation virtually always requires these lesions to be characterized as BIRADS 4a, despite the clinical knowledge that they are likely to be lactating adenomas. This sonographic appearance is due not only to the high epithelial cellularity but also to the large amount of fluid within the lumina of the true acini. Each microlobulation represents a secretion-distended acinus (Fig. 13–42). This large fluid component also explains the softness of the nodule to palpation and compression. Split-screen ultrasound images with and without compression often show 23% to 30% or more compressibility of the lesion, the greatest of any solid tumor except for lipoma (Fig. 13–43). Lactating adenomas are reported to be homogeneous. Recent experience, using the most up-to-date available equipment, has been that multiple individual cystic spaces, representing lactational lobules, can be resolved within the substance of the lactating adenoma (Fig. 13–42). The presence of a complete thin,

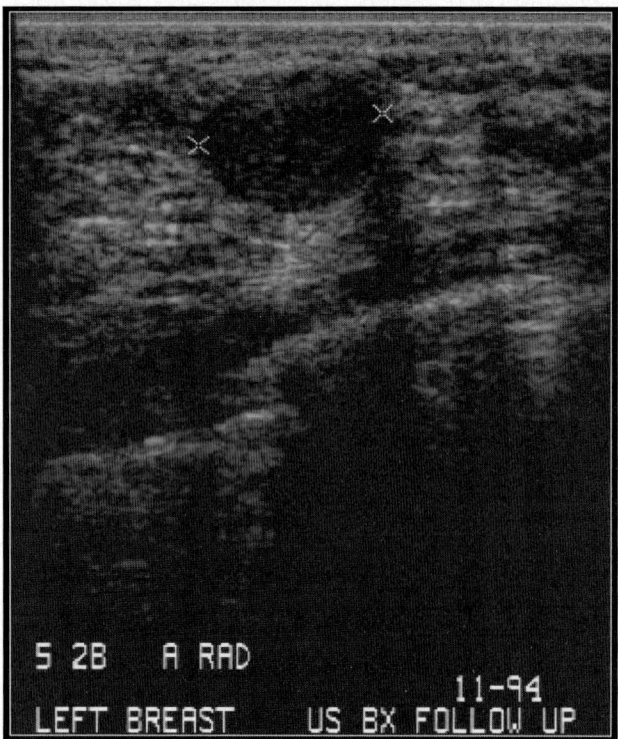

FIGURE 13–38 Tubular adenomas are usually elliptical in shape and hypoechoic and have enhanced through-transmission because they are largely composed of homogeneously distributed epithelial elements. They are indistinguishable from fibroadenomas.

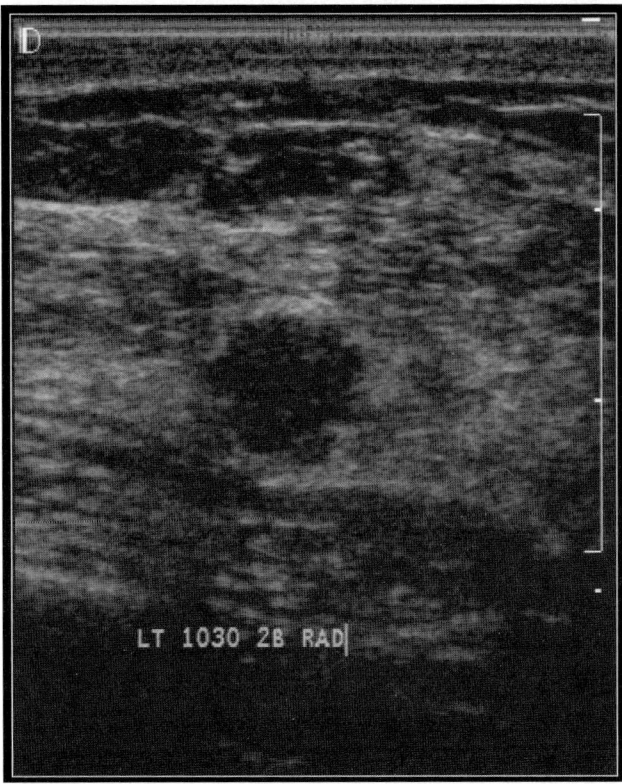

FIGURE 13–40 Like fibroadenomas, not all tubular adenomas have classical BIRADS 3 shapes and surfaces. A minority of tubular adenomas is microlobulated and therefore must be excluded from BIRADS 3 characterization and must undergo biopsy.

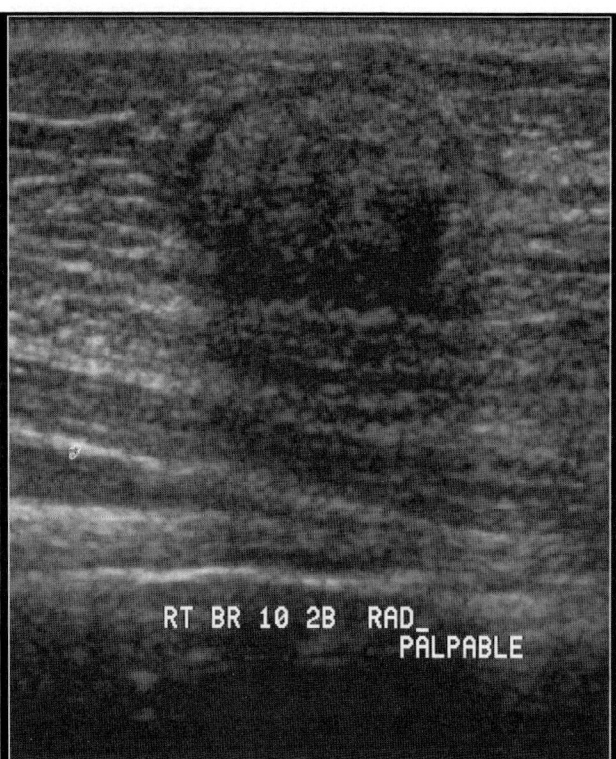

FIGURE 13–41 Most tubular adenomas have enhanced to normal through-transmission. However, this previously infarcted tubular adenoma casts a mild acoustic shadow. The infarction presumably occurred during a previous pregnancy when the lesion had been stimulated and had undergone lactational change.

echogenic capsule around lactating adenomas is more variable than for classic fibroadenomas. There are at least two possible reasons for this variability. First, lactating adenomas occur in a background of lactational lobular change. In such a background, there is very little stromal tissue that can be compressed into a pseudocapsule around the enlarging neoplasm. Second, the origins of lactating adenomas are heterogeneous. At least some of these lesions probably are not true neoplasms, instead representing foci of premature lactational change within lobular tissue early in pregnancy. Our experience has been that lactating adenomas seen in the first two trimesters of pregnancy are smaller than those seen in the third trimester or during lactation, and less frequently demonstrate a complete echogenic capsule. In some of the cases that have been followed into the third trimester of pregnancy, the foci of lactational change became indistinguishable from surrounding lactational tissue, presumably because the growth of lactational tissue caught up with the focus of premature lactational change (Fig. 13–44). Long-term follow-up in such cases has shown neither a residual sonographic nor a mammographic lesion and no residual palpable abnormality. For this reason, immediate biopsy of a solid nodule during the first two trimesters of pregnancy is not recommended if the lesion is mildly hypoechoic compared with surrounding tissues, has enhanced through-transmission and internal diffuse small cystic spaces, and is very soft and compressible, even though a complete thin, echogenic capsule is not demonstrable.

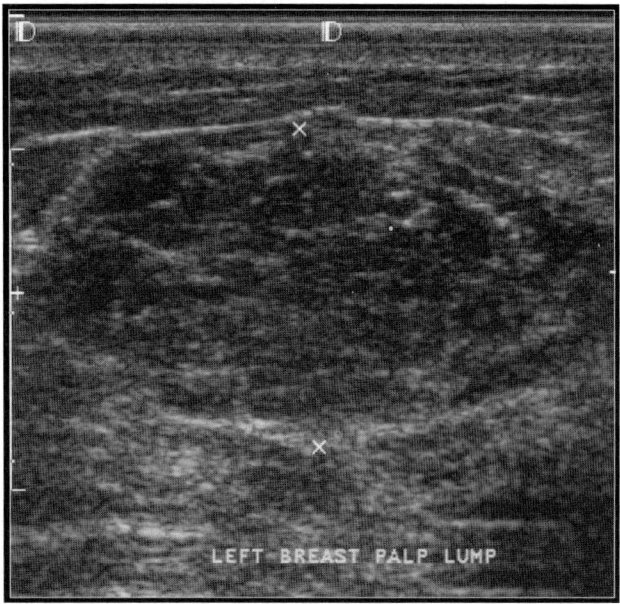

FIGURE 13–42 Despite the high likelihood that these lesions are benign from clinical information alone, almost all lactating adenomas are microlobulated, which prevents them from being characterized as BIRADS 3 and indicates the need for biopsy. The possibility of milk fistula should be mentioned to any patient undergoing core needle biopsy of a suspected lactating adenoma. Most lactating adenomas contain enough milk or secretions to demonstrate enhanced through-transmission. Although lactating adenomas have been reported to be homogeneous in echotexture, we have found virtually all to be heterogeneous. Multiple microlobules or cystic spaces each represent an acinar element distended with milk or secretions.

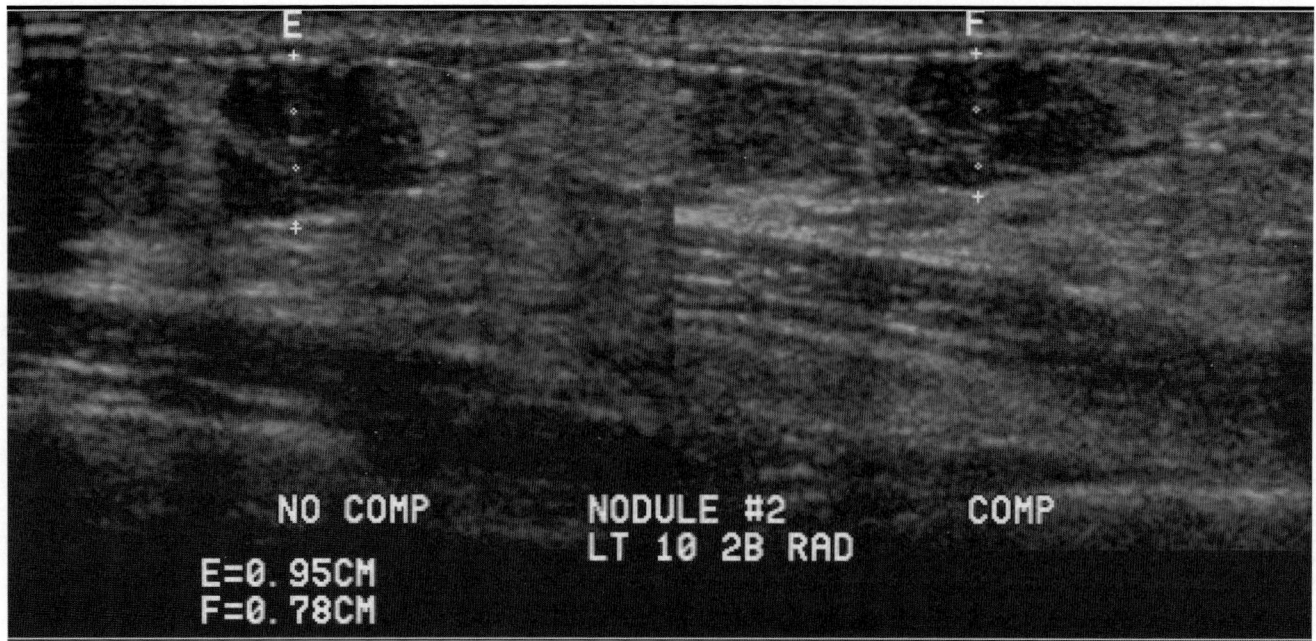

FIGURE 13–43 Because a large portion of lactating adenomas are milk or secretions within distended acini, they tend to be fairly soft and compressible.

Lactating adenomas vary in echogenicity more than any other lesions. Most lactating adenomas are hypoechoic and heterogeneous in texture. However, the milk or secretions within the dilated acini are fatty and proteinaceous and, when inspissated, can become hyperechoic (Fig. 13–45).

Acute infarction of a lactating adenoma results in findings that are indistinguishable from multiple other pathologic disorders occurring during late pregnancy or lactation. The lesion may appear to be a complex galactocele, abscess, or area of infarction of lactational breast change (Fig. 13–46). Occasionally, there may be difficulty distinguishing an infarcted lactating adenoma from a high-grade malignancy with cystic degeneration (Fig. 13–47).

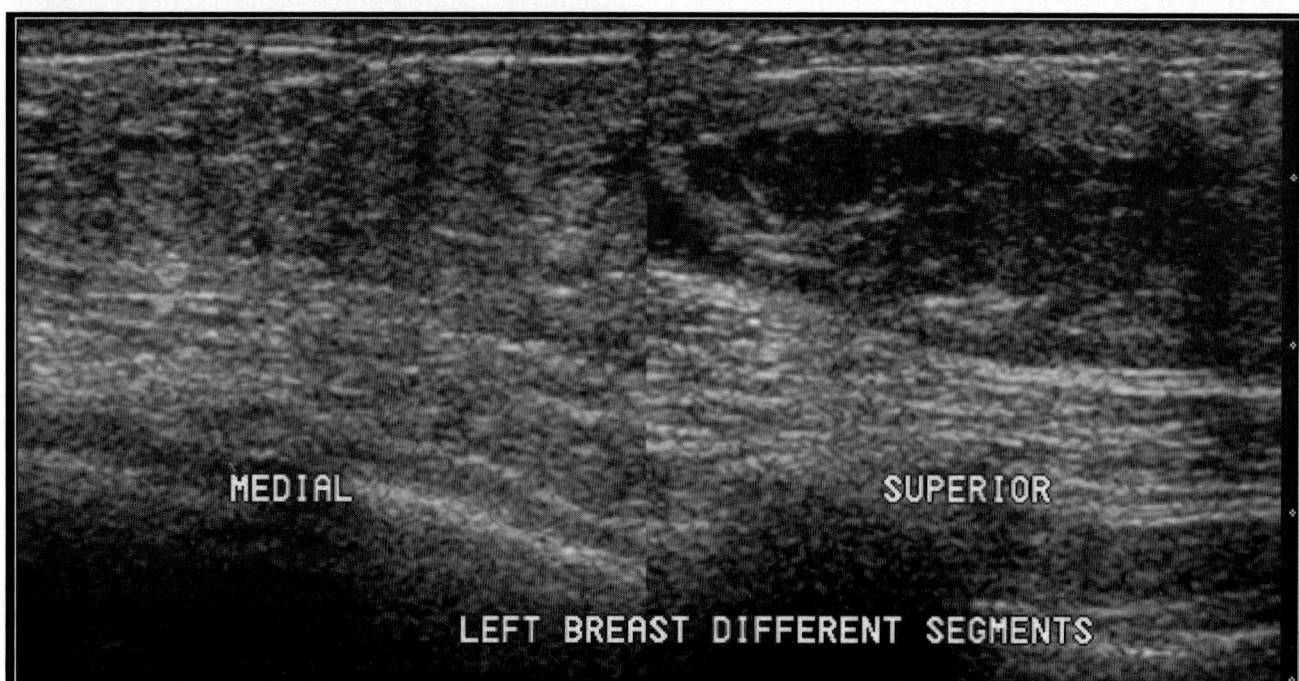

FIGURE 13–44 In some cases, it is likely that what has been diagnosed as a lactating adenoma is merely an area of focal early lactational change in breast tissue, not a true neoplasm. We have seen many cases such as this in which the lesion appeared to disappear as the surrounding tissues "caught up" and underwent lactational change late in pregnancy or during lactation.

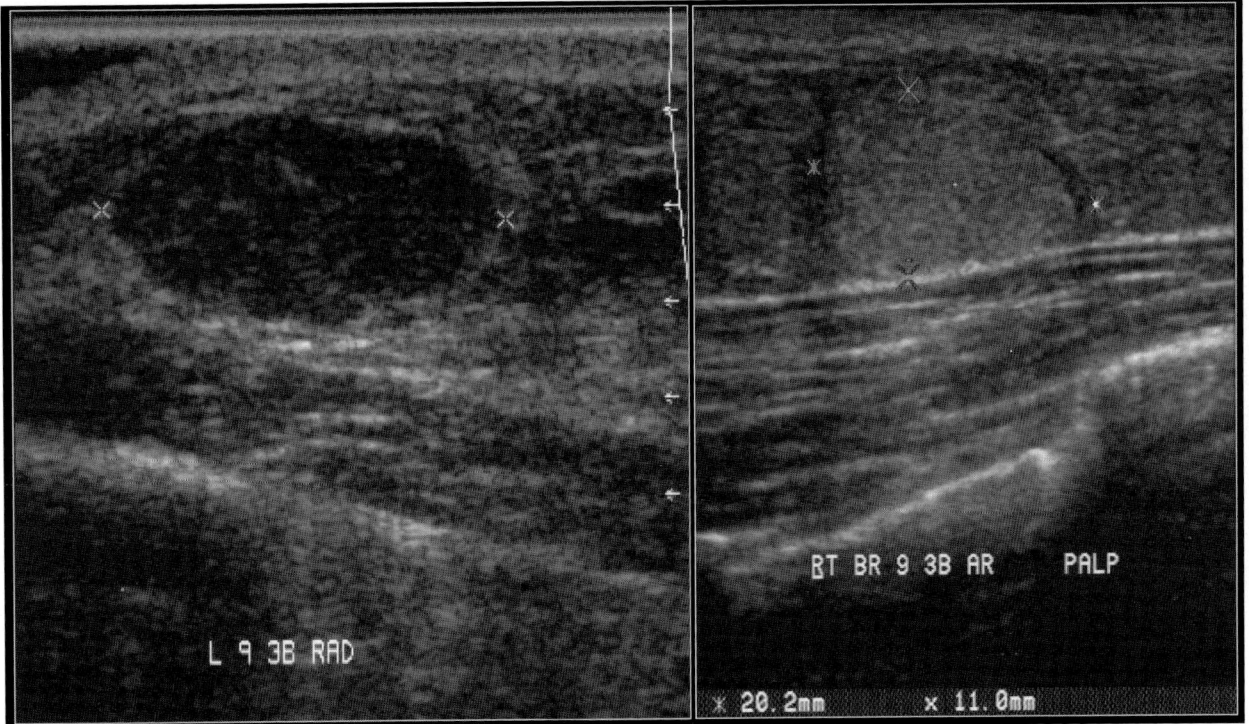

FIGURE 13–45 Not all lactating adenomas are hypoechoic. Some lactating adenomas actually appear hyperechoic (**right**). The milk or secretions contain abundant proteinaceous and fatty elements. The fatty elements of milk, when not completely emulsified within the water components, normally become echogenic. Stasis within the lesion can cause the proteins to become denatured and echogenic. Notice that both hypoechoic and hyperechoic lactating adenomas have enhanced through-transmission.

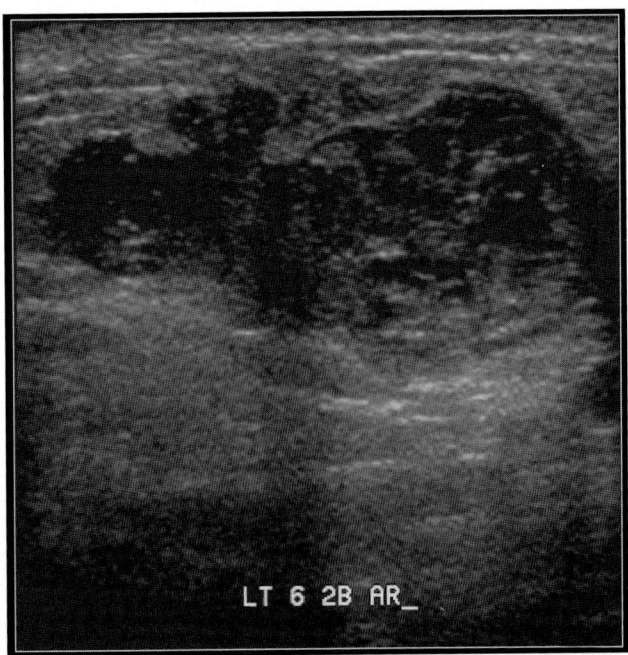

FIGURE 13–46 Lactating adenomas may undergo acute infarction. Lactating adenomas that have undergone acute infarction and liquefaction, such as this case, can mimic complicated galactoceles, puerperal abscess, or malignant nodules that have undergone cystic necrosis.

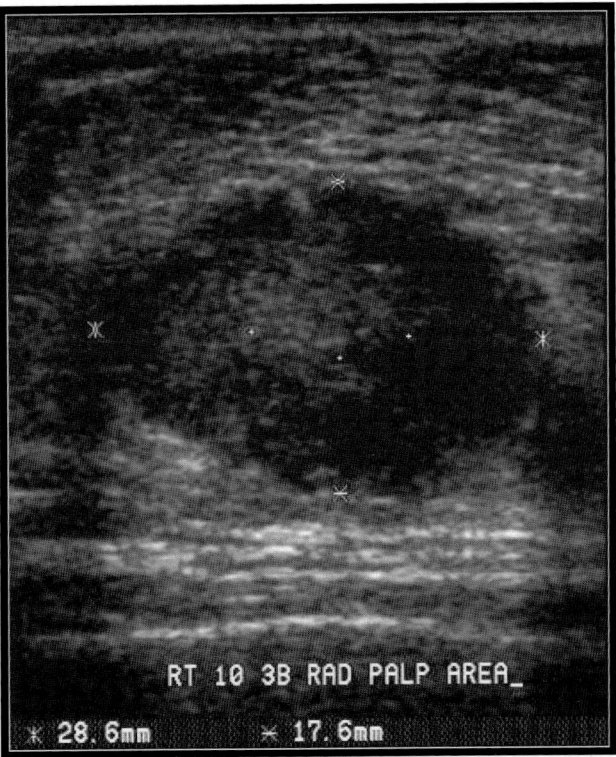

FIGURE 13–47 This high-grade invasive ductal carcinoma during pregnancy has a microlobulated appearance with enhanced through-transmission that is similar to that of lactating adenomas.

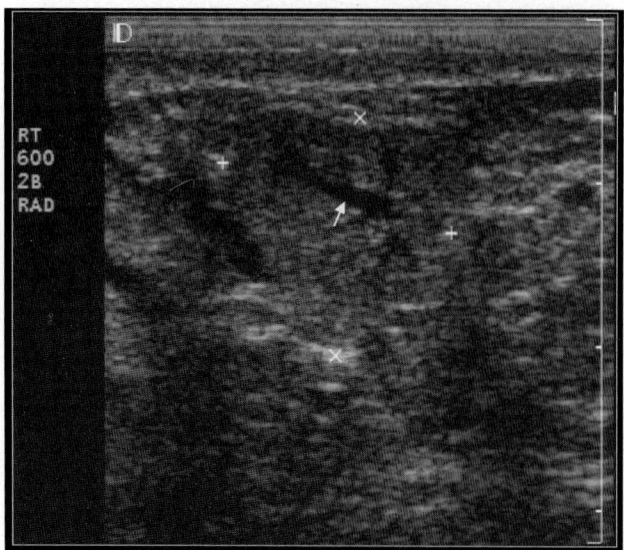

FIGURE 13–48 Preexisting fibroadenomas can undergo secretory or lactational change that can cause cystic dilation of rudimentary ducts *(arrow)*.

Lactating adenomas, because they are stimulated by the hormones of pregnancy or lactation, are almost uniformly hypervascular on color or power Doppler assessment (see Chapter 20, Fig. 20–7).

The hormones of pregnancy or lactation can occasionally stimulate secretory or lactational change within preexisting fibroadenomas. This may lead to dilated ductules and even rudimentary ducts (Fig. 13–48).

Sonographic evaluation should be similar to that for any solid nodule. Nodules not meeting strict criteria for BIRADS 3 should undergo biopsy. Almost all lactating adenomas seen during the third trimester of pregnancy or during lactation are microlobulated and therefore will be excluded from BIRADS 3 characterization. Determining whether palpable abnormalities in the first and second trimester of pregnancy are truly nodules or merely collections of lobules undergoing premature lactational change is often difficult for pathologists as well as radiologists. In such cases, conservative, very-short-interval follow-up may be considered, but because of the rapid rate of change that can occur during pregnancy or lactation, any follow-up should be performed in no more than a few weeks.

INTRAMAMMARY LYMPH NODES

General Pathologic Classification and Epidemiology

Normal and abnormal lymph nodes, including intramammary lymph nodes, are discussed and illustrated in detail in Chapter 19.

HAMARTOMAS

General Pathologic Classification and Epidemiology

Breast hamartomas are localized overgrowth of fibrous, epithelial, and fatty elements. Although hamartomas elsewhere in the body are true neoplasms of all three elements, the fibrous and glandular elements of breast hamartomas do not appear to be truly neoplastic. Most likely, these two components are normal breast elements entrapped within a lipomatous growth. Alternatively, these lesions may represent localized overgrowth of otherwise normal breast tissues. Other terms that have been used to describe breast hamartomas are adenolipofibroma, lipofibroadenoma, adenolipofibroma, and fibroadenolipoma. When there are primarily glandular and fatty elements without an associated fibrous element, the term *adenolipoma* is sometimes used.

Hamartomas primarily occur in adults during the reproductive years. These lesions have been diagnosed in patients from 15 to 88 years of age but are most common in the early 40s.

Clinical Findings

Hamartomas may present as a tender or nontender palpable lump but are now more frequently seen in asymptomatic patients, being identified on routine screening mammograms.

Hamartomas do not recur after local excision, have no special propensity to undergo malignant degeneration, and are not markers for increased relative risk for breast cancer development.

Gross Pathology

Hamartomas vary in appearance, depending on the mix of fibrous, glandular, and fatty elements. Usually, the lesions are circumscribed, firm to soft, and elliptical, spheroid, or gently lobulated in shape. The firmness depends on the prevalence of fatty elements within the lesion. Fatty components may make up only a small part of the lesion, may make up half of the lesion, or may be the predominant component. The larger the fat component, the softer and more compressible the nodule is. These tumors are often encompassed in a fibrous capsule.

Histologic Findings

Hamartomas are composed of normal lobules, fibrous tissue, and fat in varying components. All three components appear normal histologically. This fact is significant because if the pathologist does not know in advance that the radiologist or surgeon suspects the presence of a hamartoma, the pathologic diagnosis may inappropriately be reported as normal breast tissue, no diagnostic features, or nonspecific fibrocystic change. This potential dilemma is especially problematic when the excisional biopsy specimen is fragmented or when core needle or mammotomy obtains the specimen. If the appropriate histologic diagnosis of hamartoma is to be given, the pathologist must be informed that a hamartoma is suspected. Because of this problem, there is great likelihood that hamartomas are underdiagnosed histologically.

The lobules usually have a normal appearance but may show fibrocystic changes such as apocrine metaplasia and cystic dilation. There tends to be a paucity of larger ducts or branching ducts. The amount of stromal fibrous tissue varies, but it is almost always relatively hypocellular. The fat within hamartomas varies greatly in amount. Histologically, the lesion may appear to be a lipoma with a minimal amount of glandular tissue, or mostly fibrous and glandular with only a minimal amount of fatty tissue. Larger hamartomas usually have a thin capsule of compressed surrounding normal breast tissue, but this demarcation may be absent in smaller lesions.

Mammographic Findings

The mammographic findings of larger hamartomas located in entirely fatty breasts (or those located within parts of the breast that are almost entirely fatty) are definitive. The classic hamartoma is round, oval, or lobulated. The lesions show a mixture of isodense water density and fat density and are classically surrounded by a thin water-density capsule (Fig. 13–49). Lesions in which glandular and fibrous elements predominate appear to be equal to water density on mammograms, whereas those lesions in which fat predominates show more fat density on mammograms. Mammographic and palpable lesions that show classic findings of hamartoma are definitively benign (BIRADS 2) and do not need to undergo biopsy or be followed.

Routine mammograms have shown hamartomas to be much more common than earlier pathologic literature would suggest. Hamartomas have likely been underdiagnosed and inaccurately reported as normal breast tissue, accounting for the lower prevalence of these lesions in the pathologic literature.

Recent literature has suggested that hamartomas are even underdiagnosed mammographically because smaller hamartomas that are located in heterogeneously dense segments of the breast may not show classic mammographic findings. The mammographic findings described as classic and definitive occur only in larger hamartomas that displace enough normal radiographically dense tissue to be apparent or in smaller hamartomas that are completely surrounded by fat. Lesions that are not mammographically classic but that are suspected of being hamartomas may benefit from sonographic or MRI evaluation.

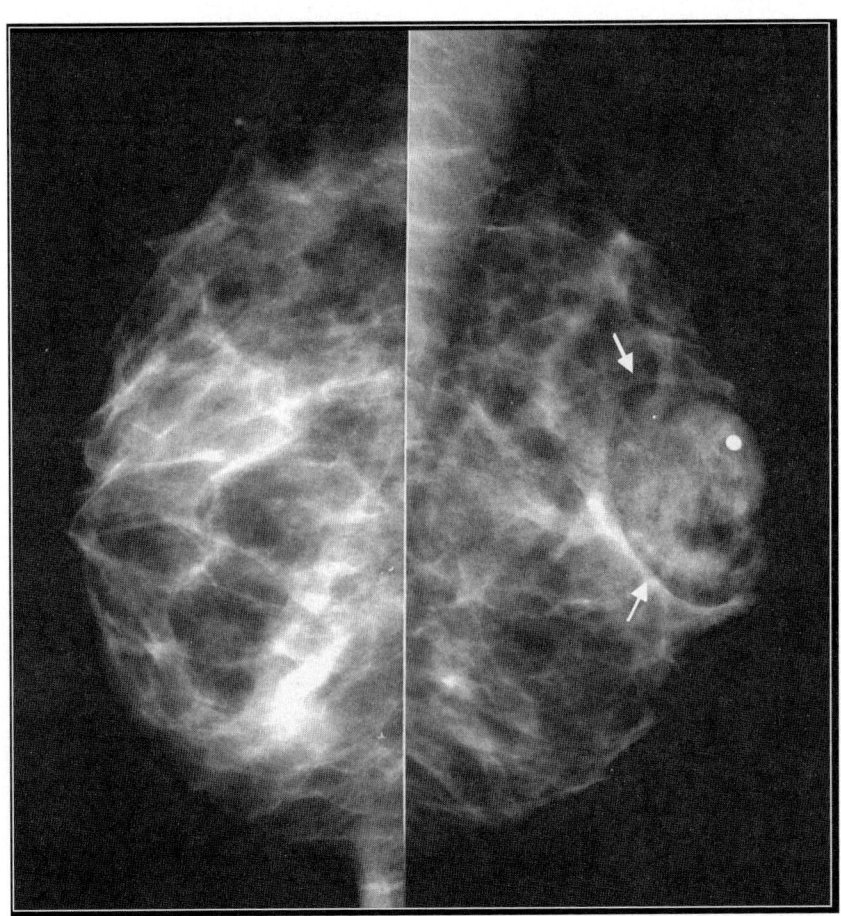

FIGURE 13–49 This classic hamartoma is mammographically definitively benign, BI-RADS 2. Classic hamartomas are typically composed of a mixture of water and fatty elements and encompassed within a thin water-density capsule.

Sonographic Findings

There is little point in performing ultrasound on mammographically classic hamartomas. These lesions, like normal intramammary lymph nodes, are definitely benign (BI-RADS 2) based on mammographic findings alone and do not require biopsy or special follow-up. However, ultrasound can be helpful in cases in which only the water-density elements of the hamartoma are identifiable on routine two-view mammograms. Also, ultrasound can be helpful and reassuring in cases in which hamartoma is suspected but in which the findings are not classic, owing to lack of a complete capsule, small size, or a relatively small fat component.

The sonographic findings of hamartomas are as variable as the histologic findings. There are reports of hamartomas being solid, homogeneously hypoechoic, and shadowing. However, our experience has been that hamartomas are usually very heterogeneous, composed of a variable mixture of isoechoic fatty or lobular elements and hyperechoic fibrous elements (Fig. 13–50). As would be expected, the relative proportions of each echotexture reflect the underlying histologic constituents. An important

point to remember is that, like normal breast tissues, isoechoic tissues may represent either fat or normal lobular (glandular) tissue. Thus, the water-density portions of the lesions on mammography may represent either fibrous tissue (hyperechoic) or lobular tissue (isoechoic). The peripheral capsule, when both present and intact, like the capsule surrounding simple cysts and simple fibroadenomas, appears as a thin, echogenic line (Fig. 13–51). However, the capsule is really a pseudocapsule of compressed breast tissue, and the thickness and echogenicity depend on the types of compressed tissues that constitute the capsule (Fig. 13–52). Because smaller hamartomas may not have a complete pseudocapsule on gross morphology, it should not be surprising that some smaller hamartomas also lack a complete capsule sonographically (Fig. 13–53). Depending on how much fat is present within the hamartoma, the lesion may be very soft and compressible. Split-screen images with and without compression often show a degree of compressibility nearly matching that of pure lipomas and lactating adenomas. Hamartomas are commonly 20% to 30% compressible, although those lesions with relatively little fat may be less compressible (Fig. 13–54). Thus, normal

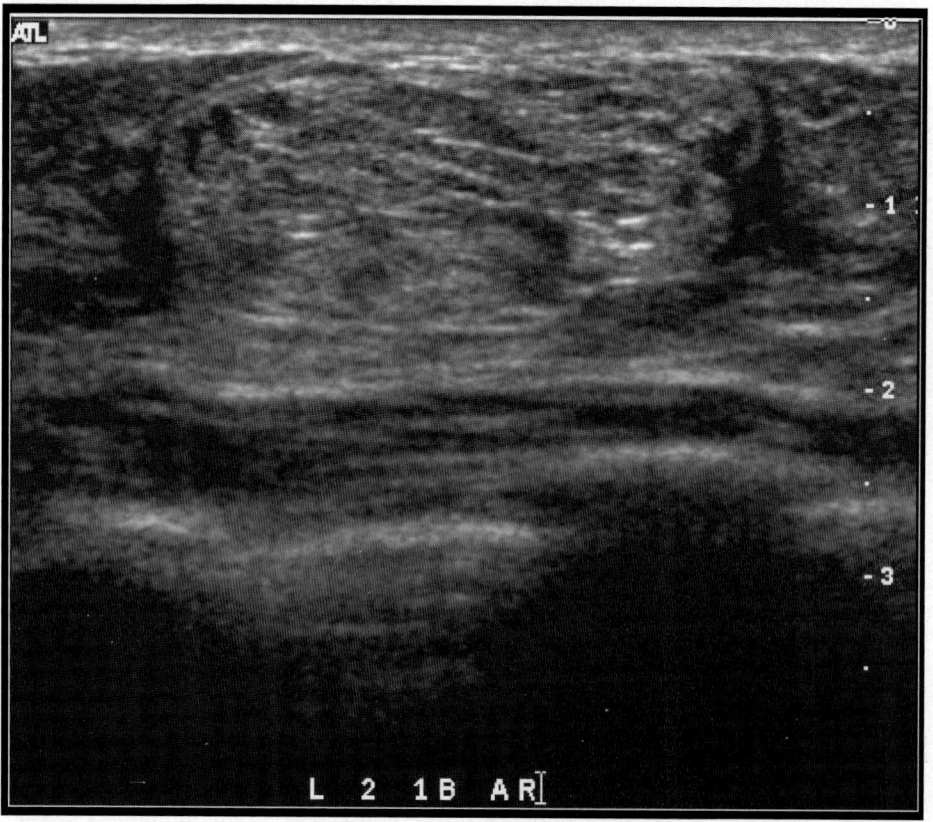

FIGURE 13–50 The classic hamartoma is sonographically similar to the classic mammographic lesion. It is comprised of a mixture of isoechoic and hyperechoic elements and surrounded by an echogenic pseudocapsule of compressed tissues that varies in thickness. The hyperechoic elements are the fibrous parts of the lesion. The isoechoic parts represent the glandular and fatty elements within the lesion.

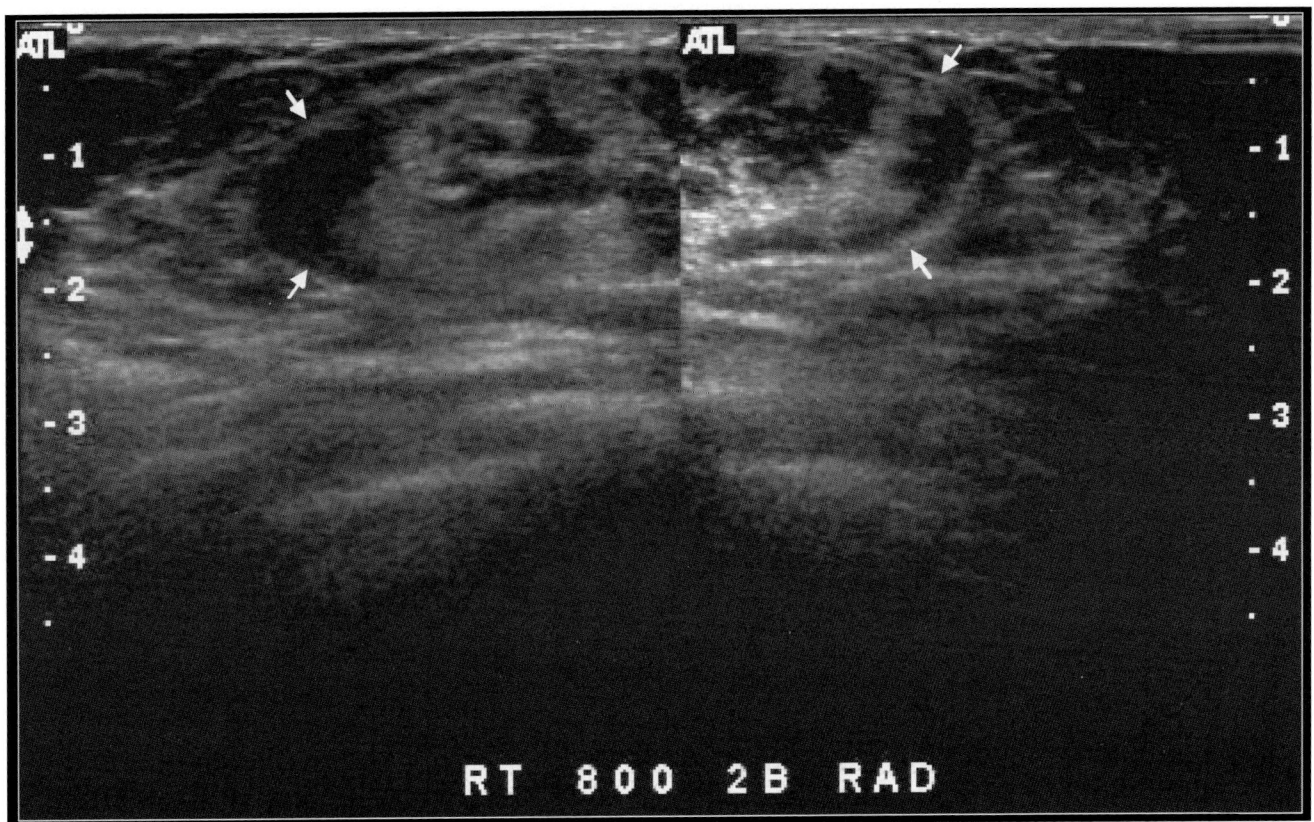

FIGURE 13–51 The classic hamartoma on ultrasound is completely encompassed in a thin, echogenic pseudocapsule *(arrows)* of compressed breast tissue. The central gray elements are glandular. The central hyperechoic elements are fibrous, and the mildly hypoechoic element just inside the capsule is fat. Not all hamartomas are classic. Thus, the capsule may be thick or partially absent.

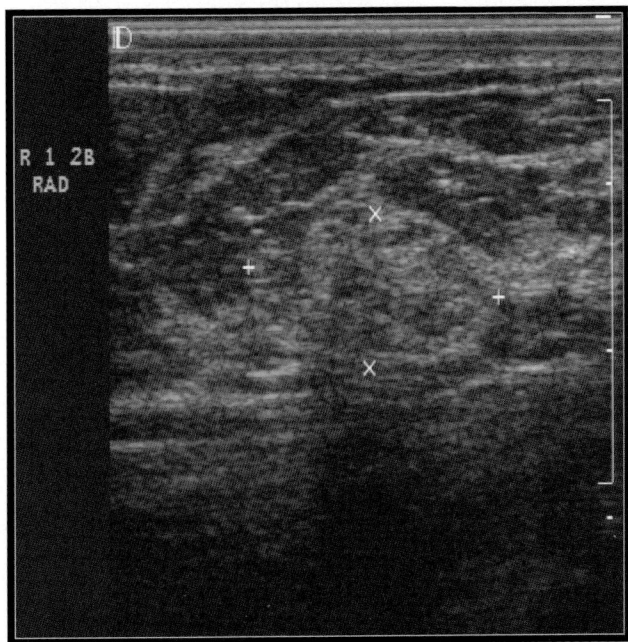

FIGURE 13–52 This hamartoma has a thick, echogenic pseudo-capsule and is composed primarily of glandular and fibrous elements.

scan pressures usually flatten the hamartoma into a wider-than-tall ellipsoid shape. A flattened target-like or multilaminated appearance is rather typical (Fig. 13–55). The center of the target-like lesion is usually isoechoic, reflecting a central collection of lobular tissue. The central glandular tissue is surrounded by a thick ring of echogenic fibrous elements, which, in turn, is surrounded by a thick isoechoic ring of fatty tissue. The fatty tissue is encapsulated within a thin, echogenic rim of fibrous tissue. Unfortunately, hamartomas often do not have a classic sonographic appearance. The target-like or multilaminated hamartoma represents a lesion in which fatty, glandular, and fibrous elements are roughly present in equal proportions. However, many hamartomas do not have a target-like or multilaminar appearance because one type of tissue or another predominates. Thus, in some cases, the fatty elements may be so dominant that the lesion is difficult to distinguish from a lipoma, both mammographically and sonographically. Such lesions are usually nearly isoechoic, fairly homogeneous, and highly compressible, just like lipomas (Fig. 13–56). In other hamartomas, adenomatous elements are so predominant that the lesion may appear sonographically similar to a fibroadenoma or adenoma—

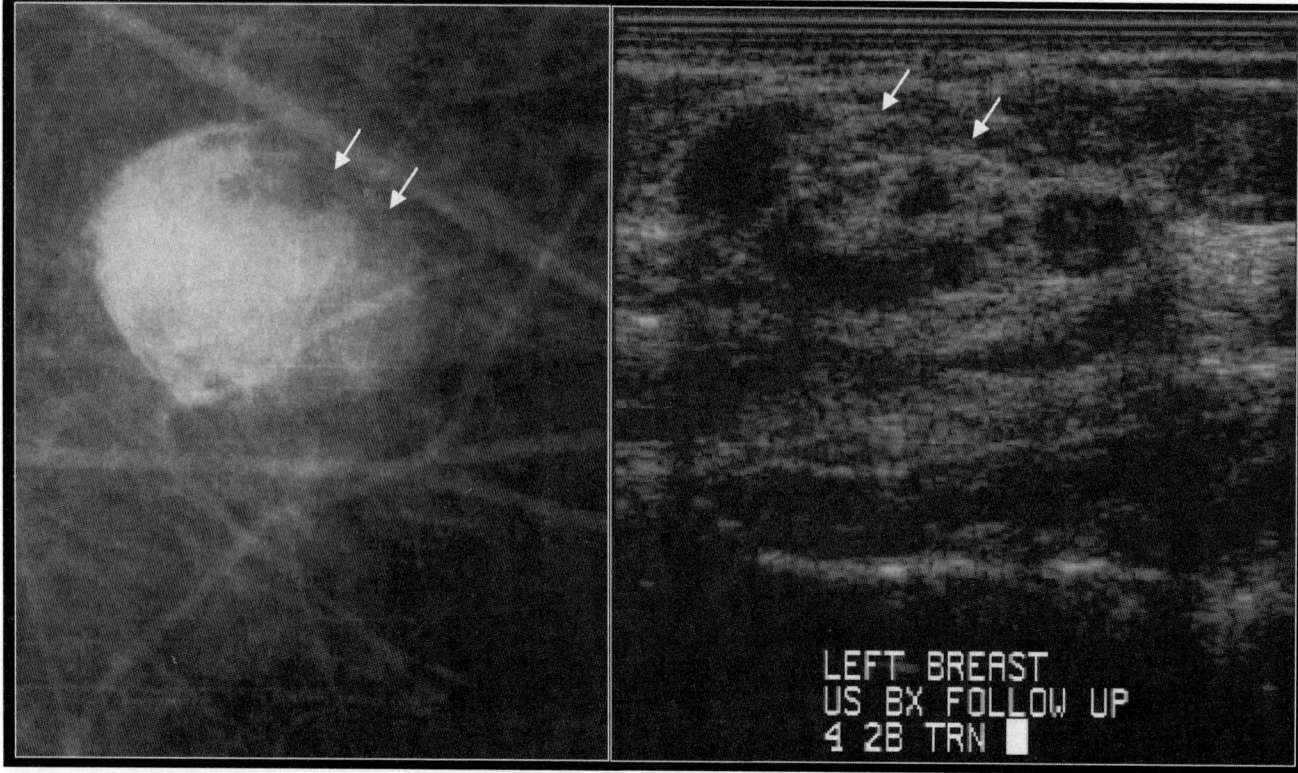

FIGURE 13–53 Smaller hamartomas are less likely to have a complete pseudocapsule of compressed breast tissue. This small hamartoma lacks a capsule along its upper margin on the mammogram and along its anterior margin sonographically *(arrows)*. That the lower portion of the nodule is water density on the mammogram indicates that the isoechoic elements are primarily glandular or adenomatous rather than fatty.

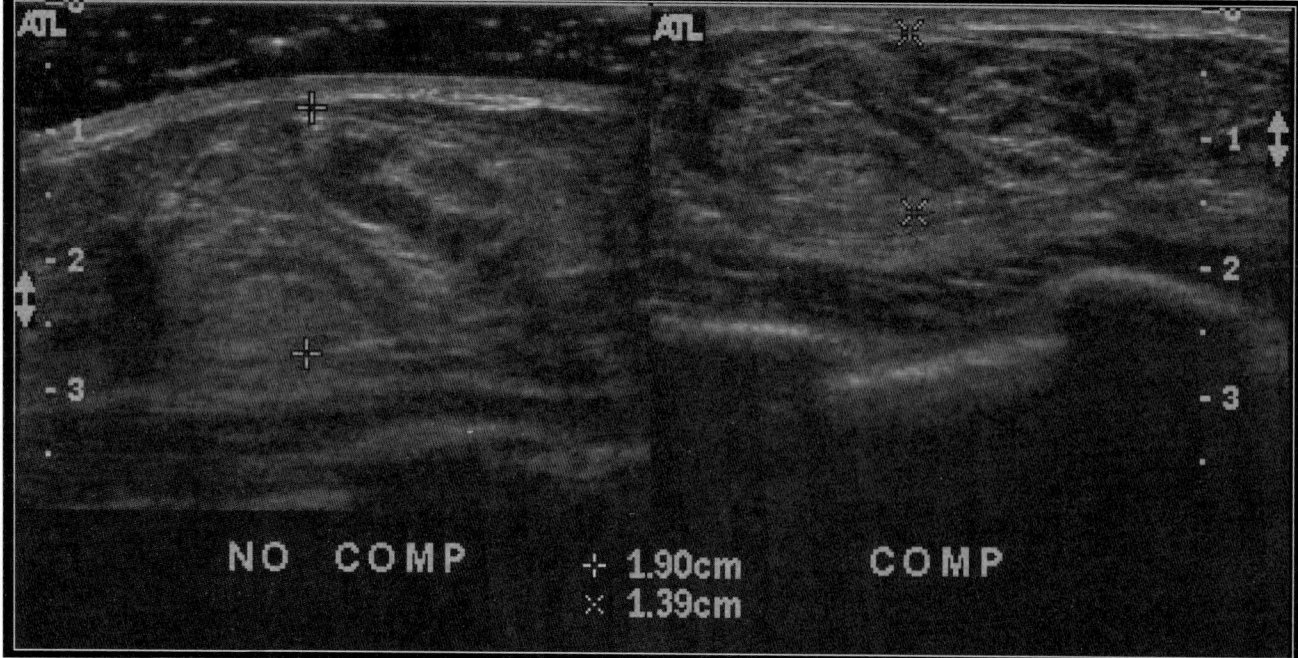

FIGURE 13–54 Because most hamartomas have significant amounts of fatty tissue, they tend to be quite soft and compressible. Most are about 30% to 35% compressible, similar to lipomas. In fact, some believe that lipomas are not true neoplasms, but instead are hamartomas that are composed almost entirely of fat.

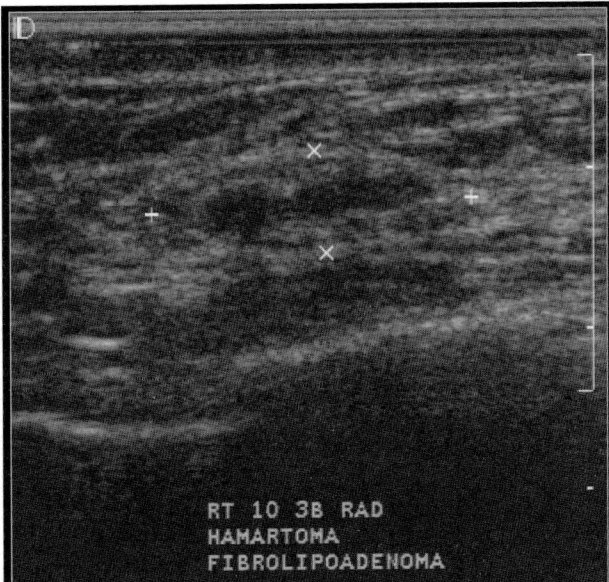

FIGURE 13–55 Many hamartomas have a targeted or multilaminar appearance. The outer echogenic line is the fibrous pseudocapsule, the isoechoic area just inside the capsule is fat, the inner echogenic ring is fibrous tissue, and the innermost isoechoic structure is glandular tissue.

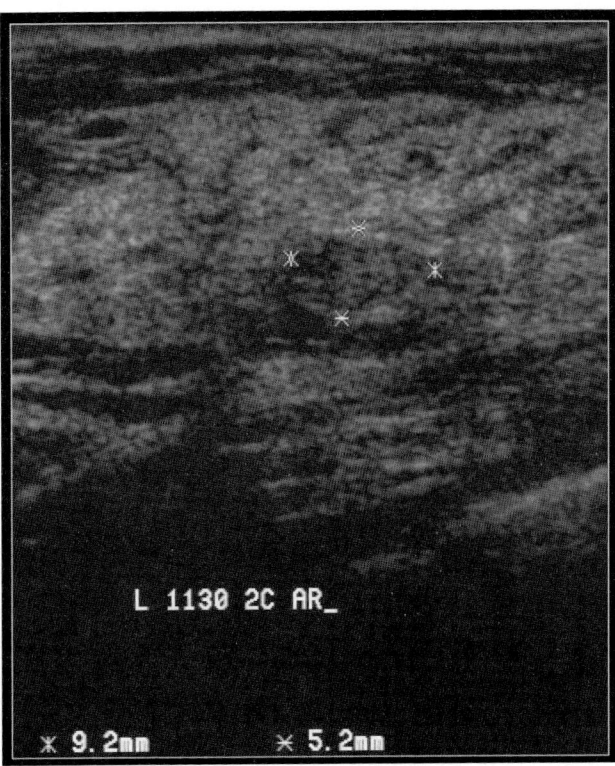

FIGURE 13–57 This homogeneously mildly hyperechoic hamartoma is composed primarily of fibrous elements.

isoechoic, elliptical, and encapsulated within a thin, echogenic capsule (Fig. 13–57). Such lesions may be mildly compressible but are less compressible than hamartomas with higher fat content. Some hamartomas that are composed of primarily fibrous and fatty elements appear to be definitively benign mammographically but not sonographically. Such lesions appear to be fairly homogeneous

and isoechoic at sonography because sonography cannot distinguish between the echogenicities of glandular tissue and fat very well. Mammography, on the other hand, shows the lesions to be mixed water and fatty density, a finding that indicates a BIRADS 2 lesion (Fig. 13–58). Fi-

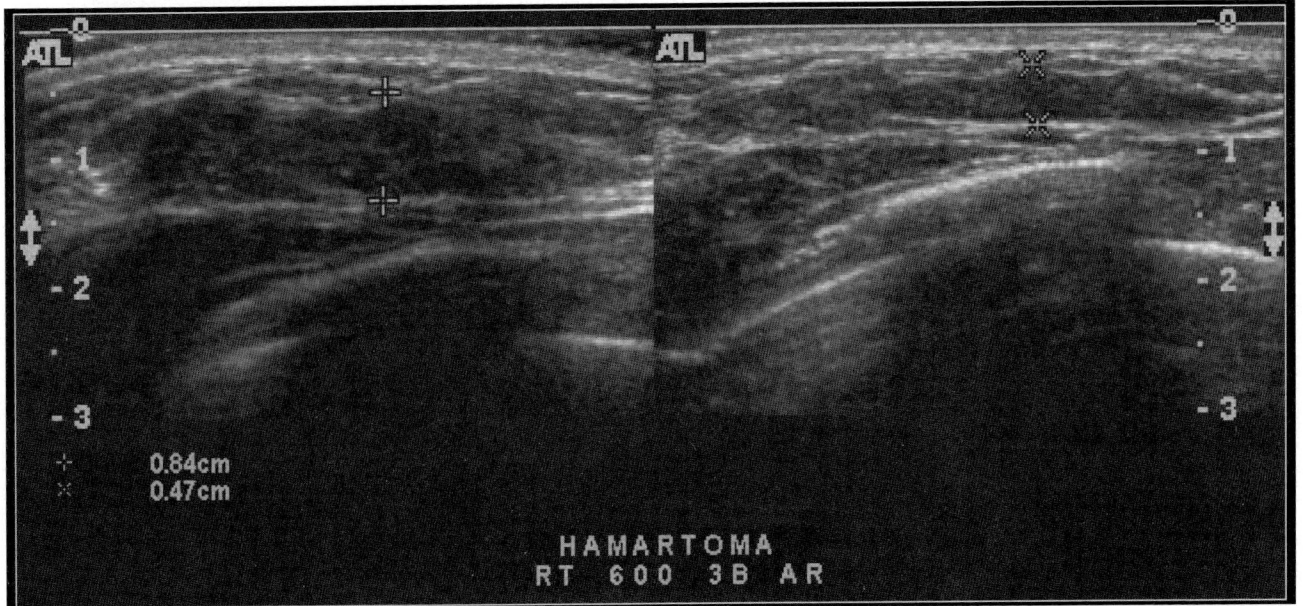

FIGURE 13–56 This homogeneously isoechoic hamartoma is composed almost entirely of fat and could easily be classified as a lipoma.

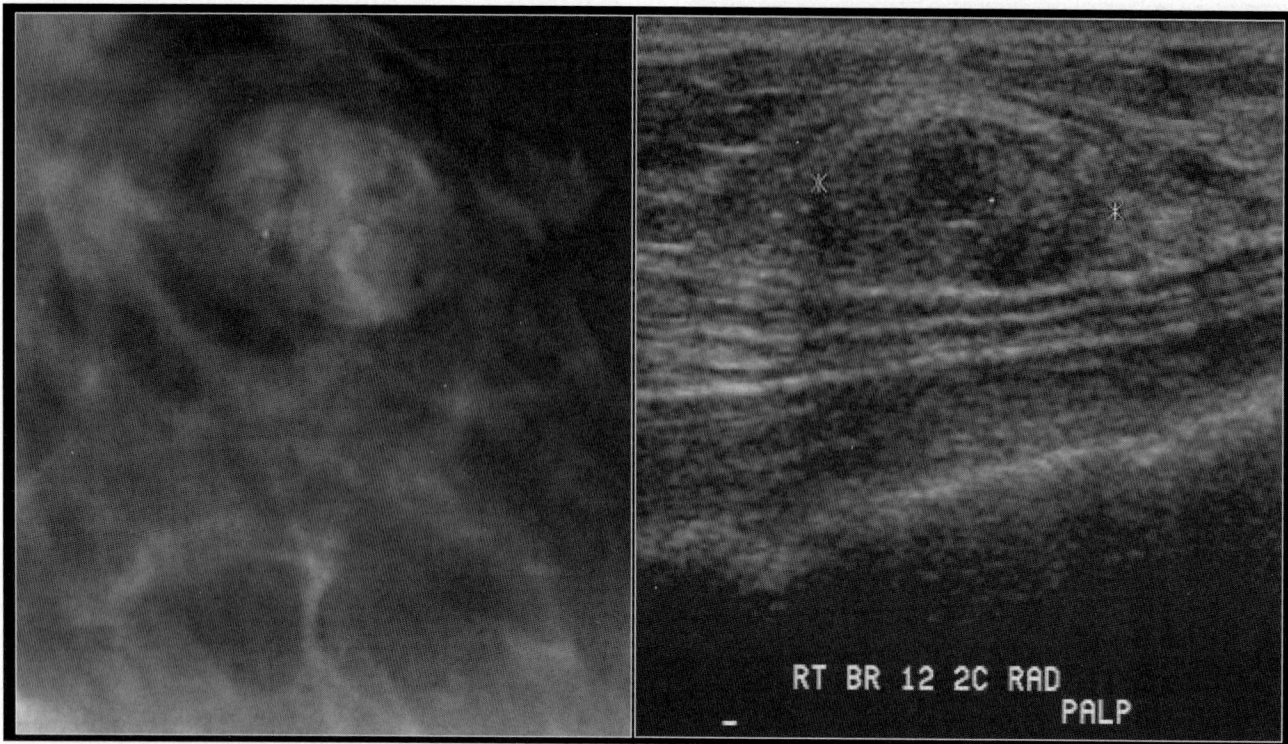

FIGURE 13–58 This nearly homogeneously isoechoic hamartoma is composed of a mixture of fatty and glandular elements but has very little fibrous component. On sonography, we cannot readily distinguish between the echogenicity of the glandular and fatty elements, but the mammogram readily shows a mixture of fat and water-density tissue. The mammographic findings are BIRADS 2, but the sonographic findings are not.

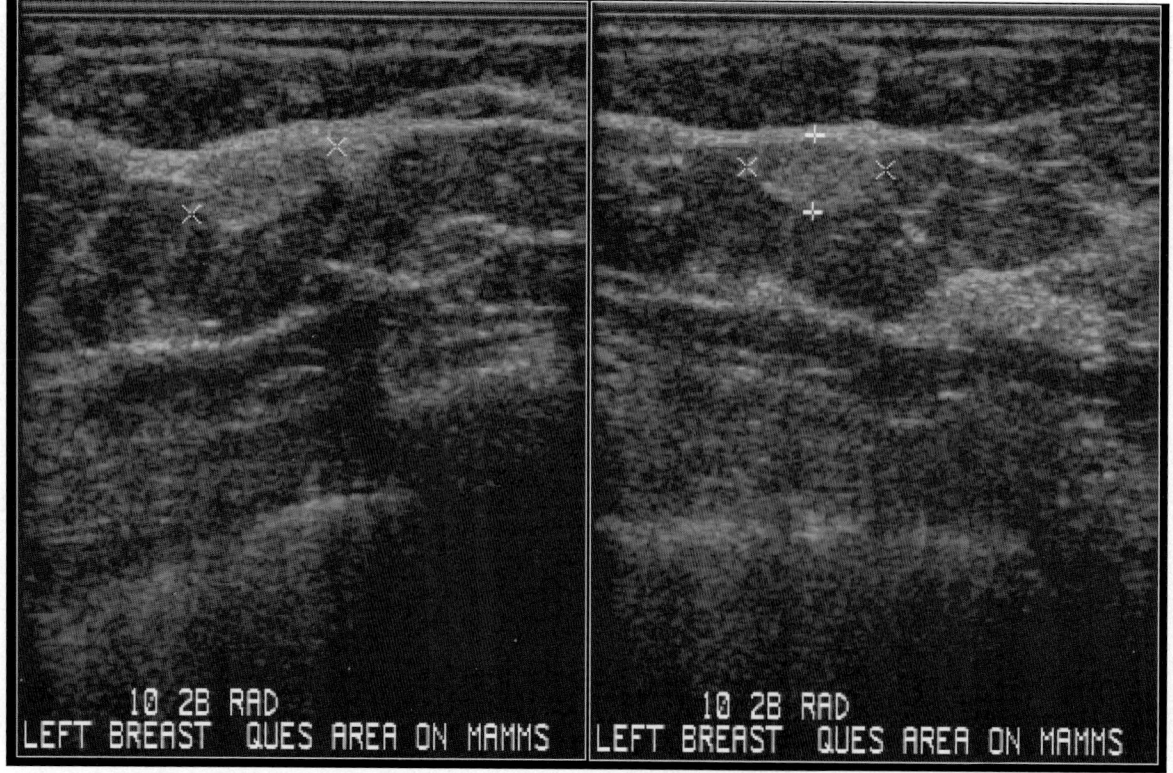

FIGURE 13–59 This homogeneously hyperechoic hamartoma contains primarily fibrous elements.

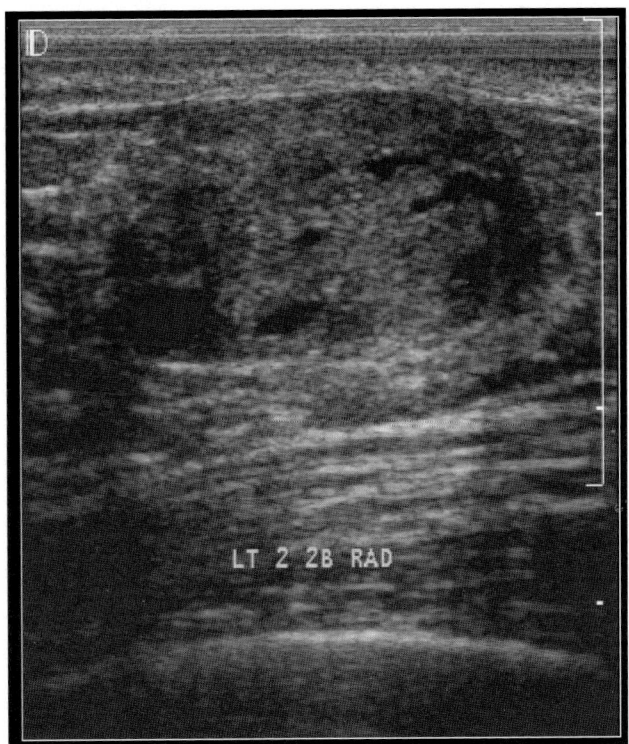

FIGURE 13–60 This isoechoic hamartoma is almost entirely composed of glandular or adenomatous elements and appears sonographically similar to an adenoma or fibroadenoma. Like fibroadenomas, the glandular elements of hamartomas may contain fibrocystic changes, including macroscopic cysts.

error is not serious because hamartomas, lipomas, and normal but prominent fat lobules are all recognizable as benign findings in most cases.

The individual components of hamartomas appear as normal fatty, fibrous, and lobular breast elements on ultrasound. Therefore, the possibility that a palpable or mammographic abnormality could be due to hamartoma must be kept in mind, or the sonographic diagnosis will be missed. The sonographer might mistakenly conclude that the palpable or mammographic abnormality is due to normal fibrofatty or fibroglandular elements. This pitfall is completely analogous to the plight of the pathologist, who diagnoses normal breast tissue or breast tissue with no diagnostic features if not informed that hamartoma is suspected. As a practical matter, however, missing the diagnosis of hamartoma is of little long-term clinical significance because these lesions are benign, usually are self-limited, and are not thought to be premalignant or to alter the patient's relative risk for breast cancer. The one circumstance in which sonographic suspicion of hamartoma may be helpful is when only the water-density elements of the hamartoma are recognized on routine two-view mammo-

nally, in some hamartomas, in which the fibrous element is predominant, the entire lesion may appear hyperechoic and may be difficult to distinguish from focal fibrous tissue (Fig. 13–59). Such lesions are more definitively benign sonographically than they are mammographically.

The adenomatous elements of hamartomas can undergo fibrocystic or benign proliferative changes. The larger the adenomatous component, the more likely this is to occur. Thus, lesions that are primarily adenomatous are those most likely to show fibrocystic change that typically appears as intralesional cystic areas and is sonographically very similar to the appearance of complex fibroadenomas that contain cysts (Fig. 13–60). In other cases of primarily adenomatous hamartomas, benign proliferative disorders such as adenosis and sclerosing adenosis may create suspicious findings that result in our having to characterize the lesion as BIRADS 4a or higher, despite the presence of fatty density on mammography (Figs. 13–61 and 13–62).

The lack of a demonstrable complete thin, echogenic capsule prevents sonographic identification of certain lesions, just as lack of a thin water-density delimiting capsule complicates definitively diagnosing hamartomas mammographically. Hamartomas that are largely composed of fat may be mistaken for lipomas or normal fat lobules. This

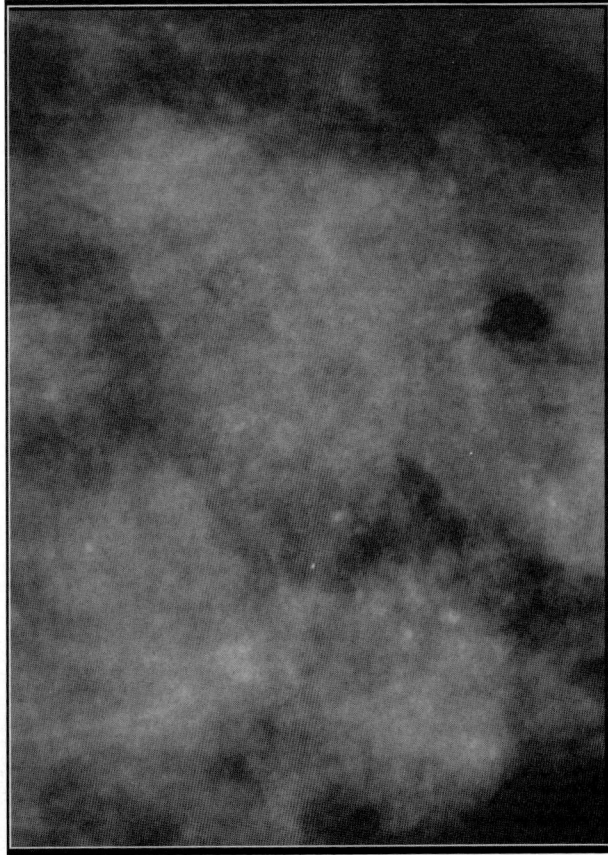

A

FIGURE 13–61 A: This large, primarily glandular hamartoma has developed extensive adenosis and contains extensive powdery calcifications. *(Continued.)*

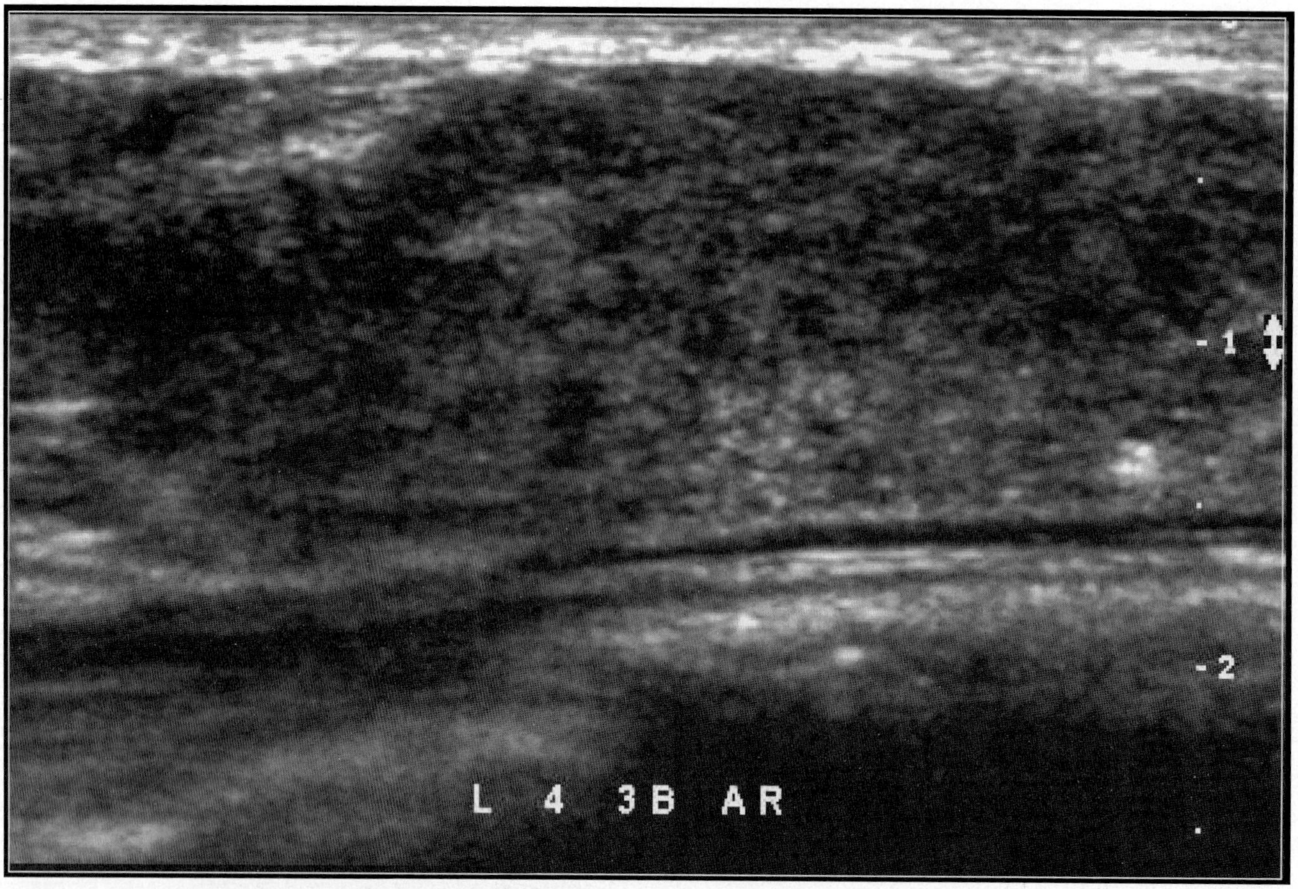

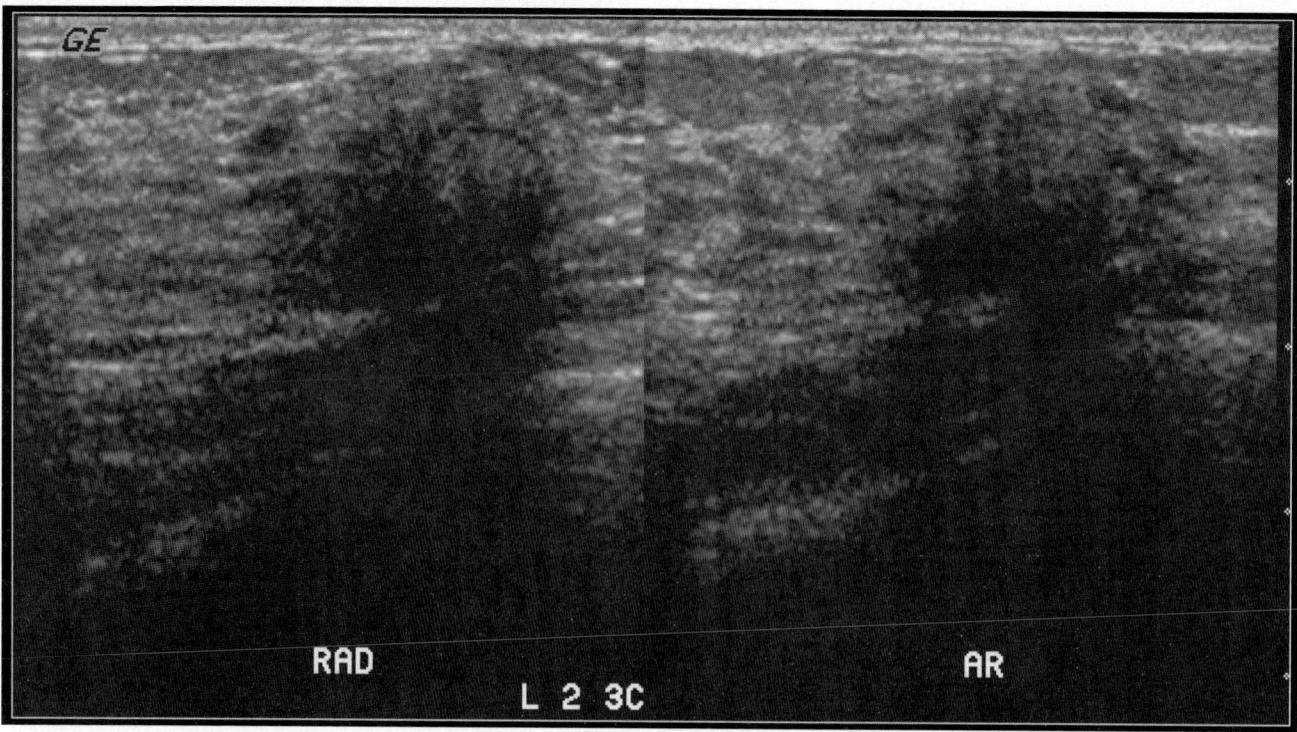

FIGURE 13–61 *(continued)* B: This large hamartoma is the same lesion shown in Fig. 13–61A. There is extensive adenosis with numerous powdery calcifications.

FIGURE 13–62 The glandular elements of this hamartoma developed severe sclerosing adenosis, which led to angular margins and acoustic shadowing, suspicious findings that require a BIRADS category of 4a or higher and demand biopsy.

grams. Such patients are referred for and undergo diagnostic ultrasound. There have been several instances in such patients in which sonography suggested the possibility of hamartoma. Subsequent additional spot compression mammograms displaced enough of the surrounding heterogeneously dense fibroglandular tissue to allow a definitive mammographic diagnosis of hamartoma to be made, thus avoiding unnecessary biopsy.

LIPOMAS

General Pathologic Classification and Epidemiology

Lipomas are benign overgrowths of adipose tissue. Breast lipomas do not differ from lipomas found elsewhere in the body and are really skin lesions rather than breast lesions. In fact, many patients with breast lipomas have lipomas elsewhere in the body. Lipomas are probably not true neoplasms, but rather variants of hamartomas that contain only fat. Occasionally, lipomas may contain small amounts of lobular (glandular) tissue and are then called *adenolipomas*. These lesions may also contain proliferating capillaries and are then called *angiolipomas*. There is also a spindle cell variety. Lipomas can occur in any tissue plane that contains fat. Most lipomas arise within the subcutaneous fat layer (premammary zone), but these lesions may also occur within the retromammary fat or within involuted fatty lobules with in the mammary zone. Lipomas occasionally arise within the chest wall muscles, and retropectoral lipomas have been described. Large lipomas can undergo fat necrosis. Breast lipomas only rarely undergo malignant degeneration to form liposarcomas and are not associated with increase relative risk for breast cancer development.

Clinical Findings

Lipomas usually present as nontender, soft, mobile, palpable lumps. Occasionally, a lipoma can be tender, especially if complicated by fat necrosis. These lesions occur nearly as commonly in males as in females and in all age groups.

Gross Pathologic Findings

Tumor size ranges from 2 to 20 cm. Lipomas are sharply delineated and usually encompassed by a thin capsule of connective tissue. The fat within lipomas is indistinguishable grossly from normal fat lobules that occur within the breast.

Histologic Findings

The adipocytes within lipomas are indistinguishable from adipocytes within normal fat lobules that occur within the breast. Therefore, the pathologist may need to know that

the surgeon or the radiologist suspects lipoma in order to make the correct diagnosis. The potential for misdiagnosis is heightened if the excisional biopsy specimen is fragmented and not intact, or if the pathologist receives core needle or mammotomy specimens. Lipomas are rarely subjected to needle biopsy. If the suspected prebiopsy diagnosis of lipoma is not communicated, however, the pathologist may assume that the target of the biopsy has been missed and that the fat obtained from the biopsy specimen is background breast tissue. Even when receiving an intact excisional biopsy specimen, the pathologist may have difficulty distinguishing between lipoma and a normal breast fat lobule. In such cases, a diagnosis of fatty pseudotumor or nodular adiposity may be given.

Pure lipomas are composed of only adipocytes. Adenolipomas contain scattered TDLUs, and angiolipomas have proliferating capillaries.

Mammographic Findings

Large lipomas, especially if surrounded by fat, have a classically benign mammographic appearance and do not require biopsy or short-interval follow-up studies. The classic lipoma is entirely fat density and has a thin, peripheral water-density capsule or water-density tissue that obscures the capsule (Fig. 13–63). However, similar to hamartomas, smaller lipomas that are surrounded by fat may be difficult to distinguish from adjacent normal fat lobules, especially if a thin water-density capsule is not seen (Fig. 13–64). Furthermore, smaller palpable lipomas that occur within heterogeneously dense breast tissue may be obscured by superimposed water-density fibroglandular elements. In such cases, there will be no mammographic evidence that the cause of the palpable abnormality is fat. Under these circumstances, a tomographic technique such as sonography, which allows simultaneous scanning and palpation in real time, can be invaluable in confirming that the palpable abnormality is merely a fat lobule or lipoma.

Large lipomas that have undergone fat necrosis may show the entire spectrum of mammographic findings that can be seen with fat necrosis. When the mammographic findings of fat necrosis are of the typically benign variety, no difficulties are encountered. If fat necrosis within a lipoma has progressed to the fibrous scarring stage, however, there may be difficulty determining mammographically whether the changes represent fat necrosis or malignant degeneration into liposarcoma.

Sonographic Findings

Lipomas with a classically benign (BIRADS 2) mammographic appearance do not require sonography for further evaluation. However, suspected lipomas that are not classic and palpable lumps occurring within a background of mammographically heterogeneously dense fibroglandular

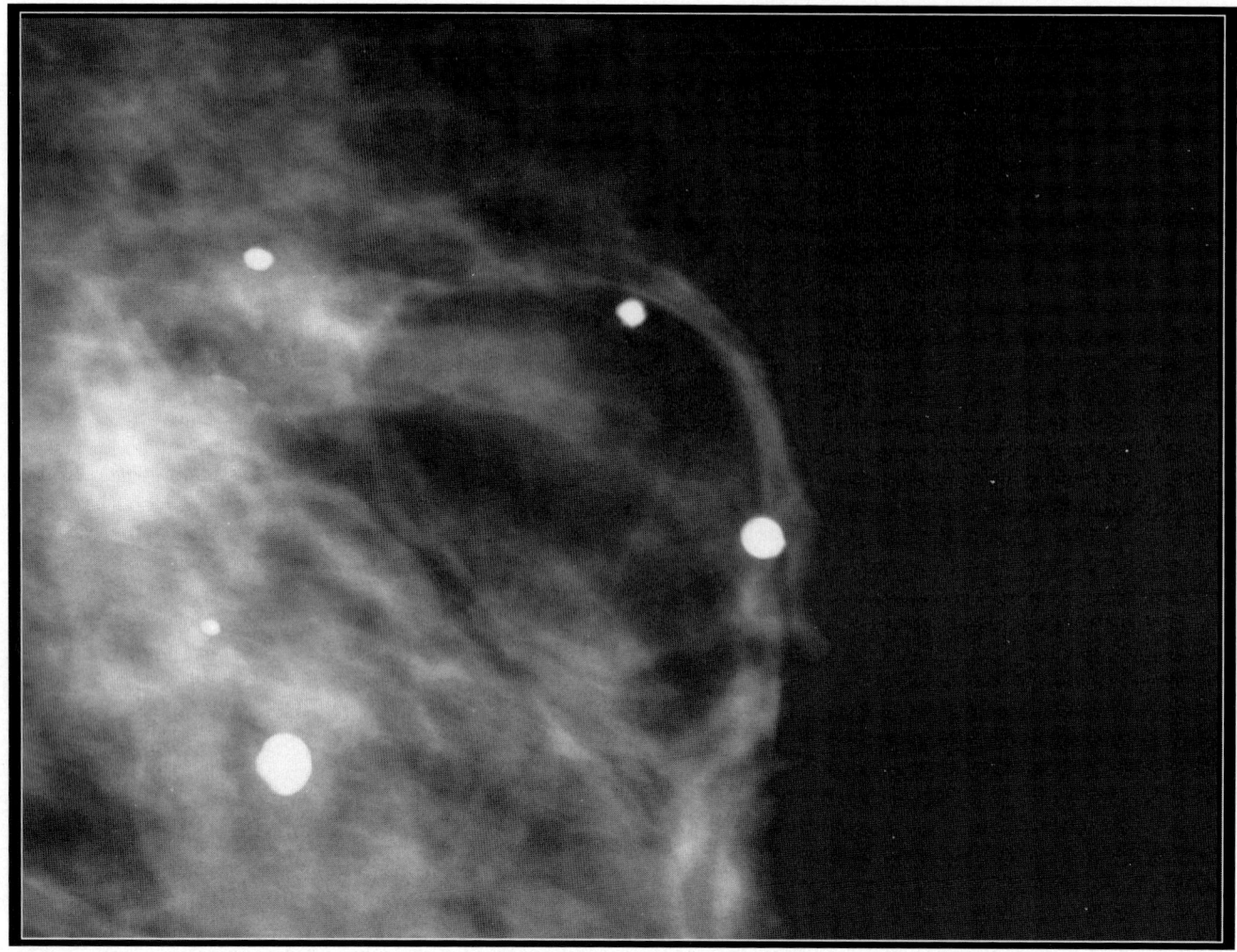

FIGURE 13–63 The classic lipoma on mammography is pure fatty density surrounded by a thin, water-density capsule. Classic lipomas on mammography are BIRADS 2, definitively benign, and do not require sonographic evaluation. However, many small lipomas that are large enough to be palpable cannot be seen mammographically but can be demonstrated sonographically.

elements require sonographic evaluation. Sonography is usually performed on lipomas presenting as palpable abnormalities associated with negative or nonspecific mammographic findings.

Lipomas typically have one of three sonographic appearances: (a) completely isoechoic with other nearby normal breast fat lobules (Fig. 13–65), (b) mildly hyperechoic with respect to other nearby normal breast fat lobules (Fig. 13–66), or (c) isoechoic with adjacent fat lobules, but having numerous thin, internal echogenic septa that course parallel to the skin line (Fig. 13–67). Regardless of the sonographic appearance, demonstration of softness is key to sonographic diagnosis. Softness may be demonstrated by deforming the lipoma with a palpating finger during scanning (Fig. 13–68) or by demonstrating compressibility in the AP dimension with the ultrasound transducer. The lat-

ter method is preferable with split-screen images taken with and without compression for documentation. Not uncommonly, lipomas can compress about 30%, although certain lesions, especially when associated with tenderness, may be less compressible (Fig. 13–69). Hyperechoic lipomas tend to be somewhat less compressible than the isoechoic variety, possibly because of edema or increased fibrous elements within the lipoma (Fig. 13–70). Lipomas that arise more deeply within the breast from the mammary zone and that are surrounded by firm, echogenic, interlobular stromal fibrous tissue may be buttressed by the surrounding tissue and therefore may be relatively incompressible.

Lipomas that are isoechoic with normal breast fatty elements may be difficult to identify and distinguish sonographically from surrounding normal breast fat if the thin, echogenic capsule cannot be demonstrated. However,

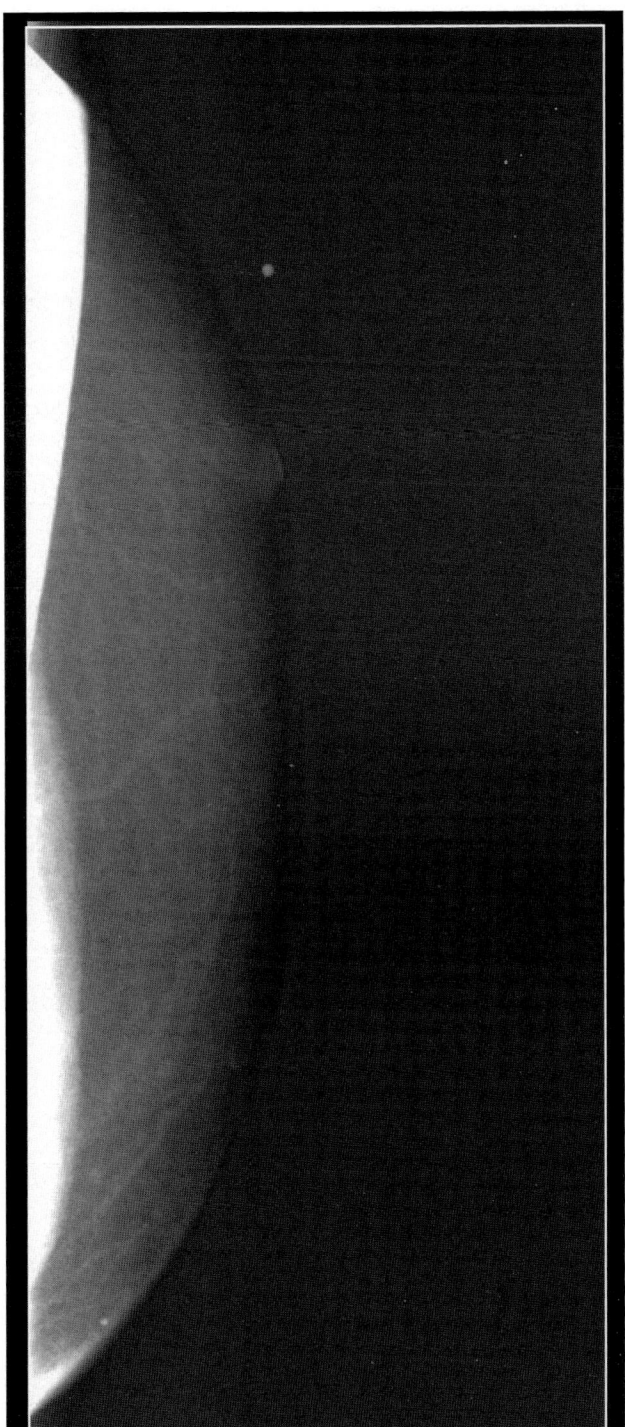

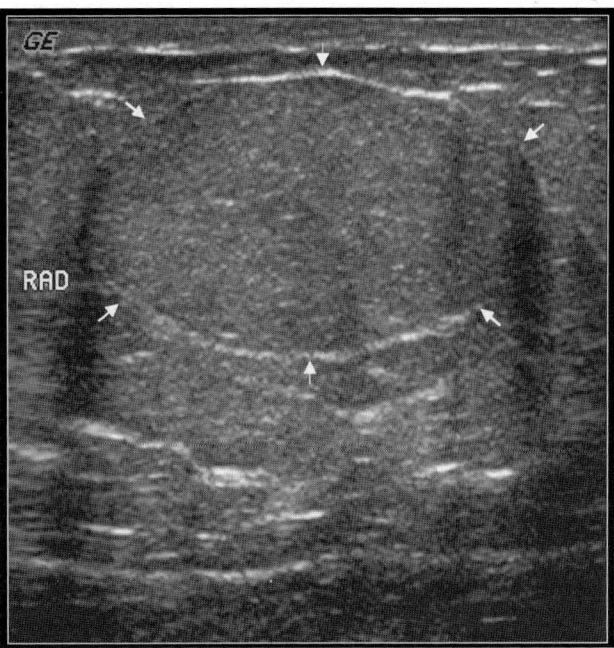

FIGURE 13–65 A large percentage of lipomas are isoechoic to surrounding fat on sonography and can be definitively diagnosed only if the thin, echogenic outer pseudocapsule *(arrows)* of compressed breast tissue can be demonstrated.

FIGURE 13–64 Small lipomas that are surrounded by fat cannot be seen mammographically unless the water-density pseudocapsule can be demonstrated.

demonstration of such a capsule is neither easy nor always possible. The capsule, like that surrounding many other benign expansile breast lesions, is essentially a pseudocapsule of compressed normal breast tissue. The larger the lesion (lipoma), the more likely there will be a sonographically demonstrable thin, echogenic capsule. Unfortunately, the larger lipomas, those most likely to have an echogenic capsule, often have diameters larger than the long-axis length of the transducer. The size discrepancy between the lesion and transducer face makes sonographic demonstration of a thin, echogenic capsule difficult. A specific attempt must be made to scan the periphery of the palpable abnormality. If the edges of a large lipoma are not scanned, it may be mistaken for normal breast fat. Smaller lipomas with maximum diameters less than the long-axis length of the probe tend to have less well-developed capsules that are more difficult to demonstrate sonographically. Thus, the capsule that surrounds both large and small lipomas can be difficult to demonstrate. One fairly consistent method of distinguishing prominent but normal fat lobules from lipomas is demonstration of a single horizontally oriented, thin, echogenic septum near the center of the normal fat lobule, but not within lipomas (Fig. 13–71). Regardless of the ability to distinguish a lipoma from a normal fat lobule in an individual case, demonstration that a palpable abnormality is unequivocally due to fat is critical. The fatty lesions that are difficult to distinguish from each other

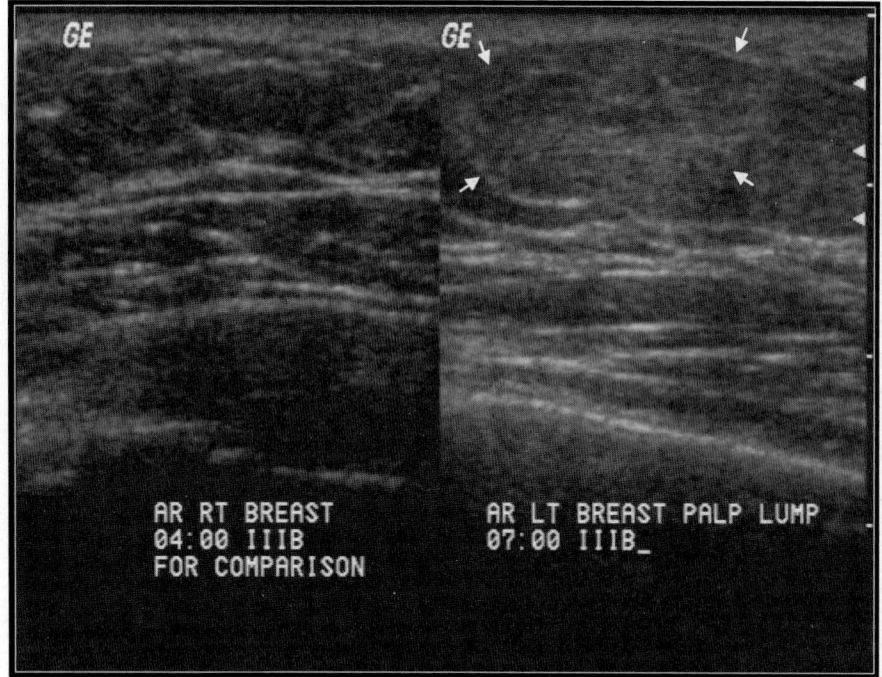

FIGURE 13–66 A significant percentage of lipomas are hyperechoic with respect to surrounding breast fat. Such lesions contain more fibrous elements than normal subcutaneous breast fat. These split-screen mirror images compare the hyperechoic lipoma on the patient's **left** *(arrows)* with the normal subcutaneous breast fat on the mirror-image location of the patient's **right.** Note that the lipoma is also thicker than the contralateral breast fat (patient's right side).

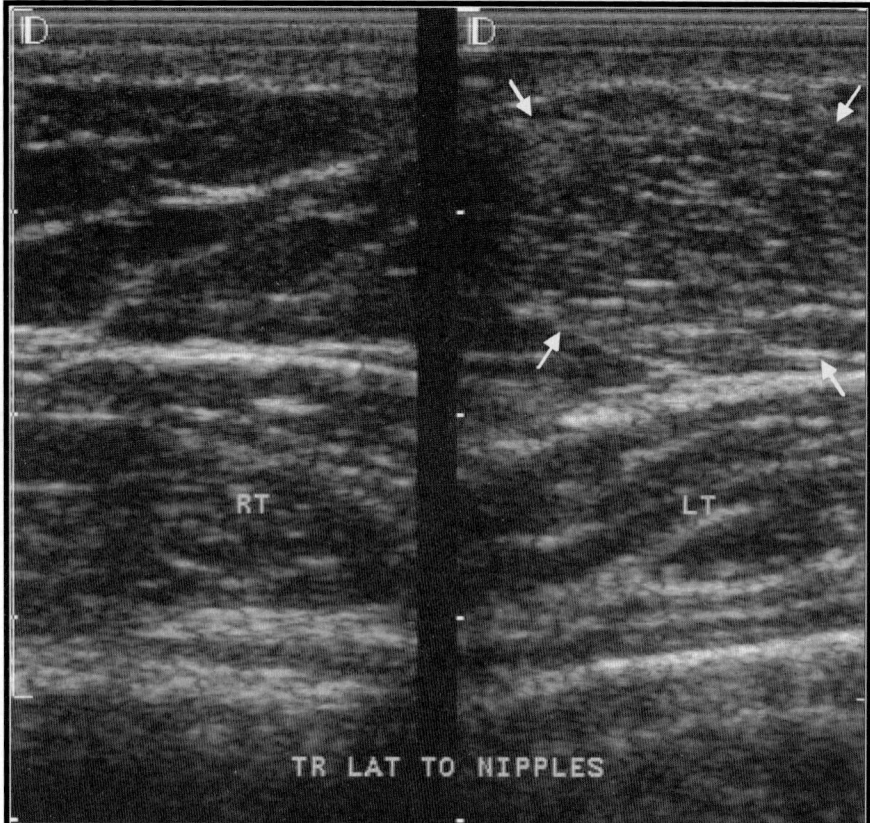

FIGURE 13–67 A small percentage of lipomas contains more numerous fibrous septations (**right image,** *arrows*) than does normal contralateral breast fat (**left image**).

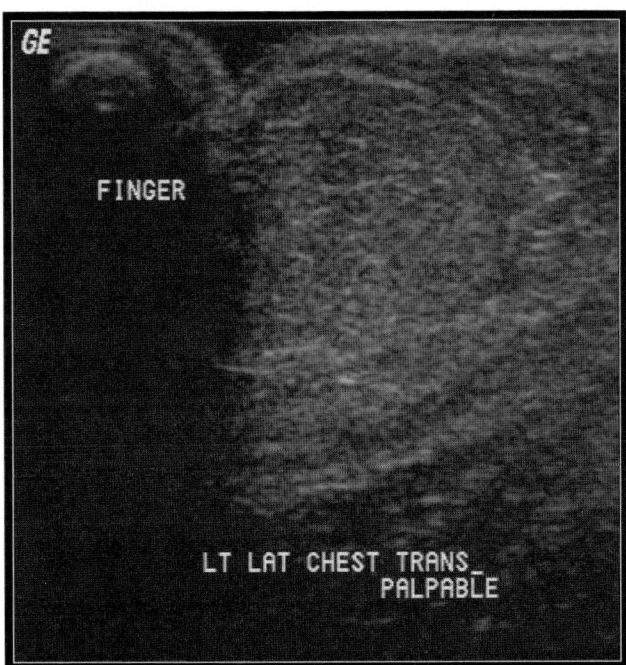

FIGURE 13–68 Lipomas are soft and easily deformable with the palpating finger.

sonographically are all definitively benign, BIRADS 2, obviating additional evaluation and the need for follow-up. Demonstrating that the lesion is soft and compressible is key to identifying the lesion as fatty.

Like lipomas, normal fat lobules occasionally cause new palpable breast abnormalities. Our experience has been that this phenomenon occurs most commonly in patients who have had rapid weight gain or loss. In such patients, some fat lobules appear to enlarge more rapidly or regress more slowly than surrounding fat lobules, thereby becoming palpable. Newly palpable fat lobules can also present after minor trauma, along the inferior mammary fold and medially in patients who wear underwire bras, and occasionally in patients with no apparent predisposing factors.

Lipomas that are mildly hyperechoic are much easier to distinguish from surrounding normal fat lobules than are isoechoic lipomas and are less likely to be missed. However, there may still be difficulty determining whether the lesion is an echogenic lipoma or merely edema within a fat lobule affected by early fat necrosis (Fig. 13–72). However, even the inability to distinguish between early fat necrosis and an echogenic lipoma in a few cases is not a major clini-

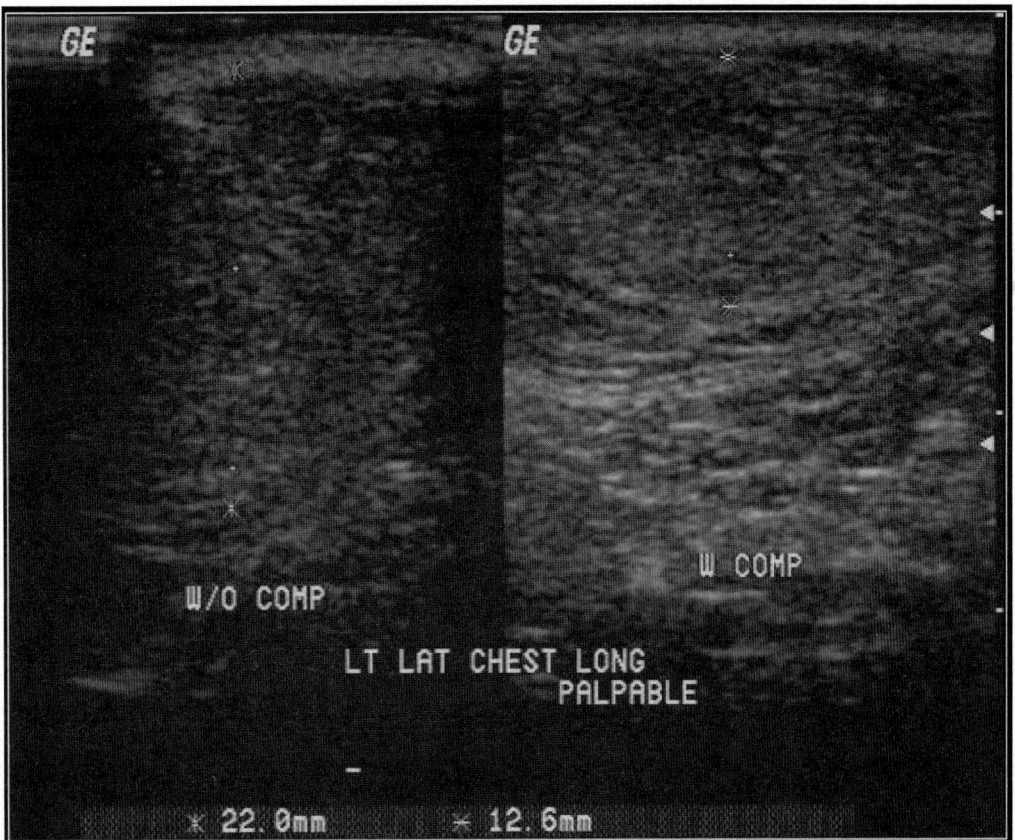

FIGURE 13–69 Lipomas are soft and compressible. Isoechoic lipomas routinely compress 30% to 50%. This isoechoic lipoma is more than 40% compressible. Hyperechoic and multiseptated lipomas are often slightly less compressible because of higher fibrous content, however, and therefore may compress less than the expected 30%.

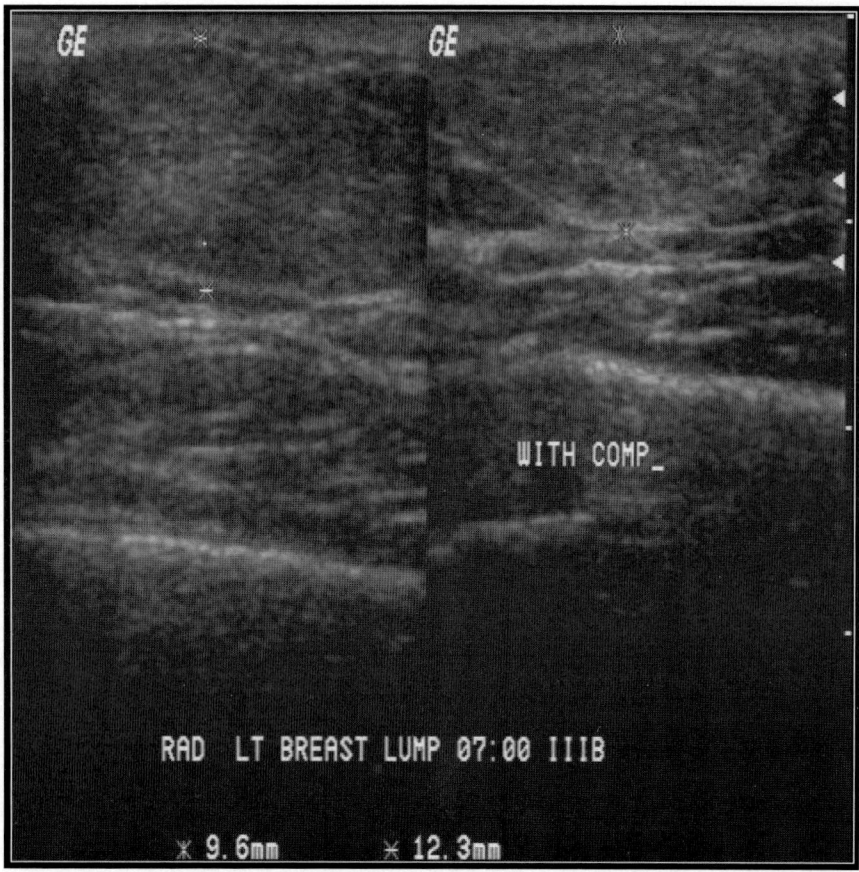

FIGURE 13–70 This hyperechoic lipoma has a higher fibrous content than do iso-echoic lipomas and thus compresses less. It is only 22% compressible. This degree of compressibility is typical for hyperechoic lipomas.

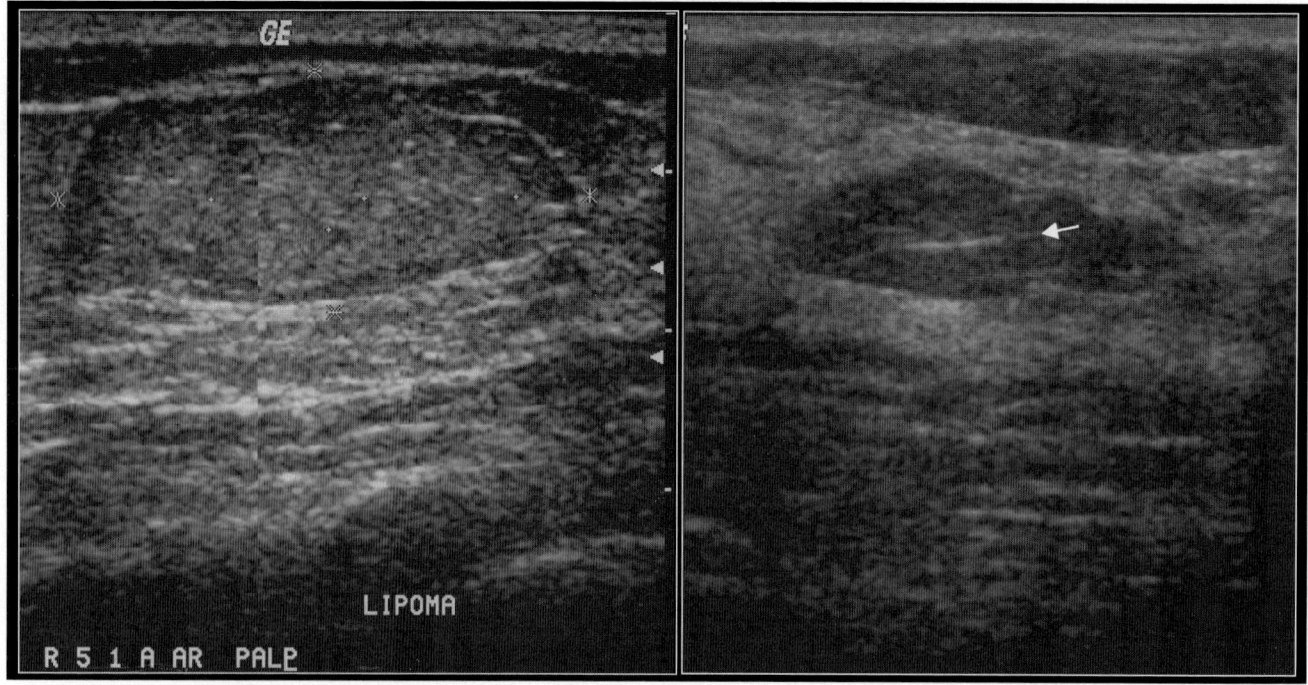

FIGURE 13–71 It may be difficult to distinguish an isoechoic lipoma (**left**) from a normal fat lob-ule (**right**). Normal fat lobules usually have a thin, echogenic fibrous septation that subdivides the lobule (**right**, *arrow*). Compressibility is not helpful because isoechoic lipomas and fat lobules are equally compressible.

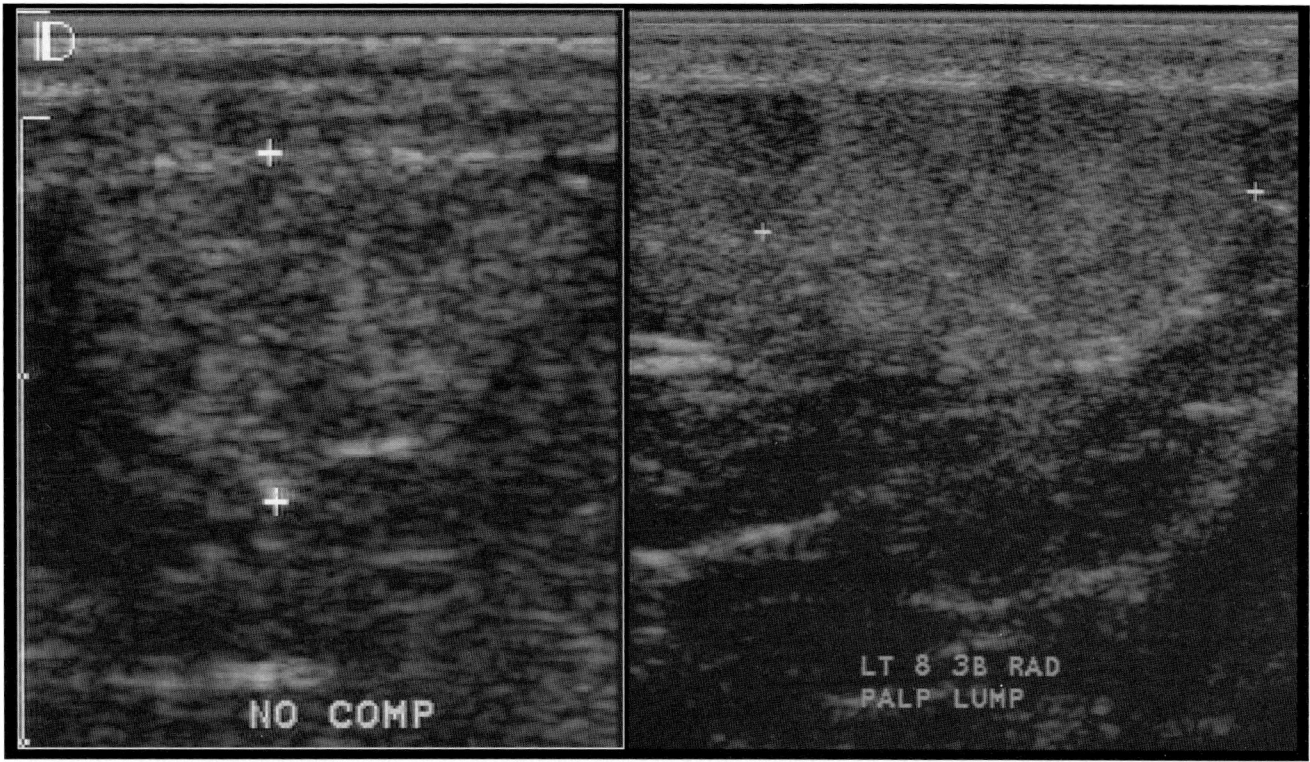

FIGURE 13–72 It may also be difficult to distinguish a hyperechoic lipoma (**left**) from an edematous fat lobule that results from early fat necrosis (**right**). Additionally, lipomas may undergo fat necrosis. Typically, the echogenic lipoma will be slightly more compressible than the edema of fat necrosis.

cal problem because both involve fat and are definitively benign (BIRADS 2). The cause of increased echogenicity within lipomas is not entirely clear. Certain lipomas can contain fibrous elements, whereas others can be edematous and show early changes of fat necrosis. In our experience, echogenic lipomas and fat lobules are more likely to be associated with tenderness than are isoechoic lipomas.

The multiseptated pattern is the least common sonographic appearance. These lesions also tend to be associated with tenderness and, like echogenic lipomas, are less compressible than the isoechoic variety.

FOCAL FIBROSIS (FIBROUS MASTOPATHY)

General Pathologic Classification, Epidemiology, and Clinical Findings

Focal fibrosis has also been termed *fibrous mastopathy, fibrous disease of the breast,* and *chronic indurative mastitis.* The term focal fibrosis provides a word picture that best fits the sonographic findings. Most American pathologists, however, probably prefer the term fibrous mastopathy.

Clinical Findings

Focal fibrosis can cause palpable lumps or can be asymptomatic and present as a focal asymmetry or nodule on mammography. It may be tender or nontender. The clinical findings are nonspecific.

Pathology

On gross inspection, focal fibrosis consists of homogenous white fibrous tissue.

Histologically, focal fibrosis represents a focal area of dense, paucicellular stromal fibrous tissue void of cellular structure, usually moderately well defined, but not encapsulated. These fibrotic lesions generally contain few, widely scattered, miniaturized ductal and lobular elements. There is no cystic dilation of the few ducts or lobules that are present. Focal fibrosis is not associated with epithelial proliferation, nor is this process associated with an increase cancer risk. Despite the term indurative mastitis that has occasionally been applied to this condition, there is no inflammation. Most common premenopausally in the fourth and fifth decades, this lesion has also been reported more commonly in diabetic women. Focal fibrosis is located most commonly in the upper outer quadrants of the breast.

Haagensen first described focal fibrosis. He emphasized that the lesion should be considered a separate entity from fibrocystic change and thought that the process represented a focal and selective stimulation of fibroblasts by estrogen. However, both the existence of focal fibrosis and its hypothesized etiology are controversial. Certain investigators consider the lesion merely to represent a variation of fibrocystic change or disorder of involution, rather than a hormonally induced fibroblastic proliferative disorder. However, its peak incidence occurring in the premenopausal years, and the association with other connective tissue disorders and with diabetes favors the process as being a true proliferative, neoplastic condition.

Focal fibrosis is probably much more common than was initially thought. When the lesion was first described, only cases that presented with dominant palpable abnormalities underwent biopsy. However, nonpalpable cases are now frequently discovered on mammography. In one series, focal fibrosis was present in up to 8% of all breast biopsies.

Focal fibrosis is not associated with an increased risk for breast cancer. The chief importance is that this lesion represents a small but significant percentage of all benign biopsies. In fact, in our study of 750 solid breast nodules presented in Chapter 12, focal fibrosis was responsible for

6.7% of all benign biopsies. Because the sonographic findings of focal fibrosis are benign with virtual certainty, sonography has the potential to prevent unnecessary biopsy of focal fibrosis.

Mammographic Findings

The mammographic findings are not specific. Focal fibrosis, when mammographically visible, creates a mass of medium to high opacity that has circumscribed to indistinct margins. Usually, the lesion has convex, rounded borders but has one or more angles or points. Occasionally, the mass is teardrop shaped. Calcifications are uncommon and when present are usually of the punctate, involutional type.

Sonographic Findings

Patients with focal fibrosis undergo sonography to characterize further either a palpable or mammographic abnormality. Like the variable mammographic findings of focal fibrosis, the sonographic findings are also variable. In some cases, the sonographic description of focal fibrosis is virtually identical to the gross pathologic description: well-circumscribed, but not encapsulated, homogenous intensely echogenic nodule. The echogenicity is identical to that of normal interlobular stromal fibrous tissue. However,

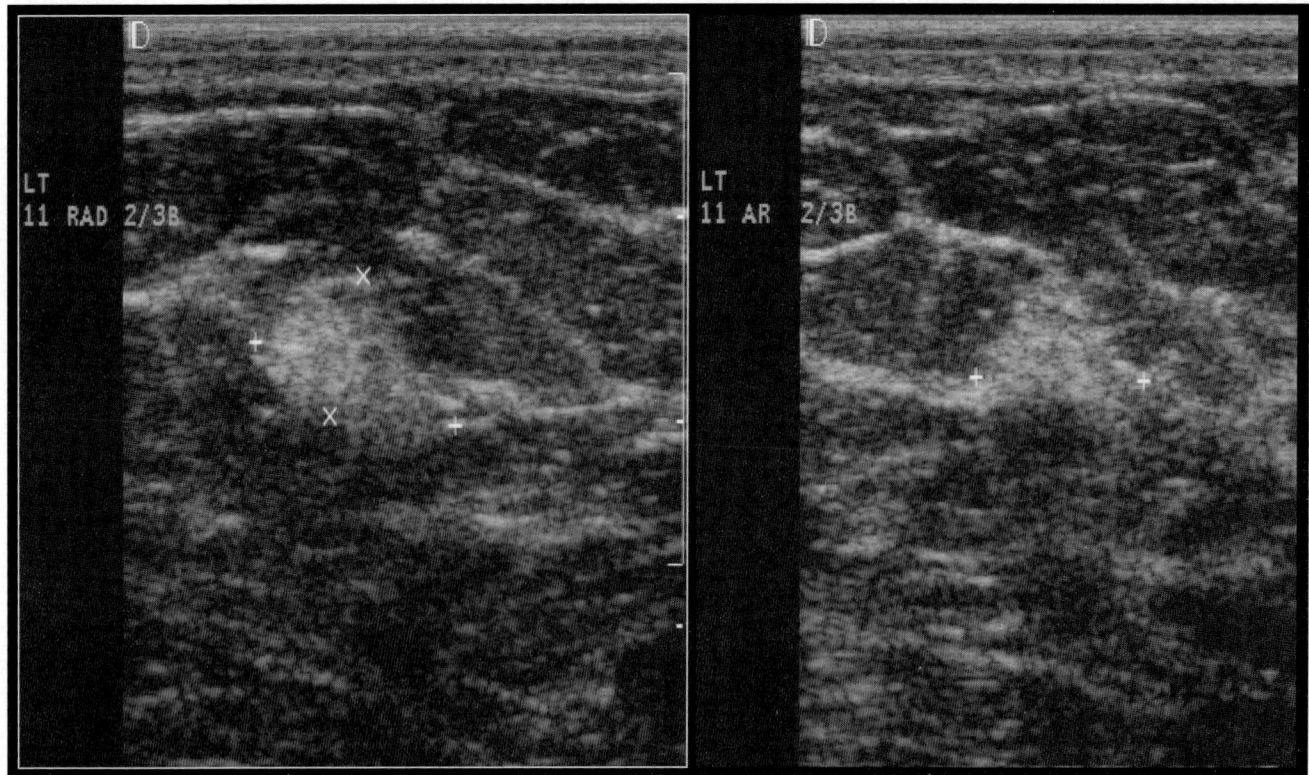

FIGURE 13–73 Focal fibrosis is purely hyperechoic and contains no prominent isoechoic ducts or lobules. According to Haagenson, focal fibrosis contains no mature lobules and only rudimentary ducts.

this variety of focal fibrous tissue is more homogeneously echogenic than is normal fibroglandular tissue (Fig. 13–73). Because the TDLUs in focal fibrosis are obliterated, atrophic, or underdeveloped histologically, it should be not be surprising that lobules are not visible within these lesions sonographically. The presence of sonographically demonstrable, normal-sized TDLUs within echogenic fibrous tissue indicates that the lesion is fibroglandular tissue, not focal fibrosis as defined by Haagensen (Fig. 13–74). However, small ducts may occasionally be demonstrable within focal fibrosis. These ducts are smaller and much less well defined than normal mammary ducts that are seen within normal fibroglandular tissue. Focal fibrosis is usually outwardly convex on the anterior and posterior borders but is often teardrop or spindle shaped because the fibrous tissue tapers into Cooper's ligaments on one or both ends (Fig. 13–73). Like other benign nodules, focal fibrosis is usually larger in horizontal axes than in the AP axis.

Purely hyperechoic malignant nodules are exceedingly rare. However, there must be no isoechoic or hypoechoic structures larger than small ducts within the echogenic tissue before the diagnosis of focal fibrosis is made. Very small, low-grade infiltrating ductal carcinomas and tubu-lar carcinomas may have a very small isoechoic or hypo-echoic central nidus surrounded by a thick, ill-defined echogenic rim (that represents the thick echogenic halo of unresolved spicules around the periphery of the nodule; see Chapter 12, Figs. 12–16). If hard-copy images are inappropriately taken along the edges (periphery) of the malignant nodule, where only the thick echogenic rim is visible, the resulting appearance may be mistaken for a purely hyperechoic nodule (see Chapter 12, Fig. 12–81). Additionally, near-field volume averaging may obscure a small hypoechoic central nidus (see Chapter 12, Fig. 12–80). Thus, the entire nodule must be evaluated in orthogonal planes before concluding that the entire composition is purely hyperechoic. The increased echogenicity must be homogeneous, and the lesion must be at least as echogenic as normal interlobular stromal fibrous tissue. Infiltrative breast malignancies that are very permeative may cause only a very subtle and ill-defined decrease in echotexture within an area of intensely echogenic fibrous tissue. Classic infiltrating lobular carcinoma, lesions in which large volumes of tissue are infiltrated by single-file columns of tumor cells, are particularly prone to create this appearance.

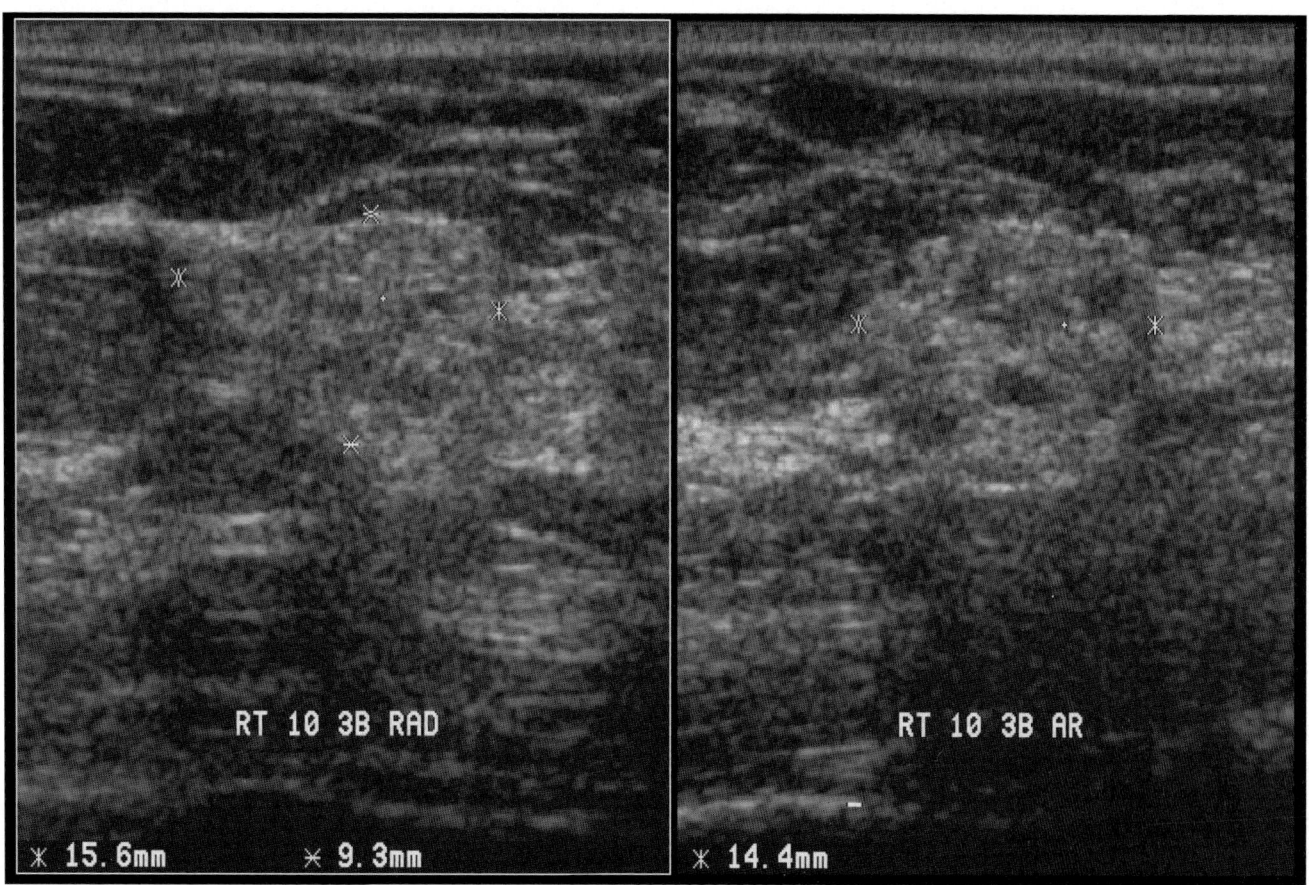

FIGURE 13–74 Fibroglandular asymmetries, unlike focal fibrosis, contain lobules and normal ducts. The isoechoic areas in these radial (RAD, **left**) and antiradial (AR, **right**) image represent prominent lobules, which do not exist in focal fibrosis.

DIABETIC MASTOPATHY (DIABETIC FIBROSIS)

General Pathologic Classification, Epidemiology, and Clinical Findings

Diabetic mastopathy usually presents in premenopausal diabetic patients about 20 years after onset of diabetes. Most patients had onset of type I diabetes before the age of 20 years. Only a few cases have been reported in patients with type II diabetes. The condition is thought to result from disorders in collagen metabolism that can occur with diabetes. The patients often have associated arthropathy that is also likely related to disordered collagen metabolism. Diabetic mastopathy is often bilateral, but not necessarily synchronous. Diabetic mastopathy most often presents as a hard, palpable, nontender lump in a premenopausal woman but may present as a focal mammographic nodule or asymmetric density. The condition is self-limiting, unlike fibromatosis; is not infiltrating; and is significant primarily because the hardness of the palpable lump is clinically worrisome and because its sonographic appearance is so suspicious that it invariably necessitates a BIRADS characterization of 4b or 5 that indicates the need for biopsy. Local resection is curative, and there is no risk for local recurrence. However, such patients often develop other foci of palpable or sonographically worrisome fibrous mastopathy in other parts of the ipsilateral breast or in the contralateral breast that require multiple additional biopsies over time. Our hope is that contrast-enhanced MRI with the rotating delivery excitation off-resonance (RODEO) sequence will enable us to differentiate diabetic mastopathy from carcinoma because diabetic mastopathy appears not to demonstrate enhancement with contrast, whereas invasive carcinoma does.

Pathology

The gross morphology is simply one of firm, well-circumscribed breast tissue.

Histologically, the mass is composed of collagenous stroma that contains more histologically normal fibroblasts than does usual stromal tissue. There are lymphocytic infiltrates centered on small vessels within the area of mastopathy, suggesting an inflammatory component. The lymphocytes in diabetic mastitis are B cells rather than the usual T cells seen in other types of mastitis.

Mammographic Findings

The mammographic findings are nonspecific. In many cases in which the patient presents with a hard palpable lump, the mammograms are homogeneously dense bilaterally, and dense tissue obscures the lesion mammographically (Fig. 13–75). In other cases, the patient may present with a nonspecific mammographic opacity for which

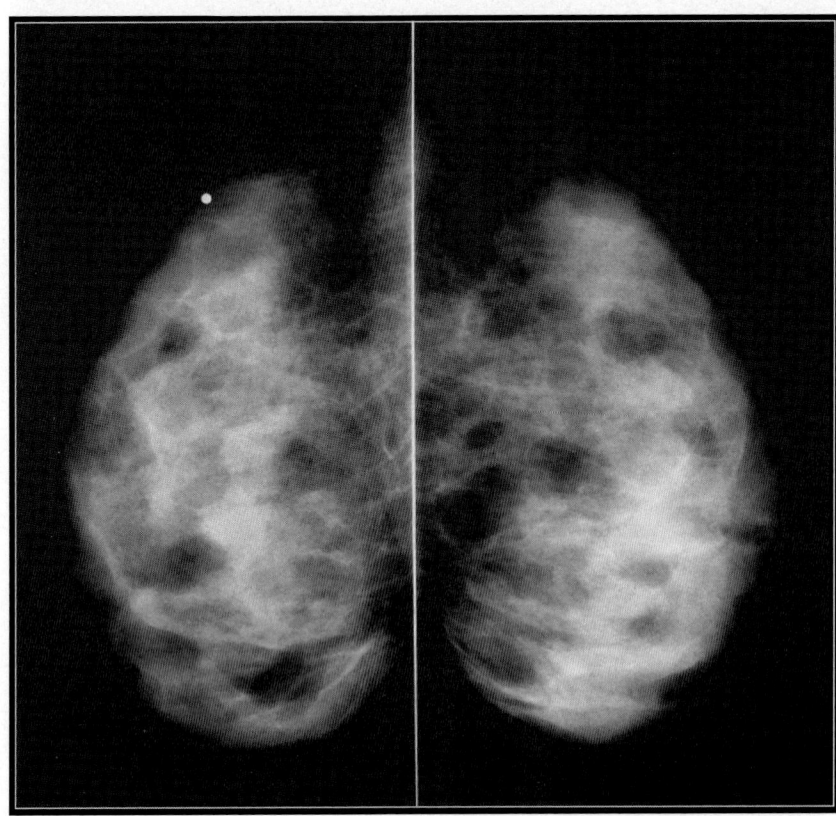

FIGURE 13–75 In many cases of diabetic mastopathy, the patient presents with a hard, palpable lump, but the mammograms show only diffusely dense tissues bilaterally. The "bb" marks the palpable lump in this patient with biopsy proved diabetic mastophy.

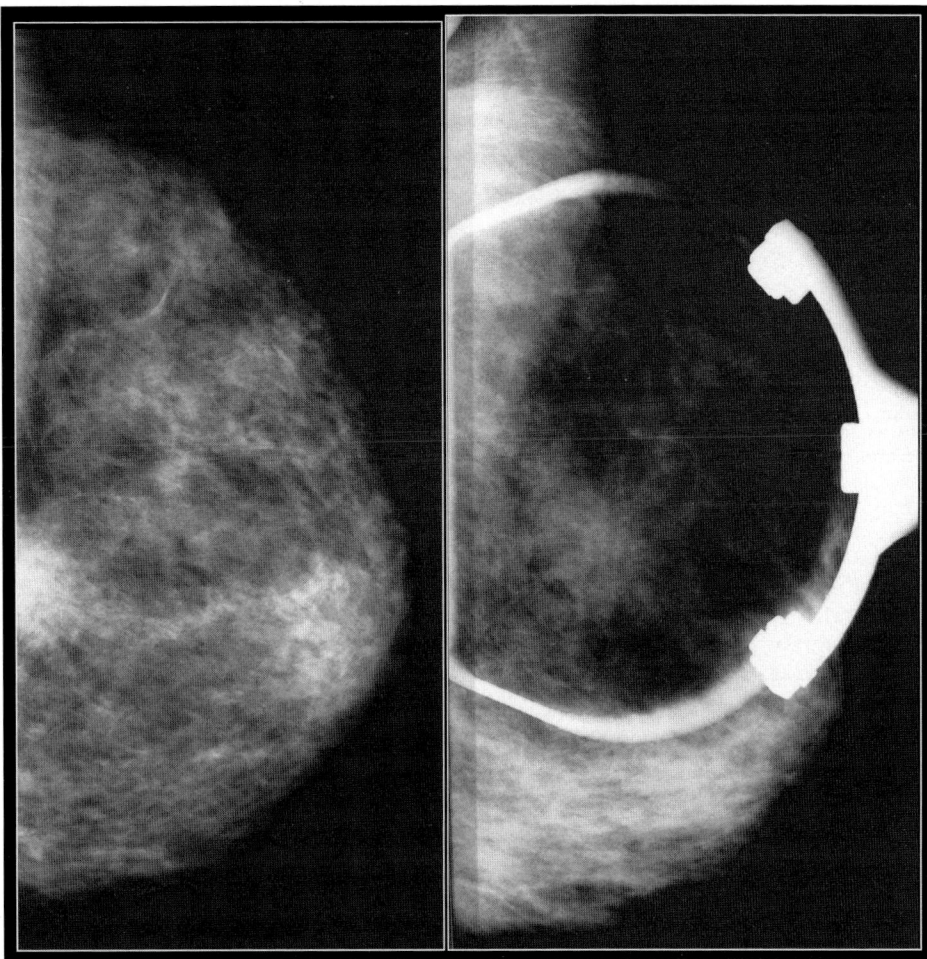

FIGURE 13–76 In other cases, the hard, palpable lump caused by diabetic mastopathy causes a nonspecific mammographic asymmetry. In fewer cases, such as this, diabetic mastopathy presents as an ill-defined or spiculated mass.

sonography is the diagnostic procedure of choice (Fig. 13–76).

Sonographic Findings

The sonographic findings are far more worrisome than the mammographic findings, especially in view of how firm the lesions are to palpation. Foci of diabetic mastopathy that are large enough to present with hard palpable lumps almost invariably have a central hypoechoic focus that has many suspicious features. It is ill-defined, angular, and microlobulated and may be taller than wide (Fig. 13–77). If often causes acoustic shadowing (Fig. 13–78). The findings are indistinguishable from those of malignant lesions at the spiculated end of the spectrum—low-grade invasive ductal carcinoma, tubular carcinoma, and invasive lobular carcinoma. Because of the ill-defined margins of the hypoechoic central focus and acoustic shadowing, the lesions are almost invariably

sonographically suspicious, and the lesion usually requires a BIRADS 4a or higher characterization and biopsy. Ultrasound-guided large core needle biopsy is an adequate alternative to excisional biopsy, especially because sonography frequently shows more areas of diabetic mastopathy than are clinically or mammographically evident.

Multifocal, multicentric, and bilateral involvement is typical of diabetic mastopathy (Fig. 13–79), which would normally be reassuring. Unfortunately, the main malignant lesion in the differential diagnosis, invasive lobular carcinoma, may also be multifocal, multicentric, and synchronously bilateral.

Diabetic mastopathy may cause multiple lesions that present not only synchronously but also on follow-up examinations over a period of time. Thus, patients with biopsy-proven diabetic mastopathy may require multiple biopsies on multiple different areas of diabetic mastopathy over time. For purposes of avoiding multiple biopsies over

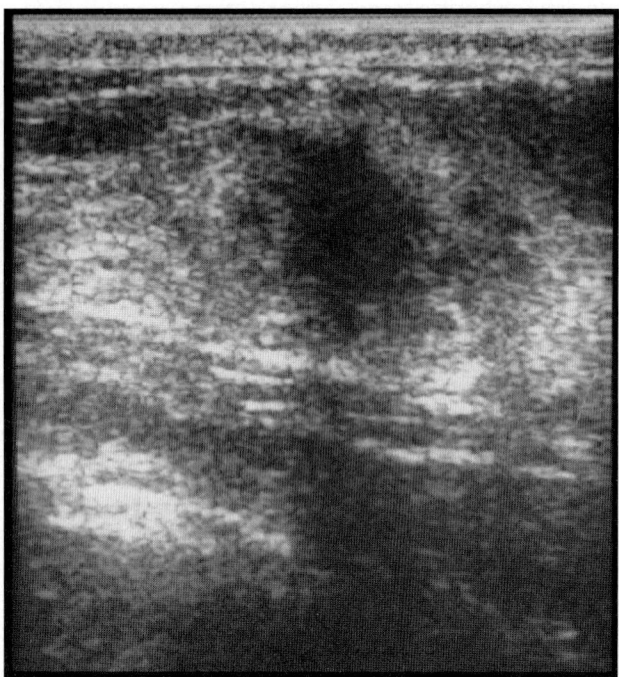

FIGURE 13–77 Diabetic mastopathy often shows numerous suspicious sonographic findings that belie its benign nature. This mass of diabetic fibrosis is markedly hypoechoic, is taller than wide, and has angular margins. It is somewhat unusual in that the sound transmission is nearly normal. Most cases of severe diabetic mastopathy cause acoustic shadowing. This mass occurred in the patient whose negative but dense mammogram is shown in Fig. 13–75.

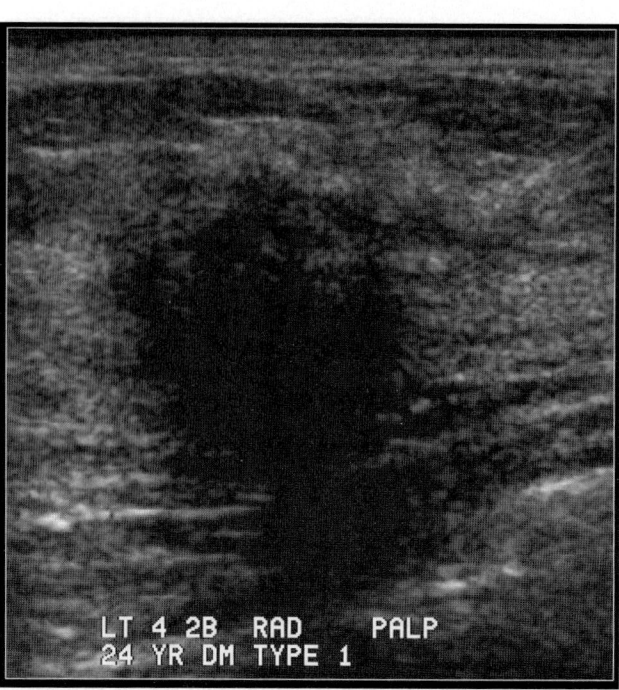

FIGURE 13–78 This palpable mass caused by diabetic mastopathy is more typical in that, in addition to being markedly hypoechoic and having angular margins, it causes acoustic shadowing. This mass caused the mammographic opacity seen in Fig. 13–76.

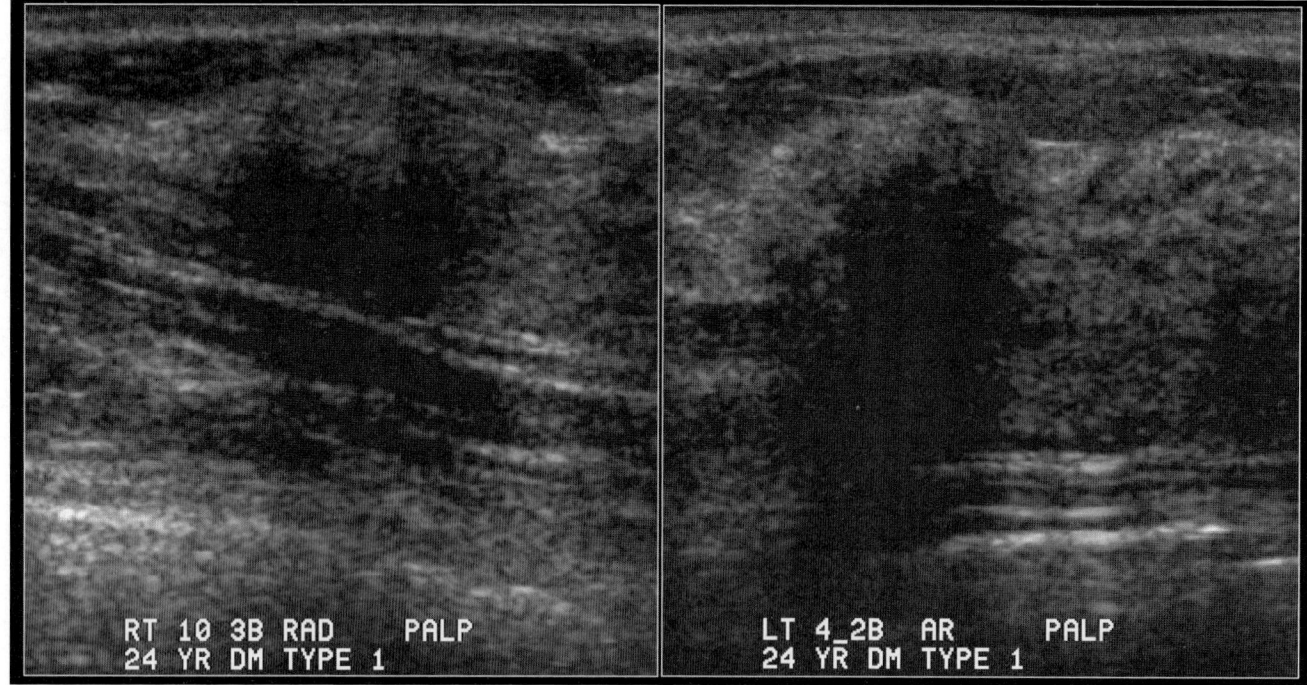

FIGURE 13–79 Multifocal, multicentric, and bilateral involvement, synchronous or sequential, is common in diabetic mastopathy. This patient had bilateral palpable and sonographically visible lesions (negative on mammography) caused by diabetic mastopathy.

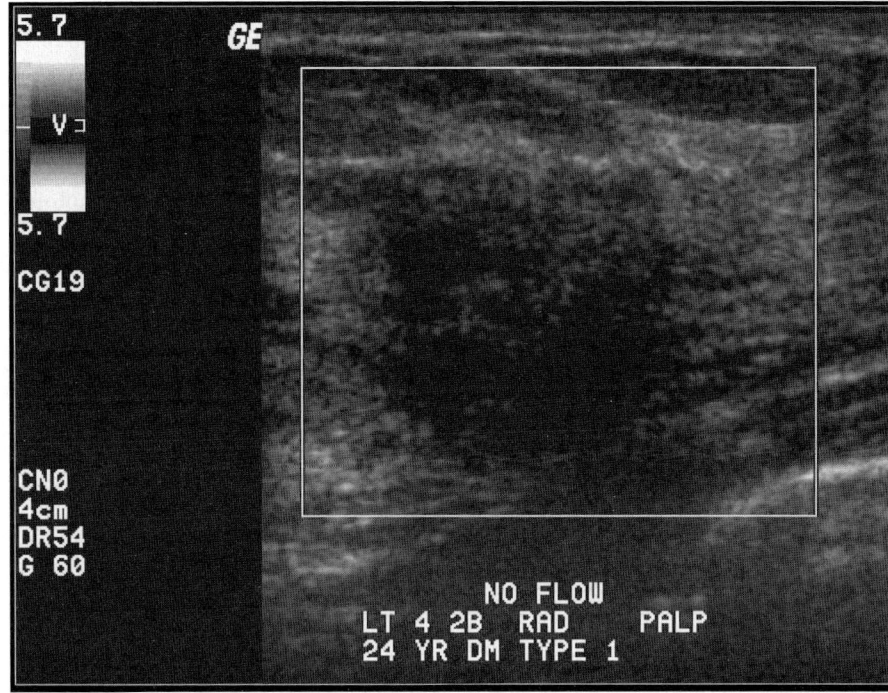

FIGURE 13–80 The sonographic appearance of diabetic mastopathy simulates the appearance of malignant nodules on the spiculated end of the spectrum, such as low-grade invasive ductal carcinoma or invasive lobular carcinoma. On a theoretical basis, color Doppler should be useful in distinguishing diabetic mastopathy, which is avascular, from carcinoma, which is more likely to show internal blood flow on color Doppler evaluation. Unfortunately, the lesions at the spiculated end of the spectrum, with which diabetic mastopathy might be confused sonographically, do not have perceptibly more flow than normal tissue or benign lesions in a large percentage of patients. Therefore, color Doppler is not very useful in making the distinction between diabetic mastopathy and spiculated carcinoma. This mass, caused by diabetic mastopathy, is avascular on color Doppler.

time, it would be helpful to have some noninvasive way other than sonographic imaging to distinguish between diabetic mastopathy and carcinoma. Doppler could be helpful because diabetic mastopathy is essentially avascular and does not have demonstrably increased flow on color Doppler, whereas many malignant nodules do (Fig. 13–80). Unfortunately, the malignant lesions that diabetic mastopathy simulates lie at the spiculated end of the spectrum and tend not to have demonstrably increased flow on unenhanced color Doppler. Perhaps sonographic contrast agents will facilitate this distinction on color or power Doppler. However, at the present time, we believe that contrast-enhanced MRI may be the most effective noninvasive way of distinguishing between diabetic mastopathy and spiculated, shadowing, invasive malignancies in patients with previously documented diabetic mastopathy who are being followed.

PSEUDOANGIOMATOUS STROMAL HYPERPLASIA

General Pathologic Classification, Epidemiology, and Clinical Findings

Pseudoangiomatous stromal hyperplasia (PASH) is a benign focal overgrowth of stromal tissue. This process occurs primarily in premenopausal women or in postmenopausal women who are undergoing combined estrogen-progesterone HRT. Similar stromal changes can occur during the postovulatory or secretory phases of the menstrual cycle.

Progesterone receptors have been found within foci of PASH. Because of the age of patients involved, the presence of similar changes during phases of the menstrual cycle in which the progesterone effect is dominant, and the presence of progesterone receptors, the process is thought to be caused by exuberant progesterone stimulation of estrogenically primed tissues. Subclinical microscopic amounts of PASH-like changes are common, being found in at least one microscopic field in up to 23% of breast biopsy specimens. Clinically apparent PASH is much less common, being reported in fewer than 100 cases in the literature to date. However, the likelihood is that clinically significant PASH is much more common than has been reported. When radiologist and pathologist are not aware of the diagnosis and do not communicate closely, the diagnosis of PASH is likely to be missed and replaced with the diagnosis of fibrocystic change or fibrosclerosis.

The first few dozen cases of PASH that were reported all presented as palpable nodules or masses. Virtually all presented as firm, mobile, nontender nodules. However, because of mammographic screening, more cases of PASH are now presenting as nonpalpable mammographic nodules or masses. In two recently reported mammographic series, about only about one-half of the mammographically detected lesions were palpable.

Pathologic Findings

The gross pathologic appearance of PASH is similar to that of fibroadenoma—a circumscribed, firm, occasionally rubbery, gray-white to gray-yellow nodule. There appears to be a capsule in certain cases, but not in others. The nodule may contain cysts.

The histologic diagnosis requires that either most of the nodule or the entire nodule be composed of PASH. The presence of microscopic amounts of affected tissue is not sufficient for the diagnosis of PASH.

The histology of PASH reveals abnormally prominent stromal elements between ducts and lobules. The stroma contains communicating slitlike spaces that simulate but do not represent vascular spaces—thus the name "pseudo-angiomatous." The spaces are formed as a result of disruption of collagen fibers and differ from true vascular channels in both contents and linings. The spaces contain mucopolysaccharide, but do not contain red blood cells, and are lined by epithelial or myoepithelial cells rather than the intima. The real histologic significance of PASH is that the pathologist may mistake the appearance of the stroma with slitlike spaces for a low-grade angiosarcoma. Additionally, the myofibroblastic or fibroblastic proliferation that occurs in PASH is similar to that which occurs within benign phyllodes tumors and fibroadenomas with cellular stroma. From cytology of very small histologic specimens, there may be difficulty determining whether PASH-like changes are isolated findings or are developing within a phyllodes tumor.

The ducts and lobules that are enveloped within PASH can undergo changes that are completely typical of fibrocystic change, including cyst formation and apocrine metaplasia. If the slitlike spaces within the collagenous stroma are not recognized, the diagnosis of fibrocystic change with fibrosclerosis, rather than PASH, may be made.

PASH is not premalignant and is not associated with an increased relative risk for breast cancer. However, there is a strong tendency for enlargement of PASH nodules to occur with time, and incomplete resection will likely lead to local recurrence. Because more cases of nonpalpable but mammographically or sonographically detected PASH are now being found, diagnosis is frequently made by stereotactically or sonographically directed core needle biopsy. A treatment dilemma has been created by enlargement of such proven cases of PASH on follow-up examinations. However, because PASH is definitively benign and not premalignant, cases diagnosed by core needle biopsy that subsequently enlarge can be managed similarly to proven fibroadenomas that subsequently enlarge.

Mammographic Findings

PASH causes a noncalcified, isodense mammographic nodule or mass in most cases that are mammographically visible. Most of these nodules are circumscribed or partially circumscribed, but a significant minority has indistinct borders. The mammographic findings are generally similar to those of fibroadenoma. However, one case of PASH pre-

senting as a high-density, spiculated nodule has been reported. In our system, all such nodules undergo sonographic evaluation before biopsy or excision.

Sonographic Findings

In a minority of cases, PASH is indistinguishable from surrounding fibroglandular tissues at sonography and is missed. However, most cases result in mildly hypoechoic, slightly heterogeneous solid nodules. About half the time, the nodule is well circumscribed and oval and is encompassed in a thin, echogenic pseudocapsule, giving it characteristics that are essentially indistinguishable from a fibroadenoma (Fig. 13–81). Similar to complex fibroadenomas, some PASH nodules contain cysts (Fig. 13–82). Other PASH nodules appear ill defined and are not encompassed in a thin, echogenic pseudocapsule. They may have other suspicious features such as being taller than wide or having angular, microlobulated margins that exclude them from BIRADS 3 classification and mandate biopsy (Fig. 13–83). Sound transmission is usually similar to that of surrounding tissues but may be slightly enhanced or

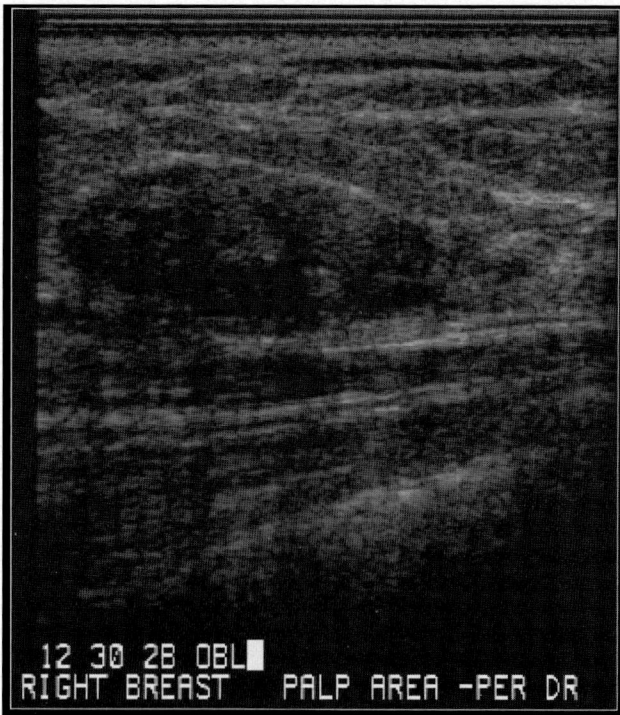

FIGURE 13–81 In about half of cases, pseudoangiomatous stromal hyperplasia causes an oval or gently lobulated nodule encompassed within a thin, echogenic capsule that is slightly heterogeneous in texture. The sonographic findings in such cases are indistinguishable from those of benign fibroadenoma and allow a BIRADS 3 classification. Thus, many such lesions are followed rather than undergoing biopsy.

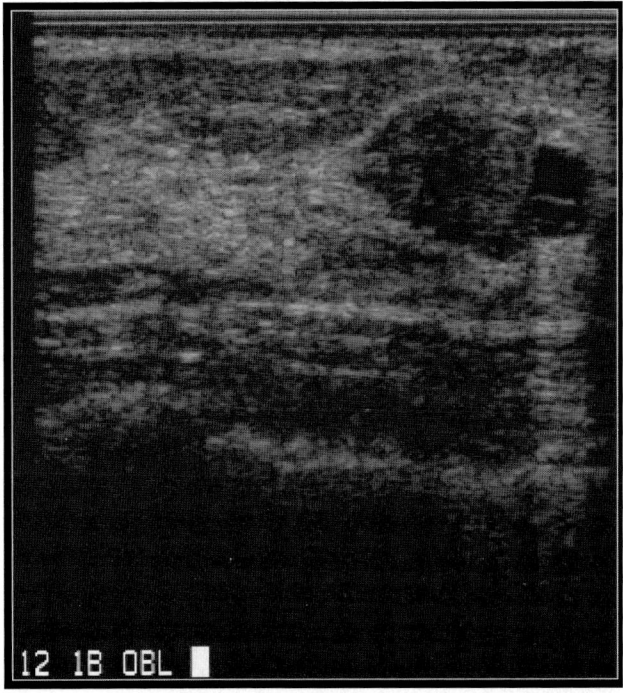

FIGURE 13–82 Solid nodules caused by pseudoangiomatous stromal hyperplasia, like complex fibroadenomas, can contain cysts.

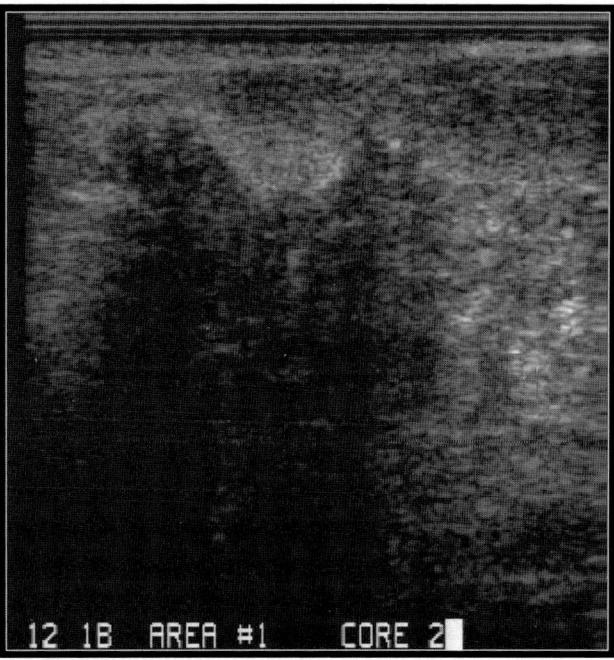

FIGURE 13–84 Although most nodules caused by pseudoangiomatous stromal hyperplasia have normal or very slightly altered sound transmission, a few cases, such as this case, cast a dense acoustic shadow as well as having angular and microlobulated margins.

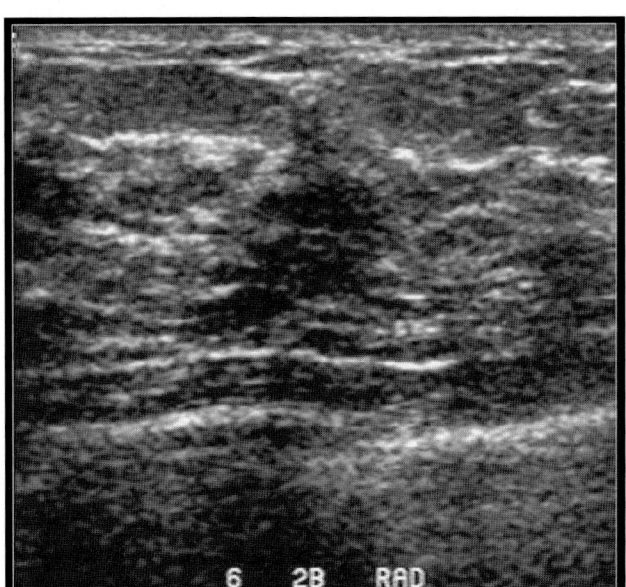

FIGURE 13–83 The other half of nodules caused by pseudoangiomatous stromal hyperplasia have suspicious features, such as being taller than wide, being microlobulated, and having angular margins that prevent the lesion from being characterized as BIRADS 3.

decreased. A few cases even have intense acoustic shadowing that, together with ill-defined, angular, and microlobulated margins, simulates the sonographic appearance of invasive lobular carcinoma (Fig. 13–84). The hyperplastic stroma is similar to that of phyllodes tumor or fibroadenoma with cellular stroma, but phyllodes tumors and cellular fibroadenomas usually have internal blood flow that is demonstrable with color Doppler, whereas PASH nodules rarely do (Fig. 13–85).

In our experience, more than half of PASH nodules that undergo biopsy are not encapsulated and have angular or microlobulated margins or other suspicious features that prevent them from being characterized as BIRADS 3 and indicate the need for biopsy. However, it is likely that many oval, encapsulated PASH nodules that can be characterized as BIRADS 3 are followed as probable fibroadenomas. Thus, the group of solid nodules caused by PASH that undergo biopsy is a highly selected subset of all PASH nodules that has suspicious features.

There are many instances in which the amount of PASH within a biopsy specimen is very small and the diagnosis of PASH is incidental. In such cases, the sonographic characteristics will reflect the pathology of the lesion within which the small amount of PASH arose. For example, foci of PASH may develop within a fibroadenoma or within a more dominant focus of fibrosclerosis. In those cases, the

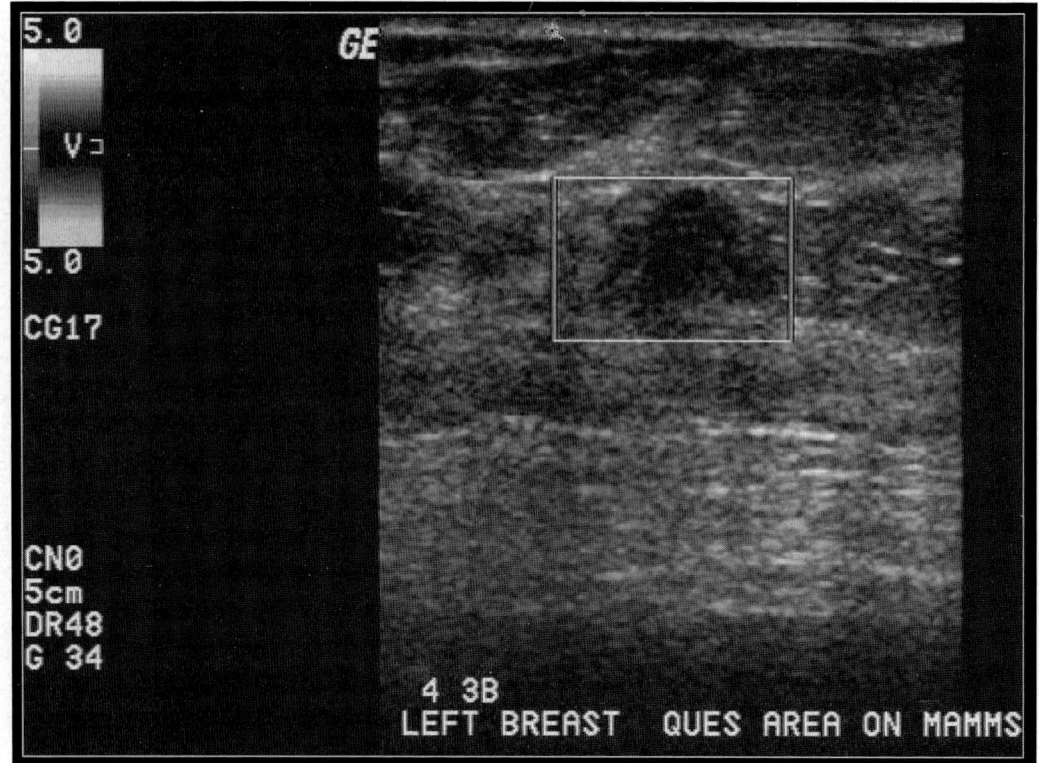

FIGURE 13–85 Although pseudoangiomatous stromal hyperplasia has fibroblasts growing within the hyperplastic stroma, a metabolically active state that is likely to require increased blood flow, we have not been able to demonstrate internal blood flow on color Doppler.

imaging features will be those of the fibroadenoma or fibrosclerosis, respectively, within which the PASH developed. The small amount of incidentally diagnosed PASH will not contribute to the imaging features of the lesion.

GRANULAR CELL TUMORS (MYOBLASTOMAS)

General Pathologic Classification, Epidemiology, and Clinical Findings

Granular cell tumor is a stromal tumor that is probably of Schwann's cell origin. Like lipomas, these lesions are not unique to the breast and can occur anywhere in the body. Only about 5% to 6% of all granular cell tumors occur within the breast. Although a patient may have more than one granular cell tumor in the body, having more than one in the breast is rare.

Granular cell tumor typically presents as a palpable or mammographic nodule or mass. Palpable lesions are firm to hard, not associated with pain, and less mobile than the typical fibroadenoma. Because these lesions are attached to surrounding tissues, dimpling of the overlying skin may occur. These tumors tend to occur in the upper inner quadrant of the breast. They are most common in women 30 to 50 years of age,, having a peak incidence in the fourth decade, but can be seen in postmenopausal women and even in males.

Pathology

Gross pathology reveals a gritty, firm, or hard nodule with irregular borders that is usually fixed to surrounding tissues. However, a minority of cases may appear smooth, circumscribed, and unattached. Most lesions are 3 cm or less in diameter.

Histologically, granular cell tumors are composed of sheets or fascicles of spindle-shaped cells that contain abundant eosinophilic granules. Because these cells invariably contain eosinophilic granules and are thought to be of Schwann's cell origin rather than muscle origin, the term *granular cell tumor* is currently preferred over the original name *myoblastoma*. A fibrous tissue background is interspersed with spindle cells. Although 99% of these tumors are histologically benign, the margins of the tumor do infiltrate adjacent breast tissues, engulfing adjacent ducts and lobules within the periphery of the tumor. Because of the infiltrating margins, granular cell tumors can be mistaken for infiltrating scirrhous breast carcinomas on both gross and histologic examination. In small biopsy specimens, such as those obtained by core needle biopsy, there may be difficulty in distinguishing granular cell tumors from invasive apocrine cell carcinoma, which also contains eosinophilic granules.

Despite the infiltrating margins, 99% of granular cell tumors are histologically benign and almost always unifocal. Wide excision is curative, but inadequate initial resection may lead to local recurrence. Granular cell tumors do not appear to be premalignant and are not associated with an increased relative risk for breast carcinoma.

Mammographic Findings

Granular cell tumors have a mammographic appearance similar to that of breast carcinoma. These tumors cause mammographic nodules that appear to be indistinctly marginated or frankly spiculated because of the infiltrating margins. There are usually no associated calcifications.

Sonographic Findings

The sonographic findings of granular cell tumors are not specific. The tumor forms a solid nodule that is usually elliptical or fusiform in shape but does not have a demonstrable thin echogenic capsule. The most unique feature of

granular cell tumors is their susceptibility to the anisotropic effect. Because of the internal fibrillar pattern, the echogenicity of the lesion varies tremendously, depending on the angle of incidence of the ultrasound beam with the internal fibrillar pattern (Fig. 13–86). Thus, when the beam is nearly perpendicular to the fibrils, the lesion appears mildly hyperechoic. However, when the beam strikes the fibrils at an oblique angle, the lesion appears hypoechoic, similar to other breast neoplasms. Only small changes in the angle of incidence can lead to great changes of echogenicity. Granular cell tumors high in fibrous content, like scirrhous breast carcinomas, may shadow intensely because of absorption (not reflection or refraction) of the ultrasound beam. Such lesions may show an anisotropic effect on sound transmission as well as echogenicity (Fig. 13–87). The sound transmission is normal or only minimally decreased when the beam strikes the fibrils at an angle of incidence nearly perpendicular to their axis but is decreased when the insonation angle is obliquely oriented. Anisotropia is commonly seen in tendons, but we know of no other breast lesion that shows such anisotropia.

Only one granular cell tumor has been seen that was completely surrounded by fat. Because these lesions are

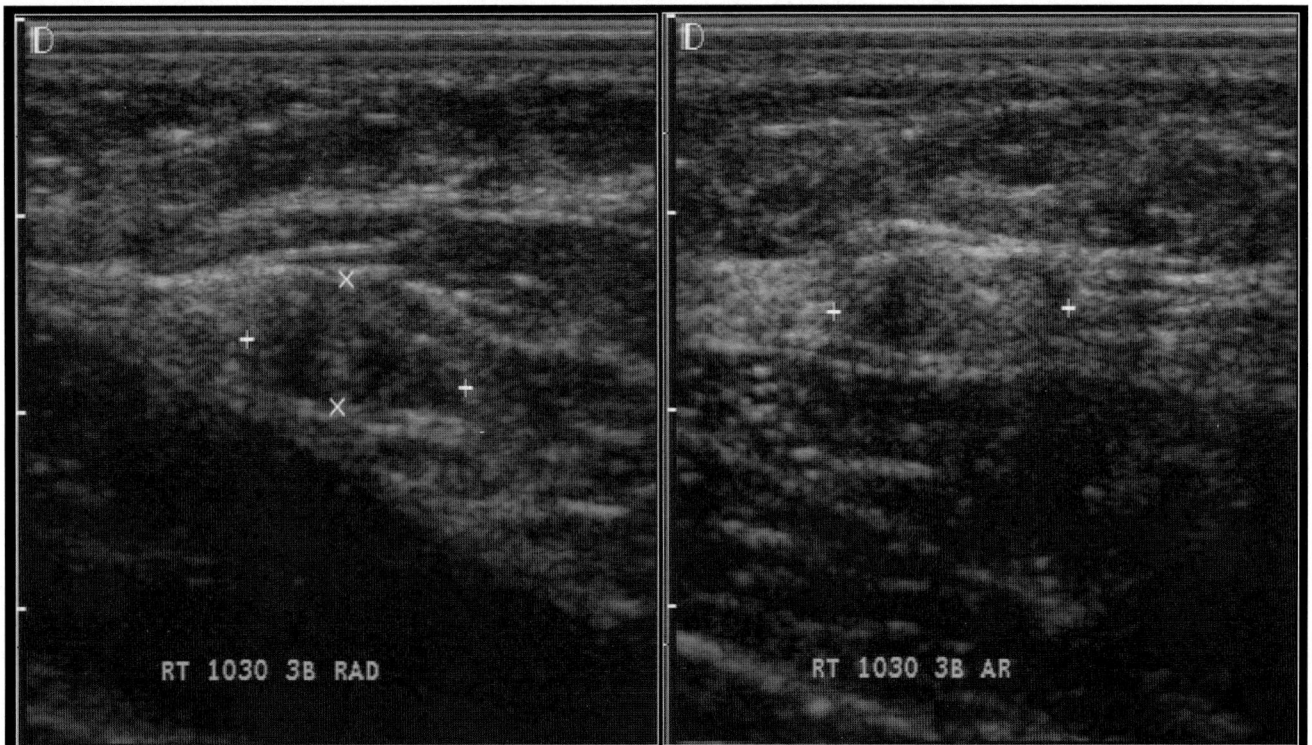

FIGURE 13–86 Granular cell tumors are composed of fibrils and therefore, like tendons, are subject to the anisotropic effect. The echogenicity varies with small changes in the angle of incidence. When the ultrasound beam strikes the internal fibrils at nearly a 90-degree angle, the lesion appears echogenic or even hyperechoic (**right**). However, when the beam strikes the fibrils at an oblique angle, the lesion appears hypoechoic (**left**). Anisotropia occurs commonly in musculoskeletal sonography, but the only lesion in the breast that demonstrates anisotropia is granular cell tumor.

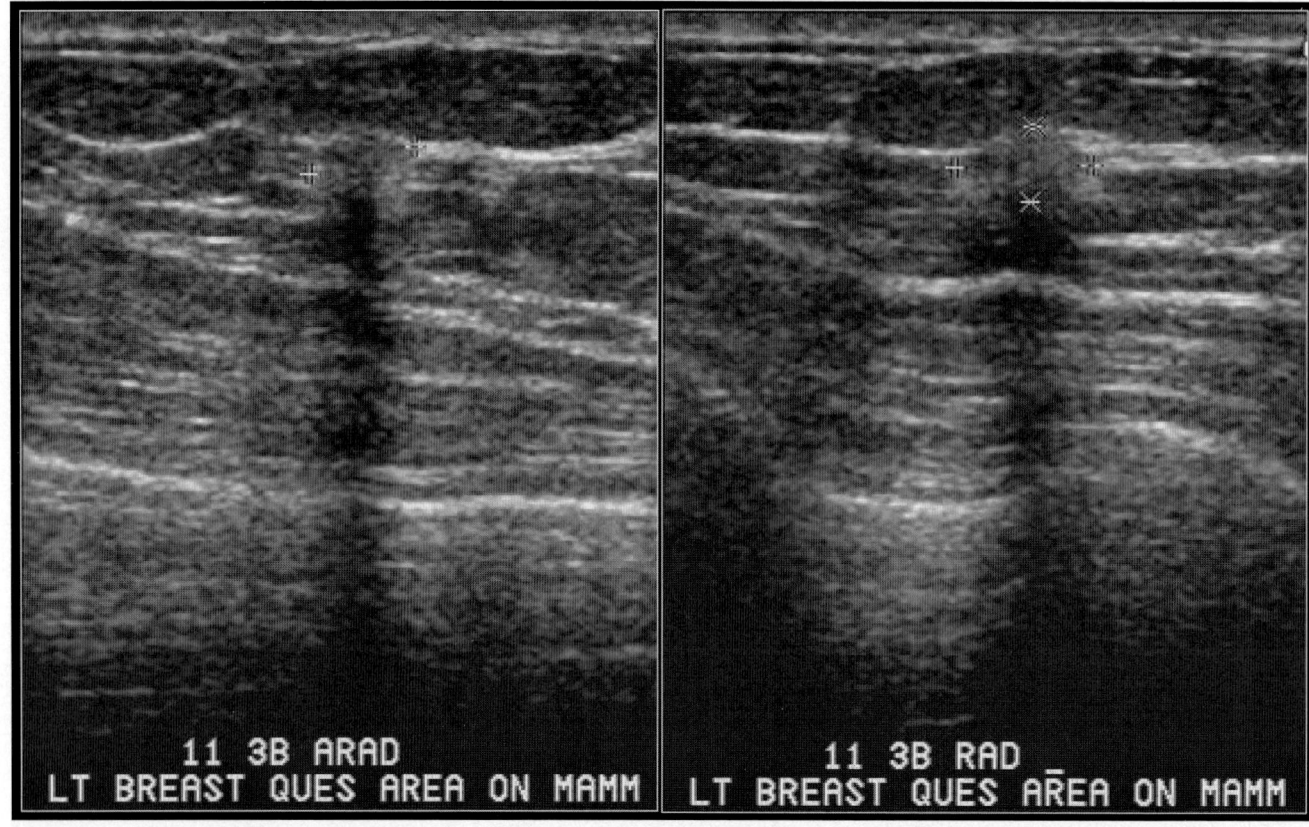

FIGURE 13–87 Anisotropia also affects the sound transmission through granular cell tumors in the breast. Scans obtained in a plane nearly perpendicular to the fibrillar pattern within the lesion show nearly normal sound transmission (**right**). However, images obtained with the beam oblique to the fibrillar pattern within the lesion show acoustic shadowing (**left**).

stromal tumors that typically occur in young women who still have abundant unregressed stromal tissue, the surrounding tissue type tends to be echogenic interlobular fibrous stroma.

Although the shape of granular cell tumors is usually elliptical and wider than tall, the presence of an infiltrating border prevents sonographic demonstration of a thin, echogenic capsule. The lack of a capsule and presence of acoustic shadowing both exclude these lesions from a probably benign (BIRADS 3) sonographic classification and necessitate biopsy.

HEMANGIOMAS

General Pathologic Classification, Epidemiology, and Clinical Findings

Hemangiomas are usually clinically inapparent and incidental findings at histology. However, larger hemangiomas may present as nonpalpable mammographic nodules. Small,

microscopically detectable perilobular hemangiomas are almost always incidental findings at histology. These lesions are relatively common, occurring in about 5% of benign biopsies and up to 11% of autopsy studies. Perilobular hemangiomas are only 2 to 4 mm in size, smaller than one low-power microscopic field, and generally imperceptible on clinical and imaging studies. Despite the name perilobular, most lesions are intralobular, being single or multiple. The major significance of perilobular hemangiomas is that these vascular tumors may be difficult to distinguish from low-grade angiosarcomas histologically, especially if there is endothelial atypia.

Macroscopic hemangiomas are larger than 4 mm, but usually less than 2 cm in diameter and rarely palpable. These lesions may present as mammographic masses and therefore necessitate ultrasound evaluation. The tumors can be classified as cavernous or capillary, depending on the size of vessels contained within. Cavernous hemangiomas are the most common type and are discussed in greater detail in Chapter 11 under the category of complex cystic lesions of the breast. Pure capillary hemangiomas are uncommon. Mixed varieties are common, however, with most cavernous hemangiomas of the breast also containing areas of capillary-sized vessels within them.

Although perilobular hemangiomas occur within the parenchyma (mammary zone), most macroscopic hemangiomas are actually subcutaneous in location rather than parenchymal. Thus, most macroscopic hemangiomas are actually skin lesions that just happen to involve the breast.

Pathology

At gross pathology, hemangiomas are dark, reddish to brown in color, and relatively soft and spongy. These masses are usually well circumscribed, although certain lesions may have peripheral vessels that grow into surrounding normal soft tissues.

As for microscopic perilobular hemangiomas, the primary significance of macroscopic hemangiomas is the potential to be confused with angiosarcoma. In addition to subtle histologic differences of these occasionally similar lesions, there are size differences. Hemangiomas are usually less than 2 cm in maximum diameter, whereas angiosarcomas are almost always in excess of 3 cm in diameter.

Neither microscopic nor macroscopic hemangiomas are palpable or otherwise clinically apparent unless the skin is directly involved.

The diagnosis of hemangioma is not possible with fine-needle aspiration biopsy but can be made with large core needle biopsy or mammotomy as well as excisional biopsy.

Mammographic Findings

Perilobular hemangiomas are not visible mammographically. Occasionally, a macroscopic cavernous or capillary hemangioma may cause a mammographic nodule. These lesions are low to medium density, round or lobulated in shape, with a circumscribed margin. Hemangiomas may contain calcifications that are, in essence, phleboliths. However, because the channels are irregular in shape, the calcifications usually do not have the classic rounded shapes expected with phleboliths forms in other parts of the body. The phleboliths associated with hemangiomas are usually amorphous or granular in appearance.

Sonographic Findings

Perilobular hemangiomas have not been reported in the sonographic literature, likely because they are too small to demonstrate sonographically. The sonographic appearance of macroscopic hemangiomas depends on the size of the vessels contained within and the presence or absence of fibrosis, scarring, thrombosis, or phleboliths. Cavernous hemangiomas may be mildly hypoechoic, isoechoic, or mildly hyperechoic and are illustrated in Chapter 11 (see

Fig. 11–130). If vessel size within the hemangioma is variable, the nodule is usually heterogeneous. Acute thrombosis causes an area of hypoechogenicity within the nodule. Phleboliths appear as punctate areas of markedly increased echogenicity that may or may not cause acoustic shadowing, depending on the diameter of the calcification relative to the beam width. Pure capillary hemangiomas have an appearance almost identical to hemangiomas of the liver—diffusely and homogeneously hyperechoic, with normal to increased sound transmission (Fig. 13–88). The shape of capillary hemangiomas of the breast is more elliptical than that of liver hemangiomas. This is because capillary hemangiomas of the breast are superficially located and soft enough to be flattened in the AP dimension by transducer pressure. Split-screen images with and without compression pressure can be helpful in distinguishing soft hemangiomas from firmer focal fibrosis, which can have an identical ellipsoid, uniformly hyperechoic appearance. Interestingly, the echogenicity of hemangiomas tends to increase as transducer pressure is increased because the interfaces between the capillaries that create the echoes are pushed closer together when the lesion is compressed (Fig. 13–89).

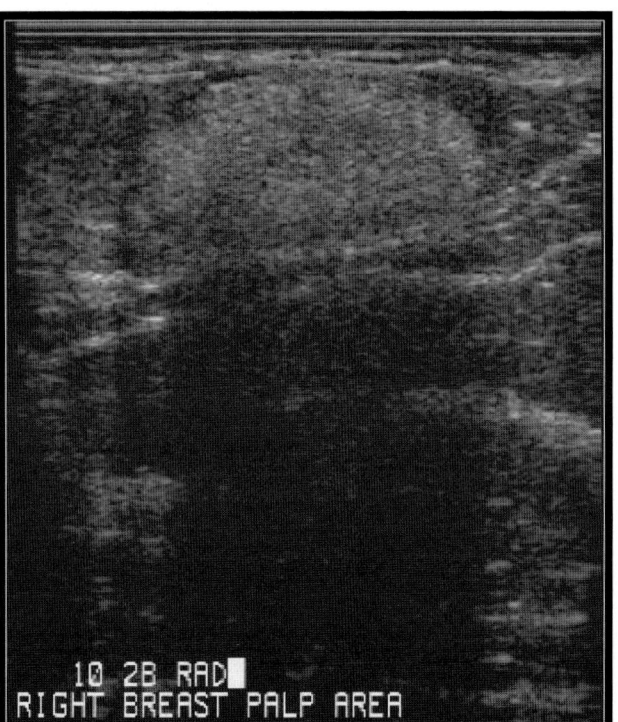

FIGURE 13–88 Pure capillary hemangiomas are well circumscribed and hyperechoic, as are hemangiomas of the liver and spleen. However, unlike hepatic hemangiomas, the hemangiomas in the breast are usually elliptical in shape because they are soft, compressible, and flattened in the anteroposterior dimension by the transducer. Hepatic hemangiomas are too deep to be compressed during scanning.

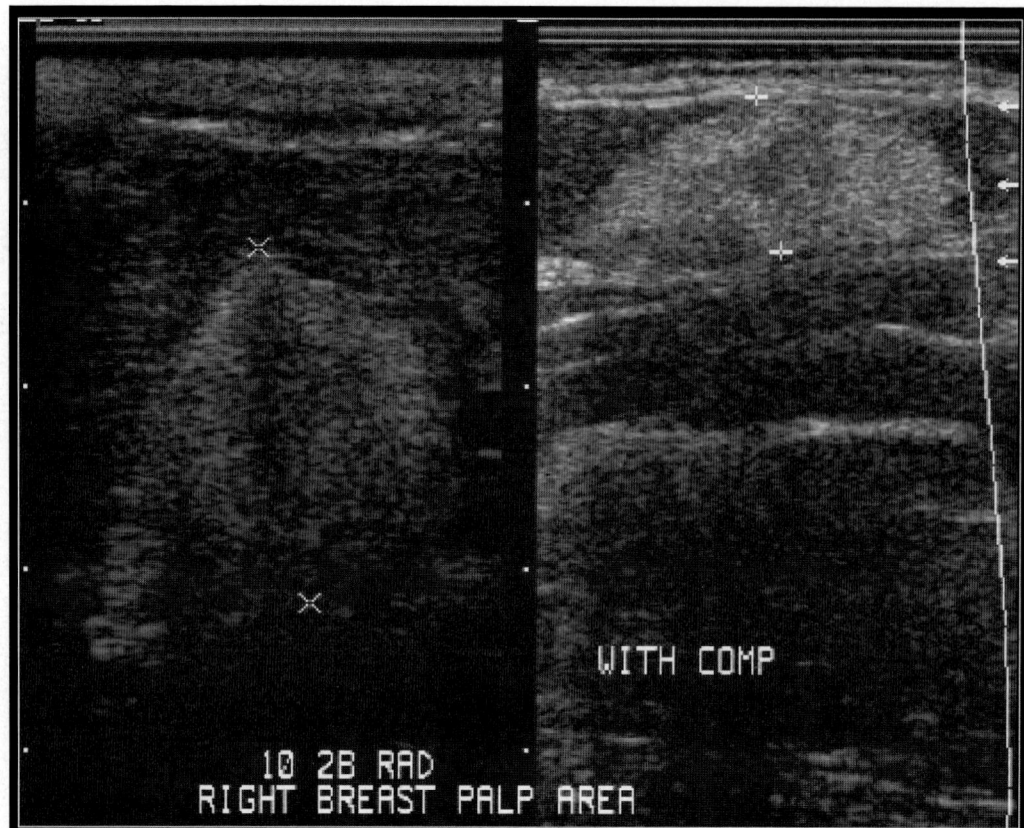

FIGURE 13–89 Hemangiomas become more echogenic as well as more elliptical in shape when compressed during scanning. The image on the **right** was obtained with very light compression pressure. Note that the lesion is more spherical in shape and less echogenic. The image on the **left** was obtained with normal scan pressure. The lesion is now both more echogenic and elliptical in shape.

FIBROCYSTIC CHANGES AND BENIGN PROLIFERATIVE DISORDERS

General Pathologic Classification, Epidemiology, and Clinical Findings

Fibrocystic change and benign proliferative disorders are virtually ubiquitous and their presentations, and their imaging appearances are myriad. Many of the well-known imaging manifestations of these processes are macroscopic simple and complex cysts. The cystic manifestations of fibrocystic change are discussed in Chapter 10. However, pathologists recognize histologic fibrocystic changes that can produce the sonographic appearance of a solid nodule. There are several different mechanisms by which fibrocystic change can create what appear to represent solid nodules during sonography. First, TDLUs can, in fact, be filled and distended with solid material by either papillary apocrine metaplastic growth or florid duct hyperplasia (papillary duct hyperplasia). Second, the TDLU can be distended by adenosis or sclerosing adenosis. Third, the "fibro" component of fibrocystic change, fibrosis, sclerosis, and hyalinization, may enlarge TDLUs. Fourth, the TDLU

can be enlarged by microcysts (<2 mm) that are too small to resolve sonographically. Fifth, even when there are macroscopic cysts, the cyst can become filled with various echogenic substances, including papillary apocrine metaplasia, papillary duct hyperplasia, foamy macrophages, various white blood cells, red blood cells, and proteinaceous debris that forms a gel-like or foamlike substance within the cyst. Solid-appearing manifestations of fibrocystic change are discussed in detail in Chapters 10 and 12.

In this section, we discuss primarily the benign proliferative disorder adenosis. In particular, we discuss presentation of sclerosing adenosis and tumoral adenosis as solid nodules. Adenosis is hyperplasia of the intralobular ductules that leads to enlargement of lobules and an increase in the number of lobules. When adenosis becomes extensive enough, the enlarged and more numerous lobules can coalesce into a solid mass termed *tumoral adenosis*. Tumoral adenosis is distinguished from adenosis or sclerosing adenosis only in extent. Tumor adenosis is to adenosis as lung consolidation is to fluffy alveolar infiltrates. Tumoral adenosis may appear as mammographic opacities and sonographic solid masses that are difficult or impossible to distinguish from DCIS or even invasive malignancy in some cases.

Mammographic Findings

Most adenosis is not mammographically visible and appears only as fluffy fibroglandular density. Adenosis may result in amorphous, powdery or punctate calcifications (Fig. 13–90). Sclerosing adenosis occasionally can cause mammographic architectural distortion (Fig. 13–91) or spiculation that is difficult to distinguish from radial scar or malignancy. Tumoral adenosis can lead to large masses or focal mammographic opacities (Fig. 13–92).

Sonographic Findings

Adenosis is visible sonographically as enlargement and increase in the number of TDLUs. The enlargement of the lobules caused by adenosis is not so much a pathologic process as a variant of normal or aberration of normal development and involution (ANDI) that creates an in-between sensitivity state between the purely hyperechoic fibrous breast and the purely isoechoic glandular breast. Normal lobules are up to 1 to 2 mm. The size of the TDLUs that

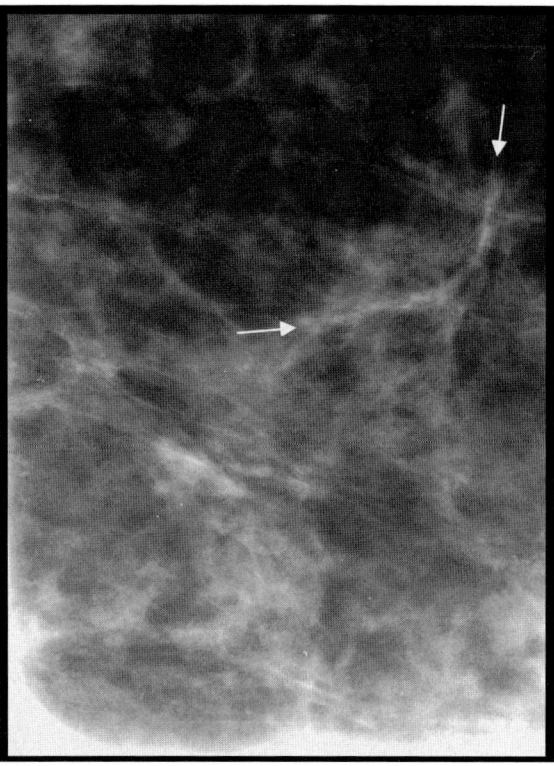

FIGURE 13–91 Sclerosing adenosis can lead to architectural distortion in some cases and frank spiculation in others. Persistence of such findings on spot compression views such as this leads to BIRADS 4 or higher classification and biopsy.

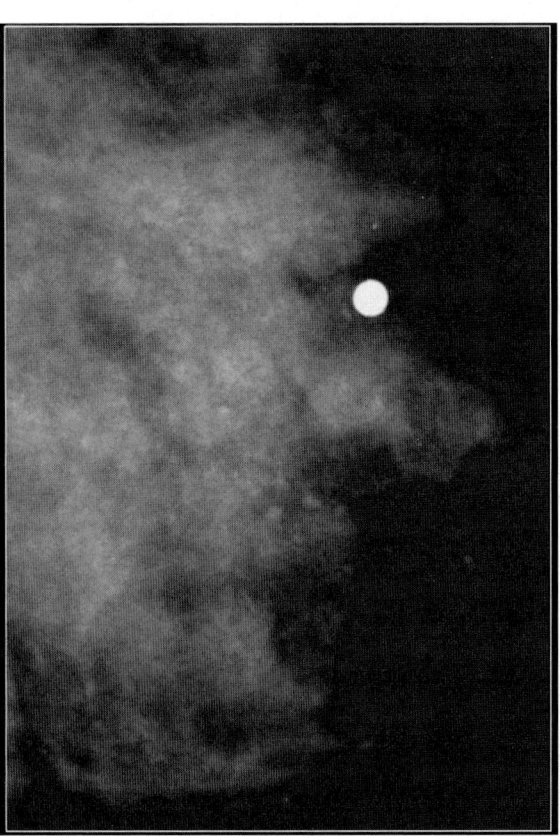

FIGURE 13–90 Typical adenosis calcifications are amorphous, powdery or punctate, and usually widely distributed. Such calcifications are typically characterized as BIRADS 3, probably benign, and followed. Occasionally low-nuclear-grade ductal carcinoma *in situ* can cause similar-appearing calcifications. They are so small that they cannot be demonstrated sonographically in some cases.

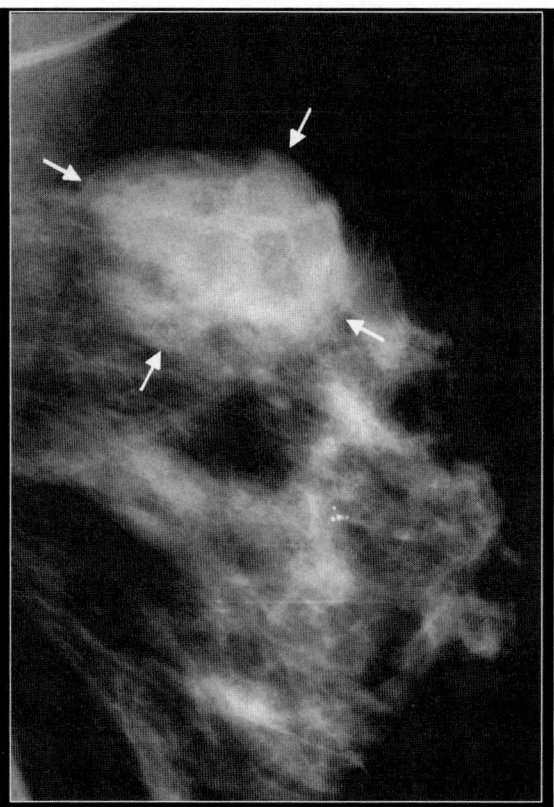

FIGURE 13–92 Tumoral adenosis can lead to focal masses or focally asymmetric mammographic opacities such as this.

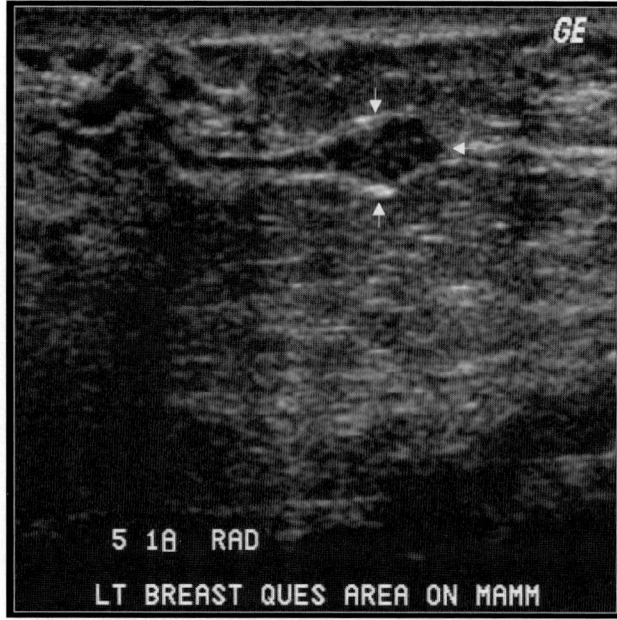

FIGURE 13–93 Sclerosing adenosis may present sonographically as a mildly enlarged terminal ductolobular unit *(arrows).*

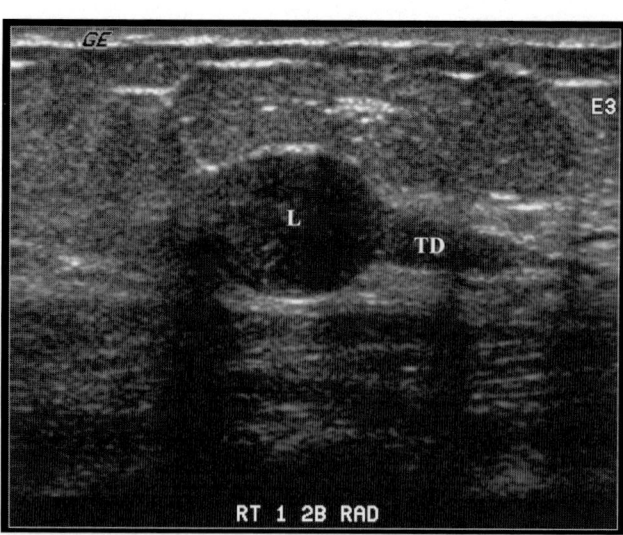

FIGURE 13–94 In other cases, sclerosing adenosis presents as severe enlargement of a terminal ductolobular unit. Note the faint calcifications that were better shown on other images. L, lobule; TD, extralobular terminal duct.

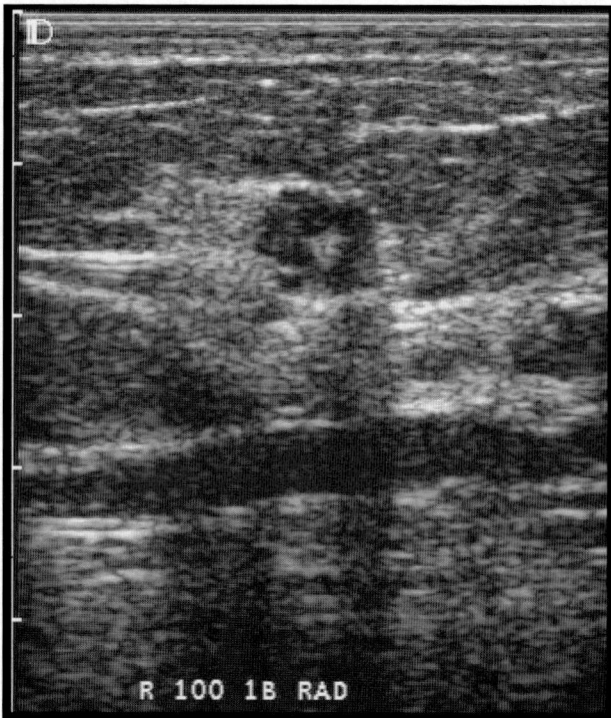

FIGURE 13–95 This case of sclerosing adenosis presents as a solid, microlobulated nodule with a hyperechoic central focus that represents sclerosis. The appearance is similar to that of radial scar or complex sclerosing lesion and some cases of intermediate-grade invasive ductal carcinoma with central necrosis and scarring. Such an appearance always demands a BIRADS 4a or higher classification and biopsy.

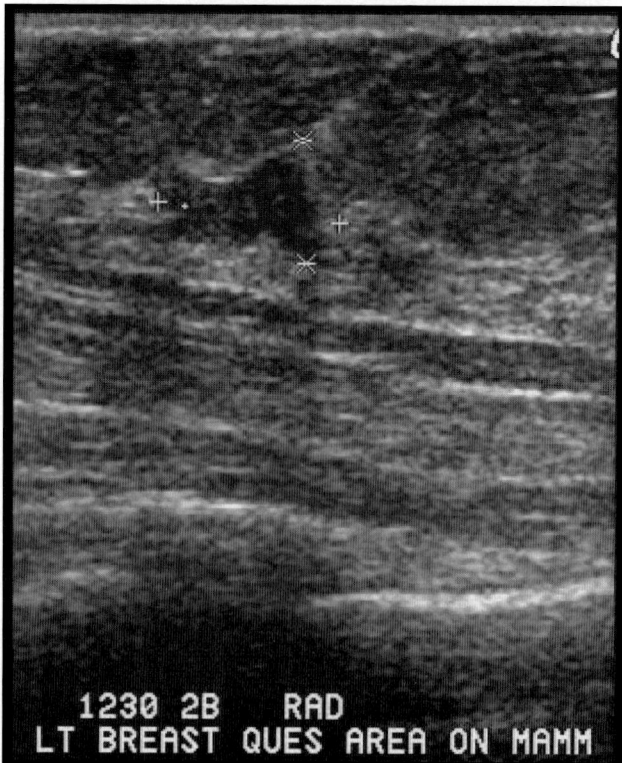

FIGURE 13–96 This case of sclerosing adenosis presents as a mildly hypoechoic solid nodule that has angular margins. The presence of angular margins indicates the need for a BIRADS 4a or higher classification and biopsy.

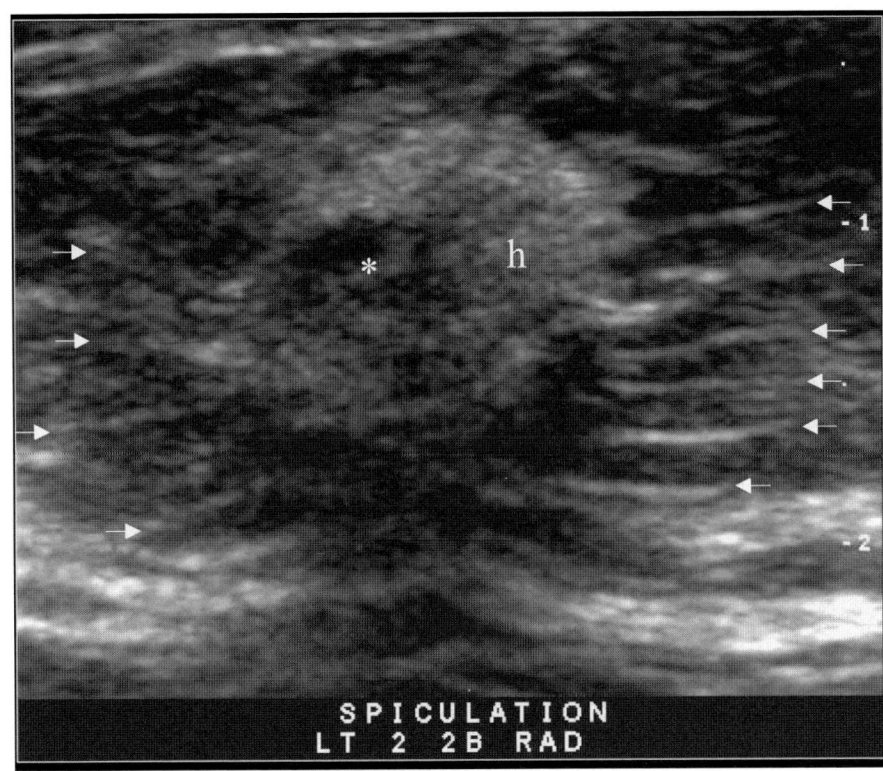

FIGURE 13–97 This case of sclerosing adenosis caused a frankly spiculated lesion. There is an ill-defined heterogeneous central nidus *(*)* and a thick, echogenic halo *(h)*, and extending into the surrounding fat are hyperechoic spiculations *(arrows)*.

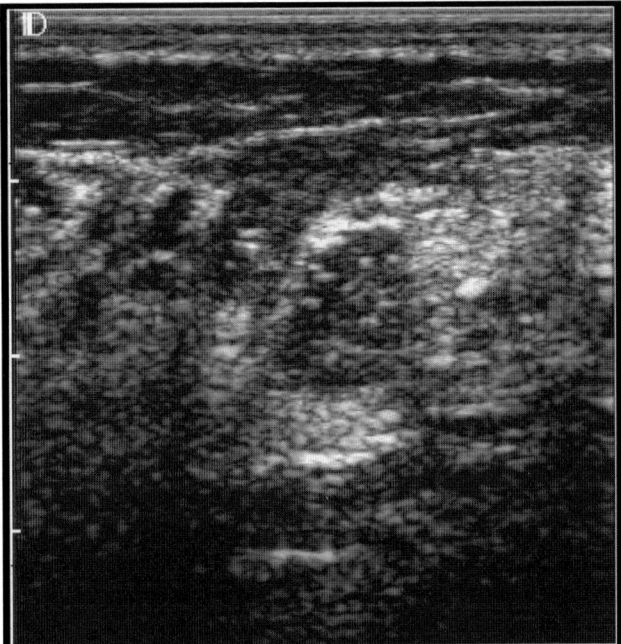

FIGURE 13–98 This case of sclerosing adenosis causes a taller-than-wide, microlobulated, angular solid nodule that contains numerous punctate echoes that represent calcifications.

are most enlarged by adenosis creates a threshold below which a solid nodule cannot be identified. TDLUs affected by adenosis may achieve diameters of 5 mm. If there are dozens of TDLUs affected by adenosis that are 5 mm in diameter in the areas of a palpable or mammographic abnormality that requires sonographic evaluation, no nodule smaller than the 5-mm TDLU can be detected or distinguished from the adenosis-affected TDLUs.

Sclerosing adenosis has a variety of sonographic appearances. It can present as a moderately (Fig. 13–93) or severely enlarged TDLU (Fig. 13–94). It can present as a microlobulated solid nodule with a central echogenic focus representing the sclerosis (Fig. 13–95). If the sclerosis is severe, the small nodule formed may be angular (Fig. 13–96) or frankly spiculated (Fig. 13–97). Although the calcifications in adenosis are generally very small, they may be large enough to cause punctate internal echoes in some cases of sclerosis adenosis (Fig. 13–98).

Tumoral adenosis is not a separate condition, but simply more extensive and confluent focal involvement with adenosis or sclerosing adenosis. It creates large isoechoic masses (usually in excess of 2 to 3 cm) that are masslike and difficult to distinguish sonographically from DCIS (usually intermediate nuclear grade) or invasive carcinoma (see Chapter 12, Fig. 12–98). The tumoral adenosis is sonographically conspicuous when surrounded by

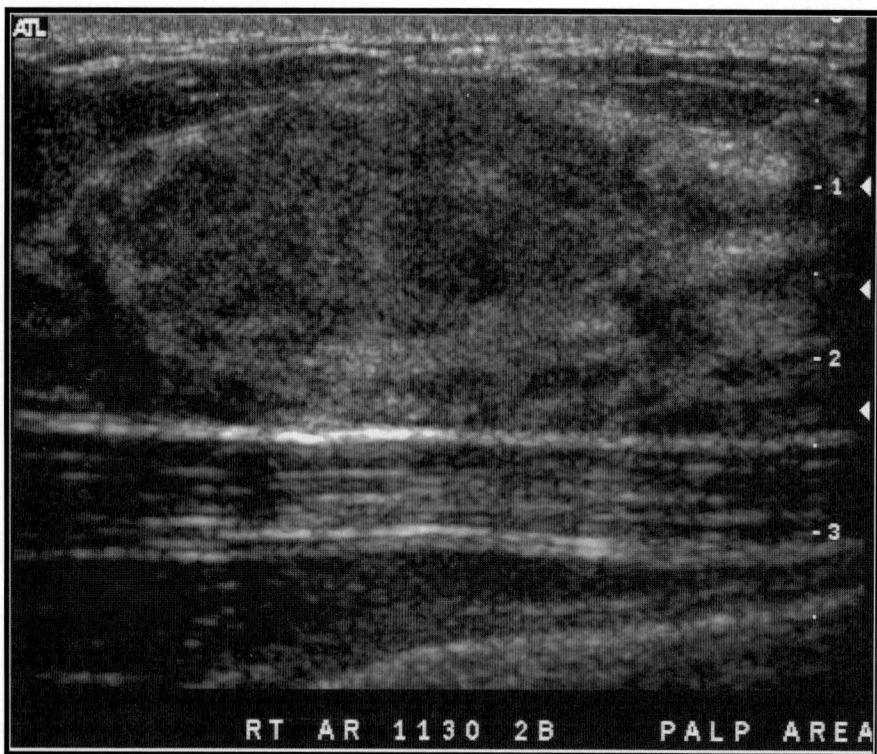

RT AR 1130 2B   PALP AREA

FIGURE 13–99 This mass of isoechoic tumoral adenosis is sonographically conspicuous because it is surrounded by hyperechoic fibrous tissue.

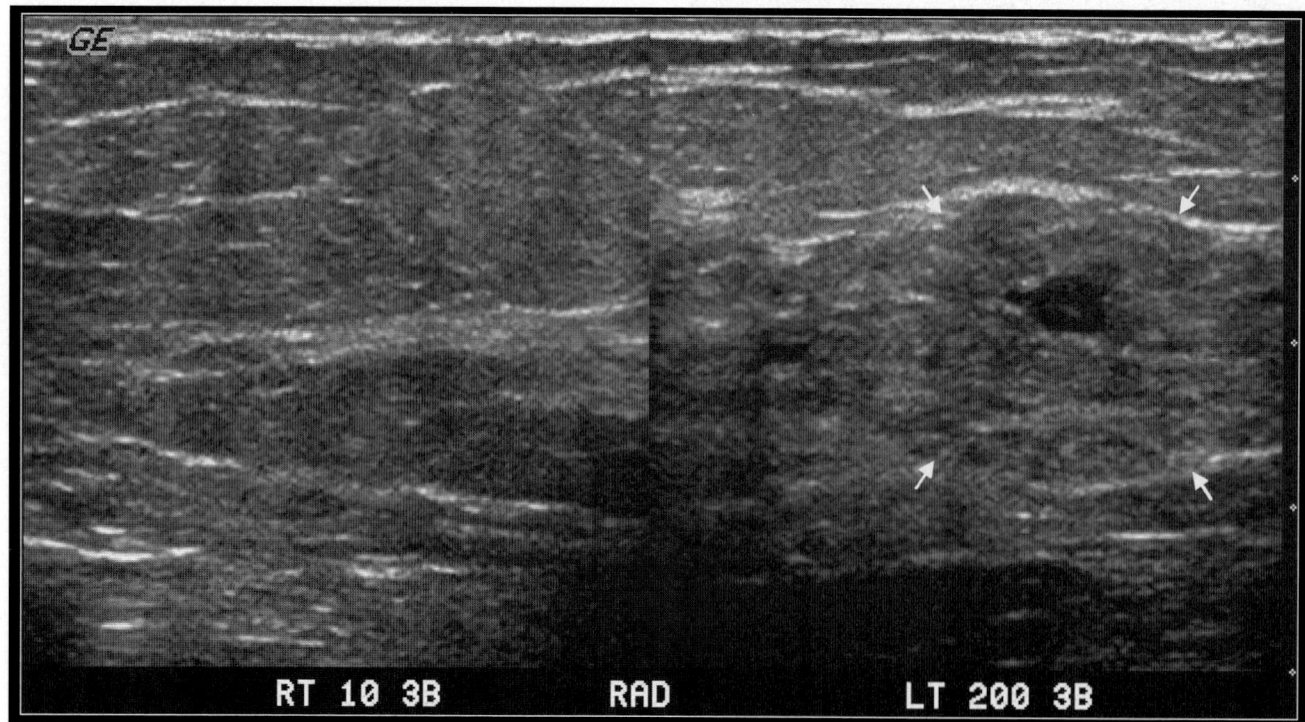

RT 10 3B   RAD   LT 200 3B

FIGURE 13–100 This mass of isoechoic tumoral adenosis *(arrows)* is sonographically inconspicuous because it is surrounded by isoechoic fat. Split-screen mirror images of the upper outer quadrants of the right breast **(left)** and left breast **(right)** show the tumoral adenosis to contain a cyst.

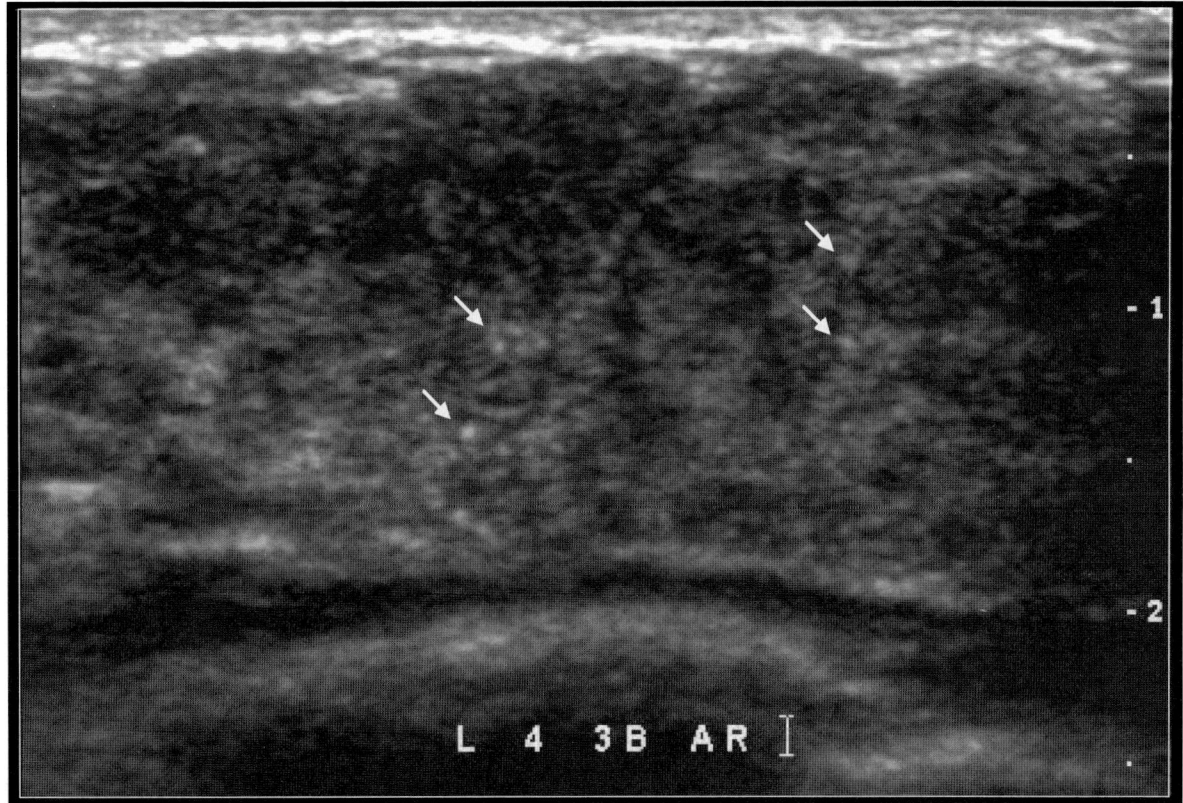

FIGURE 13-101 This mass of tumoral adenosis contains tiny punctate bright echoes that represent the powdery amorphous calcifications that are so typical of adenosis.

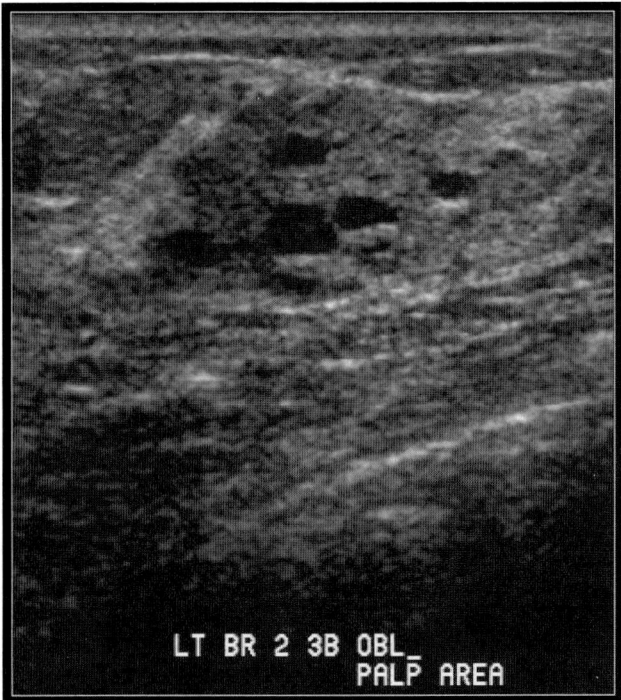

FIGURE 13-102 The isoechoic masses of tumoral adenosis are difficult to distinguish sonographically from ductal carcinoma *in situ* and some intermediate-grade invasive ductal carcinomas. However, tumoral adenosis often contains benign cysts that meet criteria for simple cysts, whereas any areas of cystic or hemorrhagic degeneration within malignant nodules are usually ill defined and complex.

hyperechoic fibrous tissue (Fig. 13–99) but may be subtle when surrounded by isoechoic fat (Fig. 13–100). Like the smaller nodules caused by sclerosing adenosis, tumoral adenosis may contain powdery amorphous calcifications or punctate calcifications (Fig. 13–101). A few features may be helpful in distinguishing tumoral adenosis from DCIS. Unlike DCIS or invasive carcinoma, tumoral adenosis may contain well-circumscribed and thinly encapsulated simple cysts (Fig. 13–102). Additionally, vocal fremitus may be helpful. DCIS tends to cause a defect in fremitus (see Chapter 20, Fig. 20–87), whereas tumoral adenosis tends to vibrate like normal tissue (see Chapter 20, Fig. 20–86). Fremitus is discussed and illustrated in Chapter 20.

SUGGESTED READINGS

Fibroadenomas

Adler DD, Hyde DL, Ikeda DM. Quantitative sonographic parameters as a means of distinguishing breast cancers from benign solid breast masses. *J Ultrasound Med* 1991;10(9):505–508.

Baker KS, et al. Carcinoma within fibroadenomas: mammographic features. *Radiology* 1990;176(2):371–374.

Blickstein I, et al. Echogenicity of fibroadenoma and carcinoma of the breast. Quantitative comparison using gain-assisted densitometric evaluation of sonograms. *J Ultrasound Med* 1995;14(9): 661–664.

Burnett SJ, et al. Benign biopsies in the prevalent round of breast screening: a review of 137 cases. *Clin Radiol* 1995;50(4):254–258.

Campbell RE, et al. Image interpretation session: 1993. Fibroadenoma of the breast. *Radiographics* 1994;14(1):209–210.

Cant PJ, et al. Non-operative management of breast masses diagnosed as fibroadenoma. *Br J Surg* 1995;82(6):792–794.

Chopier J, et al. Solid breast nodules: reliability of ultrasonographic and cytological studies. *J Radiol* 1995;76(5):263–266.

Cole-Beuglet C, et al. Fibroadenoma of the breast: sonomammography correlated with pathology in 122 patients. *AJR Am J Roentgenol* 1983;140(2):369–375.

Cyrlak D, Wong CH. Mammographic changes in postmenopausal women undergoing hormonal replacement therapy. *AJR Am J Roentgenol* 1993;161:1177–1183.

Dupont WD, et al. Long-term risk of breast cancer in women with fibroadenoma. *N Engl J Med* 1994;331(1):10–15.

Feig SA. Breast masses. Mammographic and sonographic evaluation. *Radiol Clin North Am* 1992;30(1):67–92.

Fornage BD, Lorigan JG, Andry E. Fibroadenoma of the breast: sonographic appearance. *Radiology* 1989;172(3):671–675.

Guyer PB, Dewbury KC. Sonomammography in benign breast disease. *Br J Radiol* 1988;61(725):374–378.

Guyer PB, et al. Ultrasonic attenuation in fibroadenoma of the breast. *Clin Radiol* 1992;45(3):175–178.

Hall FM. Probably benign breast nodules: follow-up of selected cases without initial full problem-solving imaging [Comment]. *Radiology* 1995;194(2):305.

Hanson CA, Snover DC, Dehner LP. Fibroadenomatosis (fibroadenomatoid mastopathy): a benign breast lesion with composite pathologic features. *Pathology* 1987;19(4):393–396.

Harper AP, et al. Ultrasound in the evaluation of solid breast masses. *Radiology* 1983;146:731–736.

Hayashi N, et al. Real-time sonography of palpable breast masses. *Br J Radiol* 1985;58(691):611–615.

Heywang SH, et al. Specificity of ultrasonography in the diagnosis of benign breast masses. *J Ultrasound Med* 1984;3(10):453–461.

Hindle WH, Alonzo LJ. Conservative management of breast fibroadenomas. *Am J Obstet Gynecol* 1991;164(6 Pt 1):1647–1651.

Holcombe C, et al. Blood flow in breast cancer and fibroadenoma estimated by colour Doppler ultrasonography. *Br J Surg* 1995; 82(6):787–788.

Husien AM. Ultrasonic attenuation of fibroadenoma of the breast [Letter; comment]. *Clin Radiol* 1992;46(3):220.

Isaacs JH. Benign tumors of the breast. *Obstet Gynecol Clin North Am* 1994;21(3):487–497.

Ishii M. The study of ultrasonographic diagnosis of breast diseases. *Nippon Igaku Hoshasen Gakkai Zasshi* 1992;52(7):1033–1035.

Ishii M. Ultrasonographic diagnosis of breast diseases: a review of diagnostic criteria of sonomammography on a real-time scanner. *Nippon Igaku Hoshasen Gakkai Zasshi* 1993;53(10):1141–1159.

Jackson VP, et al. The spectrum of sonographic findings of fibroadenoma of the breast. *Invest Radiol* 1986;21(1):34–40.

Kornguth PJ, Bentley RC. Mammographic-pathologic correlation: part 1, benign breast lesions. *J Womens Imaging* 2001;3:29–37.

Kuipjer A, Mommoer EC, van der Wall E, et al. Histopathology of fibroadenoma of the breast. *Am J Clin Pathol* 2001;115(5): 736–742.

Langer TG, Shaw de Paredes E. Evaluation of nonpalpable mammographic nodules. *Applied Radiol* 1991;4:19–28.

Leonardi M, et al. The value of ultrasonography in benign breast diseases. *Minerva Ginecol* 1993;45(3):113.116.

McDivitt RW, et al. Histologic types of benign breast disease and the risk for breast cancer. The Cancer and Steroid Hormone Study Group. *Cancer* 1992;69(6):1408–1414.

Merchant TE, et al. Fibroadenoma of the breast: in vivo magnetic resonance characterization. *Eur J Radiol* 1991;13(2):91–95.

Meyer JE, et al. Enlarging occult fibroadenomas. *Radiology* 1992; 183(3):639–641.

Nguyen J, McMullen K, Sardi A. Lobular carcinoma in situ within a fibroadenoma. *J La State Med Soc* 1991;143(10):33–35.

Pierart J, et al. Radiologic visibility of breast fibroadenomas. *Rev Med Chil* 1995;123(2):192–198.

Possover M, et al. New perspectives in color ultrasound in breast diagnosis. *Geburtshilfe Frauenheilkd* 1994;54(8):432–436.

Schepps B, Scola FH, Frates RE. Benign circumscribed breast masses. Mammographic and sonographic appearance. *Obstet Gynecol Clin North Am* 1994;21(3):519–537.

Sickles EA, et al. Benign breast lesions: ultrasound detection and diagnosis. *Radiology* 1984;151(2):467–470.

Skaane P, Engedal K. Analysis of sonographic features in the differentiation of fibroadenoma and invasive ductal carcinoma. *AJR Am J Roentgenol* 1998;170(1):109–114.

Spencer NJ, et al. Pathological-radiological correlations in benign lesions excised during a breast-screening program. *Clin Radiol* 1994;49(12):853–856.

Stavros AT, et al. Solid breast nodules: use of sonography to distinguish between benign and malignant lesions [Comments]. *Radiology* 1995;196(1):123–134.

Swisher RC, et al. Enlarging fibroadenoma in a postmenopausal woman: case report. *Radiology* 1992;184:425–426.

Tavassoli K, et al. Ultrasound diagnostic criteria in breast disease. *Panminerva Med* 1997;39(3):178–182.

Vetshev PS, et al. Ultrasound diagnosis of breast nodules. *Khirurgiia* (Mosk) 1995;(1):8–11.

Weinstein SP, Orel SG, Collazzo E, et al. Cycolosporin A-induced fibroadenomas of the breast: report of 5 cases. *Radiology* 2001; 220:465–468.

Wilson R. Management of probably benign breast lesions. *Radiology* 1995;194(3):912.

Giant Fibroadenomas, Juvenile Fibroadenomas, and Fibroadenomas with Cellular Stroma

Alagaratnam TT, Ng WF, Leung EY. Giant fibroadenomas of the breast in an oriental community. *J R Coll Surg Edinb* 1995; 40(3):161–162.

Amiel C, et al. Giant breast fibroadenoma. *J Gynecol Obstet Biol Reprod* (Paris) 1993;22(7):764–765.

Boothroyd A, Carty H. Breast masses in childhood and adolescence. A presentation of 17 cases and a review of the literature. *Pediatr Radiol* 1994;24(2):81–84.

Garcia CJ, Espinoza A, Dinamarca V, et al. Breast US in children and adolescents. *Radiographics* 2000;20(6):1605–1612.

Jonides L, Rudy C, Walsh S. Breast masses in adolescent girls. *J Pediatr Health Care* 1992;6(5):274, 287–288.

Konemer KA, Rhee K, Siegel M, et al. Gray scale sonography of breast masses in adolescent girls. *J Ultrasound Med* 2001;20: 491–496.

Reddick RL, Shin TK, Sawhney D, et al. Stromal proliferations of the breast: an ultrastructural and immuno histochemical evaluation of cystosarcoma phyllodes, juvenile fibroadenoma, and fibroadenoma. *Hum Pathol* 1987;18(1):45–49.

Remadi S, et al. Cellular (juvenile) fibroadenoma of the breast. A clinico-pathologic and immunohistochemical study of 7 cases. *Ann Pathol* 1994;14(6):392–397.

Simmons PS. Diagnostic considerations in breast disorders of children and adolescents. *Obstet Gynecol Clin North Am* 1992;19(1): 91–102.

Steinbock RT, et al. The ultrasound appearance of giant fibroadenoma. *J Clin Ultrasound* 1983;11:451–454.

West KW, et al. Diagnosis and treatment of symptomatic breast masses in the pediatric population. *J Pediatr Surg* 1995;30(2): 182–187.

Tubular Adenomas

Moross T, Lang AP, Mahoney L. Tubular adenoma of the breast. *Arch Pathol Lab Med* 1983;107(2):84–86.

Onuma H, Kasuga Y, Masuda H, et al. A case of tubular adenoma of the breast preoperatively suspected to be an advanced cancer. *Gan No Rinsho* 1989;35(1):81–85.

Soo MS, Dash N, Bentley R, et al. Tubular adenomas of the breast: imaging findings with histologic correlation. *AJR Am J Roentgenol* 2000;174:757–761.

Lactating Adenomas and Secretory Adenomas

Beharndt VS, Barbakoff D, Askin FB, et al. Infarcted lactating adenoma presenting as a rapidly enlarging breast mass. *AJR Am J Roentgenol* 2999;173(10):933–935.

Bottles K, Taylor RN. Diagnosis of breast masses in pregnant and lactating women by aspiration cytology. *Obstet Gynecol* 1985; 66[3 Suppl]:s76–s78.

Darling ML, Smith DN, Rhie E, et al. Lactating adenoma: sonographic features. *Breast J* 2000;6(4):252–256.

Eld S, Dos Santos E, Boesserie-LaCroix M, et al. Lactating adenoma: radiologic aspects. A case report. *J Radiol* 82(3):264–267.

James K, Bridger J, Anthony PP. Breast tumour of pregnancy ('lactating' adenoma). *J Pathol* 156(1):37–44.

Sumkin JH, et al. Lactating adenoma: US features and literature review. *Radiology* 1998;206(1):271–274.

Yang WT, Suen M, Metreweli C. Lactating adenoma of the breast: antepartum and postpartum sonographic and color Doppler appearances with histopathologic correlation. *J Ultrasound Med* 1997;16(2):145–147.

Complex Fibroadenomas

DuPont WD, Page DL, Parl FF, et al. Long-term risk of breast cancer in women with fibroadenoma. *N Engl J Med* 1994;331(1):10–15.

Kuijper A, Mommers EC, van der Wall E, et al. Histopathology of fibroadenoma of the breast. *Am J Clin Pathol* 2001;115(5):736–742.

Nussbaum SA, Feig SA, Capuzzi DM. Breast imaging case of the day. Fibroadenoma with microcalcification. *Radiographics* 1998; 18(1):243–245.

Page DL, Dupont WD. Anatomic markers of human premalignancy and risk of breast cancer. *Cancer* 1990;66[6 Suppl]:1326–1335.

Hamartomas (Adenomyolipomas, Myoadenolipomas, and Lipoadenomyomas), Leiomyomas, and Benign Spindle Cell Tumors

Abbit PL, de Paredes ES, Sloop FB Jr. Breast hamartoma: a mammographic diagnosis. *South Med J* 1988;81(2):167–170.

Adler DD, Jeffries DO, Helvie MA. Sonographic features of breast hamartomas. *J Ultrasound Med* 1990;9(2):85–90.

Altermatt HJ, Gebbers JO, Laissue JA. Multiple hamartomas of the breast. *Appl Pathol* 1989;7(2):145–148.

Black J, Metcalf C, Wylie EJ. Ultrasonography of breast hamartomas. *Australas Radiol* 1996;40(4):412–415.

Crothers JG, Butler NF, Fortt W, Gravelle IH. Fibroadenolipoma of the breast. *Br J Radiol* 1985;58(3):191–202.

Daya D, et al. Hamartoma of the breast, an underrecognized breast lesion. A clinicopathologic and radiographic study of 25 cases. *Am J Clin Pathol* 1995;103(6):685–689.

Fiirgaard B, Kristensen S. Muscular hamartoma of the breast: a case report. *Acta Radiol* 1992;33(2):115–116.

Garijo MF, Torio B, Val-Bernal JF. Mammary hamartoma with brown adipose tissue. *Gen Diagn Pathol* 1997;143(4):243–246.

Helvie MA, Adler DD, Rebner M, et al. Breast hamartomas: variable mammographic appearance. *Radiology* 1989;170(2):417–421.

Jones MW, Norris HJ, Wargotz ES. Hamartomas of the breast. *Surg Gynecol Obstet* 1991;173(1):54–56.

Kievit HC, et al, Magnetic resonance image appearance of hamartoma of the breast. *Magn Reson Imaging* 1993;11(2):293–298.

Kopans DB, Meyer JE, Proppe KH. Ultrasonographic, xeromammographic, and histologic correlation of a fibroadenolipoma of the breast. *J Clin Ultrasound* 1982(10):409–411.

Mallory SB. Cowden syndrome (multiple hamartoma syndrome). *Dermatol Clin* 1995;13(1):27–31.

Rege JD, et al. Mammary hamartomas—a report of 15 cases. *Indian J Pathol Microbiol* 1997;40(4):543–548.

Rosen PP, Romain K, Liberman L. Mammary cystosarcoma with mature adipose stromal differentiation (lipophyllodes tumor) arising in a lipomatous hamartoma. *Arch Pathol Lab Med* 1994; 118(1):91–94.

Scott Conner CE, et al. Changing clinical picture of mammary hamartoma. *Am J Surg* 1993;165(2):208–212.

Diabetic Mastopathy, Fibrosclerosis, Focal Fibrosis, and Stromal Fibrosis

Garstin WI, et al. Fibrous mastopathy in insulin dependent diabetics. *Clin Radiol* 1991;44(2):89–91.

Harvey SC, Denison CM, Lester SC, et al. Fibrous nodules found at large-core breast biopsy of the breast: imaging features. *Radiology* 1999;211(5):535–540.

Hermann G, Schwatz IS. Focal fibrous disease of the breast: mammographic detection of an unappreciated condition. *AJR Am J Roentgenol* 1983;140(6):1245–1246.

Revelon G, Sherman ME, Gatewood OM, et al. Focal fibrosis of the breast: imaging characteristics and histopathologic correlation. *Radiology* 2000;216(1):255–259.

Rosen EL, Soo MS, Bentley RC. Focal fibrosis: a common breast lesion diagnosed at imaging-guided core biopsy. *AJR Am J Roentgenol* 1999;173(6):1657–1662.

Sklair-Levy M, Samuels TH, Catzavelos C, et al. Stromal fibrosis of the breast. *AJR Am J Roentgenol* 2001;177:573–577.

Venta LA, Wiley EL, Gabriel H, et al. Imaging features of focal breast fibrosis: mammographic-pathologic correlation of noncalcified breast lesions. *AJR Am J Roentgenol* 1999;173(2):309–316.

Lipomas

Hall FM, Connolly JL, Love SM. Lipomatous pseudomass of the breast: diagnosis suggested by discordant palpatory and mammographic findings. *Radiology* 1987;164(2):463–464.

Smith DN, Denison CM, Lester SC. Spindle cell lipoma of the breast. A case report. *Acta Radiol* 1996;37(6):893–895.

Solvetti FM, Thorel MF, Marandino F. Breast lipomas in echography. A discussion of 3 cases and review of the literature. *Radiol Med* (Torino) 2000;99(4):281–284.

Granular Cell Tumors and Fibromyoblastomas

Ammar A, et al. Granular cell tumors of the breast. Apropos of two cases. *Arch Anat Cytol Pathol* 1994;42(3–4):188–191.

Callonnec F, et al. Granular cell tumors (Abrikossoff's tumors) of the breast. Apropos of 4 cases. *J Radiol* 1992;73(5):335–339.

Khansur T, Balducci L, Tavassoli M. Granular cell tumor. Clinical spectrum of the benign and malignant entity. *Cancer* 1987;60(2):220–222.

Kommoss F, et al. Granular cell tumor of the breast mimicking carcinoma in pregnancy. *Obstet Gynecol* 1989;73(5):898–900.

Pierre F, et al. A misleading breast tumor: a granular cell tumor of the breast. *J Gynecol Obstet Biol Reprod* (Paris) 1990;19(8):999–1005.

Rickard MT, Sendel A, Burchett I. Case report: granular cell tumour of the breast. *Clin Radiol* 1992;45(5):347–348.

Scatarige JC, et al. Acoustic shadowing in benign granular cell tumor (myoblastoma) of the breast. *J Ultrasound Med* 1987;6(9):545–547.

Siegel JR, Sanders L, Kalisher L, et al. Unusual sonographic features of granular cells tumor of the breast. *J Clin Ultrasound* 1999;18:857–859.

Tobin CE, Hendrix TM, Geyer S, et al. Breast imaging case of the day. *Radiographics* 1996;16:983–985.

van Doorn-Kaivers M, Billenkamp G. Granular cell tumor misdiagnosed as scirrhous breast cancer. *Geburtshilfe Frauenheilkd* 1992;52(1):62–64.

Vos LD, et al. Granular cell tumor of the breast: mammographic and histologic correlation. *Eur J Radiol* 1994;19(1):56–59.

Pseudoangiomatous Stromal Hyperplasia

Cohen MA, Morris EA, Rosen PP, et al. Pseudoangiomatous stromal hyperplasia: mammographic, sonographic, and clinical patterns. *Radiology* 1996;198(1):117–120.

Cyriak D, Carpenter PM. Breast imaging case of the day. Pseudoangiomatous stromal hyperplasia. *Radiographics* 1999;19(4):1086–1088.

Haagensen CD. Diseases of the breast. Philadelphia: WB Saunders, 1986:259–265.

Polger MR, Denison CM, Lester S, et al. Pseudoangiomatous stromal hyperplasia: mammographic and sonographic appearances. *AJR Am J Roentgenol* 1996;166(2):349–352.

Powell CM, Cranor ML, Rosen PP. Pseudoangiomatous stromal hyperplasia (PASH): a mammary stromal tumor with myofibroblastic differentiation. *Am J Pathol* 1995;19(3):270–277.

Hemangiomas

Carreira C, Romano C, Rodriguez R, et al. A cavernous haemangioma of breast in male: radiological-pathologic correlation. *Eur Radiol* 2001;11(2):292–294.

Courcoutsakis NA, et al. Breast hemangiomas in a patient with Kasabach-Merritt syndrome: imaging findings. *AJR Am J Roentgenol* 1997;169(5):1397–1399.

Dener C, Sengui N, Tez S, et al. Haemangiomas of the breast. *Eur J Surg* 2000;166(12):977–979.

Gembala RB, et al. Color Doppler detection of a breast perilobular hemangioma. *J Ultrasound Med* 1993;12(4):220–222.

Perugini G, et al. Cavernous hemangioma of the pectoralis muscle mimicking a breast tumor. *AJR Am J Roentgenol* 1994;162(6):1321–1322.

Webb LA, Young JR. Case report: haemangioma of the breast—appearances on mammography and ultrasound. *Clin Radiol* 1996;51(7):523–524.

Fibrocystic Changes, Benign Proliferative Changes, Adenosis, and Sclerosing Adenosis

Cyrlak D, Carpenter PM, Rawal NG. Breast imaging case of the day. *Radiographics* 1999;19:245–247.

Ichihara S, Aoyama H. Intraductal carcinoma of the breast arising in sclerosing adenosis. *Pathol Int* 1994;44(9):722–726.

Jensen RA, Page DL, Dupont WD, et al. Invasive breast cancer risk in women with sclerosing adenosis. *Cancer* 1989;64(10):1977–1983.

Kamel OW, Kempson RL, Hendrickson MR. In situ proliferative epithelial lesions of the breast. *Pathology* (Phila) 1992;1(1):65–102.

Nielsen NS, Nielsen BB. Mammographic features of sclerosing adenosis presenting as a tumor. *Clin Radiol* 1986;37(4):371–373.

Poulton TB, de Paredes ES, Baldwin M. Sclerosing lobular hyperplasia of the breast: imaging features in 15 cases. *AJR Am J Roentgenol* 1995;165(2):291–294.

MALIGNANT SOLID BREAST NODULES: SPECIFIC TYPES

GENERAL PATHOLOGY OF BREAST MALIGNANCIES

Carcinomas constitute the bulk of breast malignancies and therefore are the primary target of breast screening programs. Sarcomas of the breast, on the other hand, are rare.

Breast carcinomas arise from the epithelium of ducts or lobules. These malignancies may be classified as *in situ* or invasive (infiltrating). *In situ* carcinomas remain confined within the basement membrane of the ducts or ductules of origin, but this does not necessarily imply that *in situ* malignancies are always small and well localized. *In situ* carcinomas can spread extensively intraluminally within the duct system of the breast without actually invading through the basement membrane into surrounding fatty or fibrous stroma. Additionally, certain *in situ* lesions have a propensity to arise multifocally, multicentrically, or bilaterally.

In situ carcinomas arise within preexisting areas of ductal or lobular epithelial hyperplasia. There is a continuous spectrum of epithelial proliferation extending from usual hyperplasia through *in situ* carcinoma. Usual epithelial hyperplasias are ubiquitous and are not obligate precursors to carcinoma. However, the more florid and extensive the hyperplasia, the higher the likelihood of atypia, and the greater the risk is of eventual progression to *in situ* carcinoma. Atypical ductal hyperplasia will be discussed in detail in Chapter 15.

In situ breast carcinomas can be classified as ductal (DCIS) or lobular (LCIS). Despite the terminology, DCIS, like LCIS, usually arises within terminal ductolobular unit (TDLU). DCIS most often arises within the terminal duct of the TDLU near its junction with the lobule, whereas LCIS most often arises within the intralobular ductules (acini) of the TDLU. There is little resistance to antegrade growth of LCIS into the terminal duct (pagetoid spread) or of retrograde growth of DCIS into the ductules of the lob-

ule (cancerization of lobules). DCIS also readily grows antegradely into larger ducts. By the time of clinical or mammographic diagnosis, DCIS usually involves an entire TDLU at the minimum.

DCIS can spread extensively by simple intraductal growth (with or without grossly distending ducts) throughout one or more quadrants of the breast without invading through the basement membrane. Currently, most cases of DCIS are detected because of calcifications seen on mammograms.

DCIS represents a broad spectrum of lesions, not a single pathologic entity. Because of the heterogeneity, the imaging features and biologic behavior of DCIS vary greatly from lesion to lesion. LCIS is usually an incidental finding on biopsy done for another reason and rarely has specific clinical, mammographic, or sonographic features of its own. DCIS and LCIS can eventually evolve into invasive ductal or lobular carcinoma, but do not always do so and may take years to do so.

The term *invasive breast carcinoma* encompasses a broad spectrum of different malignant lesions that vary greatly morphologically and histologically. Invasive carcinomas can be divided into three different groups: special type, invasive lobular, and not otherwise specified (NOS). The largest group of breast invasive malignancies is classified as NOS invasive adenocarcinomas. The term *invasive duct carcinoma* is used interchangeably with NOS. Invasive duct carcinoma or NOS accounts for about 60% to 70% of all breast carcinomas in most series. Even NOS invasive carcinomas represent a heterogenous group that varies greatly in its morphology and histology. Because of the widely varied histologic features of NOS breast carcinomas, the prognosis varies greatly. However, as a group, NOS carcinomas have the worst prognosis of all breast carcinomas.

Special-type invasive carcinomas include tubular, colloid (mucinous), medullary, and invasive papillary carcinomas. As a group, special-type carcinomas have a better prognosis than NOS lesions, but the prognosis also varies amongst special-type tumors. Generally, tubular, invasive papillary, and colloid carcinomas grow more slowly, metastasize distantly less often, and have lower mortality and higher cure rates than do NOS carcinomas.

Invasive lobular carcinomas (ILC) also vary in gross and microscopic pathologic characteristics and therefore in sonographic appearance. In most instances, the infiltrative nature of the classic ILC makes it indistinguishable sonographically from low- to intermediate-grade NOS carcinomas. The prognosis for ILC is intermediate between those of NOS and tubular, invasive papillary, or colloid carcinomas, similar to the prognosis for medullary carcinomas. The diffuse pattern of infiltration of classic ILCs differs from that of other breast carcinomas and is more prone to be missed mammographically than are other types of breast carcinoma.

Metastases to the breast from other organs can produce solid breast nodules that are indistinguishable from primary malignant nodules in certain cases. However, these secondary malignancies are more often circumscribed in appearance than are primary breast carcinomas.

DUCTAL CARCINOMA *IN SITU*

General Pathologic Classification, Epidemiology, and Clinical Findings

DCIS, by definition, is a noninvasive malignancy that grows within breast ductules or ducts. The term *intraductal carcinoma* can be used interchangeably with DCIS. Although individual *in situ* carcinoma cells are indistinguishable from those of infiltrating carcinoma, they have not invaded through the basement membrane and therefore cannot metastasize.

Before screening mammography became prevalent, DCIS usually presented clinically as a palpable mass and was rare. Less than 5% of all breast malignancies were classified as DCIS. Now, however, DCIS constitutes 20% to 40% of all breast malignancies because it is detected during routine widespread mammographic screening.

DCIS represents a spectrum of noninvasive neoplasms rather than a single entity. The classification of the various types of DCIS is somewhat controversial. Traditionally, DCIS has been subdivided into comedo necrosis and noncomedo necrosis groups. Noncomedo necrosis DCIS is further subdivided into micropapillary, cribriform, and solid types. Solid-type DCIS is most frequently associated with comedo necrosis. However, the solid-type classification is probably not useful because this histologic tissue type can also be found in association with micropapillary and cribriform types of noncomedo DCIS. Each type of DCIS is then further subdivided into nuclear grade groups: low nuclear grade (LNG), intermediate nuclear grade (ING), or high nuclear grade (HNG). Comedo necrosis occurs most frequently in HNG DCIS but can occur in lower-nuclear-grade lesions as well.

The recent trend has been to combine nuclear grade with presence or absence of necrosis to determine the prognosis of DCIS and to guide treatment. HNG DCIS and lesions with necrosis display the most aggressive behavior. Such lesions are more likely to demonstrate microinvasion, are more likely to progress to grossly invasive carcinoma and to do so in a shorter time, are more likely to recur quickly after wide excision, and have a 1% to 2% positive axillary node rate (due to nondiagnosed microinvasion) than cases of LNG DCIS without necrosis. Although HNG DCIS lesions with comedo necrosis are more aggressive and appear more extensive mammographically than LNG lesions without necrosis, they are not more extensive histologically. Histologic studies have shown that LNG micropapillary and cribriform types of DCIS are 5 cm or larger in about one-half of cases, nearly the same as for HNG DCIS with comedo necrosis. The reason for this discrepancy between mammographic and histologic size of LNG DCIS is that mammographic assessment of size is based on the extent of calcifications, which, in turn, reflects the extent of necrosis. Mammographic assessment of DCIS size is less accurate for LNG DCIS than for HNG DCIS because the necrosis within which calcifications develops is much less uniformly distributed in LNG DCIS than it is in HNG DCIS. Thus, mammography more accurately reflects the true extent of HNG DCIS than it does the true extent of LNG DCIS.

The Van Nuys classification system for DCIS (Silverstein et al., 1994) identifies three different groups, based on different recurrent rates. Group 1 includes non-HNG DCIS without comedo necrosis. Group 2 includes non-HNG DCIS with comedo necrosis. Group 3 includes HNG DCIS with or without comedo necrosis. Recurrence rates are 3.8% in group 1, 11.1% in group 2, and 26.5% in group 3. Even with postlumpectomy radiation therapy, the recurrence rate for group 3 at 7 years approaches 30%. Based on these data, it has been proposed that patients with group 1 and 2 DCIS continue to undergo breast conservation therapy, whereas patients with group 3 lesions would be better treated with skin sparing mastectomy and immediate reconstruction.

That there frequently is a mixture of nuclear grades within the same lesion complicates the classification of DCIS. In such cases, the lesion is assigned the highest nuclear grade that is found within the lesion. Thus, if any necrosis is present, the lesion is assigned to the comedo necrosis group even if most of the lesion does not display comedo necrosis. If a lesion is mostly ING DCIS, but there is a small focus of HNG DCIS, the entire lesion is classified as HNG.

The degree of enlargement of ducts and ductules is greater for HNG DCIS and less for LNG DCIS. There are four mechanisms by which DCIS can enlarge the ducts: (1) lumen distention by tumor cells, (2) lumen distention by necrotic debris, (3) periductal inflammation, and (4) periductal desmoplasia. All four contributors to duct enlargement are more likely to occur and are more pronounced with HNG DCIS than with LNG DCIS. Thus, although LNG DCIS may spread just as extensively within the ductal system as does HNG DCIS, it causes lesser degrees of duct enlargement.

The occurrence of periductal desmoplastic or inflammatory reaction in a noninvasive lesion such as DCIS may seem surprising but appears to be a reaction to necrosis within the lumen. Such reaction is similar to the chemical periductal mastitis and fibrosis incited by the inspissated fatty secretions that occur in the chronic duct ectasia. Indeed, the gross "cheesy" appearance of the inspissated secretions in chronic duct ectasia so nearly resemble the necrotic debris in comedo DCIS that in Europe, chronic duct ectasia has been termed *comedo mastitis.*

HNG DCIS more frequently presents with a palpable or mammographic soft tissue mass than does LNG DCIS because it more grossly distends ductules and because it incites periductal inflammation and fibrosis.

DCIS has been reported to be multifocal in up to 60% of cases. However, Holland and colleagues (1990), using careful serial subgross sections under mammographic guidance, found that only 1% of carcinomas were truly multifocal or multicentric and that apparently remote areas of malignant involvement had, in fact, originated from spread of DCIS through contiguous ducts.

DCIS is not considered an obligate precursor to invasive carcinoma. Only 30% of all DCIS lesions are reported to progress to invasive carcinoma. However, if left untreated indefinitely, it seems likely that even LNG DCIS will eventually progress to invasive carcinoma.

Mammographic Findings

The mammographic hallmark of DCIS is calcifications. Stomper and associates (1992) found calcifications associated with DCIS in 84% of cases. In 72% of lesions, calcifications were the only finding. In another 12% of cases, there was a nodule or mass in association with calcifications. In only 10% of DCIS lesions there were soft tissue densities without calcifications. Evans et al. found calcifications in 89% of screening detected DCIS and 81% of symptomatic patients with DCIS. The percentage of DCIS presenting with calcifications has been shown to be higher in women less than 50 years of age than those 50 or older. Also, women 50 and older are more likely than those under 50 to have an associated soft tissue density, nodule, or mass caused by DCIS. This phenomenon may merely be due to the younger patients having denser breast tissues that could obscure any soft tissue density associated with DCIS.

Calcifications in DCIS can arise by different mechanisms. The calcifications in comedo DCIS are large, dense, dystrophic, and located within the necrotic debris that lies within the center of the lumen. Often, these calcifications have a characteristic linear, branching shape and a patchy pattern resembling snakeskin. The shape of these calcifications reflects the shape of the involved duct, forming a cast of the lumen—thus the term *casting calcifications.* In contrast, HNG DCIS without comedo necrosis can form dystrophic calcifications within the malignant epithelium lining the involved duct. These calcifications have a less distinctive, but still coarse, angular, granular pattern that has been described as an arrowhead, crushed stone, or broken arrowhead pattern. The calcifications in LNG and ING DCIS are typically smaller and less dense and have been described as granular or amorphous and far more difficult to distinguish from similar calcifications caused by fibrocystic change (FCC) or adenosis. A mixture of different types of calcifications can result in a pleomorphic pattern (Fig. 14–1). Granular calcifications are the most common type seen mammographically, occurring in 52% of cases of DCIS with calcifications. Casting calcifications occur in 35% of cases, and mixed or pleomorphic varieties occur in 13% of cases of DCIS. As noted earlier, the calcifications are more uniformly distributed throughout HNG DCIS than they are in LNG DCIS; therefore, the extent of calcifications more accurately reflects the true extent of HNG DCIS than it does the extent of LNG DICS.

Casting calcifications predict HNG DCIS with a high degree of certainty. Granular, punctate, and amorphous calcifications have far less predictive value. So difficult is the distinction between benign and malignant granular or amorphous calcifications that 60% to 80% of biopsies of calcifications of these types show benign breast changes.

Although the pattern of calcifications can suggest the presence and even the type of DCIS, the accuracy for predicting nuclear grade is less than 100%. Of casting calcifications, 78% are associated with comedo DCIS, whereas only 55% of granular calcifications are due to noncomedo DCIS. More important, there is difficulty determining from mammographic calcifications whether the tumor is pure DCIS or infiltrating malignancy with extensive intraductal components (EICs). Because calcifications typically occur in the DCIS components of a tumor, stereotactically guided biopsy of calcifications accurately diagnoses DCIS but tends to lead to underdiagnosis of invasion.

Mammographic findings other than calcifications can occur. These findings include a nodule or mass with or without calcifications (Fig. 14–2), a nonspecific soft tissue density, architectural distortion, asymmetric density (Fig. 14–3), or solitary or multiple abnormally prominent ducts.

DCIS associated with a soft tissue component (with or without calcifications) is most likely to occur in HNG

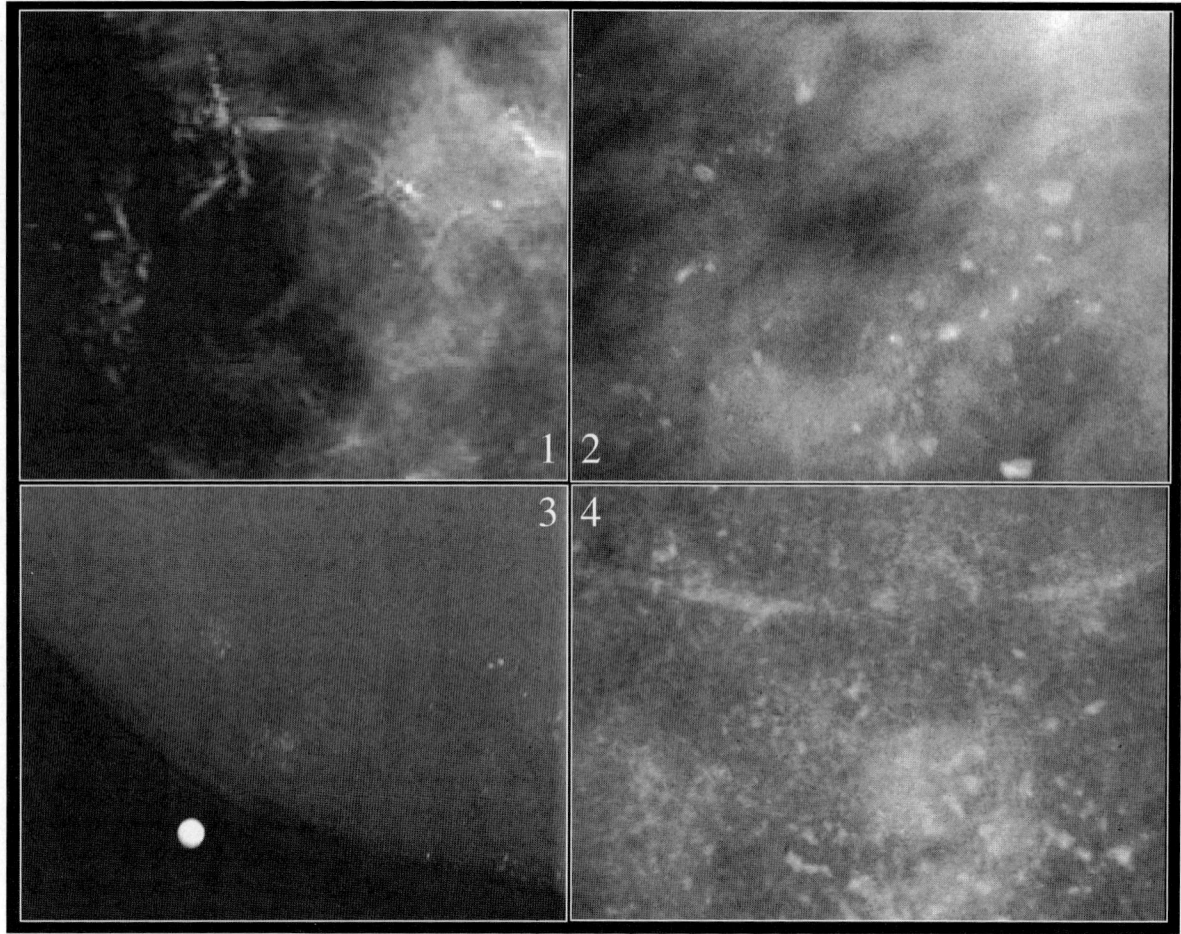

FIGURE 14–1 Most cases of ductal carcinoma *in situ* present as isolated calcifications on routine screening mammograms. Patterns of calcifications include casting calcifications *(1)*; coarse granular calcifications *(2)*; clusters of punctate and amorphous calcifications *(3)*; and pleomorphic calcifications that represent a mixture of casting, coarse granular, and amorphous calcifications *(4)*.

DCIS with comedo necrosis and that the soft tissue density is due to intense stromal reaction even in the absence of invasion.

Mammographic stereotactic guidance can be used to guide needle localization for surgical breast biopsy, large core needle biopsy, and directional vacuum-assisted biopsy (DVAB). In patients with nipple discharge and negative mammograms, galactography may be performed to identify the offending lesion. Findings of DCIS at galactography include a filling defect, duct obstruction, or focal area of narrowing of a duct lumen. Galactography can also be used to localize such lesions for surgical excision. These findings are discussed in detail in Chapter 8.

Sonographic Findings

Mammography is generally more effective than sonography for detection of DCIS because mammography is more effective at demonstrating and characterizing the microcalcifications with which DCIS presents in most cases. Most of the time, patients with suspicious calcifications go straight to stereotactically guided needle or surgical biopsy and do not undergo diagnostic breast ultrasound. However, that does not mean that sonography is completely incapable of demonstrating DCIS, or has no role in diagnosing DCIS. There are several specific circumstances in which sonography may be of benefit in the evaluation of patients with DCIS. These include the following:

- Evaluation of the 10% of patients who have soft tissue densities without calcifications
- Evaluation of patients with palpable abnormalities and negative or nonspecific mammograms
- Evaluation of the patient with nipple discharge and guiding aspiration and core needle biopsy of intracystic papillary DCIS
- Evaluation of the size of the lesion in cases of non-comedo DCIS in which the extent of calcifications on

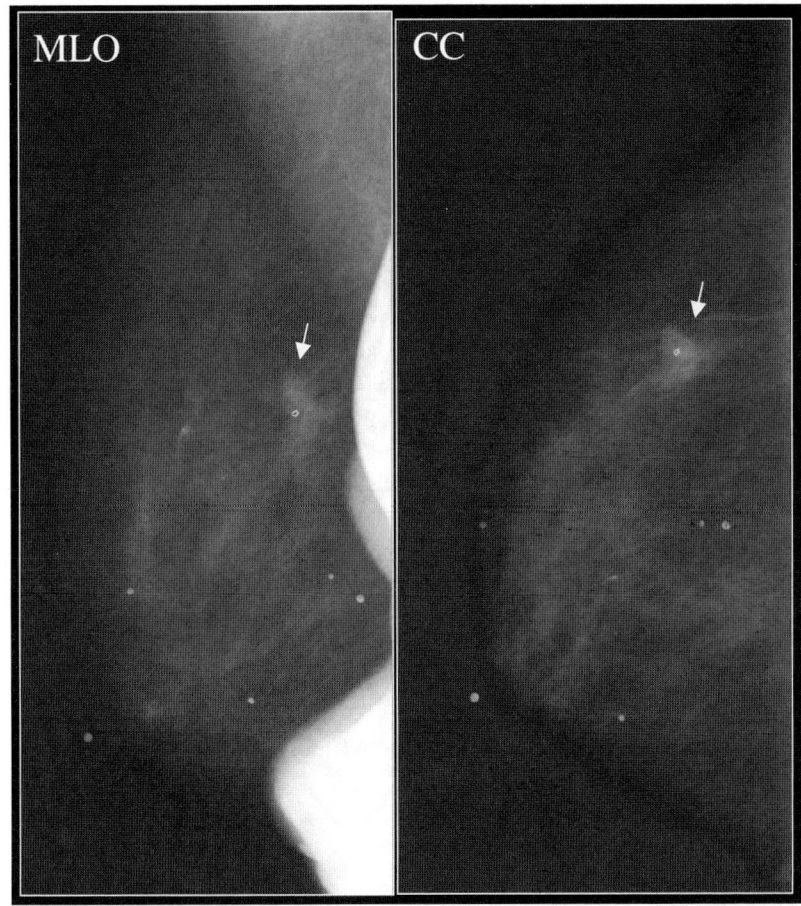

FIGURE 14–2 In a small percentage of cases, ductal carcinoma *in situ* (DCIS) presents with a nodule or mass *(arrows)* that may or may not contain calcifications. (Diagnosis was high-nuclear-grade DCIS with necrosis and periductal inflammatory and stromal response.)

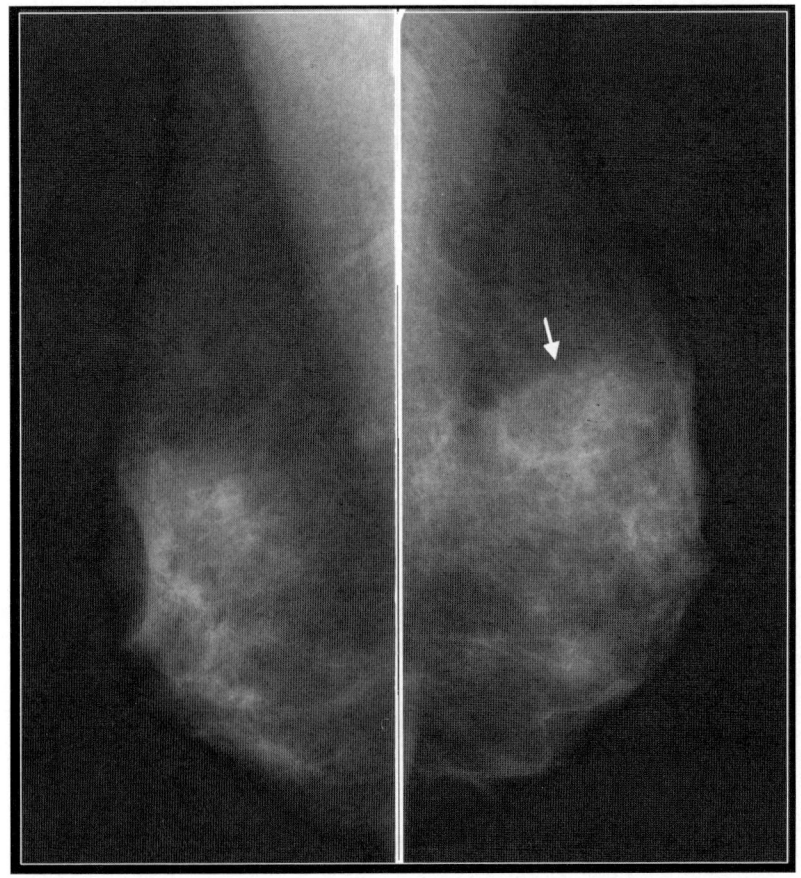

FIGURE 14–3 Occasionally, ductal carcinoma *in situ* (DCIS) may appear as a focal mammographic asymmetry *(arrow)*. (Diagnosis was intermediate-nuclear-grade DCIS).

mammography is likely to underestimate the size of the lesion

- Identification of invasive components of carcinoma when calcifications suggest pure DCIS
- Assessment of regional lymph nodes in large, HNG DCIS
- Guidance of needle localization of calcifications
- Guidance of ductography or needle localization of intraductal papillary lesions
- Guidance of core needle biopsy in the rare cases in which stereotactic biopsy is not possible

Because normal ducts and TDLUs are demonstrable, it should not be surprising that abnormally distended ducts and TDLUs in patients with DCIS can be demonstrated sonographically. The most reliable technique for demonstrating DCIS distended ducts is to scan them in a plane that is parallel to the long axis of the ducts—the internal radial plane. Teboul and Halliwell have documented the relative effectiveness of long-axis and short-axis scanning of mammary ducts as opposed to random longitudinal and transverse scan planes and appropriately termed it *ductal echography.*

As noted in Chapter 12, soft suspicious findings that suggest the presence of DCIS or DCIS components of disease are duct extension (Fig. 14–4) and branch pattern (Fig.

14–5), which indicate the presence of tumor-enlarging ducts. Microlobulations can be seen with either invasive and intraductal tumor but more frequently represents DCIS grossly enlarging ducts or TDLUs (Fig. 14–6). Microcalcifications are also soft sonographic findings that suggest DCIS and can be associated with any of the other soft findings noted earlier. The calcifications occur within the necrotic debris in the center of the lumen of involved ducts or ductules. The calcifications within DCIS are large enough to cause small bright echoes but too small to shadow. They can be identified within mildly or grossly enlarged ducts (Fig. 14–7), microlobulations resulting from tumor-filled ducts (Fig. 14–8), cancerized lobules (Fig. 14–9), amorphous sheets of isoechoic tissue (Fig. 14–10), intraductal and intracystic papillary lesions (Fig. 14–11), or invasive nodules (Fig. 14–12).

Limitations of Diagnostic Breast Ultrasound in Ductal Carcinoma In Situ

Even when the sonographic technique used is optimal, sonographic diagnosis of DCIS can be compromised by several factors. First, DCIS does not always grossly distend ducts and TDLUs. Ducts and TDLUs that are not abnormally enlarged will not be recognized sonographi-

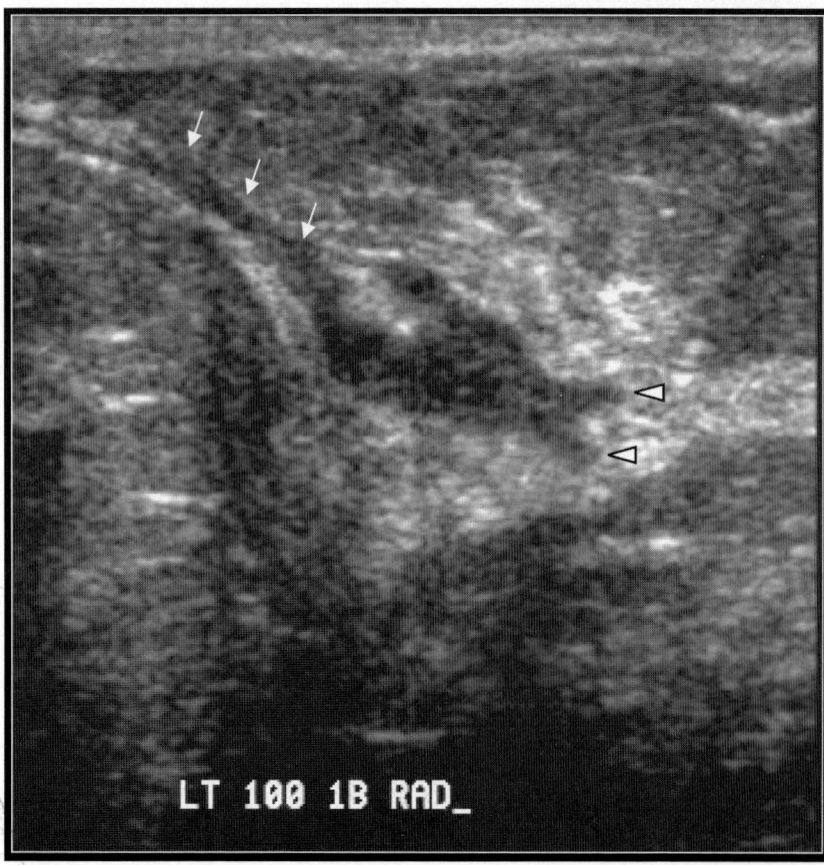

FIGURE 14–4 This mixed invasive and intraductal carcinoma has a prominent duct extension *(arrows)* that represents prominent ductal carcinoma *in situ* (DCIS) components that extend nearly to the nipple. Peripheral branches *(arrowheads)* also represent DCIS components.

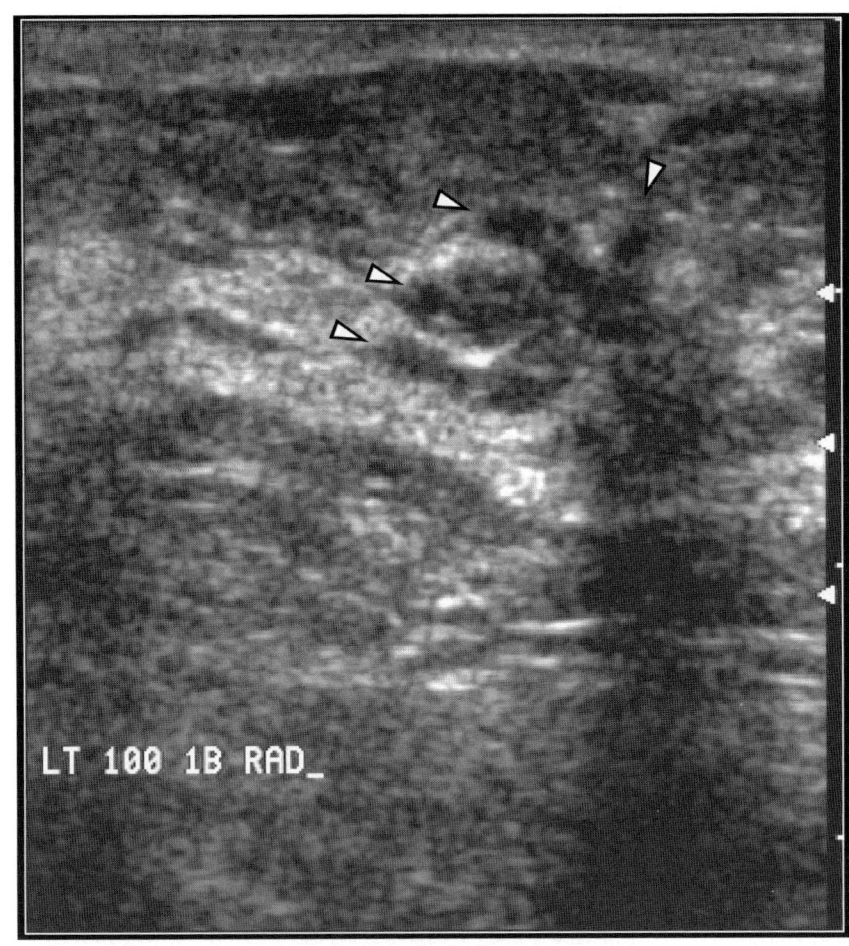

FIGURE 14–5 This mixed invasive and intraductal carcinoma has a prominent branch pattern *(arrowheads)* that indicates ductal carcinoma *in situ* (DCIS) components. Small bright echoes within the branches represent calcifications in areas of necrosis within the DCIS components.

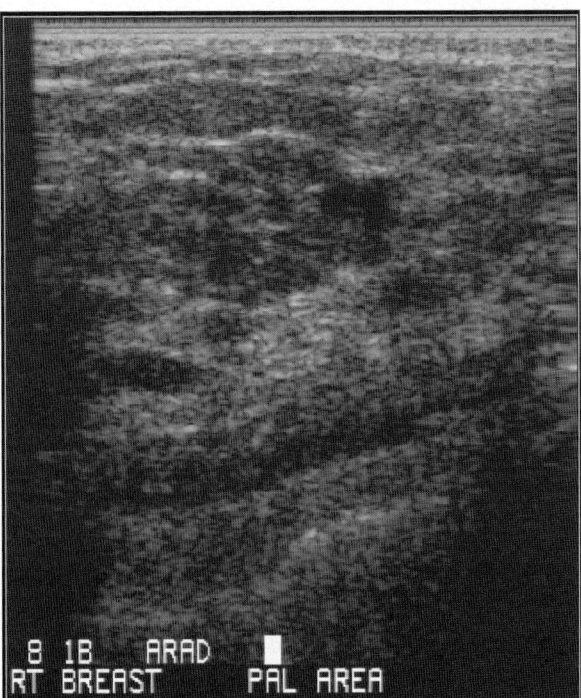

FIGURE 14–6 This pure ductal carcinoma *in situ* (DCIS) lesion is heavily microlobulated. Each of the lobulations represents a duct or ductule enlarged by DCIS.

cally as abnormal. As noted previously, HNG DCIS, especially when comedo necrosis is present, is more likely to grossly enlarge ducts enough to be sonographically recognized as being too large than are LNG and ING DCIS (Fig. 14–13). LNG and ING DCIS may not grossly enlarge the ducts or TDLUs enough for them to be sonographically distinguishable from normal ducts. Additionally, certain cases of DCIS show mixed patterns. Portions of the lesion that are HNG may demonstrate gross enlargement of ducts or TDLUs that is easily recognized sonographically, whereas in other parts of the lesion, LNG components may not enlarge ducts and TDLUs enough for them to be sonographically distinguished from normal. This can lead to sonographic underestimation of the true size of the lesion.

Second, DCIS is not the only pathologic process that can enlarge the ducts and TDLUs. Virtually the entire spectrum of benign FCC and benign proliferative disorder (BPD) or aberration of normal development and involution (ANDI) can enlarge these structures. Among the benign processes that can cause enlargement of intralobular ductules are microcysts that are too small to resolve with ultrasound and macrocysts filled with debris or papillary

(text continued on page 606)

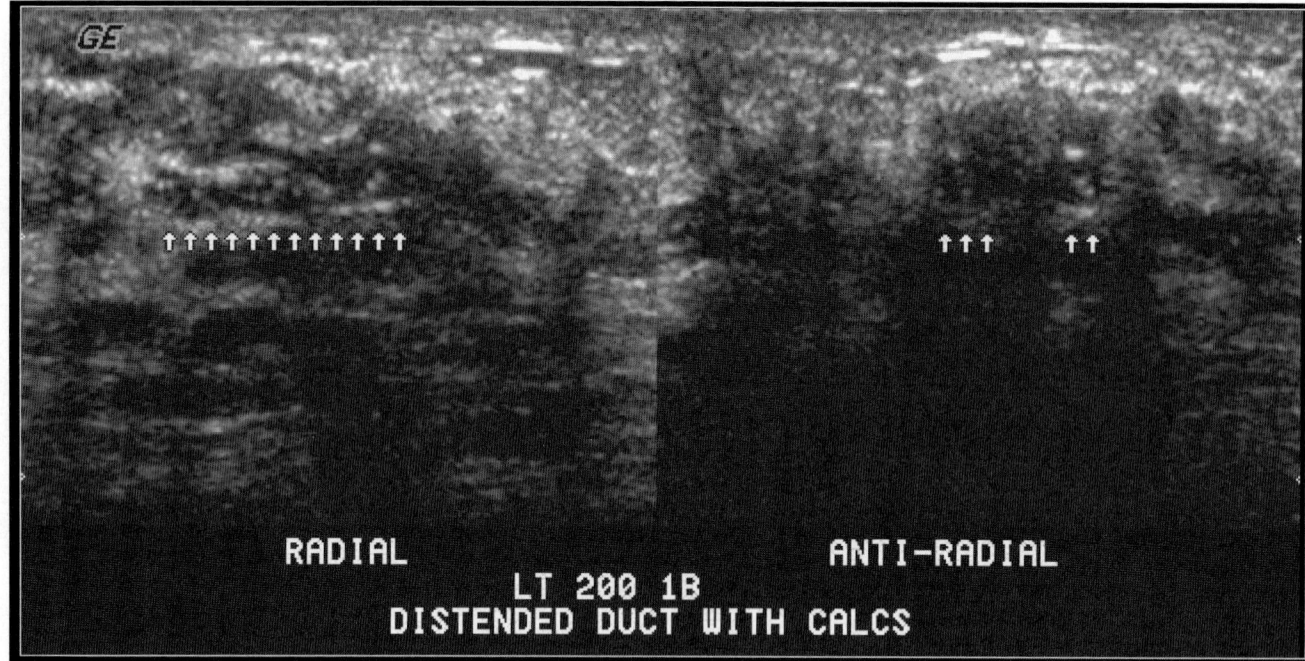

FIGURE 14–7 Ducts that are grossly distended with intermediate-nuclear-grade ductal carcinoma *in situ* contain bright echoes that represent calcifications within areas of necrosis.

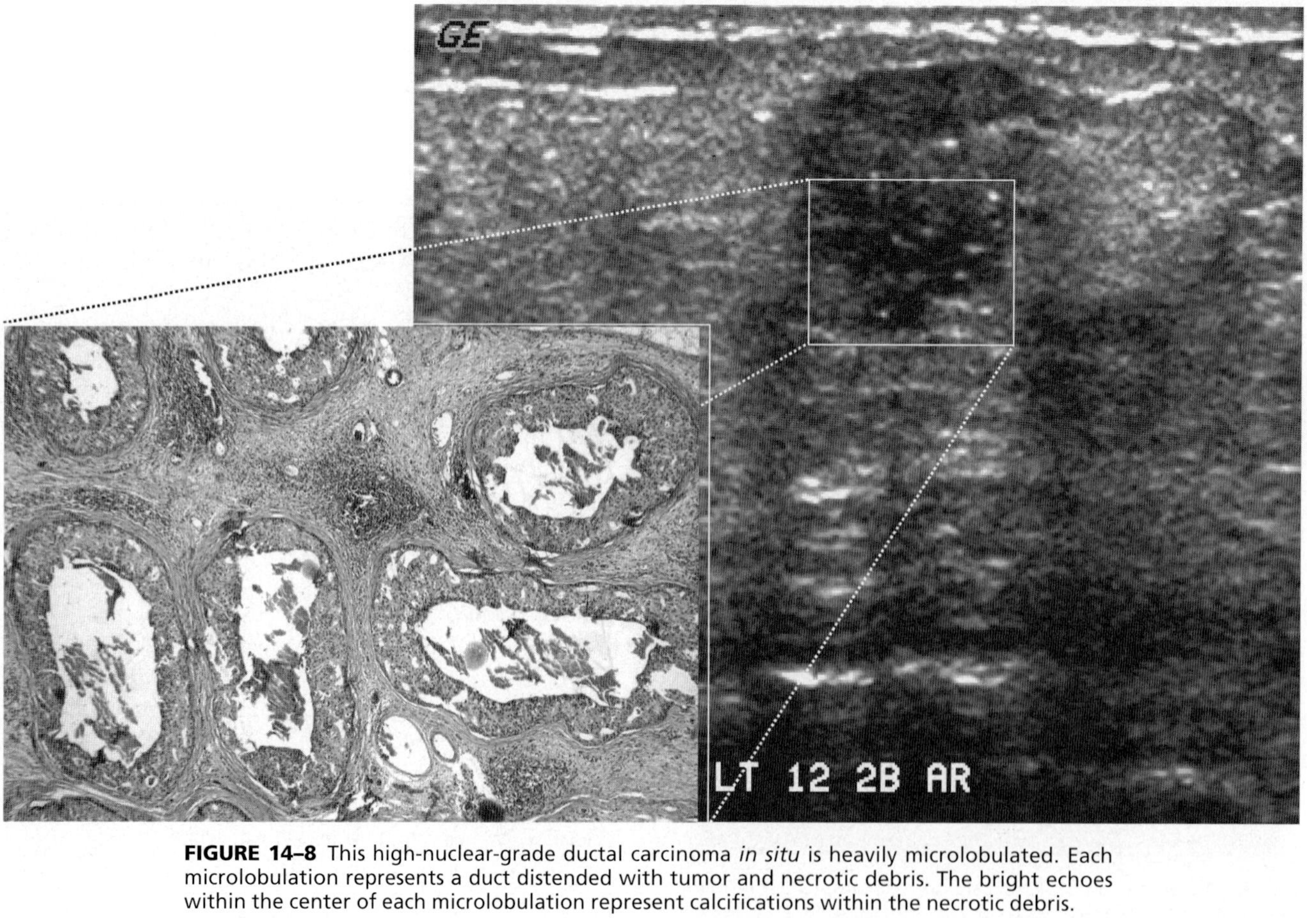

FIGURE 14–8 This high-nuclear-grade ductal carcinoma *in situ* is heavily microlobulated. Each microlobulation represents a duct distended with tumor and necrotic debris. The bright echoes within the center of each microlobulation represent calcifications within the necrotic debris.

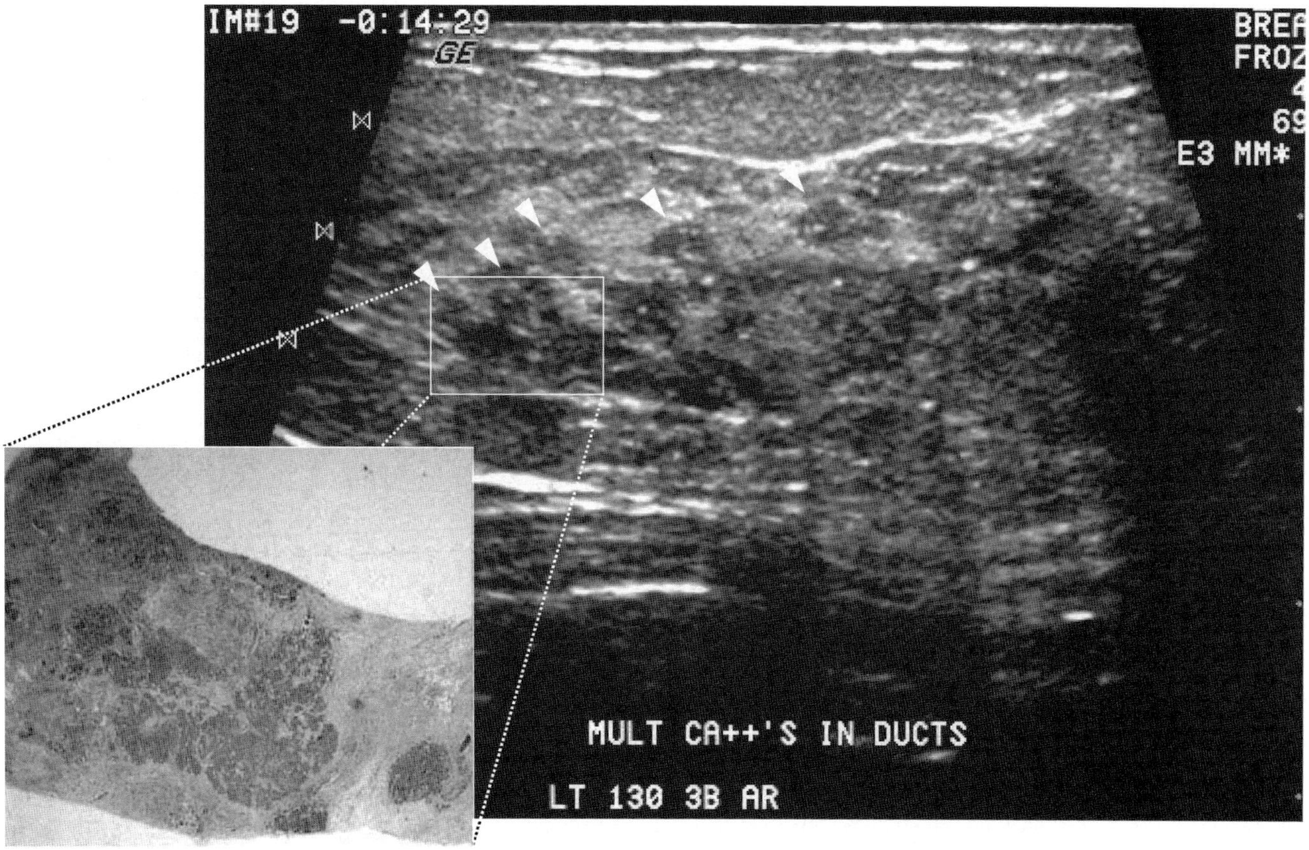

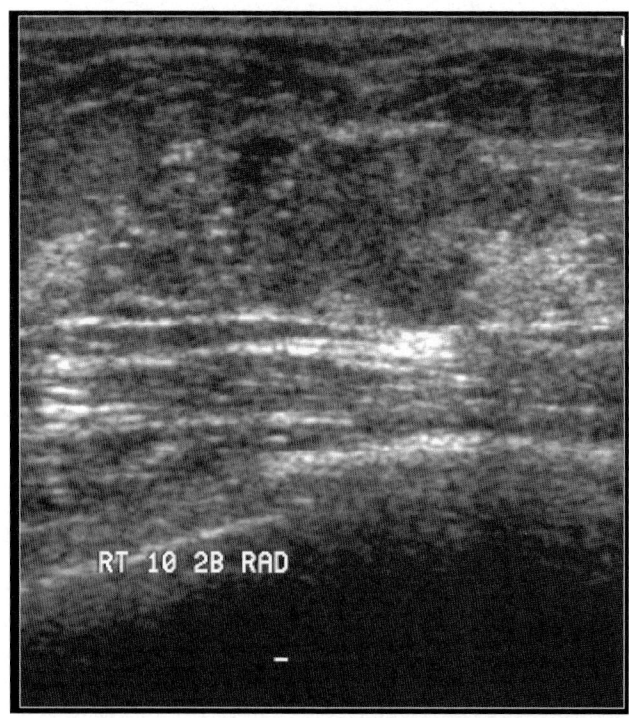

FIGURE 14–9 This extensive ductal carcinoma *in situ* has cancerized numerous lobules *(arrowheads)*. The punctate echoes that represent calcifications are present in ducts and cancerized lobules.

FIGURE 14–10 Calcifications are present within isoechoic tissue that represents intermediate-nuclear-grade ductal carcinoma *in situ* (DCIS). This appearance is indistinguishable from tumoral adenosis sonographically. However, DCIS may vibrate differently from adenosis on power Doppler fremitus.

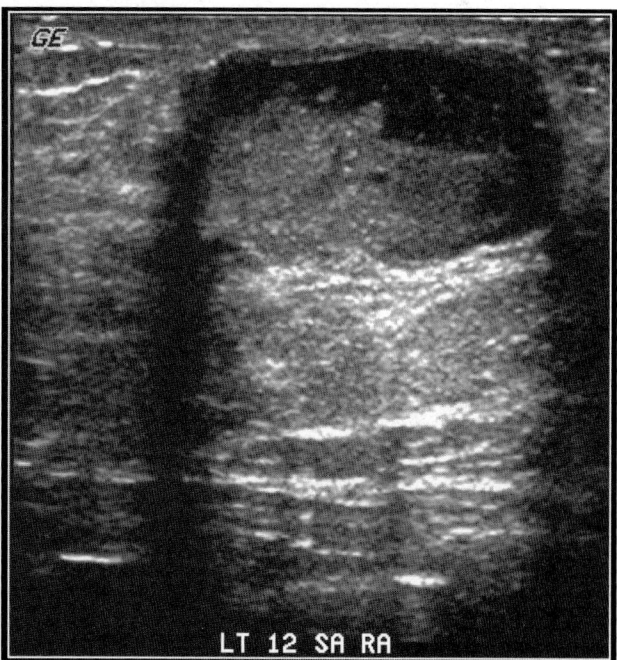

FIGURE 14–11 This intracystic mural nodule caused by low-nuclear-grade papillary ductal carcinoma *in situ* contains calcifications.

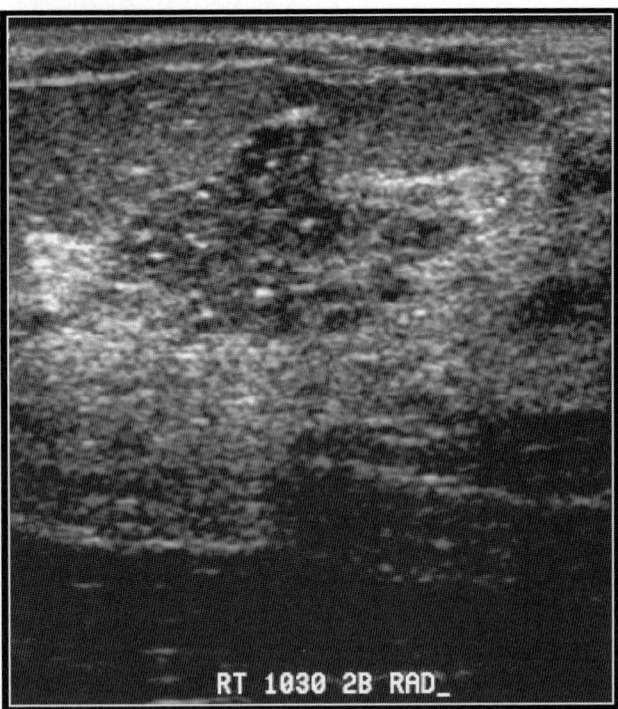

FIGURE 14–12 Bright echoes within this nodule caused by invasive ductal carcinoma represent calcifications.

growth, apocrine metaplasia, or florid ductal hyperplasia (papillary duct hyperplasia, papillomatosis) as well as stromal sclerosis.

Interpretation of the significance of enlargement of lobules is made even more difficult by the nonuniform involvement of TDLUs that results from these benign processes. TDLUs affected by FCC and BPD often vary greatly in size, not only in different lobes of the breast, but also within the same lobe. In a background of benign FCC or BPD, especially if involvement is nonuniform, the sensitivity for discriminating malignant enlargement of TDLUs will be compromised. This means that enlarged TDLUs must be interpreted within the context of the anatomy of the rest of the ipsilateral breast and the mirror-image location of the contralateral breast. If there is diffuse enlargement of TDLUs throughout both breasts, the assumption must be that similarly enlarged TDLUs in the region of clinical or mammographic interest are enlarged because of FCC or BPD. On the other hand, if the TDLUs in the area of interest are enlarged out of proportion to other TDLUs in the breast, there should be more concern. The patient's age and hormonal status should also be taken into account. In postmenopausal women who are not receiving hormone replacement therapy (HRT), lobular enlargement should

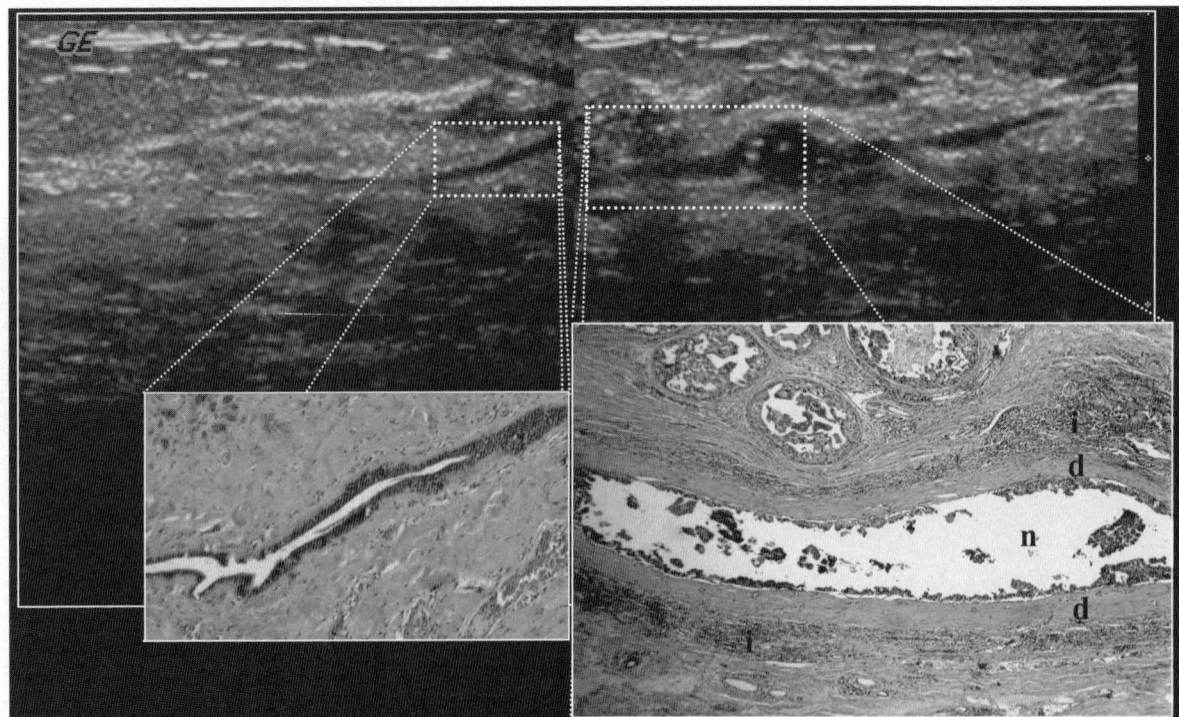

FIGURE 14–13 Split-screen mirror images obtained parallel to the long axis of a normal duct with mild usual ductal hyperplasia (**left**, patient's right side) and a duct distended with high-nuclear-grade ductal carcinoma *in situ* (**right**, patient's left side) show that apparent duct size on sonography is affected by four factors: necrosis in the center of the lumen *(n)*, tumor cell mass *(c)*, periductal desmoplasia or fibrosis *(d)*, and periductal inflammatory infiltrates *(i)*. All four contributors to duct size are more common and more extensive with higher nuclear grades. Note that the region of duct that appears large sonographically has only slightly more necrotic debris in the center of the lumen but has considerably more periductal inflammatory infiltrate than do narrower areas of the duct.

engender more concern than in a patient who is premenopausal or postmenopausal but taking HRT.

Third, diffuse enlargement of larger-order ducts may be also due to benign breast disorders that simulate DCIS. Late phases of the duct ectasia–periductal mastitis complex can be virtually identical in sonographic appearance to DCIS (Fig. 14–14). Intense periductal inflammation or fibrosis, calcification of inspissated inflammatory secretions within the lumen of the duct, and obliteration of the lumen by fibrosis all can simulate the appearance of HNG DCIS.

Fourth, focal papillary lesions within larger-order ducts are most likely benign large papillomas but could contain areas of malignant degeneration (papillary DCIS).

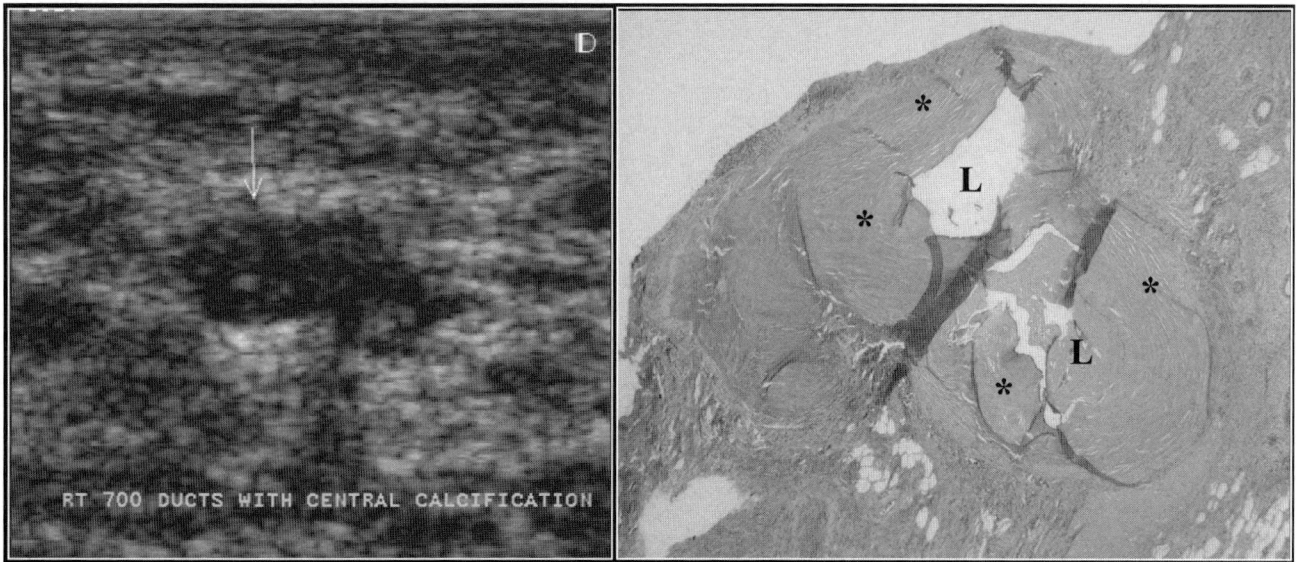

FIGURE 14–14 A: Pleomorphic calcifications resemble those of ductal carcinoma *in situ* (DCIS) but in this case result from the chronic duct ectasia—-periductal mastitis complex. **B:** Sonographic findings of the chronic duct ectasia—-periductal mastitis complex also simulate those of DCIS. The duct appears enlarged and hypoechoic and contains central necrotic debris and calcifications. However, most of what appears to be tumor within the duct is actually periductal fibrosis (*) that compresses the inspissated secretion-filled lumen *(L)*.

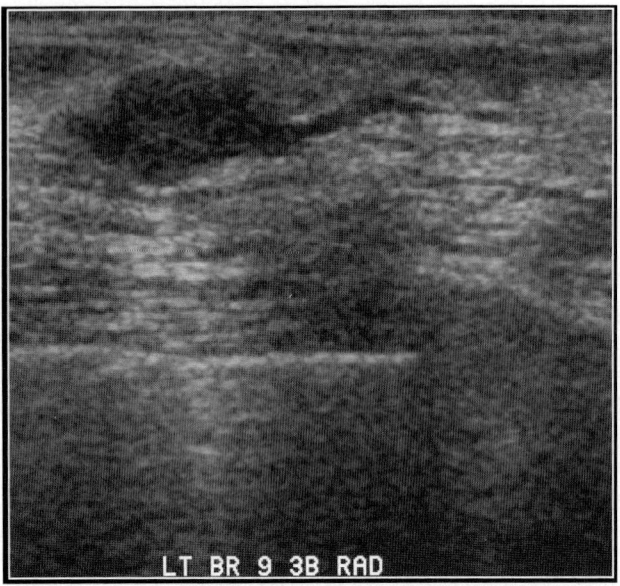

FIGURE 14–15 Many centrally located cases of ductal carcinoma *in situ* (DCIS), such as this case, arise within preexisting benign large duct papillomas. Thus, the sonographic appearances of centrally arising DCIS may be indistinguishable from those of benign papillomas. The more expansile the lesion is, the higher the risk for DCIS.

There are findings in intraductal papillary lesions that indicate an increased risk for atypia or DCIS, but these are not absolute. These findings include expansion of the duct lumen size, involvement of long segments of duct and branch ducts, and involvement of TDLUs (Fig. 14–15).

Sonography is not as sensitive as mammography for calcifications. Calcifications are generally seen sonographically only when located within an enlarged duct or TDLU or within a relatively homogeneous isoechoic or hypoechoic nodule, especially if the calcifications are the small punctate or amorphous type that can be seen in LNG DCIS. There is a limit on the size of calcifications that can be shown sonographically, even with the best current equipment and under optimal conditions. Under such conditions, calcifications as small as 200 μm can be demonstrated. However, in many cases, conditions are not ideal because of the depth of the calcifications, shadowing, or background echogenicity. In such challenging cases, even 500-μm calcifications may be difficult to identify. Because of these inherent sonographic limitations, we rely on mammography for identification and characterization of calcifications.

Indications for Ultrasound in Selected Patients with Ductal Carcinoma In Situ or with Suspected Ductal Carcinoma In Situ

Evaluation of the 10% of Patients Who Have Soft Tissue Densities without Calcifications

About 10% of patients with DCIS present with a mammographic soft tissue density but no visible calcifications. Be-

cause these particular lesions are not infiltrative, the mammographic nodules or asymmetric densities are not usually classically spiculated masses. Rather, these lesions are the indistinct or partially obscured nonspecific densities for which sonographic evaluation is ideal. Enlarged ducts and ductules, periductal inflammatory and desmoplastic reaction, and cancerization of lobules can all contribute to a soft tissue mass, individually or in combination. Sonographic evaluation of these nodules is performed just as for any other mammographic lesion. One or more of the soft suspicious sonographic findings—microlobulation, duct extension, or branch pattern—is usually present, preventing misclassification of the lesion as Breast Imaging Reporting and Data System (BIRADS) category 3.

Evaluation of Patients with Palpable Abnormalities and Negative or Nonspecific Mammograms

About 5% of DCIS cases present because of a palpable abnormality. Most of these patients have calcifications in the area of the palpable abnormality. In the minority of patients who have either a negative mammogram or a soft tissue density without calcifications in the area of the palpable abnormality, sonographic evaluation can be of benefit. In such cases, the principles for sonographic evaluation are the same as for any other palpable abnormality.

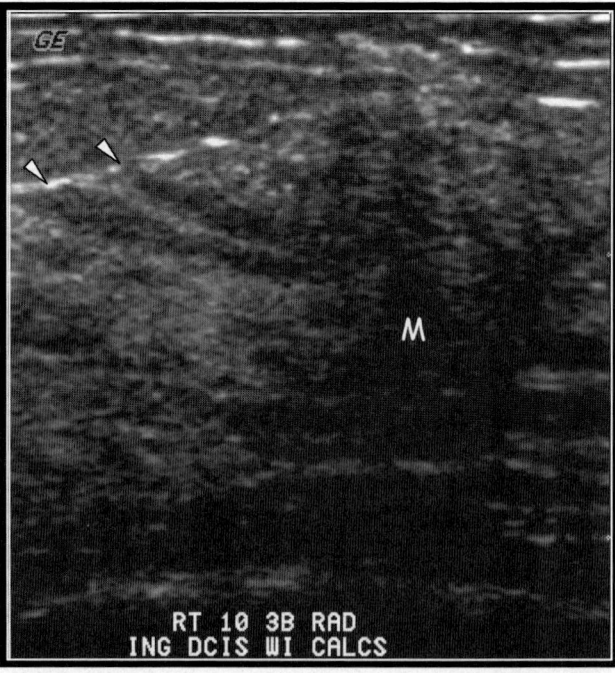

FIGURE 14–16 Although there were mammographically detectable calcifications within the main mass (M) of intermediate-nuclear-grade ductal carcinoma *in situ* (DCIS), noncalcified DCIS extends away from the main mass within long branching ducts *(arrowheads).* The DCIS within the branch pattern could not be seen mammographically because it contained no calcifications. Thus, sonography showed components of DCIS that were not visible mammographically. Bracketing wires were placed under ultrasound guidance to enable resection of both calcified and noncalcified components of the lesion.

Evaluation of the Patient with Nipple Discharge

Galactography is generally the procedure of choice for evaluating nipple discharge. However, ultrasound is also quite useful in many patients. The methods and interpretation are discussed in greater detail in Chapter 8. A small percentage of patients with nipple discharge have DCIS. The differential diagnostic problems are in discriminating between intraductal papilloma, DCIS, and ductal ectasia.

Evaluation of the Size of the Lesion in Cases of Noncomedo Ductal Carcinoma *In Situ* in which the Extent of Calcifications on Mammography Is Likely to Underestimate the True Size of the Lesion

Mammographic estimation of DCIS size is more accurate for HNG DCIS with casting calcifications than it is in cases of LNG or ING DCIS that lacks casting calcifications. Although ultrasound is not specifically performed to determine the extent of DCIS, it is often used to guide biopsy or to localize such lesions for excision. During ultrasound guidance, there is an opportunity to evaluate lesion size. Sonography may show abnormally enlarged ducts and lobules that do not contain calcifications, thereby better demonstrating the extent of the lesion than do the mammographically visible calcifications (Fig. 14–16). The extent of such lesions can be mapped out with ultrasound-guided biopsies, and the lesion can be appropriately bracketed for surgical excision by placing multiple localization wires under ultrasound guidance.

Identification of Invasive Components of Carcinoma

Although mammographically detected calcifications are a valuable sign of malignancy, they are primarily a manifestation of DCIS. Mammographically suspicious calcifications can represent either pure DCIS or the DCIS components of lesions that also contain invasive carcinoma. Stereotactically guided needle biopsy tends to target and diagnose DCIS but tends to underestimate presence of invasion. Even in patients who undergo mammographically guided needle localization excisional biopsy of calcifications, the presence of invasion may be missed if the pathologists use a random sectioning technique rather than serial sectioning for assessing the surgical specimen.

Sonography of clustered calcifications can be of value if sonography demonstrates a solid nodule with hard findings, such as spiculations, thick halo, angular margins, and acoustic shadowing, that suggest the presence of invasive malignancy (Fig. 14–17). Ultrasound-guided biopsy of the solid nodule that contains hard findings may reveal invasion when stereotactically guided biopsy of calcifications reveals only DCIS. A combination of ultrasound-guided biopsy of the mass and stereotactically guided biopsy of the calcifications offers the best opportunity to determine the true histology and extent of malignant disease.

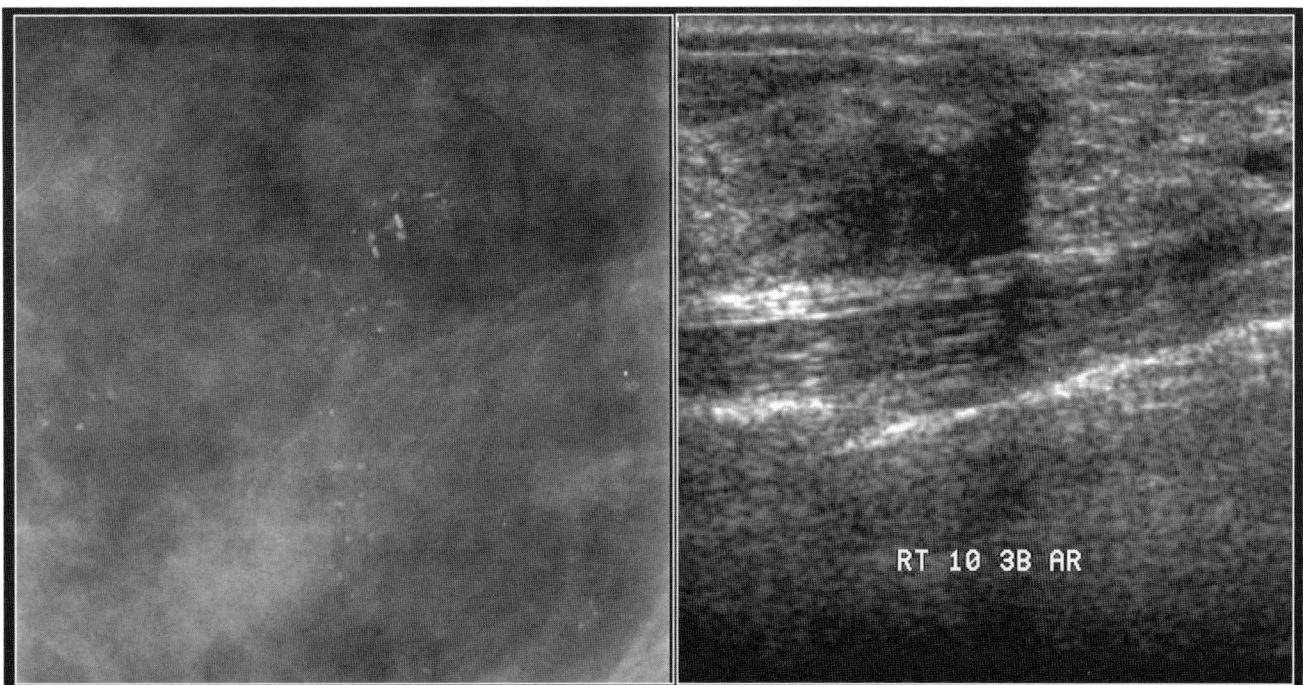

FIGURE 14–17 Clustered calcifications in a "crushed stone" pattern suggested the presence of ductal carcinoma *in situ* (DCIS), which was confirmed by stereotactic biopsy. Sonography demonstrates a solid nodule that has angular margins, a hard suspicious finding that suggests the presence of invasion. Ultrasound-guided biopsy of the solid nodule led to the correct diagnosis of intermediate-grade invasive not otherwise specified carcinoma. The combination of ultrasound and stereotactic biopsies appropriately revealed mixed invasive and intraductal disease. Without ultrasound, the stereotactic biopsy alone would have underdiagnosed the lesion as pure DCIS.

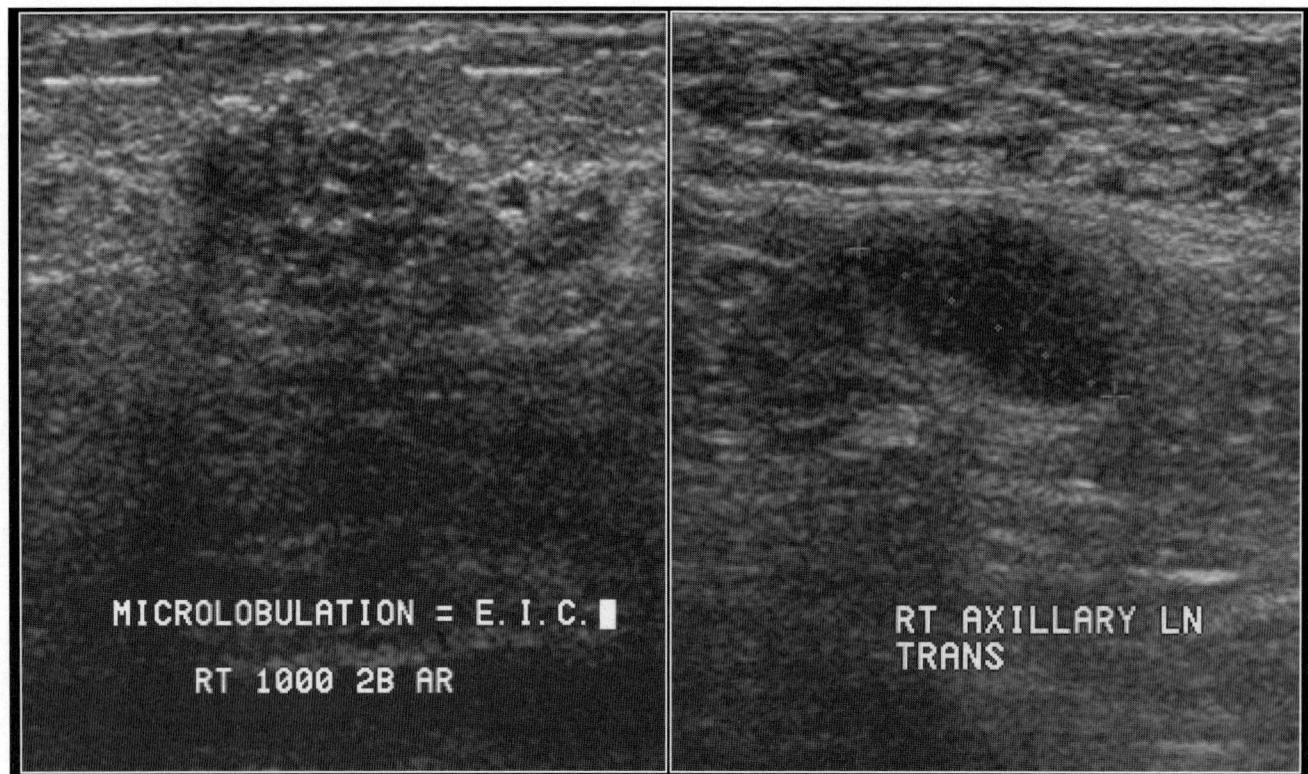

FIGURE 14–18 This heavily microlobulated solid nodule **(left)** underwent ultrasound-guided large core needle biopsy that revealed high-nuclear-grade ductal carcinoma *in situ* (DCIS). At the time of the ultrasound-guided biopsy of the primary lesion, the axillary lymph nodes were assessed, and an abnormal axillary lymph node was detected and also underwent biopsy, revealing metastatic breast carcinoma. The patient subsequently underwent lumpectomy. Random-sectioning histologic evaluation of the lumpectomy specimen initially revealed pure high-nuclear-grade DCIS. However, because the previous lymph node biopsy had revealed metastasis, it was apparent that the invasive part of the lesion had been missed both by ultrasound-guided core needle biopsy and by random sectioning of the surgically excised specimen. The specimen had to be resectioned serially and histologically evaluated in its entirety, which led to the appropriate diagnosis of microinvasion within this high-nuclear-grade DCIS.

Assessment of Regional Lymph Nodes in Patients with Bulky High-Nuclear-Grade Ductal Carcinoma *In Situ* Lesions

Stereotactic biopsy of calcification tends to underdiagnose invasion. Even random section histologic evaluation of surgically excised DCIS may underdiagnose invasion. This is why about 2% of HNG DCIS lesions have been reported to have lymph node metastases. For these reasons, we assess not only the area of calcifications (looking for signs of invasion) but also the axillary lymph nodes in cases that have mammographic calcifications suspicious for HNG DCIS (Fig. 14–18). The presence of grossly abnormal-appearing lymph nodes on sonography can be assessed with ultrasound-guided core needle biopsy or fine-needle aspiration biopsy (FNAB). Biopsy-documented metastasis to axillary lymph nodes indicates that the lesion contains invasive components and is not pure DCIS and obviates a sentinel node procedure.

Guidance of Needle Localization of Calcifications

Ultrasound can be useful in guiding needle localization for excisional breast biopsy or breast conservation surgery. Although mammographic or stereotactic guidance is usually used for needle localization biopsy of calcifications, there are certain advantages to using ultrasound for the needle localization biopsy. Many patients have a nodule, mass, enlarged solid ducts, or calcifications that are sonographically visible; thus, ultrasound-guided needle localization is possible. If a mass or the calcifications are sonographically visible, the localization is much quicker and more accurate when performed with sonography than with mammography (Fig. 14–19). Sonography of the specimen is also useful in any case in which nodules or calcifications are localized with ultrasound guidance (Fig. 14–20).

Most needle localizations for surgical excisions of microcalcifications are now performed on patients in whom a definitive diagnosis of malignancy had already been estab-

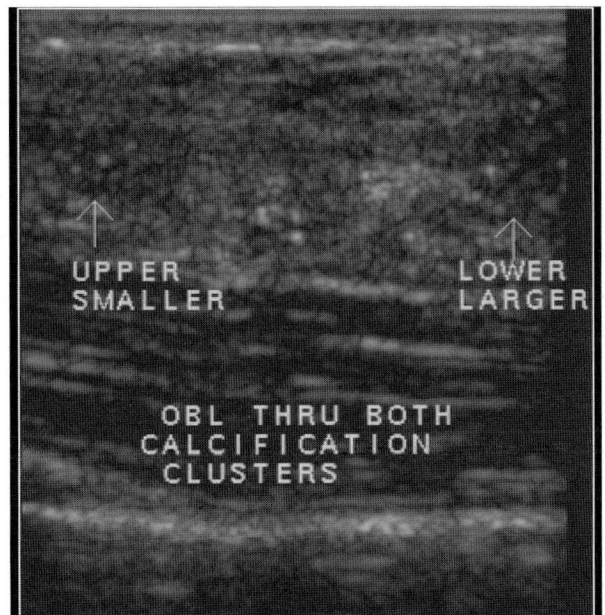

FIGURE 14–19 Even cases in which mammography shows only calcifications may benefit from sonographic evaluation and sonographically guided needle localization or biopsy. This patient had clustered granular calcifications on mammography. Sonography showed not only the cluster of calcifications seen mammographically *(lower larger cluster)* but also second *(upper smaller cluster)* and third *(arrowhead)* clusters of calcifications that were not seen mammographically. The upper and lower clusters of calcifications were bracketed with wires placed under ultrasound guidance to facilitate complete resection. Margins were clear, and histology in all three clusters was intermediate-nuclear-grade ductal carcinoma *in situ.*

lished by imaging-guided DVAB. The DVAB creates a small cavity at the site of biopsy, which fills with blood or serous fluid and which remains for several days after the biopsy procedure in most patients. These small, complex, cystic mammotomy cavities are easily found and localized sonographically. Because of the increasing success rate for localizing calcifications with ultrasound, a very brief look with ultrasound before beginning any mammographically guided needle localization of calcifications can demonstrate that ultrasound guidance of the procedure is feasible. There are several reasons to perform the needle localization under ultrasound rather than mammographic guidance, and these are discussed and illustrated in detail in Chapter 18.

Guidance of Ductography or Needle Localization of Intraductal Papillary Lesions

When sonography reveals an intraductal papillary lesion, ultrasound can be used to localize the lesion for excisional biopsy, to guide percutaneous galactography, or to guide DVAB. Ultrasound assessment of nipple discharge and ultrasound-guided interventional procedures in patients with nipple discharge or intraductal papillary lesions are discussed in detail in Chapter 8.

Guidance of Aspiration and Core Needle Biopsy of Intracystic Papillary Lesions

Sonography is the method of choice for showing intracystic papillary lesions, including intracystic DCIS. Most in-

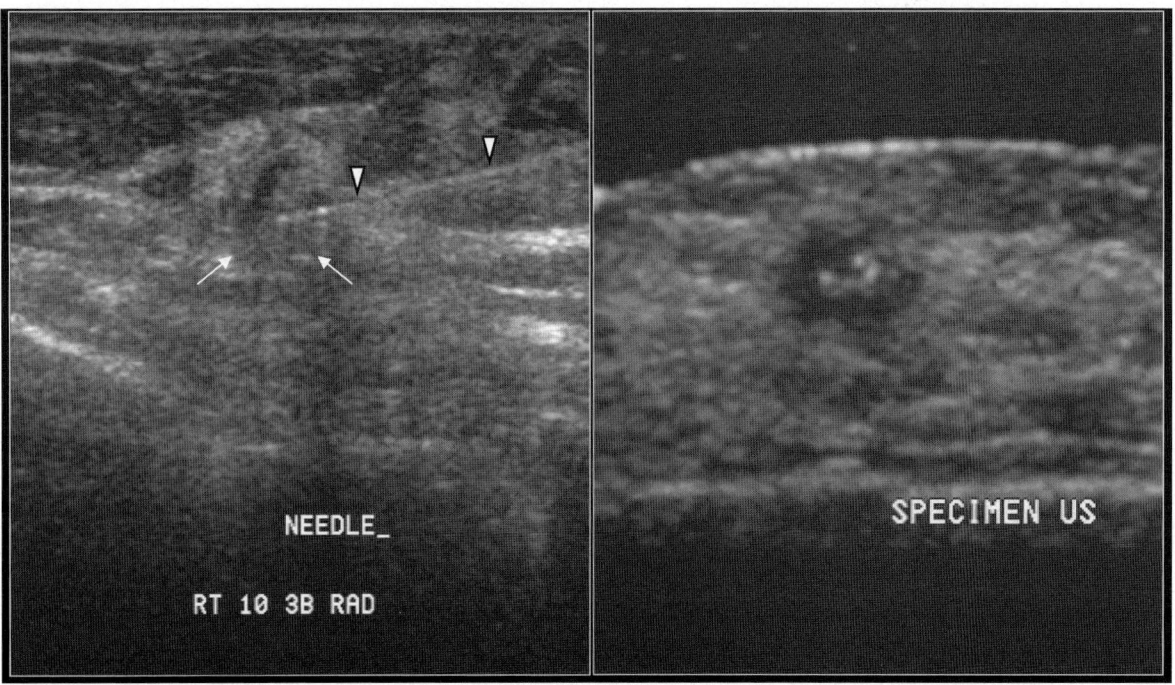

FIGURE 14–20 This patient had a suspicious cluster of punctate calcifications. Ultrasound was used to localize (*arrowheads* indicate localization needle) the calcifications for surgical excision and revealed a nodule *(arrows)* in the area of calcifications (**left**). Specimen ultrasound showed the nodule to be centered within the specimen with clear margins in all directions, including planes not shown on specimen radiography (**right**).

tracystic papillary lesions are caused by benign papillomas or papillary apocrine metaplasia, but a small fraction are caused by DCIS or various invasive malignancies. When sonographic evaluation of a complex cyst reveals a suspicious papillary lesion, ultrasound-guided needle localization for excisional biopsy or ultrasound-guided 11-gauge DVAB with deployment of a marker can be performed. In such cases, aspiration of fluid for cytology is not sufficient because of the high rate of false-negative cytologic studies and because the residual mural nodule or thick septation may no longer be identifiable after fluid is aspirated from the cyst, should that become necessary because of malignant or atypical cytology. Sonographic assessment of complex cysts is discussed in detail in Chapter 10 (Fig. 14–21).

Guidance of Core Needle Biopsy in the Rare Cases in which Stereotactic Biopsy Is Not Possible

There are rare cases in which stereotactically guided large core needle biopsy or mammotomy is not possible—when calcifications are too deep and close to the chest wall and in patients who are unable to lie prone. Ultrasound guidance can be used in at least some of these cases.

Summary

In summary, DCIS is primarily a mammographic diagnosis rather than a sonographic or clinical diagnosis. However, despite the advantages of mammography in demonstrating calcifications and detecting DCIS, there are several specific instances in which ultrasound can be useful. Ultrasound can be helpful in patients with DCIS who have associated mammographic soft tissue densities or clinically palpable abnormalities, nipple discharge, or intracystic lesions; it can help assess lesion size by showing parts of the lesion that are not calcified; it can show unsuspected foci of invasion and lymph node metastases; and it is also useful in guiding large core needle biopsy or mammotomy needle localizations for excisional biopsy in selected patients.

LOBULAR CARCINOMA *IN SITU* AND INTRAEPITHELIAL LOBULAR NEOPLASIA

LCIS is part of a spectrum of abnormalities called *intraepithelial lobular neoplasia*. This classification includes LCIS and

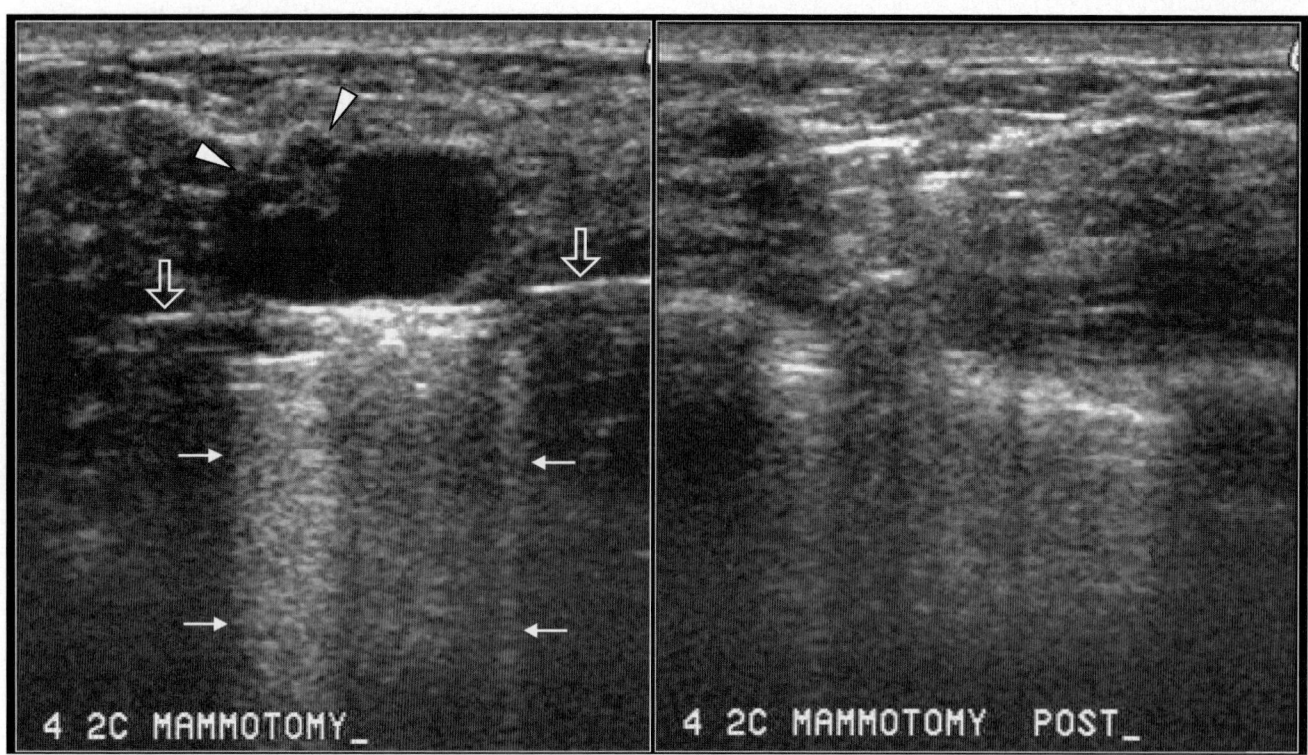

FIGURE 14–21 This patient presented with a palpable lump that was shown by sonography to be caused by a complex cyst containing a papillary mural nodule (**left**, *arrowheads*). The **left** image shows an 11-gauge directional vacuum-assisted biopsy needle *(hollow arrows)* deep to the lesion. The vacuum holes in the aperture of the needle create ring-down artifact *(arrows)* that shows the aperture to be appropriately positioned immediately deep to the lesion. The postbiopsy image **(right)** shows that all imaging evidence of the lesion has been removed. A mammotomy clip was deployed. Histologic assessment of the mammotomy specimen revealed low-nuclear-grade ductal carcinoma *in situ*. The mammotomy clip was localized mammographically a few weeks later, and lumpectomy showed no residual disease.

atypical lobular hyperplasia. Lobular neoplasia may be a direct precursor to development of invasive malignancy. However, in most instances, LCIS is a general risk marker for development of breast cancer in any part of either breast, not simply within the focus of LCIS. LCIS is multicentric about 68% of the time and bilateral in about 30% of cases. Twenty to 30% of patients with LCIS develop an invasive malignancy over a course of 15 to 20 years, almost one-half occurring in the contralateral breast. Most of these developing lesions are ILCs, but many are invasive ductal carcinomas.

Patients with this diagnosis may consider bilateral prophylactic mastectomy. Women with dense breasts who have the diagnosis of LCIS and do not undergo bilateral mastectomy may benefit from additional whole breast sonography after mammography, but the benefit of this is unproved.

Mammographic and Sonographic Findings

LCIS is usually an incidental diagnosis, made on biopsy performed to evaluate either a mammographic or palpable abnormality. In most cases, the LCIS does not cause mammographic or clinical findings. LCIS may develop within preexisting fibroadenoma or radial scars. In such cases, the imaging findings are those of the underlying fibroadenoma rather than being specific for LCIS.

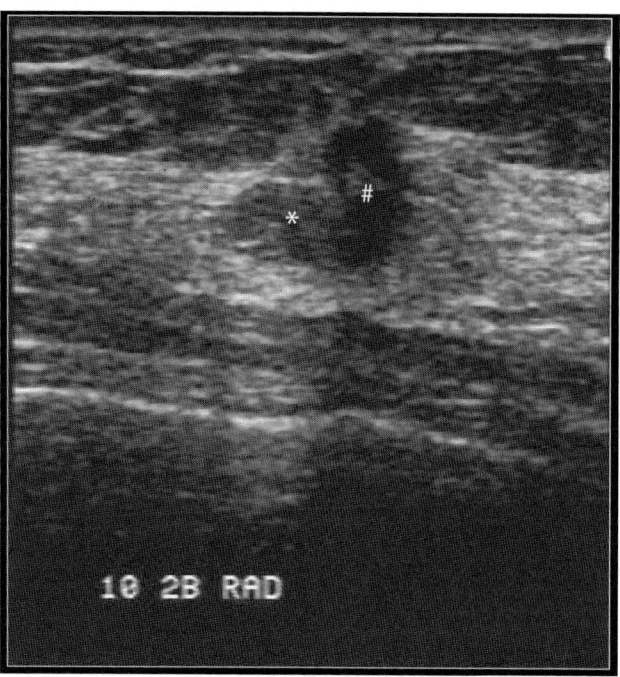

FIGURE 14–23 This bilobed solid nodule had two components: the isoechoic horizontal component *(*)* was shown to be lobular carcinoma *in situ* (LCIS) and the markedly hypoechoic, spiculated, taller-than-wide component *(#)* was shown to be invasive lobular carcinoma (ILC) that had evolved from the LCIS. Contrast-enhanced magnetic resonance imaging (MRI) was performed bilaterally to stage malignant disease and showed multiple foci of abnormal enhancement bilaterally. Second-look ultrasound and ultrasound-guided biopsies confirmed MRI suspicion of multifocal bilateral ILC. In the rare cases in which LCIS causes imaging findings, LCIS tends to be more aggressive and is more likely to have invasive carcinoma associated with it.

Although the diagnosis of LCIS is usually serendipitous, certain cases may actually cause suspicious imaging findings. The recent literature suggests that LCIS that causes imaging abnormalities may differ in significance from LCIS that is an incidental finding (Fig. 14–22). One group is an incidental finding and merely represents a generalized risk factor. On the other hand, LCIS that causes suspicious imaging findings is more pleomorphic, is more aggressive, and is more likely to be a direct precursor to development of invasive malignancy (Fig. 14–23).

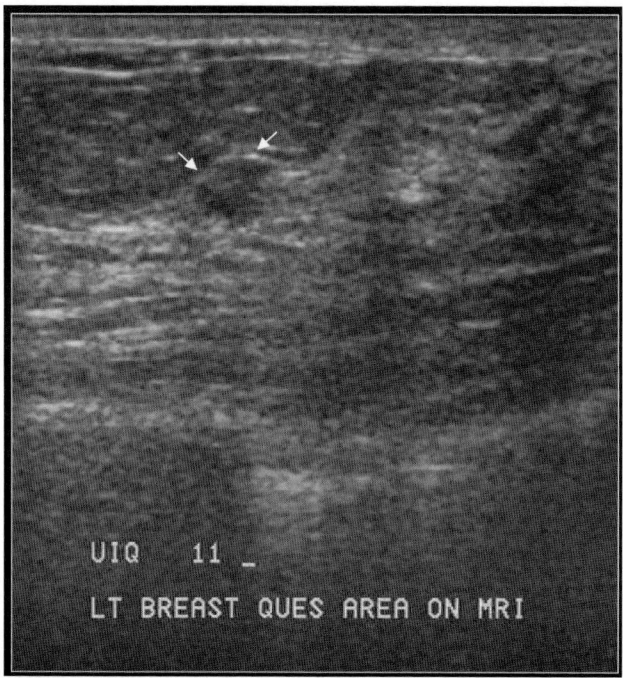

FIGURE 14–22 The 11-gauge directional vacuum-assisted biopsy of this small solid nodule with angular margins *(arrows)* showed a radial scar that contained lobular carcinoma *in situ* (LCIS) in its periphery. The diagnosis of LCIS was incidental to the magnetic resonance imaging and sonographic finding of a radial scar.

INFILTRATING DUCTAL CARCINOMA, BREAST CARCINOMA OF NO SPECIFIC TYPE, AND BREAST CARCINOMA NOT OTHERWISE SPECIFIED

General Pathologic Classification, Epidemiology, and Clinical Findings

Invasive breast carcinomas are a heterogeneous group that can be divided into three general subgroups: invasive NOS carcinomas, special-type carcinomas, and ILCs. All of the cancers that cannot be classified into special or lobular groups are lumped into the group called invasive adenocarcinoma of no special type (NST) or invasive adenocarcinoma NOS. The terms infiltrating or invasive duct carcinoma and NST or NOS carcinoma are used interchangeably. NOS carcinomas are the most common invasive breast malignancies, constituting 50% to 90% of all invasive breast cancers. These lesions generally have the worst prognosis of the various types of breast carcinoma, especially if the histologic grade is high. NOS tumors have a propensity to be intermediate to high grade.

Many invasive breast carcinomas have mixtures of histologic types. NOS invasive carcinomas can contain components of lobular carcinoma or special-type tumors, such as tubular, medullary, colloid, or papillary carcinoma. About one-half of NOS tumors contain foci of tubular carcinoma within them, and 6% of NOS tumors contain foci of ILC. In cases in which the histology is mixed special type and NOS, the prognosis is usually that of the worst component of the tumor: the NOS component.

NOS breast carcinomas also make up a very heterogeneous group of lesions. The gross morphology and histology of these lesions varies tremendously. Anatomic and histologic variables that affect sonographic appearance include the tumor cellularity, composition of extracellular matrix, host reaction to the lesion, water content, histologic grade, site of origin, presence of necrosis or scarring, whether host reaction is fibroelastotic or inflammatory, extent of DCIS components, multifocality, multicentricity, attachment to skin, and presence or absence of lymphatic invasion. To complicate the picture further, these anatomic and histologic variations do not always develop independently of each other and can be related and occur in constellations.

Site of Origin

Most NOS tumors are believed to arise within the terminal duct of the TDLU. Spread from the TDLU in which these tumors originate can then occur by DCIS components within the ductal system or by direct invasion of perilobular and periductal tissues. Most NOS carcinomas spread by both routes and thus contain combinations of intraductal (DCIS) and invasive components. Carcinomas that arise within TDLUs are considered peripheral in origin even if they arise from centrally located TDLUs that are connected directly to the subareolar portions of the lobar ducts. However, the behavior of such lesions differs from that of carcinomas that arise from peripherally located TDLUs. The resistance to extensive intraductal spread of tumor appears to be lower for centrally arising lesions than for peripherally arising lesions. Such lesions frequently have extensive intraductal components (EICs) that grow into and distend the central ducts. On the other hand, carcinomas arising from peripherally located TDLUs tend to invade the surrounding tissues more easily, involving Cooper's ligaments relatively early. If the breast tissue around the peripheral TDLU in

which invasive carcinoma has developed has become atrophic, the atrophic peripheral ducts resist intraductal spread more than do central ducts. Even when peripherally arising NOS invasive carcinomas spread intraductally, the peripheral DCIS components are less likely to distend the ducts grossly than are the DCIS components of carcinomas arising from centrally located TDLUs.

Although most NOS tumors arise within TDLUs, a few arise directly within larger ducts, usually within preexisting papillomas or foci of florid usual or atypical duct hyperplasia. These more centrally arising tumors differ in their sonographic appearance from most other NOS tumors, tending to reflect the sonographic appearance of the preexisting lesion from which they arose. Thus, an NOS carcinoma arising from a preexisting benign large duct papilloma can be grossly morphologically indistinguishable from a benign large duct papilloma. Invasive breast carcinomas that arise centrally are more likely to be low-grade NOS, to have special-type components such as invasive papillary carcinoma, and to become encysted than are carcinomas that arise peripherally within TDLUs.

Gross Morphology of Invasive Not Otherwise Specified Carcinomas

On gross pathologic examination, the borders of an NOS breast carcinoma can appear frankly spiculated or circumscribed. Because invasive NOS carcinomas can be heterogeneous, not only from nodule to nodule but also within an individual nodule, many NOS carcinomas demonstrate more than one type of margin characteristic. Part of the surface might be circumscribed, whereas other parts might be spiculated. Additionally, the gross and microscopic evidence of spiculation may differ from each other. Lesions that appear to be completely circumscribed on gross pathologic examination can show microscopic evidence of spiculation in up to one-third of NOS carcinomas.

Morphologically, most NOS breast carcinomas have irregular or microlobulated margins. Irregular or angular margins represent invasive tumor extending into surrounding tissues and frequently occur along the undersurface of the anterior mammary fascia, in periductal tissues, and at the bases of Cooper's ligaments. Microlobulations can represent fingers of invasive tumor or DCIS components that enlarge ducts or TDLUs (cancerize lobules).

Because of the high likelihood of spiculation, angular margins, or microlobulations occurring along at least part of the surface of an NOS carcinoma, there is an extremely low likelihood of its entire surface appearing circumscribed and smooth if the entire surface is carefully evaluated.

Histology of Not Otherwise Specified Tumors

NOS breast carcinomas can be graded histologically, which is important in defining prognosis and managing treatment. A modification of the system proposed by Bloom and Richardson is the most widely used. In this system, three histologic features are graded: tubule formation, nuclear pleomorphism, and hyperchromatism (or number of mitoses). Each of these factors is assigned a score from 1 to 3, with 1 representing the lowest grade and 3 the highest. Lower grades indicate better differentiation of the tumor and therefore better prognosis.

The tubule score assesses the extent of tubule formation by malignant cells. Lesions with a score of 1 are made up predominantly of well-formed tubules and are well differentiated. Lesions with a tubule score of 2 have a mixture of areas with tubule formation and areas where only cords or sheets of cells exist. Lesions with a tubular score of 3 have essentially no tubular formation and are composed entirely of sheets or cords of cells and thus are undifferentiated.

The nuclear pleomorphism score assesses size and variability of tumor cell nuclei. A score of 1 is assigned if nuclei are relatively small and similar in size and shape. A score of 2 is assigned if the nuclei vary moderately in size and shape. A score of 3 is assigned if nuclei vary greatly in size and shape, especially if there are very large, irregularly shaped nuclei.

The mitoses score assesses the numbers of mitoses per high-power field. A score of 1 is assigned if there are no mitoses. A score of 2 is assigned if there are 1 or 2 mitoses per high-power field. A score of 3 is assigned if there are 3 or more mitoses per high-power field.

The individual scores are assigned an Arabic numeral and are then summed to arrive at a total Bloom-Richardson-Scarf score of between 3 and 9. The total scores are then used to derive a histologic grade, which is assigned a Roman numeral rather than an Arabic numeral. Bloom-Richardson-Scarf scores can range from 3 to 9. Scores from 3 through 5 are considered to be low grade or histologic grade I. Total scores of 6 and 7 are considered intermediate grade or histologic grade II. Scores of 8 and 9 are considered high grade or histologic grade III.

The histologic grade often varies from one part of an NOS lesion to another. In such cases, assigning the highest grade found within the malignancy to the whole lesion is advisable. Variability of histologic grade within the lesion may account for the reported variability in grading. Random methods of biopsy, such as imaging-guided core needle biopsy, and random sectioning methods used to assess excisional biopsy specimens contribute to variability. The presence of multiple different histologic grades within a single lesion is simply a manifestation of their tendency to dedifferentiate over time, creating a polyclonal lesion. Histologic grading certainly has a subjective component, and the reported interobserver and intraobserver reproducibility of scores varies from 60% to 90%. The variability is corroborated by the wide variation in the percentage of NOS breast carcinomas in each histologic grade that has been reported in the literature: 3% to 33% of NOS lesions have been reported to be histologic grade I; 23% to 52% have been reported to be histologic grade II; and 25% to

67% have been reported to be histologic grade III. Although part of the variation is undoubtedly due to variations in patient populations, much of the variation must be due to differing interpretations of histologic data or to differences in histologic sampling. Histologic grades must be distinguished from the nuclear grades that are assigned to pure DCIS or invasive lobular carcinoma. The nuclear grade (pleomorphism) is merely one component of the histologic grade.

Compared with low-grade lesions, high-grade or histologic grade III tumors are likely to be more cellular, have larger components of hyaluronic acid in the extracellular matrix, incite more inflammatory and less desmoplastic response, have more EICs, and have more necrosis. When compared with low-grade or histologic grade I carcinomas, a larger percentage of the volume of high-grade lesions is composed of tumor cells, and a smaller percentage of the lesion is composed of extracellular matrix. The extracellular matrix of high-grade lesions tends to be composed of greater amounts of hyaluronic acid and lesser amounts of collagen than are low-grade lesions. Hyaluronic acid is a huge hydrophilic macromolecule whose three-dimensional structure includes many interstices that bind water molecules. Thus, between higher cellularity and the presence of more hyaluronic acid in the extracellular matrix, high-grade lesions contain much more water than do low-grade lesions. This affects sound transmission.

The more desmoplastic response incited by a tumor, the more likely it is to have spiculated margins; and the less desmoplasia, the more likely the margins are to be circumscribed. Because high-grade NOS carcinomas tend to have relatively little desmoplasia, they show a propensity to lie at the circumscribed rather than the spiculated end of the malignant nodule spectrum. Low-grade lesions, on the other hand, contain more desmoplasia and tend to be spiculated.

The percentage of high-grade NOS tumors is higher in younger patients than in older patients and constitutes a large percentage of interval cancers (those that develop between routine screening examinations).

High-grade NOS tumors are more likely to be tender to palpation and to elicit pain when punctured by a needle for biopsy or localization than are low-grade lesions. The presence of an inflammatory infiltrate may explain this pain and tenderness, but such lesions are also more likely to have perineural invasion, which can also lead to pain and tenderness.

The prognosis is much worse for histologic grade III tumors than for grade I tumors. Grade II tumors, of course, have a prognosis intermediate between grade I and grade III tumors. The prognosis obtained by combining histologic grade and lymph node status is more accurate than that obtained by either alone. Grade III tumors have a greater chance of lymph node involvement and distant metastases and therefore lower survival rates than do lower-grade lesions.

The histologic grade affects the appearance of these lesions on imaging studies in many ways. These variations are discussed in detail in the section on sonographic appearance.

Host Reaction to the Tumor: Stromal Reaction versus Inflammatory Reaction

Although the malignant cells of which NOS breast carcinomas are composed are epithelial in origin (adenocarcinomas), almost all lesions incite some desmoplasia or an inflammatory reaction. Some lesions incite an almost purely fibroelastotic stromal reaction, whereas others are more likely to stimulate an inflammatory response, but most incite mixtures of stromal and inflammatory responses. In general, low-grade invasive NOS carcinomas tend to have more stromal and less inflammatory reaction, whereas high-grade lesions tend to have more inflammatory and less stromal reaction.

The fibrous stromal reaction is one of the components that make the tumor firm to palpation and gross inspection, make the lesion feel larger to palpation, and lead to spiculated margins. The degree of fibrous stromal reaction does not seem to have prognostic significance when considered separately. However, lower-grade lesions tend to have relatively more stromal reaction, whereas higher-grade tumors tend to have relatively less stromal reaction. It is likely that the fibrous stromal response is an attempt by the body to "wall off" the tumor and prevent it from spreading. However, it is a slowly developing response, and high-grade lesions may grow too rapidly to allow a fibrous stromal response to occur.

A portion of the fibrosis within NOS breast carcinomas may actually represent scarring, rather than the typical desmoplastic stromal reaction. Linnell has proposed that breast carcinomas can be subdivided into two types that arise differently: (a) tubuloductal carcinoma and (b) ductal carcinoma of the comedo type. He proposes that tubuloductal lesions arise within radial scars, infiltrate early, have little pagetoid growth, do not cancerize lobules, contain smaller cells, and have a better prognosis. These tubuloductal lesions have a persistent residual central fibroelastotic scar, giving clues to the origin of these lesions. An alternative, but equally (if not more plausible) postulate for such central scars is that the scarring represents fibrosis arising from healed areas of central necrosis. The second type of lesion, the ductal carcinoma of the comedo type, arises within the TDLU, is prone to pagetoid growth and cancerization of lobules, has no scar remnants, contains large tumor cells, and has a worse prognosis.

High-grade invasive NOS carcinomas frequently contain a peripheral infiltrate of lymphocytes or plasma cells that is a poor prognostic sign. It is not clear whether the poorer prognosis is independently related to the lymphocytic infiltrates or merely a manifestation of the tendency of such infiltrates to occur in high-grade lesions. The lymphocytic infiltrate can be so dense that it can be difficult to determine whether the lesion is a primary high-grade breast carcinoma or a metastasis to an intramammary lymph node. Lesions with abundant inflammatory response are likely to be circumscribed and soft on gross inspection. The presence of lymphocytic infiltrates also directly affects mammographic and sonographic appearances, as is discussed subsequently.

The presence of inflammatory cells within the tumor should be distinguished from "inflammatory carcinoma," which represents a specific type of lesion in which dermal lymphatics are involved by tumor and with which mastitis is associated.

Necrosis

About one-third of NOS invasive breast carcinomas have necrosis within the invasive component, which must be distinguished from the necrosis that occurs within the lumina of ductules that contain DCIS. Necrosis within the invasive portion of breast carcinomas is common in high-grade NOS lesions and is very unusual in low-grade NOS lesions. The presence of necrosis within invasive components worsens prognosis, and the more extensive the necrosis, the worse the prognosis is. Necrotic NOS carcinomas are soft and usually circumscribed. Both blood flow and oxygen levels are reduced within areas of necrosis, preventing immunologic and chemotherapeutic agents from reaching the tumor cells, protecting the tumor from treatment, and contributing to worsened prognosis.

Necrosis within the invasive portions of NOS tumors may be liquefactive, hemorrhagic, or fibrotic. Liquefactive and hemorrhagic necrosis occurs most commonly in high-grade lesions. Cystic areas within such NOS lesions usually represent large areas of liquefied or hemorrhagic tumor necrosis. Necrotic fibrotic scarring occurs most commonly within intermediate-grade invasive NOS carcinomas and can be indistinguishable from the areas of fibrosis described by Linnel (discussed earlier).

Extent of Intraductal Component

About 85% of NOS breast carcinomas have a mixture of invasive and intraductal (DCIS) components. The intraductal component most often lies in the periphery of these lesions. Large amounts of intraductal tumor have been defined in three different ways. First, there is DCIS with microscopic invasion that involves of 5% to 10% of the lesion or extends less than 1 mm beyond the duct. These tumors are often inappropriately grouped with pure DCIS and likely account for most reported cases of DCIS with lymph node metastases. A second definition is EIC, which is defined as DCIS involving at least 25% of the borders of the lesion and involving the surrounding tissues. A third and final definition is *predominant intraductal component*, which is defined as

DCIS having 4 times the volume of invasive carcinoma or involving at least 80% of the total lesion. It can be difficult to determine precisely the percentage of DCIS components within a lesion, especially if the pathologist employs random rather than serial section techniques.

The extent of intraductal component is related to the grade of the lesion and the site of origin of the tumor. High-grade NOS lesions are more likely to grow rapidly and extensively within the ductal system than are low-grade lesions. Centrally arising lesions seem more prone to early and aggressive spread through the ductal system than do peripherally arising lesions.

EIC within an invasive NOS carcinoma affects the prognosis in two ways, depending on whether the patient is treated with mastectomy or breast conservation surgery. In patients who undergo mastectomy, EIC affects survival. Patients whose NOS carcinomas have EIC are less likely to have lymph node and distant hematogenous metastases, and therefore, better survival, than are NOS tumors without EIC. In patients who undergo breast conservation therapy, the presence of EIC affects local recurrence rates. Patients who have NOS tumors with EIC and who undergo breast conservation therapy have a higher risk for local recurrence than do patients whose NOS carcinomas do not have EIC. Thus, the presence of EIC worsens the prognosis for local recurrence if breast conservation therapy is performed, even though EIC improves prognosis for survival in patients who undergo mastectomy.

Most local recurrences are the result of inadequate resection of the primary tumor, not of new foci of tumor development (metachronous lesions). The presence of EIC increases the likelihood that a portion of the tumor that the surgeon is unable to detect will be surgically transected and remain within the breast after breast conservation therapy, leading to eventual local recurrence. In patients who undergo wide excision and have no evidence of EIC, the risks for local recurrence at 5 and 10 years are 2% and 3%, respectively. In patients whose tumors show evidence of EIC, the local recurrence rates at 5 and 10 years are 24% and 40%, respectively.

Local recurrence of breast cancer, although discouraging, does not necessarily imply an increased fatality rate. Local recurrence rates depend on the extent of resection, but patient survival does not. Local recurrence indicates inadequate surgical resection or aggressive biologic behavior of the tumor, but has no definite affect on patient survival as long as the local recurrence is detected and resected promptly. Mortality from breast carcinoma is dictated by systemic metastasis, not local control.

Multifocal or Multicentric Disease

Multifocal tumor is defined as multiple tumors within the same quadrant of the breast. Multicentric tumor is defined as multiple foci of tumor in different quadrants of the breast or separated by 5 cm or more. NOS carcinomas are multifocal in 25% to 50% of cases. However, in most instances, the multiple foci of invasion are merely different parts of the same lesion, connected by EICs of tumor. The subareolar region of the breast is the most common site for additional foci of invasive disease. Regardless of whether multiple foci of invasive tumor represent completely separate neoplasms or different areas of invasion within the same lesion, failure to remove all components will result in local treatment failure.

Multicentric disease is less likely to represent extensive single tumor and more likely to represent completely separate, synchronous tumors, and occurs in 15% to 20% of NOS breast carcinomas.

Synchronous bilateral invasive NOS breast carcinomas occur in 5% to 8% of patients. The risk for a new cancer forming in the contralateral breast after diagnosis of ipsilateral NOS breast cancer is about 1% per year, sixfold higher than for the general population. If there is LCIS within the tissues surrounding an invasive NOS carcinoma, the risk for contralateral disease is even greater.

Invasion of Cooper's Ligaments

NOS carcinomas that arise peripherally have a tendency to invade through the lobule or terminal duct relatively early. One of the paths of least resistance for invasion is along Cooper's ligaments toward the skin. This invasion causes the flattening or dimpling of the skin clinically. Such skin changes may only be seen with the patient placed in certain positions.

Invasion of Lymphatic Vessels and Lymph Node Metastases

Invasion of lymphatic vessels and blood vessels and along nerves can be detected histologically, but not directly, by imaging studies. Lymph vessel invasion is associated with a higher risk for axillary lymph node metastases. The presence and extent of lymph node metastasis is directly associated with larger and more poorly differentiated tumors; therefore, involvement of the lymph nodes is a marker of more aggressive tumor behavior and carries a greater likelihood of existing or subsequent systemic dissemination. Lymph node metastases and sonographic assessment of lymph nodes is discussed in detail in Chapter 19.

Mammographic Findings

In view of the large variations in gross tumor morphology and histology of invasive NOS carcinomas, it should not be surprising that the mammographic findings also vary tremendously. Mammographic findings include soft tissue densities or masses, calcifications, and architectural distortion. NOS carcinomas may present as isolated, focal, asymmetric opacities. The risk for malignancy in patients whose only mammographic finding is focal asymmetry is very low. Invasive NOS carcinomas that present as masses usually have spiculated or indistinct margins, but a small percentage can present with circumscribed margins. However, even circumscribed carcinomas are usually indistinct, angular, or microlobulated over a small portion of their surfaces on spot compression views.

About half of all invasive NOS carcinomas contain calcifications that usually lie within DICS components of the lesions. High-grade NOS lesions are more likely to contain HNG DCIS components and therefore are more likely to be associated with the casting or crushed stone types of calcifications associated with HNG DCIS. Low-grade invasive NOS lesions are more likely to have LNG or ING DCIS components and to be associated with the less abundant, punctate, or small granular calcifications that occur in LNG DCIS. As noted earlier, the extent of calcification more reliably correlates with extent of disease in high-grade lesions than in low-grade lesions.

The presence of EIC can manifest mammographically as linearly arranged calcifications that extend away from the edges of the dominant mass into surrounding tissues. EIC most commonly extends within the ducts toward the nipple (duct extension) but can also extend away from the nipple in multiple branching ducts (branch pattern). EIC can also present mammographically as an abnormally large duct extending from the mass toward the nipple without calcifications. Another manifestation of EIC might be multiple separate foci of spiculation or multiple separate nodules with calcifications bridging the space between them.

In some cases, only subtle architectural distortion is present. The distortion might manifest as straight, radiating, water-density lines representing subtle spiculation or slight bulges or angular indentations of the anterior or posterior mammary fascia.

Of course, in some patients, the mammograms will appear to be completely negative. Sonography is especially useful among patients who have palpable lumps but negative mammograms that show dense tissue in the area of the palpable lump.

Sonographic Findings of Invasive Not Otherwise Specified Lesions

Like the mammographic findings of invasive NOS breast carcinomas, the sonographic findings vary greatly and reflect the gross morphologic and histologic heterogeneity of NOS carcinomas from nodule to nodule and within individual nodules.

Site of Origin

The sonographic appearance varies with the site of involvement. Small peripheral NOS carcinomas can present as

small microlobulated lesions that represent cancerized TDLUs (Fig. 14–24). These lesions differ in appearance from DCIS lesions only in having spiculations or a thick, echogenic halo rather than a thin, echogenic capsule surrounding the lesion. The spicules may be quite long compared with the size of the lesion and are straighter than normal Cooper's ligaments (Fig. 14–25). Small peripheral invasive NOS carcinomas often have a small intraductal component that enlarges the extralobular terminal duct and are taller than wide, reflecting the orientation of the TDLU in which the lesion arose (Fig. 14–26). In some cases, DCIS components can enlarge the extralobular terminal duct component to almost the same degree as the lobule is enlarged. Tumor may extend from the extralobular terminal duct into the distal portions of the main lobar duct, where it tends to grow toward the nipple (Fig. 14–27). If the extralobular terminal duct and distal lobar duct become grossly enlarged, the lesion can have a hockey-stick appearance (Fig. 14–28). When multiple TDLUs and the peripheral segment of the lobar duct are enlarged, there may be multiple taller-than-wide components attached to a horizontally oriented duct of variable size (Fig. 14–29).

Lesions that arise in more centrally located TDLUs grow into the central lobar ducts earlier in the process and tend to have earlier and more extensive intraductal involve-

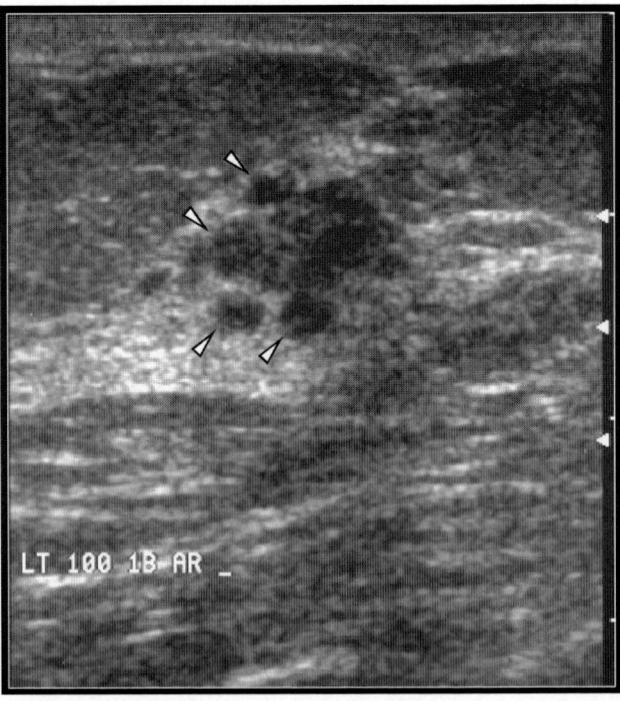

FIGURE 14–24 This mixed invasive and intraductal carcinoma is surrounded by microlobulations *(arrowheads)*. The central mass is intermediate-grade invasive not otherwise specified carcinoma, and the microlobulations represent intermediate-nuclear-grade ductal carcinoma *in situ* components that have cancerized surrounding lobules.

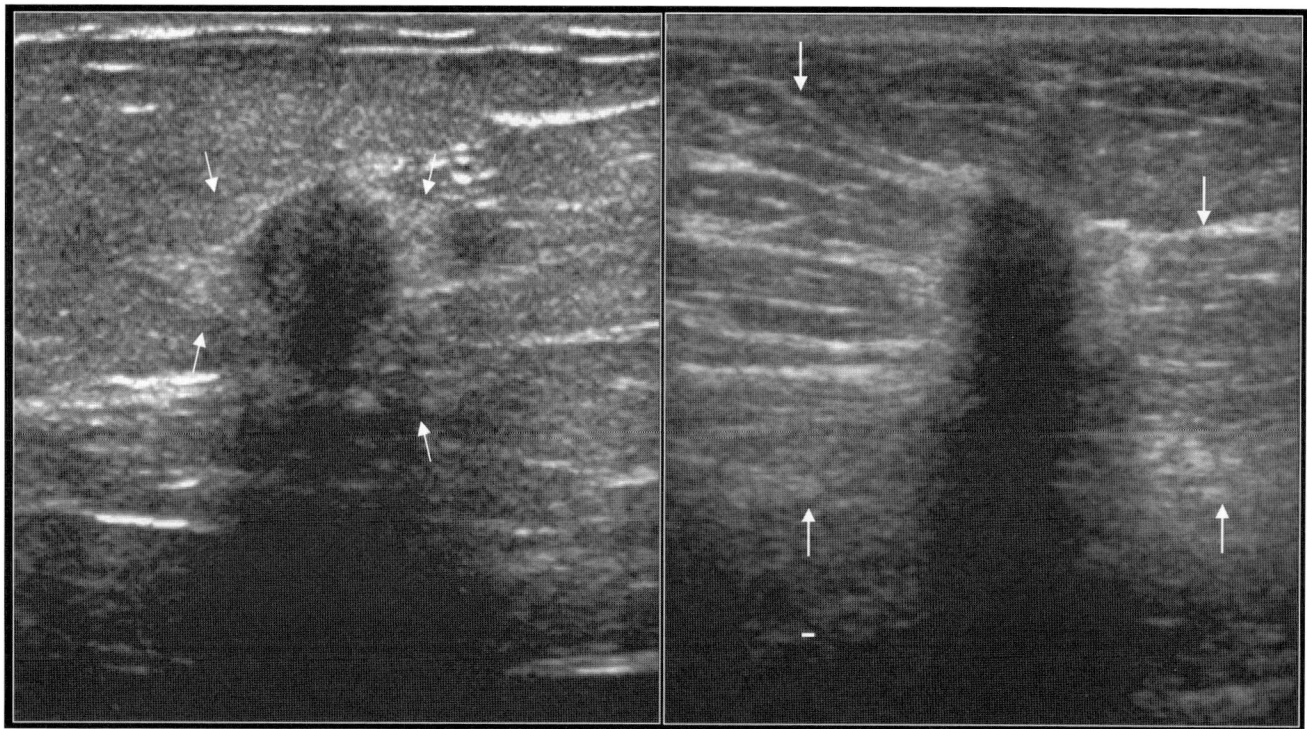

FIGURE 14–25 Early invasion rather than extensive intraductal spread typifies peripheral site of origin. These lesions are usually either frankly spiculated (**right**, *arrows*) or encompassed by a thick, echogenic halo (**left**, *arrows*). The spicules of small, peripherally arising invasive not otherwise specified carcinomas are typically long compared with the diameter of the lesion and straighter than those of radial scars.

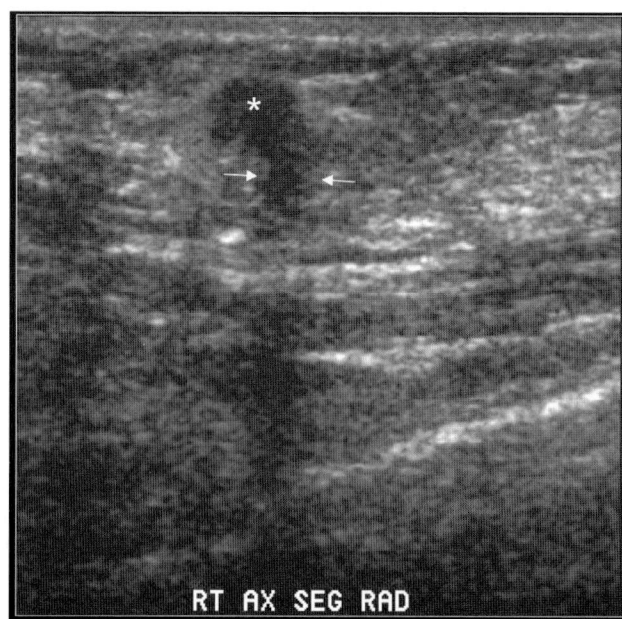

FIGURE 14–26 The extralobular ductal component *(arrow)* of the small, peripherally arising, invasive not otherwise specified carcinoma may be nearly as large as the lobular component *(*)*.

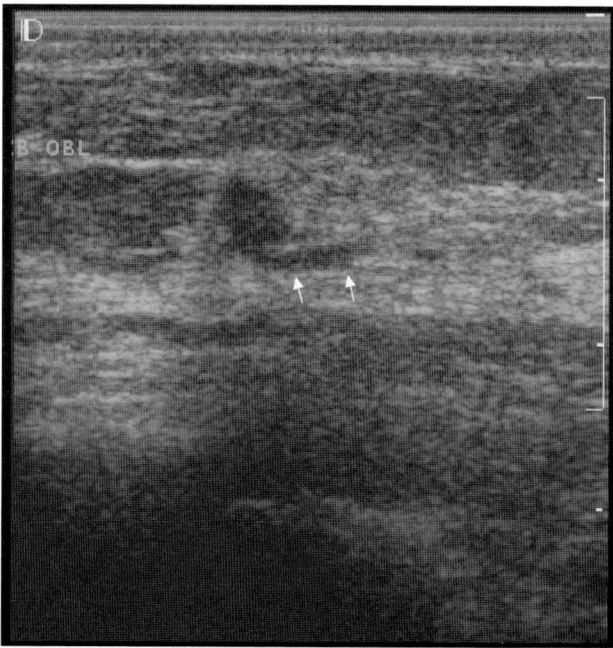

FIGURE 14–27 Even in small, peripherally arising, invasive not otherwise specified carcinomas, a small ductal carcinoma *in situ* component can reach the main lobar duct and begin growing toward the nipple *(arrows)*.

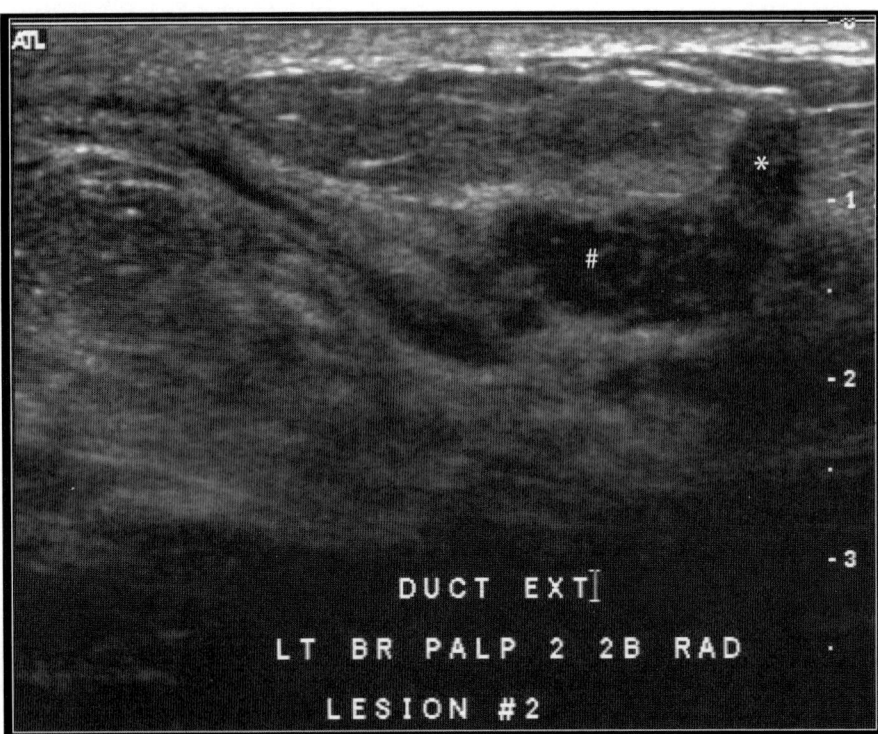

FIGURE 14–28 In later-stage peripherally arising, invasive not otherwise specified carcinomas, the ductal carcinoma *in situ* component that involves the distal end of the lobar duct can grossly enlarge the duct or invade out of the duct to create a hockey-stick shape. The vertical portion of the lesion represents the terminal ductolobular unit of origin *(*)*, and the horizontal portion represents the component involving the peripheral aspect of the lobar duct *(#)* (and in some cases periductal tissues).

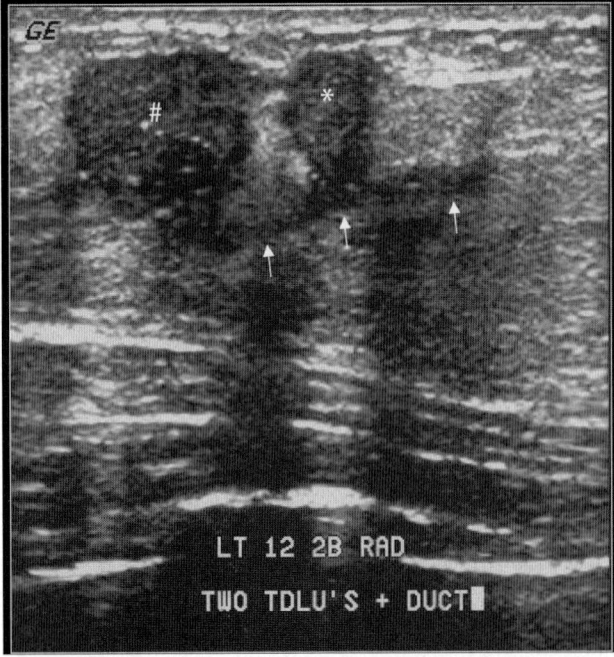

FIGURE 14–29 As a peripherally arising lesion *(#)* grows centrally within the main duct toward the nipple, it can cancerize more centrally lying terminal ductolobular units (TDLUs) *(*)*. This leads to an appearance of multiple taller-than-wide cancerized TDLUs attached to a lobar duct *(arrows)*.

ment. In such cases, the invasive component may be a relatively small taller-than-wide nodule, with a spiculated margin or a thick, echogenic halo that is connected to an abnormally large single or branching solid duct (Fig. 14–30). Such a lesion may extend all the way to the nipple (Fig. 14–31). Alternatively, the involved duct may be only minimally enlarged, but filled with calcifications extending toward the nipple. In such cases, the invasive part of the tumor usually contains calcifications similar to those within the duct (Fig. 14–32).

Margin Characteristics

Two-thirds of invasive NOS carcinomas are grossly spiculated, and one-third appear circumscribed at gross pathologic examination. Circumscribed lesions may appear to have a pseudocapsule of surrounding compressed breast tissue similar to that caused by a benign lesion such as a fibroadenoma. However, most of these grossly circumscribed NOS lesions show evidence of infiltration of surrounding tissues on microscopic examination. Furthermore, even circumscribed lesions that have a thin, echogenic pseudocapsule generally have an incomplete capsule. Careful sonographic assessment of the entire surface in radial and antiradial planes usually demonstrate infiltrative areas that are spiculated; a thick, echogenic halo; or angular margins (Fig. 14–33). In some cases, however, the lesion has a com-

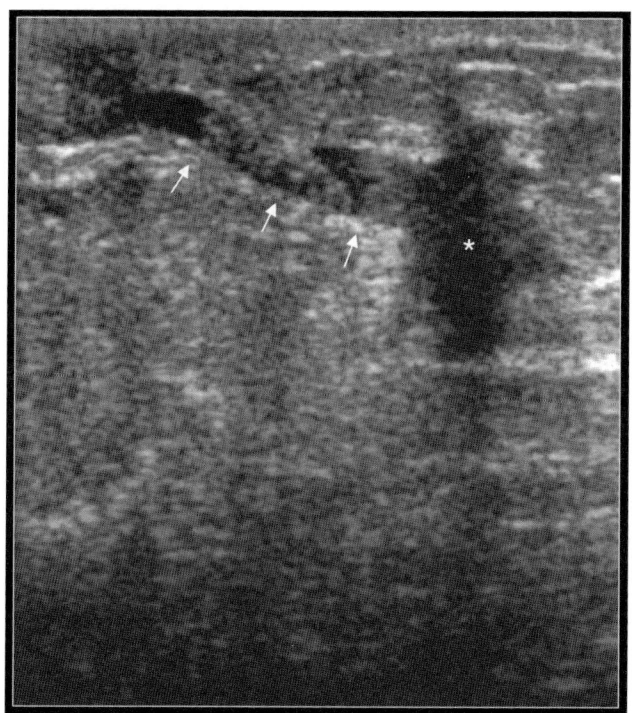

FIGURE 14–30 Centrally arising, invasive not otherwise specified carcinomas tend to have prominent lobar duct involvement by ductal carcinoma *in situ* components *(arrows)* early in the course of their development. In many cases, the length of duct involvement exceeds the diameter of the invasive site of origin *(*)*.

plete thin, echogenic capsule, but it is associated with other soft suspicious findings, such as microlobulation, branch pattern, or duct extensions.

The histopathologic basis for solid nodule margin characteristics is discussed in detail in Chapter 12 and illustrated in Figs. 12–13 to 12–22. Nodules that are spiculated on gross morphologic pathologic examination can demonstrate either discrete frank spiculation or an ill-defined thick, echogenic halo sonographically, depending on the size of the spicules and the resolution of the ultrasound equipment. In some cases, retracted Cooper's ligaments may be difficult to distinguish from spiculations. Subtle skin retraction can be difficult to appreciate in the supine position when transducer compression is employed. Upright scanning and using very light scan pressure and a standoff of acoustic gel can facilitate the sonographic demonstration of skin retraction (Fig. 14–34).

The visibility of the spicules depends on the echogenicity of the infiltrated background tissue. When the spiculated nodule is surrounded by isoechoic fat, hyperechoic spicules are visible. When the tumor nodule is surrounded by hyperechoic fibrous tissue, hypoechoic spicules are more apparent. The visibility of spiculations also depends on the orientation of the spicules relative to the sonographic beam. Hyperechoic spiculations are better demonstrated when they are oriented nearly perpendicularly to the beam, whereas hy-

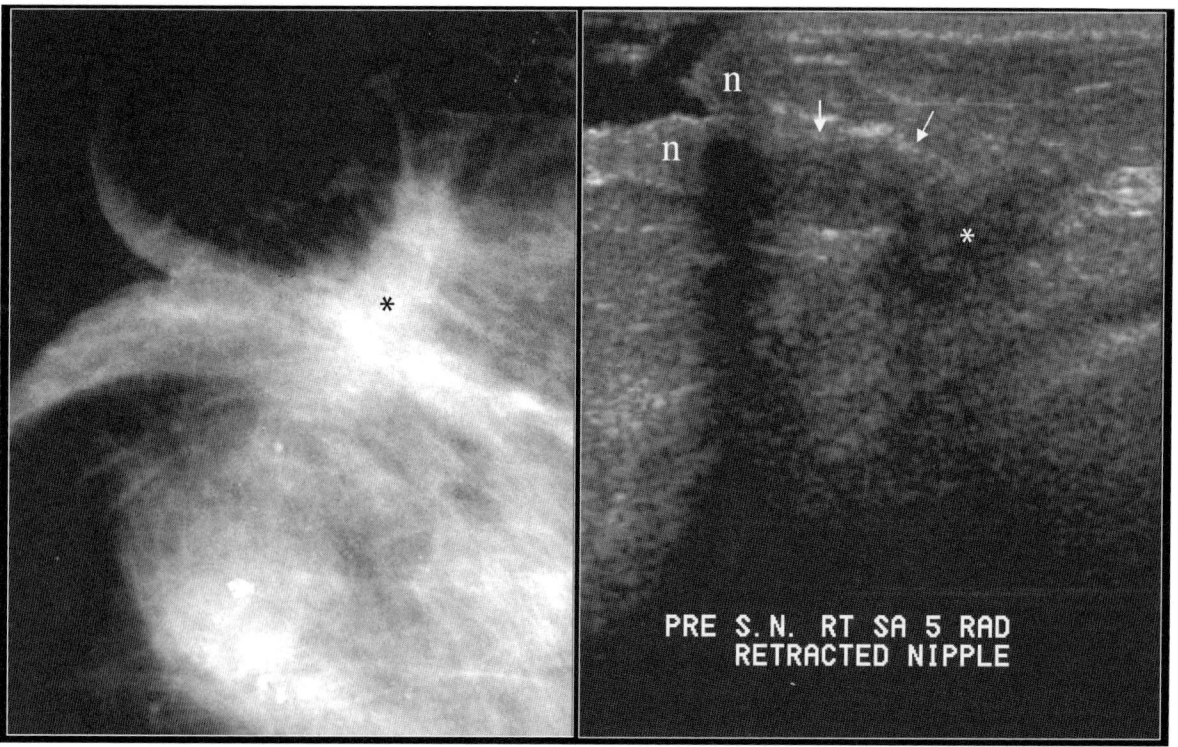

FIGURE 14–31 In centrally arising, mixed invasive and intraductal not otherwise specified lesions, the intraductal ductal carcinoma *in situ* component *(arrows)* frequently extends all the way to the nipple *(n)* from the invasive site of origin *(*)*.

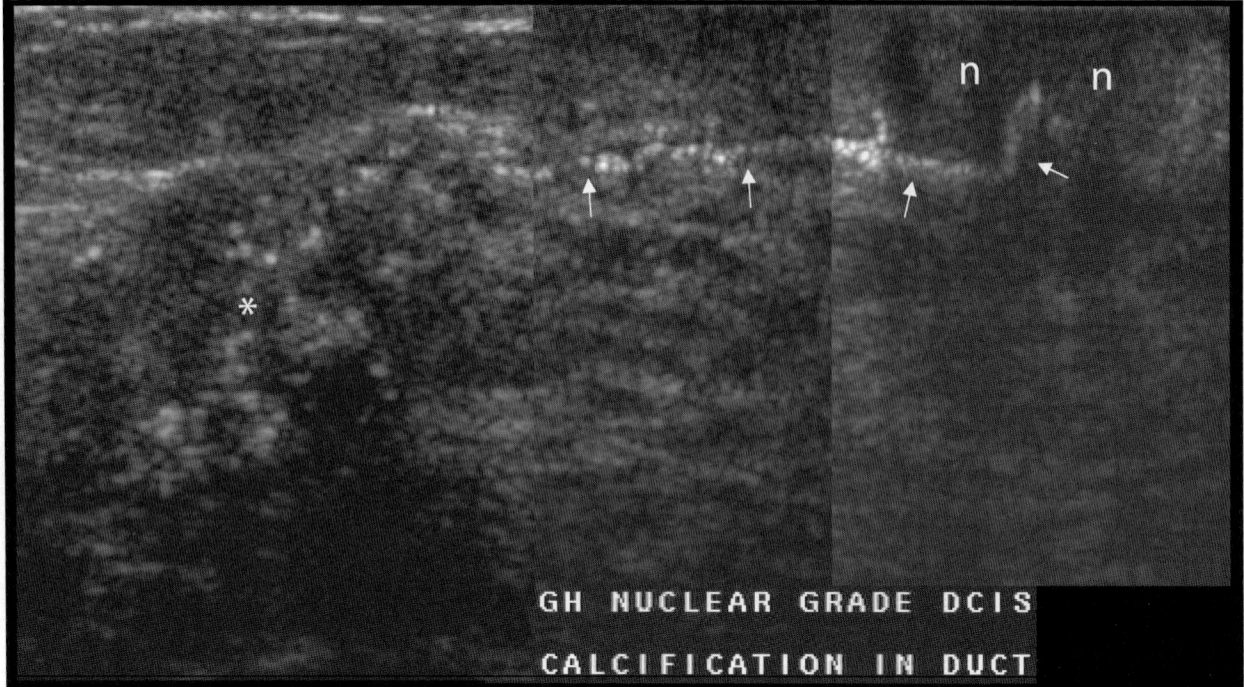

FIGURE 14–32 This large, centrally arising mixed invasive and intraductal not otherwise specified carcinoma shows dense calcifications not only within the main invasive component of the lesion *(*)* but also along the ductal carcinoma *in situ* (DCIS) component within the lobar duct *(arrows)* that extends all the way to the nipple *(n)*. Note that, unlike the case shown in Fig. 14–31, the involved lobar duct is not grossly distended by the DCIS component.

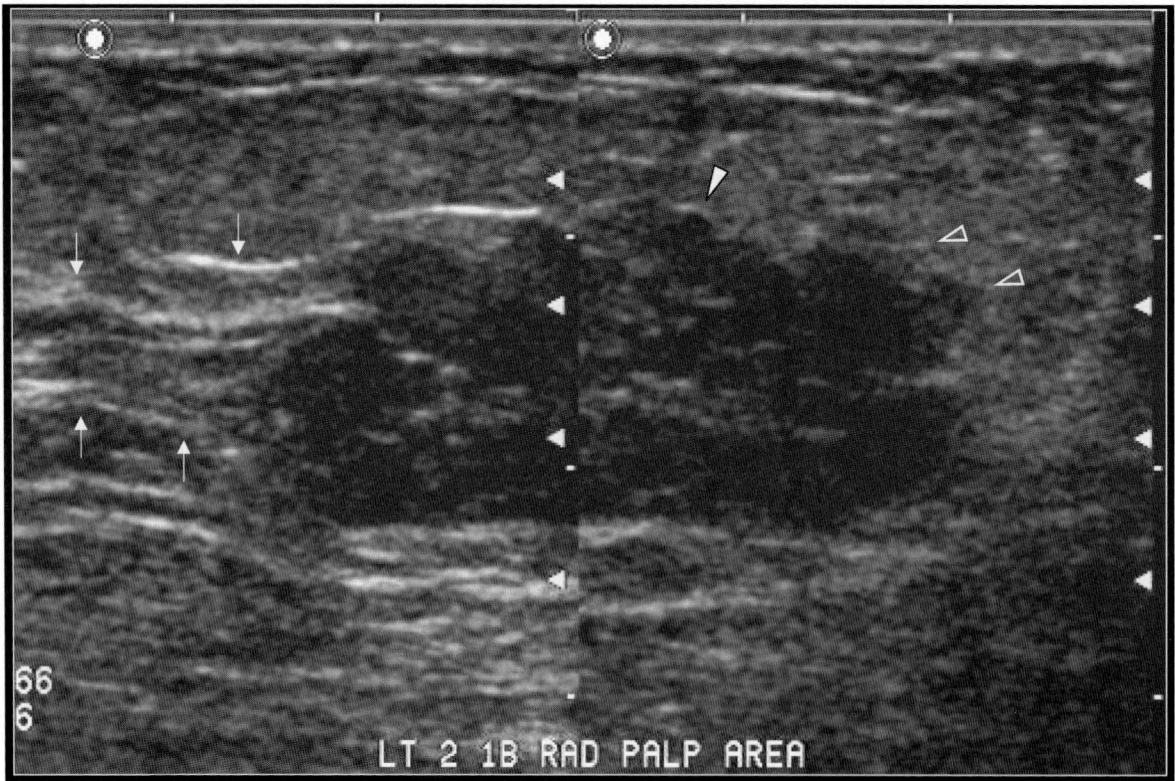

FIGURE 14–33 The surface characteristics of this mixed invasive and intraductal not otherwise specified carcinoma are a mixture of soft and hard findings. Along the left side of the lesion are spiculations *(arrows)*, a hard finding indicating the presence of invasion. Around the right three-fourths of the surface is a thin, echogenic capsule. However, other soft suspicious findings, such as microlobulation *(solid white arrowhead)*, and hard suspicious findings, such as angular margins *(hollow arrowheads)*, are present in association with the thin capsule.

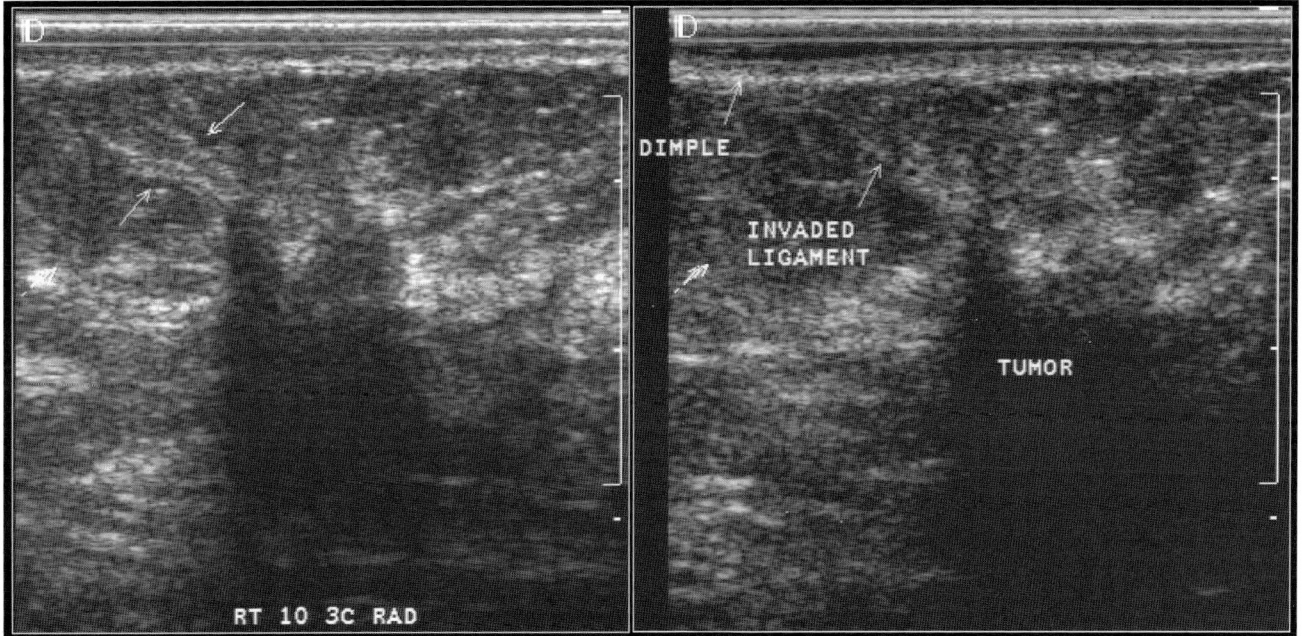

FIGURE 14–34 The normal supine scan technique with moderate compression pressure obscures subtle signs of skin dimpling. The **left** image, obtained with normal supine scan techniques, shows an invasive carcinoma nodule that has invaded the base of several Cooper's ligaments *(arrows)*, placing traction on them, but not causing visible skin dimpling. The **right** image was obtained with the patient upright and with a thin standoff of acoustic gel. Dimpling caused by traction on Cooper's ligaments *(arrow)* is now evident.

poechoic spiculations are better demonstrated when nearly parallel to the beam (Fig. 14–35). Spiculations that are very short and close together can present as an ill-defined thick, echogenic halo rather than individual spiculations. The thick, echogenic halo usually appears widest and brightest along the edges of the nodule, where the spicules are nearly perpendicular to the beam and where they make strong spicular reflectors. The halo usually appears thinnest and least echogenic on the anterior and posterior surfaces of the lesion, where the spicules are nearly parallel to the ultrasound beam and make very weak spicular reflectors (Fig. 14–36). Of course, the ability to demonstrate a thick, echogenic halo around an invasive NOS carcinoma depends on the type of tissue that surrounds the lesion. When the lesion is surrounded by fat, the hyperechoic halo is readily apparent against the isoechoic background. However, when the malignant nodule is surrounded by hyperechoic fibrous tissue, the halo is relatively inapparent and difficult to demonstrate (Fig. 14–37).

Some malignant NOS carcinomas are spiculated over part of their surfaces and circumscribed over other parts. In lesions that have mixed invasive and DCIS components, the invasion typically is most pronounced peripherally, and the intraductal components are most pronounced centrally. Thus, spiculation or a thick, echogenic halo commonly oc-

curs along the peripheral aspect of a lesion, whereas soft findings that represent DCIS components of the lesion, such as microlobulation and duct extension, lie centrally (Fig. 14–38).

Low- to intermediate-grade invasive NOS carcinomas that are high in stromal fibrous content are more likely to be frankly spiculated than are high-grade lesions. High-grade NOS lesions, on the other hand, which have less fibrous stromal reaction, are less likely to be frankly spiculated and more likely to appear circumscribed (Fig. 14–39).

In certain cases, a thick, echogenic halo represents peritumoral edema rather than unresolved spiculations. Peritumoral edema can result from intense inflammatory host response to the lesion or can be caused by lymphedema resulting from lymphatic invasion. Peritumoral edema that results from an intense inflammatory response to high-grade invasive NOS carcinomas differs from spiculations in that it is equally well seen on the anterior and posterior surfaces of the lesion and because it is amorphous rather than linear in texture. Peritumoral edema that is the result of lymphatic invasion and obstruction is more often asymmetrically distributed. Because lymphatic drainage is toward the skin, peritumoral lymphedema is typically located superficial to the lesion. Both patterns of peritumoral edema are illustrated in Chapter 12 (see Fig. 12–17).

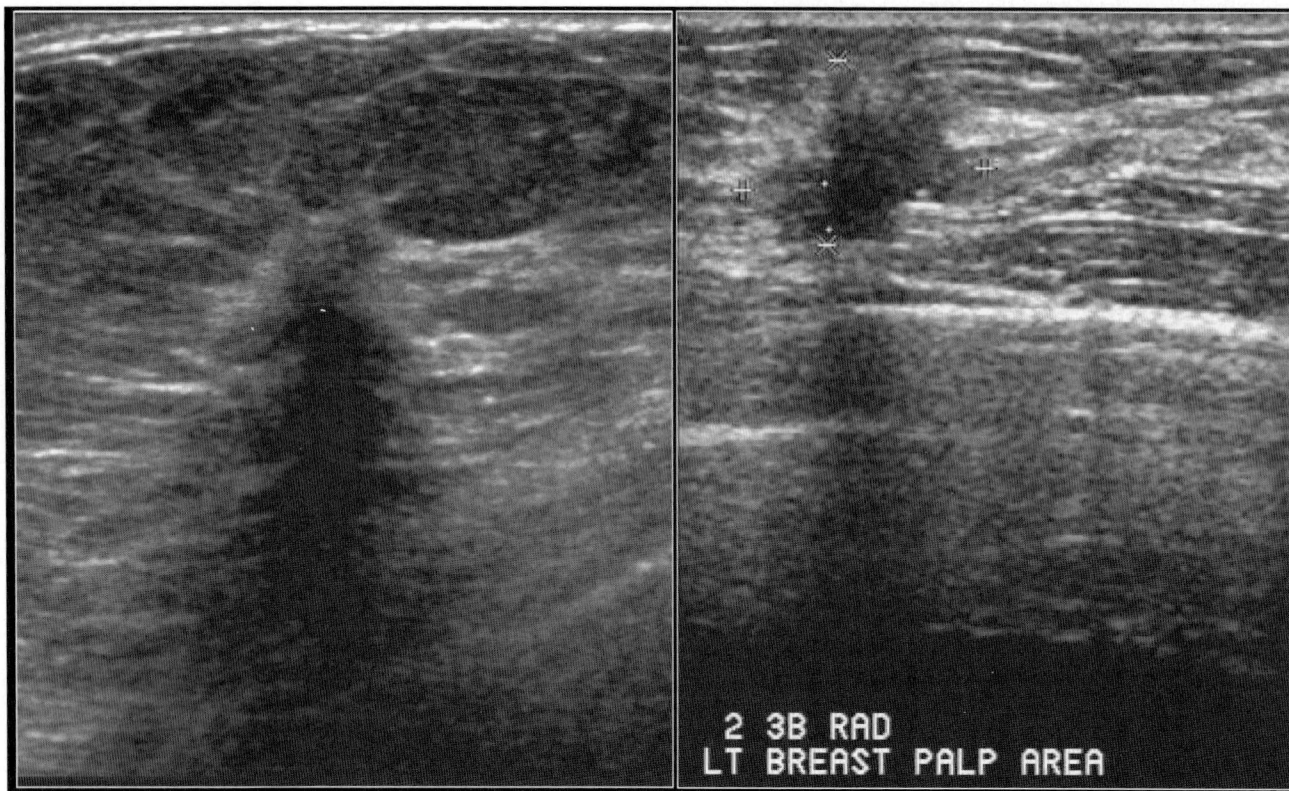

FIGURE 14–35 Frank hyperechoic spiculations are best seen around the edges of fat-surrounded lesions where they are nearly perpendicular to the beam (**left**). Frank hypoechoic spiculations are better seen in fibrous tissue–surrounded lesions where they are nearly parallel to the ultrasound beam (**right**, anterior surface of nodule).

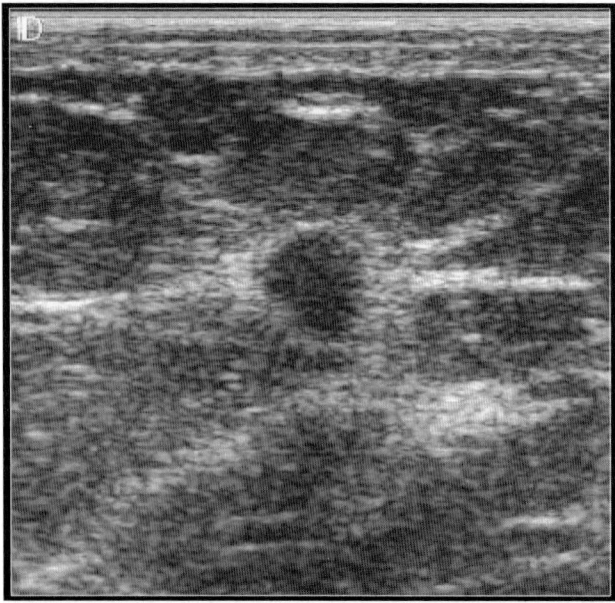

FIGURE 14–36 The thick, echogenic halo represents unresolved hyperechoic spiculations and is best seen and thickest along the edges of the nodule, where the spiculations are more nearly perpendicular to the ultrasound beam.

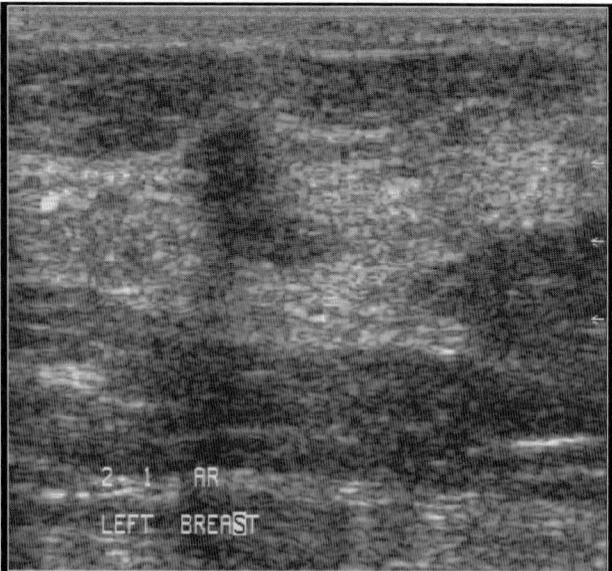

FIGURE 14–37 When invasive not otherwise specified carcinomas are surrounded by hyperechoic fibrous tissue, the thick, echogenic halo can be obscured by the equally echogenic surrounding fibrous tissue. If individual spicules are too small to resolve, neither frank spiculations nor a thick echogenic halo may be demonstrable.

Other Surface Characteristics of Invasive Not Otherwise Specified Carcinomas

Whether spiculated or not, invasive NOS carcinomas usually have angular, irregular, or microlobulated margins. Even high-grade malignant NOS carcinomas with thin, echogenic capsules usually have one or more angles in which the lesion invades the bases of Cooper's ligaments (Fig. 14–40). The histopathologic basis for angular margins is discussed and illustrated in detail in Chapter 12 (see Figs. 12–18 to 12–25).

Shape

Small invasive NOS carcinomas are frequently larger in the anteroposterior (AP) dimension than in the horizontal dimensions. The histopathologic bases for this finding are discussed and illustrated in detail in Chapter 12 (see Figs. 12–33 to 12–41). The shape of a small invasive NOS carcinoma reflects the shape of the TDLU in which it arose. Because the long axis of most TDLUs is oriented in the AP direction, most normal TDLUs appear taller than wide. A small invasive NOS carcinoma that involves only a single vertically oriented TDLU will also appear to be taller than wide (Figs. 14–26 and 14–27; see also Chapter 12, Fig. 12–40). As the malignant lesion enlarges and spreads intraductally through the horizontally ori-

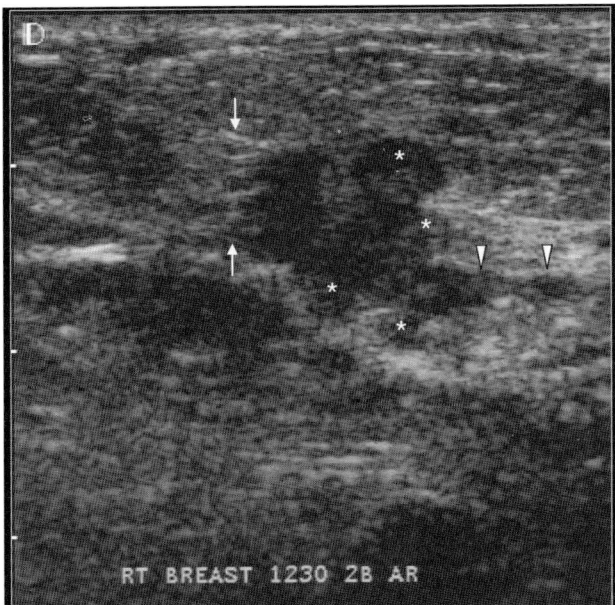

FIGURE 14–38 In mixed invasive and intraductal not otherwise specified carcinomas, the resistance to invasion appears to be lowest peripherally, and the resistance to intraductal spread appears to be lowest centrally. Thus, when there is a mixture of hard findings of invasion and soft findings suggestive of intraductal growth, the hard findings, such as spiculations *(arrows)*, tend to occur peripherally, whereas the soft findings, such as duct extension *(arrowheads)* and microlobulation (* indicates cancerized lobules), tend to occur centrally.

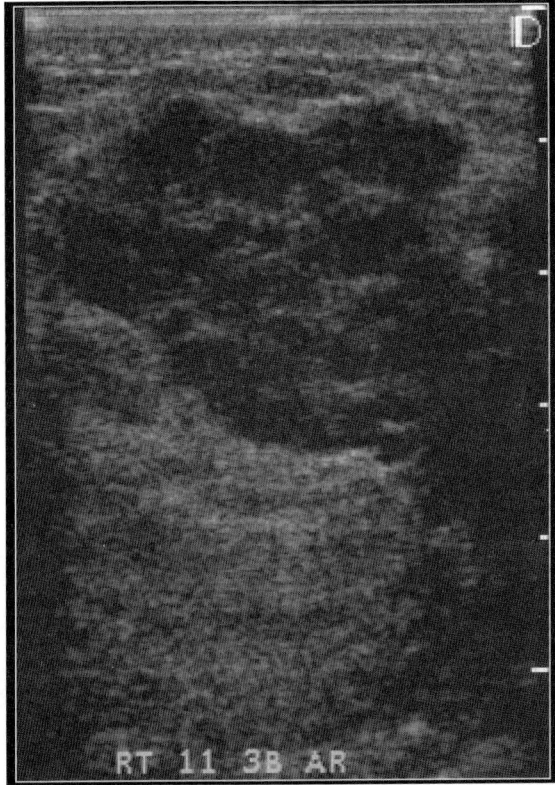

FIGURE 14–39 The higher the histologic grade of invasive not otherwise specified carcinoma, the more likely its margins are to appear well circumscribed sonographically, and the less likely it is that the lesion will appear to be frankly spiculated.

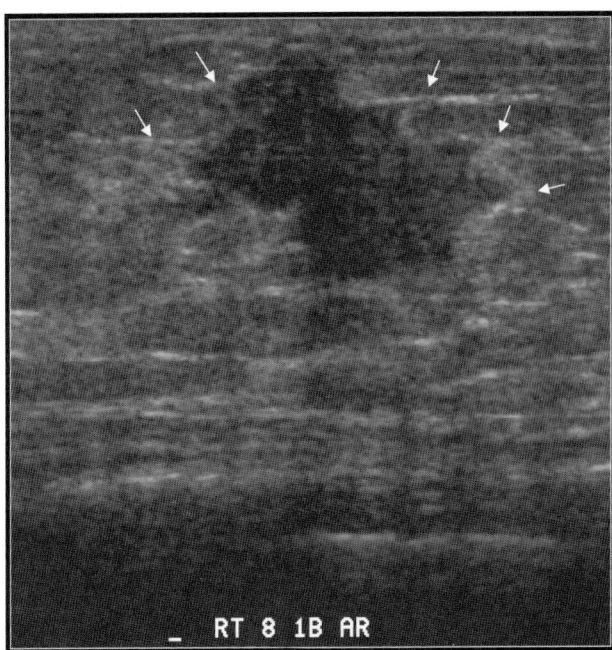

FIGURE 14–40 Invasive not otherwise specified (NOS) carcinomas of any grade tend to have angular margins. The most common location for angular margins is where Cooper's ligaments intersect the surface of the nodule *(arrows)*. Even high-grade invasive NOS carcinomas that are encompassed in thin, echogenic pseudocapsules usually have angular margins.

ented lobar ductal system, the growth axis of the lesion will change from the AP dimension to a horizontal dimension, and the lesion will have a tendency to become wider than tall (Fig. 14–28; see also Chapter 12, Fig. 12–41). Growth through the horizontally oriented ductal system explains why larger tumors are much less often taller than wide than are smaller lesions.

Duct extension from the main tumor nodule toward the nipple on radial scans usually indicates intraductal tumor growth within larger-order ducts but occasionally can be due to periductal invasive tumor with or without associated intraductal tumor. The histopathologic basis of duct extension is discussed and illustrated in detail in Chapter 12 (see Figs. 12–43 to 12–49). The loose periductal stromal fibrous tissue offers a relatively low-resistance path for growth of invasive tumor. Thus, in some cases, a duct extension might represent periductal tumor invasion rather than DCIS components. In other cases, periductal invasive NOS carcinomas surrounds DCIS components of disease within the duct lumen, creating the "duct within a duct" appearance histologically. The chief significance of this pattern is the potential by an inexperienced pathologist to mistake this growth for purely intraductal noninvasive growth. The segment of the duct involved with periductal invasion appears focally wider than the segment of duct that contains only intraductal tumor (Fig. 14–41).

Branch pattern indicates either peripherally growing fingers of invasive tumor infiltrating breast tissues around the central nidus or, less often, intraductal growth in small ducts away from the nipple. The histopathologic basis of branch pattern is discussed and illustrated in detail in Chapter 12 (see Figs. 12–43 to 12–50). Branch pattern can be caused by fingers of invasive tumor as well as by intraductal components of tumor. When the apparent branches are very small, it can be difficult to determine whether branch pattern represents DCIS or invasive components of the lesion (Fig. 14–42).

For the most part, we agree with Teboul and Halliwell that the most important shapes in the breast are those correlating with the underlying basic anatomy: the lobules, extralobular terminal ducts, larger order ducts, Cooper's ligaments, fat, and skin. Because the normal anatomic structures can be demonstrated by scanning in planes that are parallel and perpendicular to the long axes of the breast lobes, these structures can be evaluated for abnormal solid enlargement and architectural distortion, rather than simply evaluating the shape of a nodule in random planes. Even in patients in whom atrophy and regression have made normal structures inapparent, scanning in anatomic planes will allow determination of whether a nodule represents an enlarged TDLU and whether there is extension into other parts of the breast by invasion of normal structures or growth within abnormally enlarging ductal structures.

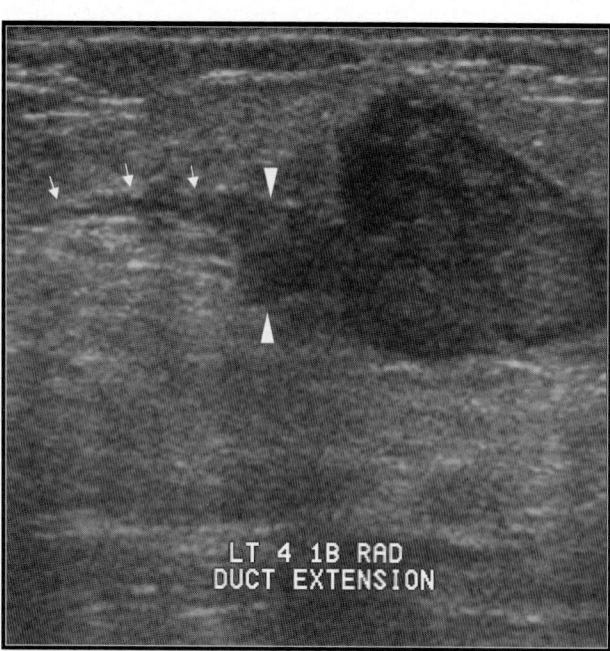

FIGURE 14–41 This intermediate-grade invasive not otherwise specified lesion has ductal carcinoma *in situ* components growing within the lobar duct toward the nipple *(arrows)*. Additionally, a portion of the duct extension is focally wider than the rest of the duct *(arrowheads)* and represents an area where carcinoma has invaded the periductal tissues. Histologically, this area showed the "duct-in-duct" appearance.

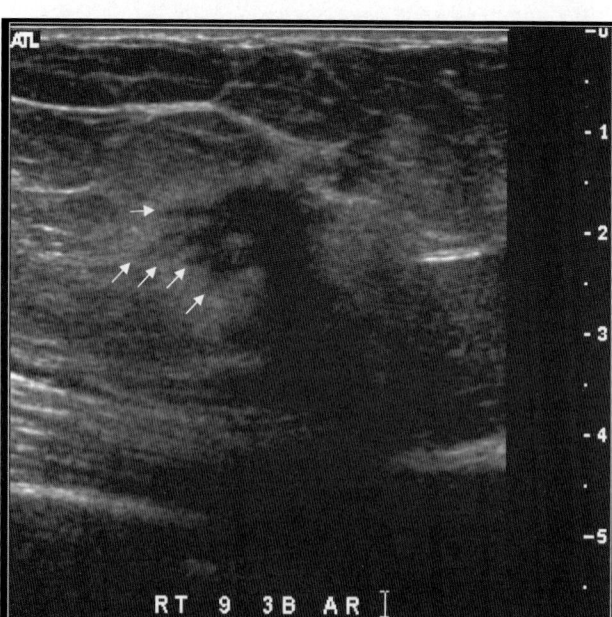

FIGURE 14–42 In mixed invasive and intraductal not otherwise specified carcinoma. branch pattern *(arrows)* suggests the presence of ductal carcinoma *in situ* elements growing into peripherally located ducts that surround the lesion.

Histologic Grade of Invasive Not Otherwise Specified Carcinoma

The histologic grade will affect the appearance of invasive NOS carcinomas, both directly and indirectly. Tumor grade directly affects sound transmission, margin characteristics, the presence or absence of duct extension, and the size of microlobulations and branch patterns. Histologic grade directly affects the sonographic appearance because high-grade lesions are often larger, are infiltrated by lymphocytes, have areas of necrosis, and are far more likely to have abundant blood flow that is demonstrable by color or power Doppler. (Doppler assessment of histologic grade is discussed in Chapter 20.) The differences in sonographic appearance owing to tumor grade occur reliably enough for sonography to suggest histologic grade of the lesion.

Suspicion that the lesion is of high histologic grade can be useful to the radiologist, the surgeon, and even the oncologist. Sonographic appearances indicating that the lesion is high grade suggest the need to look closely for multifocal or multicentric lesions, EICs, and lymph node metastases. Sonographic suspicion of multicentricity, EICs, and positive axillary nodes can all be verified by ultrasound-guided core needle biopsies performed at the same time the primary lesion undergoes biopsy; that is, the extent of malignant disease can be mapped out before surgery with carefully targeted, ultrasound-guided needle biopsies. Armed with a more thorough knowledge of the extent of tumor, the surgeon and oncologist can better decide on the need for preoperative or postoperative adjuvant therapy, the extent of surgery, and the need for axillary dissection.

The tendency for high-grade lesions to be more cellular, to have more hyaluronic acid in the extracellular matrix, and to incite lymphoplasmacytic rather than fibroelastotic host response compared with low-grade lesions results in greater water content and in better sound transmission through high-grade NOS carcinomas than through low-grade lesions. In fact, most high-grade NOS carcinomas have enhanced through-transmission (Fig. 14–43). Cystic or hemorrhagic necrosis that commonly occurs in high-grade invasive NOS carcinomas also contributes to enhanced through-transmission.

Low-grade NOS carcinomas are less cellular, have more collagen and less hyaluronic acid in the extracellular matrix, incite more desmoplastic and less inflammatory response, and contain less water than do high-grade NOS lesions. Low-grade NOS carcinomas most often cause acoustic shadowing and are associated with thick, echogenic halos or frank spiculation (Fig. 14–44). Low-grade NOS carcinomas are less prone than high-grade lesions to undergo cystic or hemorrhagic necrosis.

Intermediate-grade lesions have histologic features that lie between those of high-grade and low-grade NOS carcinomas. Intermediate-grade invasive NOS carcinomas have the most variable sound transmission and are the least

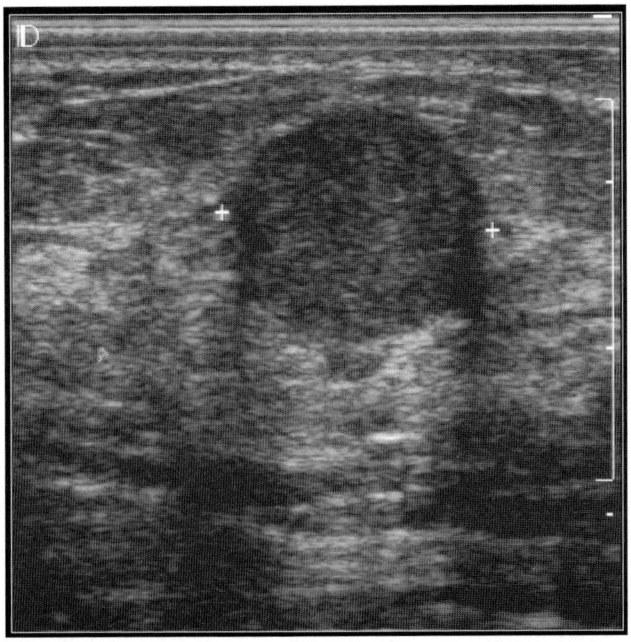

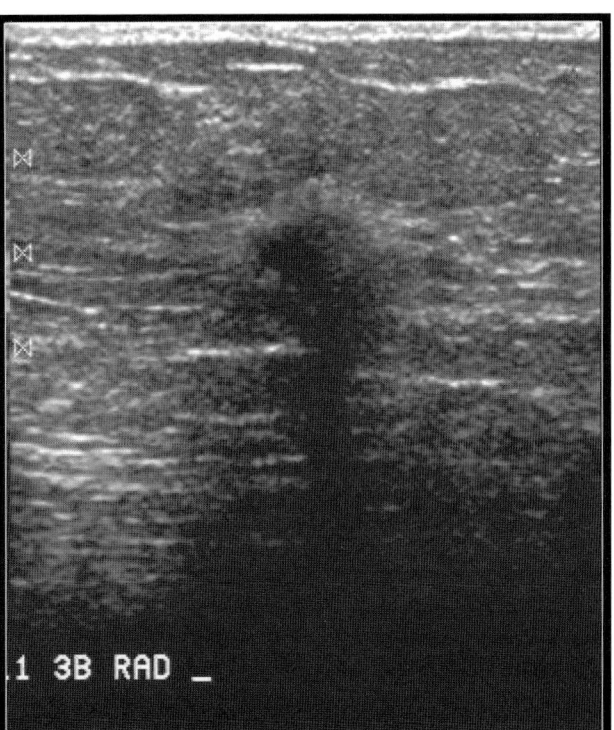

FIGURE 14–43 Because high-grade invasive not otherwise specified carcinomas are highly cellular and have little desmoplasia, they typically demonstrate enhanced sound transmission.

FIGURE 14–44 Low-grade invasive not otherwise specified carcinomas larger than 15 mm in diameter typically cast acoustic shadows because of the relatively large amounts of desmoplasia present within them.

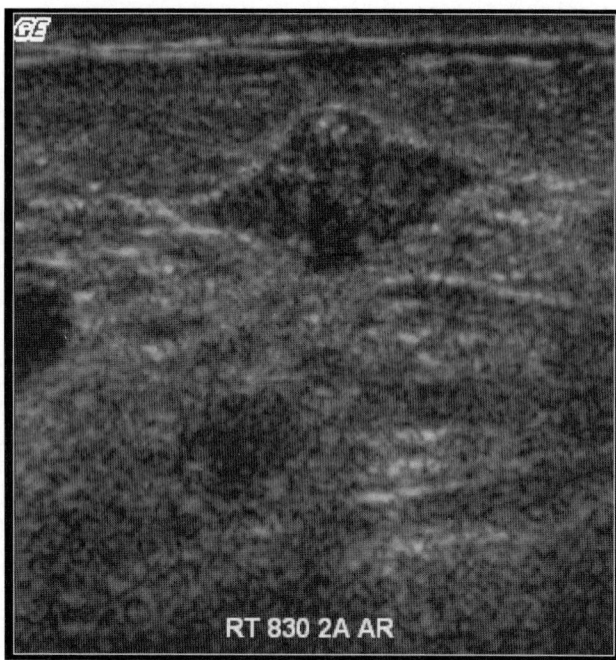

FIGURE 14–45 Intermediate-grade invasive not otherwise specified (NOS) carcinomas most commonly have normal sound transmission, but many cast acoustic shadows. The sound transmission characteristics of intermediate-grade invasive NOS carcinomas overlap those of low-grade lesions.

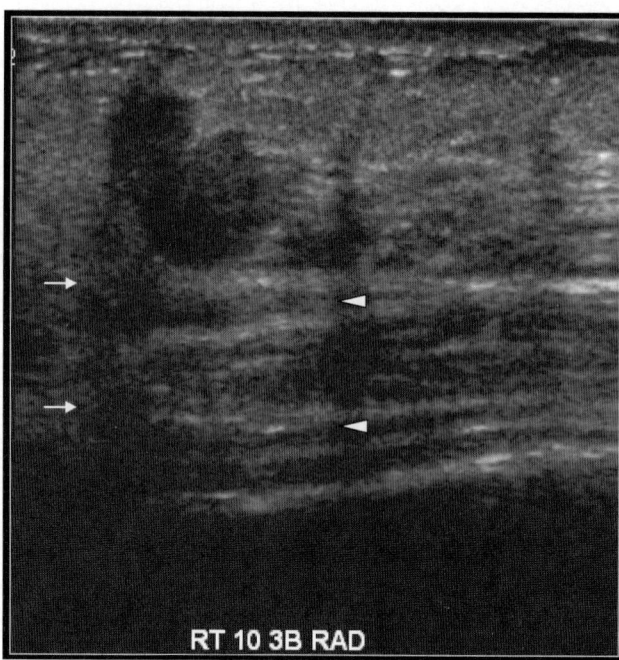

FIGURE 14–46 Intermediate-grade invasive not otherwise specified carcinomas frequently exhibit mixed sound transmission, containing foci of normal, increased *(arrowheads)*, and decreased sound transmission *(arrows)*.

reliably graded based on the degree of sound transmission. Most intermediate lesions have transmission similar to surrounding tissues (Fig. 14–45), but many cause acoustic shadowing similar to that of low-grade lesions. A few may even demonstrate enhanced through-transmission. Furthermore, it is not unusual for intermediate-grade invasive NOS carcinomas to show mixed sound transmission. Small foci exhibiting enhanced through-transmission, acoustic shadowing, and normal sound transmission may all coexist in the same lesion (Fig. 14–46).

The presence of enhanced through-transmission more than doubles the risk that the lesion is high grade, and the presence of acoustic shadowing halves the risk for the lesion being high grade (Figs. 14–47 and 14–48). The presence of enhanced through-transmission is a stronger predictor that invasive NOS carcinoma is high grade than acoustic shadowing is a predictor of low grade. Acoustic shadowing is not very useful in distinguishing between low- and intermediate-grade invasive NOS because many intermediate-grade invasive NOS carcinomas cast acoustic shadows.

Unfortunately, the maximum diameter of the invasive NOS carcinomatous nodule confounds the ability of sound transmission to predict the histologic grade. Apparently, a malignant nodule must reach a critical size before the histologic features that affect sound transmission cause their characteristic effects on sound transmission. In our experience, that critical size appears to be a maximum diameter of 1.5 cm. This means that low-grade lesions 1.5 cm or greater in maximum diameter cause the expected acoustic shadowing in a very high percentage of cases, but lesions less than 1.5 cm in diameter often have normal sound transmission. High-grade invasive NOS carcinomas 1.5 cm or greater in diameter demonstrate enhanced through-transmission in a very high percentage of cases, but high-grade lesions less than 1.5 cm in diameter tend to have normal through-transmission. Intermediate-grade invasive NOS carcinomas less than 1.5 cm in diameter tend to have either normal through-transmission or to cause acoustic shadowing, whereas intermediate-grade lesions 1.5 cm in diameter usually show mixed patterns of sound transmission.

The margins of the nodule also are affected by tumor grade. The classic appearance of spicules and the thick, ill-defined halo are largely related to the presence of desmoplastic reaction that is typically associated with low- and intermediate-grade lesions. High-grade lesions tend to have less prominent spiculations mammographically or sonographically even though they may be spiculated microscopically. High-grade lesions are more likely to appear grossly circumscribed on imaging studies.

The histologic grade of the invasive NOS carcinoma affects the relative sizes of the thick, echogenic halo and the central hypoechoic tumor nidus. Low-grade invasive NOS

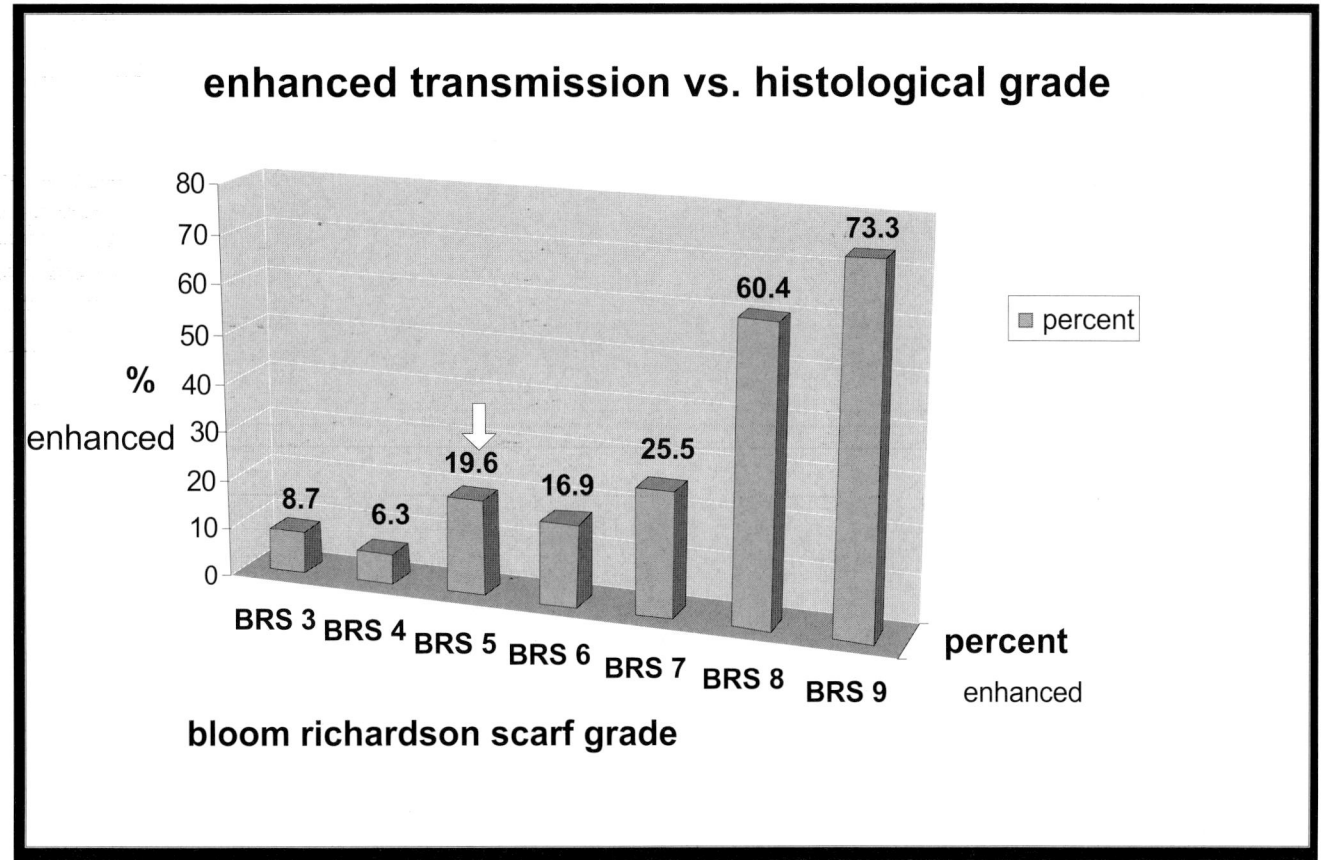

FIGURE 14–47 This bar graph shows percentage of invasive not otherwise specified carcinomas that have enhanced through-transmission for each Bloom-Richardson-Scarf (BRS) histologic grade. Note that as the BRS grade of the lesion increases, the chances of its demonstrating enhanced through-transmission increase. The increase is most marked for BRS grade 8 and 9, which are high-grade lesions. Note also that BRS grade 5 lesions *(hollow arrow)* have sound transmission more similar to intermediate-grade (BRS 6 and 7) than to low-grade lesions (BRS 3 and 4). BRS 5 lesions are considered intermediate grade histologically.

carcinomas have relatively prominent thick, echogenic halos in comparison to the hypoechoic central tumor nidus, whereas intermediate-grade lesions tend to have larger central tumor nodules in comparison to the thick, echogenic halos. High-grade NOS carcinomas tend to have thin, echogenic capsules (Fig. 14–49). It is common for the thick, echogenic halo to be wider than the diameter of the central nidus in low-grade lesions. Additionally, the uniformity of the thickness of the halo is affected by the grade of the lesion. A uniformly thick, echogenic halo is more typically of a low-grade invasive ductal carcinoma, whereas variable thickness of the halo or involvement of only part of the tumor margin by spiculations or thick halo favors the lesion being intermediate or high grade. As an invasive NOS carcinoma enlarges, it tends to dedifferentiate and develop clones of higher-grade tumor cells. The halo around the lower-grade portions of the lesion tends to be thicker, whereas the halo around the less differentiated, higher-grade portions of the lesion tends to be relatively thinner.

The histologic grade also affects the sonographic appearance of microlobulations and branch patterns. Most invasive NOS carcinomas have DCIS components that can manifest as microlobulations, duct extension, or branch pattern. In most cases, the nuclear grade of the DCIS components is similar to the histologic grade of the invasive component of the invasive NOS lesions. Thus, high-grade invasive NOS carcinomas tend to have HNG DCIS components, and low-grade invasive NOS carcinomas tend to have LNG DCIS components. As noted in the DCIS section, HNG DCIS is more likely to enlarge ducts and TDLUs grossly than is LNG DCIS. HNG DCIS components have more tumor cells and necrosis within the lumen and also incite more periductal fibrotic stromal or inflammatory reaction than do LNG DCIS components. Thus, the soft suspicious findings that represent the DCIS components of high-grade invasive NOS carcinomas (microlobulations and branch pattern) tend to be larger than those associated with low-grade NOS carci-

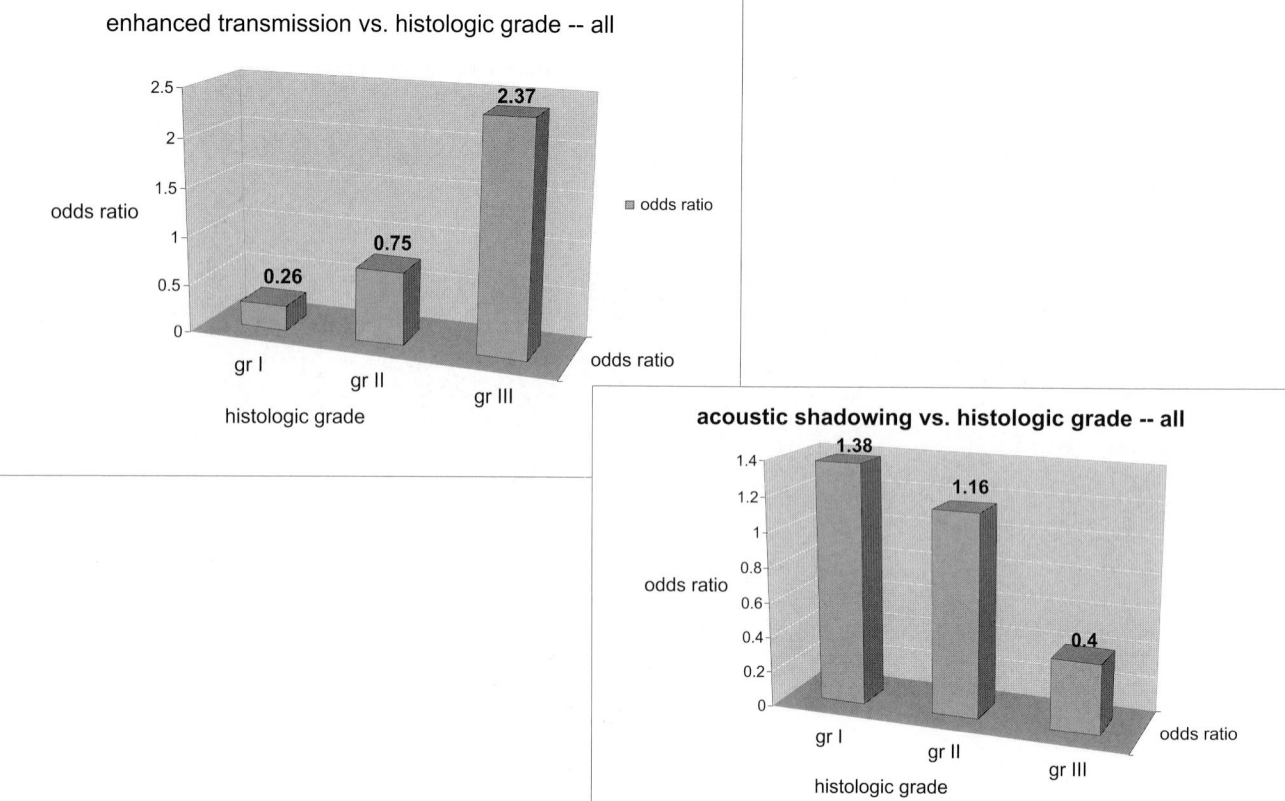

FIGURE 14–48 These bar graphs show the odds ratio of a lesion being high grade versus enhanced through-transmission (**upper left**) and acoustic shadowing (**lower right**). Note that the presence of enhanced sound transmission is a much stronger predictor of an invasive NOS carcinoma being high grade than shadowing is a predictor of such a lesion being low grade. The presence of enhanced through-transmission more than doubles the risk (over prevalence of 27%) that a lesion is high grade (**upper left**). Acoustic shadowing, on the other hand, reduces the risk for a lesion being high grade to less than half. The presence of acoustic shadowing only increases the risk for a lesion being low grade by a factor of 1.38 because many lesions that cause acoustic shadowing are intermediate grade.

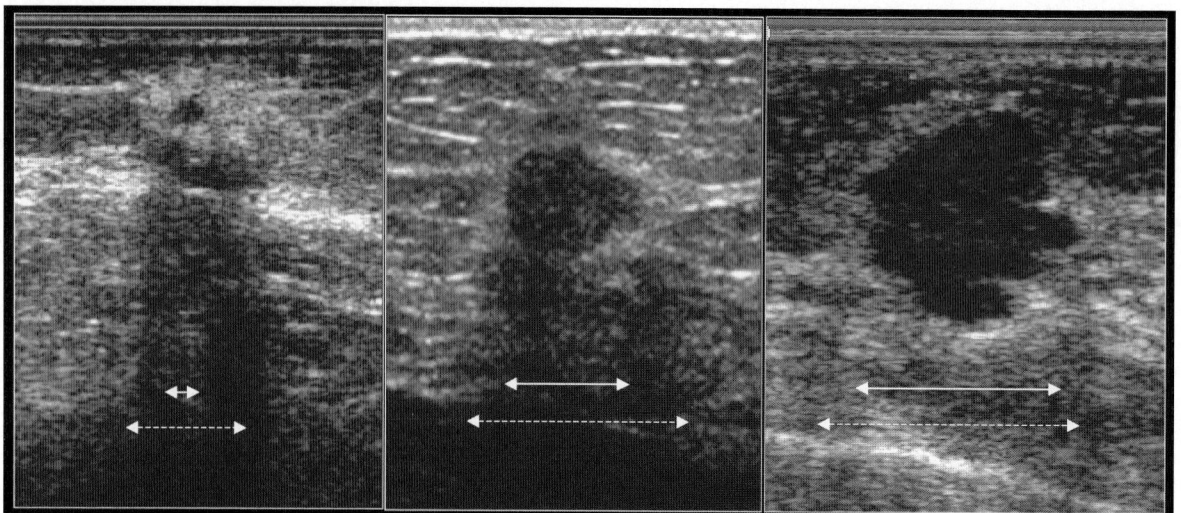

FIGURE 14–49 The thicker the echogenic halo relative to the size of the hypoechoic central tumor nidus, the greater the chances that an invasive not otherwise specified carcinoma is low grade. Lesions with very thick halos and a very small central tumor nidus are typically low grade (**left**). Lesions in which the halo is less thick than the diameter of the central nidus tend to be intermediate grade (**middle**). High-grade lesions have thin, echogenic capsules or echogenic haloes that are relatively thin in comparison to the central hypoechoic tumor nidus (**right**, *solid line* indicates central nidus size, *dotted line* indicates size of lesion including thick, echogenic halo).

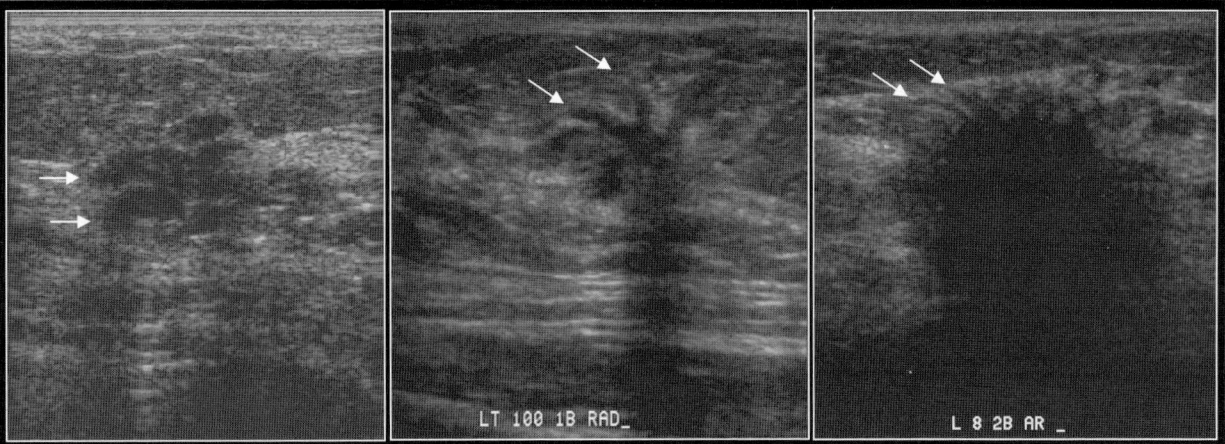

FIGURE 14–50 The size of branch pattern is correlated with the histologic grade of invasive not otherwise specified carcinomas. Large branch patterns suggest the presence of high-nuclear-grade ductal carcinoma *in situ* components and high-grade invasive lesions (**left**). Intermediate-sized branch ducts suggest the presence of an intermediate-grade lesion (**middle**). Very small branches suggest the presence of a low-grade lesion (**right**).

nomas. The size of branch pattern correlates with the histologic grade of invasive NOS carcinoma. Large branching ducts suggest a high-grade lesion, very small ducts that are difficult to distinguish from spiculations suggest the presence of a low-grade lesion, and intermediate-sized ducts suggest the presence of an intermediate-grade lesion (Fig. 14–50). Large microlobulations suggest the presence of a high-grade lesion, small microlobulations suggest the presence of a low-grade lesion, and intermediate-sized microlobulations suggest an intermediate-sized lesions (Fig. 14–51).

The higher the histologic grade of the invasive NOS carcinoma, the more likely prominent duct extensions are to occur. However, the diameter of the duct extension does not reflect the histologic grade of the lesion because duct extension so often involves the lactiferous sinus portion of the lobar duct, which is so distensible that even low-grade DCIS components of invasive NOS carcinoma can distend the duct to several millimeters in diameter.

In summary, several sonographic features are affected by the histologic grade of the lesion. The histologic grade of invasive NOS carcinomas affects sound transmission; spicula-

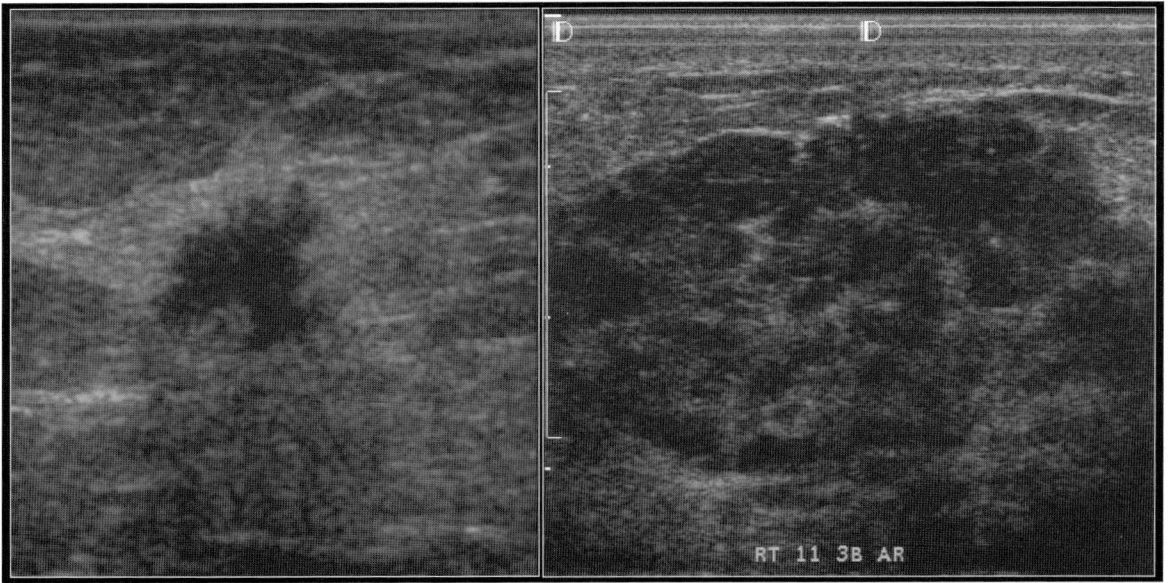

FIGURE 14–51 The size of microlobulations correlates with the histologic grade of invasive not otherwise specified carcinomas. Small microlobulations suggest the presence of low-nuclear-grade ductal carcinoma *in situ* components and low-grade invasive components (**left**). Large microlobulations suggest the presence of a high-grade lesion (**right**).

tions; thick, echogenic halo; size of branch pattern and microlobulations; and Doppler demonstrable vascularity. A thorough understanding of the histopathologic basis of these findings can help us to assess the histologic grade of the lesion as well as characterizing lesions into BIRADS categories.

Fibrous Stromal Reaction—Desmoplasia

The degree of desmoplastic response affects several sonographic features of invasive NOS carcinomas—echogenicity, sound transmission, spiculation, and thick, ill-defined, echogenic capsule.

Desmoplastic NOS lesions transmit sound poorly and cast acoustic shadows of varying degrees. In general, the greater the desmoplastic response within and surrounding a lesion, the more uniform and intense will be the shadowing. Lesions with a large component of desmoplastic reaction are typically markedly hypoechoic with respect to fat. This phenomenon is paradoxical because normal interlobular stromal fibrous tissue is hyperechoic. In some markedly hypoechoic lesions, intense shadowing contributes to the apparent hypoechogenicity. The sonographic appearance of frank spiculation or the presence of a thick, ill-defined echogenic capsule around an invasive NOS carcinoma is also strongly correlated with the presence of marked desmoplastic reaction in the periphery of the nodule.

Although most invasive NOS carcinomas incite a degree of fibrous stromal reaction, the desmoplasia is most pronounced in lower-grade lesions and least pronounced in higher-grade lesions. Therefore, the presence of marked hypoechogenicity, intense shadowing, and a very prominent, thick, ill-defined echogenic capsule or frank spiculations tends to be associated with low-grade (grade I) NOS carcinomas.

Desmoplasia directly affects the hardness and compressibility of NOS carcinomas. Lesions that have intense desmoplastic response are usually of lower grade and are relatively noncompressible. Intermediate-grade lesions, which have intermediate degrees of desmoplasia, are often minimally compressible (up to about 10%). However, high-grade lesions, which are very cellular, have little desmoplastic response, and are prone to cystic necrotic change, may compress up to 15%, similar to the compressibility of cellular or myxoid fibroadenomas (Fig. 14–52).

The presence of desmoplasia is inversely related to the amount of blood flow that is demonstrable within the lesion using color Doppler. Desmoplasia requires very little blood flow. Invasive NOS carcinomas with large components of desmoplasia usually have either no demonstrable internal flow or very little internal flow. Whatever flow is present is usually along the periphery of the nodule, where tumor cells are most numerous and tumor growth is most active. A contributing factor to the lack of demonstrable internal flow is acoustic shadowing, which may prevent demonstration of what little central flow is present.

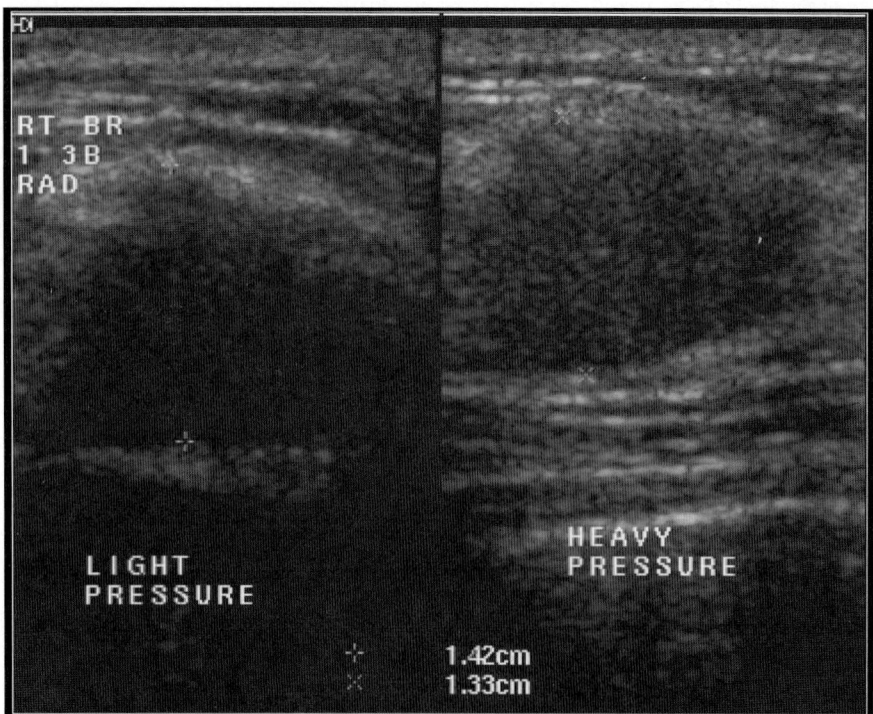

FIGURE 14–52 High-grade invasive not otherwise specified (NOS) carcinomas, such as this lesion, can be partially compressible because they have relatively little desmoplasia. This high-grade invasive NOS carcinoma compressed 6%.

Inflammatory Infiltrates

The presence of lymphocytic (or plasma cell) infiltrates also affects several sonographic features of invasive NOS carcinomas, including echogenicity, sound transmission, and capsular characteristics. Inflammation and desmoplasia represent different types of host response to the tumor and appear to be inversely proportional to one another in amount. Lesions that have abundant lymphocytic infiltrate usually have relatively smaller amounts of desmoplasia, whereas lesions that have abundant desmoplasia tend to have less abundant inflammatory response. It seems that the type of reaction incited depends on the degree of tumor cell differentiation. Desmoplasia tends to predominate in low- to intermediate-grade NOS lesions, whereas lymphocytic infiltrates tend to predominate in high-grade or intermediate-grade lesions. Normal epithelial and myoepithelial cells can stimulate growth of the supporting stromal elements. Well-differentiated, low-grade, invasive NOS lesions appear to maintain this ability to a certain degree, which is manifested as desmoplasia. These low-grade tumors may also be closer (in regard to antigen characteristics) to normal epithelial cells, may not be recognized as immunologically foreign and therefore are less likely to stimulate a cell-mediated lymphocytic immune response. High-grade lesions, being less well differentiated, may lose the ability to stimulate supportive stromal growth and may have fewer antigens in common with normal epithelial elements, thereby appearing more foreign and inciting a greater lymphocytic immune response. Furthermore, the earlier access of high-grade lesions to the lymphatic and vascular systems may lead to an earlier and more intense systemic immune response to the tumor. Finally, the presence of necrosis likely releases large amounts of antigen, inciting a more intense host immune response.

Intense lymphocytic reaction contributes to the hypoechogenicity of and sound transmission through certain high-grade invasive NOS carcinomas. This is not surprising because lymphomas, pure collections of lymphocytes, can appear to be nearly anechoic (pseudocystic appearance) and have enhanced sound transmission.

Because breast cancers are heterogeneous, and the histologic grade of the lesion may vary from location to location within the lesion, the distribution of lymphocytes within invasive NOS breast carcinomas may not be uniform, leading to heterogeneous echogenicity and variable sound transmission. In most invasive NOS breast carcinomas, the lymphocytic host response is most intense in the periphery of the lesion and can give rise to peritumoral inflammatory echogenic edema that can simulate the thick, echogenic halo caused by unresolved hyperechoic spiculations.

Tumor Necrosis

Invasive NOS carcinomas are prone to central ischemia and necrosis. Tumor sizes above 2 mm require tumor neovascularity to enable continued growth. The areas of rapid growth in malignant nodules lie in the periphery of the lesion, so this is where most of the neovascularity develops. The centers of growing malignant lesion are less well vascularized. Rapidly growing carcinomas may outgrow their blood supply, precipitating necrosis, which is most likely to occur in the less well-vascularized interior of the lesion.

Necrosis most commonly occurs in rapidly growing high-grade invasive NOS carcinomas, but it can occur in intermediate-grade lesions. The type of necrosis and its sonographic appearance varies with the histologic grade of the lesion. Acute liquefactive necrosis occurs most commonly in high-grade invasive NOS breast carcinomas, whereas chronic necrosis that heals with echogenic fibrous scarring is more typical of intermediate-grade lesions. Areas of necrosis within low-grade lesions are uncommon and are usually too small to be detectable sonographically.

At sonography, acute tumor necrosis within high-grade invasive NOS carcinomas is usually manifested as areas of cystic or hemorrhagic change within the interior of the solid mass that contribute to enhance sound transmission (Fig. 14–53). The areas of cystic change within such lesions are usually relatively small compared with the total volume of the mass, so there should be little chance of confusing such a lesion for a simple cyst. However, in rare

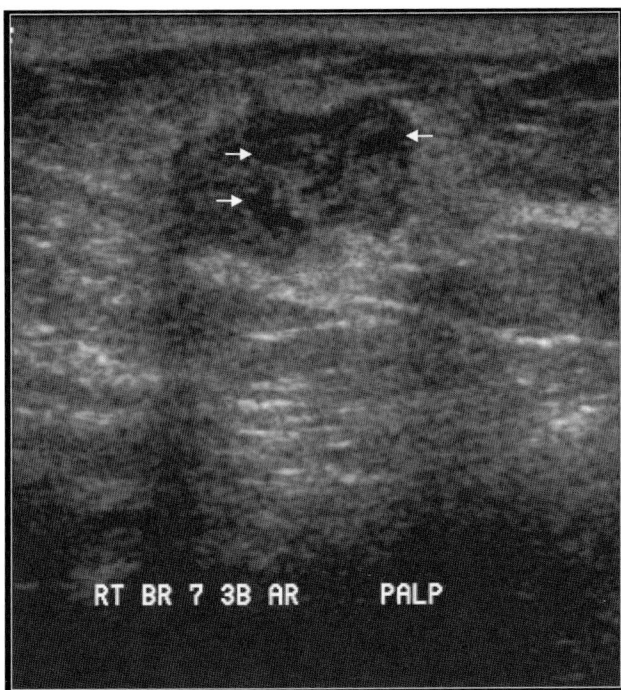

FIGURE 14–53 Areas of cystic necrosis *(arrows)* within invasive not otherwise specified (NOS) carcinomas are more likely to occur in rapidly growing high-grade lesions. This high-grade invasive NOS carcinoma also has an echogenic halo of peritumoral edema.

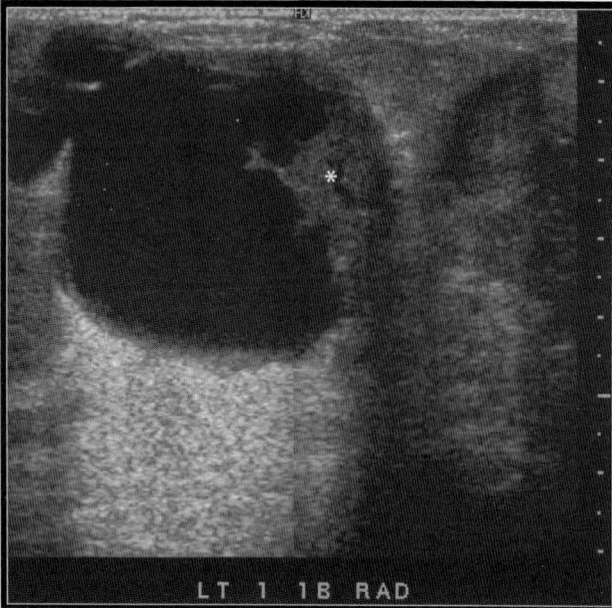

FIGURE 14–54 This high-grade invasive not otherwise specified carcinoma has undergone extensive necrosis, leaving residual tumor only along one wall *(*)*.

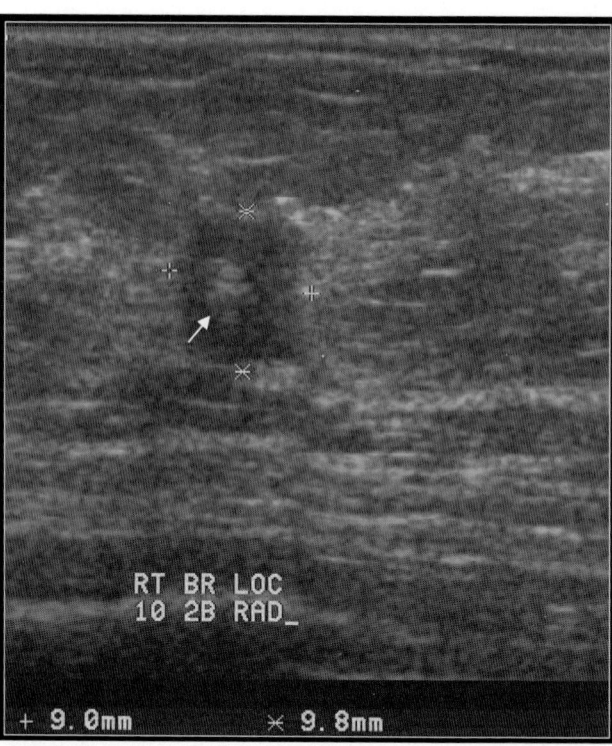

FIGURE 14–56 A radial scar with hyperechoic central fibroelastosis *(arrow)* surrounded by peripheral hypoechoic florid benign proliferative changes can simulate an intermediate-grade invasive not otherwise specified carcinoma with a hyperechoic central scar.

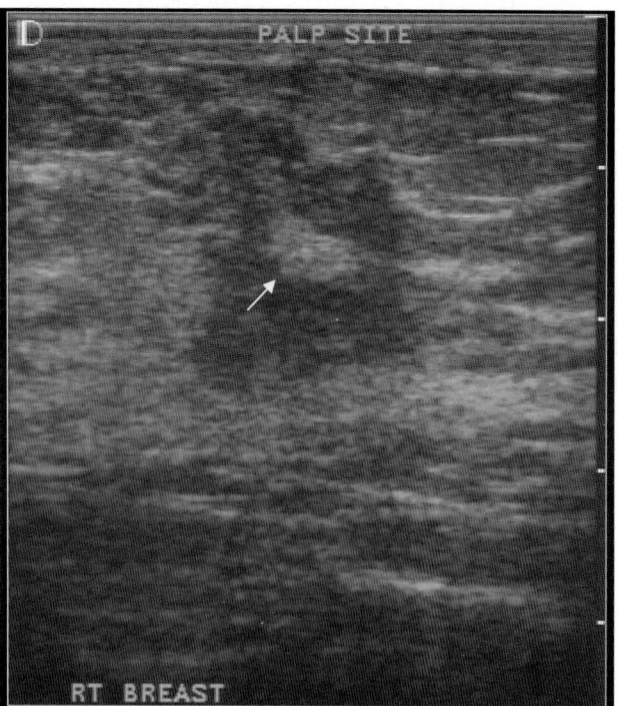

FIGURE 14–55 The necrosis within intermediate grade invasive not otherwise specified carcinomas is manifest by hyperechoic central scars *(arrow)* rather than the areas of cystic or hemorrhagic necrosis.

cases, virtually the entire tumor may undergo necrosis, leaving a large central cystic cavity and viable tumor only in the periphery (Fig. 14–54). When almost the entire lesion is necrotic, there may be enough floating debris that areas of cystic necrosis have the same echogenicity as the surrounding, markedly hypoechoic, solid components. Color Doppler may be helpful in such cases because blood flow frequently can be shown within hypoechoic solid parts of the tumor, but not within the areas of cystic degeneration (see Chapter 20, Figs. 20–32 and 20–95).

Areas of chronic necrosis that heal with fibrous scarring most commonly occur in intermediate-grade NOS breast carcinomas. Typically, the scar is centrally located, hyperechoic, and surrounded by a hypoechoic to isoechoic solid mass demonstrating hard suspicious features. When large, the appearance is classic for intermediate-grade NOS breast carcinoma (Fig. 14–55). When the lesion containing the hyperechoic central scar is small, the lesion will be indistinguishable from a radial scar that contains abundant proliferative change in the periphery (Fig. 14–56). Linnel has postulated that the group of invasive breast carcinomas classified as tubuloductal carcinomas arise within radial scars, which usually retain a remnant of the central scar. This could explain hyperechoic scars in some intermediate-

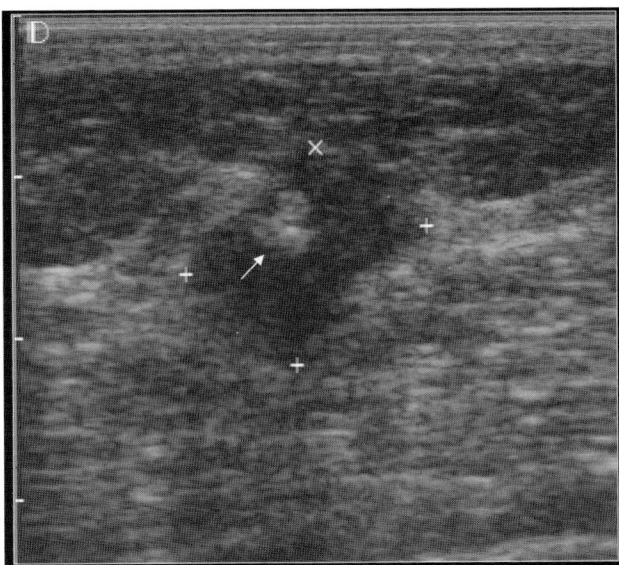

FIGURE 14–57 The compressed and distorted mediastinum *(arrow)* of a tumor-filled lymph node can simulate the appearance of the central fibrotic scar on an intermediate-grade invasive not otherwise specified carcinoma.

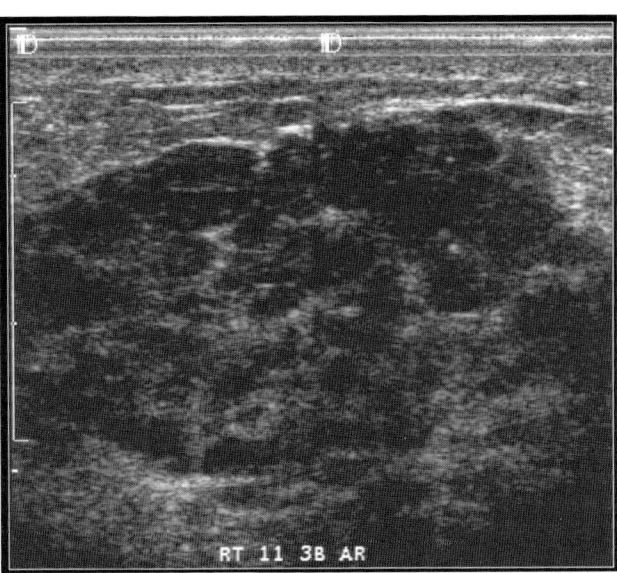

FIGURE 14–58 Heavy surface or internal lobulations suggest the presence of extensive intraductal components of tumor.

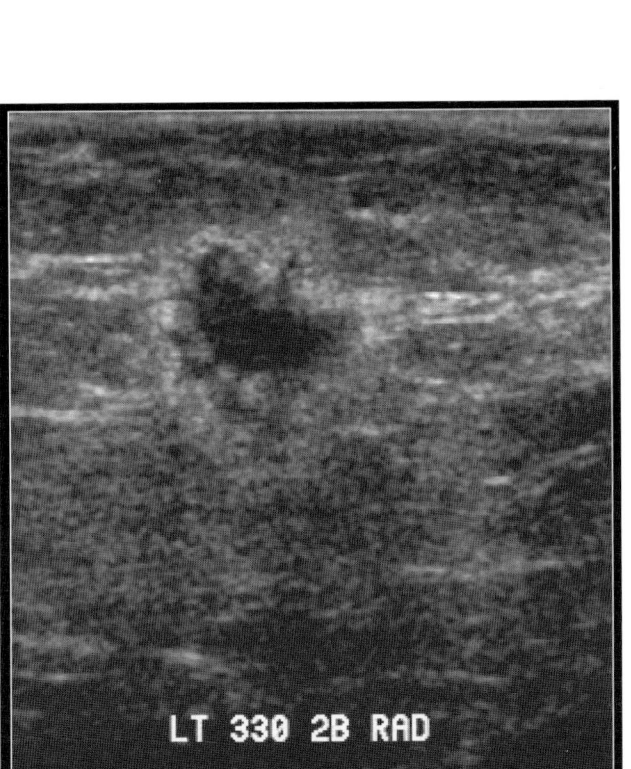

FIGURE 14–59 Heavy microlobulation that extends away from the main nodule into surrounding tissues suggests an increased likelihood of extensive intraductal components of tumor. In this case, the microlobulations represent cancerized lobules.

grade carcinomas. The central scar in small lesions may simulate the echogenic hilum of an intramammary lymph node that contains metastatic disease (Fig. 14–57).

Extensive Intraductal Component and Multifocal or Multicentric Lesions

Most invasive NOS carcinomas contain a mixture of invasive and intraductal (DCIS) components. EICs can lie within the substance of the invasive portion of the lesion, but more extensive components involve the surface of the lesion and extend from the nodule into surrounding ducts and lobules.

Invasive NOS carcinomas with EIC have two main sonographic appearances. They can present with heavy internal and surface microlobulations (Fig. 14–58) or with a mixture of hard and soft suspicious findings. Usually, the dominant invasive nodule demonstrates hard findings, and prominent soft findings lie on the surface or extend into surrounding tissues. The soft findings that are manifestations of EIC include microlobulations extending into surrounding tissues (Fig. 14–59), long duct extensions (Fig. 14–60), and extensive branch pattern (Fig. 14–61). The presence of numerous calcifications also increases the likelihood of EIC, especially when the calcifications can be shown to lie within microlobulations that represent DCIS-filled ducts containing central necrosis (Fig. 14–62). Such calcifications are usually readily visible mammographically.

High-grade invasive ductal carcinomas are more likely to have EIC than are low-grade lesions, and the DCIS

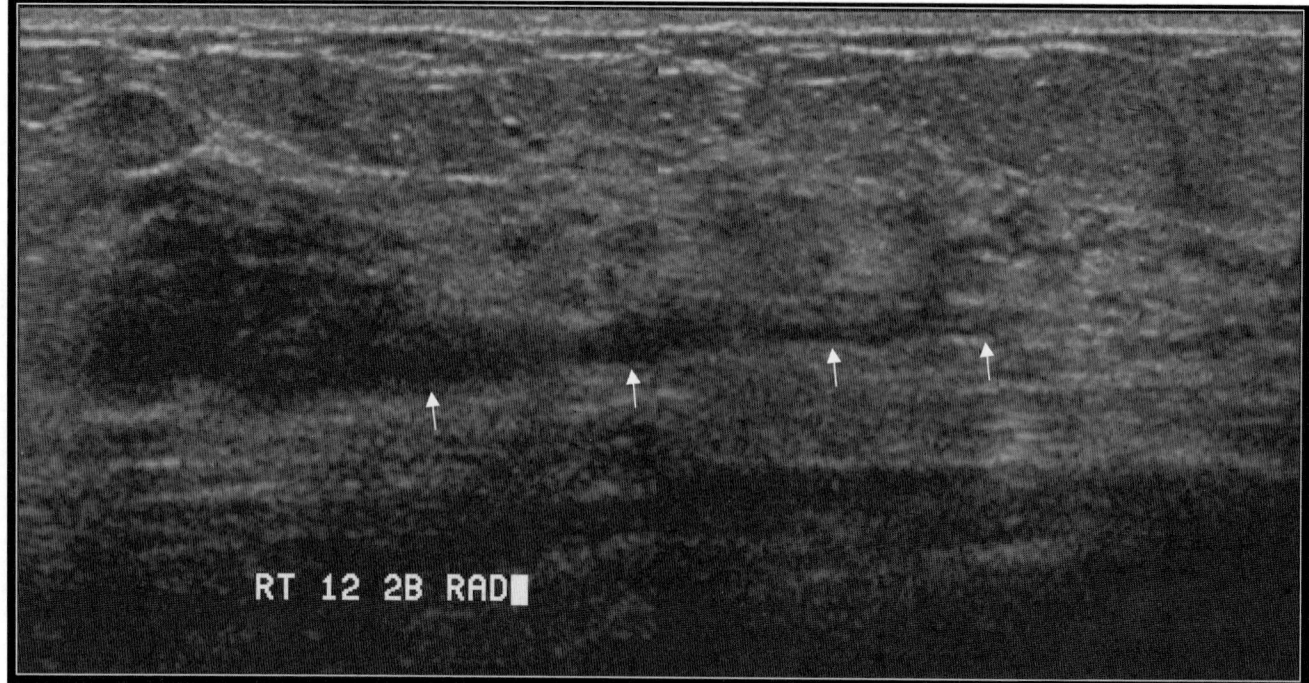

FIGURE 14–60 Long duct extensions suggest the presence of extensive intraductal components of tumor. Transection of the duct will result in positive margins and an increased likelihood of local recurrence.

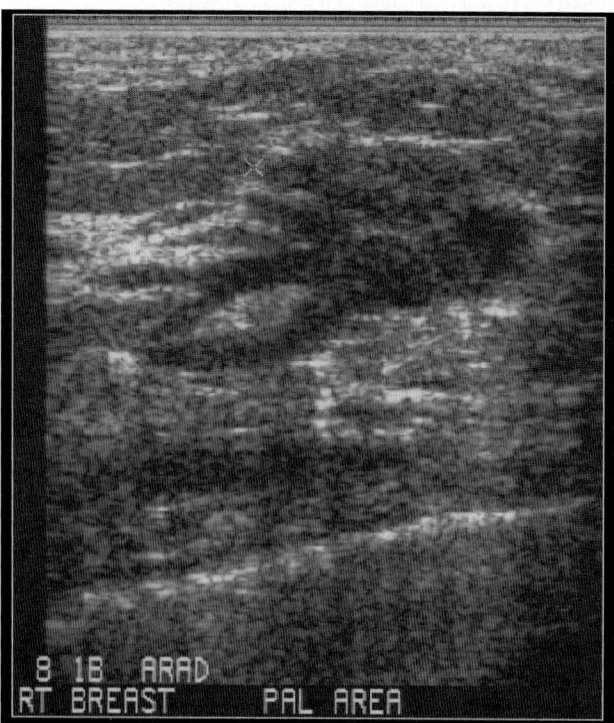

FIGURE 14–61 The presence of extensive branch patterns suggests the presence of extensive intraductal components.

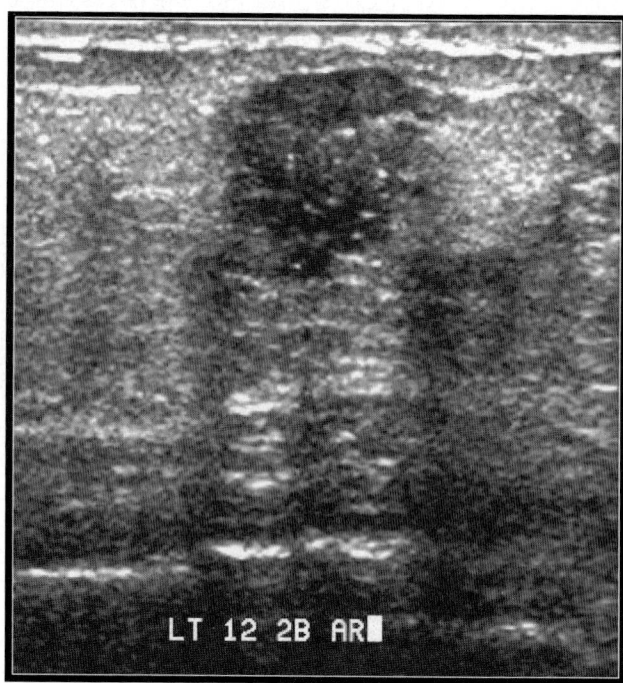

FIGURE 14–62 Numerous microcalcifications suggest the presence of extensive intraductal components, particularly when each calcification lies within a microlobulation. In this case, the microlobulations within which the calcifications lie each represent a duct distended with DCIS. Within the center of each DCIS distended duct is necrosis within which the calcifications form.

components of high-grade lesions are more likely to enlarge the ducts grossly enough to be sonographically detectable than are those of low-grade lesions. Furthermore, the calcifications associated with the DCIS components of high-grade lesions are more likely to be coarse enough to be sonographically detectable than are the smaller calcifications associated with the DCIS components of low-grade lesions. The ducts that are involved with LNG DICS components of low-grade invasive NOS carcinomas may not distend the ducts enough to result in sonographically detectable duct extension, branch pattern, surface microlobulations, or calcifications. Thus, sonography is more likely to detect EIC associated with high-grade lesions than with low-grade lesions.

Preoperative detection of EIC is important because intraductal components may not be detected by the surgeon at the time of lumpectomy and thus may be inadvertently transected. This results in positive margins. If the positive margins are detected, re-resection of the residual disease is necessary, increasing the number of surgeries necessary to extirpate the malignancy completely. On the other hand, if the positive margins are not detected, local recurrence will eventually happen. Preoperative detection of EIC, mapping of its extent with imaging-guided biopsies, and appropriate multiwire localizations can help minimize the

number of surgeries necessary to rid the patient of tumor, minimize the chances of local recurrence, and aid in decisions about postoperative radiation and chemotherapy.

In many cases, the presence of multifocal NOS carcinoma can be demonstrated sonographically. Showing the extent of disease on a single view often requires extended field of view or split-screen combined images. In most cases, multiple different foci of invasion are connected by bridges of DCIS that are visible as duct extensions or branch patterns of variable length (soft finding). By carefully examining duct extensions and branch patterns extending away from the primary invasive lesions (index lesion), additional foci of invasion (hard findings) may be more readily demonstrated sonographically. The points of low resistance for invasion within extensive DCIS appear to be from cancerized lobules and from branch points of the duct (Fig. 14–63). Even though careful serial section histologic studies strongly suggest that most foci of multifocal invasive carcinoma are connected by DCIS components, all or parts of the DCIS bridges may not be sonographically detectable if they do not grossly distend the ducts or if DCIS within the connecting bridge necrosed and regressed (Fig. 14–64). The grossly enlarged connecting bridges of HNG DCIS between multiple high-grade invasive lesions are more likely to be demonstrable

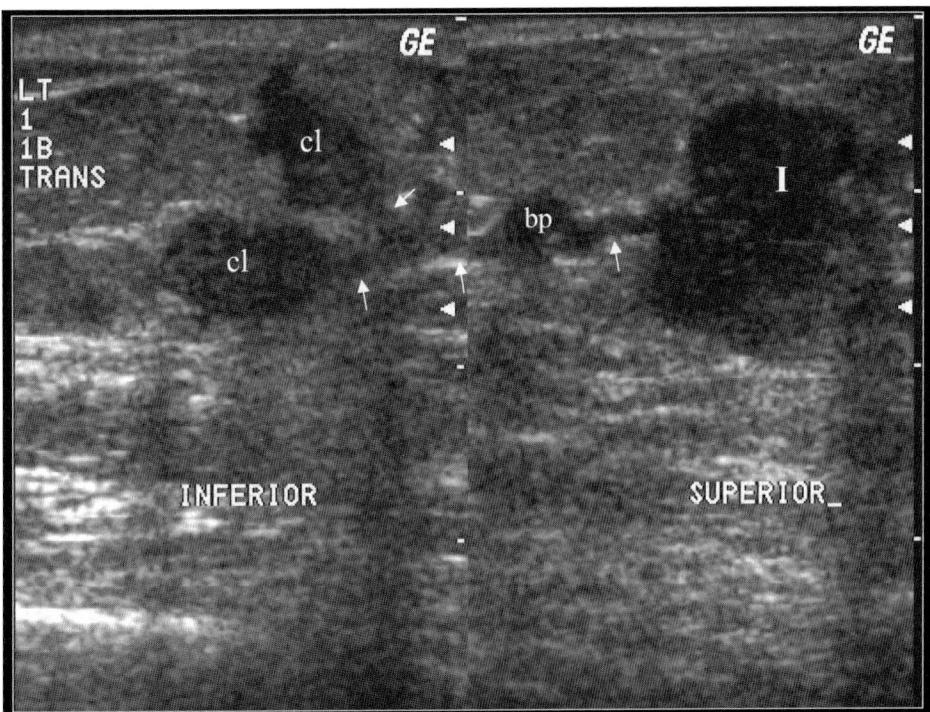

FIGURE 14–63 Combined split-screen images were necessary to show the extent of this multifocal lesion. There are four foci of invasion that arise from the primary or index lesion *(I)*, from two cancerized lobules *(cl)*, and a branch point in the duct *(bp)*. Note the Y-shaped bridge of ductal carcinoma *in situ (arrows)* that connects the multiple foci of invasion. Branch points in ducts and cancerized lobules appear to be sites of low resistance to invasion.

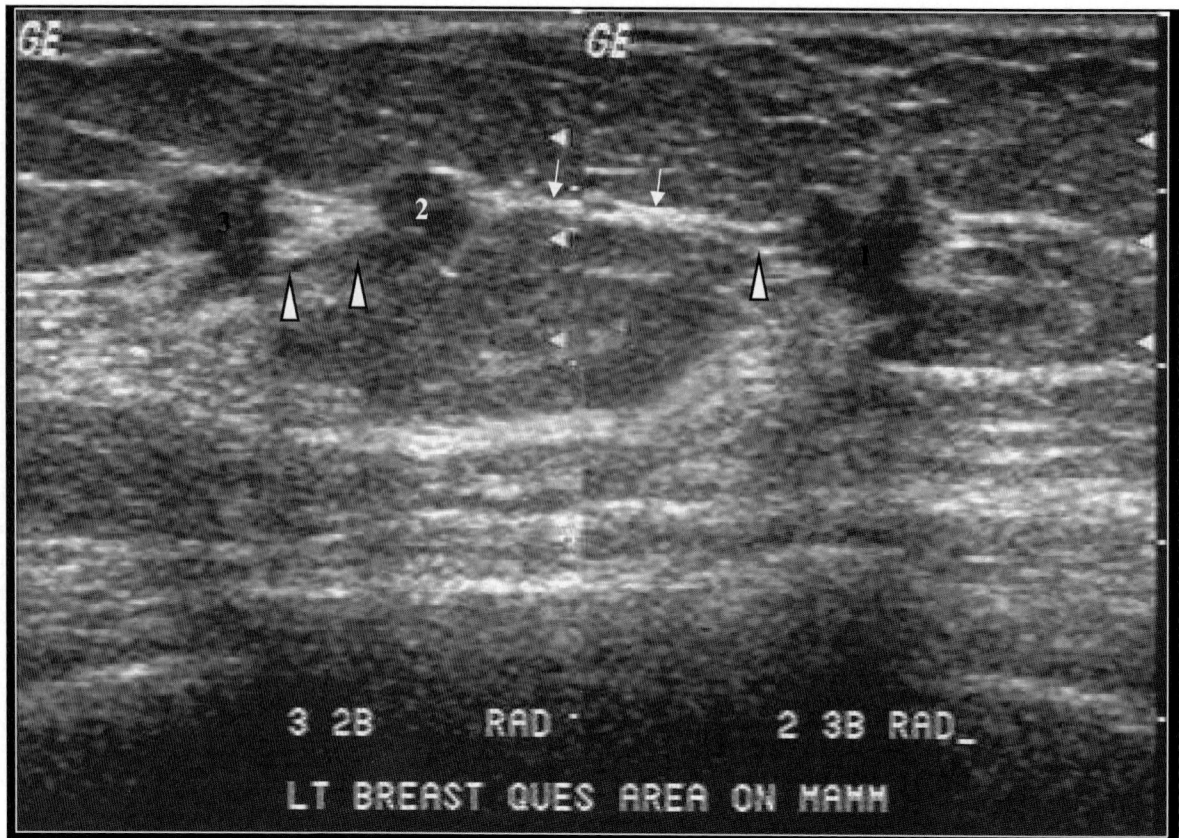

FIGURE 14–64 Ductal carcinoma *in situ* (DCIS) components that connect the multiple foci of invasion either can be too small to detect or have undergone necrosis and regressed. In such cases, only fibrous tissue or Cooper's ligaments can be seen between foci of invasion. In this case, split-screen combined images show a residual DCIS bridge between invasive foci 2 and 3 *(arrowheads)* but only a partial DCIS bridge between lesions 1 and 2. The DCIS between lesions 1 and 2 has either undergone necrosis and regressed or does not enlarge the duct enough for it to be sonographically demonstrable *(arrows, between invasive foci 1 and 2)*. Each focus of invasion appears to have arisen from a cancerized terminal ductolobular unit.

than are the much less enlarged bridges of LNG DCIS between multiple low-grade foci of invasive NOS carcinoma. In other cases, the DCIS bridge that connects invasive foci may persist but is too tortuous too demonstrate on a single image. Power Doppler vocal fremitus can aid in demonstrating multiple foci of invasion and is discussed and illustrated in Chapter 20 (see Figs. 20–91 and 20–92).

Multicentric carcinoma represents multiple foci of tumor that lie in different quadrants of the breast or are 5 cm or more apart. Multicentric carcinoma is more likely to represent completely separate foci of tumor that are not connected by DCIS than is multifocal carcinoma. Additionally, multicentric carcinoma is more likely to be of different histologic types than is multifocal carcinoma (Fig. 14–65). The presence of multifocal carcinoma is more readily detected during targeted assessment of a palpable lump or mammographic lesion than is multicentric carcinoma. Routine preoperative detection of multicentric carcinoma requires that whole breast evaluation with ultrasound or magnetic resonance imaging be performed in all patients who have solid nodules that are characterized as BIRADS 4b or 5 and who will undergo biopsy.

Involvement of Cooper's Ligaments

About two-thirds of invasive NOS tumors arise within TDLUs that lie in the anterior aspect of the mammary zone just deep to the anterior mammary fascia. In older patients, these lesions can appear to arise within the subcutaneous fat because the surrounding fibrous stroma has regressed, leaving the TDLU entrapped within a Cooper's ligament. The TDLUs and small ducts that lie within Cooper's ligaments are the last elements to regress completely with age. Thus, in patients with extensive atrophy, a large percentage of all residual peripheral ducts and TDLUs may lie within Cooper's ligaments. Additionally, a small fraction of TDLUs can actually develop ectopically in very superficial locations within the anteriorly positioned Cooper's ligaments. These intraligamentous TDLUs are surrounded by more fat and less stromal fibrous tissue than

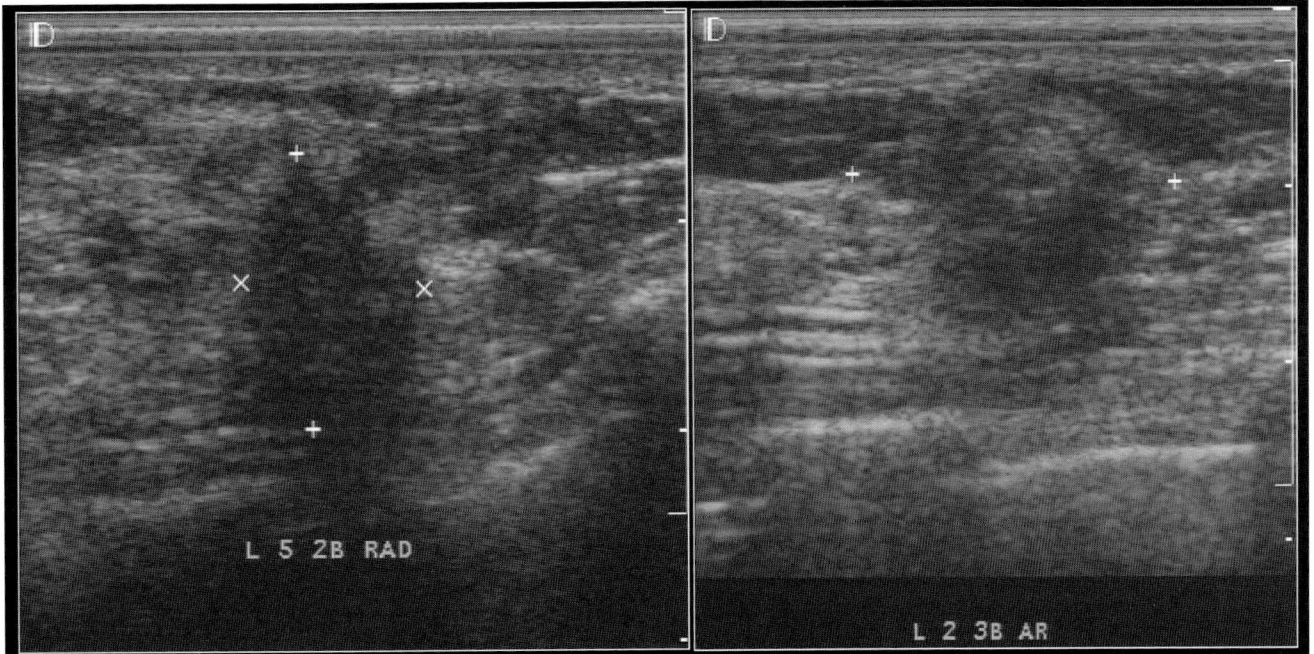

FIGURE 14–65 Multicentric carcinoma occurs in different quadrants of the breast or at distances of more than 5 cm apart. Multicentric disease usually represents completely separate lesions that are not connected by ductal carcinoma *in situ* elements. All the invasive foci of multifocal disease have similar histology, but the histology of multicentric lesions often differs. This patient had an intermediate-grade invasive not otherwise specified carcinoma in the upper outer quadrant at the 2:00 position (**right**) and an invasive lobular carcinoma, classic type, in the lower inner quadrant at 5:00 (**left**).

are the TDLUs that lie more deeply within the mammary zone. The estrogen levels within fat that surrounds intraligamentous TDLUs may be higher than they are within the stromal fibrous tissue that surrounds more deeply located TDLUs. Thus, intraligamentous TDLUs may be subject to more persistent estrogenic stimulation than are more deeply located TDLUs, making intraligamentous TDLUs more prone to malignant degeneration. The paths of low resistance for tumor growth appear to differ between deeply located fibrous-surrounded TDLUs and superficial fat-surrounded TDLUs. DCIS that arises in deeply located fibrous-surrounded TDLUs spreads easily through the ductal system. On the other hand, DCIS that arises in superficially located, fat-surrounded TDLUs, where surrounding fibrous stromal and ductal elements have regressed, cannot spread easily through the ductal system and are prone to early invasion into surrounding fat. Once invasion has occurred, one of the paths of lowest resistance of growth for such tumors is toward the skin within the potential space between the two leaves of anterior mammary fascia that form Cooper's ligaments.

Invasion of Cooper's ligaments can be shown sonographically in several ways. First, malignant ligamentous involvement can be seen as a hypoechoic angular widening of the deep part of the ligament (Fig. 14–66). Second, it may present as an abnormal echogenic or hypoechoic

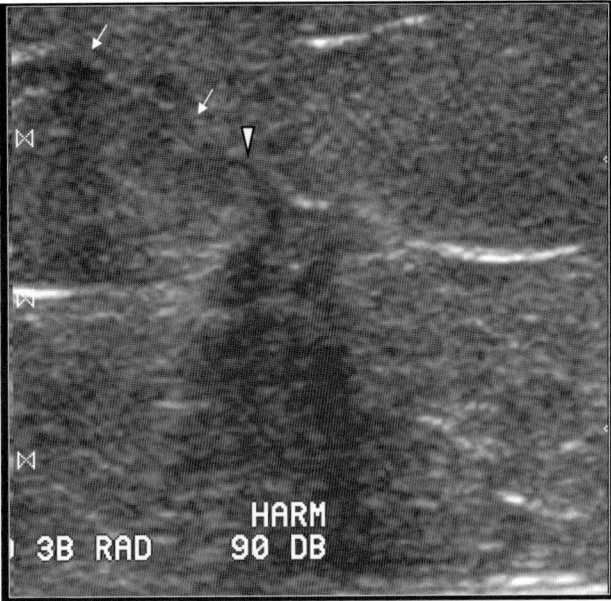

FIGURE 14–66 Early involvement of Cooper's ligament by invasive not otherwise specified carcinoma presents as an angular hypoechoic extension *(arrowhead)* of the nodule into the base of the ligament *(arrows)*. Invasion into Cooper's ligaments causes most angular margins.

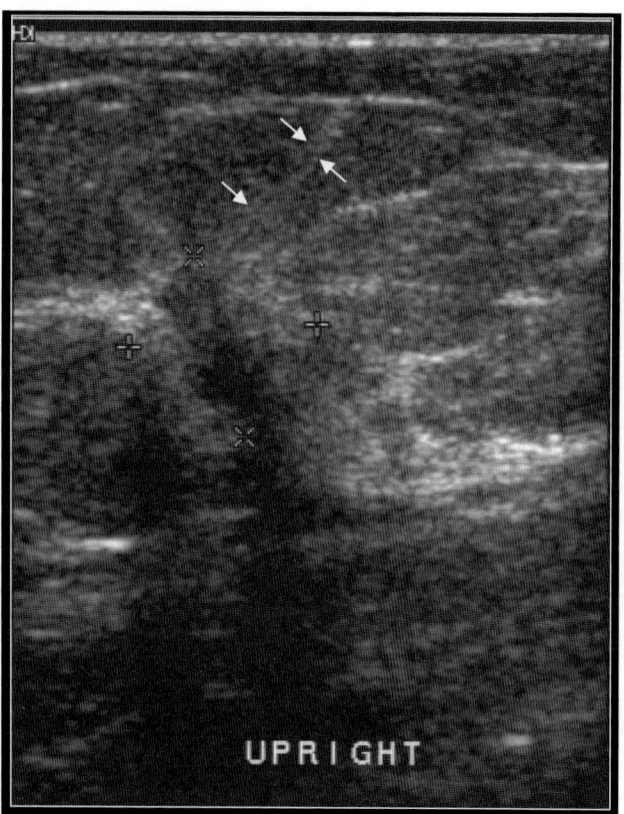

FIGURE 14–67 Invasion and traction on Cooper's ligaments can cause echogenic thickening and straightening of the ligaments *(arrows)*.

thickening and straightening of the ligament (Fig. 14–67). The skin at the site of ligamentous attachment can be flattened or dimpled. Dimpling is difficult to detect in the supine patient when moderate compression is applied during scanning. It is more apparent when using very light compression and a glob of gel as an acoustic standoff and when the patient is in the upright position with the arms extended above the head (Fig. 14–34). Direct invasion of Cooper's ligaments is a route by which cancer can reach the skin, and Cooper's ligament invasion that is not recognized preoperatively, resulting in its transection during surgery, contributes to local recurrences within the subcutaneous fat or skin (Fig. 14–68).

Lymphatic or Vascular Invasion

Lymphatic or vascular invasion is a difficult histologic diagnosis that cannot be directly identified sonographically. The pathologist is usually unable to distinguish small blood vessels from lymphatic vessels, and sectioning artifacts can push tumor cells into vessels. There is an associated increased risk for lymph node and distant metastasis and a worse prognosis.

When vascular invasion is severe and results in obstruction of vascular channels, lymphedema can occur. The end stage of such a process is the classic inflammatory carcinoma, which is discussed later in this chapter. In less severe cases, edema may be limited and may not reach the skin surface, involving only the immediate areas surround-

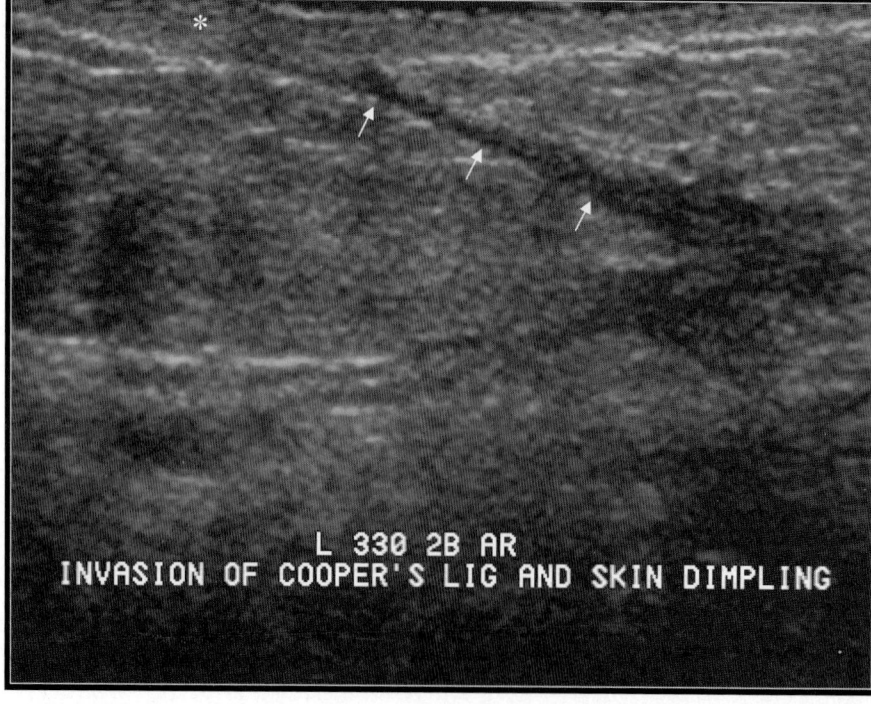

FIGURE 14–68 Invasive not otherwise specified carcinoma can grow farther up Cooper's ligaments toward the skin, causing hypoechoic widening of the ligament *(arrows)*. Such thickening is associated with skin dimpling and can even cause skin thickening by direct invasion or by lymphatic obstruction and edema *(*)*. A standoff of acoustic gel and scanning in the upright position with the arms elevated facilitate the sonographic demonstration of skin dimpling.

ing the NOS tumor nodule. Although tumor-filled lymphatic channels cannot be directly demonstrated sonographically, the lymphedema caused by severe lymphatic invasion and obstruction can be detected sonographically if the lesion is surrounded by fat. Peritumoral edema manifests as hyperechogenicity of the fat surrounding the invasive lesion. Peritumoral lymphedema typically occurs between the lesion and the skin because the direction of lymphatic drainage from the tumor is toward the subdermal lymphatic network, then to the periareolar network, and finally to the axillary lymph nodes. Identification of the typical lymphedema pattern around a suspicious solid nodule that is characterized as BIRADS 4 or 5 warrants sonographic evaluation of axillary lymph nodes. Peritumoral edema as one of the causes of a thick, echogenic halo is discussed and illustrated in Chapter 12 (see Fig. 12–17).

Special-Type Invasive Breast Carcinomas

MEDULLARY CARCINOMA

General Pathologic Classification, Clinical Findings, and Epidemiology

Medullary carcinoma of the breast is a special-type tumor that is relatively uncommon, constituting 5% or less of all breast carcinomas in most series. Medullary carcinoma is more common in younger patients and in Japanese and black patients. It makes up more than 10% of all breast carcinomas in patients younger than 35 years of age. Medullary carcinomas occur bilaterally in 3% to 18% of patients and are multicentric in fewer than 10% of cases.

Medullary carcinomas often present as rapidly enlarging, clinically "mobile" lumps but may also be asymptomatic and discovered at mammography. In our experience, medullary carcinomas are frequently associated with tenderness because of the intense inflammatory response that they incite.

At gross pathologic examination, medullary carcinomas are circumscribed, ovoid or lobulated, mobile, and firm to palpation, but not as firm as most NOS carcinomas. Medullary carcinomas that have undergone extensive necrosis may even be soft to palpation. These lesions are less frequently attached to surrounding tissues than are most other invasive breast malignancies and can even appear to be encapsulated. The gross characteristics of medullary carcinomas are more similar to those of fibroadenomas than they are to those of usual invasive NOS carcinoma. Because of rapid growth, medullary carcinomas are often quite large at the time of presentation. The average size is about 2 to 3 cm. Medullary carcinomas are frequently multilobulated or microlobulated internally and on the nodule's surface.

Pure medullary carcinomas have a prognosis intermediate between NOS carcinomas and other lower-risk special-type carcinomas such as tubular, mucinous, or invasive papillary carcinoma. The 5-year survival rate is 89%. However, nodes are positive in 42%.

Only carcinomas that meet strict histologic criteria should be classified as medullary carcinomas. Lesions that do not meet all of the strict criteria and have atypical features should be classified as *atypical medullary carcinoma*, which are probably variants of NOS carcinoma rather than true medullary carcinomas. A more appropriate term for such lesions is *invasive NOS carcinoma with medullary features*. The distinction between pure medullary carcinoma and atypical medullary carcinoma is important because their prognoses differ. The prognosis of atypical medullary carcinomas is the same as the prognosis of invasive NOS carcinomas, not the better prognosis of pure medullary carcinomas.

Pure medullary carcinomas must meet the following strict histologic criteria: the margins of the lesion must be histologically circumscribed (with a thin capsule of compressed breast tissue) around most of the periphery of the lesion, and infiltration into surrounding tissues can be present in only one location. In addition, two or more areas of direct invasion of surrounding tissues exclude a lesion from classification as pure medullary carcinoma and require the diagnosis of invasive NOS carcinomas with medullary features. Intraductal components in the periphery of the lesion that involve small ducts and lobules frequently create a multilobulated or microlobulated surface. Pure medullary carcinomas must be composed of at least 75% syncytial growth. Only a small part of the tumor may be composed of tubules, cords, or papillary growth. The malignant epithelial cells must be of high or intermediate nuclear grade. Lesions in which the malignant cells are low nuclear grade should be excluded from classification as pure medullary carcinoma. The mitotic rate should also be high. There must be only minimal desmoplastic stromal response. The scant fibrovascular stroma within medullary carcinomas is usually quite loose. There must be at least moderate to severe infiltration by lymphocytes or plasma cells, usually within the loose stroma, but occasionally dispersed directly within the sheets of malignant cells.

Lymphoplasmocytic infiltrates should also involve 75% or more of the periphery of the lesion in addition to involving the center of the nodule. Although direct invasion of tumor cells into surrounding tissues is very limited in pure medullary carcinomas, the lymphoplasmocytic infiltrates often infiltrate into surrounding tissues. This infiltration can make the margins of the lesion appear grossly ill defined rather than circumscribed and can cause peritumoral edema. The degree of lymphoplasmocytic infiltration may be so extensive that germinal centers form, making the distinction between medullary carcinomas and metastasis of high-grade NOS carcinoma to intramammary lymph nodes difficult. This distinction is especially troublesome when the lesion arises within the axillary segment of the breast, where intramammary lymph nodes are most frequently located. The lymphoplasmacytic reaction is not just limited to the primary lesion but can also occur within the regional lymph nodes. Axillary lymph nodes are frequently enlarged in patients with medullary carcinoma, even when the lymph nodes do not contain metastatic deposits. The intense lymphoplasmacytic reaction associated with medullary carcinomas probably represents a pronounced host immunologic response to the tumor and likely accounts for the better prognosis of medullary carcinomas in comparison to NOS lesions.

Additional common histologic features that are frequently present, but not required for the diagnosis of medullary carcinoma, include necrosis and hemorrhage, especially within larger lesions. Both necrosis and hemorrhage can progress to cyst formation within the lesion.

Atypical medullary carcinomas do not meet strict criteria for pure medullary carcinoma and have any of several the following atypical features:

- Less than 75% syncytial growth pattern and more than 25% tubule formation or papillary growth pattern
- More than one focus of invasion in the periphery
- Mild rather than moderate or pronounced lymphoplasmocytic infiltrate
- Low-grade rather than intermediate- to high-grade nuclear cytology

Mammographic Findings

Because of the circumscribed growth pattern, medullary carcinoma presents mammographically as circumscribed nodules that can be similar in appearance to fibroadenomas. Medullary carcinomas are more likely to be multilobulated or even microlobulated than fibroadenomas, a reflection of the intraductal components of tumor along the periphery of medullary carcinomas. Some medullary carcinomas have indistinct margins, owing to dense lymphocytic infiltrates that extend from the periphery of the nodule into surrounding tissues. Calcifications within medullary carcinomas are uncommon.

Sonographic Findings

The sonographic appearance of medullary carcinoma accurately reflects the underlying gross tumor morphology and the histologic components of the lesion.

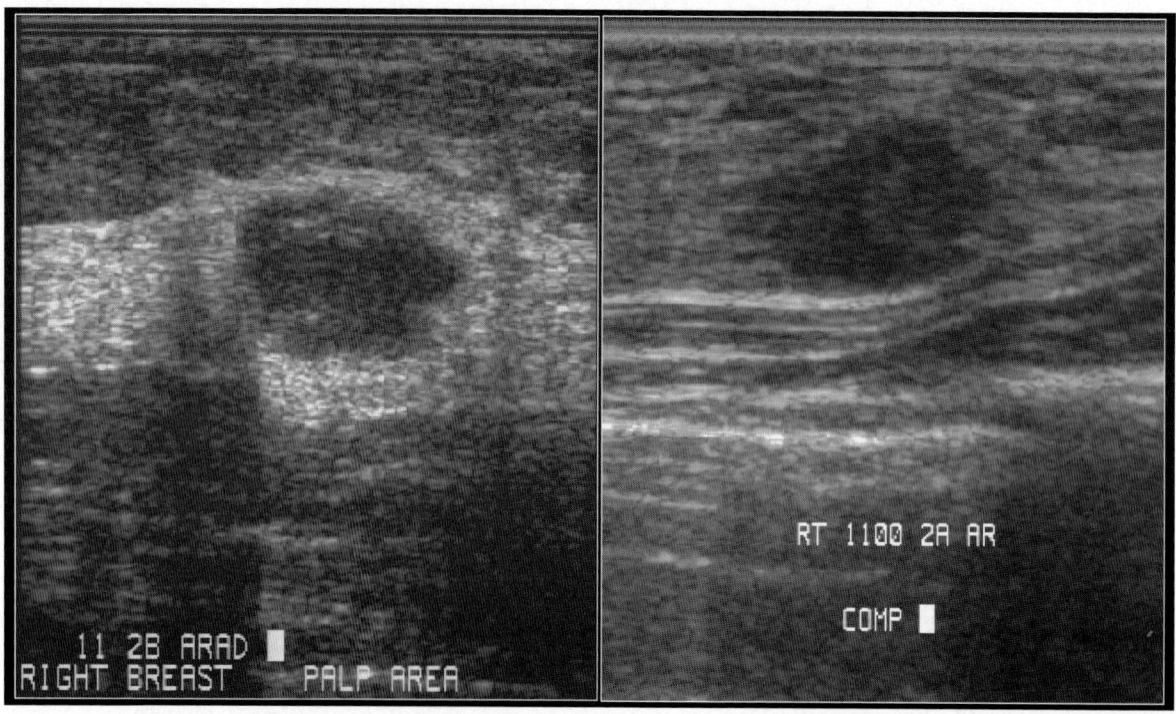

FIGURE 14–69 Medullary carcinomas invariably demonstrate enhanced through-transmission **(left).** The presence of enhanced through-transmission is so consistent that the diagnosis is probably atypical medullary carcinoma **(right)** or invasive ductal carcinoma with medullary features rather than pure medullary carcinoma if sound transmission is normal or decreased.

The most reliable finding is enhanced through-transmission. Because of the highly cellular syncytial growth pattern, the paucity of desmoplastic dense fibrous stromal reaction, the presence of moderate to severe lymphoplasmocytic infiltrates, and the frequent presence of areas of cystic necrosis and hemorrhage, all medullary carcinomas show enhanced through-transmission. In fact, the presence of enhanced through-transmission is so universal that absence of acoustic enhancement should raise serious questions about the diagnosis of pure medullary carcinoma. Such cases almost represent atypical medullary carcinomas rather than pure medullary carcinomas, and the prognosis of such cases is similar to that of invasive NOS carcinomas (Fig. 14–69).

Most medullary carcinomas are markedly hypoechoic in comparison to fat. These lesions may be so hypoechoic that there may be a pseudocystic appearance similar to that of lymphoma of the breast. However, there is usually abundant internal blood flow in such lesions; thus, color Doppler will be helpful in avoiding mischaracterizing the lesion as cystic (see Chapter 20, Fig. 20–25). The more marked the lymphoplasmocytic infiltrate, the more hypoechoic is the lesion. Small areas of necrosis or hemorrhage within the lesions contribute to the hypoechogenicity but may also create heterogeneous echogenicity. Larger areas of

necrosis or hemorrhage can create macroscopic areas of cystic change within the lesions that are detectable sonographically. A mildly hypoechoic appearance also results when the lymphoid infiltrates are limited to the periphery of the lesion. Internal necrosis that has not yet become cystic may cause some heterogeneous echoes centrally (Fig. 14–69, left).

Because medullary carcinomas are usually circumscribed on both gross pathologic and histologic examination, the lesions are also well circumscribed sonographically. Medullary carcinomas usually have a sonographically demonstrable thin, echogenic capsule surrounding most of the lesion. Because the presence of a thin, echogenic capsule is an important indicator of benignity, there is a risk for falsely classifying a medullary carcinoma as BIRADS 3 if the entire surface area of the nodule is not inspected carefully and if the shape of the nodule is not considered. Evaluation of the entire nodule is important because medullary carcinomas usually have one area of invasion on the surface of the nodule. Thus, medullary carcinomas will usually have one area along the surface where the thin, echogenic capsule is absent, where the margins are angular, or where there is a partial, thick, ill-defined halo (Fig. 14–70). Furthermore, the presence of small components of intraductal tumor on the surface of the nodule frequently causes mi-

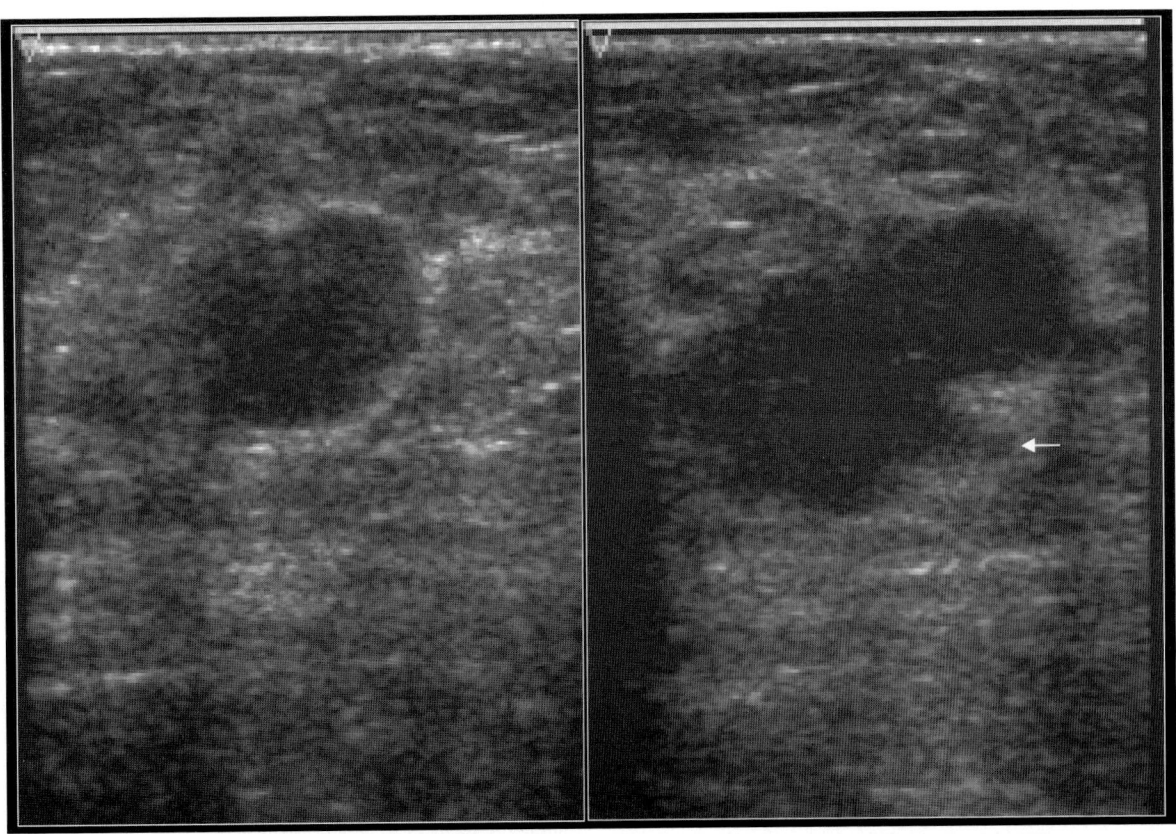

FIGURE 14–70 Although medullary carcinomas are classic circumscribed cancers and are frequently well circumscribed and thinly encapsulated over most of their surfaces **(left)**, most have at least one area of invasion and angularity **(right**, different area in the same lesion shown on the left).

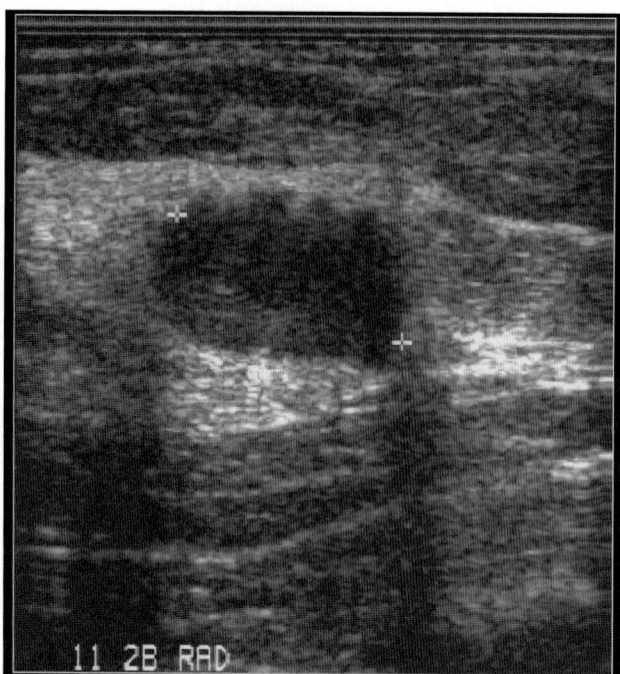

FIGURE 14–71 Because medullary carcinomas frequently have intraductal components of tumor, at least a portion of the well-circumscribed surface often shows microlobulation.

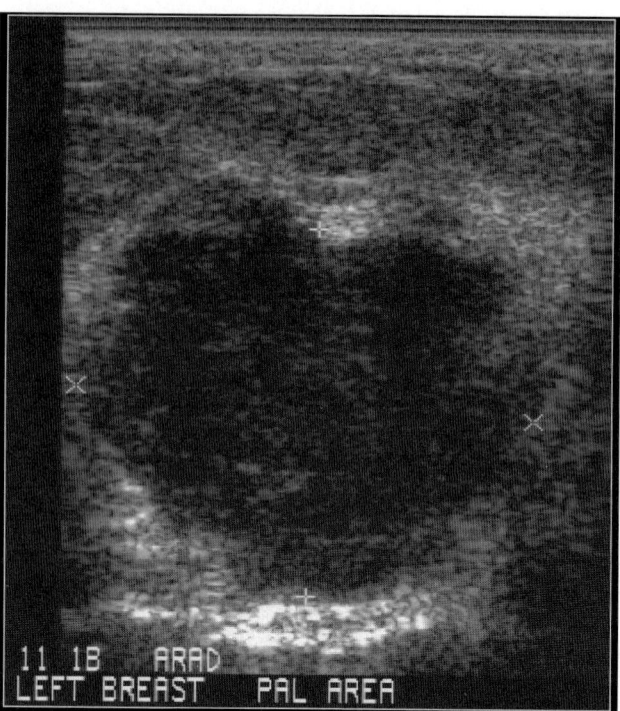

FIGURE 14–72 The intense lymphoplasmacytic response to medullary carcinoma can cause a thick, echogenic halo of peritumoral edema.

crolobulation of the tumor surface. This margin characteristic is readily demonstrable sonographically and should prevent false characterization of these lesions as probably benign (Fig. 14–71). Internal microlobulation is also frequently demonstrable sonographically. The intraductal components may also give rise to duct extension and branch pattern, just as do invasive NOS carcinomas. Furthermore, because medullary carcinoma arises from the same sites as NOS carcinomas, and early growth is typically along the axis of the TDLU, small medullary carcinomas have a tendency to be taller than wide, just as do NOS lesions. Finally, although medullary carcinoma tumor cells tend to push rather than invade surrounding tissues, the lymphocytic infiltrates in the periphery of such lesions frequently do infiltrate into surrounding tissues. This histologic behavior results in an ill-defined, thick, echogenic halo that represents peritumoral edema (Fig. 14–72).

In our experience, virtually all medullary carcinomas demonstrate at least one suspicious finding that prevents the lesions from inappropriately being characterized as BI-RADS 3. Assessment of only the presence of a thin, echogenic capsule without taking shape into account, however, could lead to mischaracterization of medullary carcinomas into the BIRADS 3 category.

Although false-negative sonographic classification of medullary carcinomas as BIRADS 3 should not occur very often, there may be difficulty distinguishing medullary carcinoma from certain other benign and malignant breast nodules. Lesions that can appear similar to med-

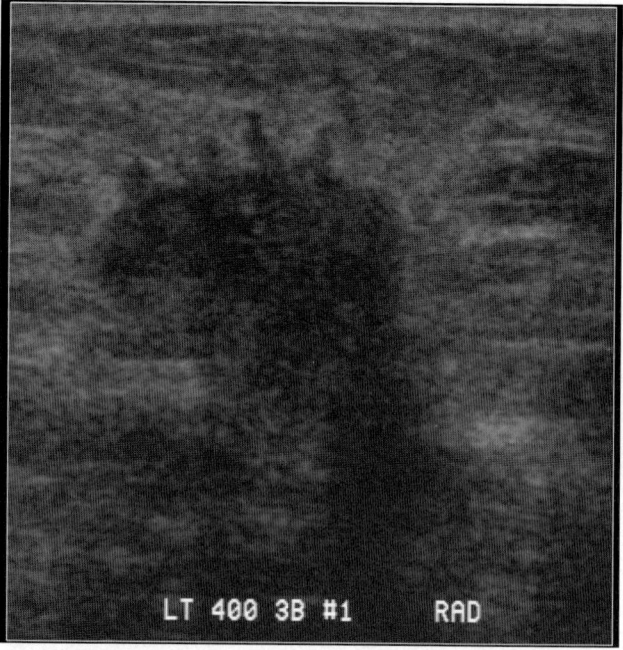

FIGURE 14–73 This atypical medullary carcinoma has two features that strongly suggest that it cannot be a pure medullary carcinoma. First, it has multiple angles, indicating multiple areas of invasion. A pure medullary carcinoma should have no more than one area of invasion. Second, it causes acoustic shadowing, a finding indicating the presence of too much desmoplasia for this lesion to be a pure medullary carcinoma. This lesion was initially misdiagnosed histologically as a pure medullary carcinoma with random sectioning technique, but discordant sonographic findings instigated reassessment histologically.

ullary carcinomas sonographically are high-grade invasive NOS carcinoma, lymphoma, phyllodes tumor, and large fibroadenoma with cellular stroma (juvenile or giant fibroadenoma).

The findings of atypical medullary carcinomas vary, depending on how many atypical features are exhibited and how far the lesions deviate from meeting strict criteria for pure medullary carcinoma. Atypical medullary carcinomas that almost meet criteria for pure medullary carcinoma and have few atypical features can be sonographically indistinguishable from pure medullary carcinomas. On the other hand, atypical medullary carcinomas that have many atypical features can appear indistinguishable from invasive NOS carcinomas. The most consistently present sign of classic pure medullary carcinomas is enhanced through-transmission. Thus, lack of enhanced sound transmission or the presence of acoustic shadowing indicates with virtual certainty that the lesion cannot possibly be a pure medullary carcinoma (Fig. 14–73).

COLLOID CARCINOMA (MUCINOUS CARCINOMA)

General Pathologic Classification, Clinical Findings, and Epidemiology

Colloid carcinoma has also been called *mucinous carcinoma, gelatinous carcinoma,* and *mucous carcinoma.* Colloid carcinoma is a relatively uncommon special-type carcinoma, with pure colloid carcinomas constituting about 2% of all breast carcinomas. These lesions are more common in older women than in younger women. Seven percent of all breast carcinomas in women 75 years of age or older are colloid carcinomas, whereas only 1% of carcinomas in women 35 years of age or younger are of the colloid type. The average age of women diagnosed with colloid carcinoma is 63 years. About one-half of all colloid carcinomas present as palpable abnormalities. The other half are asymptomatic and diagnosed on mammograms.

Colloid carcinoma occurs in pure and mixed forms. Pure colloid carcinoma has variously been defined as at least 50% or at least 75% colloid pattern, with the remainder of the lesion showing other patterns. The most widely used definition is a carcinoma, of which at least 75% is composed of a colloid pattern. The mixed colloid carcinoma contains less than 75% colloid pattern, with other patterns accounting for more than 25% of the volume of the lesion. The mixed form of colloid carcinoma should be considered and termed an *invasive NOS carcinoma that contains foci of colloid carcinoma* or an *invasive NOS carcinoma with colloid features.* Mixed colloid lesions occur in younger women, are larger, and are more likely to be palpable than are pure mucinous carcinoma. Mixed colloid carcinomas also account for about 2% of all carcinomas.

The gross morphology of colloid carcinomas depends on whether they are pure or mixed. Pure colloid carcinomas are circumscribed, smooth, lobulated, and firm to soft, depending on the percentage of the tumor composed of mucin. The larger the percentage of mucin, the softer the lesion is to palpation. Although the lesions are circumscribed, a capsule is usually not identified. The gross findings of pure colloid carcinoma are very similar to the gross findings in myxoid fibroadenomas. Mixed colloid carcinomas are more likely to infiltrate surrounding tissues than are pure colloid carcinomas and therefore are more likely to be ill defined and attached to surrounding tissues on gross examination. Mixed colloid carcinomas also contain more fibrous stromal reaction (desmoplasia) than pure colloid carcinomas and therefore are much firmer when palpated. Pure colloid carcinomas tend to be smaller than the mixed colloid varieties. The mean diameter of pure colloid carcinomas is 1.2 cm, whereas the mean diameter for mixed mucinous carcinomas is 3.6 cm. The difference in size between smaller pure and larger mixed colloid carcinomas is so pronounced that most lesions larger than 5 cm represent mixed colloid carcinomas.

On microscopic examination, there is abundant extracellular mucin surrounding malignant epithelial cells as well as varying amounts of intracellular mucin. The relative proportions of tumor cells and mucin vary from tumor to tumor but are usually relatively uniform throughout an individual lesion. Most of the malignant epithelial cells are located in the periphery of the lesion. In certain cases, the mucin is so abundant and the tumor cells so sparse that the rare cells identified appear to be floating in a sea of mucin. Often, several high-power fields have to be searched to find the individual tumor cells. The percentage of extracellular mucin in pure colloid carcinoma averages 83.5%, ranging from 40% to 99.8%. The percentage of mucin mixed colloid carcinoma is less—a mean of 68.3% and a range from 32% to 97%.

Colloid carcinomas contain DCIS in 75% of cases. The DCIS components of colloid carcinoma, like those of medullary carcinoma, usually lie in the periphery of the lesion and contribute to microlobulation, duct extensions, and branch patterns.

Pure colloid carcinomas contain moderately well-differentiated malignant epithelial cells and minimal amounts of desmoplasia and inflammation. Necrosis, cystic change, calcifications, and lymphatic invasion are rare.

The distinction between pure and mixed colloid carcinoma is important clinically because of the greatly different prognoses. Pure colloid carcinoma has a relatively favorable prognosis in comparison to NOS carcinomas. The prognosis of mixed colloid carcinomas, on the other hand, is worse than for pure colloid lesions and only minimally better than for invasive NOS carcinomas. Pure colloid carcinomas have positive nodes in only 6%, mixed colloid carcinomas in 36%, and NOS carcinomas in 43%

of cases. The 10-year disease-free survival rate after mastectomy in pure colloid carcinoma is 90%, whereas for mixed colloid carcinomas, it is only 60%. Despite the relatively favorable prognosis for patients who have pure colloid carcinomas, follow-up must be maintained for a longer time before the assumption of cure can be made. About half the recurrences and half the cancer deaths in patients with pure colloid carcinoma occur more than 10 years after diagnosis and initial treatment.

The histologic differential diagnosis of colloid carcinomas includes pure colloid carcinoma, mixed colloid carcinoma, infiltrating lobular carcinoma, and mucocele-like lesions. Infiltrating lobular carcinomas differ from colloid carcinoma in that they have intracellular mucin but do not contain abundant extracellular mucin. There is a broad spectrum of mucocele-like lesions, including both benign and malignant conditions. Mucous-filled benign cysts and ducts occur. These lesions can be associated with usual or atypical ductal hyperplasia or with DCIS. In all of these cases, pools of mucin that simulate the pools of extracellular mucin in pure mucinous carcinoma can be identified. The distinction between benign mucin-containing lesions and invasive pure colloid carcinoma can be especially difficult on FNAB because few or no cells on a background of mucin may be obtained. Even myxoid fibroadenomas can be difficult to distinguish from colloid carcinoma on FNAB.

Mammographic Findings

Most pure colloid carcinomas are well circumscribed and lobulated or microlobulated, or multinodular. A few of these lesions may appear to have an indistinct margin, primarily owing to surrounding fibroglandular elements. Pure colloid carcinomas are seldom frankly spiculated and contain calcifications in less than 5% of cases.

Mixed colloid carcinomas are often ill defined or angular in shape and may even be frankly spiculated. Calcifications are more likely to occur in mixed lesions than in pure colloid carcinomas but are still uncommon. On gross pathologic examination, mammographic nodules caused by mixed colloid carcinomas are larger than those caused by pure mucinous carcinoma, and a maximum diameter or more than 3 cm favors mixed over pure colloid carcinoma.

Sonographic Findings

The sonographic appearance of colloid carcinoma varies with the maximum diameter of the lesion. In lesions with maximum diameters of 1.5 cm or less, the background echogenicity is nearly isoechoic to fat, making them difficult to identify (Fig. 14–74). Even when detected, the presence of a well-circumscribed thin, echogenic capsule in such small colloid carcinomas can also make them difficult to distinguish from fibroadenomas. Although the overall echogenicity of small colloid carcinomas is isoechoic with

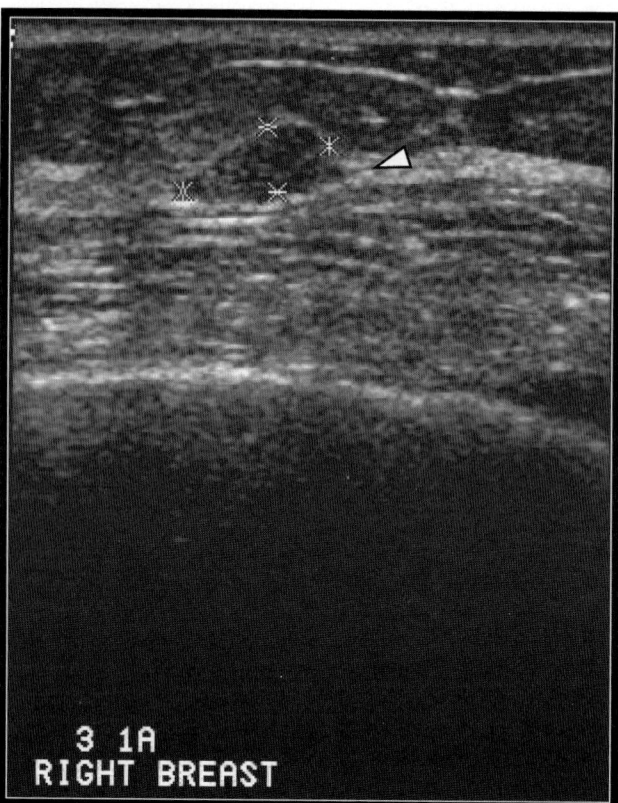

FIGURE 14–74 Small colloid carcinomas (<1.5 cm) are isoechoic with fat, well circumscribed, and usually thinly encapsulated. Careful inspection will usually show one or more angular margins *(arrows)*. Because the lesions are isoechoic with fat, they are among the easiest of malignant nodules to miss.

fat, the echotexture of such lesions is usually slightly coarser and more heterogeneous than that of fat—an appearance that can be described as "salt and pepper." They may even appear to be slightly hyperechoic with respect to surrounding fat, but not as hyperechoic as and more heterogeneous than normal interlobular stromal fibrous tissue. The shape is highly variable, but small mucinous carcinomas are often taller than wide and have surface microlobulations (Fig. 14–75). Prominent duct extensions or branch pattern are rare in pure mucinous carcinoma. A thin, echogenic capsule surrounds most of the lesion, but typically, there is at least a portion of the margin that appears to have a thick, echogenic halo that represents either edema or tiny unresolved spicules (Fig. 14–76). Frank spiculation is rarely demonstrable. Colloid carcinomas do not cause acoustic shadowing. However, whether the lesion demonstrates normal or enhanced through-transmission depends on the maximum diameter of the lesion. Colloid carcinomas larger than 1.5 cm in maximum diameter virtually always manifest enhanced through-transmission, but colloid carcinomas smaller than 1.5 cm in maximum diameter can demonstrate either normal or enhanced through-transmission (Fig. 14–77).

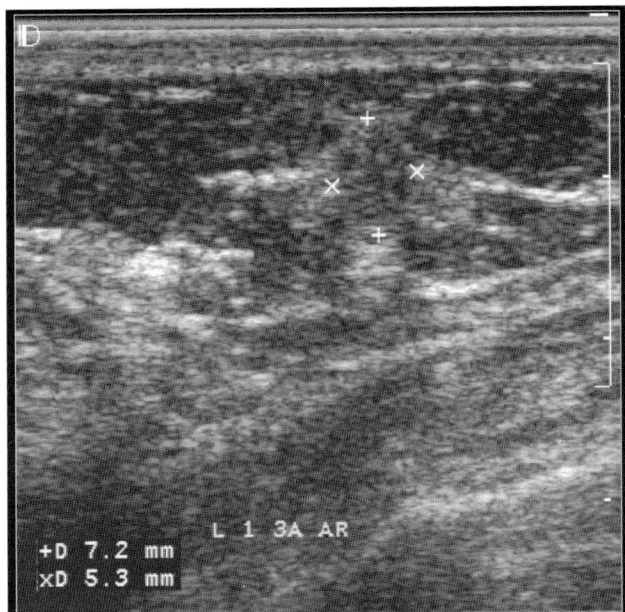

FIGURE 14–75 Although small colloid carcinomas are typically isoechoic with fat, echotexture is slightly more heterogeneous, causing a "salt-and-pepper" appearance. Small colloid carcinomas can even appear to be slightly hyperechoic with respect to fat, but not as hyperechoic as normal interlobular stromal fibrous tissue. Like other types of small carcinomas, colloid carcinomas are frequently taller than wide.

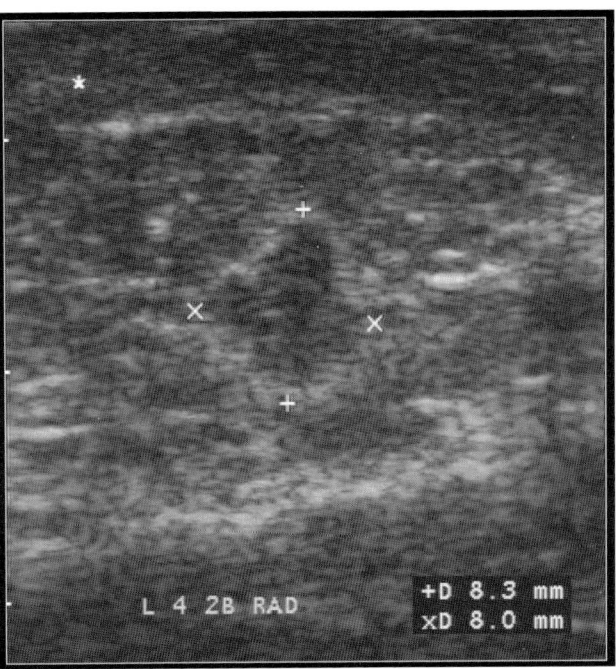

FIGURE 14–76 Although mucous-containing portions of the lesion are generally encompassed by a thin, echogenic capsule, frankly invasive portions of the lesion demonstrate thicker, less well-defined capsules or thick, echogenic halos. This small colloid carcinoma is also taller than wide.

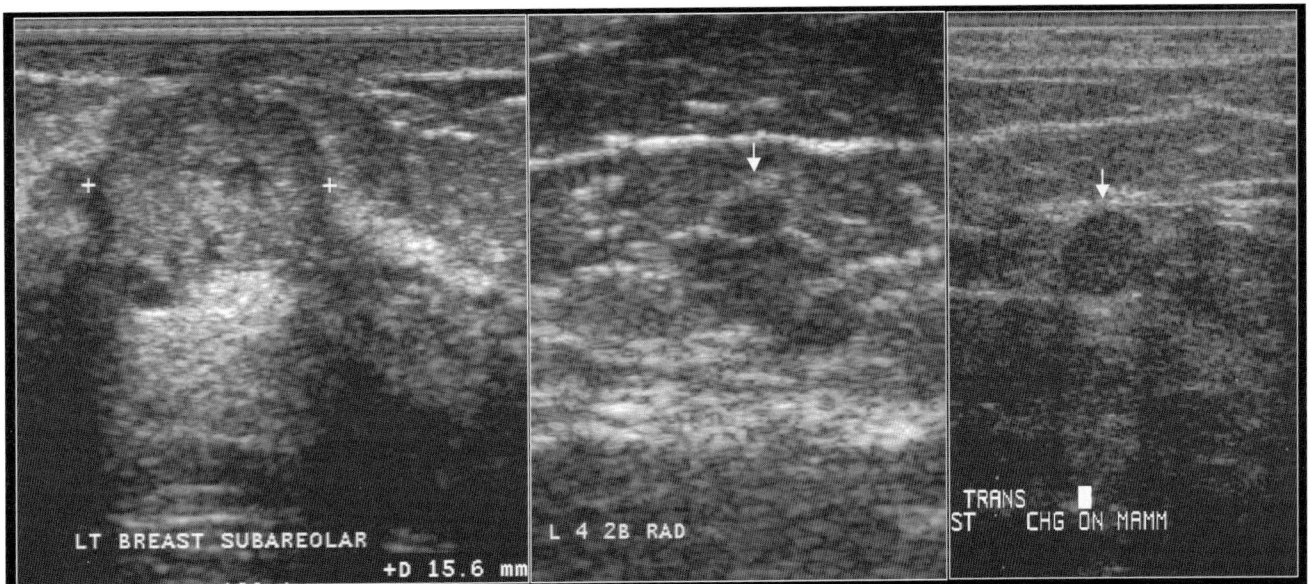

FIGURE 14–77 Large pure colloid carcinomas that are 1.5 cm in maximum diameter or greater always demonstrate enhanced through-transmission (*left*). Small colloid carcinomas that are less than 1.5 cm in maximum diameter, however, can show normal (**middle**) or enhanced (**right**) sound transmission.

The sonographic differential diagnosis for pure colloid carcinoma includes normal fat lobules, lipomas, and certain fibroadenomas (usually those with cellular or myxoid stroma). Fat lobules and lipomas are far more compressible than colloid carcinomas, usually compressing more than 30%. Even soft pure colloid carcinoma virtually never compresses more than 15%. Fibroadenomas with myxoid change are usually flatter, much more compressible, less microlobulated, and far less likely to have a thick, echogenic halo around any part of the lesion.

The appearance of invasive NOS carcinomas with colloid components is far more variable and less predictable than that of pure colloid carcinoma and depends on the percentage of tumor that is colloid and the type of NOS elements that make up the bulk of the noncolloid portion of the lesion. The sonographic appearance can vary from one almost identical to pure mucinous carcinoma to one that is identical to various types of NOS lesions. Obviously, the more NOS components, the more the lesion will approximate NOS lesions in appearance. Compared with pure mucinous lesions, mixed mucinous carcinomas are more likely to be hypoechoic and to have angular margins, frank spiculation, acoustic shadowing, duct extensions, branch pattern, and a complete thick, echogenic halo. For purposes of determining prognosis and adjudicating histologic results of ultrasound-guided core needle biopsy, the pres-

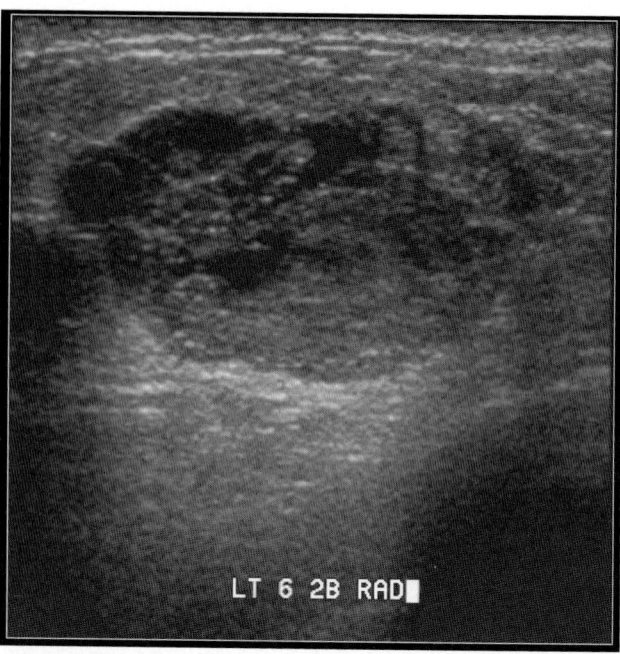

FIGURE 14–79 Pure colloid carcinomas rarely undergo cystic degeneration. Internal cystic changes, especially in lesions larger than 3 cm, strongly suggest that the lesion is an invasive not otherwise specified carcinoma with colloid changes rather than a pure colloid carcinoma.

ence of acoustic shadowing or evidence of spiculation strongly suggests that the lesion must actually represent an invasive duct carcinoma with colloid features rather than a pure colloid carcinoma (Fig. 14–78). Cystic change in pure colloid carcinomas is rare and, together with a diameter of 3 cm or greater, should raise questions about the diagnosis of pure colloid carcinoma. Such lesions are more likely invasive NOS carcinomas with colloid features (Fig. 14–79).

TUBULAR CARCINOMA

General Pathologic Classification, Clinical Findings, and Epidemiology

Tubular carcinomas are uncommon, constituting only 2% of all breast carcinomas, but are more common in pure mammographic screening series, making up to 10% of mammographically detected carcinomas. Mixed varieties or tubular carcinomas constitute another 3% to 8% of carcinomas. These mixed lesions are usually low- to intermediate-grade invasive NOS carcinomas that contain foci of tubular carcinoma. Pure tubular carcinoma occurs in younger patients, with a median age in the late 40s. The median age for mixed tubular lesions is greater, being similar to the age peak for invasive NOS carcinoma. The demographics are likely merely a manifestation of an individual tubular carcinoma's tendency to become less differentiated over time.

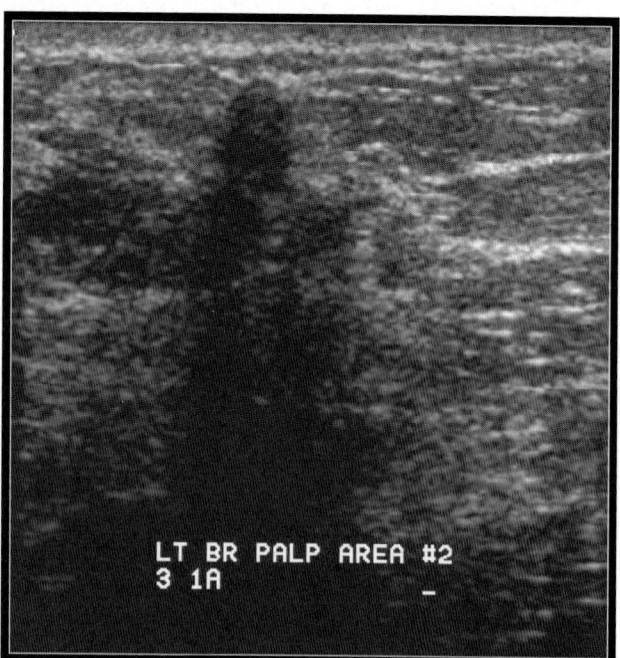

FIGURE 14–78 Colloid carcinomas virtually never cast acoustic shadows. The presence of a shadow, as in this case, or spiculation suggests that the lesion is actually an invasive not otherwise specified carcinoma with colloid features rather than a pure colloid carcinoma. A histologic diagnosis of pure colloid carcinoma in such a case represents nonconcordance between imaging and histologic findings and indicates the need for either histologic reassessment or rebiopsy.

Tubular carcinomas are defined as highly differentiated invasive carcinomas that form well-defined tubules (containing epithelium, but no myoepithelium) and that have abundant desmoplastic fibrous stromal reaction between the tubules.

Although tubular carcinoma has been considered a special-type tumor, the recent trend has been to classify it merely as a low-grade invasive NOS carcinoma because there is a continuous spectrum from pure tubular carcinoma to mixed NOS carcinoma with tubular features, depending on the percentage of the lesion that displays tubular features. The definition of pure tubular carcinoma varies and requires that from 50% to 90% of the lesion be composed of tubular carcinoma. Based on prognosis, at least 75% tubular features is the most widely applied and appropriate criterion for the definition of pure tubular carcinoma. The less than 25% invasive, NOS portion of the lesion that is not histologically pure tubular carcinoma should be low grade. If the nontubular portion of the lesion is intermediate or high grade, the lesion should be considered an NOS carcinoma with foci of tubular carcinoma, even if the nontubular portion of the lesion makes up less than 25% of the lesion.

The prevalence of bilateral and multicentric pure tubular carcinomas is controversial. Some studies report a very low prevalence, whereas other reports suggest a high prevalence. There may be two groups of patients with tubular carcinomas: one with unifocal lesions, and another with multicentric and bilateral disease. There may also be a genetic basis for this phenomenon. Certain patients with tubular carcinoma have LCIS in the surrounding tissues. These are the patients more likely to have multicentric or bilateral disease. This group of patients may also have mixed tubular and ILCs, the so-called tubulolobular carcinoma. The risk for multicentricity and bilaterality, therefore, appears to be related to the presence or absence of LCIS in the tissues surrounding the pure tubular carcinoma, as opposed to simply the presence of the pure tubular carcinoma.

Tubular carcinomas have a propensity to arise in TDLUs that lie far peripherally in the breast and may arise from the center of radial scars or complex sclerosing lesions. There are several practical implications of this far peripheral origin. First, tubular carcinomas are frequently surrounded by fat and therefore are readily visible at small sizes on mammograms. Second, there is early invasion and attachment to fat, making these lesions immobile. Third, there is a propensity for early involvement of Cooper's ligaments, just as there is for ILC. Even though these lesions are detected mammographically at such small sizes that they are not palpable, careful physical examination reveals a subtle skin dimpling over the lesion due to traction on Cooper's ligaments in about 15% of cases. Fourth, the ducts draining the affected TDLU are often atrophic, and EIC rarely occurs in association with pure tubular carcinoma.

At gross pathologic examination, pure tubular carcinomas are hard, gritty, stellate, or ill-defined lesions that are firmly attached to surrounding tissues and that are often less than 1 cm in maximum diameter. Mixed tubular lesions, on the other hand, are more likely to be more than 1 cm in maximum diameter. Such lesions are likely longer standing and may have begun as pure tubular lesions but evolved into less differentiated lesions over time. Because of a high content of elastic tissue within the center of the lesion, often retraction of the center of the lesion on cut surfaces produces a depressed, puckered appearance compared with surrounding tissues.

At histology, the tubular epithelium within tubular carcinoma closely resembles that of normal ductules, showing only mild atypia. However, the tubules in tubular carcinoma are only a single layer thick and are devoid of the myoepithelial elements and basement membrane seen within normal ductules. The tubules may be round but are often compressed and angulated into bizarre shapes by the surrounding desmoplastic stroma. The lobular architecture that is seen in sclerosing adenosis is absent in tubular carcinoma. All tubular carcinomas incite a marked desmoplastic response. The fibrous stroma within tubular carcinoma differs from normal interlobular stromal fibrous tissue, being more cellular, having denser collagen, and containing more peritubular elastic tissue. Tubular carcinomas do not incite an intense inflammatory response, generally do not contain areas of necrosis, and rarely invade lymphatics. Tubular carcinomas have DCIS components in 75% of cases, usually of the cribriform or micropapillary type. The DCIS components associated with tubular carcinoma tend to be within the center of the lesion, unlike other special-type lesions such as medullary and mucinous carcinoma, in which the DCIS components of the lesion tend to be present within the periphery. Tubular carcinomas can have LCIS, rather than DCIS, within or surrounding them. Such lesions may also have mixed areas of infiltrating lobular carcinoma within them or around them.

The prognosis of pure tubular carcinomas is very favorable in comparison to invasive NOS carcinoma. Deaths from pure tubular carcinomas less than 1 cm in maximum diameter are rare. The 15-year disease-free survival rate of patients with pure tubular carcinoma smaller than 1 cm is nearly 100%. Small mixed tubular carcinomas, those that have a maximum diameter of 1 cm or less, have a prognosis similar to that of pure tubular carcinoma. However, mixed tubular carcinomas larger than 1.5 cm in maximum diameter have a 15-year survival of 72%, similar to that of low-grade invasive NOS carcinomas.

Pure tubular carcinomas are associated with positive axillary lymph nodes in fewer than 10% of patients. In the small percentage of cases in which axillary lymph nodes are positive, usually only 1 or 2 low axillary nodes are involved. Mixed tubular carcinomas, however, have positive lymph nodes in almost 40% of cases. The prognosis for axillary lymph node metastases, local recurrence, and disease-free survival of any individual mixed tubular carcinoma is determined by the extent and histologic grade of the nontubular component of the lesion rather than by the tubular component.

Mammographic Findings

Only 30% to 40% of tubular carcinomas present as palpable lumps. The other 60% to 70% are nonpalpable lesions that are detected on routine screening mammograms. Tubular carcinomas usually present mammographically as small, fat-surrounded, spiculated or ill-defined, peripherally located noncalcified nodules. Screening-detected lesions are typically quite small, averaging only 8 mm in diameter. Palpable lesions are usually larger, averaging about 12 mm in diameter. Only about 10% to 15% of pure tubular carcinomas have associated calcifications.

Tubular carcinomas may be difficult to distinguish mammographically from radial scars or complex sclerosing lesions. Tubular carcinomas generally have mammographically dense centers (white star appearance), whereas radial scars generally have relatively lucent centers (black star appearance). In any individual case, however, distinguishing

radial scar from tubular carcinoma can be difficult or impossible. In fact, in some cases, tubular carcinomas and radial scars coexist. Some believe radial scars represent common sites of origin for tubular carcinomas. Thus, many radiologists, surgeons, and pathologists recommend complete surgical excision of spiculated lesions that are diagnosed histologically as radial scars or complex sclerosing lesions to make sure that they do not contain tubular carcinoma.

Sonographic Findings

There are two main divergent sonographic manifestations of tubular carcinomas that depend largely on the maximum diameter of the lesion. Small tubular carcinomas that are less than 1.5 cm in maximum diameter invariably are either spiculated or encompassed by thick, echogenic halos and have angular margins. These small lesions can be either isoechoic or mildly hypoechoic and often taller than wide in shape. The sound transmission varies greatly, with dense acoustic shadowing in some and normal sound transmission in others (Fig. 14–80). A few very small lesions cause intense shadowing. In fact, if a very small spiculated lesion shadows so intensely as to make identification of the poste-

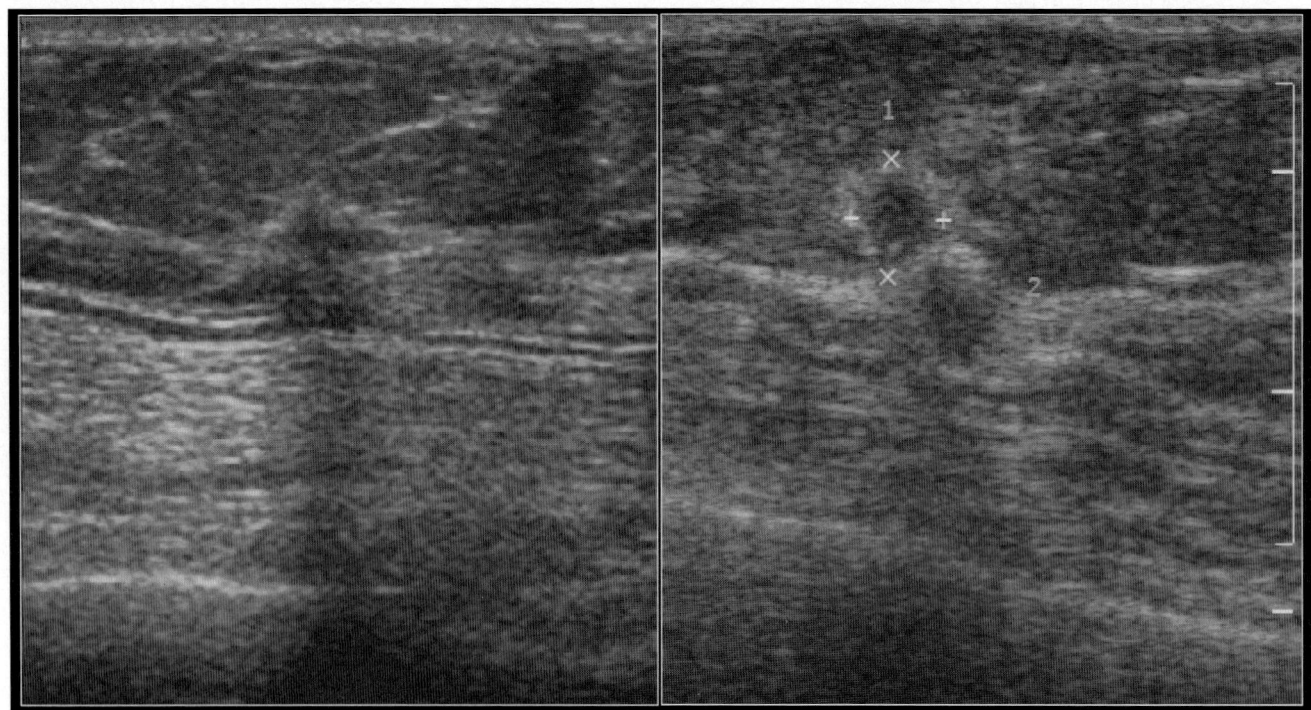

FIGURE 14–80 The sonographic appearance of tubular carcinomas varies greatly with size. Small tubular carcinomas that are less than 1.5 cm in maximum diameter are usually isoechoic to only mildly hypoechoic, have angular margins, and are either frankly spiculated or encompassed by a thick, echogenic halo **(left)**. Tubular carcinomas can be multifocal, isoechoic, and taller than wide **(right)**. The sound transmission of small tubular carcinomas varies. Certain small tubular carcinomas cast acoustic shadows **(left)**, but many demonstrate normal sound transmission **(right)**.

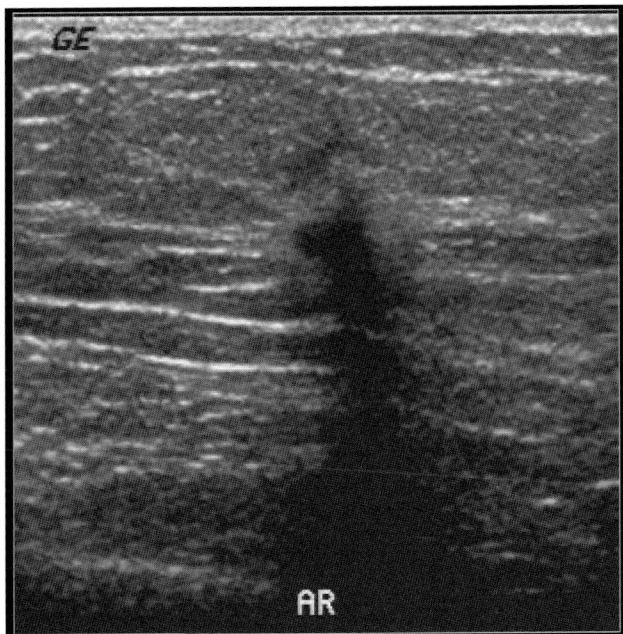

FIGURE 14–81 Although many small tubular carcinomas are isoechoic and have normal sound transmission, some have appearances similar to larger tubular carcinomas. They are markedly hypoechoic and cast intense acoustic shadows. Such lesions presumably contain more desmoplasia than do nonshadowing lesions of the same size. When a small lesion that has a maximum diameter less than 1 cm shadows intensely, tubular carcinoma should be the first entity in the differential diagnosis.

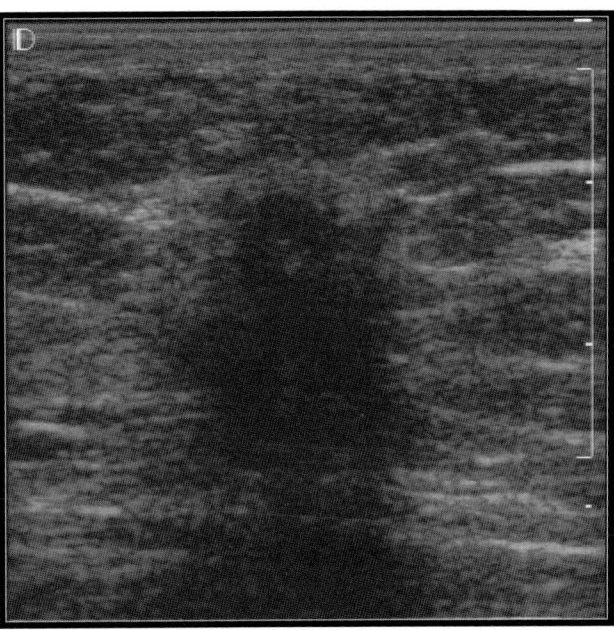

FIGURE 14–82 Tubular carcinomas that are greater than 1.5 cm in maximum diameter are typically markedly hypoechoic, have angular margins, are either frankly spiculated or encompassed by a thick, echogenic halo, and cause acoustic shadowing.

rior margin difficult, the lesion is likely a pure tubular carcinoma (Fig. 14–81). Tubular carcinomas that are larger than 1.5 cm in maximum diameter have a more characteristic and uniform sonographic appearance. They are more hypoechoic, cast strong acoustic shadows, are spiculated or encompassed by a thick, echogenic halo, and have angular margins. They are less often taller than wide than are smaller lesions (Fig. 14–82). Desmoplasia within the tumor causes the acoustic shadowing. Although all tubular carcinomas have abundant desmoplastic reaction, some small tubular carcinomas do not shadow because they apparently lack a critical mass of desmoplasia necessary to cause shadowing. On the other hand, all large tubular carcinomas have achieved a critical mass of desmoplasia and therefore cast acoustic shadows. Pure tubular carcinomas can demonstrate either normal sound transmission or acoustic shadowing, but they never demonstrate enhanced through-transmission. Thus, a histologic diagnosis of pure tubular carcinoma should be questioned in any lesion that demonstrates enhanced through-transmission.

Both small and large pure tubular carcinomas incite enough of a desmoplastic response that they always manifest frank spiculations or a thick, echogenic halo. The thickness of the spiculation or hyperechoic halo surrounding tubular carcinoma is remarkable in comparison to the central nidus. In very small lesions, the echogenic halo may

contribute far more to the maximum diameter of the lesion than does the small central nidus.

Because the DCIS components of pure tubular carcinomas tend to be located within the center of the lesion, rather than on the surface, they tend not to affect the shape or surface characteristics of the lesion. Tubular carcinomas are less often heavily microlobulated and less often demonstrate duct extension and branch pattern than invasive NOS carcinomas. Microlobulations that do occur in pure tubular carcinomas usually represent fingers of invasive tumor rather than intraductal components of tumor.

The location of pure tubular carcinomas is another clue to the histology. The peripheral location, within areas of the breast in which surrounding fibroglandular elements regressed, leaving only fat surrounding the lesion, is typical of pure tubular carcinomas. Tubular carcinomas often appear to arise within a Cooper's ligament, and often there is evidence of straightening and retraction of such ligaments (Fig. 14–83).

Mixed tubular lesions may appear identical to tubular carcinomas but have a wider spectrum of appearances that parallels those of invasive NOS carcinomas (Fig. 14–84).

The sonographic appearance of tubular carcinomas can be simulated by small infiltrating lobular carcinomas, low-grade invasive NOS carcinomas with or without foci of tubular carcinoma, and radial scars or complex sclerosing lesions. Additionally, fibrous scarring due to surgery and fat necrosis can cause angular hypoechoic shadowing lesions. Benign lesions that simulate malignancy are dis-

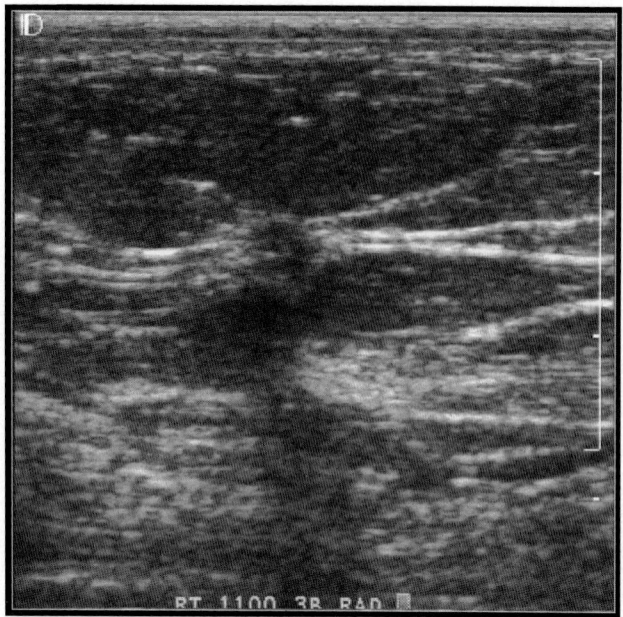

FIGURE 14–83 Tubular carcinomas are frequently completely surrounded by fat and located within Cooper's ligaments or other echogenic fascia layers. Because of the location of these lesions, they exert pronounced effects on the echogenic ligaments, retracting and straightening them out of proportion to the size of the lesion. Notice how much retraction of tissues this small tubular carcinoma creates.

cussed in more detail and illustrated in Chapters 18 and 21. ILCs, like tubular carcinomas, arise peripherally and involve Cooper's ligaments very early but are often much larger, are less likely to be taller than wide, are more ill-defined, and more typically have surrounding fibrous tissue rather than surrounding fat. Low-grade invasive NOS lesions can be indistinguishable from tubular carcinoma but are also usually larger and are more likely to be surrounded by fibrous tissue. Because the intraductal elements of NOS lesions tend to be found in the periphery of the nodule rather than centrally located, NOS lesions are more likely than tubular carcinomas to show evidence of duct extension, branch pattern, and microlobulation. Radial scars are virtually never distinguishable from very small tubular carcinomas sonographically. Radial scars are almost never palpable, but most tubular carcinomas are nonpalpable as well. Not only are tubular carcinomas and radial scars difficult to distinguish from each other, but also tubular carcinomas may arise from radial scars. Recent literature recommends that all areas of suspected radial scar must undergo resection rather than large core needle biopsy. Surgical scars can have findings similar to tubular carcinoma in scan planes parallel to the scar. However, these findings are usually obviously linear scars in scan planes performed perpendicular to the scar. Additionally, fibrous scarring due to

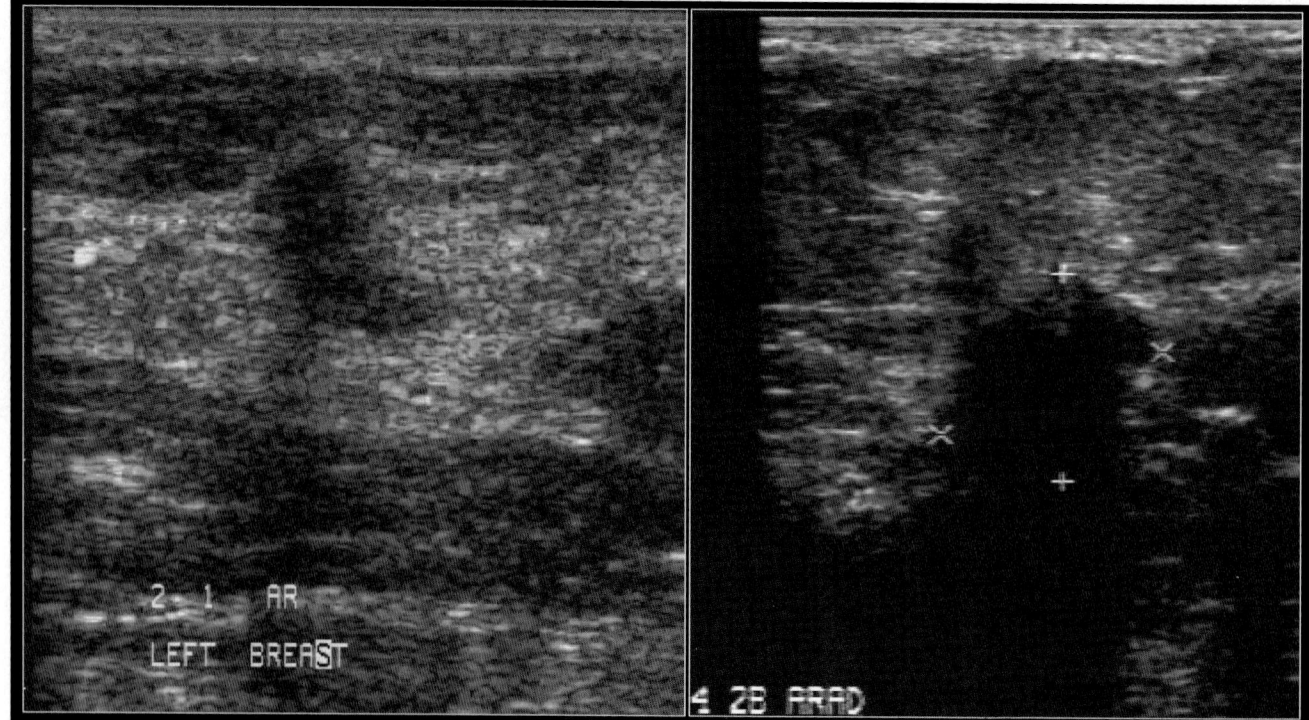

FIGURE 14–84 Low-grade invasive not otherwise specified carcinomas with tubular features are sonographically indistinguishable from pure tubular carcinomas. The sonographic findings in such lesions, like those of pure tubular carcinomas, depend on the size of the lesion. Small lesions tend to have normal sound transmission, whereas larger lesions (<1.5 cm) tend to cast acoustic shadows.

surgery or fat necrosis is usually mildly compressible, and shadowing may disappear when greater scan compression pressure is applied. Tubular carcinomas are typically very hard and incompressible.

INVASIVE PAPILLARY CARCINOMA

General Pathologic Classification, Clinical Findings, and Epidemiology

Invasive papillary carcinomas are uncommon, representing only 1% to 2% of all breast carcinomas. The peak incidence occurs in postmenopausal women between the ages of 63 and 67 years. In men, the invasive papillary carcinoma constitutes a slightly larger percentage of all breast cancers.

Papillary carcinoma is defined as carcinoma having a predominantly papillary pattern, frequently showing foci of papillary DCIS. Areas of tubular carcinoma and cribriform or solid DCIS can be present within papillary carcinomas. There is typically a fibrovascular stromal core or stalk through which the papillary carcinoma receives an abundant blood supply.

About half of papillary carcinomas arise peripherally within TDLUs from areas of florid duct hyperplasia, and half arise centrally, usually within preexisting large duct papillomas. Malignancies that arise from papillomas frequently contain a mixture of papillary carcinoma and benign papilloma. For this reason, many pathologists are reticent to assess the histology of papillary lesions from core needle specimens. Papillary carcinomas are more prone to develop in patients who have multiple peripheral papillomas than in those with single central papillomas. The premalignant potential of multiple central papillomas is uncertain, but one might assume that such lesions have a malignant potential between that of a single central papilloma and the risk for multiple peripheral papillomas.

Invasive papillary carcinomas can present as palpable lumps, as mammographic lesions, or with nipple discharge, which is frequently bloody. The incidence of nipple discharge in patients with papillary carcinoma is 22% to 34%.

At gross pathology, most papillary carcinomas are 2 to 3 cm in size. These lesions are soft, well circumscribed, and frequently encapsulated by a band of fibrosis. Such lesions are also referred to as being encysted, even if there is no fluid around the papillary carcinoma. In most cases, the capsule of such lesions is actually the duct wall or cyst wall within which the lesion is encysted, but in other cases, the capsule represents reactive fibrosis. Papillary carcinomas are often reddish or dark brown in color, stained by hemorrhage of varying ages. When papillary carcinomas occur within a cyst, there are usually clots as well a mural nodule within the cyst. Hemorrhage is thought to occur secondary to infarction or torsion of papillae.

Histologic examination reveals a "frond-forming" lesion with low-grade malignant epithelial cells on the surface of the papillae. Papillary carcinomas typically contain complex glandular spaces as well as larger cystic spaces, which are responsible for the characteristic soft and compressible presentation. There is usually a mixture of invasive papillary and papillary DCIS components. The intraductal (DCIS) components are typically found in the periphery of the lesion. The foci of invasion may be very small and involve only fibrovascular stroma within the lesion, not affecting the periphery of the lesion. When the lesion is encysted, DCIS components extend beyond the cyst into the surrounding soft tissue in almost half the cases. As is the case for invasive NOS lesions, local recurrences are seen more commonly in papillary carcinomas in which EIC extends into surrounding tissues than in lesions in which intraductal components are sparse.

The pathologist may have difficulty distinguishing a benign papilloma from papillary carcinoma, especially when the papillary carcinoma arises within a preexisting papilloma. Associated hemorrhage, chronic inflammation, infarction, and fibrosis can make the margins very irregular and can make determining whether a papillary carcinoma is purely intraductal or invasive. This is especially true of lesions that lie within the nipple or immediately deep to the nipple.

The prognosis for pure invasive papillary carcinoma is relatively good. Assessing data about prognosis is difficult because many studies have not distinguished between invasive papillary carcinoma and papillary DCIS. However, death from invasive papillary carcinoma is rare, and lymph node metastases occur in only about 1% of cases, usually involving only one or two low axillary lymph nodes. Further, invasive papillary carcinomas tend to be slow growing. Because of slow growth, recurrences of papillary carcinoma after local resection tend to occur late—after 5 years.

As is the case with other special-type tumors, there are pure and mixed forms of papillary carcinoma. Although lesions that meet criteria for pure papillary carcinoma have the very good prognosis noted earlier, mixed lesions should be considered to be invasive NOS carcinomas with foci of papillary carcinoma and have a prognosis that is similar to that of the NOS component of the tumor.

Mammographic Findings

The mammographic findings of papillary carcinoma depend on whether the lesion is found within a cyst, whether it is causing nipple discharge, and the relative proportions of DCIS and invasive tumor.

Intracystic papillary carcinomas present as mammographic nodules. These nodules are typically spherically shaped (because the cyst is under tension), well circumscribed, and of high mammographic opacity owing to the presence of intracystic hemorrhage. In lesions in which there is gross invasion of surrounding tissues, the margin on which the invasion is occurring may be indistinct or spiculated. When the lesion contains EIC, there may be calcifications within the intracystic mural nodule or within the intraductal components that extend into the surrounding tissues. Extensions of intraductal tumor into surrounding tissues, like invasion, may cause indistinct margins. In the past, pneumocystography was employed to demonstrate the presence of intracystic papillary lesions, but now high-quality ultrasound makes diagnostic pneumocystography unnecessary.

Lesions that are not within a cyst may present mammographically as a nodule or calcifications. The nodule is frequently "knobby," multinodular, or microlobulated and less often spheroid or elliptical in shape. The more extensive the papillary DCIS components, the more likely there will be associated calcifications and that the distribution of calcifications parallels the distribution of DCIS components. In lesions with gross invasion, the invaded margins may appear indistinct or frankly spiculated.

Papillary carcinomas that cause nipple discharge may be mammographically detectable only on galactography, causing a variety of abnormalities, including (a) a small intraductal papillary lesion that does not fill the duct, (b) a larger intraductal papillary lesion that completely obstructs but does not expand the duct, (c) an expansile and obstructive intraductal papillary lesion, and (d) an irregular partial or complete encasement of a duct.

Sonographic Findings

The sonographic findings of invasive papillary carcinoma, like the mammographic findings, depend on the gross morphology of the lesion.

Intracystic papillary carcinomas can present as mural nodules or thickened septations within cysts. Thickened cyst walls, thick isoechoic septations, and mural nodules must be analyzed very carefully because they are far more frequently caused by FCC with papillary apocrine metaplasia, intracystic clots, or echogenic lipid levels than by intracystic papillomas or papillary carcinomas. The method of sonographically assessing such complex cysts is discussed and illustrated in detail in Chapter 10 (see Figs. 10–25 to 10–34). The most reliable of these imaging findings is the presence of a duct extension from the nodule toward the nipple (Fig. 14–85). Intracystic papillomas, intracystic papillary DCIS, and invasive intracystic papillary carcinoma are not reliably distinguishable from each sonographically; therefore, suspicious intracystic papillary lesions must undergo histologic evaluation.

Invasive papillary carcinomas that are not contained within cysts appear as intraductal nodules, enlarged lobules, or solid nodules. Larger solid nodules caused by papillary carcinoma that do not lie within cysts have two different appearances, depending on whether the lesions arise centrally or peripherally. Lesions that arise peripherally usually originate within TDLUs involved with papillary ductal hyperplasia (papillomatosis). These lesions are

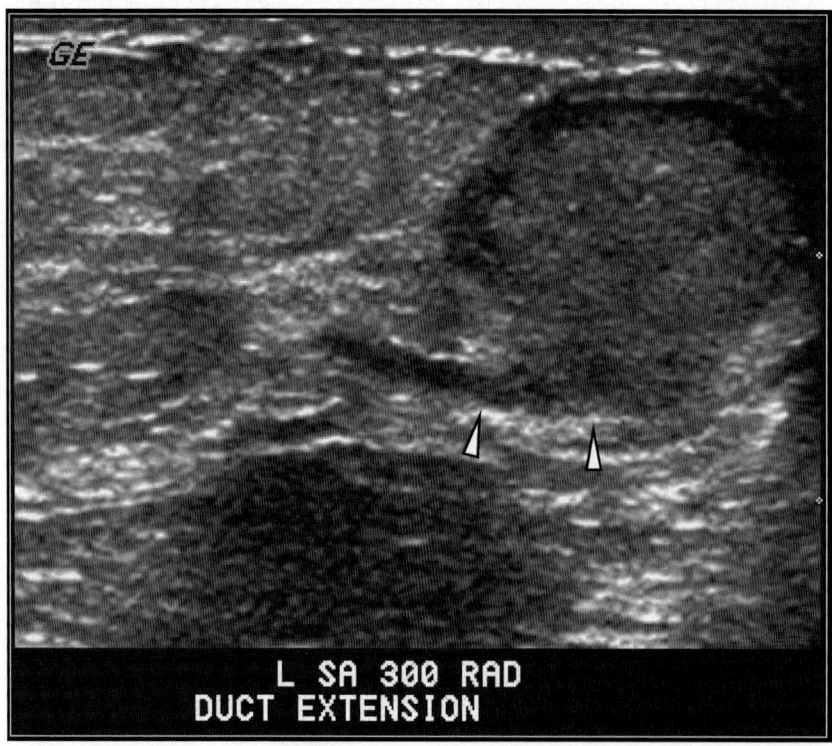

FIGURE 14–85 Intracystic invasive papillary carcinomas often have intraductal components that form a ductal extension toward the nipple *(arrowheads).*

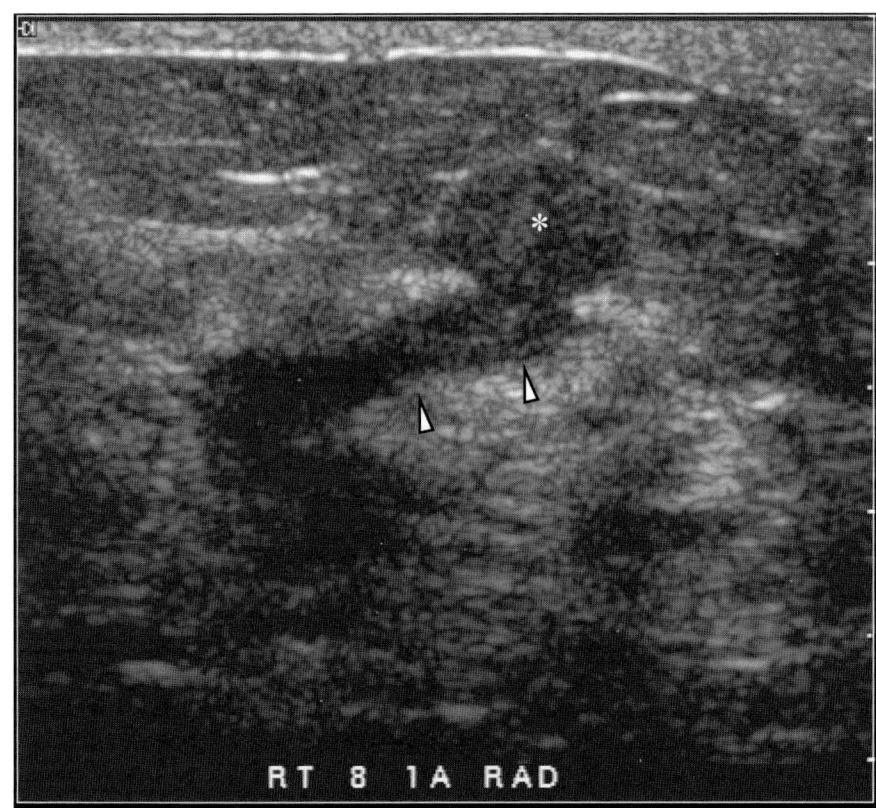

usually circumscribed, are multilobulated or microlobulated in shape, and may have the appearance of grossly abnormally enlarged TDLUs (Fig. 14–86). Intracystic invasive papillary carcinomas are usually hypoechoic and have enhanced through-transmission, likely due to the abundant glandular spaces and cyst and the loose fibrovascular stroma of these lesions. They are usually relatively soft. Split-screen compression images often show compressibility of 15% or more. There may be punctate calcifications within the nodule (Fig. 14–87). When invasive papillary carcinomas have DCIS elements, and when several ducts and lobules are involved, there may be obvious microlobulation, duct extension, or branch patterns (Fig. 14–88). Centrally arising lesions usually have more pronounced duct extension than do peripheral lesions. When the invasive component involves the periphery of the tumor, the margins of the nodule may be angular and spiculated or can have a thick, echogenic halo. However, the invasion frequently occurs centrally, into the internal fibrovascular stroma, and therefore does not affect the outer margins of the lesion. For this reason, the lack of angular margins or absence of a thick, echogenic halo does not exclude invasive carcinoma in these lesions.

Invasive papillary carcinomas that arise centrally and that do not form cysts or cause nipple discharge typically

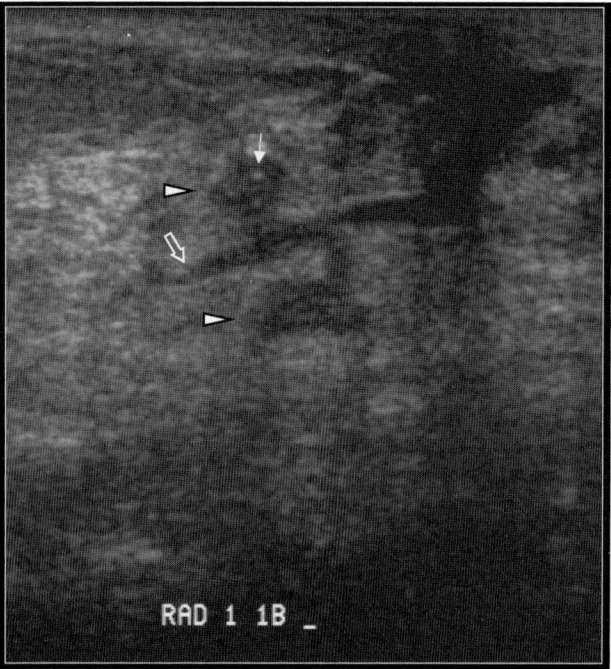

FIGURE 14–87 Papillary carcinomas may have associated punctate calcifications *(arrow)* that usually occur within the ductal carcinoma *in situ* (DCIS) components of the lesion. This lesion has extensive DCIS components that involve two terminal ductolobular units *(arrowheads)* and distal portions of the lobar duct *(hollow arrow)*.

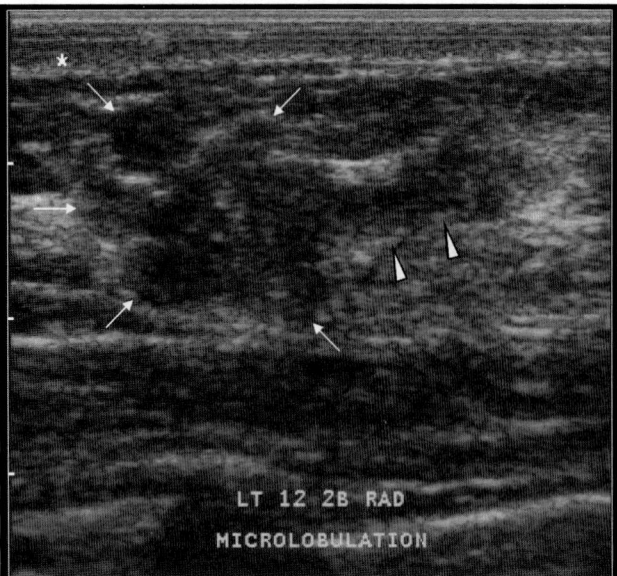

FIGURE 14–88 This large, peripherally arising invasive papillary carcinoma involves the distal end of the lobar duct *(arrowheads)* and several terminal ductolobular units *(arrows)*. It contains multiple punctate calcifications. The through-transmission is less than usual for an invasive papillary carcinoma.

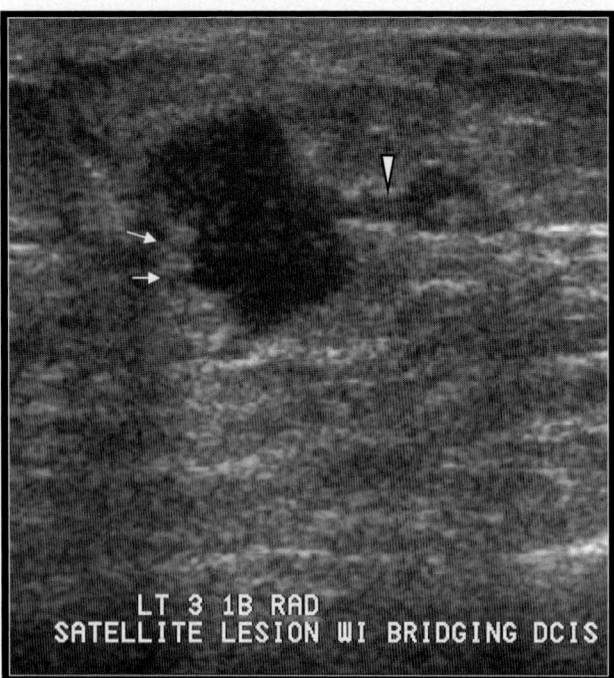

FIGURE 14–89 Centrally located invasive papillary carcinomas frequently have prominent duct extensions of ductal carcinoma *in situ* elements *(arrowheads)* that are best shown in the radial plane. Note the angular margins on the invasive component of the lesion *(arrows)*.

present as solid nodules. Like peripherally arising papillary carcinomas, such lesions are usually well circumscribed, markedly hypoechoic, and soft and demonstrate enhanced through-transmission. Because these lesions almost certainly arise within preexisting large duct papillomas, intraductal components of the lesion are almost certain to be growing along the large-order ducts within which the papilloma arose. Thus, radial scans will demonstrate large duct extensions (Fig. 14–89) and can show extensive branch pattern and microlobulation. As is the case for peripheral lesions, when there is invasion of the outer margin of the lesion, that margin can appear angular, and the lesion can have a thick, echogenic halo or spiculations around it. Calcifications can occur within the central part of the lesion or within duct extensions.

Intraductal solid nodules of variable sizes are most likely to be detected in patients who present with nipple discharge. Malignant intraductal nodules have the same spectrum of sonographic appearances as benign large duct papillomas that are discussed and illustrated in detail in Chapter 8 (see Figs. 8–36 to 8–40). However, malignant intraductal nodules tend to be longer and larger, expand the duct more (Fig. 14–90), and are more likely to involve

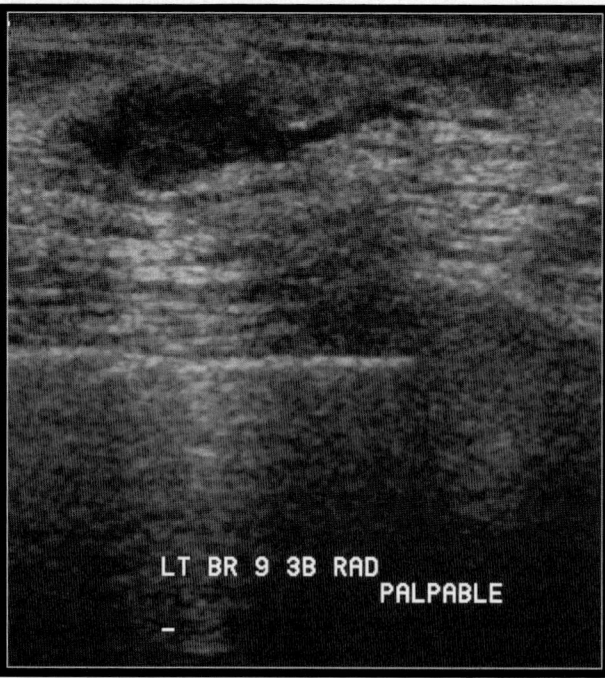

FIGURE 14–90 This centrally arising invasive papillary carcinoma grossly expands a centrally located lobar duct. The histology showed a mixture of benign and invasive malignant papillary elements, suggesting strongly that the carcinoma arose from a preexisting benign large duct papilloma. Invasion was inward, into the fibrovascular core, rather than outward, making margin assessment less valuable than it is for other types of carcinomas. The degree of duct expansion, the length of duct involved, the involvement of branch ducts, and expansion of terminal ductolobular units are better indicators of risk than are margin characteristics for most intraductal papillary lesions.

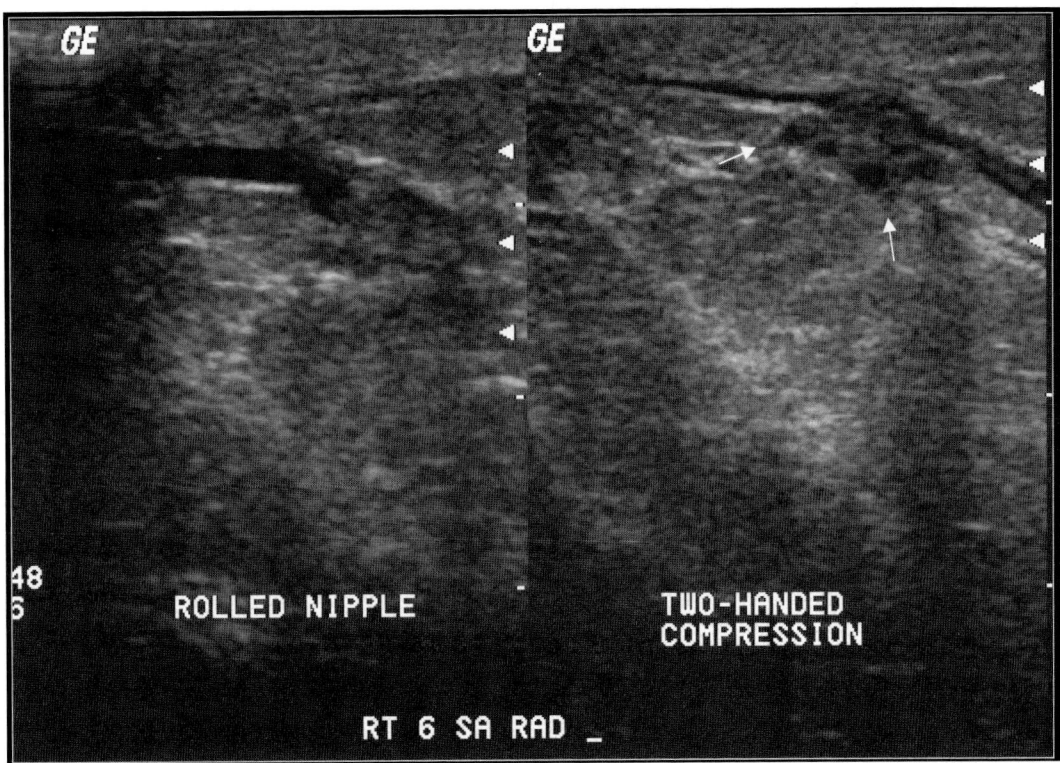

FIGURE 14–91 Extension of an intraductal lesion through the echogenic duct wall is a worrisome finding in intraductal papillary lesions of any size. This small, centrally located invasive papillary carcinoma also arose from a preexisting benign large duct papilloma. However, sonography shows the lesion invading through the posterior duct wall. The disruption of the posterior wall of the duct is better seen when the lesion is compressed with the transducer **(right)**. Note that the component that has invaded through the posterior wall of the duct has angular interfaces *(arrows)* with the surrounding tissues.

distal branch ducts than do benign intraductal papillary lesions. Centrally arising invasive papillary carcinomas that arise from preexisting benign large duct papillomas may erode through the duct wall (Fig. 14–91).

Color Doppler is invaluable in the evaluation of papillary lesions, particularly intracystic lesions. The use of color Doppler in such lesions is illustrated in Chapter 20. All true papillary lesions of the breast—benign papillomas, papillary DCIS, and invasive papillary carcinoma—have prominent fibrovascular cores. In many instances, color or power Doppler can be used to show flow within the fibrovascular stalk that feeds these lesions (see Chapter 20, Fig–20–2). However, because papillary lesions are so soft and compressible, use of too much transducer pressure while performing color Doppler may completely interrupt the flow of blood into the nodule and prevent color Doppler from demonstrating the fibrovascular stalk (see Chapter 20, Fig. 20–14). One subtle difference between the vascular stalk of malignant and benign intracystic papillary lesions is that benign papillomas are generally fed by a single arborizing vessel, whereas malignant intracystic papillary carcinoma more often incites the formation of multiple feeding vessels (see Chapter 20, Fig. 20–31). Color Doppler or power Doppler vocal fremitus can also be useful in distinguishing the intra-cystic papillary lesion from complicating echogenic hemorrhage into the surrounding cyst fluid and adherent clot (see Chapter 20, Figs. 20–32 and 20–93).

INVASIVE LOBULAR CARCINOMA

Pathology, Clinical Findings, and Epidemiology

ILC is the second most common invasive breast malignancy. Depending on the strictness of definition and whether invasive lobular variants are included, ILC accounts for 5% to 15% of all invasive breast malignancies.

ILC can be classified as either classic (pure) or variant. Variant types include solid and alveolar lobular carcinomas. Some also include tubulolobular carcinoma as a variant; ILCs that have mixtures of these types are classified as mixed or pleomorphic. Variant types differ from classic ILCs not only in histology but also in biologic behavior and prognosis.

ILCs are slightly more common in elderly women but occur throughout the same age ranges as invasive NOS carcinomas. The mean age at diagnosis is between 45 and 56 years.

When an ILC does cause a palpable abnormality, the lesion is usually an ill-defined mass or vague thickening rather than a well-defined nodule. At times, ILC causes innumerable small, hard nodules or a diffuse granularity within the breast that feels like grains of rice or small pebbles. However, in many cases, even large ILCs do not cause palpable abnormalities. Of all invasive malignancies, ILC is the least likely to result in a palpable mass or nodule and therefore the most likely to have a falsely negative clinical examination. The subtleness of clinical findings associated with ILC reflects the diffusely infiltrating nature of the lesion.

Like the clinical findings, the gross pathology of ILC is variable. Certain lesions develop as a well-defined, hard, fixed mass, similar to the mass cause by scirrhous invasive NOS carcinomas. In other cases, ILC causes an ill-defined area of induration within the biopsy specimen. In the few cases in which infiltration is very diffuse and there is no associated desmoplastic response, even very large ILCs may not be palpable within the resected specimen. The size range of ILC is similar to that for NOS carcinomas, but a precise diameter can be difficult to measure in the diffusely infiltrating form.

The histology of ILCs reflects two features: (a) cytology and (b) pattern of infiltration. Classic or pure ILC is a diffusely infiltrative lesion. Pure classic ILC is composed of small, only mildly atypical cells that diffusely infiltrate surrounding fibrous tissue in single rows or columns. The cells are similar to those seen in LCIS and have few mitoses. This histologic pattern of single-file infiltration has been described as "Indian file" or "single file," the latter a more politically correct term. In cases of ILC that are paucicellular, there may be large spans of normal stroma between columns of tumor cells. In such cases, needle biopsy, especially FNAB, may miss the tumor cells. There are cases in which the tumor cells grow in concentric rings around the ducts in a pattern that has been termed *targetoid*. ILC tends to be less destructive than invasive NOS carcinoma. The tumor cells in ILC tend to grow along and between normal structures without destroying background tissue. Thus, the stromal fibrous tissue within which are interspersed columns of tumor cells is infiltrated but otherwise normal breast tissue. In fact, the lack of destruction and absence of desmoplastic response associated with diffusely infiltrating lesions often results in a lack of a central tumor nidus and accounts for the lack of a well-defined palpable mass and the high rate of falsely negative clinical exams and mammograms in patients with diffusely infiltrating classic ILC.

Solid and alveolar variants of ILC have similar cytology but differ in the pattern of infiltration. Solid-type ILC grows in sheets rather than in single-file columns. Alveolar-type ILC grows in a pattern of small nodules. Both of these variant types of ILC are more likely to have a central nidus that is palpable and to cause mammographic or sonographic masses than is classic ILC. Mixed or pleomorphic varieties can have a mixture of two or more of these patterns of infiltration. Classic or pure ILC must have a dif-fusely infiltrating single-file pattern in 70% or more of the lesion. An ILC containing less than 70% classic pattern must be classified as mixed or pleomorphic. In some cases, it can be difficult to distinguish mixed or pleomorphic ILC from NOS carcinoma.

A high percentage of ILCs have associated LCIS within the lesion or within the surrounding tissues. LCIS most commonly occurs with classic ILC, in which 90% of lesions have associated LCIS, but also occurs less frequently in solid and alveolar variants, in which 50% to 60% of cases have associated LCIS.

The incidence of bilaterality or multicentricity in ILC is high. Reported incidences of bilaterality vary from 6% to 47%. The highest risk for multicentricity and bilaterality occurs with classic ILC and reflects the underlying risk in the 90% of cases that have associated LCIS components. Additionally, classic ILC may show pagetoid growth within ducts, and this intraductal growth, if extensive, may contribute to multifocality of the lesion.

The prognosis of ILC is controversial. There are researchers who have reported a better prognosis for ILC than for invasive NOS carcinoma, but others have found ILC and NOS carcinoma to have the same prognosis. There is high likelihood that if only pure or classic ILC is considered and strictly defined, the prognosis is slightly better than for NOS carcinomas but worse than for tubular carcinomas. Solid and alveolar variants and mixed or pleomorphic forms of ILC appear to have prognoses similar to that of NOS and worse than that of classic ILC. As is the case for NOS carcinomas, size and lymph node status are the primary determinants of prognosis in patients with ILC. Multicentricity and bilaterality complicate assessment of prognosis based on size. Nuclear grade also affects prognosis. Typically, ILCs are not graded using the Bloom-Richardson-Scarff histologic grade but are assigned nuclear grades similar to those assigned to DCIS.

The pattern of hematogenous metastases from ILC is peculiar and differs from that of other breast cancers. ILC is more prone to metastasize to gut, peritoneum and retroperitoneum, gynecologic organs, and leptomeninges than are other types of breast cancer.

Mammographic Findings

The mammographic findings of ILC are nonspecific. The most common finding is an asymmetric density with or without architectural distortion. Less common is a spiculated or indistinctly marginated mass. Only about 10% of cases have associated calcifications. Most ILCs do not have high mammographic opacity because of the diffuse infiltrating pattern into normal tissues. Rather, these lesions are isodense with surrounding breast tissues. This fact should not be surprising because the lesions are, in fact, composed mainly of normal breast tissue within which are widely scattered columns of infiltrating tumor cells. Unfortunately, many ILCs do not cause any mammographic abnormality. Even very large, diffusely infiltrating ILCs may be missed in mammographically opaque breasts. A disproportional percentage of falsely negative mammograms are due to diffusely infiltrating lesions, and ILC accounts for slightly more than half of such lesions.

Sonographic Findings

Sonography may be even more important in diagnosing ILC than other types of breast carcinoma because mammography is more frequently false negative in cases of ILC than in other types. The sonographic findings of ILC vary greatly, as do the pathologic and mammographic findings. The sonographic findings range from no detectable lesions at all to masses that have appearances similar to infiltrating NOS carcinomas. However, the rate of false-negative sonograms is much lower than the rate of false-negative mammograms. Sonographic detectability depends on whether the ILC forms a central mass and the relative proportion of the lesion that is diffusely infiltrating. Lesions that do not form a central tumor mass and that are entirely composed of diffusely infiltrating elements are most likely to be missed sonographically, especially if the lesions are paucicellular and the single-file columns of tumor cells are widely separated by normal stromal fibrous tissue. Such lesions are also

the most likely to be missed by clinical examination and mammography. Sonography usually detects, but is prone to underestimate, the size of lesions that manifest abundant epithelial growth centrally but have diffusely infiltrating elements in the periphery. The variant lesions, by virtue of their pattern of growth, are more likely to form a dominant tumor that is readily detectable by sonography.

Certain cases of ILC form masses that simulate NOS carcinomas. These lesions are usually mildly to moderately hypoechoic, have angular or ill-defined margins, and demonstrate moderate to severe degrees of acoustic shadowing (Fig. 14–92). Because ILC generally does not incite much desmoplastic response, the shadowing is likely caused by alteration in the axes of normal stromal fibrous tissue planes by columns of infiltrating tumor cells rather than by desmoplasia. Even when ILC forms a discrete hypoechoic central tumor nidus, the diffusely infiltrating peripheral components of tumor may rise to a halo around the central nidus that appears isoechoic or only slightly less echogenic than normal interlobular stromal fibrous tissue (Fig. 14–93). The echotexture of both the central hypoechoic tumor nidus and the surrounding isoechoic or mildly hyperechoic halo around classic ILC lesions is usually heterogeneous because of the tendency of ILC to infiltrate around normal structures without destroying them (Fig. 14–94). The bright echoes giving rise to the heterogeneous

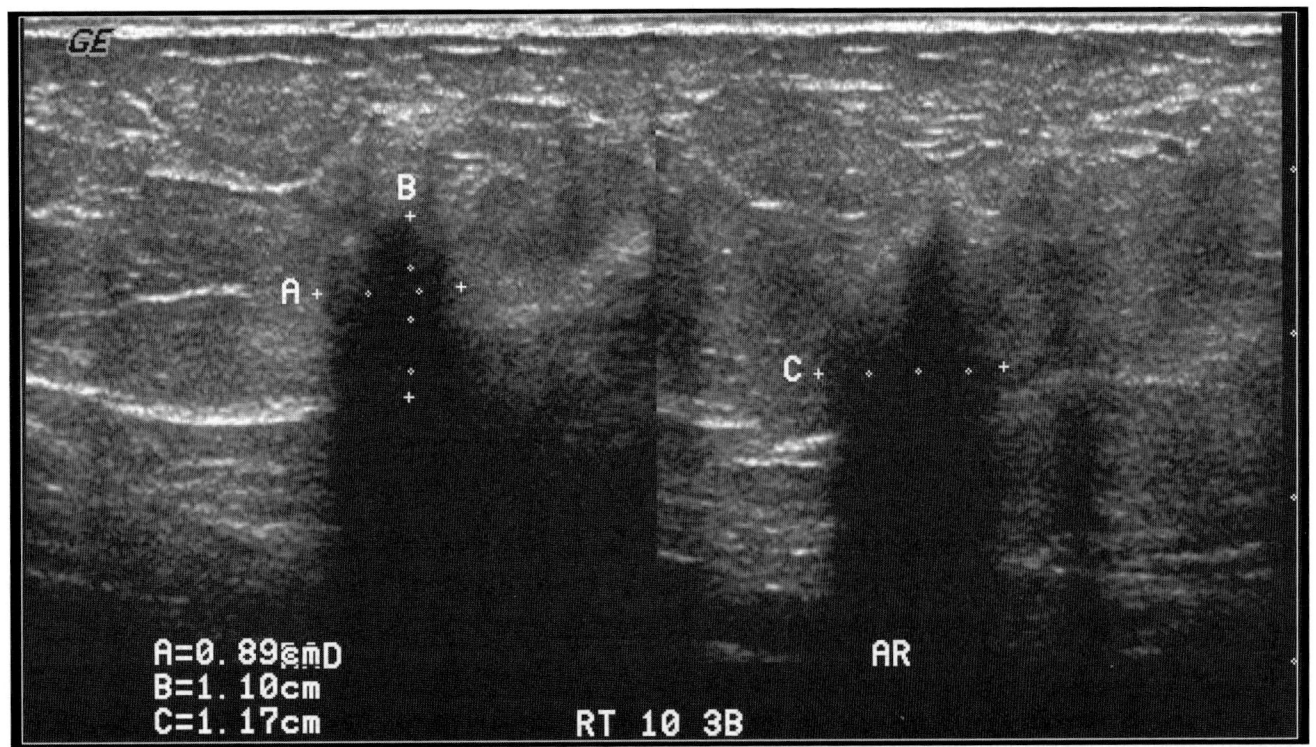

FIGURE 14–92 Invasive lobular carcinoma that forms a discrete mass has a sonographic appearance that simulates low-grade invasive not otherwise specified carcinoma. The lesion is hypoechoic, has angular and ill-defined margins, and causes intense acoustic shadowing.

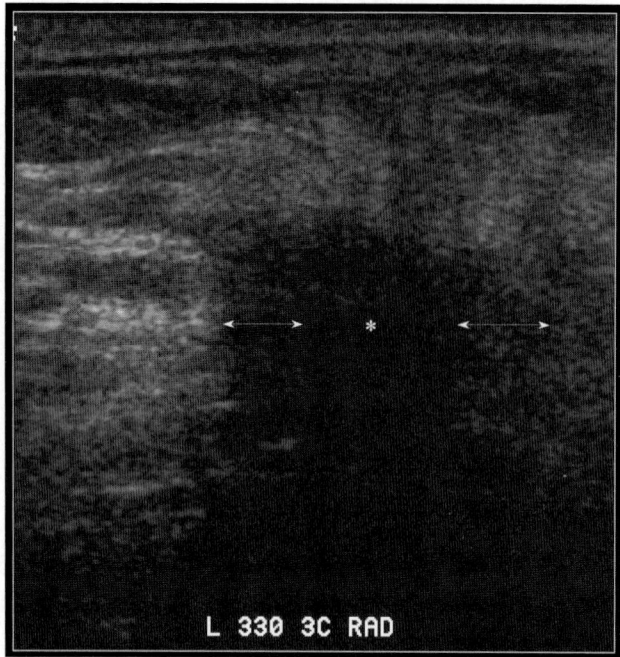

FIGURE 14–93 This invasive lobular carcinoma forms a discrete, markedly hypoechoic mass centrally *(*)* but has a mildly hypoechoic thick halo around the central nodule *(double-headed arrows)* that represents a peripheral zone of diffuse infiltration.

FIGURE 14–94 The echotexture of invasive lobular carcinoma (ILC) is heterogenous because of its tendency to infiltrate around normal structures such as vessels and ducts without destroying them. The bright internal echoes within ILC arise from interfaces between tumor and residual normal structures such as ducts and vessels.

echotexture are likely caused by normal stromal, ductal, lobular, and vascular structures that have been encased, but not destroyed, by tumor cells.

Even diffusely infiltrating classic ILC lesions that do not form a discrete central tumor mass can cause very subtle

changes that are detectable sonographically. An ill-defined area of decreased echogenicity within normally more hyperechoic stromal fibrous tissue (gray rather than white fibrous tissue) can be the only finding in such cases (Fig. 14–95). Awareness that such areas may represent diffusely infiltrat-

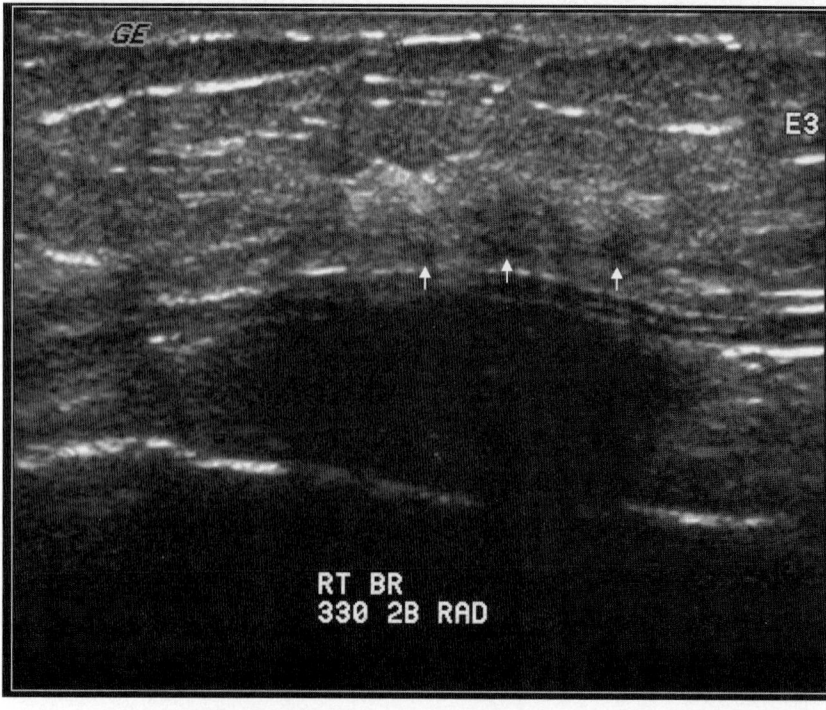

FIGURE 14–95 In cases of diffusely infiltrating classic invasive lobular carcinoma (ILC), the only sonographic finding can be a subtle decrease in echogenicity *(arrows)* of the normally intensely hyperechoic interlobular stromal fibrous tissue. This lesion is multifocal, a common occurrence in classic ILC.

ing neoplasm (ILC or NOS lesions can have a diffuse infiltrating pattern) can help prevent false-negative studies. However, such findings are not specific for diffusely infiltrating malignancy and can be seen in a variety of benign and malignant conditions that cause enlargement and coalescence of numerous TDLUs, including a variety of FCCs (e.g., apocrine metaplasia, microcysts, mucous formation, fibrosclerosis), adenosis and sclerosing adenosis, florid duct hyperplasia, pseudoangiomatous stromal hyperplasia (PASH), atypical ductal or lobular hyperplasia, and DCIS.

Power Doppler vocal fremitus can be helpful in distinguishing diffusely infiltrating malignancies from benign FCCs, benign proliferative changes, or ANDIs (see Chapter 20, Figs. 20–86 and 20–87).

An ill-defined area of partial acoustic shadowing is another finding that can occur as the result of diffusely infiltrating ILC (Fig. 14–96). In some cases, the profile of the area of shadowing is rather typical of classic diffusely infiltrating ILC. When two or three adjacent Cooper's ligaments are involved, the hypoechoic or shadowing area can assume a shape similar to the profile of a suspension bridge—a finding we have termed the *Golden Gate sign* (Fig. 14–97). When more numerous and more closely spaced Cooper's ligaments are involved, the shadowing profile resembles that of a picket fence (Fig. 14–98).

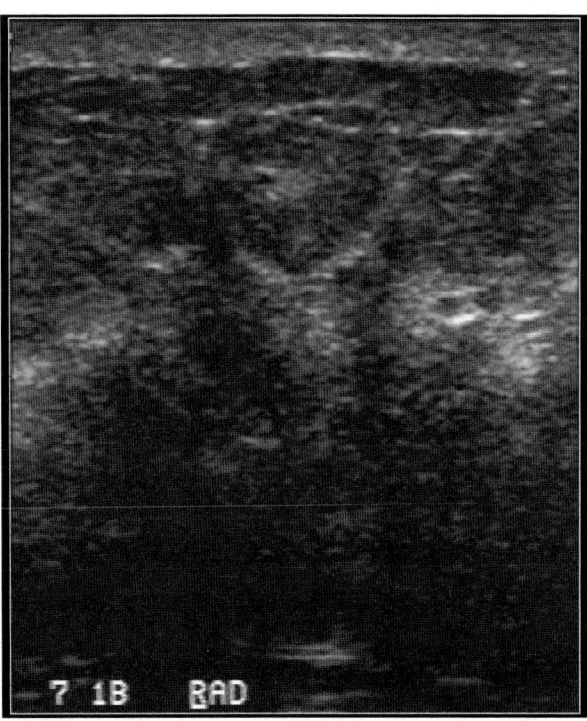

FIGURE 14–96 Ill-defined acoustic shadowing is another finding that may be caused by diffusely infiltrating classic invasive lobular carcinoma.

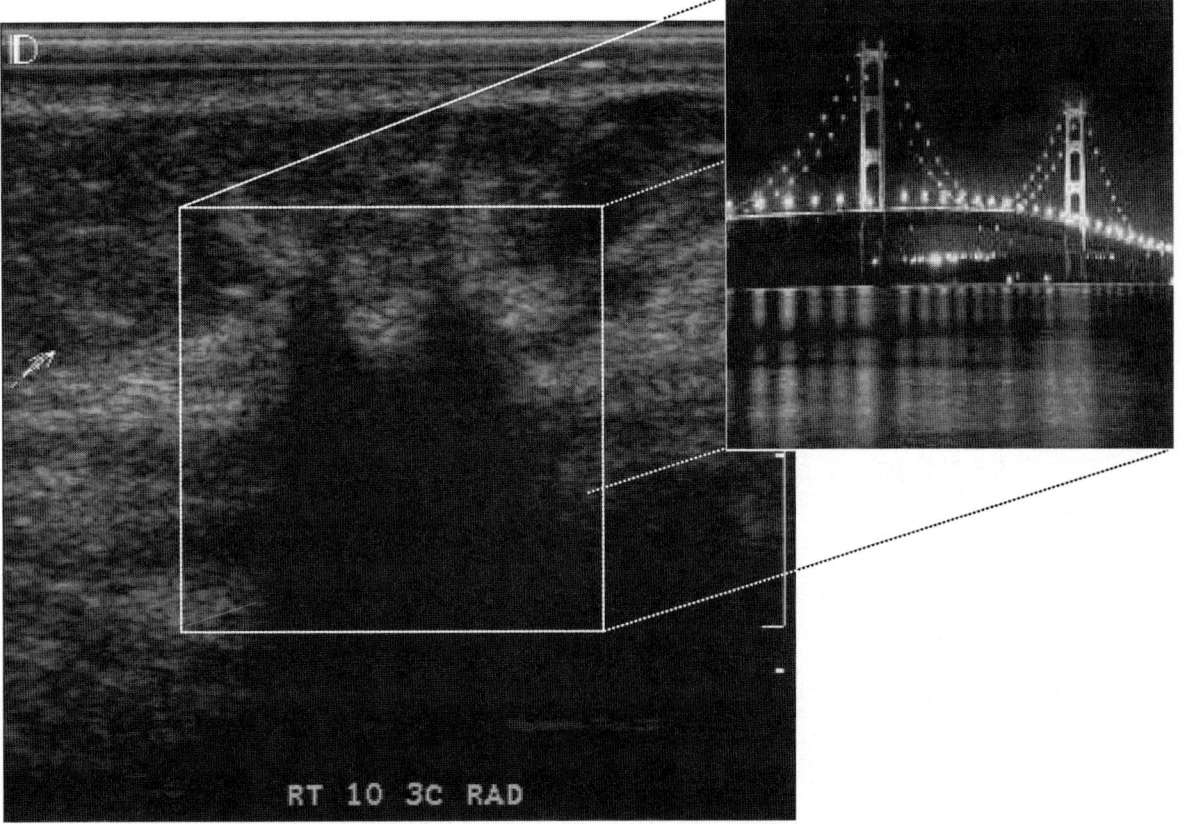

FIGURE 14–97 Because of its propensity to spread horizontally and involve the bases of multiple Cooper's ligaments, the shape of the leading edge of the shadow caused by invasive lobular carcinoma (ILC) shows two or more peaks that resemble the profile of a suspension bridge. We have termed this characteristic ILC shadow profile the "Golden Gate" sign.

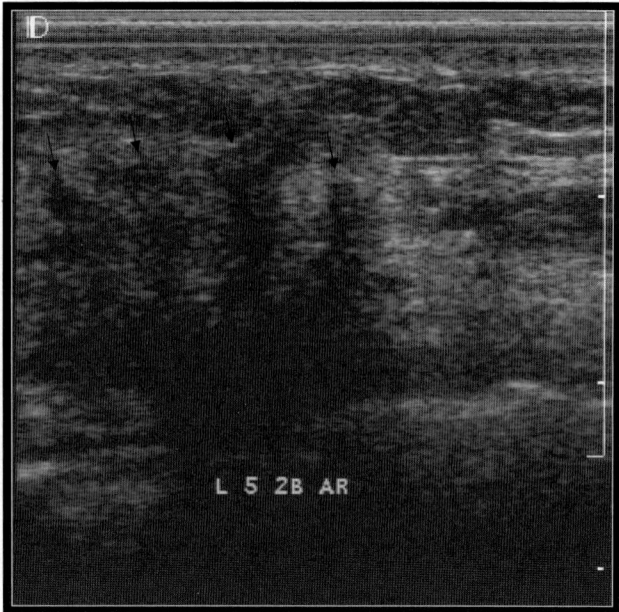

FIGURE 14–98 Invasive lobular carcinoma that involves the base of numerous, more closely spaced Cooper's ligaments can have a picket fence appearance. *(arrows)*

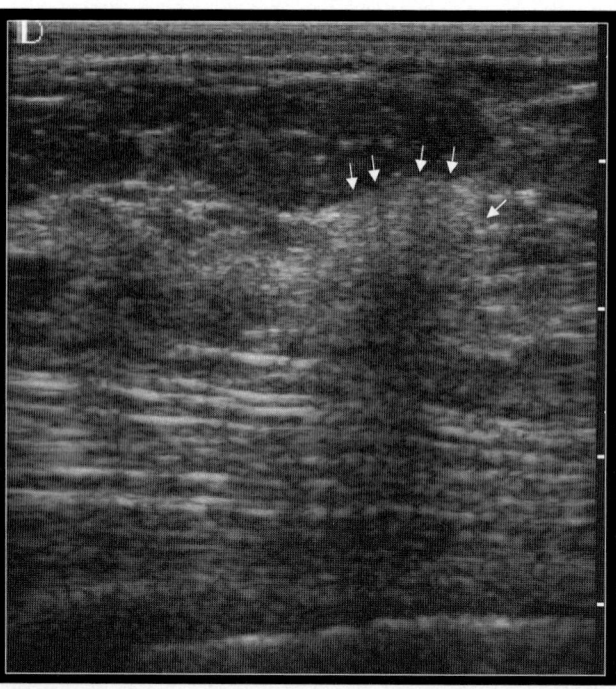

FIGURE 14–99 Classic invasive lobular carcinoma that lies within hyperechoic fibrous tissue can demonstrate hypoechoic spicules of diffuse infiltration *(arrows)*.

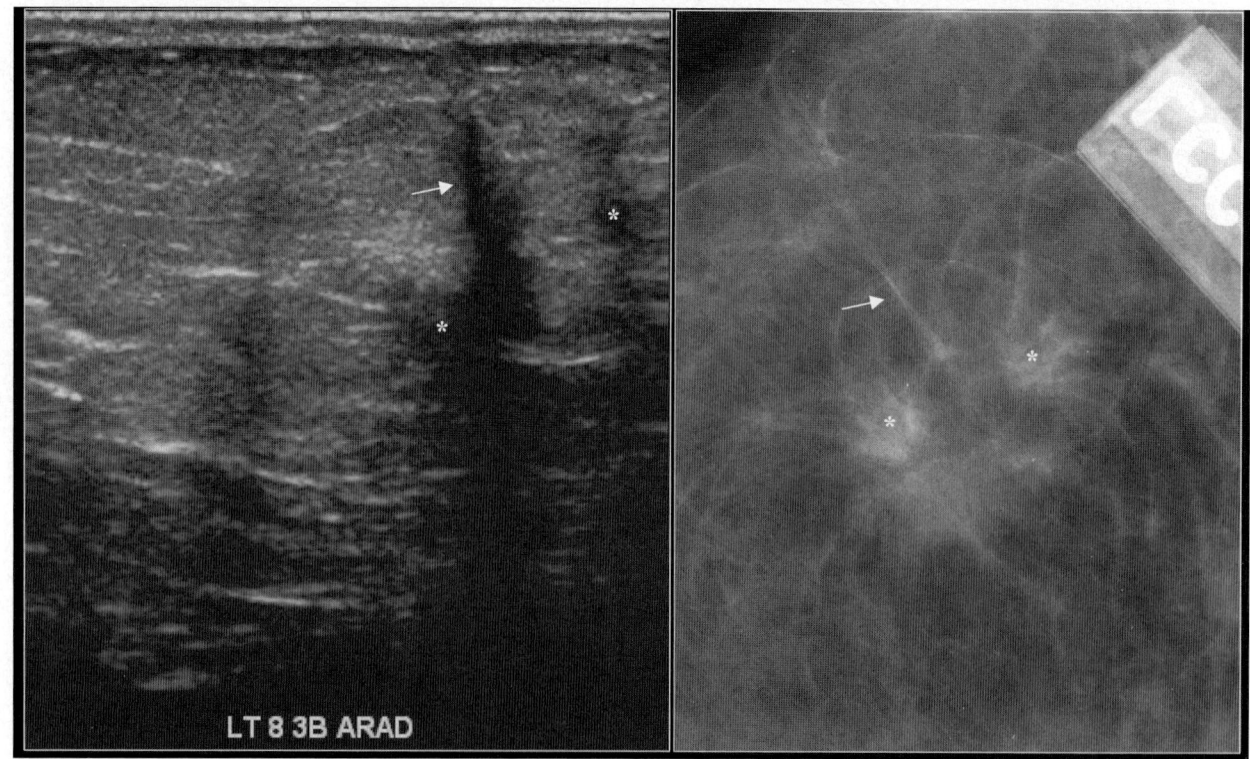

FIGURE 14–100 Cooper's ligaments that are invaded by classic invasive lobular carcinoma (ILC) may appear hypoechoic, widened, and straightened *(arrows)*. Multiple discrete tumor nidi are also present *(*)*.

Like subtle hypoechogenicity, ill-defined shadowing is also a nonspecific finding. Shadowing can be artifactual, arising in critical angle phenomena tissue planes that are oriented steeply obliquely to the ultrasound beam. Such critical angle shadowing can be minimized by vigorous compression with the transducer that forces obliquely oriented tissue planes into horizontal planes. The shadowing caused by diffusely infiltrating malignant lesions, on the other hand, is unlikely to be significantly decreased or eradicated by compression. Shadowing can also be caused by benign sclerosing breast processes such as radial scar and fibrosclerosis, but shadowing that arises from these lesions usually cannot be ablated by compression. Diabetic mastopathy may also cause one or more areas of ill-defined acoustic shadowing.

Careful assessment for subtle architectural distortions and alterations in echogenicity can help to detect diffusely infiltrating classic ILCs. ILC originates within TDLUs that are distended by LCIS. From there, it diffusely infiltrates between collagen fibers into surrounding fibrous tissues, along and around ducts, and into Cooper's ligaments. Careful analysis of ductal and lobular anatomy can reveal the central nidus of the tumor to be enlargement of small ducts or TDLUs that are surrounded by architectural distortions. Fine, subtly hypoechoic spicules of tumor can extend into surrounding hyperechoic fibrous tissue (Fig. 14–99). Invaded Cooper's ligaments can appear thickened, straightened, and abnormally hypoechoic centrally (Fig. 14–100). With very light compression and an acoustic gel standoff, skin retraction by an affected Cooper's ligament can be demonstrated. Some lesions grow intraductally toward the nipple (pagetoid spread), giving rise to sonographically visible duct extensions (Fig. 14–101). However, the pagetoid spread of classic ILC seldom enlarges ducts enough for this finding to be sonographically demonstrable.

The variant types of ILC, which typically create better-defined masses histologically, also form better-defined masses sonographically. Alveolar variant of ILC presents as a discrete solid nodule that either has frank spiculations or a thick, echogenic halo. Such an appearance simulates that of low- to intermediate-grade NOS carcinomas (Fig. 14–102). The solid variant of ILC typically presents as a circumscribed hypoechoic solid nodule with enhanced sound transmission that more closely resembles high-grade invasive NOS carcinomas (Fig. 14–103).

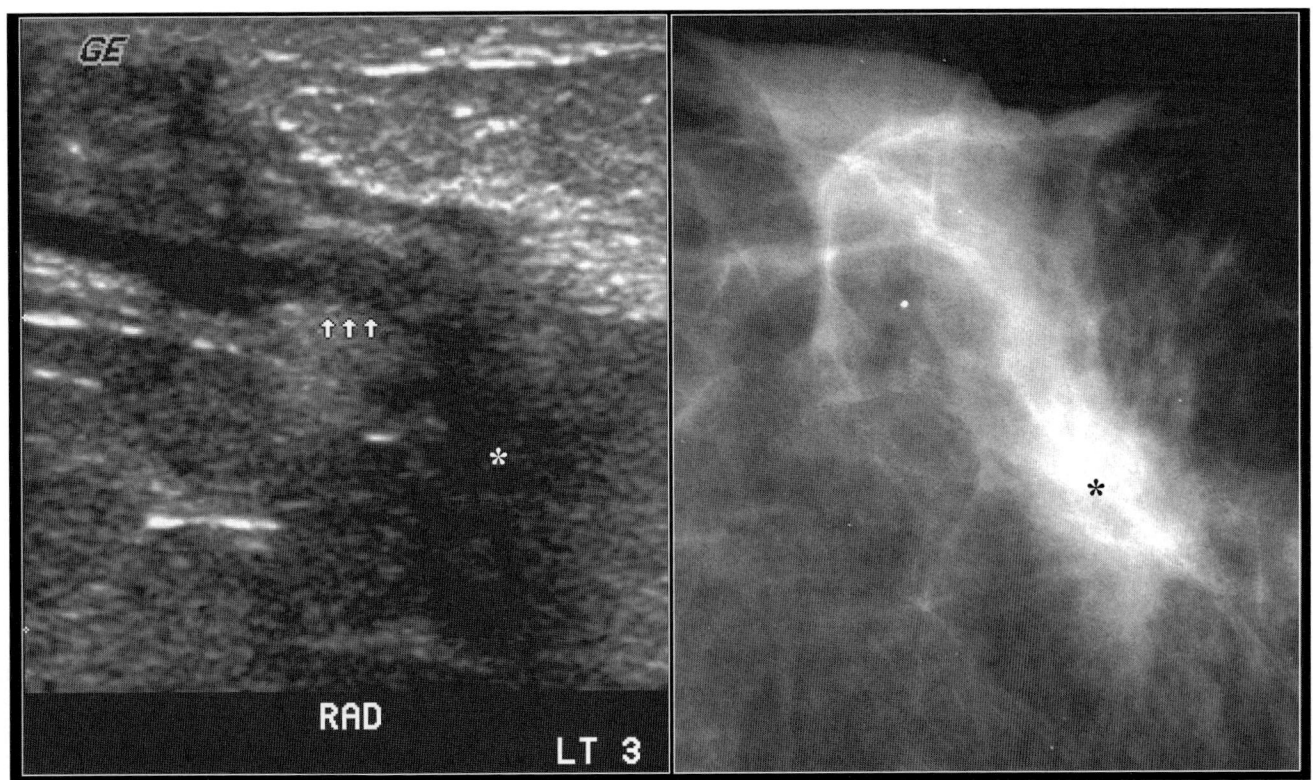

FIGURE 14–101 Classic invasive lobular carcinoma (ILC) can spread intraductally toward the nipple (*arrows* indicate pagetoid spread, * indicates classic ILC part of lesion). However, it is unusual for pagetoid spread of classic ILC to cause this degree of duct enlargement.

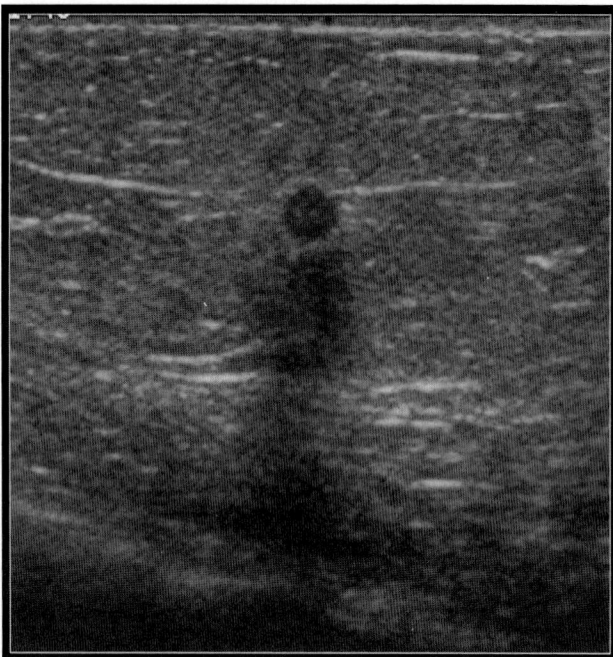

FIGURE 14–102 Alveolar variant of invasive lobular carcinoma creates better-defined nodules that are either frankly spiculated or encompassed by a thick, echogenic halo. The sonographic appearance is similar to that of small low-grade not otherwise specified and tubular carcinomas.

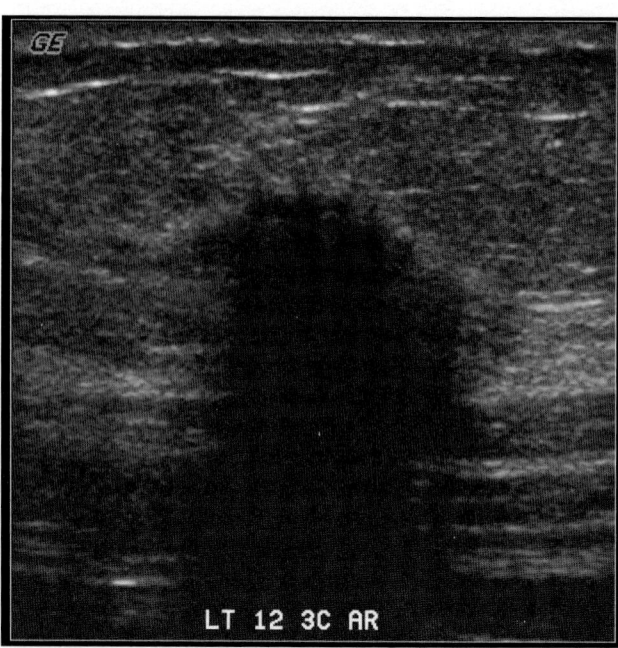

FIGURE 14–104 Tubulolobular carcinomas that are larger than 1.5 cm in maximum diameter tend to be markedly hypoechoic, cause intense acoustic shadowing, and are either frankly spiculated or encompassed by a thick, echogenic halo. The appearance is similar to that of large low-grade invasive not otherwise specified carcinomas, tubular carcinomas larger than 1.5 cm, and some classic invasive lobular carcinomas.

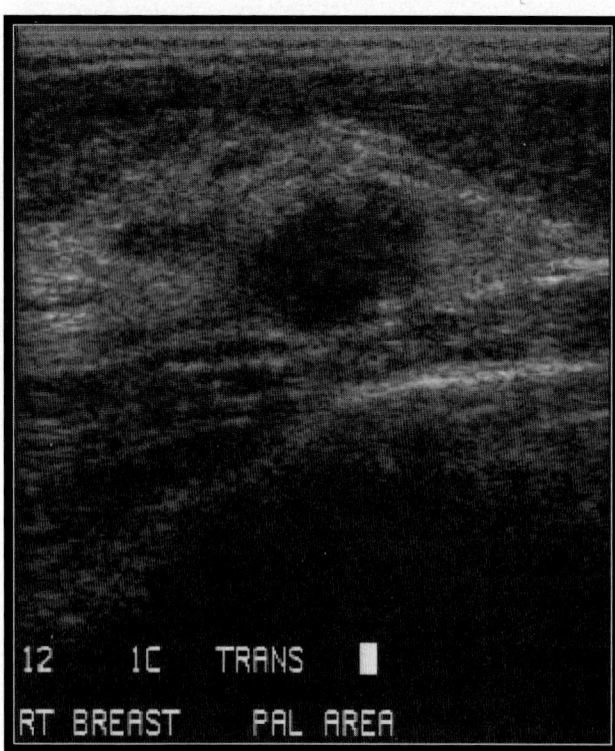

FIGURE 14–103 The solid variant of invasive lobular carcinoma creates circumscribed masses that have normal or enhanced through-transmission and that resemble high-grade invasive not otherwise specified carcinomas.

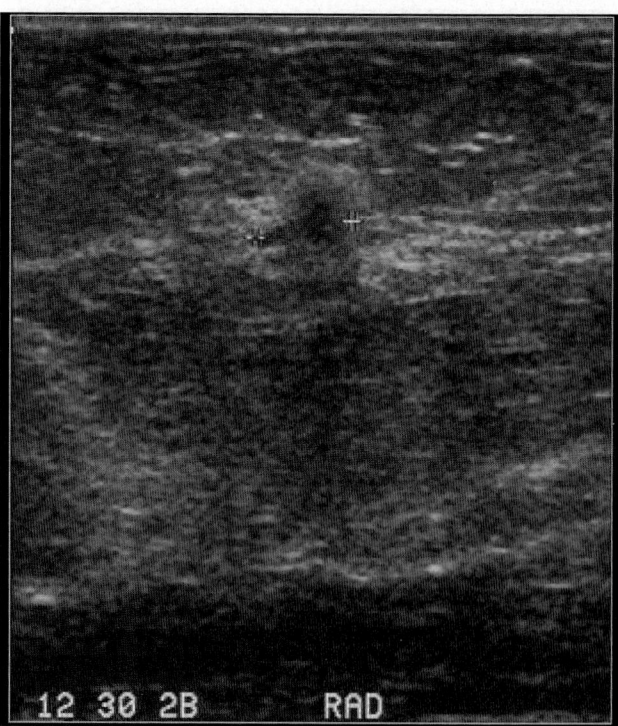

FIGURE 14–105 Small tubulolobular carcinomas that are less than 1.5 cm in diameter often appear isoechoic or only mildly hypoechoic, have angular margins, and are either frankly spiculated or encompassed within a thick, echogenic halo. Sound transmission can be either normal or decreased. The sonographic appearance is similar to that of small low- to intermediate-grade invasive not otherwise specified or tubular carcinomas that are less than 1.5 cm in maximum diameter.

TUBULOLOBULAR CARCINOMA

Whether tubulolobular carcinoma is a special type of invasive NOS of carcinoma or a variant of ILC is controversial. Histologically, tubulolobular carcinoma forms tubules within areas of ILC. The distribution of tubules and single-file ILC within the lesion is highly variable. The prognosis of such a lesion is better than for classic ILC but worse than for pure tubular carcinoma. Like tubular carcinoma, tubulolobular carcinoma can contain DCIS elements.

The lesions are grossly firm to palpation and usually are not large (less than 2 cm in most cases).

The mammographic features are nonspecific, but more similar to those of tubular carcinoma than to those of ILC.

The sonographic appearances of tubulolobular carcinoma, like those of pure tubular carcinoma, vary with the maximum diameter of the lesion. Lesions larger than 1.5 cm in maximum diameter typically appear to be markedly hypoechoic, have angular margins, cast acoustic shadows, and are either frankly spiculated or are surrounded by thick, echogenic halos (Fig. 14–104). Lesions that have maximum diameters less than 1.5 cm can have appearances identical to larger lesions, but more typically are isoechoic and have angular margins and thick, echogenic halos (Fig. 14–105). The greater the percentage of tubular carcinoma within the lesion, the more likely the lesion is to be markedly hypoechoic and cause acoustic shadowing.

Other Uncommon and Rare Forms of Invasive Primary Breast Cancer

There are numerous uncommon and rare forms of primary invasive breast cancer. These tumors are rarely seen or reported in regard to sonographic appearance. In most instances, these lesions manifest multiple suspicious features that require a BIRADS 4a or higher characterization, but the sonographic features are not specific enough to allow distinction between these rare lesions and the far more common invasive NOS, ILC, or special-type carcinomas. These lesions include the following:

- Invasive cribriform carcinoma
- Secretory carcinoma
- Squamous cell carcinoma
- Salivary gland–type carcinomas
- Adenoid cystic carcinoma
- Mucoepidermoid carcinoma
- Pleomorphic (mixed cell) carcinoma
- Signet ring carcinoma
- Lipid-rich carcinoma
- Clear cell carcinoma
- Carcinoma with sarcomatous metaplasia
- Carcinoma with spindle cell metaplasia
- Myoepithelioma
- Carcinoid
- Carcinosarcoma

METAPLASTIC CARCINOMA (CARCINOMA WITH SARCOMATOUS METAPLASIA, CARCINOSARCOMA)

Metaplastic carcinoma is rare, representing only 0.2% of all breast malignancies. It is a mixture of high-grade NOS or anaplastic carcinomatous and metaplastic sarcomatous elements. The proportion of the lesion that is sarcomatous varies from 10% to 96% of the mass. The types of sarcomatous element also vary widely. Loose or tight spindle cells and fibrosarcomatous, chondroid, and osteoid elements are common. Myxoid and fibromyxoid types also occur, and individual lesions can contain mixtures of sarcomatous elements. Additionally, the metaplastic elements can evolve from one type to another over time. For example, we have seen chondroid sarcomatous elements progress to osteoid sarcomatous elements after induction chemotherapy. Because there are both carcinomatous and sarcomatous elements, the term *carcinosarcoma* has also been used to describe these lesions.

Metaplastic carcinomas occur in the same age groups as invasive NOS carcinomas and ILC. Metaplastic carcinomas have a very poor prognosis, even worse than that of high-grade NOS carcinomas. The more anaplastic the carcinomatous elements are and the higher the percentage of the lesion that is sarcomatous, the worse the prognosis. Regional lymph node metastases are generally from the carcinomatous element, but hematogenous metastases can arise from both carcinomatous and sarcomatous elements.

Most metaplastic carcinomas form large, firm masses. Because they grow so rapidly, they are typically quite large (often more than 5 cm) and adherent to surrounding structures at the time of discovery.

Mammographic Findings

Mammographically, the lesions appear to be large, high-density, circumscribed but lobulated masses. Calcifications are uncommon, but ossification can occur within osteoid sarcomatous elements.

Sonographic Findings

Sonographically, metaplastic carcinomas are large solid lobulated masses that frequently have areas of cystic or hemorrhagic necrosis. The border is microlobulated and angular in most cases. The mixture of carcinomatous and sarcomatous elements and the varying types of sarcoma usually result in the texture being markedly heterogeneous, even in areas of the tumor where there are no cystic changes (Fig. 14–106). The margins are well circumscribed and encompassed by a thin, echogenic pseudocapsule of compressed breast tissue in most cases, placing these lesions at the circumscribed end of the malignant spectrum. Some cases can incite an intense enough peritumoral inflammatory response to create a thick, echogenic halo of peritumoral edema. Most lesions demonstrate enhanced through-transmission, but some transmit sound normally. However, lesions that contain osteoid sarcomatous elements tend to create intense acoustic shadows (Fig. 14–107). Carcinomatous elements within the lesion can contain DCIS components that spread intraductally, giving rise to prominent duct extensions in some cases (Fig. 14–108). Metaplastic carcinomas are very active metabolically and therefore are hypervascular on color Doppler, except within areas of necrosis.

SARCOMAS OF THE BREAST

Pathology, Clinical Findings, and Epidemiology

Sarcomas of the breast include those arising from phyllodes tumors—usually mixed cell types; those arising from breast stroma—pure or mixed; angiosarcoma; fibrosarcoma; liposarcoma; malignant fibrous histiocytoma; chondrosarcoma; and osteosarcoma. Pure sarcomas of the breast (except for malignant phyllodes tumors) are quite rare. They are not as common as carcinomas with sarcomatous metaplasia. Pure sarcomas can arise from a preexisting mesenchymal tumor (such as a phyllodes tumor), a hamartoma, or normal underlying breast stroma. Lesions arising from normal breast stroma are even less common than those arising within a preexisting mesenchymal tumor are. Because of the paucity of reports describing the sonographic appearance of breast sarcomas (other than those arising from phyllodes tumors), a thorough discussion is beyond the scope of this book. Most sarcomas have malignant sonographic features that require a BIRADS 4a or higher classification. As is the case for breast carcinomas, breast sarcomas can appear to be either circumscribed or spiculated. Most have normal to enhanced through-transmission, are very vascular on color Doppler, and are quite heterogeneous internally (Fig. 14–109). However, the

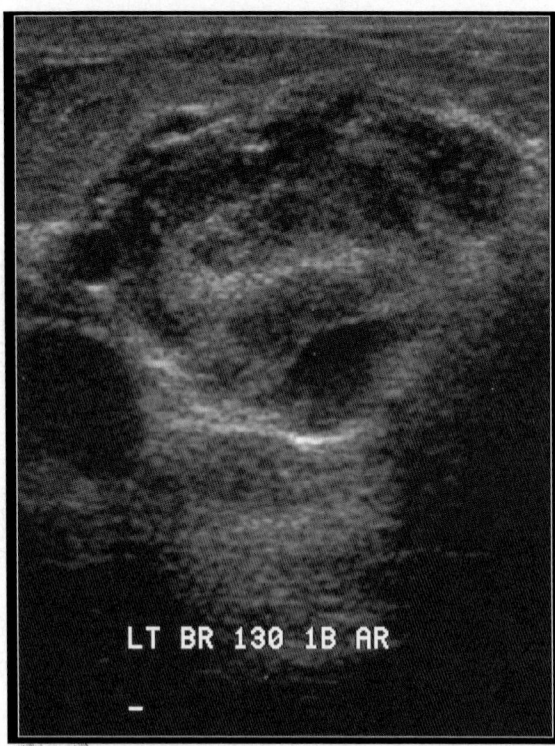

FIGURE 14–106 Metaplastic carcinomas (invasive carcinoma with sarcomatous metaplasia) present as large, circumscribed, very heterogeneous solid masses that frequently have areas of cystic degeneration. Sound transmission is usually enhanced but occasionally can be normal. The marked heterogeneity is a hallmark of these lesions and arises from the mixture of carcinomatous and sarcomatous elements and the frequent presence of hemorrhagic and cystic necrosis.

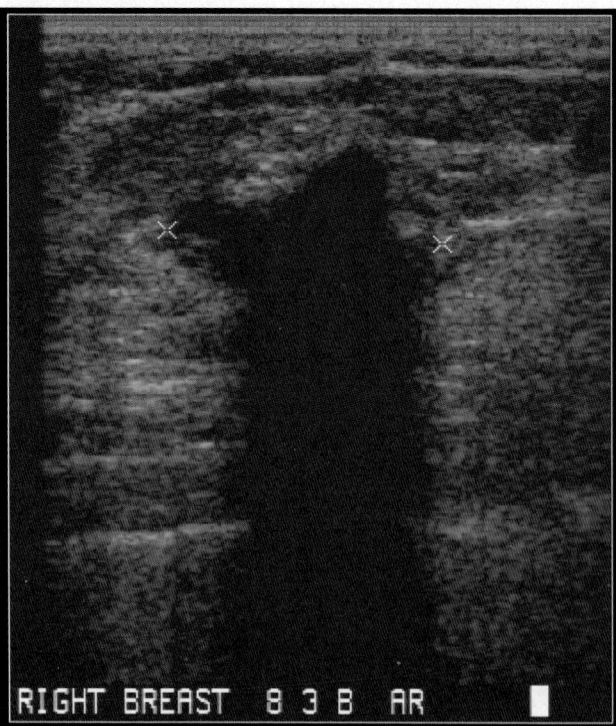

FIGURE 14–107 Most metaplastic carcinomas have enhanced sound transmission, a few have normal transmission, but a rare metaplastic carcinoma that contains ossified osteoid matrix, such as this lesion, can cause intense acoustic shadowing.

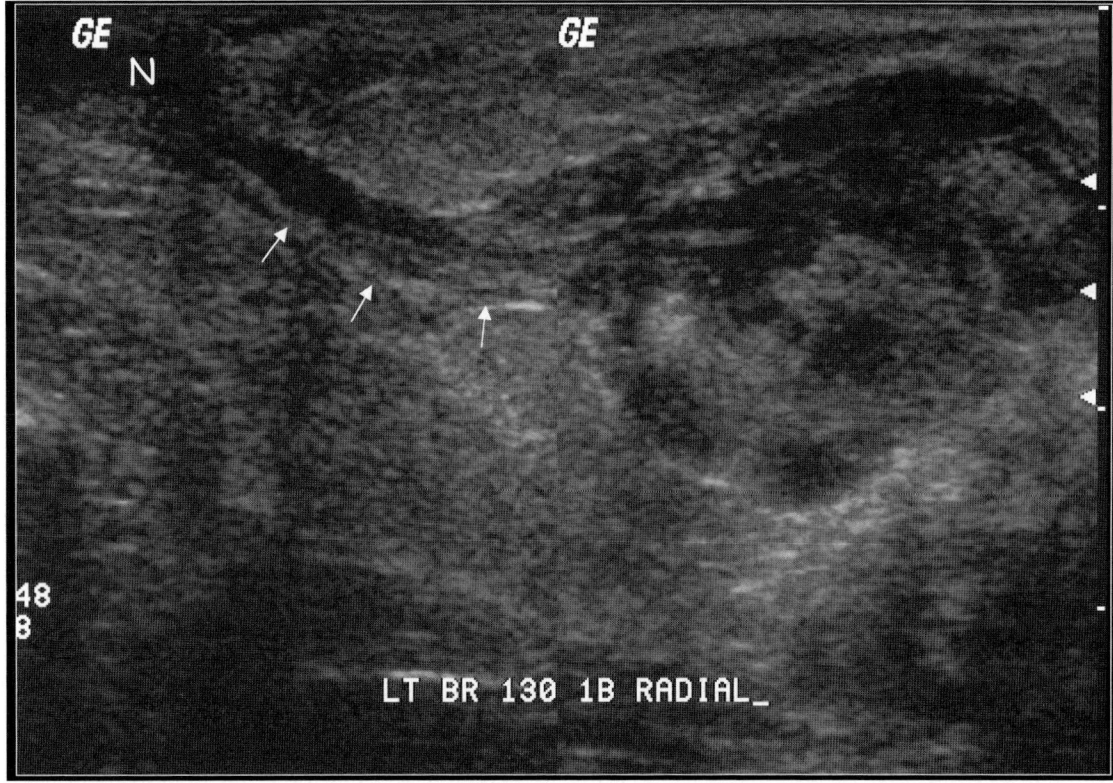

FIGURE 14–108 Ductal carcinoma *in situ* components of the carcinomatous element of metaplastic elements of metaplastic carcinomas can grow intraductally toward the nipple *(N)*, creating prominent duct extensions *(arrows)*.

features present are not specific enough to allow distinction of sarcomas from typical invasive NOS carcinomas.

Sarcomas are important mainly because such lesions lie within the differential diagnosis of more common benign entities with which they can be confused histologically. For example, benign PASH can be mistaken histologically for the far less common angiosarcoma. Aggressive treatment by mastectomy, which is appropriate for angiosarcoma, would be completely inappropriate for the patient with PASH. On the other hand, angiosarcomas sometimes appear so benign histologically that they may be confused with benign hemangiomas histologically. Hemangiomas are usually asymptomatic incidental findings at histologic examination.

Phyllodes tumors, which can be either benign or malignant, and which may be considered premalignant, are discussed in Chapter 15.

METASTATIC BREAST NODULES FROM NONBREAST PRIMARIES

Pathology, Clinical Findings, and Epidemiology

Metastases to the breast from nonbreast primary malignancies are a relatively rare occurrence. In most instances, sec-

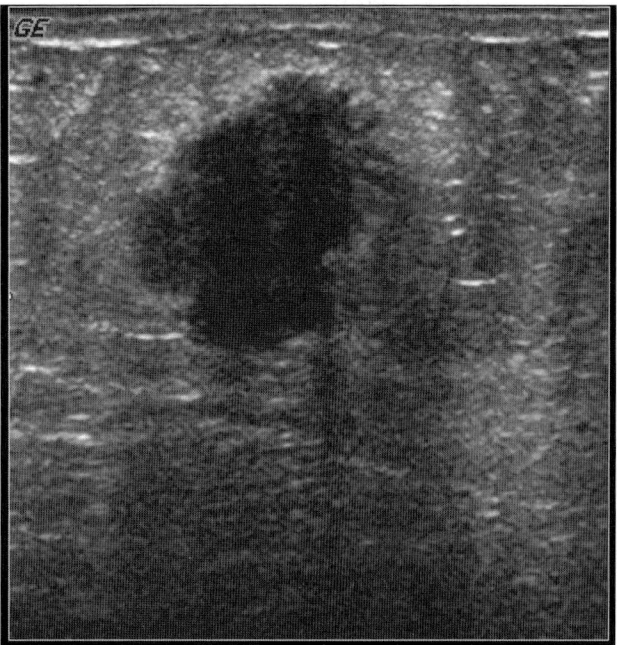

FIGURE 14–109 This fibrosarcoma of the breast is markedly hypoechoic, taller than wide, and frankly spiculated and has normal to slightly increased sound transmission. The findings are suspicious and prevent the lesion from being characterized as BIRADS 3, but do not help distinguish it from carcinoma.

ondary involvement of the breast is part of widely disseminated metastatic disease that occurs late in the course of the primary disease, and the diagnosis of metastatic disease to the breast is usually not in question. However, in a small percentage of patients (25% to 40%), mammographic or clinical evidence of a breast mass (or masses) may be the initial presenting finding of metastatic disease. In such cases, the diagnosis of metastatic disease may not be obvious based on clinical, mammographic, sonographic, or histologic findings.

Metastases to the breast can arise from any primary malignancy. However, the most common primaries that metastasize to the breast in adult patients are melanoma, lung carcinoma, ovarian carcinoma, and carcinoid tumors arising from the gastrointestinal tract. Other tumors reported to metastasize to the breast are medullary carcinomas of the thyroid, renal carcinoma, and gastric carcinoma. In men, prostate carcinoma can metastasize to the breast. In children, neoplasms of small round cells, such as rhabdomyosarcoma, neuroblastoma, Ewing's sarcoma, and medulloblastoma, can metastasize to the breast.

Metastases to the breast most often present as a single palpable or mammographic mass. Despite breast metastases usually being a late manifestation of widely disseminated disease, only about 15% of cases of metastases to the breast initially present as multiple nodules in one or both breasts. Later, as the disease progresses, the percentage of multiple nodules increases to about 25%.

The histology of metastases to the breast usually reflects the primary cells of origin well enough that the pathologic diagnosis is obvious. However, in cases in which the cells are very undifferentiated, or in which the histology of the primary tumor is similar to histology that might be found in breast primary malignancies, the pathologist may have difficulty in distinguishing primary breast carcinoma from metastases to the breast. In such cases, evaluation of ancillary findings and tumor markers may be helpful in assessment. Because most breast carcinomas have a DCIS component, the presence of intraductal components favors the lesion being primary breast carcinoma rather than a metastasis to the breast. However, because not all primary invasive breast carcinomas have intraductal components, the lack of intraductal tumor does not completely exclude a breast primary. Furthermore, an occasional metastasis from a nonbreast primary, once established in the breast, can spread through the ductal system as well as through lymphatic vessels within the breast. Second, metastases to the breast tend to displace and surround normal breast structures rather than to expand and distort them from within, as do primary invasive breast malignancies (with the exception of pure ILC). In addition, metastatic lesions can occur in areas of the breast that are devoid of surrounding atypical or even benign proliferative change. Primary invasive breast malignancies, on the other hand, tend to occur within a sea of surrounding benign or atypical proliferative change. Finally, the pathologist may

find it helpful to assess the tissue for estrogen and progesterone receptors. The presence of such receptors, common in many primary invasive breast malignancies, would be rare in metastatic lesions except those arising from ovary or prostate. Of course, the absence of such receptors would not totally exclude a breast primary because there are invasive breast malignancies that are devoid of such receptors.

Metastatic lesions to the breast tend to be highly cellular and usually do not incite the desmoplastic response that most primary breast malignancies do. Instead, metastases are more prone to incite an intense inflammatory response. The histologic features of metastases resemble the sonographic features of primary breast carcinomas that lie at the circumscribed end of the spectrum and usually differ in appearances from spiculated primary breast cancers.

In rare cases, nonbreast metastases to the breast can stimulate such an intense an inflammatory response that clinical findings simulate those caused by inflammatory primary breast carcinomas. In such cases, there is usually evidence of tumor emboli within lymph vessels, just as in inflammatory primary invasive carcinoma of the breast.

Mammographic Findings

Metastasis to the breast from nonbreast primary carcinomas presents as a single nodule in 75% to 85% of cases and as multiple or bilateral nodules in 15% to 25%. Most nonbreast metastatic nodules are rounded, ovoid, or lobulated in shape. The margins are usually circumscribed, but some are all of the margin may be indistinct. A smaller percentage of nonbreast breast metastases have irregular, jagged, or angular margins. Because they do not stimulate a desmoplastic response, metastases of nonbreast origin rarely are frankly spiculated. In cases with extensive lymphatic involvement, there may be evidence of skin thickening similar to that seen with inflammatory primary invasive carcinoma of the breast.

Palpable metastases to the breast that are mammographically visible are similar in size mammographically and clinically because of the absence of desmoplastic response. Primary breast carcinomas with desmoplasia generally appear to be larger on palpation than on mammography. Metastatic nodules to the breast rarely demonstrate calcifications, except for medullary carcinoma of the thyroid or ovarian carcinoma metastases.

The mammographic findings of metastases to the breast are not specific. Circumscribed spherically or elliptically shaped metastatic nodules can be mammographically indistinguishable from cysts or fibroadenomas. Metastatic nodules that have indistinct or angular margins can be indistinguishable from circumscribed invasive primary breast malignancies or lymphoproliferative lesions. The presence of multiple nodules, especially if bilateral, would favor metastases to the breast over primary breast carcinoma but would not completely exclude the possibilities of synchronous multicentric and bilateral breast primary malignancies or metastatic spread of a single breast primary to other parts of the same breast or contralateral breast.

Sonographic Findings

The sonographic findings of metastases to the breast from nonbreast primaries reflect their histology. Because they are highly cellular and do not incite much desmoplastic response, most metastases have sonographic characteristics similar to circumscribed primary breast carcinomas. Individual metastatic nodules are usually spherical, elliptical, or lobulated in shape. They are usually circumscribed but may have one or more angular margins (a sign of infiltration into surrounding tissues). Because these lesions do not incite a classic desmoplastic response, they are not frankly spiculated, nor do they demonstrate classic thick, echogenic halos in most cases. However, because metastases can incite an intense inflammatory response and obstruct lymphatics, some nonbreast metastases to the breast appear to be encompassed within an ill-defined area of increased echogenicity that represents peritumoral inflammatory edema or lymphedema (Fig. 14–110). Additionally, because of high cellularity and lack of desmoplasia, most metastatic lesions appear to be mildly to markedly hypoechoic and have normal or enhanced through-transmission. Nonbreast metastases to the breast rarely cause acoustic shadowing.

The sonographic findings of metastases to the breast are usually easily distinguished from those of fibroadenoma. However, a small metastatic nodule from a primary lung carcinoma caused one of the false-negative studies in our initial series (1995) of 750 solid breast nodules. Considering the relative rarity of metastatic lesions to the breast, this suggests that metastatic lesions are more likely to simulate benign lesions than are primary invasive breast carcinomas.

The sonographic findings of metastatic lesions to the breast are also unlikely to simulate those of low- to intermediate-grade NOS carcinomas, tubular carcinomas, or ILCs, which lie at the spiculated end of the malignant spectrum. The chief sonographic differential diagnostic concern is therefore between primary breast carcinomas that lie at the circumscribed end of the spectrum (high-grade NOS lesions or certain special-type carcinomas such as medullary, colloid, or invasive papillary carcinoma) and nonbreast metastases to the breast. All of the lesions within the differential diagnosis have similar gross histologic characteristics: high cellularity and relative lack of desmoplastic response that result in generally similar sonographic characteristics. Thus, just as the pathologist needs to look for *in situ* components to distinguish metastatic lesions from primary breast carcinoma histologically, sonographers must look for soft suspicious findings such as duct extension, branch pattern, microlobulations, and calcifications that suggest the presence of DCIS components to make the same distinction sonographically. However, as is the case

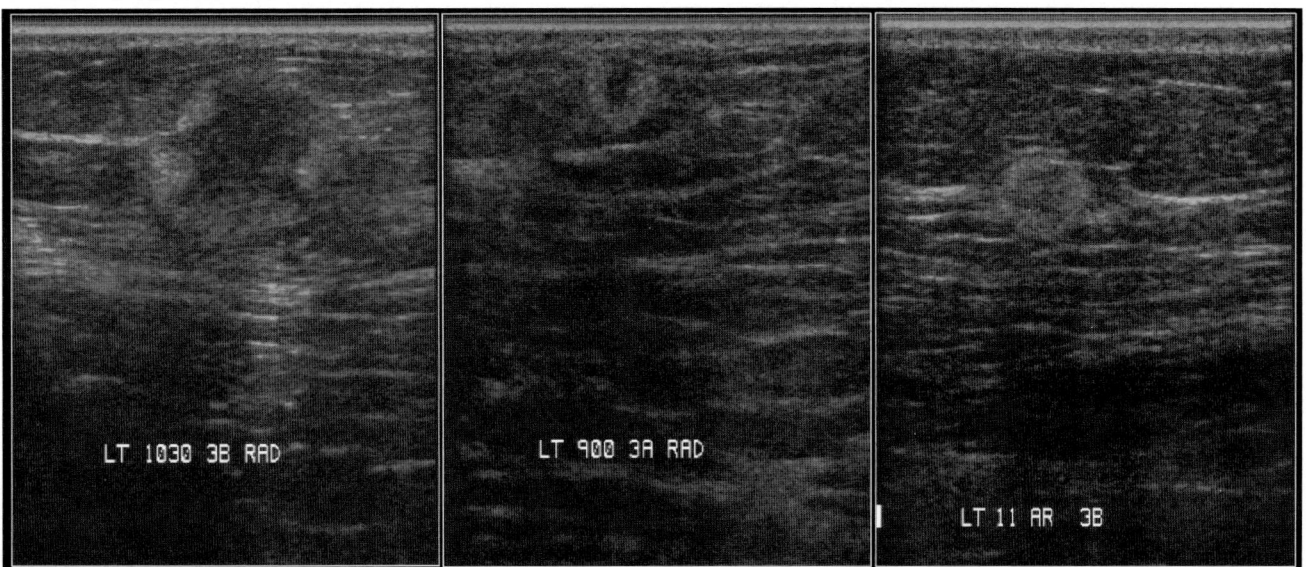

FIGURE 14–110 Although most metastases are circumscribed, these carcinoid lung cancer metastases incited intense peritumoral inflammatory edema that created a thick, echogenic halo around each metastasis. The **left** lesion has angular margins, the **middle** lesion is taller than wide and angular, and the **right** lesion also has angular margins. Thus, even though most metastases are circumscribed, most also have other suspicious features that prevent them from being characterized as BIRADS 3.

for histologic assessment of *in situ* components, lack of sonographic evidence of intraductal component does not completely exclude the presence of a primary invasive breast carcinoma because not all primary invasive breast nodules show sonographic evidence of DCIS components.

As is the case mammographically, the presence of multiple widely scattered solid nodules, especially bilaterally distributed, would favor metastatic disease, but would not completely exclude multicentric synchronous breast cancer or metastatic spread of a breast cancer. Demonstration of DICS bridges between individual nodules, indicating the presence of EIC, would favor multifocal or multicentric primary breast cancer over multicentric metastatic disease.

Doppler findings in metastases to the breast also overlap with those of circumscribed primary breast malignancies. Many metastases to the breast appear hypervascular on color Doppler. This appearance should not be surprising because most metastatic lesions arrive in the breast by hematogenous spread. Hematogenous spread implies that the lesions have a high potential to stimulate angiogenesis. Lesions strongly able to stimulate angiogenesis are also those most capable of creating sufficient neovascularity to be detectable with color Doppler. In addition to tumor neovascularity, the inflammatory host response generated by such lesions tends to lead to inflammatory hyperemia.

BREAST MASSES OF HEMATOPOIETIC OR LYMPHOPROLIFERATIVE ORIGIN

Pathology, Clinical Findings, and Epidemiology

Breast neoplasms of hematopoietic or lymphoproliferative origin are rare. However, the exact proportion primary to the breast varies with the cell type and with the method of detection. Lymphoproliferative breast lesions that present as palpable lumps usually represent secondary involvement of the breast in patients with widely disseminated systemic disease. On the other hand, lymphoproliferative disease within the breast that is asymptomatic and presents solely by mammography is more likely to be a primary breast lesion. Lymphoproliferative lesions that can primarily or secondarily involve the breast include non-Hodgkin's lymphoma (NHL), Hodgkin's lymphoma, leukemia, and myeloma or plasmacytoma.

NON-HODGKIN'S LYMPHOMA

Pathology, Clinical Findings, and Epidemiology

NHL of the breast is rare. This disease represents less than 0.5% of all breast malignancies and about 2% of all extranodal lymphomas. To be considered primary to the breast, there must be no evidence of lymphoma elsewhere in the body except in the regional lymph nodes draining the breast. The axillary lymph nodes contain NHL in about one-third of cases of primary breast lymphoma.

The age range is similar to that of primary invasive breast cancer, spanning from 15 to 86 years and averaging 55 years of age. In primary cases, there is a single nodule in about 70% of cases; there are multiple nodules in about 9% of cases, clinical findings similar to inflammatory carcinoma in 9%, and no findings in the remainder of cases. In primary cases, the incidence of bilaterality is about 10%, but in secondary cases, there is bilateral involvement up to 25% of the time.

NHL most commonly presents as a palpable mass that often enlarges rapidly and usually is not tender. Because of the rapid growth, these masses can be quite large at the time of diagnosis and frequently contain areas of necrosis. In other cases, there may be diffuse enlargement, edema, or erythema of the breast. In 9% of cases, there are no clinical findings, and the lesions are detected only on routine mammography.

Seventy-one percent of NHLs of the breast are of the diffuse type, whereas 29% are of the nodular type. About one-half of lesions are histiocytic, 25% are poorly differentiated, 20% are mixed, and 5% to 10% are well defined or Burkitt's lymphoma. Almost all NHLs are of the B-cell type. T-cell breast lymphomas are rare.

Like most metastases, NHLs are highly cellular lesions that incite essentially no desmoplastic reaction. Lymphomas have a population of uniform, small, round neoplastic cells centrally, but often have a rim of reactive, non-neoplastic, heterogeneous lymph cells surrounding them. These reactive cells sometimes even form lymphoid follicles that can contribute to the multilobulated surface appearance of these lesions.

NHL cells tend to proliferate most actively and densely within and immediately around the ducts and lobules. These neoplastic cells frequently grow into the lumina of the ducts and ductules within the lobules, disrupting the normal epithelial structure. The presence of these small round lymphoma cells within and around the lobules and ducts of the breast can make it difficult for the pathologist to distinguish NHL from LCIS and ILC without the use of leukocyte markers. Medullary carcinoma, which usually has an associated dense lymphocytic or plasmocytic infiltrate, can also have an appearance that occasionally simulates lymphoma. Finally, pseudolymphoma can be confused with lymphoma clinically, mammographically, sonographically, and histologically. Pseudolymphoma is a benign condition in which a dense infiltrate of non-neoplastic lymphocytes develops, containing normal lymphoid follicles, and displacing normal breast tissue. The etiology of pseudolymphoma is uncertain but most likely represents an unusually intense reaction to either inflammation or trauma. These infiltrates can develop rapidly and are most common in the stomach and lung but can occur in the breast.

The prognosis of NHL of the breast depends on whether the lesion is secondary or primary. The prognosis is poor for NHL of the breast that is a manifestation of disseminated disease, but better for primary breast lymphoma. Primary NHL of the breast has a 40% to 50% disease-free survival rate 4 years after local resection and postoperative radiation therapy.

Mammographic Findings

The mammographic findings of breast lymphoma are nonspecific. In most patients, there is a circumscribed or partially circumscribed, noncalcified mass that can be spherical, elliptical, or multilobulated. The circumscription reflects the lack of desmoplastic reaction. In the few cases in which the margins are ill defined or indistinct, they are not frankly spiculated. The mass is often quite large. The benign peripherally located lymphocytic infiltrate and the associated peripheral edema contribute to the apparent lesion size. In certain instances, there are multiple masses. In a few cases, there is evidence of hazy increased density and skin thickening without retraction, with or without a discrete underlying mass. These mammographic findings reflect inflammatory edema and lymphedema associated with lymphatic obstruction. About 12% of patients have mammographic evidence of axillary lymphadenopathy associated with the other mammographic findings.

Sonographic Findings

The sonographic findings of NHL of the breast are typical of any lesion that is highly cellular and has a paucity of desmoplastic reaction. In cases in which breast involvement is secondary to systemic disease, the pattern of involvement generally strongly suggests NHL. In addition to known disease elsewhere in the body, patients with secondary breast involvement frequently have bilateral axillary lymph node involvement (Fig. 14–111). Even in some cases of primary breast lymphoma, the mass may be recognized as an abnormally enlarged intramammary or axillary lymph node, suggesting the diagnosis (Fig. 14–112). NHL of the breast can occur in males or females.

In many cases, however, the mass is either not a lymph node or is so distorted that it is unrecognizable as a lymph node. The location of such nodules is often where intramammary lymph nodes occur uncommonly. In most cases, these lymphomatous nodules are circumscribed and encompassed by a thin, echogenic capsule (Fig. 14–113). However, as the lymphomatous nodule enlarges, the likelihood of peritumoral inflammatory edema or lymphedema that causes a thicker, ill-defined echogenic halo around the nodules increases (Fig. 14–114). Because these lesions tend to enlarge rapidly, they are often quite large by the time the patient presents for sonography. The nodule is usually

(text continued on page 674)

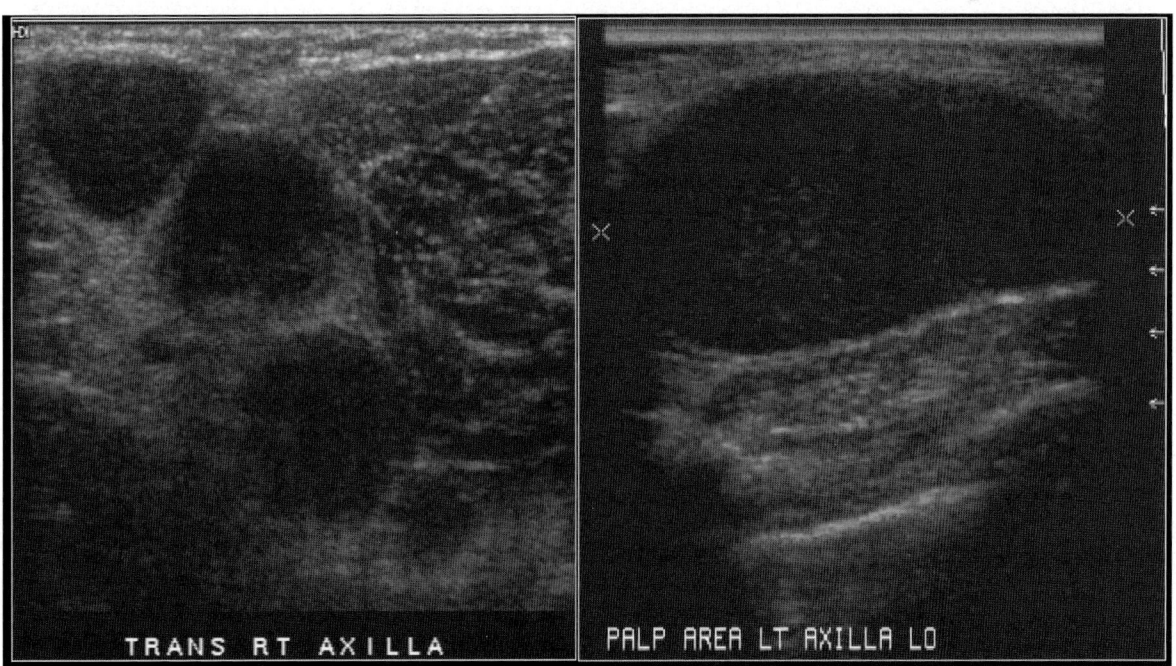

A

FIGURE 14–111 A: This patient presented with a palpable lump in the left axilla. Sonography showed markedly abnormal lymph nodes. Evaluation of the right axillary lymph nodes showed them to be abnormal as well. Because of bilateral involvement, evaluation of the abdomen was performed. *(Continued.)*

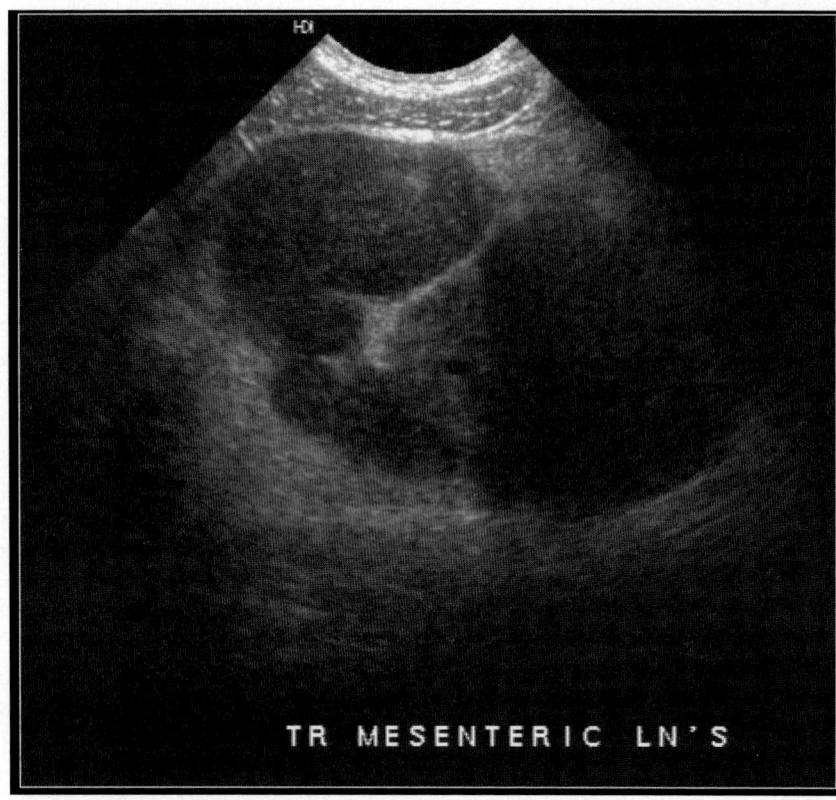

FIGURE 14–111 (continued) B: In addition to abnormal axillary lymph nodes bilaterally, this patient had severe mesenteric lymphadenopathy. The presence of bilateral axillary lymphadenopathy suggests that non-Hodgkin's lymphoma (NHL) breast involvement is part of disseminated disease rather than primary disease in the breast and indicates a need to search for evidence of NHL elsewhere in the body.

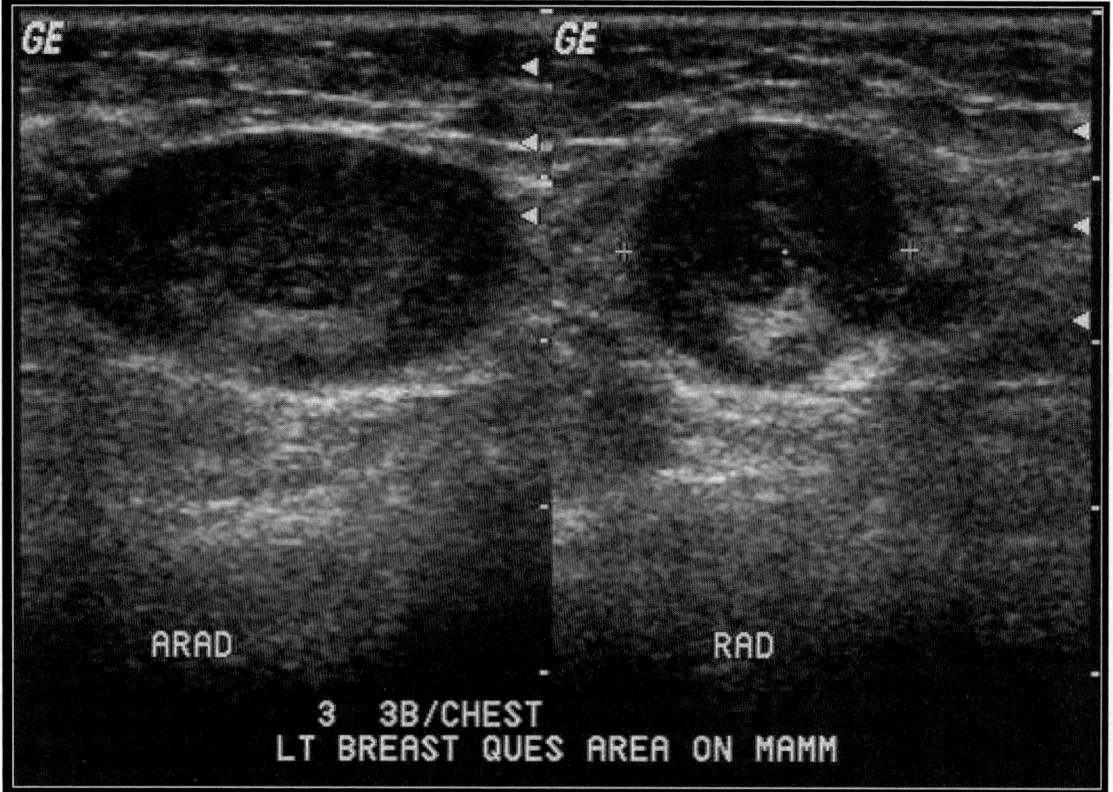

FIGURE 14–112 A: In cases of primary breast lymphoma, the nodule may be recognizable as an abnormal intramammary lymph node. *(Continued.)*

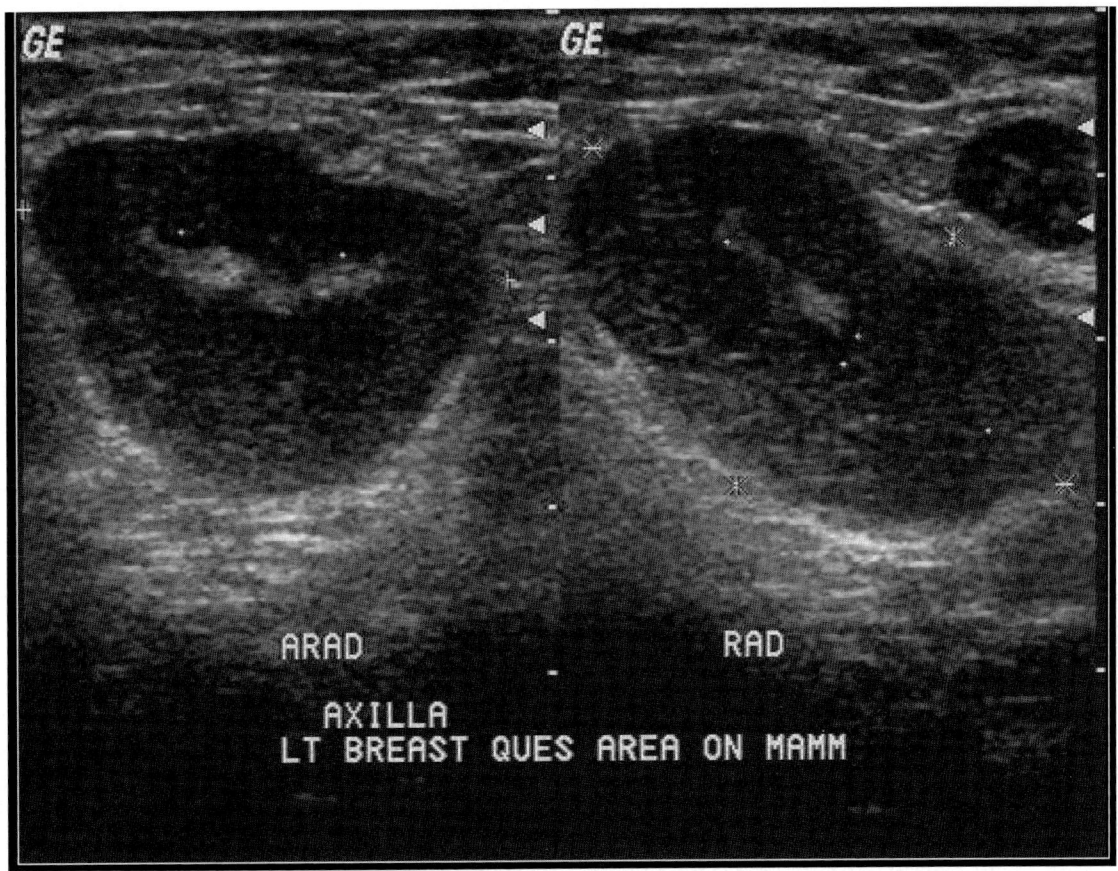

B

FIGURE 14–112 *(continued)* **B:** When an abnormal intramammary lymph node is detected, the axillary lymph nodes should also be assessed. The lymphomatous intramammary lymph node shown in the image in part **A** was associated with axillary lymphadenopathy.

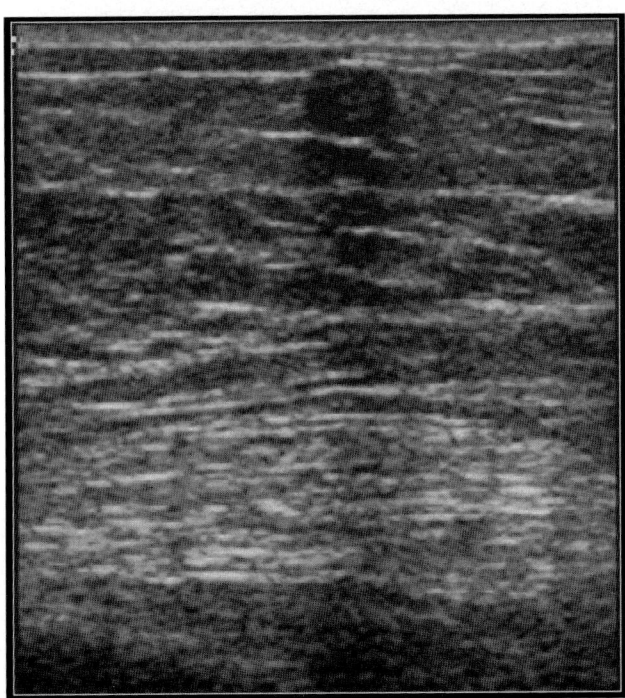

FIGURE 14–113 Non-Hodgkin's lymphoma nodules in the breast that cannot be recognized as intramammary lymph nodes are generally well circumscribed and encompassed by a thin, echogenic capsule.

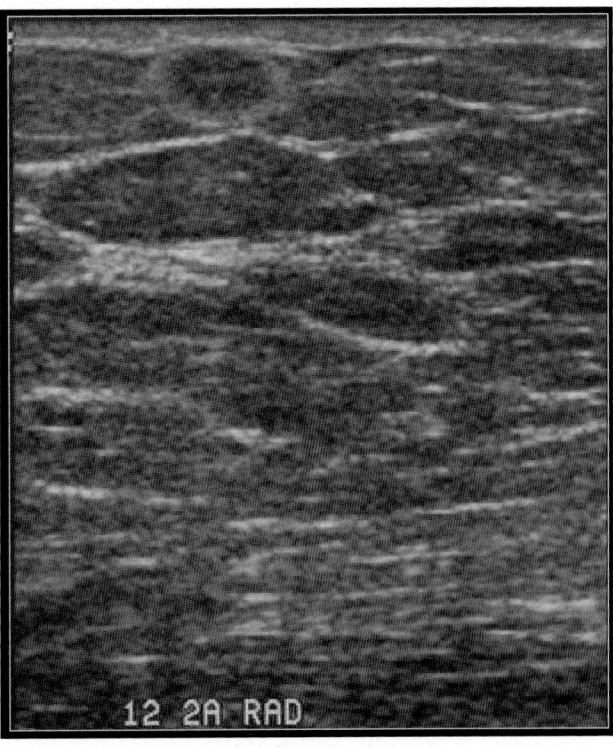

FIGURE 14–114 As non-Hodgkin's lymphoma nodules in the breast enlarge, they are likely to develop an ill-defined, thick, echogenic rim of inflammatory edema or lymphedema.

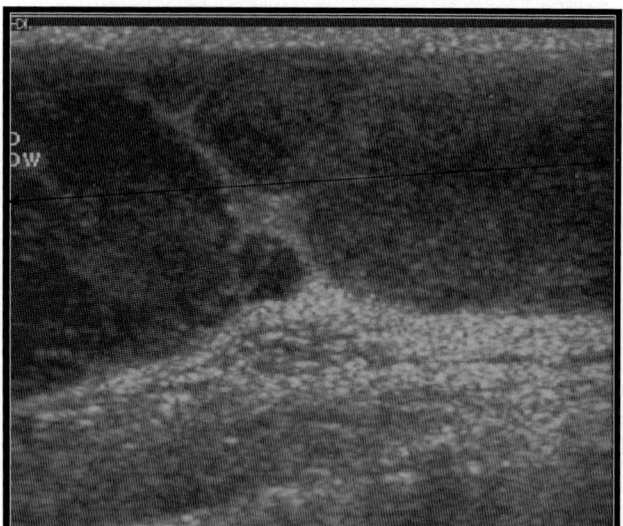

FIGURE 14–115 Large lymphomatous nodules tend to be multilobulated because the lymphocytic reactive peripheral infiltrates incited by the lesion tend to form lymphoid follicles.

multilobulated, reflecting the benign lymphoid infiltrates with lymphoid follicles that tend to form along the periphery of the central neoplastic lymphomatous mass (Fig. 14–115). The sound transmission deep to breast lymphomas is usually enhanced. The lesions are typically hypoechoic and

homogeneous in internal echotexture. In fact, lymphomas can appear to be nearly anechoic, and together with their usual enhanced sound transmission, they can appear pseudocystic (Fig. 14–116). Areas of cystic necrosis within the mass can contribute to the pseudocystic appearance. Lymphomas that have not undergone extensive central liquefactive necrosis are usually hypervascular, and demonstration of internal flow with color Doppler may be helpful in distinguishing between nearly anechoic lymphomatous tissue and cysts (Fig. 14–116). Lymphomas tend to be quite soft, soft enough that excessive compression during color Doppler assessment can shut off flow to these lesions. Therefore, very light compression should be used when evaluating these lesions with color or power Doppler.

The sonographic appearance is not specific for lymphoma but rather is typical of any highly cellular lesion associated with relatively little desmoplastic reaction. The extensive lymphocytic infiltrates also contribute to the marked hypoechogenicity and enhanced through-transmission. The rapid enlargement is also not specific because all highly cellular lesions with lymphocytic infiltrates tend to enlarge rapidly and to be large at the time of initial diagnostic studies. Other lesions that share some or all of these clinical, sonographic, and histologic features and must be included in the sonographic differential diagnosis include medullary carcinoma, high-grade NOS lesions, metaplastic

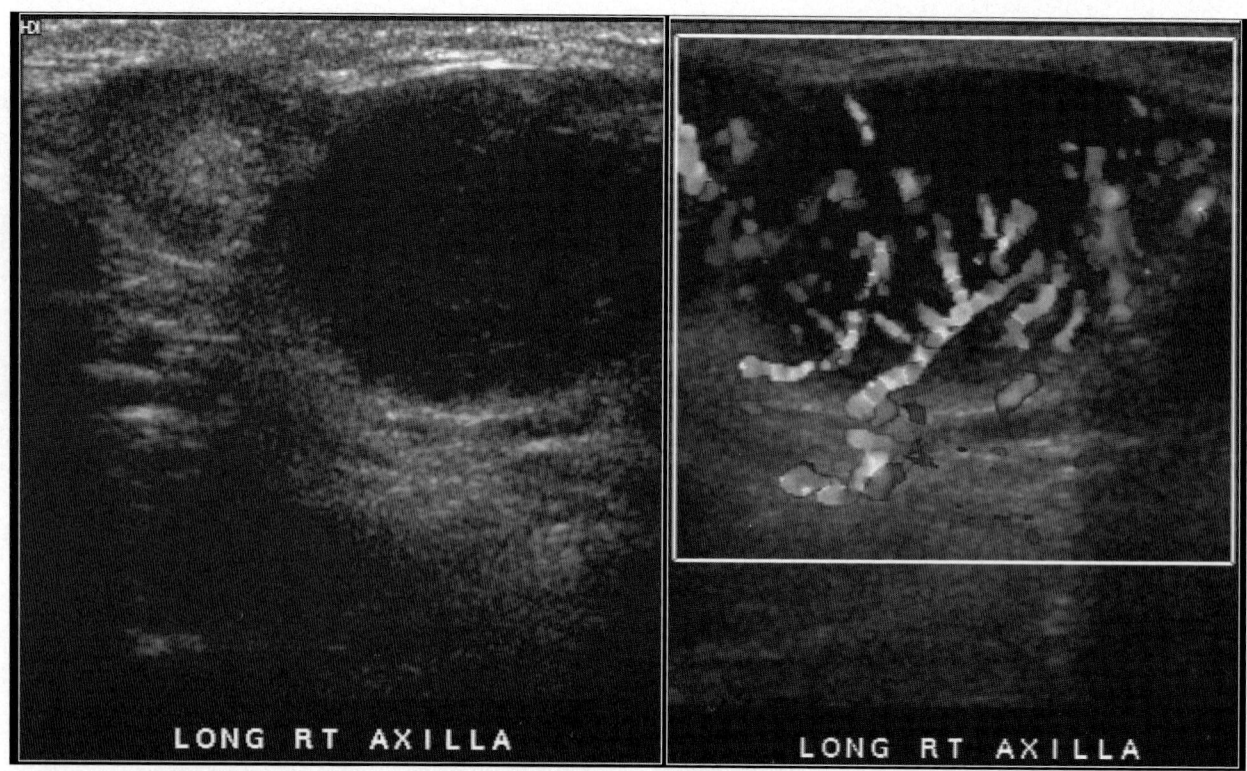

FIGURE 14–116 Lymphomatous breast nodules usually demonstrate enhanced sound transmission and can appear to be so nearly anechoic that they appear to be cystic (pseudocystic appearance, **left**). Color or power Doppler is very helpful in avoiding mischaracterizing lymphomas as cystic because pseudocystic lymph nodes are generally markedly hypervascular (**right**).

carcinoma, and phyllodes tumors. All of these other neoplasms also tend to be hypervascular on Doppler exam because of their rapid growth and high metabolic needs that demand high blood flow.

HODGKIN'S LYMPHOMA

Pathology, Clinical Findings, and Epidemiology

Hodgkin's lymphoma involves the breast even more rarely than does NHL. Breast involvement by Hodgkin's disease is usually part of systemic disease and represents a direct extension from lymph node disease involving the internal mammary or axially lymph nodes. The histologic differential diagnosis is similar to that for NHL.

Mammographic and Sonographic Findings

The mammographic and sonographic findings do not differ from those of NHL.

PLASMACYTOMA

Pathology, Clinical Findings, and Epidemiology

Plasmacytoma of the breast is very rare. Breast involvement is usually secondary to underlying systemic disease. Only a few cases of primary extramedullary plasmacytoma of the breast have been reported, and these usually preceded ultimate disseminated bone marrow involvement (multiple myeloma).

Histologically, there is a proliferation of a mixture of mature and immature plasma cells that compresses, displaces, and effaces normal breast ducts and lobules. The pathologist must distinguish the plasma cell infiltrates in plasmacytoma from those seen in plasma cell mastitis, a variant of periductal mastitis associated with chronic ductal ectasia. The presence of only mature plasma cells, dilated ducts with inspissated secretions, and intraductal or periductal fibrosis can help the pathologist distinguish plasma cell mastitis from plasmacytoma.

Treatment is targeted primarily at systemic disease. Local excision with postoperative radiation is used for treating the breast component of disease.

Mammographic and Sonographic Findings

The findings are similar to those for lymphoma. The lesions, which typify plasmacytomas, do not often reach the size of those associated with NHLs.

LEUKEMIA

Pathology, Clinical Findings, and Epidemiology

Leukemic involvement of the breast is usually secondary to known preexisting disseminated disease. Rarely, breast involvement presents before evidence of systemic disease is known, but in all cases is followed by hematologic evidence of the disease within less than a year.

Acute granulocytic leukemia is the most common form of leukemia to involve the breast and tends to occur in younger patients than does breast involvement by the other lymphoproliferative neoplasms, often affecting young adults and even children. As is the case for NHL of the breast, the small round leukemic cells, if they grow within ducts and lobules and disrupt the normal epithelium, can simulate the findings seen in classic infiltrating lobular carcinoma or even LNG DCIS.

The soft tissue masses associated with acute granulocytic leukemia, including breast masses, have been called *granulocytic sarcomas*. On gross pathologic examination, these masses often have a greenish color, owing to the actions of myeloperoxidase, and have been called *chloromas*.

Mammographic and Sonographic Findings

These lesions have been infrequently reported but have findings similar to those for NHL.

Tumor Patterns that Do Not Reflect a Specific Cell Type

There are tumor patterns that can occur with several different histologic invasive breast malignancies. These include inflammatory and intracystic malignancies of the breast.

INFLAMMATORY CARCINOMA OF THE BREAST

Pathology, Clinical Findings, and Epidemiology

Inflammatory carcinoma of the breast represents a clinical constellation of findings that occurs in association with breast carcinoma. Inflammatory carcinoma usually occurs in association with high-grade invasive NOS lesions but can occur with other primary breast carcinomas and even with primary or secondary lymphomas. Clinically, inflammatory carcinoma is defined as evidence of erythema, warmth, and edema involving more than one-third of the skin of the breast in association with an underlying invasive breast malignancy. In about 80% of cases, the pathologist can find evidence of tumor emboli within the dermal lymphatics. For this reason, researchers have advocated not classifying a breast carcinoma as inflammatory unless there is evidence of tumor emboli within the dermal lymphatics. However, other researchers have advocated adherence to the original description of inflammatory carcinoma, being based solely on the clinical skin findings. There have been some patients in whom the pathologist identifies dermal lymphatic tumor emboli but who do not show evidence of skin inflammation. Such cases have variously been classified as inflammatory carcinoma, occult inflammatory carcinoma, or dermal lymphatic carcinomatosis of the breast. There is obviously no uniform agreement on the definition of inflammatory breast carcinoma.

Patients who have inflammation over less than one-third of the breast, in association with carcinoma, should be considered to have breast carcinoma with an inflammatory component rather than as inflammatory carcinoma. Patients who first present with inflammation should be considered to have primary inflammatory breast carcinoma. Patients who do not have inflammation when first diagnosed with breast cancer, but who develop the findings later, should be considered to have secondary inflammatory carcinoma.

Inflammatory breast carcinoma is relatively uncommon, representing only about 1% of all breast carcinomas. Pregnant and lactating women appear to have a higher risk for inflammatory carcinoma than do other women, suggesting a possible hormonal influence. Clinically, the onset of erythema and edema can be rapid and is often associated with pain. There is a discrete palpable mass or lump in association with diffuse hardening or induration of the breast in about 75% of patients. The other 25% of patients, however, have diffuse induration without a discrete mass. Patients without a palpable mass are more likely to have diffuse carcinoma involving the entire breast and have a worse prognosis than those who have a discrete mass. The skin thickening and edema associated with inflammatory carcinoma is usually most severe in the dependent portions of the breast, where the classic *peau d'orange* appearance may be present. A significant percentage of patients with inflammatory carcinoma have nipple inversion or flattening. Many patients also have palpable axillary lymphadenopathy.

Because of the rapid onset, patients who have a palpable lump may be suspected of having mastitis with an abscess rather than inflammatory carcinoma. Patients who do not have a discrete mass may be suspected of having mastitis rather than inflammatory carcinoma. Thus, in any patient with mastitis, an index of suspicion for inflammatory carcinoma must be maintained in order not to miss cases of inflammatory carcinoma that simulate mastitis.

Even at gross pathologic examination, a small but significant proportion of cases do not have a discrete palpable mass. The absence of a mass suggests the presence of diffuse carcinoma.

Occasionally, the diagnosis can be made simply with a skin biopsy showing tumor emboli within the dermal lymphatics. However, dermal involvement is not present in all cases, and biopsy of the palpable or mammographic mass or blind biopsies of indurated portions of the breast may be necessary to verify the suspected diagnosis.

On histologic examination, the underlying tumor is usually a very poorly differentiated, high-grade invasive NOS carcinoma. The tumor is usually centrally located, often quite large, and either multicentric or diffuse. Diffusely invasive carcinomas can involve the entire breast. The periphery of underlying malignancy has a rim of lymphocytic infiltrate, as do most high-grade NOS lesions. Regardless of whether the lymphocytic rim is associated with inflammation, there is little evidence of inflammatory infiltrates within the skin and subcutaneous tissues, despite the presence of clinical signs of inflammation. Rather, there is evidence of edema and vascular dilation without associated inflammatory infiltrate. The hyperemia is diffuse throughout the tumor and surrounding breast tissues. Most patients with inflammatory carcinoma have gross disease within the axillary lymph nodes and frequently also have metastases to the internal mammary lymph nodes.

The prognosis of inflammatory carcinoma in patients who are treated only with lumpectomy or mastectomy is poor. The survival rate after local treatment only is 5% or less at 5 years. Aggressive radiation and chemotherapy regimens have improved survival rates to 35% to 55%.

Mammographic Findings

Only a small percentage of patients have completely normal mammograms. This phenomenon occurs in patients with extremely dense breast tissue in some cases, but in other cases represents the presence of a diffusely infiltrating malignancy involving virtually the entire breast. The mammogram is abnormal in most patients with inflammatory carcinoma. All patients show evidence of hazy increased opacity, thickening of Cooper's ligaments, and skin thickening. Most patients show evidence of a mass with or without calcifications. Slightly fewer than 20% of patients have mammographic evidence of axillary lymphadenopathy. In patients who have evidence of edema, but no mass, the findings may be indistinguishable from mastitis. Even in those patients with an ill-defined mass, the distinction between nonpuerperal mastitis with abscess formation and inflammatory carcinoma can be difficult without the aid of ultrasound.

Sonographic Findings

The sonographic findings of inflammation associated with carcinoma are similar to those caused by inflammation of any etiology. The skin is thickened and increased in echogenicity, and it loses the clear delineation from underlying subcutaneous fat. The subcutaneous fat becomes more echogenic, and the difference between the echogenicities of fat and the normally more echogenic fibroglandular elements decreases or disappears. Cooper's ligaments appear wider and less well defined. Anatomic landmarks within echogenic fibroglandular tissue become ill defined, limiting the ability to demonstrate ducts and lobules. Split-screen imaging of mirror-image locations of the contralateral breast can accentuate the alterations in echotexture caused by the inflammatory edema (Fig. 14–117). Sometimes, dilated veins and lymphatic channels are demonstrable within the edematous subcutaneous fat. However, most

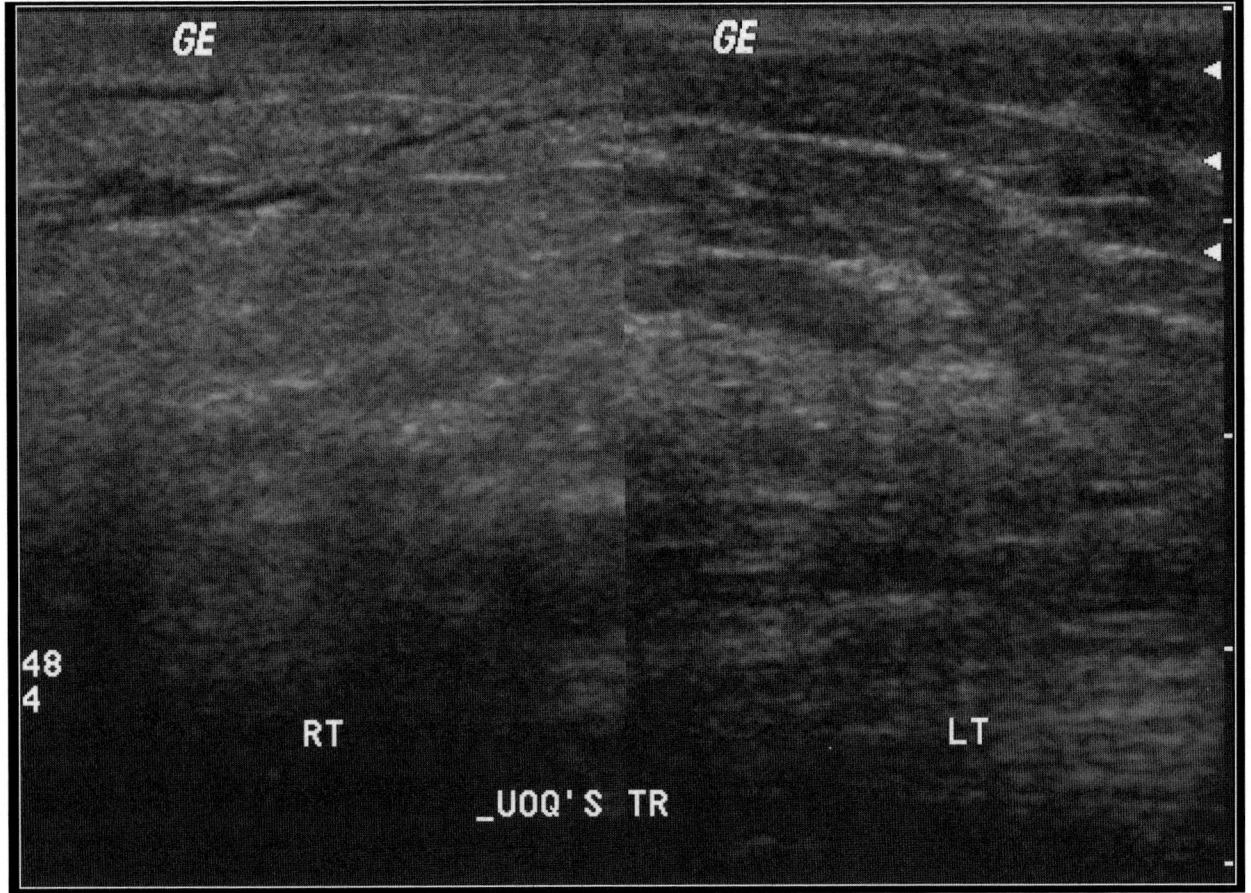

FIGURE 14–117 Split-screen mirror-image locations in the right and left breast accentuate the alterations in echogenicity in the right breast caused by inflammatory carcinoma. On the right side, the skin is thickened, the fat is hyperechoic, and the distinction between fat and fibrous tissue and Cooper's ligaments is markedly diminished. There are exudative effusions coursing along Cooper's ligaments. These are sheets of fluid, not dilated lymphatics. Sound penetration is diminished, in some cases so severely that use of a lower-frequency transducer is necessary to achieve adequate penetration.

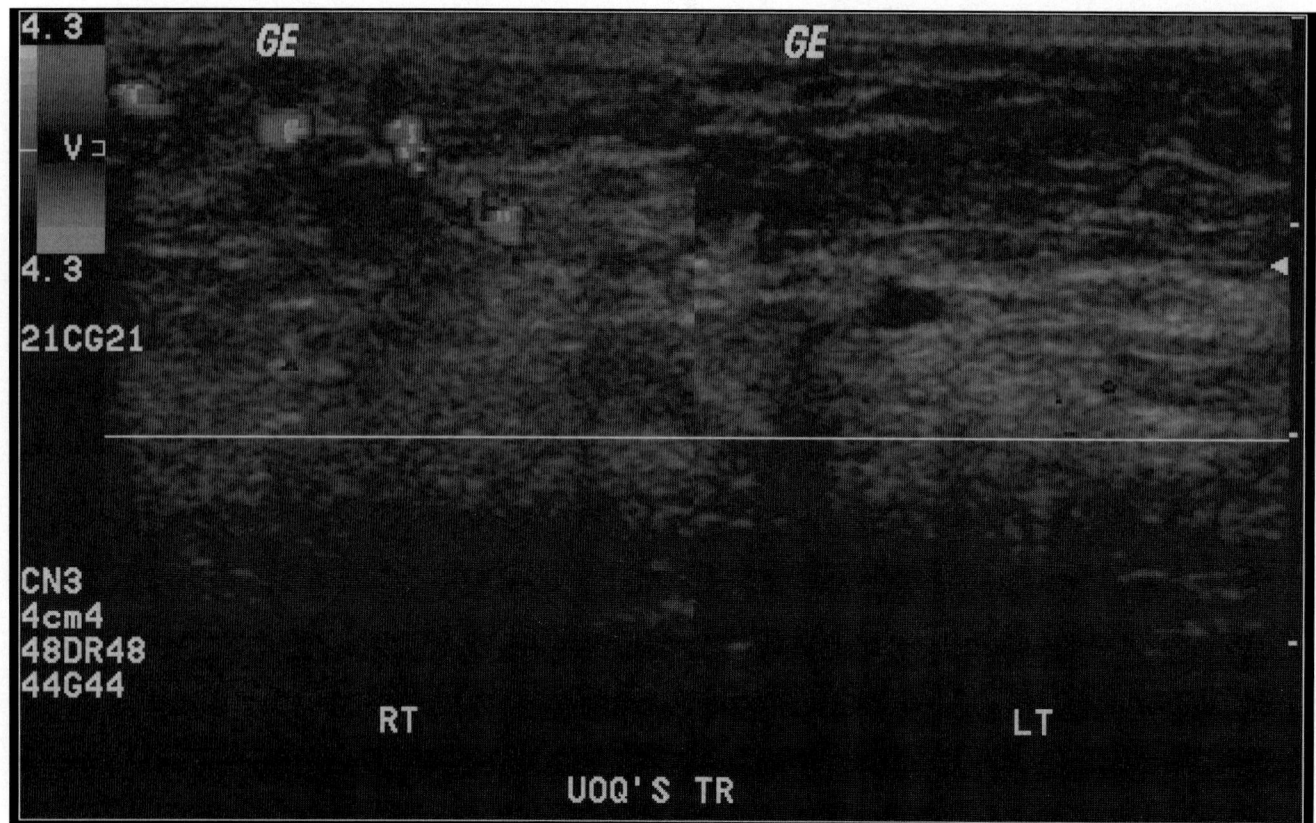

FIGURE 14–118 Split-screen mirror-image color Doppler scans show hyperemia in association with the edema on the patient's right side.

of the structures that have previously been interpreted as dilated lymphatic channels are, in fact, merely sheets of interstitial fluid rather than dilated lymphatic channels. The dilated veins, however, are real and are a manifestation of marked neoplastic and inflammatory hyperemia. The hyperemia, like the edema, can be accentuated by comparing it with the amount of blood flow in the mirror-image location of the unaffected contralateral breast (Fig. 14–118). All of these findings can be seen in acute infectious mastitis and are not specific for inflammatory carcinoma unless the malignancy causing the inflammation can be demonstrated. Inflammatory carcinomas of the breast show the most markedly increased blood flow patterns on color Doppler of all breast neoplasms.

The edema that enlarges and thickens the entire breast decreases sound transmission. The combination of increased breast thickness and decreased sound transmission often limits the ability of the normally used 10- to 12-MHz ultrasound transducers to penetrate to the chest wall adequately to identify the underlying malignancy. Suspected inflammatory carcinoma is one of the few cases in which lower-frequency transducers (5 MHz) may be necessary to obtain adequate penetration and optimally demon-

strate the underlying carcinoma in patients with suspected inflammatory carcinoma (Fig. 14–119).

The underlying malignant mass in patients with inflammatory carcinoma is often quite large (more than 5 cm) and multifocal (Fig. 14–120). Because the surrounding fat is abnormally echogenic, the malignant mass appears relatively hypoechoic in comparison. The underlying malignancy is usually a very cellular, high-grade NOS lesion with little desmoplastic response, a combination of histologic findings that are usually associated with enhanced through-transmission of sound. However, because of the highly attenuating edema in and around the tumor and general difficulty penetrating to the chest wall, these lesions often paradoxically cast an acoustic shadow. Occasionally, a large malignant mass that has undergone cystic necrosis may be difficult to distinguish from an immature abscess associated with mastitis. When the underlying malignancy is diffusely infiltrating, it will have very ill-defined margins (Fig. 14–121). The echogenic halo around spiculated lesions that represents either spiculations or peritumoral edema is relatively inapparent and difficult to demonstrate because the surrounding edematous fat is equally echogenic. In patients with diffuse infiltrating

(text continued on page 681)

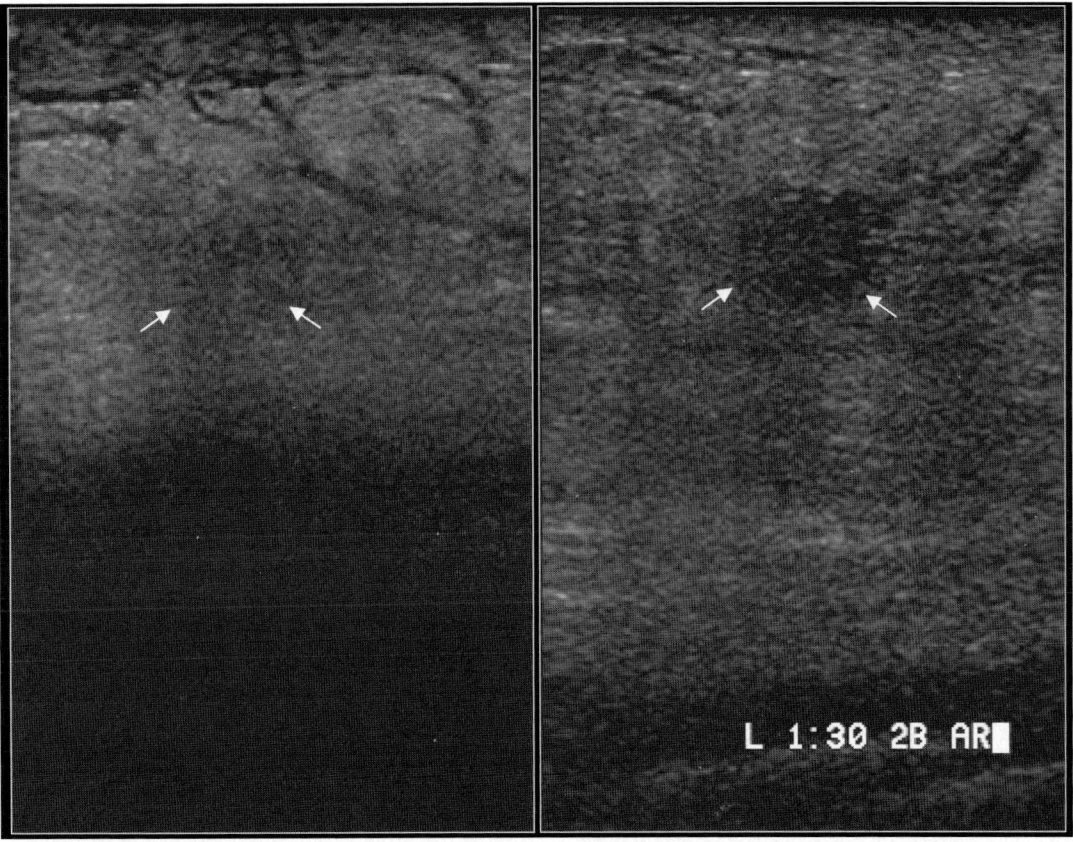

FIGURE 14–119 In this patient with inflammatory carcinoma, the severe edema decreased sound transmission so much that carcinoma could not be seen with the 10-MHz transducer that we usually use for breast ultrasound (**left**, *arrows*). By using a 5-MHz transducer, the carcinoma is better shown (**right**, *arrows*).

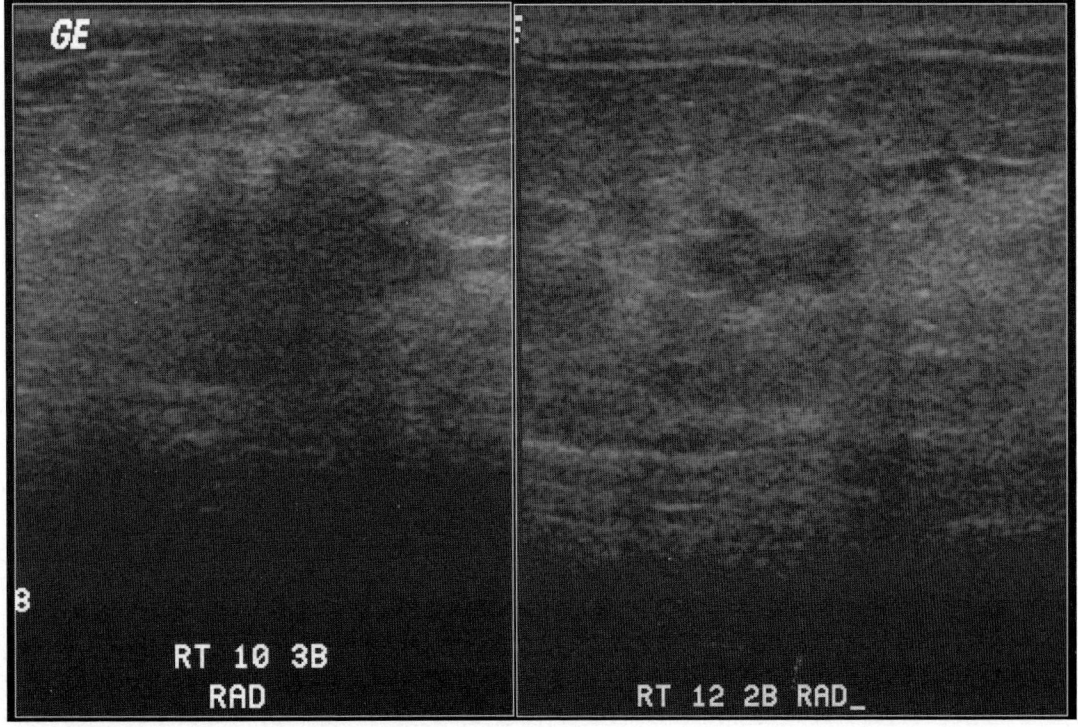

FIGURE 14–120 Inflammatory carcinoma is frequently associated with either a very large malignant mass or, as in this case, multifocal disease.

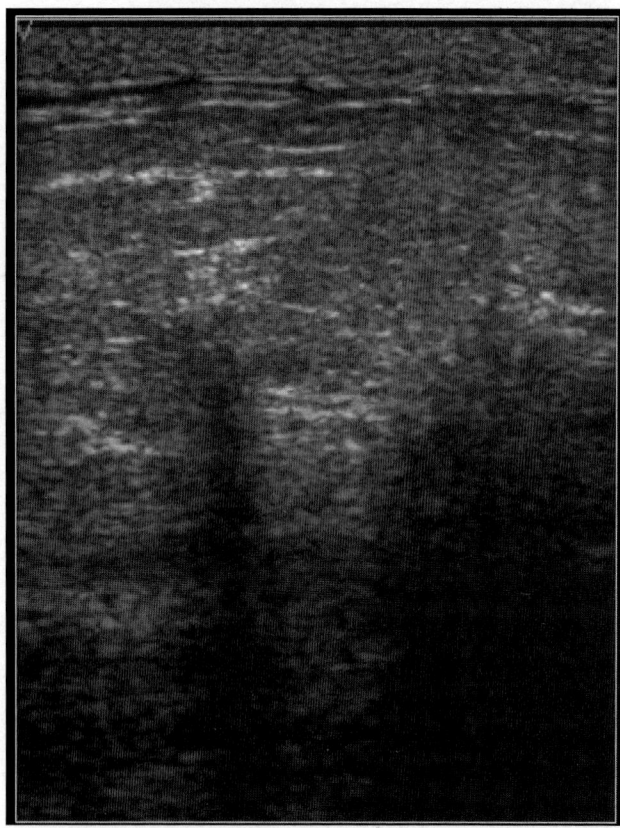

FIGURE 14–121 The malignant nodule underlying the inflammation is often diffusely infiltrating and has ill-defined margins. The scattering of the ultrasound beam caused by edema contributes to the poor definition of such masses.

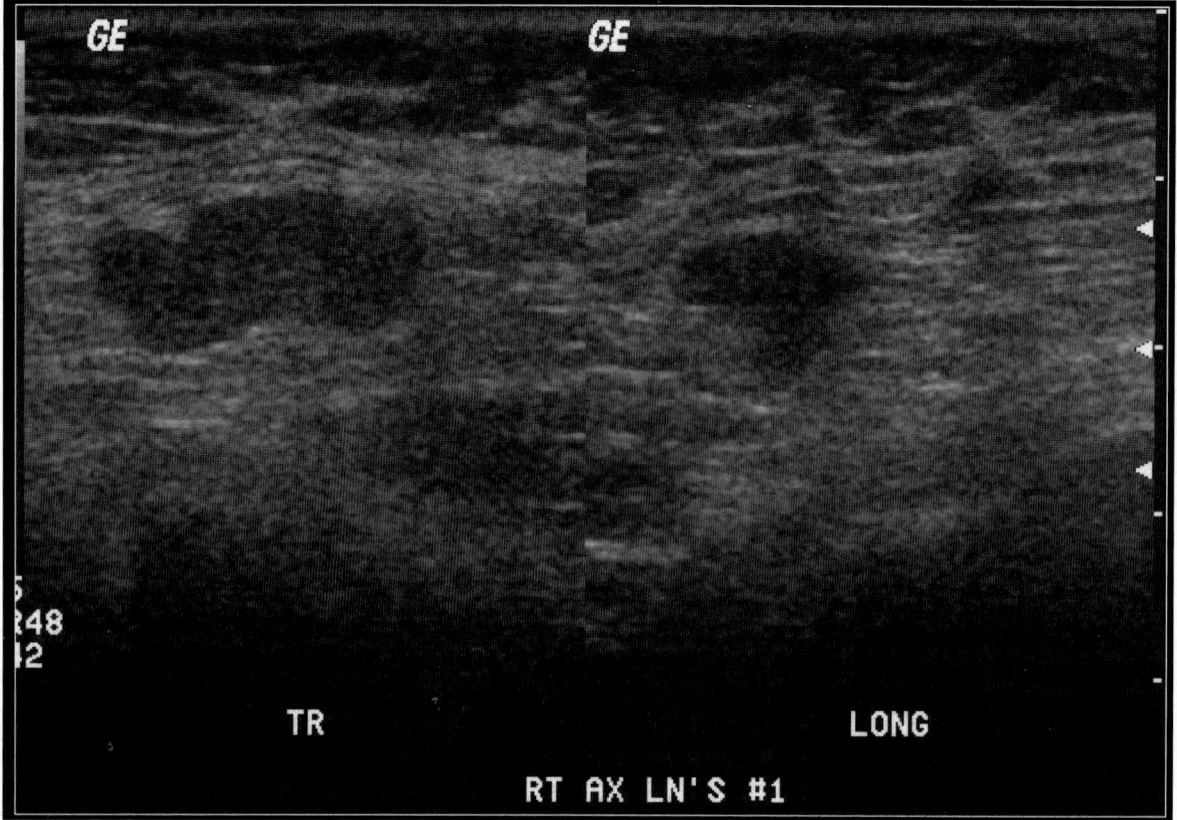

FIGURE 14–122 Although mammographic evidence of axillary lymphadenopathy occurs in a relatively small percentage of patients with inflammatory carcinoma, it is sonographically demonstrable in almost all of these patients.

lesions that involve the entire breast, there may be no sonographically demonstrable mass.

Abnormally large intramammary and axillary lymph nodes are more commonly demonstrable with ultrasound than they are mammographically (Fig. 14–122). This is not at all surprising in light of the high percentage of these patients showing histologic evidence of lymphatic tumor emboli. However, axillary lymph nodes can also be enlarged in patients who have mastitis and abscess rather than inflammatory carcinoma. Ultrasound-guided biopsy of enlarged axillary lymph nodes may yield a definitive diagnosis of inflammatory carcinoma in patients in whom a discrete breast mass is not demonstrable.

INTRACYSTIC CARCINOMA

Pathology, Clinical Findings, and Epidemiology

Intracystic carcinomas are rare, constituting less than 0.5% of all breast carcinomas in women and 5% to 7.5% of all breast malignancies in men.

Similar to inflammatory carcinomas, intracystic carcinomas do not represent a single histologic cell type. Additionally, some intracystic malignancies are *in situ*, whereas others are invasive. Therefore, modifying descriptors that refer to the invasiveness and cell type must be used in conjunction with the term intracystic carcinoma. For example, the term invasive papillary intracystic carcinoma would be more appropriate than intracystic carcinoma alone.

Intracystic malignancies form in one of three ways: (a) a papillary lesion can become encysted within a duct, by a combination of secretion and obstruction, causing the duct to dilate cystically around the lesion; (b) a carcinoma can secondarily invade the fibrous wall of a preexisting adjacent benign cyst; or (c) a large, rapidly growing lesion can undergo extensive cystic necrosis.

Patients with intracystic carcinoma of the first type tend to be postmenopausal, having an average age at diagnosis of 65 years. These lesions are usually also quite large and bulky, averaging 5 cm in diameter. These papillomatous lesions probably arise from preexisting large duct papillomas that have undergone malignant degeneration and therefore tend to occur centrally, relatively near the nipple. Intracystic papillomas, which can have a similar appearance on gross pathologic inspection, tend to occur in younger patients (mean age of 43 years) and are usually smaller, averaging 1.5 cm in diameter. The most common gross pathologic appearance is that of a large mural nodule, arising from one wall of the cyst and filling a variable volume of the cyst. These papillary lesions can also appear as thick septations or eccentric wall thickenings. The invasive or DCIS components of the solid part of the lesion can extend beyond the confines of the cyst. Distinguishing intra-

cystic papillary lesions from benign fibrocystic disease is discussed in detail in Chapter 10 and earlier in this chapter in the discussion of invasive papillary carcinoma. Not all intracystic malignancies are invasive papillary carcinoma, and any cell type can present as an intracystic lesions.

The cysts in which the second type of intracystic carcinoma occur are usually large. Tumor within the wall creates only subtle small areas of thickening or mural nodules. These intracystic malignancies occur in younger patients, especially during pregnancy.

The third type of cystic malignancies are not truly intracystic malignancies. Rather, they are usually high-grade solid malignant masses that have undergone more than the usual degree of central tumor necrosis.

The prognosis of intracystic malignancies is generally better than for NOS carcinomas as a whole, probably because so many are pure DCIS and do not extend beyond the wall of the cyst. However, intracystic DCIS and intracystic invasive malignancies that extend well beyond the confines of the cyst into surrounding tissue have a prognosis similar to that of noncystic lesions of the same cell type and invasiveness.

Mammographic Findings

The mammographic findings are nonspecific. Intracystic malignancies usually present as spherically or elliptically shaped high-density masses. The mass margins can be circumscribed, partially circumscribed, or indistinct, depending on whether invasive or DCIS components infiltrate beyond the cyst wall into surrounding tissues. Mammography cannot determine whether the lesion is cystic or solid unless pneumocystography is performed. However, sonography can show everything that pneumocystography can, plus more. Ultrasound is also less expensive and less invasive. Thus, ultrasound is always indicated.

Sonographic Findings

The sonographic appearance of intracystic malignancies depends on the method of formation.

Intracystic papillary malignancies that arise in preexisting large duct papillomas frequently have large cystic components and appear as papillary nodules, thick isoechoic septations (Fig. 14–123), or eccentric wall thickening (Fig. 14–124). Such lesions are typically hypervascular and are fed by many vessels (Fig. 14–125). Although the bulk of the solid components of such lesions lies within the cyst, either invasive (Fig. 14–126) or intraductal components (Fig. 14–127) of the lesion can extend into surrounding tissues.

A malignant solid nodule can grow into a preexisting cyst in two ways. First, an invasive malignancy can directly invade the wall of the adjacent cyst (Fig. 14–128). Second,

(text continued on page 685)

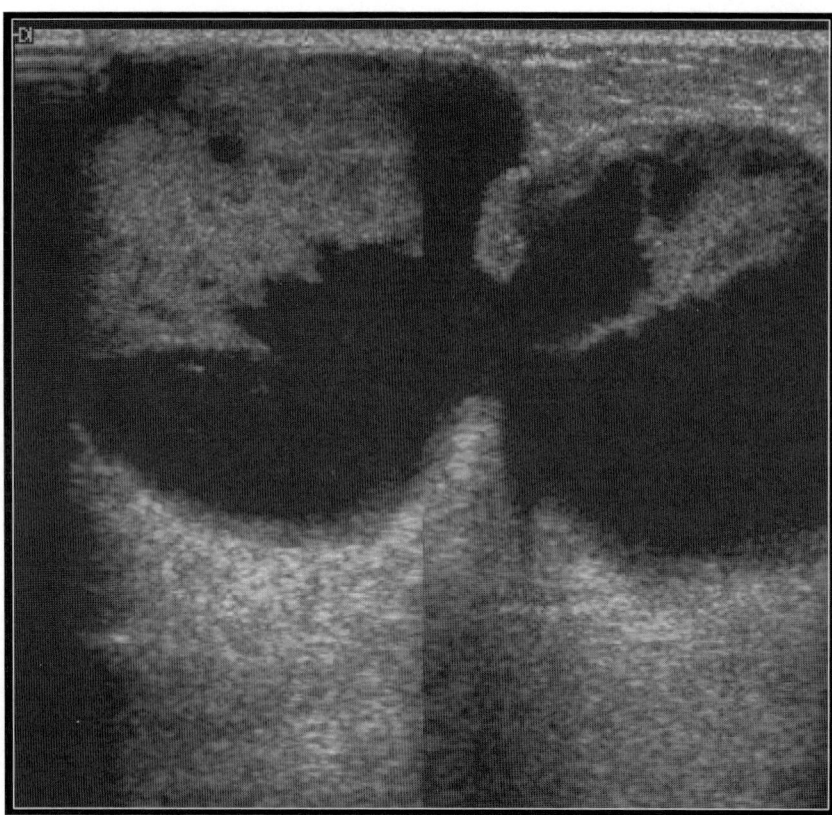

FIGURE 14–123 Intracystic malignancies that arise from preexisting, centrally located large duct papillomas tend to have large cystic components with mural nodules or thick, isoechoic septations.

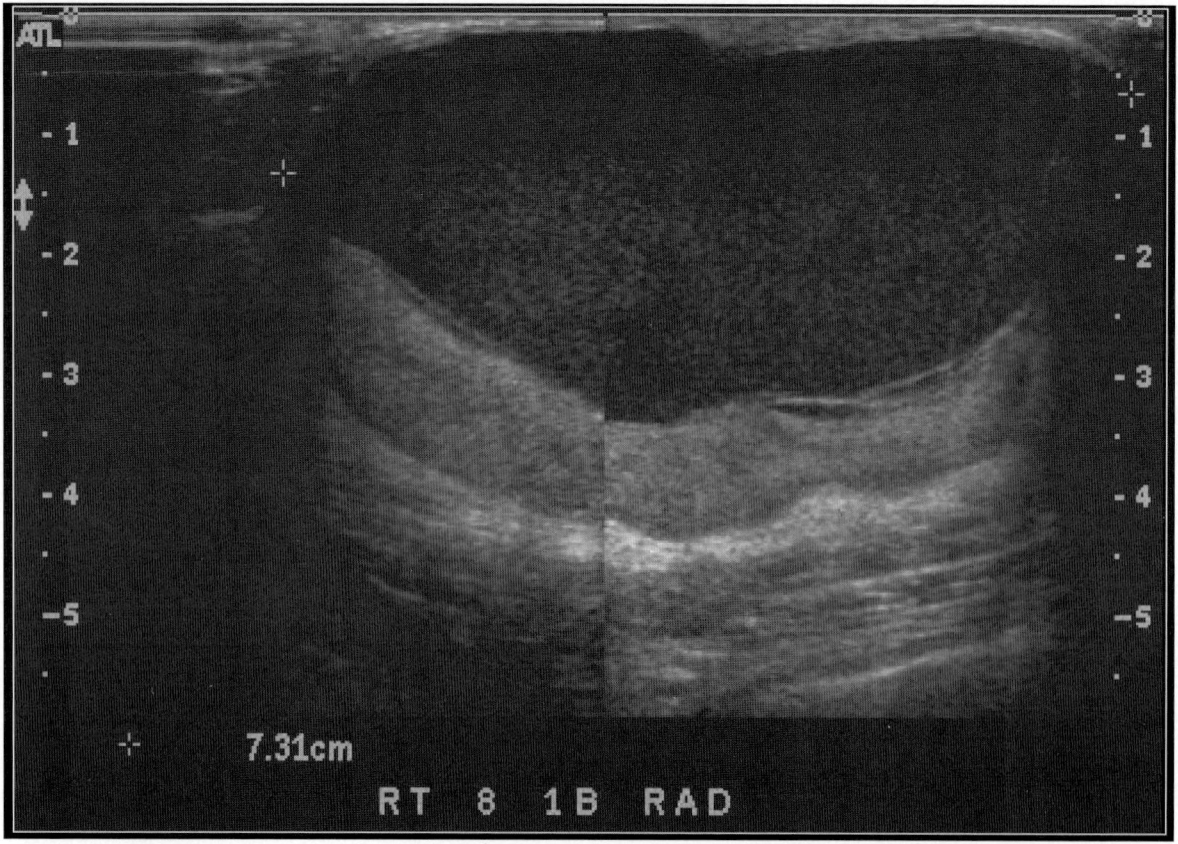

FIGURE 14–124 Other intracystic malignancies that arise from preexisting, centrally located large duct papillomas have large cystic components with eccentric wall thickening.

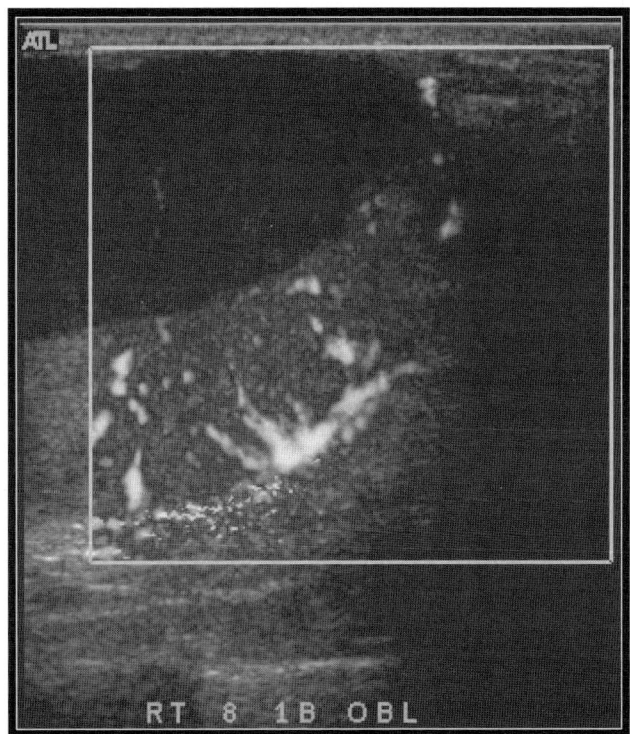

FIGURE 14–125 Intracystic malignancies are frequently very vascular and are fed by multiple arteries. The vessels help distinguish this eccentric wall thickening from layered debris and papillary apocrine metaplasia.

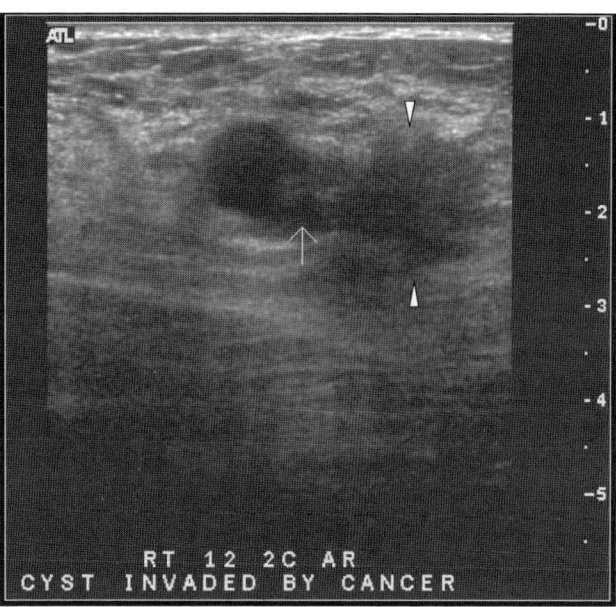

FIGURE 14–126 Invasive intracystic malignancies usually have invasive components that extend outside the cyst into surrounding tissues (*arrow* indicates intracystic component, *arrowheads* indicate extracystic component).

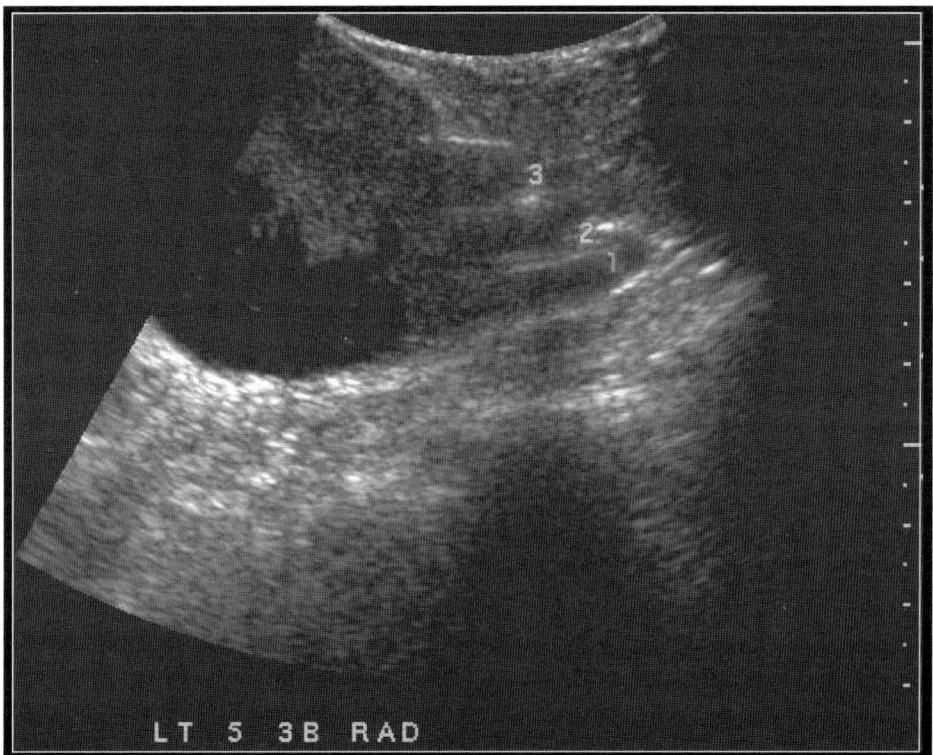

FIGURE 14–127 In addition to invading surrounding tissues, intracystic malignancies can have ductal carcinoma *in situ* components that extend intraductally into surrounding tissues and can manifest with soft findings such as branch pattern *(numbered branches)*.

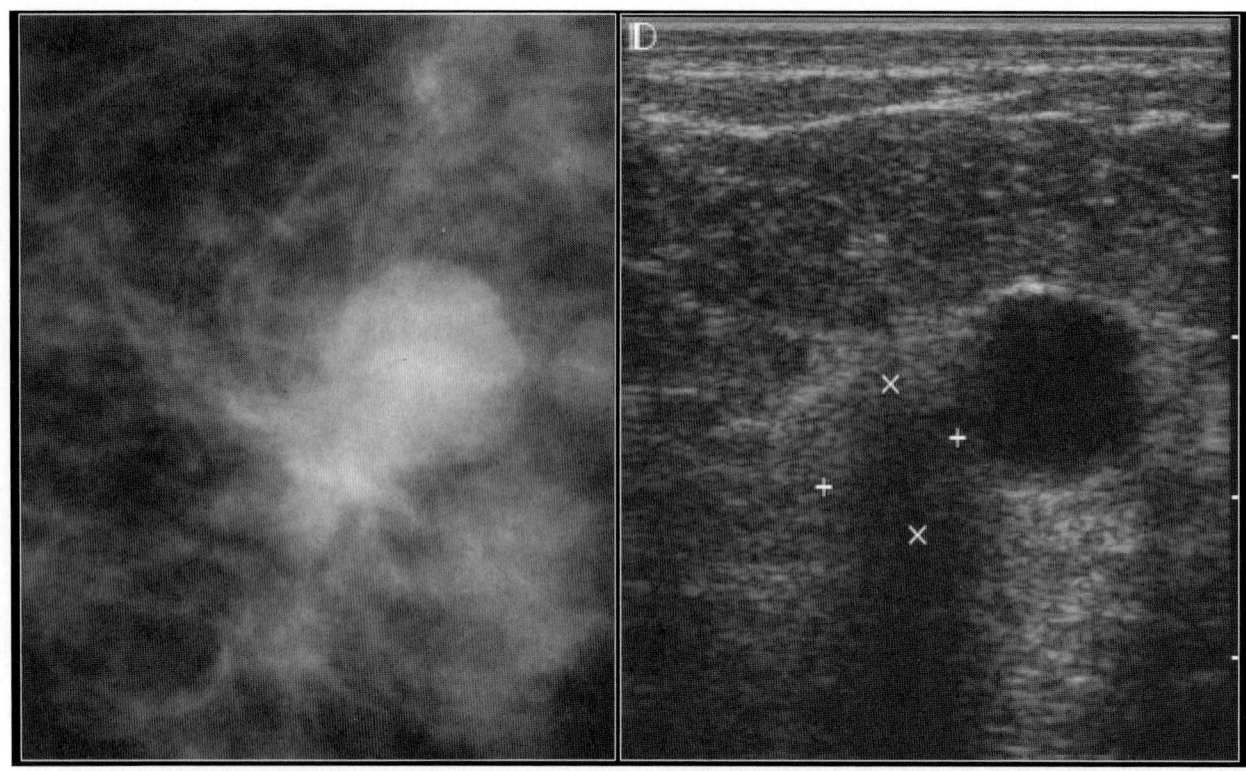

FIGURE 14–128 An invasive malignancy can arise next to a cyst and secondarily invade the cyst wall rather than forming inside a cyst or secondarily developing a cyst around it. This small tubular carcinoma invades into one wall of a preexisting cyst.

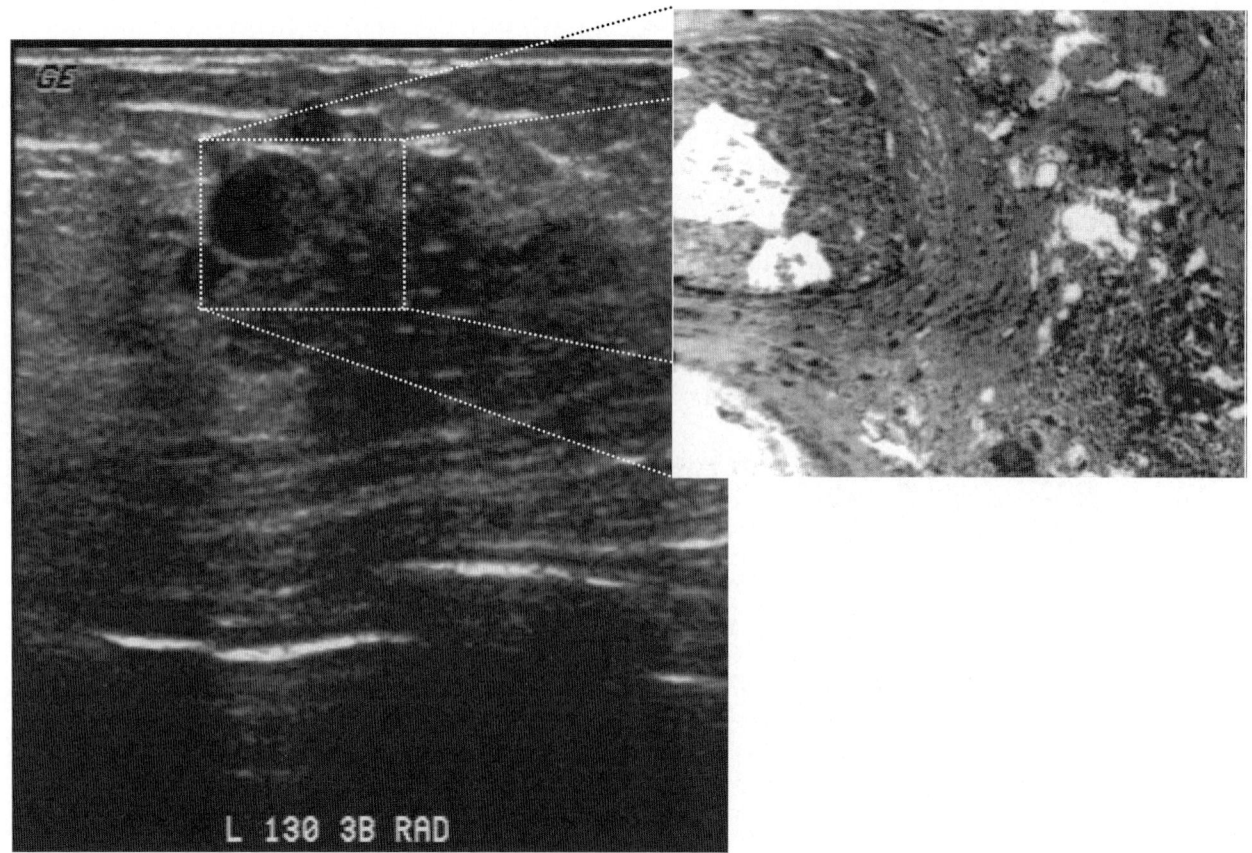

FIGURE 14–129 This mixed invasive and intraductal not otherwise specified carcinoma has ductal carcinoma *in situ* elements that have become encysted.

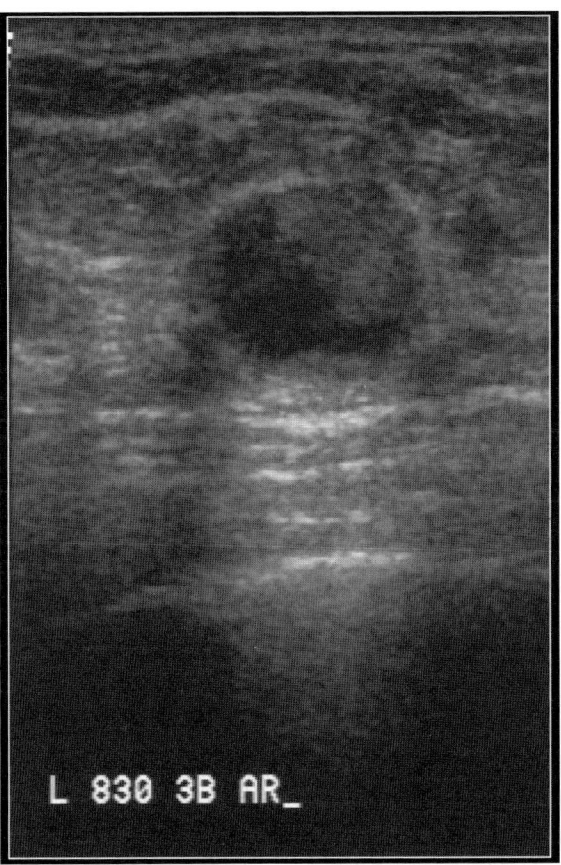

FIGURE 14–130 This rapidly growing, high-grade invasive not otherwise specified carcinoma has undergone enough cystic or hemorrhagic necrosis to appear cystic.

DCIS components of a mixed invasive and intraductal lesion or pure DCIS can grow into a cyst through the duct from which the cyst formed (Fig. 14–129).

Finally, high-grade, very rapidly growing invasive carcinomas (Fig. 14–130) or pure DCIS can undergo enough extensive cystic or hemorrhagic necrosis to appear cystic (Fig. 14–131). Extensive necrosis in pure DICS often presents as a cluster of complex microcysts.

Ultrasound-guided 11-gauge DVAB is the best method of establishing the diagnosis in lesions suspected of being intracystic malignancies. Fluid cytology is too inaccurate to be relied on in such cases. With ultrasound-guided 11-gauge DVAB, the likelihood of removing all imaging evidence of a lesion is high, so that some method of localizing the biopsy site is necessary; therefore, a marker should always be deployed after DVAB in case the histology is malignant or atypical and later surgical excision of the biopsy site is necessary. Obviously, ultrasound-guided needle localization of the intracystic lesion for surgical excision is also possible and will be the procedure of choice when DVAB is not available. Some pathologists hesitate to distinguish benign from malignant papillary lesions with less than a complete surgical excision.

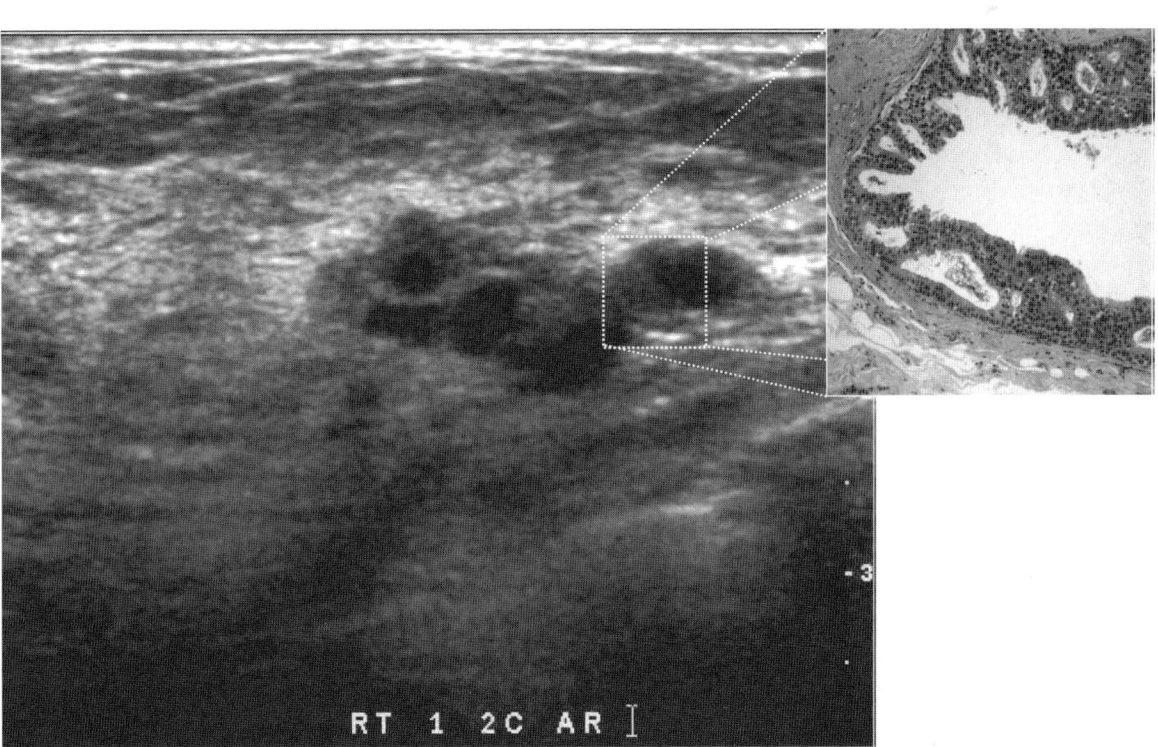

FIGURE 14–131 Very rapidly growing high-nuclear-grade ductal carcinoma *in situ* may have so much central necrosis that it appears to be mostly cystic, usually presenting as clustered complex microcysts.

SUGGESTED READINGS

General Information

Bloom HJG, Richardson WW. Histologic grading and prognosis in breast cancer. *Br J Cancer* 1957;11:359–377.

Harper AP, et al. Ultrasound in the evaluation of solid breast masses. *Radiology* 1983;146(3):731–736.

Richter K, Heywang-Kobrunner SH. Sonographic differentiation of benign from malignant breast lesions: value of indirect measurement of ultrasound velocity. *AJR Am J Roentgenol* 1995;165(4): 825–831.

Rizzato G, Chersevani R, Abbona M, et al. High resolution sonography of breast carcinoma. *Eur J Radiol* 1997;24(1):11–19.

Skaane P, Engedal K. Analysis of sonographic features in the differentiation of fibroadenoma and invasive ductal carcinoma. *AJR Am J Roentgenol* 1998;170(1):109–114.

Stavros AT, et al. Solid breast nodules: use of sonography to distinguish between benign and malignant lesions. *Radiology* 1995; 196(1):123–134.

Teboul M, Halliwell M. Anatomy of the breast. In *Atlas of Ultrasound and Ductal Echography of the Breast: The Introduction of Anatomic Intelligence into Breast Imaging.* Cambridge, MA: Blackwell Science; 1995:49–82.

Ductal Carcinoma *In Situ*

Graversen HP, et al. In situ carcinomas of the female breast. Incidence, clinical findings and DBCG proposals for management. *Acta Oncol* 1988;27(6A):679–682.

Gufler H, Buitrago-Tellez CH, Madjar H, et al. Ultrasound demonstration of mammographically detected microcalcifications. *Acta Radiol* 2000;41(3):217–221.

Hashimoto BE, Kramer DJ, Picozzi VJ. High detection rate of breast ductal carcinoma in situ calcifications on mammographically directed high resolution sonography. *J Ultrasound Med* 2001;20(5): 501–508.

Lennington WJ, et al. Ductal carcinoma in situ of the breast. Heterogeneity of individual lesions. *Cancer* 1994;73(1):118–124.

Moon WK, Im JG, Koh YH, et al. US of mammographically detected clustered calcifications. *Radiology* 2000;217(3):849–854.

Schoonjans JM, Brem RF. Sonographic appearance of ductal carcinoma in situ diagnosed with ultrasonographically guided large core needle biopsy: correlation with mammographic and pathologic findings. *J Ultrasound Med* 2000;19(7):449–457.

Sener SF, Candela FC, Paige ML, et al. Limitations of mammography in the identification of noninfiltrating carcinoma of the breast. *Surg Gynecol Obstet* 1988;167:135–140.

Lobular Carcinoma *In Situ*

Davis N, Baird RM. Breast cancer in association with lobular carcinoma in situ. Clinicopathologic review and treatment recommendation. *Am J Surg* 1984;147:641–645.

Frykberg ER. Lobular carcinoma in situ of the breast. *Breast J* 1999;5(5):296–303.

Georgian-Smith D, Lawton T. Calcifications of lobular carcinoma in situ of the breast: radiologic-pathologic correlation. *AJR Am J Roentgenol* 2001;176:1255–1259.

Cancer Size

Fornage BD, Toubas O, Morel M. Clinical, mammographic, and sonographic determination of preoperative breast cancer size. *Cancer* 1987;60(4):765–771.

Meden H, Neues KP, Roben-Kampken S, et al. A clinical, mammographic, sonographic and histologic evaluation of breast cancer. *Int J Gynaecol Obstet* 1995;48(2):193–199.

Rahusen FD, Taets van Amerongen AH, et al. Ultrasound-guided lumpectomy of nonpalpable breast cancers: a feasibility study looking at the accuracy of obtained margins. *J Surg Oncol* 1999; 72(2):72–76.

Tresserra F, Feu J, Grases PJ, et al. Assessment of breast cancer size: sonographic and pathologic correlation. *J Clin Ultrasound* 1999; 27(9):485–491.

Extensive Intraductal Components

Boyages J, Recht A, Connolly JL, et al. Early breast cancer: predictors of breast recurrence for patients treated with conservative surgery and radiation therapy. *Radiother Oncol* 1990;19(1):29–41.

Healey EA, Osteen RT, Schniktt SJ, et al. Can the clinical and mammographic findings at presentation predict the presence of an extensive intraductal component in early stage breast cancer? *Int J Radiat Oncol Biol Phys* 1989;17(6):1217–1221.

Holland R, Connolly JL, Gelman R, et al. The presence of an extensive intraductal component following limited excision correlates with prominent residual disease in the remainder of the breast. *J Clin Oncol* 1990;8(1):113–118.

Kamio T, Hamano K, Kameoka S, et al. Ultrasonographic diagnosis of breast cancer with intraductal spreading of cancer cells. *Nippon Geka Gakkai Szsshi* 1996;97(5):338–342.

King JM. A practical approach to breast ductal carcinoma in situ and tumors with extensive intraductal component. *Pathology* 1994; 26(2):90–93.

Krishnan L, Jewell WR, Krishnan EC, et al. Breast cancer with extensive intraductal component: treatment with immediate interstitial boost irradiation. *Radiology* 1992;183(1):273–276.

Lindley R, Bulman A, Parsons P, et al. Histologic features predictive of an increased risk of local recurrence after treatment of breast cancer by local tumor excision and radical radiotherapy. *Surgery* 1989;105(1):13–20.

Satake H, Shimamoto K, Sawaki A, et al. Role of ultrasonography in the detection of intraductal spread of breast cancer: correlation with pathologic findings, mammography and MR imaging. *Eur Radiol* 2000;10(11):1726–1732.

Stomper PC, Connolly JL. Mammographic features predicting an extensive intraductal component in early-stage infiltrating ductal carcinoma. *AJR Am J Roentgenol* 1992;158(2):269–272.

Paget's Disease of the Nipple

Burke ET, Braeuning MP, McLelland R, et al. Paget disease of the breast: a pictorial essay. *Radiographics* 1998;18:1459–1464.

Iekda DM, Helvie MA, Frank TS. Paget disease of the nipple: radiologic-pathologic correlation. *Radiology* 1993;189:89–93.

Sawyer RH, Asbury DL. Mammographic appearances in Paget's disease of the breast. *Clin Radiol* 1994;49:185–188.

Multifocal and Multicentric Carcinoma

Berg WA, Gilbreath PL. Multicentric and multifocal cancer: wholebreast US in preoperative evaluation. *Radiology* 2000;214(1): 59–66.

Leopold KA, Recht A, Schnitt SJ, et al. Results of conservative surgery and radiation therapy for multiple synchronous cancers of one breast. *Int J Radiat Oncol Biol Phys* 1989;16(1):11–16.

Tobin CE, Henrix TM, Resnikoff LB, et al. Breast imaging case of the day. Multicentric intraductal papillary carcinoma. *Radiographics* 1996;16(3):720–722.

Inflammatory Carcinoma

Dershaw DD, Moore MP, Liberman L, et al. Inflammatory breast carcinoma: mammographic findings. *Radiology* 1994;190(3):831–834.

Jalyesimi IA, Buzdar AU, Hortobagyi G. Inflammatory breast cancer: a review. *J Clin Oncol* 1992;10(6):1014–1024.

Tubular Carcinoma of the Breast

Cyrlak D, Carpenter PM, Rawal NB. Breast imaging case of the day. *Radiographics* 1999:19:813–816.

Elson BC, Helvie MA, Frank TS, et al. Tubular carcinoma of the breast: mode of presentation, mammographic appearance, and frequency of nodal metastases. *AJR Am J Roentgenol* 1993;161:1173–1176.

Leibman AJ, Lewis M, Kruse B. Tubular carcinoma of the breast: mammographic appearance. *AJR Am J Roentgenol* 1993;161:1134–1135.

Mitnick JS, Gianutsos R, Pollack AH, et al. Tubular carcinoma of the breast: sensitivity of diagnostic techniques and correlation with histopathology. *AJR Am J Roentgenol* 1999;172:319–323.

Tukel S, Kocak S, Aydintug S, et al. Radial scar and tubular carcinoma of the breast. *Australas Radiol* 1997;41(2):190–192.

Vega A, Garijo F. Radial scar and tubular carcinoma. Mammographic and sonographic findings. *Acta Radiol* 1993;34:43–47.

Medullary Carcinoma of the Breast

Cheung YC, Chen SC, Lee KF, et al. Sonographic and pathologic findings in typical and atypical medullary carcinomas of the breast. *J Clin Ultrasound* 2000;28(7):325–331.

Meyer JE, Amin E, Lindfors KK, et al. Medullary carcinoma of the breast: mammographic and US appearance. *Radiology* 1989;170:79–82.

Rigaud C, Theobald S, Noel P, et al. Medullary carcinoma of the breast. A multicenter study of its diagnostic consistency. *Arch Pathol Lab Med* 1993;117:1005–1008.

Colloid Carcinoma of the Breast

Cardenosa G, Doudna C, Eklund GW. Mucinous (colloid) breast cancer: clinical and mammographic findings in 10 patients. *AJR Am J Roentgenol* 1994;162:1077–1079.

Chopra S, Evans AJ, Pinder SE, et al. Pure mucinous breast cancer-mammographic and ultrasound findings. *Clin Radiol* 1996;51(6):421–424.

Conant EF, Dillon RL, Palazzo J, et al. Imaging findings in mucin-containing carcinomas of the breast: correlation with pathologic features. *AJR Am J Roentgenol* 1994;163:821–824.

Memis A, Ozdemir N, Parildar M, et al. Mucinous (colloid) breast cancer: mammographic and US features with histologic correlation. *Eur J Radiol* 2000;35(1):39–43.

Weaver MG, Abdul-karim FW, al-Kaisi N. Mucinous lesions of the breast. A pathologic continuum. *Pathol Res Pract* 1993;189:873–876.

Wilson TE, Helvie MA, Oberman HA, et al. Pure and mixed mucinous carcinoma of the breast: pathologic basis for differences in mammographic appearance. *AJR Am J Roentgenol* 1999;165:285–289.

Invasive Papillary Carcinoma of the Breast

Kenlson MH, el Yousef SJ, Goldberg RE, et al. Intracystic papillary carcinoma of the breast: mammographic, sonographic, and MR appearance with pathologic correlation. *J Comput Assist Tomogr* 1987;11:1074–1076.

Liberman L, Feng T, Susnik B. Case 35: intracystic papillary carcinoma with invasion. *Radiology* 2001;219:781–784.

McCulloch GL, Evans AJ, Yeoman L, et al. Radiological features of papillary carcinoma of the breast. *Clin Radiol* 1997;52(11):865–868.

Mercado CL, Hamele-Bena D, Singer C, et al. Papillary lesions of the breast: evaluation with stereotactic directional vacuum-assisted biopsy. *Radiology* 2001;221:650–655.

Mitnick JS, Vazquez MF, Harris MN, et al. Invasive papillary carcinoma of the breast: mammographic appearance. *Radiology* 1990;177:803–806.

Schneider JA. Invasive papillary breast carcinoma: mammographic and sonographic appearance. *Radiology* 1989;171:377–379.

Soo MS, Williford ME, Walsh R, et al. Papillary carcinoma of the breast: imaging findings. *AJR Am J Roentgenol* 1995;164(2):321–326.

Tobin CE, Hendrix TM, Resnikoff LB, et al. Breast imaging case of the day. *Radiographics* 1996;16:720–722.

Invasive Lobular Carcinoma

Bazzocchi M, Facecchia I, Zuiani C, et al. Diagnostic imaging of lobular carcinoma of the breast: mammographic, ultrasonographic, and MR findings. *Radiol Med* (Torino) 2000;100(6):436–443.

Butler RS, Venta LA, Wiley EL, et al. Sonographic evaluation of infiltrating lobular carcinoma. *AJR Am J Roentgenol* 1999;172(2):325–330.

Cawson JN, Law EM, Kavanagh AM. Invasive lobular carcinoma: sonographic features of cancers detected in a BreastScreen program. *Australas Radiol* 2001;45(1):25–30.

Evans N, Lyons K. The use of ultrasound in the diagnosis of invasive lobular carcinoma of the breast less than 20 mm in size. *Clin Radiol* 2000;55(4):261–263.

Gill HK, Berg WA. Case 39: invasive lobular carcinoma. *Radiology* 2001;221:132–136.

Helvie MA, Paramagul C, Oberman HA, et al. Invasive lobular carcinoma. Imaging features and clinical detection. *Invest Radiol* 1993;28(3):202–207.

Hollingsworth AB, Taylor LD, Rhodes DC. Establishing a histologic basis for false negative mammograms. *Am J Surg* 1993;166:643–647.

Krecke KN, Gisvold JJ. Invasive lobular carcinoma of the breast: mammographic findings and extent of disease at diagnosis in 184 patients. *AJR Am J Roentgenol* 1993;161:957–960.

Lambie RW, Hodgden D, Herman EM, et al. Sonomammographic detection of lobular carcinoma not demonstrated on xeromammography. *J Clin Ultrasound* 1983;11:495–497.

Mendelson EB, Harris KM, Doshi N, et al. Infiltrating lobular carcinoma: mammographic patterns with pathologic correlation. *AJR Am J Roentgenol* 1989;153:265–271.

Paramagul CP, Helvie MA, Adler DD. Invasive lobular carcinoma: sonographic appearance and role of sonography in improving diagnostic sensitivity. *Radiology* 1995;195(1):231–234.

Rissanen T, Tikkakoski T, Autio AL, et al. Ultrasonography of invasive lobular breast carcinoma. *Acta Radiol* 1998;39(3):285–291.

Schnitt SJ, Connolly JL, Recht A, et al. Influence of infiltrating lobular histology on local tumor control in breast cancer patients treated with conservative surgery and radiotherapy. *Cancer* 1989;64:448–454.

Silverstein MJ, Lewinsky BS, Waisman JR, et al. Infiltrating lobular carcinoma. Is it different from infiltrating duct carcinoma? [Comment]. *Cancer* 1994;74:986–987.

Skaane P, Skjorten F. Ultrasonographic evaluation of invasive lobular carcinoma. *Acta Radiol* 1999;40(4):369–75.

Tubulolobular Carcinoma of the Breast

Fisher ER, Gregoiro RM, Redmond C, et al. Tubulolobular invasive breast cancer: a variant of lobular invasive cancer. *Hum Pathol* 1977;8(6):679–683.

Green I, McCormick B, Cranor M, et al. A comparative study of pure tubular and tubulolobular carcinoma of the breast. *Am J Surg Pathol* 1997;21(6):653–657.

Linnell F, Ljungberg O. Breast carcinoma. Progression of tubular carcinoma and a new classification. *Acta Pathol Microbiol Scand* 1980;88:59–60.

Carcinoma with Sarcomatous Metaplasia (Metaplastic Carcinoma)

Evans HA, Shaughnessy EA, Nikiforov YE. Infiltrating ductal carcinoma of the breast with osseous metaplasia: imaging findings with pathologic correlation. *AJR Am J Roentgenol* 1999;172:1420–1422.

Sarcomas of the Breast

Elson BC, Ikeda DM, Andersson I, et al. Fibrosarcoma of the breast: mammographic findings in five cases. *AJR Am J Roentgenol* 1992; 158(5):993–995.

Tassin GB, Fornage BD, Sneige N. Primary multifocal angiosarcoma of the breast: sonographic evaluation with pathologic correlation. *J Ultrasound Med* 1990:481–483.

Lymphomoproliferative Neoplasms of the Breast

Coll D, Spence L, Cardenosa G. Plasmacytoma of the breast: mammographic and sonographic findings (on the AJR viewbox). *AJR Am J Roentgenol* 1999;173:1135.

Liberman L, Giess C, Dershaw D, et al. Non-Hodgkin lymphoma of the breast: imaging characteristics and correlation with histopathologic findings. *Radiology* 1994;192:167.

Memis A, Killi R, Sebnem O, et al. Bilateral breast involvement in acute lymphoblastic leukemia: color Doppler sonography findings. *AJR Am J Roentgenol* 1995;165:1011.

Mendelson EB, Doshi N, Brabb BC, et al. Pseudolymphoma of the breast: imaging findings. A case report. *AJR Am J Roentgenol* 1994;162:617–619.

Whitfill, CH, Feig SA, Webner D. Breast imaging case of the day. *Radiographics* 1998;18:1038–1042.

Zack JR, Trevisan SG, Gupta M. Primary breast lymphoma originating in a benign intramammary lymph node. *AJR Am J Roentgenol* 2001;177:177–178.

Metastases of the Breast

Bohman LG, Bassett LW, Gold RH, et al. Breast metastases from extramammary malignancies. *Radiology* 1982;144:309–312.

Rizzatto LE, Giuseppetti GM, Dini G, et al. Metastatic tumors in the breast: sonographic findings. *J Ultrasound Med* 1985;4(2): 69–74.

Soo MS, Williford ME, Elenberger CD. Medullary thyroid carcinoma metastatic to the breast: mammographic appearance.

Yang WT, Metrewell C. Sonography of nonmammary malignancies of the breast. *AJR Am J Roentgenol* 1999;172:343–348.

Yang WT, Muttarak M, Ho LW. Nonmammary malignancies of the breast: ultrasound, CT, and MRI. *Semin Ultrasound CT MR* 2000;21(5):375–394.

ATYPICAL, HIGH-RISK, PREMALIGNANT, AND LOCALLY AGGRESSIVE LESIONS

There are several different types of lesions that, although not frankly malignant, indicate increased risk for the patient (Table 15–1). The high-risk lesion may be premalignant, may have a high incidence of synchronous malignant change, or may merely be an indicator in mildly to moderately increased generalized risk for subsequent development of malignancy in any part of either breast. High-risk lesions can recur locally and can be difficult to diagnose histologically.

ATYPICAL DUCTAL HYPERPLASIA

General Histologic Classification, Clinical Findings, and Epidemiology

There is a continuous spectrum of epithelial proliferative disorders ranging from usual ductal hyperplasia (UDH), to florid or papillary duct hyperplasia (PDH), to atypical ductal hyperplasia (ADH), to ductal carcinoma *in situ* (DCIS), to invasive duct carcinoma [not otherwise specified (NOS) carcinoma]. The normal epithelium in the ducts and lobules of the breast contains two layers: epithelium and myoepithelium. In UDH, both layers become hyperplastic, and the number of cell layers is greater than the normal two. In mild UDH, the proliferation of epithelium and myoepithelium generally results in three or four layers of cells. Moderate UDH results in five or more layers. In florid duct hyperplasia or PDH, the hyperplastic epithelial-myoepithelial elements tend to grow in papillary formations or to fill completely and distend ductal and acinar spaces. Certain cases of PDH may begin to form fibrovascular cores and thus may be impossible to distinguish from papillomas.

We must begin by discussing the benign end of the spectrum in which ADH lies. Classification as UDH does not indicate the site of origin of the hyperplasia; this lesion is more commonly found within lobules than within the terminal ducts. What UDH does indicate is a pattern of cellular proliferation that differs from other patterns of proliferation such as those of lobular hyperplasia or apocrine metaplasia and hyperplasia. However, different types of hyperplasia commonly coexist. For example, apocrine metaplasia and UDH occur together quite commonly.

UDH, whether mild, moderate, or florid, is characterized histologically by the variability of the nuclear appearance and the preservation of distinct epithelial and myoepithelial layers.

Because of the overlap in histologic findings between ADH and DCIS, some propose that both lesions be classified as *intraepithelial neoplasia*.

There are no gross or clinical findings that are characteristic of ADH. In fact, the histologic diagnosis of ADH is often serendipitous. The biopsy in which the diagnosis of ADH is established is usually performed because of a palpable or mammographic lesion that is caused by a coexisting benign or malignant breast condition. Thus, the gross pathologic findings usually reflect the coexisting condition for which the biopsy was performed and are not those of ADH.

Histologically, ADH differs from UDH in several ways. First, there is less variability of cells and nuclei in ADH than in UDH. The cells in ADH appear relatively uniform in size and shape in comparison to those in UDH. The nuclei in ADH are hyperchromatic and also uniform. The cells fill and distend the duct lumen, often forming bridges and spaces similar to the spaces in cribriform DCIS or papillae similar to those of micropapillary DCIS. The spaces may show areas of necrosis and dystrophic calcification. ADH involves the lobules and terminal ducts to the greatest degree but can also involve central ducts. Most centrally occurring cases of ADH likely arise within preexisting benign large duct papillomas.

The prevalence of ADH has been reported to be low, about 3%. However, the prevalence of ADH is much higher

689

TABLE 15–1. HIGH-RISK, BUT NOT FRANKLY MALIGNANT, SOLID BREAST LESIONS

Atypical
  Atypical ductal hyperplasia (ADH)
  Atypical lobular hyperplasia (ALH)

Premalignant
  ADH and ALH
  Phyllodes tumor (PT)
  Juvenile papillomatosis

Risk markers for ipsilateral or contralateral invasive breast
  cancer development
  ADH and ALH
  Juvenile papillomatosis
  Complex fibroadenoma (FAC)

Histologically ambiguous lesions or benign lesions that can be
  mistaken for malignant
  ADH versus ductal carcinoma *in situ* (DCIS)
  Benign PT versus malignant PT
  Radial scar (RS)

Locally aggressive benign lesions
  PT

High risk for associated atypical or invasive malignancy
  RS and complex sclerosing lesions

among patients who undergo biopsy for nonpalpable, mammographic lesions than for palpable lesions. This is especially true if the only mammographic finding is calcifications. In such series, up to 16% to 17% of all benign biopsies may show atypia, about 75% of which is associated with ADH and 25% with atypical lobular hyperplasia (ALH).

As we progress through the spectrum from UDH to ADH, the premalignant risk increases. Mild UDH increases the risk for cancer development in the same or contralateral breast by about twofold. PDH increases the risk slightly more, approaching threefold. ADH about doubles the risk for cancer development over UDH to about 4 to 5 times the baseline. ADH in association with a positive first-degree family history almost doubles the risk for cancer development over ADH associated with a negative family history—in the range of 8 to 10 times that of baseline risk.

The increased risk for cancer development associated with ADH is not limited to the site from which ADH is diagnosed, but rather is generalized, including distant areas of the ipsilateral breast as well as the contralateral breast. Therefore, some investigators have questioned whether ADH is truly a premalignant lesion. However, studies have shown ADH to be present within the periphery of excised *in situ* and invasive malignant lesions in about 70% to 80% of cases. The presence of ADH in the periphery of such lesions strongly suggests that ADH does have direct premalignant potential and that both DCIS and invasive carcinomas probably arise within areas of preexisting foci of ADH (at least for low- to intermediate-grade malignancies). The significance of ADH in the periphery of malig-

nant lesions is still controversial, and other investigators disagree with the theory that ADH in the periphery indicates that a malignant lesion arose from preexisting ADH.

Mammographic Findings

The mammographic findings of ADH are nonspecific. In most cases, these findings are represented by microcalcifications in the absence of any other mammographic abnormalities. In occasional cases, increased soft tissue density due to associated fibrosis, adenosis, or sclerosing adenosis might also be seen. Occasionally, architectural distortion or frank spiculation may be seen (with or without associated calcifications) when the ADH develops in the periphery of a radial scar or with severe sclerosing adenosis. In a few cases, where ADH develops within a large preexisting centrally located intraductal papilloma, there may be an associated nodule.

Until recently, the literature suggested that the diagnosis of ADH obtained on biopsies of nonpalpable mammographic lesions was usually serendipitous because the mammographic abnormalities were caused by associated or underlying conditions rather than ADH. In fact, this theory holds true in just over half of cases, usually those in which the mammographic finding is calcifications only. In such cases, the calcifications represent associated adenosis or sclerosing adenosis rather than the ADH. This is also true in cases in which ADH arises within an underlying spiculated lesion, such as a radial scar. However, recently there have been reports that in slightly fewer than half of the cases of ADH diagnosed because of calcifications alone, the calcifications actually lie within the focus of ADH. The calcifications, like those found in association with low- to intermediate-grade DCIS, develop in the necrotic spaces within the ADH, similar to the spaces seen in cribriform or micropapillary DCIS.

Sonographic Findings

As is true of the mammographic findings, the sonographic findings often represent those of the underlying lesion within which the ADH develops. The sonographic find-

TABLE 15–2. SONOGRAPHIC APPEARANCES OF ATYPICAL DUCTAL HYPERPLASIA

Peripheral origin [arises within terminal ductolobular units
  (TDLU) or radial scar]
  Enlarged TDLUs
  Enlarged terminal duct with or without TDLU
  Radial scar

Central origin (arises within papilloma)
  Intraductal nodule (within fluid-filled duct)
  Solid ductal appearance
  Nodule

ings of ADH vary, depending on whether the atypical cells arise within a peripheral or central location and on the appearance of the preexisting benign lesion within which the cells develop (Table 15–2).

Sonographic Appearance of Peripherally Located Atypical Ductal Hyperplasia

ADH usually arises peripherally within TDLUs. This pattern of involvement often is identifiable sonographically as an abnormally enlarged TDLU (Fig. 15–1) or cluster of TDLUs (Fig. 15–2). In such cases, ADH almost always arises within areas of preexisting PDH, and the lobular enlargement is merely a reflection of the underlying PDH, which tends to affect the lobule to a much greater degree than the terminal duct. However, TDLU enlargement is nonspecific. Diffuse lobular enlargement throughout the breasts in a premenopausal woman is usually attributable to benign fibrocystic change or benign proliferative disorders without atypia. Adenosis, sclerosing adenosis, PDH, apocrine metaplasia, and fibrocystic change with microcysts can all cause lobular enlargement. However, ADH and low-nuclear-

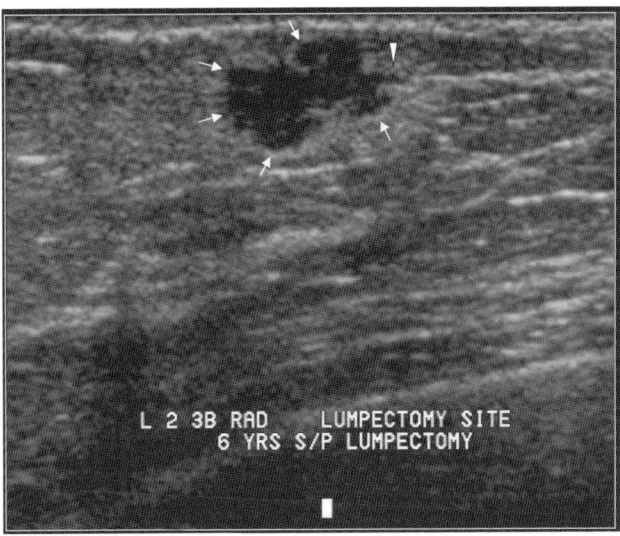

FIGURE 15–2 More severe, peripherally arising atypical ductal hyperplasia (ADH) may present as abnormal enlargement of a cluster of terminal ductolobular units (*arrowhead* indicates distal end of lobar duct; *arrows* indicate enlarged lobules). This finding is also nonspecific and can be seen in a variety of fibrocystic or benign proliferative disorders or in ductal carcinoma *in situ*. In patients with ADH, the enlargement usually reflects the florid or papillary duct hyperplasia within which the atypia developed.

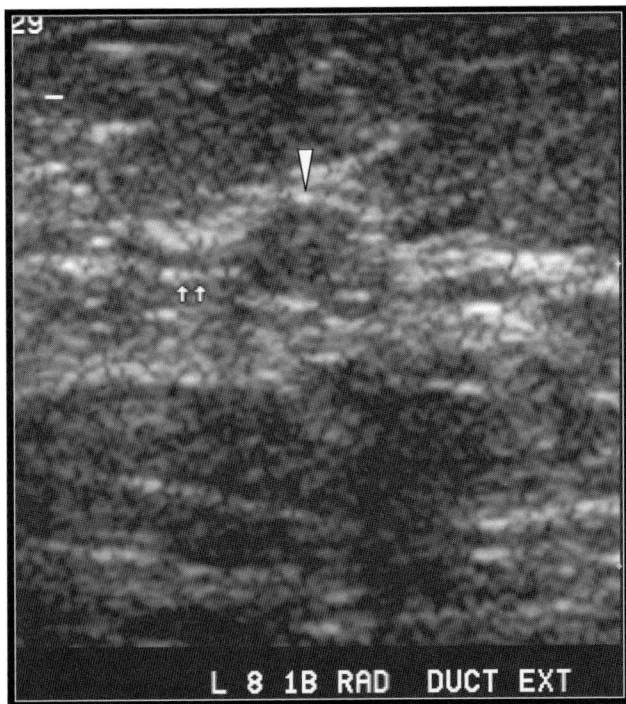

FIGURE 15–1 Atypical ductal hyperplasia (ADH) that arises peripherally may present as a terminal ductolobular unit (TDLU) that is disproportionately enlarged in comparison to other TDLUs in the same segment of the breast, a very nonspecific finding that can be seen in a variety of fibrocystic and benign proliferative disorders. In most cases of ADH, the enlargement is caused by the underlying florid duct hyperplasia (*small arrows* indicate extralobular terminal duct; *arrowhead* indicates enlarged lobule).

grade DCIS tend to enlarge a single TDLU or a group of TDLUs out of proportion to other lobules within the same segment of the breast. Disproportionate lobular enlargement indicates an increased risk for ADH or low-nuclear-grade DCIS in the postmenopausal patient who is not receiving hormone replacement therapy. In cases of ADH that present with mammographically visible calcifications, sonography may show mildly enlarged lobules (Fig. 15–3) or peripheral ducts (Fig. 15–4) that contain calcifications. This, too, is a nonspecific finding, because ductal calcifications in mildly enlarged ducts are frequently seen with PDH, and chronic duct ectasia and lobular calcifications are frequently seen with adenosis and papillary apocrine metaplasia. However, even though the findings of ADH are nonspecific, most cases of ADH present with at least one suspicious findings that requires a characterization of BIRADS 4a or higher.

The second appearance of peripheral ADH simply reflects the appearance of a preexisting radial scar within which the ADH has developed. Sonographically, this lesion may be difficult or impossible to distinguish from a small tubular carcinoma or low-grade invasive NOS carcinoma. The appearance varies greatly with the amount of proliferative change in the periphery of the lesion. Because this appearance of ADH is really the appearance of a radial scar and is not specific for ADH, the sonographic appearance of ADH in radial scars is discussed and illustrated in greater detail later in this chapter in the section on radial scars.

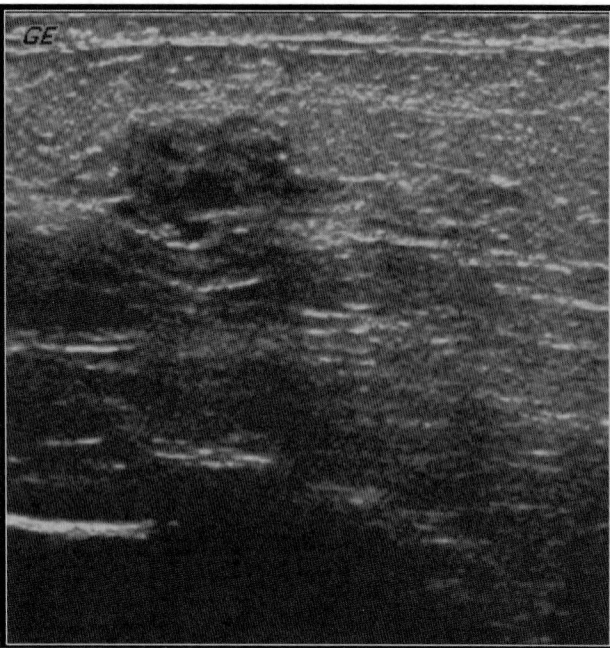

FIGURE 15–3 When peripherally arising atypical ductal hyperplasia presents as mammographic calcifications, sonography may show clustered calcifications in an enlarged terminal ductolobular unit, a nonspecific finding. Similar findings can occur with papillary apocrine metaplasia, florid duct hyperplasia, adenosis, or ductal carcinoma *in situ*.

Sonographic Appearance of Centrally Arising Atypical Ductal Hyperplasia

As is the case for peripherally arising ADH, the sonographic appearance of centrally arising ADH merely reflects the appearance of the underlying benign condition within which the ADH arose. Centrally arising ADH almost always arises within preexisting large duct papillomas or areas of PDH and therefore is usually indistinguishable from benign large duct papillomas. Papillomas and ADH have three main presentations:

1. An intraductal solid nodule of variable size and length within a fluid-filled duct (Fig. 15–5)
2. A solid-appearing duct (Fig. 15–6)
3. A nodule with characteristics that suggest an intraductal location
A. Duct extension (Fig. 15–7)
B. Branch pattern (Fig. 15–8)

Although lesions with these appearances indeed represent benign intraductal papillomas, a large enough percentage of them contain ADH or DCIS to warrant biopsy of them all. In fact, of central lesions resembling benign large duct papillomas, the risk for DCIS is 6% and the risk for ADH is 7%.

Although the sonographic findings of both peripherally and centrally arising ADH are nonspecific, one or more suspicious findings are usually present and prevent

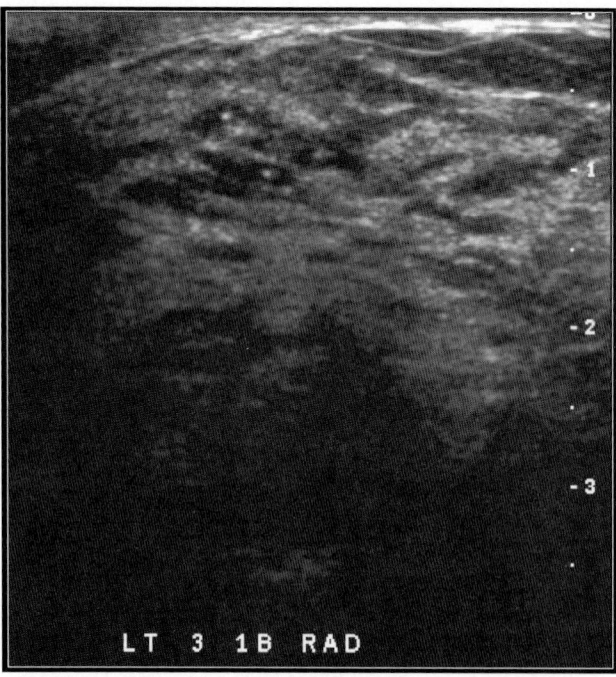

FIGURE 15–4 When peripherally arising atypical ductal hyperplasia presents as mammographic calcifications, sonography may show calcifications in mildly enlarged ducts. This finding is nonspecific and can be seen in florid duct hyperplasia, chronic duct ectasia–periductal mastitis complex, and ductal carcinoma *in situ*.

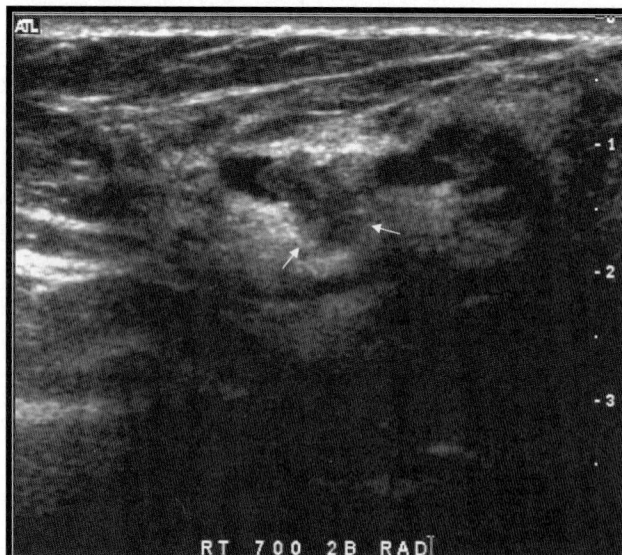

FIGURE 15–5 Centrally arising atypical ductal hyperplasia (ADH) often arises within a preexisting benign large duct papilloma. The sonographic features of such lesions are simply those of the papilloma in which the ADH arose. In this case, the ADH arose within an intraductal nodule in an ectatic, fluid-filled duct. One side branch is involved and expanded *(arrows)*. The more expansile, the longer, and the more it involves branch ducts, the more likely a papilloma is to contain ADH or ductal carcinoma *in situ*.

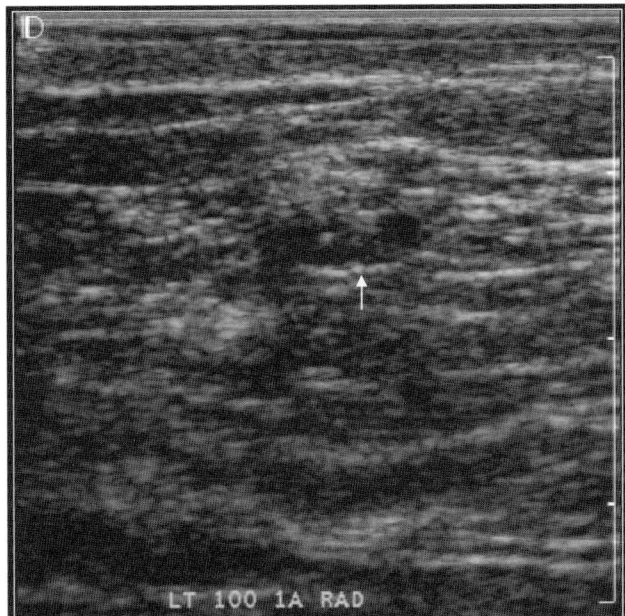

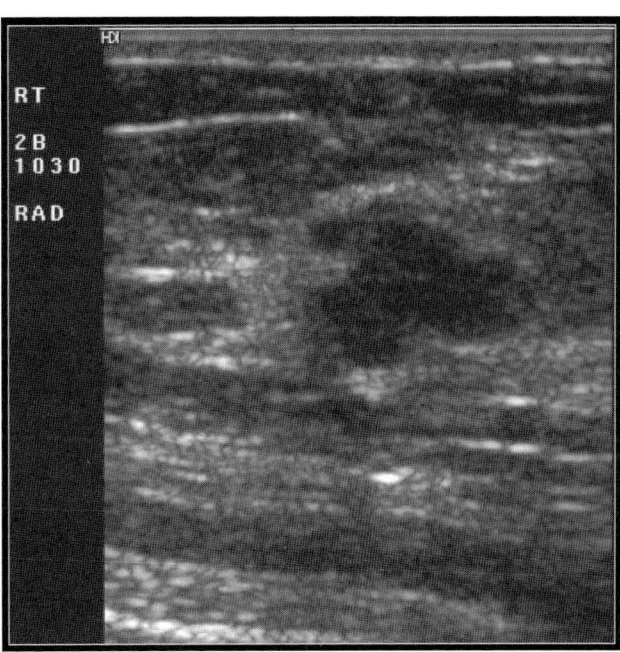

FIGURE 15–6 Centrally occurring atypical ductal hyperplasia may present as a solid tubular structure *(arrow)*, an intraductal papillary lesion in which the associated duct ectasia and secretions have regressed. This nonspecific finding could also be seen in benign large duct papilloma and ductal carcinoma *in situ*. This lesion also contains a single punctate echo that represents a calcification within the mildly enlarged solid duct.

FIGURE 15–8 Centrally arising ductal carcinoma *in situ* (DCIS) may present as a nodule with branch pattern. This nonspecific finding can also be seen with large duct papillomas and DCIS. The combination of duct extension and branch pattern in this horizontally oriented nodule gives the characteristic "lazy Y" appearance of intraductal lesions that involve branch ducts.

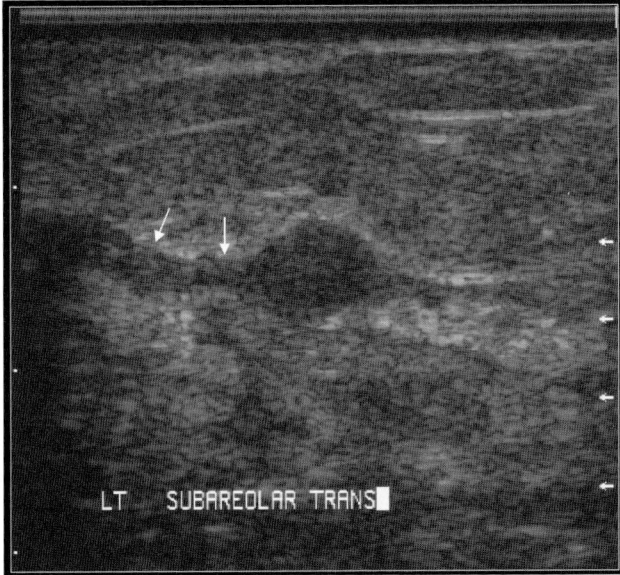

FIGURE 15–7 Centrally arising atypical ductal hyperplasia may present as a nodule with a prominent duct extension *(arrows)*. This finding can also be seen in benign large duct papillomas and ductal carcinoma *in situ* (DCIS). Note that the nodule greatly expands the ducts. The greater the degree of expansion of the duct, the higher is the risk for atypia or DCIS.

ADH from being characterized as BIRADS 3. ADH most commonly manifests soft suspicious sonographic findings that can also be seen with DCIS: duct extension, branch pattern, or microlobulation. When ADH arises within radial scars, hard suspicious findings, such as angular margins, spiculation, or thick, echogenic halo, are present. In fact, 30 of 32 cases of ADH identified sonographically had suspicious sonographic features that required a BIRADS 4a or higher characterization. Microlobulation occurs in 47% of cases of ADH, duct extension occurs in 52%, branch pattern in 35%, sonographically visible calcifications in 13%, spiculation or thick, echogenic halo in 17%, and angular margins in 27%. The incidence of calcifications in sonographically detected ADH is low because most cases of ADH that presented with just calcifications underwent stereotactic biopsy without being evaluated sonographically.

In summary, the sonographic findings of ADH are those of the underlying proliferative conditions in which it arises—usually PDH or radial scar for peripheral lesions and intraductal papilloma for central lesions. The sonographic findings of both peripheral and central ADH are usually suspicious and require a BIRADS 4a or higher classification 94% of the time. The suspicious features warrant biopsy based on the strict criteria presented in Chapter 12.

ADH exists when there are certain cytologic or histologic patterns of DCIS that are not fully developed. The features of DCIS that are present are therefore usually incomplete. Even if complete, these features may not be uniformly present throughout the specimen. Thus, there are cases of ADH that differ from DCIS only quantitatively, but not qualitatively. Because of the nonuniform distribution of DCIS features within such lesions, a random sampling technique such as core biopsy may miss or underestimate the extent of such change. For this reason, histologic diagnoses of ADH obtained from core needle biopsy specimens should be followed up with excisional biopsy. A significant percentage of cases that are diagnosed as ADH on core biopsy sample will be upgraded to DCIS after excisional biopsy, which more accurately reflects the true extent of DCIS features. Directional vacuum-assisted biopsy (DVAB) with an 11-gauge needle obtains larger cores than does 14-gauge core needle biopsy and decreases the risk for underdiagnosing malignancy, but does not reduce that risk to zero. The need for surgical reexcision after a diagnosis of ADH obtained with 11-guage DVAB is more variable than after 14-guage core needle biopsy. If the mammotomy specimen contains only a small focus of atypia that is not near the margins of the mammotomy specimen, surgical reexcision is generally not necessary. However, if the atypical focus within the specimen is large or extends to the margin of the mammotomy cores, surgical reexcision should still be performed.

ATYPICAL LOBULAR HYPERPLASIA

General Pathologic Findings, Clinical Findings, and Epidemiology

ALH, like ADH, is defined as the presence of several, but not all, cytologic and histologic features of lobular carcinoma *in situ* (LCIS) or a very limited degree of atypia (involving only one TDLU). Like ADH, ALH lies along a continuous spectrum from benign lobular hyperplasia, to ALH, to LCIS. As is the case for ductal hyperplasia, ALH most commonly involves the lobule and less commonly involves the ducts. The term lobular, therefore, denotes the pattern of cell proliferation rather than the location of proliferation, a pattern that distinguishes this condition from UDH and apocrine metaplasia.

Like ADH, ALH is considered to be both a premalignant lesion as well as an indicator of generalized increased risk for breast cancer development. This increased risk exists in the entirety of both breasts and is not localized to the immediate vicinity in which LCIS is diagnosed. ALH is considered to be premalignant because of the potential to develop into invasive lobular carcinoma, and ALH is frequently found in tissues surrounding LCIS and invasive lobular carcinoma. However, like ADH, ALH is not an obligate precursor to malignancy. All cases of ALH do not progress to malignancy. ALH not only increases the risk for future development of LCIS and invasive lobular carci-

noma but also increases the risk for DCIS and invasive NOS carcinoma. ALH increases the relative cancer risk fourfold to fivefold. In patients with positive first-degree family histories, ALH increases the risk sixfold to eightfold.

There are no gross pathologic findings specific for ALH. In fact, ALH is almost always an incidental finding within a tissue specimen obtained to evaluate a palpable or mammographic finding caused by an unrelated abnormality that occurred in the same vicinity.

Histologically, benign hyperplasia and ALH should be distinguished from adenosis, in which the numbers of lobules and the numbers of ductules within the lobules is increased, but in which the two-layered, epithelial-myoepithelial lining of the ductules is normal. In lobular hyperplasia, there is an increase in the number of cell layers to three or more. In severe cases, there is filling and distention of the ductules and lobules. The cells of ALH are more uniform in size and have more uniform and hyperchromatic nuclei than do those in benign lobular hyperplasia. The cells that are involved in lobular hyperplasia are smaller than those in both UDH and ADH. Additionally, ALH much less often contains central spaces with necrosis and dystrophic calcification than does ADH.

Mammographic Findings

There are no mammographic findings specific for ALH. The diagnosis of ALH obtained from biopsies performed because of mammographic abnormalities is usually incidental and serendipitous. Like ADH, the lesion is often discovered on biopsies for calcifications in surrounding areas of adenosis or sclerosing adenosis. However, unlike ADH, the calcifications are very rarely within the actual area of ALH. This is because ALH is much less likely to have spaces containing necrosis and calcifications than is ADH. ALH is more likely to involve multiple TDLUs in multiple different areas of the breast than is ADH.

Sonographic Findings

The diagnosis of ALH obtained from biopsies of sonographic lesions, like the diagnosis of ALH obtained from biopsies performed for mammographic lesions, is usually an incidental finding. The sonographic abnormalities for which a biopsy showing ALH is performed are usually adenosis, sclerosing adenosis, PDH, or papillary apocrine metaplasia (Fig. 15–9).

ALH can directly cause sonographic findings in certain cases. However, the positive sonographic finding that ALH causes is a completely nonspecific enlargement of TDLUs that can be seen in numerous other benign and malignant conditions. The tendency for ALH to involve multiple TDLUs in different parts of both breasts makes it difficult to distinguish ALH from underlying benign causes of generalized TDLU enlargement.

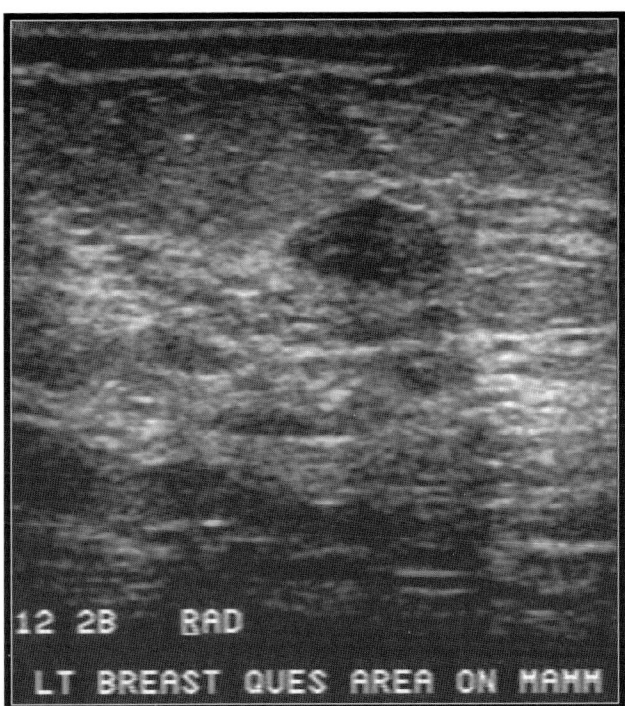

FIGURE 15–9 The diagnosis of atypical lobular hyperplasia (ALH) is usually incidental. In this case, the biopsy was performed to evaluate a complex cyst with a mural nodule caused by papillary apocrine metaplasia (PAM). The imaging findings that precipitated the biopsy were caused by the PAM, not the ALH.

ALH also has a propensity to develop within fibroadenomas. Unfortunately, in most cases, the ALH that develops within a fibroadenoma or complex fibroadenoma, but does not change its sonographic appearance and therefore is not detectable.

LOBULAR CARCINOMA *IN SITU*

LCIS is discussed and illustrated in Chapter 14.

PHYLLODES TUMOR

General Pathologic Findings, Clinical Findings, and Epidemiology

Johannes Muller originally described phyllodes tumors in 1838 as "cystosarcoma phyllodes" because he interpreted the lesion as a malignant sarcoma. *Phyllodes* means leaflike and is an apt description of the pattern of stromal growth. There are often clefts like distorted cystic spaces between the leaflike stromal growths, accounting for the *cysto* portion of the name. The term cystosarcoma phyllodes, which implies malignancy in all cases, has now been replaced with the term *phyllodes tumor*, which appropriately does not de-

finitively indicate whether the lesion is benign or malignant. In the past, these lesions have incorrectly been called giant fibroadenomas. That term should be abandoned. A giant fibroadenoma is a large, often juvenile, fibroadenoma that should not be confused with a phyllodes tumor.

Phyllodes tumors may be either benign or malignant. According to the literature, roughly two-thirds of phyllodes tumors are benign, and one-third are malignant. In our highly screened patient population, most phyllodes tumors are benign, probably because we are diagnosing them much earlier than in the past. However, even histologically benign phyllodes tumors may be locally aggressive and can recur locally if not completely resected. Larger lesions that occur in smaller breasts and phyllodes and in younger patients are more likely to be inadequately resected and to recur locally.

Phyllodes tumors are rare, constituting less than 1% of all breast tumors and about 2% to 3% of all fibroepithelial lesions. The peak incidence of phyllodes tumors is between ages 45 and 49 years, about 10 years later than the peak incidence of fibroadenomas, but phyllodes tumors can occasionally occur in teenagers. Phyllodes tumors are more common in women of Mexican descent, especially if born and raised in Mexico. This fact suggests an environmental influence on phyllodes tumor growth in addition to a familial tendency for phyllodes tumor formation. Latin American women with phyllodes tumors also tend to be diagnosed at an earlier age than are other women.

According to the literature, about 80% of patients with phyllodes tumors present with a palpable mass, and about 20% are detected during routine mammographic breast cancer screening. However, in our highly screened patient population, the percentage of mammographically detected phyllodes tumors is much higher. For palpable phyllodes tumors, there is often a history of rapid enlargement over a short period of time after initial detection. This behavior is compatible with relatively rapid estimated doubling times, in certain cases being more rapid than those of breast carcinomas. The doubling time has been estimated at 116 days for benign phyllodes tumors and 36 days for malignant phyllodes tumors. Patients with very large and rapidly growing lesions may have markedly prominent veins visible within the skin lying over the lesion because of the marked vascularity of such lesions. Such rapidly growing lesions have a tendency to undergo internal cystic necrosis or hemorrhage and may even develop ulceration of the skin overlying the lesion. Because of the marked vascularity of such lesions, necrosis is often accompanied by hemorrhage into the tumor. Internal hemorrhage probably accounts for the very rapid enlargement over a few days reported in certain lesions.

Malignant phyllodes tumors rarely metastasize through the lymphatic system to axillary lymph nodes. Like other sarcomas, these malignancies are more prone to hematogenous spread to lungs, liver, and other distant locations.

At gross pathology, phyllodes tumors may be quite large—up to 15 cm. Phyllodes tumors usually present as a discrete mass that is lobulated and can be either soft or hard, depending on the degree of cystic degeneration and hemorrhage. Grossly infiltrating malignant phyllodes tumors may be fixed to surrounding tissues and are also more likely to show extensive necrosis and hemorrhage. When the lesion is incised, the internal structure reveals the leaflike polypoid structure and concave clefts that histologically characterize phyllodes tumors.

Histologically, phyllodes tumors, like fibroadenomas, are composed of a mixture of stromal and epithelial elements, but stroma of phyllodes tumors is far more cellular than the stroma of most fibroadenomas. Although the stromal proliferation is the dominant histologic feature, the presence of epithelial elements is necessary for the stromal overgrowth to occur. The epithelium exerts a field effect that potentiates stromal overgrowth. Certain phyllodes tumors may arise from preexisting fibroadenomas, but this concept is difficult to prove conclusively. Origin of a phyllodes tumor within a preexisting hamartoma has been documented, but hamartomas are unlikely to be very common sites of origins for phyllodes tumors. Most phyllodes tumors probably arise *de novo*. The histology of phyllodes tumors is similar to that of an exaggerated intracanalicular fibroadenoma. The overgrown stromal elements form polypoid leaflike structures (from which the term phyllodes is derived) that indent cystlike spaces. The stroma is markedly hypercellular, especially in the areas surrounding the ducts, owing to the potentiating field effect of the duct epithelium on the surrounding stroma. The margins of benign phyllodes tumors are pushing rather than infiltrating, thus creating a pseudocapsule of compressed breast tissue in the periphery of the lesion that is similar to that seen surrounding fibroadenomas. Malignant phyllodes tumors have frankly infiltrating borders similar to those seen in breast carcinomas. Occasionally, epithelial elements may become hyperplastic, but the epithelial hyperplasia rarely progresses to carcinoma. Carcinomatous epithelial change is likely rare because the rapid growth of the phyllodes tumor causes the lesion to be discovered and undergo resection before such epithelial degenerative change can occur.

Malignant phyllodes tumors have the potential to metastasize distantly through the bloodstream and to kill the patient, but benign phyllodes tumors are unlikely to kill the patient. Therefore, great effort has been made in attempting to distinguish between malignant and benign phyllodes tumors based on imaging and histologic characteristics. Unfortunately, distinguishing benign from malignant phyllodes tumors by either mammographic or sonographic criteria has been difficult and unsuccessful in series of phyllodes tumors that have been reported in the literature. In fact, distinguishing between benign and malignant phyllodes tumors histologically is even difficult. No single cytologic or histologic feature enables the pathologist to distinguish benign from malignant phyllodes tumor conclusively. The difficulty is accentuated by the commonly pronounced variation in histology from one part of the lesion to another. This problem is so difficult, in fact, that the recommendation has been made that phyllodes tumors be classified into three groups—benign, borderline malignant, and frankly malignant—rather than just benign and malignant. Others have argued against the borderline classification. A panel of histologic findings is usually relied on to characterize phyllodes tumors as either benign or malignant. Benign lesions have (a) clearly defined margins, (b) absence of marked cytologic atypia, and (c) fewer than 5 mitoses per high-power field. On the other hand, malignant phyllodes tumors have (a) microscopically invasive margins, (b) marked cytologic atypia of the hyperplastic stromal cells, (c) more than 5 mitoses per high-power field, and (d) marked stromal overgrowth with few epithelial elements. Unfortunately, even histologic classification using multiple features is not perfect. Lesions that have been classified histologically as benign have been documented to metastasize and kill. The presence of necrosis is considered to be a secondary finding suggestive of malignant change. Malignant change, when present, occurs within the hyperplastic stromal cells, resulting in sarcomatous lesions; fibrosarcoma, liposarcoma, and rhabdomyosarcoma are the most likely.

Histologically, the diagnosis of phyllodes tumor is usually not as difficult as the distinction between benign and malignant phyllodes tumors. However, occasionally the histologic diagnosis of phyllodes tumor can be difficult, usually with small specimens, such as those obtained by 14-gauge core needle biopsy. The lesions most often confused with phyllodes tumor are intracanalicular fibroadenoma with highly cellular stroma and carcinoma with sarcomatous metaplasia (also called *carcinosarcoma* or *metaplastic carcinoma*).

Because of the propensity to recur locally, the treatment of phyllodes tumor is wide excision. However, adequate excision will vary with the size of the lesion and the size of the breast in which the lesion develops and with whether or not the lesion is malignant. In cases in which the lesion is small, a lumpectomy with a 1-cm margin may be adequate. In lesions that are 3 cm or larger, a segmentectomy may be necessary. In very large lesions and in those that are histologically infiltrating or frankly malignant, mastectomy may be the best choice. Because the distant spread of malignant phyllodes tumor is hematogenous rather than through the lymphatic system, axillary dissection is unlikely to be helpful and in most cases is unnecessary.

Mammographic Findings

Most phyllodes tumors appear as circumscribed, lobulated, high-density masses. Calcifications are not common but, when present, are often quite large and coarse. The mammographic findings of benign phyllodes tumors are nonspecific and are similar to those seen in large cysts, fibroadenomas, and even circumscribed carcinomas. Malignant phyllodes tumors that have grossly invasive margins tend to appear ill defined or indistinct but usually are not frankly spiculated. However, a significant percentage of malignant phyllodes tumors have circumscribed rather than ill-defined borders mammographically. Thus, the gross appearance of the margins on mammography has not been a good predictor of benign versus malignant behavior of phyllodes tumors. The only mammographic feature that has been found to correlate with the presence of malignant phyllodes tumor is maximum diameter. Liberman and colleagues (1996) have found that phyllodes tumors with a maximum diameter of 3 cm or more are statistically significantly more likely to be malignant than those that are smaller than 3 cm.

Sonographic Findings

The sonographic appearance of phyllodes tumors accurately reflects their gross morphologic and histologic features. Phyllodes tumors are solid nodules or masses sonographically. In most cases, the margins are well circumscribed, and in most cases, there is even a complete, well-circumscribed, thin, echogenic external capsule that is demonstrable, reflecting the grossly circumscribed morphology of most phyllodes tumors (Fig. 15–10). Unfortunately, some malignant phyllodes tumors also have a sonographically demonstrable capsules, so that demonstration of a capsule does not enable us to distinguish completely between benign and malignant phyllodes tumors. However, many malignant phyllodes tumors do have angular or irregular margins and should be suspected of being malignant based on their margin characteristics (Fig. 15–11). Phyllodes tumors are usually mildly to moderately hypoechoic with surrounding fat and rarely have internal, sonographically visible calcifications. Phyllodes tumors rarely give rise to acoustic shadowing. Enhanced through-transmission is common and reflects the high stromal cellularity of phyllodes tumors and their lack of associated desmoplastic response (Fig. 15–12). The frequent presence of cystic necrosis probably also contributes to the enhanced through-transmission and may give rise to small cysts, 3 to 10 mm in diameter, that are demonstrable in slightly more than half of cases (Fig. 15–13). These cysts may be round but often appear flattened in the anteroposterior dimension at sonography. The flattened appearance reflects the slitlike nature of the cystic spaces that occur between the leaflike stromal proliferations occurring in phyllodes

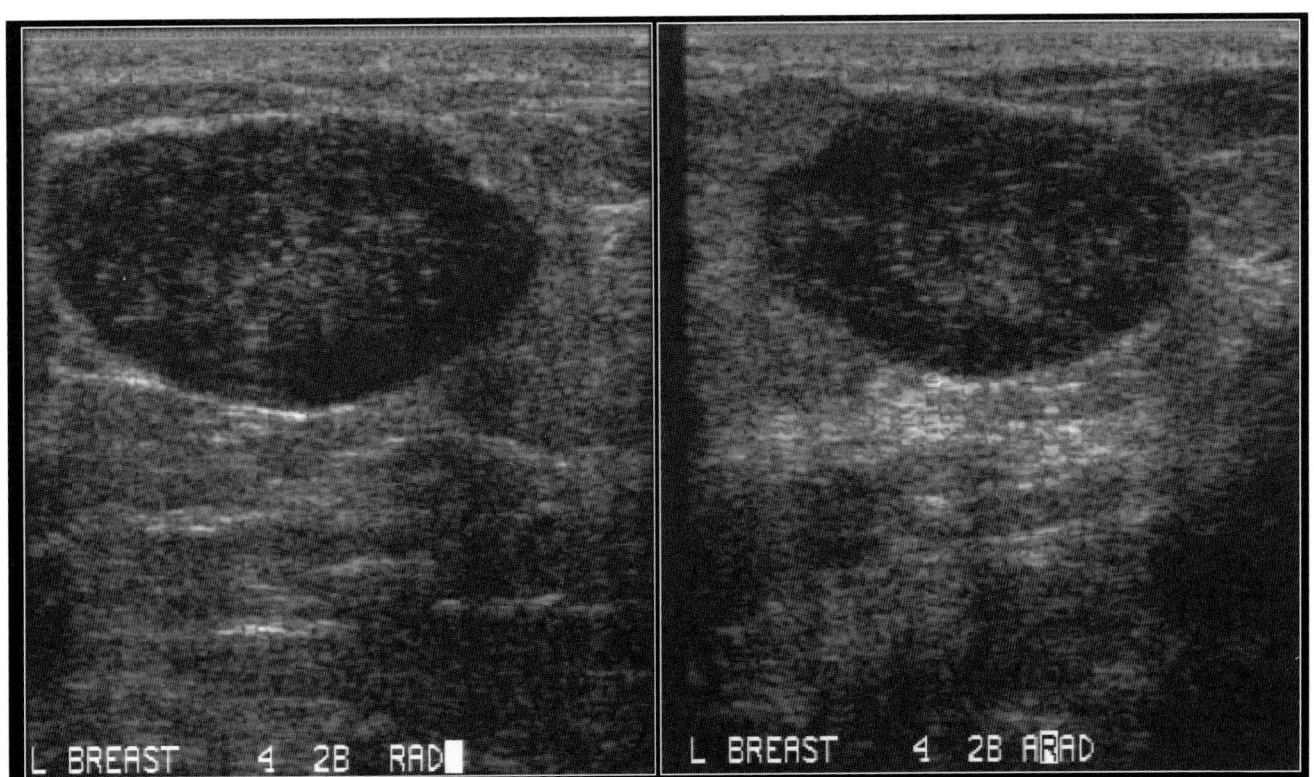

FIGURE 15–10 Most benign phyllodes tumors are well circumscribed and are completely encompassed by a thin, echogenic capsule, just as are most fibroadenomas. Most benign phyllodes tumors are mildly to moderately hypoechoic.

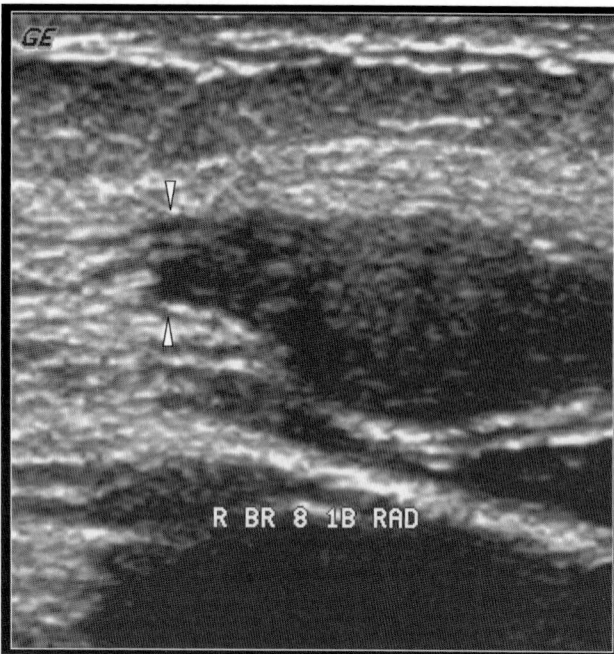

FIGURE 15–11 Malignant phyllodes tumors tend to have at least some margins that are ill defined, angular, or spiculated *(arrowheads)*.

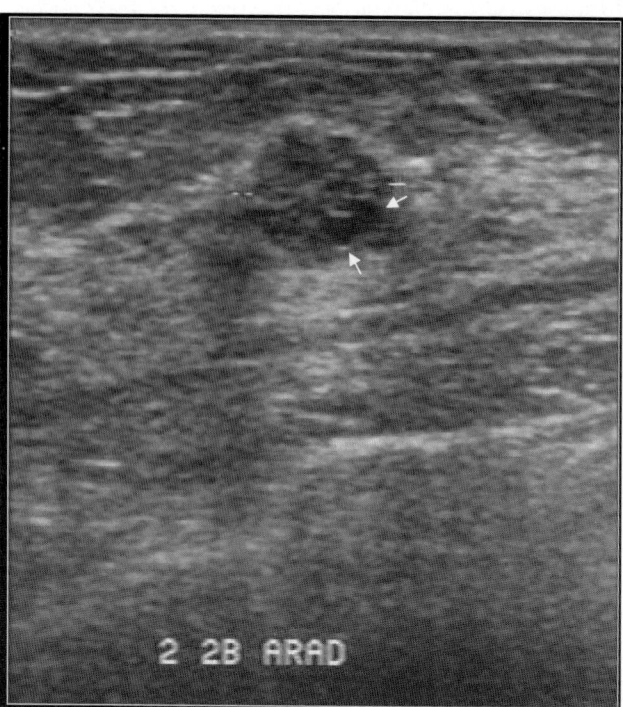

FIGURE 15–13 About one-half of all cases of benign phyllodes tumors have small cysts *(arrows)* 3 to 10 mm in diameter. These are round, but the cystic spaces are more typically flattened and slitlike.

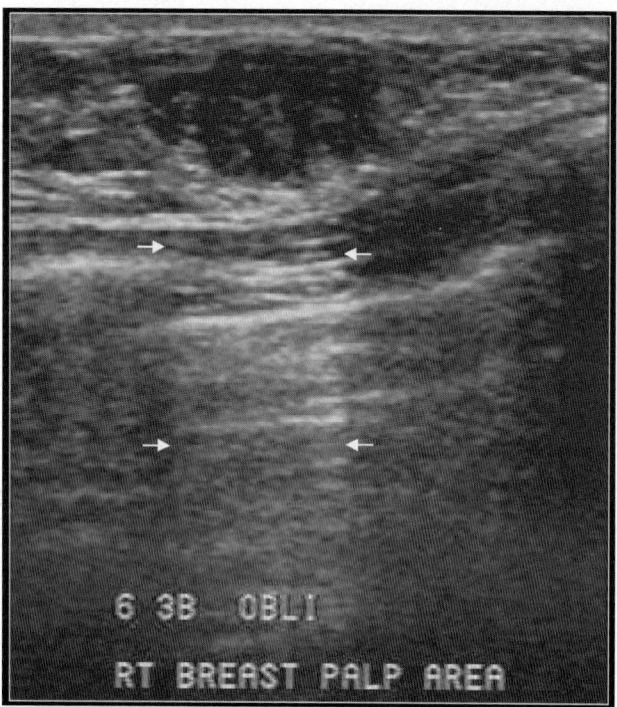

FIGURE 15–12 Most benign and malignant phyllodes tumors demonstrate enhanced through-transmission, primarily as the result of highly cellular stroma.

tumors. Although these slitlike spaces are oriented randomly in all directions within the lesions, only those spaces that are most nearly perpendicular to the beam, the horizontally oriented cystic slits, are well seen sonographically. The slits that are oriented more nearly parallel to the beam are poorly demonstrated. Because of this phenomenon, most phyllodes tumors appear to have horizontally oriented echogenic striations. When the slit is wide and the axial resolution of the transducer high, anechoic fluid can be demonstrated within the slit (Fig. 15–14). In most cases, the slit is too narrow, the axial resolution of the transducer is inadequate to demonstrate fluid, and the slit appears only as an echogenic line (Fig. 15–15). Horizontal striations, reflecting the presence of clefts that are oriented perpendicular to the ultrasound beam, are so characteristic of the internal echotexture of benign phyllodes tumors that we always raise the question of phyllodes tumor and recommend biopsy, even in patients whose solid nodules would otherwise be characterized as BIRADS 3 (Fig. 15–16). Certain intracanalicular fibroadenomas that have cellular stroma can also demonstrate internal horizontal linearity. This should not be surprising because these lesions are similar to phyllodes tumors morphologically and histologically. As is the case for mammographic masses, there is evidence that lesions larger than 3 cm in maximum

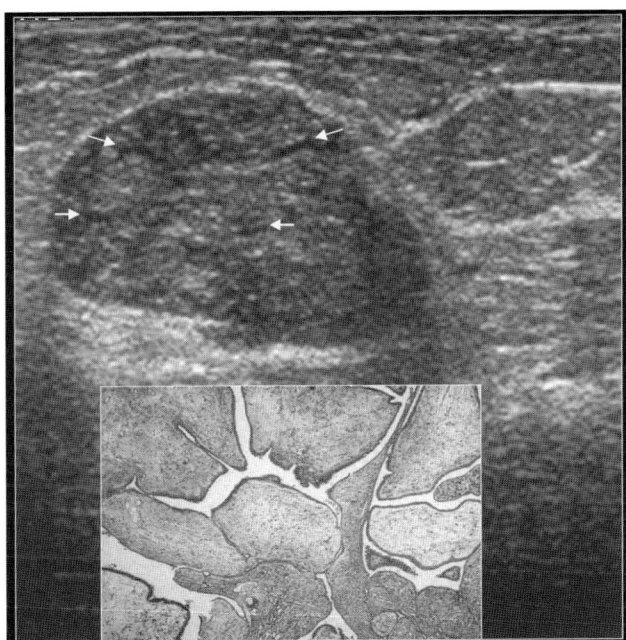

FIGURE 15–14 The cystic spaces within benign phyllodes tumors (PTs) are generally within slitlike clefts. These clefts are oriented in all directions randomly. However, because the axial resolution of the ultrasound beam is invariably better than lateral resolution, sonography tends to demonstrate well only the clefts that have their long axes oriented nearly perpendicular to the beam. This creates an internal echotexture in PTs that appears to have only horizontally oriented slits *(arrows)*.

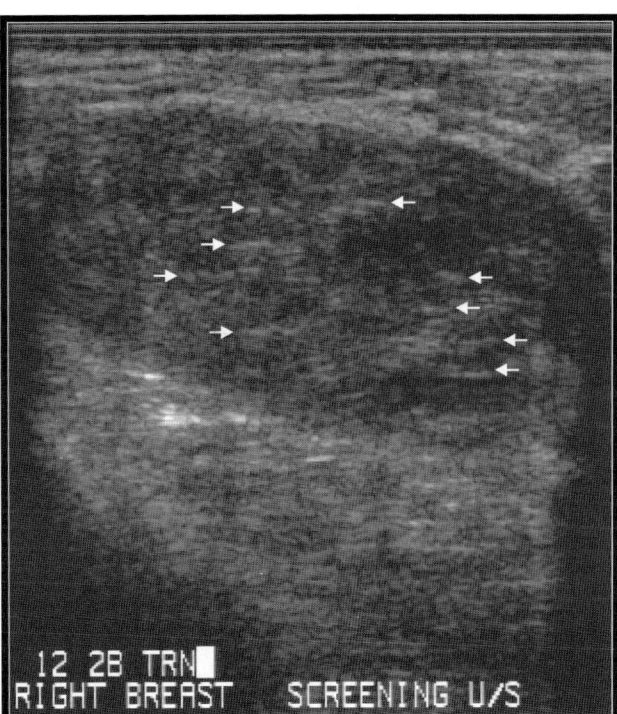

FIGURE 15–15 In most cases, the clefts within the phyllodes tumor are too narrow to resolve sonographically as fluid-filled slits, and show up merely as elongated linear echoes *(arrows)* that are oriented perpendicular to the beam. These horizontal striations can be seen in a small percentage of intracanalicular fibroadenomas but are quite characteristic of phyllodes tumors. Horizontal linear striations are the sonographic finding that we have found to be most useful in trying to distinguish phyllodes tumor from fibroadenoma.

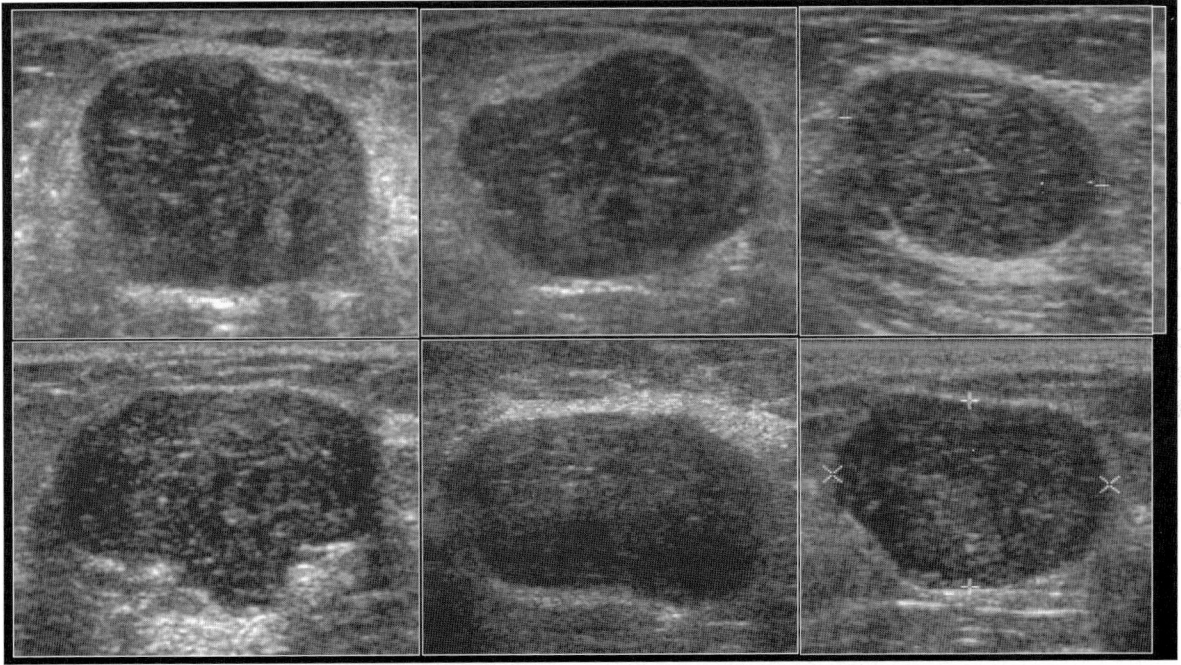

FIGURE 15–16 All six of these lesions are histologically proven benign phyllodes tumors (PTs), and all six demonstrate variable degrees of horizontally oriented linear echoes that reflect the presence of clefts that lie perpendicular to the ultrasound beam. Horizontal striations are so characteristic of the internal echotexture of benign PTs that their presence suggests that the lesion is a PT, not a fibroadenoma and warrant recommendation for biopsy, even when the nodule would otherwise be characterized as BIRADS 3. Horizontal striations can occasionally be seen in intracanalicular fibroadenomas that have cellular stroma, lesions that are similar to PTs morphologically and histologically.

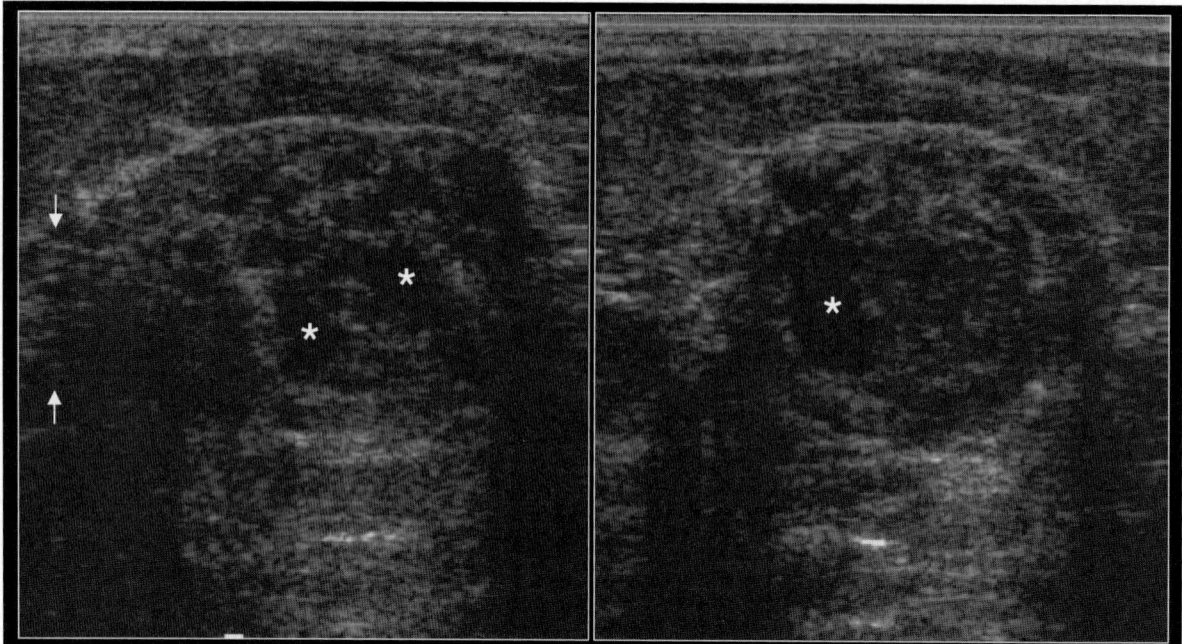

FIGURE 15–17 The larger the phyllodes tumor, the more likely it is to be malignant. Cystic spaces larger than 3 mm in maximum diameter *(*)* are also associated with increased risk for the phyllodes tumor being malignant. Note that the left border of this large (>3 cm) phyllodes tumor appears to be spiculated *(arrows)*.

diameter have a threefold to fourfold increased relative risk for malignancy. Lesions larger than 8 cm in maximum diameter are almost certainly malignant. Phyllodes tumors that contain cystic areas larger than 3 mm are also more likely to be malignant (Fig. 15–17). Such large cystic spaces correspond to areas of necrosis or hemorrhage histologically. Because histologic evidence of necrosis is more likely to be found in malignant lesions and is associated with higher local recurrence rate and increased risk for distant metastases, the sonographic finding of large cystic spaces within a solid nodule shown to be a phyllodes tumor at biopsy is similarly worrisome. Necrosis may lead to fibrous scarring as well as cystic change, and this can cause markedly coarse and heterogeneous echotexture throughout the lesion. Thus, markedly heterogeneous echotexture should also be considered suspicious for malignant phyllodes tumor (Fig. 15–18).

The sonographic differential diagnosis of phyllodes tumor varies with the morphologic and gross histologic composition of the lesion. Malignant phyllodes tumors with grossly infiltrating borders are relatively hypoechoic, often contain large cystic spaces, have angular margins, demonstrate enhanced through-transmission, and can appear similar to medullary carcinoma or high-grade invasive NOS carcinoma. Circumscribed elliptically shaped or lobulated phyllodes tumors can be indistinguishable from large fibroadenomas with cellular stroma or fibroadenomas with extensive myxoid change. Smaller, circumscribed

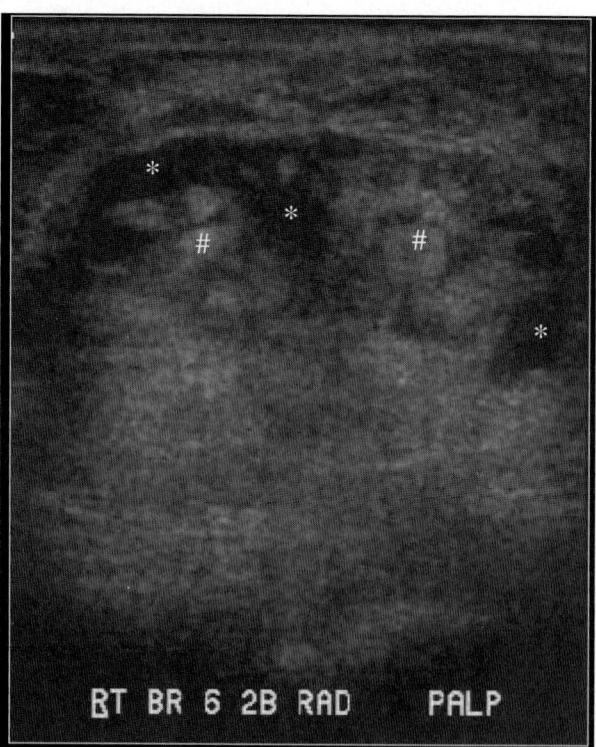

FIGURE 15–18 Internal echotexture that is markedly more heterogeneous than normal is highly correlated with extensive necrosis, a finding that has a strong associated with malignant phyllodes tumors. This large malignant phyllodes tumor with extensive necrosis shows areas of both cystic necrosis *(*)* and necrosis with hyperechoic fibrosis *(#)*.

phyllodes tumors with internal cysts can be difficult to distinguish from complex fibroadenomas that contain apocrine metaplasia and internal cysts. The cysts in phyllodes tumors are more likely to appear slitlike than those of complex fibroadenomas, presenting as horizontal striations rather than spherical or elliptical, as do the cystic spaces within complex fibroadenomas.

JUVENILE PAPILLOMATOSIS

General Pathologic Classification, Clinical Findings, and Epidemiology

Juvenile papillomatosis usually presents in the second or third decade of life as a discrete palpable lesion with clinical findings similar to those of a fibroadenoma. However, this lesion can occur as late as the fifth decade. The palpable abnormality is usually unilateral and unicentric but can be multicentric and bilateral.

The significance of juvenile papillomatosis as a risk marker for breast cancer development is controversial. There are investigators who believe the implications of juvenile papillomatosis are similar to those associated with ADH, with increased risk bilaterally. Others believe the lesion is premalignant. Still others believe that juvenile papillomatosis does not confer additional risk to the patient. In about 25% of patients with juvenile papillomatosis, there is a strong first-degree family history of breast cancer. It has been suggested that juvenile papillomatosis can represent an unusually early manifestation of genetic predisposition for breast cancer development, such as that associated with the presence of the *BRCA1* gene, but this relationship is not proved.

At gross pathology, there are often multiple cysts associated with various fibrocystic and proliferative changes. The gross appearance of multiple small cysts and intervening proliferative changes causes a gross focal breast appearance similar to that of Swiss cheese, leading to the term *Swiss cheese disease* to describe the gross appearance of this disease process.

Histologically, there are usually multiple small cysts associated with UDH of various degrees. In most cases, duct hyperplasia is florid and papillary. In about 10% of cases, the ductal hyperplasia is atypical, a finding associated with increased relative risk for cancer development. Fibrosis, papillary apocrine metaplasia, adenosis, sclerosing adenosis, and radial scars are often associated with juvenile papillomatosis. It is because of the relatively frequent presence of associated ADH that juvenile papillomatosis is considered a high-risk condition.

Mammographic Findings

Because juvenile papillomatosis often occurs in adolescents and women younger than 30 years of age, the patient may be evaluated with sonography first, without undergoing mammography. In those who do undergo mammography, the study is often negative because the dense breast tissue present in young women obscures the pathology. In cases in which mammography is performed and is not normal, the abnormalities are usually nonspecific, reflecting only the presence of small cysts or associated fibrocystic changes. Calcifications caused by sclerosing adenosis or architectural distortion due to a radial scar may be present.

Sonographic Findings

Juvenile papillomatosis is uncommon, and ultrasound descriptions of the disease are even less common. Because juvenile papillomatosis is a peripheral rather than a central form of florid duct hyperplasia, the disease does not have the typical appearance of central large duct papillomas. One reported lesion was described as an ill-defined solid mass with multiple small cystic spaces peripherally. We have seen only a few proven cases that accurately fit the description of Swiss cheese disease. In those cases, there were numerous small cysts involving the periphery of a single lobe (Fig. 15–19). The individual cysts were

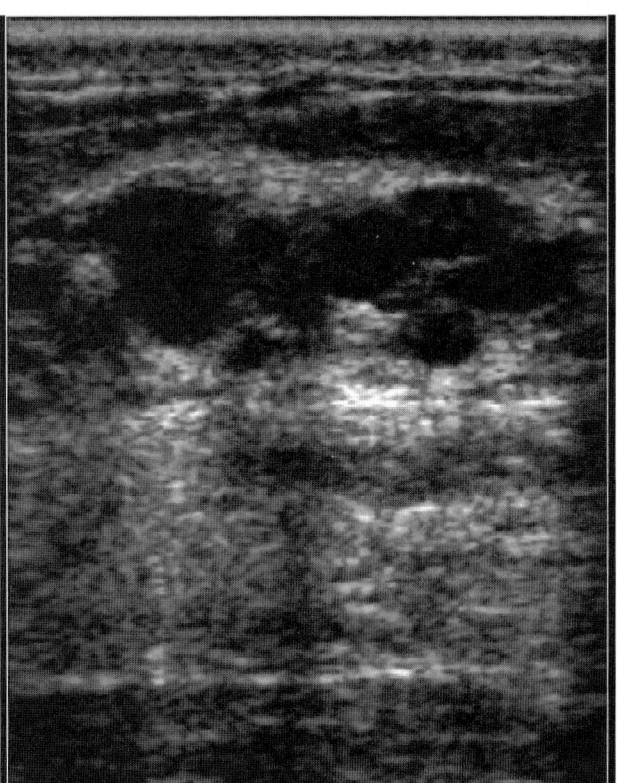

FIGURE 15–19 Clusters of cysts with proliferative changes creating isoechoic thickening between cysts in juvenile papillomatosis give the appearance of Swiss cheese.

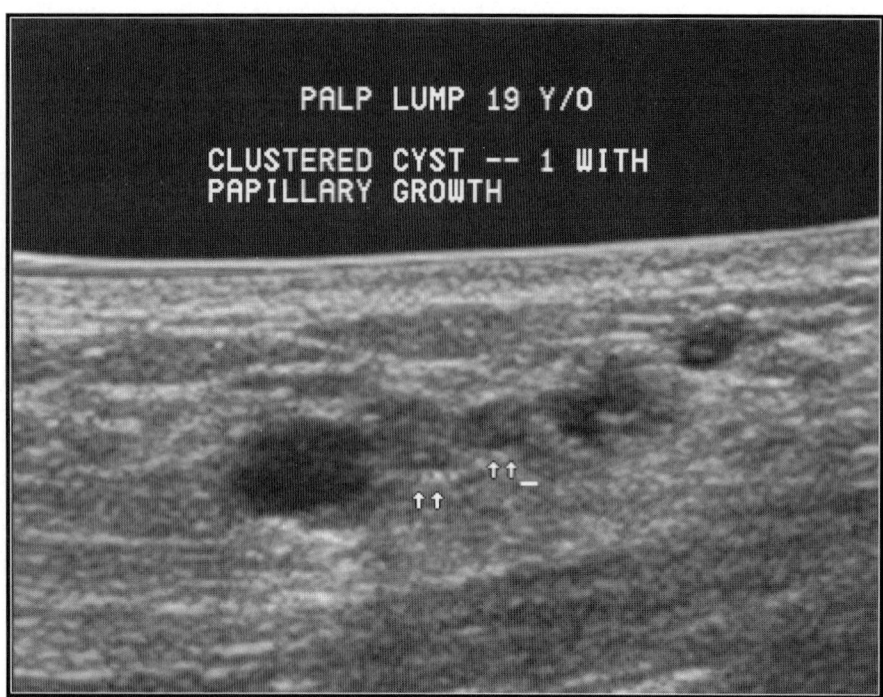

FIGURE 15–20 This cluster of cysts in a 19-year-old with juvenile papillomatosis contains some simple and some complex cysts. The echogenic material within the complex cysts (*arrows*) was caused by a mixture of papillary apocrine metaplasia and florid duct hyperplasia. There was no atypia.

too small to be palpable, but the cluster of cysts and the associated hyperplastic elements caused the palpable abnormality that precipitated the workup. Because of the numerous small cysts, the palpable lumps had a coarse, granular feeling. Some of the numerous small cysts are simple, but many are complex, containing papillary excrescences representing PDH in certain cases and papillary apocrine metaplasia in others (Fig. 15–20). The appearance of clusters of cystic lesions in a patient older than 30 years of age would not be at all suspicious for juvenile papillomatosis. In fact, fibrocystic change commonly has this sonographic appearance. It is the occurrence of clusters of simple and complex cysts in a patient younger than 30 years of age that should raise suspicion. Although fibroadenomas commonly occur in patients younger than 30 years of age, cysts are much less common in this age group. In certain cases, the solid components are so dominant that the palpable abnormality appears to be solid and that only microcysts, some containing calcifications, can be seen (Fig. 15–21). In other cases, benign proliferative changes progress to ADH with or without the presence of an associated radial scar. Although such lesions generally have more solid components and less cystic change, an absolute distinction between cases of juvenile papillomatosis that contain atypia and cases that do not is not possible sonographically (Fig. 15–22).

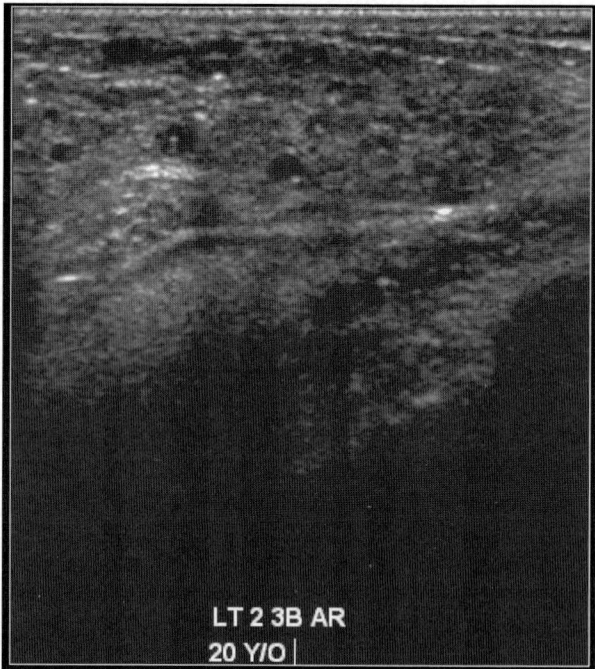

FIGURE 15–21 This 21-year-old patient presented with a palpable lump that sonography showed corresponded to focally prominent glandular tissue containing cysts. Many of the cysts contain milk of calcium. Biopsy showed the entire spectrum of fibrocystic and benign proliferative changes, including florid duct hyperplasia, papillary apocrine metaplasia, cysts, and sclerosing adenosis. The calcifications occurred both within cysts and in areas of sclerosing adenosis.

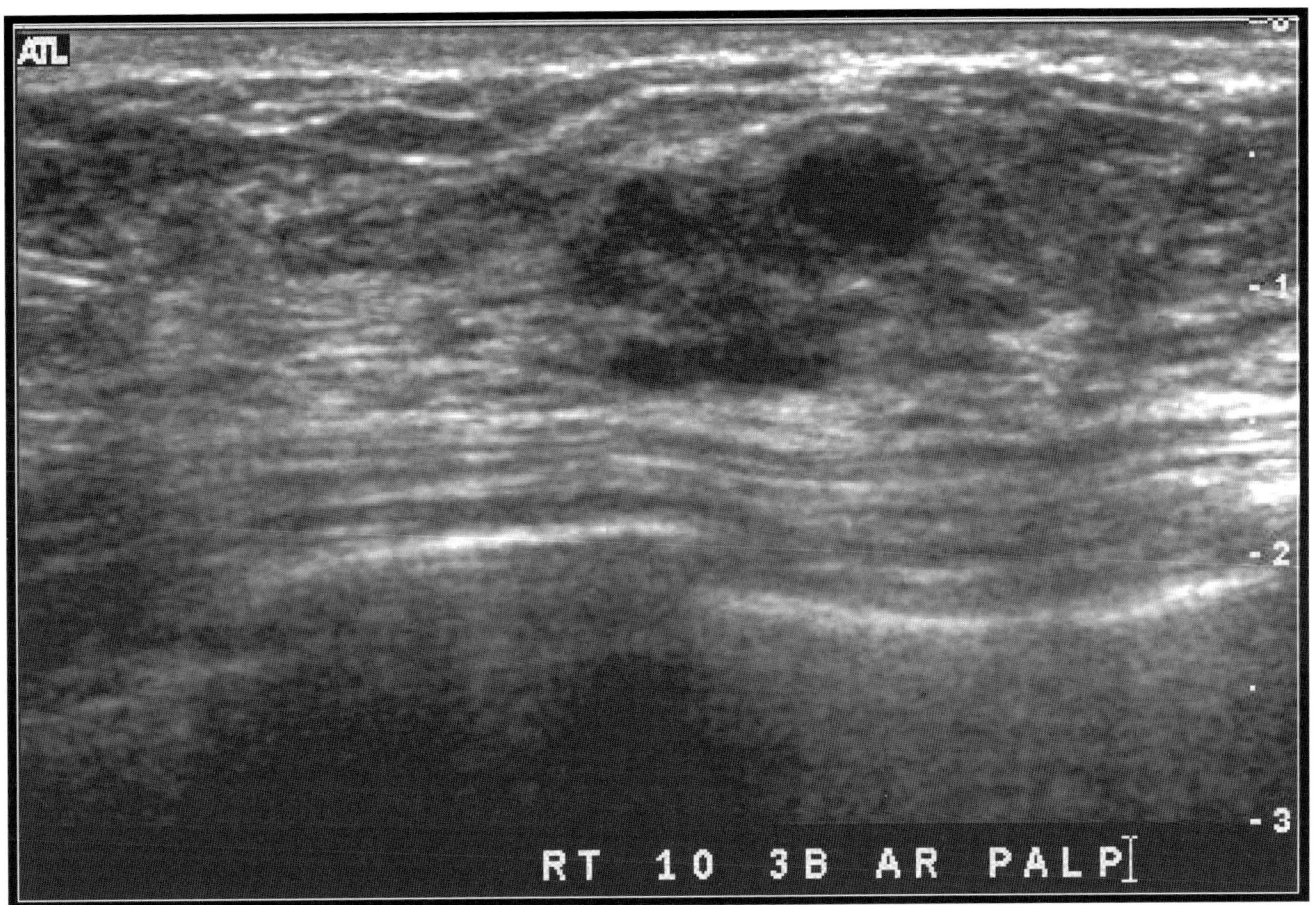

FIGURE 15–22 This 19-year-old patient presented with a palpable lump. Sonography showed a microlobulated mixed cystic and solid nodule that at biopsy was shown to be juvenile papillomatosis. The microlobulated structures corresponded to foci of papillary duct hyperplasia and papillary apocrine metaplasia developing within a radial scar. Some of the papillary duct hyperplasia was atypical. This is an example of juvenile papillomatosis that is associated with a radial scar and in which atypical duct hyperplasia had developed.

RADIAL SCARS AND COMPLEX SCLEROSING LESIONS

General Pathologic Findings, Clinical Findings, and Epidemiology

Radial scars, like other lesions discussed in this chapter, are controversial. Radial scars and complex sclerosing lesions of the breast are significant because they simulate spiculated breast carcinomas on gross pathologic examination and on mammograms (primarily tubular carcinoma). However, these lesions are also significant because they may either be premalignant or have a high association with atypia or low-nuclear-grade DCIS. Many different terms have been used to describe these lesions, including *sclerosing papillomatosis, sclerosing papillary proliferation, infiltrating epitheliosis, nonencapsulated sclerosing lesion, indicative mastopathy, obliterative mastopathy scleroelastic lesion, complex compound heteromorphic lesion, benign sclerosing ductal proliferation,* and *radial sclerosing lesion.* There are pathologists who term such

lesions less than 1 cm in diameter as radial scars and those lesions 1 cm and greater as complex sclerosing lesions. Radial scars are so small that they are often found as incidental findings in biopsy specimens obtained for other reasons. As a practical matter, lesions large enough to be imaged should probably more appropriately termed complex sclerosing lesions. Most, however, do not distinguish between radial scars and complex sclerosing lesions, considering them all to be radial scars, regardless of size.

Radial scars are relatively common. Depending on the thoroughness of histologic sampling of mastectomy specimens, small radial scars less than 1 cm in diameter can be found in 2% to 28% of patients. Most of these lesions are too small to be mammographically visible. Radial scars are often multifocal and bilateral. When multiple, these lesions are frequently asymmetrically distributed and vary in their stages of development.

Most small radial scars are incidental findings at pathologic examination. Larger lesions, which may be several centimeters in maximum diameter, are more often detected as spiculated lesions on screening mammograms. Despite the apparent large size, only a small percentage of radial scars or complex sclerosing lesions are palpable.

Radial scars have two different appearances on gross pathologic examination: a frankly spiculated lesion or a "puckered" nodule. These two appearances are thought to represent opposite ends of the temporal spectrum. The puckered nodular appearance, much like that of a drawn pursestring, is thought to represent an early phase of the lesion in which the peripheral parenchymal proliferative processes, adenosis, and duct hyperplasia predominate. The spiculated lesions are thought to represent a later stage of the disease, in which the central elastosis predominates, but the surrounding proliferative processes have regressed. The elastosis tends to have a yellowish or whitish chalky appearance.

On microscopic examination, radial scars are composed of a central core of fibrosis and elastosis surrounded by proliferating ducts and lobules arranged in a radiating or spiculated fashion. There are bands of elastotic tissue that radiate out from the central core and pull the proliferating ducts and lobules toward the center of the lesion, resulting in the radiating orientation. Within the central elastosis, ducts are distorted and compressed. In the periphery, there are alternating bands of fibroelastosis and parenchyma. The peripheral bands of elastosis pull the parenchymal elements toward the central scar, creating the puckered appearance. The parenchyma is involved by various proliferative and sclerotic processes, including adenosis, sclerosing adenosis, PDH, apocrine metaplasia, and cyst formation. In certain cases, cyst formation with or without papillary apocrine metaplasia in the periphery is the dominant feature. PDH may progress to frank papilloma formation. In a few cases, there are abundant inflammatory cells surrounding the parenchymal elements. In almost half of cases, the peripheral parenchymal components are involved by a sclerosing process, such as sclerosing adenosis or sclerosing duct hyperplasia.

The etiology of radial scars is unknown. Certain investigators believe that radial scars originate from focal areas of inflammation, but others believe that radial scars are the culmination of burned-out sclerosing proliferative processes.

Both the central and peripheral processes of radial scars may simulate malignant processes on histologic examination. The compressed distorted ducts within the central area of elastosis may simulate tubular carcinoma. The PDH in the periphery of the lesion may be difficult to distinguish from low-nuclear-grade DCIS in certain cases. The presence of myoepithelial and epithelial layers and the presence of a basement membrane in radial scars should distinguish the lesions from tubular carcinoma, which lacks a myoepithelial layer.

The significance of radial scars is controversial. There is literature reporting that radial scars are direct precursors to tubular carcinomas. Other investigators believe that radial scars, like ADH and LCIS, are nonspecific indicators of increased risk for cancer development, both ipsilaterally and contralaterally. Tabar and colleagues report a 10% to 30% risk for associated ADH, low-nuclear-grade DCIS, or tubular carcinoma in association with radial scars. However, there are also researchers who report that radial scars are simple, straightforward, benign processes that are significant only because they simulate spiculated malignancies mammographically and on gross pathologic examination.

Even the recommended method for biopsy of suspected radial scars is controversial. Because early atypical or malignant changes may involve only a small part of the lesion, and because neither mammography nor sonography is able to help us determine in which part of the lesion the early atypical or malignant change is developing, some have recommended against using random sampling biopsy techniques such as core needle biopsy. Core biopsy may miss the areas containing atypia or DCIS, resulting in false-negative diagnoses. These physicians also point out that core biopsy may lead to false-positive diagnoses because confusion between the histology of tubular carcinoma and radial scars may be greater in the smaller the core specimens compared with excisional lumpectomy samples. Therefore, these investigators recommend that all lesions suspected of being radial scars be completely surgically excised. Others, primarily those who believe that radial scars are strictly benign sclerosing processes, believe that large core needle biopsy (14 gauge) is adequate to establish definitively the diagnosis of radial scars, to exclude malignancy, and to avoid a false-positive diagnosis of tubular carcinoma. A compromise viewpoint is that 14-gauge core needle biopsy of radial scars is inadequate but that 11-gauge DVAB can remove most or all of the lesion, allow complete histologic evaluation of all tissues removed and therefore minimize both the underdiagnosis of atypical carcinoma or DCIS and the false positive diagnosis of tubular carcinoma. This viewpoint has recently been further refined, based on the size of the lesion. If the radial scar is small and all imaging evidence of the lesion is removed using 11-gauge DVAB, it has been suggested that excision is not necessary. If the lesion is large and imaging suggests that part of the lesion remains after 11-gauge DVAB, then excision is necessary. Although this refined, compromise viewpoint seems compelling to some, others still believe that complete excision is the only rational method of dealing with radial scars.

Mammographic Findings

Most radial scars are detected as incidental nonpalpable spiculated lesions on screening mammography that simulate spiculated breast carcinomas such as tubular carcinoma (Fig. 15–23).

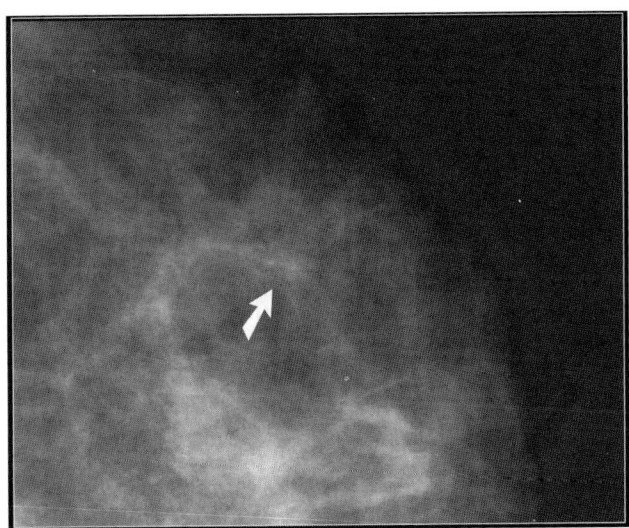

FIGURE 15–23 This small radial scar forms a spiculated lesion that has a radiopaque center rather than a fatty center. This makes the lesion mammographically indistinguishable from a small spiculated malignancy such as tubular carcinoma.

There are several subtle differences between the mammographic appearances of radial scars and breast carcinomas, but there is enough overlap that an absolute distinction between the two is not possible by mammography alone. First, radial scars often have a degree of fat density within the central nidus (black star), whereas spiculated carcinomas usually have a high-density central nidus (white star) that does not contain fat density. However, a few radial scars can present with high-density centers, and more important, certain spiculated malignant nodules can contain fat density within the central nidus. Second, the spiculations in radial scars are often very long in comparison to the size of the central nidus, are gently curved, are thicker than malignant spiculations, and contain alternating fat and water-density components. The spiculations around carcinomas are usually straight, thin, high-density structures that are proportionate in length to the size of the central nidus. Unlike the spiculations in radial scars, malignant spiculations do not contain bands of alternating fat and water density. However, some radial scars have short, straight spiculations, and some malignant lesions have curving spiculations with alternating fat and water density.

Clinical findings can be helpful, but unfortunately, there is also overlap in the clinical features of radial scars and tubular carcinoma. Spiculated malignancies larger than 1 cm are frequently palpable, whereas radial scars much larger than 1 cm seldom are palpable. However, in one reported series of complex sclerosing lesions, 25% of the lesions were palpable.

The presence of calcifications is more frequently associated with spiculated malignant nodules than with radial scars but can be seen in both. Spiculated invasive malignancies often contain both central and peripheral calcifications, whereas radial scars contain peripheral calcifications within areas of associated sclerosing adenosis.

Although the mammographic differences are definitive enough to allow distinction between radial scars and spiculated malignancy in some cases, overlap causes errors in many others. Errors in distinction occur often enough that biopsy and histologic confirmation are always necessary, even when mammographic findings strongly favor radial scars over spiculated breast carcinoma.

Sonographic Findings

Because most radial scars are detected as incidental findings on mammograms, and because they usually require evaluation with additional mammographic views and stereotactically guided biopsy, most radial scars are never evaluated sonographically. However, sonography can be useful in guiding needle localization or 11-gauge DVAB for excisional biopsy in these cases; thus, many radial scars are evaluated with ultrasound for purposes of preoperative surgical localization or for guiding 11-gauge DVAB. Additionally, radial scars that do not have classic mammographic findings or that are palpable may be evaluated sonographically rather than mammographically.

Unfortunately, like the mammographic findings, the sonographic findings of radial scars are not definitive or specific enough to allow absolute distinction between radial scar and spiculated malignant nodules. The sonographic findings caused by radial scars depend on the amount of peripheral proliferative change present. Radial scars that are dominated by the central fibroelastosis and in which the peripheral proliferative changes have regressed are difficult to identify and may even be missed by sonography. On the other hand, lesions in which the peripheral proliferative changes dominate are easier to identify and are less often missed sonographically. These lesions correspond to the puckered nodule gross morphologic appearance discussed earlier.

The sonographic appearance of small radial scars in which the peripheral proliferative elements have largely regressed, leaving only the central fibroelastosis, varies with the echogenicity of the tissue within which the lesion lies. Small, fat-surrounded, spiculated radial scars appear to be small isoechoic to mildly hypoechoic solid nodules with angular margins that are either frankly spiculated or encompassed within a thick, echogenic halo. The thick, echogenic halo represents unresolved spiculations and is thickest and best seen along the edges of the lesion, where the spicules are perpendicular to the beam, an appearance identical to small spiculated malignant nodules (Fig. 15–23). When surrounded by intensely echogenic fibrous tissue, very small radial scars in which central fibroelastosis predominates can actually appear

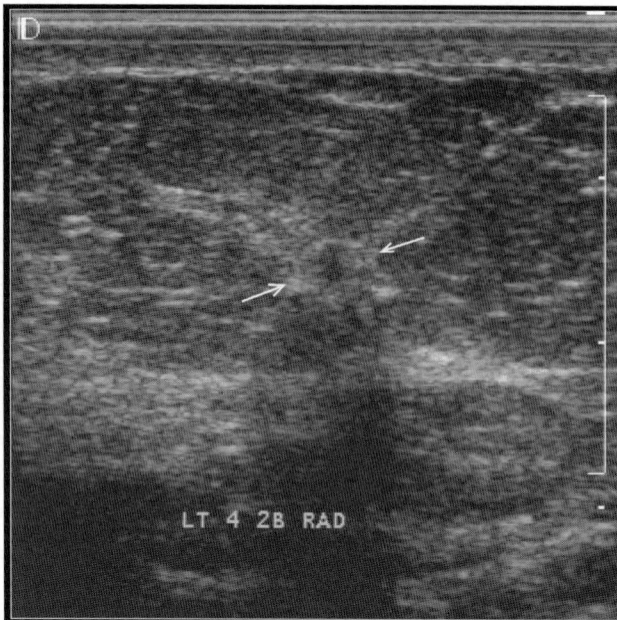

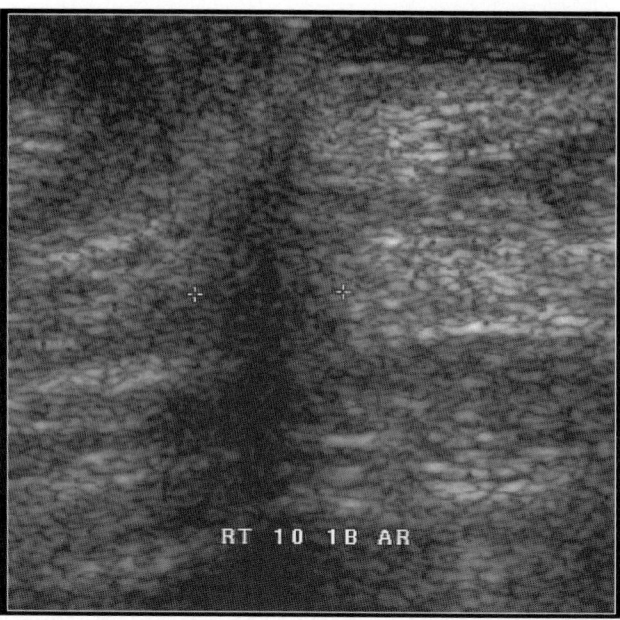

FIGURE 15–24 Larger, fat-surrounded, spiculated radial scars in which the peripheral proliferative elements have regressed and only the central fibroelastotic scar remains appear to form iso-echoic to mildly hypoechoic solid nodules that have angular margins and are either frankly spiculated or encompassed by a thick, echogenic halo *(arrows)*. The appearance is indistinguishable from that of small low-grade invasive not otherwise specified or tubular carcinomas. The mammogram of this radial scar is shown in Figure 15–23.

FIGURE 15–26 Spiculated radial scars in which the peripheral proliferative elements have regressed and only the central fibroelastotic scar remains, whether surrounded by fat or fibrous tissue, often cast mild to moderate acoustic shadows.

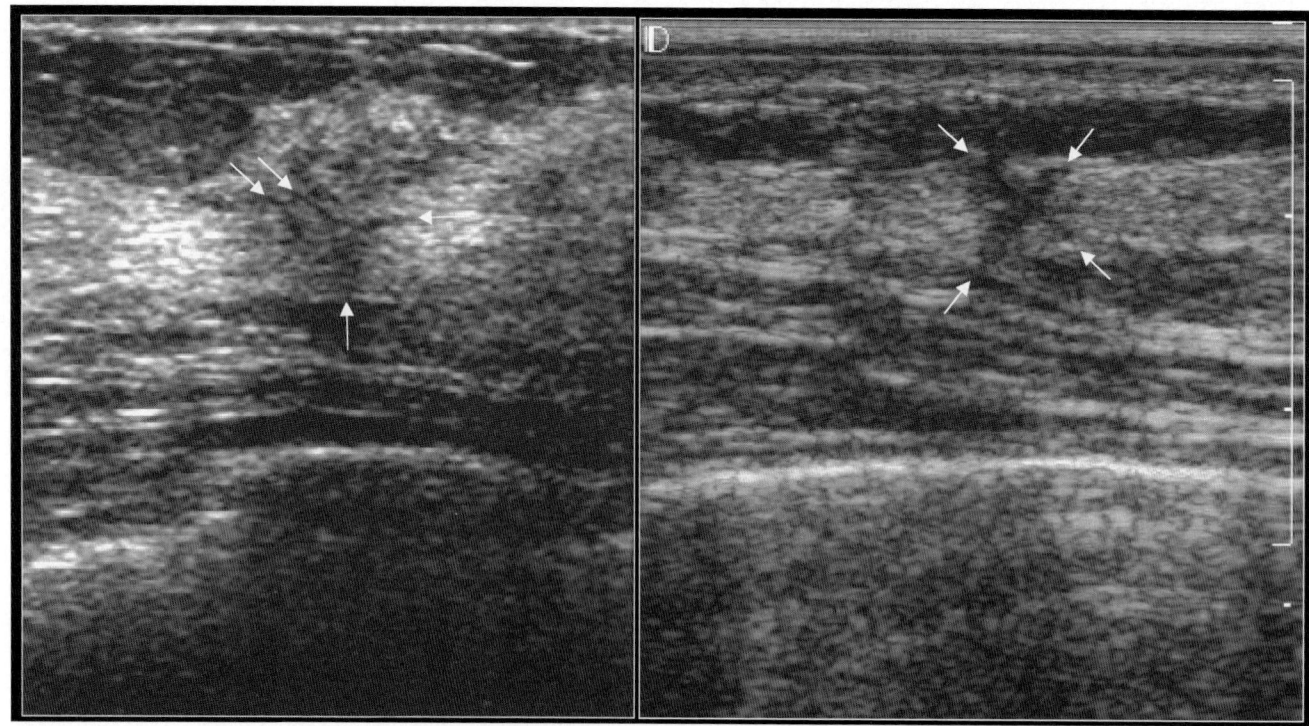

FIGURE 15–25 Spiculated radial scars in which the peripheral proliferative elements have regressed and only the central fibroelastotic scar remains, when surrounded by hyperechoic fibrous tissue, appear to by hypoechoic stellate lesions *(arrows)*. These lesions are very small- **(left)** and medium-sized **(right)** radial scars that are surrounded by hyperechoic fibrous tissue.

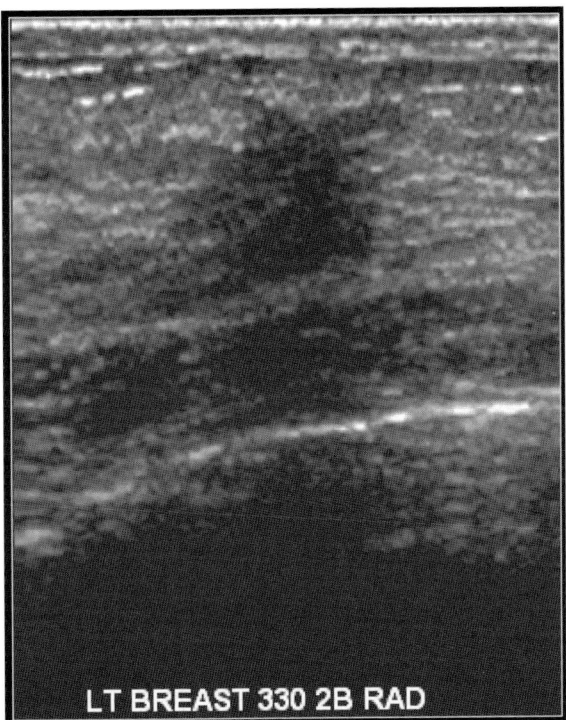

FIGURE 15–27 "Puckered" radial scars in which the peripheral proliferative elements are more pronounced than is the central fibroelastotic scar appear to be isoechoic to hypoechoic solid nodules that are microlobulated and have angular margins. Unlike the spiculated form of radial scars, frank spiculations, thick, echogenic halos, and acoustic shadowing are usually absent from puckered lesions.

hypoechoic when not surrounded by abundant proliferative changes (Fig. 15–24). The central fibroelastosis may appear mildly hypoechoic, angular, or spiculated (Fig. 15–25). The spiculated form of radial scars often causes faint to moderate acoustic shadowing (Fig. 15–26). Spiculated radial scars in which peripheral proliferative elements have regressed are never palpable.

The appearance of a radial scar in which the peripheral proliferative changes predominate, lesions that correspond to the puckered gross pathologic appearance, differs greatly from that of the spiculated form of radial scars. Puckered radial scars isoechoic solid nodules that are mildly hypoechoic to isoechoic, have angular margins, may be spiculated, and usually transmit sound as well as or better than normal tissue (Fig. 15–27). This appearance is similar to that of intermediate-grade invasive NOS carcinomas. Because of the abundant hyperplastic and proliferative change in the periphery of such lesions, acoustic shadowing is less common than it is for the spiculated variety of radial scars in which proliferative change has regressed. In some cases, the central fibroelastotic scar causes a central focus of hyperechogenicity within the solid nodule, similar to the central fibrotic scar seen in some intermediate-grade invasive NOS carcinomas (Fig. 15–28). The proliferative changes in puckered radial scars are most pronounced during times when lobular proliferation normal occurs (i.e., during pregnancy, lactation, the late teens, and early 20s)

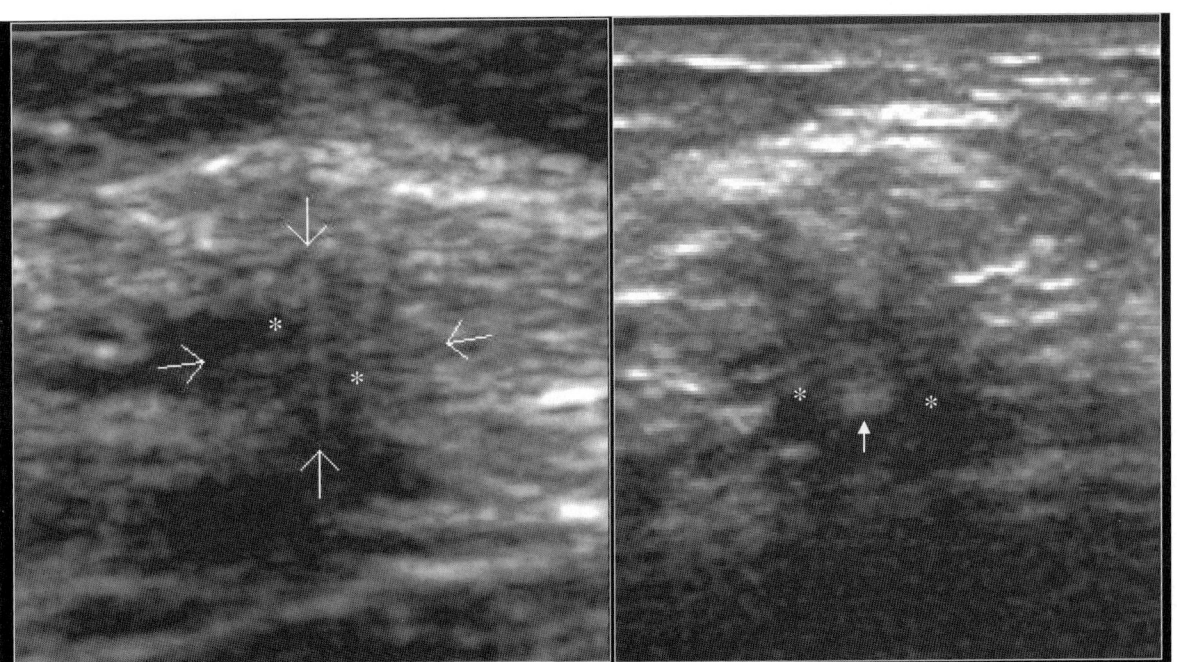

FIGURE 15–28 In some cases of the puckered form of radial scar, there is a bright echo within the center of the solid nodule. The hypoechoic components *(*)* of the nodule represent the peripheral proliferative elements, and the hyperechoic central focus *(arrows)* represents the fibroelastotic scar. The radial scar shown on the left is very small, has very little peripheral proliferative change, and has a very small central scar (fibroelastosis). The radial scar shown on the right is larger, has more peripheral proliferative change, and has a larger central scar.

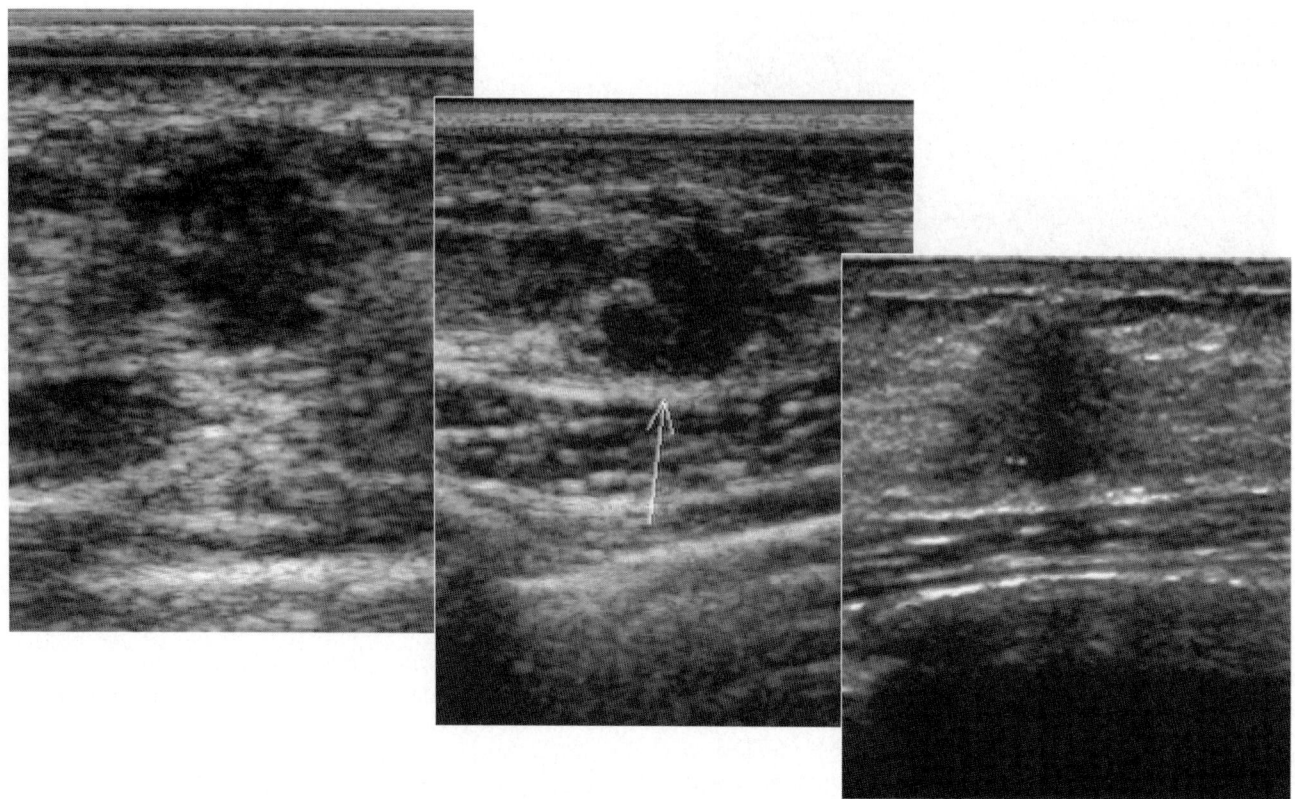

FIGURE 15–29 During times of life when lobular proliferation and stimulation are the greatest, the peripheral proliferative changes dominate the sonographic appearance, and radial scars invariably take the puckered solid nodule form. The radial scar on the **left** occurred during pregnancy, the radial scar in the **middle** occurred during lactation, and the radial scar on the **right** occurred during the late teens, all times of rapid lobular proliferation. Note that the markedly stimulated radial scars during pregnancy and lactation (**left** and **middle**) demonstrate enhanced sound transmission.

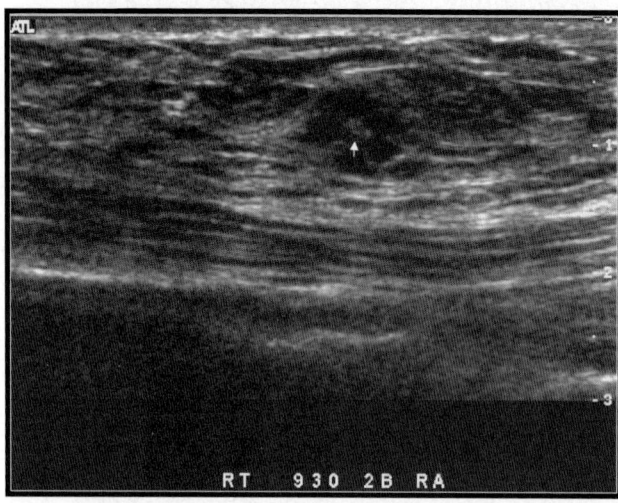

FIGURE 15–30 In the puckered form of radial scars, when fibrocystic change with apocrine metaplasia is the dominant proliferative change, multiple small cysts may form in the periphery of the radial scar. This appearance is termed apocrine "blebbing." The central scar is hyperechoic *(arrow).*

(Fig. 15–29). Radial scars in which fibrocystic changes predominate may have a relatively small central nidus surrounded by numerous simple and complex cysts—a finding that corresponds to the histologic condition termed apocrine "blebbing" (Fig. 15–30). The radial scars that present as palpable lumps are those in which the peripheral proliferative or fibrocystic changes predominate. This type of radial scar is most likely to occur at times in life when dense surrounding breast tissue can obscure it mammographically or in patients in whom we try to avoid mammography (during pregnancy and lactation, and when younger than 30 years of age); thus, this type of radial scar is most likely to be evaluated sonographically.

ADH and DCIS can arise from radial scars. Sonographically, there is little to distinguish radial scars that contain ADH or DCIS from other radial scars that contain abundant proliferative changes. In general, the isoechoic proliferative changes in radial scars that contain ADH or DCIS tend to be more pronounced than for radial scars that contain only benign proliferative changes, but the difference is very subjective (Figs. 15–31 and 15–32). Fur-

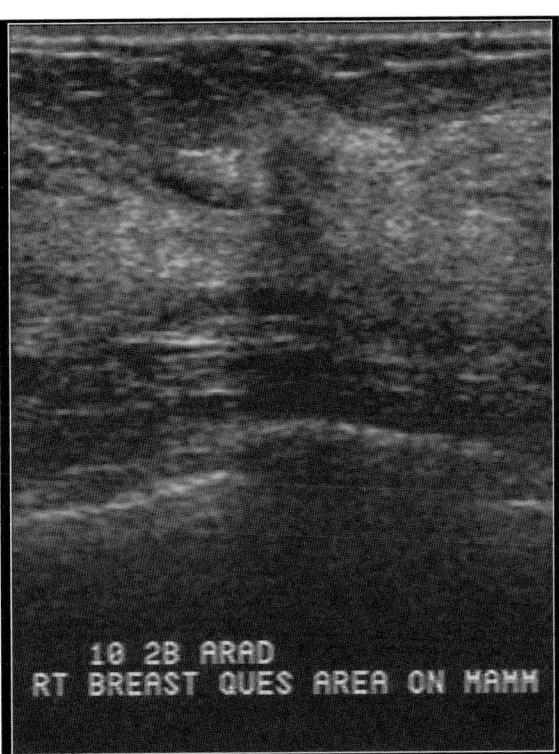

FIGURE 15–31 This spiculated form of the radial scar contained atypical ductal hyperplasia (ADH) at biopsy. There are no sonographic findings that distinguish between radial scars with ADH and those without ADH.

thermore, the peripheral proliferative changes that occur in radial scars during pregnancy, lactation, and the late teens or early 20s can rival the amount of peripheral isoechoic tissue seen with ADH or DCIS.

SUGGESTED READINGS

Generalized Risk Factors for Breast Cancer Development

Afek A, Shibi R, Kopolovitz G. Benign and premalignant breast lesions—clinico-pathological correlation. *Harefuah* 1997;133(9): 375–378.

Arthur JE, et al. The relationship of "high risk" mammographic patterns to histological risk factors for development of cancer in the human breast. *Br J Radiol* 1990;63(755):845–849.

Bodian CA, et al. Prognostic significance of benign proliferative breast disease. *Cancer* 1993;71(12):3896–3907.

Bodian CA, et al. Reproducibility and validity of pathologic classifications of benign breast disease and implications for clinical applications. *Cancer* 1993;71(12):3908–3913.

Contesso G, et al. Anatomopathological problems of mastopathies at risk. *Arch Anat Cytol Pathol* 1994;42(5):211–216.

Dupont, WD, Page DL. Risk factors for breast cancer in women with proliferative breast disease. *N Engl J Med* 1985;312(3):146–151.

Dupont WD, et al. Breast cancer risk associated with proliferative breast disease and atypical hyperplasia. *Cancer* 1993;71(4):1258–1265.

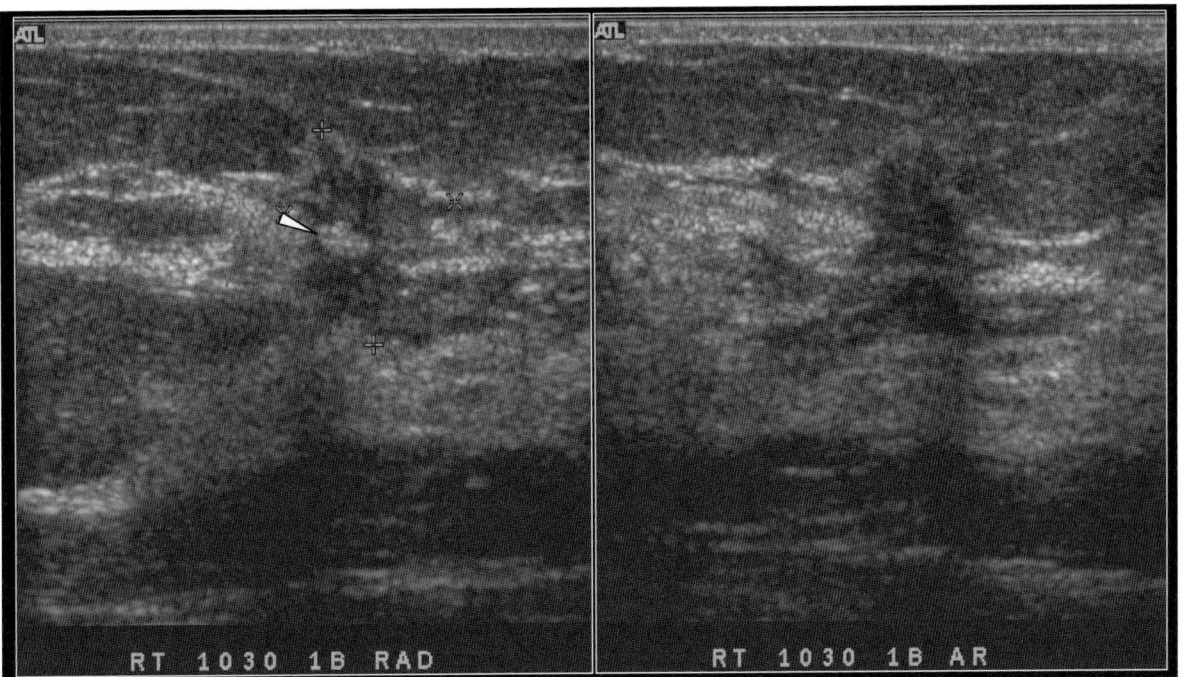

FIGURE 15–32 Ductal carcinoma *in situ* developed within this large radial scar. Notice the central hyperechoic structure that corresponds to the fibroelastotic scar *(arrowhead)*. The only feature that might help distinguish this from an uncomplicated radial scar is that the amount of peripheral proliferative change is much greater than usually seen in even the puckered form of radial scar. However, benign radial scars that occur during pregnancy, lactation, or the late teens and early 20s can have similar degrees of proliferative change.

Gozzi G, et al. High-risk focal breast lesions in echography and mammography. *Radiol Med* (Torino) 1989;78(6):603–666.

Jacquemier J, et al. Breast tissue: estrogen receptors. Immunohistochemical and biochemical analysis of normal and hyperplastic tissue and carcinoma in situ. Apropos of 86 cases. *Bull Cancer* (Paris) 1987;74(2):129–149.

London SJ, et al. A prospective study of benign breast disease and the risk of breast cancer [published erratum appears in *JAMA* 1992; 267(13):1780]. *JAMA* 1992;267(7):941–944.

Marcus JN, et al. Pathology and heredity of breast cancer in younger women. *Monogr Natl Cancer Inst* 1994;(16):23–34.

Page DL, Dupont WD. Anatomic markers of human premalignancy and risk of breast cancer. *Cancer* 1990;66(6 Suppl):1326–1335.

Urbanski S, et al. The association of histological and radiological indicators of breast cancer risk. *Br J Cancer* 1988;58(4):474–479.

Tabor L. *Teaching Atlas of Mammography, Third edition.* New York: Thieme;1993.

Walker RA. The pathology of "precancerous" breast disease. *Pathol Annu* 1994;29(Pt 2):75–97.

Weber J, et al. Borderline lesions of the breast: clinical and radiological study of 20 cases. *J Belge Radiol* 1990;73(2):89–96.

Atypical Ductal Hyperplasia, Papillary Duct Hyperplasia, Atypia, and Ductal Carcinoma *In Situ* in Papillary Lesions

al-Kaisi N. The spectrum of the "gray zone" in breast cytology. A review of 186 cases of atypical and suspicious cytology. *Acta Cytol* 1994;38(6):898–908.

Bardales RH, Suhrland MJ, Stanley MW. Papillary neoplasms of the breast: fine-needle aspiration findings in cystic and solid cases. *Diagn Cytopathol* 1994;10(4):336–341.

Bartow SA, et al. Prevalence of benign, atypical, and malignant breast lesions in populations at different risk for breast cancer. A forensic autopsy study. *Cancer* 1987;60(11):2751–1260.

Brem RA, Behrndt VS, Sanow L, et al. Atypical ductal hyperplasia: histologic underestimation of carcinoma in tissue harvested from impalpable breast lesions using 11-guage stereotactically guided directional vacuum-assisted biopsy. *AJR Am J Roentgenol* 1999; 172(5):1405–1407.

Brown TA, et al. Atypical hyperplasia in the era of stereotactic core needle biopsy. *J Surg Oncol* 1998;67(3):168–173.

Cardenosa G, Eklund GW. Benign papillary neoplasms of the breast: mammographic findings. *Radiology* 1991;181(3):751–755.

Carter BA, Page DL, Schuyler P, et al. No elevation in long-term breast cancer risk for women with fibroadenomas that contain atypical hyperplasia. *Cancer* 2001;92(1):30–36.

Helvie MA, et al. Atypical hyperplasia of the breast: mammographic appearance and histologic correlation. *Radiology* 1991;179(3): 759–764.

Hoshi K, et al. Pathological characterization of atypical ductal hyperplasia of the breast. *Gan To Kagaku Ryoho* 1995;1:36–41.

Hughes DE, Orr JD, Smith NM. Intraduct papillomatosis of the breast in a peripubertal male. *Pediatr Pathol* 1994;14(4):561–565.

Jackman RJ, et al. Stereotactic large-core needle biopsy of 450 nonpalpable breast lesions with surgical correlation in lesions with cancer or atypical hyperplasia. *Radiology* 1994;193(1):91–95.

Jensen RA, et al. Invasive breast cancer risk in women with sclerosing adenosis. *Cancer* 1989;64(10):1977–1983.

Kamel OW, Kempson RL, Hendrickson MR. In situ proliferative epithelial lesions of the breast. *Pathology* 1992;1(1):65–102.

Liberman L, et al. Atypical ductal hyperplasia diagnosed at stereotactic core biopsy of breast lesions: an indication for surgical biopsy. *AJR Am J Roentgenol* 1995;164(5):1111–1113.

Liberman L. Clinical management issues in percutaneous core breast biopsy. *Radiol Clin North Am* 2000;38(4):791–807.

Mariuzzi GM, et al. Quantitative study of ductal breast cancer progression. Morphometric evaluation of phenotypical changes occurring in benign and preinvasive epithelial lesions. *Pathol Res Pract* 1994;190(11):1056–1065.

McDivitt RW, et al. Histologic types of benign breast disease and the risk for breast cancer. The Cancer and Steroid Hormone Study Group. *Cancer* 1992;69(6):1408–1414.

Moriya T, et al. Significance of proliferative breast lesions around breast cancers. *Gan To Kagaku Ryoho* 1995;1:42–45.

Page DL, et al. Atypical hyperplastic lesions of the female breast. A long-term follow-up study. *Cancer* 1985;55(11):2698–2708.

Page DL, Dupont WD. Premalignant conditions and markers of elevated risk in the breast and their management. *Surg Clin North Am* 1990;70(4):831–851.

Page DL, Dupont WD. Anatomic markers of human premalignancy and risk of breast cancer. *Cancer* 1990;66[6 Suppl]:1326–1335.

Page DL, Jensen RA, Simpson JF. Premalignant and malignant disease of the breast: the roles of the pathologist. *Mod Pathol* 1998; 11(2):120–128.

Rubin E, et al. Proliferative disease and atypia in biopsies performed for nonpalpable lesions detected mammographically. *Cancer* 1988; 61(10):2077–2082.

Stomper PC, et al. Atypical hyperplasia: frequency and mammographic and pathologic relationships in excisional biopsies guided with mammography and clinical examination. *Radiology* 1993; 189(3):667–671.

Tavassoli FA, Norris HJ. A comparison of the results of long-term follow-up for atypical intraductal hyperplasia and intraductal hyperplasia of the breast. *Cancer* 1990;65(3):518–529.

Tavassoli FA. Ductal carcinoma in situ: introduction of the concept of ductal intraepithelial neoplasia. *Mod Pathol* 1998;11(2):140–154.

Watanabe K. Evaluation of atypical ductal hyperplasia. *Gan To Kagaku Ryoho* 1995;1:26–31.

Phyllodes Tumors

Aranda FI, Laforga JB, Lopez JI. Phyllodes tumor of the breast. An immunohistochemical study of 28 cases with special attention to the role of myofibroblasts. *Pathol Res Pract* 1994;190(5):474–481.

Bernstein L, Deapen D, Ross RK. The descriptive epidemiology of malignant cystosarcoma phyllodes tumors of the breast. *Cancer* 1993;71(10):3020–3024.

Buchberger W, et al. Phylloides tumor: findings on *mammography, sonography,* and aspiration cytology in 10 cases. *AJR Am J Roentgenol* 1991;157(4):715–719.

Cabaret V, Delobelle-Deroide A, Vilain MO. Phyllodes tumors. *Arch Anat Cytol Pathol* 1995;43(1–2):59–72.

Chua CL, Thomas A. Cystosarcoma phyllodes tumors. *Surg Gynecol Obstet* 1988;166(4):302–306.

Cohn-Cedermark G, Rutqvist LE, Rosendahl I, et al. Prognostic factors in cystosarcoma phyllodes. A clinicopathologic study of 7 patients. *Cancer* 1991;68(9):2017–2022.

Cole-Bueglet C, Soriano R, Kurtz AB, et al. Ultrasound, x-ray mammography, and histopathology of cystosarcoma phyllodes. *Radiology* 1983;146(2):481–486.

Cosmacini P, et al. Mammography in the diagnosis of phyllodes tumors of the breast. Analysis of 99 cases. *Radiol Med* (Torino) 1991;82(1–2):52–55.

Cosmacini P, et al. Phyllodes tumor of the breast: mammographic experience in 99 cases. *Eur J Radiol* 1992;15(1):11–14.

Dietrich CU, et al. Cytogenetic findings in phyllodes tumors of the breast: karyotypic complexity differentiates between malignant and benign tumors. *Hum Pathol* 1997;28(12):1379–1382.

Dragj F, Sabolla L, Campani R, et al. Diagnostic imaging of phyllodes tumors: preliminary observations. *Radiol Med* (Torino) 1996; 91(5):585–589.

Hines JR, Murad TM, Beal JM. Prognostic indicators in cystosarcoma phyllodes. *Am J Surg* 1987;153(3):276–280.

Jorge Blanco A, Vargas Serrano B, Rodriguez Romero R, et al. Phyllodes tumors of the breast. *Eur Radiol* 1999;9(2):356–360.

Kahan Z, et al. Recurrent phyllodes tumor in a man. *Pathol Res Pract* 1997;193(9):653–658.

Leveque J, et al. Malignant cystosarcomas phyllodes of the breast in adolescent females. *Eur J Obstet Gynecol Reprod Biol* 1994;54(3):197–203.

Liberman L, et al. Benign and malignant phyllodes tumors: mammographic and sonographic findings. *Radiology* 1996;198(1):121–124.

Lu YJ, et al. Phyllodes tumors of the breast analyzed by comparative genomic hybridization and association of increased 1q copy number with stromal overgrowth and recurrence. *Genes Chromosomes Cancer* 1997;20(3):275–281.

McGregor GI, Knowling MA, Este FA. Sarcoma and cystosarcoma phyllodes tumors of the breast—a retrospective review of 58 cases. *Am J Surg* 1994;167(5):477–480.

Modena S, et al. Phyllodes tumor of the breast: problems of differential diagnosis and therapeutic approach from an analysis of 17 cases. *Eur J Surg Oncol* 1993;19(1):70–73.

Nishimura R, et al. Malignant phyllodes tumour with a noninvasive ductal carcinoma component. *Virchows Arch* 1998;432(1):89–93.

Page JE, Williams JE. The radiological features of phylloides tumour of the breast with clinico-pathological correlation. *Clin Radiol* 1991;44(1):8–12.

Rajan PB, Cranor ML, Rosen PP. Cystosarcoma phyllodes in adolescent girls and young women: a study of 45 patients. *Am J Surg Pathol* 1998;22(1):64–69.

Reddick RL, et al. Stromal proliferations of the breast: an ultrastructural and immunohistochemical evaluation of cystosarcoma phyllodes, juvenile fibroadenoma, and fibroadenoma. *Hum Pathol* 1987;18(1):45–49.

Reinfuss M, Mitus J, Stelmach A. Phyllodes tumor of the breast. *Strahlenther Onkol* 1995;171(1):5–11.

Rowell MD, et al. Phyllodes tumors. *Am J Surg* 1993;165(3):376–379.

Sawney N, Garrahan N, Douglas-Jones AG, et al. Epithelial-stromal interactions in tumors. A morphologic study of fibroepithelial tumors of the breast. *Cancer* 1992;70(8):2115–2120.

Schon G, et al. Giant cystosarcoma phylloides: mammographic and sonographic findings in an unusual case. *Aktuelle Radiol* 1994;4(1):41–43.

Stebbing JF, Nash AG. Diagnosis and management of phyllodes tumour of the breast: experience of 33 cases at a specialist centre. *Ann R Coll Surg Engl* 1995;77(3):181–184.

Steinbock RT, et al. The ultrasound appearance of giant fibroadenoma. *J Clin Ultrasound* 1983;11(10):451–454.

Ward RM, Evans HL. Cystosarcoma phyllodes. A clinicopathologic study of 26 cases. *Cancer* 1986;58(10):1182–2289.

Yeh IT, Francis DJ, Orenstein JM. Ultrastructure of cystosarcoma phyllodes and fibroadenoma—a comparative study. *Am J Clin Pathol* 1985;84(2):131–136.

Radial Scars

Adler DD, Helvie MA, Oberman HA, et al. Radial sclerosing lesion of the breast: mammographic features. *Radiology* 1990;176(3):737–740.

Azavedo E, Svane G. Radial scars detected mammographically in a breast cancer screening programme. *Eur J Radiol* 1992;15(1):18–21.

Bonzanini M, et al. Cytologic features of 22 radial scar/complex sclerosing lesions of the breast, three of which associated with carcinoma: clinical, mammographic, and histologic correlation. *Diagn Cytopathol* 1997;17(5):353–362.

Cohen MA, Sferiazza SJ. Role of sonography in evaluation of radial scars of the breast. *AJR Am J Roentgenol* 2000;174(4):1075–1078.

Ciatto S, et al. Radial scars of the breast: review of 38 consecutive mammographic diagnoses. *Radiology* 1993;187(3):757–760.

Finlay ME, Liston JE, Lunt LG, et al. Assessment of the role of ultrasound in the differentiation of radial scars and stellate carcinoma of the breast. *Clin Radiol* 1994;49(1):52–55.

Frouge C, et al. Mammographic lesions suggestive of radial scars: microscopic findings in 40 cases. *Radiology* 1995;195(3):623–625.

Mitnick JS, Vazquez MF, Harris MN, et al. Differentiation of radial scar from scirrhous carcinoma of the breast: mammographic-pathologic correlation. *Radiology* 1989:173(12):697–700.

Nielsen M, Christensen L, Andersen J. Radial scars in women with breast cancer. *Cancer* 1987;59(5):1019–1025.

Orel SG, et al. Radial scar with microcalcifications: radiologic-pathologic correlation. *Radiology* 1992;183(2):479–482.

Poulton TB, de Paredes ES, Baldwin M. Sclerosing lobular hyperplasia of the breast: imaging features in 15 cases. *AJR Am J Roentgenol* 1995;165(2):291–294.

Rosen PP. Subareolar sclerosing duct hyperplasia of the breast. *Cancer* 1987;59(11):1927–1930.

Sloane JP, Mayers MM. Carcinoma and atypical hyperplasia in radial scars and complex sclerosing lesions: importance of lesion size and patient age. *Histopathology* 1993;23(3):225–231.

Vega A, Garijo F. Radial scar and tubular carcinoma: mammographic and sonographic findings. *Acta Radiol* 1993;34(1):43–47.

Wallis MG, et al. Complex sclerosing lesions (radial scars) of the breast can be palpable. *Clin Radiol* 1993;48(5):319–320.

Juvenile Papillomatosis

Batchelor JS, Farah G, Fisher C. Multiple breast papillomas in adolescence. *Surg Oncol* 1993;54(1):64–66.

Hsieh SC, Chen KC, Chu CC, et al. Juvenile papillomatosis of the breast in a 9-year-old girl. *Pediatr Surg Int* 2001;17(2):206–208.

Kersschot EA, et al. Juvenile papillomatosis of the breast: sonographic appearance. *Radiology* 1988;169(3):631–633.

Nonomura A, et al. Secretory carcinoma of the breast associated with juvenile papillomatosis in a 12-year-old girl. A case report. *Acta Cytol* 1995;39(3):569–576.

Rosen PP, et al. Juvenile papillomatosis and breast carcinoma. *Cancer* 1985;55(6):1345–1352.

Rosen PP. Papillary duct hyperplasia of the breast in children and young adults. *Cancer* 1985;56(7):1611–1617.

Taffurelli M, et al. Juvenile papillomatosis of the breast. A multidisciplinary study. *Pathol Annu* 1991;1:25–35.

16

EVALUATION OF THE MALE BREAST

There are three basic categories of diseases of the male breast:

1. Gynecomastia and other benign conditions involving ducts and periductal fibrous stroma
2. Primary breast malignancy
3. Conditions that arise from tissues other than ducts and periductal stromal tissue, including:
   a. Lesions arising within skin or subcutaneous tissues
   b. Lesions arising from blood vessels (including hematogenous metastases), lymphatics, or nerves
   c. Lesions arising from the lymphoreticular system

USE OF SONOGRAPHY IN DISEASE TO ASSESS THE MALE BREAST

The incidence of breast cancer in males is too low to justify routine screening mammography. Thus, all imaging of the breast in the male is diagnostic. Most male patients present with palpable abnormalities that may or may not be painful or tender, but a few present with nipple discharge. Despite the relatively small size of male breasts, mammography is usually technically possible and is useful in distinguishing between gynecomastia and breast carcinoma. However, mammography's advantage over sonography in demonstrating calcifications is much less important in males than in females because microcalcifications occur much less frequently in male breast cancers than in female cancers. Therefore, sonography is frequently used to assess breast complaints in males, either in addition to mammography or instead of mammography. Sonography is just as effective for evaluation of palpable lumps in the male patient as it is in the female patient. Sonography is also effective in evaluating the cause of nipple discharge in most male and female patients. Although technically adequate diagnostic mammograms can be obtained in most males, in cases in which there are suspicious findings and biopsy becomes necessary, stereotactically guided biopsy is much more difficult in males than in females because of the small breast size in males. Such cases usually require sonographic rather than stereotactic guidance of the biopsy.

The small breast size that can make mammography and stereotactically guided biopsy technically difficult facilitates adequate penetration of the breast with high-frequency ultrasound. Near-field, high-frequency, high-resolution ultrasound is just as effective in evaluating palpable abnormalities in the male breast as it is in evaluating lumps in the female breast. The breast pathologies of mammary ductal and stromal processes in males are very similar to those abnormalities in females; thus, the sonographic features that reflect the gross morphology and histology of ductal and stromal pathology are similar. However, unlike females, males do not have fully developed lobules; therefore, classic lobular processes such as fibrocystic change and adenosis rarely occur in the male breast. Most pathologic lesions in the male breast arise either from ducts and periductal stomal elements or from overlying subcutaneous tissues, skin, and whole-body support structures like the vascular, lymphatic, and neural systems.

The sonographic suspicious and reassuring findings and the evaluation algorithm are similar in males and females. Therefore, once a lesion has been sonographically characterized as BIRADS 4 or higher, biopsy should be performed. Because of technical difficulties with stereotactically guided interventional procedures in the small male breast, most interventional procedures in males are performed with ultrasound guidance.

GYNECOMASTIA

Etiology

Gynecomastia is the most common disease process of the male breast and is the most frequent cause of palpable abnormalities. Gynecomastia means "woman-like breasts" and comes from the Greek roots *gyne* meaning women and *mastos* meaning breasts. Histopathologically, gynecomastia represents a benign proliferation of subareolar ductal and periductal stromal tissues. The degree of ductal and periductal stromal stimulation varies with the degree and duration of stimulation. The more pronounced and longer the duration of stimulation, the more likely it is that periductal stroma fibrous tissue will be laid down. There are numerous potential causes of gynecomastia, but all have a similar underlying mechanism—an imbalance between estrogenic and testosterone effects at the level of breast tissues.

Both males and females produce androgens and estrogens, and there is free and continuous interconversion of certain estrogens and androgens. Males normally produce androgens and estrogens in a 100:1 ratio, but in the circulation, it is an even higher 300:1 ratio.

How estrogenic effects increase and the testosterone effects decrease at the level of breast tissues is not fully understood. Increased circulating estrogens, decreased circulating androgens, increase in circulating estrogens to a greater extent than androgens are increased, cross hormone receptor sensitivity with other hormones or other substances that mimic estrogens, blockage of androgen-binding globulin, blockage of testosterone receptor sites, increased sensitivity of breast tissue receptor sites to estrogen, and decreased sensitivity of androgen receptor sites to androgen all appear to contribute.

A brief review of sex hormone metabolism helps to understand the potential mechanisms for development of gynecomastia. Although most of the final maximally biologically active sex hormones are produced in the gonads, prohormones are produced in the pituitary and adrenal glands, and active final forms of the hormones can be produced in many peripheral tissues of the body, particularly within the liver and in adipose tissue. The sex hormones are produced from cholesterol, a 27-carbon molecule. From cholesterol, 6 carbon atoms are cleaved to form pregnenolone, which is the precursor of all adrenal and sex hormones. From pregnenolone, progesterone and 17-α-progesterone are sequentially formed. Within the adrenal glands, progesterones are converted to androstenedione and dehydroepiandrosterone (DHEA). Androstenedione is released from the adrenal into the bloodstream and is carried by the androgen-binding protein to the testis, where it is converted within Leydig's cells to testosterone. Testosterone can be converted to dihydrotestosterone (DHT) in Sertoli's cells or in peripheral tissues. Sertoli's cells also produce circulating binding protein for testosterone that testosterone binds to while circulating in the bloodstream. Only free testosterone that is not bound to testosterone-binding globulin is free to enter peripheral tissue cells, where it exerts its secondary sex characteristic effects. The globulin that binds testosterone will also accept estradiol into its receptor. Thus, high levels of estradiol can displace or block testosterone from attaching,

resulting in an elevation of levels of unbound, metabolically active testosterone within the blood. Dihydrotestosterone is 10 times more active in its androgenic effects than is testosterone, which, in turn, is many times more active than is androstenedione. Thus, androstenedione, a popular anabolic steroid supplement among serious athletes and bodybuilders, is really a prohormone with little direct effect. The metabolic pathways of androgens are illustrated in Figs. 16–1 and 16–2.

Paradoxically, elevated levels of unbound testosterone within the circulation can directly elevate estrogen levels by a process termed *aromatization,* which is the main mechanism by which testosterone is metabolized. Aromatase, the enzyme that facilitates aromatization, is present within testicular cells, the ovary, and many other tissues (including liver and adipose tissue). Aromatase converts testosterone directly to estradiol and also converts androstenedione to estrone. Although estrone exhibits much less estrogen than does estradiol, estrone is readily converted to its more active metabolite, estradiol, within peripheral tissues. Thus, increased amounts of either exogenous or endogenous androgens can be aromatized to estradiol, and paradoxically cause gynecomastia. Even normal levels of testosterone can lead to abnormally high levels of estradiol if aromatase activity is supernormal. Cross hormone effects (hyperthyroidism, hyperprolactinemia), some medications and drugs, and paraneoplastic syndromes, and congenital etiologies can all elevate aromatase activity.

Gynecomastia can result from abnormalities at any point during the formation or metabolism of androgens and estrogens. Tables 16–1 and 16–2 list various disorders, supplements, medications, and drugs that can cause gynecomastia and the suspected mechanisms by which they lead to gynecomastia. Some of these entities act at only one point, whereas others are multifactorial and act at more than one level. In some cases, the exact mechanisms by which estrogen-to-androgen ratios are altered are not well understood.

At certain times in life, gynecomastia can be considered to be physiologic, occurring in a significant percentage of patients transiently because of transient endogenous estrogen-to-androgen ratio imbalances. Physiologic gynecomastia occurs occasionally in newborns (increased estrogen levels) and in more than half of boys at puberty (increased free testosterone levels).

Newborn male and female babies may have breast enlargement caused by exposure to high levels of maternal estrogens *in utero* and from breast-feeding. Gynecomastia in the newborn can be associated with duct ectasia and galactorrhea, which has been called "witch's milk." This process usually resolves spontaneously over a few weeks but can last for 1 or 2 years. The spontaneous regression of transient gynecomastia of the newborn can take longer in breast-fed babies who have additional exposure to estrogenic substances in breast milk.

metabolic pathway to sex hormones in adrenal cortex and testes

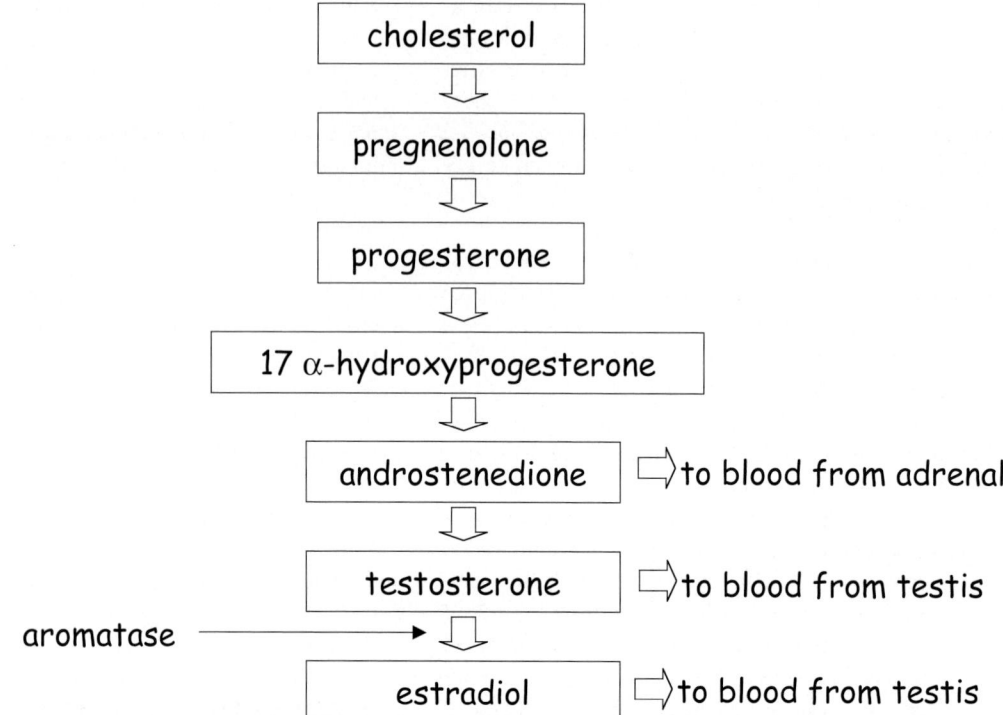

FIGURE 16–1 The metabolic pathway for testosterone begins with cholesterol and ends in the process of aromatization, which converts testosterone to estradiol. Disorders in this pathway that result in elevation of estradiol levels in comparison to testosterone levels lead to gynecomastia.

The most common cause of gynecomastia is puberty. Physiologic pubertal gynecomastia affects up to 60% of young males and is usually self-limited, spontaneously resolving over a few months to 2 or 3 years. The etiology of pubertal gynecomastia is multifactorial. It is related to a sudden surge in sex hormone production. The production of testosterone increases 30-fold, but the production of estradiol also increases 3-fold. The timing of the increases in estradiol and testosterone production may be critical. At least in some boys, it appears that the 3-fold increase in estradiol production precedes the much larger increased in testosterone production. This not only increases free estradiol levels but also competes with testosterone for sites on gonadal steroid-binding globulin, displacing some testosterone, which then undergoes aromatization to form even more free estradiol. Eventually, testosterone production catches up to and greatly exceeds estradiol production, restoring estrogen-to-androgen ratios to normal. Additionally, it appears that the rapid increase in testosterone production precedes both increases in the number of peripheral tissues testosterone receptor sites and increases in

the production of testosterone-binding globulin by months to years. The relative paucity of peripheral receptor sites and testosterone-binding globulins leads to elevated free testosterone blood levels, which, in turn, leads to increased aromatization and estradiol production. As the teenage male ages, the number of testosterone receptor sites and the amount of testosterone-binding globulin eventually increase enough to bind most of the testosterone produced, reducing excess unbound testosterone levels, decreasing aromatization, and finally, decreasing estradiol levels. As the estradiol levels fall, the estrogenic stimulation of the breasts diminishes, and the pubertal gynecomastia resolves spontaneously in most cases.

Physiologic gynecomastia also occurs during andropause and in old age, and like physiologic pubertal gynecomastia, it has a multifactorial etiology. Testosterone production normally decreases with age, and the number and avidity of tissue testosterone-binding sites also decreases. Furthermore, individuals tend to gain weight and body fat with age. Adipose tissue contains high levels of aromatase. Thus, the more adipose tissue

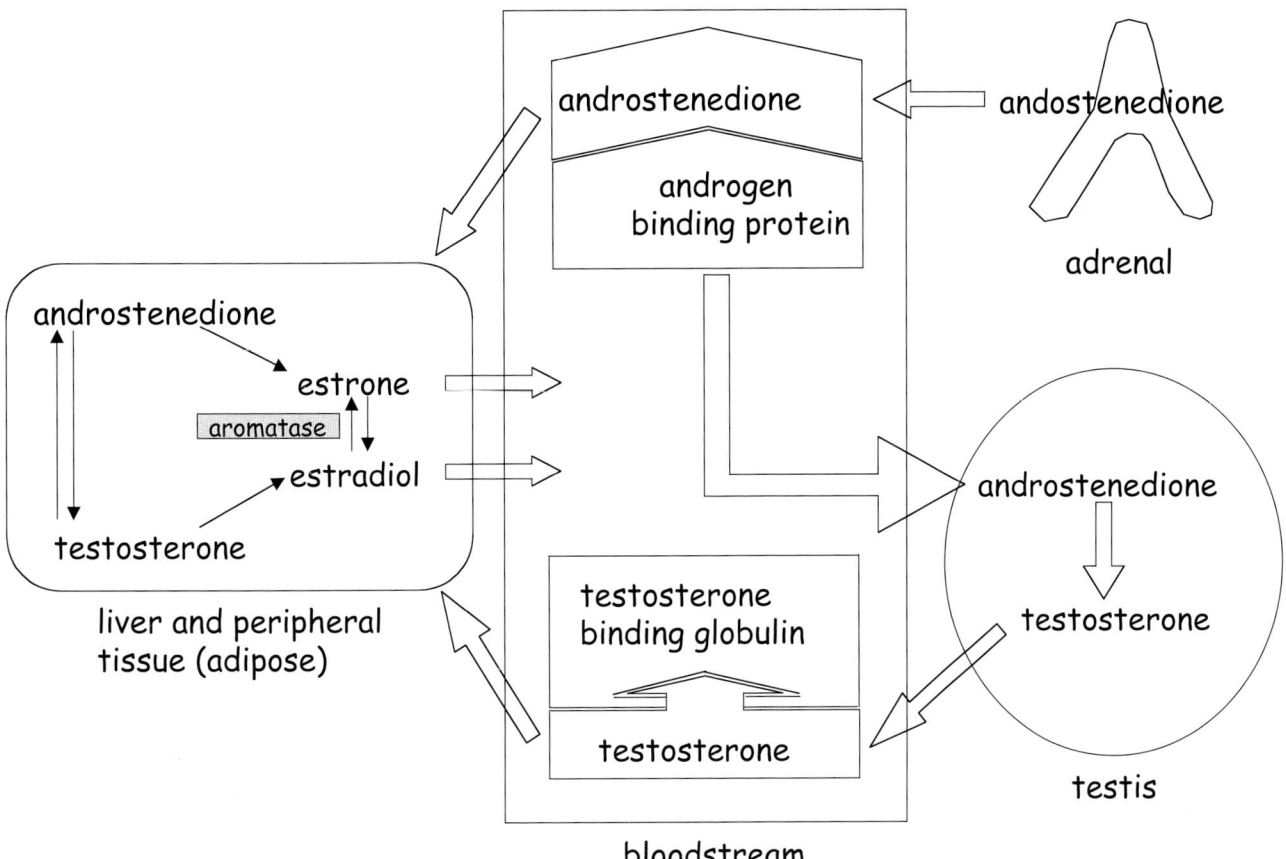

FIGURE 16–2 This figure illustrates the pathways followed by androstenedione and testosterone from the adrenals and testes through the bloodstream to the testis, liver, and peripheral tissues. Anything that interferes with this pathway can decrease testosterone levels, but increased levels of intrinsic or extrinsic testosterone or increased aromatase activity can result ultimately in increased estradiol levels to above normal. Finally, a deficiency of testosterone receptor sites or inhibition or blocking of these sites can prevent testosterone from exerting its effects.

one has, the more testosterone aromatization and estradiol production there is.

In addition to physiologic gynecomastia, older men are also more likely to have multiple reasons for pathologic gynecomastia. Older men are more likely to require medications that are known to cause gynecomastia. Liver dysfunction becomes more common with age, and metabolism of estradiol into inactive metabolites can be adversely affected. Finally, treatment of prostate cancer by orchiectomy and administration of estrogens can contribute to gynecomastia.

Gynecomastia is less common in the age group between the teenage years and old age and usually is pathologic in this age group. The most common etiology for gynecomastia in this young adult and middle age group is medications, nutritional supplements, and ingestion of anabolic steroids, typically in athletes and bodybuilders. Unfortunately, the use of steroids is far more widespread than realized. Many of these patients deny use of such substances, especially in professional or competitive athletics, in which steroid use is outlawed. In addition to athletes and bodybuilders, many men now take supplements such as androstenedione that are marketed as over-the-counter treatments for erectile dysfunction. Such patients may be too embarrassed to admit using such substances. Finally, many men take DHEA or pregnenolone as dietary supplements. The compounds have been marketed as "master hormones" that regulate the body, increase energy and resistance to disease, improve sexual function, and lengthen life. These patients are generally unaware that both substances can eventually be metabolized to testosterone and can subsequently undergo aromatization to estradiol, leading to gynecomastia; thus, there is a high probability that they will not offer a history of using such substances. These men need to be queried very specifically about use of supplements, including pregnenolone and DHEA. Generally, the risk for gynecomastia is much higher with DHEA than with pregnenolone.

TABLE 16–1. CAUSES OF GYNECOMASTIA

Physiologic gynecomastia
  Newborns and infants
  Pubertal
  Andropause and old age

Pathologic gynecomastia
  Decreased testosterone production
    Congenital primary testicular failure
      Defects in testosterone synthesis, Klinefelter's syndrome, hermaphroditism, anorchia, Kallmann's syndrome, 5α-reductase deficiency
    Acquired primary testicular failure
      Torsion, trauma, infection, surgical or chemical castration
    Secondary testicular failure
      Hypothalamic disease, pituitary disease
    Defective or absent testosterone receptor sites or testosterone resistance
      Renal failure, severe chronic illnesses, human immuno-deficiency virus, androgen insensitivity syndrome
    Antiandrogenics or androgen inhibitors
      Finasteride, flutamide, cyproterone acetate, etomidate
  Increased free estradiol blood levels
    Exogenous estrogen
      Creams, phytoestrogens in food, and estrogen mimics in environment
    Crossover effects from other hormones that are abnormally increased
      Hyperthyroidism and hyperprolactinemia
    Enhanced estrogen
    Paraneoplastic syndromes—human chorionic gonadotropin (hCG) production
      Carcinomas of lung, liver, kidney, and stomach; extra-gonadal choriocarcinoma
    Paraneoplastic syndromes—eutopic hCG production
      Choriocarcinoma of testis
    Decreased metabolism of estradiol
      Liver disease
    Competition for gonadal steroid-binding globulin sites
      Spironolactone, ketoconazole
    Increased aromatization
      Congenitally increased aromatase activity
      Hermaphroditism
      Acquired increased aromatase in peripheral tissues
        Obesity, refeeding after starvation, hyperthyroidism
      Increased testicular production of aromatase
        Sertoli's cell tumors, sex cord tumors, Leydig's cell tumors, germ cell tumors
      Increased adrenal production of aromatase
        Adrenal tumors
    Exogenous hormone ingestion
      Androgens, anabolic steroids, human growth hormone (hGH), hCG, pregnenolone, dehydroepiandrosterone (DHEA)

Illegal drugs

Medications

Idiopathic

TABLE 16–2. MEDICATIONS AND DRUGS ASSOCIATED WITH GYNECOMASTIA

Illegal abuse drugs
  Alcohol
  Marijuana (phytoestrogen)
  Heroin and methadone
  Amphetamines
  Cocaine

Hormones and prohormones
  Androgens
  Anabolic steroids
  Pregnenolone
  Dehydroepiandrosterone (DHEA)
  Estrogens
  Growth hormone
  Human chorionic gonadotropin
  Prolactin

Antiandrogens and androgen inhibitors
  Finasteride
  Ranitidine
  Cyproterone acetate

Cardiovascular drugs—angiotensin-converting enzyme (ACE) inhibitors, calcium channel blockers
  Amiodarone
  Captopril
  Digitoxin
  Diltiazem
  Enalapril
  Methyldopa
  Nifedipine
  Reserpine
  Spironolactone
  Verapamil

Antiulcer drugs
  Cimetidine
  Ranitidine
  Omeprazole

Antibiotics
  Ethionamide
  Isoniazid
  Ketoconazole
  Metronidazole

Psychoactive pharmaceuticals
  Diazepam
  Haloperidol

Genetic disorders that lead to gynecomastia may first become manifest in this age group (Table 16–1).

Clinical Findings

Gynecomastia typically presents as a unilateral or bilateral palpable subareolar thickening or lump that is often tender. Unilateral gynecomastia is more likely to present as a discrete lump or mass than is bilateral gynecomastia and therefore is more likely to be confused clinically with breast cancer. Because of the asymmetry and more masslike clinical presentation of unilateral gynecomastia, it is far more likely to be assessed with mammography or sonography than is bilateral gynecomastia. Despite the term *unilateral gynecomastia*, such cases almost always represent markedly asymmetric bilateral gynecomastia.

Early or florid phases of gynecomastia can be painful (mastodynia) or exquisitely tender. Over time, the tenderness usually gradually diminishes, even if the palpable abnormality persists. Other patients present with nipple discharge. These patients usually are in the florid or early phase of the process and have associated duct hyperplasia or duct ectasia. Males with duct ectasia can develop any of the complications of the duct ectasia–periductal mastitis complex that affect females, including periductal mastitis, subareolar abscess formation, nipple retraction, and fistula formation.

Gynecomastia must be distinguished from pseudogynecomastia. Pseudogynecomastia occurs in obese men in which the breasts become enlarged solely because of fat deposition in the breasts. There is no evidence of benign ductal and fibrous periductal stromal overgrowth. It may be difficult to distinguish between true gynecomastia and pseudogynecomastia by clinical findings alone in some patients, but mammography and sonography can readily do so.

Generally, treatment or removal of the cause of gynecomastia within 6 months of its onset results in complete regression of all signs and symptoms. However, when the etiology persists for 6 months to a year, signs and symptoms are more likely to regress only partially. When the underlying causes of gynecomastia persist for more than a year, the palpable and visible abnormalities of gynecomastia are likely to persist indefinitely, even though pain and tenderness tend to resolve eventually.

Diagnostic Testing

Physiologic gynecomastia generally does not require any laboratory or imaging testing. A careful history that includes past and current illnesses and a complete list of drug abuse, medications, and nutritional supplements should ferret out a cause in most cases. Physical examination of the scrotum will help in cases of testicular tumors, atrophy, or hypoplasia.

When an underlying etiology for gynecomastia cannot be identified from the history and physical examination, laboratory and imaging other than breast ultrasound is warranted. Additionally, in cases in which breast size is greater than 5 cm, there is an acutely tender lump of recent onset, or there are associated signs of malignancy such as hard, fixed lymphadenopathy, one might consider additional testing. Standard liver and renal function tests identify chronic underlying diseases that increase peripheral aromatization. If there are other signs of feminization,

testosterone, luteinizing hormone (LH), estradiol, and DHEA levels should be assessed. If there are no signs of feminization, free testosterone, LH, follicle-stimulating hormone (FSH), prolactin, β-human chorionic gonadotropin (β-hCG), and estradiol levels are required. If serum estradiol is elevated, a scrotal ultrasound should be performed. If β-hCG levels are elevated, chest x-ray or chest computed tomography (CT) and scrotal ultrasound should be obtained. If prolactin is elevated, CT or magnetic resonance imaging of the sella of the brain is indicated. If a paraneoplastic syndrome of any sort is suspected, extensive imaging workup with CT scans may be warranted.

Treatment

Physiologic gynecomastia that occurs in the newborn and at puberty seldom requires any treatment. The metabolic events that alter estrogen-to-androgen ratios resolve spontaneously soon enough that gynecomastia seldom progresses beyond the proliferative phase. Regression is usually spontaneous and complete.

When the cause or causes of gynecomastia do not spontaneously resolve promptly, medical or surgical treatment may be warranted. The first step in medical treatment should be to discontinue offending medications, drugs, or supplements. The next step should be to treat conditions in which elevated levels of other hormones have crossover effect on estrogen receptors. Hyperthyroidism frequently causes gynecomastia and can be treated with radioactive iodine. Associated liver and renal disease can be treated medically in some cases.

In cases in which medications cannot be discontinued, an attempt can be made to manipulate hormone levels. This can be accomplished by raising DHT levels or by decreasing estradiol levels. DHT levels can be raised by direct administration of DHT. DHT is the most biologically active endogenous androgen and is a metabolite of testosterone that is formed one step beyond the aromatization step and therefore cannot be converted to estradiol. Thus, administration of DHT can beneficially alter the estrogen-to-androgen ratio and make gynecomastia regress. Unfortunately, DHT has so many other serious side effects (liver damage, baldness, prostate hypertrophy, and possibly prostate carcinoma) that it is rarely used for any indication.

Estradiol levels can be reduced in several ways. Antiestrogen therapies can be tried. These include clomiphene (simulates release of pituitary gonadotropins), tamoxifen and other selective estrogen receptor modulators (SERMs), and danazol (synthetic steroid with antiestrogenic properties). Some of these are very weak estrogens that avidly bind to estrogen receptor sites in the tissues, blocking the more biologically active estradiol molecules from attaching to the sites. In others, the antiestrogen mechanism is more complex or less well understood.

Decreasing aromatization can lower estradiol levels and cause gynecomastia to regress. In obese patients, weight loss may decrease the amount of aromatase, thereby decreasing aromatization of testosterone to estrogen within adipose tissues and also decreasing the amount of free estradiol available to stimulate breast tissues. Certain pharmaceutical agents can directly inhibit aromatase. D_1-Testonelactone was the first aromatase inhibitor, but it had some undesirable side effects. Newer agents purported to have fewer side effects include letrozole, anastrozole, fadrozole, fromestane, exemestane, and D-indole methane. Athletes and bodybuilders who refuse to discontinue anabolic steroids are experts in the effectiveness of the various antiestrogens and often use them prophylactically to prevent gynecomastia while continuing to use anabolic steroids of various types. Many athletes and bodybuilders know far more about sex hormone metabolism and gynecomastia than do their physicians. Most of what they have learned has come from Internet sites. Unfortunately, whereas the volume of information on the Internet is superb, the veracity may not be.

Zinc appears to facilitate development of testosterone receptor sites, decreasing free testosterone blood levels and therefore decreasing aromatization and estradiol production. Zinc may also facilitate production of testosterone-binding globulin by Sertoli's cells. Furthermore, zinc deficiency increases estrogen receptor sites in the peripheral tissues, including breast tissue; therefore, zinc deficiency may facilitate the development of gynecomastia.

The effectiveness of medical treatments of gynecomastia depends on its histologic phase when therapy is initiated. Complete regression of gynecomastia is the rule during its proliferative phase. Complete resolution of pain, tenderness, and secretions, but only partial regression of the palpable lump and visible enlargement, should be expected in cases in which gynecomastia has progressed to the mixed phase. Medical treatment is ineffective in patients whose gynecomastia has progressed to the quiescent phase. In general, the longer gynecomastia has persisted, the less likely medical treatment is to be completely successful. Patients whose gynecomastia has progressed to the fibrous or quiescent phase who wish treatment for cosmetic reasons must undergo surgery.

Histology

Gynecomastia can be divided into three phases histologically. The first phase, the florid or active phase, is characterized by ductal epithelial and myoepithelial proliferation and hyperplasia. The third phase, the fibrous phase, is characterized by the deposition of dense, collagenous periductal fibrous tissue. This has also been called the quiescent phase because the process is usually inactive during this phase. The second phase, the mixed or transitional phase, occurs between the first florid and third fibrous phases and is characterized by a mixture of proliferative ductal and periductal fibrous changes. The duration of each phase varies, depending on the sensitivity of breast tissue to estrogenic stimulation and the degree to which the estrogen-to-androgen ratios are elevated. Generally, the florid phase lasts a few months, and deposition of significant amounts of dense periductal fibrous tissue ensues at about 6 months. If the underlying cause of gynecomastia resolves or is treated, the patient may never progress to the quiescent phase. The quiescent phase occurs in patients whose underlying cause for gynecomastia persists untreated long enough for amounts of periductal fibrous tissue to be laid down. After 1 year, the volume of dense periductal fibrous tissue commonly exceeds the volume of ductal tissue, and successful treatment of the underlying cause results in regression of the ducts, but not of the fibrous tissue, ushering in the fibrous or quiescent phase. The clinical findings discussed in the preceding section correspond to the histologic phases.

During florid and mixed phases, there are variable degrees of usual duct hyperplasia (UDH) present. When the underlying cause of estrogen-to-androgen ratio imbalance is severe or long-standing, UDH can become florid or papillary, and in some instances, it may involve into papillomas, atypical ductal hyperplasia, or even ductal carcinoma *in situ* (DCIS).

UDH may result in hypersecretion and duct ectasia. The duct ectasia is generally mild and transient, especially in physiologic gynecomastia. However, when the underlying cause for alteration in the estrogen-to-androgen ratio imbalance is long-standing and severe, duct ectasia may persist and become severe. Severe duct ectasia in males is subject to all the same complications as it is in females. Chronic duct ectasia can lead to periductal mastitis, periductal fibrosis, cholesterol granuloma formation, and acute and chronic subareolar abscess formation.

Mature lobules are rarely seen in males. Gynecomastia is a manifestation of estrogen effect, whereas lobules are a manifestation of progesterone effect. Progesterone levels generally are not elevated enough in patients with gynecomastia to stimulate lobular formation and maturation. However, in severe and long-standing cases of gynecomastia, a few immature lobules may develop. Additionally, in cases in which prohormones are taken or elevated by intrinsic causes, lobular development may be more extensive.

If the underlying cause of gynecomastia is treated or resolves spontaneously, the gynecomastia tends to resolve spontaneously soon after, preventing progression to the second or third phases. Rapid and spontaneous complete regression during proliferative or early mixed phases occurs most commonly in adolescents. In adults, the causes of gynecomastia are more likely to be long-standing, and gynecomastia is more likely to have time to progress to the late mixed or quiescent phases. The deposition of dense fibrous tissue is permanent, so that gynecomastia that has reached the fibrous phase generally never completely resolves without surgical excision.

Mammographic Findings

Mammography is effective at distinguishing pseudogynecomastia from true gynecomastia. In pseudogynecomastia, the entire breast is fatty, and there are no prominent water-density tissues in the subareolar regions of the breast. In gynecomastia, there is a triangular area of water-density tissue radiating out from the nipple into the breast tissues that represents the stimulated subareolar ducts and variable amounts of periductal fibrous tissue (Fig. 16–3). Although this triangle can be symmetric, it frequently extends farther into the upper outer quadrants of the breast than it does to the medial and inferior quadrants of the breast. The sides of this density are usually straight or concave, whereas the deep margin appears serrated because the ducts diverge widely enough more deeply in the breast for fat to insinuate itself between the ducts. More superficially, the ducts and their enveloping periductal fibrous tissue are so closely packed that the mammographic density appears fairly homogeneous. The size of the subareolar water-density tissue is proportionate to the severity and degree of stimulation. Generally, the tissue appears most prominent in the proliferative and early mixed phases and less prominent in late mixed and quiescent phases.

In most cases, mammography is effective at distinguishing a neoplastic nodule or mass from gynecomastia. However, when gynecomastia is markedly asymmetric and

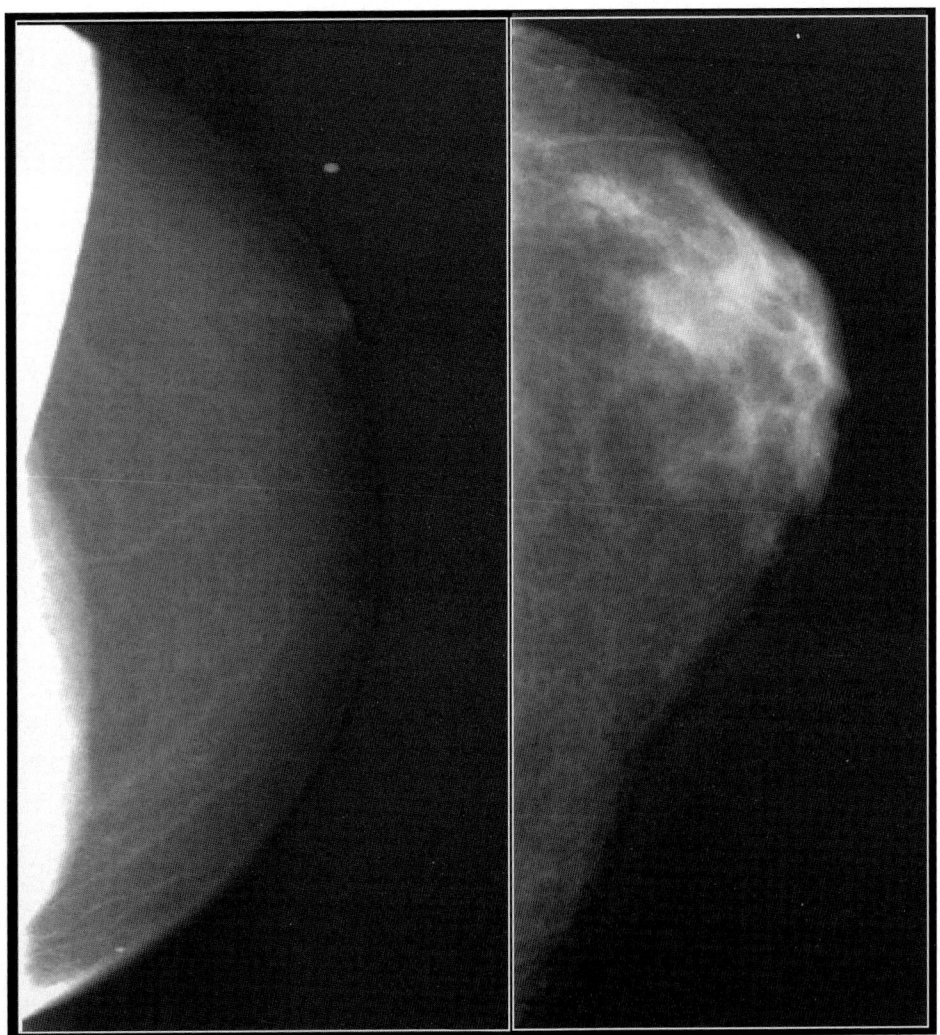

FIGURE 16–3 Mammography and ultrasound can distinguish pseudogynecomastia from true gynecomastia, but the clinical exam often cannot. In pseudogynecomastia, the breasts are enlarged entirely by fatty tissues, and the subareolar ducts and the periductal stroma are not stimulated and enlarged (**left**). Gynecomastia typically forms a deltoid-shaped water density that radiates out from the nipple, usually eccentrically laterally toward the upper outer quadrants. The lateral margins of the water-density ducts and periductal stromal tissue are usually straight or concave. The deep margin is irregular, with fat lobules interspersed between ducts (**right**).

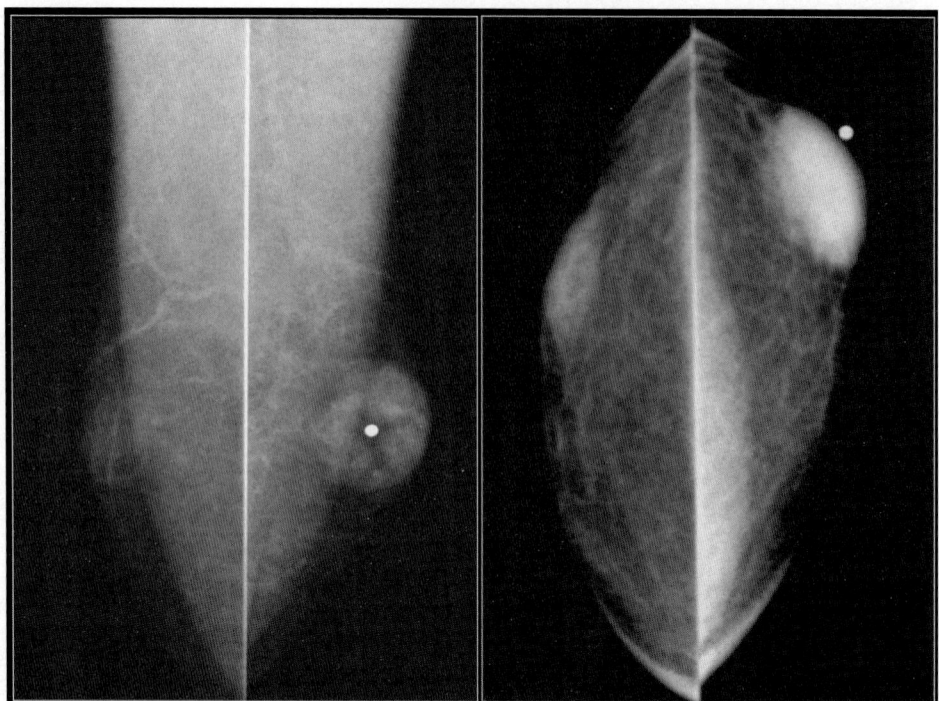

FIGURE 16–4 Markedly asymmetric or unilateral gynecomastia more frequently has convex margins than does bilaterally symmetric gynecomastia. Convex margins make it more difficult to distinguish between gynecomastia and neoplasm mammographically. Sonography is generally more useful than mammography in such patients.

florid, the cluster of subareolar ducts can have convex outward margins that simulate a mass and require additional evaluation with sonography (Fig. 16–4). In such cases, ultrasound is usually more effective than mammography in distinguishing between neoplasm and gynecomastia.

Because the detection of calcification, for which mammography is generally more sensitive than sonography, is not as important in males as it is in females, sonography rather than mammography can be used as the first diagnostic imaging examination.

Sonographic Findings

The sonographic appearance of gynecomastia correlates directly with the histologic phase of the process. In the proliferative phase, hypoechoic prominent subareolar ducts and variable degrees of edematous periductal stromal fibrous tissue dominate the sonographic appearance. Proliferative phase gynecomastia invariably appears nearly completely hypoechoic (Fig. 16–5). When scanned from a straight anterior approach, the sonographic appearance can demonstrate multiple suspicious sonographic features, including marked hypoechogenicity, angular margins, and branch pattern. Additionally, the cluster of stimulated subareolar

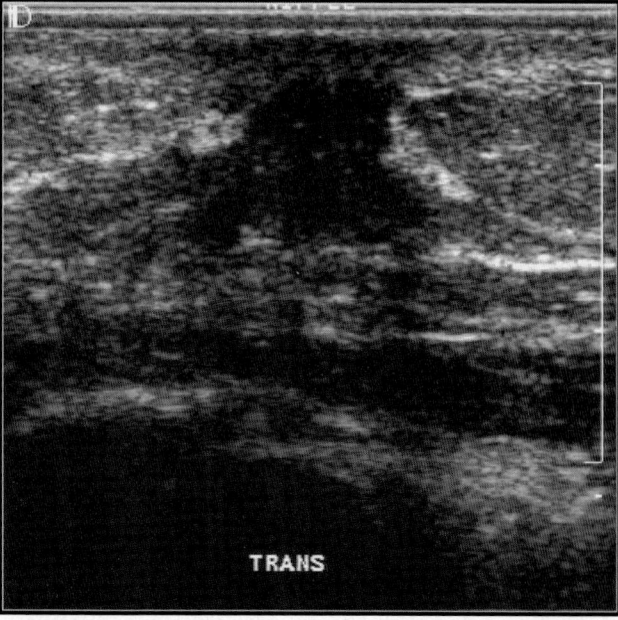

FIGURE 16–5 The sonographic appearance of proliferative-phase gynecomastia is dominated by hypoechoic, markedly enlarged, and stimulated subareolar ducts.

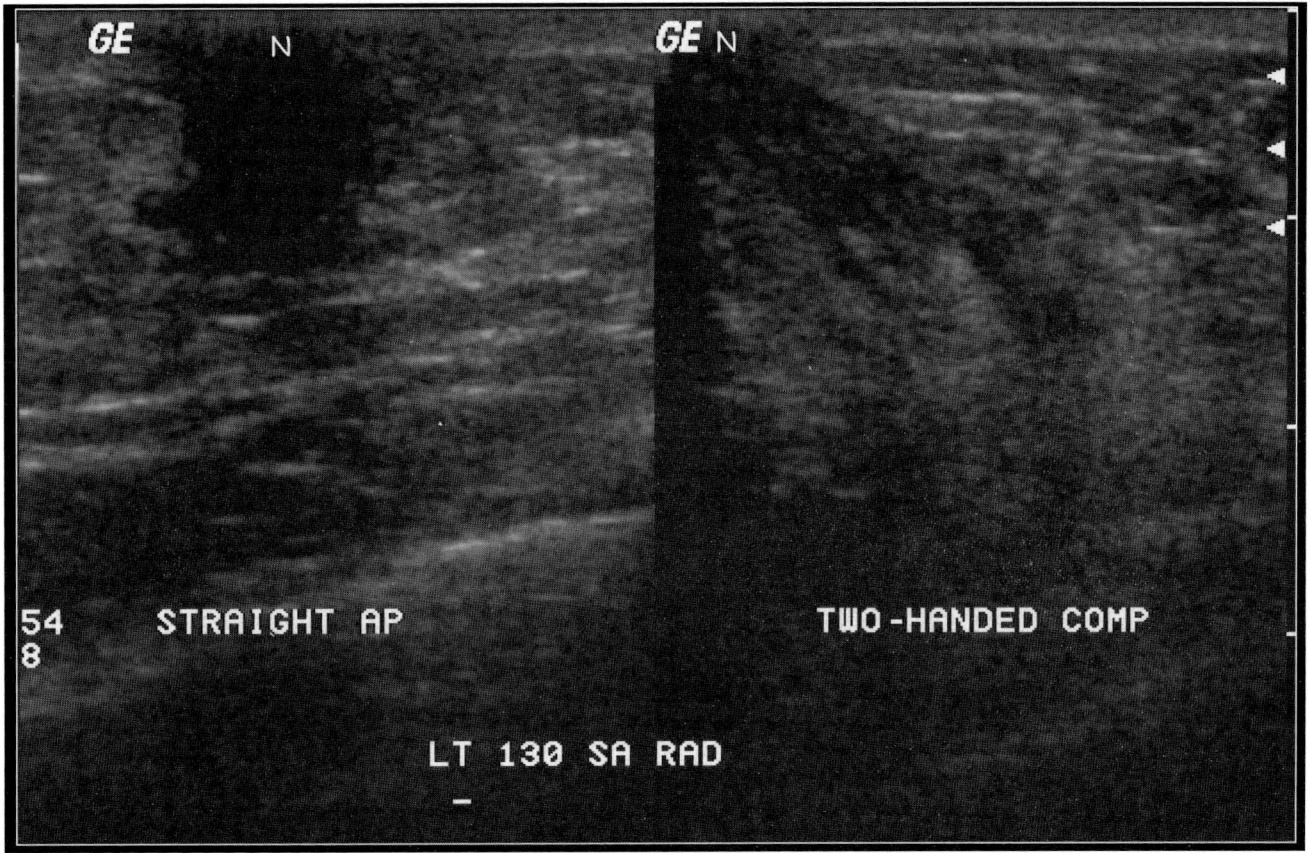

FIGURE 16–6 When scanned from straight anteriorly, the proliferative phase of gynecomastia can be very difficult to distinguish from a malignant subareolar mass. It is markedly hypoechoic, taller than wide, has angular margins and branch pattern, and sometimes has microlobulation. The individual ducts are poorly defined and cannot be identified as separate structures because they are oriented nearly parallel to the ultrasound beam and make poor specular reflectors (**left**). However, when viewed during the two-handed compression maneuver, the same subareolar ducts are viewed at an angle of incidence of nearly 90 degrees, and the ducts are compressed, allowing individual ducts to be well demonstrated and eradicating the worrisome masslike appearance (**right**). The sonographic appearance of proliferative gynecomastia from an anterior approach would have to be characterized as suspicious, BIRADS 4. The appearance during the two-handed compression maneuver can be characterized as benign gynecomastia, BIRADS 2. N, nipple.

ducts often appears taller than wide. Because the stimulated ducts lie parallel to the beam and are weak spicular reflectors when oriented in that way, they cannot be identified sonographically as ducts and appear masslike. To assess the subareolar ducts in the male, one must use a special maneuver, the two-handed compression technique, which we developed to better assess the subareolar ducts in females who present with nipple discharge (Fig. 16–6).

Physiologic gynecomastia of newborns and physiologic pubertal gynecomastia usually resolve quickly enough that they are typically seen only in the proliferative phase. The sonographic appearance of newborn gynecomastia is identical in male and female infants and is illustrated and discussed in Chapter 4. The active phase of physiologic pubertal gynecomastia is very similar to the sonographic appearance of premature thelarche in girls in physiology,

histologic features, and sonographic appearance. Both pubertal gynecomastia and premature thelarche reflect primarily estrogenic stimulation of the subareolar ducts and periductal stromal tissues. Additionally, both pubertal gynecomastia and premature thelarche may affect the breasts asymmetrically (Fig. 16–7). Not until establishment of regular ovulation and mature corpus lutea does the female breast develop mature lobules that differentiate it sonographically from the male breast with gynecomastia.

The sonographic appearance of mixed phase reflects the presence of both prominent hypoechoic ducts and markedly hyperechoic dense periductal fibrous tissues (Fig. 16–8). The hyperechoic fibrous tissue enables the sonographer to identify individual ducts, even from an anterior approach, and results in a less suspicious appearance than that of proliferative phase gynecomastia, but the two-

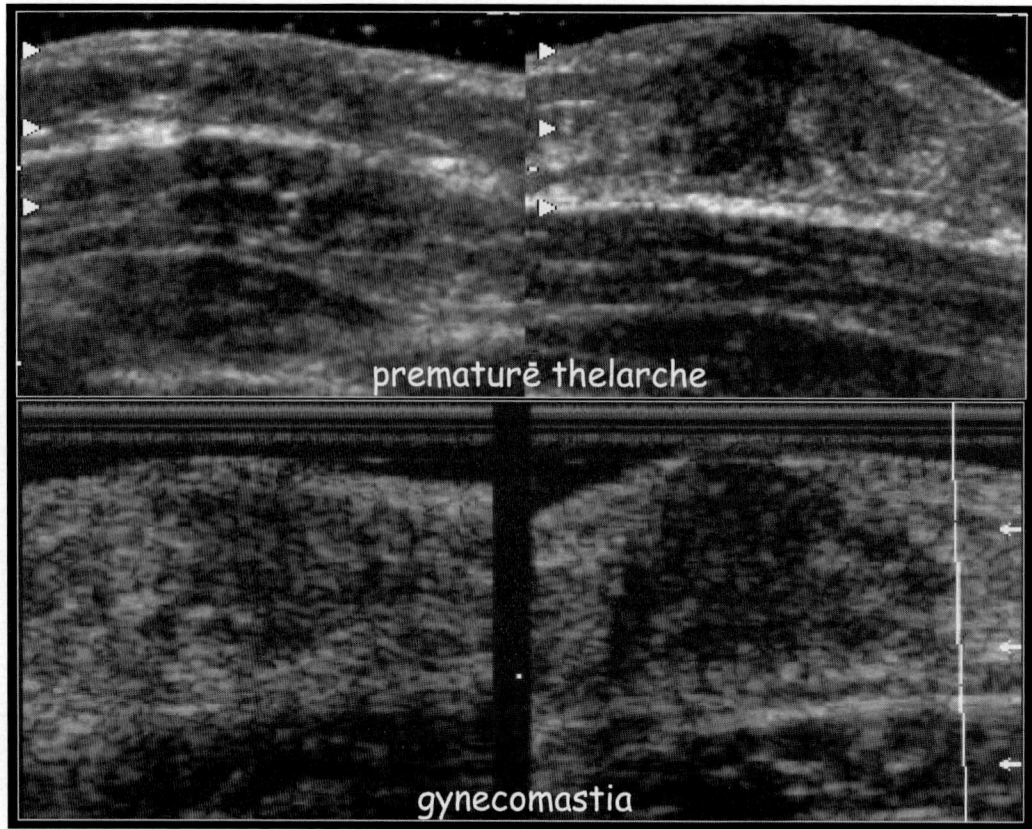

FIGURE 16–7 The sonographic appearances and histology of physiologic gynecomastia of puberty are very similar to those of premature thelarche. Both demonstrate estrogen-stimulated and enlarged ducts and periductal stromal elements but lack findings of mature lobules because of absence of progesterone effects.

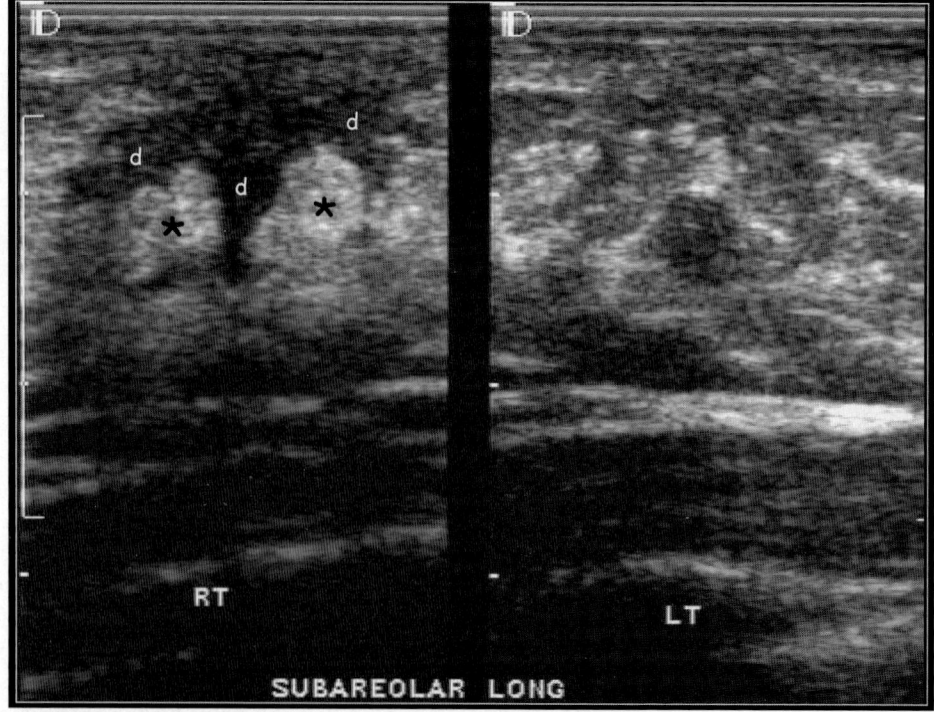

FIGURE 16–8 Mixed-phase gynecomastia is characterized by enlarged hypoechoic ducts *(d)* with interposed hyperechoic fibrous tissues *(*)*. Although occurring after the proliferative phase, mixed-phase gynecomastia is still active and tender. The enlarged hypoechoic ducts often contain duct hyperplasia. Like the proliferative phase, the mixed phase can be markedly asymmetric.

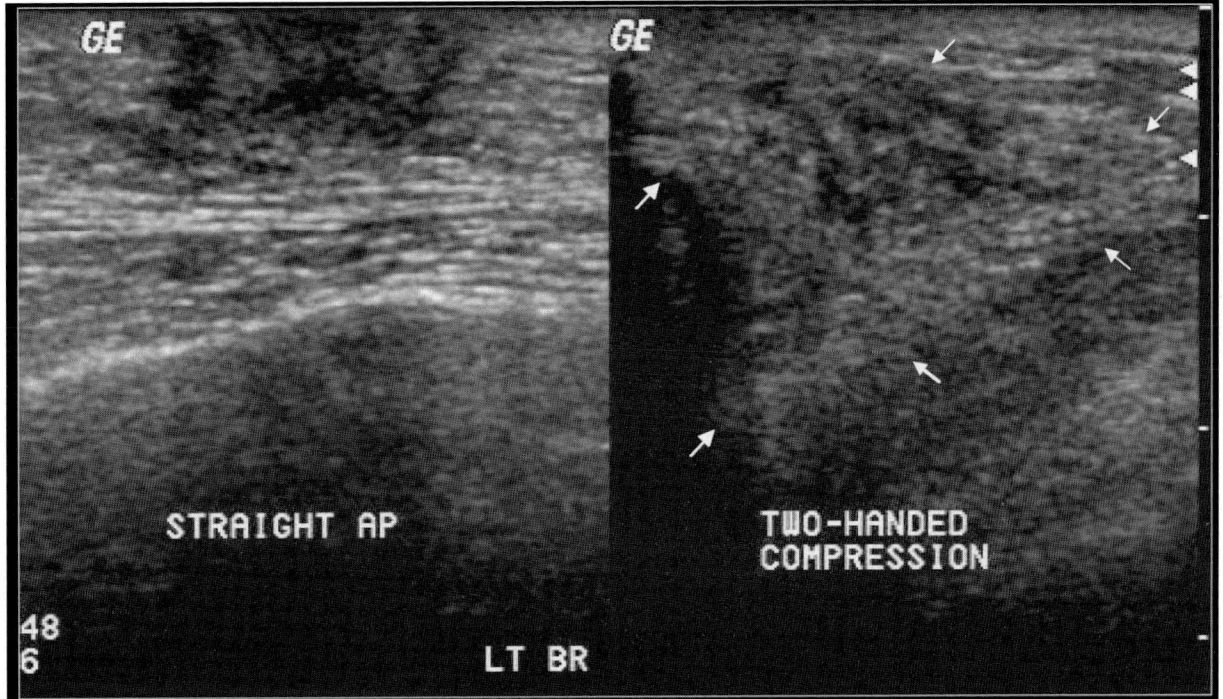

FIGURE 16–9 The two-handed compression maneuver may not be necessary in every case of mixed-phase gynecomastia, but in many cases, it can be very helpful. Note the individually resolved hypoechoic ducts surrounded by a trapezoidal collection of hyperechoic periductal stromal fibrous tissue *(arrow)*.

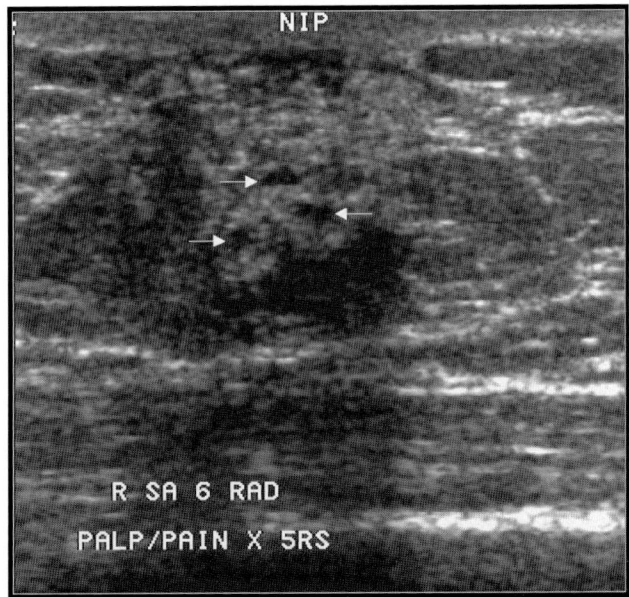

FIGURE 16–10 Hyperechoic periductal stromal fibrous tissue dominates the sonographic appearance of the quiescent phase of gynecomastia. In some cases, such as this, small residual ducts can be seen *(arrows)*. In others, ducts are not visible. Although ducts can regress if the cause of elevated estrogen-to-androgen level resolves, the hyperechoic fibrous elements that are laid down generally are permanent.

handed compression technique is helpful in enough cases that we still use it routinely. As is the case for proliferative phase gynecomastia, the two-handed compression technique enables the sonographer or sonologist to look at the subareolar ducts at an angle of incidence that is more nearly perpendicular to the long axis of the ducts and also compresses the ducts (Fig. 16–9).

The quiescent phase of gynecomastia is dominated by hyperechoic fibrous tissue. The prominent hypoechoic subareolar ducts have regressed and may be sonographically invisible; but more typically, they are visible but small (Fig. 16–10). The two-handed compression maneuver generally adds little in the evaluation of quiescent phase gynecomastia. In patients who have quiescent gynecomastia and who later become obese, fat lobules may be interspersed within the fibrous tissue, simulating the appearance of some lipomas (Fig. 16–11).

Ductal growth in the proliferative phase of gynecomastia is metabolically active enough to cause hyperemia that is easily demonstrable with color Doppler (Fig. 16–12). There may also be demonstrable hyperemia early in mixed phase gynecomastia. Color Doppler shows no evidence of increased blood flow during the quiescent phase of gynecomastia. The degree of hyperemia on color Doppler directly correlates with the degree of ductal stimulation and hyperplasia.

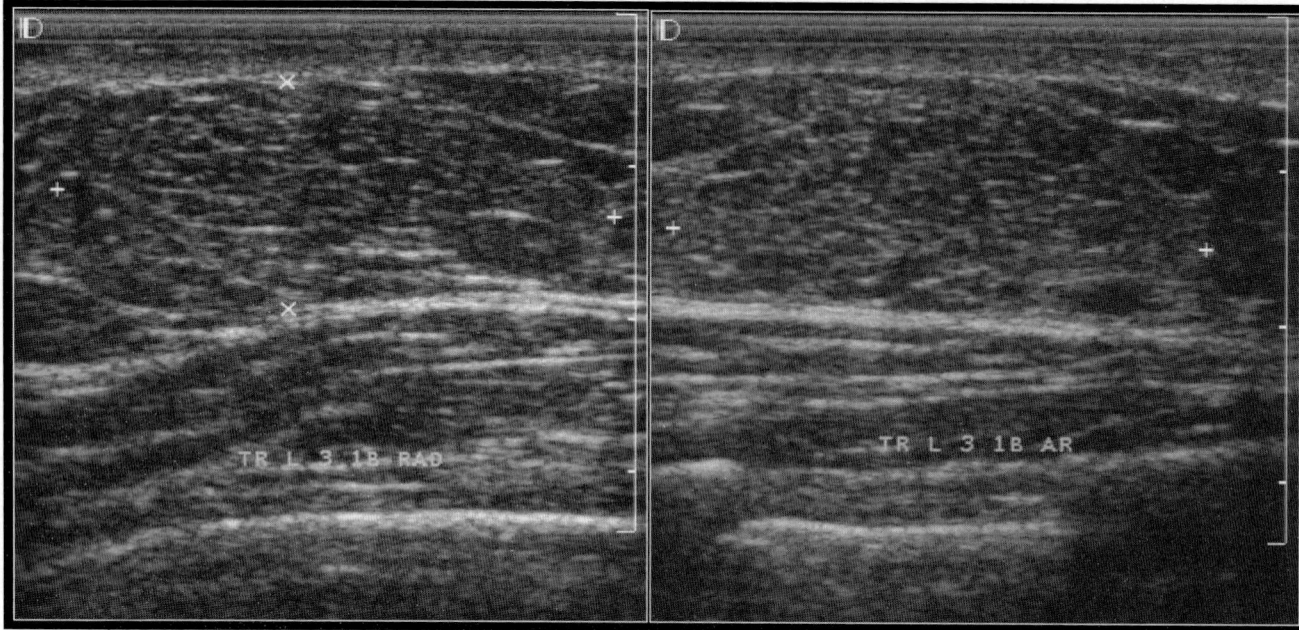

FIGURE 16–11 This patient with quiescent-phase gynecomastia has gained much weight since the cause of his gynecomastia was cured. He has no residual prominent ducts, but fat lobules that lie between the residual hyperechoic fibrous elements have expanded, pushing the fibrous elements apart. Some lipomas can have a very similar appearance.

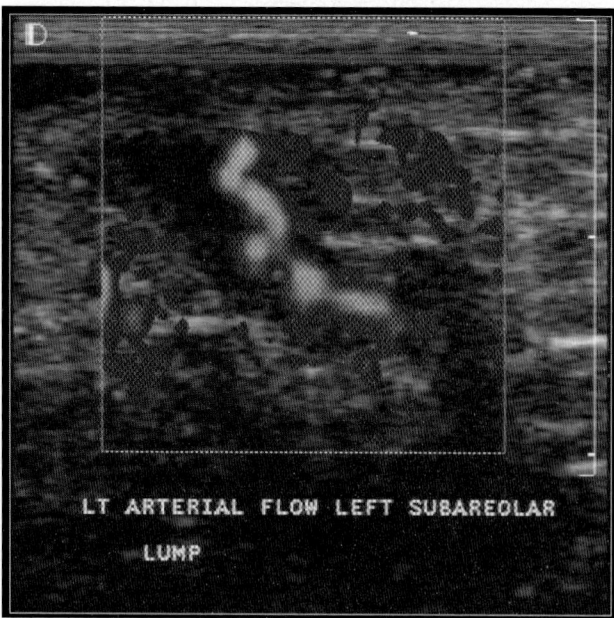

FIGURE 16–12 The enlarged hypoechoic ducts in proliferative and mixed phases of gynecomastia are metabolically very active and frequently associated with visibly increased flow by color and power Doppler.

Most patients who appear to have unilateral gynecomastia clinically actually have markedly asymmetric bilateral involvement that is demonstrable by mammography and sonography (Fig. 16–13). However, in rare circumstances, sonography confirms the clinical suspicion of unilateral gynecomastia to be truly unilateral (Fig. 16–14).

During the mixed and proliferative phases of gynecomastia, when duct hyperplasia is severe, duct ectasia may develop. The hyperplastic duct epithelium secretes fluid into the duct lumen, causing it to dilate. The degree of duct ectasia is usually mild to moderate (Fig. 16–15). As in women, duct ectasia can cause nipple discharge but is more often asymptomatic. It is highly likely that duct ectasia is underdiagnosed during sonography from a straight anterior approach because individual ducts are poorly demonstrated owing to an angle of incidence too close to 0 degrees. In our experience, duct ectasia is often only demonstrable during the two-handed compression maneuver (Fig. 16–16).

In males who do have duct ectasia, any of the complications of the duct ectasia–periductal mastitis complex that are seen in females can occur, including rupture of the ducts that leads to periareolar abscess (Fig. 16–17), fistulous tracts, and nipple retraction.

(text continued on page 727)

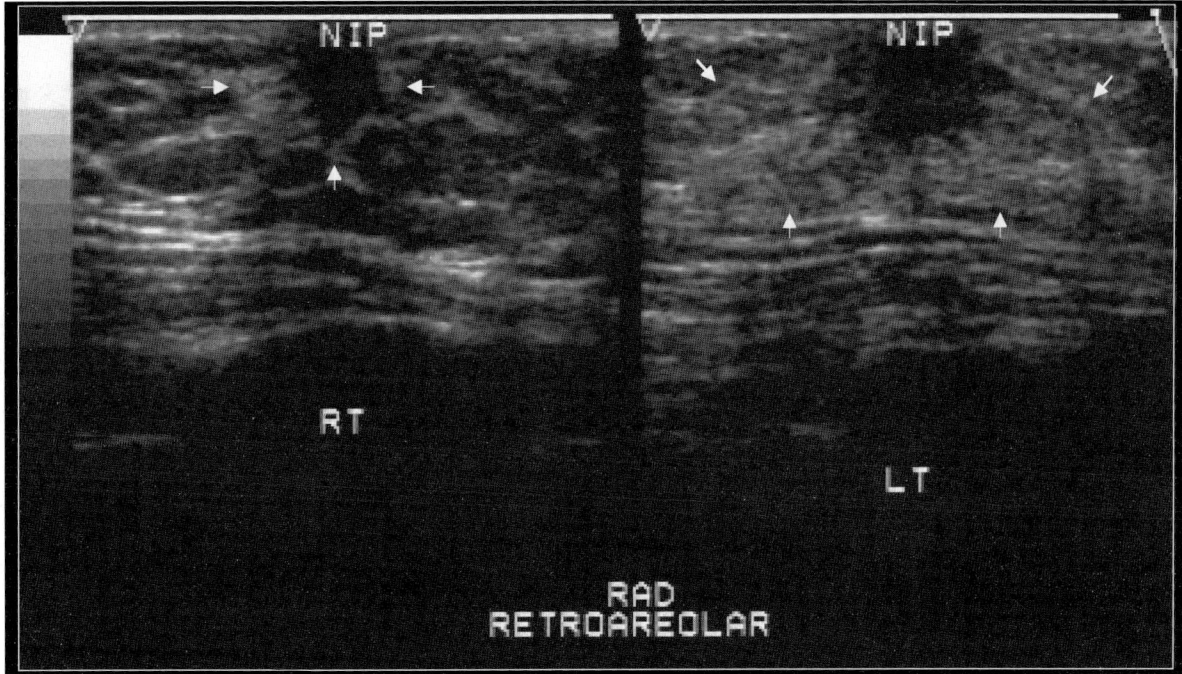

FIGURE 16–13 Most patients who appear clinically to have unilateral gynecomastia actually have markedly asymmetric bilateral gynecomastia *(arrows)* that can be shown by sonography and mammography. This patient appeared to have unilateral gynecomastia clinically but actually had markedly asymmetric bilateral mixed-phase gynecomastia *(arrows)* shown by sonography.

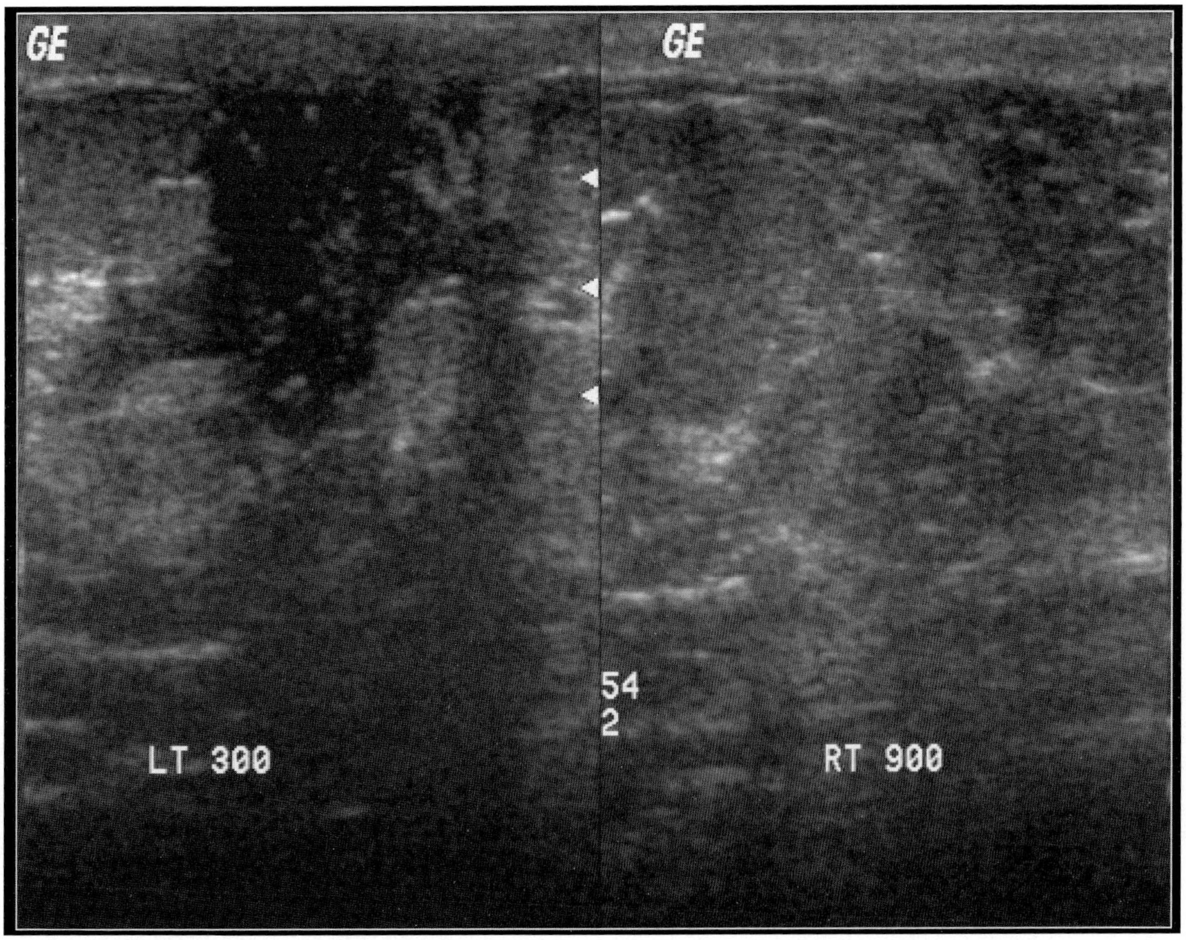

FIGURE 16–14 Although most cases of clinically apparent unilateral gynecomastia are actually caused by asymmetric bilateral gynecomastia, rare cases of true unilateral gynecomastia do occur. This patient has florid proliferative-phase ducts on the left and no visible ducts on the right.

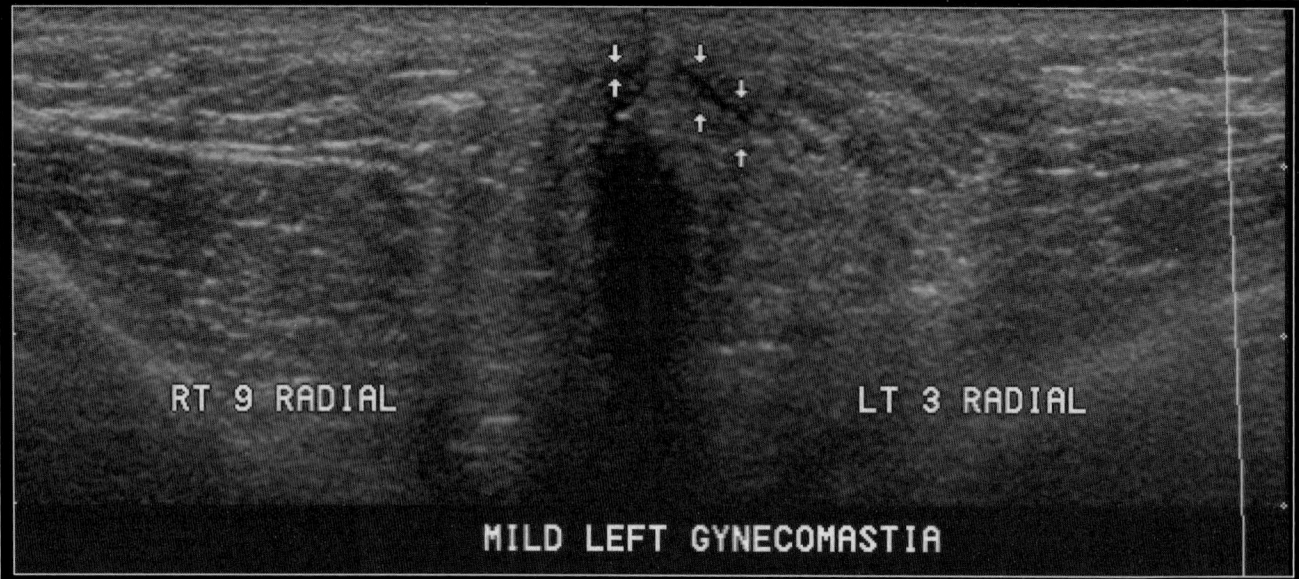

RT 9 RADIAL   LT 3 RADIAL

MILD LEFT GYNECOMASTIA

FIGURE 16–15 Mild to moderate duct ectasia occasionally occurs in association with gyneco-mastia and, as in women, may or may not cause nipple discharge. The mild duct ectasia in this man did not cause secretions.

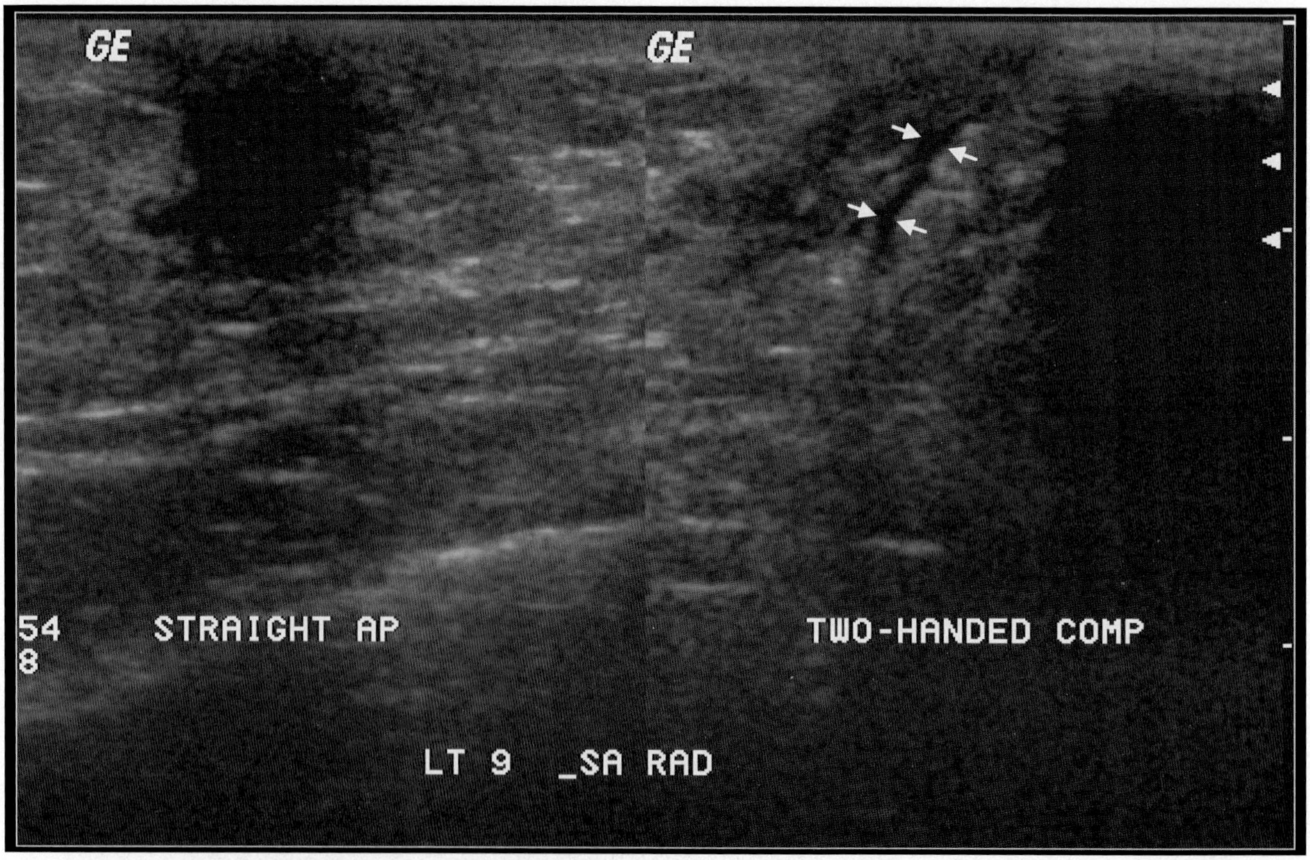

GE   GE

54
8   STRAIGHT AP   TWO-HANDED COMP

LT 9 _SA RAD

FIGURE 16–16 The incidence of duct ectasia is likely to be much higher than the published fig-ures but underdiagnosed by sonography. The ectatic duct in this patient cannot be seen when a traditional anterior approach is used (**left**). However, the improved angle of incidence created by the two-handed compression technique (**right**) readily allows us to demonstrate the moderately ectatic, fluid-filled duct (arrows).

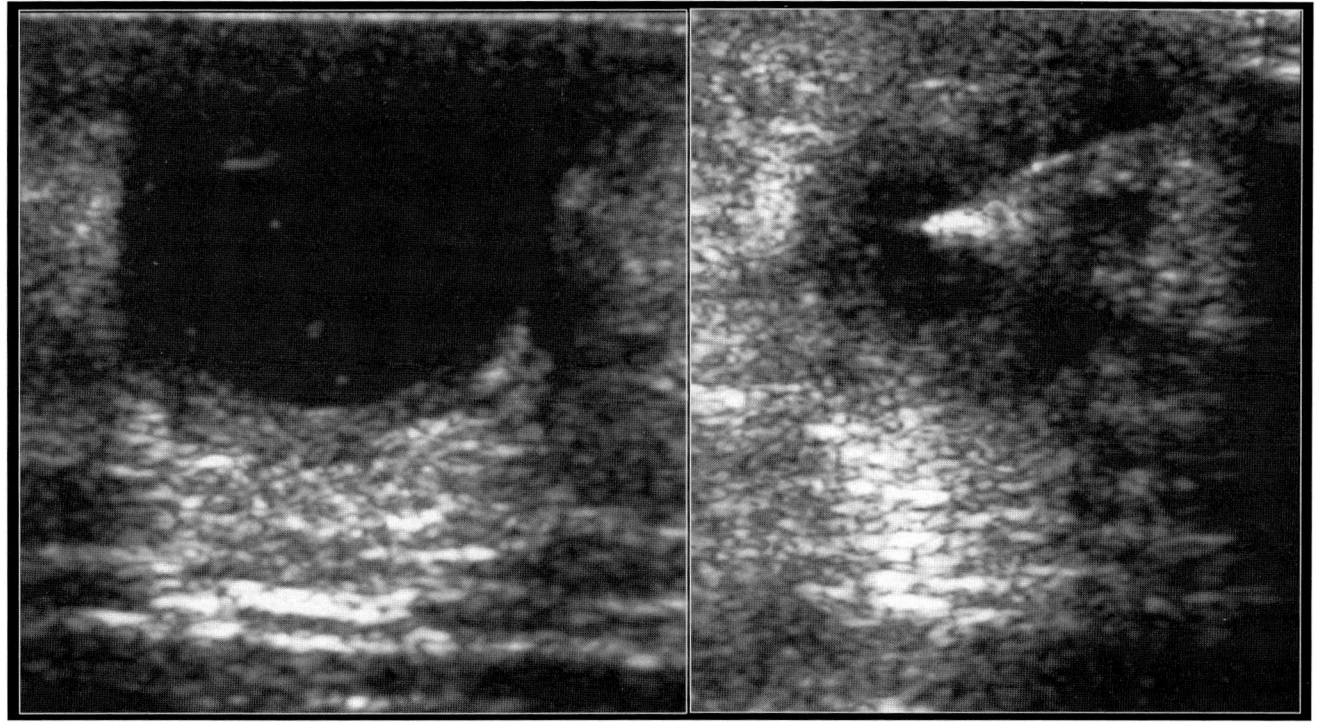

FIGURE 16–17 Sonography showed the mass to be caused by a subareolar abscess, a complication of duct ectasia (**left**). Aspiration was performed (**right**) and showed purulent fluid that revealed *Staphylococcus aureus* on Gram stain and culture. The patient had proliferative-phase gynecomastia with duct ectasia on the contralateral side.

OTHER BENIGN CONDITIONS ARISING FROM MALE DUCTS AND PERIDUCTAL STROMAL FIBROUS TISSUES

Benign tumors arising from ducts and periductal stroma tissue of the male breast are rare. Benign lesions arising from the stimulated ducts in the male breast include intraductal and intracystic papillomas. Their sonographic features are similar to the features of papillomas in the female breast. Intraductal papillomas are discussed in greater detail in Chapter 8, and intracystic papillomas are discussed in greater detail in Chapter 10. Rare cases of juvenile papillomatosis have also been reported in the male breast. The sonographic appearances are similar to those in females and are discussed in greater detail in Chapter 15. Benign lesions that arise from periductal stromal elements that have been reported in males include fibrosclerosis, diabetic mastopathy, and pseudoangiomatous stromal hyperplasia. The sonographic appearances of such rare lesions are similar to the appearances in females and are discussed in greater detail in Chapter 13.

Lesions that normally arise from lobules, such as fibroadenomas, most fibrocystic changes, and phyllodes tumors, have been reported in males but occur even more rarely than benign lesions of ductal and periductal stromal because mature lobules rarely develop in the male breast.

Only when the underlying cause for hormonal imbalance is severe and prolonged do males develop lobules and lesions of lobular origin.

BENIGN LESIONS THAT ARISE FROM SKIN AND SUBCUTANEOUS, VASCULAR, LYMPHATIC, AND NEURAL TISSUES

Skin, subcutaneous tissue, blood vessels, nerves, and lymphatic tissues are present everywhere in the body. The lesions that arise from these structures can involve any part of the body, including the breast. Such lesions generally are not any more likely to arise in the breast than they are elsewhere in the body. Because the male breasts constitute only very a small percentage of the body, only a small percentage of such lesions involve the breast—generally 5% or 6%. The histology of such lesions is generally similar, regardless of the part of the body in which they arise. As is always the case, the sonographic features merely reflect the gross morphology and histology of the lesion. Thus, a lesion that arises within the subcutaneous fat of the male breast, such as a lipoma, looks identical histologically and sonographically to a lipoma that arises from the subcutaneous tissues of the back, arm, or leg. Similarly, the histology and sonographic features of skin and subcutaneous lesions, such as sebaceous cysts and lipomas, are nearly identical in males and females.

Skin lesions that are as common in the male breast as in the female breast include sebaceous cysts, moles, and epidermal inclusion cysts. These are skin lesions that have incidentally occurred within the skin overlying the male breast, not true breast lesions. Nevertheless, certain patients with such lesions do present to the breast radiologist for diagnosis, requiring that the breast radiologist recognize and understand such lesions. Sebaceous cysts in the area of the male breast most commonly occur in the presternal and parasternal areas (Fig. 16–18) and near the axilla. An acoustic standoff pad or a thick dollop of acoustic gel is usually necessary to demonstrate sebaceous cysts adequately (Fig. 16–19). The sonographic features of sebaceous cysts are discussed in greater detail in Chapter 10.

Subcutaneous lesions that involve the male breast include lipomas and fat necrosis. After gynecomastia, lipomas are the second most common male breast lesion that a sonographer will see. Lipomas are nearly as common in the male breast as in the female breast. There are slight differences in lipomas in males and females. First, male breast stroma contains very little fat; hence, lipomas in males almost all arise from the subcutaneous fat rather than from the mammary zone. In women, lipomas can arise within the mammary zone, retromammary fat, or subcutaneous fat. As in the female breast, lipomas in the male breast can be isoechoic, hyperechoic, or mixed in echogenicity. For

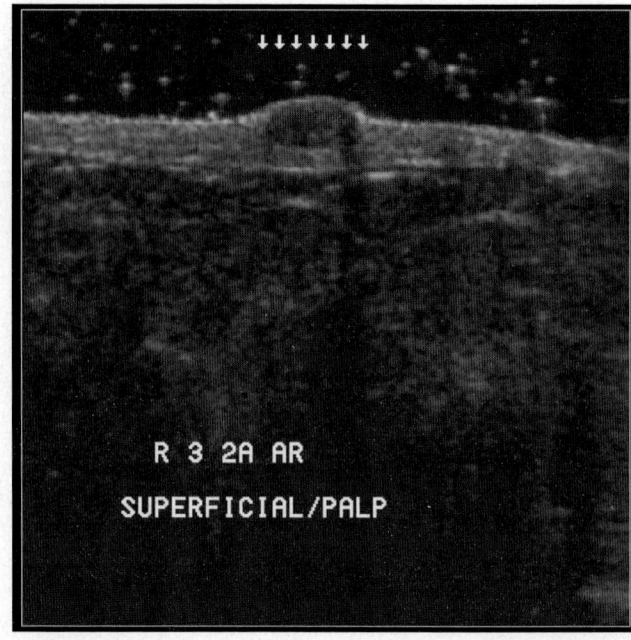

FIGURE 16–19 As in women, demonstration of sebaceous cysts and other skin lesions usually requires an acoustic standoff pad or, as in this case, a standoff of a thick layer of acoustic gel.

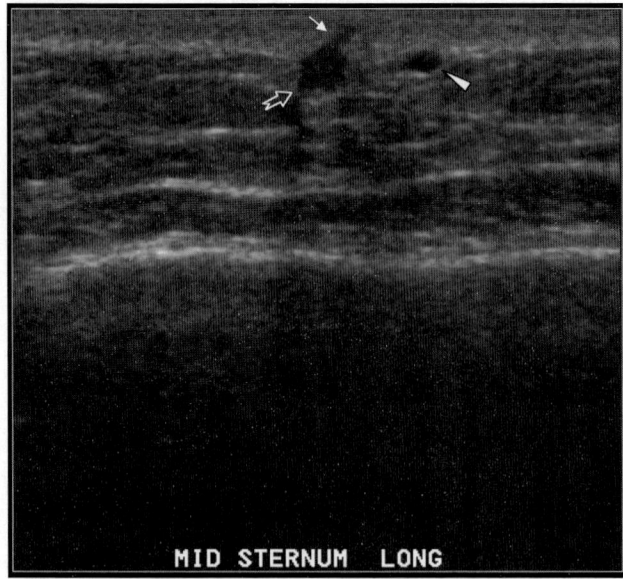

FIGURE 16–18 Sebaceous cysts and epidermal inclusion cysts are skin lesions that can occur in the breast and therefore occur relatively commonly in males as well as females. The thickened and obstructed hair follicle *(hollow arrow)* into which this epidermal cyst *(arrowhead)* drains is visible as a hypoechoic line coursing obliquely through the skin. A normal vein is visible next to the cyst *(arrowhead)*.

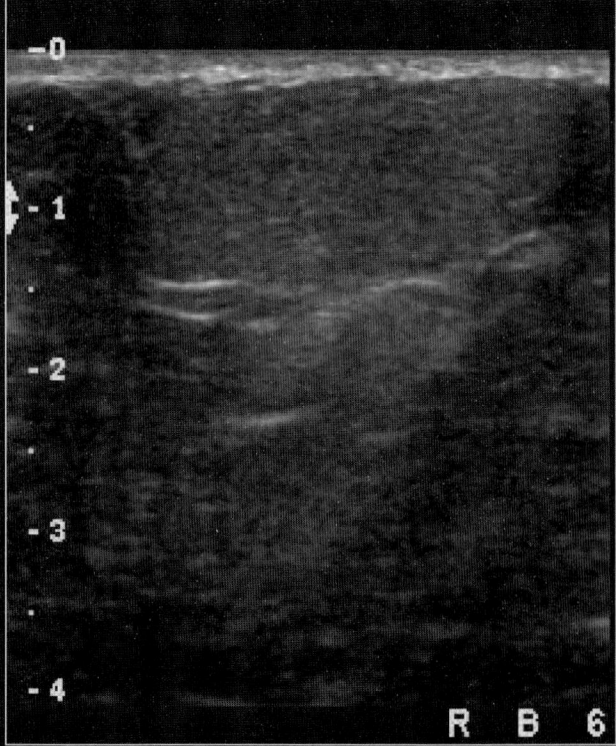

FIGURE 16–20 Lipomas in males are usually mildly hyperechoic compared with surrounding subcutaneous fat.

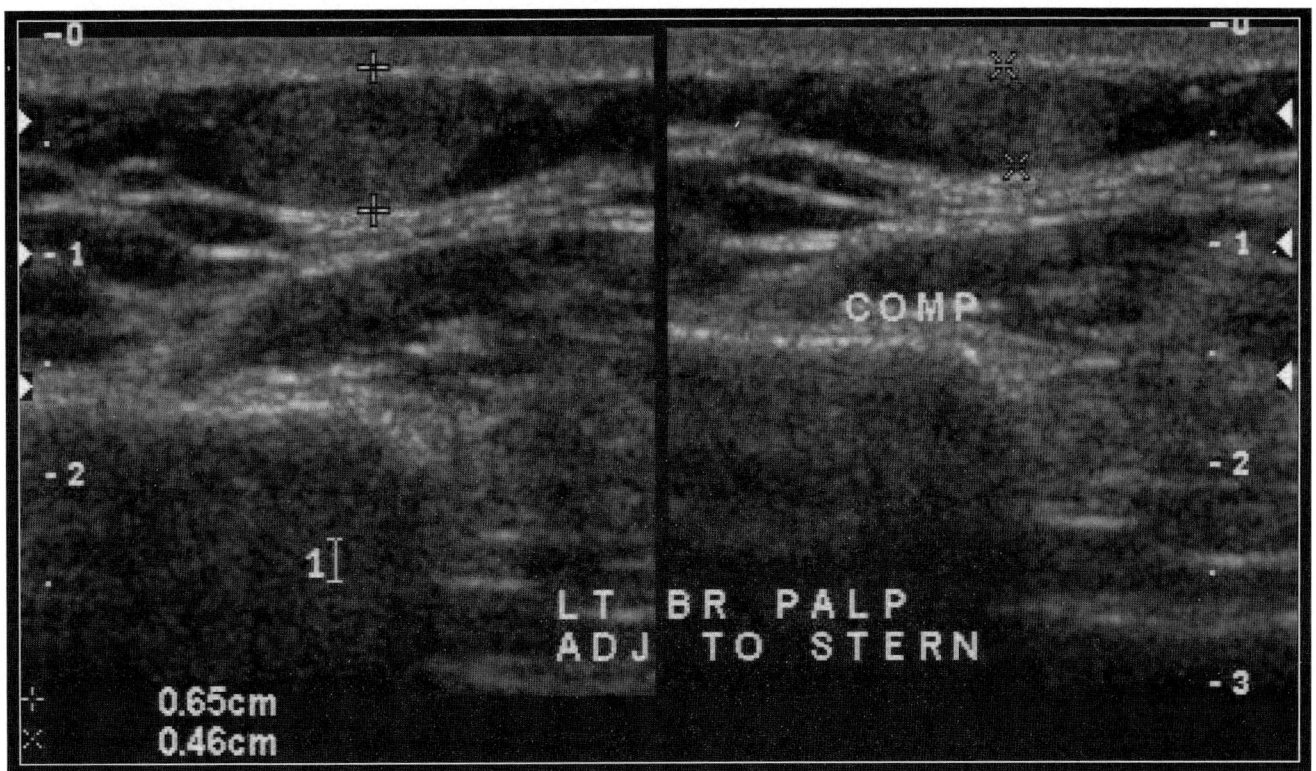

FIGURE 16–21 The hyperechoic subcutaneous lipomas that we generally see in males have higher fibrous content and therefore are slightly less compressible than are isoechoic lipomas. Hyperechoic lipomas tend to be slightly less than 30% compressible, whereas isoechoic lipomas can be compressed much more than 30%. Split-screen images obtained without **(left)** and with **(right)** vigorous compression with the transducer show this hyperechoic lipoma to be 29% compressible.

reasons that are not clear, a much larger percentage of lipomas in the male breast appear to be hyperechoic (Fig. 16–20). Hyperechoic lipomas generally contain more fibrous components than do isoechoic lipomas. Isoechoic lipomas are generally soft enough that they can be readily be compressed more than 30% in virtually all cases; however, because of higher fibrous content, the hyperechoic lipomas seen in the male breast sometimes compress less than 30% (Fig. 16–21). Nevertheless, the appearance of hyperechoic lipomas is so characteristic that they can readily be characterized as Breast Imaging Reporting and Data System (BIRADS) category 2 even if they compress slightly less than 30%. Multiple lipomas are common. Patients who have one lipoma frequently have additional lesions elsewhere in the body or elsewhere in the breast (Fig. 16–22). Lipomas are also discussed in Chapter 13.

Fat necrosis is less common within the subcutaneous fat of the male breast than it is within the female breast because males far less frequently undergo lumpectomy and biopsy than do females. Breast surgery is the most common cause of fat necrosis. However, nonsurgical breast trauma is more common in males than in females. Males suffer more direct blows from contact sports, assaults, and motor vehi-

cle crashes than do females. Seat-belt injuries can cause fat necrosis in both male and female breasts (Fig. 16–23). The subcutaneous fat that surrounds implanted pacemakers frequently undergoes fat necrosis. The sonographic appearances of fat necrosis vary greatly over time and are discussed in greater detail in Chapters 11 and 18.

Hamartomas can occur in males as well as in females. The histologic and sonographic appearances vary as greatly in males as they do in females. Hamartomas are discussed in greater detail in Chapter 13.

Vascular lesions that have been reported in the male breast include: pseudoaneurysms, arteriovenous fistulas, arteriovenous malformations, cavernous and capillary hemangiomas, venous malformations (see the color images in Chapter 20, Figs. 20–71 and 20–72), and superficial venous thrombosis. These appear similar in all parts of the body and in males and females. Some of these lesions are discussed in Chapters 11 and 13.

Lymphatic lesions include normal intramammary and axillary lymph nodes, inflamed or reactive intramammary or axillary lymph nodes, and lymphangioma (cystic hygroma). Cystic hygromas frequently involve the axillary

(text continued on page 732)

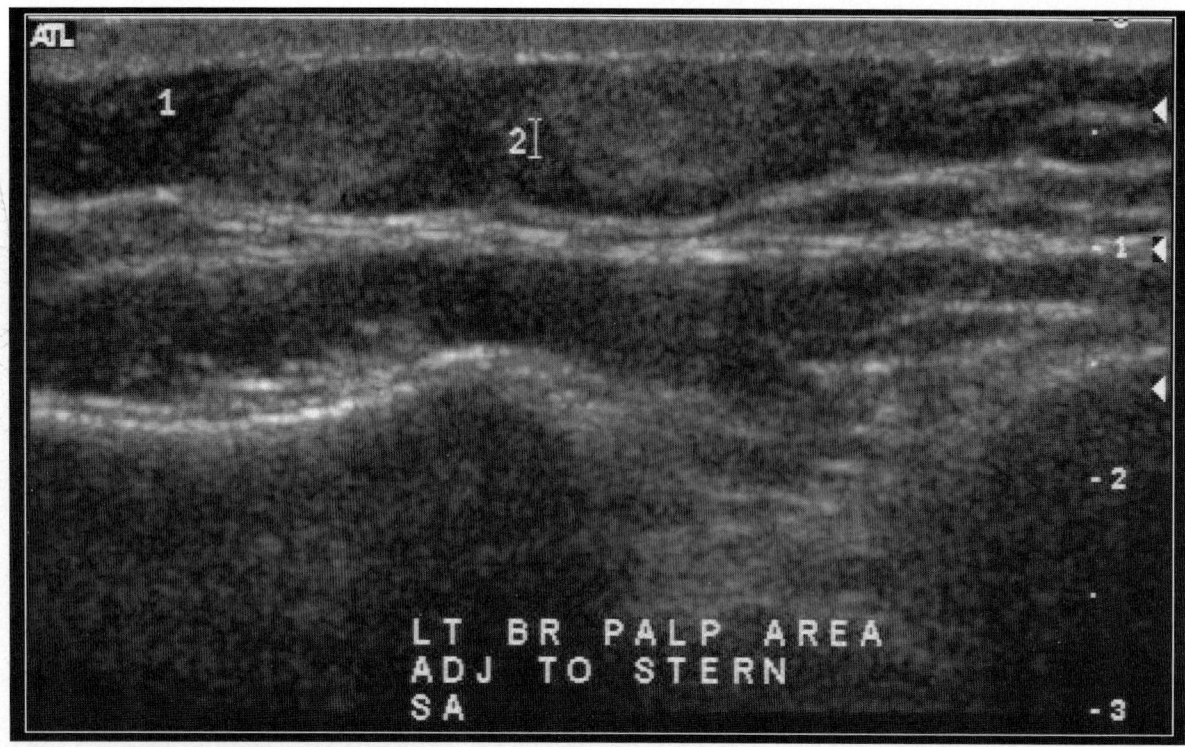

FIGURE 16–22 Both male and female patients frequently have multiple lipomas.

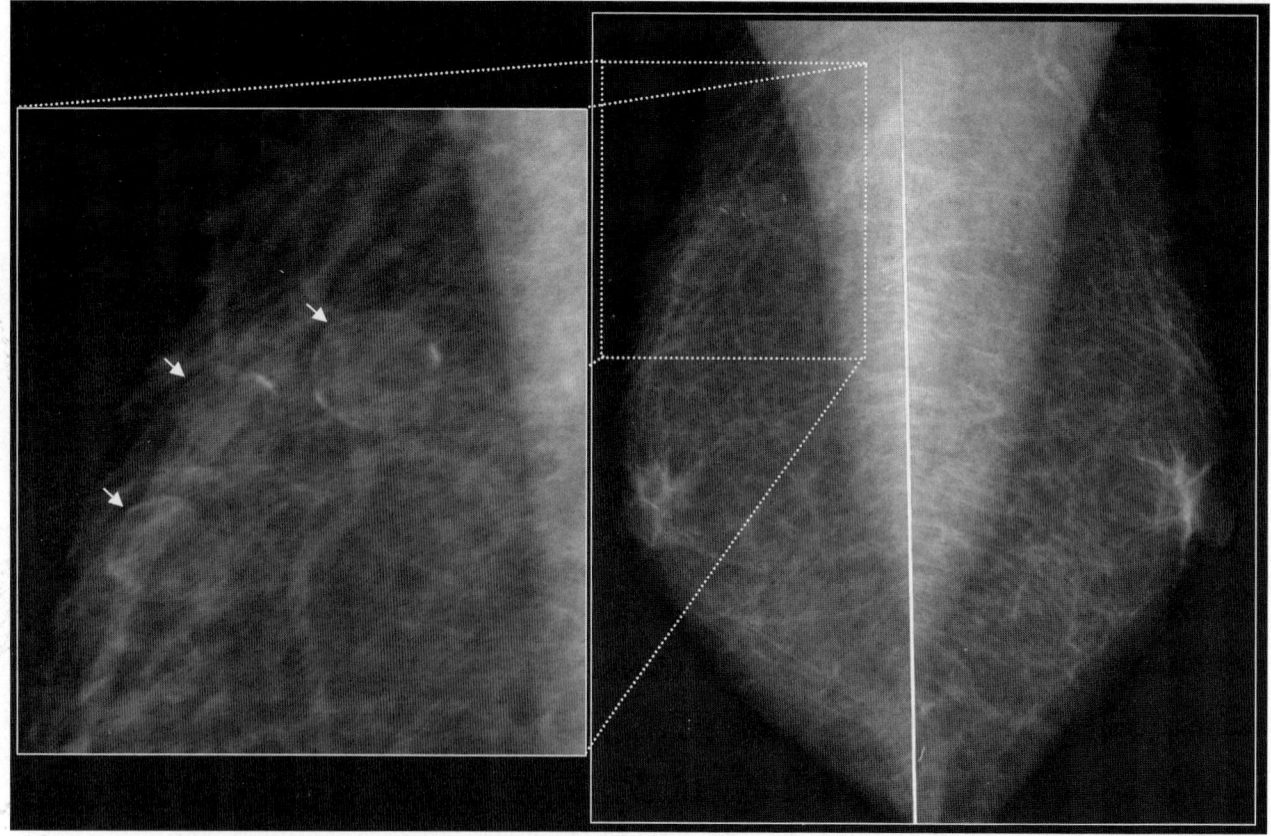

A

FIGURE 16–23. A: As in females, fat necrosis can occur. In this patient, a seat-belt injury occurred during a motor vehicle crash that was severe enough to cause ecchymosis. Over 2 years, this evolved into fat necrosis that manifested as palpable lumps and classic mammographic eggshell calcifications around lipid cysts, just as it would in females. Three calcified lipid cysts are linearly *(arrows)* arranged parallel to the line of the seat-belt injury and are best seen in the magnified view on the left. Before being seen for ultrasound, the patient had forgotten about his old injury and did not associate the old injury with the new palpable lumps. *(Continued.)*

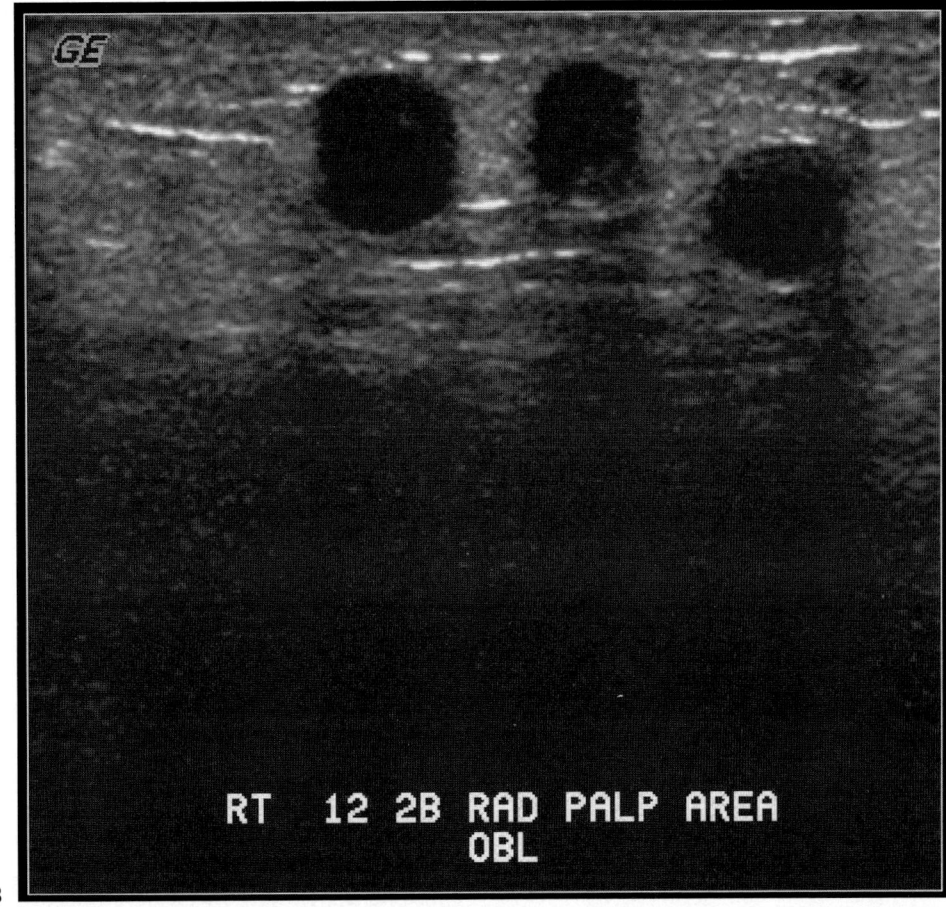

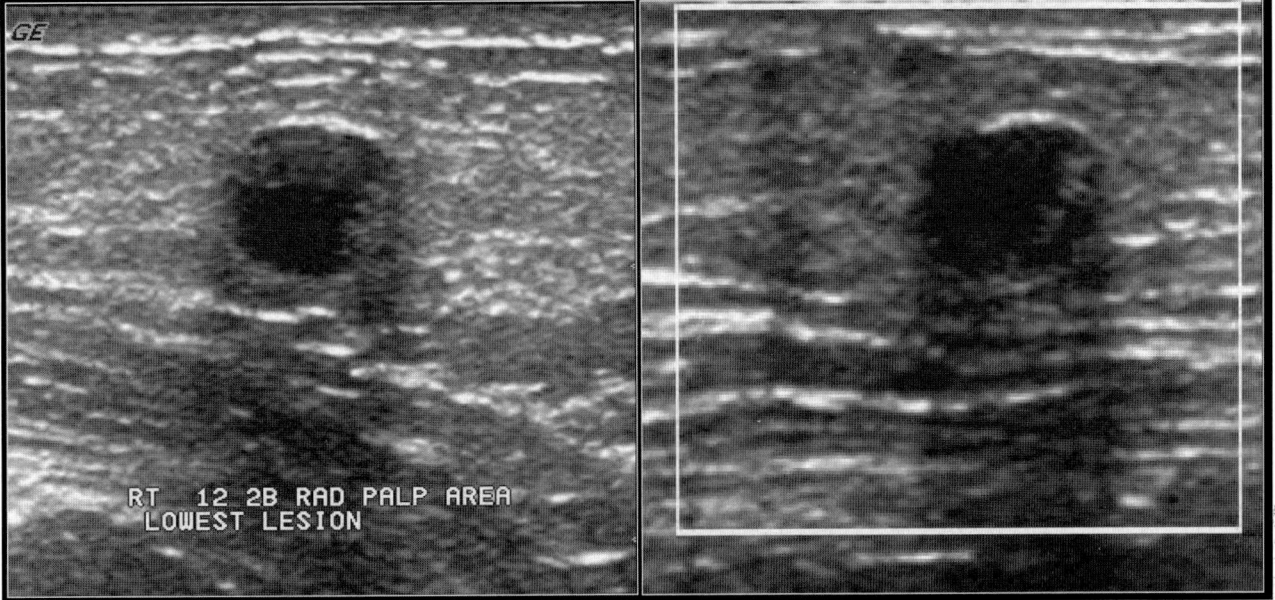

FIGURE 16–23. *(continued)* **B:** Sonography demonstrated that the three linearly arranged calcified lipid cysts caused the palpable lumps. There is little acoustic shadowing in comparison to the degree of calcification on the mammograms. **C:** A magnified view of one of the calcified lipid cysts shows a mural nodule along the wall on the right side of the image that could be mistaken for an intracystic tumor. Color Doppler shows no fibrovascular stalk, a finding that favors fat necrosis. The mural nodule is caused by adherent chronic hematoma.

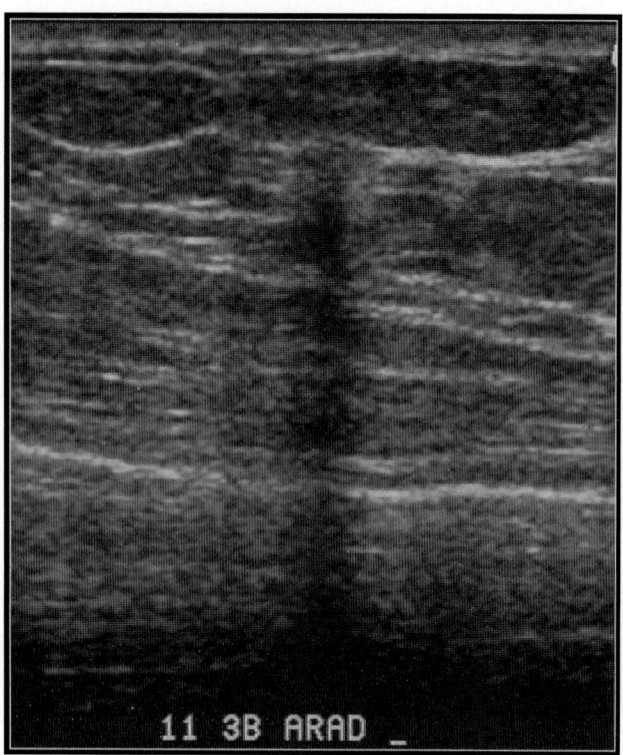

FIGURE 16–24 This granular cell tumor, a lesion of Schwann's cell origin, arose within the upper outer quadrant of the breast in a male.

region in both males and females at birth. Such lesions often appear to regress completely clinically, but in these cases, sonography may show subclinical persistence. Lymph nodes are discussed in detail in Chapter 19, and lymphangiomas are discussed in Chapter 11.

Lesions of neural origin that can involve the breast include neurofibromas and granular cell tumors. Granular cell tumors, which were originally thought to be myofibroblastomas, are now thought to arise from Schwann's cells of the neural sheath. The histology and sonographic features of such lesions are similar in males and females (Fig. 16–24). Most granular cell tumors are benign, but a few are malignant. Even benign granular cell tumors may be locally aggressive; thus, wide excision is the treatment of choice in both males and females. Granular cell tumors are also discussed in Chapter 13. The breast may have also multiple neurofibromas in neurofibromatosis.

CARCINOMA OF THE MALE BREAST

Risk Factors

Carcinoma of the male breast is rare, with about 1,400 new cases reported each year in the United States, resulting in 300 deaths. Male breast cancer accounts for less than 1% of all malignancies in males as well as less than 1% of all breast cancers. The mean age of diagnosis is between 60 and 64 years, 6 to 11 years later than found in females. Less than 1% of male breast cancers occur before the age of 30 years, and less than 6% are found before the age of 40 years. The incidence in the United States and Europe is 1 case in 100,000 male years and, unlike the incidence of breast cancer in females, has been stable over the past few decades. The incidence varies with race and ethnic background. The incidence is higher in Jewish, Egyptian, and West African black males and is lower in Japanese males. Bilateral breast cancer occurs in less than 20% in males. A multitude of risk factors, including genetic, hormonal, and environmental etiologies, play roles in the development of male breast cancer. A positive family history increases the risk twofold to fourfold. Certain genetic and chromosomal conditions are associated with increased risk for breast cancer; these include Klinefelter's syndrome (XYY chromosomes), Kallmann's (hypogonadotrophic hypogonadism) syndrome, and Cowden's syndrome (multiple hamartoma syndrome associated with germline mutations in the *PTEN* tumor suppressor gene).

The underlying common thread in different populations that are at increased risk for breast cancer is prolonged and severe elevation of the estrogen-to-androgen ratios. Thus, the factors that predisposed toward gynecomastia also increase the risk for developing breast cancer. However, despite similar underlying causes, it has been difficult to prove that there is a direct progression from gynecomastia to breast cancer. Additionally, the correlation between gynecomastia and breast cancer is weaker than one might expect because of the short duration and rapid and often spontaneous resolution of gynecomastia in such a large percentage of males. If only males whose underlying cause for imbalance in the estrogen-to-androgen ratio is chronic and severe were considered, it is likely that there would be a high correlation. The longer the duration of gynecomastia and the imbalance in estrogen-to-androgen ratios, the more likely breast cancer is to develop. Thus, it seems likely that gynecomastia indicates an increased risk for development of breast cancer only if the underlying cause is long-standing.

Chronic diseases that result in elevation of estrogen levels and that have been associated with increased risk for breast cancer include cirrhosis, schistosomiasis, and malnutrition. The high incidence of breast cancer in Egyptian males is likely due to cirrhosis associated with schistosomiasis, and the high incidence of breast cancer in West African black males is likely due to starvation and nutritional cirrhosis.

The relationship between estrogens and androgens appears to have a significant influence on the development of male breast cancer. Klinefelter's patients with XXY karyotype and elevated estradiol-to-testosterone ratio owing to chronically elevated FSH levels have a reported 3% risk and a 20-fold increased incidence of breast cancer. Patients with Klinefelter's syndrome are more likely than most other males to have bilateral breast cancer and malignancies of unusual cell types, including lymphomas.

Bilateral breast cancer has been described in both transsexual and prostate cancer patients after long-term estrogen administration. Bilateral metastases to the breast have also been reported in patients with prostate cancer treated with diethylstilbestrol (DES).

Causes of prolonged decrease in testosterone production also appear to increase the risk for breast cancer in males. Thus, males with testicular atrophy for any reason are at increased risk for breast cancer. Torsion and infarction, orchitis, severe testicular trauma, and undescended testes can all cause testicular atrophy and therefore increase the risk for breast cancer. Vascular compromise after bilateral inguinal herniorrhaphy is relatively common, and an increased incidence of breast cancer in males has actually been demonstrated in patients who have undergone inguinal herniorrhaphy.

Some studies have shown that being obese for 10 years or more increases the risk for breast cancer in males. Long-term use of digoxin, methyldopa, and serotonin uptake inhibitors also increases the risk for breast cancer in males.

Hormonal disorders other than imbalances of estrogen-to-androgen ratios may increase the risk for breast cancer in males. Bilateral benign papillomas and bilateral invasive papillary carcinomas have been reported in males with severe and prolonged hyperprolactinemia caused by pituitary adenomas, after administration of prolactin-elevating or prolactin-mimicking drugs, after serious head trauma, and after irradiation of the brain.

Occupational exposures have also been implicated in the development of breast cancer in males. Workers exposed to long-term elevations in environmental temperatures, such as blast furnace and steel workers, have an increased frequency of breast cancer. It is postulated that elevated temperatures suppress normal testicular function. Chronic exposure to electromagnetic fields in telephone linemen, electrical power workers, and electricians exposed before the age of 30 years with a latency of 30 years also have a higher incidence of breast cancer. The development of breast cancer in males exposed to ionizing radiation for intrathoracic tumors or gynecomastia has been reported.

Diseases that suppress the immune system may increase the risk for breast malignancy of all types. Patients with acquired immunodeficiency syndrome (AIDS) have more primary and metastatic breast malignancies. Malignancies that arise from skin, subcutaneous tissues, vessels, nerves, and lymphatics are also more common in patients with AIDS, including Kaposi's sarcoma and lymphoma.

There is some debate about whether the prognosis of breast cancer in males is worse than that in females. Factors that determine prognosis—maximum tumor diameter, axillary lymph node status, and involvement of critical structures such as nipple, skin, and chest wall—are similar to those in females. When matched for stage of cancer, the prognosis for males and females appears to be similar. However, males tend to present at a later stage than do females for two reasons. First, males are less aware and concerned about breast cancer and wait longer to see their doctors. Second, because the male breast is smaller than the female breast, involvement of the nipple, skin, chest wall, and lymph node tends to occur when the lesions are smaller than in females.

Clinical Findings

Males who develop breast cancer are likely to have underlying long-standing gynecomastia. It may be clinically difficult to distinguish asymmetric gynecomastia from breast cancer. Most males with breast cancer present with a painless palpable hard nodule that most commonly lies subareolarly and less frequently lies in the upper outer quadrant. Asymmetric gynecomastia is more often tender and lies directly deep to the nipple, but in long-standing gynecomastia, the situation in which breast cancer is most likely to develop, tenderness has usually resolved long before breast cancer develops. Gynecomastia often extends into the upper outer quadrant of the breast and, like carcinoma, can appear to be slightly eccentric in location with respect to the nipple. The lump caused by breast cancer has usually been present for a minimum of 6 months before presentation because males tend to wait longer to seek medical attention than do females with palpable lumps. Because most male breast carcinomas arise within central ducts rather than peripheral lobules, serosanguinous or frankly bloody discharge occurs more frequently in males than in females. Because the male breast is smaller than the female breast, nipple and skin retraction occur at smaller lesion sizes than in females and are present in a larger percentage of males. Unilateral gynecomastia is not fixed to surrounding structures except in patients with chronic duct ectasia–periductal mastitis complex, who can have nipple discharge, nipple retraction, and ulceration that simulate malignant changes. A few males may present with nipple ulceration due to Paget's disease of the nipple. This is more frequently pigmented than in females.

Up to one-third of males with breast cancer report recent trauma to the chest, but it is unlikely that this causes breast cancer because the time interval is too short. It is far more likely that the trauma is incidental and merely drew attention to the palpable preexisting carcinoma.

In about half of cases, there are already palpable axillary lymph nodes at the time of presentation. It is likely that breast cancer of males invades the lymphatics at a smaller size than in females because the richest network of lymphatic lies in the periareolar region where almost all male breast cancers occur. In a small percentage of these cases, there is lymphedema or full-blown signs of inflammatory carcinoma.

Histology

Histologically, almost all male breast malignancies are carcinomas, and most are invasive ductal not otherwise specified (NOS) carcinomas, just as in females. However, pure ductal carcinoma *in situ* (DCIS) and extensive intraductal components are less common than in females and, when present, are usually of the papillary type (occasionally cribriform) and intracystic. Although the bulk of pure DCIS lies within cysts, there are usually elements that extend well outside the cyst into surrounding ducts. Pure DCIS in males is usually low to intermediate grade. High-grade and comedo DCIS tend to occur only when associated with invasive elements. Lobular carcinomas are extremely rare, not a surprising fact given that lobule formation in males is uncommon. Invasive lobular carcinomas do occur in transsexuals who take high-dose estrogens long-term and in males being treated for prostate cancer with DES.

Interestingly, estrogen receptors are identified in 85% of all male breast carcinomas, a larger percentage than in females. Although not yet proved, it is likely that estrogen receptor–positive male breast cancers, like those in females, respond better to hormonal treatment with SERMS or aromatase inhibitors. Tumors that have high apolipoprotein D content have a better prognosis than those with low apolipoprotein D content.

As in females, a small percentage of malignant male breast lesions are sarcomas, but these usually originate in whole-body organ systems rather than in breast tissues proper. Lymphoproliferative neoplasms, such as non-Hodgkin's lymphomas, are the most common sarcomas. Sarcomas that arise from vascular, neural, adipose, or fibrous elements within the subcutaneous fat, skin, or chest wall are even more rare.

Metastases to the male breast do occur, most commonly from prostate carcinoma, especially in patients treated with DES. Bilateral primary breast carcinomas have also been reported in these patients, and it can be difficult to distinguish bilateral metastases from bilateral primary tumors clinically, on imaging studies, and histologically. The presence of estrogen receptors in primary breast carcinomas or positive immunohistochemical markers for prostate-specific antigen (PSA) in prostatic carcinoma metastases may be the only findings that enable distinction between the two. Occasional cases of bladder cancer metastases to the male breast have been reported.

Mammographic Findings

The mammographic appearance of breast cancer in males is similar to that of invasive NOS carcinoma in females in most cases. Male breast cancers most frequently appear to be angular or spiculated masses. Although most are roughly subareolar, the position is usually slightly eccentric with respect to the nipple. Because the percentage of male cancers that are invasive papillary and intracystic is higher than in females, a slightly larger percentage of male cancers will appear to be circumscribed. Circumscribed masses are less reassuring in males than females because males far less often develop BIRADS 3 lesions of lobular origin—cysts and fibroadenomas—than do females. Thus, every circumscribed mammographic mass in males should be assumed to be an intracystic neoplasm and should be aggressively investigated with sonography.

The presence of calcifications is less common in males than in females because calcifications occur mainly in DCIS components of tumor. Breast cancer in males far less frequently is pure DCIS or has DCIS components than does breast cancer in females. Breast calcifications that occur in males are typically less numerous, coarser, and are more likely to lie in the tissues surrounding the mass than within the mass than is the case in females.

Skin and nipple retraction are more common than in breast cancers that occur in females. Enlarged axillary lymph nodes and signs of generalized edema (skin thickening and hazy increased density) are present more often than in female breast cancers.

Bilateral mammograms should always be performed because the risk factors that predispose to development of cancer on one side also increase the risk contralaterally.

In rare patients with nipple discharge, galactography can be helpful, but we believe that sonography should be equally useful in such patients.

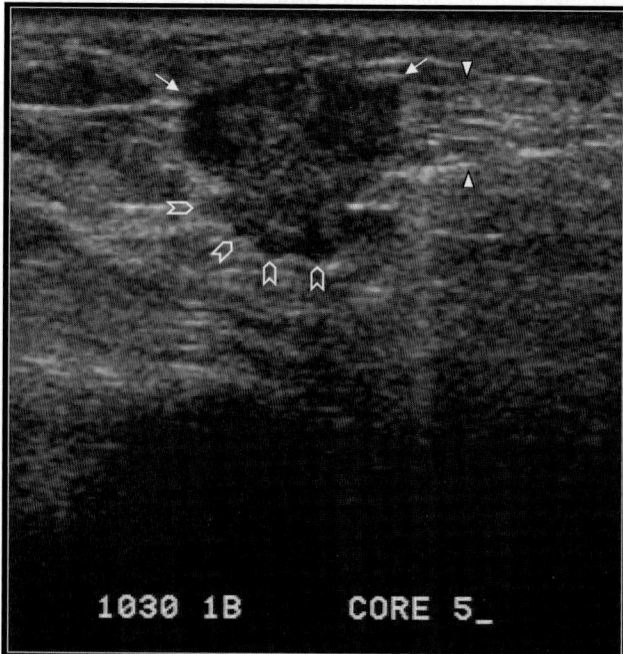

FIGURE 16–25 This invasive breast cancer in a male with long-standing gynecomastia due to cirrhosis has several hard suspicious findings indicating invasion. It is taller than wide, has a microlobulated deep margin *(hollow arrows)*, angular margin along its upper edges *(arrows)*, and spiculations *(arrowheads)*. These features are similar to those seen in invasive not otherwise specified carcinomas in females.

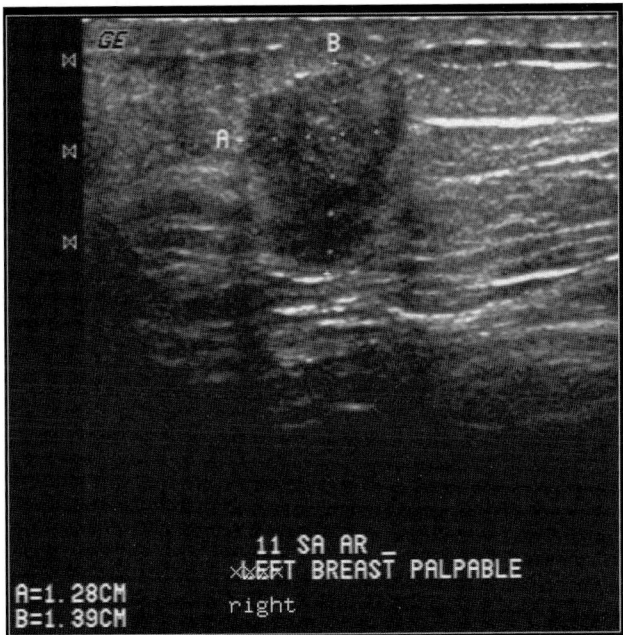

FIGURE 16–26 This invasive not otherwise specified carcinoma in a male is taller than wide and has a thick, echogenic halo that is visible along its sides.

Ultrasound will often be used, even when mammographic findings are definitively malignant, to guide interventional procedures. Biopsy is technically easier and more likely to be successful with sonographic guidance than with stereotactic biopsy in most cases because of small breast size.

Sonographic Findings

Carcinomas of the male breast have sonographic characteristics similar to carcinomas of the same cell type found in the female breast as described in Chapters 12 and 14. The chief differences between male and female invasive ductal carcinomas are the sites of origin and the extent of DCIS components. Most invasive NOS carcinomas in females arise peripherally within terminal ductolobular units and only secondarily involve the central ducts. Most male invasive NOS carcinomas arise within subareolar ducts, and thus, are centrally located. Most of the suspicious findings in invasive NOS carcinomas in males are hard findings that indicate invasion, such as angular margins; thick, echogenic halo or spiculations; and acoustic shadowing (Figs. 16–25 to 16–27). DCIS components are less common in invasive NOS carcinomas in males than in females. For this reason, soft findings that indicate the presence of intraductal (DCIS) components, such as duct extension, branch pattern, calcifications, and microlobulations, occur less commonly than they do in the female breast (Fig. 16–28). As noted earlier, because the male breast is smaller than the female breast, even small male breast cancers can invade skin, nipple, and chest wall (Fig. 16–29).

Pure DCIS is much less common in males than in females and is usually of the papillary type and intracystic. Invasive intracystic papillary carcinomas is difficult to distinguish from pure intracystic DCIS and benign intracystic papillomas mammographically or sonographically because the invasion is usually inward, into the fibrovascular stalk, rather than outward. Thus, the surface characteristics of the lesion are not affected by invasion, and surface characteristics cannot be used to characterize the lesion.

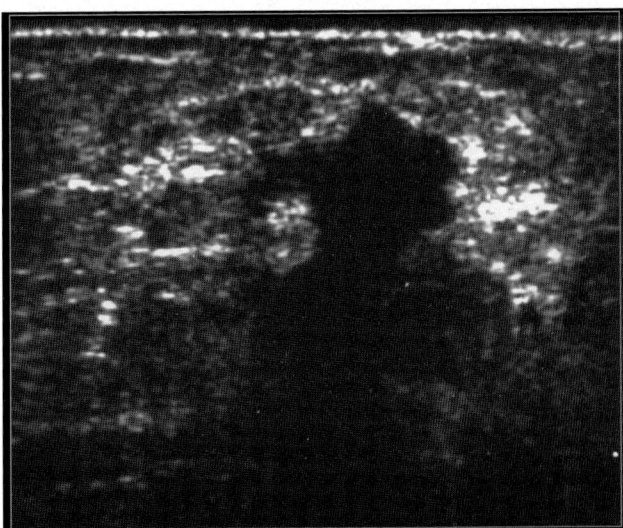

FIGURE 16–27 This invasive ductal carcinoma in a male has angular margins and casts a dense acoustic shadow indicating abundant desmoplasia.

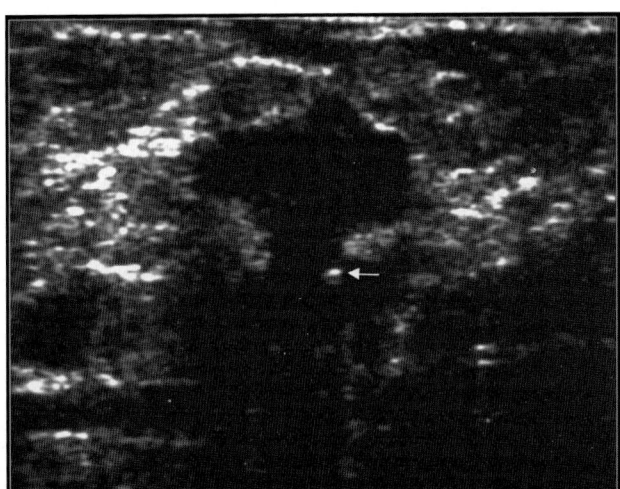

FIGURE 16–28 Ductal carcinoma *in situ* components and calcifications occur less commonly in invasive not otherwise specified carcinomas in males than in females but can be seen in certain cases of male breast carcinomas *(arrow)*.

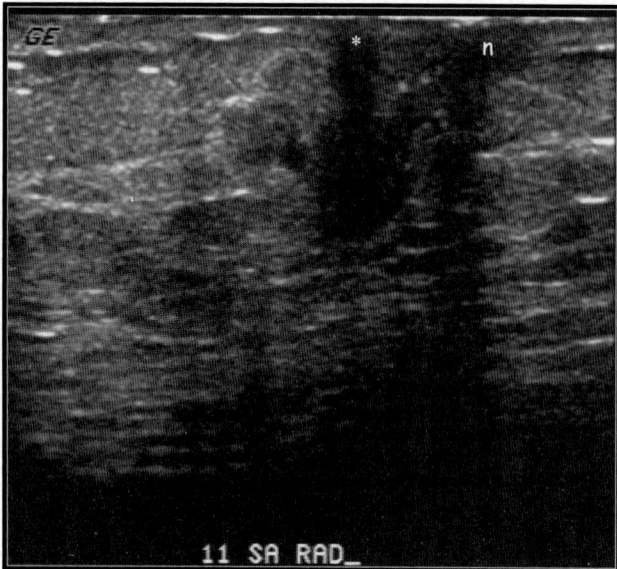

FIGURE 16–29 Even small breast carcinomas in males can invade the skin *(*)*, nipple *(n)*, and chest wall because of the smaller size of the male breast.

The mammographic appearance is usually that of a well-circumscribed nodule representing the cyst that surrounds the malignant mural nodule. One wall can be irregular or indistinct, but the irregularity is easy to miss if it does not project in tangent on one view of the mammograms (Fig. 16–30). Sonography is superior to mammography for characterization of discrete masses in the male breast and shows a mural nodule with angular margins and an absent thin, echogenic capsule at its point of attachment (Fig. 16–31). In some cases, DCIS is associated with severe duct ectasia and bloody nipple discharge (Fig. 16–32).

The sonographic appearances of other, less common primary breast carcinomas are similar to the appearances of the same histologic lesions in females. The appearance of other types of carcinomas are discussed and illustrated more extensively in Chapter 14.

Lymphoma affects the male breast with about the same frequency that it affects the female breast. In certain groups of males, particularly those with human immunodeficiency virus infection, lymphomatous breast involvement is actually more common than in females. As in females, lymphomatous involvement of the breast may be primary, or it may be secondary to disseminated lymphoma (Fig. 16–33). Large primary lymphomas may have a pseudocystic appearance (Fig. 16–34). Other sarcomas, such as fibrosarcoma (Fig. 16–35), liposarcoma, rhabdomyosarcoma, and hemangiosarcomas, are exceedingly rare in the male breast.

Metastases to the male breast most frequently arise in the prostate (especially if the patient has been treated with

(text continued on page 739)

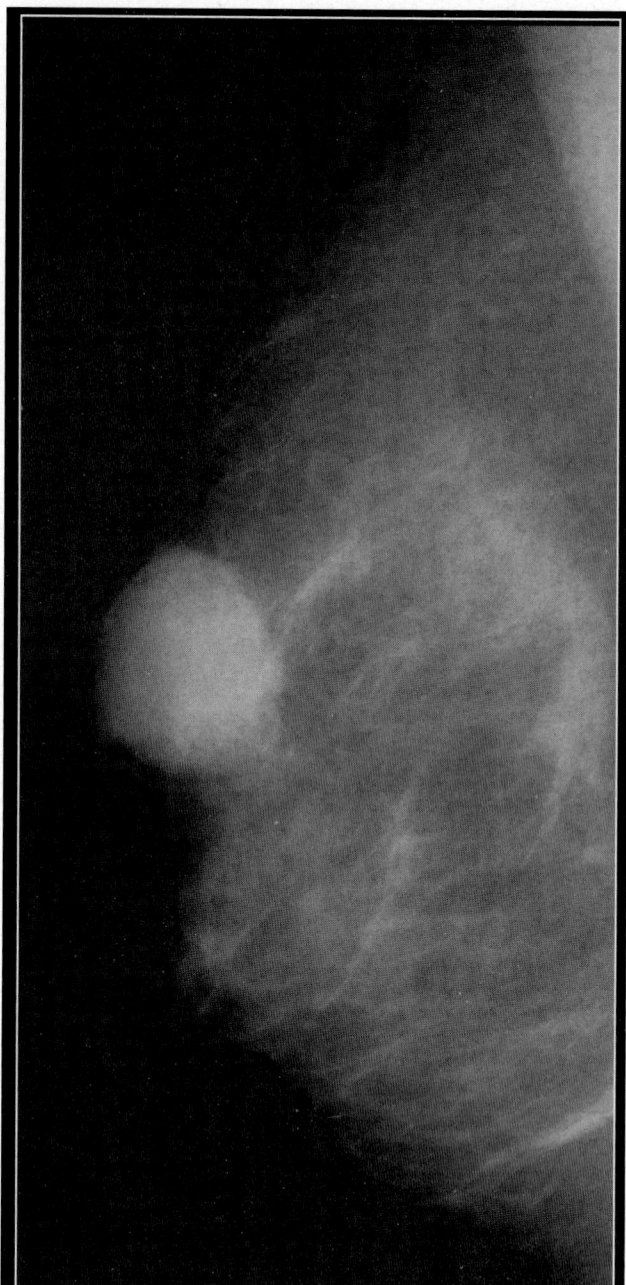

FIGURE 16–30 Intracystic papillary carcinomas are more common in males than in females because most breast carcinomas in males arise within central ducts, whereas most breast carcinomas in females arise peripherally. Intracystic papillary lesions usually appear as completely or partially circumscribed masses on mammography. Circumscribed nodules are reassuring in females, but not males, because most circumscribed lesions in females represent cysts or fibroadenomas that arise within lobules. Males do not usually have lobules, and most circumscribed nodules in males represent cysts that contain papillary lesions. Thus, sonographic evaluation is essential in all circumscribed nodules that occur in males.

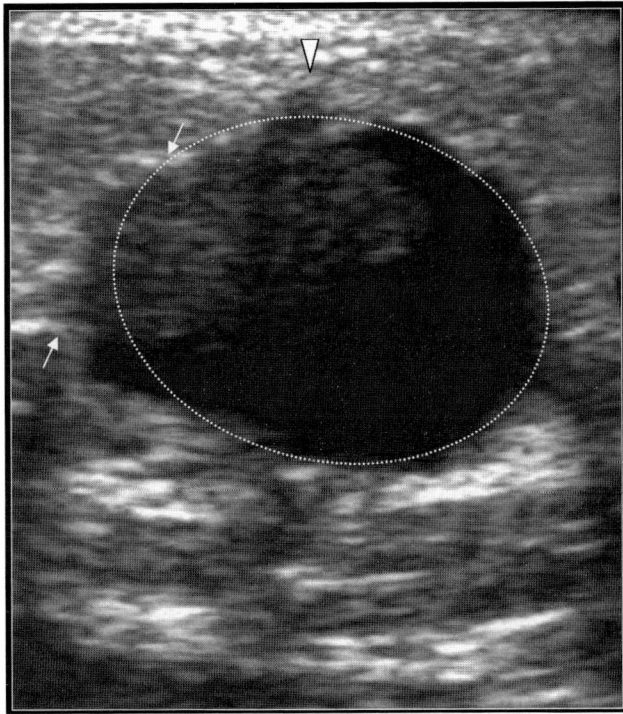

FIGURE 16–31 Sonography of the lesion shown in Fig. 16–30 shows a complex cyst with a mural nodule that proved to be caused by ductal carcinoma *in situ*. Note that all along the attachment of the mural nodule to the wall of the cyst, there are angular margins, and the thin, echogenic capsule is absent *(arrow)*. Note also that the lesion grows beyond the confines of the oval cyst anteriorly *(arrowhead)* as well as along the area with angular margins *(arrow)*. These are suspicious findings and require BIRADS 4a or higher classification and biopsy.

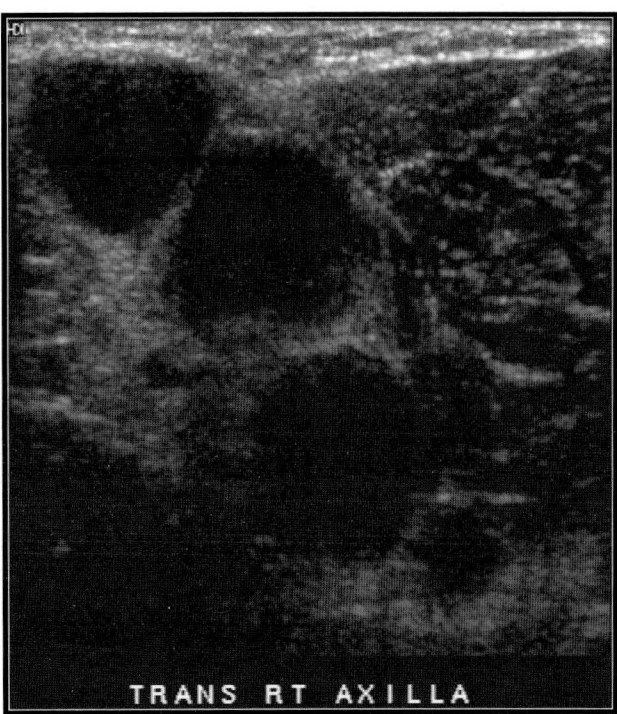

FIGURE 16–33 This lymphoma developed in a young adult male with acquired immunodeficiency syndrome. It was widely disseminated and involved the right breast and the right axillary lymph nodes secondarily.

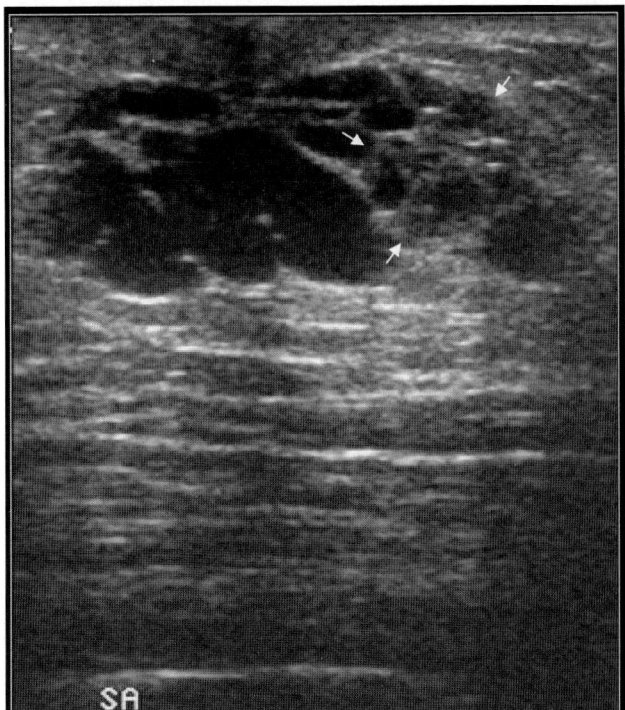

FIGURE 16–32 This male presented with bloody discharge. Sonography shows severe duct ectasia that contains intraductal papillary lesions and thickening of the duct walls *(arrows)*. Ultrasound-guided 11-gauge directional vacuum-assisted biopsy revealed low- and intermediate-grade ductal carcinoma *in situ* with micropapillary features.

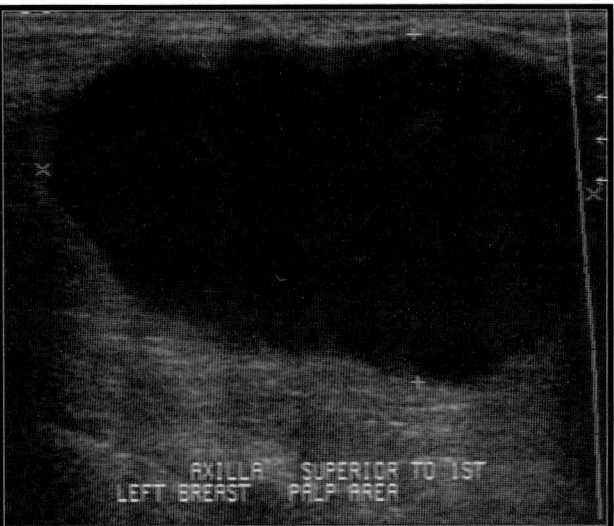

FIGURE 16–34 This large pseudocystic lymphoma was primary to the right axilla. No disease outside of the breast and axilla could be detected by computed tomography or positron-emission tomography scans.

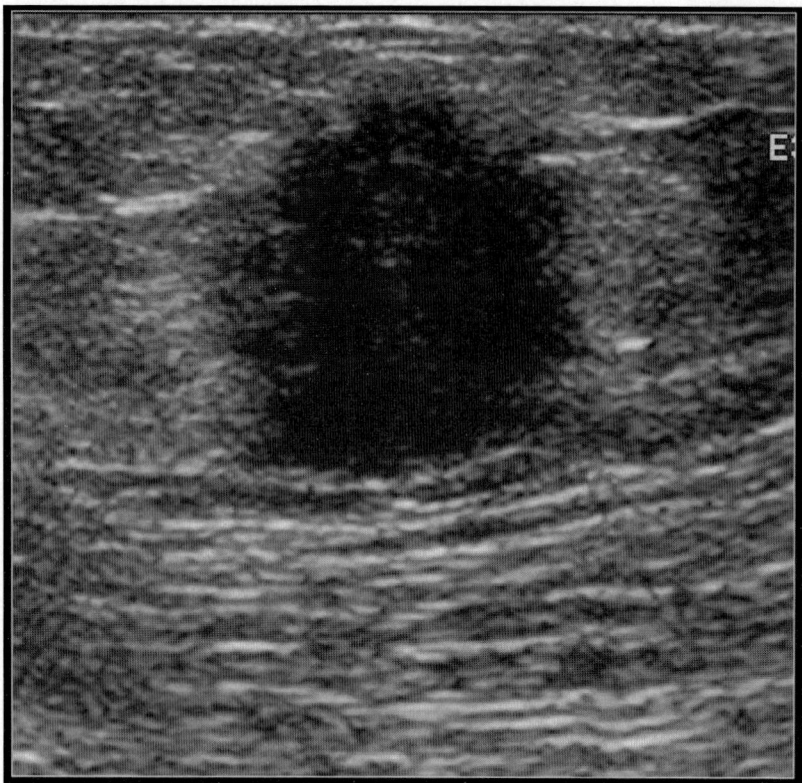

FIGURE 16–35 This palpable fibrosarcoma arose within the subcutaneous fat of the left breast in a middle-aged man. Its appearance is similar to that of fibrosarcoma in any other part of the body. It has many suspicious hard findings indicating invasion, such as angular margins; thick, echogenic halo; taller-than-wide shape; and a markedly hypoechoic echotexture. These findings are similar to those in invasive not otherwise specified carcinomas and prevent distinction between carcinoma and sarcoma sonographically. There were no enlarged axillary lymph nodes by sonography. The presence of enlarged lymph nodes would have been in favor of carcinoma and against sarcoma because sarcomas metastasize hematogenously far more readily than they do to lymph nodes.

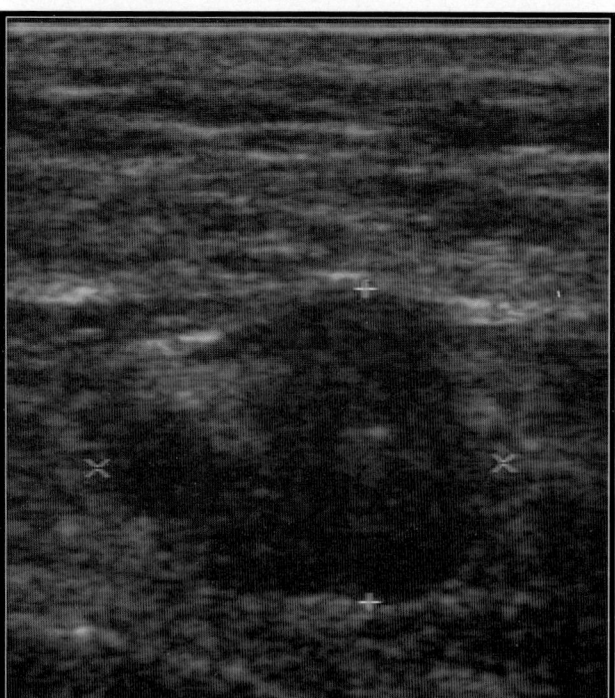

FIGURE 16–36 This metastasis to the breast originated from prostatic carcinoma in an elderly man who was being treated with diethylstilbestrol. Its sonographic appearance is indistinguishable from that of primary breast cancer. Its histology was similar to that of breast cancer, but histochemical analysis showed high prostate-specific antigen levels.

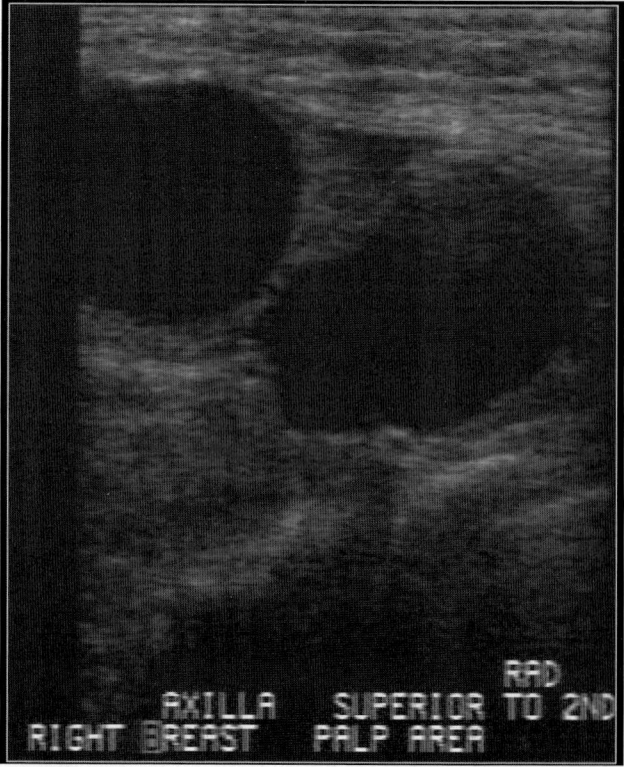

FIGURE 16–37 These axillary lymph node metastases in a middle-aged man are from an unknown primary. Whole breast sonography was performed and did not demonstrate a primary breast carcinoma.

DES) and are difficult to distinguish from primary invasive NOS carcinoma sonographically and histologically (Fig. 16–36). The presence of estrogen receptors in such lesions favors them being primary breast carcinomas, and histochemical evidence of PSA favors the lesion being of prostate origin. Metastases to the axillary lymph nodes in males can originate anywhere but often arise in the skin of musculoskeletal system of the arm or shoulder. Metastases to axillary lymph nodes occur frequently in malignant melanoma. In some cases, there is no known primary (Fig. 16–37). In such cases, it is very important to scan the entire breast to try to identify an occult breast primary. Of course, sonography can be used to guide biopsy of the nodes to try to identify the cell type and deduce the organ of origin.

SUGGESTED READINGS

General

Appelbaum AH, Evans GFF, Levy KR, et al. Mammographic appearance of male breast disease. *Radiographics* 1999;19:599–568.

Buchberger W, Penz T, Strasser K, et al. The radiological diagnosis of the male breast. Mammography, sonography and pathohistological correlation. *Rofo Fortschr Geb Rontgenstr Neuen Bildgeb Verfahr* 1991;155(3):260–266.

Cole-Bueglet C, Schwartz GF, Kurtz AB, et al. Ultrasound mammography for male breast enlargement. *J Ultrasound Med* 1982;1(8):301–305.

Jellins J, Kossoff G, Reeve TS. The ultrasonic appearance of pathology in the male breast. *Ultrasound Med Biol* 1975;2(1):43–44.

Stewart RA, Howlett DC, Hearn FJ. Pictorial review: the imaging features of male breast disease. *Clin Radiol* 1997;52(10):739–744

Volpe CM, Raffetto JD, Collure DW, et al. Unilateral male breast masses: cancer risk and their evaluation and management. *Am Surg* 1999;65(3):250–253.

Gynecomastia

Carlson HE. Gynecomastia. *N Engl J Med* 1980;303:795–799.

Conway GS, MacConnell T, Wells G, et al. Importance of scrotal ultrasonography in gynaecomastia. *BMJ* 1988;297(6657):1176–1177.

Emory TH, Charboneau JW, Randall RV, et al. Occult testicular interstitial-cell tumor in a patient with gynecomastia: ultrasonic detection. *Radiology* 1984;151(2):474.

Hendry WS, Garvie WH, Ah-See AK, et al. Ultrasonic detection of occult testicular neoplasms in patients with gynaecomastia. *Br J Radiol* 1984;57(679):571–572.

Ismail AA, Barth JH. Endocrinology of gynaecomastia. *Ann Clin Biochem* 2001;38(Pt 6):596–607.

Rissanen TJ, Makarainen HP, Kallioinen MJ, et al. Radiography of the male breast in gynecomastia. *Acta Radiol* 1992;33(2):110–114.

Ulmas J. Gynecomastia-like lesions in the female breast. *Arch Pathol Med* 2000;124(6):844–847.

Wigley KD, Thomas JL, Bernardino ME, et al. Sonography of gynecomastia. *AJR Am J Roentgenol* 1981;136(5):927–930.

Benign Lesions of Ductal or Stromal Origin other than Gynecomastia

Ansah-Boateng Y, Tavassoli FA. Fibroadenoma and cystosarcoma phyllodes of the male breast. *Mod Pathol* 1992;5(2):114–116.

Badve S, Sloane JP. Pseudoangiomatous hyperplasia of male breast. *Histopathology* 1995;26(5):463–466.

Bettini U. Angiohamartomas of the male breast. *Arch De Vecchi Anat Patol* 1965;45(2):681–703.

Cavazza A, Nigrisoli E, Tinterri C, et al. Male diabetic mastopathy: description of a case. *Pathologica* 1997;89(2):159–162.

Cesur Y, Caksen H, Demirtas I, et al. Bilateral galactocele in a male infant: a rare cause of gynecomastia in childhood. *J Pediatr Endocrinol Metab* 2001;14(1):107–109.

Chan KW, Lau WY. Duct ectasia in the male breast. *Aust N Z J Surg* 1984;54(2):173–176.

Giltman LI. Solitary intraductal papilloma of the male breast. *South Med J* 1981;74(6):774.

Hunfield KP, Bassler R, Kronsbein H. "Diabetic mastopathy" in the male breast—a special type of gynecomastia. A comparative study of lymphocytic mastitis and gynecomastia. *Pathol Res Pract* 1997;193(3):197–205.

Magro G, Sidoni A, Bisceglia M. Solitary fibrous tumour of the breast: distinction from myofibroblastoma. *Histopathology* 2000;37(2):189–191.

Mansel RE, Morgan WP. Duct ectasia in the male. *Br J Surg* 1979;66(9):660–662.

Martorano N, Raya PJL, Anorbe ME, et al. Intracystic papilloma in the male breast: ultrasonography and pneumocystography diagnosis. *J Clin Ultrasound* 1993;21(1):38–40.

McClure J, Banerjee SS, Sandilands DG. Female type cystic hyperplasia in a male breast. *Postgrad Med J* 1985;61(715):441–443.

Nielsen VT, Andreasen C. Phyllodes tumour of the male breast. *Histopathology* 1987;11(7):761–762.

Sara AS, Gottfried MR. Benign papilloma of the male breast following chronic phenothiazine therapy. *Am J Clin Pathol* 1987;87(5):649–650.

Silverman JF, Raso DS, Elsheikh TM, et al. Fine-needle aspiration cytology of a subareolar abscess of the male breast. *Diagn Cytopathol* 1998;18(6):441–444.

Sund BS, Topstad TK, Nesland JM. A case of juvenile papillomatosis of the male breast. *Cancer* 1992;70(1):126–128.

Weinstein SP, Conant EF, Orel SG, et al. Diabetic mastopathy in men: imaging findings in two patients. *Radiology* 2001;219(3):797–799.

Benign Lesions Arising in Skin, Subcutaneous Tissues, Nerves, Lymphatics, and Blood Vessels

Aqel NM, Al-Sewan M, Collier DS. Intramammary lymph nodes as a cause of bilateral breast enlargement in a man. *Histopathology* 1999;35(6):580–581.

Carreira C, Romero C, Rodriguez R, et al. A cavernous hemangioma of the breast in male: radiological-pathological correlation. *Eur Radiol* 2001;11(2):292–294.

Cooper RA, Ramamurthy L. Epidermal inclusion cysts in the male breast. *Can Assoc Radiol J* 1996;47(2):92–93.

Dockery WD, Singh HR, Wilentz RE. Myofibroblastoma of the male breast: imaging appearance and ultrasound-guided core biopsy diagnosis. *Breast J* 2001;7(3):192–194.

Kondo-Moria A, Murata S, Murakami T, et al. Bilateral areolar sebaceous hyperplasia in a male. *J Dermatol* 2001;28(3):172–173.

Lee S, Morimoto K, Daseno S, et al. Granular cell tumor of the male breast: report of a case. *Surg Today* 2000;30(7):658–662.

Ormandi K, Lazar G, Toszegi A, et al. Extra-abdominal desmoid mimicking malignant male breast tumor. *Eur Radiol* 1999;9(6):1120–1122.

Pauwels P, Sciot R, Croiset F, et al. Myofibroblastoma of the breast: genetic link with spindle cell lipoma. *J Pathol* 2000;191(3):282–285.

Schwarz IS, Marchevsky A. Hemangioma of the male breast. *Am J Surg Pathol* 1987;11(9):739.

Talwar S, Prasad N, Gandhi S, et al. Haemangiopericytoma of the adult male breast. *Int J Clin Pract* 1999;53(6):485–486.

Cancer of the Male Breast

Ambrogetti D, Ciatto S, Catarzi S, et al. [The combined diagnosis of male breast lesions: a review of a series of 748 consecutive cases.] *Radiol Med* (Torino) 1996;91(4):356–359.

Anan H, Okazaki M, Jufimitsu R, et al. Intracystic papillary carcinoma in the male breast. A case report. *Acta Radiol* 2000;41(3):227–229.

Andre S, Ronseca I, Pinto AE, et al. Male breast cancer: a reappraisal of clinical and biologic indicators of prognosis. *Acta Oncol* 2001;40(4):472–478.

Berge T. Metastases to the male breast. *Acta Pathol Microbiol Scand* 1971;79(5):491–496.

Camus MG, Joshi MG, Mackarem G, et al. Ductal carcinoma in situ of the male breast. *Cancer* 1994;74(4):1289–1293.

Cappabianca S, Grassi R, D'Alessandro P, et al. Metastasis to the male breast from carcinoma of the urinary bladder. *Br J Radiol* 2000;73(876):1326–1328.

Ciatto S, Iossa A, Bonardi R, et al. Male breast carcinoma: review of a multicenter series of 150 cases. Coordinating Center and Writing Committee of FONCAM (National Task Force for Breast Cancer), Italy. *Tumori* 1990;76(6):555–558.

Clark JL, Nguyen PL, Jaszcz WB, et al. Prognostic variables in male breast cancer. *Am Surg* 2000;66(5):502–511.

Crichlow RW, Galt SW. Male breast cancer. *Surg Clin North Am* 1990;70(5):1165–1177.

Cutili B, Dilhuydy JM, DeLafonatna B, et al. Ductal carcinoma in situ of the male breast. Analysis of 31 cases. *Eur J Cancer* 1997;33(1):35–38.

Demers P. Occupational exposure to EM fields and breast *cancer* in men. *Am J Epidemiol* 1991;134:340–348.

Desai DC, Brennan EJ, Carp NZ. Paget's disease of the male breast. *Am Surg* 1996;62(12):1068–1072.

Digenis AG, Ross CB. Carcinoma of the male breast: a review of 41 cases. *South Med J* 1990;83(10):1162–1167.

Emoto, A, Nasu N, Mimata H, et al. A male case of primary bilateral breast cancers during estrogen therapy for prostate cancer. *Nippon Hinyokika Gakkai Zasshi* 2001;92(7):698–701.

Erren TC. A meta-analysis of epidemiologic studies of electric and magnetic fields and breast cancer in women and men. *Bioelectromagnetics* 2001;[Suppl 5]:S105–S119.

Ewertz M, Holmberg L, Tretli S, et al. Risk factors for male breast cancer: a case-control study from Scandinavia. *Acta Oncol* 2001;40:467–471.

Fackenthal JD, Marsh DJ, Richardson AL, et al. Male breast cancer in Cowden syndrome patients with germline PTEN mutations. *Med Gent* 2001;38(3):159–164.

Fallentin E, Rothman L. Intracystic carcinoma of the male breast. *J Clin Ultrasound* 1994;22(2):118–120.

Forloni F, Giovilli M, Pecis C, et al. Pituitary prolactin-secreting macroadenoma combined with bilateral breast cancer in a 45 year-old male. *J Endocrinol Invest* 2001;24(6):454–459.

Fujikawa T, Sonobe M, Nishimura S, et al. A case of mucinous carcinoma of the male breast with unusual ultrasonographic findings mimicking phyllodes tumor. *Breast Cancer* 1998;5(1):83–86.

Goss PE, Reid C, Pintilie M, et al. Male breast carcinoma: a review of 229 patients who presented to the Princess Margaret Hospital during 40 years: 1955–1996. *Cancer* 1999;85(3):629–639.

Haga S, Watanabe O, Shimizu T, et al. Breast cancer in a male patient with prolactinoma. *Surg Today* 1993;23(3):251–255.

Hayes R, Cummings B, Miller RA, et al. Male Paget's disease of the breast. *Cutan Med Surg* 2000;4(4):208–212.

Hecht JR, Winchester DJ. Male breast cancer. *Am J Clin Pathol* 1994;102[4 Suppl]:S1–S2.

Hendricx TM, Tobin CE, Resnikoff LB, et al. Breast imaging case of the day. *Radiographics* 1996;16(2):452–455.

Hittmar AP, Lininger RA, Tavassoli FA. Ductal carcinoma in situ (DCIS) in the male breast: a morphologic study of 84 cases of pure DCIS and 30 cases of DCIS associated with invasive carcinoma—a preliminary report. *Cancer* 1998;83(10):2139–2149.

Humphreys M, Lavery P, Morris C, et al. Klinefelter syndrome and non-Hodgkin's lymphoma. *Cancer Genet Cytogenet* 1997;97(2):111–113.

Imoto S, Hasebe T. Intracystic papillary carcinoma of the breast in male: case report and review of the Japanese literature. *Jpn J Clin Oncol* 1998;28(8):517–520.

Jackson VP, Gilmor RL. Male breast carcinoma and gynecomastia: comparison of mammography with sonography. *Radiology* 1983;149(2):533–536

Karamanakos P, Apostolopoulos V, Fafouliotis S, et al. Synchronous bilateral primary male breast carcinoma with hyperprolactinemia. *Acta Oncol* 1996;35(6):757–759.

Koe M, Oztas S, Erem MT, et al. Invasive lobular carcinoma of the male breast: a case report. *Jpn J Clin Oncol* 2001;31(9):444–446.

Mabuchi K. Risk factors for male breast cancer. *J Natl Cancer Inst* 1985;74:371.

Madden CM, Reynolds HE. Intracystic papillary carcinoma of the male breast. *AJR Am J Roentgenol* 1995;165(4):1011–1012.

Mansouri H, Jalil A, Chouhou L, et al. A rare case of angiosarcoma of the breast in a man: case report. *Eur J Gynaecol Oncol* 2000;21(6):603–604.

Miranda EG, Iravani S, Doll DC. Unusual presentations of malignancy. Case 2: breast plasmacytoma in a patient with HIV virus. *J Clin Oncol* 2001;19(13):3290–3291.

Mouthon L, Cohen R, Martin A, et al. Breast adenocarcinoma complicating Kallman's syndrome. PMID: 11711277.

Munitz V, Illana J, Sola J, et al. A case of breast cancer associated with juvenile papillomatosis of the male breast. *Eur J Surg Oncol* 2000;26(7):715–716.

Murata T, Kuroda H, Nakahama T, et al. Primary non-Hodgkin malignant lymphoma of the male breast. *Jpn J Clin Oncol* 1996;26(4):243–247.

Nakamura S, Ishida-Yamamoto A, Takahashi H, et al. Pigmented Paget's disease of the male breast: report of a case. *Dermatology* 2001;202(2)134–137.

Olsson H, Ranstam J. Head trauma and exposure to prolactin-elevating drugs as risk factors for male breast cancer. *J Natl Cancer Inst* 1988;80(9):679–683.

Ozet A, Yavuz AA, Komurcu S, et al. Bilateral male breast cancer and prostate cancer: a case report. *Jpn J Clin Oncol* 2000;30(4):188–190.

Pollan M, Gustavsson P, Floderus B. Breast cancer, occupation, and exposure to electromagnetic fields among Swedish men. *Am J Intern Med* 2001;39(3):276–285.

Pritchard TJ. Breast cancer in male to female transsexuals. A case report. *JAMA* 1988;259:2278–2280.

Ravandi-Kahani F, Hayes TG. Male breast cancer: a review of the literature. *Eur J Cancer* 1998;34(9):1341–1347.

Rosen PP, Oberman HA. *Atlas of tumor pathology: tumors of the mammary gland.* Washington, DC: Armed Forces Institute of Pathology, 1993:281–291.

Rosenblatt KA. Breast cancer in men: aspects of familial aggregation. *J Natl Cancer Inst* 1991;83:849–854.

Sashiyama H, Abe Y, Miyazawa Y, et al. Primary non-Hodgkin's lymphoma of the male breast: a case report. *Breast Cancer* 1999;6(1): 55–58.

Scheidbach H, Dworak O, Schumucker B, et al. Lobular carcinoma of the breast in an 85 year-old man. *Eur J Surg Oncol* 2000;26(3): 319–321.

Schlappack OK. Report of two cases of male breast cancer after prolonged estrogen treatment. *Cancer Detect Prevent* 1986;9:319–322.

Steinta R. Male breast cancer in Israel: selected epidemiology aspects. *Isr J Med Sci* 1981;7:816–821.

Tochika N, Takano A, Yoshmot T, et al. Intracystic carcinoma of the male breast: report of a case. *Surg Today* 2001;31(9):806–809.

Tukel S, Ozcan H. Mammography in men with breast cancer: review of the mammographic findings in five cases. *Australas Radiol* 1996;40(4):387–390

Wallace WA, Balsitis M, Harrison BJ. Male breast neoplasia in association with selective serotonin re-uptake inhibitor therapy: a report of three cases. *Eur J Surg Oncol* 2001;27(4):429–431.

Yan Z, Hummel P, Waisman J, et al. Prostatic adenocarcinoma metastatic to the breasts: report of a case with diagnosis by FNAB. *Urology* 2000;55(4):590.

Yang WT, Whitman GJ, Yuen EH, et al. Sonographic features of primary breast cancer in men. *AJR Am J Roentgenol* 2001;176(2): 413–416.

Yildirim E, Bergeroglu U. Male breast cancer: a 22-year experience. *Eur J Oncol* 1998;24(6):548–552.

ULTRASOUND-GUIDED NEEDLE PROCEDURES IN THE BREAST

Steve H. Parker

Ultrasound-guided interventional procedures in the breast include the following:

- Cyst aspiration
- Abscess drainage
- Ductography
- Needle localization
- Fine-needle aspiration biopsy (FNAB)
- Automated large core needle biopsy
- Directional vacuum-assisted biopsy (DVAB; mammotomy)
- Magnetic resonance imaging (MRI)–directed second-look ultrasound and biopsy
- Radiofrequency (RF) interventions
- Sentinel node analysis
- Therapy and *in situ* ablation

Ultrasound is generally the modality of choice for interventional procedures in almost all nodules and masses, whether palpable or mammographically visible. Obviously, ultrasound must be the modality that guides intervention in nodules seen only with ultrasound. In lesions that are both mammographically and sonographically visible, ultrasound is still usually the guidance modality of choice because it is faster than mammographic guidance, uses no ionizing radiation, is more accurate than mammographic guidance, and virtually never requires repositioning of the interventional device or the patient. With ultrasound guidance, unlike with mammographic guidance, the guidance is real-time, is three-dimensional (3-D), and does not require "guestimation" of needle position or movement of the nodule secondary to needle advancement, changes of patient position, or breast compression. The lesion types that are the exceptions to ultrasound being the modality of choice for guidance of interventional procedures are (a) microcalcifications unassociated with a mass, (b) very small nodules deeply located in large fatty breasts, and (c) suspicious mammographic asymmetries that are not reliably identified on diagnostic ultrasound. In these instances, stereotactic mammographic guidance is necessary.

There are at least four real-time methods of guiding interventional procedures of the breast:

- Freehand guidance
- Needle guidance
- UltraGuide
- Mammosound

We strongly prefer the freehand guidance method. This is performed without the constraints of a needle guide, and the needle is inserted and advanced under the long axis of the ultrasound transducer. The physician holds the transducer in one hand and the interventional instrument in the other hand, continually adjusting each in order to visualize the needle or probe in real time as it advances through the breast to its target (Fig. 17–1). Most find it easiest to hold the transducer in the nondominant hand and the interventional device in the dominant hand. In this way, the dominant hand makes most of the finer real-time adjustments to keep the interventional device in line with the transducer. Naturally, it is best if one is ambidextrous enough to hold either instrument in either hand to allow for utmost flexibility in approach to the lesion. This technique requires the most skill and experience of the various guidance possibilities.

Before performing freehand ultrasound-guided procedures in the breast, it is prudent for physicians to master the technique with practice on phantoms. A simple Jell-O phantom can be made with peas and grapes imbedded within clear gelatin. The advantage of this phantom is that one can visualize with the naked eye (and compare to the ultrasound image) the accuracy of needle progress and ultimate targeting. Another popular phantom is the turkey-breast phantom. To prepare this phantom, one makes several incisions with a scalpel in a thawed turkey breast and implants olives or capers (depending on how challeng-

Steve H. Parker, MD, FACR, Sally Jobe Breast Center, Greenwood Village, CO.

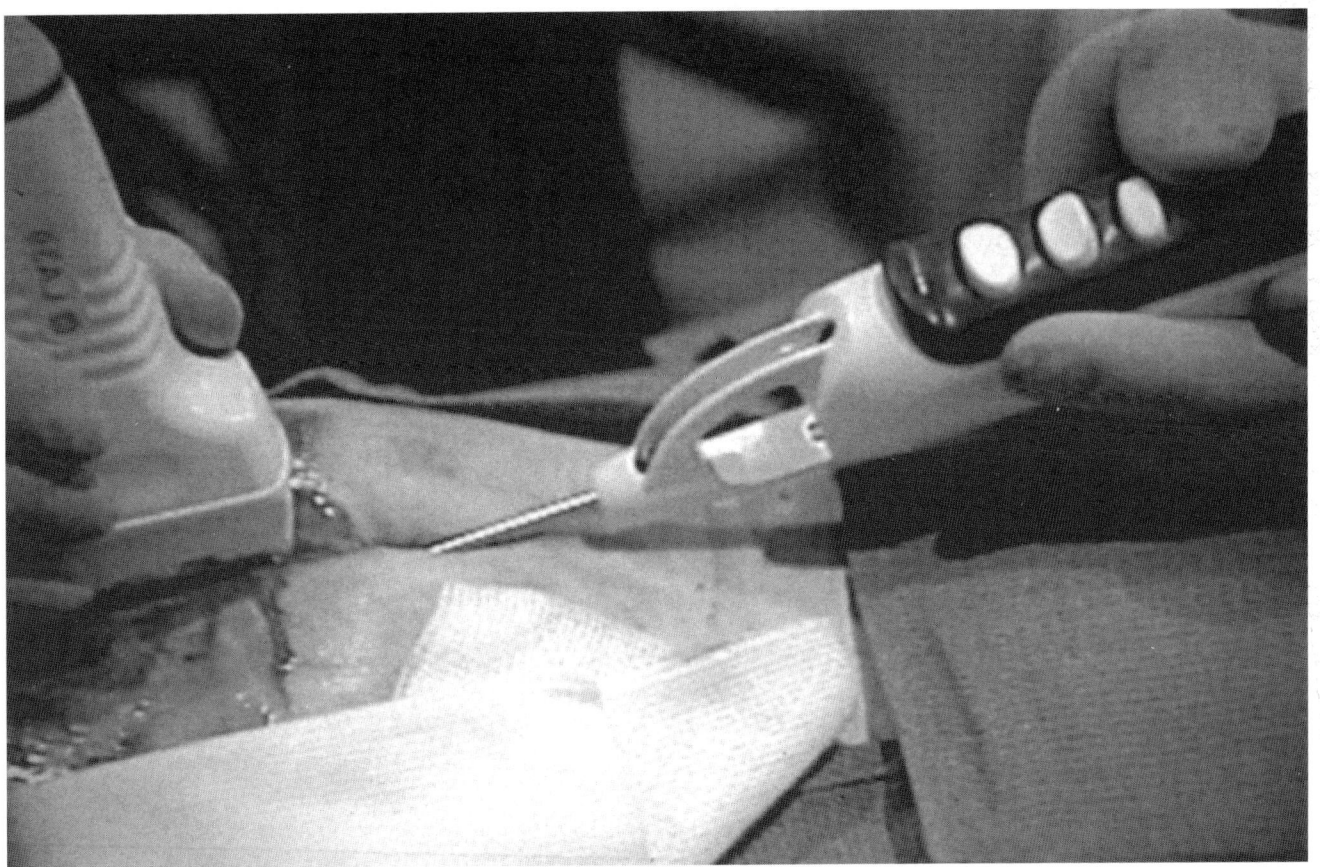

FIGURE 17–1 Freehand ultrasound guidance. The transducer is held in one hand, and the interventional device is held in the other. Most operators find it easiest to hold the transducer in the nondominant hand.

ing the phantom is to be) into these incisions. This creates a more realistic feel for the physician, and the operator cannot "cheat" and look at the needle with the naked eye.

The freehand approach can be performed in several different manners. Some advocate the short-axis approach, whereby the needle enters the breast alongside the middle of the ultrasound transducer. This gives a more direct route to the lesion; however, this small advantage is outweighed by significant disadvantages. First, one is unable to see the position or angle of the needle as it passes through more superficial tissues on its way to the deeper lesion. Therefore, although the lesion has been located with ultrasound and one can confirm that some part of the needle is in the lesion, little real-time feedback is available as the needle is advanced to the lesion. We can see when some part of the needle has entered the lesion, but often we do not know whether this is the tip of the needle or the barrel of the needle, with the tip of the needle having passed deep to the lesion. Furthermore, because one does not really have real-time guidance of the needle into the lesion, it is difficult to guide the needle into specific parts of the nodule to ensure thorough canvassing of the lesion. Additionally, the needle's angle of approach is steep, making it difficult to per-

form biopsy of lesions near the chest wall or immediately anterior to an implant, especially with a "long-throw" core biopsy gun. Using a DVAB device is even more problematic with this approach.

The long-axis approach with a steep angle of entry offers better guidance of the needle before it actually penetrates the lesion than does the short-axis approach, but it still does not show the needle as well as does the long-axis shallow approach. It does minimize the length of the needle's path through intervening superficial tissues, but the steepness of the needle prevents it from being a strong specular reflector. This makes it more difficult to see the needle shaft well. In some instances, only the echo at the tip of the needle is seen using this approach, sometimes making it little better than the short-axis approach. The angle of the needle is more of a problem for deeply located lesions than for superficial lesions. The skin entry point and the lesion depth determine the angle of approach to a lesion. The closer to the end of the transducer the skin entry point is placed and the deeper the lesion, the steeper the angle of approach. Therefore, for superficial lesions, one can enter immediately adjacent to the end of the transducer, resulting in a shorter distance to the lesion and a relatively shallow angle of approach and allowing for good needle visualization.

For deeper lesions, a skin entry point 1 to 2 cm from the end of the transducer will result in a more shallow angle of approach than a skin entry point right next to the transducer, resulting in better needle visualization. Thus, the deeper the lesion, the further from the end of the transducer one should place the skin entry point of the needle. Also, the position of the lesion along the transducer face depends on its depth. Deeper lesions are scanned so that the lesion is displayed at the far end of the probe from the puncture site. Superficial lesions are displayed toward the end of the probe nearer the puncture site. This strategy allows a fairly shallow needle angle for both deep and superficial lesions. Positioning deep lesions at the end of the transducer near the puncture site would result in a steep needle angle, causing the needle to be seen relatively poorly.

If one is approaching a lesion with a steep angle, levering the needle hub downward as it passes next to the lesion results in a shallower angle, with an angle of incidence nearly perpendicular to the ultrasound beam and parallel to the ultrasound transducer. This enables us to see the shaft of the needle as well as the echo from the tip of the needle. Seeing the entire needle and the direction that it is pointing before it approaches the lesion enables us to make corrections in the position of the probe and needle to keep it exactly on target. Another advantage of this approach is that as the needle tip is levered anteriorly, it pulls lesions away from the chest wall. Thus, there are multiple maneuvers that need to be kept in mind when performing ultrasound-guided interventions in order to best see the needle and ensure the most accurate targeting.

Needles used for interventional breast procedures pass more easily through fatty and glandular tissues than through densely echogenic fibrous tissues, which can be very hard and rubbery. Such tissue can deflect the needle tip or act as a blunt wedge, continually pushing the lesion away from the advancing needle or causing the lesion to "roll off the tip" of the needle. When a lesion lies deep to echogenic fibrous tissue, we scan circumferentially around the lesion, looking for a needle approach that avoids intervening echogenic fibrous tissue (or at least minimizes the amount of fibrous tissue through which the needle must pass).

Another possible guidance approach is to use a needle guide. Use of a mechanical needle guide, however, needlessly complicates an ultrasound-guided procedure. These devices restrict the angle at which the needle is inserted and do not allow for real-time changes in angle or direction of the needle after it has entered the breast. On the other hand, with freehand guidance, one can make unlimited changes in needle angle and direction in order to approach the lesion more accurately. Two available technologies allow for needle guidance without the restrictions of a mechanical guide. The UltraGuide is a virtual needle guide system whereby the projected path of the needle is displayed on the ultrasound screen without the encumbrances of a physical needle guide. To accomplish this task, a small magnetic field is created around the breast by a magnet in the UltraGuide console (Fig. 17–2A, B). A sensing lead is placed on the transducer, and another lead is placed on the proximal aspect of the needle being used for the intervention. The relative relationship of the two leads is then displayed on the monitor by projecting the expected trajectory of the needle path as two parallel dotted lines de-

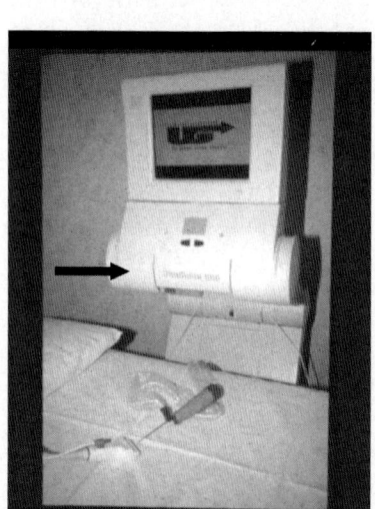

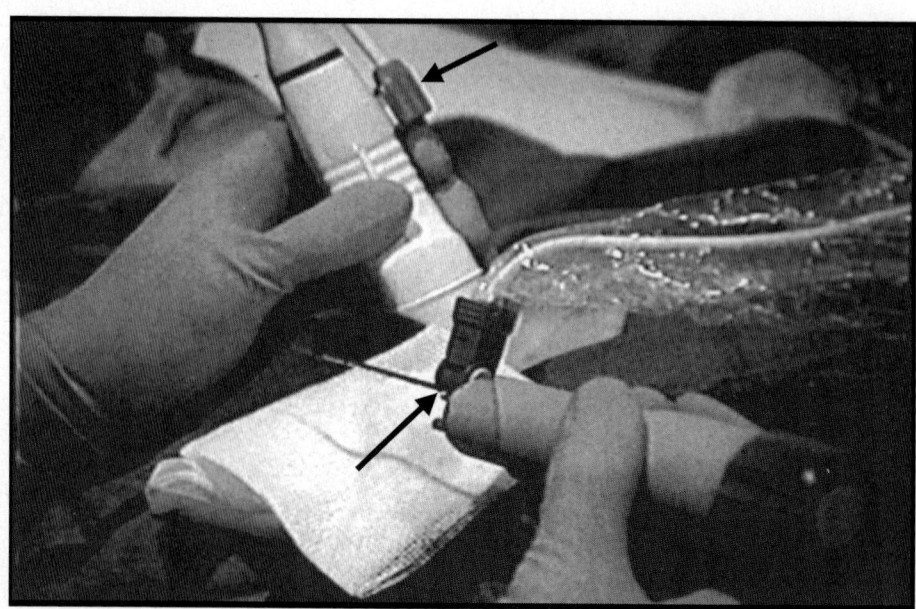

A

B

FIGURE 17–2 UltraGuide ultrasound guidance. **A:** The base of the console contains a magnet *(arrow)* creating a magnetic field over the patient. **B:** Leads on the transducer and needle *(arrows)* allow for calculation of the relative position of each. *Continued.*

scribing the expected corridor through which the needle will pass (Fig. 17–2C, D). This trajectory continually readjusts as the needle-transducer positions are changed.

Another ultrasonographic approach to a "virtual" needle guide for lesions seen mammographically is a tech-

nology known as Mammosound (Fig. 17–3A). The Mammosound is a prone digital stereotactic biopsy table with integrated and correlated automated ultrasound. The patient is placed on the stereotactic table in the same manner as for a stereotactic biopsy with the breast in compression. A digi-

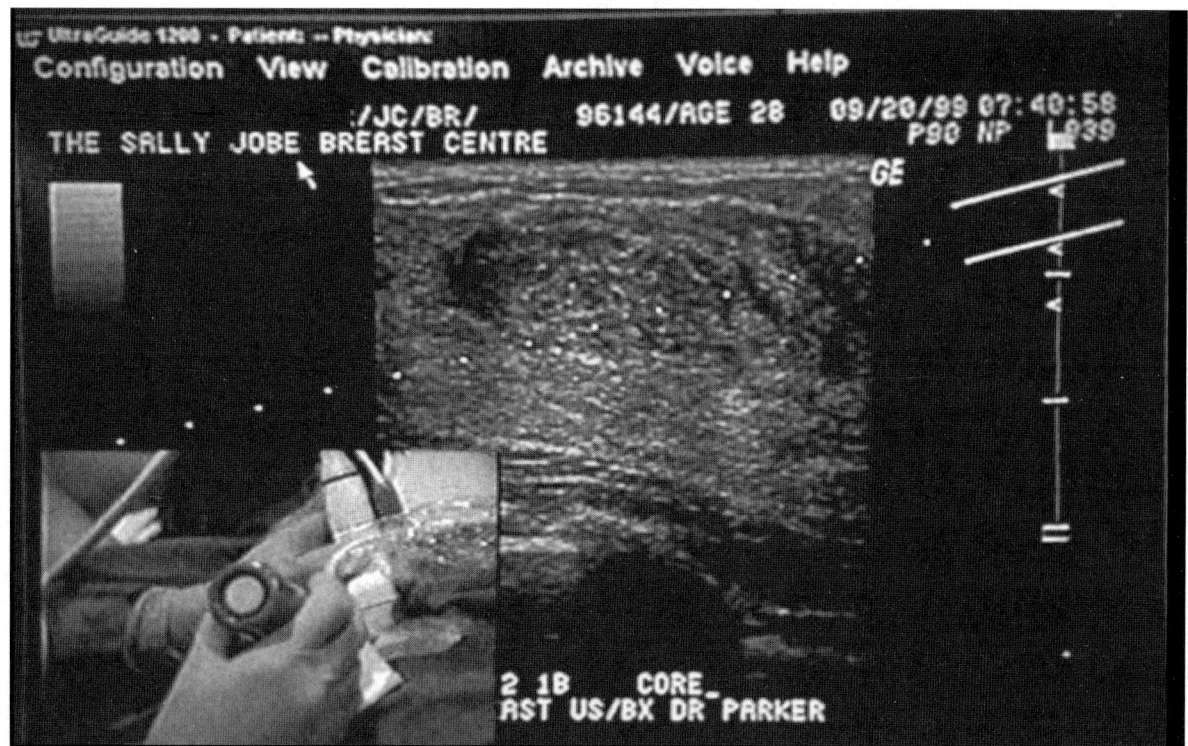

C

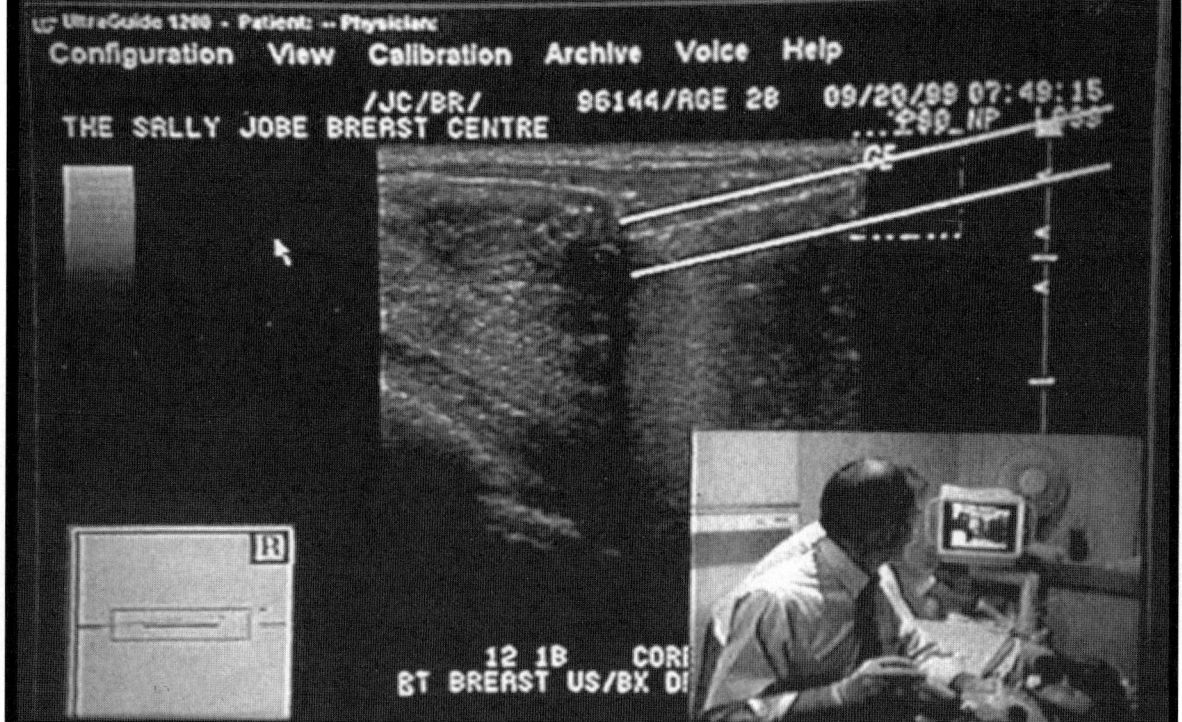

D

FIGURE 17–2 *(continued)* **C:** The expected needle path is then displayed on the monitor. **D:** The needle can be observed coursing toward the lesion between the needle path indicators.

tal scout image of the mammographic lesion is obtained and subsequently targeted. Automated ultrasound scanning of that region of the breast is then automatically accomplished through an aperture in the compression plate. The best ultrasound image of the lesion is then chosen and displayed next to the digital scout image of the lesion (Fig.

17–3B). Targeting on the ultrasonographic lesion results in the X, Y, and Z coordinates corresponding to the lesion (similar to the coordinates produced for a stereotactic biopsy). These coordinates are transmitted to the stage holding the biopsy instrument mounted on a "lateral" arm that is positioned orthogonal to the plane of compression and

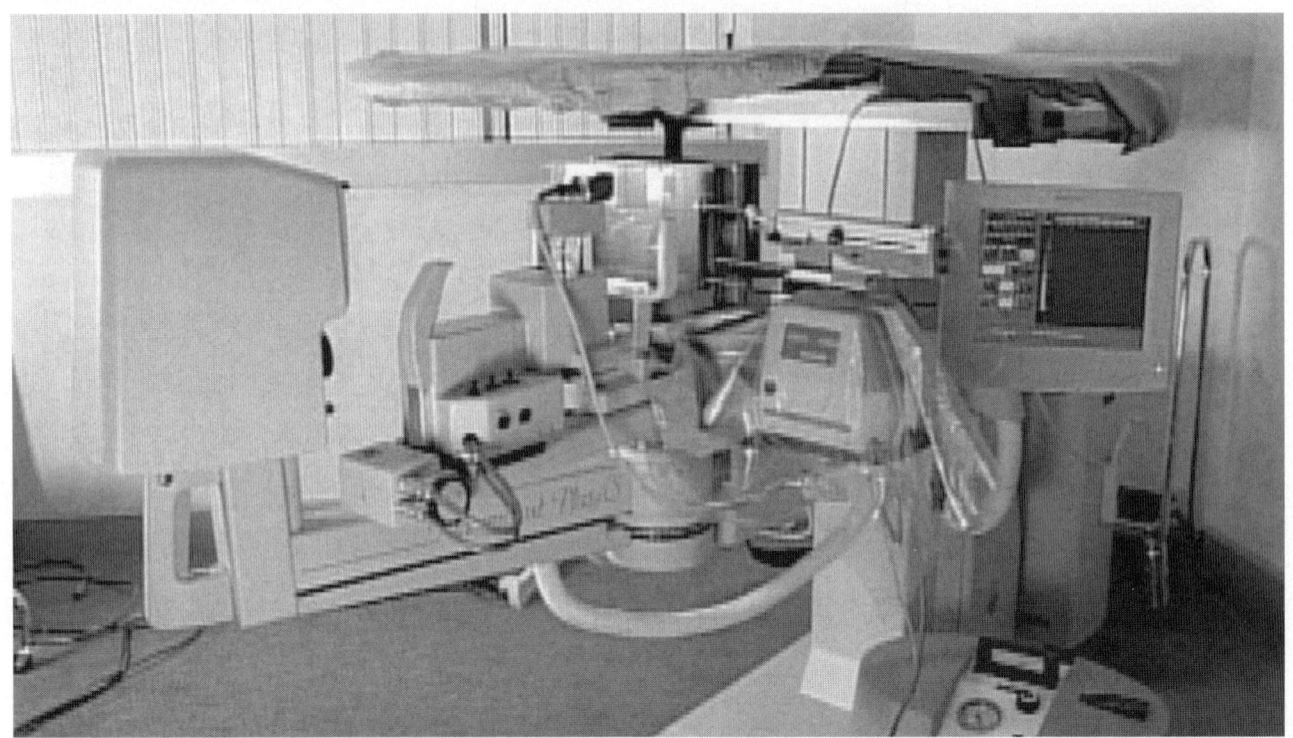

A

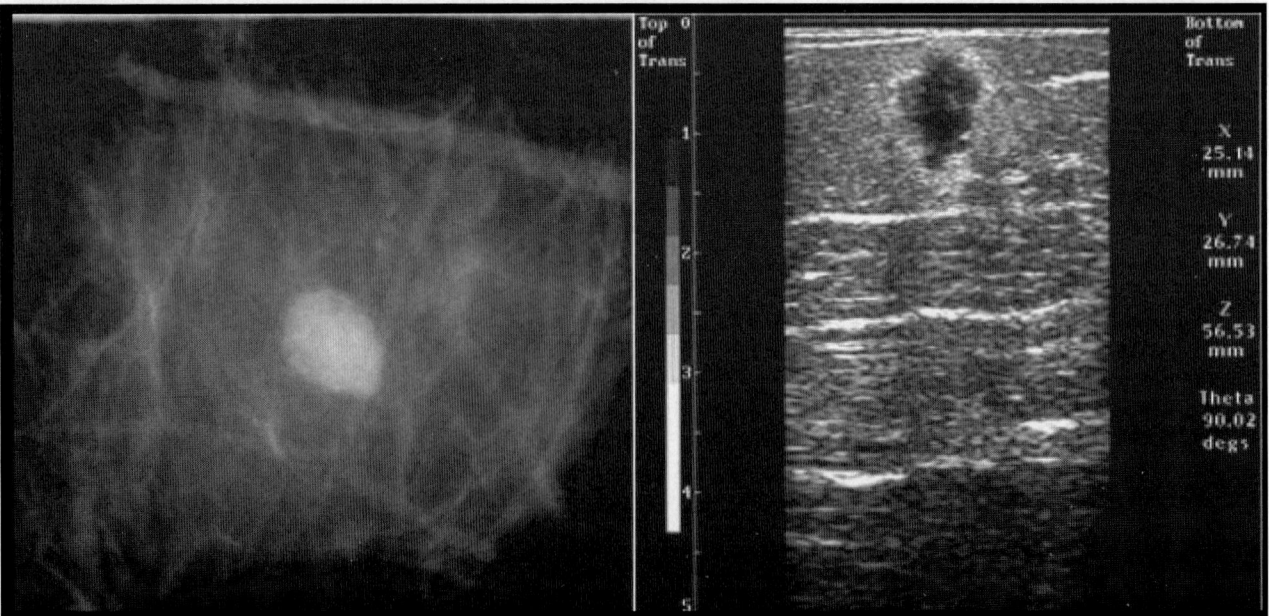

B

FIGURE 17–3 Mammosound ultrasound guidance. **A:** The Mammosound consists of a prone, digital stereotactic table with integrated, correlational ultrasound capability. **B:** After the digital mammographic scout image is obtained and the lesion targeted, automated ultrasound scanning is accomplished, and the best correlative image is chosen. (*Continued.*)

therefore also to the ultrasound transducer face. The needle is automatically moved to the appropriate trajectory (according to the X and Y coordinates), and the transducer automatically rotates in line with that trajectory to allow for real-time imaging of the needle as it is advanced to the designated depth (Z axis) (Fig. 17–3C). When the needle is at the appropriate depth, real-time monitoring of the progress of the biopsy (vacuum-assisted excisional biopsy) can be performed (Fig. 17–3D). After the ultrasonographic evidence of the lesion has been removed, a metallic marker is placed in the cavity, and the needle removed.

These last two approaches to ultrasound-guided interventions should appeal most to physicians who are uncomfortable with the freehand technique.

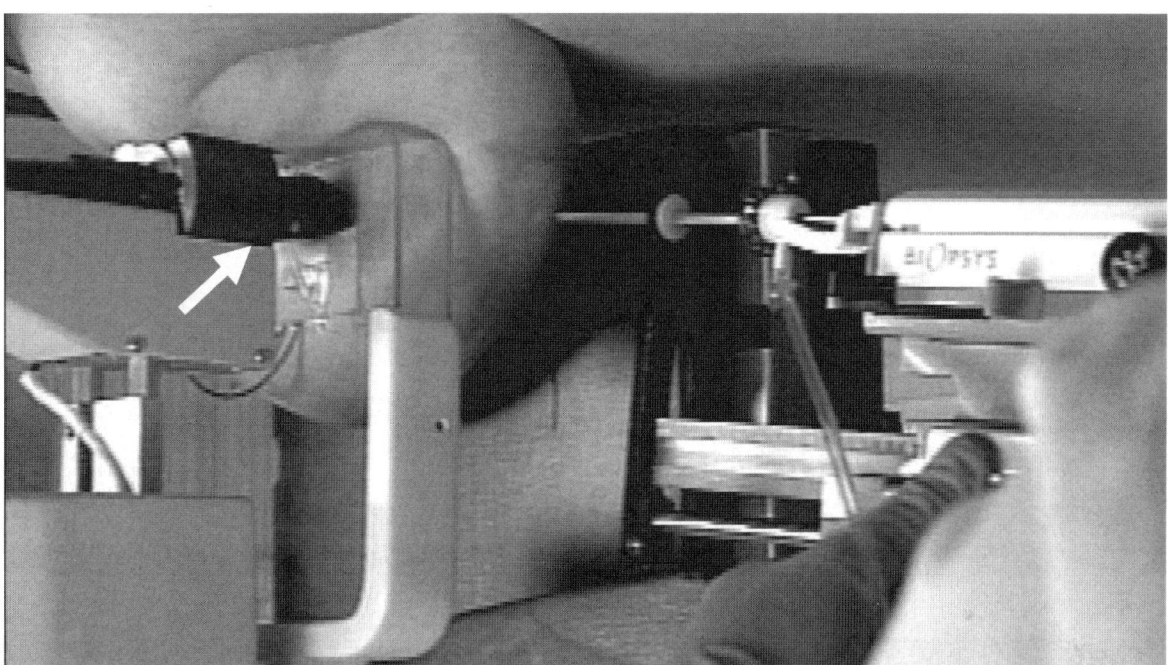

C

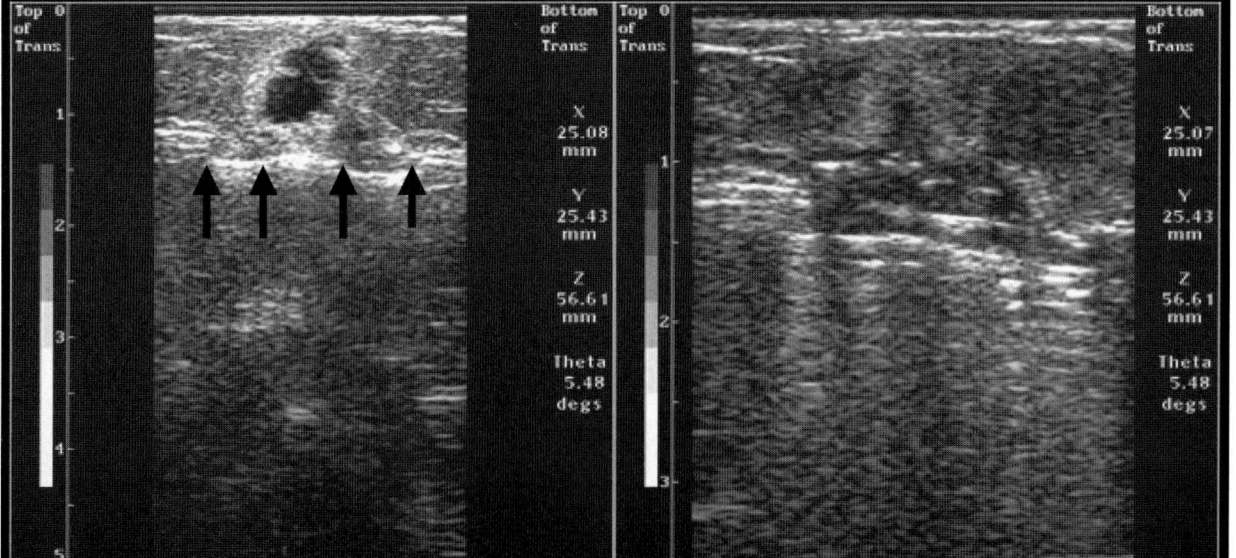

D

FIGURE 17–3 *(continued)* **C:** After the ultrasonographic lesion is targeted, the lateral arm holding the Mammotome in place is automatically aligned on the proper trajectory, and the ultrasound transducer *(arrow)* automatically rotates to align its long axis along the expected path of the probe. **D:** The probe is advanced to the designated depth, and the progress of the probe can be monitored in real time. Once the probe is at the appropriate depth, the cutter is opened, and minor adjustments can be made to center the aperture *(arrows)* under the center of the lesion. The biopsy proceeds until all or almost all the ultrasonographic evidence of the lesion has been removed.

CYST ASPIRATION

Aspiration of simple cysts is not necessary for diagnostic purposes. Cysts meeting strict criteria for simple cysts have virtually no chance of being malignant or infected. Aspiration may be helpful for the following:

- Relief of pain or tenderness
- Relief of anxiety
- Improvement of clinical examination
- Improvement of diagnostic mammograms
- Recurrence of cyst after previous aspiration

We use two different methods of sonographically guided breast cyst aspirations: a 21-gauge Vacutainer system with a red-topped vacuum tube, or if the fluid appears thick, a 16-gauge hypodermic needle attached to a 6-mL syringe. One can observe in real time the complete evacuation of the cyst and ensure that no solid component remains after the aspiration (Fig. 17–4). There is no need to perform diagnostic pneumocystography on breast cysts that have undergone ultrasound examination. There is nothing inside these cysts that pneumocystography will show that ultrasound will not also show. Some investigators have injected air into recurrent cysts in hopes of drying the secreting cyst wall epithelium and preventing recurrence. We prefer to subject recurrent cysts to ultrasound-guided mammotomy to prevent recurrence and to obtain definitive histology at the same time in order to ensure that there is no associated malignancy responsible for the cyst recurrence. Likewise with complex cysts that have mural nodules, thickened internal septations, or irregularly thickened outer walls, we perform ultrasound-guided mammotomy to ensure that these complex cysts do not contain malignancy. If one were merely to aspirate the cyst, the resultant cytology could be falsely negative even in the face of an intracystic or adjacent carcinoma. If one were to perform a standard 14-gauge, automated core biopsy on the complex cyst, then the cyst decompression that results from the first pass might make further passes difficult and potentially inaccurate. On the other hand, when performing ultrasound-guided mammotomy, no part of the complex cyst or adjacent tissue is left unsampled.

ABSCESS DRAINAGE

Complex cysts and fluid collections should be aspirated and drained if there is suspicion of inflammation or infection. In such cases, the fluid will appear grossly yellowish and frankly purulent. The fluid should be sent for Gram stain and culture and sensitivity, but generally not for cytology. If the fluid is purulent, we usually place a 5- or 6-French one-stick abscess drainage catheter within the abscess under ultrasound guidance (Fig. 17–5). After evacuating and irrigating the cavity, the patient is sent home

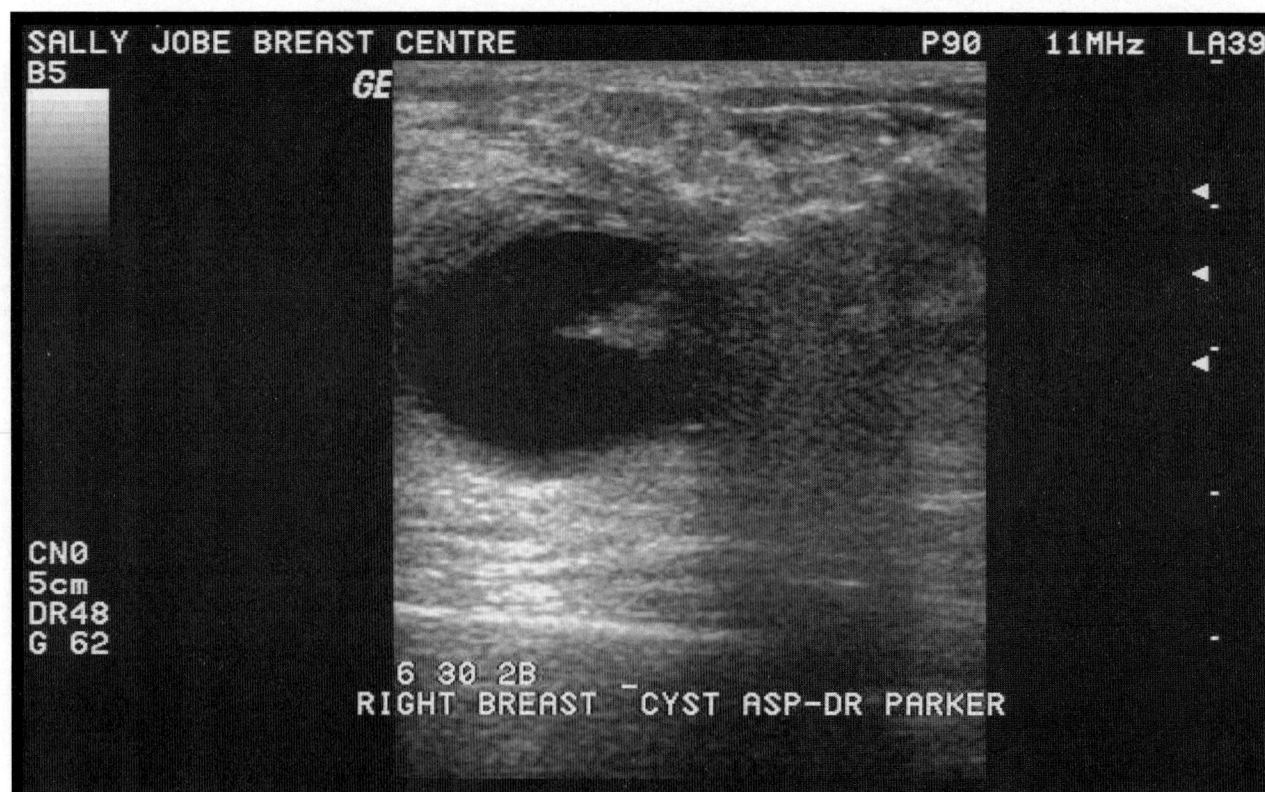

A

FIGURE 17–4 Ultrasound-guided cyst aspiration. **A:** A 21-gauge Vacutainer needle is advanced into the cyst. (*Continued.*)

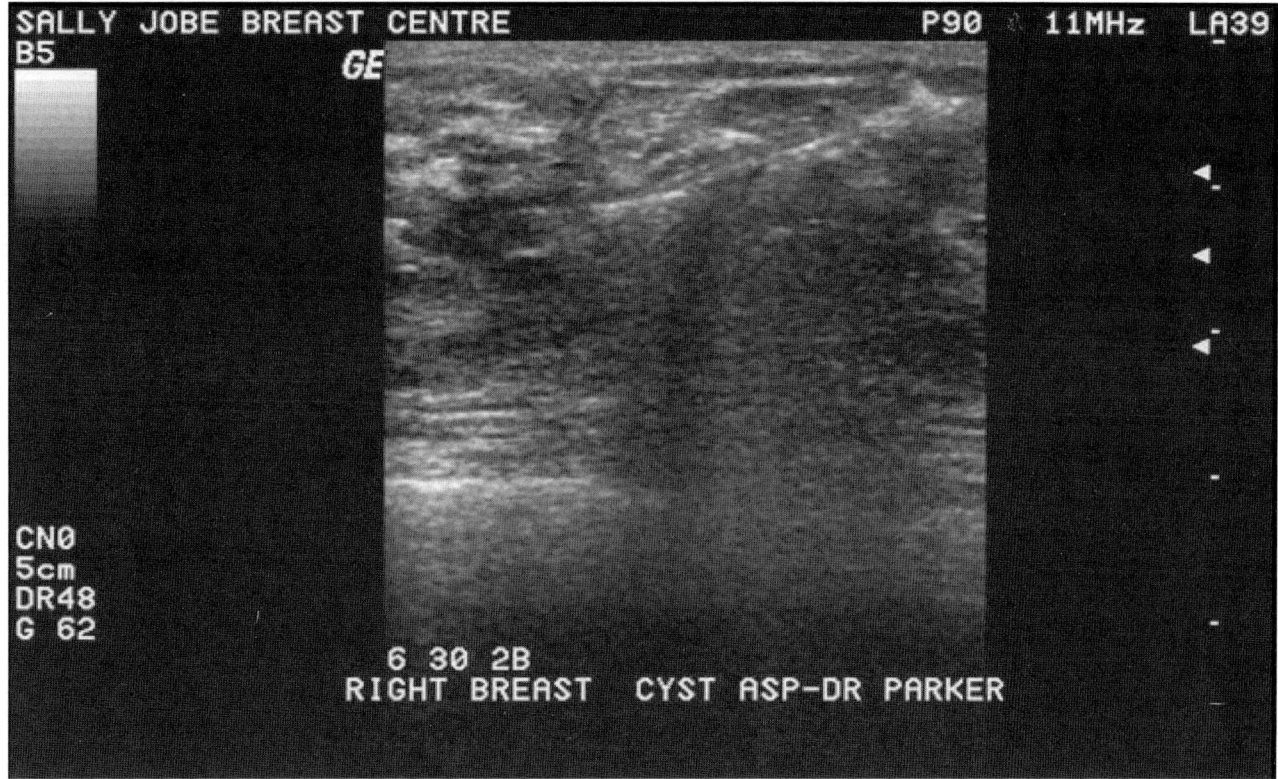

FIGURE 17–4 *(continued)* **B:** Aspiration continues until the cyst is entirely evacuated, with no solid component remaining.

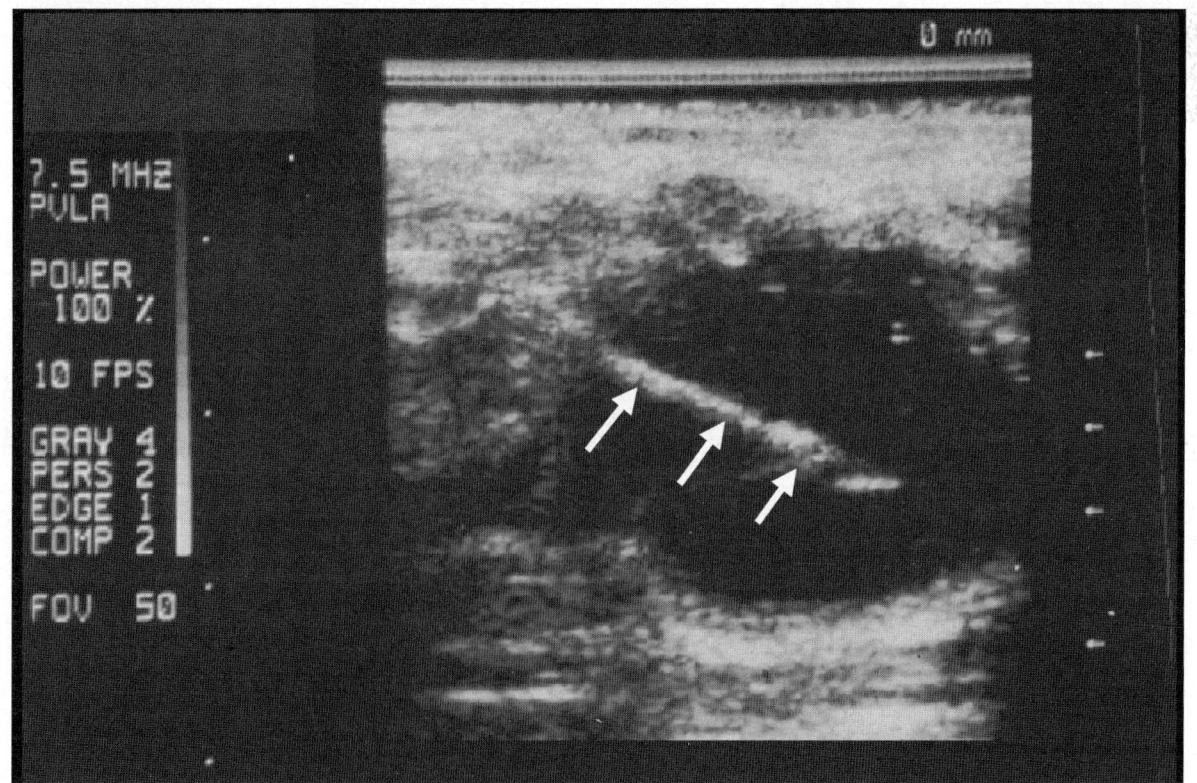

FIGURE 17.5 Ultrasound-guided abscess drainage. **A:** A one-stick drainage catheter is inserted into the abscess *(arrows).* *(Continued.)*

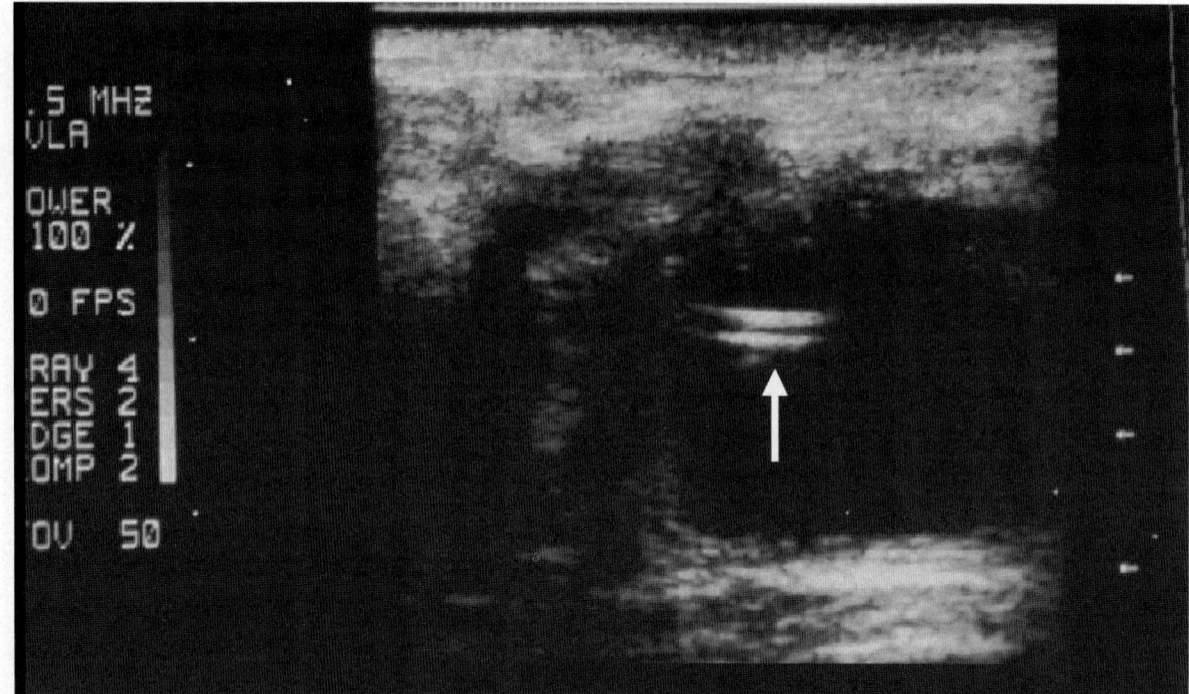

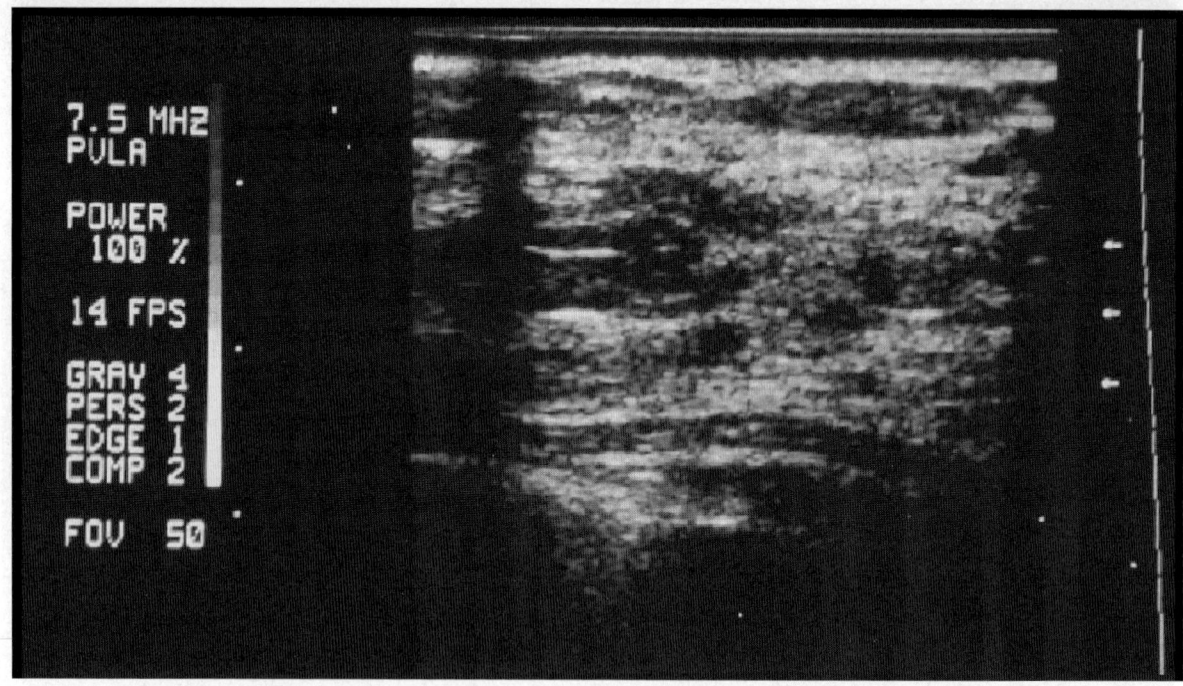

FIGURE 17.5 *(continued)* **B:** The catheter *(arrow)* is advanced over the trocar and the trocar removed. **C:** The catheter is left to drain for 48 to 72 hours before being pulled.

with the catheter in place to collect drainage. Because most
breast infections are caused by staphylococci, we usually
prescribe dicloxacillin for the 2 to 3 days while we await
the culture results. The patient should return to have the
catheter pulled in 48 to 72 hours. At this time, the culture
results are reviewed and antibiotics changed, if necessary.

DUCTOGRAPHY

Ultrasound can be used for ductography in two ways.
First, if attempted duct cannulation is unsuccessful, ultrasound can be used to guide insertion of a 25-gauge needle
into the ectatic duct at the trigger point for the patient's

discharge. Radiopaque contrast can then be instilled through this needle and mammograms performed demonstrating any filling defect. This may be unnecessary if the ultrasound identifies an obvious intraductal lesion before cannulating the duct and instilling contrast. The other means by which ultrasound can be used in the setting of ductography is to identify an intraductal lesion found by conventional ductography and to perform an ultrasound-guided mammotomy of that intraductal lesion (Fig. 17–6).

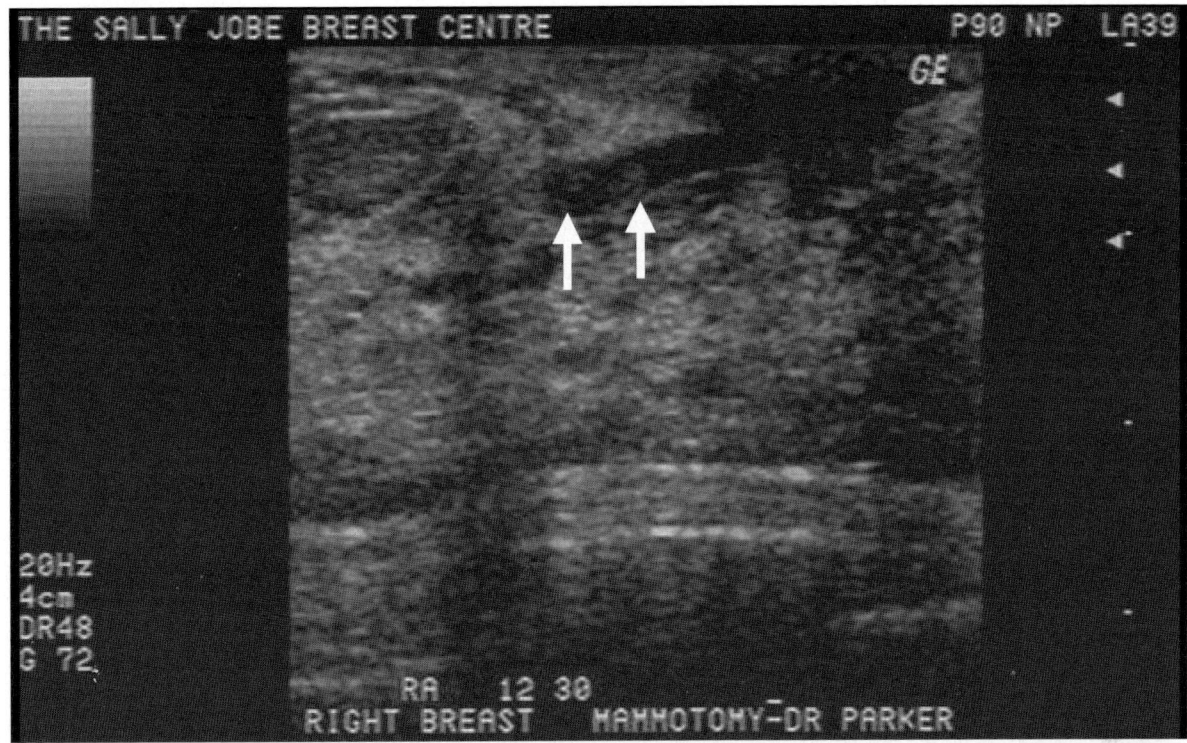

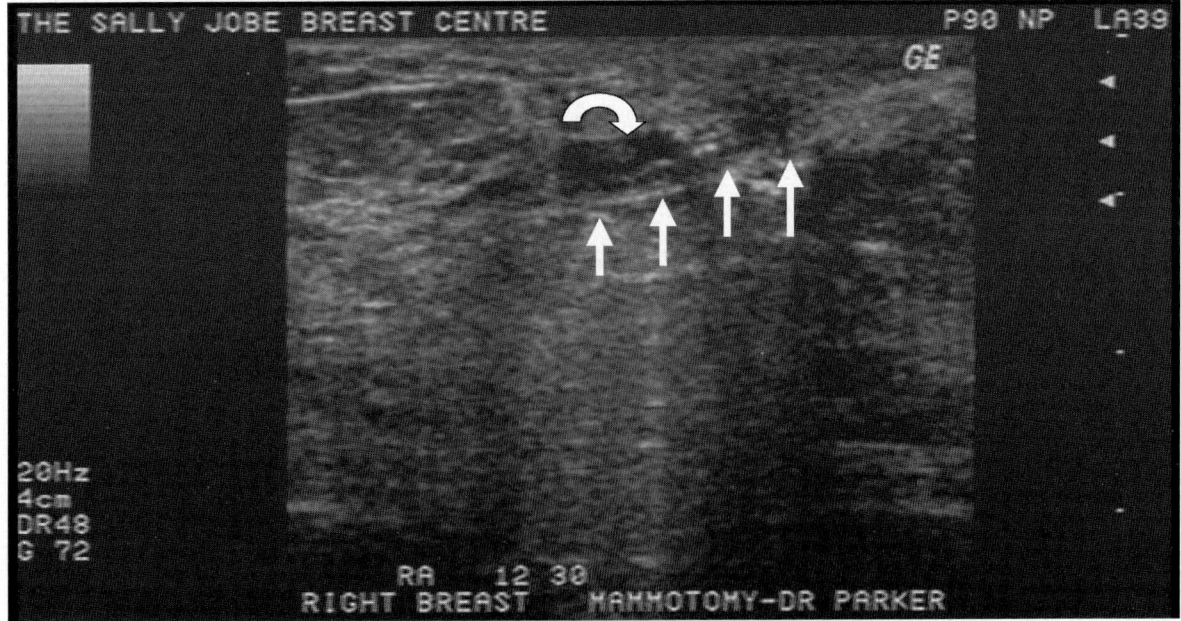

FIGURE 17.6 Ultrasound-guided mammotomy of benign papilloma. **A:** After an intraductal lesion is identified on ductography in a patient with a nipple discharge, an ultrasound is performed to verify the intraductal lesion *(arrows)*. **B:** An ultrasound-guided mammotomy *(straight arrows)* can then be performed to confirm histologically that the lesion is a benign intraductal papilloma *(curved arrow)* and, most of the time, eliminate the patient's discharge.

NEEDLE LOCALIZATION

Ultrasound-guided needle localizations are faster and easier to perform than mammographic localizations. Any ultrasonographically visible lesion that requires surgical excision (usually a malignancy that previously underwent biopsy because there should be no need to perform surgical biopsy of any undiagnosed breast lesion) should be localized using ultrasound guidance. Using a postbiopsy marking system that can be seen with ultrasound as well as mammography

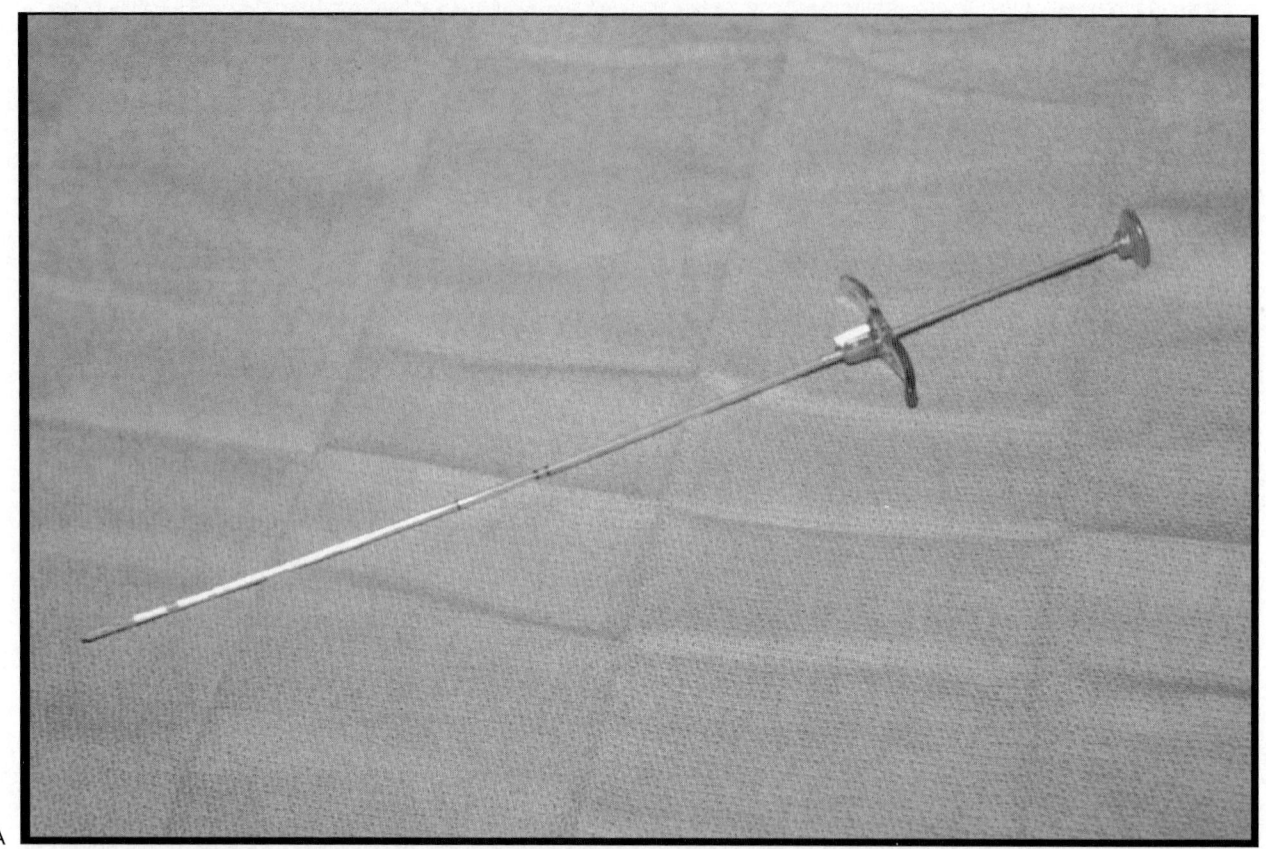

A

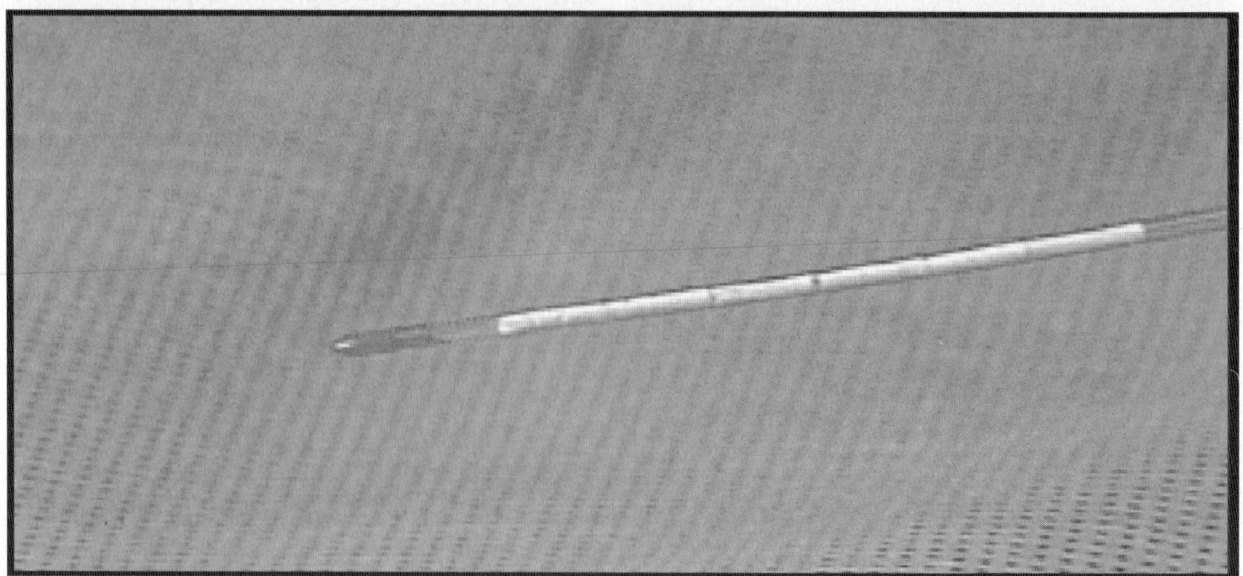

B

FIGURE 17.7 SenoRx GelMark postbiopsy marking system. **A, B:** The GelMark consists of seven catheter-delivered gelatin pledgets, with the center pledget containing a metallic marker. The gelatin pledgets can be seen with ultrasound, and the metallic marker can be seen mammographically. (*Continued.*)

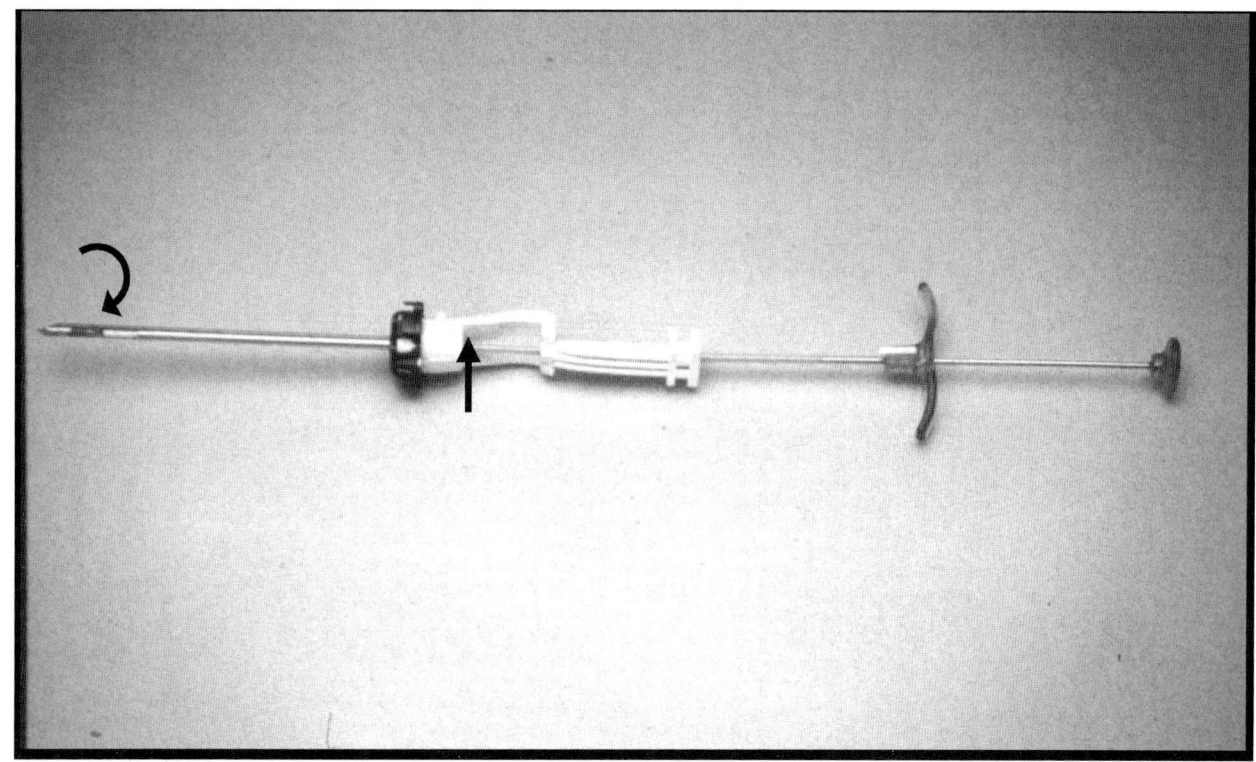

C

FIGURE 17.7 *(continued)* **C:** The GelMark catheter is inserted through the distal aspect of the Mammotome probe *(straight arrow)* so that the aperture on the GelMark catheter and the aperture of the probe are aligned *(curved arrow)*. The GelMark can be used following an ultrasound-guided or stereotactically guided mammotomy.

(such as the SenoRx GelMark system) allows one to perform virtually all localizations with ultrasound guidance—even ductal carcinoma *in situ* (DCIS) lesions previously diagnosed with stereotactic biopsy (Fig. 17–7). Typically, the localization is performed using some form of needle and hookwire combination whereby a wire is left at the site of the lesion. These standard hookwires are associated with several problems, however. They can be difficult to advance through dense breasts. They can bend off target as they are advanced. They are difficult to palpate and can be pulled out inadvertently. A new multiwire localization device, the SenoRx Anchor Guide, addresses these deficiencies (see later in the section on RF devices).

BIOPSY

Ultrasound-guided breast biopsy is usually reserved for solid breast lesions (with the exception of certain complex or recurrent cysts, as noted previously). Naturally, if there is any question about whether or not a breast lesion is cystic or solid, a quick ultrasound-guided aspiration should be performed with a 16-gauge hypodermic needle. If the lesion does not aspirate, then one should proceed to an ultrasound-guided breast biopsy. There are three general cat-

egories of ultrasound-guided breast biopsy: FNAB, automated large core biopsy, and DVAB (mammotomy).

Fine-Needle Aspiration Biopsy

FNAB of the breast has been performed for almost a century. It has been used with ultrasound guidance for more than 20 years. Despite this long history, the technique was never able to replace open surgical biopsy of the breast reliably. Because FNAB relies on cytology instead of histology, it could never match the definitive diagnoses provided by surgical histology. Because of the considerable false-negative findings rate and occasional false-positive results, appropriate follow-up and treatment could not be carried out without further intervention or uncertainty. Therefore, at least in the United States, FNAB has fallen out of favor in most locales.

Automated Large Core Biopsy

To obtain histologic breast diagnoses in a nonsurgical fashion, techniques were developed in the 1980s to automate and adapt different types of core biopsy needles. Presently, the choice of what kind of ultrasound-guided, histologic biopsy to perform is largely dictated by the size of the

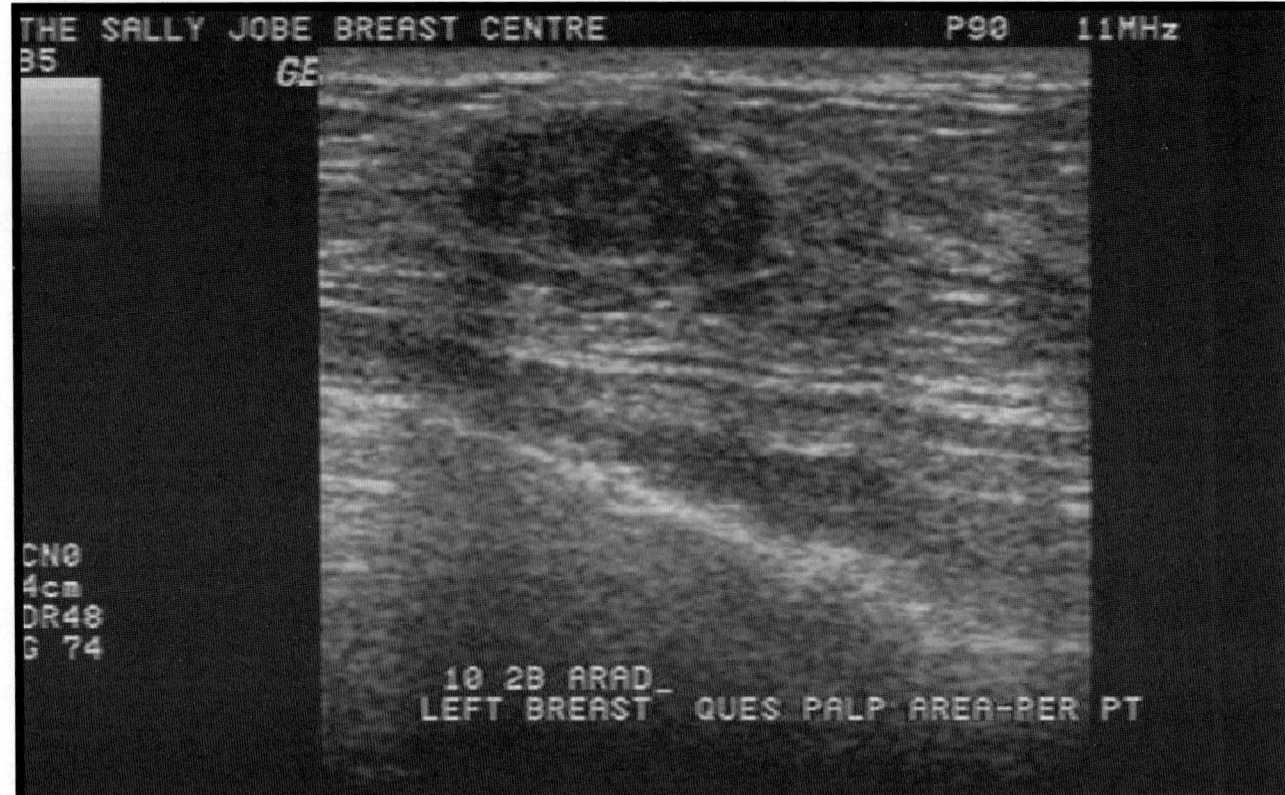

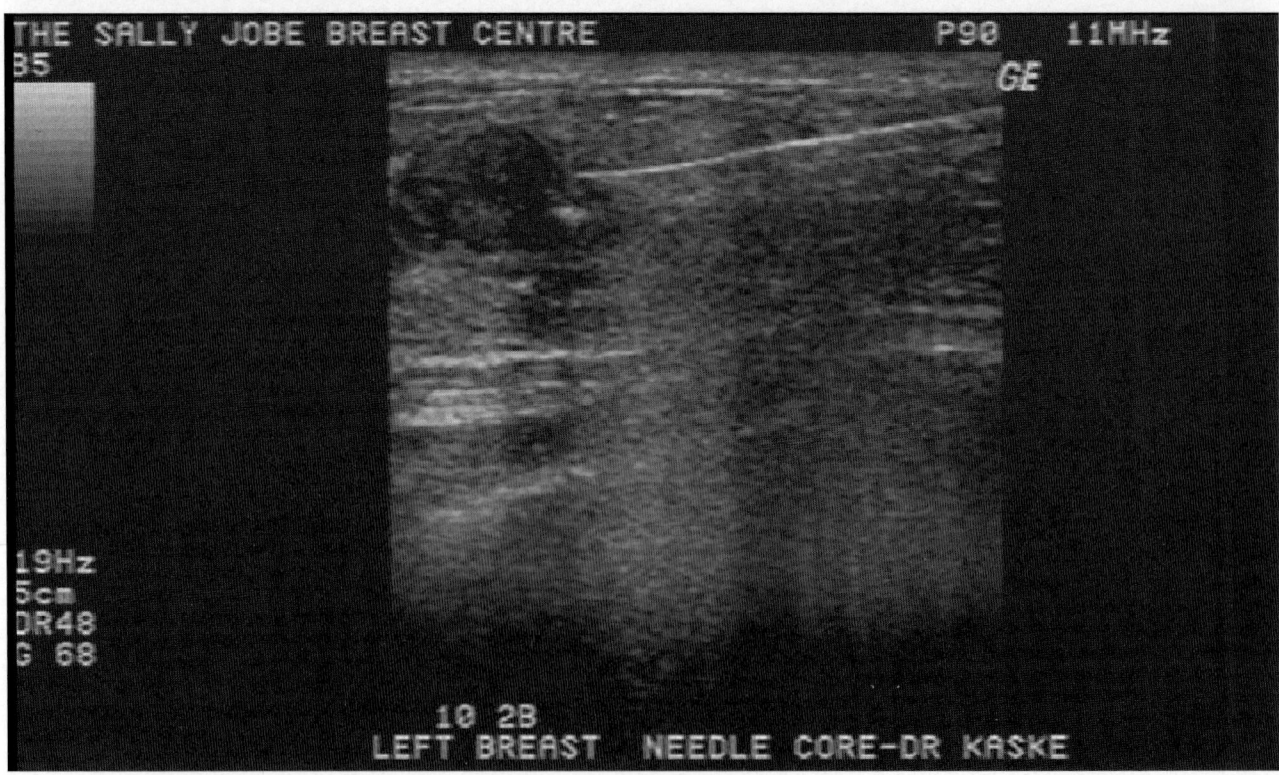

FIGURE 17.8 Ultrasound-guided 14-gauge automated core biopsy. **A:** Lesions 1.5 cm or larger generally undergo biopsy using an automated core biopsy device, such as the Monopty. **B:** The needle is advanced to the periphery of the lesion, and five samples are sequentially obtained.

lesion. Because a review of our 12-year experience in performing imaging-guided breast biopsy has revealed no false-negative findings following 14-gauge automated core biopsy of masses larger than 1.5 cm, we continue to use this method for larger masses (Fig. 17–8). We usually obtain five large core needle specimens from a solid mass. Rather than obtaining these randomly, and risking oversampling in some areas of the nodule and undersampling in other areas, we systematically biopsy the center of the lesion, then the anterior aspect, followed by similar peripheral biopsies in the posterior, medial, and lateral aspects of the lesion. One can use a 13-gauge thin-wall coaxial needle and reorient the coaxial needle accordingly between passes, or one can make multiple insertions at the appropriate different angles with the 14-gauge automated core needle alone.

Directional Vacuum-Assisted Biopsy (Mammotomy)

Because our data have shown that false-negative diagnoses do occur after 14-gauge automated core biopsy of small masses (<1.5 cm), we prefer to use the ultrasound-guided mammotomy technique for these lesions in order to eliminate any potential for sampling error. As noted earlier, we

also use this technique for biopsy of recurrent or suspicious complex cysts. The original technique involved using an articulated arm to hold the Mammotome in place after the probe was positioned (Fig. 17–9A). More recently, a hand-held Mammotome has become available that has largely supplanted the articulated arm approach (Fig. 17–9B). A similar technique is used regardless of which of the two types of ultrasound mammotomy equipment is employed. The Mammotome is advanced under real-time guidance to a position just posterior to the lesion. The aperture of the probe is opened, and minor adjustments are made to position the center of the aperture beneath the center of the lesion (Fig. 17–9C). The tissue acquisition sequence is then begun, acquiring tissue at the 10:30, 12:00, and 1:30 positions until all or almost all visualized evidence of the lesion is removed. A metallic marker is then placed within the resultant biopsy cavity. We prefer the SenoRx GelMark post-biopsy marking device because it is visible with both ultrasound and mammography (Fig. 17–9D–F). This is very useful in the preoperative localization setting because it is generally easier and faster to perform localizations with ultrasound than to use stereotactic mammography as the guidance modality. For lesions between 1.5 and 2.5 cm that are considered most likely benign but that the patient

(text continued on page 758)

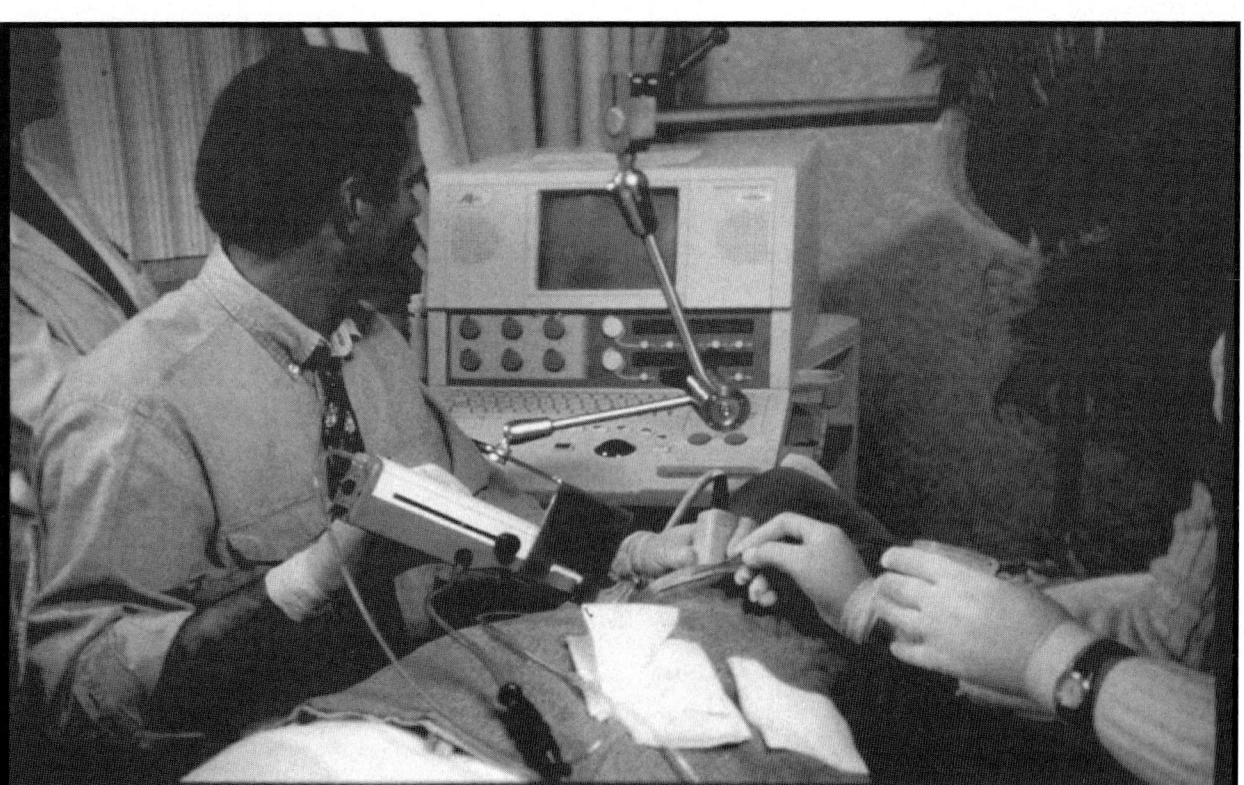

A

FIGURE 17.9 Ultrasound-guided mammotomy. **A:** The articulated arm version of the Mammotome creates a stable platform from which the biopsy can be carried out. (*Continued.*)

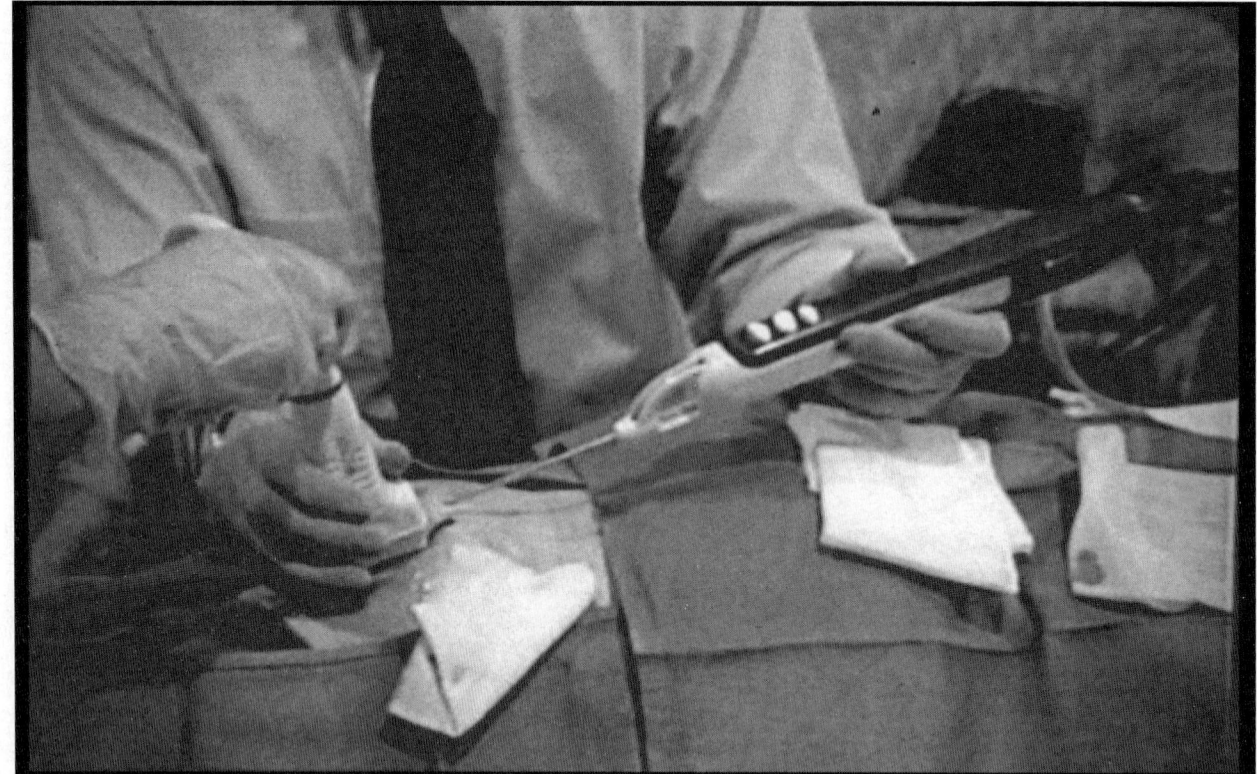

B

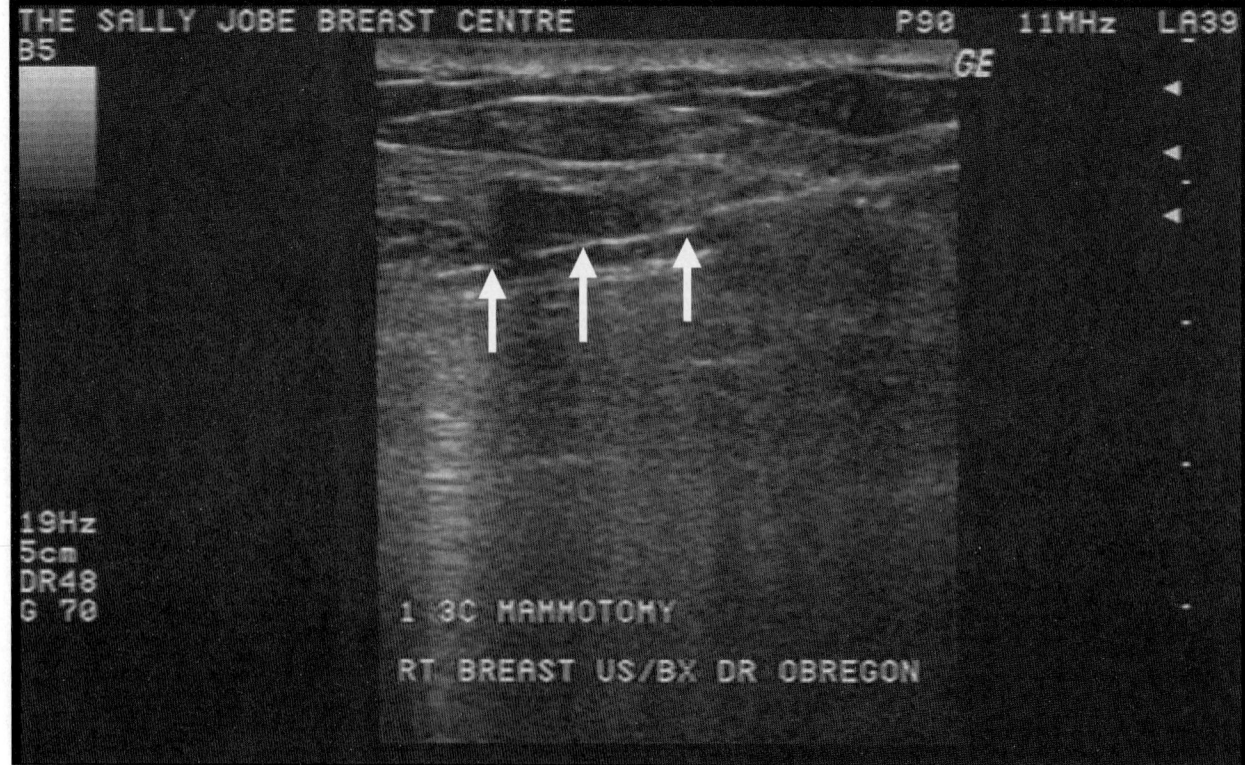

C

FIGURE 17.9 *(continued)* **B:** The hand-held version of the Mammotome allows for continuous freehand guidance. **C:** Regardless of the Mammotome used, the principle is the same—advance the probe posterior to the lesion and center the aperture *(arrows)* under the center of the lesion.

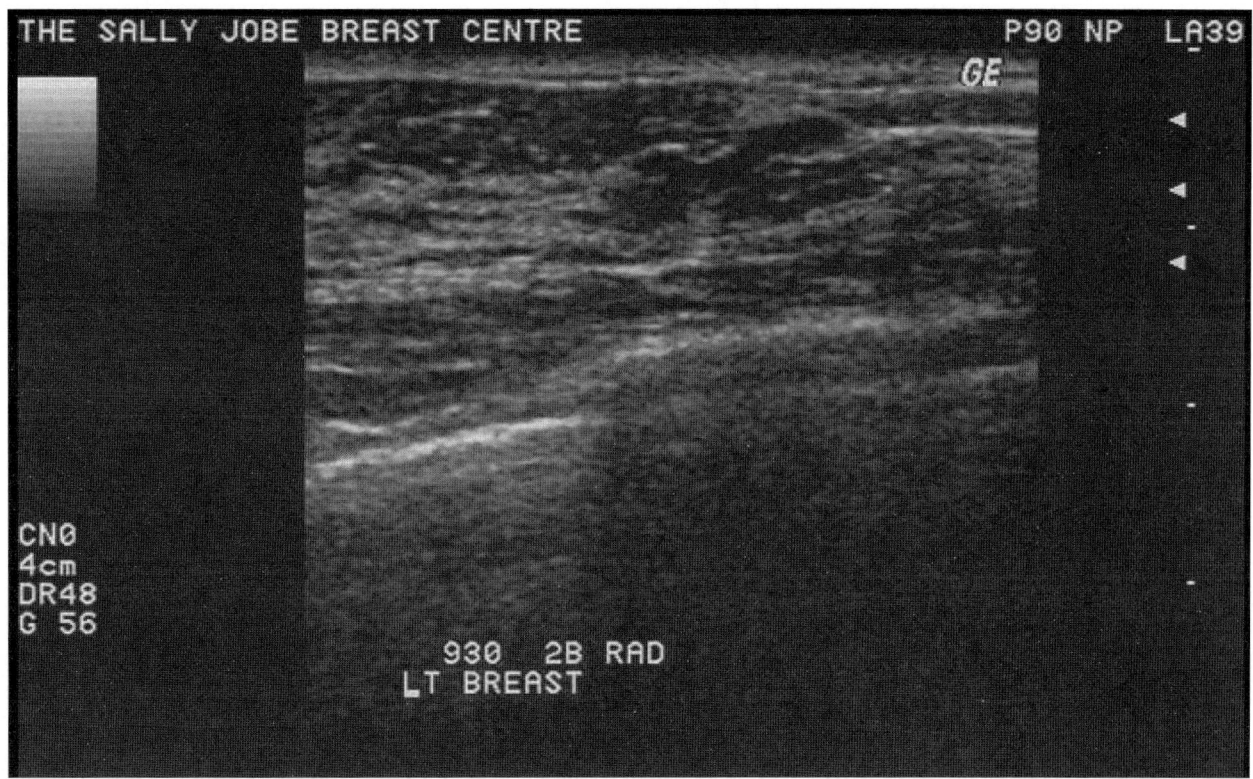

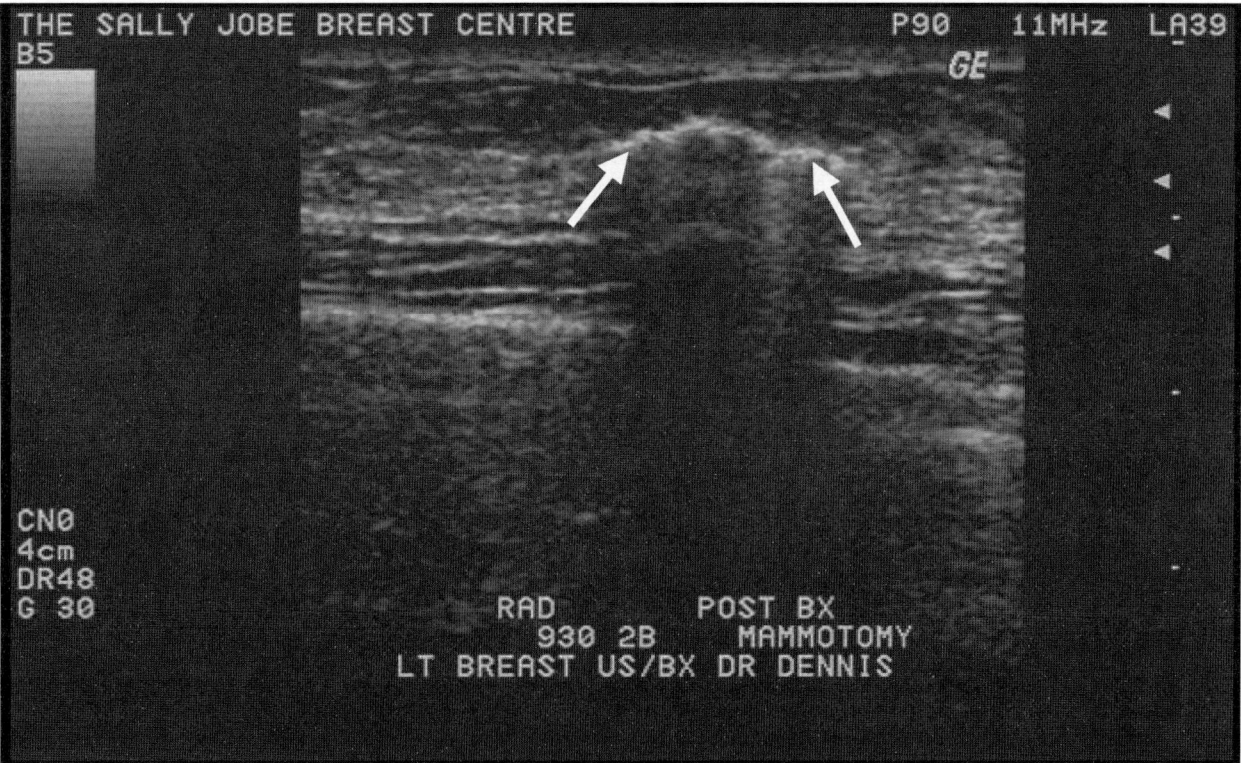

FIGURE 17.9 *(continued)* **D, E:** A breast lesion before and after mammotomy with placement of echogenic GelMark gelatin pledgets *(arrows)* in resultant biopsy cavity. *(Continued.)*

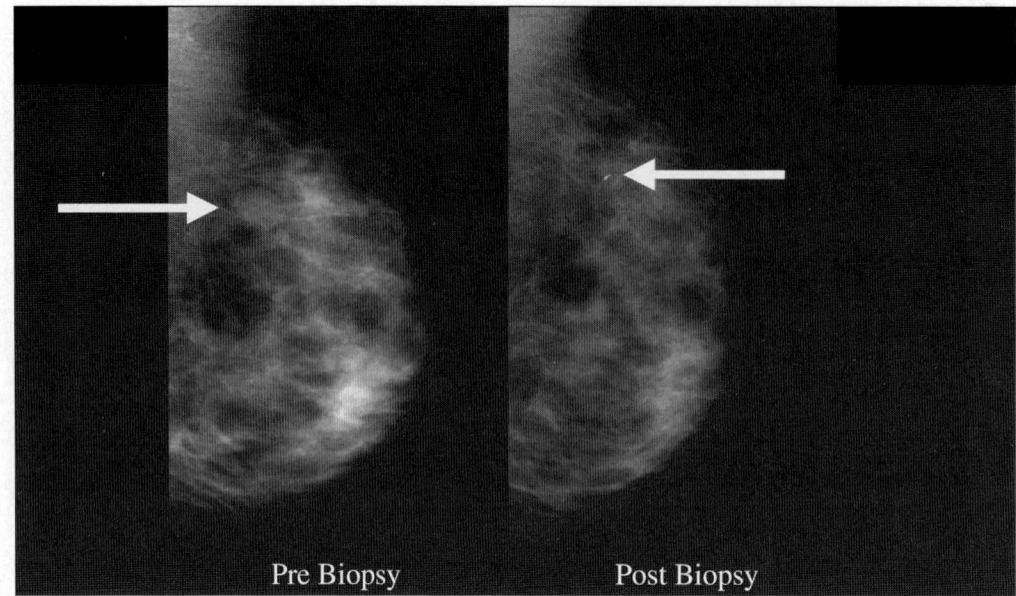

Pre Biopsy   Post Biopsy

F

FIGURE 17.9 *(continued)* **F:** Prebiopsy and postbiopsy mammograms showing breast lesion and subsequent postbiopsy metallic marker within the center gelatin pledget *(arrow)*.

would prefer to have removed, we use an 8-gauge hand-held Mammotome. We perform these biopsies when the patient is insistent that the lesion be removed and would go to surgery otherwise. Another, less frequent use of the Mammotome is for foreign body extraction. We have removed a piece of retained localization wire following needle-localized surgical excision and postbiopsy Mammotome clips that the patient desired to have removed. The technique is the same for targeting and removing a breast lesion under ultrasound or stereotactic guidance.

MAGNETIC RESONANCE IMAGING–DIRECTED SECOND-LOOK ULTRASOUND AND BIOPSY

As high-resolution breast MRI has become more common, it is apparent that there needs to be a means by which the areas of MRI enhancement can be further defined. Because the specificity of MRI (whether or not one employs a dynamic technique to determine temporal enhancement patterns) is not sufficient to eliminate biopsy of enhancing regions, we use targeted ultrasound (so-called second-look ultrasound) to evaluate carefully the location of the MRI enhancement. If the ultrasound of that specific location is at all abnormal (even subtly so), we proceed with an ultrasound-guided mammotomy of that region (Fig. 17–10). If the ultrasound is completely normal, we do not proceed with biopsy. In this way, we use ultrasound as a filter to improve the specificity of breast MRI.

Most of the breast MRIs that we perform are in the setting of a newly diagnosed breast cancer. The function of the

MRI, then, is to determine the true extent of the cancer and whether it is multifocal, multicentric, or in the contralateral breast. Since 1996, our data have been very consistent. We have found the malignancy to be multifocal (larger than expected but still within the same quadrant) in 30% of the patients and multicentric (malignancy in a different quadrant than the known cancer) in 5% of the patients. In addition, unsuspected contralateral cancer is found in 5% of the patients. Without breast MRI and second-look ultrasound and biopsy, many of these patients would return in a few years with "recurrent" cancer. With breast MRI, one can eliminate these cases by treating the otherwise unsuspected disease at the initial presentation of the first cancer. Other uses for breast MRI include screening for high-risk patients (including those with a core needle or mammotomy diagnosis of atypical ductal hyperplasia, lobular carcinoma in situ, or atypical lobular hyperplasia), patients with adenocarcinoma in their axillary node with an unknown primary, postlumpectomy patients with questionable or involved margins, and follow-up of patients undergoing neoadjuvant chemotherapy.

RADIOFREQUENCY DEVICES

A new family of instruments is now being developed and introduced that uses RF energy to penetrate and cut breast tissue. Many of these instruments can be used with ultrasound guidance. When the RF energy is applied, it results in some interference ("snow") in the ultrasound image.

(text continued on page 762)

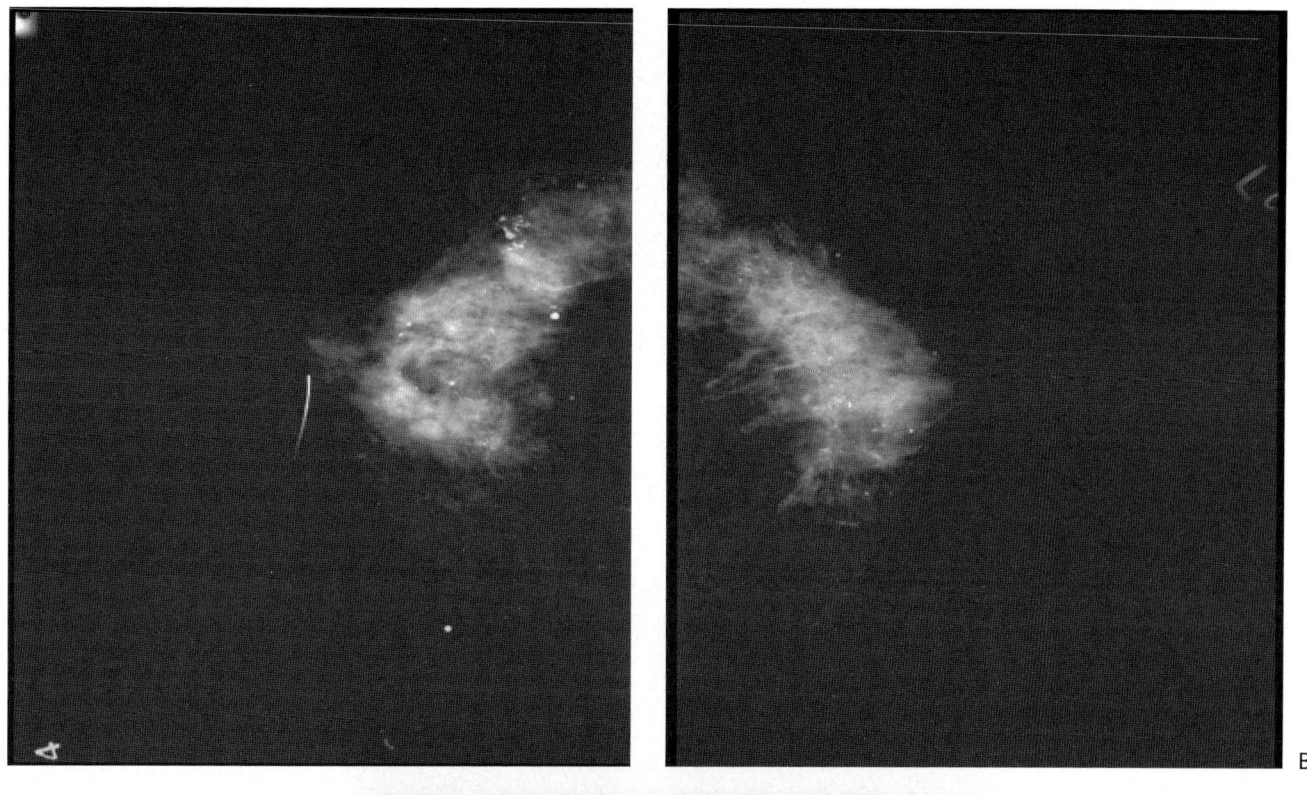

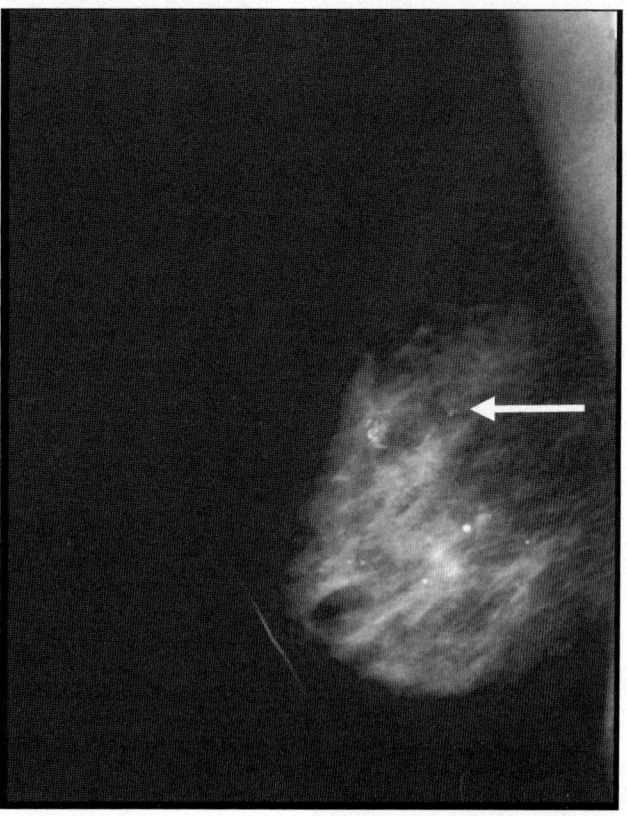

FIGURE 17.10 Breast magnetic resonance imaging (MRI) in newly diagnosed breast cancer. **A:** Right breast craniocaudal view demonstrates a very dense breast with numerous calcifications. **B:** Left breast craniocaudal view demonstrates similar findings. **C:** Right breast mediolateral oblique (MLO) view was noted to have questionable new calcifications in the 12:00 position *(arrow).* These underwent stereotactic biopsy, which revealed ductal carcinoma *in situ* (DCIS). *(Continued.)*

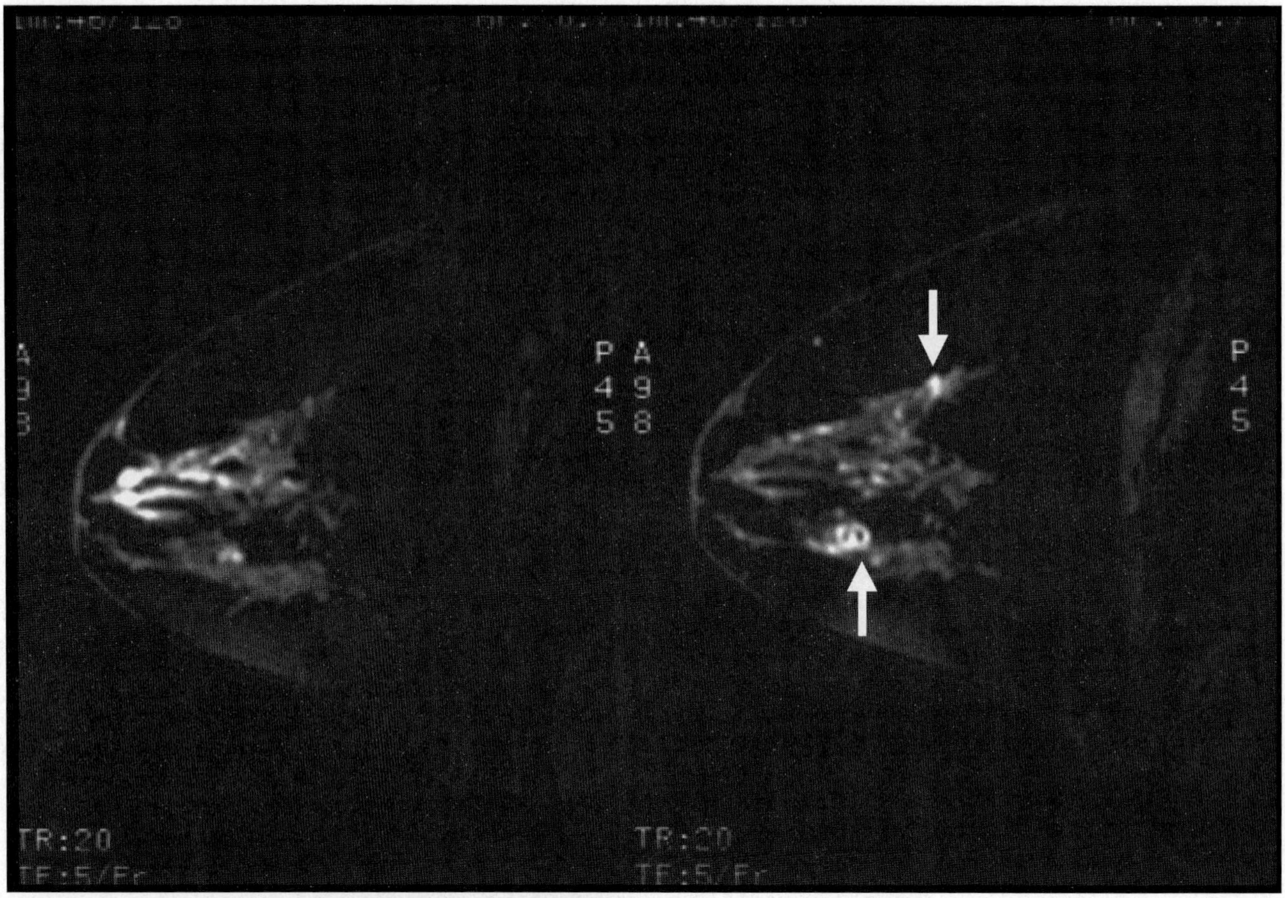

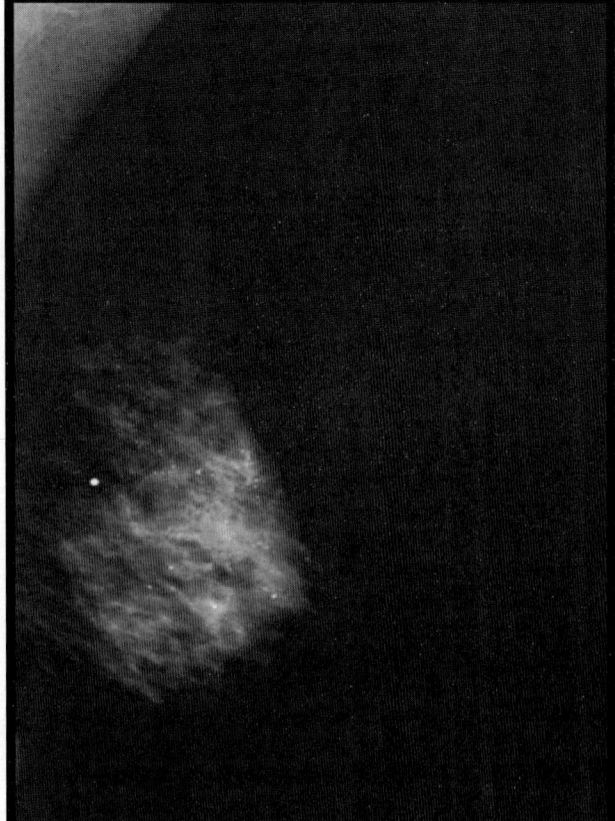

D

E

FIGURE 17.10 *(continued)* **D:** Subsequent right breast MRI demonstrated enhancement of the 12:00 DCIS *(arrow)* and also enhancement at 6:00 *(arrow).* Second-look ultrasound and ultrasound-guided biopsy of the lesion found at 6:00 revealed infiltrating lobular carcinoma. **E:** Left breast MLO view did not demonstrate any new calcifications or masses. *(Continued.)*

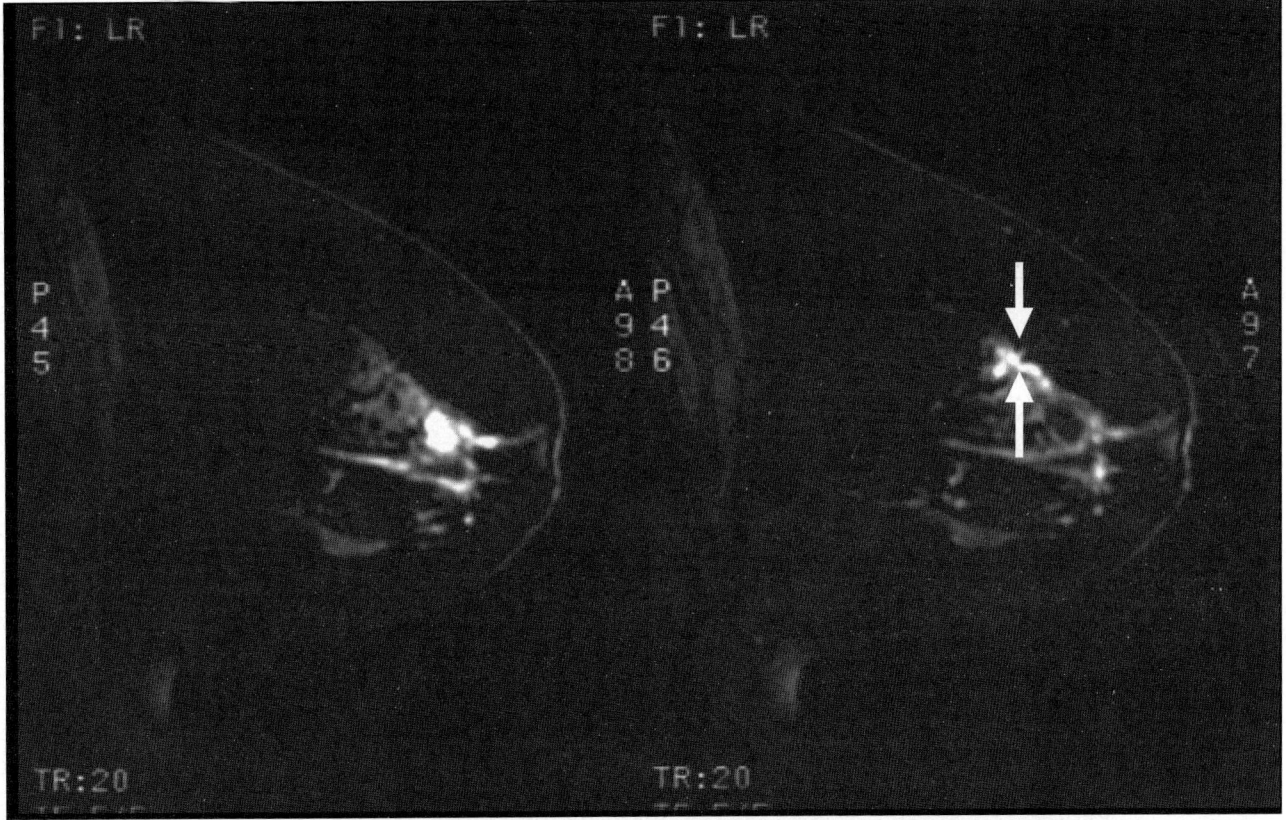

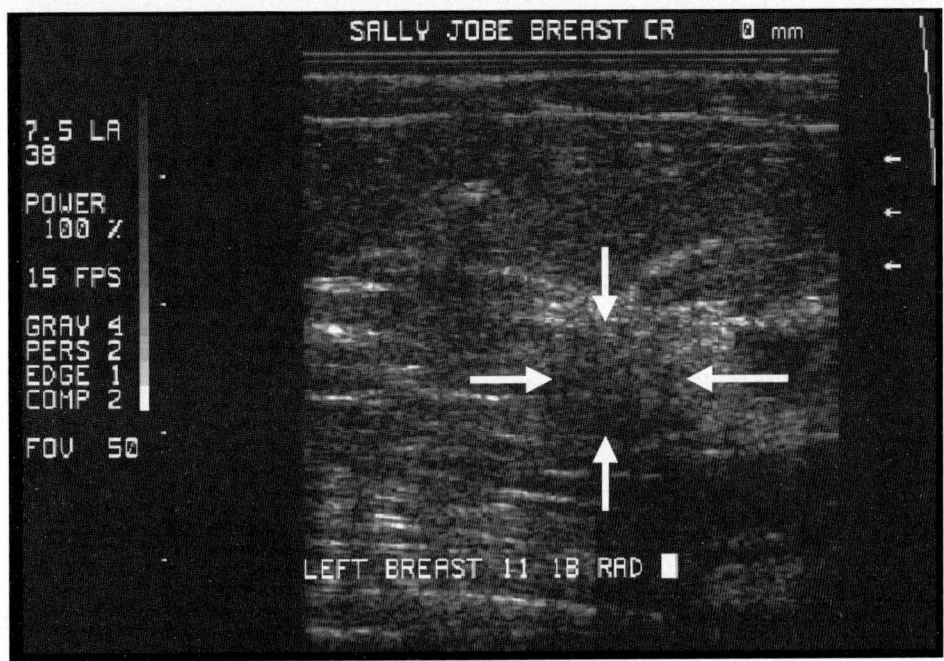

FIGURE 17.10 *(continued)* **F:** Left breast MRI demonstrated enhancement in the 11:00 position *(arrows)*. **G:** Second-look ultrasound of the 11:00 region demonstrated a vague hypoechoic region *(arrows)*. *(Continued.)*

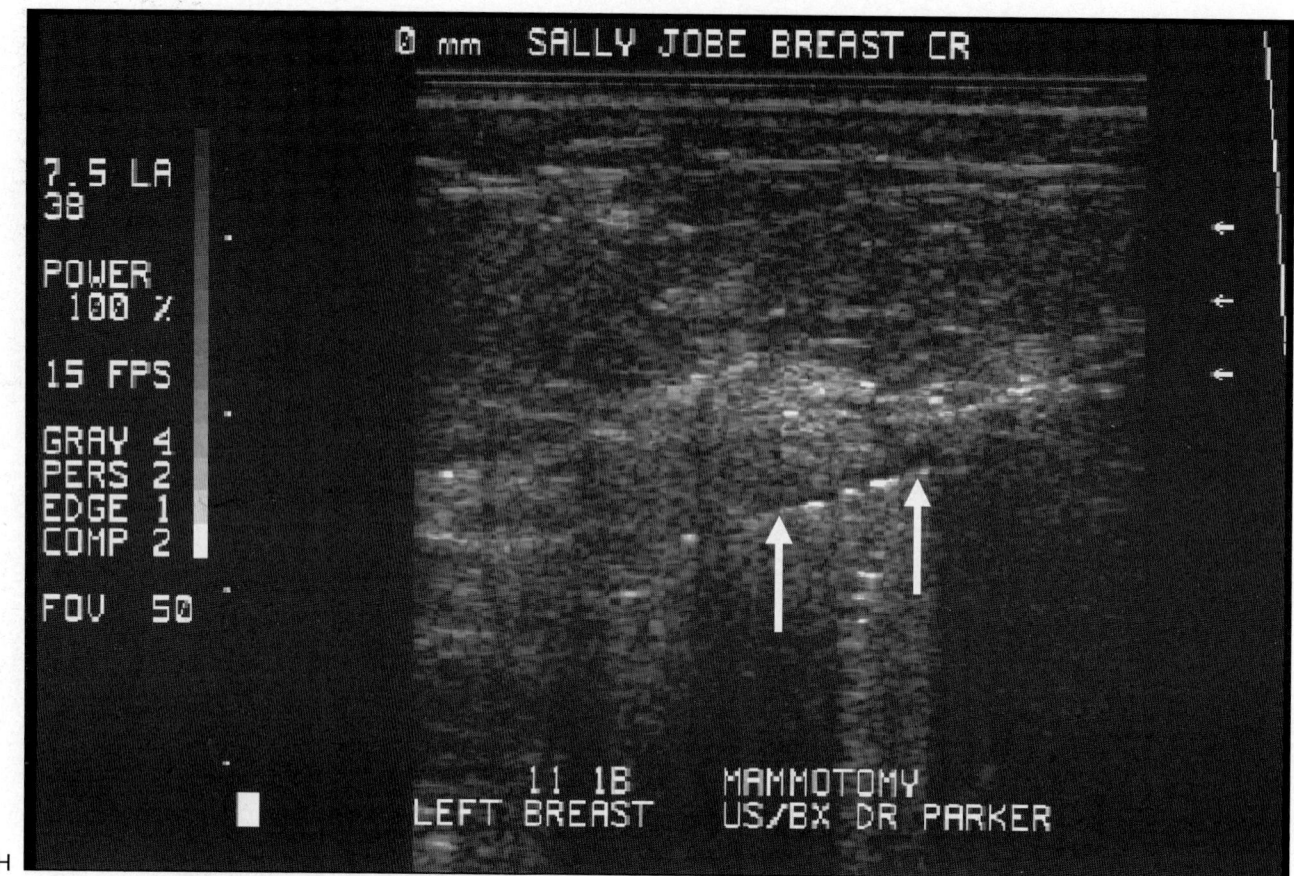

FIGURE 17.10 *(continued)* **H:** Ultrasound-guided mammotomy *(arrows)* revealed contralateral infiltrating lobular carcinoma.

Therefore, it is best if the energy is pulsed to allow for visualization of the instrument as it is advanced through the breast. The simplest instrument of this type is an RF introducer, the SenoRx Easy Guide, designed to penetrate dense breast tissues easily and provide a cannula or port through which a Mammotome probe or even a 14-gauge core needle can be advanced to perform the biopsy (Fig. 17–11). As mentioned earlier, a multiwire localization device, the SenoRx Anchor Guide, is now available that also uses RF energy (Fig. 17–12A). The tip of the device uses RF energy to penetrate the breast tissue easily and accurately under ultrasound guidance. Once the device is centered within a lesion, multiple (12) RF energized wires are extruded from the device to surround the lesion (Fig. 17–12B). These wires are palpable to the surgeon but are not sharp. Therefore, the surgeon can more accurately excise the lesion and surrounding tissue without taking out an unnecessarily large amount of tissue or taking too little tissue, risking "dirty" margins (Fig. 17–12C). In fact, a preliminary study revealed that use of the Anchor Guide resulted in significantly fewer lumpectomies with involved margins than when standard localization wires were used. Another RF device, the SenoCor, has been introduced by SenoRx, which allows for a substantially greater amount of tissue to be harvested per pass than either the automated core needle or the Mammotome (Fig. 17–13). In addition, it automatically bivalves each core (like a hotdog bun). This is important because many pathologists perform only three sections of core biopsy material, which, in an 11-gauge sample, leaves a significant amount of the core sample unstudied. The Senocor, on the other hand, forces the pathologist to review the equivalent of six sections. Therefore, the material submitted is more thoroughly sectioned and evaluated. A final RF product is Neothermia's En Bloc device, which involves RF penetration, and a web of RF energized wires that "basket" the lesion for percutaneous removal (Fig. 17–14).

(text continued on page 769)

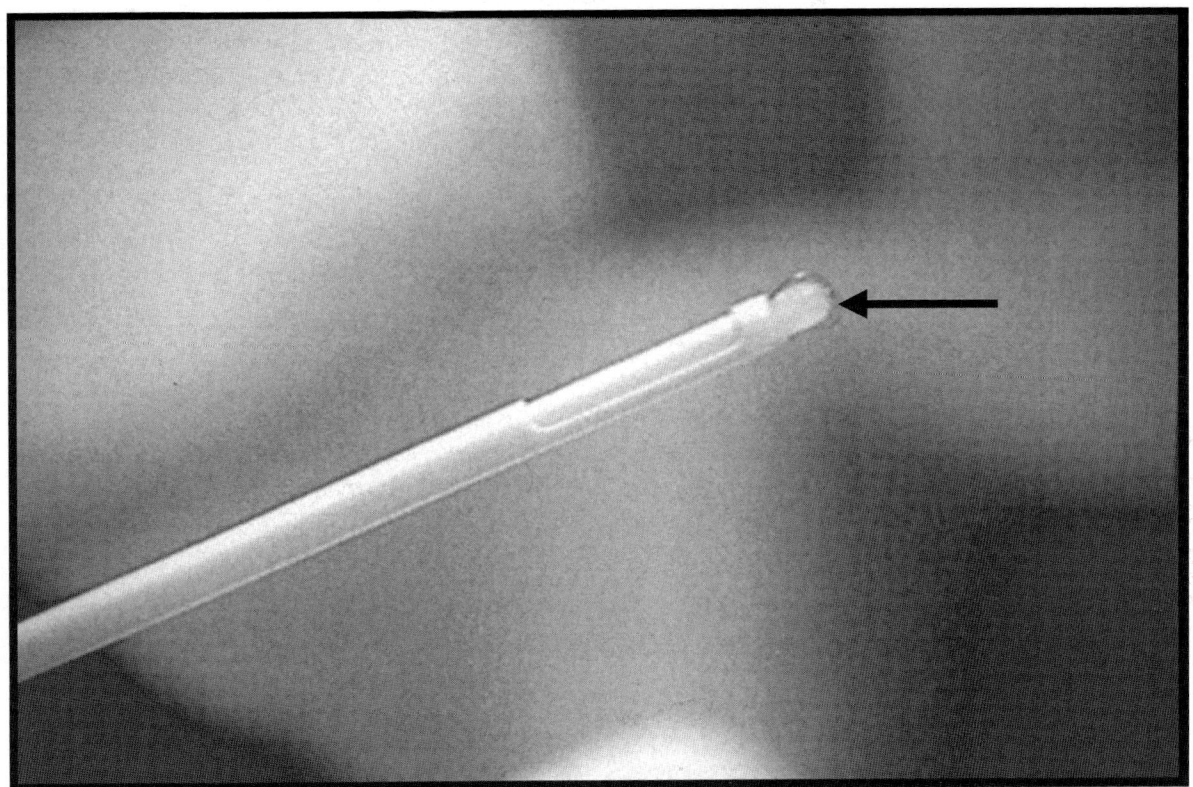

A

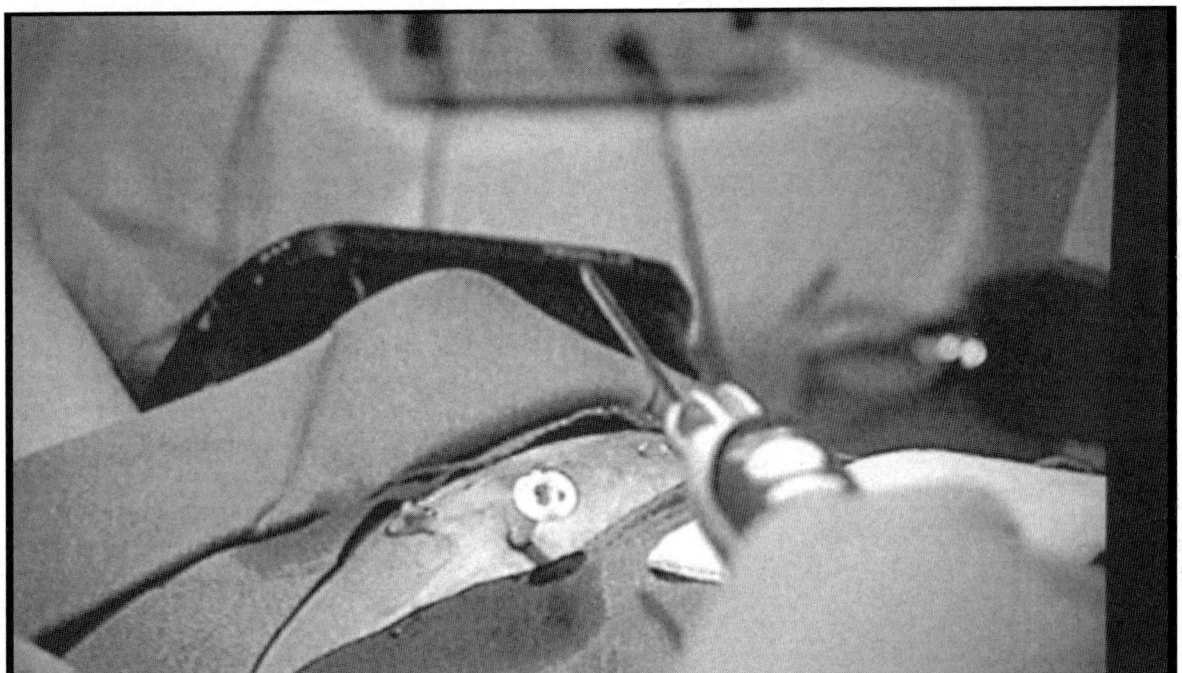

B

FIGURE 17.11 Radiofrequency (RF) introducer—the Easy Guide. **A:** The Easy Guide has an RF wire at its tip, which glides through even dense breast tissue *(arrow)*. **B:** Once in place with its aperture just posterior to the lesion to undergo biopsy, the inner trocar is removed, leaving the cannula within the breast. *(Continued.)*

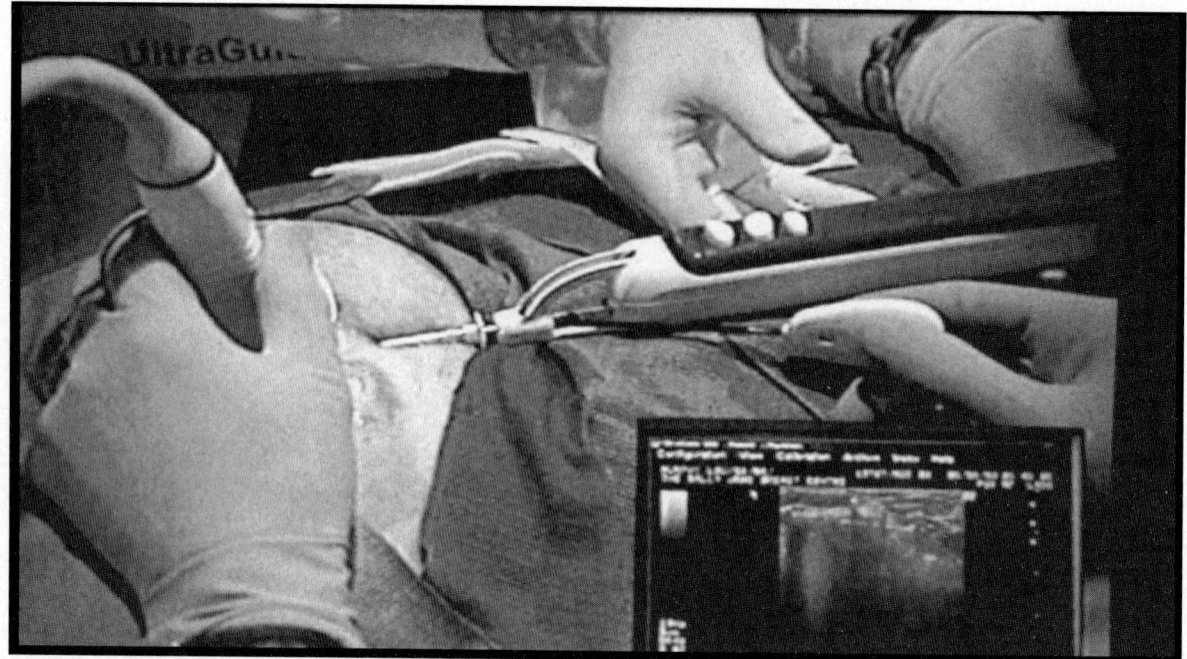

FIGURE 17.11 *(continued)* **C:** The Mammotome can then be advanced into that cannula with its aperture matching that of the Easy Guide. The biopsy can then proceed as usual.

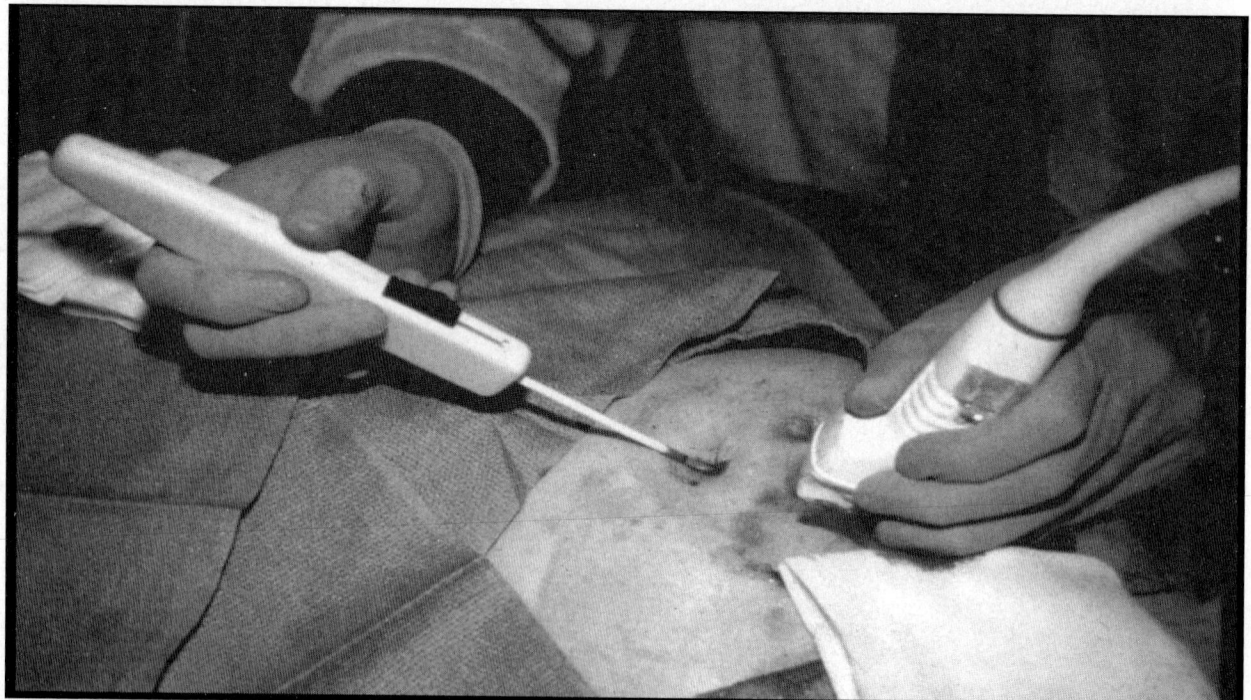

FIGURE 17.12 Radiofrequency (RF) multiwire localization device—the Anchor Guide. **A:** The Anchor Guide also has an RF tip, which allows the device to be easily advanced through the lesion to be removed. Once centered within the lesion, the RF energy is switched to the multiple wires to be extruded from the device. After the wires are extruded, the handle is detached from the needle portion of the device. (*Continued.*)

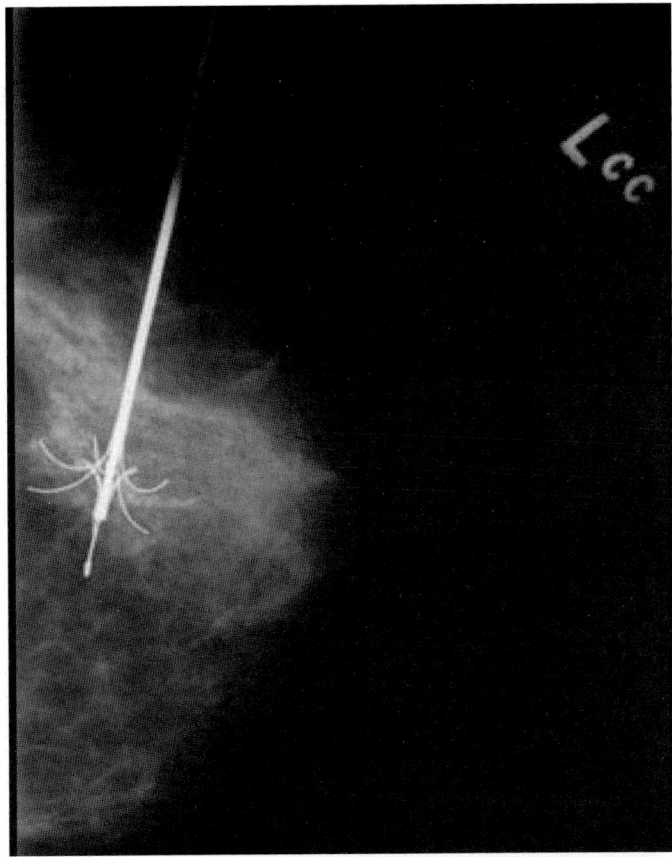

B

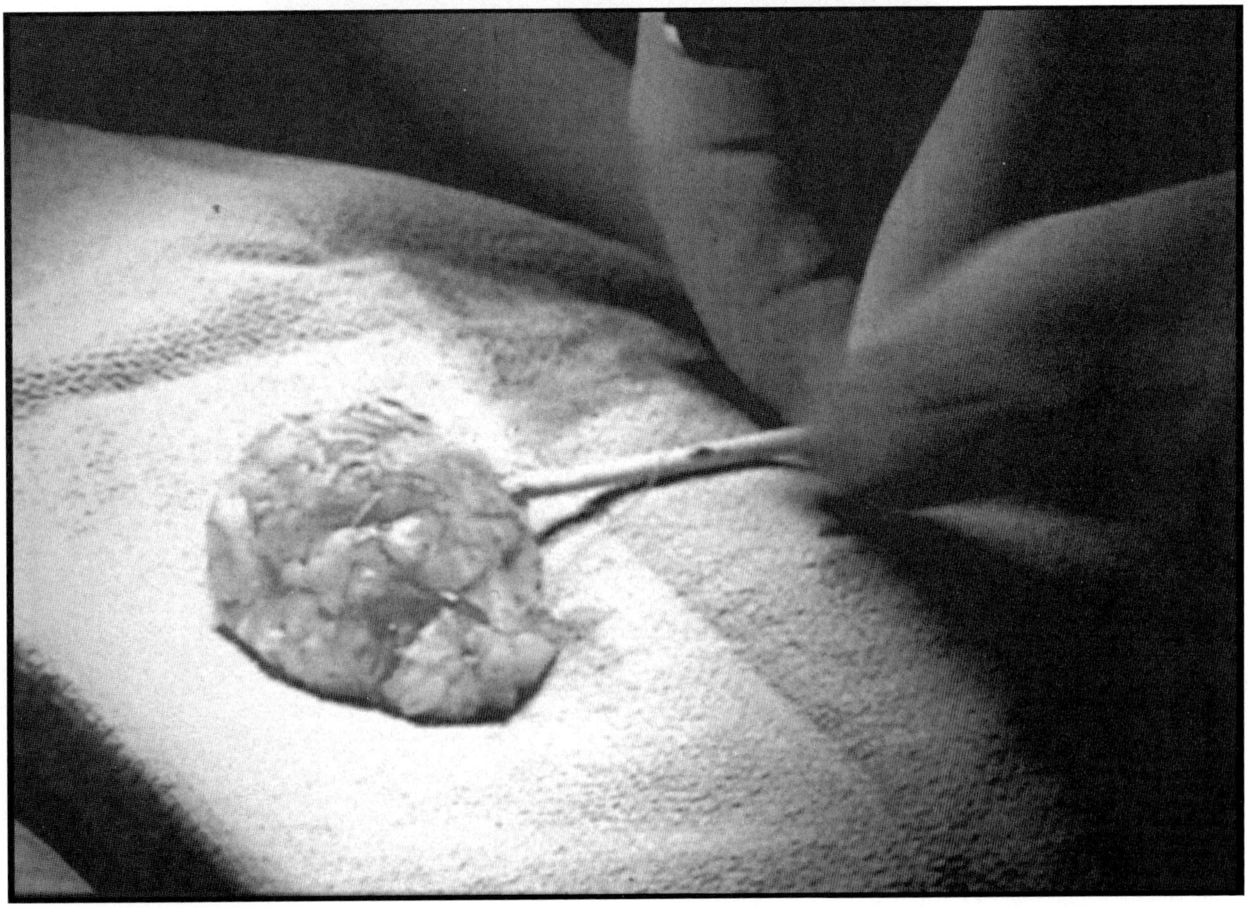

C

FIGURE 17.12 *(continued)* **B:** Postlocalization mammogram shows the wires extended from the device and surrounding the density corresponding to the lesion. **C:** Lumpectomy specimen with Anchor Guide device still contained within it.

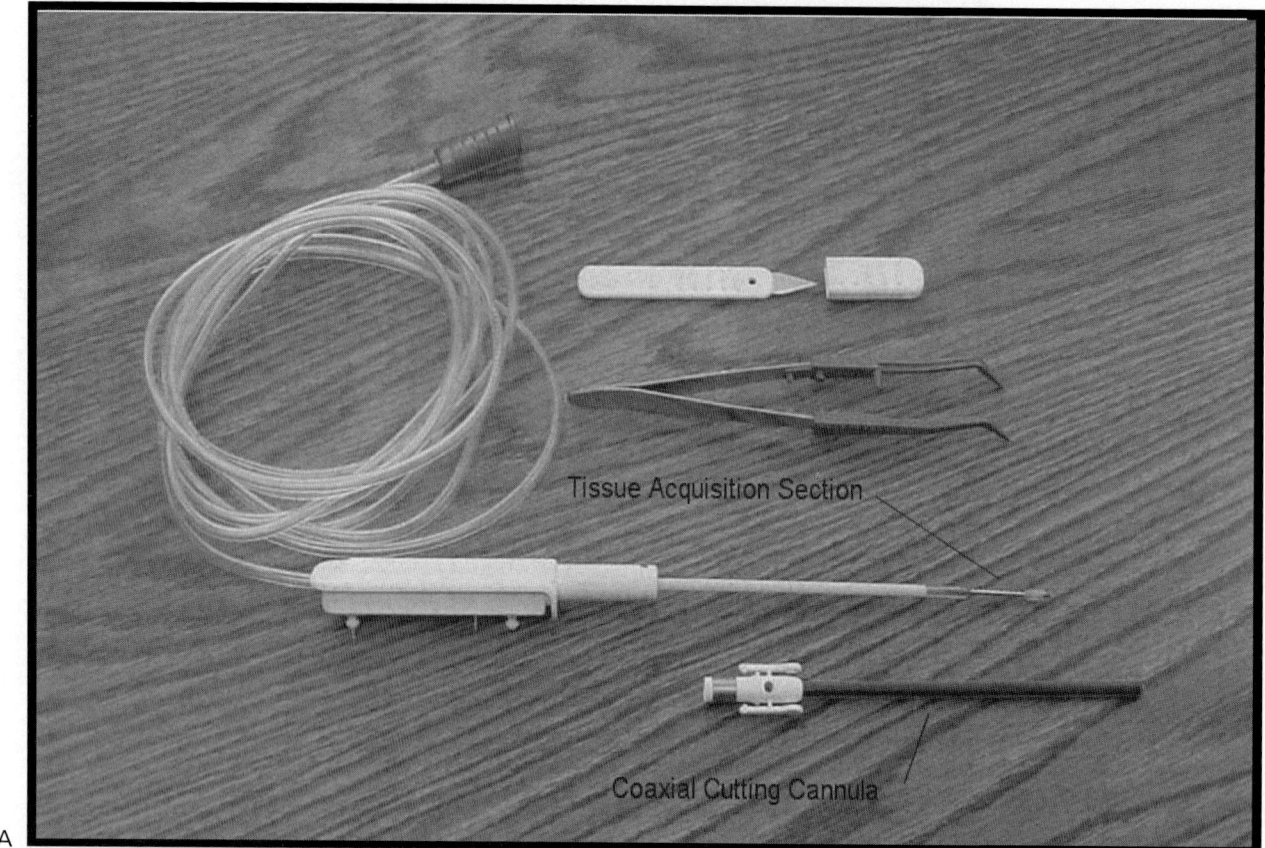

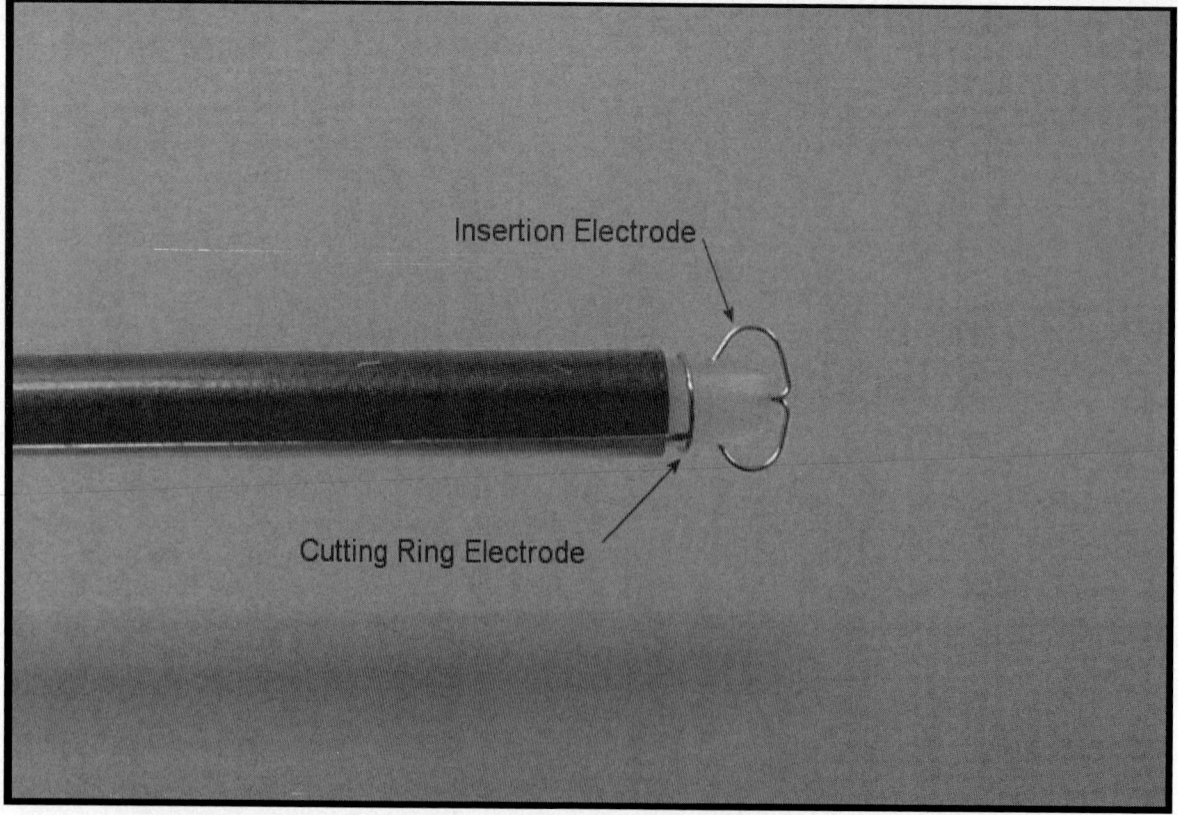

FIGURE 17.13 Radiofrequency (RF) core biopsy device. **A:** The Senocor uses both RF and vacuum to obtain tissue. **B:** The tip has an RF wire similar to the Easy Guide, which allows smooth introduction into the lesion to undergo biopsy. (*Continued.*)

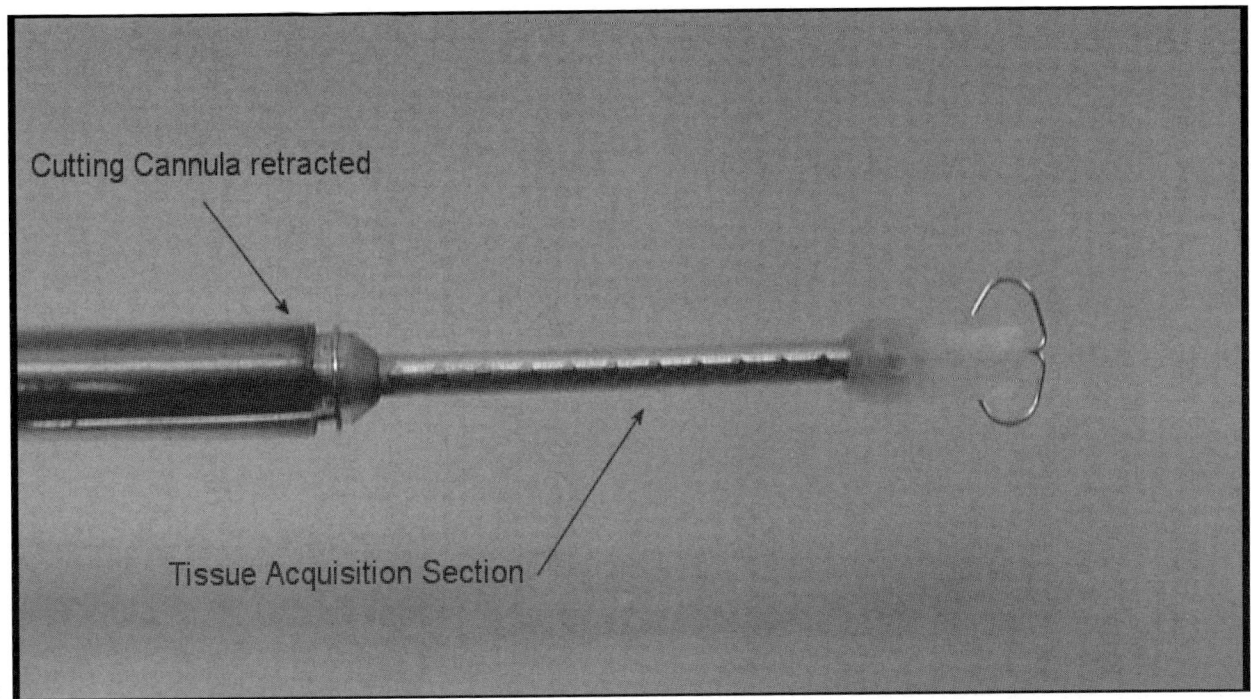

C

FIGURE 17.13 *(continued)* **C:** Vacuum holes along the specimen collection region of the inner trocar pull tissue concentrically around the trocar. The outer cannula has a cutting wire positioned circumferentially around its end that advances over the trocar, obtaining a large core of breast tissue and sectioning (bivalving) it at the same time.

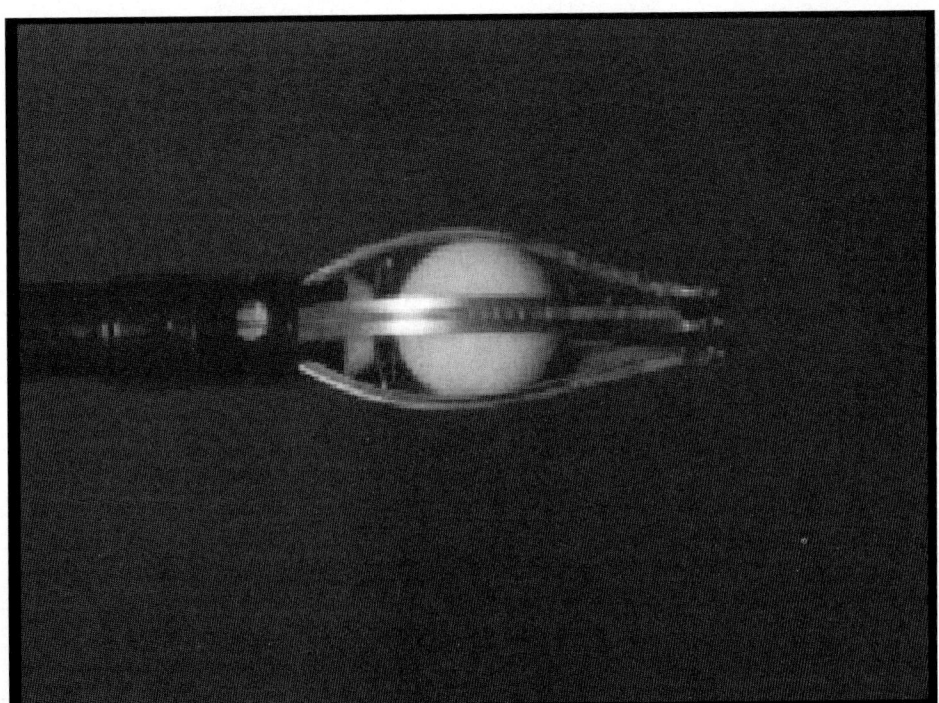

A

FIGURE 17.14 Radiofrequency (RF) excisional biopsy device. **A:** The instrument *en bloc* is advanced under ultrasound or stereotactic guidance through an incision to the periphery of the breast lesion, and multiple RF wires "basket" a volume of tissue. (*Continued.*)

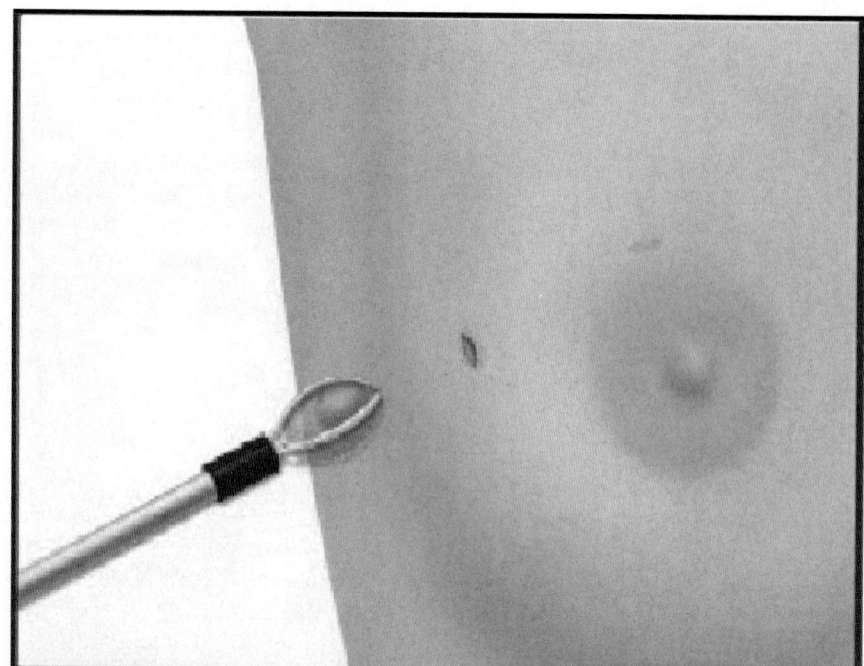

B

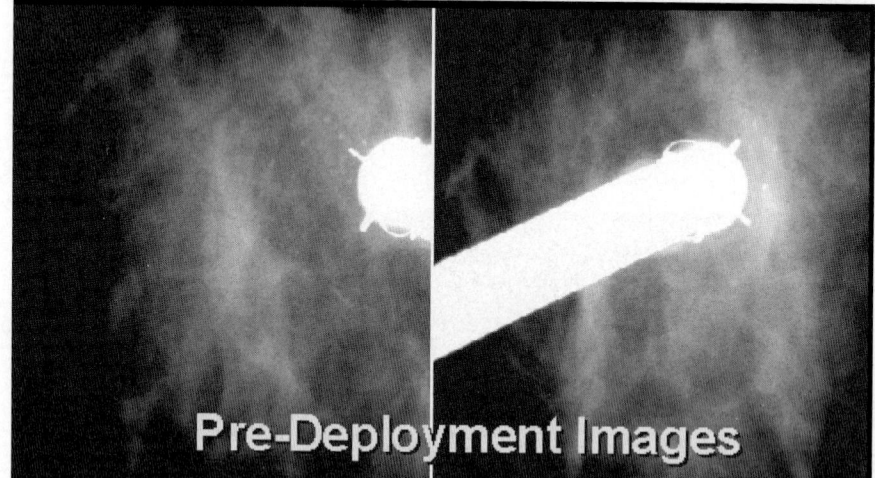

Pre-Deployment Images

C

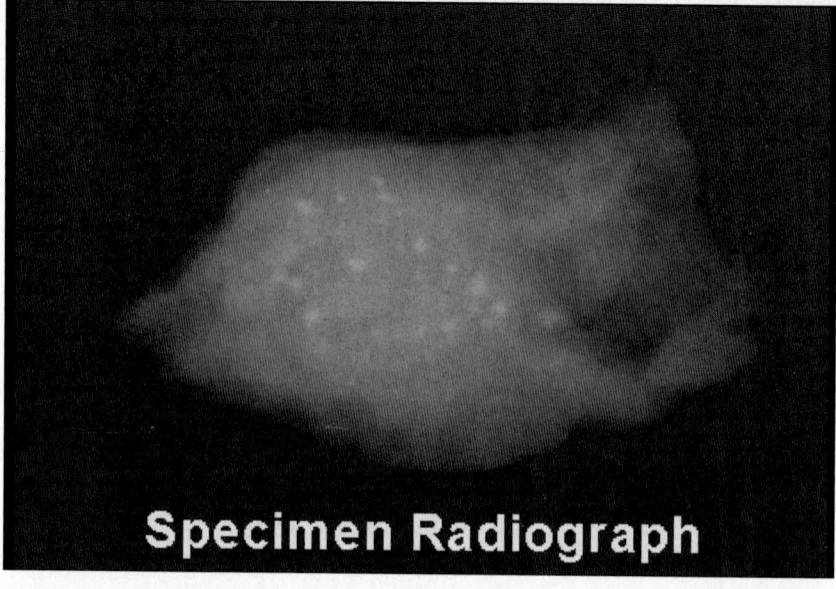

Specimen Radiograph

D

FIGURE 17.14 *(continued)* **B:** The specimen is then removed intact through the skin incision. **C:** Stereotactic localization using the device. **D:** Specimen radiograph of resultant tissue.

SENTINEL NODE ANALYSIS

Sentinel node analysis represents a major advance in breast cancer surgery. Rather than subjecting a patient to a full axillary node dissection as was done routinely in the past, the patient now only has a few nodes removed after they have been labeled with a radionuclide. This results in little or no morbidity as compared with the full axillary dissection. We use ultrasound in two aspects of sentinel node analysis. First, we ultrasonographically screen the axilla of patients with possible infiltrating carcinomas at the time of the original diagnostic workup and ultrasound-guided breast biopsy of the breast mass. If there is an ultrasonographically abnormal axillary node seen at the time of the biopsy of the mass, then that node is also subjected to ultrasound-guided core biopsy (Fig. 17–15A, B). If that node is shown to harbor metastases, then the patient is not scheduled for sentinel node analysis but rather a standard axillary dissection. If the axillary nodes are ultrasonographically or histologically normal (after core biopsy), then the patient is scheduled for sentinel node analysis at the time of her lumpectomy or mastectomy. This is important for two reasons. First, if axillary metastases are proven before breast cancer surgery, sentinel node analysis is not performed, and a second operation to complete the axillary dissection can be avoided. Second, the most common cause of false-negative sentinel nodes is a result of malignancy within the sentinel node that obstructs lymphatic flow to that node. As a result of this tumor "dam," the lymphatic flow containing the radionuclide tracer is diverted around the true sentinel node to a normal node, which then is erroneously identified as the sentinel node, resulting in a false-negative finding. Identifying macroscopically metastatic lymph nodes with ultrasound (the nodes most likely to cause a tumor dam and subsequent false-negative result) before surgery allows one to screen out these potential false-negative findings before sentinel node analysis and to proceed directly to standard axillary dissection.

We also use ultrasound to help localize the sentinel node on the day of surgery. First, we use ultrasound guidance to place the radionuclide (1 mCi of technetium-99m–labeled, filtered sulfur colloid in 4 mL of sterile saline) just anterior to the tumor in the plane between the deep subcutaneous fat and the mammary zone containing the lesion (Fig. 17–16A, B). In this way, the radionuclide is placed adjacent to the tumor but is in an anatomic region rich in lymphatics. Lymphoscintigraphy is performed about 1 hour after injection of the radionuclide, and the technologist marks the skin overlying the activity in the axilla (Fig. 17–16C). The patient's axilla is then scanned with ultrasound in an alternating fashion with a hand-held scintillation counter (Fig. 17–16D–F). An ultrasonographically visible node is virtually always detected

(text continued on page 775)

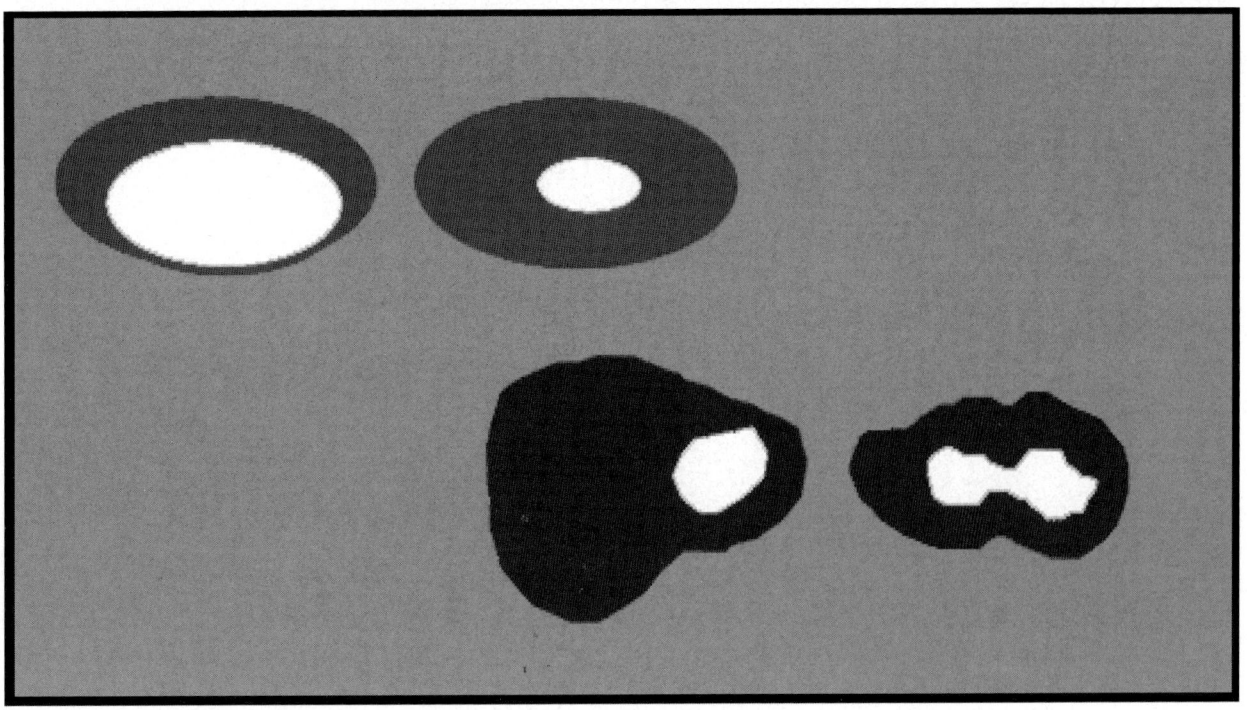

FIGURE 17.15 Axillary ultrasound and biopsy. **A:** Graphic depiction of normal and abnormal axillary nodes. Before a patient is deemed eligible for sentinel node analysis, the axilla is scanned to detect any ultrasonographically abnormal nodes. Abnormal nodes (**bottom two images**) should be differentiated from normal nodes (**top two images**). (*Continued.*)

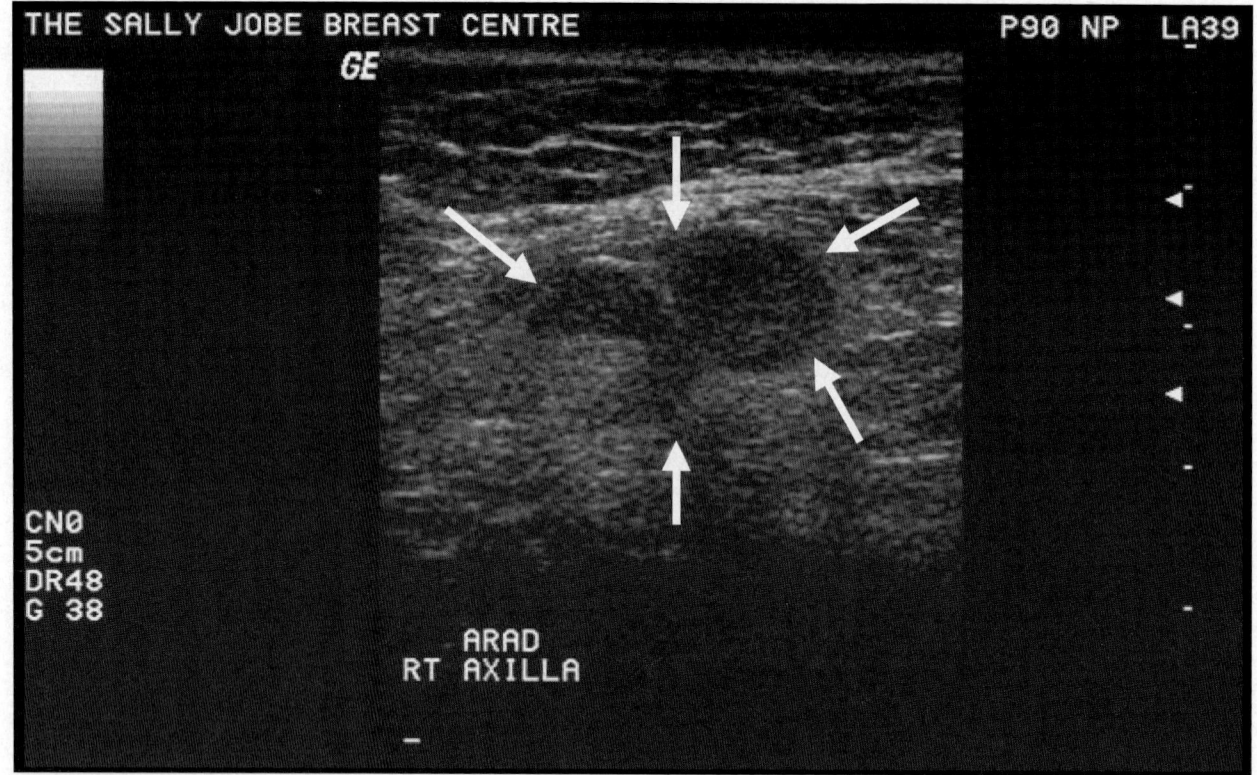

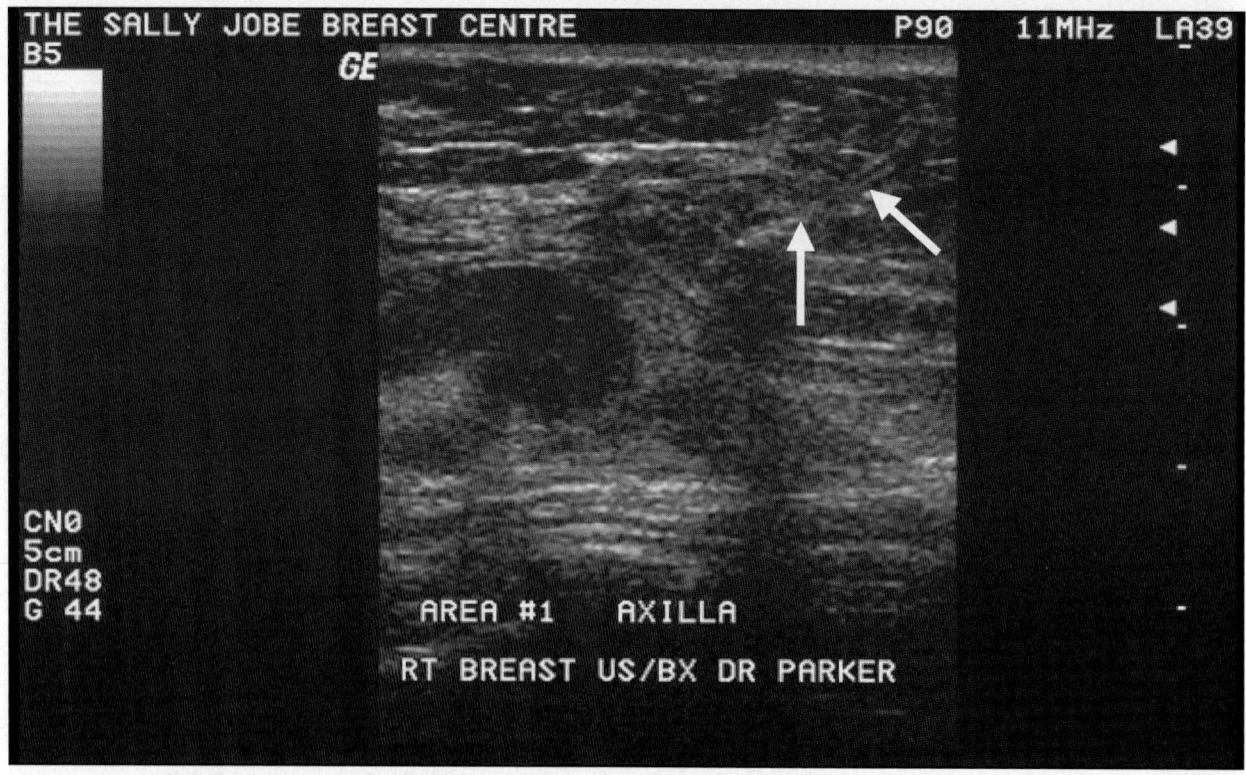

FIGURE 17.15 *(continued)* **B:** Actual ultrasound of abnormal (metastatic lymph node) *(arrows).*
C: The node is then subjected to ultrasound-guided automated core biopsy *(arrows).*

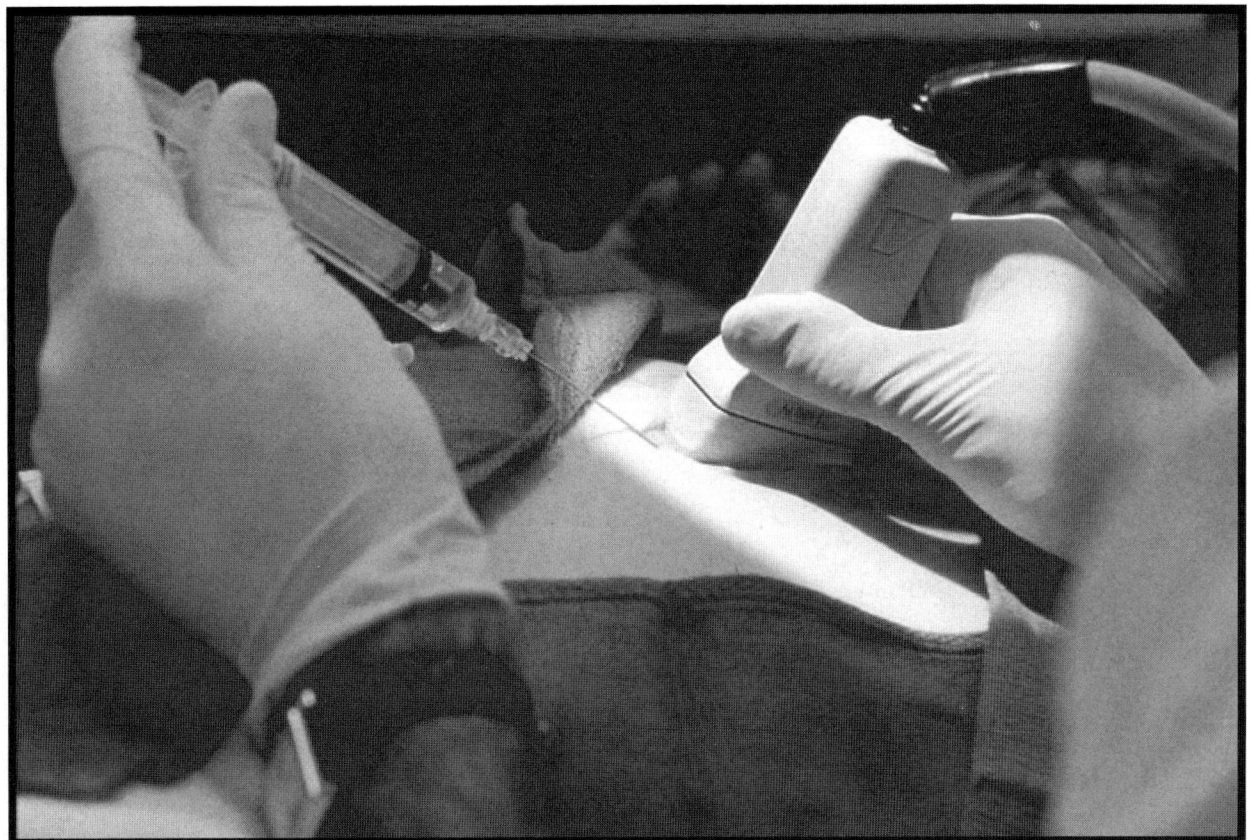

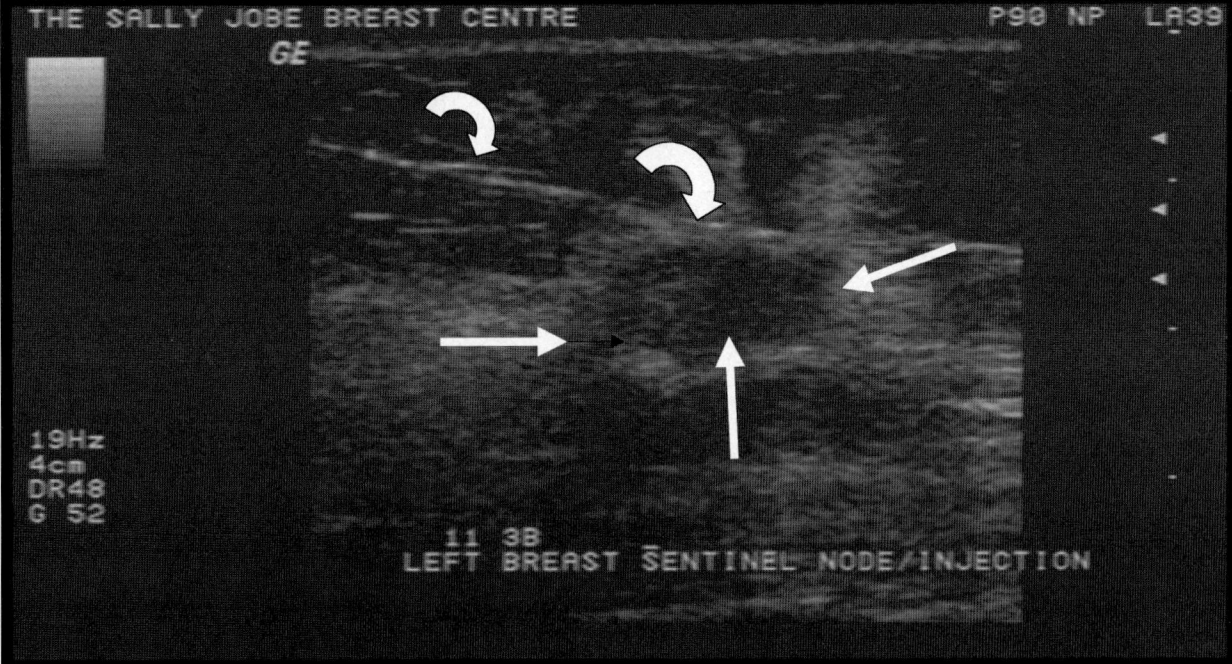

FIGURE 17.16 Sentinel node analysis. **A:** The radionuclide is injected under real-time observation. **B:** Using a 20-gauge spinal needle *(curved arrows)*, the radionuclide is placed just anterior to the tumor in the plane between the subcutaneous fat and the mammary zone containing the tumor *(straight arrows)*. *(Continued.)*

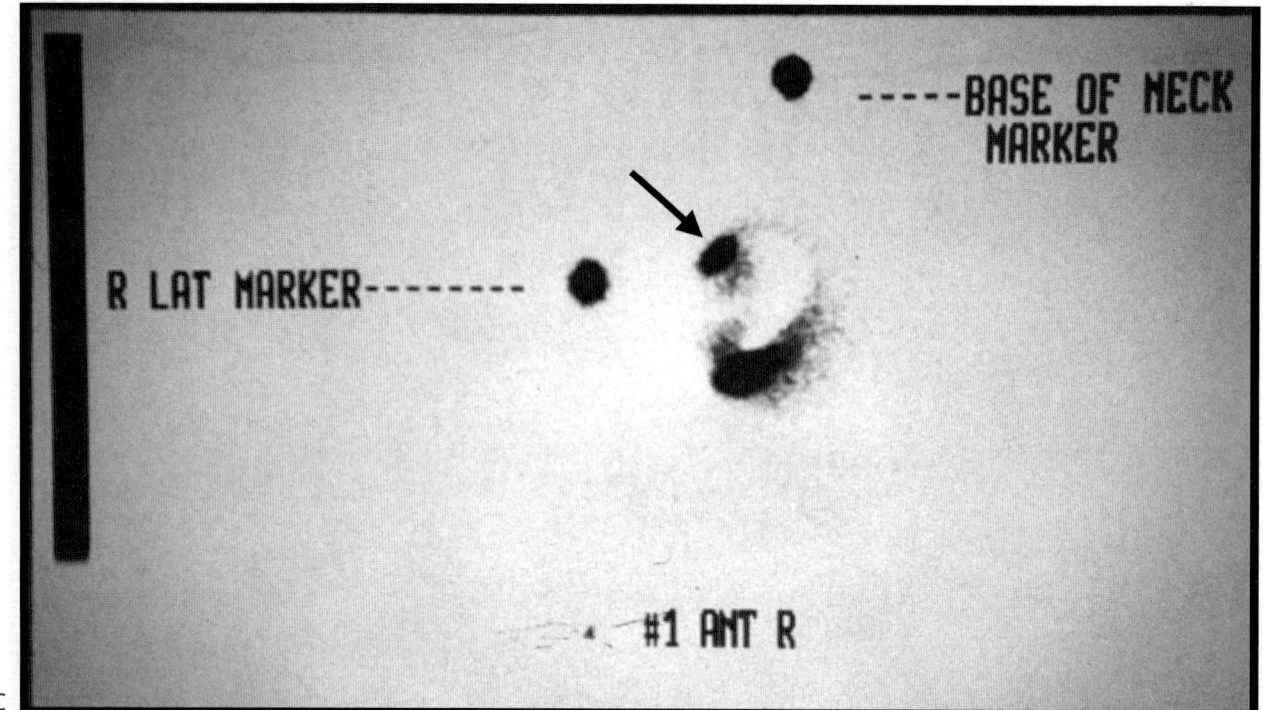

C

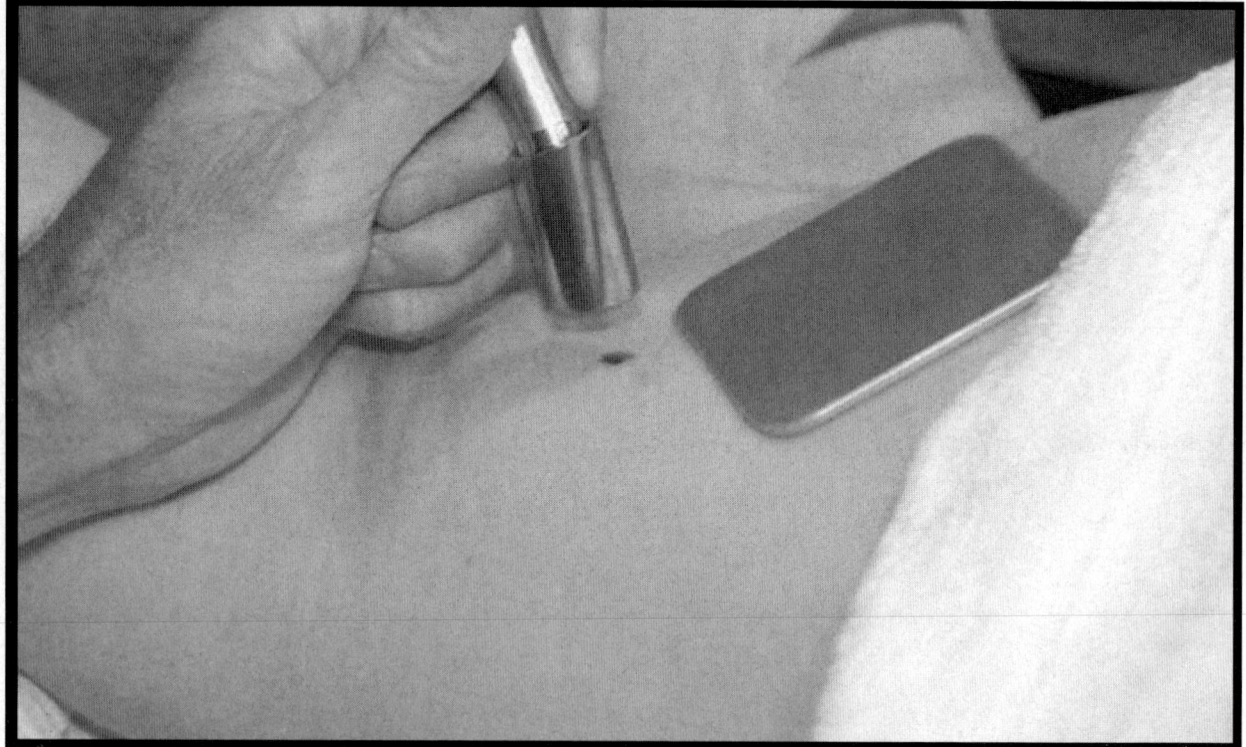

D

FIGURE 17.16 *(continued)* **C:** Lymphoscintigraphy is performed about 1 hour later, and the focal activity in the axilla corresponding to the sentinel node is identified *(arrow)*. The overlying skin is marked. **D:** A hand-held scintillation counter is used to confirm the skin mark. *(Continued.)*

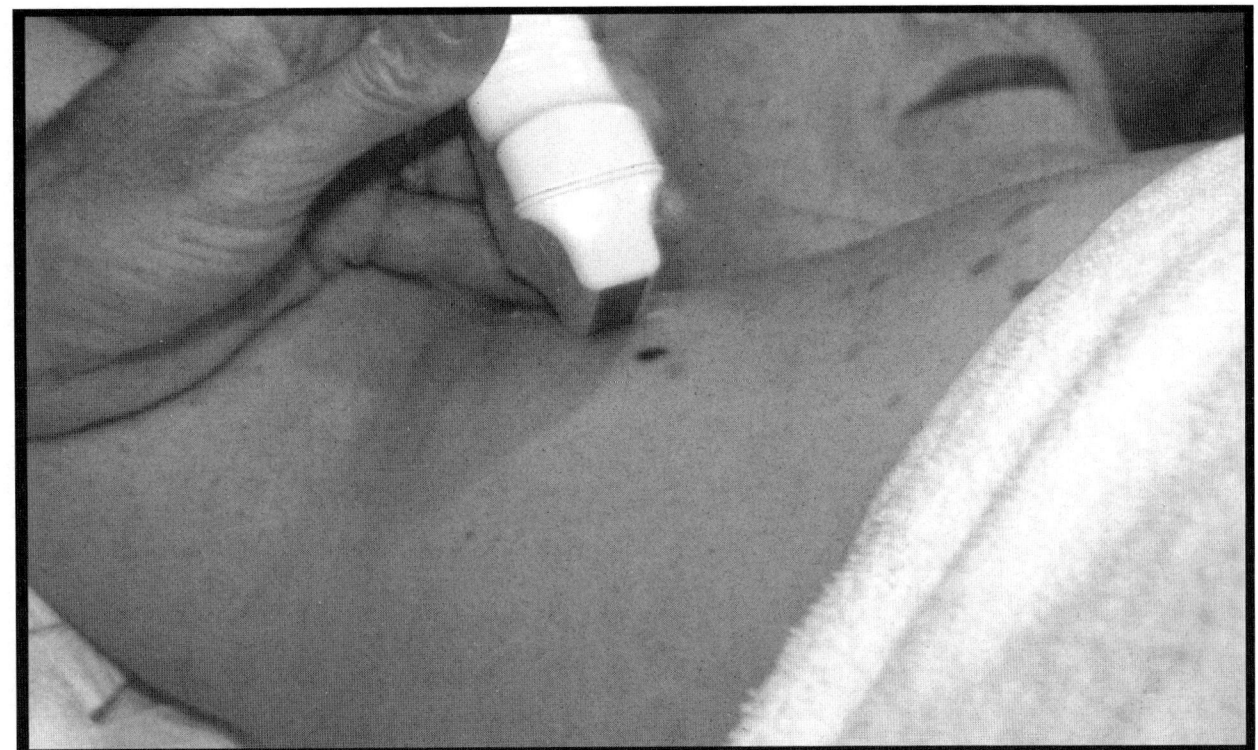

E

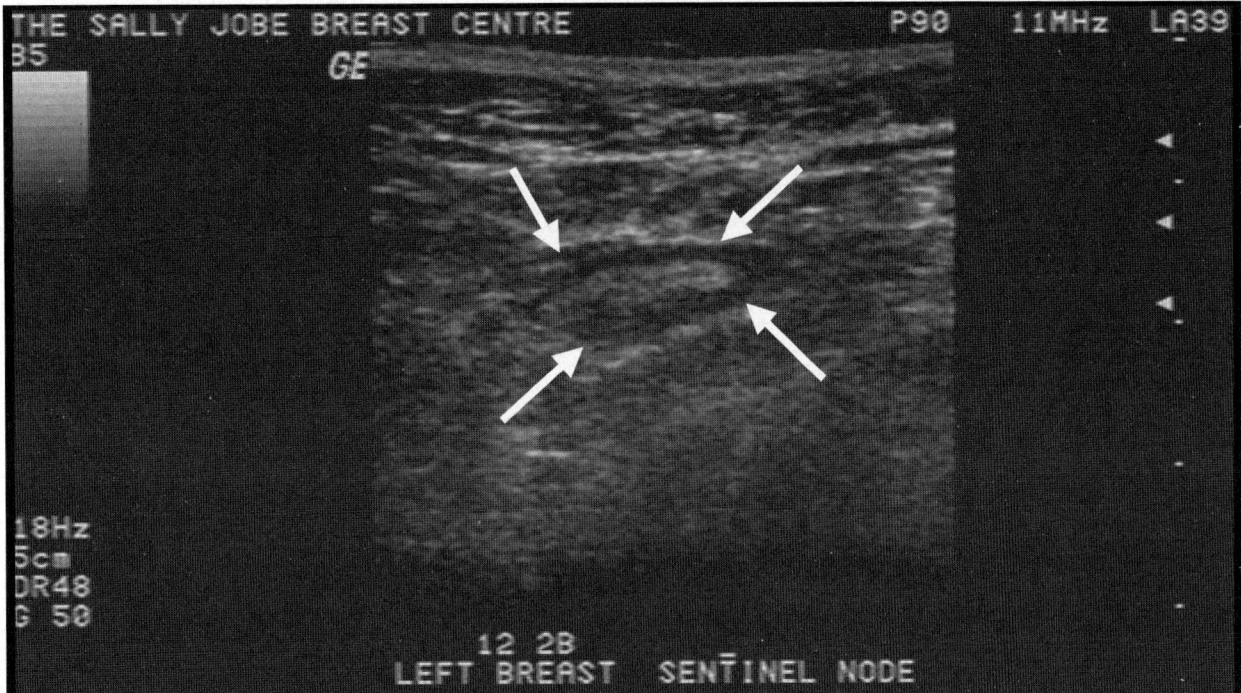

F

FIGURE 17.16 *(continued)* **E:** Ultrasound of the axilla is subsequently performed over the skin mark. **F:** The sentinel node is ultrasonographically visualized *(arrows)*. *(Continued.)*

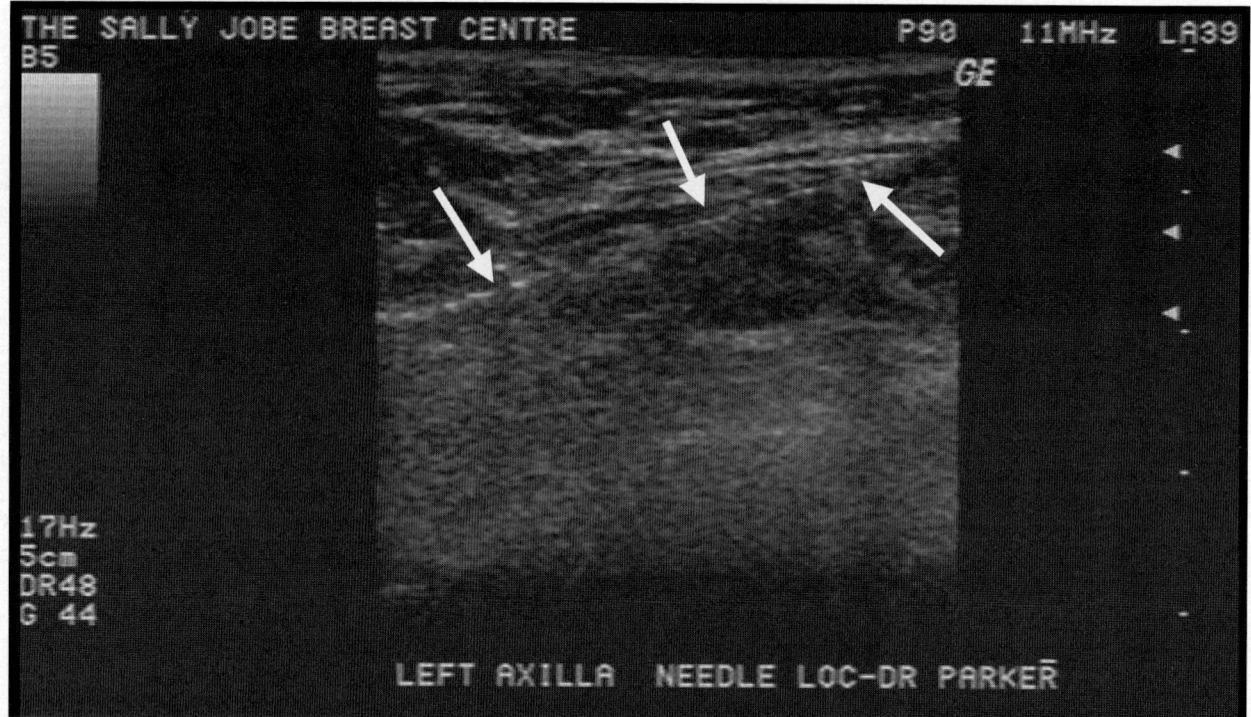

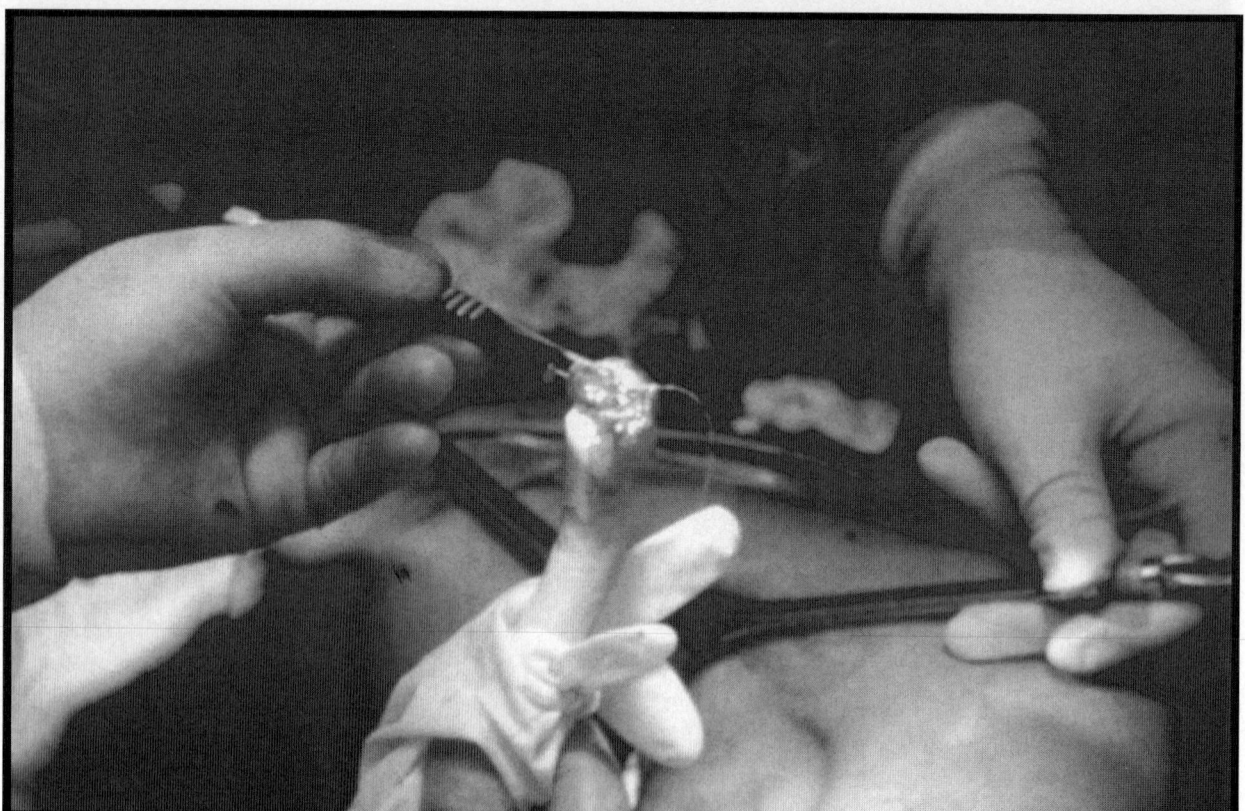

FIGURE 17.16 *(continued)* **G:** A localization wire is placed through the node under ultrasound guidance *(arrows)*. **H:** The surgeon excises the node following the localization wire and double-checks the activity with an intraoperative scintillation counter after the node is removed.

corresponding to the area of increased scintillations in the axilla. The presumed sentinel node identified by ultrasound is then wire-localized under ultrasound guidance at the same time that the primary breast carcinoma is wire-localized (Fig. 17–16G). The surgeon then only has to dissect down along the wire to reach the sentinel node. Once the node is removed, the surgeon can double-check the radioactivity with a hand-held scintillation counter in the operating room (Fig. 17–16H). Naturally, the surgeon should check in the axillary bed for any further "hot" nodes (>10% of the activity of the hottest node on a 10-second count). Any other hot nodes will be in the immediate vicinity of the localized node. We have found that this approach can substantially shorten the procedure time in the operating room and provide the surgeon with a way to double-check the sentinel node.

BREAST CANCER THERAPY AND *IN SITU* ABLATION

With the introduction of new instruments for breast biopsy and the advent of RF devices for use in the breast, there is a growing desire to migrate these technologies to minimally invasive breast cancer therapy. It is clear that ultrasound will be instrumental in the guidance of these therapeutic devices in most instances. Thus far, it has been difficult to predict margin status and adequacy of percutaneous removal and ablation, and no current minimally invasive instrument is approved for therapy by the U.S. Food and Drug Administration. Most promising for overcoming these obstacles are the RF instruments, such as the SenoRx Anchor Guide with automated wire cutter and the Neothermia En Bloc device (Figs. 17–14 and 17–17). It is likely that some form of percutaneous lesion removal, perhaps combined with *in situ* ablation, will be forthcoming. Just as the past decade has seen many exciting changes and improvements in breast cancer diagnosis (thanks in large part to ultrasound-guided interventions), health-care professionals involved in breast care can look forward to many more exciting changes in the realm of ultrasound-guided breast cancer therapy during the next decade.

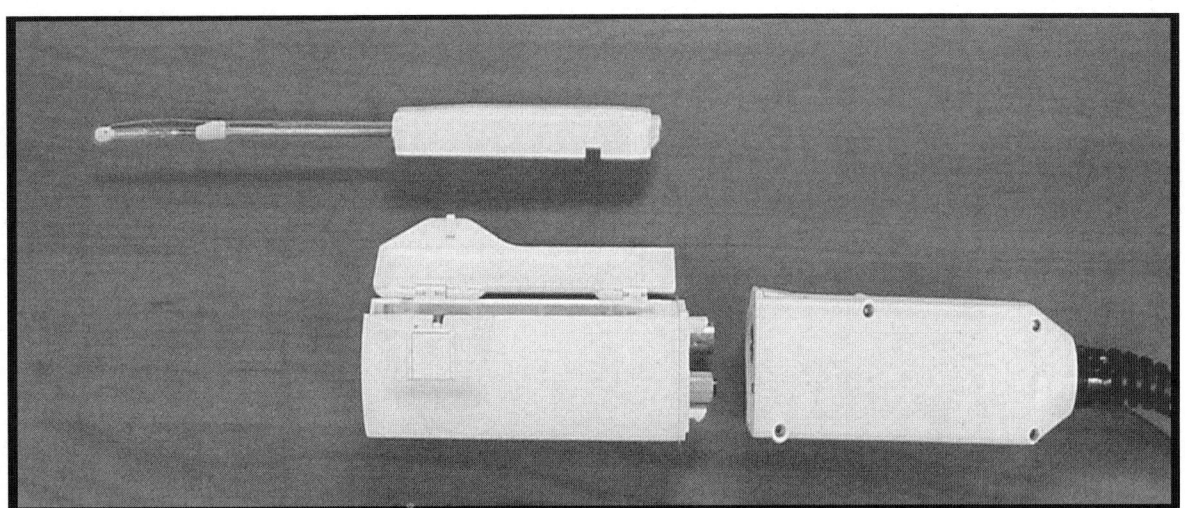

A

FIGURE 17.17 Radiofrequency localization and excision device. **A:** This device is similar to the Anchor Guide, with the addition of a cutting wire, which rotates around the volume of tissue to be excised. (*Continued.*)

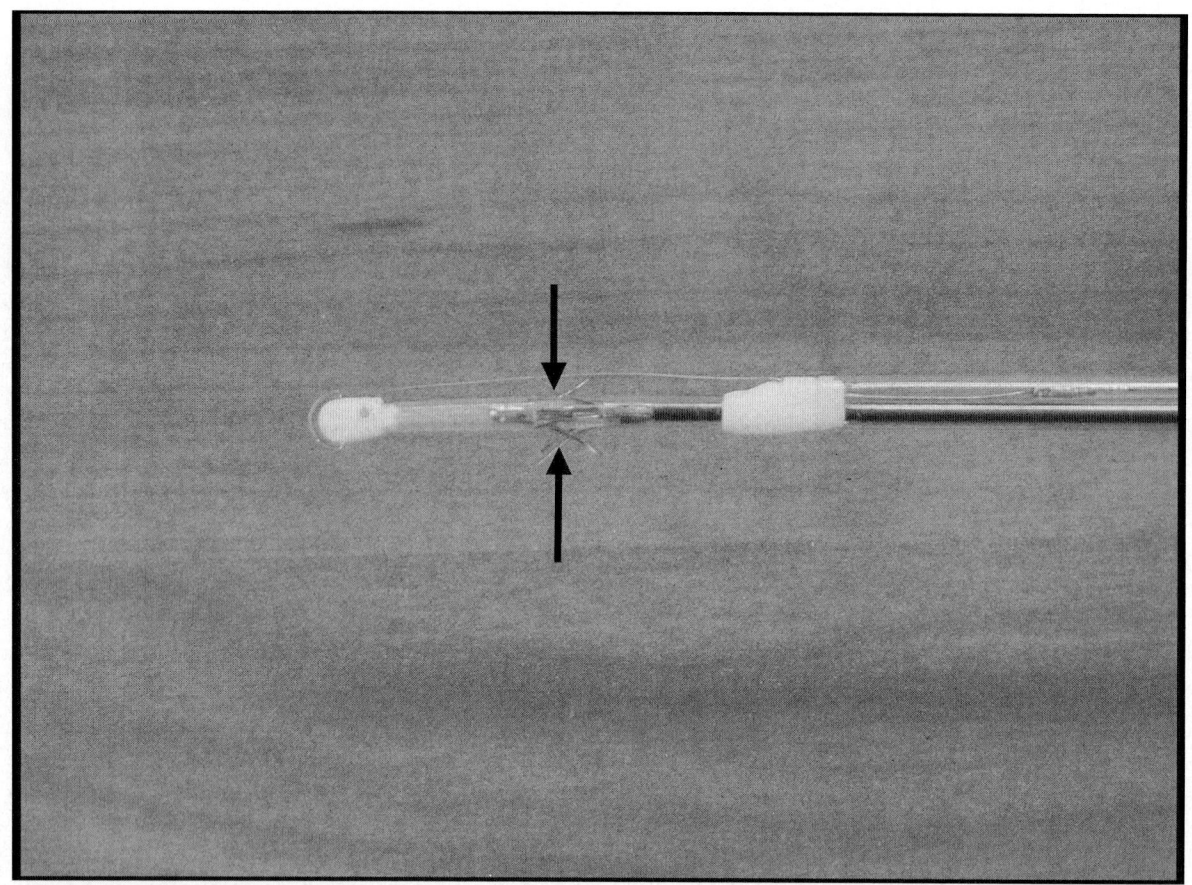

B

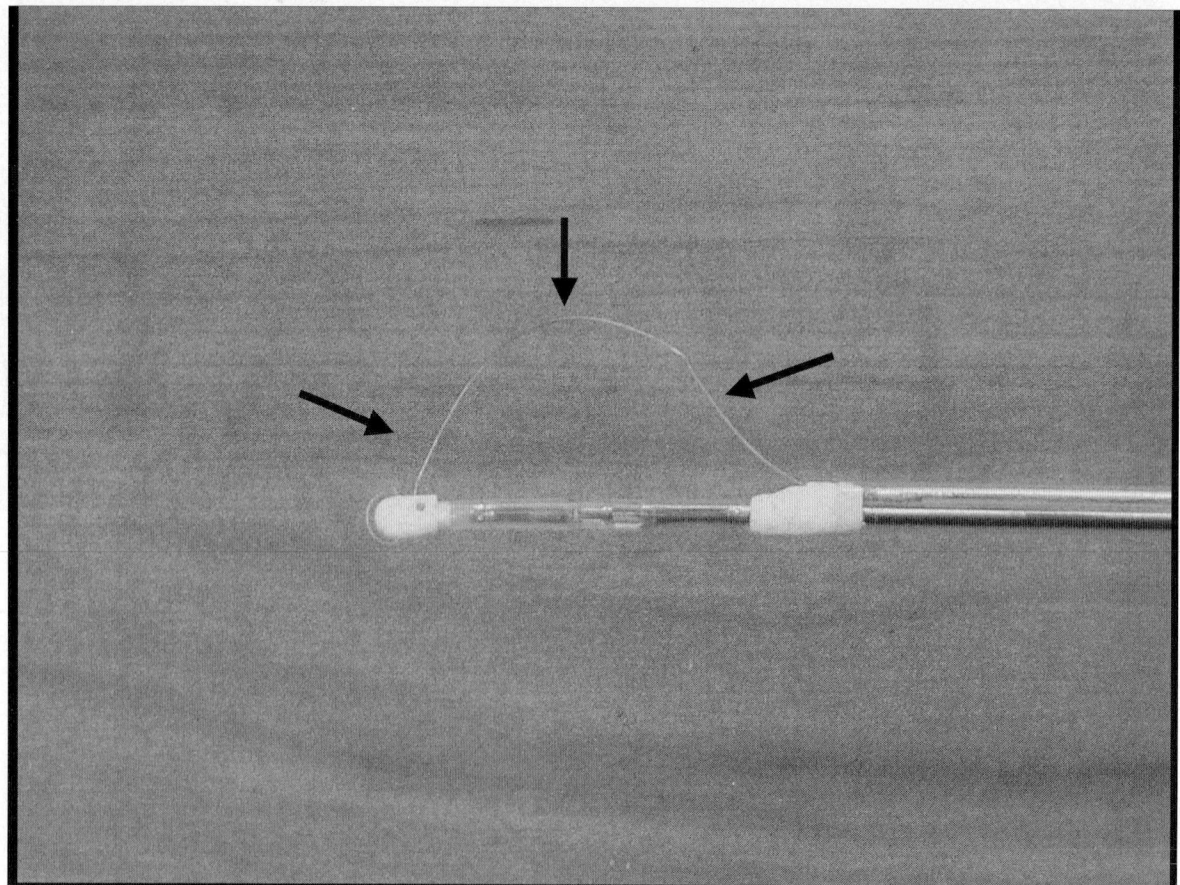

C

FIGURE 17.17 *(continued)* **B:** Anchoring wires *(arrows)* deployed after device is centered within lesion to be removed. **C:** Cutting wire rotates around lesion to excise appropriate volume of tissue around lesion *(arrows)*.

SUGGESTED READINGS

Dennis DA, Parker SH, Kaske TI, et al. Incidental treatment of nipple discharge caused by benign intraductal papilloma through diagnostic Mammotome biopsy. *AJR Am J Roentgenol* 2000;174: 1263–1268.

Parker SH, Burbank F. A practical approach to minimally invasive breast biopsy. *Radiology* 1996;200:11–20.

Parker SH, Dennis MA, Kaske TI. Identification of the sentinel node in patients with breast cancer. *Radiol Clin North Am* 2000;38: 809–823.

Parker SH, Dennis MA, Stavros AT, et al. Ultrasound-guided mammotomy: a new breast biopsy technique. *J Diagn Med Sonogr* 1996;12:113–118.

Parker SH, Jobe WE. Large-core breast biopsy offers reliable diagnosis. *Diagn Imaging* 1990;Oct:90–97.

Parker SH, Jobe WE, Dennis MA, et al. US-guided automated large-core breast biopsy. *Radiology* 1993;187:507–511.

Parker SH, Kercher JM, Dennis MA. Sonographically guided Mammotome extraction of retained localization wire. *AJR Am J Roentgenol* 1999;173:903–904.

Parker SH, Klaus AJ, McVey PJ, et al. Sonographically guided directional vacuum-assisted breast biopsy using a handheld device. *AJR Am J Roentgenol* 2001;177:405–408.

Parker SH, Stavros AT, Dennis MA. Needle biopsy techniques. *Radiol Clin North Am* 1995;33:1171–1186.

Perez-Fuentes JA, Longobardi IR, Acosta VF, et al. Sonographically guided directional vacuum-assisted breast biopsy. *AJR Am J Roentgenol* 2001;177:1459–1463.

18

SONOGRAPHIC EVALUATION OF THE IATROGENICALLY ALTERED BREAST

When we think of the altered breast, we tend to think only of the postlumpectomy or postmastectomy patient. However, iatrogenic alterations of the breast include far more than just lumpectomy and mastectomy. Table 18–1 lists iatrogenic alterations of the breast. Each affects the sonographic appearance of the breast in different ways.

Ultrasound is often used to evaluate postsurgical breasts for indications that are usually similar to those in nonoperated patients—evaluation of palpable lumps or focal mammographic abnormalities. In such cases, iatrogenic alterations might cause the palpable lump or mammographic abnormality or might merely represent incidental findings. Incidental iatrogenic alterations can represent significant complications of medical interventions but are often expected and clinically insignificant. One of the chief goals for sonography in the patient who has undergone lumpectomy, partial mastectomy, or segmentectomy for treatment of breast cancer is early detection of recurrent or residual breast carcinoma. Early detection of local recurrence is important because many patients with local recurrence may still be cured by salvage mastectomy. Iatrogenic alterations of the breast in cancer treatment patients can simulate recurrent tumor in some cases and mask recurrence in others, complicating detection of recurrent neoplasm. Detecting and appropriately recognizing iatrogenic alterations in the breast enables the sonologist to (a) identify significant complications, (b) minimize overinterpreting the findings as recurrent neoplasm and causing unnecessary biopsy, and (c) minimize the underinterpreting findings caused by recurrent tumor as merely being expected iatrogenic alterations.

ALTERATIONS CAUSED BY INTERVENTIONAL NEEDLE PROCEDURES

Hematomas and seromas can occur as undesirable complications of all needle procedures, including needle local-ization, cyst aspiration, fine-needle aspiration biopsy, large core needle biopsy, and 11-gauge directional vacuum-assisted biopsy (DVAB, mammotomy). Hematomas form relatively frequently within the lumen of aspirated cysts, particularly if the cyst wall is inflamed and hyperemic (Fig. 18–1). In general, the larger the needle and the more tissue removed, the greater the risk for hematoma formation, but even 25-gauge needles used for anesthetic injection can cause bleeding in certain patients. Hematomas can form in the tissues surrounding a solid nodule that has undergone core needle biopsy, especially in high-grade lesions that are hypervascular (Fig. 18–2). Hematoma formation is an undesirable result of a needle procedure, but it rarely requires surgical treatment, percutaneous drainage, or other intervention. The hematoma is usually small enough that it resolves spontaneously. Scarring, fat necrosis, and architectural distortion are exceedingly rare with all needle procedures, except for 11-gauge DVAB, which occasionally leads to such permanent sequelae. Hematomas that occur as complications of needle procedures are not diagnostic dilemmas. They usually occur immediately, and their formation can usually be observed in real-time ultrasound when the procedure is performed with ultrasound guidance. Seeing the hematomas forming acutely during the biopsy procedure can actually be an advantage because the ultrasound transducer can be used as a compression device to control bleeding under real-time guidance. Sonography can also be used to guide thrombin injection into the bleeding site to minimize hematomas formation. In cases in which the hematoma forms after the procedure, conservative treatment usually suffices. Ice packs, elastic wraps, and gauze packing of sports bras are routinely employed to minimize hematoma formation after biopsy procedures. Hematomas that form from arterial bleeders are essentially spontaneously thrombosed pseudoaneurysms. Radiologists who have ablated femoral artery with compression or ultrasound-guided thrombin injection should be familiar with

TABLE 18–1. IATROGENIC ALTERATIONS OF THE BREAST

Post–interventional needle procedures
    Post–11-gauge directional vacuum-assisted biopsy (DVAB)
    Post–14-gauge large core needle biopsy
    Fine-needle aspiration biopsy (FNAB)
    Cyst aspiration
    Needle localization

Post–cancer surgery
    Postlumpectomy—primary closure
    Postlumpectomy—cavity left open
    Postmastectomy
    Post–axillary dissection

Post–reconstructive surgery

Postaugmentation

Post–reduction mammoplasty

Radiation therapy
    Preirradiation localization
        For brachytherapy
        For external radiation booster dose
    Postirrradiation

Postchemotherapy

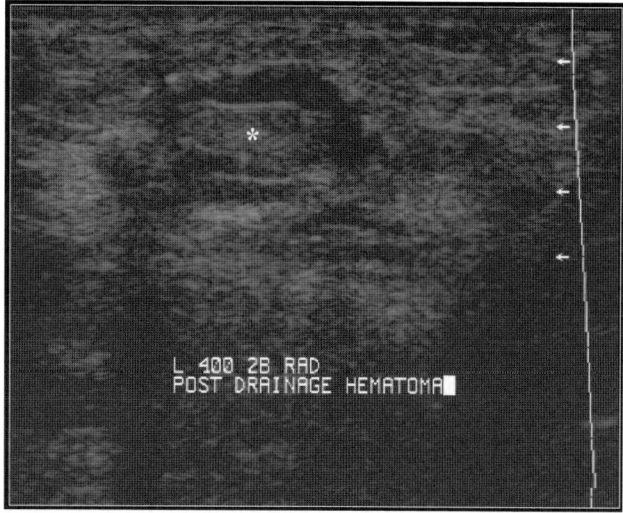

FIGURE 18–1 This acute intracystic hematoma *(*)* formed immediately after ultrasound-guided aspiration of the cyst.

the appearance of spontaneously or iatrogenically thrombosed pseudoaneurysms. A pseudoaneurysm thromboses from its periphery toward its center, and the characteristic finding in most cases is a thick, hyperechoic wall that represents the peripheral thrombosis (Fig. 18–3). The hyperechogenicity of the outer wall distinguishes hematomas from the isoechoic wall thickening that exists in inflamed cysts, cysts that contain papillary apocrine metaplasia, or cysts that contain papillomas or carcinomas. As the hematomas evolve over time and become chronic, the thick, hyperechoic outer clot tends to become isoechoic and can also become thinner. Unlike spontaneous hematomas, hematomas that form within surgical cavities or cavities created by large core DVAB needles tend not to have the thick, echogenic outer walls. Rather than being spontaneously thrombosed pseudoaneurysms, these hematomas simply fill a potential space that has been left behind by a surgeon or radiologist (Fig. 18–4).

The larger the needle, the higher is the risk for a hematoma developing. However, 11-gauge DVAB actually has some advantages in preventing hematomas over other types of needles. First, vacuum can be applied during and

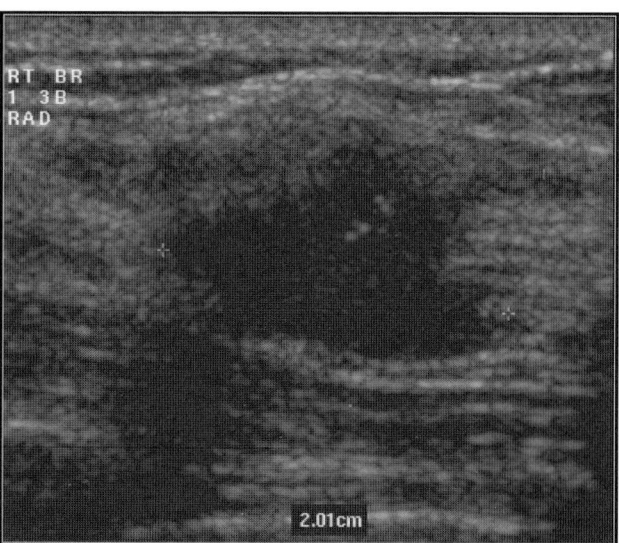

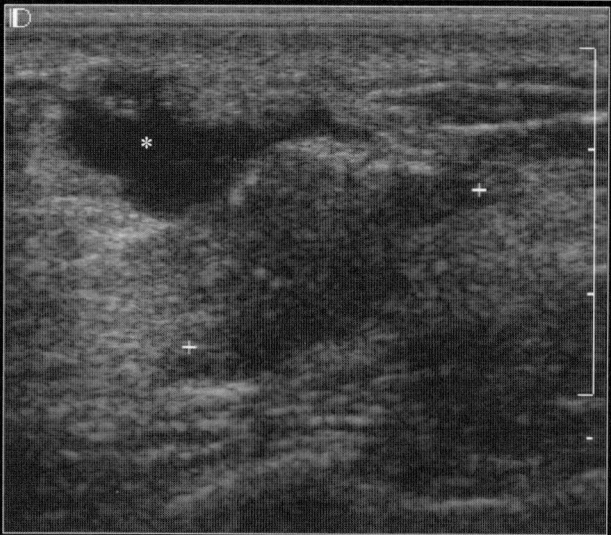

FIGURE 18–2 A: This is an intermediate-grade invasive not otherwise specified carcinoma immediately before ultrasound-guided large core needle biopsy. **B:** The fluid collection anterior to the nodule is an unintended acute postbiopsy hematoma *(*)*.

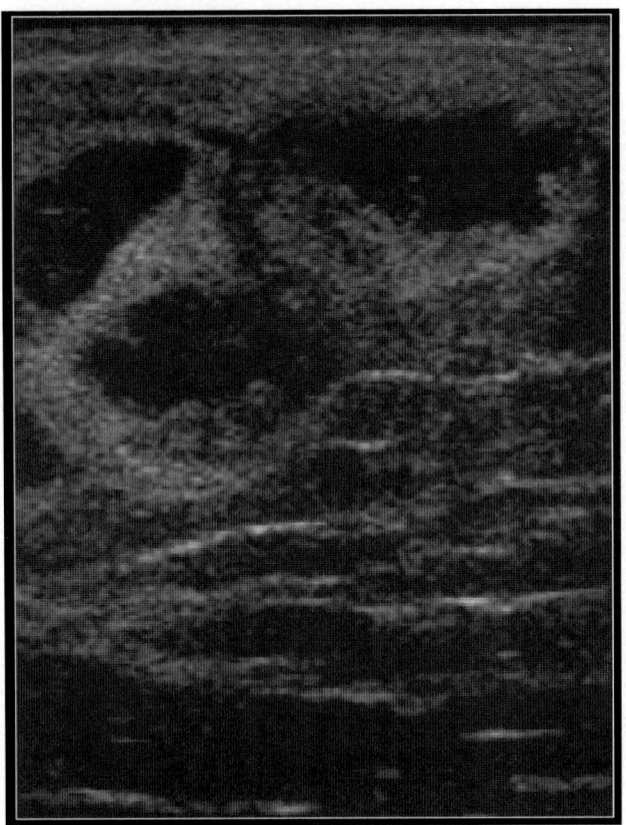

FIGURE 18–3 Acute spontaneous or posttraumatic hematomas tend to have thick hyperechoic outer walls that represent spontaneous acute thrombosis. The hematoma appears similar to a spontaneously thrombosing pseudoaneurysm, which thromboses from the periphery toward the center. In fact, one could say that all hematomas represent spontaneously thrombosed pseudoaneurysms.

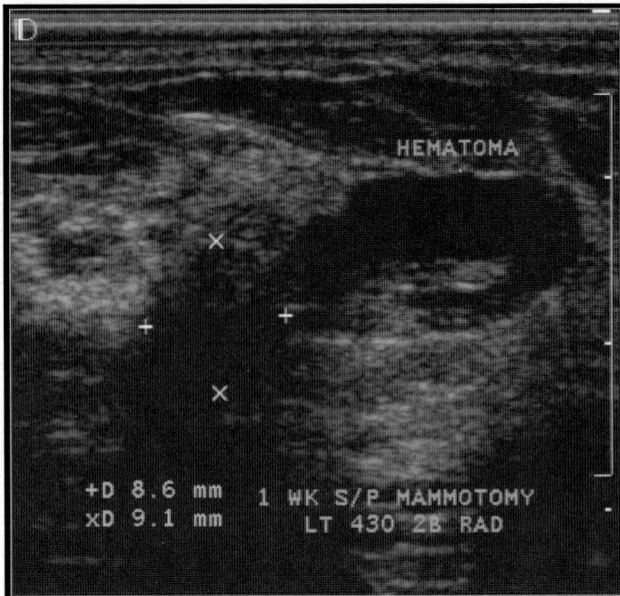

FIGURE 18–4 Hematomas that form within surgical cavities or cavities created by directional vacuum-assisted biopsy (as in this case) generally do not have the thick, echogenic outer wall that spontaneous or posttraumatic hematomas do. Rather than being spontaneously thrombosed pseudoaneurysms, these hematomas simply fill a potential space that has been left behind by a surgeon or radiologist.

at the end of the procedure to evacuate blood from the mammotomy cavity. Second, epinephrine-containing lidocaine can be instilled through the needle into the cavity during the procedure to constrict vessels and control bleeding. Thrombin can also be injected through the needle into the mammotomy cavity to control bleeding. Finally, Gelfoam pledgets that contain a metallic marker that can be inserted into the cavity to mark it for later localization can aid in tamponading bleeding. At this time, thrombin-impregnated collagen or Gelfoam markers are not available yet.

Although hematomas and seromas are generally considered to be very undesirable complications of needle procedures, the small hematomas or seromas that form within the cavity created by the 11-gauge DVAB can be used to localize the cavity for surgical excision at a later time. This becomes necessary when all imaging evidence of the lesion has been removed by the DVAB and when the histology is malignant or atypical. A metallic sidewall clip has been developed to help localize the cavity in such cases. However, the sidewall clip is generally visible sonographically only in a small percentage of cases; therefore, preoperatively localizing it usually requires mammographic guidance. However, the seroma or hematoma that forms within the mammotomy cavity can usually be identified and localized under sonographic guidance. Sonographic localization of the seroma or hematoma within the DVAB cavity offers several advantages over mammographic localization of a sidewall clip. First, the clip can migrate, but the cavity cannot. Second, sonographic guidance is easier, quicker, and statistically more likely to be close to any residual tumor that is eccentrically located in one wall of the seroma. The sidewall clip is placed eccentrically into one of the cavity walls and is just as likely to be placed on the wall opposite from the residual disease as it is on the same wall. If mammographically guided needle localization is performed and a needle position that is within 1 cm of the clip is accepted, and if the residual malignancy lies on the opposite wall of a 1-cm mammotomy cavity from the clip, the localizing needle can be as far as 2 cm from the residual disease. However, if sonographic localization is performed and the needle is precisely placed into the center of the 1-cm cavity seroma, the needle will never be more than 0.5 cm from the residual malignancy (Figs. 18–5 and 18–6). Additionally, sonography may be able to identify residual neoplasm along the wall of the mammotomy seroma or hematoma. In such cases, the residual disease, rather than the center of the cavity, can be localized (Fig. 18–7). Finally, methylene blue dye can be injected into the mammotomy seroma or hematoma, staining all of its walls and making the

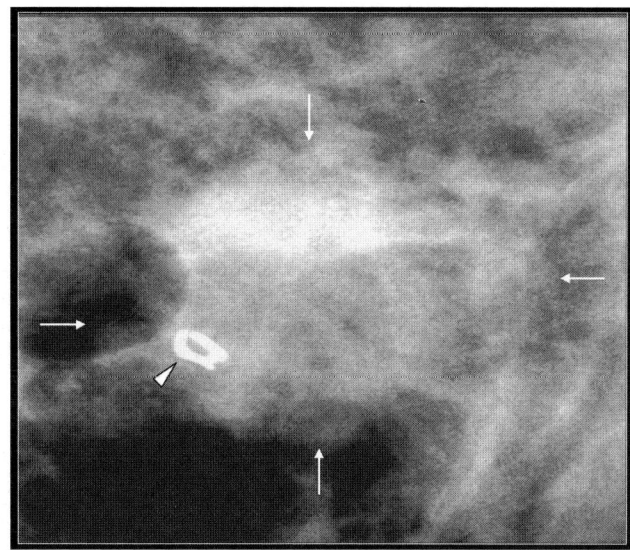

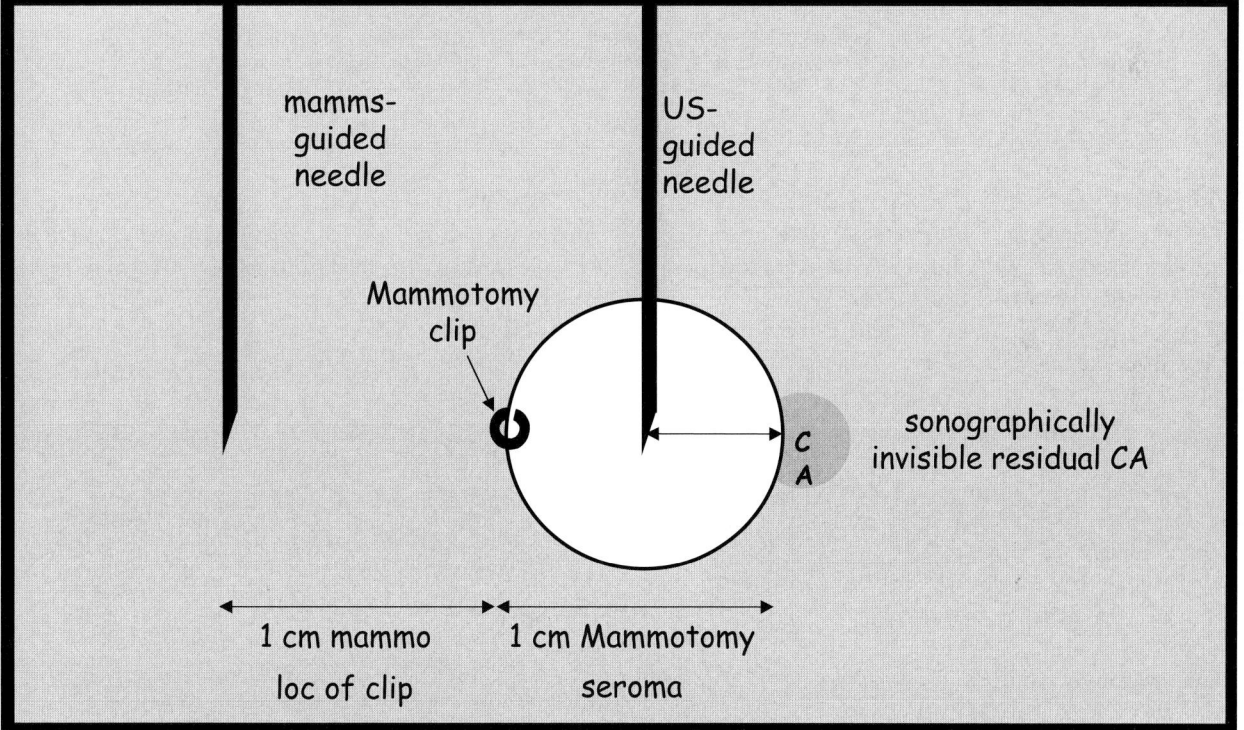

FIGURE 18–5 A: The mammotomy clip is deployed in one of the sidewalls of the mammotomy cavity, not in the center of the cavity. The oval mammotomy cavity *(arrows)* is filled with blood and serum, and the clip *(arrowhead)* lies along the inferior left edge of the seroma in about the 8:00 position. **B:** This figure illustrates the theoretical advantage to localizing the center of the seroma within the mammotomy cavity rather than the mammotomy clip. If the seroma within the mammotomy cavity is 1 cm in diameter, if there is a small focus of residual carcinoma along one wall of the seroma, and if the center of the cavity is localized under ultrasound guidance, the farthest from the residual disease that the needle can be is 0.5 cm. The mammotomy clip might be attached to any wall of the lesion, and any residual disease is just as likely to lie on the wall opposite the clip as it is to lie on the same wall. In at least one-fourth of cases, the clip is on the opposite wall of the seroma from the residual disease. If ultrasound-guided localization of the mammotomy clip is performed, the needle will be 1 cm from the residual disease in about 25% of cases. If a mammographic localization of the mammotomy clip is performed and a needle position plus or minus 1 cm from the clip is accepted, the tip of the needle might be as far as 2 cm from the residual disease. Thus, not only is sonographic localization of the seroma within the mammotomy cavity much quicker and technically easier than the mammographic localization of the clip, but also in a significant minority of cases, it more accurately localizes the residual disease.

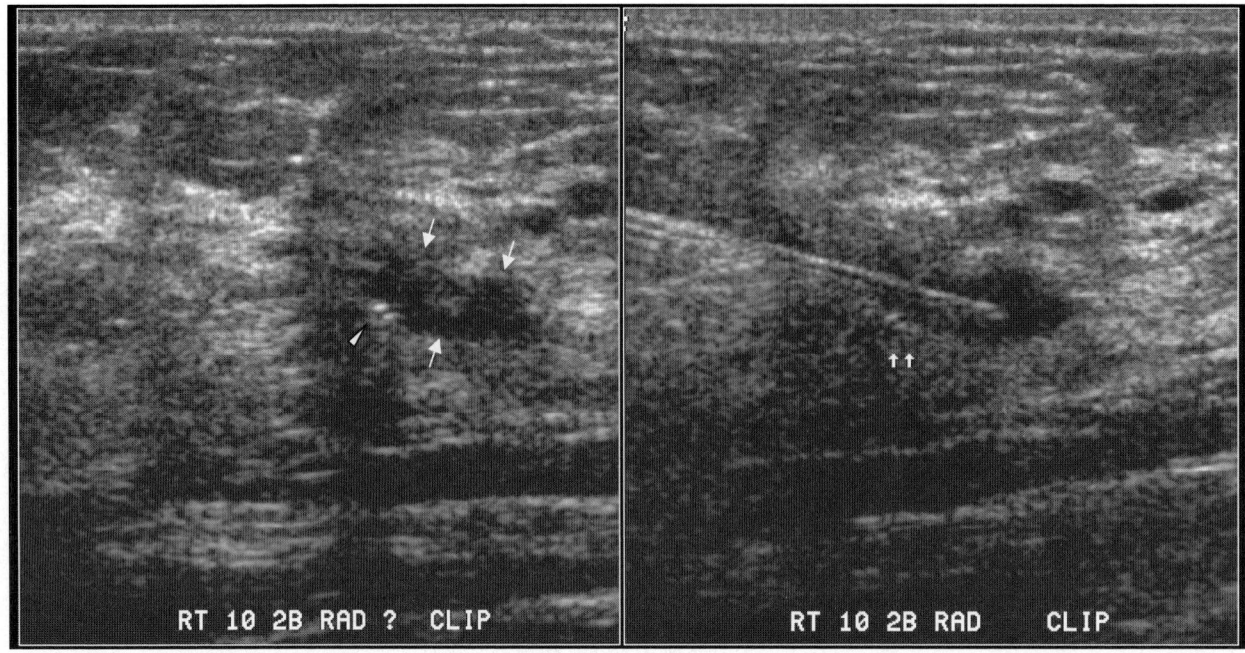

FIGURE 18–6 The seroma within the oval, stereotactically guided mammotomy cavity is readily demonstrable. In this view, **(left)**, the mammotomy clip *(arrowhead)* can be seen along the inferior left edge of the seroma *(arrow)*, not within the center of the seroma. The ultrasound-guided needle placement is to the center of the seroma parallel to its long axis **(right)**, not to the mammotomy clip *(arrows)*.

location and extent of the cavity more apparent to the surgeon. The accuracy of clip placement tends to be less accurate for stereotactically guided DVAB than for sonographically guided DVAB because the cavity created by stereotactically guided biopsy tends to be elongated and elliptical in shape rather than spherical. Stereotactic biopsy is performed with the breast in compression. The cavity created while the breast is compressed is nearly spherical, but once compression is released, the cavity becomes elongated along the axis of compression (Fig. 18–8). Although the dimensions of the cavity in planes that lie perpendicular to the axis of compression remain only about 1 cm wide, the di-

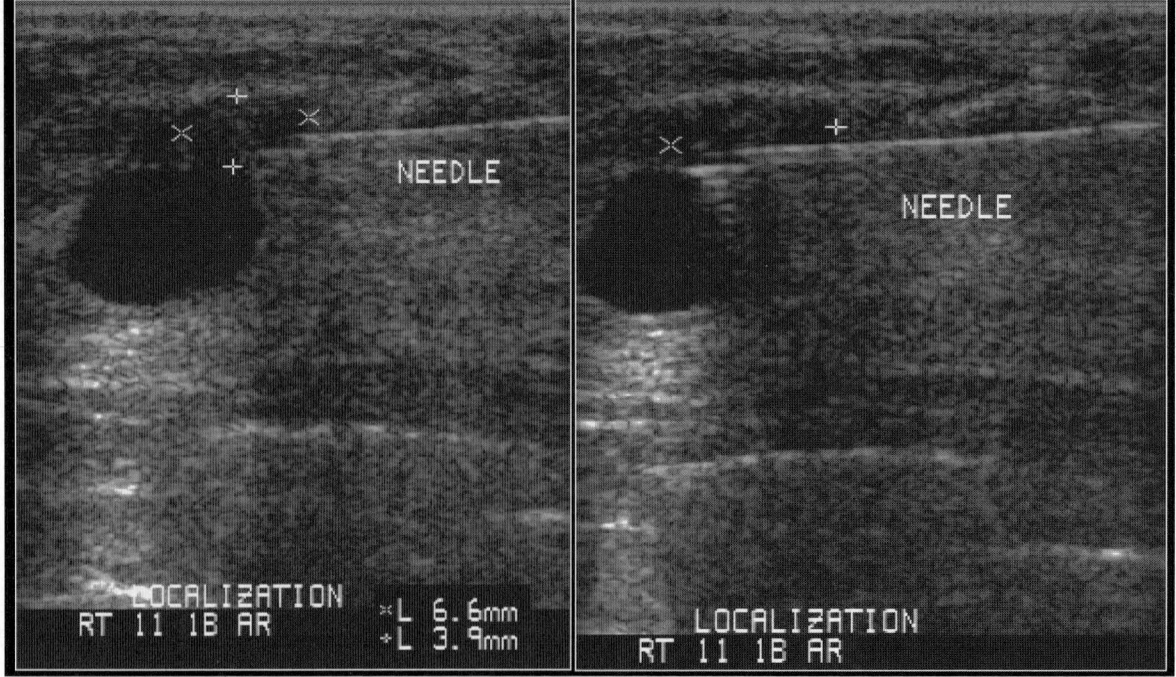

FIGURE 18–7 When residual tumor can be identified along a wall of the mammotomy cavity, **(left,** *calipers)* ultrasound-guided localization of the residual disease is preferable to localizing the cavity **(right)**.

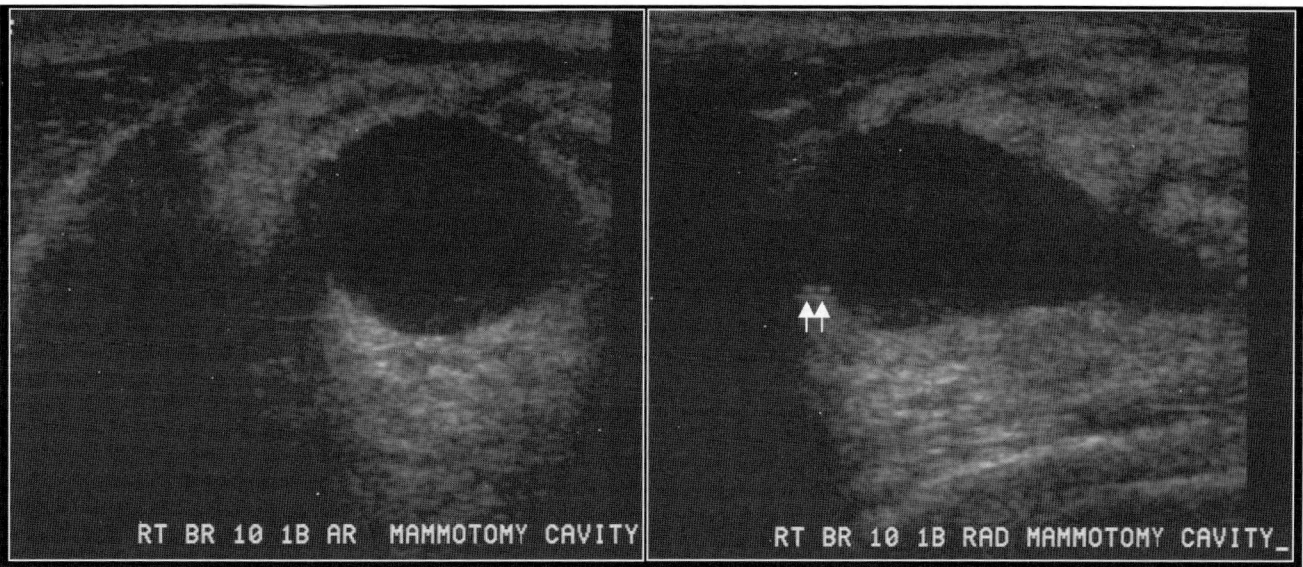

FIGURE 18–8 Although ultrasound-guided directional vacuum-assisted biopsy (DVAB) usually creates a spherically shaped mammotomy cavity, stereotactically guided DVAB usually creates an elongated cavity. The stereotactically guided biopsy is performed while the breast is being compressed. In compression, the cavity is spherical in shape, but when compression is released, the cavity elongates. Note that this stereotactic mammotomy cavity is nearly 4 cm long and that the clip lies at one end *(arrows)*, whereas any residual disease is just as likely to lie along the opposite end of the cavity from the clip as it is along the same wall as the clip. Because of the elongation of the cavity once compression is released, a mammotomy clip can lie several centimeters farther from the clip after stereotactic biopsy than it can after ultrasound-guided biopsy. For this reason, deploying markers in the center of the cavity is preferable to deploying clips eccentrically along the wall of the cavity.

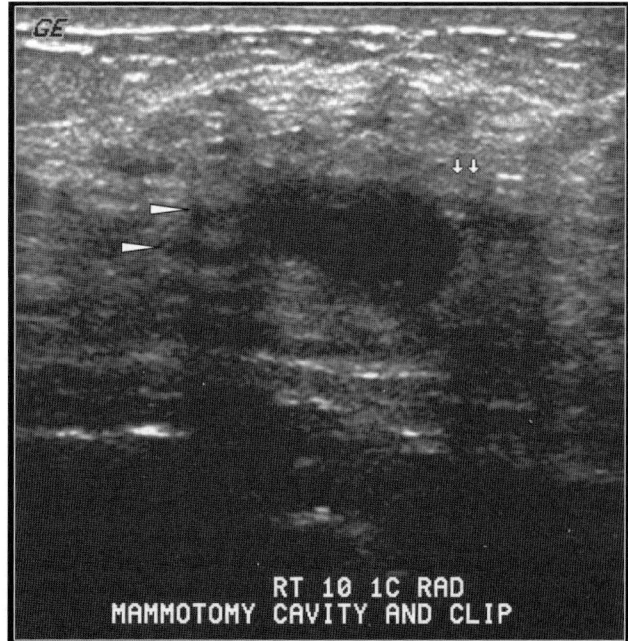

FIGURE 18–9 The two bright echoes that represent the mammotomy clip lie along the upper right edge of the mammotomy cavity *(small arrows)*. On the opposite end of the cavity, about 2 cm away from the clip, lie residual components of the ductal carcinoma *in situ (arrowheads).*

mension of the cavity that was parallel to the axis of compression can expand to 3 or 4 cm after compression is released. Thus, a sidewall clip that lies less than 1 cm from residual disease while the breast is in compression, in some cases, can lie as far as 3 or 4 cm from the residual disease when compression is released (Fig. 18–9).

The seroma or hematoma within the mammotomy cavity gradually resolves over weeks, usually 3 to 6 weeks. Once the seroma has resolved and the mammotomy cavity can no longer be identified sonographically, the chances of identifying the mammotomy clip sonographically become very slim. Occasionally, a markedly hyperechoic clip that is completely surrounded by isoechoic fat may be sonographically visible even after the seroma or hematoma has resolved. However, clips that are surrounded by nearly equally hyperechoic and heterogeneous fibrous tissue can seldom be identified sonographically once the hematoma has resolved. Mammographic localization of the mammotomy clip then becomes the only way to localize the mammotomy cavity and any potential residual malignancy or atypia. Additionally, in a few cases, distinguishing the mammotomy cavity seroma from numerous surrounding cysts has been so difficult that attempts at sonographic localization had to be abandoned in favor of mammographic localization.

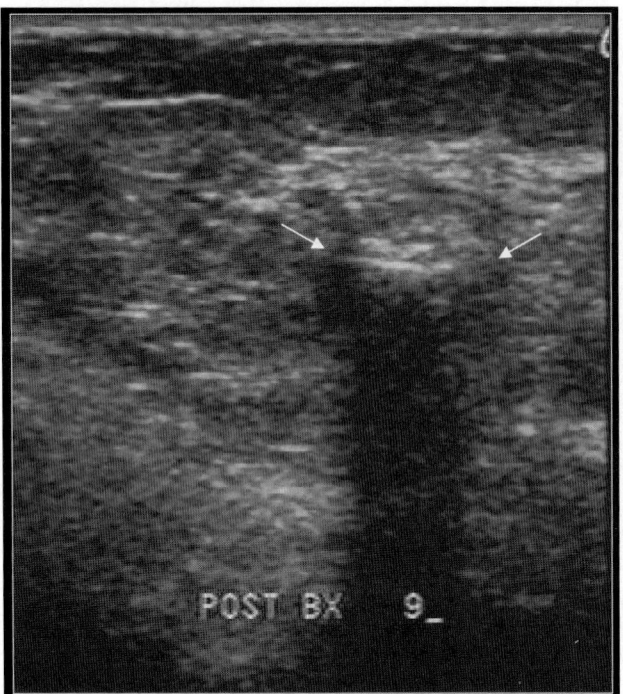

FIGURE 18–10 The gel foam pledgets that have been placed into the center of the directional vacuum-assisted biopsy cavity appear hyperechoic *(arrows)* on ultrasound, enabling them to be used as a sonographic marker. Their echogenicity gradually decreases over a few weeks until they are no longer echogenic enough to be used as a sonographic marker. The center pledget contains a metal clip that can be localized with mammographic guidance after the pledgets have become sonographically invisible.

Because of the eccentric location and variability in location of the mammotomy clip relative to any residual disease that may be present, Gelfoam pledget markers have been developed to localize the DVAB cavity. These pledgets can be place through the cannula into the center of the cavity. The pledgets are initially quite echogenic and cast an acoustic shadow that enables them to be localized with ultrasound for a few weeks after placement (Fig. 18–10). Over time, the pledgets absorb water and are absorbed, becoming sonographically invisible. However, one of the pledgets also contains a permanent metallic marker that allows the cavity to be localized indefinitely with mammographic guidance. Localizing echogenic pledgets that lie within the center of the mammotomy cavity is very much analogous to localizing the center of a mammotomy seroma or hematoma and enjoys the same advantages over mammographic localization of an eccentrically located clip attached to one wall of the cavity. Preliminary studies show that the pledgets migrate less often and over shorter distances than do sidewall clips.

Arteriovenous fistulas and pseudoaneurysms are vascular complications of large core needle biopsies that have been reported in a few instances, but we have not seen these complications. They usually result from biopsy of a sizable artery in the vicinity of the lesion. Color Doppler before biopsy can identify these vessels, and a route of entry that avoids the arteries can be chosen.

Any breast interventional needle procedure can lead to infection and abscess formation. Cysts can become secondarily infected when aspirated. The sonographic findings of inflamed and infected cysts are discussed in detail in Chapter 10, and the Doppler findings are discussed in Chapter 20. Cysts that become infected secondary to aspiration can be treated with single or repeated aspirations and antibiotics. Seromas and hematomas that are complications of interventional needle procedures can also become secondarily infected and can then evolve into abscesses and, like infected cysts, can be treated with single or multiple aspirations and antibiotics if unilocular. However, either percutaneous placement of a drain tube or surgical incision and drainage might become necessary if the abscess is multilocular. Abscesses that are complications of interventional procedures are similar to abscesses of other causes in sonographic appearances. Abscesses are discussed in Chapter 11.

The appearance of an infected hematoma generally differs slightly from that of an uninfected hematoma. Both infected and noninfected postbiopsy hematomas have thick walls and may have adherent clot and fibrinous septations. However, as noted previously, the thick wall in an acute or subacute hematoma is usually formed by hyperechoic, clotted blood, whereas the wall of an infected hematoma usually is isoechoic (Figs. 18–11). The wall of an acute hematoma is avascular, whereas the wall of an infected hematoma is usually hyperemic on Doppler evaluation.

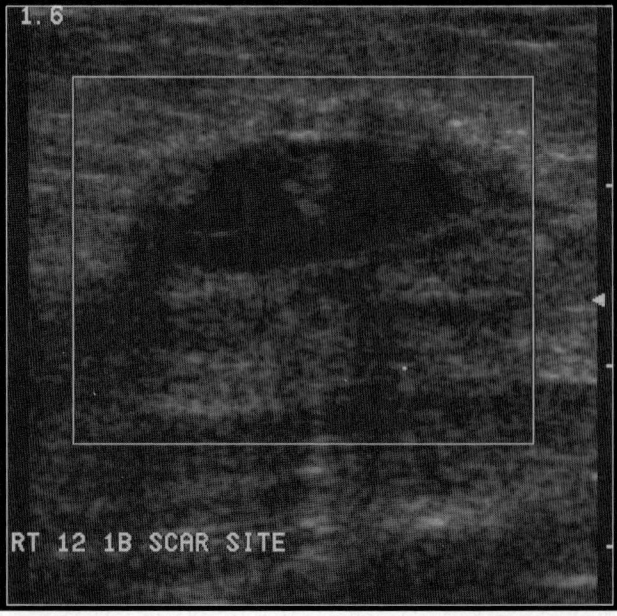

FIGURE 18–11 The walls of an infected hematoma are usually thick and isoechoic rather than hyperechoic. The thickened infected walls frequently have Doppler demonstrable hyperemia, although this case did not.

POST–CANCER SURGERY ALTERATIONS

The most significant diagnostic problem for the breast imager in assessing the breast after lumpectomy, partial mastectomy, or segmentectomy is in distinguishing between recurrent carcinoma and fat necrosis and exuberant scarring. Postoperative alterations can be subdivided into early and late changes. Early abnormalities include edema, hematoma, seroma, mastitis, and abscess formation. Late changes include lipid cyst formation with or without calcifications, foreign-body granulomas, epidermal inclusion cysts, fat necrosis, exuberant scarring, and tumor recurrences. Exuberant scar formation can occur with or without associated fat necrosis. Exuberant scar and the fibrotic phase of fat necrosis can be difficult to distinguish from recurrent carcinoma in some cases.

Postsurgical Skin Alterations

Surgical procedures typically cause thickening of the skin. The skin within and around the incision is edematous immediately after surgery. The periincisional edema usually resolves quickly. The edema within the incisional scar re-

solves more slowly but, in some cases, can persist indefinitely. The thickened skin within the incision scar appears mildly to moderately hypoechoic with respect to normal surrounding skin. Subtle skin changes may be difficult to demonstrate without an acoustic standoff (Fig. 18–12). Over time, the skin thickness and echogenicity usually return to nearly normal. However, in our experience, by comparing the periincisional areas to skin in other parts of the breast or to the mirror-image location in the contralateral breast, mild skin thickening can usually be shown to persist indefinitely (Fig. 18–13). Keloids cause even more pronounced skin thickening and hypoechogenicity (Fig. 18–14), but keloids are obvious clinically and do not require sonography for diagnosis. Very old skin scars may become thinned and hypoechoic in comparison to normal skin, especially if there has been significant weight gain that has led to stretching of the skin.

In addition to direct postsurgical changes to the skin, sonography can demonstrate subtle indirect changes to the skin such as dimpling and retraction that can be caused by either recurrent tumor or postsurgical scarring. A standoff of acoustic gel is usually necessary to demonstrate subtle skin retraction (Fig. 18–15). An acoustic standoff pad will

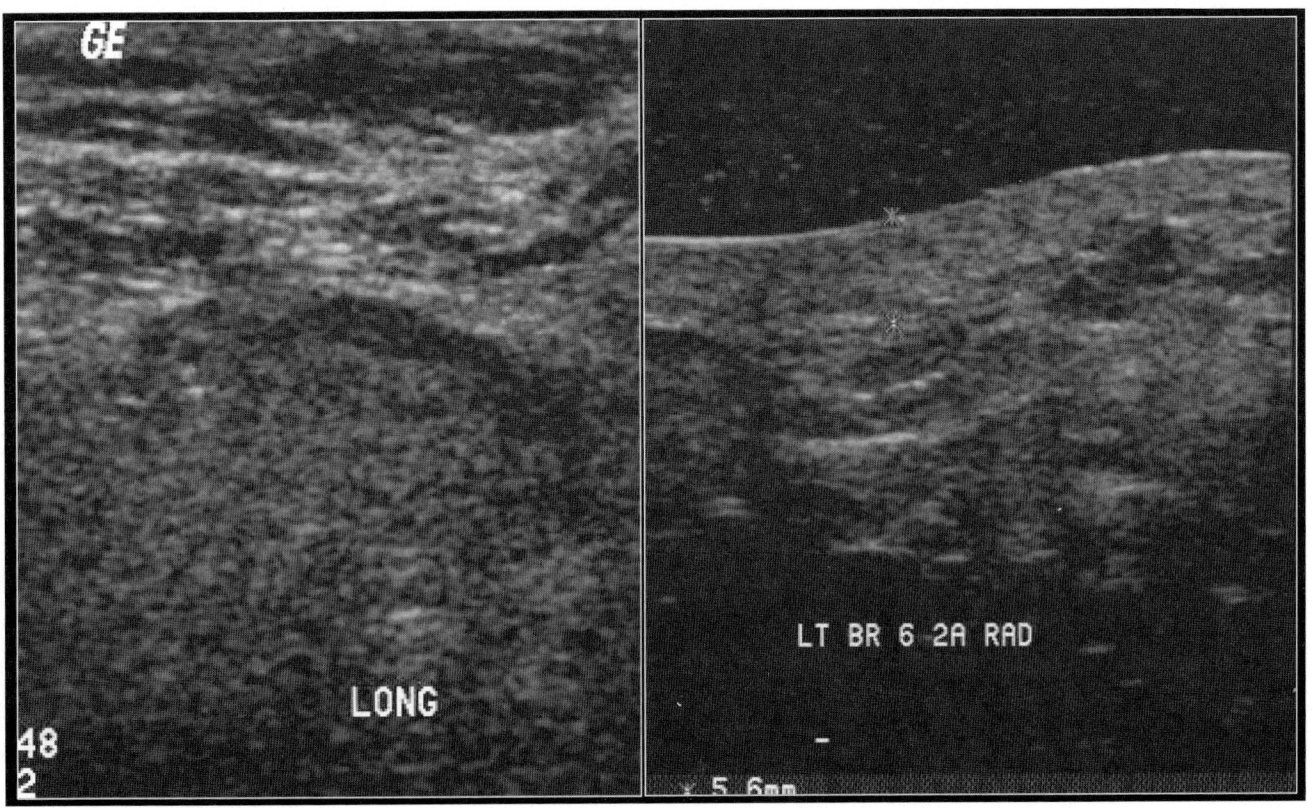

FIGURE 18–12 The skin thickening within the incision cannot be appreciated when scanned without an acoustic standoff of gel (**left**). Severe skin thickening can be demonstrated when it is scanned through a standoff of acoustic gel (**right**). Normal skin thickness is about 1.5 to 2 mm.

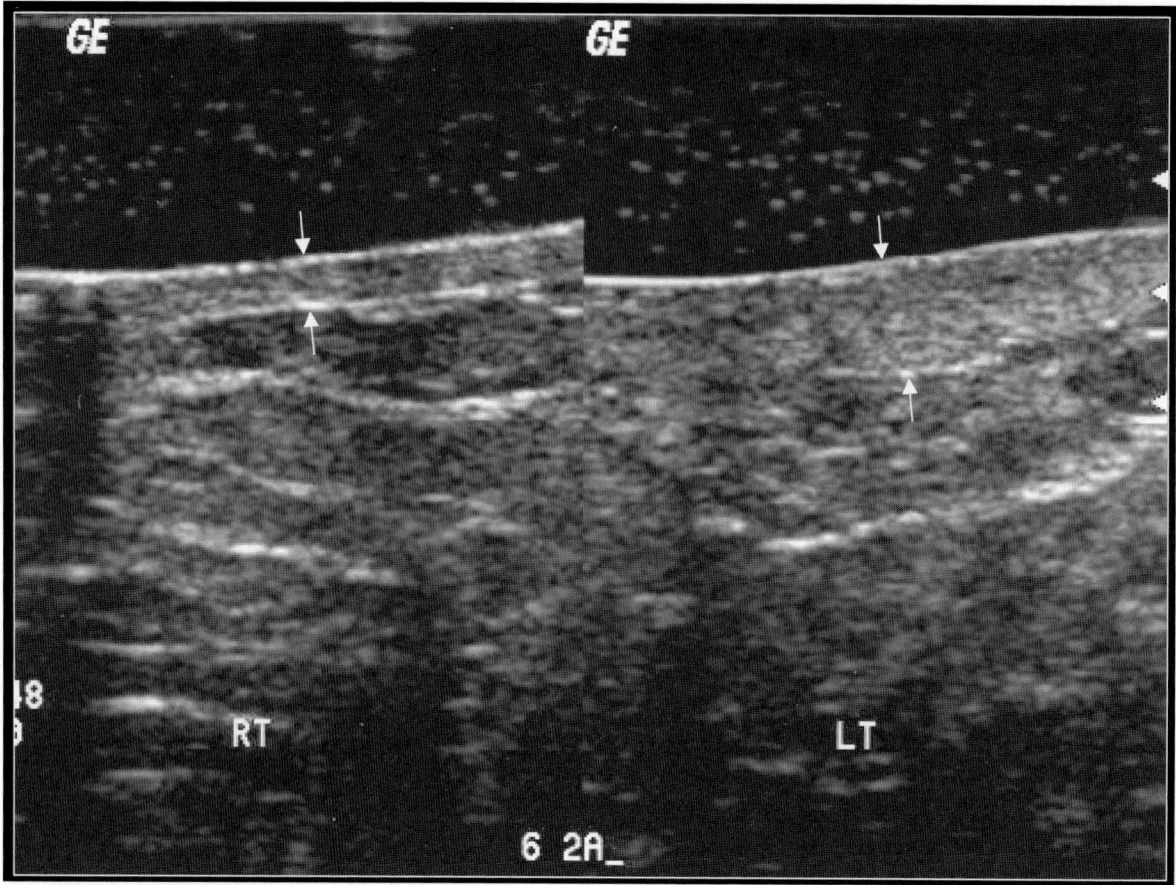

FIGURE 18–13 The chronic persistent skin thickening within the incision (**right**) is best appreciated when compared with the mirror-image location on the contralateral side (**left**) using split-screen imaging.

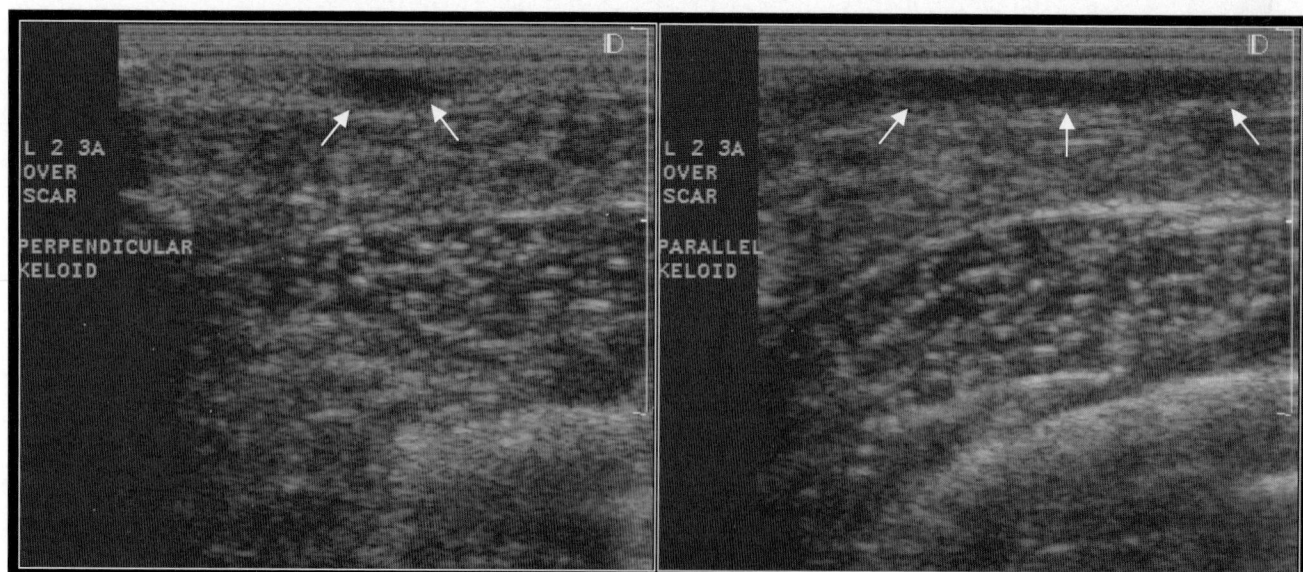

FIGURE 18–14 Keloids cause focal, markedly hypoechoic thickening of the skin *(arrows)*. The sonographic findings can be worrisome, but the clinical findings are straightforward and reassuring.

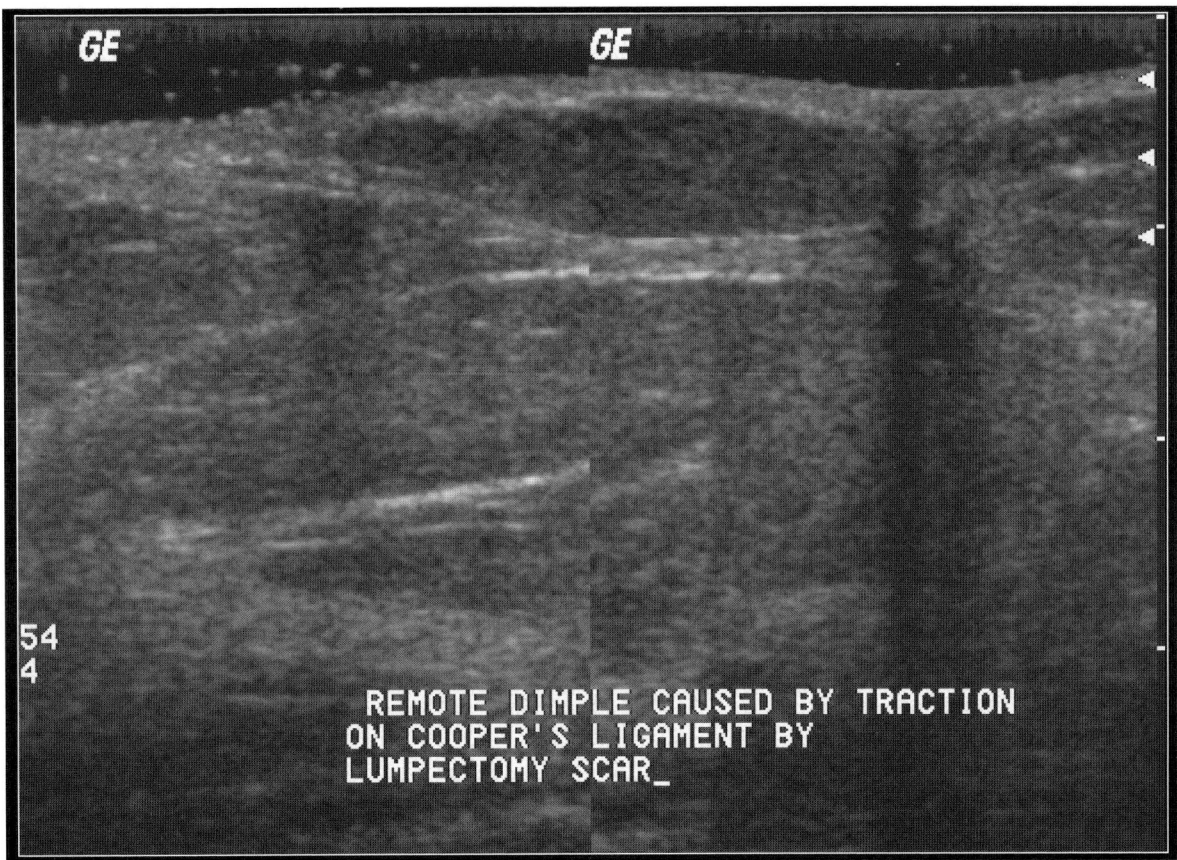

FIGURE 18–15 A standoff of acoustic gel is usually necessary to demonstrate subtle skin retraction associated with surgical scars. Without the standoff, compression of the skin by the transducer obscures these changes.

not work for this purpose because it too compresses the breast, obscuring the subtle skin indentation.

Distinguishing between recurrent tumor and postsurgical direct or indirect changes to the skin can be difficult or even impossible in certain cases. Foreign-body granulomas can form within either the skin or subcutaneous tissues and usually have the appearance of elliptically shaped isoechoic to mildly hypoechoic nodules with Breast Imaging Reporting and Data System (BIRADS) category 3 or 4a characteristics (Fig. 18–16).

Epidermal inclusion cysts vary in appearance. Early in their development, they appear to be spherical isoechoic to mildly hypoechoic, encapsulated nodules. Later, the contents of epidermal inclusion cysts tend to become hyperechoic. The hyperechoic internal nodule can appear multilaminated, representing multiple layers of keratin, can form a dense central nodule that shadows and has an appearance similar to ovarian cystic teratomas, or can form mural nodules that can be difficult to distinguish from recurrent intracystic carcinoma (Fig. 18–17). Epidermal inclusion cysts are discussed in detail in Chapter 10.

Postlumpectomy Alterations in Deeper Breast Tissues

The fatty and parenchymal elements of the breast also become edematous after surgery. Edematous fat and loose periductal stromal tissues become thickened and hyperechoic. Edema within the normally hyperechoic interlobular stroma fibrous tissue and Cooper's ligaments makes them appear less echogenic than normal (Fig. 18–18). If the edema is severe enough, fat and loose stromal tissues can become so echogenic that they are difficult to distinguish from adjacent abnormally hypoechoic edematous interlobular stromal fibrous elements and Cooper's ligaments. Thus, severe edema can make the breast appear thickened and featureless, obscuring normal anatomic structures and tissue planes (Fig. 18–19).

Edema also decreases sound transmission, making it difficult to penetrate to the chest wall using the high-frequency transducers normally employed for breast ultrasound. Thus, sonographic evaluation of severe postsurgical edema and ecchymosis may require switching to a lower-frequency transducer than we normally use for breast ultrasound.

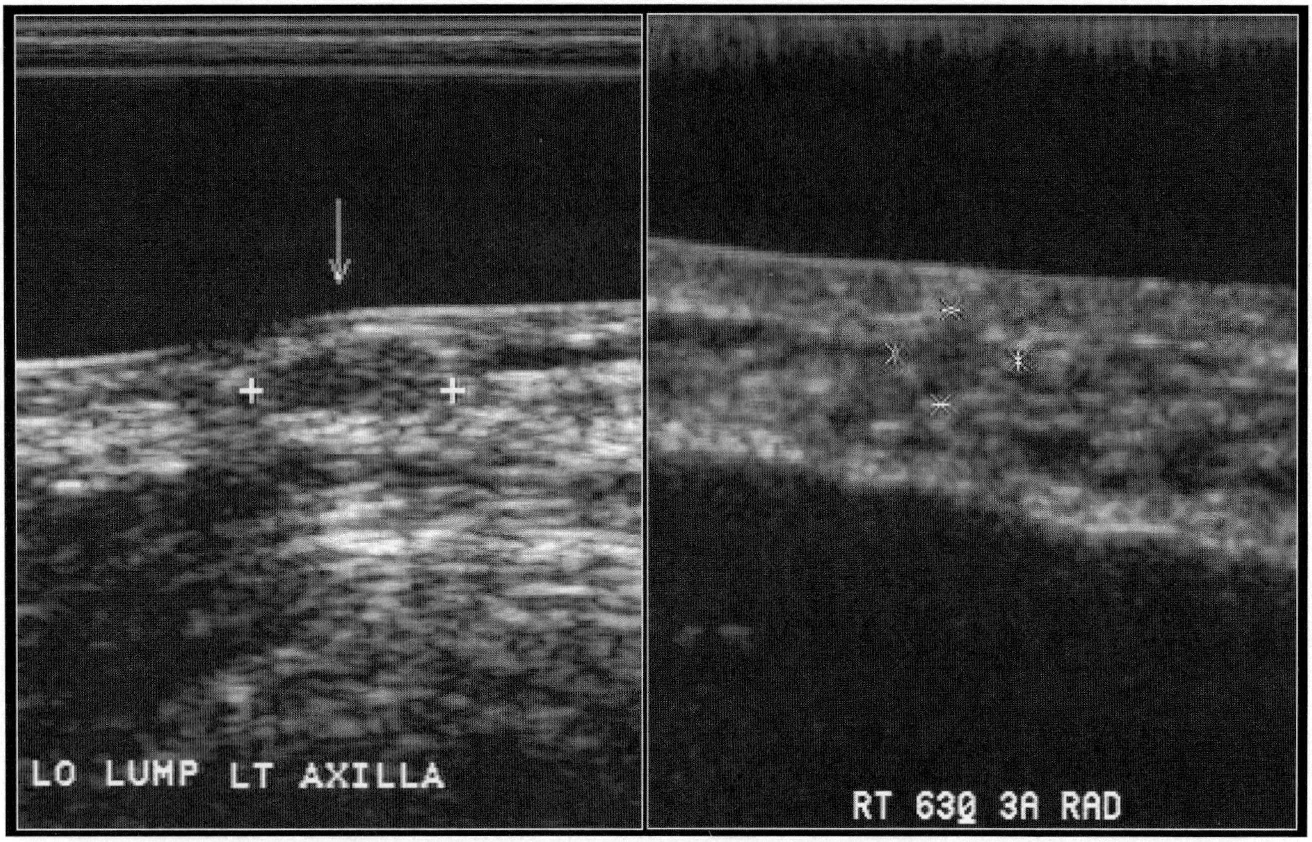

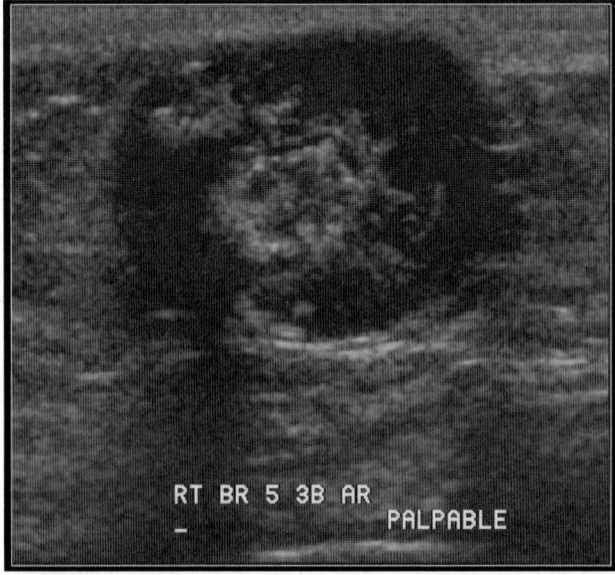

FIGURE 18–16 This foreign-body granuloma within the skin or superficial subcutaneous tissues just deep to the skin can have BIRADS 3 appearances similar to fibroadenomas (**left**) or can have suspicious features such as angulation that make them more difficult to distinguish from recurrent carcinoma (**right**).

FIGURE 18–17 This postsurgical epidermal inclusion cyst contains a central nodule of keratin that simulated recurrent intracystic neoplasm. The central keratin nodule is avascular, whereas recurrent tumor nodule would be vascular in most cases.

As is the case for most postsurgical complications, postsurgical edema can be difficult to distinguish sonographically and clinically from edema caused by recurrent or residual tumor. Even when there is an apparent mass within the edematous area of the breast, it can be difficult to distinguish exuberant scar or fat necrosis from recurrent tumor (Fig. 18–20). In such cases, assessment of the axillary and internal mammary lymph nodes can be helpful. Lymphadenopathy suggests that the edema is neoplastic in origin unless there is infection that might have caused reactive lymphadenopathy. Absence of lymphadenopathy is of less value because recurrent or residual tumor can cause edema by lymphatic invasion or inflammation without having associated lymphadenopathy.

In addition to edema and ecchymosis that can occur in and around the surgical site, patients can develop hematomas or seromas as undesirable complications or as the desired effect of not suturing the lumpectomy cavity closed. Regardless of whether the hematoma is an unplanned complication or a desired effect of leaving the lumpectomy cavity open, the histologic, morphologic, and sonographic features of hematomas evolve over time.

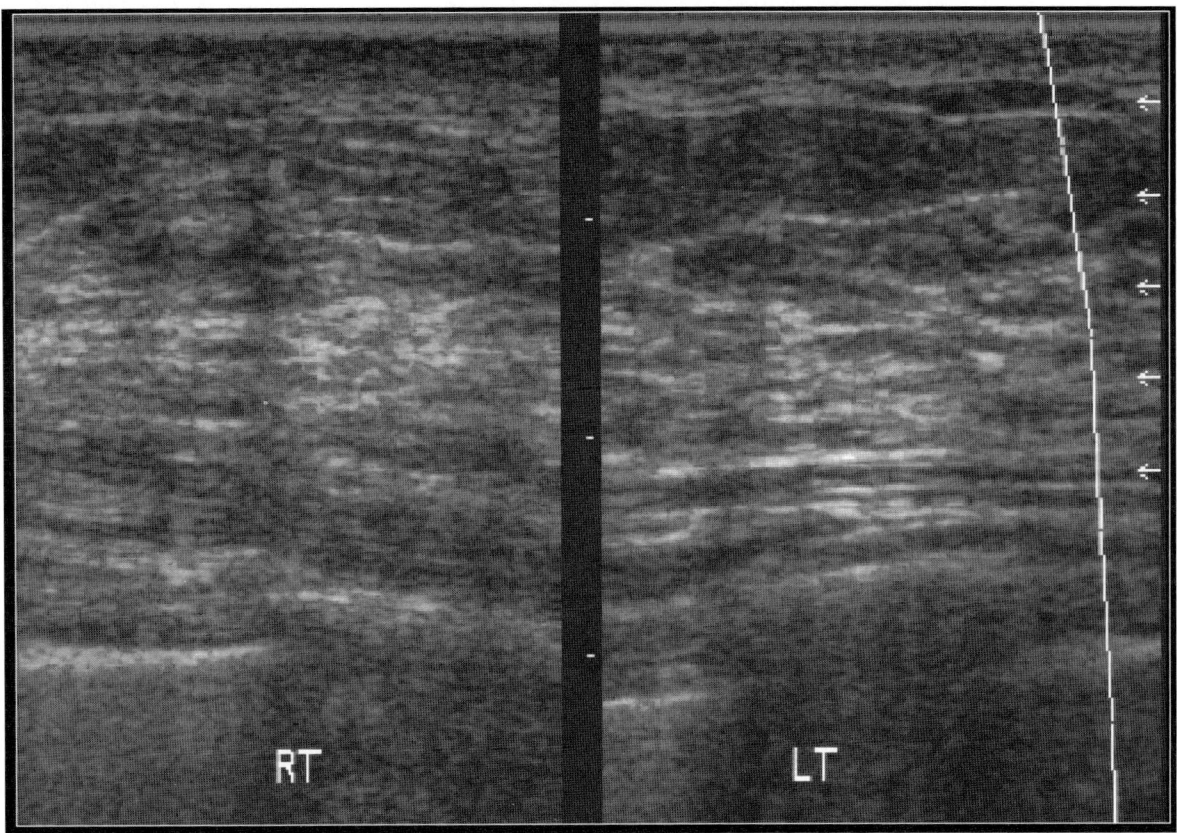

FIGURE 18–18 Postoperative edema thickens the skin and makes it less echogenic, makes fat more echogenic, and thickens and makes normally hyperechoic fibrous tissue less echogenic. Additionally, the ducts and lobules within the mammary zone become less distinct and visible. The right breast shows these changes (**left**). In the severest cases, the breast may appear amorphous, with little or no recognizable internal structure. The patient's left breast is normal (**right image**).

A mixture of liquid blood or blood breakdown products, clot, and fibrin fills the central cavity. The variety of different liquid contents makes the echogenicity of the fluid contents highly variable. Clot within a hematoma can be freely mobile and floating or may be adherent to one wall, having the appearance of a mural nodule. Fibrinous adhesions within the hematoma or seroma can either be resorbed over time or can persist as permanent fibrous septations. Clotting in the periphery of the hematoma can make the outer wall appear thick and echogenic, but inflammatory reaction to blood breakdown products often causes the outer wall to appear isoechoic. The size and shape of the hematoma conform to the size and shape of the surgical cavity. However, hematoma or seroma size and shape are also affected by whether the cavity was primarily closed surgically. The sonographic features of hematomas and seromas are discussed in Chapter 11.

The chief difference between postoperative hematomas or seromas and spontaneous or posttraumatic hematomas is the shape of the lesion. Posttraumatic or spontaneous hematomas are usually rounded and roughly spherical, elliptical, or lobulated in shape, whereas hematomas forming within surgical cavities, such as those created by lumpectomy or segmentectomy, are more often angular and elongated, conforming to the shape of the surgical cavity.

The shape and size of the seroma or hematoma that develops within a lumpectomy cavity depends on whether or not the surgical cavity is sutured closed at the time of surgery. The cavity can be primarily sutured closed or intentionally left open to accumulate blood and serum. For diagnostic biopsies, in which clear margins are not an imperative, the margins are usually small, the resection cavity is usually small, and the surgeon generally sutures the cavity closed at the completion of the procedure (*primary closure*). However, in cancer treatment surgery, the goal is to achieve clear margins, which generally means resecting enough tissue to obtain a 1-cm tumor-free zone around the malignant nodule. The amount of tissue removed *when there is known cancer* is larger than the amount resected

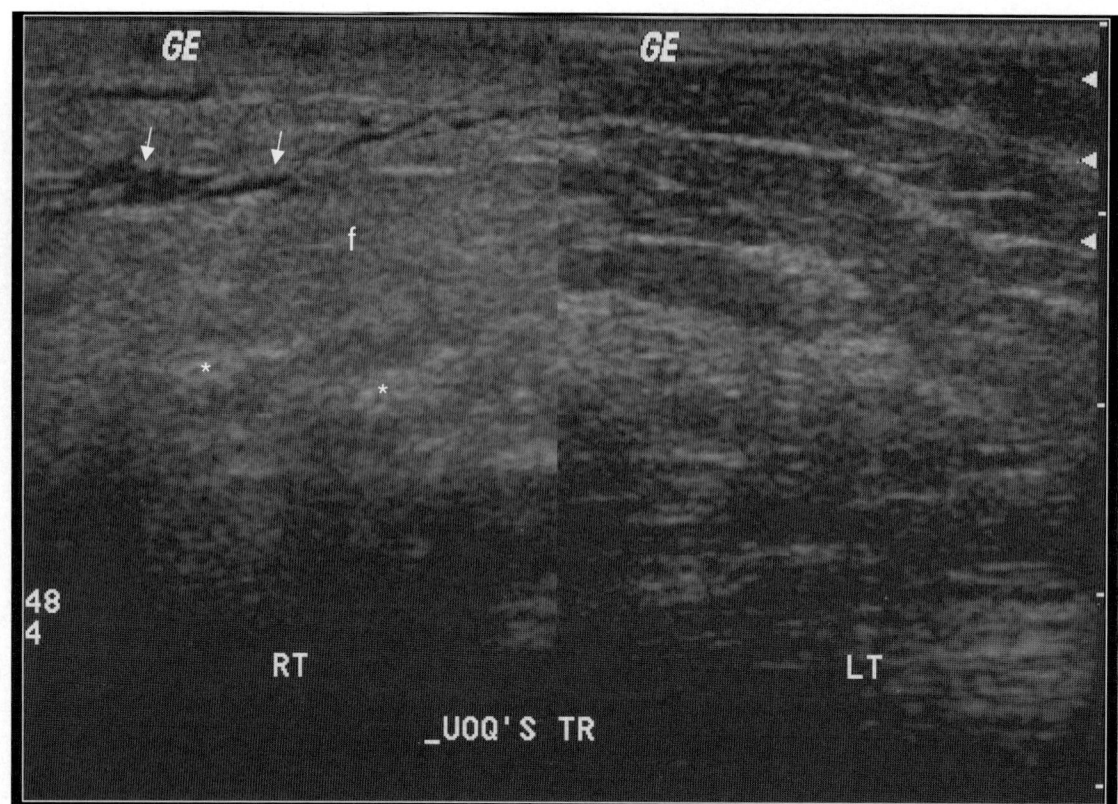

FIGURE 18–19 Edema in the right breast (**left**) is so severe and the fat *(f)* has become so hyperechoic that it is barely distinguishable from hyperechoic fibrous elements *(*)*. Serous effusions are accumulating along the surfaces of Cooper's ligaments *(arrows)*. Penetration to the chest wall using standard 12-MHz transducers is no longer adequate, and it is necessary to use a lower frequency to achieve adequate penetration to the chest wall. The patient's left breast is normal (**right image**).

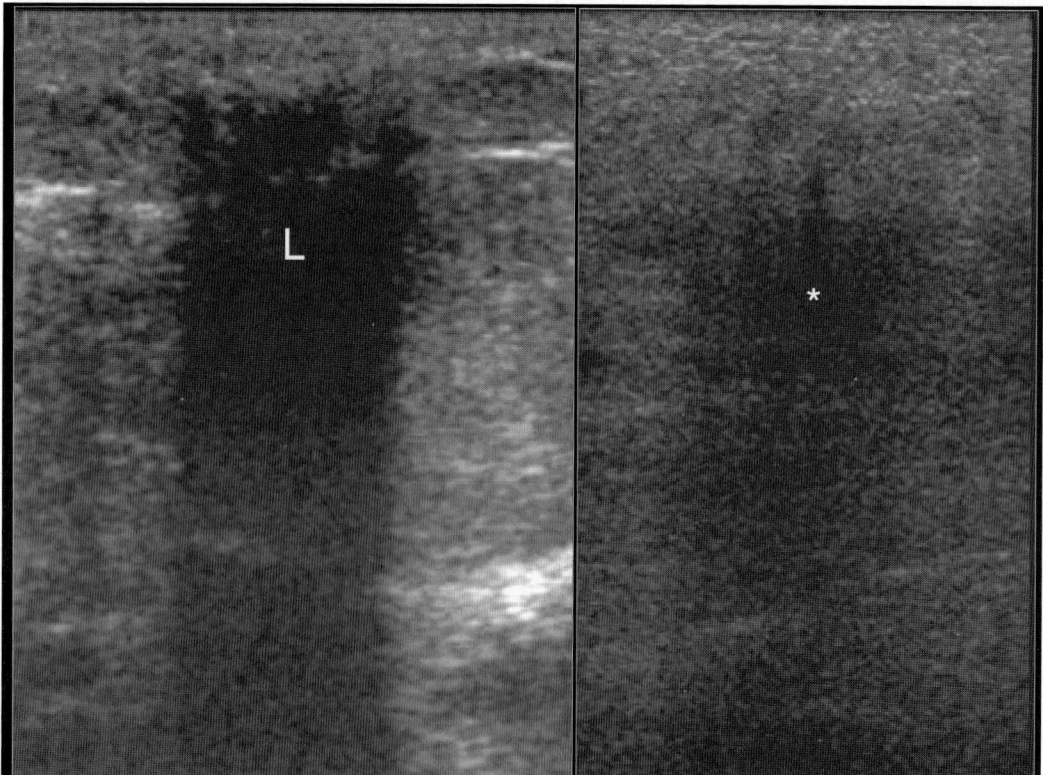

FIGURE 18–20 It can be difficult to distinguish between severe postsurgical edema and edema caused by inflammatory carcinoma. The **left** image shows edema around a lumpectomy cavity *(L)* that is causing severe acoustic shadowing. The **right** image shows severe lymphedema and inflammatory edema in a patient with inflammatory carcinoma. The image is degraded by the severity of the edema, but the malignant mass causing the edema is barely visible *(*)*.

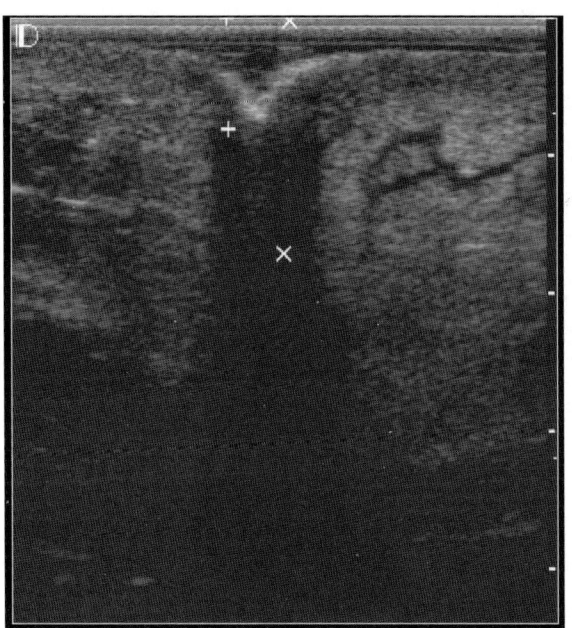

FIGURE 18–21 This patient had a large lesion and relatively small breast size. Lumpectomy with primary closure was performed and resulted in severe retraction of the skin that was obvious clinically but could not be well demonstrated sonographically without a standoff of acoustic gel.

when performing a diagnostic biopsy. The surgeon must then decide whether to suture the cavity closed. The size of the lesion, the width of the margins, and the size of the breast must all be taken into account. As in the case for diagnostic biopsies, if the lesion is very small and the breast size large, the surgeon has the option of suturing the cavity closed at the completion of the surgery. However, in cases in which the volume of tissue that must be resected is large in comparison to the breast size, primarily closing the cavity might cause indentation and deformity of overlying skin (Fig. 18–21). In such cases, the surgeon might elect to leave the cavity open so that it will accumulate blood and serum, in hopes of minimizing the deformity of overlying breast tissues and skin (Fig. 18–22).

It does appear that leaving the cavity open to accumulate serum and blood minimizes immediate skin indentation and deformity (Fig. 18–23). In many, if not most, patients, it also appears that the long-term cosmesis is improved. However, in a few patients, the chronic hematoma or seroma within the lumpectomy site progresses through the stages of fat necrosis to the fibrosis phase and retractile scar or cicatrix formation. The retraction of the scar in such cases can lead to severe deformities that might be similar in

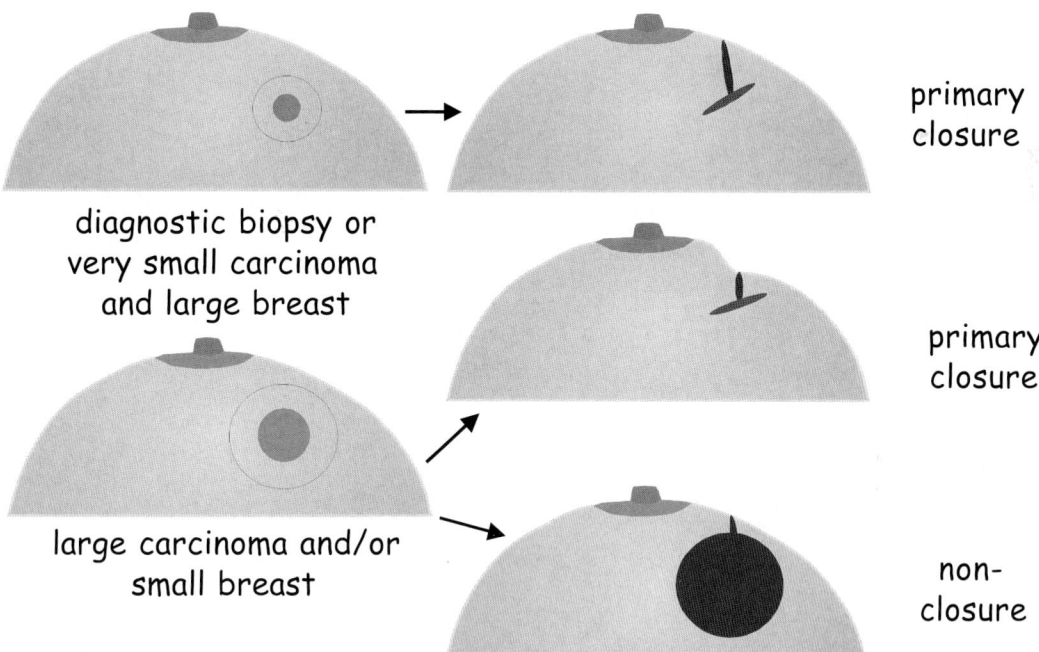

FIGURE 18–22 This figure illustrates primary closure of the lumpectomy cavity versus leaving it open to accumulate serum and blood. When surgery is diagnostic or when cancer surgery is for a very small lesion in a women with average to large breast size, it is possible to suture the surgical cavity closed at the completion of the surgery with little risk for deforming the overlying skin (**upper right**). For surgical excision of known cancer, wider margins are desirable (about 1 cm). If the lesion is large or the woman's breast size is small, suturing the surgical cavity closed (primary closure) at the end of the procedure may result in deformity of the overlying skin (**middle right**). To avoid deforming the overlying skin, the surgeon may choose to leave the surgical cavity open to accumulate blood and serum in hopes of preventing deformity of the overlying skin (**lower right**). Alternatively, some are trying to place collagen in the lumpectomy cavity. Whether or not the lumpectomy cavity is primarily closed greatly affects the sonographic appearances and the difficulties in interpreting the findings.

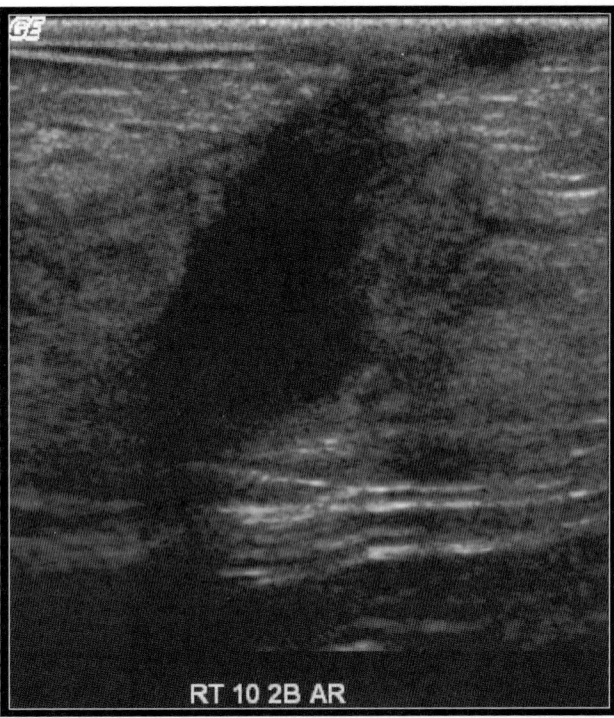

RT 10 2B AR

FIGURE 18–23 This large lumpectomy cavity was left open to accumulate serum and blood. Using very light scan pressure in order not to obscure skin retraction, it does appear that leaving the cavity open was effective in preventing skin retraction in the acute postsurgical period.

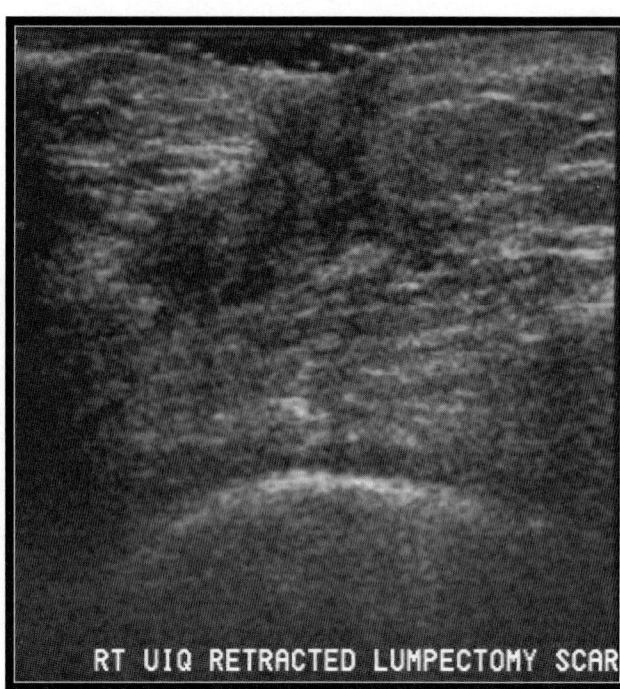

RT UIQ RETRACTED LUMPECTOMY SCAR

FIGURE 18–24 This lumpectomy cavity was left open. Early on, the cosmetic result was good. Later, however, the patient developed exuberant scarring and fat necrosis within the lumpectomy site that led to late retraction. Thus, a good early cosmetic result from leaving the lumpectomy cavity open does not guarantee a good late result. Note that a thin standoff of acoustic gel was necessary to demonstrate the skin retraction adequately on sonography.

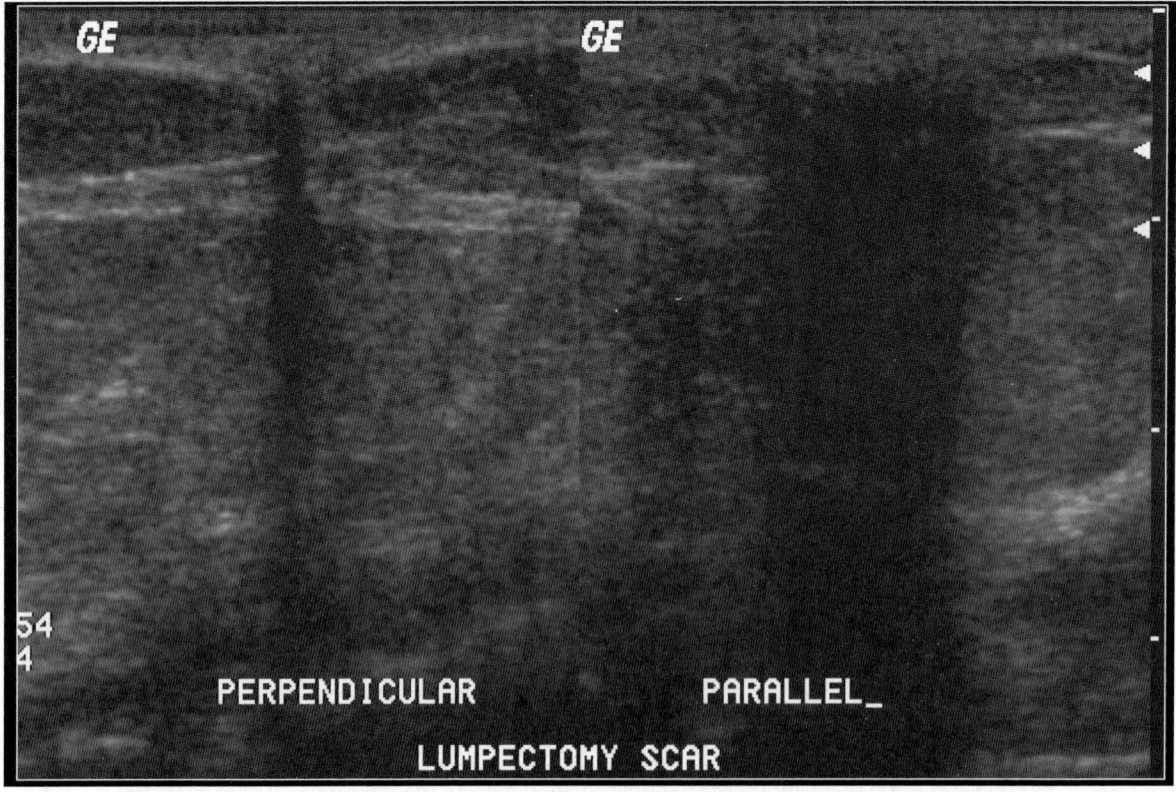

PERPENDICULAR   PARALLEL

LUMPECTOMY SCAR

FIGURE 18–25 The **left** image, obtained perpendicular to the long axis of the scar, shows the typical appearance of a lumpectomy cavity that was sutured closed at the time of surgery. The **right** image, obtained parallel to the long axis of the same lumpectomy cavity, appears more suspicious. The short-axis view (perpendicular to scar) is the key to excluding recurrent tumor, not the long-axis view (parallel to scar).

degree or worse than those would be achieved by primary closure (Fig. 18–24). Patients who have undergone postoperative radiation therapy appear to be more prone to late severe scar retraction.

The sonographic appearances of lumpectomy cavities that have been primarily closed differ from those that have been left open (Figs. 18–25 and 18–26). The key to distinguishing a cavity that has been left open from one that has been closed is its short-axis view, the one obtained perpendicular to the lumpectomy scar (Fig. 18–27). The sonographic appearance of a lumpectomy cavity in its short axis, the plane that lies perpendicular to the long axis of the incision, differs between lumpectomy cavities that have been left open and those that have been primarily closed. The short-axis view of the lumpectomy cavity that has been primarily closed appears as a linear area of hypoechogenicity within the breast tissue. The short-axis view of a lumpectomy cavity that has been left open, however, appears three-dimensional and masslike. The long-axis view that is obtained parallel to the long axis of the scar, on the other hand, appears similar in cases in which the cavity has been closed and left open. In fact, the sonographic appearance of a lumpectomy cavity that is obtained parallel to its long axis can be suspicious, regardless of whether or not the cavity was closed, because of hypoechogenicity and

critical angle shadowing (Figs. 18–28). The short axis of the primarily closed lumpectomy cavity is not always straight (Fig. 18–25). It can be obliquely oriented, curved, or complex and branching, depending on the surgical approach, the direction of tumor extensions discovered at surgery, and re-resection of positive margins that may have been necessary (Fig. 18–29).

It is important to use every diagnostic tool and technique available to help distinguish between recurrent tumor and the nonclosed lumpectomy cavity. One technique that may help is to assess the compressibility of the structure. The blood or serum within the open lumpectomy cavity can be as echogenic as recurrent tumor but usually remains partially compressible. Thus, obtaining split-screen images with and without compression and showing that the structure is more than 10% to 15% compressible favors it being a chronic hematoma, seroma, or lipid cyst within the lumpectomy cavity (Fig. 18–30). Recurrent tumor would usually be less than 10% compressible. Second, Doppler may be helpful. Chronic hematomas, seromas, lipid cysts, and fat necrosis are avascular after about 6 months, whereas recurrent tumor often has vascularity that is demonstrable with color or power Doppler (Figs. 18–31 and 18–32). It is helpful to obtain a pulsed Doppler spectral arterial waveform in addition

(text continued on page 797)

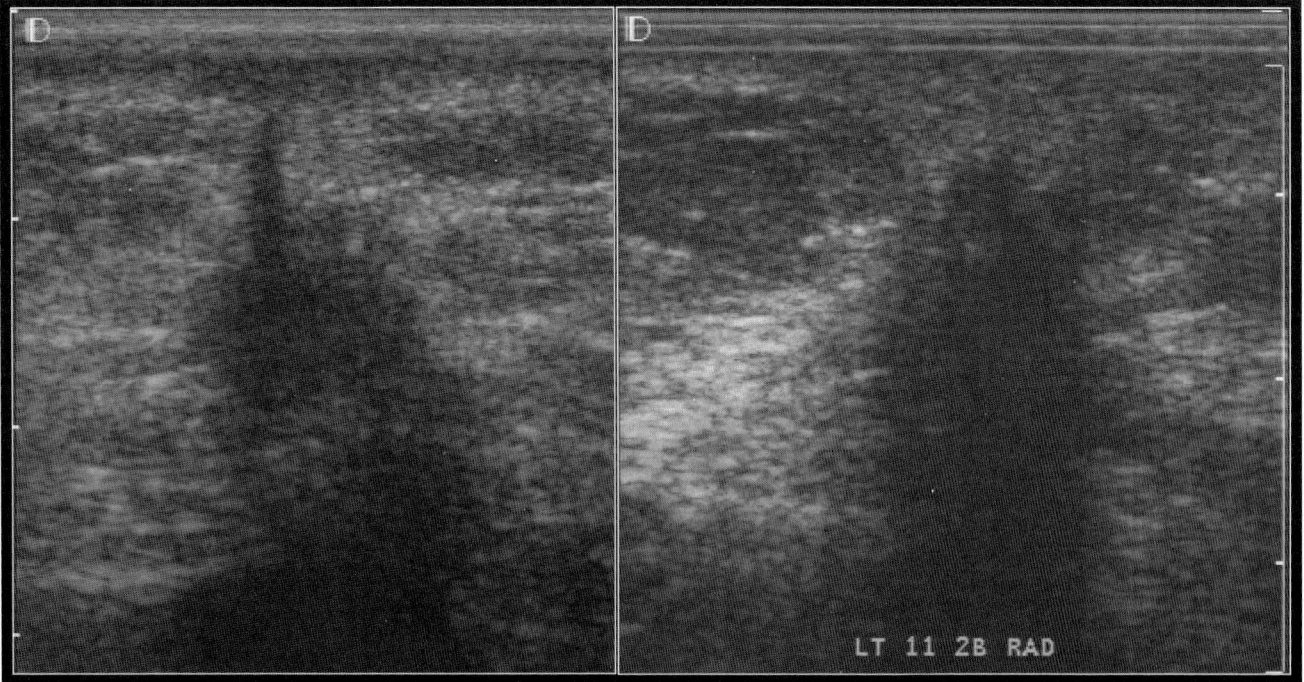

FIGURE 18–26 The **left** image was obtained in a plane that was perpendicular to the long axis of a lumpectomy cavity that was not sutured closed at the time of surgery. The **right** image was obtained in a plane that was parallel to the long axis of the same cavity. In both views, the cavity appears masslike and worrisome for recurrent tumor. The price for the better cosmetic result of leaving the cavity open is less certainty on sonography about whether or not there is recurrent tumor.

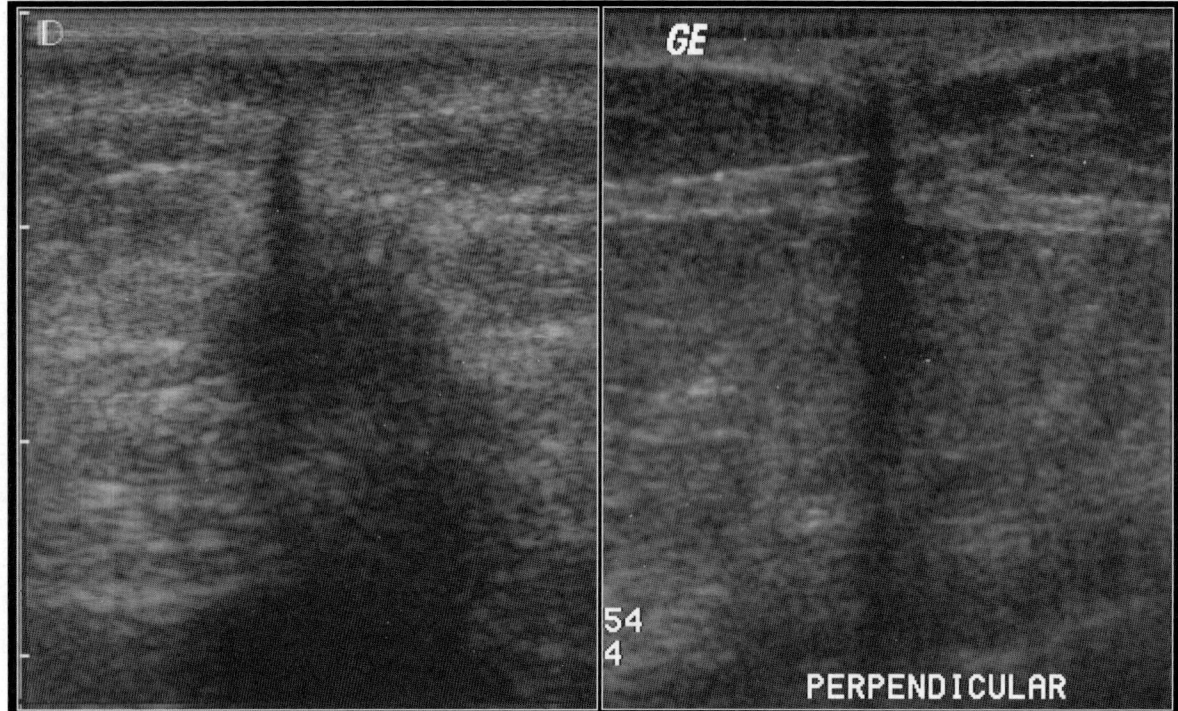

FIGURE 18–27 Images obtained in planes that are perpendicular to the long axis of the scar enable us to distinguish the primarily closed cavity from one that was left open. The **left** image shows the short axis of a cavity that was left open. The cavity appears masslike and is difficult to distinguish from recurrent tumor sonographically. The **right** image, obtained perpendicular to the long axis of a primarily closed lumpectomy cavity, appears linear. It is not masslike in its appearance and does not simulate recurrent tumor.

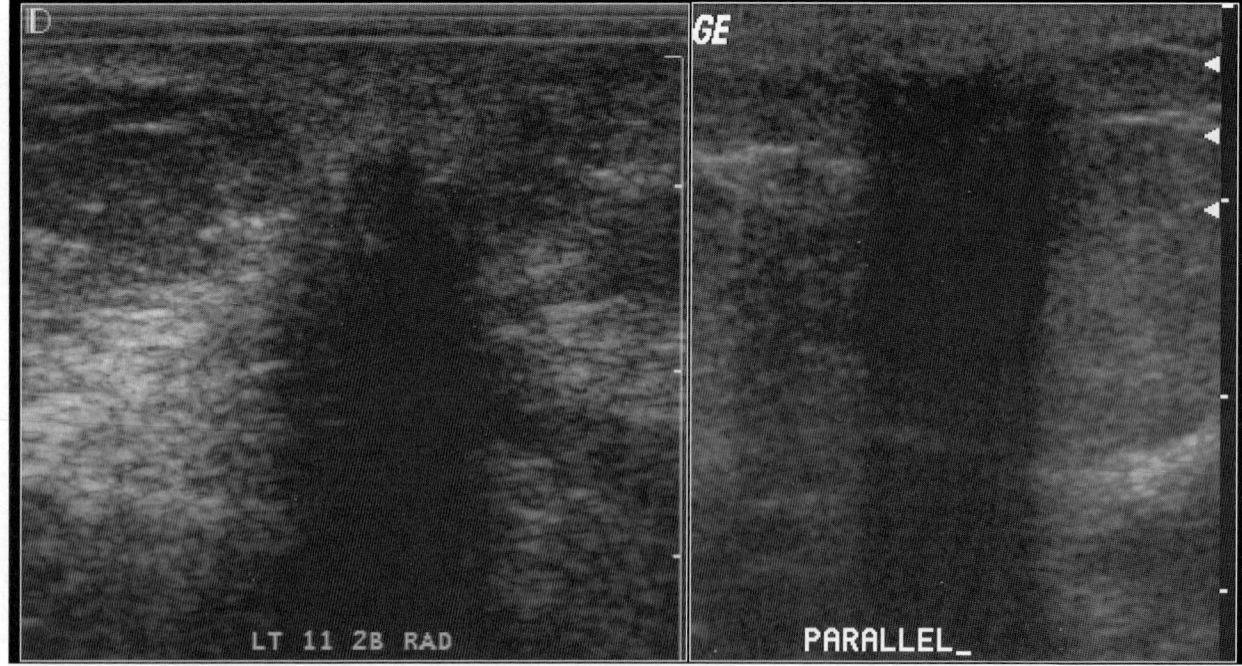

FIGURE 18–28 When the lumpectomy scar is scanned in a plane that is parallel to the long axis of the scar, it is impossible to determine whether the cavity was primarily closed. Only scanning perpendicular to the scar can show this. The **left** image was obtained parallel to the long axis of a lumpectomy cavity that was left open, whereas the **right** image was obtained parallel to the long axis of a lumpectomy cavity that was primarily closed.

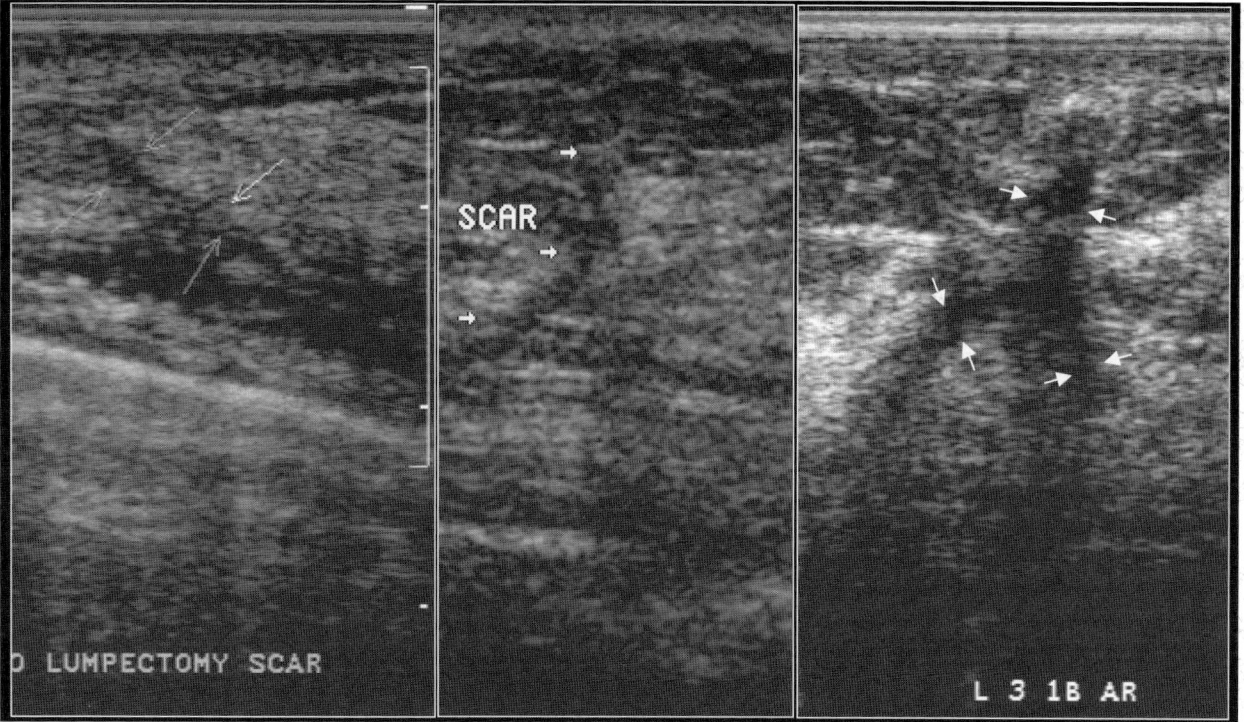

FIGURE 18–29 When the surgeon chooses a periareolar approach rather than direct cut-down approach to the lesion or when the surgeon enters the breast along the course of the localization wire, the linear scar is generally obliquely oriented (**left**). When the lesion extent in one direction was unexpectedly large or when the localization wire and skin mark were slightly off target, the linear scar appears curved (**middle**). When the surgeon encounters unexpected multifocal disease or extensive intraductal components or must re-resect positive margins, the short-axis shape of the lumpectomy scar can be quite complex and may have a branching pattern (**right**).

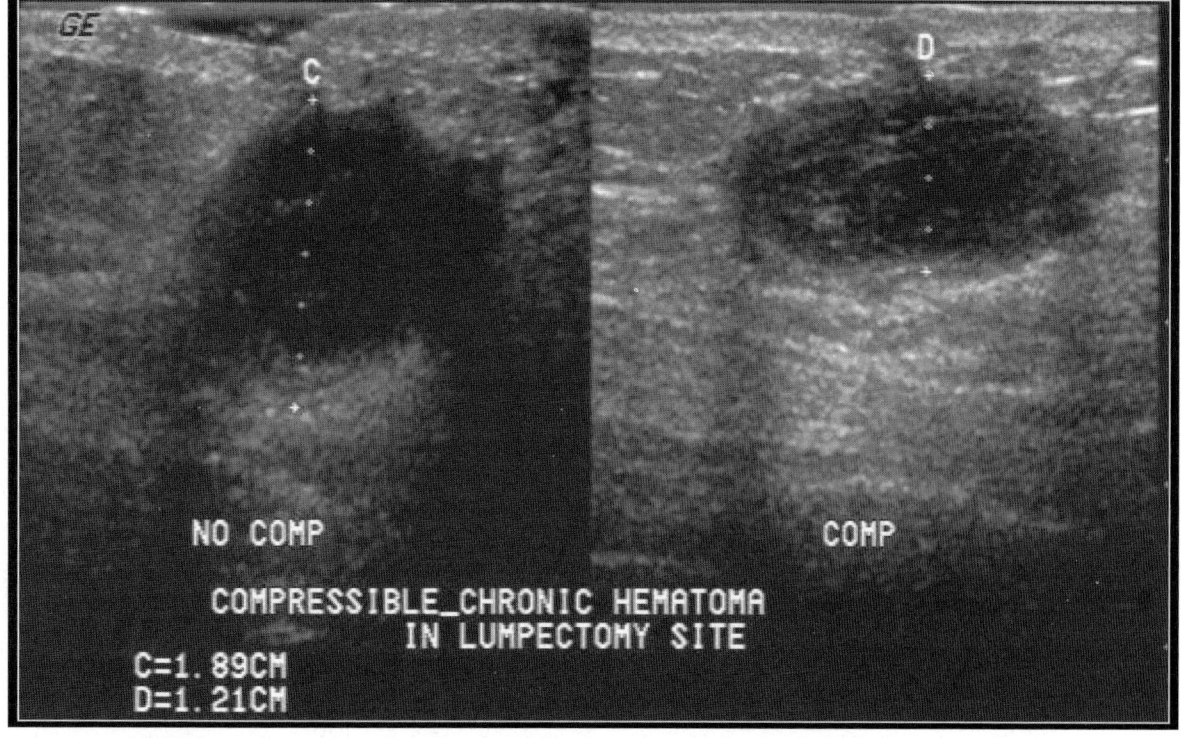

FIGURE 18–30 Dynamic compression maneuvers may be helpful in assessing the lumpectomy cavity that has been left open to accumulate blood and serum. Although the echogenicity of the blood and serum within the cavity may be similar to the echogenicity of recurrent tumor, the accumulated echogenic fluids are relatively soft and compressible, whereas recurrent tumor is not. Compressibility becomes less reliable over time as fluid is replaced by scar and fat necrosis, but in some cases, soft and compressible echogenic lipid cysts may persist indefinitely.

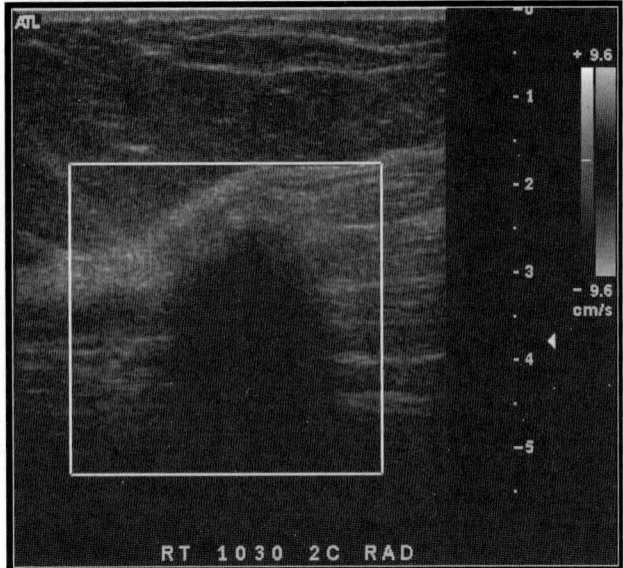

FIGURE 18–31 The fibrous phase of fat necrosis and exuberant scarring are usually avascular, whereas recurrent tumor frequently has internal blood flow that is readily demonstrable by color or power Doppler. This area of severe fat necrosis has no demonstrable blood flow within it.

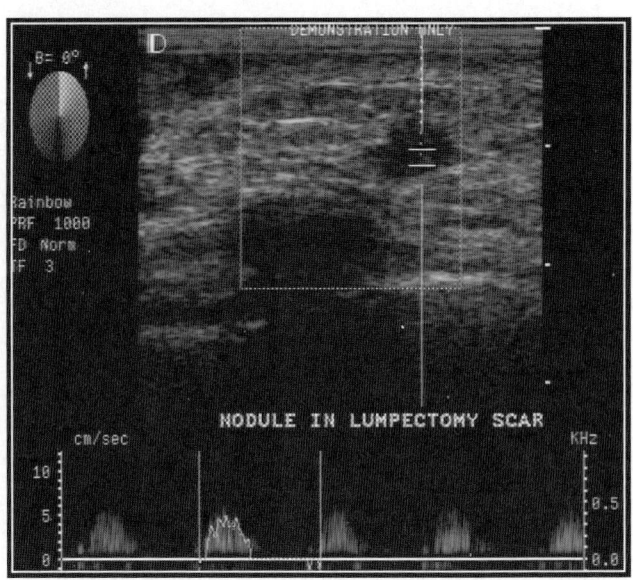

FIGURE 18–33 It is helpful to perform pulsed Doppler spectral analysis on apparent flow within a nodule suspected to be recurrent tumor in order to make sure that the apparent flow is not artifactual. Demonstration of an arterial waveform within the lesion is strong evidence for recurrent tumor rather than exuberant scar or fat necrosis.

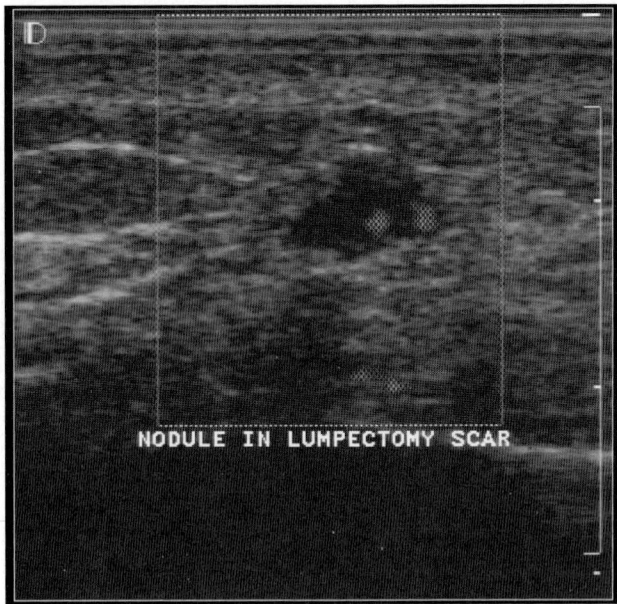

FIGURE 18–32 This small recurrent tumor nodule has demonstrable internal flow on color Doppler. As is always the case with Doppler, a positive study is more valuable than a negative study because some recurrent tumors do not have demonstrable blood flow.

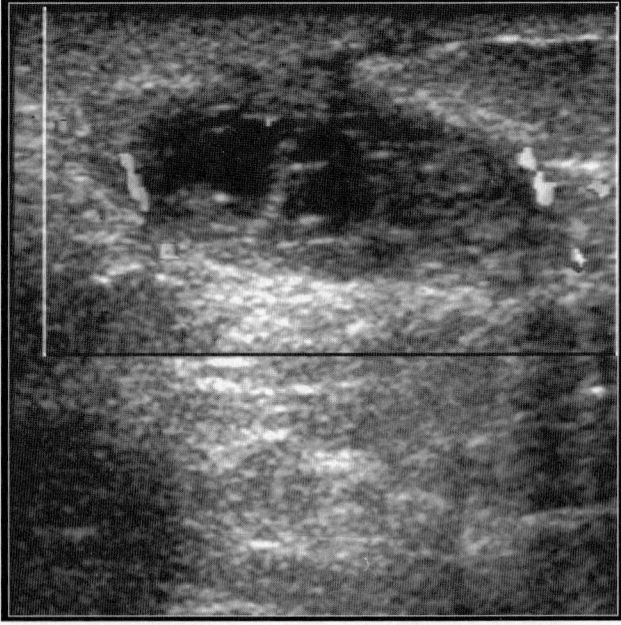

FIGURE 18–34 Only in a very small percentage of cases is there demonstrable blood flow within the walls of the surgical cavity more than 6 months after surgery in the absence of recurrent tumor. This patient still had flow within the walls of the cavity nearly a year after surgery. However, she had developed a postoperative infection, and the flow likely represented continued low-grade inflammation. The magnetic resonance image showed a pattern of enhancement in the walls of the cavity more typical of granulation tissue than recurrent tumor, and ultrasound-guided directional vacuum-assisted biopsy of the hyperemic areas showed no evidence of neoplasm.

to color or power Doppler to ensure that the signal is not artifactual (Fig. 18–33). As is always the case, a positive Doppler study is more valuable than a negative study because some recurrent carcinomas may not have demonstrable flow by color or power Doppler. Granulation tissue that develops within the walls of the lumpectomy cavity can have demonstrable blood flow in the first 6 months after lumpectomy, but as the granulation tissue progresses to fibrosis, the flow usually abates. Only in a small percentage of cases does blood flow persist in the walls of a benign lumpectomy cavity for more than 6 months after surgery, usually when there is chronic low-grade inflammation (Fig. 18–34). Therefore, Doppler is generally reliable for distinguishing between recurrent tumor and lumpectomy complications only 6 months or more after surgery. In certain cases, even after using every sonographic tool and technical trick available, the distinction between an open lumpectomy cavity and recurrent tumor may not be possible. Power Doppler vocal fremitus is not helpful in distinguishing a complex unclosed lumpectomy cavity from recurrent carcinoma because both cause defects in normal vibration (Figs. 18–35). In such cases, spot compression mammograms may be more reassuring, especially if the contents of the lumpectomy cavity are lipid. Such lipid cysts are definitively benign (BIRADS 2) mammographically but commonly appear far more suspicious sonographically, demonstrating solid masses with suspicious features such as acoustic shadowing, angular margins, microlobula-

tions, and marked hypoechogenicity (Fig. 18–36). In other cases, the complicated unclosed lumpectomy cavity can have a complex cystic appearance, with suspicious features such as mural nodules, thick and isoechoic septations, and irregularly thickened and isoechoic outer walls, whereas mammography demonstrates a definitively benign (BIRADS 2) lipid cyst (Fig. 18–37). The sonographic and mammographic findings in lipid cysts are discussed in detail in Chapters 10 and 11. Assessment of the postlumpectomy breast is one of the few circumstances (other than isolated calcifications) in which we rely entirely on the mammographic findings when the sonographic and mammographic findings are discordant. In such cases, the mammogram is truly reassuring, whereas the sonogram is falsely suspicious and worrisome. Stable serial mammographic findings, even in the absence of a lipid cyst, are also reassuring. When sonographic findings are suspicious and mammographic findings are not definitively benign, old mammograms are unavailable to document stability, or there is change or question of change mammographically, we generally proceed straight to ultrasound-guided biopsy. Contrast-enhanced high-spatial-resolution fat-suppression magnetic resonance imaging (MRI), technetium-sestamibi studies, or positron-emission tomography (PET) scans are also possible means of solving this difficult problem, but all are more expensive and less definitive than ultrasound-guided large core needle biopsy or ultrasound-guided DVAB.

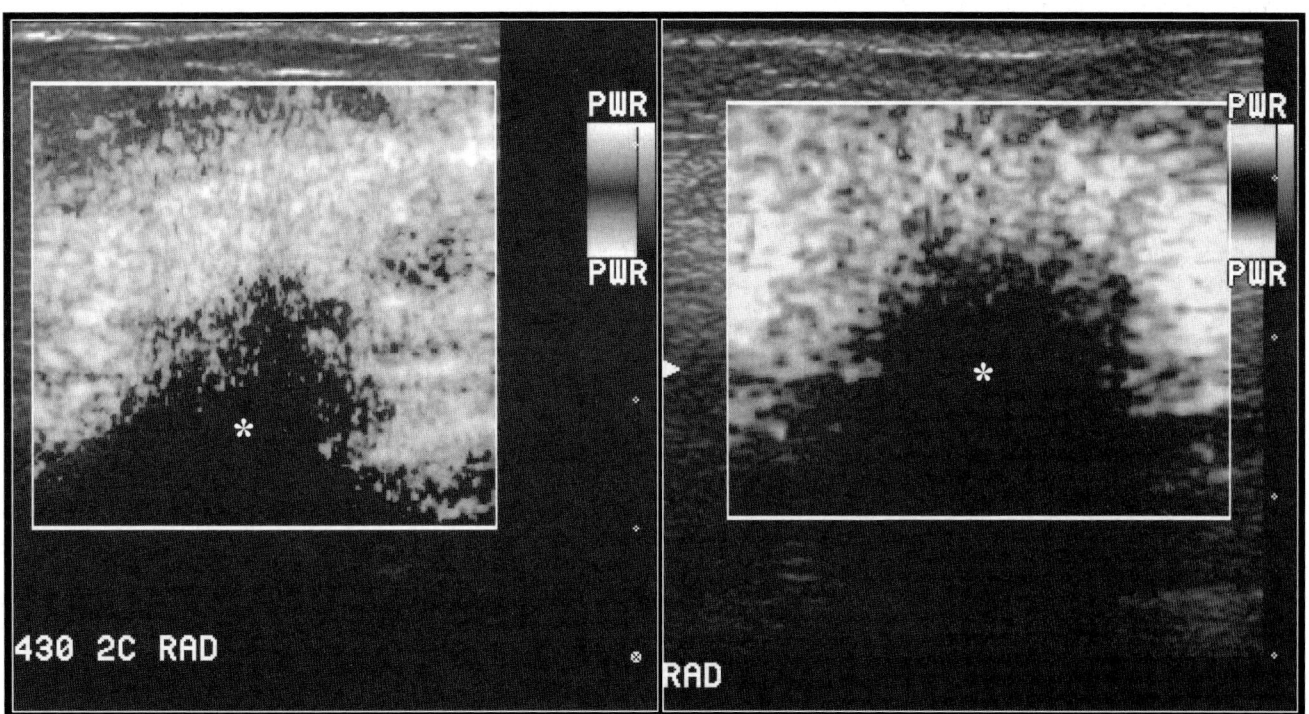

FIGURE 18–35 Power Doppler vocal fremitus helps little in distinguishing between exuberant scarring with fat necrosis (**left**) and recurrent tumor (**right**). Both the benign and malignant entities caused pronounced defects in the acoustic vibratory artifact (histology of recurrent tumor was invasive tubulolobular carcinoma).

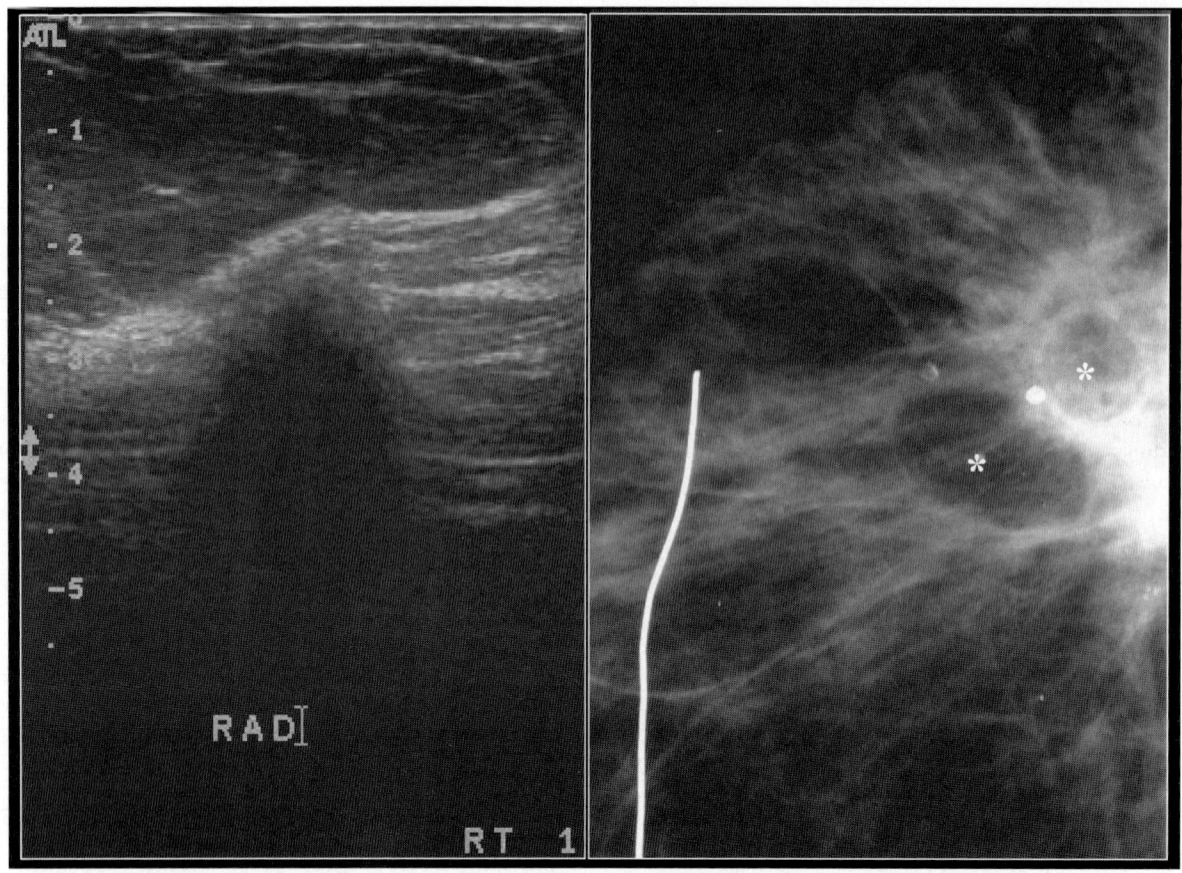

FIGURE 18–36 The sonographic appearances of exuberant scarring or fat necrosis within the lumpectomy site is often more suspicious sonographically than on spot compression mammograms. Sonographically, this fibrotic phase of fat necrosis appears to be a markedly hypoechoic, spiculated mass that causes intense acoustic shadowing, findings that require a BIRADS 5 classification. The spot compression mammogram, on the other hand, shows two lipid cysts (*) centered with the area that appears to be recurrent carcinoma on sonography.

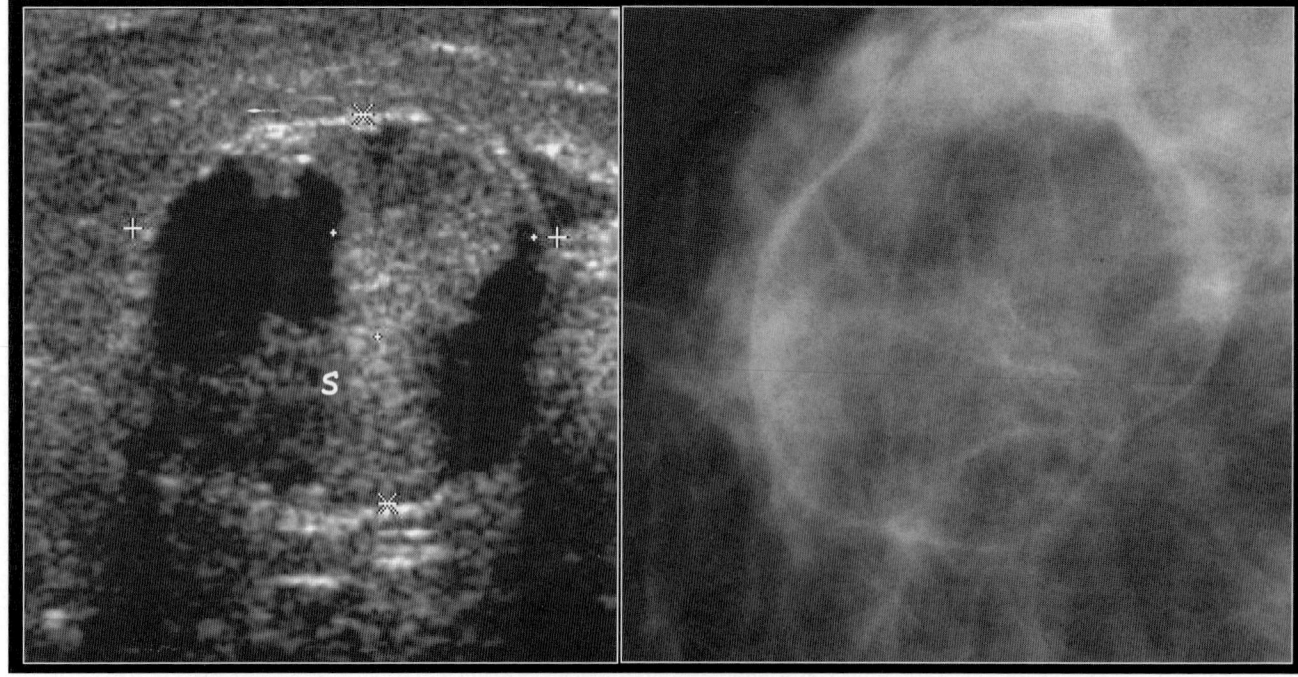

FIGURE 18–37 This chronic lipid cyst within a lumpectomy cavity has a suspicious isoechoic septation (s) on sonography. Spot compression mammograms show it to be a definitively benign lipid cyst. The suspicious septation is not visible mammographically.

Recently, surgeons have attempted to minimize deformity by filling the lumpectomy cavity with collagen at the end of the procedure. This does appear to minimize the deformity to the overlying skin, but it causes a water-density angular mass that can simulate carcinoma both on mammography and sonography (Fig. 18–38). Obtaining a postoperative mammogram to demonstrate the baseline appearance of the collagen-filled lumpectomy cavity and having it available for comparison on all follow-up studies is important in avoiding false-positive interpretation of the collagen as a mass. The collagen has no demonstrable blood flow on color Doppler (Fig. 18–39) and does not enhance on MRI. However, in the weeks immediately after lumpectomy, the granulation tissue in the walls of the lumpectomy cavity can show enhancement on contrast-enhanced MRI, simulating the ringlike peripheral enhancement pattern seen in many larger invasive carcinomas.

Fat necrosis is a complex ischemic process that has traumatic and inflammatory elements as well as some signs that suggest foreign-body reaction. Fat necrosis is dynamic, evolving through multiple phases over time. Because ischemia appears to be a key element, factors that increase the likelihood of ischemia increase the risk for postoperative fat necrosis. Large fatty breasts, long excisions, extensive resections, and radiation all increase the risk for operative and postoperative ischemia and therefore increase the likelihood of fat necrosis. Inflammation alone can cause changes that are similar to those caused by fat necrosis, but more frequently, it exacerbates and extends areas of fat necrosis that already exist.

Patients whose lumpectomy cavities are left open to accumulate blood and serum appear to be more prone to develop fat necrosis than those whose cavities are primarily closed. There is a very complicated association between hematomas, seromas, lipid cysts, and fibrous phases of fat necrosis. Hematomas and seromas have three possible outcomes: (a) complete resolution; (b) complete or partial persistence as chronic hematomas or seromas; or (c) evolution into a lipid cyst or fibrosis. The reasons for varying outcomes are not completely clear. However, the larger the

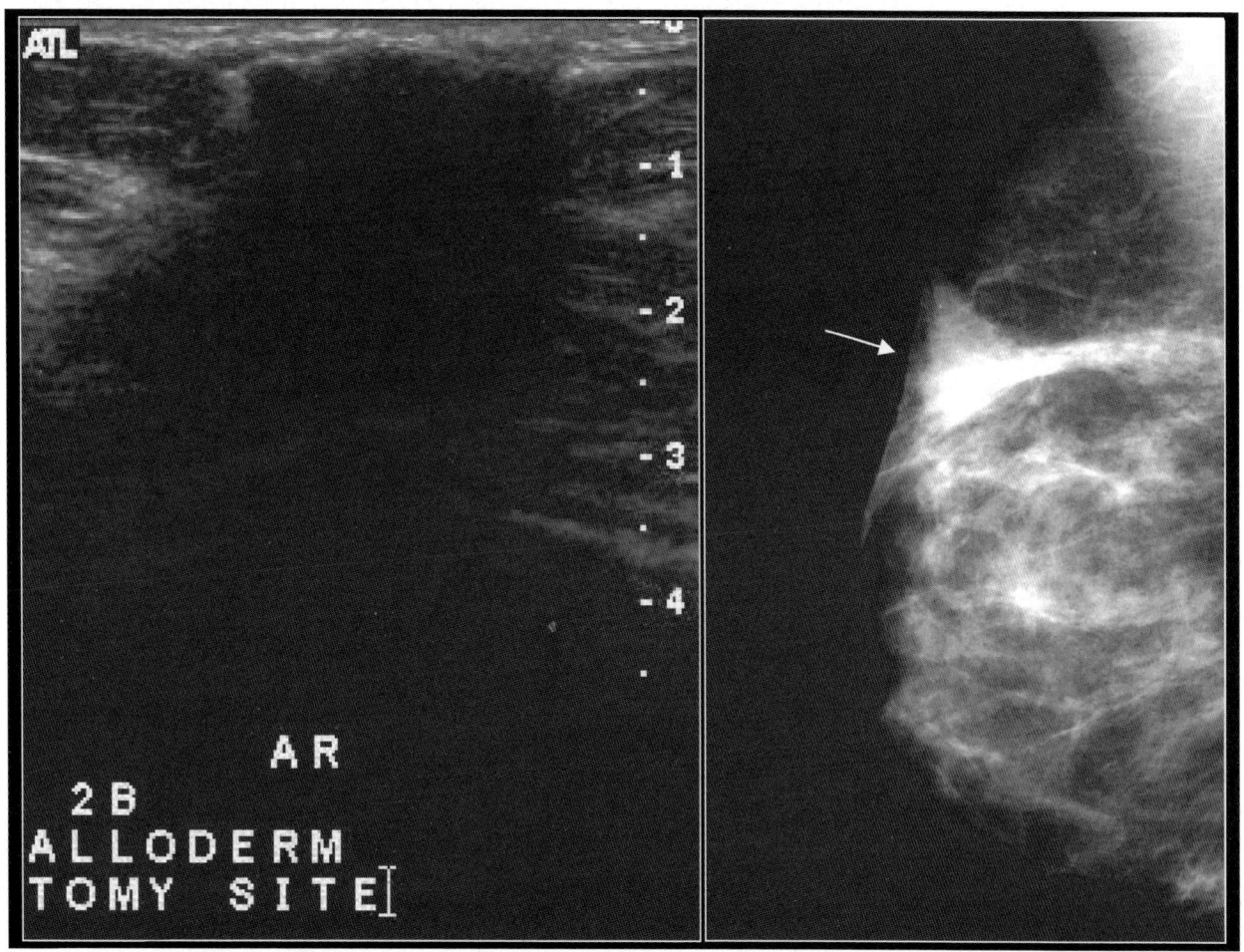

FIGURE 18–38 This patient had collagen placed in her lumpectomy cavity at the completion of surgery to try to prevent deformity of the overlying skin. The collagen has a very suspicious appearance sonographically.

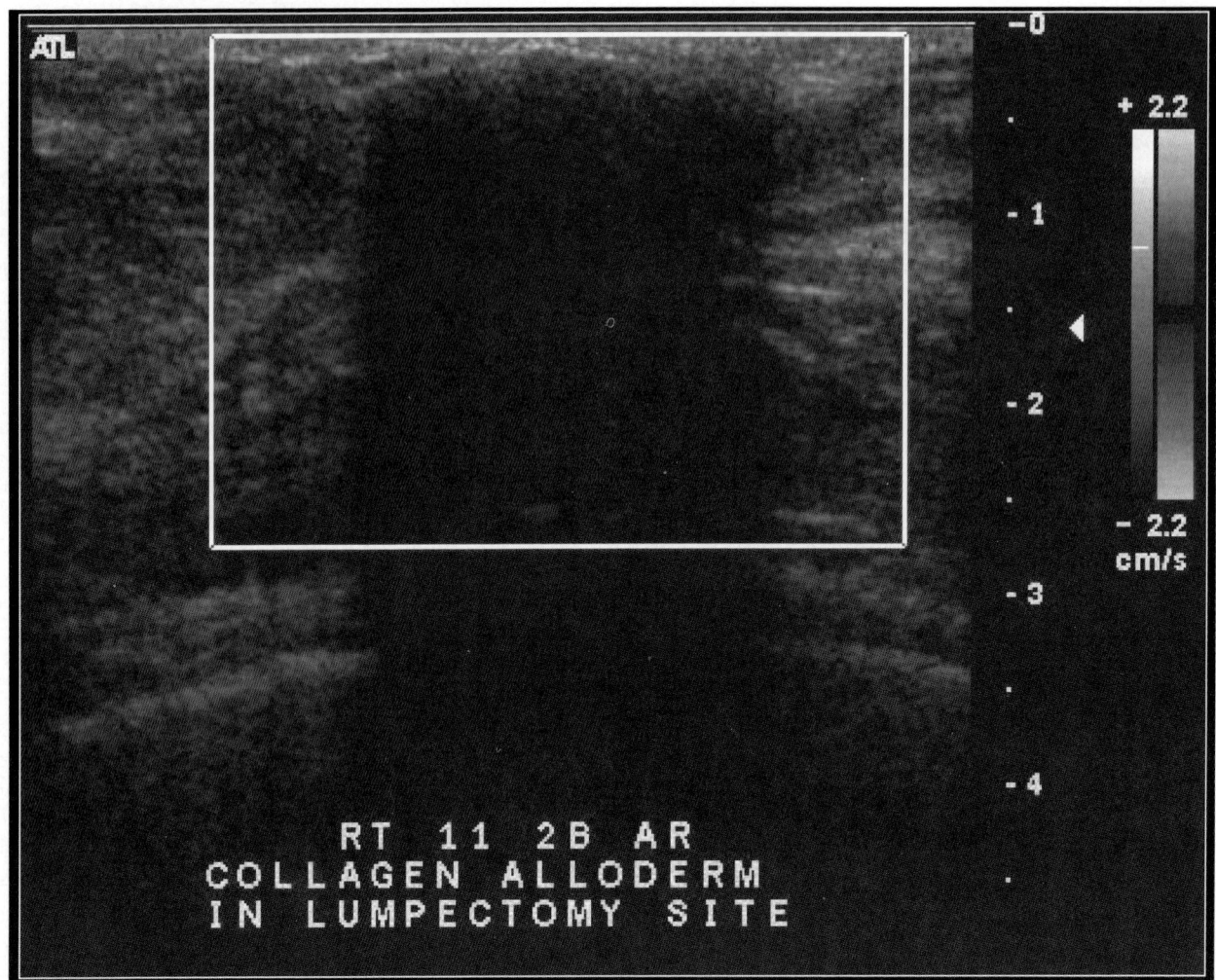

FIGURE 18–39 There is no color Doppler–demonstrable flow within the collagen filling the lumpectomy cavity.

hematoma or seroma and the greater the injury of surrounding tissues, the less likely the lesion is to resolve completely. The evolution of a hematoma or seroma into a lipid cyst is likely related to the extent of the injury to such tissues as well as to the breakdown products that arise within the hematoma or seroma and the type of tissues surrounding the lumpectomy cavity. Some of the liquid fats that eventually replace the blood or serum within the cavity likely originate from lipids within the cell membranes and cytosol of red blood cells (RBCs). These lipid RBC breakdown products tend to be less well resorbed than are the water components of the RBCs and thus persist within the lumpectomy cavity after the water-soluble components are resorbed. Lipids from RBCs are insufficient to explain all of the liquid fatty contents of lipid cysts, especially when the original fluid within the lumpectomy cavity was serum, not blood. Thus, most of the liquid fatty contents must originate within fatty tissues that surround the lumpec-

tomy cavity. It is likely that the traumatic surgical insult that formed the lumpectomy cavity also causes ischemia, necrosis, and liquefaction of surrounding fat. The breakdown products that arise from the blood and serum within the lumpectomy cavity cause a chemical inflammation that exacerbates the necrotic process in the tissues surrounding the lumpectomy cavity. The fatty acids released when adipose tissue is liquefied further inflame adjacent tissues, spreading the process. Some of the liquefied fat seeps into the lumpectomy cavity and persists long after water components of the hematoma or seroma are resorbed, contributing to its evolution from hematoma or seroma to lipid cyst.

Fat necrosis evolves through several stages. The first phase is edema of fat. The sonographic changes during the edematous phase of fat necrosis are nonspecific and can be seen in edema of any etiology. When fat necrosis is severe enough, adipose cells break down and liquefy. The liquefied fat then is either ingested by macrophages or walled off within by surrounding inflammation and fibrosis. These walled-off deposits of lipid breakdown products form lipid cysts (oil cysts). Saponification and deposition of calcium salts lead to classic "eggshell" calcifications within the wall of the lipid cyst. The mammographic findings of lipid cysts vary, depending on the maturity. The key mammographic findings of mature lipid cysts are classically benign (BI-RADS 2) findings that require no additional evaluation—spherically or elliptically shaped fatty densities that are often surrounded by eggshell calcifications. However, not all lipid cysts are mammographically classic. The mammographic findings of early, less mature lipid are nonspecific and can require additional evaluation.

Like the mammographic appearances, the sonographic appearances of lipid cysts vary with the stage of development. Early in the course of development, before the water components have been resorbed, lipid cysts can appear to be simple cysts. Later, when water components have been partially resorbed, lipid cysts may have fat–fluid levels. Fat–fluid levels within cysts are more frequently seen and more easily demonstrated on sonography than they are mammographically. It is important to scan the patient in upright or lateral decubitus positions to cause the fat–fluid interface to shift and to differentiate the lipid layer from reverberation echoes and intracystic papillary lesions. Sonographic evaluation of fat–fluid levels is discussed in detail in Chapter 10. Fat–fluid levels are not specific sonographic signs of fat necrosis and can occur in fibrocystic change and in galactoceles. In later phases, when the water component of the lipid cyst has been completely resorbed, the cyst becomes completely filled with lipid contents that are often echogenic. The lipid contents can be so echogenic that they make the lipid cyst appear to be solid on sonography. Foamy macrophages, cell debris, and the interfaces between incompletely emulsified tiny fat globules and small amounts of water within the cyst all contribute to the echogenicity of the contents of lipid cysts. Artifact that arises from calcification in the wall of the lipid cyst also can contribute to its apparent echogenicity. As the calcification within the lipid cyst wall progresses, the lipid cyst wall becomes progressively more hyperechoic. As the amount of calcium in the wall of the lipid cyst increases, the sound transmission decreases. Densely calcified lipid cysts can be difficult to distinguish sonographically from densely calcified fibroadenomas but usually form classically benign eggshell calcifications mammographically.

Lipid cysts represent only one stage in the development of fat necrosis. In areas of fat necrosis where lipid cyst formation does not occur, mastitis, foreign-body granuloma formation, and fibrosis occur. Early on, all of these processes increase the echogenicity of fat in a fashion similar to that caused by edema of any other cause. However, eventually all of these pathologic processes other than lipid cyst tend to progress to end stages of dense fibrosis. The end-stage ap-

pearance of fibrosis resulting from fat necrosis is identical to and indistinguishable from the fibrosis of postoperative scarring that occurs in the absence of fat necrosis. Fat necrosis simply adds to the degree of postsurgical fibrotic scarring. The more extensive the fibrosis, the greater the chances that the scar will retract surrounding tissues, leading to severe architectural distortion and spiculation that is mammographically and sonographically difficult to distinguish from recurrent spiculated carcinoma. The fibrosis caused by postoperative radiation contributes to the fibrosis caused by scar formation and end-stage fat necrosis in some patients. The mammographic and sonographic findings in various stages of fat necrosis are discussed and illustrated in detail in Chapter 11. The mammographic and sonographic findings in lipid cysts are discussed and illustrated in detail in Chapters 10 and 11. Our main concern in this chapter is in trying to distinguish fat necrosis in the lumpectomy site from recurrent breast carcinoma, which is discussed further in the section on recurrent carcinoma later in this chapter.

Postmastectomy Alterations

Today, most mastectomies that are performed are simple or modified radical mastectomies. Radical mastectomies, in which the pectoralis muscle is removed, are generally no longer performed. However, some living patients might have had a radical mastectomy in the distant past. Axillary dissection is usually performed along with mastectomy in patients who have invasive breast carcinoma and in selected patients with high-nuclear-grade ductal carcinoma *in situ* (DCIS). Axillary dissection is usually not performed in patients who undergo mastectomy for pure low- or intermediate-nuclear-grade DCIS. Mastectomies are performed for disease that is too extensive to be treated with breast-conserving therapy because the lesion is too large, multifocal, or multicentric or because the size of the breast is too small in comparison to lesion size. Lesions larger than 5 cm are generally considered too large for lumpectomy, regardless of the patient's breast size, but there are exceptions. Additionally, patients whose lesions are too large for breast-conserving surgery but who are insistent on not having mastectomy can undergo a trial of induction chemotherapy to try to make the lesion regress to a size that is small enough for lumpectomy. Patients with direct invasion of skin or nipple are also usually treated with mastectomy, although some surgeons perform segmentectomy with nipple resection in such cases. Patients who have high-nuclear-grade DCIS or DCIS of lower nuclear grades that has associated necrosis may have lower recurrence rates and better cosmesis with skin-sparing mastectomy and immediate reconstruction than with lumpectomy. Preoperative high-spatial-resolution MRI with contrast enhancement and fat-suppression algorithms, together with second-look ultrasound and ultrasound-guided biopsies to map out the extent of disease preoperatively, have been invaluable in deciding whether to treat with mastectomy or breast-conserving surgery.

In certain cases, mastectomy is performed for nonmedical reasons. Patients from remote rural areas and foreign patients often choose mastectomy over lumpectomy with 5 weeks of postoperative radiation therapy. Other patients might have mastectomy rather than lumpectomy because they are not well enough to undergo external radiation therapy or have contraindications to it. Brachytherapy of the lumpectomy site will likely change this patient viewpoint because it takes only a few extra days. Yet other patients may choose mastectomy simply because they do not want to worry about the slightly higher risks of local recurrence associated with lumpectomy.

The sonographic findings after mastectomy are similar to those after lumpectomy, but more extensive. The mastectomy incision is much longer than any lumpectomy incision, and thus its scar is longer. As is the case for lumpectomy scars, the orientation of the scan plane relative to the axis of the scar greatly affects its sonographic appearances. Scanning the scar parallel to its long axis may show sonographically suspicious hypoechogenicity, shadowing, and architectural distortion. Scanning the scar perpendicular to its long axis, however, is usually quite reassuring, showing only a hypoechoic line that generally involves only the skin. The skin within the scar may be permanently thickened or stretched and thinned and is usually slightly less echogenic than normal skin. Mastectomy cavities are not left open to accumulate blood and serum. In fact, drains are placed to ensure that blood and serum do not become entrapped within the scar. The mastectomy cavity does not appear to extend as deeply as lumpectomy scars because the surrounding breast tissue and subcutaneous fat have been completely removed. The skin usually lies directly on the chest wall musculature. The surgical cavity is essentially only a potential space in most patients. Only when the drain malfunctions or is removed too early does fluid collect within the mastectomy site. Hematoma and seromas that do collect in the mastectomy site tend to be very elongated in a direction that is parallel to the long axis of the scar (Figs. 18–40 and 18–41). Sonography using extended field of view is helpful in demonstrating such long fluid collections.

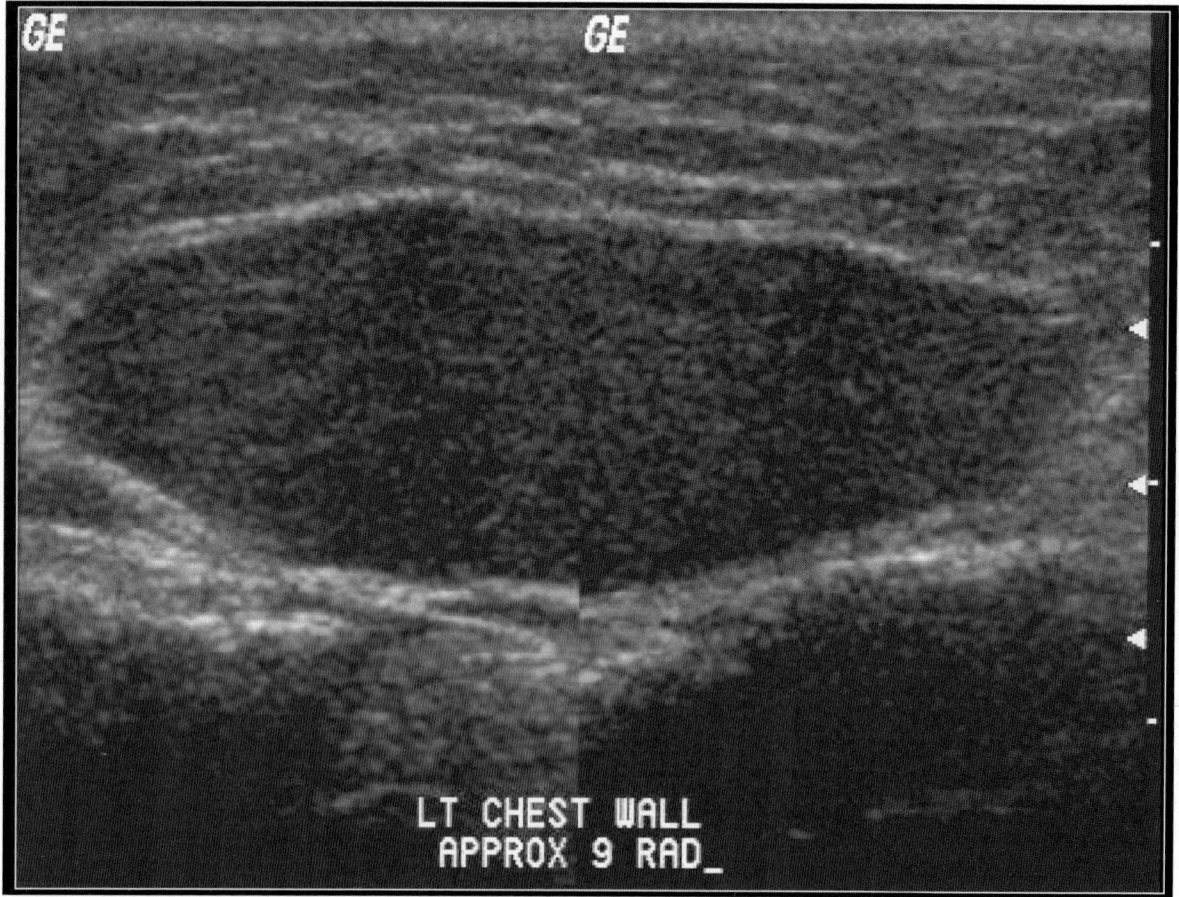

FIGURE 18–40 Hematomas are not allowed to accumulate within mastectomy surgical beds intentionally. In fact, drains are placed to make sure that they do not accumulate. However, drains may malfunction, fall out, or be removed too early, allowing hematomas to accumulate within the surgical site. Such hematomas are usually quite elongated in a direction that is parallel to the long axis of the mastectomy scar.

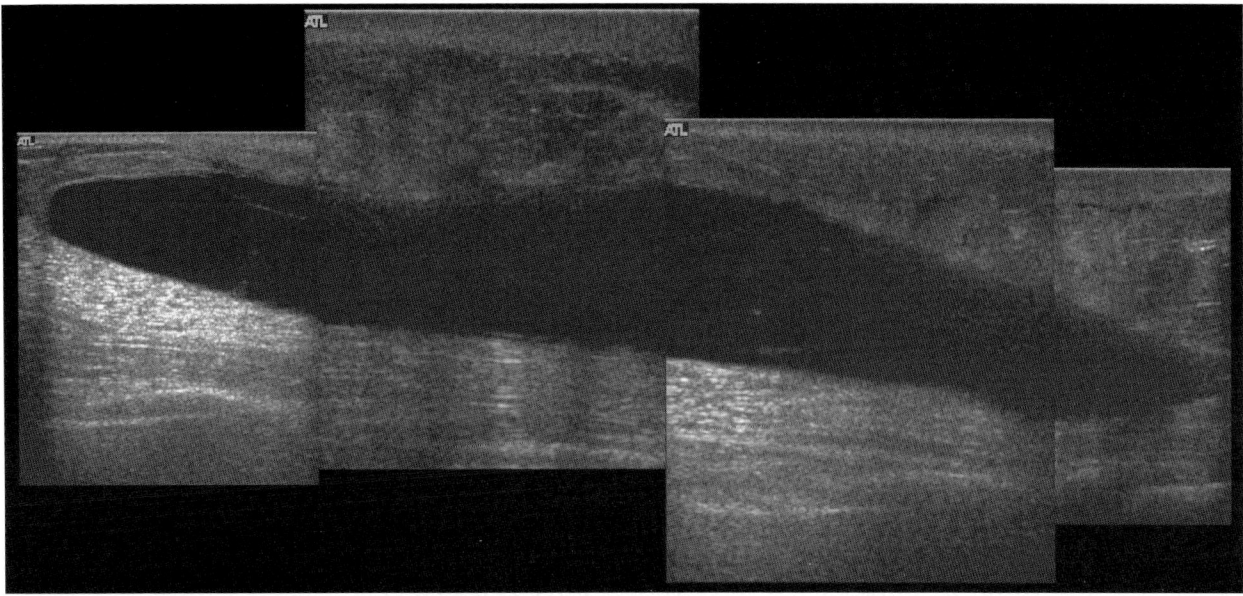

FIGURE 18–41 Seromas, like hematomas, are not allowed to accumulate within mastectomy surgical beds intentionally. In fact, drains are placed to make sure that they do not accumulate. However, drains may malfunction, fall out, or be removed too early, allowing hematomas to accumulate within the surgical site. Such seromas are usually quite elongated in a direction that is parallel to the long axis of the mastectomy scar.

Fat necrosis tends to be less of a problem after mastectomy than with lumpectomy because the blood is drained and because the fatty tissues that are involved by fat necrosis in lumpectomy patients are surgically removed. Although fat necrosis within a mastectomy scar is uncommon, exuberant scars can form in the absence of fat necrosis, especially if the chest wall undergoes postmastectomy radiation treatments. In some cases, these exuberant scars might become palpable and require sonographic evaluation.

Many patients now undergo skin-sparing simple mastectomy and immediate reconstruction. Others require gradual inflation of expanders before undergoing permanent augmentation implantation. Expanders and permanent augmentation implants are subject to all the same complications as any other implant. Periimplant hematomas, seromas, and infection occur acutely (Figs. 18–42 and 18–43). Implant rupture, capsular contracture, or delayed infection can occur. Implant complications are discussed in greater detail in Chapter 9.

Mastectomy reduces the chances of local recurrence but does not completely eliminate the risks. Thus, diagnostic imaging evaluation for local recurrence is occasionally necessary. Mammography generally cannot project the lumpectomy scar, where recurrences are most likely, away from the superimposed chest wall tissues and thus does not evaluate the mastectomy scar well. Sonography is more effective for evaluation of mastectomy scars for recurrent malignant disease. Recurrences of carcinoma are discussed in later sections.

Post–Axillary Dissection Alterations

The changes in the axilla that result from axillary dissection are analogous to those following mastectomy. The surgical site is primarily closed, drains are placed, and fluid collections are not intentionally allowed to accumulate. Changes from sentinel node procedures are much less severe than those of axillary dissection and frequently are not sonographically detectable.

As is the case in the mastectomy site, hematomas and seromas are an undesired complication of axillary dissection (Figs. 18–44 and 18–45). Additionally, fat necrosis may occur in the axillary dissection site with or without associated hematoma or seroma (Fig. 18–46).

Sonographic assessment of the axilla may be necessary in patients who develop a palpable lump after axillary dissection in order to rule out recurrent disease in lymph nodes that were not removed and in patients who develop lymphedema of the ipsilateral arm or breast. Lymphedema is a known and relatively common complication of axillary dissection but can also be caused by tumor in residual axillary lymph nodes. Patients who have evidence of perinodal invasion at the time of axillary dissection are especially prone to axillary recurrences. Sonographically demonstrable lymphadenopathy and solid masses indicate recurrent tumor, whereas the lack of demonstrable lymphadenopathy or a mass favors the lymphedema merely being a complication of the surgical procedure (Fig. 18–47). In a few patients who have undergone axillary dissection and had

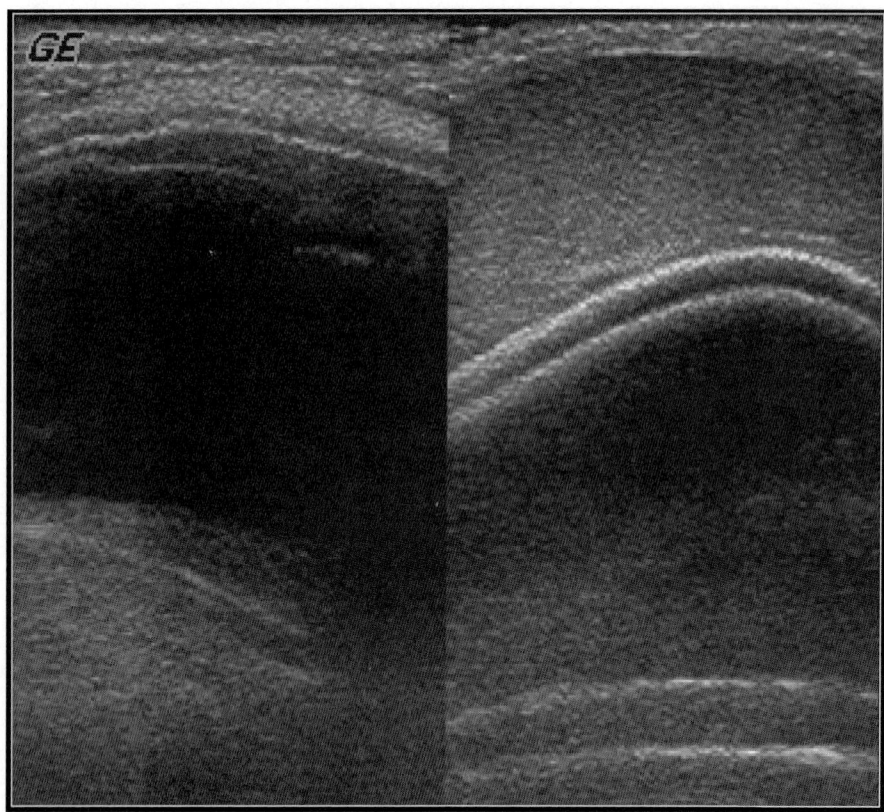

FIGURE 18–42 Expanders and implants used to reconstruct the breast after mastectomy are subject to the same acute complications as augmentation implants. In this case, an acute hematoma has formed around the left expander **(right)**.

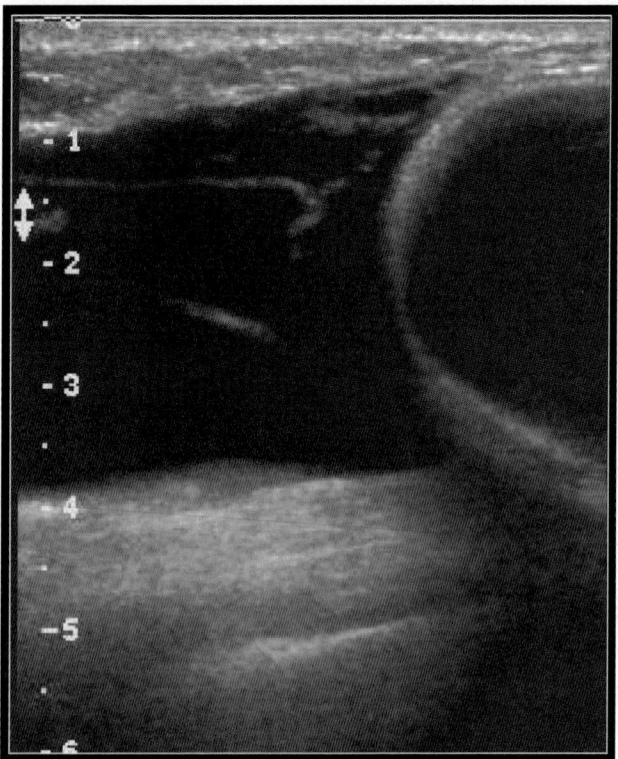

FIGURE 18–43 Expanders and implants used to reconstruct the breast after mastectomy are subject to the same acute complications as augmentation implants. In this case, a seroma that contains multiple fibrinous adhesions has developed around the expander.

postoperative axillary and breast radiation therapy, exuberant scar and the fibrotic phase of fat necrosis can develop and can be difficult to distinguish from recurrent tumor (Fig. 18–48). As is the case for the fibrotic phases of fat necrosis in the lumpectomy site, color Doppler is helpful because most metastases to the breast are hypervascular and have demonstrable flow on color or power Doppler, whereas fat necrosis and exuberant scar are usually avascular after 6 months (Fig. 18–49). Of course, seroma, chronic hematoma, or lymphocele can cause palpable lumps, with or without associated lymphedema that must be distinguished from recurrent axillary tumor.

In patients who have undergone only sentinel node procedure, the chances of residual or recurrent disease in the axilla might be slightly increased. The sentinel lymph node is falsely negative in less than 10% of cases, but in those cases, sonographic assessment of the axilla might be particularly important. Assessment of the regional lymph nodes of the breast is discussed in detail in Chapter 19.

Recurrent Carcinoma

The most important reason to understand thoroughly the range of sonographic appearances of the lumpectomy cavity and axillary dissection scars and associated fat necrosis is to better distinguish them from recurrent tumor. Unfortunately, local recurrences remain relatively common. The risk for recurrence depends on many factors. The two most

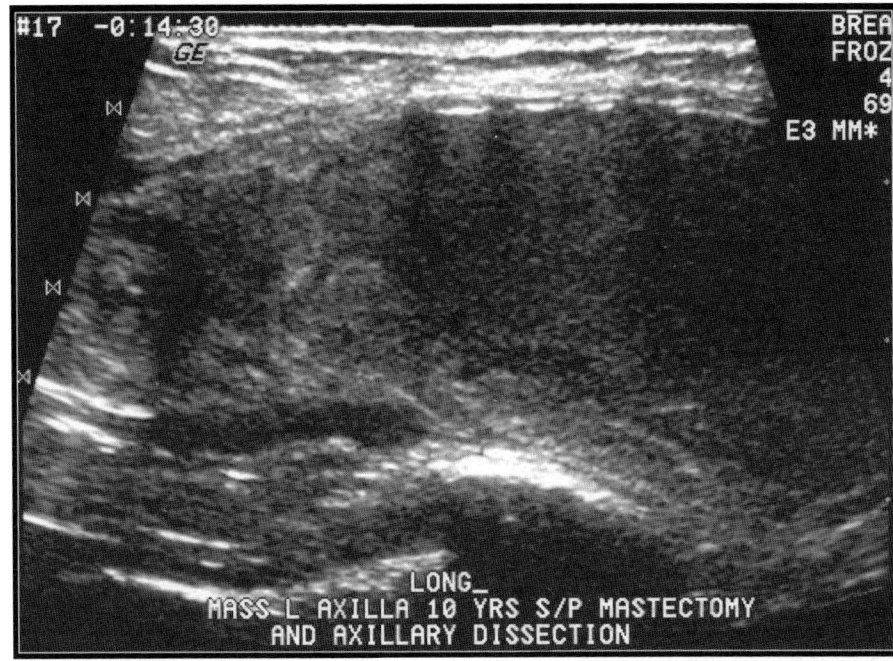

FIGURE 18–44 A large acute hematoma complicates the axillary dissection site in this patient.

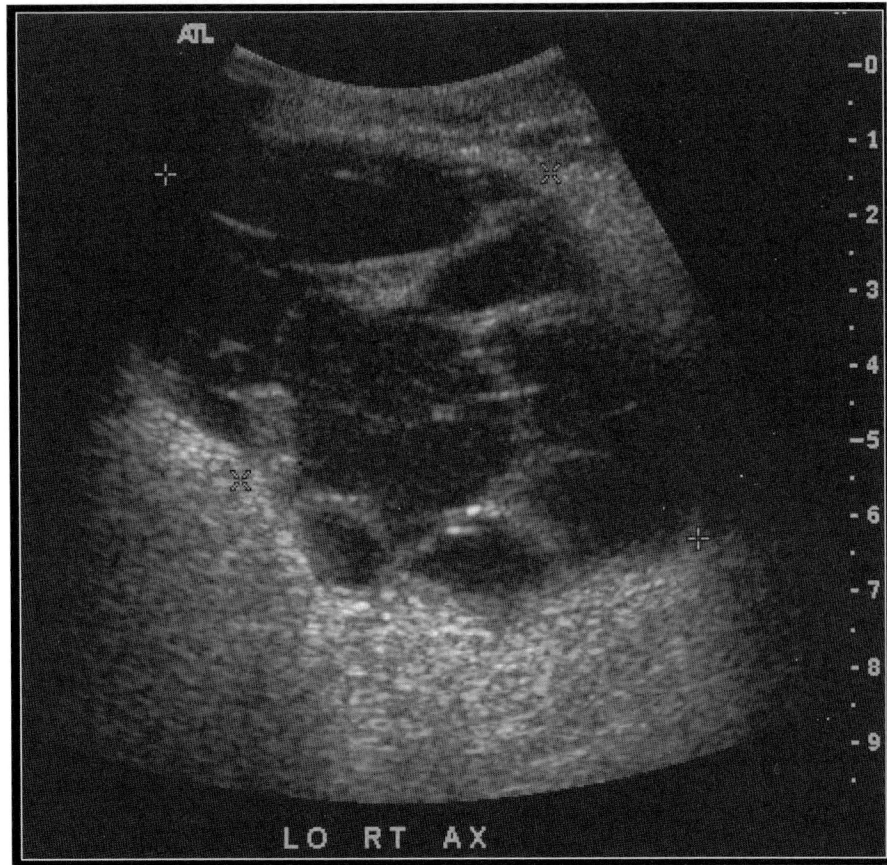

FIGURE 18–45 This large multiseptated seroma formed acutely within the axillary dissection site.

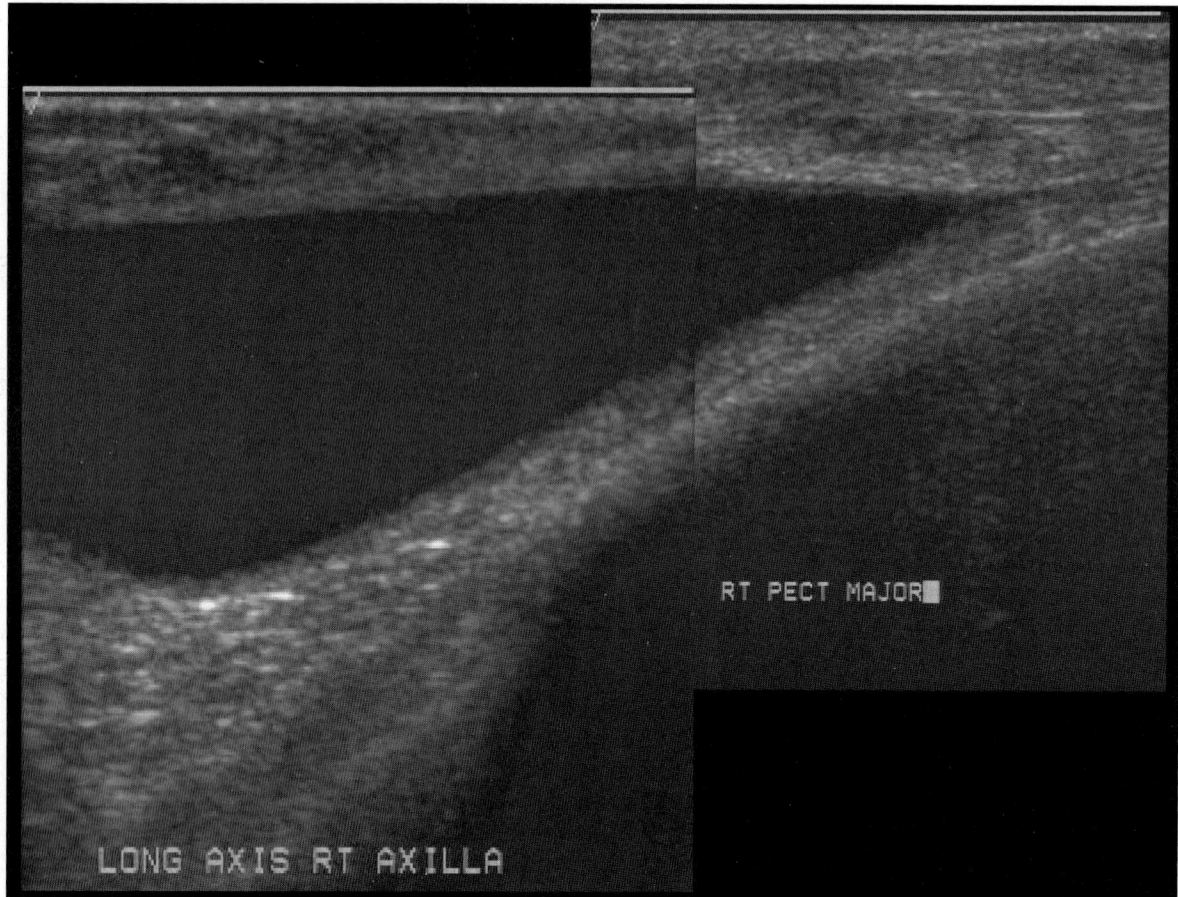

RT PECT MAJOR

LONG AXIS RT AXILLA

FIGURE 18–46 One type of fluid collection that can develop in an axillary dissection site, but not in a lumpectomy or mastectomy site, is a lymphocele. This large lymphocele accumulated gradually over a few months after axillary dissection. The patient presented for sonographic evaluation because of arm swelling and a fluctuant axillary mass.

important factors in patients with invasive not otherwise specified (NOS) carcinomas are positive margins at the time of surgery and the presence of extensive intraductal components of tumor. The two most important factors of pure DCIS are high nuclear grade and the presence of necrosis. Micropapillary DCIS is also prone to local recurrences because it is frequently more extensive than imaging studies suggest and is impalpable at the time of surgery. Postoperative radiation, adjuvant chemotherapy, and estrogen suppression with selective estrogen receptor modulators (SERMS; e.g., tamoxifen, raloxifene) or aromatase inhibitors are used to try to minimize the chances of local recurrences and are effective in many cases.

It is essential to understand why and where local recurrences occur in order to maximize the chances of recognizing them early. Local recurrences *are rarely truly recurrences.* Rather, they usually represent *residual disease* that was not recognized and resected at the time for surgery and that has not been controlled by the immune system, radiation, or chemotherapy. The problem is complex because the surgeon cannot resect disease that he or she does not know about and

the radiologist cannot identify microscopic disease for the surgeon prospectively with current imaging resolution. Contrast-enhanced MRI with high-resolution fat-suppression sequences such as rotating delivery excitation off-resonance (RODEO) has been invaluable at more accurately staging breast cancer preoperatively, but has high false-positive rates. Second-look ultrasound, performed after a positive MRI, has been helpful in sorting out the false-positive findings and in mapping out the extent of the lesion with selective ultrasound-guided biopsies. Second-look ultrasound has also been invaluable in learning to better determine extent of disease preoperatively and to detect recurrent disease with ultrasound. It is not completely clear that removal of all disease is effective or even desirable. At some point, we may have to consider removing only the bulk of the malignancy, especially the central ischemic focus, and then stimulating the immune system to handle residual disease. The problem with chemotherapy and radiation therapy (to a lesser extent) is that they tend to suppress rather than stimulate the immune system. Hormonal manipulation with SERMs or aromatase inhibitors in estrogen receptor–positive lesions,

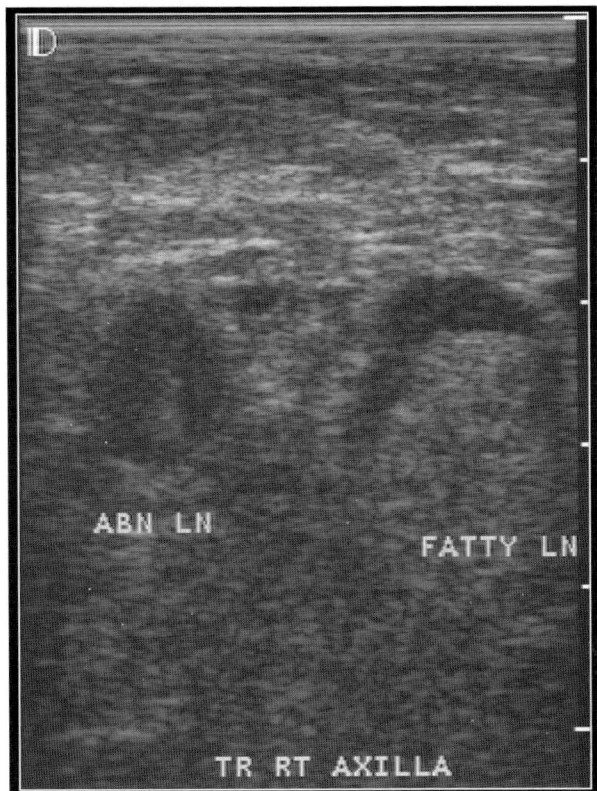

FIGURE 18–47 This patient presented to ultrasound because of ipsilateral arm and breast swelling that developed 18 months after lumpectomy without axillary dissection or radiation. Sonography showed a grossly abnormal lymph node immediately adjacent a normal-appearing node, a finding that strongly favors metastatic disease. Scan of the swollen breast also showed recurrent tumor arising from a duct lying between the nipple and the lumpectomy cavity (shown in Fig. 18–52).

administering trastuzumab (Herceptin) in trastuzumab-positive tumors, employing antimucin antibodies and anticlonal antibodies, and using angiogenesis inhibitors all promise better tumor-specific targeting that, together with generalized stimulation of the immune system with diet and nutritional supplements, appear to be a more rational approach than our current approach. However, although the future holds promises of better diagnosis and treatment and reduction in the risk for local recurrences, the reality of today is that we must be as aggressive as possible in determining the extent of disease and whether or not the lesion can be completely resected at lumpectomy with a combination of MRI, second-look ultrasound, and carefully selected ultrasound-guided biopsy mapping of lesions extent. Then, we must accurately communicate the information to the surgeon, accurately localize the lesion preoperatively or intraoperatively for the surgeon. The surgeon must then attempt to resect all known disease within the limits of breast-conserving surgery. Finally, the surgeon must appropriately orient the specimen, and the pathologist must ink and examine the specimen's margins to determine whether they contain tumor or are clear. There are many points in this algorithm at which something can go wrong, causing residual local disease to be left in the breast. This is the main reason for postsurgical radiation therapy. (Although adjuvant chemotherapy may help in preventing local recurrences, its main role is to suppress disseminated disease, not necessarily to control locoregional disease.) The key to early, sensitive, and accurate detection of recurrent disease as a result of failures in this complex algorithm is to understand its weaknesses—why and where residual disease is missed.

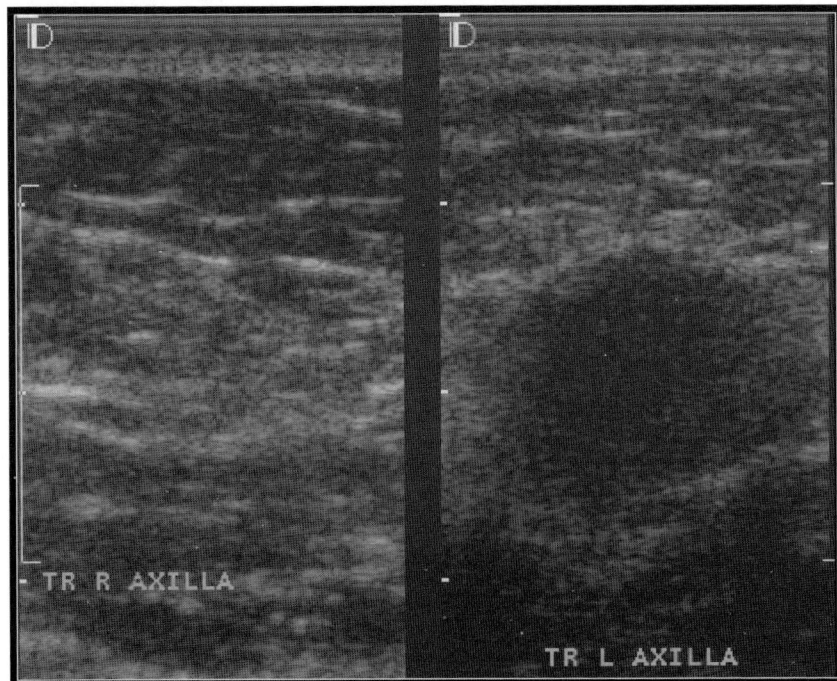

FIGURE 18–48 This patient presented with ipsilateral arm swelling months after lumpectomy and axillary dissection. Sonography showed a large hypoechoic mass that at biopsy proved to be extensive fat necrosis with no evidence of tumor.

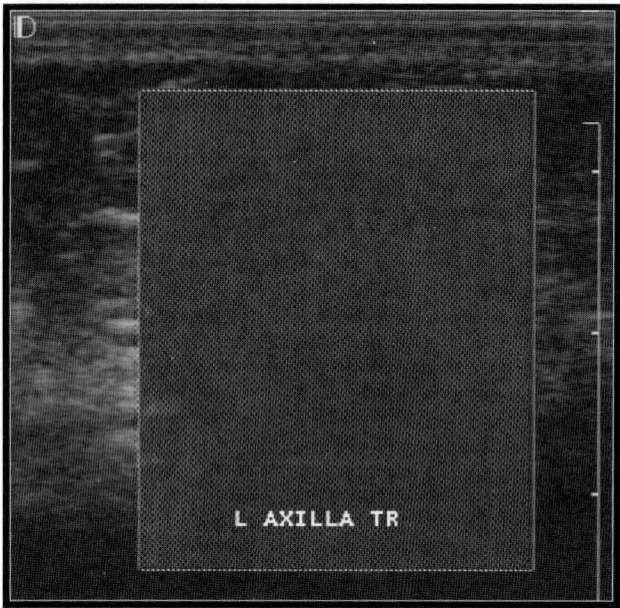

FIGURE 18–49 Power Doppler showed no blood flow within the axillary mass shown in the previous figure, a finding more compatible with fat necrosis than with recurrent tumor within the axilla.

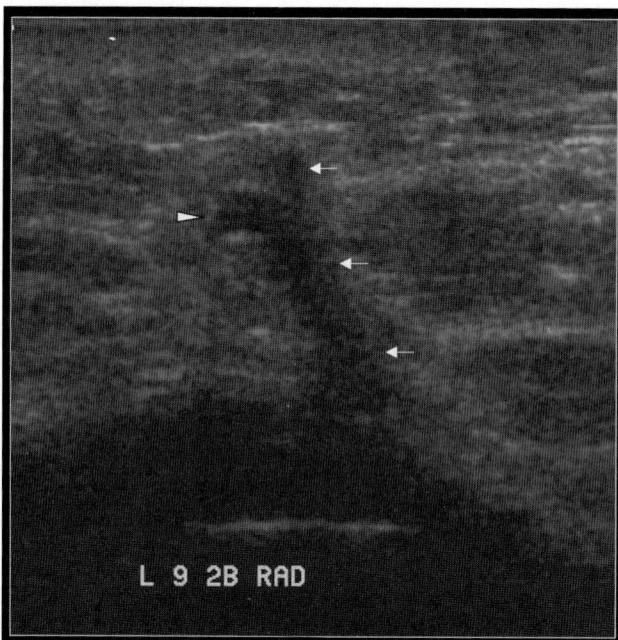

FIGURE 18–50 This local recurrence *(arrowhead)* occurred in the walls of the lumpectomy cavity *(arrows)*, a common site for recurrence.

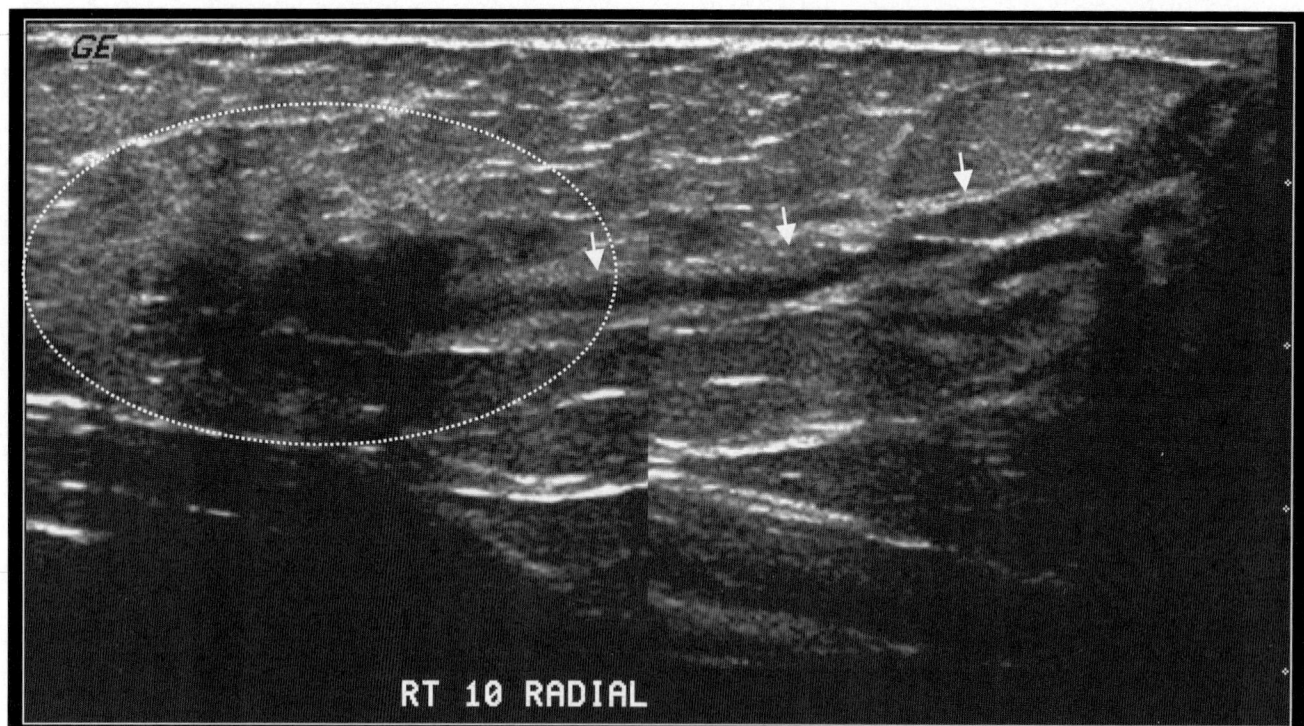

FIGURE 18–51 Local recurrences more commonly arise from central than peripheral ducts because there is very little resistance to intraductal growth within the lobar ducts, and central duct extensions can be several centimeters long *(arrows)*. Unless these are imaged and mapped with biopsies, such long duct extensions will likely be transected at surgery, leading to positive margins. If the surgeon does not know preoperatively that such extensive intraductal components are present, his wide excision *(dotted oval* indicates 1-cm margins) will likely transect the ductal carcinoma *in situ* in the lobar duct. There is about a 10% to 15% chance that the positive margin will be missed by both the surgeon and the pathologist, leading to an eventual "local recurrence."

Most local recurrences after breast-conserving surgery occur in and around the lumpectomy site (Fig. 18–50). Recurrences tend to occur in the lobar ductal system in which the lesion arises, Cooper's ligaments, skin, and chest wall. Recurrences arising with the ductal system most commonly involve the large central ducts and are the result of previously undetected and unresected extensive DCIS components of the lesion (Figs. 18–51 and 18–52). Recurrences in Cooper's ligaments are usually the result of unresected microscopic foci of invasive tumor (Fig. 18–53). Remember that angular margins are most commonly seen at points where Cooper's ligaments intersect the surface of the malignant nodule because the anterior mammary fascia is absent there, creating a path of low resistance to invasion (Fig. 18–54). Skin recurrences usually arrive there through invasion of Cooper's ligaments (Figs. 18–55 and 18–56) or through invaded lymphatic channels that tend to drain superficially from the malignant nodule to the skin and then to the periareolar network of lymphatics (Fig. 18–57). An eccentrically located, ill-defined, thick, echogenic halo that lies between the main body of the lesion and the skin that represents peritumoral edema resulting from lymphatic invasion suggests an increased risk for lymphatic spread to the skin (Fig. 18–58). Chest wall invasion can result from direct invasion or from invaded lymphatic channels along the deep surface of lesions that tend to drain medially to the internal mammary lymph nodes (Fig. 18–59). The chest wall can also be involved through perinodal invasion from internal mammary lymph nodes (Fig. 18–60) or from Rotter's lymph nodes that are located between the pectoralis major and pectoralis minor muscles. Additionally, axillary recurrences are also relatively common, usually within lymph nodes, but occasionally within the fat in patients who had evidence of perinodal invasion at the time of axillary dissection. Axillary lymph node recurrences are more common in patients who had positive nodes at the time of axillary dissection (Fig. 18–61) but also can occur in a small percentage of low-grade invasive malignancies (such as tubular carcinoma) and in high-nuclear-grade DCIS with undiagnosed microscopic invasion. Axillary lymph node recurrences also occur in a small percentage of patients who had negative sentinel lymph node procedures (Fig. 18–62).

Detection of residual tumor in the walls of the lumpectomy cavity can be complicated by chronic hematoma, scar tissue, and fat necrosis within the site that resembles recurrent tumor sonographically. Doppler can be helpful after 6 months because scar tissue and fat necrosis are usually avascular after that time. However, in our experience, contrast-enhanced MRI with a high-spatial-resolution fat-suppression sequences such as RODEO better distinguishes recurrent or residual tumor from granulation tissue, scar, and fat necrosis. Even within the first 6 months after lumpectomy, when the granulation tissue in the walls of the cavity shows some contrast enhancement on MRI,

(text continued on page 813)

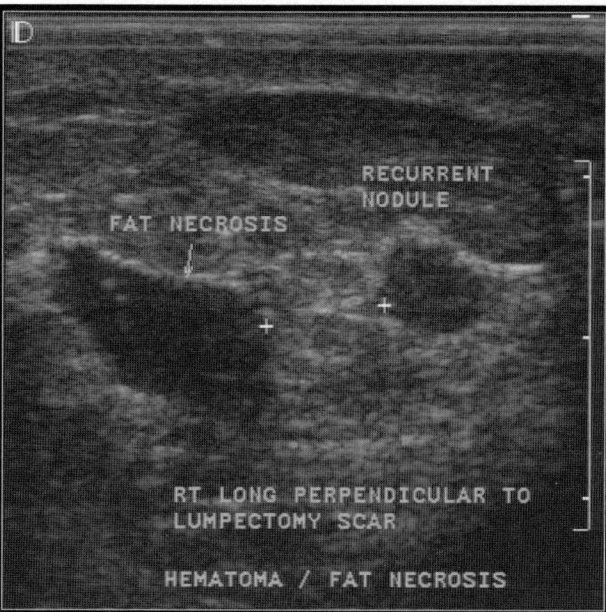
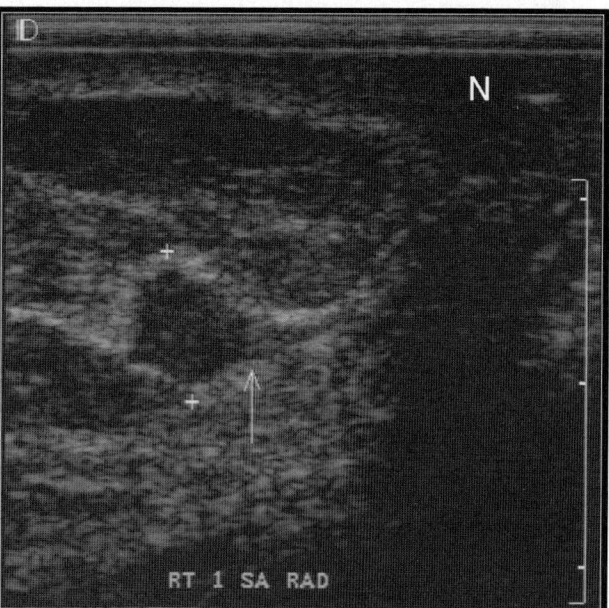

A · B

FIGURE 18–52 A: In this patient with ipsilateral arm and breast swelling 18 months after lumpectomy, a recurrent tumor nodule can be seen between the lumpectomy cavity *(arrow labeled fat necrosis)* and the nipple. This patient also had a sonographically abnormal axillary lymph node (shown in Fig. 18–47). **B:** This radial view of the recurrent tumor nodule shows a duct extension *(arrow)* toward the nipple *(N)*, suggesting that the recurrence has arisen from unresected extensive intraductal components that lie within the central lobar ducts.

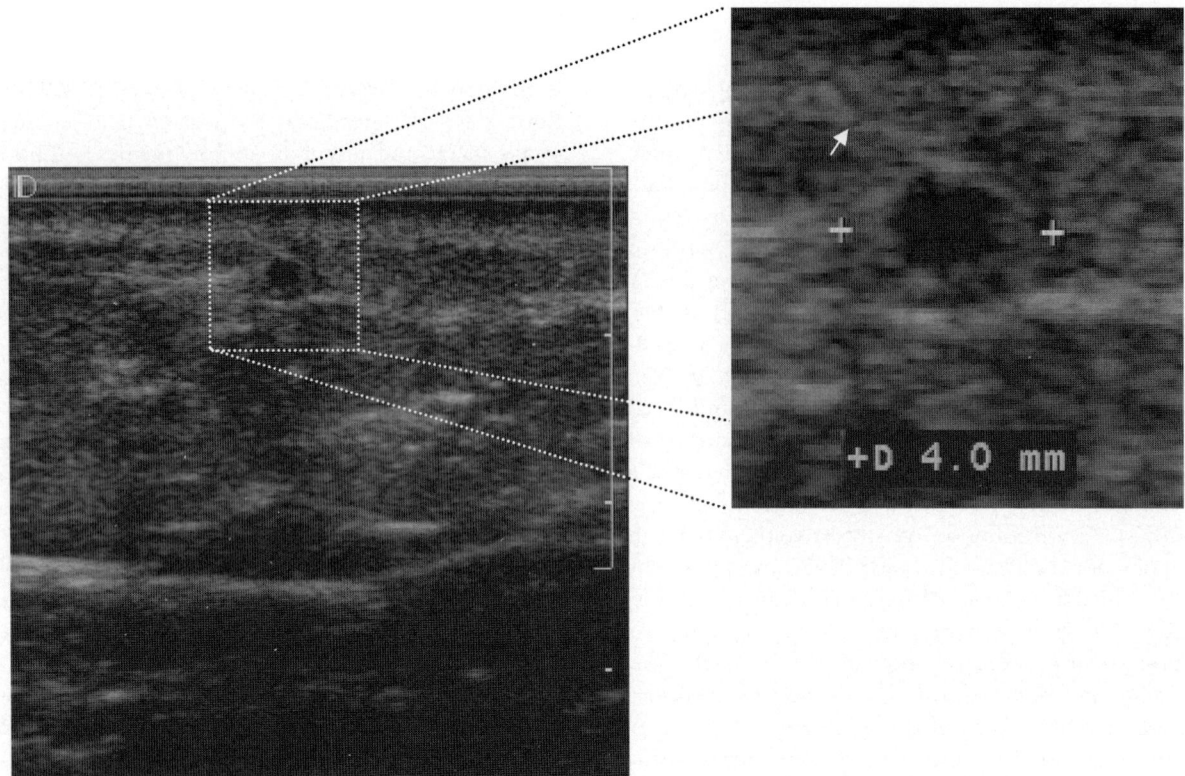

FIGURE 18–53 Another common site for local recurrences is within Cooper's ligaments *(arrow)*, which represent a path of low resistance for invasive carcinoma. Cooper's ligaments are also one of the routes that invasive carcinoma uses to gain access to the skin.

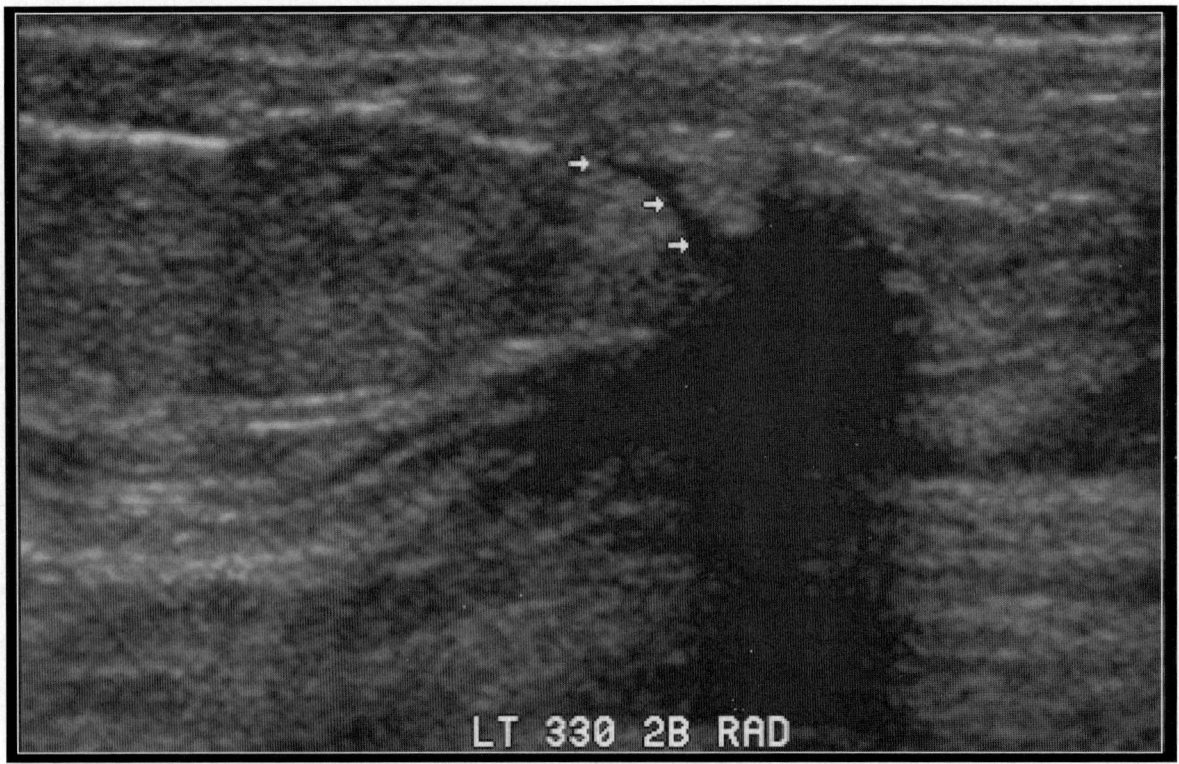

FIGURE 18–54 The points at which Cooper's ligaments intersect the surface of tumors are points of low resistance to invasion because the relatively thick and tough anterior mammary fascia is absent at the bases of the ligaments. It is at these points that cancer enters the ligaments and grows toward the skin. Subclinical growths of invasive tumor are frequently transected within the ligaments *(arrows)* in an attempt to save the overlying skin, accounting for the recurrences in Cooper's ligaments.

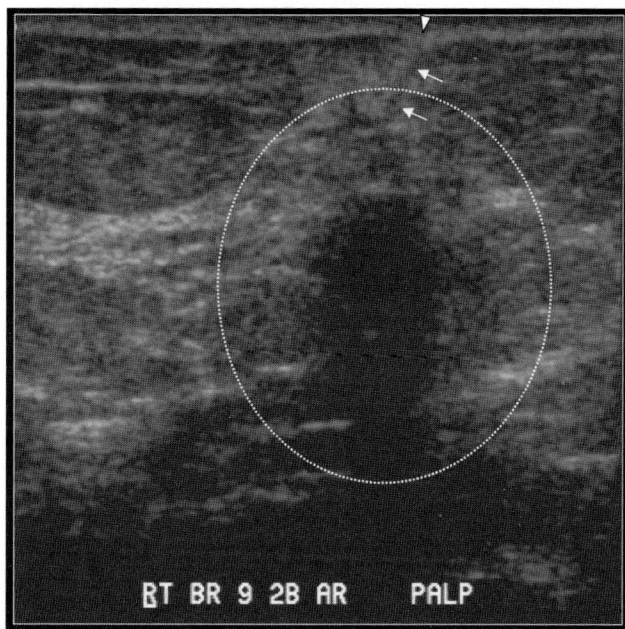

FIGURE 18–55 In this patient, the ligament is widened and edematous but has a subtle band of hypoechogenicity within it that represents invasive carcinoma *(arrows)*. Note the subtle retraction on the undersurface of the skin *(arrowhead)*. A wide excision (1-cm margin, *white dotted oval*) could easily transect the disease within the ligament, leading to an eventual ligamentous local recurrence.

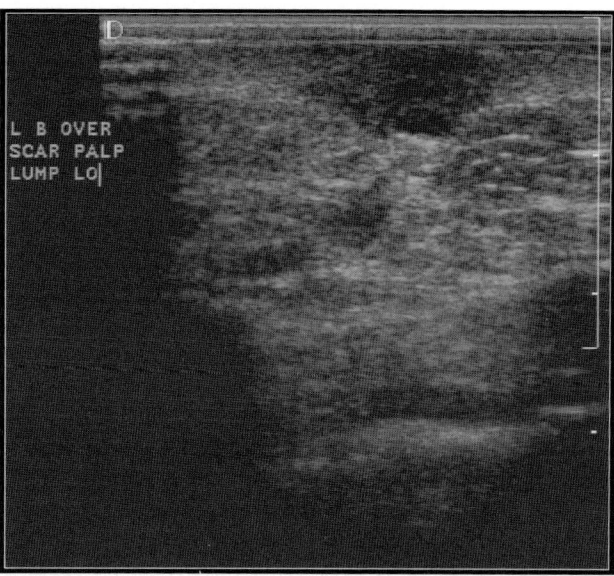

FIGURE 18–57 This local recurrence occurred within the skin. Biopsy revealed tumor within the dermal lymphatics, suggesting that the skin metastasis arrived in the skin by lymphatic invasion rather than growth up Cooper's ligaments.

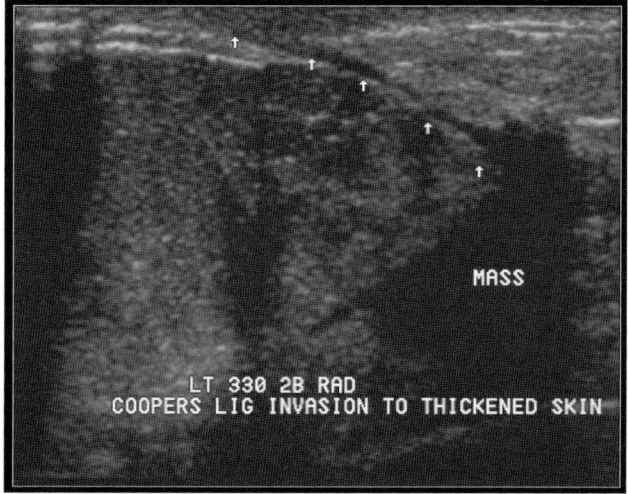

FIGURE 18–56 The involvement of the abnormally thickened skin through Cooper's ligament is larger and more obvious in this patient than in the previous case.

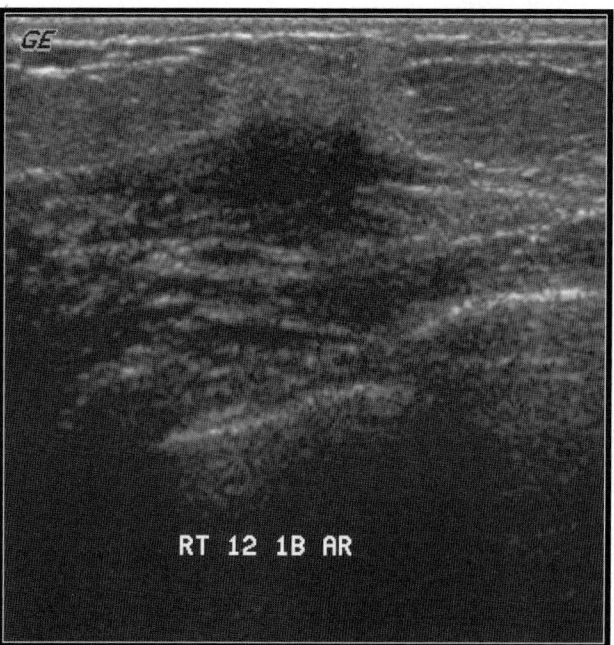

FIGURE 18–58 This intermediate-grade invasive not otherwise specified carcinoma has a fuzzy echogenic halo that lies superficial to it. This pattern of thick halo is typical of lymphedema caused by invasion of lymphatic channels. The superficial location of peritumoral edema is a manifestation of the direction of lymphatic drainage. Lymph drainage from most of the breast is superficially to the dermal net, then to the periareolar region, and finally to the axillary lymph nodes. Obstruction of these superficially draining lymphatics leads to the superficial location of the edema and suggests an increased risk for spread of tumor to the skin through the lymphatics.

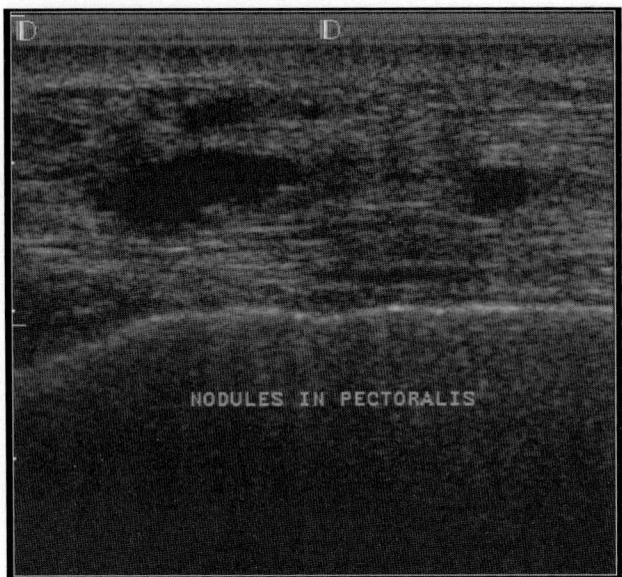

NODULES IN PECTORALIS

FIGURE 18–59 This patient developed multiple local recurrences within the pectoralis muscle. Such recurrences can occur when the muscle is directly invaded or when the malignant nodule is adherent to the muscle but can also occur by lymphatic channel invasion and from Rotter's node, which lies between the pectoralis major and minor muscles.

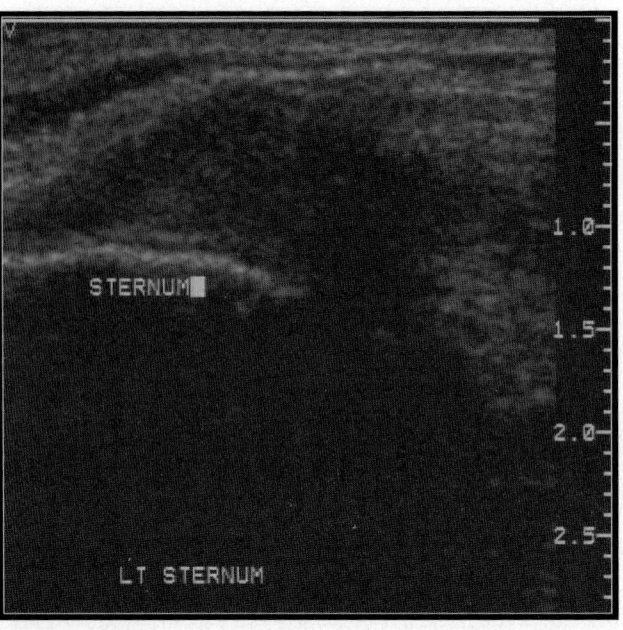

STERNUM

LT STERNUM

FIGURE 18–60 This parasternal chest wall recurrence likely arose from metastatic deposits in the internal mammary chain.

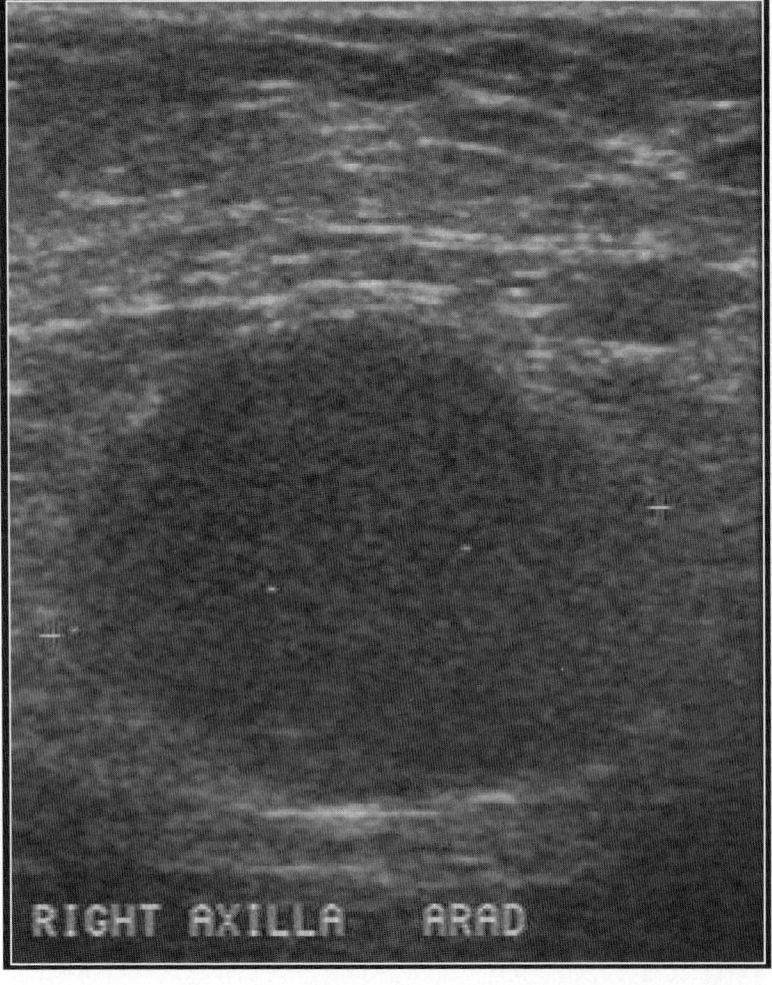

RIGHT AXILLA   ARAD

FIGURE 18–61 This axillary lymph node is grossly enlarged and distorted by recurrent breast cancer. The patient had undergone full axillary dissection and had numerous positive lymph nodes.

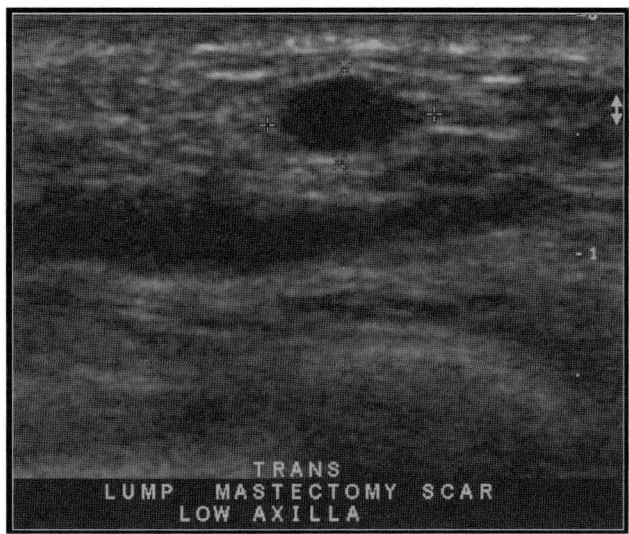

FIGURE 18–62 This mildly abnormal lymph node underwent biopsy that showed metastatic low-grade breast carcinoma in a patient that had a negative sentinel lymph node procedure. This is one of the 5% of cases in which the sentinel node procedure may be falsely negative.

its appearance differs from that of recurrent carcinoma. The thickness of the granulation tissue is usually fairly thin and uniform along the walls of the cavity, whereas the contrast enhancement associated with recurrent tumor is usually less uniform in thickness and frequently nodular in appearance. Sonography may be useful in a second-look role, guiding needle biopsy of nodular areas of enhancement.

Patients with local recurrences can have malignant disease simultaneously in many or all of the high likelihood sites noted earlier (Fig. 18–63).

The following sonographic findings in the index lesion before lumpectomy predict an increased risk for local recurrence:

1. Long duct extensions, extensive branch pattern, and very heavy microlobulation suggest the presence of extensive intraductal components, a known risk factor for local positive margins and local recurrence. The recurrent carcinoma can be DCIS or invasive carcinoma arising from an area of residual DCIS. Findings that suggest the presence of extensive intraductal components are discussed and illustrated in detail in Chapters 12 and 14.

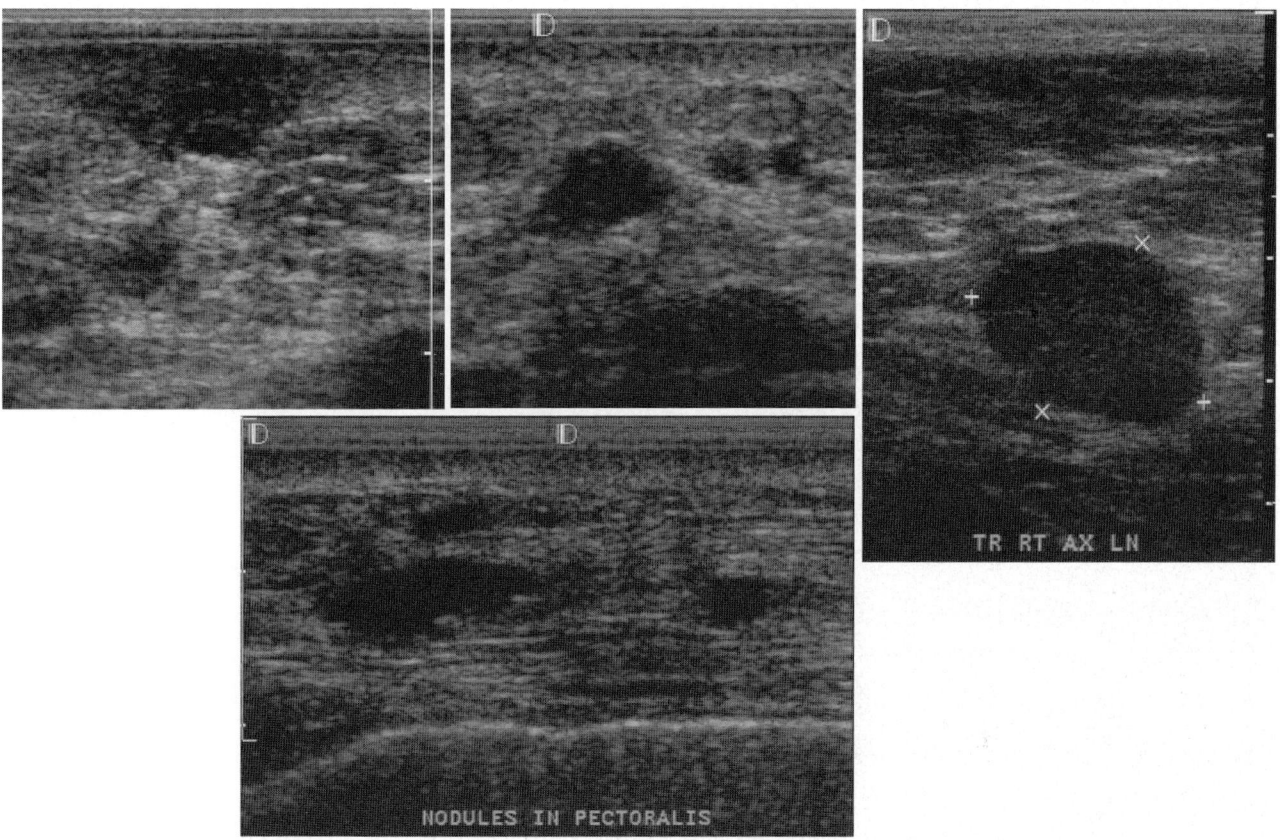

FIGURE 18–63 In certain cases, local recurrences occur in multiple sites. This patient had recurrent tumor in the skin, subcutaneous tissues, chest wall, and lymph nodes.

2. Angular margins that lie on the superficial surface of the nodule usually represent invasion of carcinoma into bases of Cooper's ligaments. Although the angles formed at the bases of the ligament represent macroscopic invasive malignant disease, it is easy to conceive of microscopic components of invasive tumor extending even more superficially into the ligament toward the skin. These microscopic growths of invasive carcinoma within Cooper's ligaments that are neither visible nor palpable might be transected in the process of trying to avoid resecting the skin overlying the malignant nodule. It is also likely that many apparent recurrences within the subcutaneous fat arise from residual disease in Cooper's ligaments.

3. An eccentrically superficially located thick, echogenic halo caused by peritumoral edema predicts an increased risk for skin recurrence by tumor with lymphatic vessels, which drain toward the subdermal net in most patients.

4. Large, deep malignant nodules that are attached to the chest wall predict a higher risk for chest wall recurrence. Even nodules that lie in the deep one-third of the medial breast, but that are not fixed to the chest wall, can lead to chest wall recurrences through lymphatic channel involvement. Such lesions tend to drain to the internal mammary lymph nodes through deep lymphatic vessels that lie near or within the chest wall. Chest wall recurrences can arise from the lymphatic channels or the internal mammary lymph nodes. Pa-tients who have enlarged Rotter's lymph nodes (lying between the pectoralis major and pectoralis minor muscles) have an increased risk for chest wall recurrence.

5. The presence of abnormally enlarged axillary lymph nodes that have angular margins suggests that there is perinodal invasion and indicates and increased risk for axillary recurrence. The presence of four or more grossly enlarged lymph nodes also suggests a higher risk for recurrence. The presence of internal mammary lymphadenopathy also is associated with more aggressive lesions, abnormal pathways of lymphatic flow, and fairly extensive axillary lymphadenopathy in most cases. Because about 5% to 10% of patients have variations in lymphatic flow or multiple sentinel nodes, axillary lymph node metastases may be missed in 5% to 10% of patients. Thus, patients who undergo sentinel node procedures rather than axillary dissections have an increased risk for axillary recurrences. The sonographic appearances of perinodal invasion of lymph node metastases are discussed and illustrated in greater detail in Chapter 19.

The pattern of local recurrences is slightly different for patients who have undergone mastectomy. Most of the subcutaneous tissues and Cooper's ligaments have been removed; thus, recurrences in these structures are fewer. The nipple and all of the ducts have been removed; thus, recurrences should not arise from the ducts. However, recurrences in the skin occur more often and earlier, as do chest

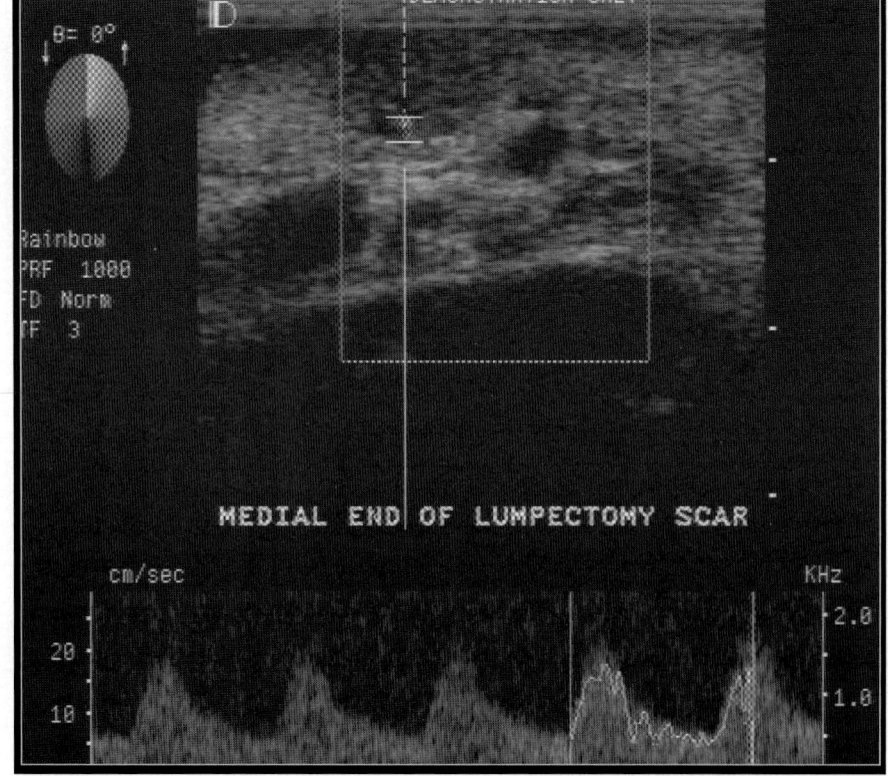

FIGURE 18–64 Pulsed Doppler spectral analysis is useful in confirming that subtle color signals within suspected recurrent nodules are real blood flow signals rather than color artifacts.

wall recurrences. Axillary recurrences are more likely than in lumpectomy simply because the lesions treated with mastectomy are usually larger and at a more advanced stage or of higher grade than the lesions removed by lumpectomy. Such lesions tend to be more aggressive and involve the lymph nodes in a higher percentage of patients.

As noted in the earlier section on the complicated lumpectomy cavity, one of the best ways to distinguish local recurrences from postsurgical complications is color or pulsed Doppler spectral analysis. Recurrent tumor nodules frequently have demonstrable flow on color Doppler, whereas postsurgical complications rarely have demonstrable blood flow (see Chapter 20, Figs. 20–64 and 20–65). Pulsed Doppler spectral analysis is helpful in determining whether color signals represent real arterial feeders or artifacts (Fig. 18–64).

POST–RECONSTRUCTIVE SURGERY ALTERATIONS

There are several different reconstructive procedures for the breast that are performed after cancer surgery in order to make an anatomically abnormal structure appear more nearly normal. This distinguishes them from cosmetic procedures, which are designed to make normal anatomic structures look better.

Although the trend in the past few decades has been toward performing breast-conserving therapy with lumpectomy, lumpectomy with nipple resection, quadrantectomy, and segmentectomy, it is still necessary to perform mastectomy under certain circumstances:

- Some cases of DCIS that are too extensive for mastectomy
- Centrally located breast cancer that involves the nipple–areolar complex
- Invasive carcinomas that are too large for lumpectomy or segmentectomy
- Multicentric carcinoma
- Recurrent carcinoma after lumpectomy
- Patients who are unable or unwilling to undergo postoperative radiation therapy

There are four main types of mastectomies that have been performed over the years: (a) radical mastectomy, (b) modified radical mastectomy, (c) simple mastectomy, and (d) skin-sparing mastectomy. The radical mastectomy involves resection of the pectoralis muscle as well as all breast tissue; all overlying skin, including the nipple; and axillary dissection. Radical mastectomies are seldom performed today. Modified radical mastectomy preserves the pectoralis muscle but removes all breast tissue and overlying skin and includes axillary dissection. A simple mastectomy removes all breast tissue and overlying skin, but does not include axillary dissection. Skin-sparing mastectomy re-

moves all breast tissue, the skin at the cancer site, and the nipple, but preserves the rest of the skin and may or may not include axillary dissection. Thus, radical, modified radical, and simple mastectomies differ in the extent of deep tissue removed, but all involve extensive resection of skin, which makes myocutaneous flaps the only reliable method of reconstruction. Skin-sparing mastectomy, on the other hand, allows for other options, including implants.

Reconstructive surgery can be performed at the time of cancer surgery or can be performed later. The trend in recent years is to perform immediate reconstruction in patients with stages 0, 1, and 2a who will not need postoperative radiation or immediate postoperative chemotherapy. In the past, immediate reconstruction was taboo because of concerns about increasing the risks for and preventing diagnosis of local recurrences. However, recent data show no increase in recurrence rates. Implants that are used to reconstruct breasts will usually be placed subpectorally for a better looking and feeling result and to reduce the risk for capsular contracture after mastectomy from nearly 100% to about 30%. However, implants are seldom used in patients who need postoperative radiation therapy because radiation increases the risks for capsular contracture. The sonographic appearances and complications in permanent implants are discussed in greater detail in Chapter 9. Temporary implants called *expanders* are also used in mastectomy patients. These implants are placed in the wound in a collapsed state. After the incision heals, it is gradually expanded over a matter of weeks with repeated injections of saline to stretch the skin over the lesion enough to accept either larger permanent implants or autologous transplanted tissue. Expanders have appearances similar to implants. Some expanders (Becker expanders) are double lumen; these are unusual in that the silicone gel compartment is outer lumen, whereas the saline compartment is inner lumen. Expanders are subject to the same acute complications as are permanent implants: hematoma, seroma, and infection (Figs. 18–42 and 18–43). However, because they are not permanent, they are not subject to chronic complications. After the skin has been stretched adequately, the expanders are removed, and definitive reconstruction is performed.

The most widely used reconstructions today are autologous myocutaneous flaps—latissimus dorsi flaps and transverse rectus abdominis myocutaneous (TRAM) flaps. The latissimus dorsi flap is more appropriate in size for repair of partial mastectomy defects that include large lumpectomies, lumpectomies with nipple resection, quadrantectomy, and segmentectomy. TRAM flaps are used to reconstruct the breast after complete mastectomy.

There has always been concern that myocutaneous flaps would increase the risk for local recurrence and obscure recurrences. However, recent studies have shown neither of these to occur. It has now been shown that local recurrences rarely occur in the transplanted autologous tissues and that local recurrences that do occur tend to arise within (a) the native breast skin that was spared at the time of mastectomy, (b) the axilla, or (c) the chest wall. Furthermore, distant metastases exist at the time of local recurrences in 75% of cases. We are seldom called on to image myocutaneous flaps for local recurrences because skin recurrences are clinically obvious and the risks for systemic disease are so high that total-body imaging such as PET scanning is usually required. Palpable lumps within the reconstructed breast sometimes require sonographic imaging, but usually represent exuberant scar or fat necrosis (Fig. 18–65). In other cases, sonography may be required to assess abnormal foci on PET scanning or foci of abnormal contrast enhancement seen on MRI.

Color duplex sonography is sometimes called on preoperatively to help the surgeon to decide whether to sacrifice the inferior or superior epigastric artery when performing a TRAM flap reconstruction. The rectus abdominis muscle is supplied by the inferior epigastric artery, a branch of the external iliac artery, and the superior epigastric artery, a continuation of the internal mammary arteries, which arise from the subclavian arteries. To swing the flap free so that it can be implanted into the breast, either the superior or inferior epigastric artery must be sacrificed. The relative contributions of the inferior and superior epigastric arteries to the blood supply of the rectus muscle vary from patient to patient. In some patients, the inferior epigastric artery is dominant; in others, the superior epigastric artery is dominant; in still others, the contributions are nearly equal. The surgeon desires to sacrifice the artery that contributes the least blood flow to the myocutaneous flap in order to ensure the best blood supply, improve the chances of success, and minimize complications. These arteries are easy to see on the B-mode image and color Doppler. Sizes and blood flow velocities and resistivity indices can be measured, and volume flows can be estimated, helping the surgeon to make his decision. Perforator branches of the superior and inferior epigastric arteries also supply the skin and subcutaneous tissues over the anterior abdominal wall. Color duplex sonography can be used to "map" these perforators so that the surgeon does not transect them while performing the flap and so that enough perforators are included in the flap to minimize the risk for extensive fat necrosis.

Proline mesh is usually implanted in the anterior abdominal wall after the flap is swung superiorly onto the chest wall to minimize the risk for hernia. Sonography may also be used after TRAM flap surgery to assess the anterior abdominal wall for hernia or complications involving the implanted mesh.

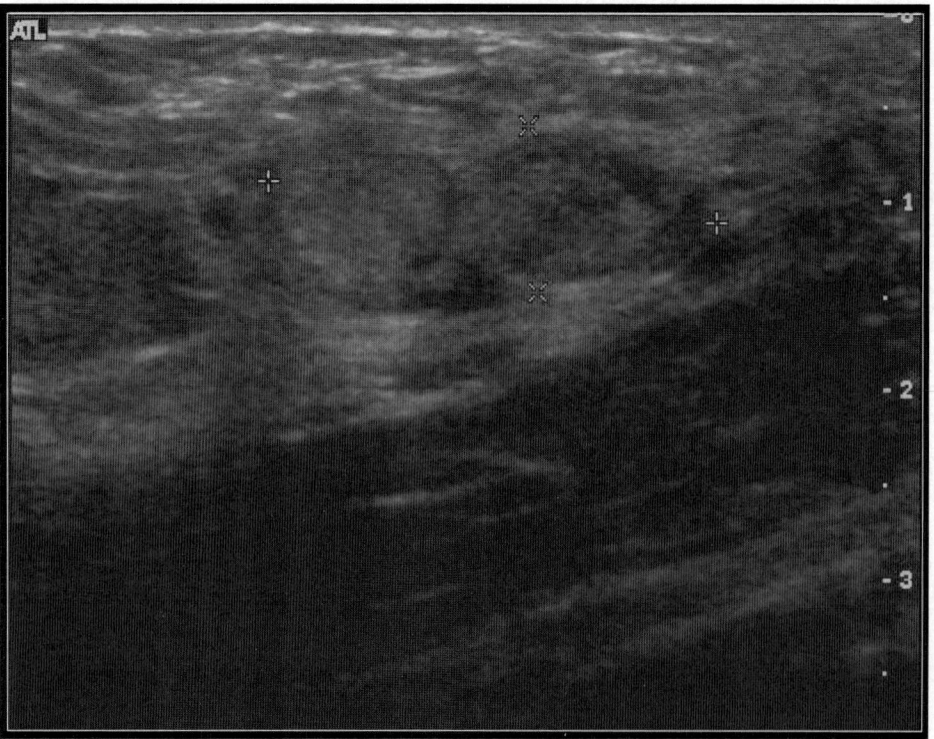

FIGURE 18–65 Tumor recurrences within transverse rectus abdominis myocutaneous (TRAM) flaps are rare. As in this case, most of the palpable lumps within such reconstruction sites represent complications of surgery such as fat necrosis.

POST–AUGMENTATION MAMMOPLASTY ALTERATIONS

The findings of normal and abnormal augmentation mammoplasties are discussed in detail in Chapter 9 and are not discussed at all in this chapter.

POST–REDUCTION MAMMOPLASTY ALTERATIONS

Two types of surgery can be used to reduce breast size and to minimize ptosis: reduction mammoplasty and mastopexy. In reduction mammoplasty, a wedge of tissue is removed from the inferior aspect of the breast. In mastopexy, on the other hand, some skin is removed, and the skin tightened, but no breast tissue is removed. Mastopexy is performed to improve ptosis of the breast. Both reduction mammoplasty and mastopexy are usually performed bilaterally but are occasionally performed unilaterally on the side that is contralateral to a mastectomy and reconstruction in order to make the size of the two breasts more symmetric.

The surgical incision for reduction mammoplasty usually lies parallel to the inframammary fold, has a linear component extending superiorly from the 6:00 position,

and sometimes is associated with a keyhole incision used to move to nipple and areola more superiorly. Reduction mammoplasty reduces the amount of inferiorly located breast parenchyma, shifts the profile of the breast superiorly, and displaces the areola and nipple to a more esthetically pleasing superior position.

The mammographic findings after reduction mammoplasty are similar to those after lumpectomy but frequently are far more extensive. Most reductions are performed to treat macromastia, and in most cases, the markedly enlarged breasts also are extensively fatty. The abnormally large size, extensive fatty content, and attenuated blood supply make such breasts particular prone to vascular compromise, especially after surgery. Thus, the most extensive and severe cases of fat necrosis that we see tend to occur in patients who have undergone reduction mammoplasty.

The mammographic and sonographic findings in patients who have undergone reduction mammoplasty are nonspecific manifestations of extensive scarring and fat necrosis. These findings are similar to those seen in patients after lumpectomy but are more extensive and widespread. Mammographically, the findings include architectural distortions that are usually most severe inferior to the nipple, where the largest volumes of tissue have been removed. Lipid cysts and eggshell calcifications are frequently extensive (Fig. 18–66).

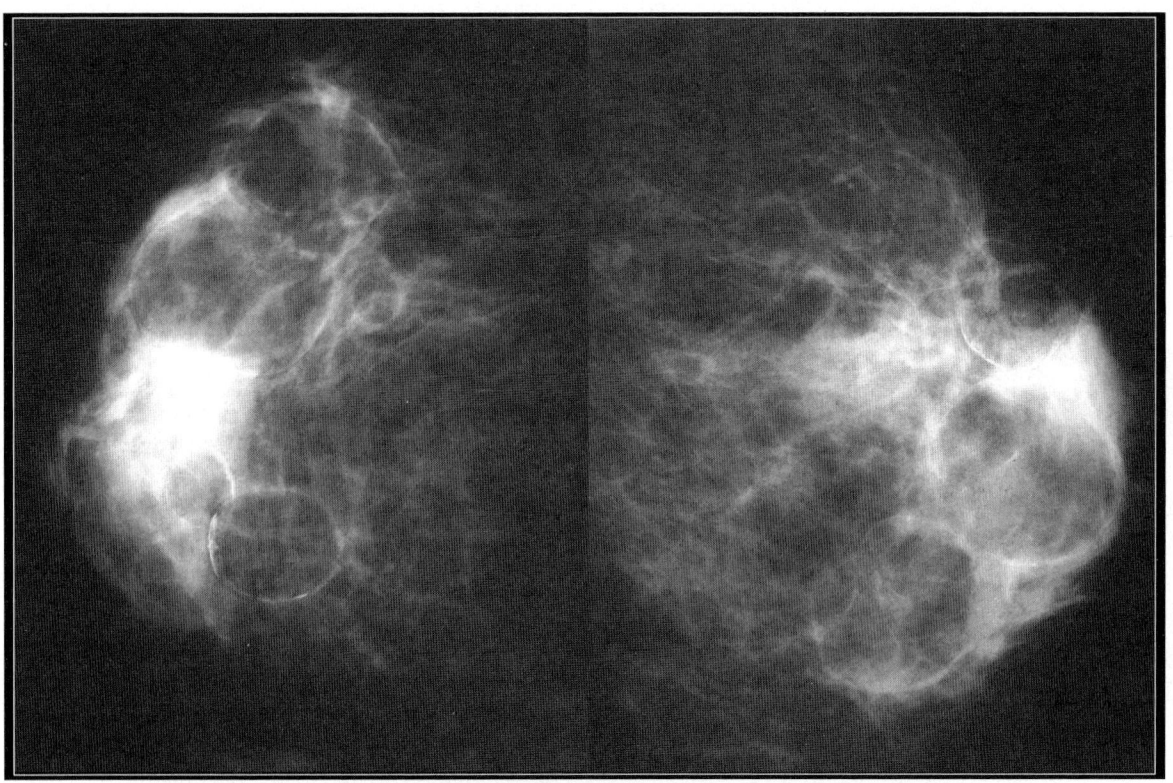

FIGURE 18–66 Bilateral postreduction mammoplasty craniocaudal views show extensive fat necrosis bilaterally manifested by multiple benign lipid cysts, some of which are beginning to develop calcifications within their walls. The most extensive and severe changes of fat necrosis that we see are invariably in patients who have undergone reduction mammoplasty.

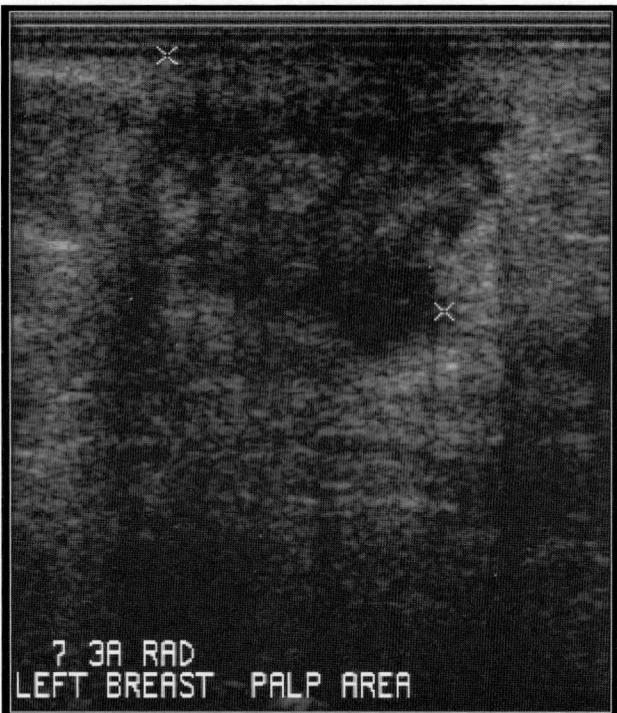

FIGURE 18–67 The contents of this lipid cyst make it appear to be solid and suspicious sonographically. Mammography showed this to be a classic lipid cyst (BIRADS 2).

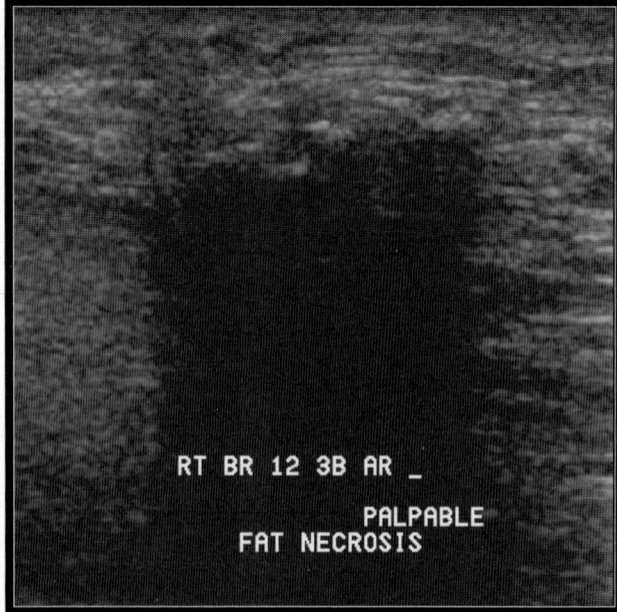

FIGURE 18–68 This mammographically benign calcified lipid cyst demonstrated suspicious findings of acoustic shadowing and angular margins on sonography.

Spiculated masses occur in some cases; in most cases, however, less specific findings of architectural distortion occur. These architectural distortions often appear linear in only one plane on spot compression views. In fact, the presence of numerous, widely scattered, large, noncalcified lipid cysts occurs only in patients who have undergone reduction mammoplasty.

The sonographic findings in postmastectomy patients often appear to be considerably more suspicious than the associated mammographic findings. The contents of lipid cysts often appear echogenic sonographically, making them appear falsely solid (Fig. 18–67). Calcified lipid cysts that appear definitively benign on the mammograms may have the appearance of suspicious shadowing masses sonographically (Fig. 18–68). Other lipid cysts can appear to be complex sonographically, containing falsely suspicious features such as mural nodules, thick and isoechoic septations, or irregularly thickened isoechoic walls (Fig. 18–37). Thus, in our experience, sonography tends to overestimate the BI-RADS categories of many findings in post–reduction mammoplasty patients. Although sonography is generally superior to mammography for characterizing most breast lesions, the opposite is true in this group of patients. Suspicious sonographic findings in patients who have undergone reduction mammoplasty should be carefully correlated with spot compression mammograms before recommending biopsy. Findings of fat necrosis are discussed in Chapter 11 and earlier in this chapter.

RADIATION THERAPY–INDUCED ALTERATIONS

Sonography is used in two different roles in patients who have undergone or will undergo radiation therapy: (a) to help localize the lumpectomy cavity for external radiation therapy booster doses or to guide brachytherapy before treatment, or (b) to assess the postirradiation breast.

Pretreatment Assessment

Localizing the Lumpectomy Cavity for Radiation Therapy Booster Doses

Radiation therapy after breast cancer surgery is used to reduce the risk for local recurrence, especially in patients at high risk for recurrences, such as those with positive margins at surgery, extensive intraductal components, or skin, nipple, or chest wall attachment. Complications from radiation limit the dose that can be delivered to the whole breast, chest wall, and axilla, but higher radiation booster doses can be delivered to small areas of the breast that are at especially high risk for local recurrence if highly critical structures such as the pericardium can be avoided. Most recurrences occur in the walls of the lumpectomy cavity and the immediately surrounding tissues. Thus, it makes sense to deliver higher radiation doses to the cavity and surrounding tissues if possible. Some have used the skin incision to target external booster doses, but the skin is often a poor guide to the actual site of the lumpectomy cavity deeper within the breast. Desire to make the skin incision periareolar or within the tension lines of the breast and the finding of more extensive tumor than expected often result in the surgeon "tunneling obliquely" under the skin to the site of the lesion. Thus, lumpectomy scars and cavities are often obliquely oriented with respect to the skin, and the deeper portions of the lumpectomy cavity can lie several centimeters away from the skin incision (Fig. 18–69).

Visual inspection of the skin incisional scar cannot determine the orientation of the lumpectomy cavity, but sonography can. The ultrasound machine can be rolled into the radiation therapy suite, and the patient can be scanned on the radiation therapy table in the same position that she will be in for therapy. The transducer angulation necessary to include the skin scar, subcutaneous incision, and entire lumpectomy cavity can be determined. The transducer can then be placed inside the booster cone, allowing both the transducer and cone to be appropriately placed and oriented. Once the cone position and orientation are determined, the transducer is removed, the radiation therapy cone is attached to the machine, and its position and angle are recorded for the remainder of booster treatments.

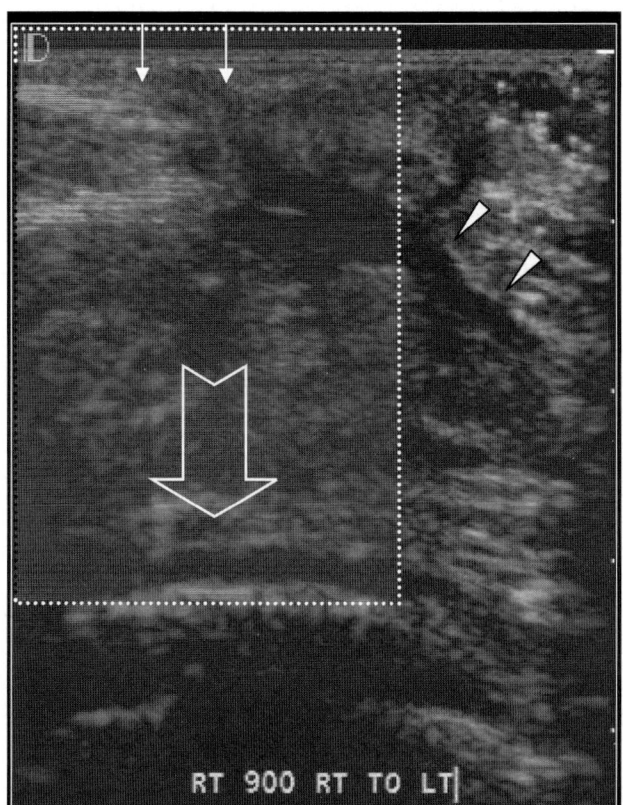

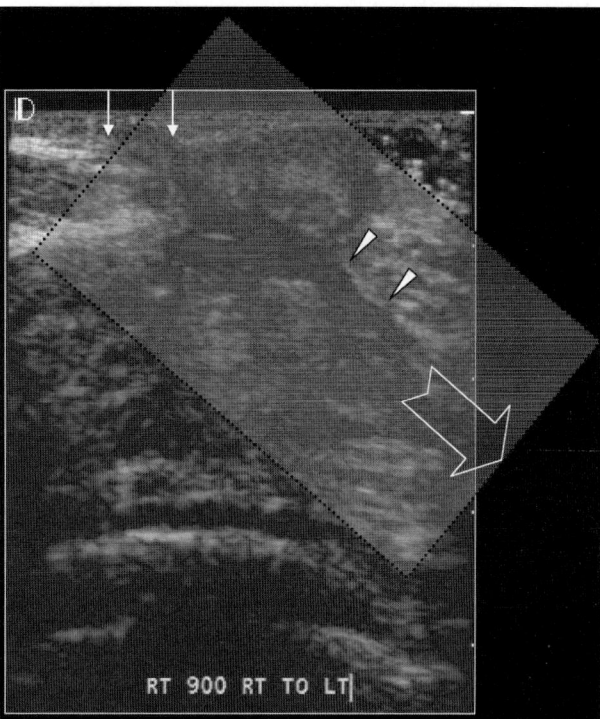

A   B

FIGURE 18–69 A: External booster doses of radiation that are centered on the skin scar and delivered in a straight anteroposterior direction might fail to deliver radiation to the area of the breast where local recurrence is most likely—the walls of the lumpectomy cavity—because lumpectomy cavities do not necessarily extend straight posteriorly from the skin into the breast. The *arrow* marks the visible skin scar. The *semitransparent shaded rectangle* represents the beam of therapeutic radiation delivered from a straight anterior approach and centered on the skin scar. Note that some of the lumpectomy cavity has been excluded from the booster dose beam *(arrowheads)*. This represents a potentially undertreated area in which local recurrence is more likely. **B:** Using ultrasound guidance in the radiation therapy suite, the booster beam can be centered on and oriented parallel to the axis of the obliquely oriented lumpectomy cavity, correctly delivering the booster dose to the walls of the lumpectomy cavity rather than the breast tissue deep to the skin scar.

Guiding Administration of Brachytherapy

Because most local recurrences occur in and in the immediate vicinity of the lumpectomy site, an alternative approach to external whole breast irradiation is to deliver a higher dose of radiation only to the localized area that is at high risk for recurrence with brachytherapy, sparing the rest of the breast, chest wall, and axilla from radiation. This minimizes complications and maximizes the chances of local control. It also has the advantage of requiring only a few days rather than the 5 weeks or longer for external radiation treatments and is a more suitable form of radiation therapy for patients referred from rural areas, other cities, or foreign countries who want to be at home and in familiar surroundings as soon as possible. It also is less expensive than external-beam therapy.

One approach is to use ultrasound before therapy to localize the lumpectomy cavity. Iodinated contrast can then be injected into the cavity under ultrasound guidance. Once the cavity is outline by contrast, it can be localized stereotactically as well as sonographically. Hollow catheters can be placed under stereotactic guidance through a compression plate that contains a grid of regularly spaced holes to allow for even spacing of catheters and uniform radiation dose delivery.

Most recently, a new and much simplified approach to brachytherapy has been developed. A catheter with a collapsed inflatable balloon can be placed in the lumpectomy cavity at the completion of lumpectomy. The balloon can then be filled with liquid radioactive material and left inflated long enough to deliver the desired dose to the cavity walls and surrounding tissues, and then deflated and removed at the completion of treatment. No imaging localization is required. This approach is so rational, efficient, and inexpensive compared with other methods that it is likely to replace other forms of brachytherapy and possibly many uses of external-beam radiation.

Post–Radiation Therapy Alterations

Post-operative radiation therapy is used primarily to prevent local recurrence in patients with stage I or II breast carcinoma. However, radiation and chemotherapy can be used together as the primary treatment in stage III breast carcinomas that are considered inoperable.

The histopathologic findings of radiation changes progress through phases. Early on, there is edema and mastitis. The edema and mastitis resolve over a matter of months in most patients but can progress to fibrosis in others. Chronic radiation changes include lobular atrophy and fibrosis. The TDLUs lose epithelial cells but maintain myoepithelial cells. With atrophy, the thickness of the fibroglandular elements of the breast regresses more rapidly than it normally would over time. The radiation also causes a chronic vasculitis that can lead to small vessel occlusion and is responsible for delayed complications such as tissue and osteonecrosis and skin ulceration.

The imaging findings of acute or early radiation-induced changes are dominated by edema. The mammogram may show only thickening of the skin, enlargement of the breast, and hazy increased density, mammographic findings typical of edema and mastitis of any cause (Fig.

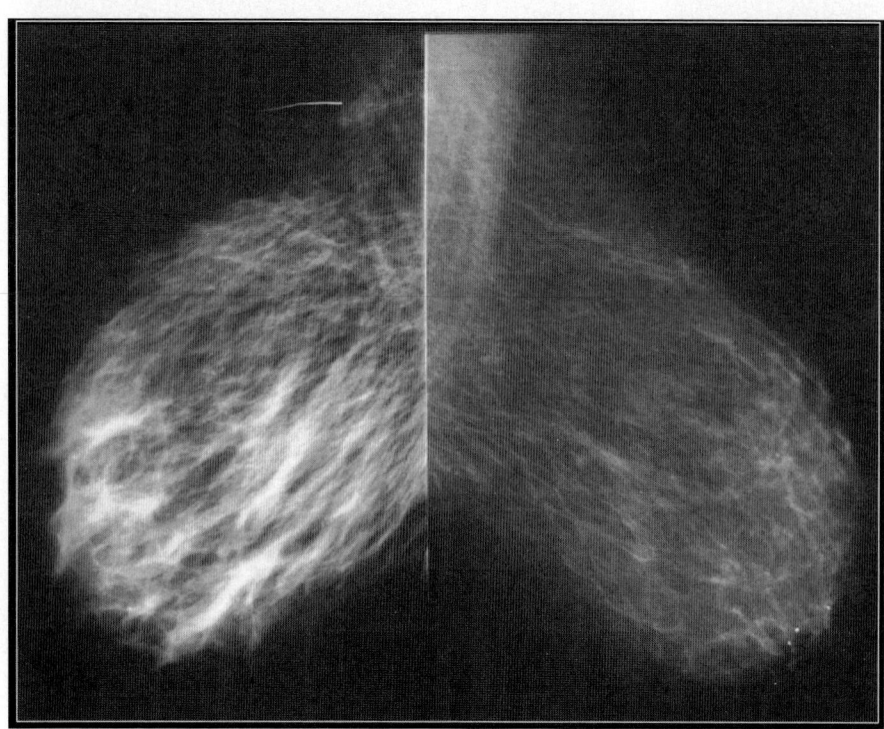

FIGURE 18–70 Acute radiation mastitis causes generalized edema (**left**) that is indistinguishable from edema of other causes. The unirradiated left breast (**right image**) is normal.

18–70). Sonographically, the edema caused by acute radiation mastitis is indistinguishable from the edema caused by mastitis, trauma, lymphatic obstruction, and inflammatory carcinoma. Radiation causes alterations in the sonographic appearance of the skin, which becomes thicker and less echogenic than normal. Normal breast skin is 2 mm or less in thickness, but acute radiation alterations may increase the thickness to well over 3 mm. The fat and loose stromal tissue that surrounds ducts and lies within lobules becomes hyperechoic. Cooper's ligaments and interlobular stromal fibrous tissues, on the other hand, become less thickened and less echogenic than normal. The combination of increasing echogenicity in fat and loose stromal tissues and decreasing echogenicity in the normally hyperechoic interlobular stromal fibrous tissue and Cooper's ligaments makes it more difficult to distinguish them from each other. These changes are all far more evident when compared with the mirror-image contralateral location on split-screen images (Figs. 18–71 and 18.72). When edema is very severe, the relative echogenicities of Cooper's ligaments and fat may reverse because of accumulation of edema with Cooper's ligaments (Fig. 18–73). In certain cases, effusions may form along Cooper's ligaments, owing to surface tension (Fig. 18–74). In cases in which radiation changes are most severe, anatomic distinction between tissues may become nearly completely obscured, and the breast becomes featureless (Fig. 18–75). The breast also becomes thicker, and the combination of thicker breast tissue and edema can prevent adequate penetration with the high-frequency (7.5 to 12 MHz) transducers that we normally use for breast ultrasound. In such cases, it may be necessary to use a 5-MHz linear transducer.

The degree of acute radiation edema varies greatly from patient to patient. In some patients, it is quite severe, whereas in others, there may be virtually no radiation edema. It can also vary from one part of the breast to another, especially in cases in which targeted booster doses are given or in which brachytherapy has been used (Fig. 18–73). In the past, uneven distribution of radiation dosage may have been responsible for some variations in the distribution and severity of edema, but with modern techniques and computer modeling, this is less of a problem than it used to be.

The sonographic signs of radiation edema begin to regress after about 6 months and are nearly gone by 12 to 18 months in some patients (Fig. 18–76). In others, the edema can progress to fibrosis. Interruption of normal lymphatic drainage by axillary dissection likely contributes to the slower resolution or persistence of edema in certain cases. Chronic edema usually causes milder changes in the appearance of the breast than does the acute phase of radiation mastitis. In patients with chronic radiation-induced edema, the fat remains mildly hyperechoic, and the skin remains mildly thickened. Ducts and lobules appear less well defined than before radiation. Slight persistent hyperechogenicity of loose stromal tissues and radiation-induced atrophy decrease their conspicuity. Although it has been reported that all sonographic evidence of altered echogenicity resolves spontaneously in most patients, we have not found this to be true. In fact, in our experience, slight alterations of echogenicity due to edema or fibrosis persist in most patients. However, this cannot be easily appreciated when only the irradiated side is evaluated.

(text continued on page 824)

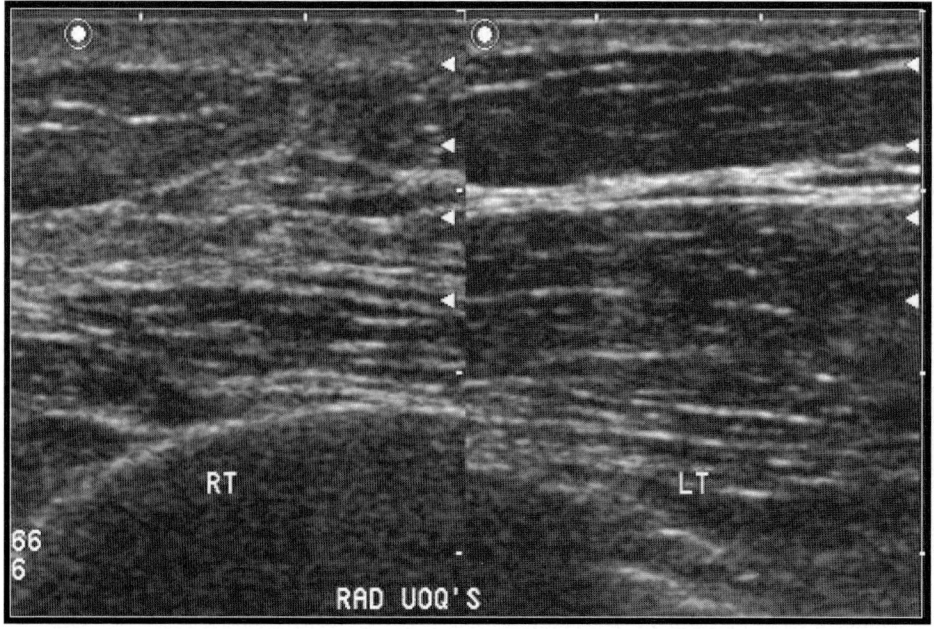

FIGURE 18–71 Moderate postirradiation mastitis in the right breast (**left**) causes the skin to be thicker and less echogenic, increases the echogenicity of the subcutaneous fat, and thickens and makes normally hyperechoic fibrous tissue less echogenic. The distinction between fibrous and fatty elements is diminished. These changes are not at all specific for radiation edema and can be seen with edema of any etiology. Split-screen mirror images accentuate the changes. The unirradiated patient's left breast has normal echogenicity for comparison.

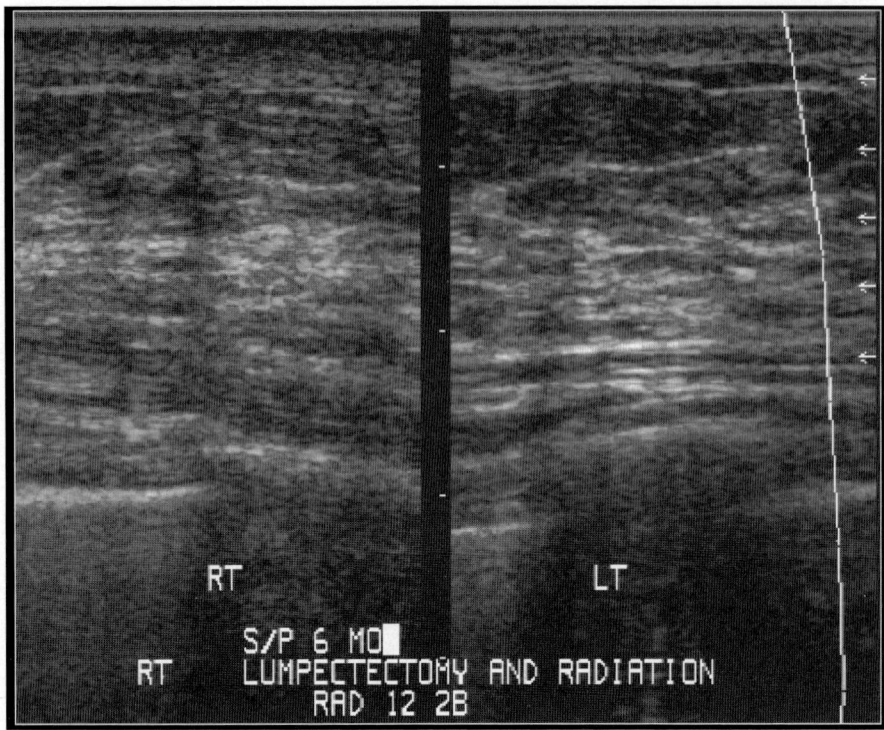

RT   LT

S/P 6 MO
RT   LUMPECTOMY AND RADIATION
RAD 12 2B

FIGURE 18–72 Split-screen mirror images of the irradiated right breast (**left image**) and nonirradiated left breast (**right image**). The normally isoechoic loose stromal tissue that surrounds ducts and lies within terminal ductolobular units that makes them visible within a background of hyperechoic interlobular stromal fibrous tissue becomes more echogenic. This decreases the contrast between ducts and lobules and surrounding fibrous tissue, making the ducts and lobules more difficult to demonstrate (right breast, **left**).

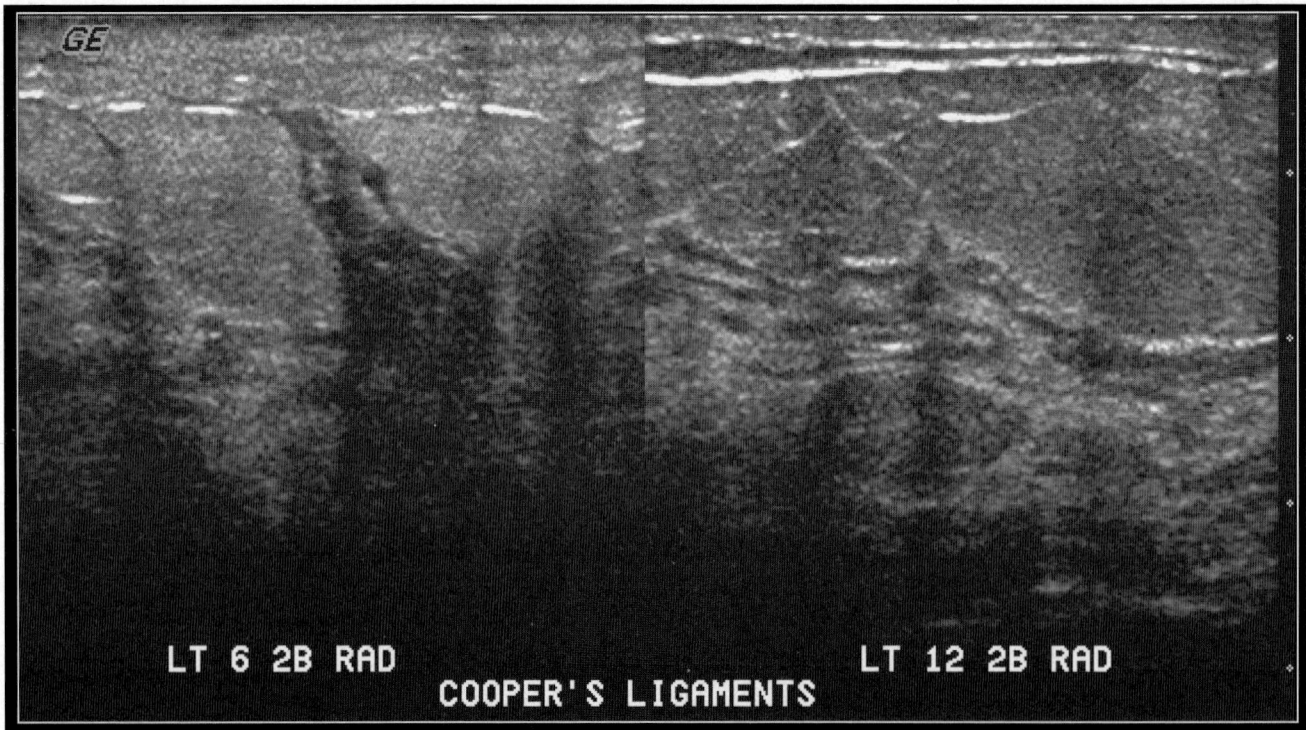

LT 6 2B RAD   LT 12 2B RAD
COOPER'S LIGAMENTS

FIGURE 18–73 When radiation edema is very severe, fluid may begin to accumulate within Cooper's ligaments, making them less echogenic than the adjacent severely edematous fat (**left**). Note that the edema is localized to the area of the booster dose and that the 12:00 area in the same breast has much less severe edema (**right**).

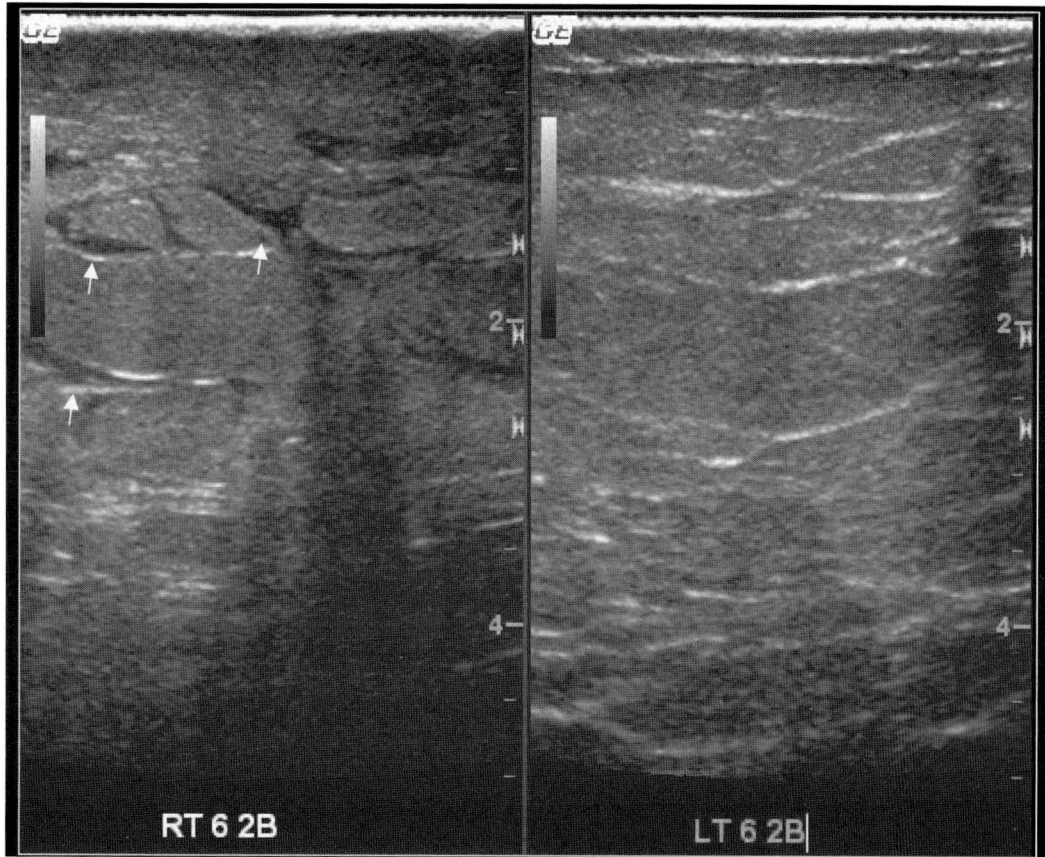

FIGURE 18–74 These split-screen mirror images compare the 6:00 locations of the irradiated right breast and the nonirradiated left breast. In the most severe cases of radiation edema, effusions can form along the surface of Cooper's ligaments (right breast, **left**, *arrows*).

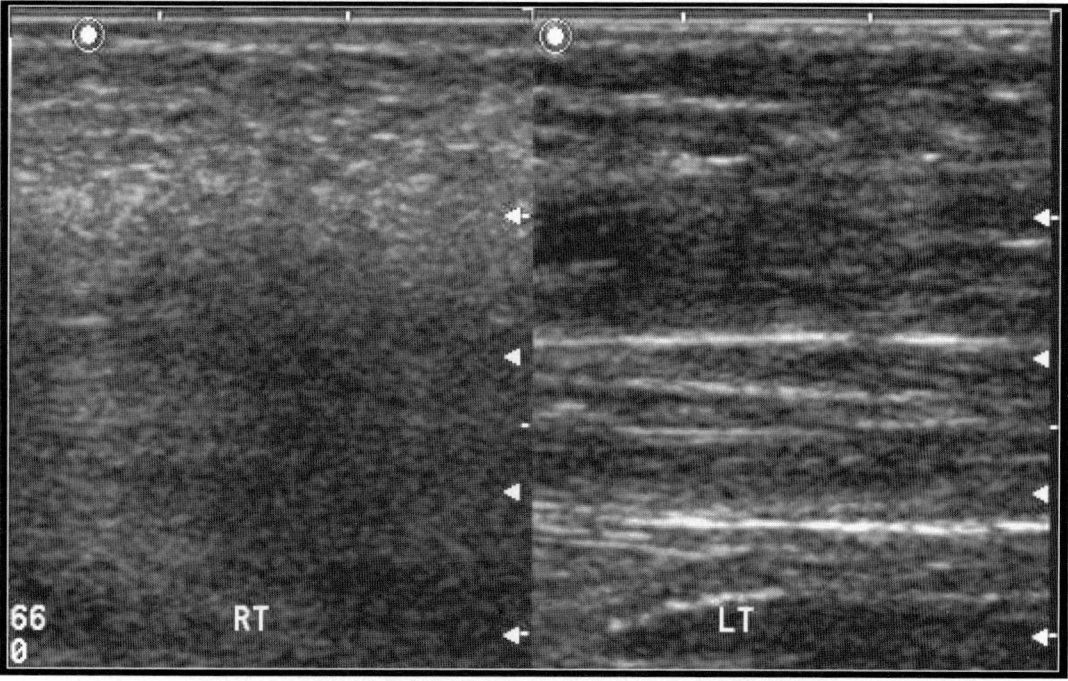

FIGURE 18–75 These split-screen mirror images compare the normal-appearing nonirradiated left breast with the severely edematous irradiated right breast. In severe cases of radiation edema, the distinction between fibrous and fatty elements may be completely lost, and the breast may appear "featureless" (right breast, **left**).

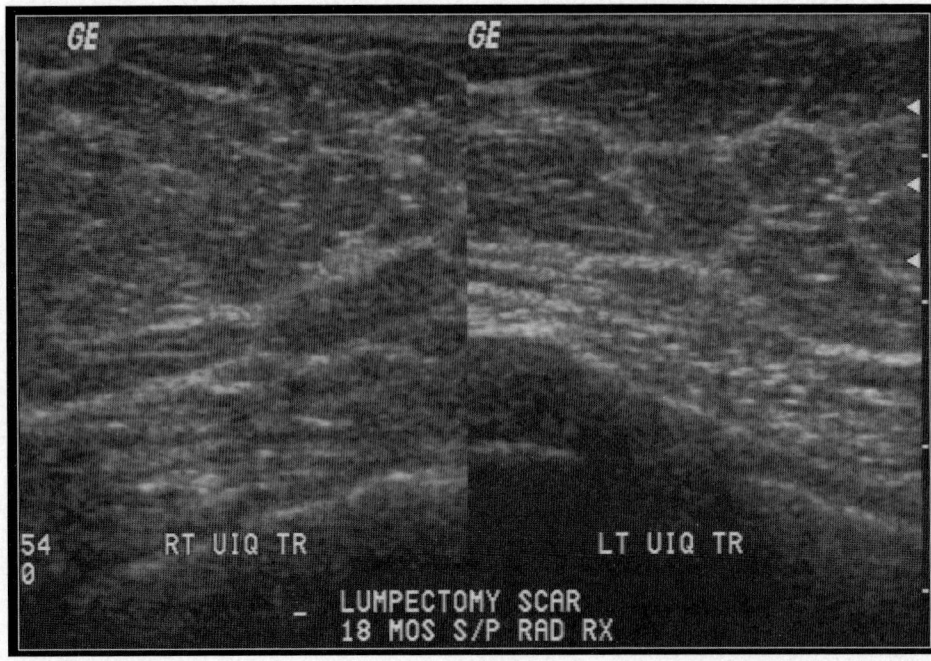

FIGURE 18–76 In some patients, radiation edema will regress nearly completely.

Time–gain curves and total gain settings are usually changed to make the breast tissues appear to have normal echogenicity, obscuring the chronic radiation changes. However, split-screen imaging of mirror-image locations of the irradiated and nonirradiated breast performed without altering scan parameters reveals mild permanent skin thickening and hyperechogenicity of the fat that cannot be appreciated with unilateral scanning (Fig. 18–77). The sonographic findings of radiation fibrosis are indistinguishable from those of mild persistent edema except for breast thickness. Edematous breasts are thickened, whereas fibrotic breasts are usually normal or thinned in comparison with the mirror-image location in the contralateral breast.

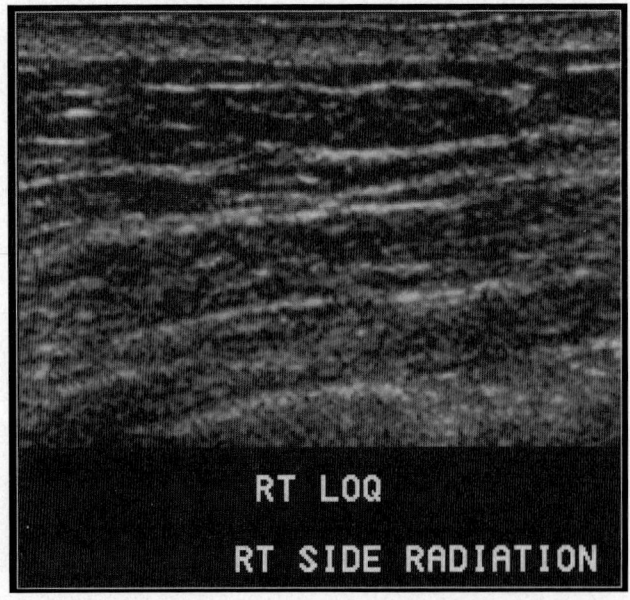

FIGURE 18–77 A: In other cases, the radiation edema or fibrosis will appear to have regressed completely if only the ipsilateral side is scanned. The gain settings have been decreased to make the echogenicity of fat appear normal. (*Continued.*)

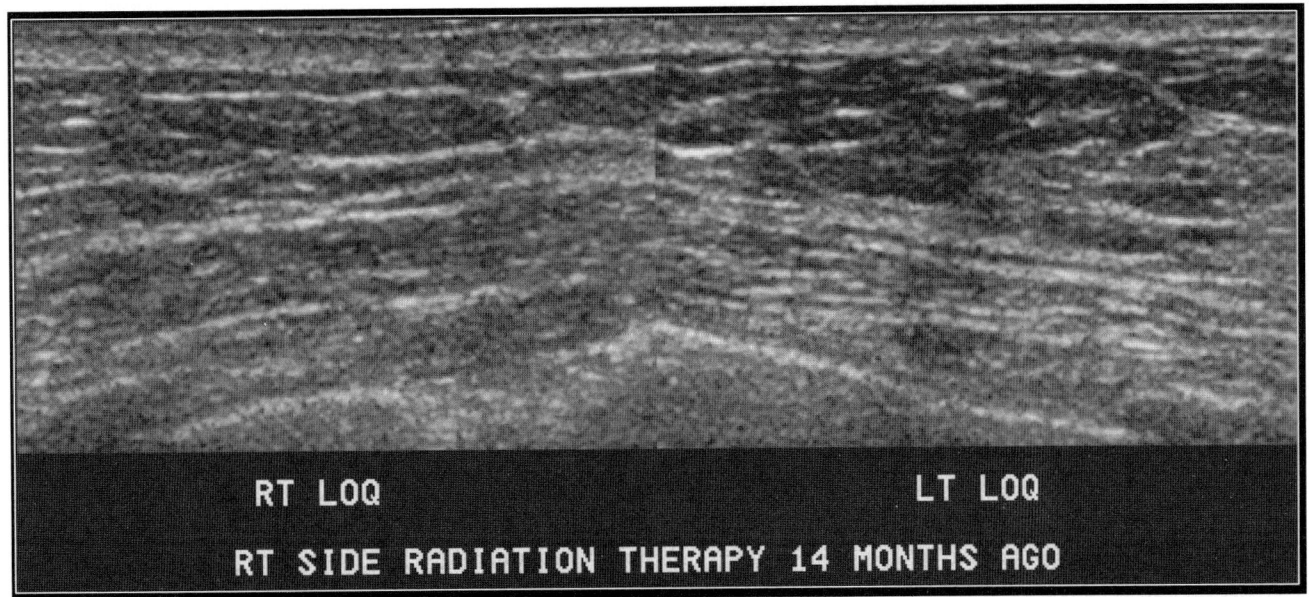

RT LOQ   LT LOQ

RT SIDE RADIATION THERAPY 14 MONTHS AGO

FIGURE 18–77 *(continued)* **B:** The split-screen mirror images compare the echogenicities of the upper outer quadrants in the irradiated right breast with the nonirradiated left breast. When the area shown in the previous image is compared to the mirror-image location in the contralateral breast, subtle persistent skin thickening and hyperechogenicity of fat are evident (right side, **left**).

POSTCHEMOTHERAPY ALTERATIONS

Chemotherapy can be used as an adjuvant to try to decrease the risk for local recurrence and systemic dissemination; it may be used to induce shrinkage of the primary tumor to attempt breast conservation therapy; and in some cases of inoperable carcinoma, it may be used as the primary treatment (usually in conjunction with radiation). Diagnostic imaging can be used to assess the effectiveness of chemotherapy in patients undergoing induction chemotherapy before attempted resection of tumor and in patients undergoing chemotherapy as the primary treatment. Sonography and contrast-enhanced high-spatial-resolution fat-suppression MRI are generally better than mammography for assessing the effect of chemotherapy on tumor size.

Although MRI seems to be more sensitive for certain types of invasive carcinoma and some DCIS components than is sonography, sonography is usually quite good for assessing the size of invasive carcinoma. Additionally, color duplex sonography allows assessment of tumor vascularity, which may regress during chemotherapy even before there is a detectable decrease in tumor size.

The chemotherapy-induced ultrasound image alterations that can occur in a tumor fall into one of four categories:

No Change in Tumor Size on Chemotherapy

A certain percentage of lesions show no response or even grow on chemotherapy (Fig. 18–78). In general, the higher the grade of the lesion, the more sensitive the carcinoma cells are to chemotherapy, but other factors also affect response. One difficulty is that imaging cannot determine whether detectable residual tumor is viable. Sonographically demonstrable residual carcinoma might represent only residual desmoplasia, extracellular matrix, necrosis, and reactive fibrosis, and might contain no living carcinoma cells.

Partial Regression of Tumor Size

Some lesions regress partially, but do not completely resolve. In such cases, it is important to assess the lesion with estimated volume calculations rather than diameters. Measuring diameters tends to underestimate the degree of response. For instance, a spherically shaped invasive NOS carcinoma that decreases from 3.0 to 2.4 cm in diameter has decreased by only 20% in diameter. However, its volume decreases 54%, from 15.6 to 7.2 mL. A good response to chemotherapy is variously defined as either a 50% or a 75% decrease in volume. Thus, in our hypothetical tumor, what appears to be a poor response by diameter measurements is actually a good response by percentage volume reduction (Fig. 18–79).

Most invasive NOS carcinomas contain DCIS components. In our experience, for reasons that are not entirely clear, the invasive parts of mixed lesions have responded better to chemotherapy than have the DCIS components (Fig. 18–80). As is the case for invasive malignant nodules that show no regression in size, the presence of a residual nodule or duct extension does not tell us with certainty

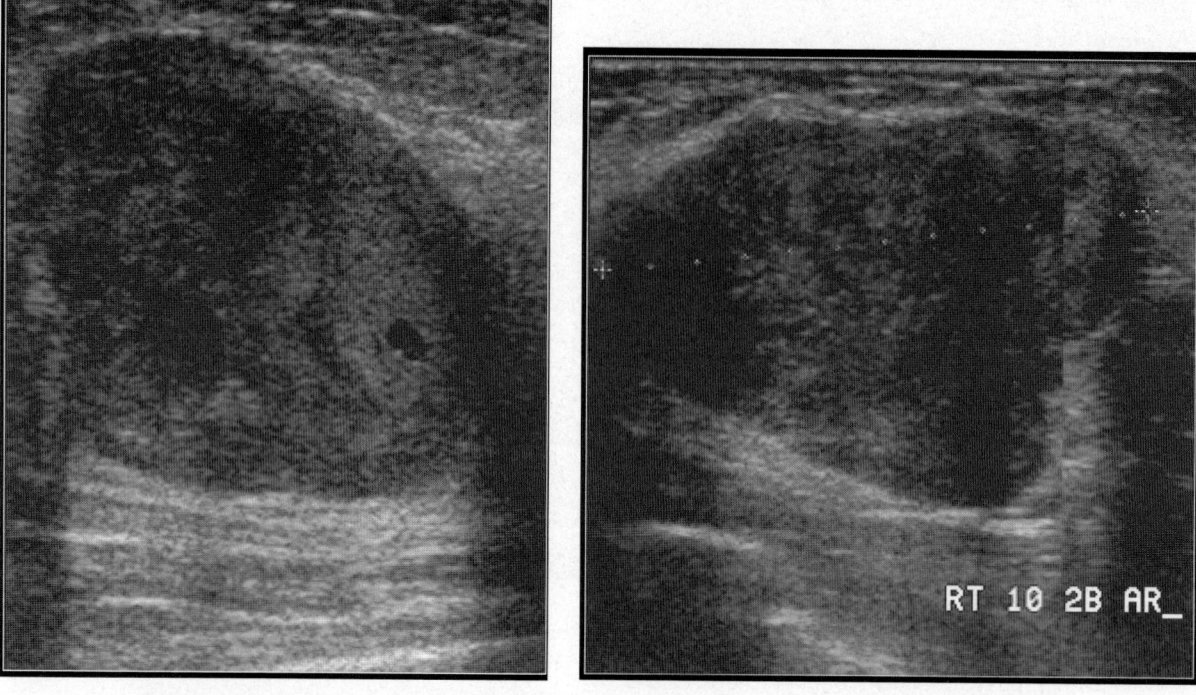

FIGURE 18–78 A: This metaplastic carcinoma was determined to be too large for the lumpectomy the patient desired; thus, the patient was given a trial of induction chemotherapy. **B:** Unfortunately, the metaplastic carcinoma did not respond at all to chemotherapy and enlarged during treatment.

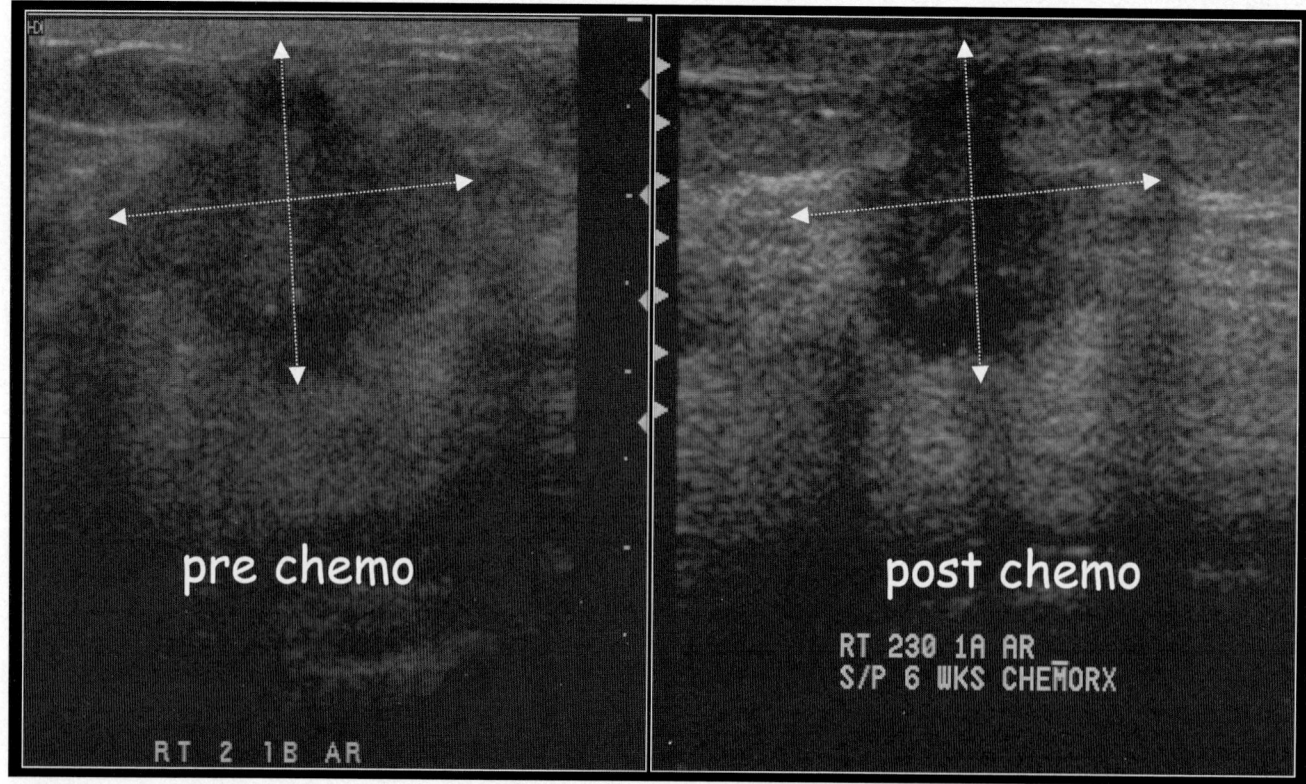

FIGURE 18–79 Before chemotherapy (**left**) and after 6 weeks of chemotherapy (**right**), antiradial plane images show a decrease in mean diameter of only 19% that would be considered a poor response. However, the estimated tumor volume has decreased by 69%, which is considered a good response.

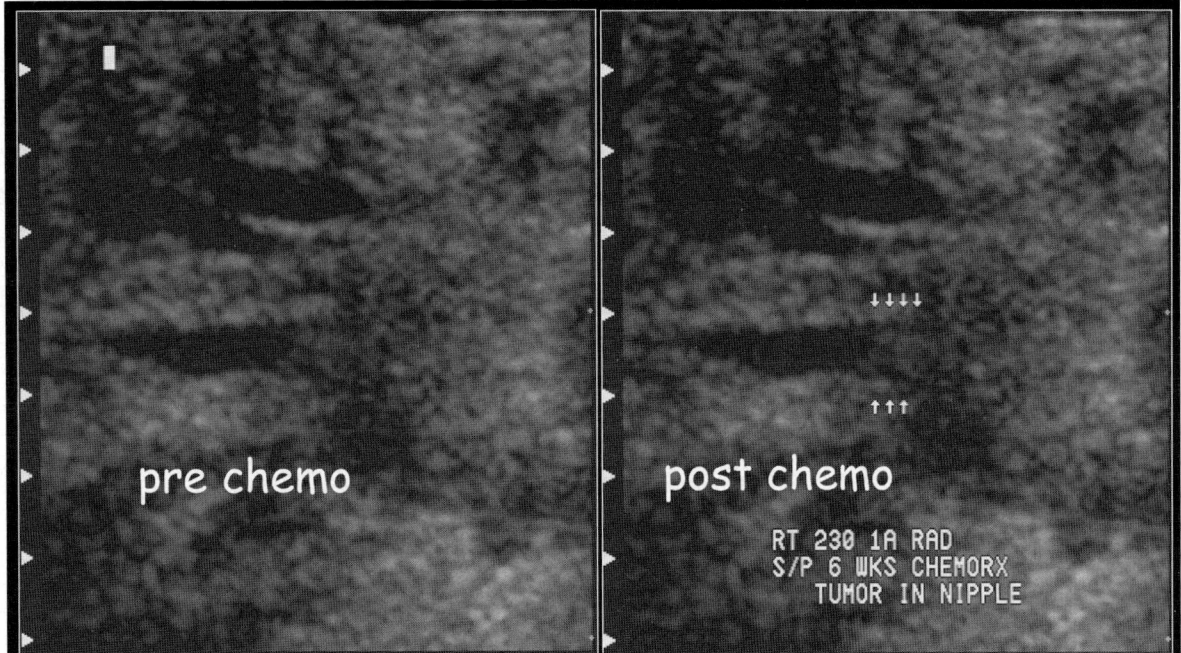

FIGURE 18–80 This is the same malignant nodule shown in Fig. 18–79. Note that despite the 69% decrease in the volume of the invasive component of tumor during chemotherapy, the intraductal component appears unchanged. It is possible that the intraductal component is no longer viable, but simply has not been resorbed; however, in many instances, we have seen invasive components of tumor regress, whereas duct extensions and branch patterns extending into the surrounding ducts remain unchanged. Intraductal components of tumor appear to respond less well to induction chemotherapy than do invasive components.

whether there is residual viable tumor. The residual enlargement of the duct might be the result of extensive necrosis of all tumor cells within the duct.

Complete Regression of Tumor

Complete chemotherapy-induced regression of a primary invasive breast cancer used to be a rare occurrence. However, with modern multidrug regimens in use today, complete regression has been reported in as many as 20% of cases (Fig. 18–81). Even lymph node metastases may completely resolve in such cases (Fig. 18–82). In many cases, a central area of distortion remains even when there is no histologic evidence of tumor (Fig. 18–83). This is because a large percentage of the volume of invasive carcinomas is composed of extracellular matrix—largely hyaluronic acid and collagen, which may be resorbed very slowly even after the tumor cells that stimulate formation of extracellular matrix have been killed.

Even when all sonographic evidence of the lesion has completely disappeared, the area formerly inhabited by the lesion must be surgically removed because it may contain malignancy that is too small to have been detected by sonography. The completely regressed lesion will not be palpable and thus will require image-guided localization. However, the nodule is also no longer visible sonographically or mammographically. Under such circumstances, the only choice is to try to identify anatomic landmarks

that are present around the tumor bed, such as ducts, fibrous ridges, and Cooper's ligaments and to localize the landmarks rather than the lesion itself under ultrasound guidance. Such an approach is not very satisfactory. A better approach is to appreciate in advance that all imaging evidence of the lesion may disappear during induction chemotherapy and to place a metallic marker in the lesion under ultrasound guidance before beginning chemotherapy. Then, if the lesion completely disappears, the clip can be localized under mammographic or stereotactic guidance to facilitate excision and histologic evaluation of the tumor bed.

The new anti-neoplastic agents that are being developed with the aid of genomic and proteomic information technology are likely to be far more specific in their effects than the current generation of chemotherapeutic agents. The new agents will kill tumor or prevent its growth without injuring normal cells, whereas the current generation of agents are toxic to both normal calls and tumor cells. The use of these new agents, in combination with generalized stimulation of the immune system by immunomodulators, monoclonal antibodies, C-mucin blockers, and antiangiogenesis agents, will likely expand the role of chemotherapy well beyond its current limits and cause complete regression in a much larger percentage of cases than current agents achieve. The role of imaging in following tumor response to such agents will likely become much more important than it is now.

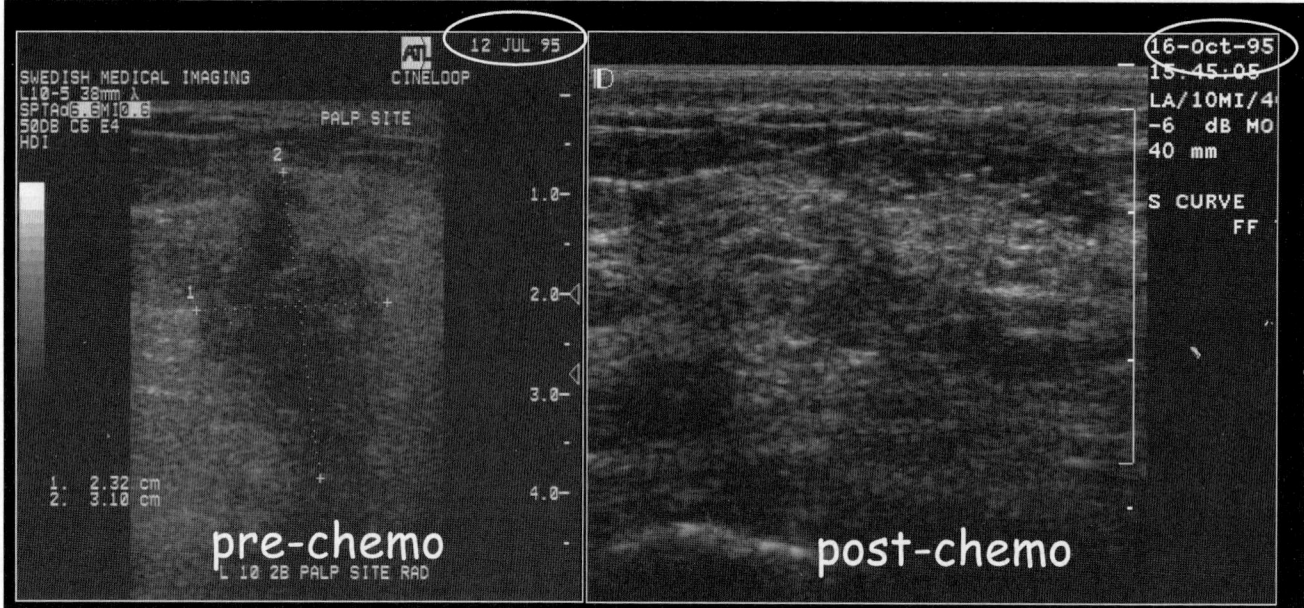

FIGURE 18–81 With today's chemotherapeutic regimens, up to 20% of lesions regress completely, making it hard to localize them for resection at the completion of therapy. For this reason, radiopaque markers should be placed along the margins of the tumor under imaging guidance before initiating chemotherapy.

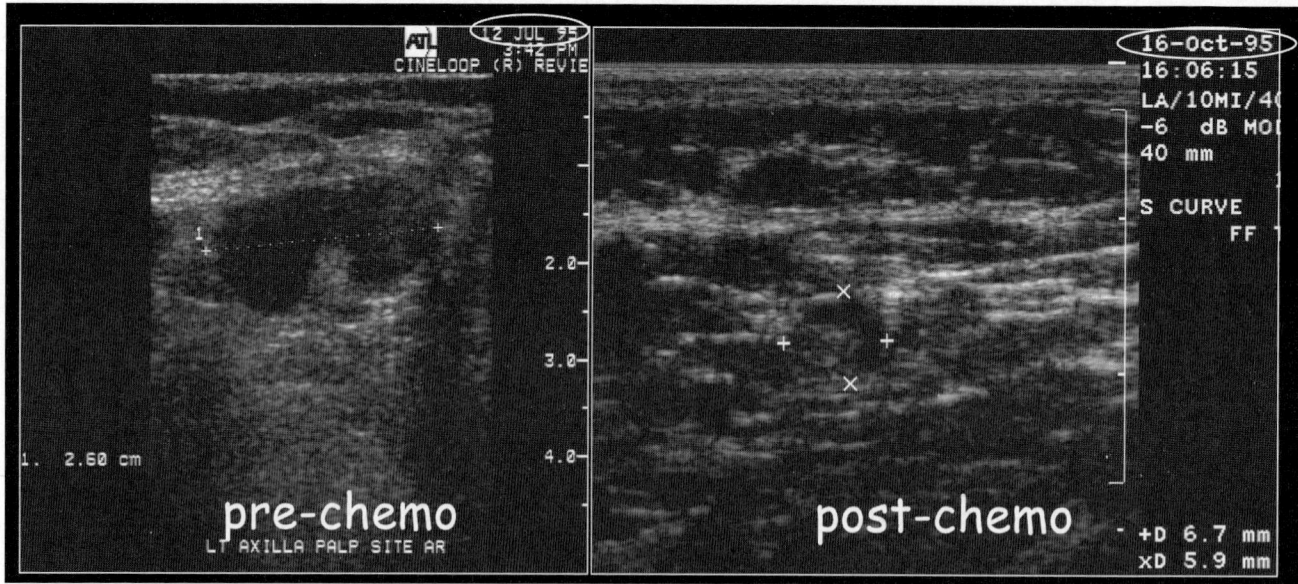

FIGURE 18–82 Metastases to lymph nodes can also regress completely during chemotherapy. The node shown on the left was proved to contain breast cancer metastases by ultrasound-guided large core needle biopsy. At the end of chemotherapy, the sonographic appearance of the lymph node had returned to normal, and no metastatic tumor could be found in any axillary lymph nodes at axillary dissection. Decrease in the size of lymph nodes during chemotherapy should be interpreted with caution, however, because even normal lymph nodes are sensitive to chemotherapy and can decrease slightly in size.

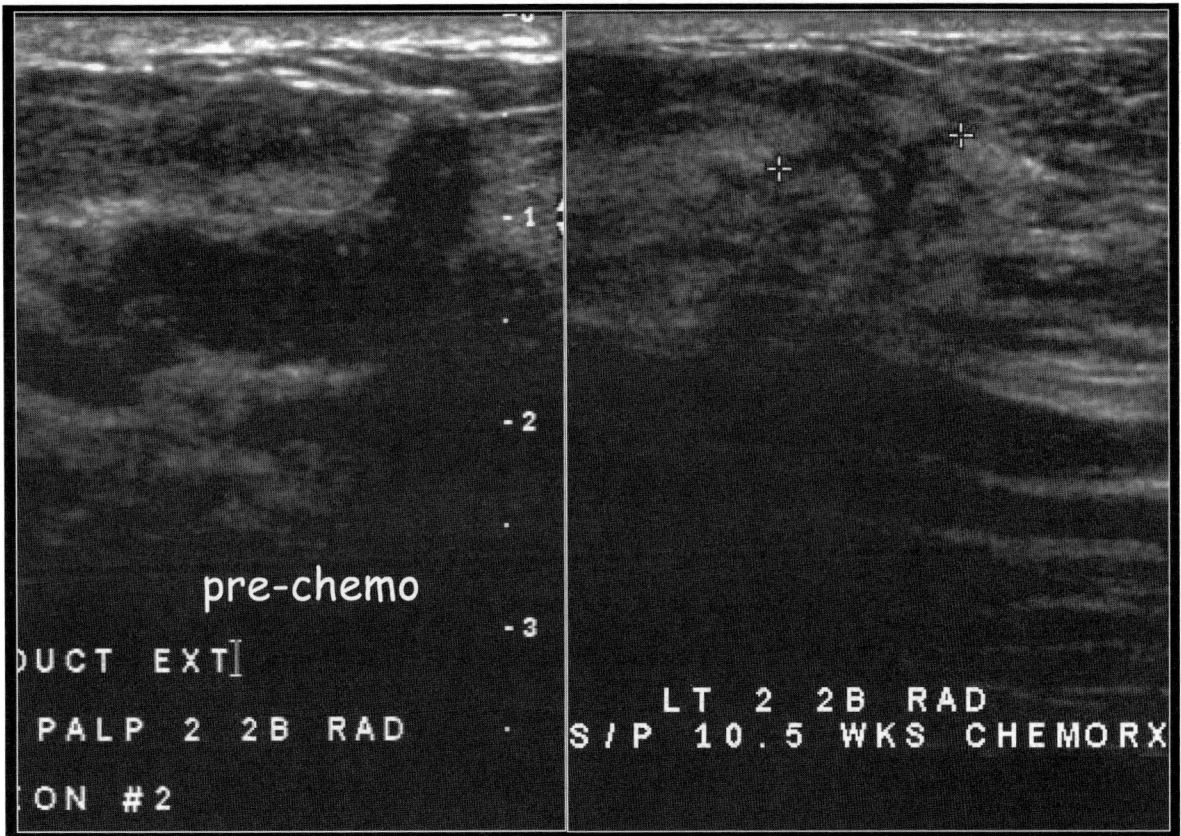

FIGURE 18–83 This large lesion was shown to be an intermediate-grade invasive ductal carcinoma by ultrasound-guided large core needle biopsy. Because of small breast size, the surgeon did not want to perform breast-conserving surgery without first trying to shrink the tumor with chemotherapy **(left)**. At the completion of chemotherapy, only a stellate-shaped residual nidus was visible *(calipers)*. At surgery, no viable tumor was found, and the hypoechoic area corresponded to scarring **(right)**. The chemotherapy had completely killed the tumor.

Alteration in the Histology of the Lesion, Independent of Size Changes

Carcinoma essentially represents a dedifferentiation of cells, and the higher the histologic grade of the lesion, the more dedifferentiated it becomes. As noted in Chapters 12 and 14, the sonographic features are affected by the histologic grade of the lesion. Effective chemotherapy not only can cause a malignant nodule to shrink, but it tends to kill the higher-grade clones of cells within a polyclonal lesion more effectively than it kills lower-grade cells for a variety of reasons. Thus, an invasive carcinoma that contains a majority of high-grade carcinoma cells and a minority of intermediate-grade carcinoma cells before chemotherapy might contain only intermediate-grade tumor cells after chemotherapy. Because high-grade invasive carcinoma is associated with enhanced sound transmission, it should not be surprising if the sound transmission through such a lesion changed during chemotherapy. Thus, a lesion that is mostly high grade and shows enhanced through-transmission before chemotherapy that becomes intermediate grade

after chemotherapy might have normal or decreased sound transmission after chemotherapy (Fig. 18–84). The change in histologic grade and sound transmission can change independently of changes in size. Thus, histologic grade may decrease, and sound transmission may change even though the tumor does not decrease in size (Fig. 18–85).

Not only can induction chemotherapy decrease the histologic grade of some lesions, but also it can completely change the cell type in others. Carcinoma with sarcomatous metaplasia (metaplastic carcinoma, carcinosarcoma; see Chapter 14) is particularly prone to this phenomenon. Metaplastic carcinomas can contain very unusual cell types for breast lesions, such as chondroid and osteoid metaplastic sarcomatous elements. We have observed immature chondroid elements within a metaplastic carcinoma evolve into mature ossified osteoid elements during induction chemotherapy (Fig. 18–86).

In addition to inducing imaging alterations within the malignant nodule, chemotherapy can cause Doppler-detectable changes in blood flow that precede imaging findings. Much of the tumor mass is not actually living tumor

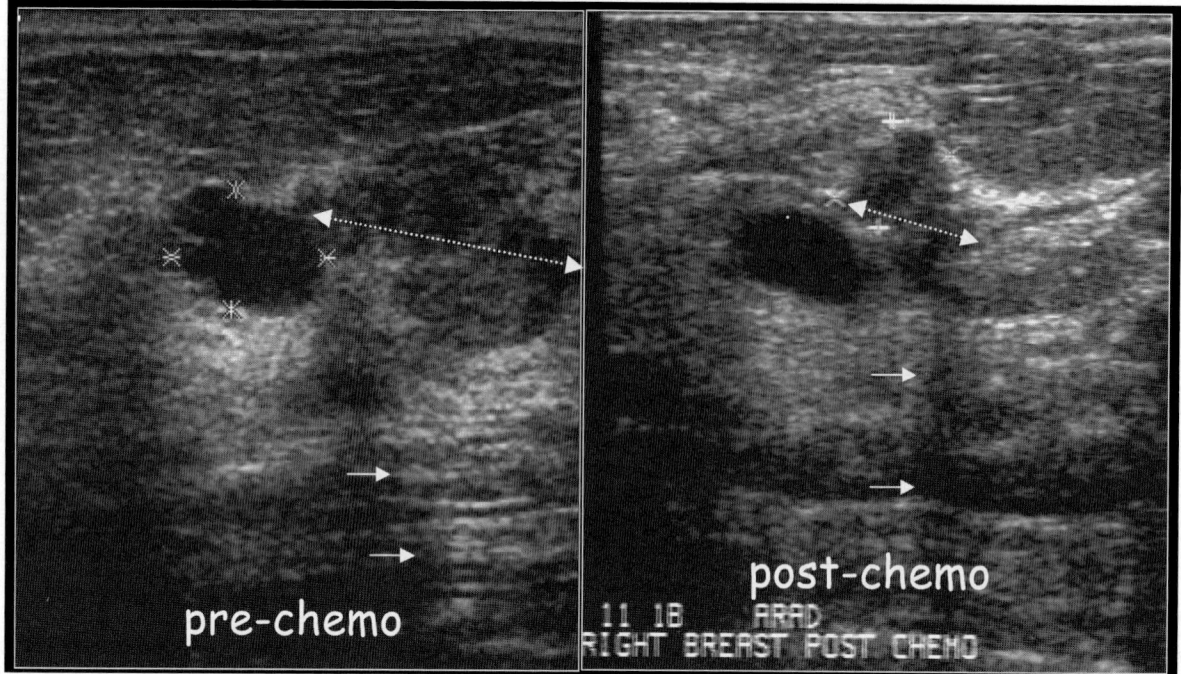

FIGURE 18–84 In some cases, the histologic grade of the tumor decreases during chemotherapy while the lesion regresses in size. The **left** image shows a nodule next to a cyst that ultrasound-guided large core needle biopsy proved to be a high-grade invasive ductal carcinoma. Note the enhanced sound transmission (**left**, *arrows*) that typically corresponds to high-grade lesions. The **right** image shows the lesion after chemotherapy. It has decreased in size and now casts a weak acoustic shadow that is more typically seen with low-grade lesions. At surgery, only low- and intermediate-grade components of tumor remained. The high-grade components had either become more differentiated or had been killed and replaced by lower-grade components.

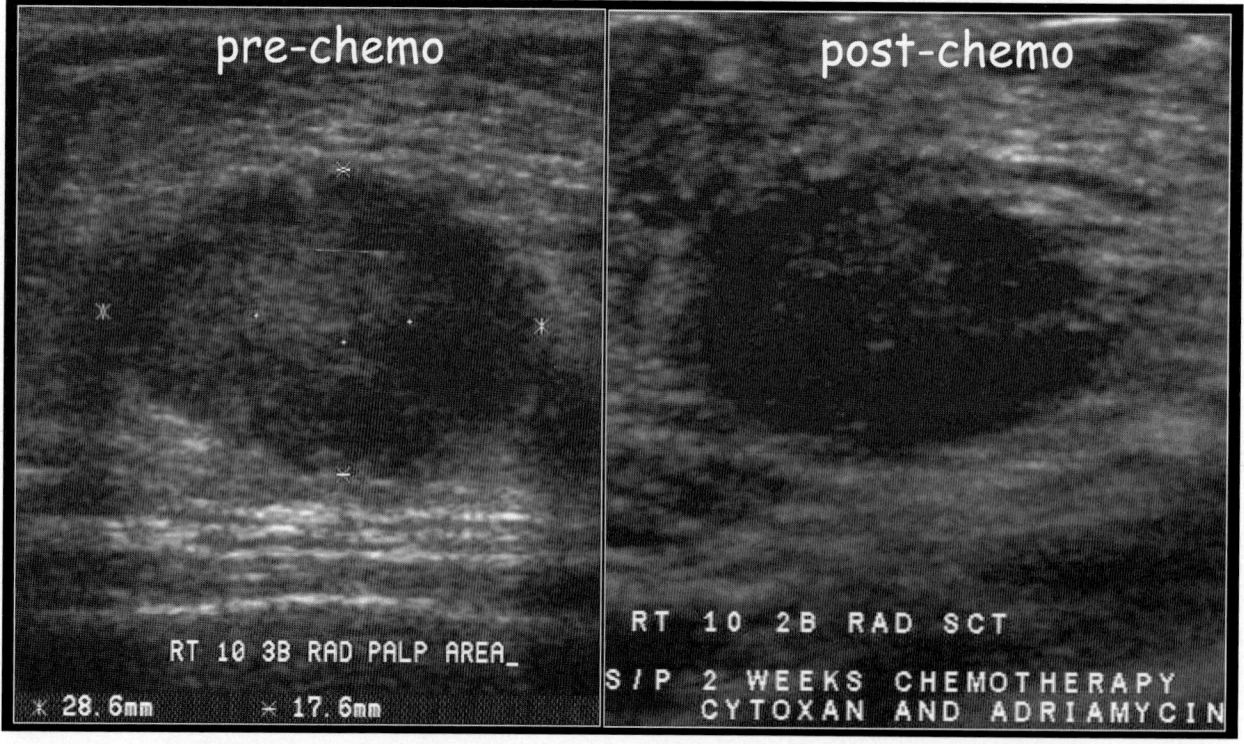

FIGURE 18–85 This high-grade invasive ductal carcinoma showed markedly enhanced through-transmission before beginning chemotherapy (**left**). The prechemotherapy histology was obtained by ultrasound-guided large core needle biopsy. After chemotherapy (**right**), the lesion had decreased very little in size, but the sound transmission had decreased to normal from enhanced. At surgery, the histologic grade of the lesion had decreased from high to intermediate grade even though the lesion had shrunk very little.

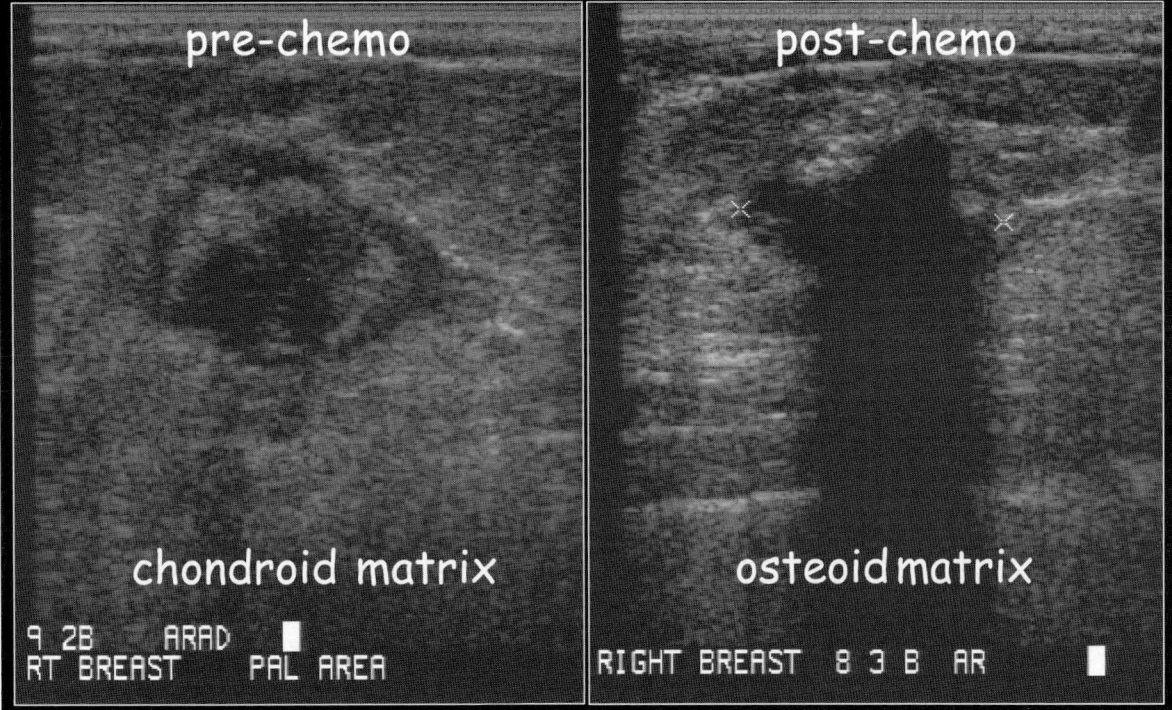

FIGURE 18–86 In some cases, the histology of the lesion changes even more dramatically during chemotherapy. This metaplastic carcinoma had immature chondroid components that were shown by ultrasound-guided large core needle biopsies performed before initiating chemotherapy **(left)**. The scan performed at the end of chemotherapy showed a slight decrease in size but a dramatic change in sound transmission. The lesion now caused intense acoustic shadowing. At surgical excision, it was found that the immature chondroid components of the lesion had become mature osteoid components. Mature bone had formed within the lesion, accounting for the dense acoustic shadowing that appeared after chemotherapy.

cells but rather is amorphous extracellular matrix or desmoplasia. Chemotherapy might kill the tumor cells within the mass but cannot remove them or the extracellular matrix that surrounds them. Thus, even if all tumor cells are killed, it may appear that the size of the lesion has not decreased on the sonographic image. However, the metabolic requirements and need for blood flow in a malignant nodule both decrease if the tumor cells are killed or injured. Furthermore, the dead or injured tumor cells cannot secrete angiogenesis factors. This leads to a decrease in the number of vessels and amount of blood flow to the tumor.

In addition to tumor flow, many malignant nodules incite inflammatory hyperemia. High-grade lesions are particularly prone to attract innumerable lymphocytes and plasma cells that secrete substances that cause vasodilation and inflammatory hyperemia. These lymphocytes and plasma cells are among the most sensitive cells in the body to chemotherapy and may also be killed or injured by chemotherapy. Thus, chemotherapy may reduce blood flow to malignant nodules in two completely different ways: (a) by killing tumor cells and decreasing tumor neovascularity, and (b) by killing or injuring lymphocytes and plasma cells and reducing inflammatory hyperemia

in and around the nodule. The net result is that chemotherapy can cause a Doppler-demonstrable decrease in flow long before the image can detect a decrease in the size of the tumor. This decrease in flow is more likely to be appreciable on the periphery of the lesion. In many tumors, the blood flow inside the substance of the nodule is sparse because of necrosis or because the internal tumor vessels are extrinsically compressed by the ever-increasing hyaluronic acid in the extracellular matrix of the tumor. Ultrasound contrast agents may increase the sensitivity of Doppler for chemotherapy-induced changes in flow to malignant nodules.

SUMMARY

Iatrogenic alterations of the breast are numerous and varied in their histologic and sonographic features. When the alterations are the result of treatment for breast cancer, it is important to distinguish iatrogenic alterations in normal anatomy from recurrent tumor. In some cases, this is not possible with imaging studies alone, and biopsy is necessary. In other cases, sonography is prone to characterize the alterations into falsely high BIRADS categories compared with mammography. This is particularly likely to happen when there is exuberant scar or fat necrosis. If the mammographic findings are definitively benign in such cases, they should be relied on more than the sonographic findings. Patients who may have fat necrosis and who have suspicious findings sonographically should undergo spot compression mammography, and mammograms should be compared with prior films before recommending biopsy based on the sonographic findings alone. Patients who have undergone lumpectomy without primary closure of the lumpectomy cavity and patients who have undergone reduction mammoplasties are particularly prone to develop fat necrosis and exuberant scarring severe enough to result in false-positive sonography findings.

Women who have undergone breast surgery, radiation therapy, or chemotherapy are at least as likely as the general population to develop additional breast problems requiring diagnostic breast sonography. The complaints with which these patients present may be secondary to iatrogenic alterations or recurrent tumor, or may be the result of completely new and unrelated breast lesions. It is important not to assume that a new clinical problem is merely an iatrogenic alteration or recurrent tumor. One must keep in mind the possibility that the lesion causing the problem for which the patient presents might be new and completely unrelated to the previous malignant nodule or to iatrogenic alterations created when the malignant lesion was treated.

The role of ultrasound in the iatrogenically altered patient is to accomplish the following:

- Detect and correctly characterize acute or chronic iatrogenic alterations
- Detect recurrent carcinoma
- Detect new and unrelated abnormalities

The role of ultrasound in monitoring the effectiveness of chemotherapeutic regimens is still evolving. The importance of sonography is likely to expand as chemotherapeutic agents become more specific, safer, and more widely used. If improvements in nonsurgical treatment of breast cancer improve enough to lead to a decrease in the role of surgery, the need to monitor nonsurgical treatment with sonographic and other imaging will be increased.

Doppler might show decrease in vascularity of malignant nodules as a response to chemotherapeutic agents well before imaging can show decrease in size of the lesion. Ultrasound contrast agents may give an even larger advantage to Doppler in assessing early response to therapy. Use of antiangiogenesis agents will likely increase the importance of Doppler even more.

SUGGESTED READINGS

Recurrent Carcinoma

Buchberger W, Hamberger L, Schon G, et al. Mammography and sonography in the diagnosis of recurrence after breast-conserving therapy of breast cancer. *Rofo Geb Rontgenstr Neuen Bildgeb Verfahr* 1991;154:650–656.

Dershaw DD, McCormick B, Cox L, et al. Differentiation of benign and malignant local tumor recurrence after lumpectomy. *AJR Am J Roentgenol* 1990;155:35–38.

Giess CS, Keating DM, Osborne MP, et al. Local tumor recurrence following breast-conservation therapy: correlation of histopathologic findings with detection methods and mammographic findings. *Radiology* 1999;212:829–835.

Lee CH, Carter D. Detecting residual tumor after excisional biopsy of impalpable breast carcinoma: efficacy of comparing preoperative mammograms with radiographs of the biopsy specimen. *AJR Am J Roentgenol* 1995;164:81–86.

Moore MM, Whitney LA, Cerilli L, et al. Intraoperative ultrasound is associated with clear lumpectomy margins for palpable infiltrating ductal breast cancer. *Ann Surg* 2001;233:761–768.

Philpotts LE, Lee CH, Haffty BG, et al. Mammographic findings of recurrent breast cancer after lumpectomy and radiation therapy: comparison with primary tumor. *Radiology* 1996;201:767–771.

Rahusen FD, Taets van Amerongen AH, van Diest PJ, et al. Ultrasound-guided lumpectomy of nonpalpable breast cancers: a feasibility study looking at the accuracy of obtained margins. *Surg Oncol* 1999;72:72–76.

Rissanen TJ, Makarainen HP, Mattila SI, et al. Breast cancer recurrence after mastectomy: diagnosis with mammography and ultrasound. *Radiology* 1993;188:463–467.

Shaikh N, LaTrenta G, Swistel A, et al. Detection of recurrent breast cancer after TRAM flap reconstruction. *Ann Plast Surg* 2001;47:602–607.

Postsurgical Breast and Fat Necrosis

Balu-Maestro C, Bruneton JN, Geoffray A, et al. Ultrasonographic post-treatment follow-up of breast cancer patients. *J Ultrasound Med* 1991;10:1–7.

Brenner RJ, Pfaff JM. Mammographic changes after excisional biopsy for benign disease: serial findings standardized by regression analysis. *AJR Am J Roentgenol* 1996;167:1047–1052.

Gerlach B, Holzgreve W. Breast ultrasound in pre-and postoperative patients. *Ultrasound Q* 1995;13:27–40.

Harrison RL, Britton P, Warren R, et al. Can we be sure about a radiological diagnosis of fat necrosis? *Clin Radiol* 2000;55:119–123.

Mendelson EB. Imaging the post-surgical breast. *Semin Ultrasound CT MR* 1989;10:154–170.

Preradiation Therapy Guidance

Leonard C, Harlow CL, Coffin C, et al. Use of ultrasound to guide radiation boost planning following lumpectomy for carcinoma of the breast. *Int J Oncol Biol Physiol* 1993;27:1193–1197.

Postirradiation Follow-Up

Calkins AR, Jackson VP, Morphis JG, et al. The sonographic appearance of the radiated breast. *J Clin Ultrasound* 1988;16:409–415.

Dershaw DD, Shank B, Reisinger S. Mammographic findings after breast cancer treatment with local excision and definitive irradiation. *Radiology* 1987;164:455–461.

Edeiken BS, Fornage BD, Bedi DG, et al. US-guided implantation of metallic markers for permanent localization of the tumor bed in patients who undergo preoperative chemotherapy. *Radiology* 1999;213:895–900.

Grant EG, Richardson JD, Cigtay OS, et al. Sonography of the breast: findings following conservative surgery and irradiation of the breast for early carcinoma. *Radiology* 1983;147:535–539.

Harris KM, Costa-Greco MA, Baratz AB, et al. The mammographic features of the postlumpectomy, postirradiation breast. *Radiographics* 1989;9:253–268.

Hassell PR, Olivotto IA, Mueller HA, et al. Early breast cancer: detection of recurrence after conservative surgery and radiation therapy. *Radiology* 1990;176:731–735.

Leucht WJ, Rabe DR. Sonographic findings following conservative surgery and irradiation for breast carcinoma. *Ultrasound Med Biol* 1988;14[Suppl 1]:27–41.

Peters ME, Fagerholm MI, Scanlan KA, et al. Mammographic evaluation of the postsurgical and irradiated breast. *Radiographics* 1988;8:873–899.

Wratten C, Kilmurray J, Wright S, et al. Pilot study of high-frequency ultrasound to assess cutaneous edema in the conservatively managed breast. *Int J Cancer* 2000;90:295–301.

Chemotherapy Follow-Up

Balu-Maestro C, Bruneton JN, Geoffray A, et al. Ultrasonographic post-treatment follow-up of breast cancer patients. *J Ultrasound Med* 1991;10:1–7.

Dash N, Chafin SH, Johnson RR, et al. Usefulness of tissue marker clips in patients undergoing neoadjuvant chemotherapy for breast cancer. *AJR Am J Roentgenol* 1999;173:911–917.

Forouhi P, et al. Ultrasonography as a method of measuring breast tumour size and monitoring response to primary systemic treatment. *Br J Surg* 1994;81(2):223–225.

Gawne-Cain ML, Smith E, Darby M, et al. The use of ultrasound for monitoring breast tumour response to pro-adjuvant therapy. *Clin Radiol* 1995;50:681–686.

Kuerer HM, Singletary SE, Busdar AU, et al. Surgical conservation planning after neoadjuvant chemotherapy for stage II and operable stage III breast carcinoma. *Am J Surg* 2001;182:601–608.

Lagalla R, Caruso G, Finazzo M. Monitoring treatment response with color and power Doppler. *Eur J Radiol* 1998;[Suppl 2]:S149–156.

Poplak SP, Maurer HL. Reduction in size of a breast mass due to concurrent chemotherapy: pitfalls in mammographic follow-up. *AJR Am J Roentgenol* 1996;167:392–393.

Reynolds HE, Kesnefsky MH, Jackson VP. Tumor marking before primary chemotherapy for breast cancer. *AJR Am J Roentgenol* 1999;173:919–920.

Seymour MT, Moskovic EC, Walsh G, et al. Ultrasound assessment of residual abnormalities following primary chemotherapy for breast cancer. *Br J Cancer* 1997;76:371–376.

19

EVALUATION OF REGIONAL LYMPH NODES IN BREAST CANCER PATIENTS

IMPORTANCE OF LYMPH NODE METASTASIS FROM BREAST CANCER

The presence of lymph node metastasis, maximum diameter, and histologic grade are the three most important indicators of prognosis in breast cancer patients. As the number and level of lymph nodes involved with metastasis increases, the prognosis worsens.

Lymph node metastasis is partially dependent on size and histologic grade. The larger the maximum diameter and the higher the histologic grade of invasive breast carcinoma, the higher are the risks for lymph node metastasis.

Normal Lymphatic Drainage of the Breast

The lymphatics from most of the breast drain into the axillary lymph nodes. The medial-most portions of the breast drain through the chest wall into the internal mammary lymph nodes.

The axillary lymph nodes are divided into three levels. Low axillary lymph nodes (level 1) lie lateral to the pectoralis minor muscle; the mid-axillary lymph nodes (level 2 nodes) lie directly deep to the pectoralis minor muscle; and the high or apical axillary lymph nodes (level 3 or subclavicular nodes) lie medial and superior to the upper medial edge of the pectoralis minor muscle. Rotter's lymph nodes lie at the same level as level 2 or mid-axillary lymph nodes, but instead of lying deep to the pectoralis minor muscle, they lie between the pectoralis major and minor muscles (Fig. 19–1).

The internal mammary lymph nodes lie between the pleura and the intercostal muscles in the first through third intercostal spaces within 1 to 2 cm of the lateral sternal borders. These nodes lie adjacent the internal mammary artery and veins, which are readily identifiable with color Doppler sonography. The internal mammary lymph nodes

are also located immediately adjacent to perforating branches of the internal mammary arteries that pass outwardly through the intercostal muscles to supply the breast and the perforating veins that course parallel to the arteries, carrying blood back to the internal mammary vein. Normal internal mammary lymph nodes are smaller than corresponding axillary lymph nodes and are rarely larger than 0.6 cm in maximum diameter.

Up to 28% of patients can have lymph nodes that lie within breast tissue. These are intramammary lymph nodes. Like axillary lymph nodes, intramammary lymph nodes can become inflamed and can be involved by metastatic disease. Intramammary lymph nodes most commonly occur in the upper outer quadrant or axillary segment of the breast but may occur in any other quadrant.

Breast Cancer Lymph Node Metastases

Although certain breast cancers spread distantly through the bloodstream very early in their development, most spread by local invasion, intraductal growth, and the lymphatic system in a stepwise and predictable fashion before distant hematogenous metastasis occurs. Breast cancer metastases most commonly involve the axillary lymph node group. Lymphatic spread usually occurs to the low axillary lymph nodes first. Involvement of mid-axillary and high axillary lymph nodes usually occurs only after the low axillary lymph nodes are involved. For this reason, only the low axillary and mid-axillary lymph nodes are evaluated by axillary dissection, whether associated with segmental resection (lumpectomy), simple mastectomy, or modified radial mastectomy. Only during radical mastectomy or when level 1 and 2 nodes are grossly involved are high axillary lymph nodes removed. Radical mastectomy is generally no longer performed in the United States. If low axillary and mid-axillary lymph nodes evaluated at axillary dissection

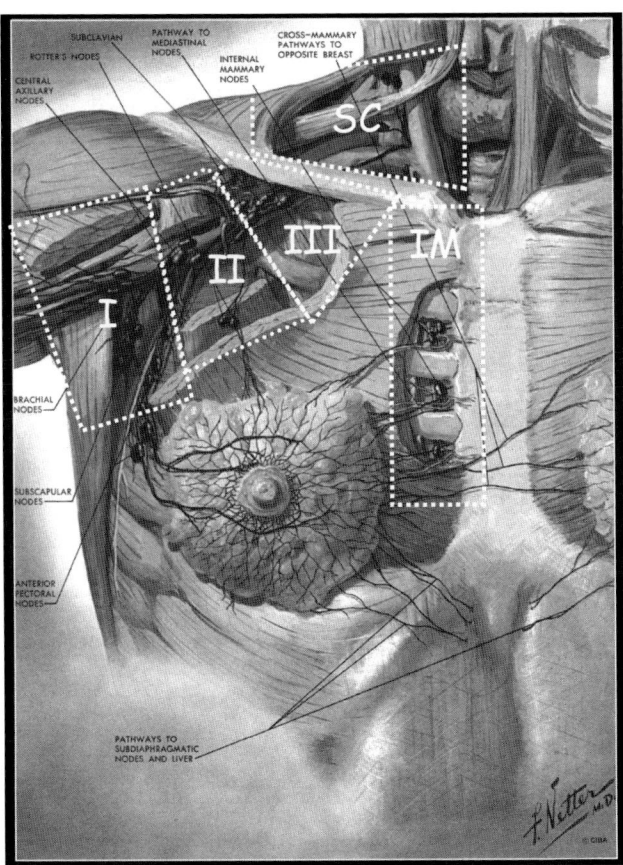

FIGURE 19–1 The regional lymph node chains that are of importance in breast cancer patients are the axillary lymph nodes, the internal mammary lymph node chain, and the supraclavicular chain. Most of the breast drains preferentially to the axillary lymph nodes. The far medial and chest wall areas preferentially drain toward the internal mammary chains. The axillary chain is divided into levels by the pectoralis minor muscle. Nodes that lie inferior and lateral to the pectoralis minor are level 1 nodes or low axillary nodes. Nodes that lie directly behind the pectoralis muscle are level 2 or mid-axillary nodes. Nodes that lie superior and medial to the pectoralis muscle are level 3 nodes or high axillary nodes. The level 3 nodes are also called *infraclavicular* or *subclavicular* nodes. Metastases to supraclavicular nodes are considered distant metastases because they must first pass through level 3 axillary nodes or internal mammary nodes and usually the internal jugular nodes before arriving in the supraclavicular chain. Metastases to internal mammary nodes involve the first three interspaces, most commonly to the second interspace.

are negative for metastasis, it is assumed that the high axillary lymph nodes are also negative. If mid-axillary lymph nodes do contain metastasis, radiation therapy, systemic therapy, or both are undertaken, rather than performing radical mastectomy and level 3 dissection.

Recently, the concept of the sentinel lymph node has been emphasized. In the systematic and stepwise progression of most breast cancers, the first lymph node to which metastasis occurs is termed the sentinel lymph node. The sentinel lymph node is usually a level 1 lymph node, but oc-

casionally it can be an intramammary node or a level 2 node. In a very small percentage of cases, the sentinel lymph node can be an internal mammary lymph node. The sentinel node is usually a single lymph node, but there may be a cluster of two, three, or four sentinel lymph nodes. Injecting technetium-labeled sulfur colloid into the breast enables us to identify the sentinel lymph node preoperatively with radionuclide imaging or intraoperatively using gamma probes. Injecting blue dye alone or in conjunction with radionuclide facilitates detection of the sentinel lymph nodes intraoperatively. If the sentinel lymph node does not contain metastatic disease, there is about a 95% chance that there are no metastases in higher axillary lymph nodes, allowing formal axillary dissection to be avoided. If the sentinel lymph node is positive for metastasis, level 1 and 2 axillary dissection usually follows. Performing sentinel node analysis minimizes morbidity from axillary procedures that are primarily used for staging rather than treatment of cancer. Positive ultrasound-guided large core needle biopsy of a morphologically abnormal sentinel lymph node can indicate the need for formal axillary dissection and can obviate a sentinel node surgical procedure.

Most of lymphatic drainage of the breast preferentially drains toward the axillary lymph nodes. Even most medial breast cancers spread initially to the axillary lymph nodes first. The internal mammary lymph nodes can contain metastases in up to 20% of patients, but in most of these patients, extensive metastases to axillary lymph nodes have occurred first. Isolated metastasis to internal mammary lymph nodes with complete sparing of the axillary nodes occurs in less than 10% of patients. Most patients with isolated internal mammary lymph node metastases have large and deeply located medial primary breast carcinomas, but even cancers that are located far laterally in the breast can metastasize to internal mammary lymph nodes when extensive axillary lymph node metastases (tumor dam) or previous surgery disrupts the normal routes of lymphatic drainage through the axilla. There are lymphatic channel connections between right and left internal mammary lymph node chains; thus, spread of metastases to the contralateral internal mammary lymph nodes can occur. The internal mammary lymph nodes drains superiorly to internal jugular and supraclavicular lymph nodes, posteriorly into mediastinal or hilar lymph nodes, or superficially into intramammary lymph nodes that lie in the far medial aspect of the breast just superficial to the chest wall musculature.

The risk for metastasis to internal mammary lymph nodes, like that of axillary lymph nodes, increases with increasing size of the primary tumor. In small breast carcinomas, the prevalence of positive internal mammary lymph nodes is much lower than 10%. Internal mammary lymph node metastases, like axillary lymph node metastases, can involve only one or a few nodes. Only a single intercostal space is involved in 43% of cases. Two interspaces are involved in 26% of cases, three interspaces in 22% of cases, and four or more interspaces in 9% of cases. When only a single interspace is involved, it is most commonly the second (60%). The third and first interspaces are the next most commonly involved (26% and 14%, respectively). Internal mammary lymph node metastases in the fourth or lower interspaces seldom occur in the absence of extensive metastases within the first three interspaces. The surgical removal of internal mammary lymph nodes is tedious and has a higher morbidity than does axillary dissection. Because of the relative uncommonness of internal mammary lymph node metastasis and the difficulty of surgery, internal mammary lymph node dissection has been largely abandoned. Furthermore, internal mammary lymph nodes seldom undergo biopsy, so we seldom have histologic confirmation of the suspected diagnosis. The absence of histologic data concerning the presence or absence of internal mammary lymph node metastases is undoubtedly a confounding factor in accurately determining the prognosis of some breast cancer patients. Evaluation of internal mammary lymph nodes requires imaging studies, including lateral chest radiography, computed tomography scans, magnetic resonance imaging (MRI), sonography, lymphoscintigraphy, or positron-emission tomography scans. Radiation therapy, rather than surgery, is usually counted on to control suspected (but not histologically proved) internal mammary node metastases.

Breast carcinoma can also spread to supraclavicular lymph nodes but does not do so directly. Supraclavicular lymph nodes are generally involved only after internal jugular or subclavian lymph nodes are involved. For this reason, supraclavicular nodal metastases, unlike those to axillary and internal mammary nodes, are considered distant metastases. The prognosis is worse in patients with supraclavicular lymph node metastasis than it is in patients with only axillary lymph node metastasis.

In cases in which extensive metastasis within an intramammary lymph node destroys the normal lymph node architecture, it can be difficult for the pathologist to distinguish between metastasis and a second primary tumor (multifocal disease). This distinction is especially difficult when the primary tumor contains abundant lymphocytes, such as occurs in medullary carcinoma and some high-grade invasive not otherwise specified lesions. Metastasis to an intramammary lymph node has an effect on prognosis similar to that of metastasis to a single low axillary lymph node.

Certain lymph node metastases can invade directly through the lymph node capsule into the perinodal soft tissues. Extracapsular invasion by breast cancer metastases occurs more frequently when lymph node metastases are larger and more numerous. Surprisingly, extracapsular invasion does not have a statistically significant impact on survival prognosis, but it does increase the risk for axillary recurrences. Extracapsular extension from internal mammary lymph nodes or Rotter's lymph nodes can lead to chest wall and pericardial invasion.

The histology of lymph node metastases is similar to that of the primary tumor in about 85% of cases. In some instances, however, the lymph node metastases may be less differentiated and of higher histologic grade than the primary, especially if the cell population in the primary tumor is heterogeneous and polyclonal.

HISTOLOGY OF THE NORMAL LYMPH NODE

Although the sonographic appearance of lymph nodes bears some resemblance to that of the kidneys, their anatomy differs greatly. The vascular supply of both kidneys and lymph nodes enters and exits through the hilum, and the effluent from both kidneys and lymph nodes exits through the hilum. Then the differences begin. The first major difference is that in lymph nodes, afferent lymphatic channels do not enter the lymph node from the hilum, but rather from the periphery, through the capsule of the lymph node. After the lymphatic fluid from the afferent lymphatic channel has penetrated the lymph node capsule, it flows into the subcapsular sinus and then centrally through the cortical sinuses and toward the lymph node mediastinum, where it enters the medullary sinusoids (Fig. 19–2). From the medullary sinusoids, the lymphatic fluid collects into afferent lymphatic channels that exit the lymph node through the hilar notch of the lymph node, similar to the way that the collecting system exits the kidney. Thus, lymphatic flow within the lymph node is from peripheral to central. This pattern of flow affects the sonographic appearance of metastases to lymph nodes. Unlike afferent lymphatic channels, the normal arteries that feed and the normal veins that drain the lymph node enter and exit the lymph node only through the hilum. No arteries or veins normally penetrate the lymph node capsule. The development of transcapsular arterial branches occurs in lymph nodes that bear metastases.

The cells that line the lymphatic channels differ from those that line the collecting system of the kidneys. Instead of being lined by epithelium, the lymph node sinusoids are lined by macrophage-like reticuloendothelial cells.

In the cortex, between the subcapsular and cortical sinusoids, lie the primary follicles that contain developing lymphocytes of B-cell origin. When stimulated by antigens, the primary follicles enlarge and develop germinal centers of activated B cells. Lying between the follicles and enveloping them are T-cell–type lymphocytes. There are also lymphatic tissues in the mediastinum of the lymph node. Between the medullary sinusoids lie medullary cords that contain lymphocytes and plasma cells. Fibrous septations divide the lymph node cortex

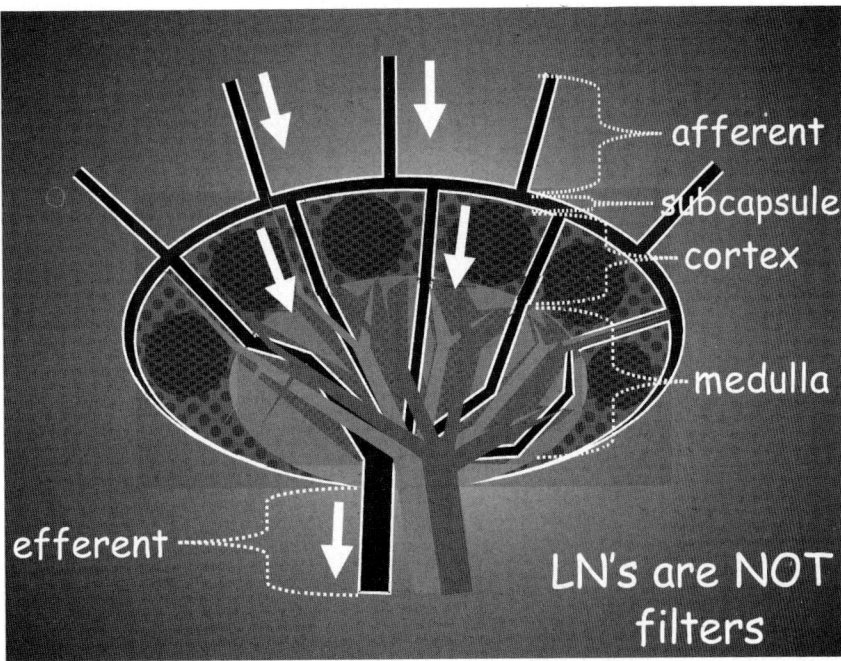

FIGURE 19–2 The lymph node consists of a cortex and a mediastinum. The cortex contains sub-capsular and cortical sinusoids and lymphatic tissue that includes lymphoid follicles. The medulla consists of medullary sinuses and medullary cords that contain lymph tissue. Lymph fluid enters the lymph node through afferent lymphatic channels that penetrate the capsule, dumping lymphatic fluid into the subcapsular sinuses. From the subcapsular sinuses, the lymph flows through the cortical sinusoids to the medullary sinuses and finally into the efferent lymphatic channels that exit the lymph node through the hilar notch. The lymph node is usually supplied by a single artery and drained by a single vein that enter and exit the hilar notch. Blood vessels do not normally enter or exit the lymph node through the capsule that surrounds the cortex. The amount of fat within the mediastinum varies greatly.

into compartments and pass from the capsule centrally toward the mediastinum.

CHANGES IN LYMPH NODES OVER TIME

Over time, the histology of lymph nodes tends to change. Repeated episodes of inflammation and infection and age-related decreases in responsiveness of the immune system tend to lead to atrophy, thinning, and scarring of both cortical and medullary elements within the lymph node. As the medullary and cortical elements become thinner, the amount of fat within the lymph node mediastinum increases. Thus, aging tends to increase the fatty component of lymph nodes within the mediastinum and decreases the medullary cord and cortical components. Frequently, fatty infiltration progresses faster than medullary and cortical atrophy occur, resulting in enlargement of the outer diameters of the lymph node, despite the thinning of the cortex and medulla. Atrophy leads to fairly uniform thinning of cortex and medulla, but scarring may lead to asymmetric thinning. The temporal changes within lymph nodes occur so consistently, particularly within major regional lymph node chains such as the axillary and inguinal chains, that by late adulthood, all of the lymph nodes may be histologically and morphologically abnormal, showing evidence of atrophy and scarring. Thus, the only classically normal lymph nodes that we might see tend to occur in children and adolescents.

FUNCTIONS OF LYMPH NODES

Like the anatomy, the functions of lymph nodes differ greatly from those of the kidney. The main function of the kidney is filtration—either passive or active. The lymph node is not truly a filter, but rather is an antigen-recognition and antibody-production structure. Antigens can be held within the lymph node to allow enough time for initiation of the antibody-recognition and antibody-production process to begin, but antigens can eventually pass through the sinusoids within the lymph node and exit the node through the efferent lymphatics. Although the lymph node should not be thought of as a filter *per se*, strands of collagen within the sinusoids can attach to antigenic structures passing though the sinusoids, temporarily slowing their passage through the lymph nodes. The level of the sinusoids at which certain antigens are slowed by these collagen fibers varies. Metastases tend to be delayed and ultimately implant within the subcapsular and cortical sinusoids, whereas foreign bodies, such as droplets of silicone gel and carbon particles, tend to accumulate within the medullary sinusoids. Thus, metastatic disease tends to affect the cortex, whereas foreign bodies affect primarily the medulla of the lymph node. The cortical implantation site of lymph node metastases from breast cancer creates important morphologic changes that can be detected sonographically and that help us immensely in assessing lymph nodes for metastatic disease.

ULTRASOUND APPEARANCE OF NORMAL LYMPH NODES

Despite the great anatomic differences, lymph nodes simulate miniature kidneys sonographically. Both are elliptical in shape, both have relatively hypoechoic cortex, and both have relatively hyperechoic hila or mediastina. Both the normal lymph node and the normal kidney are flattened

and C shaped in their short axes. The opening in the C is where the cortex of both lymph nodes and kidney is absent—the hilum (Fig. 19–3). On color or power Doppler, both usually have a single feeding artery that enters through the hilar notch. The artery that feeds a normal lymph node can often be demonstrated with color or power Doppler, but the vein often cannot (Fig. 19–4). However, it is here that the similarities end. The relative thickness of the cortex and hila differs between lymph nodes and kidneys. The cortex of normal lymph nodes is relatively thinner than that of normal kidneys. It could be said that the cortex of the normal lymph node is similar to the thickness of the cortex of a kidney that has undergone severe central atrophy and is affected by severe renal sinus lipomatosis. If the cortical thickness of a lymph node appears similar to the cortical thickness of a normal kidney in a child or adolescent, then the lymph node cortex is mildly diffusely thickened, usually owing to inflammation (Fig. 19–5). The renal medulla, manifested as the renal pyramids, lies within and is enveloped by the renal cortex and thus lies within the hypoechoic parenchymal layer of the kidney, not the hilum or mediastinum of the kidney. The medullary sinuses and cords of the lymph node, on the other hand, lie central to

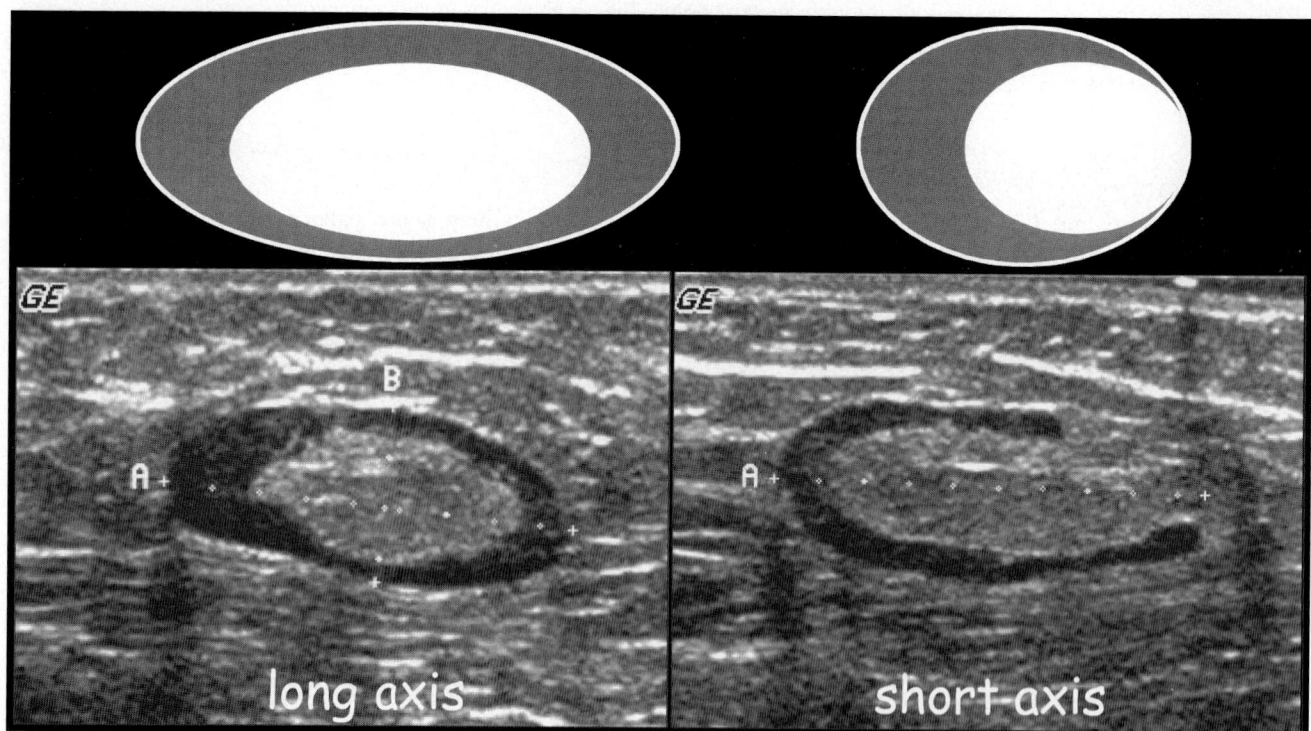

FIGURE 19–3 Normal lymph nodes are elliptical in shape in long axis and C shaped in short axis. The cortex, composed largely of lymphatic tissue and fluid-filled cortical sinuses that are oriented roughly parallel to the ultrasound beam, is mildly to moderately hypoechoic. The mediastinum, which contains alternating medullary cords and sinusoids that have innumerable interfaces, appears isoechoic to hyperechoic, depending on the amount of fat relative to medullary tissues. In the short axis, the cortex is absent at the hilar notch.

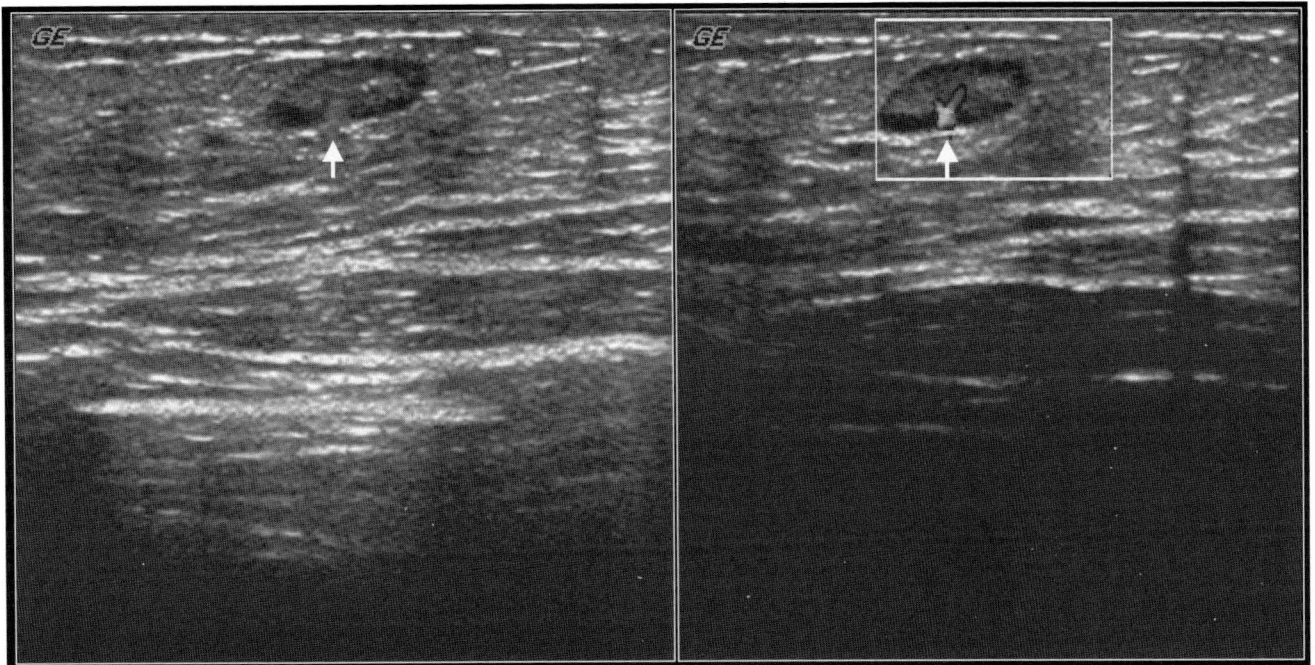

FIGURE 19–4 Normal lymph nodes are fed by a single artery that enters through the hilar notch that is demonstrable by color or power Doppler. The vein that drains the normal lymph node is usually not demonstrable with Doppler.

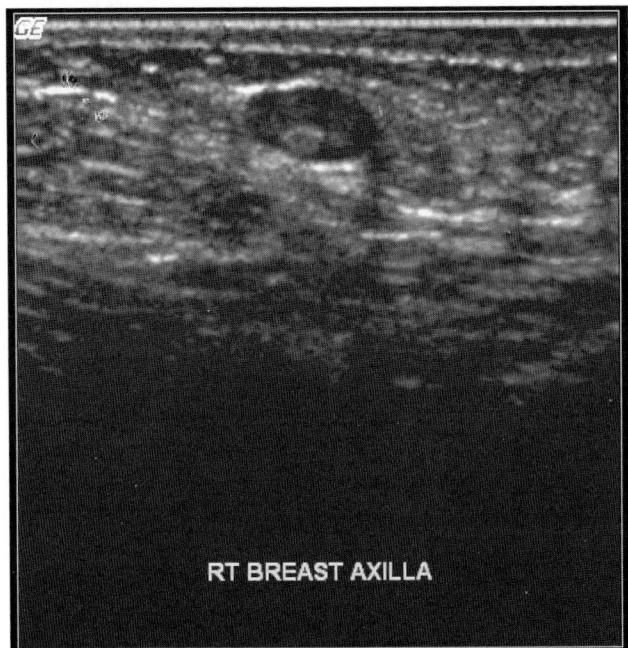

FIGURE 19–5 The cortex of normal lymph nodes is generally thinner than the cortex of a normal kidney. When the lymph node cortex appears as thick as the cortex of a normal kidney, as in this case, the node is usually inflamed or reactive.

the lymph node cortex, within the mediastinum of the lymph node. The renal pyramids, composed of well-hydrated collecting tubules that are oriented parallel to the ultrasound beam and thus make poor specular reflectors, are markedly hypoechoic relative to the renal cortex. Unlike the hypoechoic renal medulla, the medullary portions of the lymph node are hyperechoic. The innumerable interfaces between the medullary cords and medullary sinuses, many of which are perpendicular to the ultrasound beam, thus making strong specular reflectors, give rise to the echogenicity in the periphery of the lymph node mediastinum. The collecting system of the lymph nodes, the efferent lymphatics that exit from the mediastinum of the lymph node through the hilar opening, never become distended enough to be seen sonographically.

The sonographic appearance of normal lymph nodes varies with the relative sizes of the cortex and mediastinum and with the degree of fatty infiltration of the mediastinum (Fig. 19–6). In general, the larger the outer diameter of a normal lymph node, the greater is the fat content of the mediastinum and the greater are the atrophy or stretching and thinning of the cortex. The degree of fatty replacement and cortical thinning tend to increase with age as a result of repeated episodes of inflammation, scarring, atrophy, and

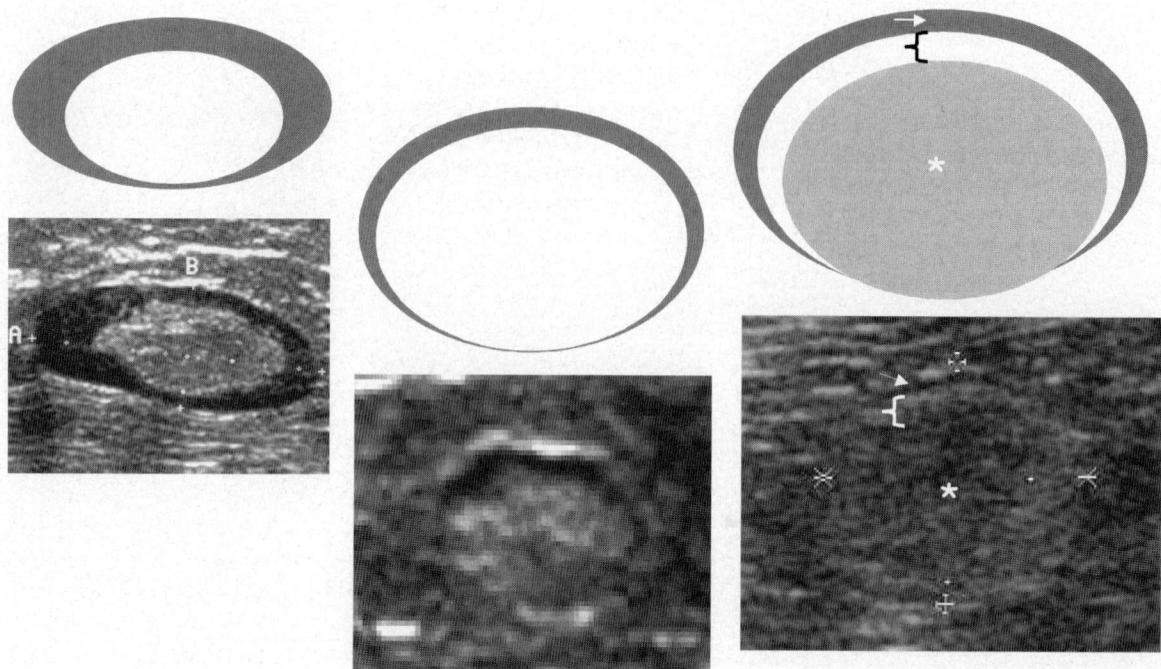

FIGURE 19–6 There is a spectrum of normal lymph node appearances depending on the degree of cortical atrophy and fatty infiltration of the hilum. The **left** nodal appearance is the most frequently seen in young people. As the patient ages, the cortex tends to become thinner, and the echogenic hilum tends to enlarge (**middle**). In some cases, cortical atrophy is severe *(arrow, right)*, fatty infiltration of the hilum is so extensive that most of the mediastinum assumes the isoechoic texture of fat *(*)*, and the hyperechoic medulla is atrophic and compressed and is visible as a thin echogenic layer *(bracket)* that lies just inside the cortex (**right**).

weight gain. Lymph nodes that have normal uniform cortical thickness and relatively small, uniformly echoic mediastina (because their mediastina are entirely composed of echogenic medullary cords and sinuses) tend to be seen in young individuals who have had few episodes of inflamma-tion and few opportunities for atrophy and scarring to have occurred (Fig. 19–7). As the patient ages, cortical and medullary scarring and atrophy lead to progressive thinning of the cortex (Fig. 19–8). With aging, fat also tends to infiltrate the mediastinum, beginning at the hilar opening

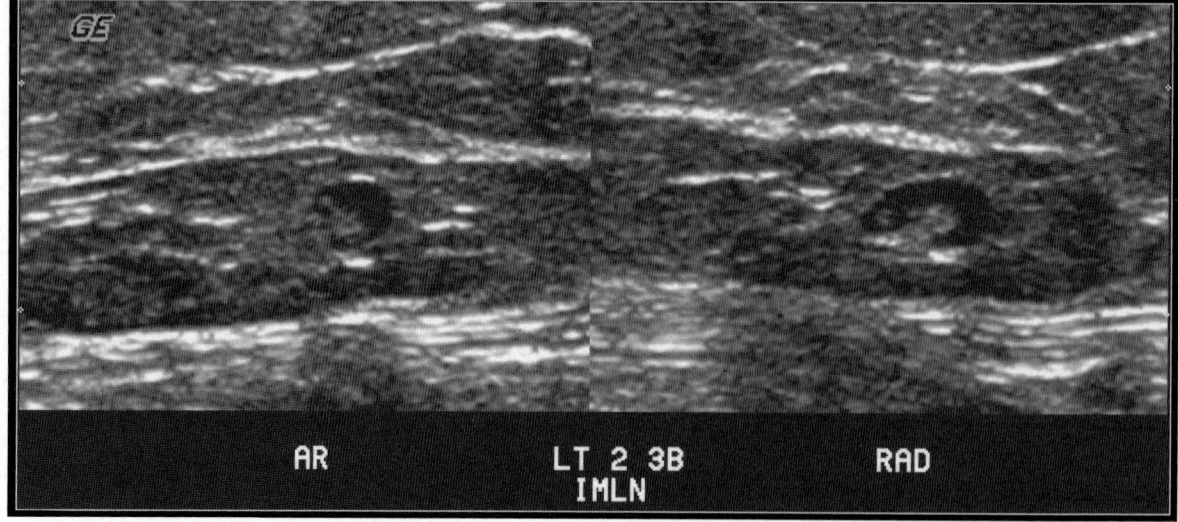

FIGURE 19–7 Lymph nodes in young patients have undergone few episodes of inflammation and scarring and have the classic reniform appearance. The cortex is relatively thick and hypoechoic, and the mediastinum is relatively small and uniformly echogenic.

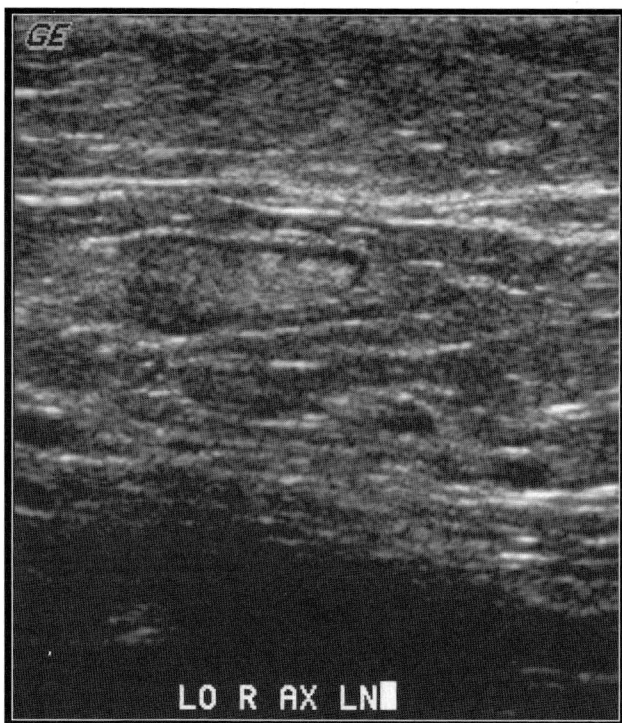

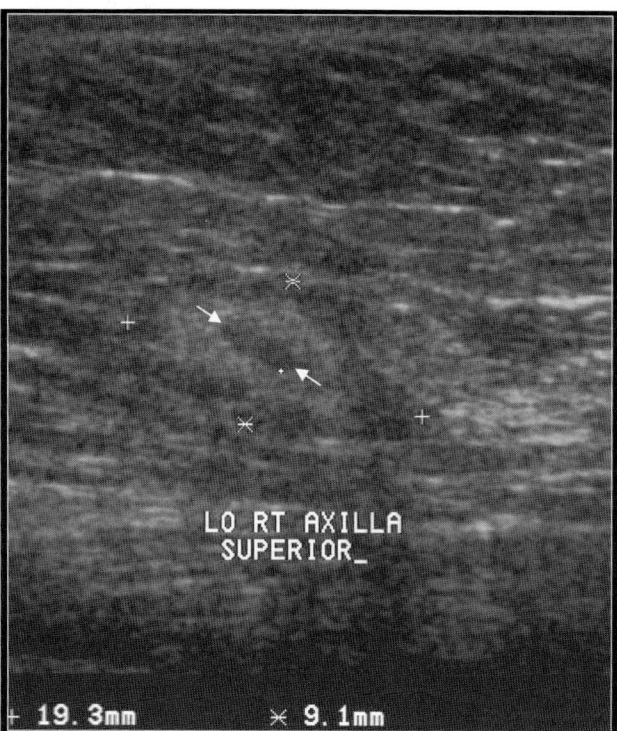

FIGURE 19–8 With repeated episodes of inflammation and scarring that invariably occur with aging, the cortex atrophies and becomes thinner, and the echogenic mediastinum becomes relatively larger.

FIGURE 19–9 Fat infiltrates the mediastinum. Early on, only a small amount of isoechoic fat may be present near the hilar notch in the short axis, and a focus of isoechogenicity *(arrows)* surrounded by the echogenic medulla is present in the long axis.

and progressing peripherally toward the cortex, relegating the hyperechoic medullary cords and sinuses to the periphery of the mediastinum. The portion of the mediastinum near the hilar notch that has been replaced by fat appears to be isoechoic with fat rather than hyperechoic (Fig. 19–9). As fatty infiltration progresses and the echo-producing medulla is pushed toward the periphery, the mediastinum becomes progressively less echogenic (Fig. 19–10). In cases in which cortical and medullary atrophy are the most severe and fatty replacement of the mediastinum is extensive, nearly the entire mediastinum of the lymph node can appear to be replaced by isoechoic fat, leaving only a very thin layer of residual hyperechoic medulla that lies along the undersurface of the markedly thinned cortex (Fig. 19–11).

In cases in which atrophy and scarring have made the cortex so nearly isoechoic with surrounding fat that it is difficult to identify sonographically, coded harmonics can be helpful. Lymph node cortex that appears to be nearly isoechoic with surrounding fat on fundamental imaging frequently appears markedly hypoechoic and more conspicuous with coded harmonics (Fig. 19–12). This makes identifying and evaluating lymph nodes easier, quicker, and more accurate.

As noted earlier, the age-related processes of atrophy and scarring within lymph nodes are so universal that most breast-related lymph nodes in middle-aged or elderly

women will show sonographic abnormalities. The most common finding indicating scarring is irregularity in the thinning of the lymph node cortex. When the cortex is so severely scarred and focally atrophic that segments of cortex are not sonographically visible, there is no diagnostic dilemma. Clearly, the node process is old, and the abnormal segment of cortex is the part that is abnormally thinned or absent (Fig. 19–13). However, in a case in which the cortex is only mildly thinned focally, there may be a diagnostic dilemma. It can be difficult to determine whether the thin or thick portions of the cortex are abnormal. (Fig. 19–14). This creates a dilemma because focal thickening of the cortex is an important morphologic feature of metastasis, which is discussed later.

Paradoxically, as the degree of cortical and medullary atrophy and fatty mediastinal replacement increases, the outer diameter of the lymph node may increase greatly. Such lymph nodes may be greater than 2 cm in shortest diameter but of no clinical or sonographic concern. Thus, size is often a poor criterion for judging the normalcy of a lymph node.

Shape can also be important. Normal lymph nodes are elliptical in shape. Abnormal lymph nodes tend to become more rounded and nearly circular in shape. However, fatty infiltration can cause a lymph node to become more rounded in addition to enlarging it. Thus, shape also has limitations.

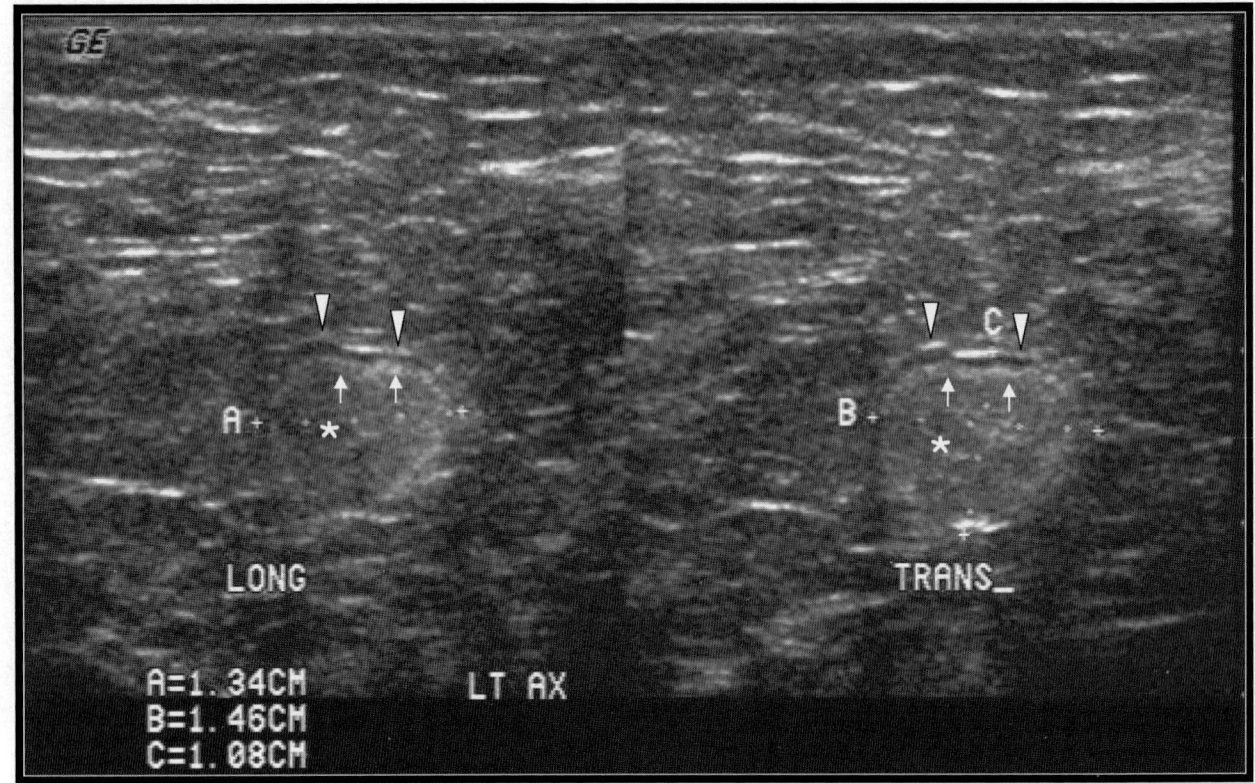

FIGURE 19–10 As fatty infiltration of the mediastinum progresses, most of the fatty replaced mediastinum *(*)* becomes isoechoic or nearly isoechoic with the fat that surrounds the lymph node. The atrophic echogenic medulla *(arrows)* persists as a thin, hyperechoic band just deep to the hypoechoic cortex *(arrowheads)*. Fatty replacement of the mediastinum that is particularly extensive not only can enlarge the node but also can make the node nearly spherical in shape, similar to the shape caused by extensive metastatic replacement.

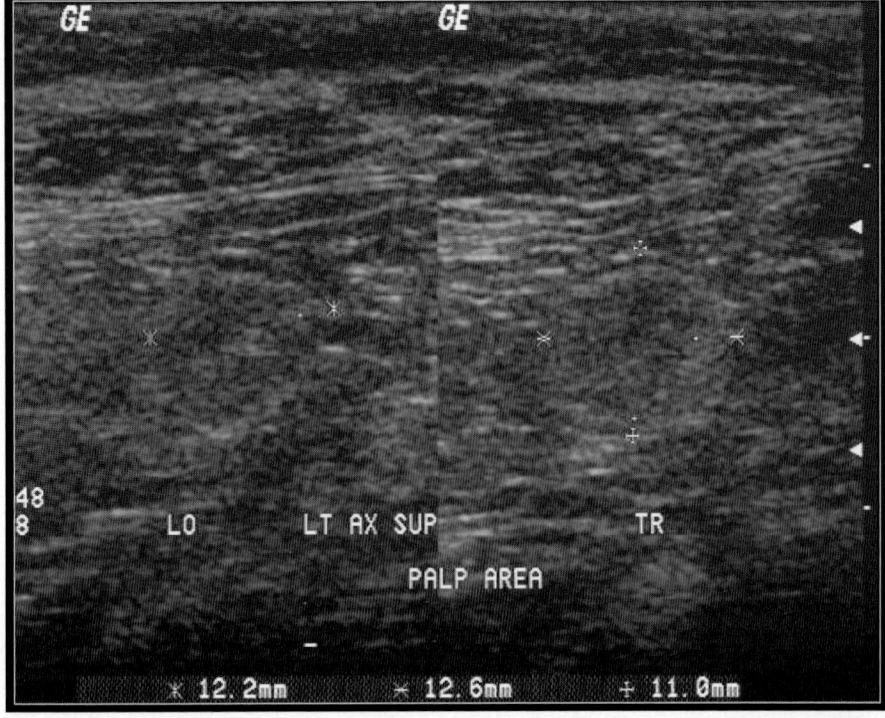

FIGURE 19–11 The most severe cases of fatty infiltration are associated not only with marked thinning of the medulla and cortex but also with enlargement and rounding of the lymph node.

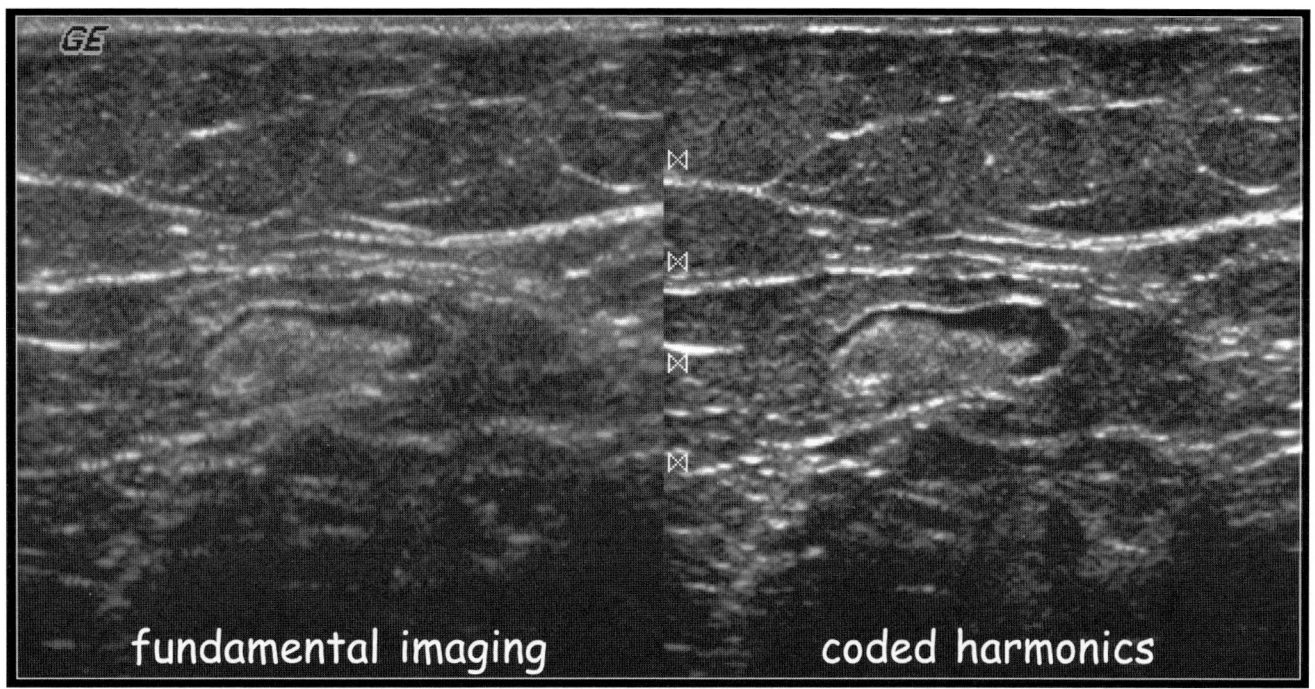

fundamental imaging   coded harmonics

FIGURE 19–12 Coded harmonics (**right**) makes the cortex of lymph nodes appear relatively more hypoechoic and conspicuous than it appears with fundamental imaging (**left**).

Because size and shape have limitations, assessing morphologic features of the cortex, mediastinum, and capsule tends to be far more important in assessing the normalcy or lymph nodes. Morphologic assessment of lymph nodes is discussed later in this chapter.

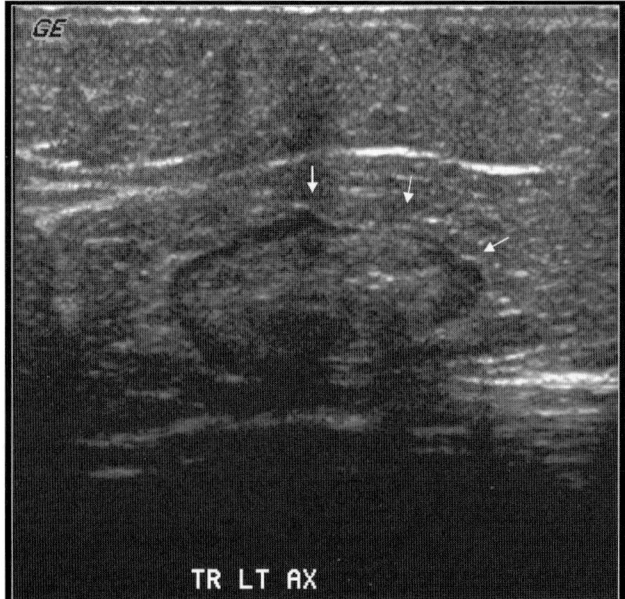

TR LT AX

FIGURE 19–13 As patients age, the chances of significant scarring of the lymph node increase. This usually manifests as focal thinning or absence of the cortex *(arrows)*.

Lymph nodes in which there has been abundant fatty replacement of the lymph node mediastinum have classically benign mammographic appearances that enable BI-RADS 2 characterization and eliminate the need for diagnostic sonography. However, in younger patients, in whom the mediastinum contains relatively greater amounts of water-density structures (blood vessels, efferent lymphatic vessels, medullary cords, and medullary sinuses) and relatively less fat, the fatty mediastinum can be difficult to demonstrate mammographically. Sonography does not depend on the presence of fat to demonstrate the definitively benign echogenic lymph node mediastinum. Instead, it shows the echogenic interfaces between the different water-density elements within the mediastinum. Thus, in many cases in which mammography has difficulty showing or completely fails to show a definitively benign fatty mediastinum, sonography easily shows a classically benign hyperechoic mediastinum that better enables us to characterize the nodule as BIRADS 2 (Fig. 19–15).

The morphologic features of superficially located lymph nodes are usually easier to assess than are the morphologic features of smaller and more deeply located lymph nodes. With current top-of-the-line equipment, normal intramammary and at least some normal low (level 1) axillary lymph nodes can be identified in all patients. Normal internal mammary lymph nodes and level 2 and 3 axillary lymph nodes tend to be smaller and more deeply located and can be demonstrated in some patients. Normal

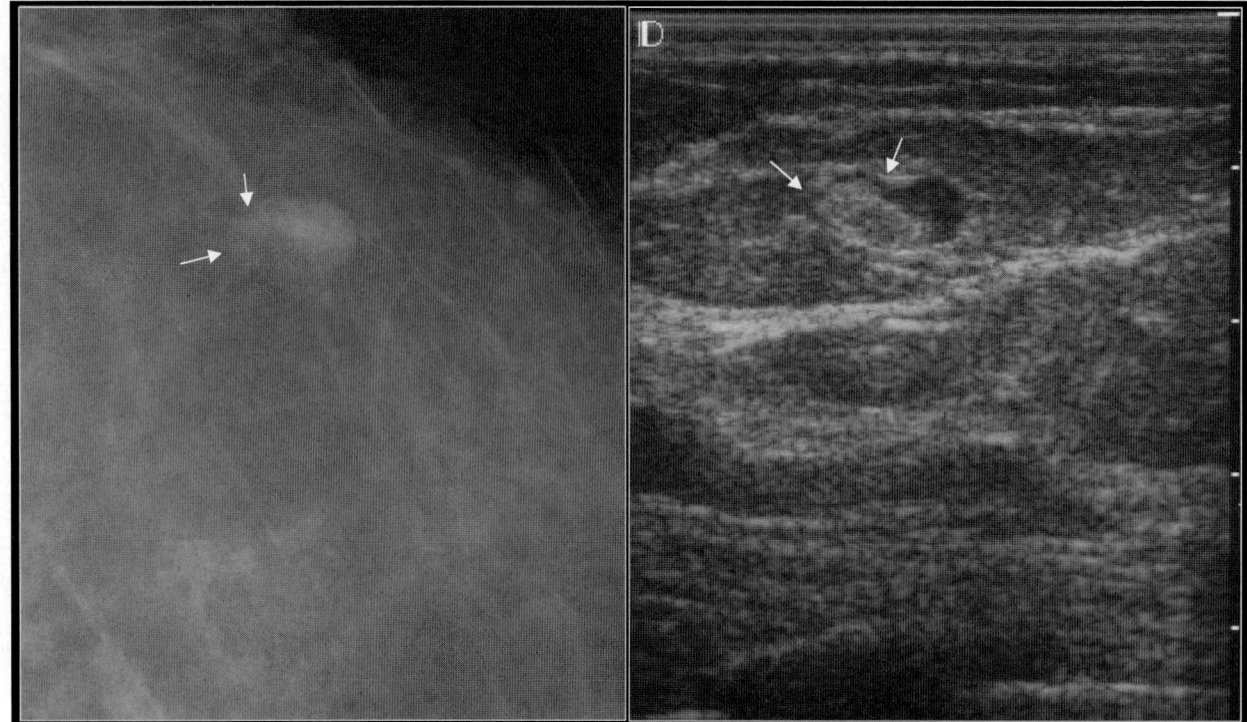

FIGURE 19–14 When cortical scarring *(between arrows)* occurs in a lymph node with normal thickness, it can be difficult to determine whether the thick or thin part of the cortex is abnormal. Does this lymph node have a segment of cortex that is abnormally thickened (**right edge**), or does it have normal cortical thickness with a segment of cortex that is abnormally thinned (**left edge**)? Biopsy revealed a benign but scarred lymph node.

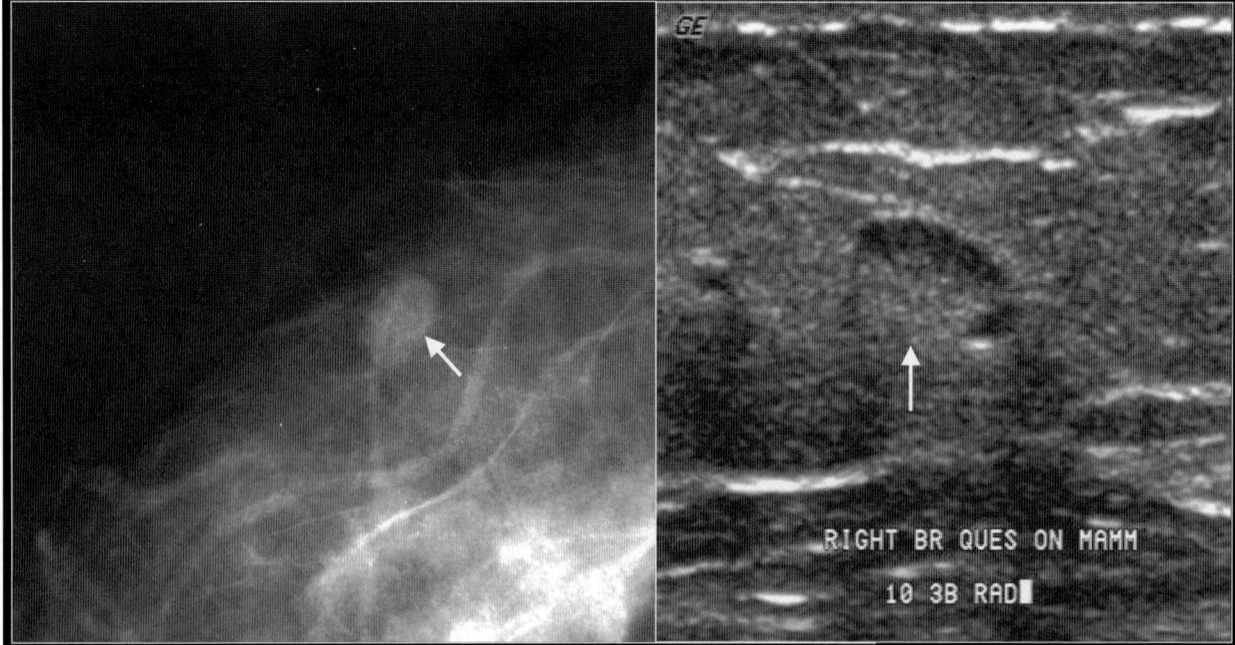

FIGURE 19–15 The classic fatty mediastinum that enables a BIRADS 2 classification of normal intramammary lymph on mammography may be far easier to see sonographically than it is mammographically in young patients in whom there is little fatty infiltration of the mediastinum.

supraclavicular lymph nodes can be identified sonographically in most patients.

Axillary Lymph Nodes

The pectoralis minor muscle, the important landmark for assessment of level of axillary lymph nodes, can be identified in all patients (Fig. 19–16). Normal level 2 or midlevel axillary lymph nodes are difficult to demonstrate, but abnormally enlarged lymph nodes lying at levels 2 and 3 can be demonstrated sonographically (Fig. 19–17). Normal-sized Rotter's nodes, which lie in the tissue plane between the pectoralis major and pectoralis minor muscles, can be demonstrated in some patients (Fig. 19–18). Color or power Doppler may be necessary to distinguish Rotter's nodes from vessels that lie within the same tissue plane. As is the case with level 2 and 3 axillary lymph nodes, Rotter's nodes can more consistently be demonstrated when abnormally enlarged. Identifying Rotter's nodes can be important because metastases to these nodes can give rise to chest wall invasion.

Internal Mammary Lymph Nodes

It has been written that normal internal mammary lymph nodes are not sonographically visible and that any visible internal mammary lymph nodes must be abnormally enlarged. With current equipment and techniques, this is

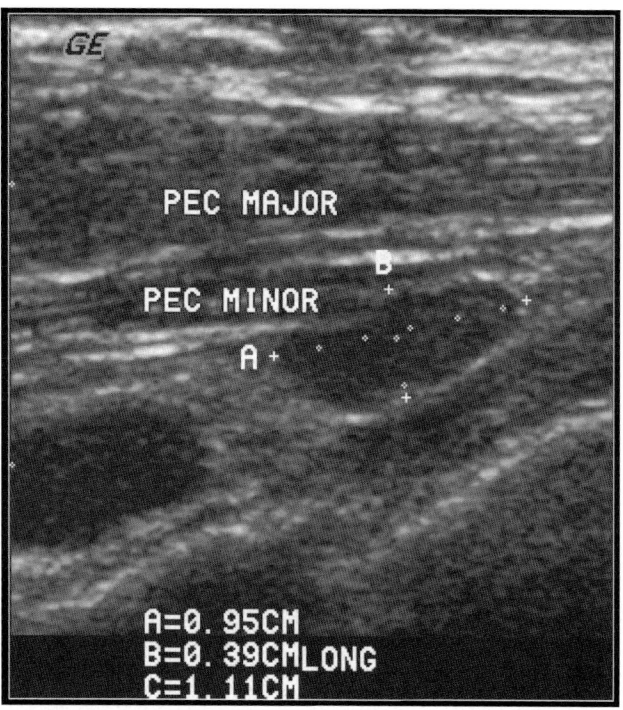

FIGURE 19–17 Normal level 2 nodes are only occasionally seen, but abnormally enlarged level 2 nodes can routinely be identified.

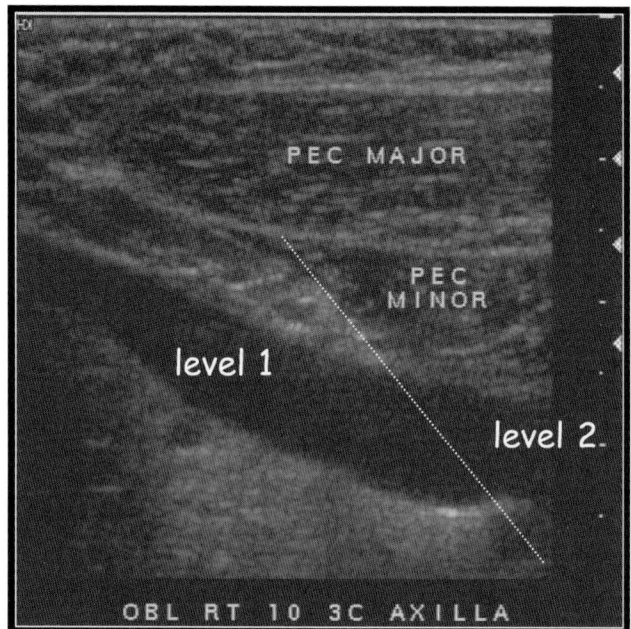

FIGURE 19–16 The pectoralis minor muscle, the landmark for determining the level of axillary lymph nodes, is sonographically visible just posterior to the pectoralis major muscle. Level 1 nodes lie inferior and lateral to the pectoralis minor muscle, and level 2 nodes lie directly posterior to the pectoralis minor muscle.

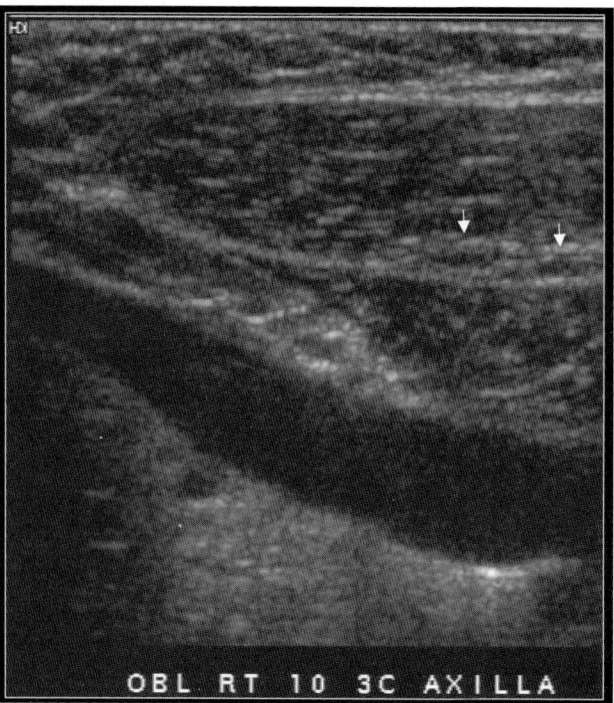

FIGURE 19–18 Normal-sized Rotter's lymph nodes *(arrows)* that lie between the pectoralis major and minor muscles can be demonstrated occasionally.

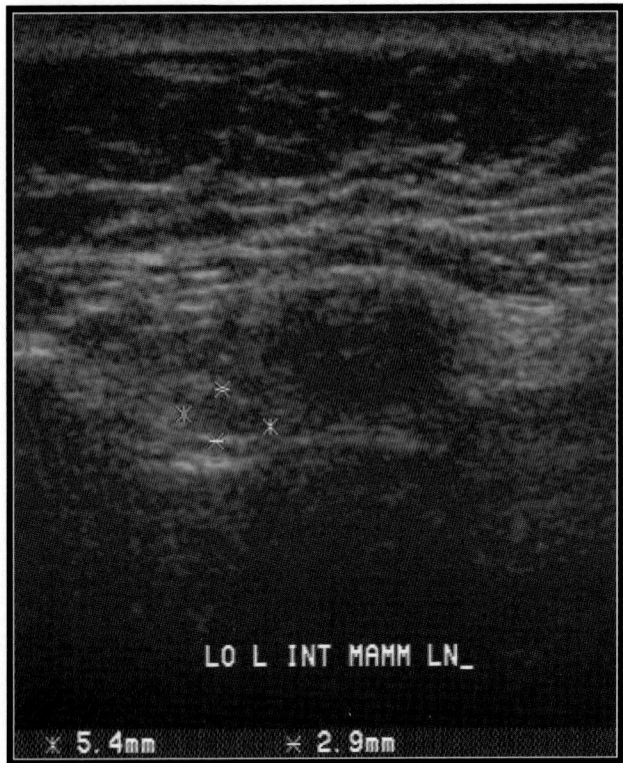

FIGURE 19–19 Internal mammary lymph nodes are smaller than axillary lymph nodes, usually 5 mm or less in maximum diameter. They can lie anywhere along the craniocaudal axis of the interspace but can be identified most frequently just superior to the costal cartilage at the inferior end of the interspace *(calipers)*. Because of the depth and small size, cortex and mediastinum can seldom be distinguished from each other in normal internal mammary lymph nodes.

no longer true. In some patients, we can identify normal internal mammary lymph nodes (Fig. 19–19). They are much smaller than most axillary lymph nodes, averaging about 4 to 6 mm in maximum diameter. Because of incoherence of the beam caused by the musculature and tendons of the chest wall and the lens effect of the costal cartilages, the internal structure of the internal mammary lymph nodes cannot be shown as well as can that of axillary and internal mammary lymph nodes. The echogenic mediastinum and lymph node capsule can seldom be distinguished from each other. Thus, morphologic evaluation of internal mammary lymph nodes is less valuable than it is for larger and more superficially located axillary nodes. We have to rely more heavily on size than morphology when assessing internal mammary lymph nodes. Both coded harmonics and real-time compounding have been immensely helpful in demonstrating internal mammary lymph nodes. Coded harmonics helps because by suppressing speckle, it makes the cortex appear more hypoechoic than surrounding chest wall tissues (Fig. 19–20). Real-time compounding helps in several ways. It suppresses speckle, shows the lymph node capsule better by minimizing critical angle phenomena, and steers under costal cartilages to minimize their lens effects (Fig. 19–21). The internal mammary lymph nodes can lie anywhere along the interspaces between the costal cartilages in the craniocaudal direction, but we most frequently find normal-sized internal mammary lymph nodes along the upper edge of the third costal cartilage in the second interspace.

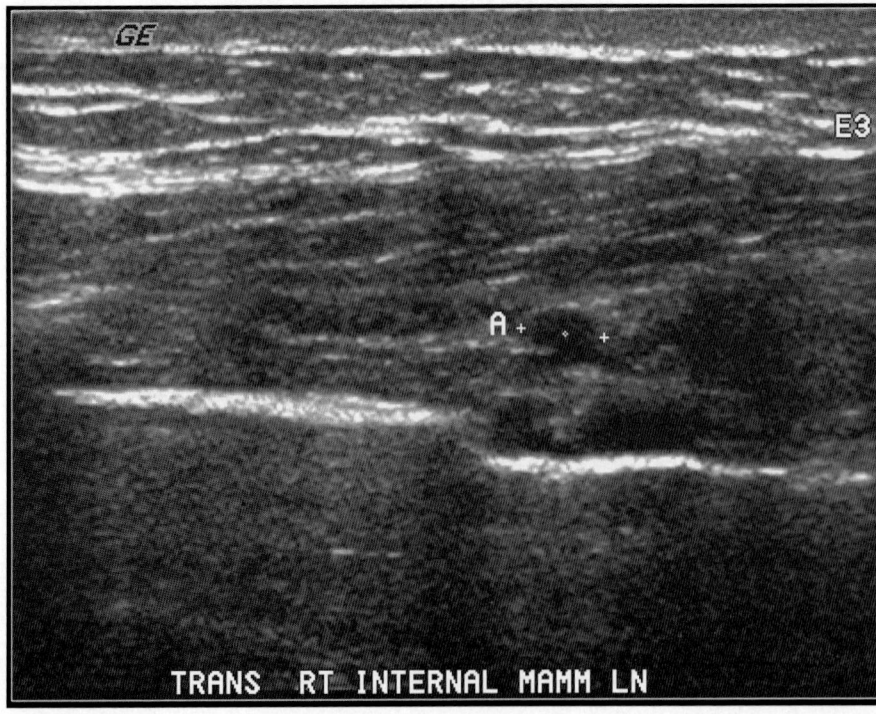

FIGURE 19–20 By making the internal mammary node appear more hypoechoic, high-frequency coded harmonics can help make identifying internal mammary lymph nodes easier when penetration is adequate *(calipers)*.

Color or power Doppler can be very useful in identifying internal mammary lymph nodes. Doppler may help in three different ways. First, the internal mammary lymph nodes lie near the internal mammary vessels along the deep and lateral edges of the sternum. Identifying the internal mammary artery and vein enables us to begin our search in the correct geographic area (Fig. 19–22). Second, it can help distinguish internal mammary lymph nodes from tortuous internal mammary veins, which can simulate lymph nodes on B-mode images (Fig. 19–23). The internal mammary veins can be surprisingly dilated and tortuous in some patients, particularly patients who have cor pulmonale or other causes of elevated right atrial end-diastolic pressure. Third, power Doppler vocal fremitus may be helpful in identifying internal mammary lymph nodes because they vibrate differently from chest wall muscles and tendons (Fig. 19–24).

The internal mammary lymph nodes can contain metastases in cases in which there are large medial primary lesions, deep lesions that involve the chest wall (chest wall lymphatics tend to drain medially to internal mammary lymph nodes). However, internal mammary lymph nodes are most frequently involved with lesions in the upper outer quadrant that are associated with extensive axillary lymph node metastases that apparently block the normal route of lymphatic drainage and cause collateral drainage through the internal mammary lymph node system (Fig. 19–25).

Intramammary Lymph Nodes

Intramammary lymph nodes are common. They most frequently present as incidental findings detected on screening mammography. In cases in which the fatty mediastinum is well demonstrated mammographically, no further evaluation is necessary. However, when the mammogram does not show a clear-cut fatty hilum, sonography can be helpful because it can frequently show the classic echogenic lymph node mediastinum when mammography cannot (Fig. 19–15). Internal mammary lymph nodes can also present as palpable lumps that require sonography.

Most intramammary lymph nodes lie within the upper outer quadrant of the breast or within the axillary segment of the breast, but they can occur in any quadrant as well as in the subareolar area (Fig. 19–26).

The area of the breast outside the upper outer quadrants where we most frequently see normal intramammary lymph nodes sonographically, but not on mammography, is the extreme medial aspect of the breast. These intramammary lymph nodes lie near the lateral edge of the sternum in a

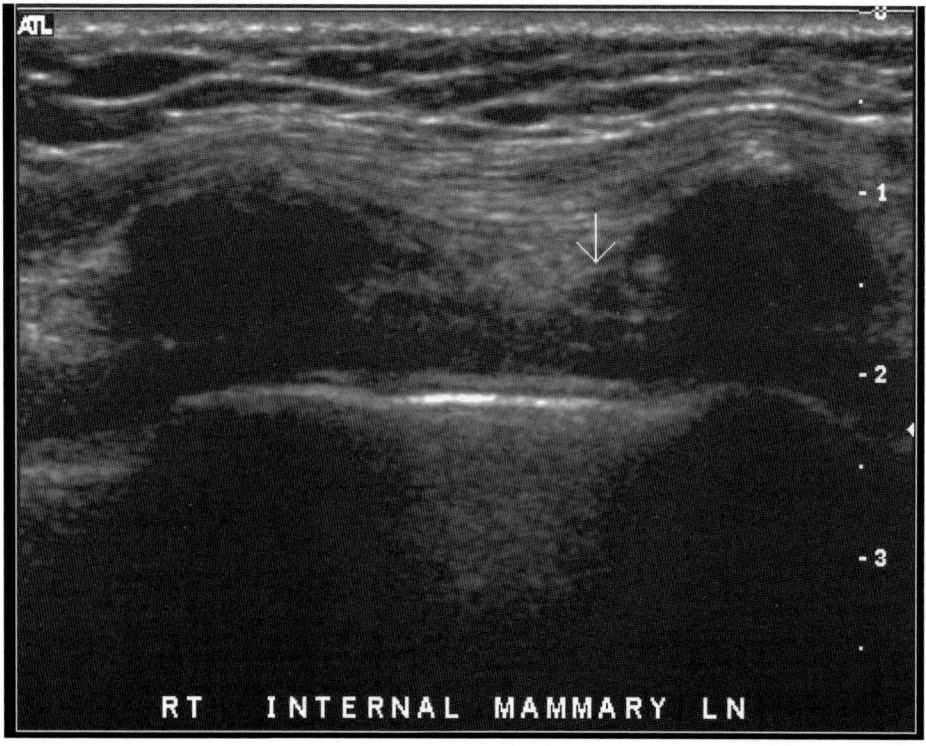

FIGURE 19–21 Real-time compounding can help demonstrate the thin, echogenic capsule that surrounds normal internal mammary lymph nodes *(arrow).*

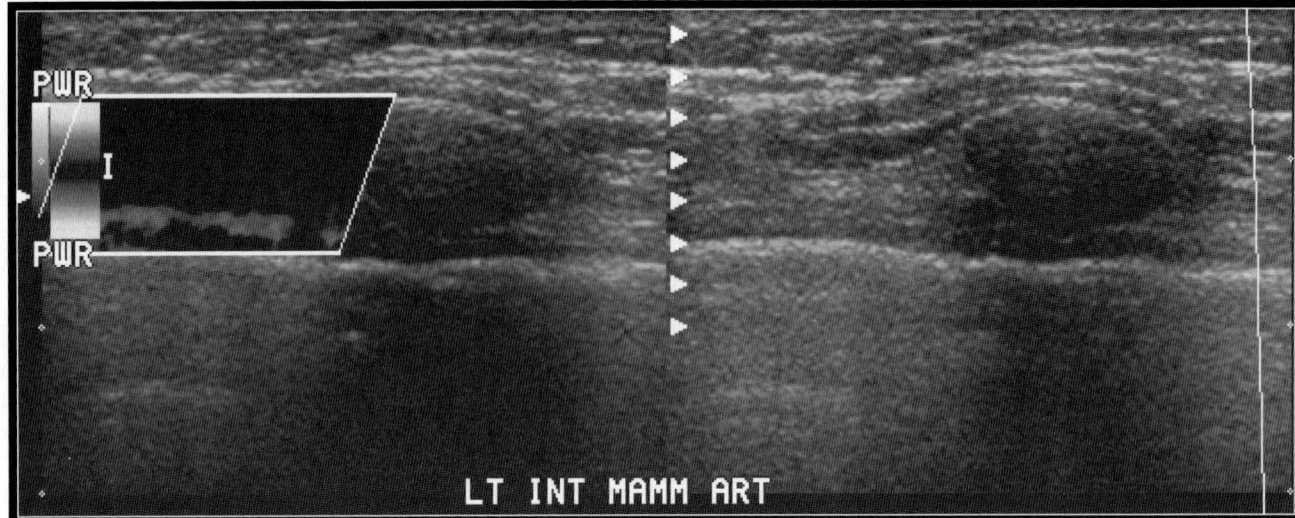

FIGURE 19–22 Color Doppler or power Doppler may aid in finding internal mammary lymph nodes by identifying the course of the internal mammary artery and veins. The internal mammary lymph node chain lies parallel to the artery and vein.

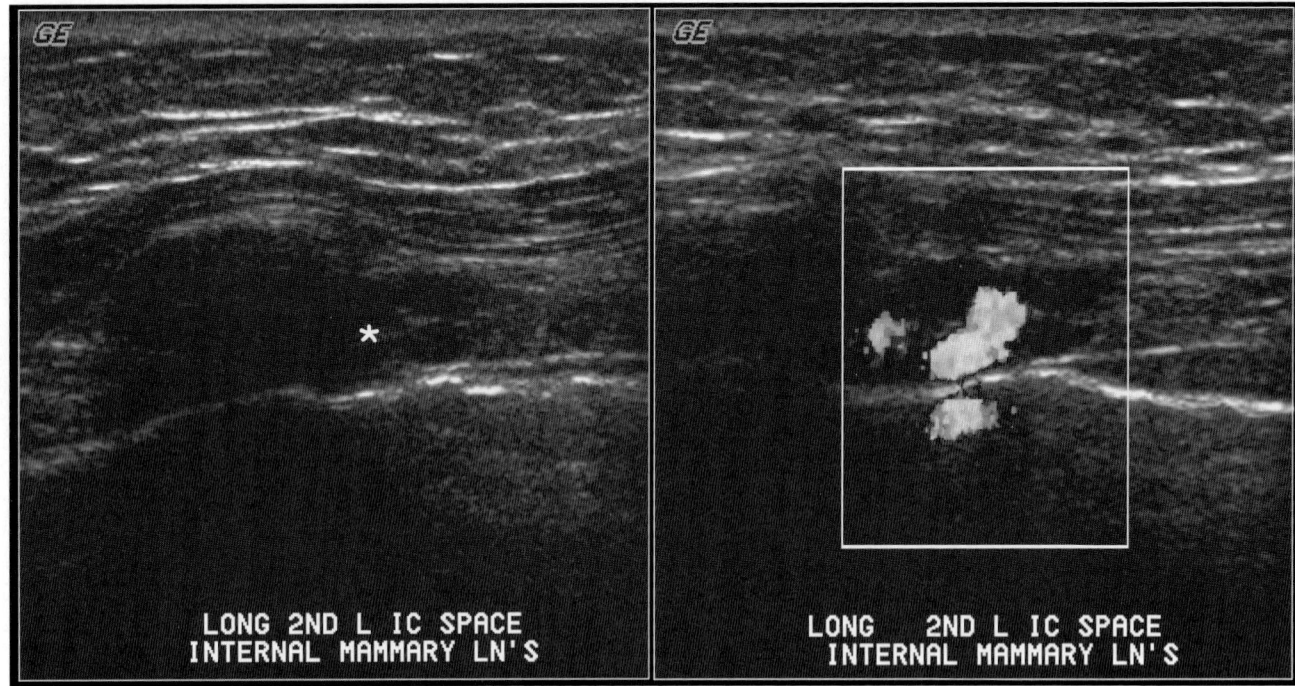

FIGURE 19–23 Color Doppler or power Doppler may help to distinguish hypoechoic internal mammary lymph nodes from prominent tortuous internal mammary veins (*). This distinction may be difficult using only the B-mode image.

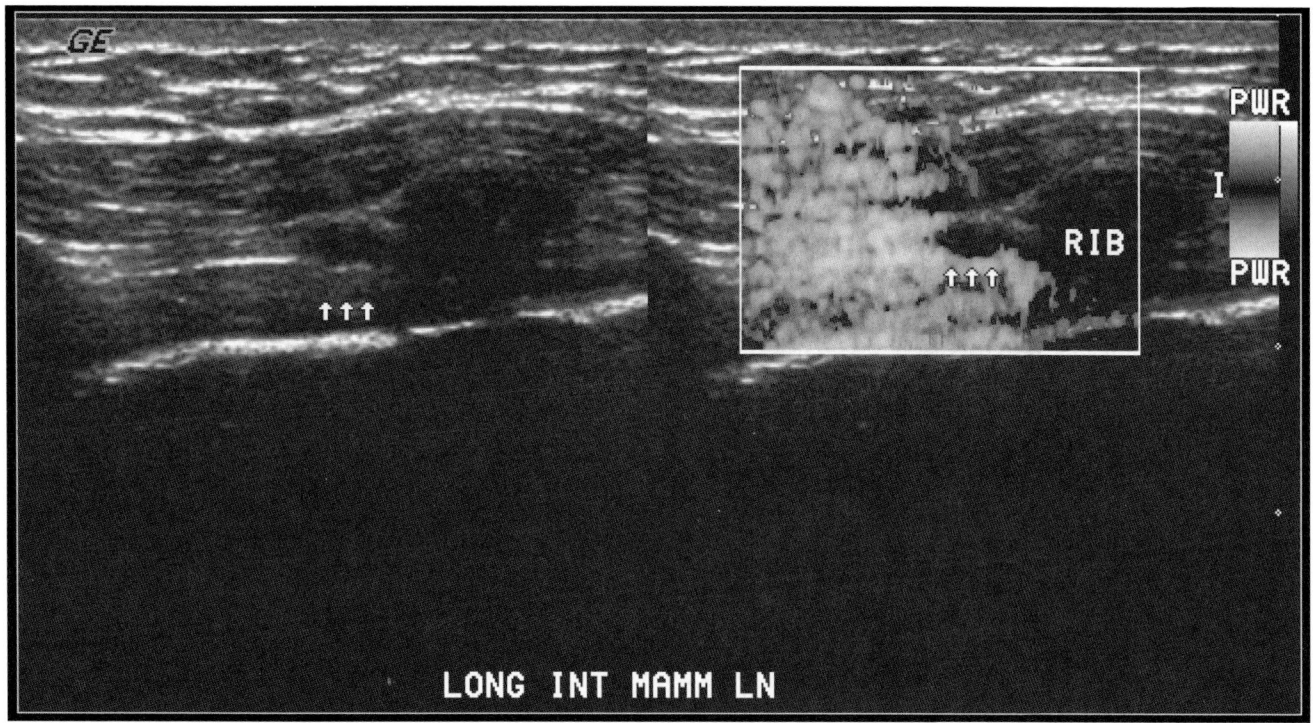

FIGURE 19–24 Internal mammary lymph nodes vibrate much less than the surrounding muscles and tendons in the chest wall during the power Doppler vocal fremitus maneuver, creating a defect in the acoustic vibratory artifact *(arrows)*.

chain that is roughly parallel to the internal mammary chain. They most frequently present as palpable lumps in very thin and small-breasted women (Fig. 19–27). To our knowledge, they have not been reported in the literature, possibly because they lie so superficially that they are difficult to visualize without an acoustic standoff or 1.5-dimensional array transducer (Fig. 19–28). We have not seen reports of these lymph nodes in the anatomic or histologic literature, and they are only rarely visible mammographically because they lie too close to the chest wall to be visible on mammograms in most patients (Fig. 19–29). We have termed these far medial intramammary lymph nodes medial *external mammary lymph nodes* because they lie roughly parallel to the internal mammary lymph nodes, but superficial to the chest wall. Most of these medial external mammary lymph nodes have been sonographically normal, but we have seen silicone granulomas, lymphoma (Fig. 19–30), and metastases (Fig. 19–31) within these nodes.

It should be remembered that the entire spectrum of diseases that affect axillary lymph nodes can affect intramammary lymph nodes in any location. Thus, intramammary nodes may be inflamed or involved with various neoplastic processes, including breast cancer metastases and lymphoma. It is also important to remember that an intramammary lymph node can be the sentinel lymph

(text continued on page 853)

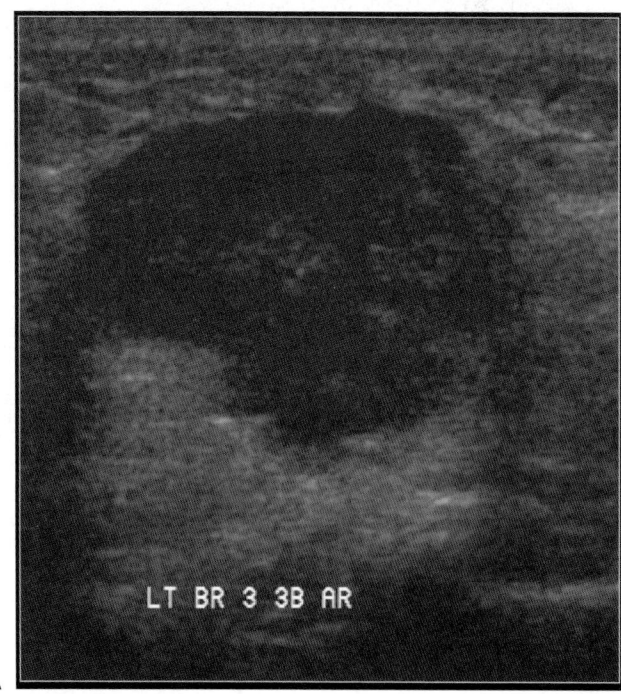

FIGURE 19–25 A: Internal mammary lymph nodes most frequently occur with laterally located lesions that have extensive axillary lymph node metastases. This high-grade invasive ductal carcinoma lies in the far lateral aspect of the breast. *(Continued.)*

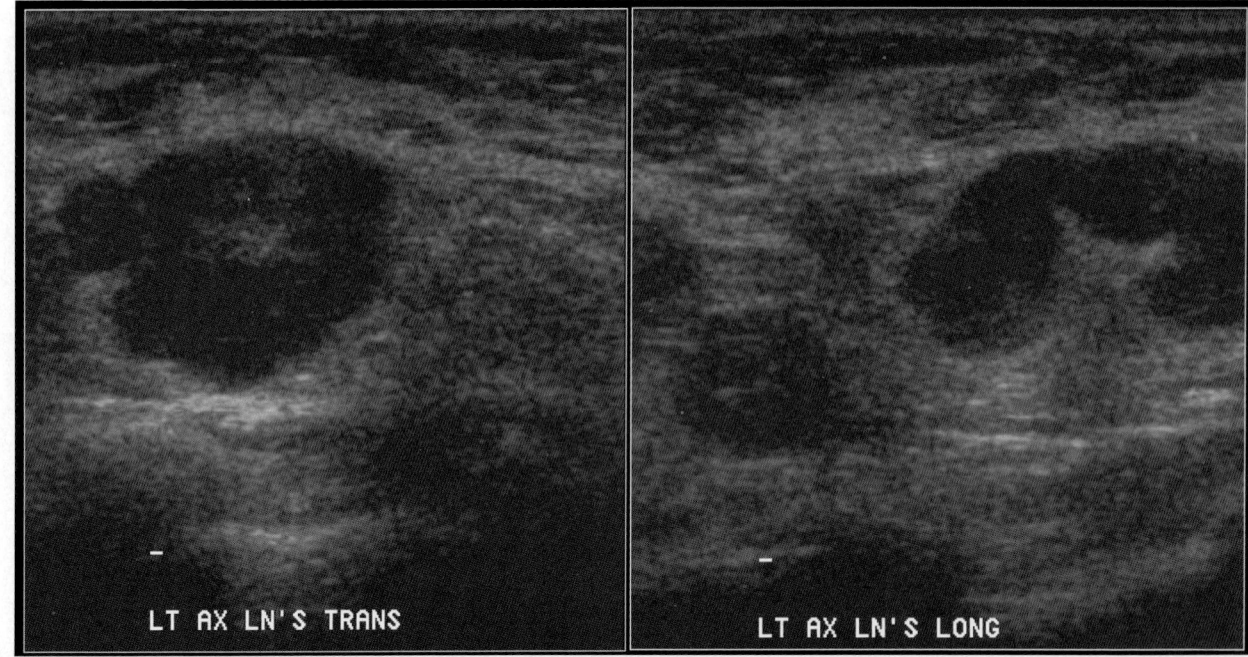

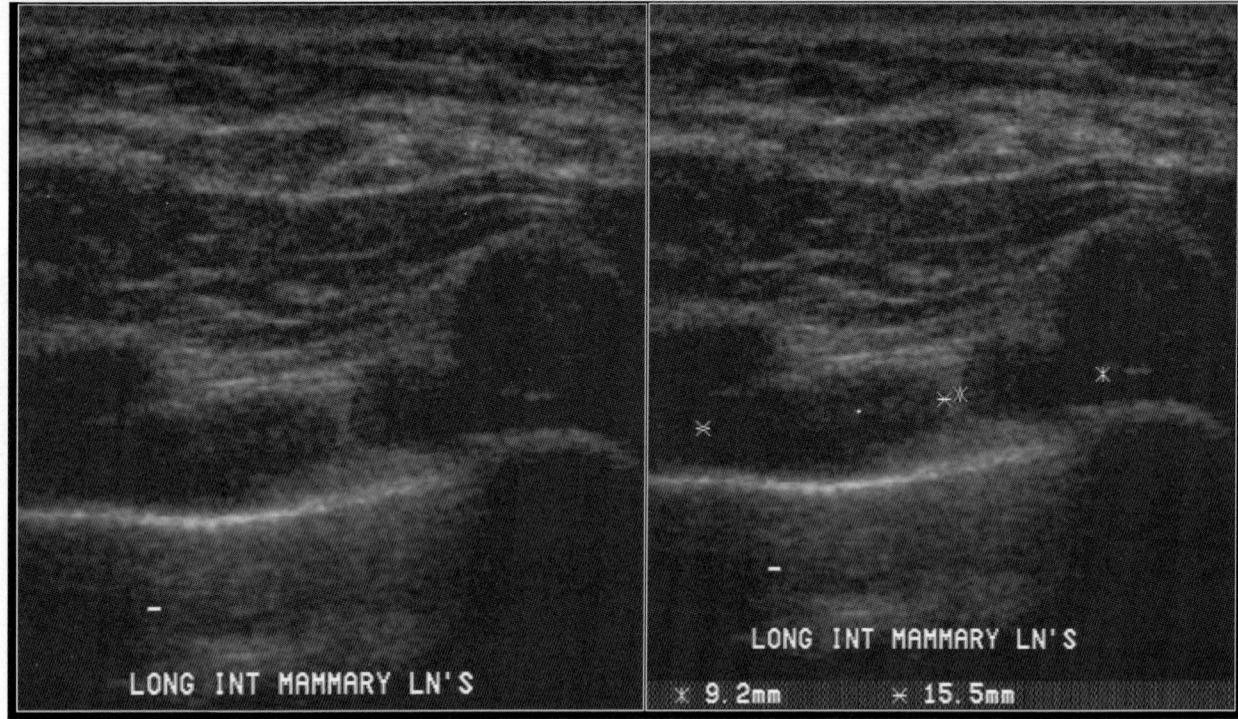

FIGURE 19–25 *(continued)* **B:** The lesion shown in Fig. 19–26B was associated with severe axillary lymphadenopathy. Extensive axillary metastases create a so-called tumor dam, blocking the normal lymphatic drainage pattern and increasing the likelihood of collateral flow through the internal mammary lymph node chain. **C:** The primary lesion shown in Fig. 19–26A and the metastasis-laden axillary lymph nodes shown in Fig. 19–26B were associated with extensive internal mammary lymph node metastases *(calipers)*.

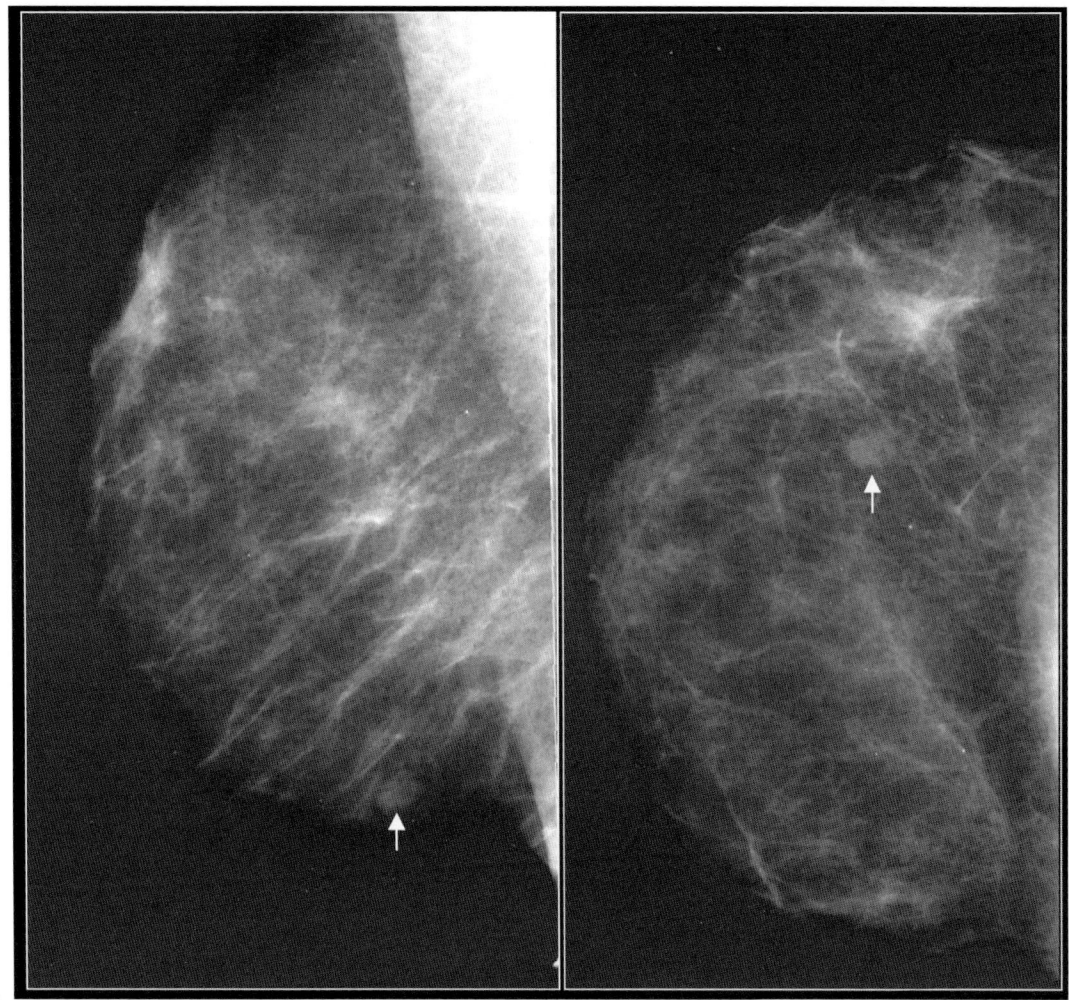

A

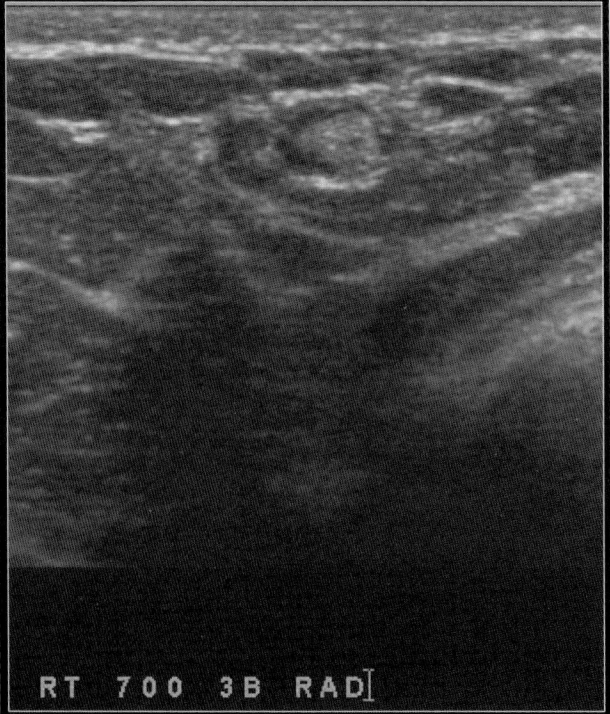

B

FIGURE 19–26 A: Although intramammary lymph nodes most commonly occur in the upper outer quadrants, they can occur in any part of the breast. This intramammary node lies near the 7:00 position, far inferiorly in the right breast. **B:** This sonographically normal (BIRADS 2) intramammary lymph node (shown mammographically in Fig. 19–26A) lies at 7:00 in the right breast.

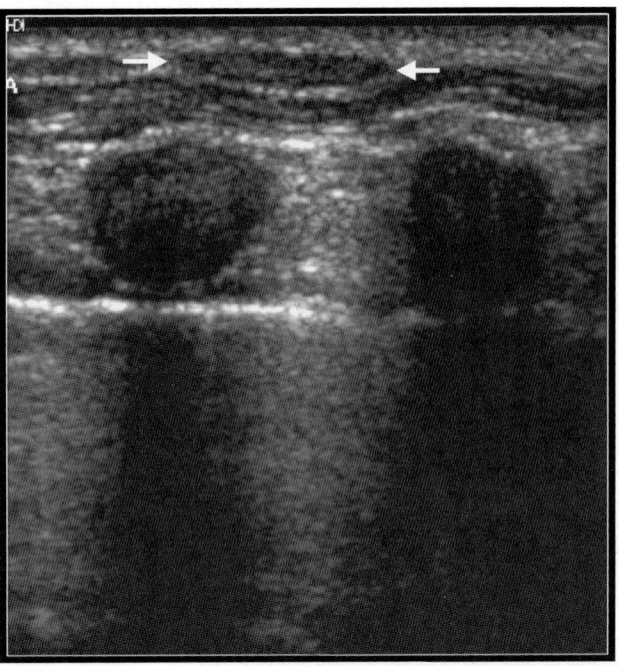

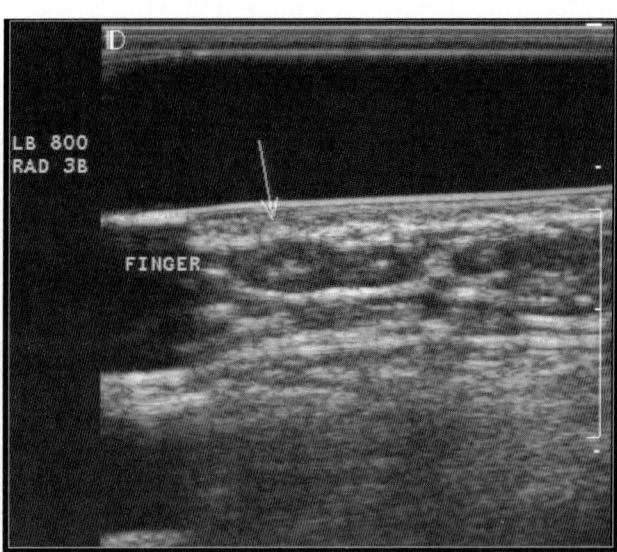

FIGURE 19–28 External mammary lymph nodes lie so superficially that they can be difficult to demonstrate without an acoustic standoff.

FIGURE 19–27 Intramammary lymph nodes that lie far medially in the breast usually present as palpable lumps in thin women with small breasts. There is a chain of such lymph nodes that lies parallel to the internal mammary lymph nodes that we have termed the medial *external mammary lymph nodes.*

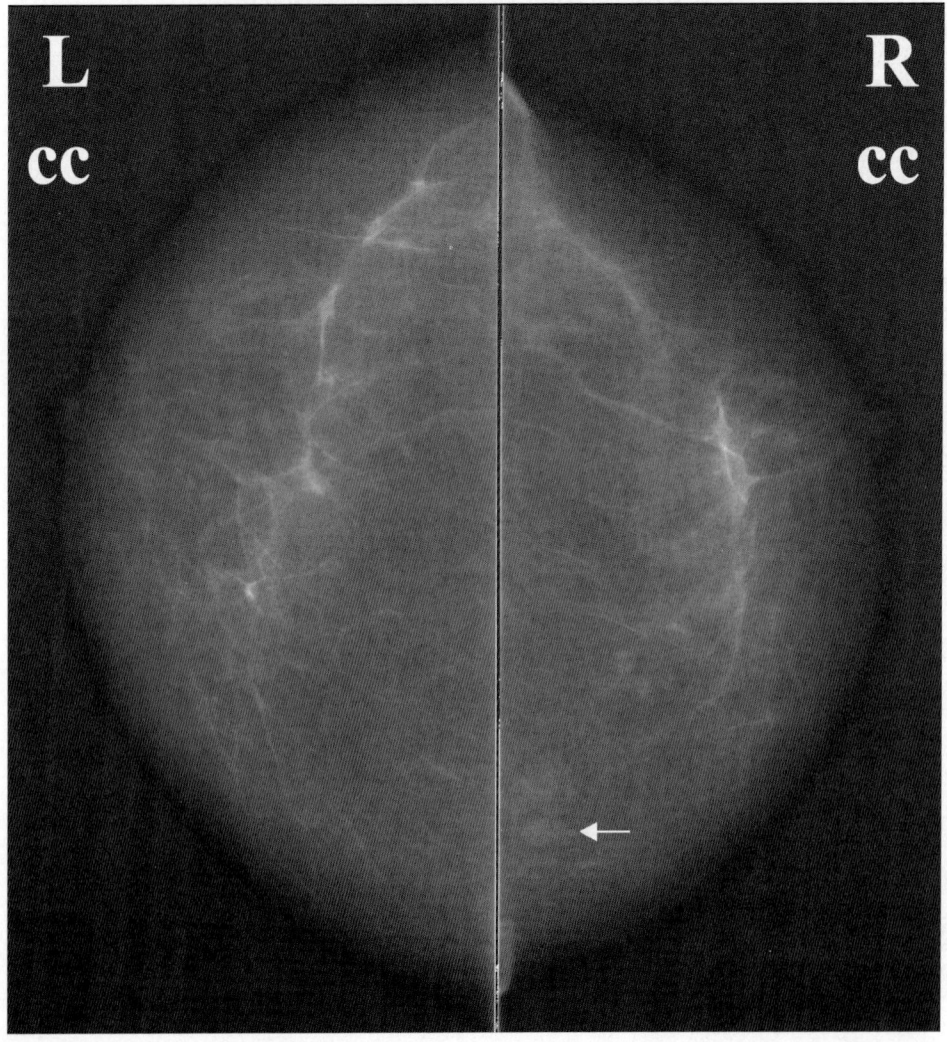

FIGURE 19–29 Medial external mammary lymph nodes are not mammographically demonstrable very often because they lie so close to the chest wall in women with small breasts that mammographic compression cannot project them far enough away from the chest wall for them to be visible mammographically. The few cases in which we have seen them occurred in patients with larger fatty breasts.

node (Fig. 19–32). Intramammary lymph nodes that are replaced with metastasis are more prone than larger axillary lymph nodes to have a pseudocystic appearance, particularly when the primary breast lesion is high-grade invasive ductal carcinoma or medullary carcinoma. Either color Doppler or power Doppler are essential in such cases in avoiding false characterization of the metastatic lymph nodes as a cyst (see the color images in Chapter 20, Fig. 20–26). For reasons that are unclear, medullary carcinoma can stimulate hyperplasia in intramammary and axillary lymph nodes that causes them to be enlarged and indistinguishable from metastasis containing lymph nodes.

Supraclavicular Lymph Nodes

Supraclavicular nodes are seldom evaluated unless there is a palpable lump or mass and unless there is suspicion of recurrent metastatic breast carcinoma (Fig. 19–33). In such

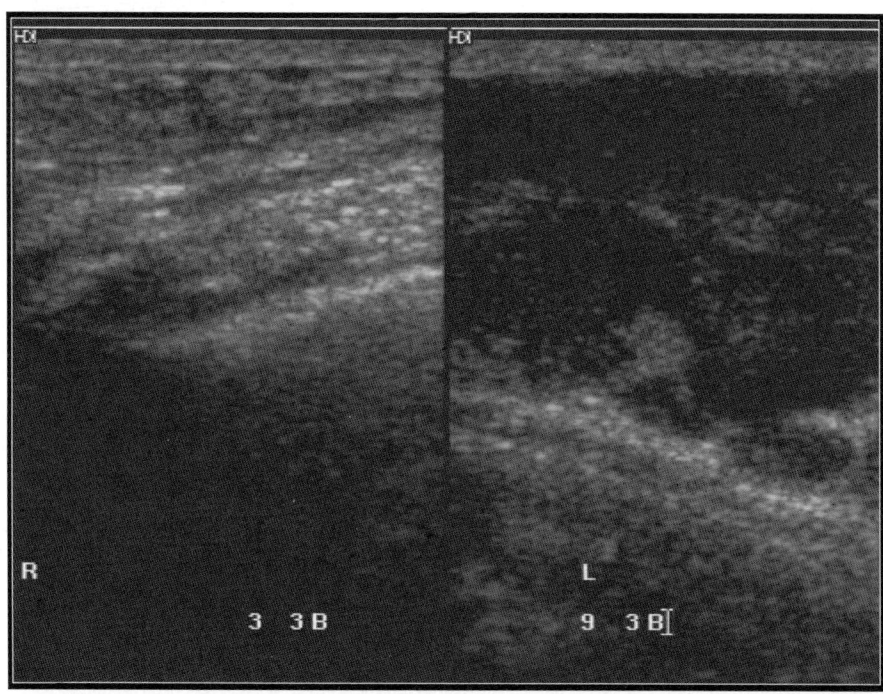

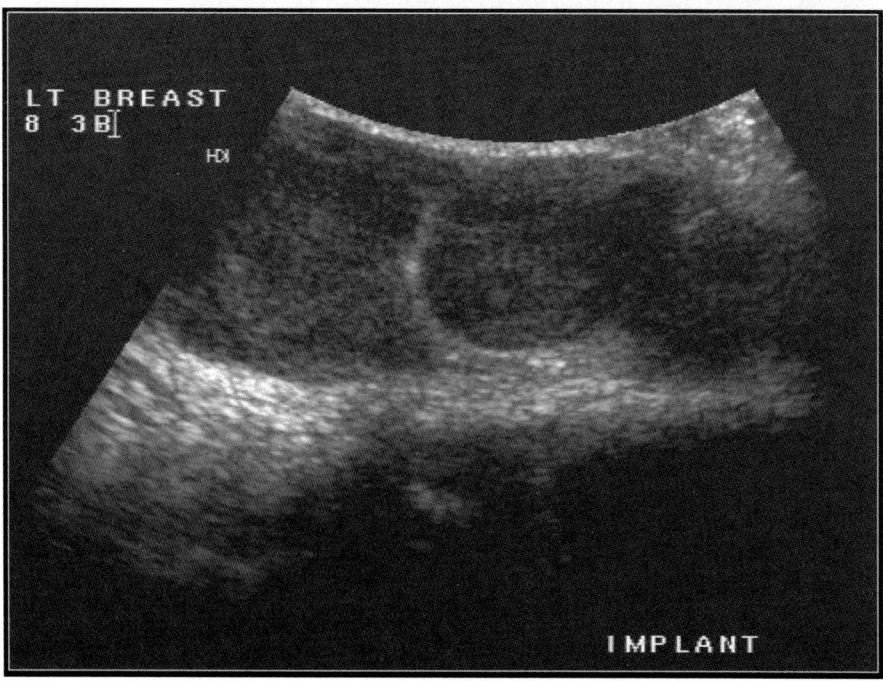

FIGURE 19–30 A: Split-screen images of the extreme medial mirror-image areas in the right and left breast show a large hypoechoic mass on the **left**. **B:** Long-axis view through the mass shows multiple masses that represent lymphomatous involvement of the external mammary lymph node chain.

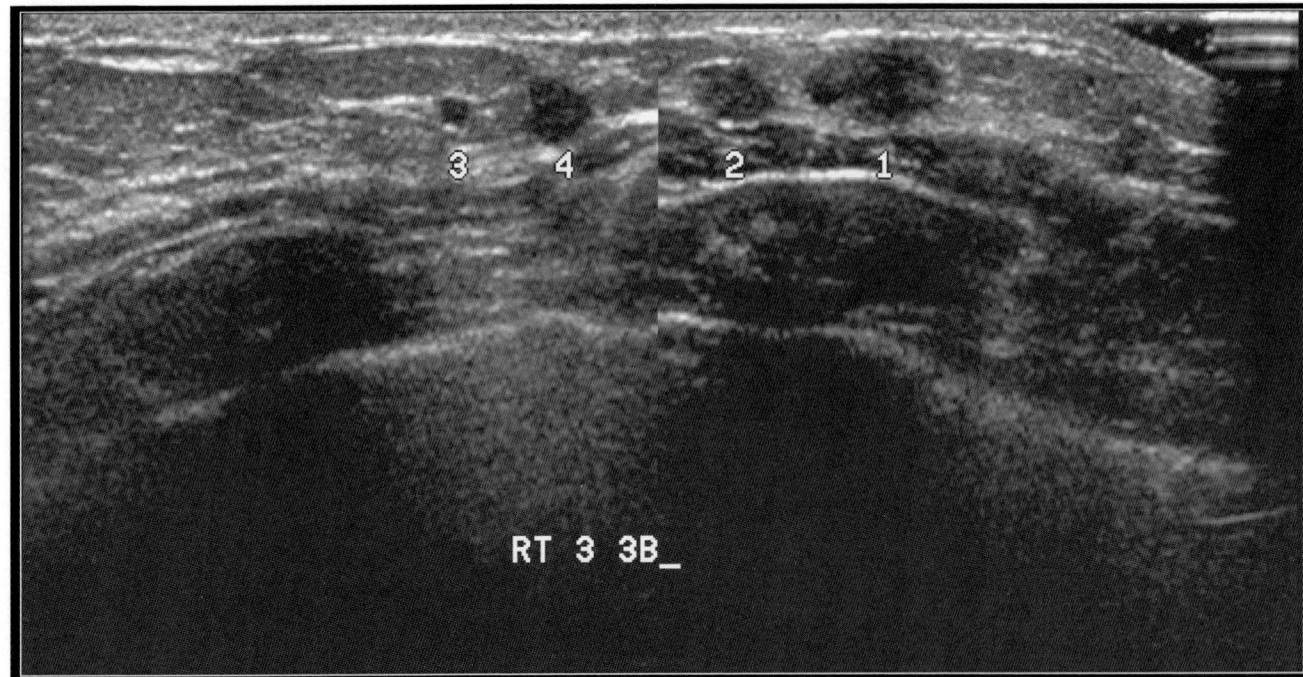

FIGURE 19–31 This patient with breast cancer has multiple metastases in the medial external mammary lymph node chain.

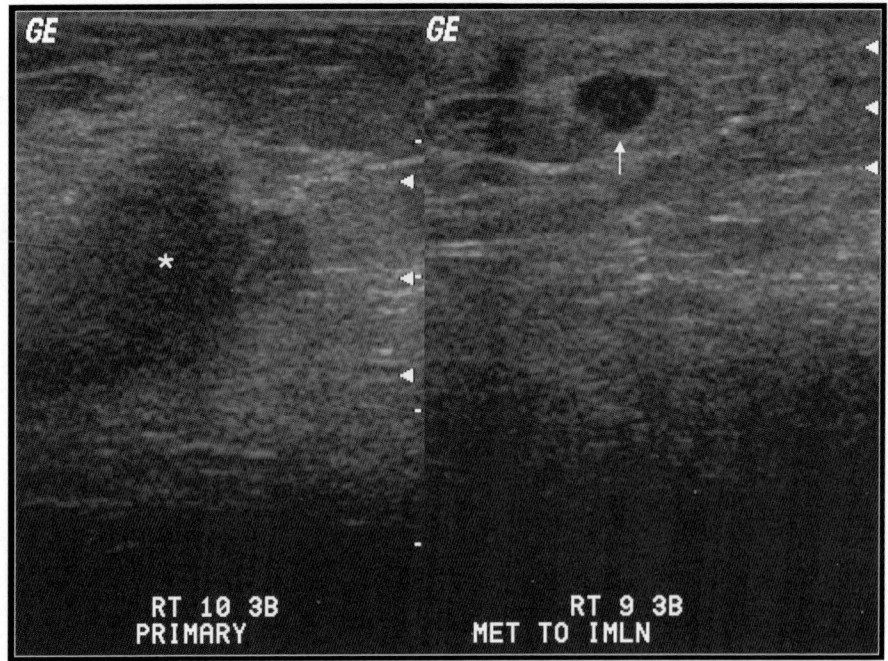

FIGURE 19–32 The sentinel lymph node may be an intramammary lymph node *(arrow)* (* indicates primary breast carcinoma).

cases, enlargement of supraclavicular nodes must be assumed to represent metastatic breast cancer until proved otherwise. This is especially true of Doppler flow studies that are suspicious for neoplasm. Ultrasound-guided biopsy frequently is used to verify the suspicion.

SONOGRAPHIC ASSESSMENT OF ABNORMAL LYMPH NODES

There are three different levels at which we evaluate lymph nodes. The first level is to determine whether the nodule is a lymph node or some other type of nodule. The second level is to determine whether the lymph node is sonographically normal. The third and most difficult level is to determine whether the findings that make a lymph node to appear abnormal are caused by inflammation or neoplasm. Several different sonographic and Doppler findings can be employed to aid in the assessment of inflammation versus malignancy and are listed in Table 19–1.

Size: Maximum Diameter

A diameter greater than 1 cm has been suggested as the sign of an abnormal axillary lymph node. This is too small if the maximum diameter is used to assess the lymph node. Many normal axillary lymph nodes are more than 1 cm in maximum diameter. If a minimum diameter of 1 cm is used, this measurement is more useful, but is still not as good as morphologic assessment of the node. Normal lymph nodes tend to be elliptical and flattened in the dimension that lies in a plane perpendicular to the chest wall. If a 1-cm cutoff value is used, it should only be used for this shortest dimension of the lymph node (Fig. 19–34). Even then, many normal fatty replaced lymph nodes will exceed 1 cm in shortest diameter (Fig. 19–35), and some metastatic-containing nodes that are morphologically abnormal, particularly internal mammary and intramammary nodes, will be less than 1 cm (Fig. 19–36). Of all the criteria, size appears to be the least useful unless the lymph node is grossly enlarged. Additionally, although size may be of some help in distinguishing between normal and abnor-

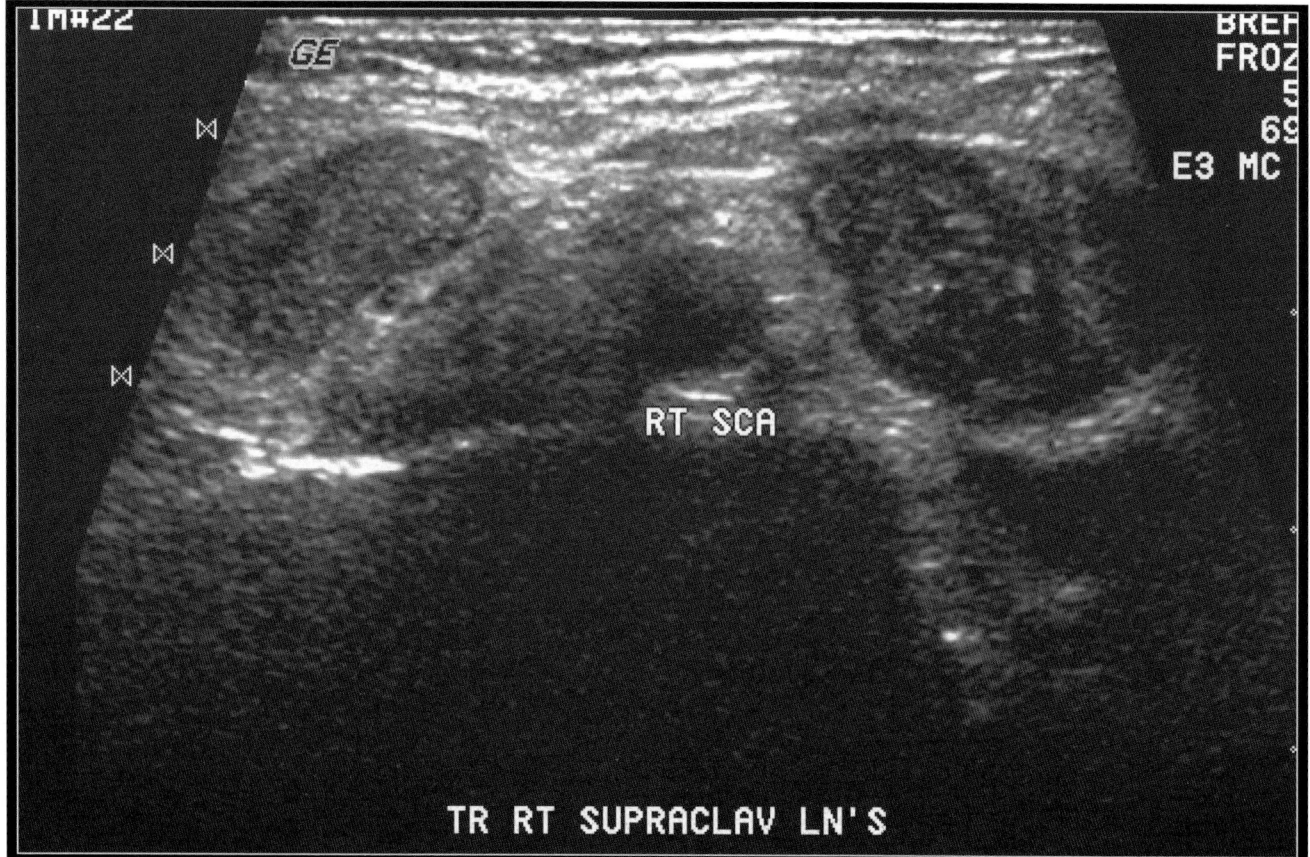

FIGURE 19–33 Metastases to supraclavicular lymph nodes are considered distant metastases. This patient has multiple grossly enlarged and distorted supraclavicular nodes.

TABLE 19–1. SONOGRAPHIC FINDINGS OF ABNORMAL LYMPH NODES

Size—enlarged diameter

Shape—rounding

Echogenicity—markedly hypoechoic cortex

Morphologic abnormalities
   Cortical thickening—uniform versus eccentric
   Hilar compression—uniform versus eccentric
   Hilar indentation—convex "rat bit"
   Hilar displacement
   Hilar obliteration
   Loss of echogenic outer capsule and angular margins

Relationship between adjacent lymph nodes

Right-to-left symmetry or asymmetry

Color Doppler flow pattern

Pulsed Doppler spectral analysis waveform pattern

mal lymph nodes, it is of minimal value in distinguishing between inflammatory and neoplastic enlargement, except in the dimension that leads to a change in lymph node shape and leads to abnormal rounding of the lymph node. What differs in fatty replaced nodes and metastatic nodes that are abnormally enlarged by any defined diameter is the thickness of the cortex. Because metastatic disease is a subcapsular and cortical process, morphologic assessment of the cortex is more solidly based in the histology of lymph node metastases than is the size of the lymph node.

Shape: Abnormal Rounding

Normal lymph nodes are elliptically shaped, having long and short axes. They also tend to be rotated into an orientation during sonographic compression that places the flattened or short axis perpendicular to the chest wall (see Chapter 6, Fig. 6–13). Inflammatory enlargement tends to enlarge the lymph node proportionately in all planes, leading to elliptically shaped enlargement. Neoplastic involvement, on the other hand, is more likely to enlarge the lymph node disproportionately in its shortest plane, leading to abnormal "rounding" of the lymph node. In the most severely involved lymph nodes, the shape may be nearly spherical (Fig. 19–37). In severe cases of necrotizing

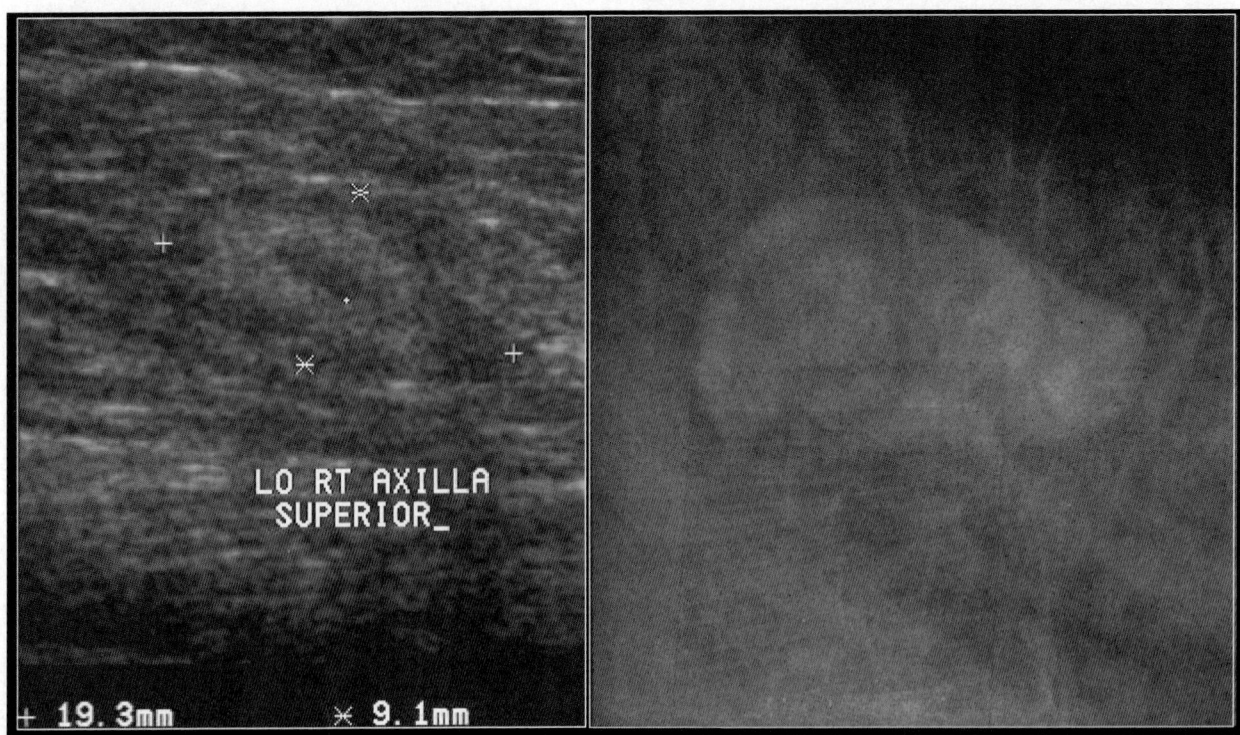

FIGURE 19–34 This normal lymph node has a maximum diameter of more than 1 cm but has uniform cortical thickness and is morphologically and histologically normal. If a 1-cm diameter criterion is used to assess the normalcy of a lymph node, it should be applied only to the shortest diameter of the node. The shortest diameter usually lies perpendicular to the chest wall during sonography and is less than 1 cm, a normal measurement, in this patient.

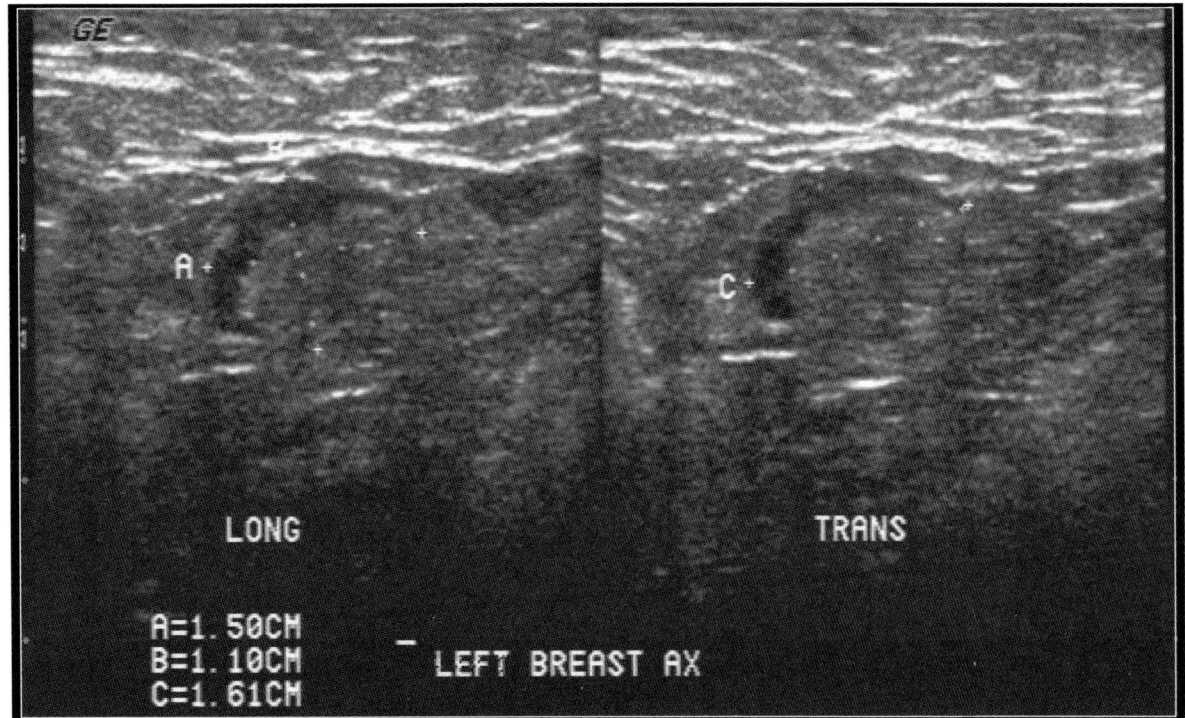

FIGURE 19–35 Many normal lymph nodes that have extensive fatty replacement within the mediastinum have minimum diameters greater than 1 cm. The fatty replacement not only enlarges the nodes but also makes them slightly rounder and less elliptical in shape.

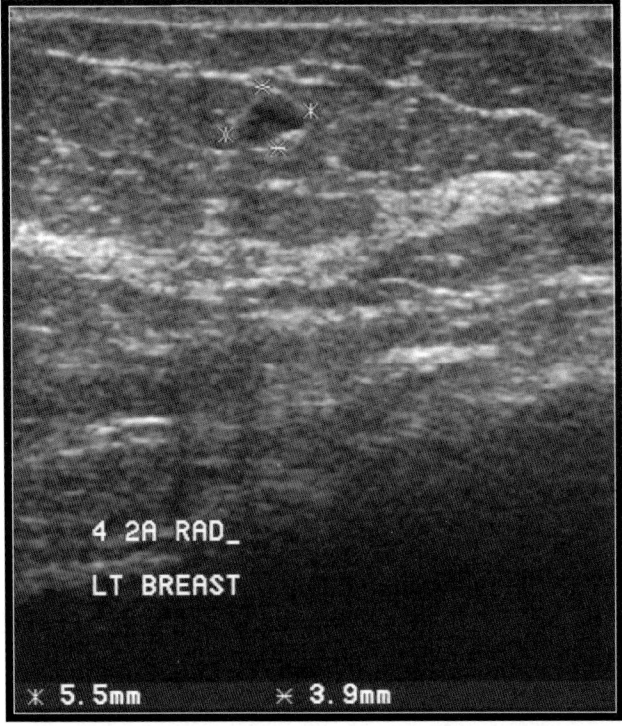

FIGURE 19–36 Some metastasis-containing lymph nodes can have maximum diameters of less than 1 cm. This is particular likely to happen with intramammary and internal mammary nodes than contain metastatic disease.

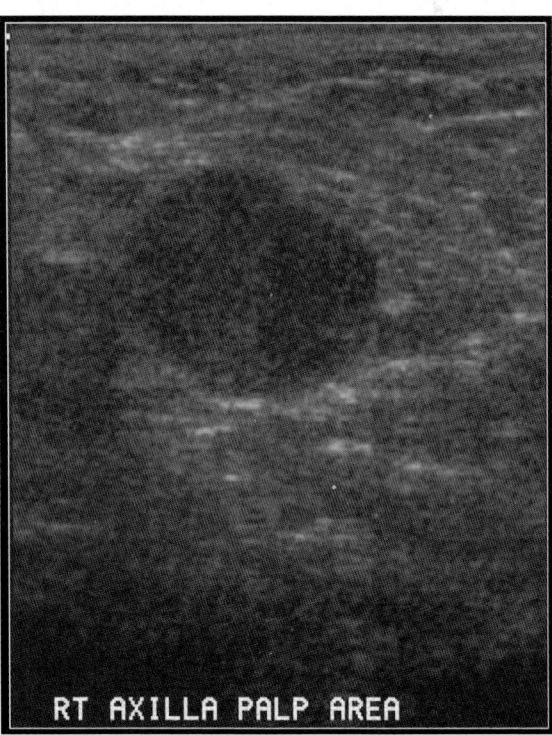

FIGURE 19–37 Lymph nodes that are extensively replaced with metastasis become rounder. In severe cases, they may be nearly spherical in shape.

lymphadenitis, however, the lymph nodes can also become spherical in shape. Even fatty replaced nodes may be rounded and nearly spherical in shape (Fig. 19–10). What differs in fatty replaced nodes and metastatic nodes that are abnormally rounded is the thickness of the cortex. Because metastatic disease is a subcapsular and cortical process, morphologic assessment of the cortex is more solidly based in the histology of lymph node metastases than is shape of the lymph node.

Echogenicity: Marked Hypoechogenicity of the Cortex

The cortex of abnormal lymph nodes tends to become markedly hypoechoic. It may become so hypoechoic that it appears nearly anechoic, causing the lymph node to assume a pseudocystic appearance that can be distinguished from a true cyst only by demonstrating internal vessels with color Doppler. Although such pseudocystic involvement of the lymph node cortex is more typical of neoplastic than inflammatory involvement, it may occur in severe cases of

inflammation, especially in cases of necrotizing lymphadenitis. The decrease in echogenicity is merely a manifestation of the high cellularity and homogeneity of the abnormal lymph node, whether the high cellularity reflects mainly lymphoid hyperplasia, metastasis with lymphoid hyperplasia, or metastatic tumor cells. Additionally, high-frequency coded harmonics tends to make even the cortex of completely normal lymph nodes appear markedly hypoechoic. Thus, hypoechogenicity is of most value in distinguishing the cortex from the mediastinum of the lymph node, facilitating morphologic assessment of the cortex.

Morphologic Changes in the Lymph Node

Morphologic changes in the lymph nodes that help us distinguish inflamed nodes from those that contain metastases are summarized in collage form in Figs. 19–38 and 19–39. The morphologic assessment of lymph nodes appropriately focuses most of the attention on the cortex of the lymph node. Foreign bodies tend to accumulate in the medullary sinuses of the lymph node, affecting the medi-

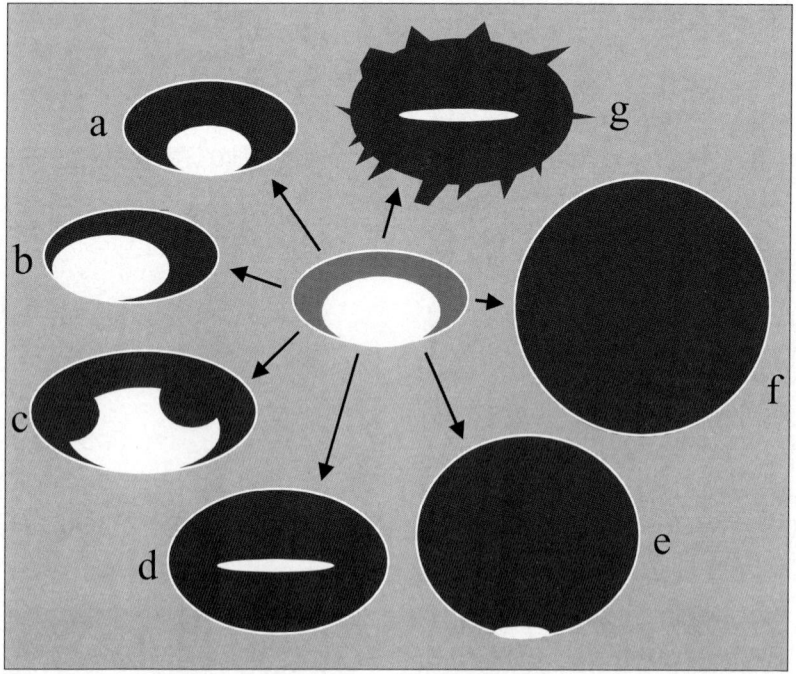

FIGURE 19–38 This figure shows the spectrum of abnormal lymph nodes. In the center is an illustration of a normal lymph node. **A:** A lymph node with uniformly mildly thickened cortex that is typical of inflamed or reactive nodes. **B:** eccentric cortical thickening, which favors metastatic disease. **C:** Convex indentations of the mediastinum (rat bites) that favor metastatic disease. **D:** Severe compression of the mediastinum to a slitlike configuration that can occur in metastatic disease or severely inflamed lymph nodes. **E:** Severe eccentric compression and displacement of the mediastinum to the edge of the node that favors metastatic disease. **F:** Complete mediastinal obliteration and rounding of the lymph node that favors metastatic disease but that can also occur in cases of severe necrotizing lymphadenitis. **G:** Perinodal invasion by metastasis. The outer thin, echogenic capsule of the lymph node has been destroyed and cannot be identified and the lymph node has angular margins.

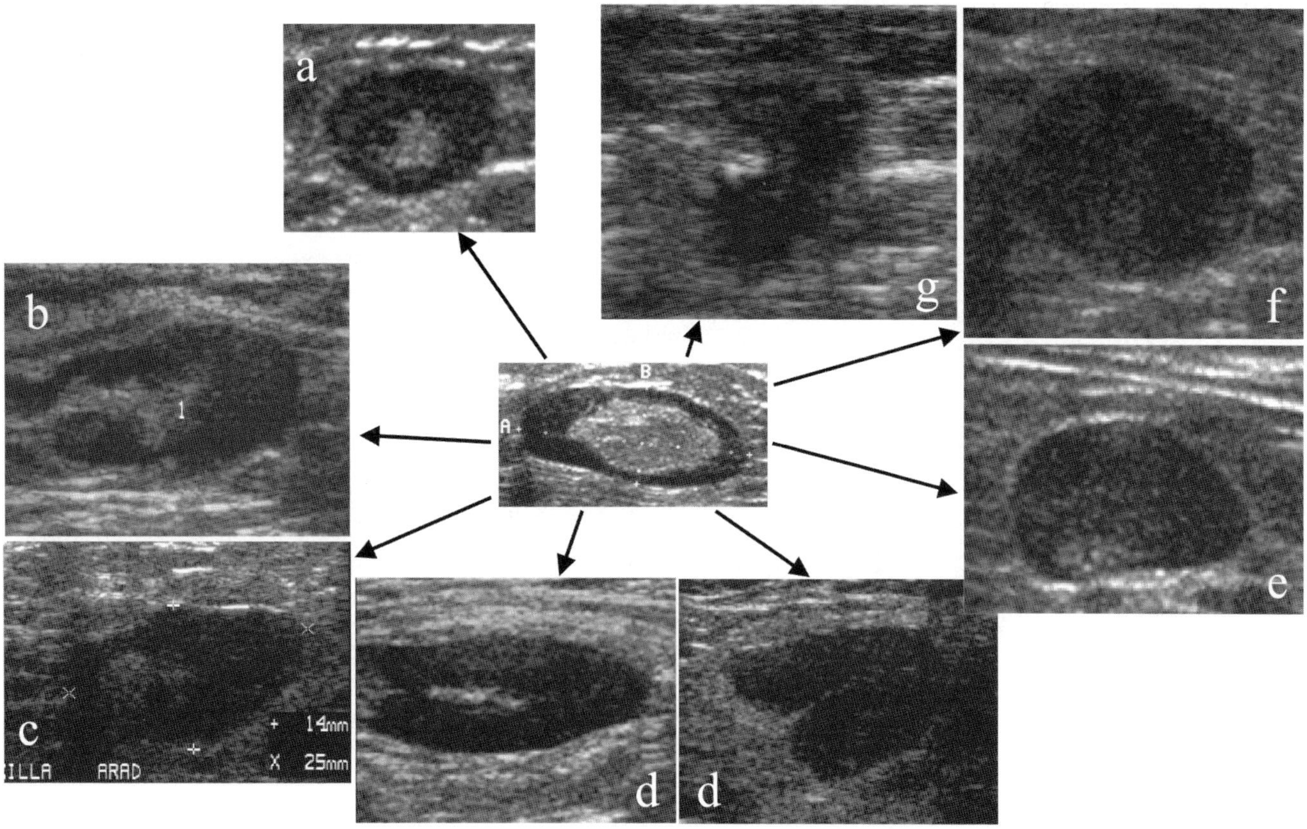

FIGURE 19–39 Range of abnormal sonographic LN appearances. This figure shows the spectrum of abnormal lymph nodes. In the **center** is a normal lymph node. **A:** A lymph node with uniformly mildly thickened cortex that is typical of inflamed or reactive nodes. **B:** Eccentric cortical thickening that favors metastatic disease. **C:** Convex indentations of the mediastinum (rat bites) that favor metastatic disease. **D:** Severe compression of the mediastinum to a slitlike configuration that can occur in metastatic disease or severely inflamed lymph nodes. **E:** Severe eccentric compression and displacement of the mediastinum to the edge of the node that favors metastatic disease. **F:** Complete mediastinal obliteration and rounding of the lymph node that favors metastatic disease but that can also occur in cases of severe necrotizing lymphadenitis. **G:** Perinodal invasion by metastasis. The outer thin, echogenic capsule of the lymph node has been destroyed and cannot be identified, and the lymph node has angular margins.

astinum first, and then affecting the cortex only late in the process (Fig. 19–40). Metastases, on the other hand, affect the subcapsular sinuses and cortical sinuses first, affecting the lymph node from the cortex inwardly (Fig. 19–41). The mediastinum is displaced and compressed inward by the thickening cortex. The out margins of the node can also be affected. Tumor deposits in the subcapsular sinuses tend to create focal outward bulges or lobulations in the outer contour of the lymph node. Tumor deposits in the more deeply located cortical sinusoids tend to create convex inward indentations into the mediastinum. Both processes lead to eccentric widening of the cortex early and to diffuse widening later on. Subcapsular deposits can invade through the capsule of the lymph node and can stimulate neovascularity that enters the node through abnormal routes. Thus, cortical changes are key to diagnosing lymph node metastases.

Eccentric Cortical Thickening

Metastatic cells enter the lymph node through the capsule through the afferent lymphatic and tend to lodge in the subcapsular and cortical sinuses of the lymph node. Early metastatic involvement of subcapsular and cortical sinuses is eccentric. Thus, early metastases can cause eccentric thickening and hypoechogenicity within the lymph node cortex (Fig. 19–42) and focal bulges of the cortex outwardly into surrounding perinodal fat or inwardly into the hyperechoic lymph node mediastinum (Fig. 19–43). Inflammation also affects the cortical thickness but tends to do so

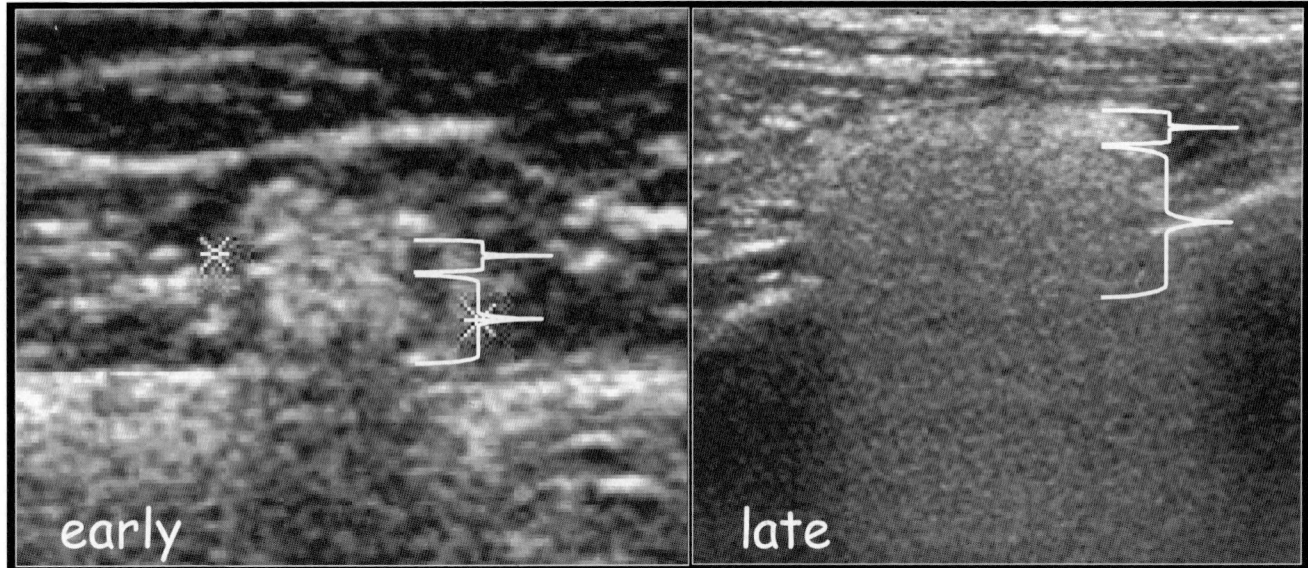

FIGURE 19–40 Foreign bodies such as silicone gel accumulate within the medullary sinuses first and only later fill the cortical sinuses. Early accumulation **(left)** within the medullary sinuses leads to little detectable change in echogenicity within the mediastinum *(large bracket)* but is evident because of the incoherent acoustic shadowing deep to the mediastinum. At this point, the cortex is still spared *(small bracket)*. Later, as more silicone gel accumulates **(right)**, the mediastinum assumes the classic "snowstorm" appearance *(large bracket)*. The cortex is also involved and has become hyperechoic *(small bracket)*.

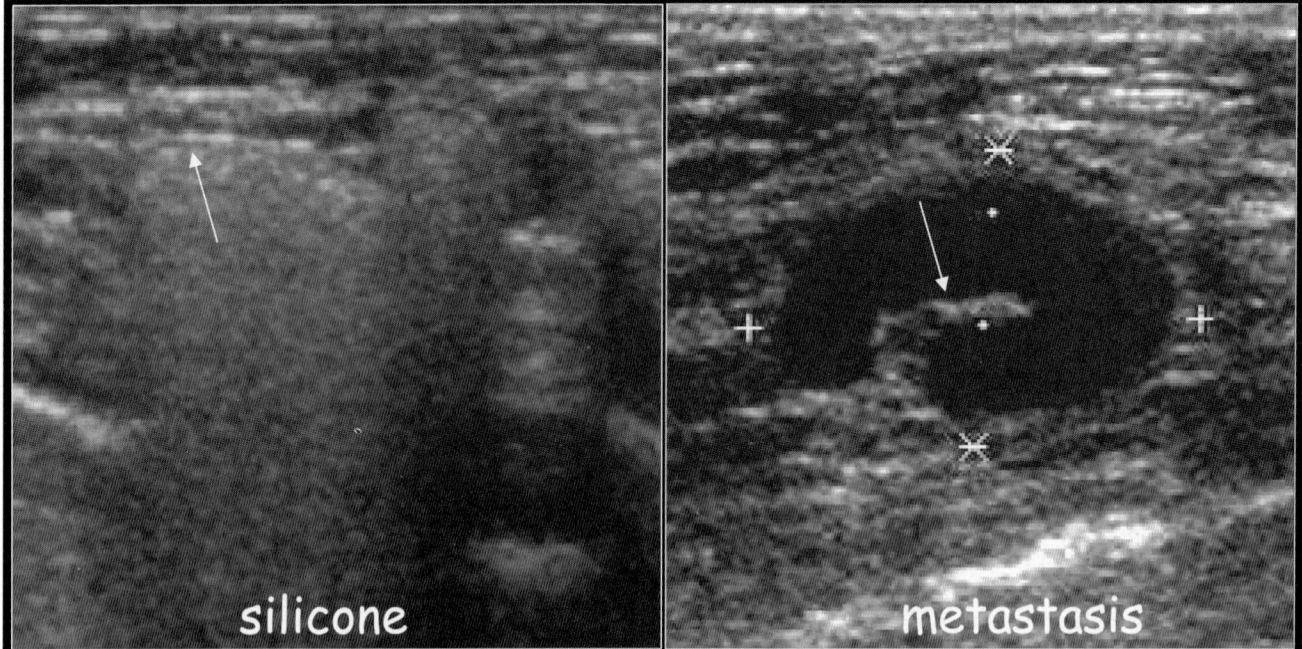

FIGURE 19–41 Foreign bodies such as silicone granulomas affect the lymph node from the mediastinum outwardly **(left)**. Tumor and infection, on the other hand, affect the lymph node from the subcapsular portion of the cortex inwardly **(right)**. Thus, analysis for metastasis requires attention to the cortex. The attention given to the mediastinum primarily concerns the effects of thickened cortex on the mediastinum.

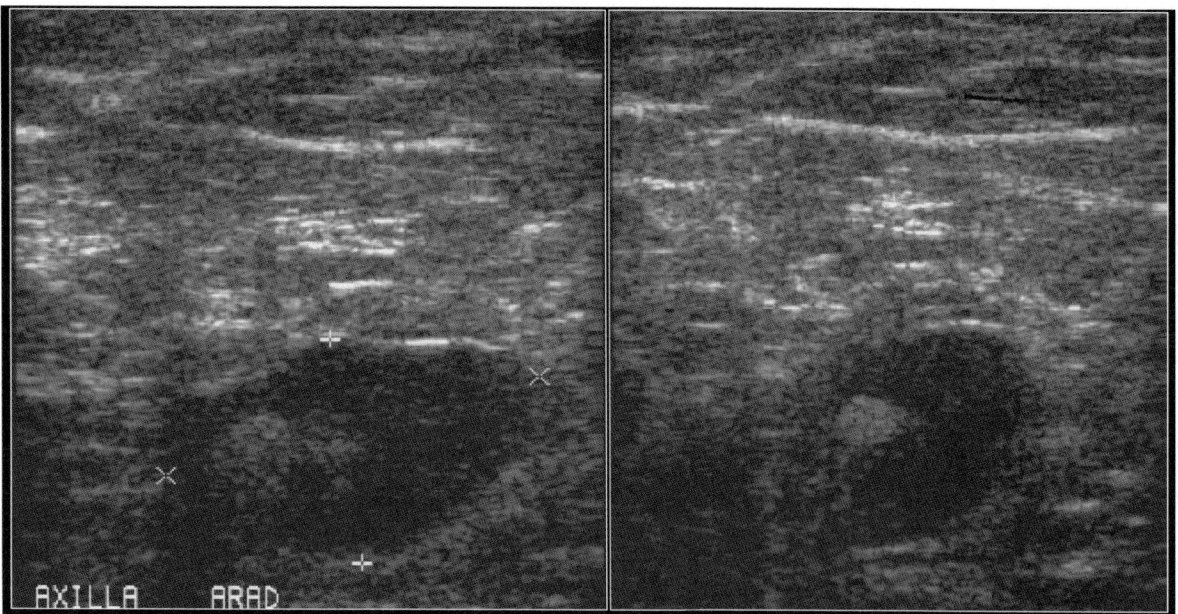

FIGURE 19–42 The hallmark of lymph node metastasis that has not completely replaced the involved lymph node is eccentric hypoechoic cortical thickening. Note that the cortex of this metastatic lymph node is eccentrically thickened and hypoechoic in both views (**left**, long-axis view; **right**, short-axis view).

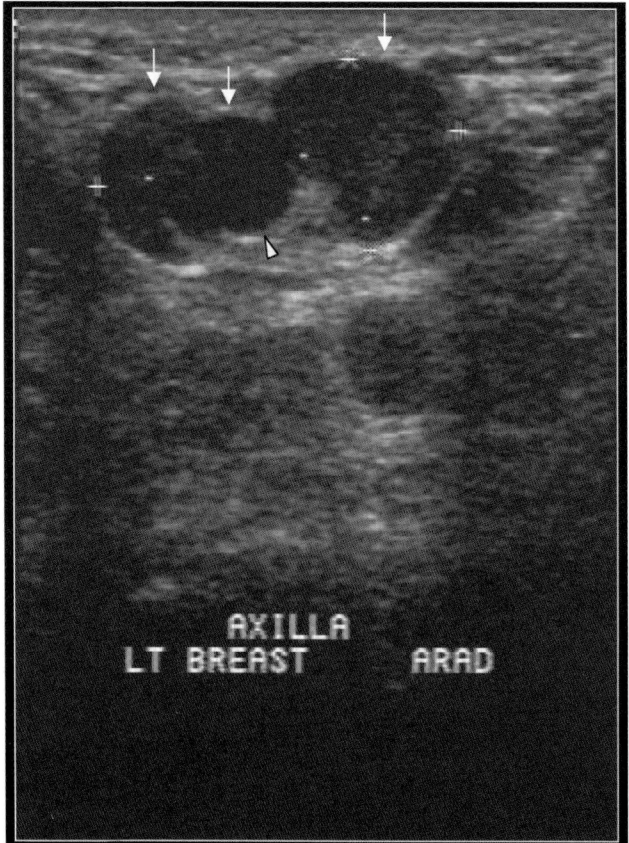

FIGURE 19–43 Eccentric cortical thickening may bulge outwardly, creating a lobulated outer contour *(arrows)* of the lymph node. Inflammation usually does not do this. Note that the echogenic mediastinum is also indented *(arrowhead)*, compressed, and displaced to the posterior edge of the node.

more uniformly (Fig. 19–44). Eccentric cortical thickening can occur in inflammation, when part of the cortex that has not been scarred thickens, but parts of the cortex that have been scarred cannot thicken (Fig. 19–45). In some lymph nodes that do not have a thickened cortex, a portion of cortex can be asymmetrically thinned and atrophic, simulating asymmetric thickening due to metastatic disease (Figs. 19–13 and 19–14). Late or severe metastatic involvement of the lymph node eventually tends to affect the entire cortex, causing more nearly uniform cortical thickening.

Eccentric Mediastinal Compression

The asymmetric cortical thickening caused by early metastatic disease can cause asymmetric compression of the hyperechoic lymph node mediastinum (Fig. 19–46). The more uniform cortical thickening caused by inflammation, on the other hand, tends to result in uniform compression of the mediastinum (Fig. 19–47). However, later on, metastases may involve the entire cortex and lead to more uniform compression of the mediastinum (Fig. 19–48).

Convex Inward Focal Compression of the Mediastinum—"Rat Bites"

Early metastatic deposits that lodge in the deep cortical sinusoids rather than the subcapsular sinusoids can cause focal thickening of the inner cortex of the lymph node that manifests as convex inward indentation of the hyperechoic lymph node mediastinum by hypoechoic cortex (Fig. 19–49). Such

(text continued on page 864)

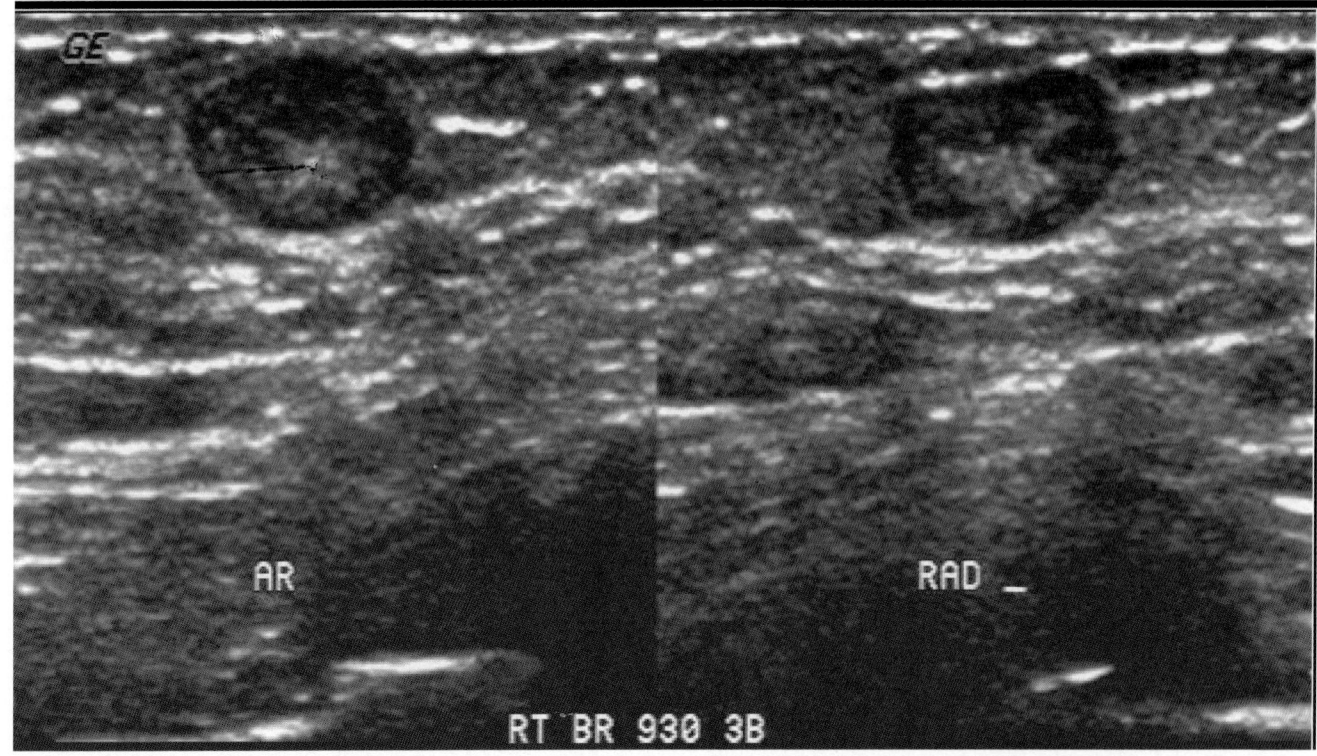

FIGURE 19–44 The cortical thickening caused by inflammation is usually more uniform than that caused by metastatic disease. Note that enlarged follicles in inflamed nodes can create convex indentations of the mediastinum similar to those caused by metastatic disease. However, the indentations are smaller, more numerous, more echogenic, and more evenly distributed than are those caused by metastases.

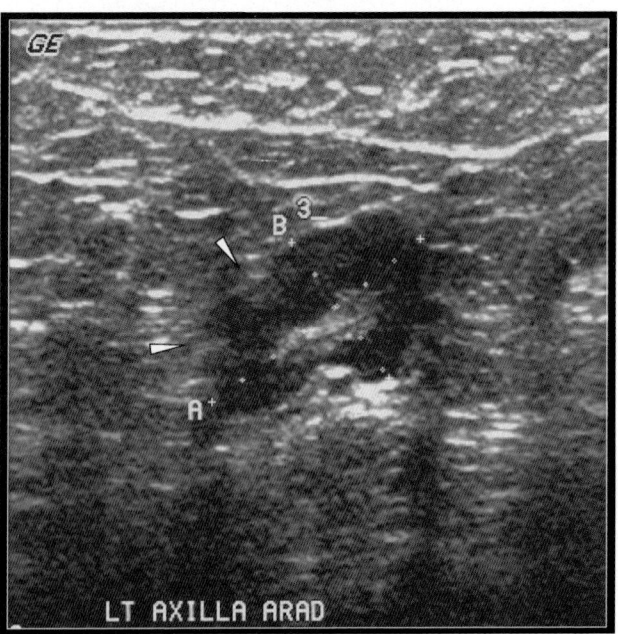

FIGURE 19–45 Occasionally, an inflamed lymph node that has previously undergone scarring will appear to have eccentrically thickened cortex because of the presence of thinner, scarred areas of cortex (*arrowheads*). Such nodes may be impossible to distinguish from metastatic nodes by sonography alone.

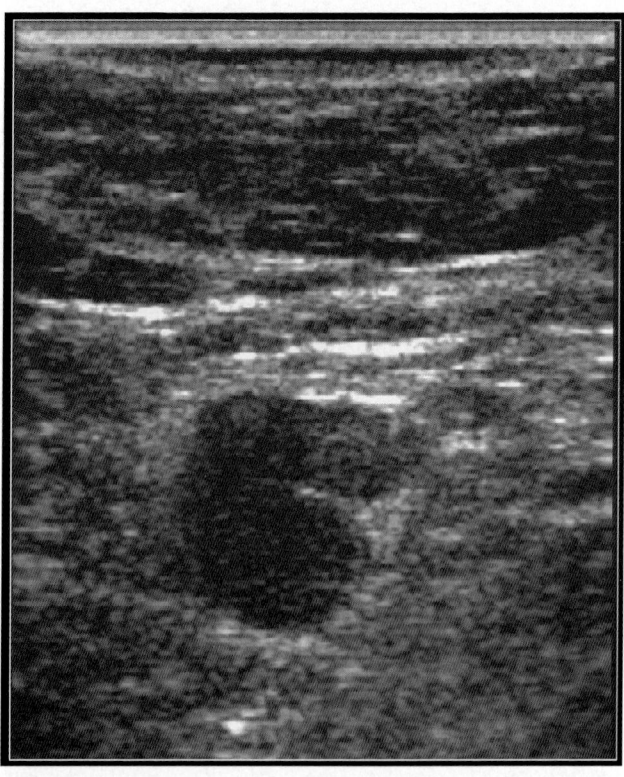

FIGURE 19–46 Metastases severely and eccentrically compress this lymph node mediastinum. It is compressed more from posteriorly than from anteriorly.

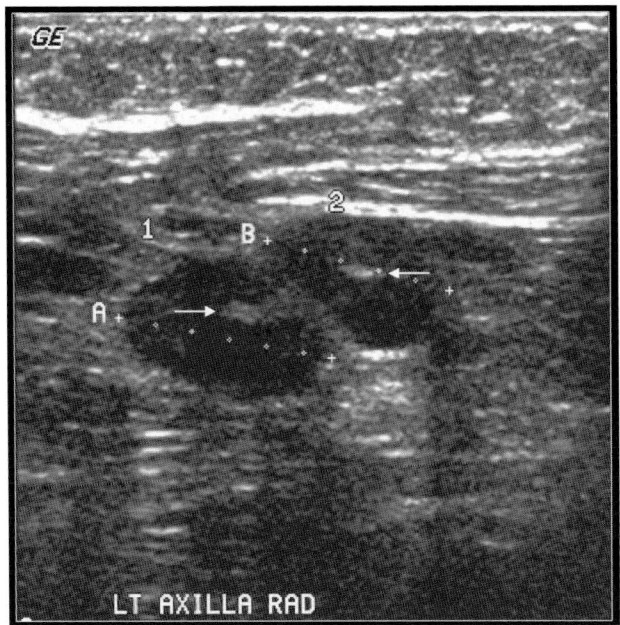

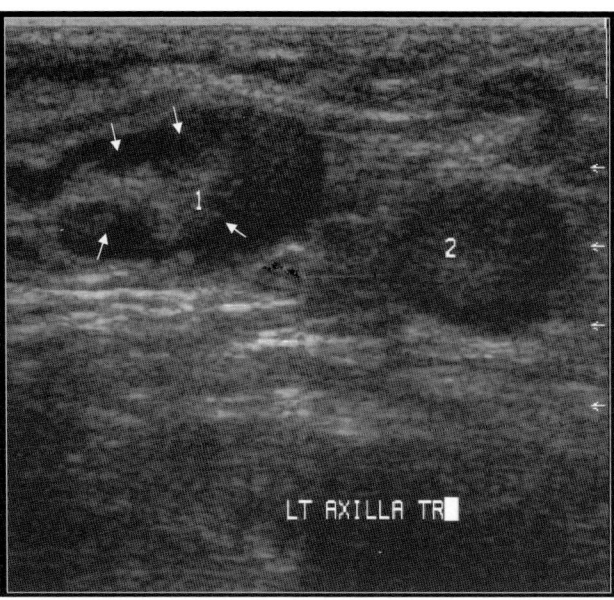

FIGURE 19–47 In severely inflamed lymph nodes, the mediastinum may also be so severely compressed that it becomes slit-like *(arrows)*. Inflammation usually compresses the mediastinum more symmetrically than does metastatic disease.

FIGURE 19–49 Convex inward nonuniform and eccentric indentations of the mediastinum ("rat bites") are characteristic of metastatic disease involving the deep cortical sinusoids *(arrows)*.

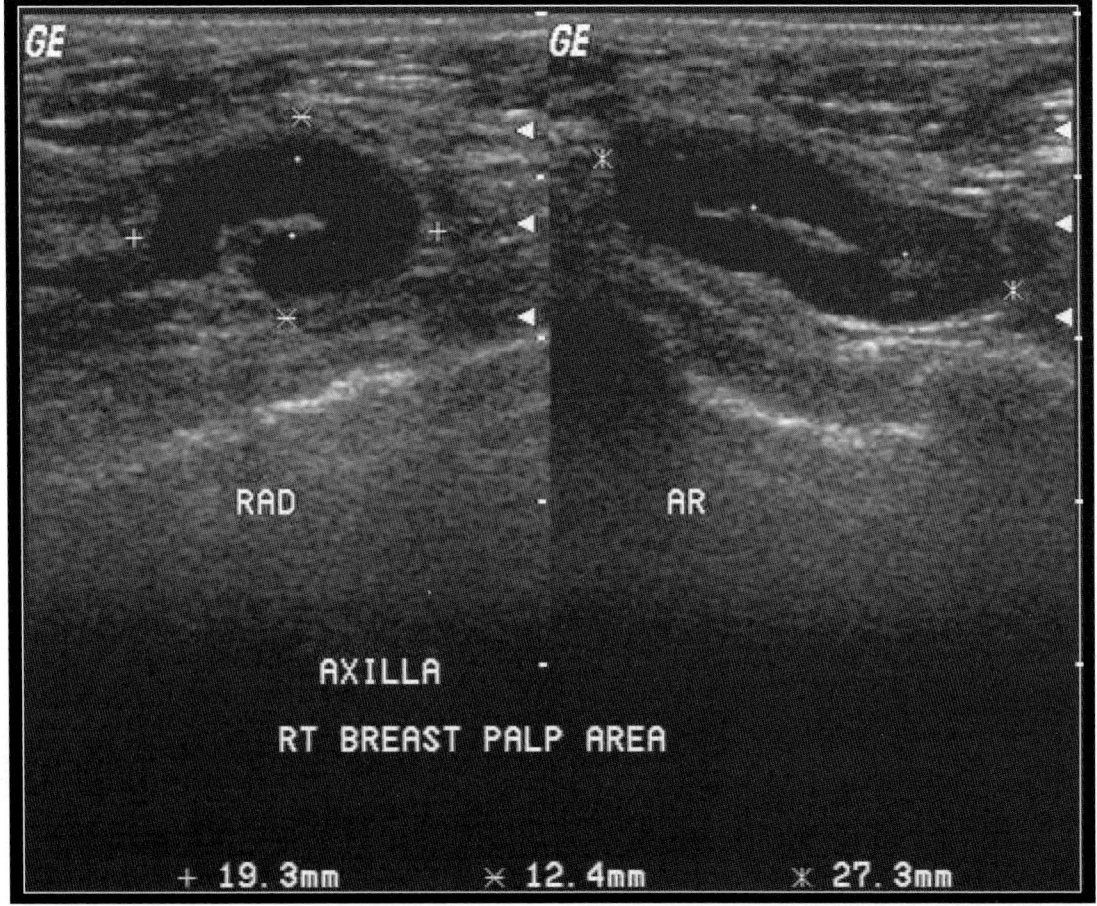

FIGURE 19–48 Asymmetric cortical thickening and asymmetric compression of the mediastinum are features of metastatic disease that has not completely replaced the lymph node cortex. In cases in which the cortex is completely replaced by metastasis, the cortical thickening and mediastinal compression can become more symmetric.

convex inward indentations of mediastinum can occur when inflammation causes severe enlargement of follicles, but like inflammatory cortical thickening and mediastinum compression, the inflammatory convex indentations of the mediastinum tend to be multiple, smaller, and uniform because all of the follicles develop germinal nodules and become enlarged (Fig. 19–44).

Mediastinal Displacement

Severe concentric or nearly concentric compression of the mediastinum by thickened cortex may make the residual hyperechoic mediastinal tissues appear slitlike (Figs. 19–46 and 19–48). Compression of such severe degree, although more typical of neoplasm, can also occur in severely inflamed lymph nodes (Fig. 19–47). Severe eccentric cortical thickening can completely displace the lymph node mediastinum to one edge of the lymph node or even completely out of the lymph node (Fig. 19–50). This appears to be a specific finding for metastatic disease because such eccentric mediastinal displacement rarely occurs in inflammatory conditions.

Mediastinal Obliteration

In the most severely abnormal lymph nodes, the mediastinal echoes can become completely obliterated and nonidentifiable because of complete compression or because of complete displacement outside the node (Fig. 19–51). Such severe involvement is more typical of metastatic disease than of inflammatory involvement, but can also occur in cases of severe necrotizing lymphadenitis (Fig. 19–52).

Loss of Thin, Echogenic Outer Capsule and Presence of Angular Margins

The loss of the thin, echogenic outer capsule of the lymph node and the presence of angular margins strongly suggests the presence of perinodal invasion, a finding that is not seen with inflammation (Fig. 19–53). Other lymph nodes that are affected by perinodal invasion can be frankly spiculated (Fig. 19–54). Because perinodal invasion fixes lymph nodes to surrounding tissues, the node cannot be rotated into a horizontal orientation by sonographic compression, causing the rare finding of a lymph node that is taller than wide.

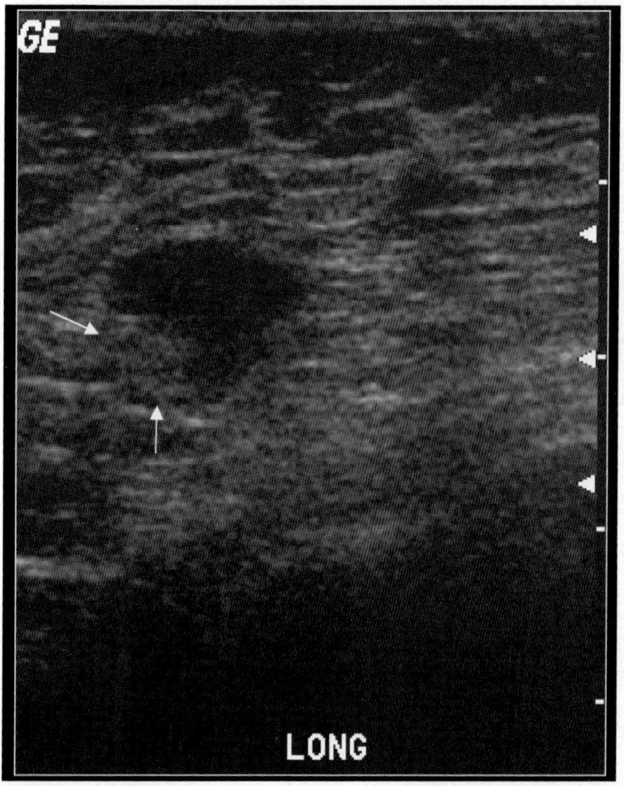

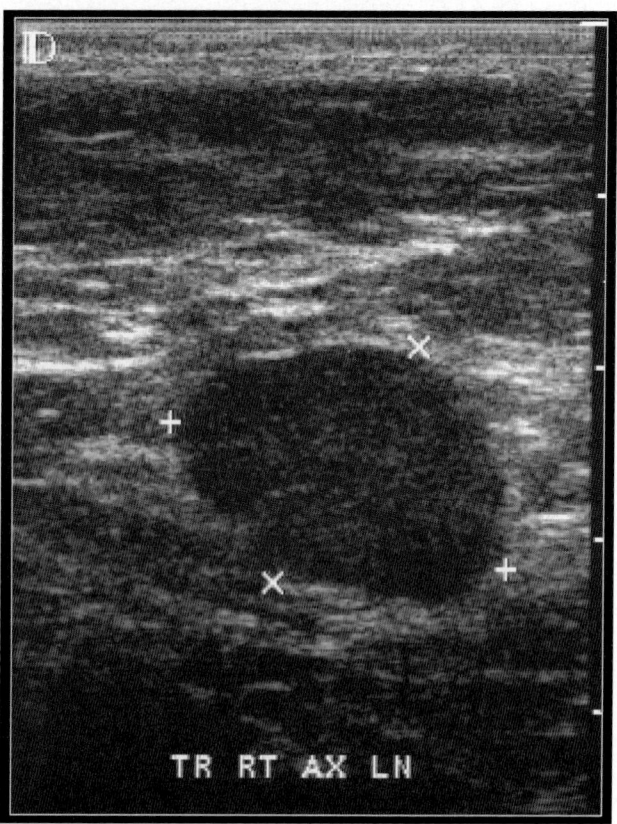

FIGURE 19–50 Extensive replacement of lymph node cortex by metastatic tumor may so eccentrically compress the mediastinum that it is pushed to the edge of the node *(arrows)* or even outside the node into surrounding tissues.

FIGURE 19–51 The hilum may be completely obliterated and not identifiable in lymph nodes that have been completely replaced by tumor.

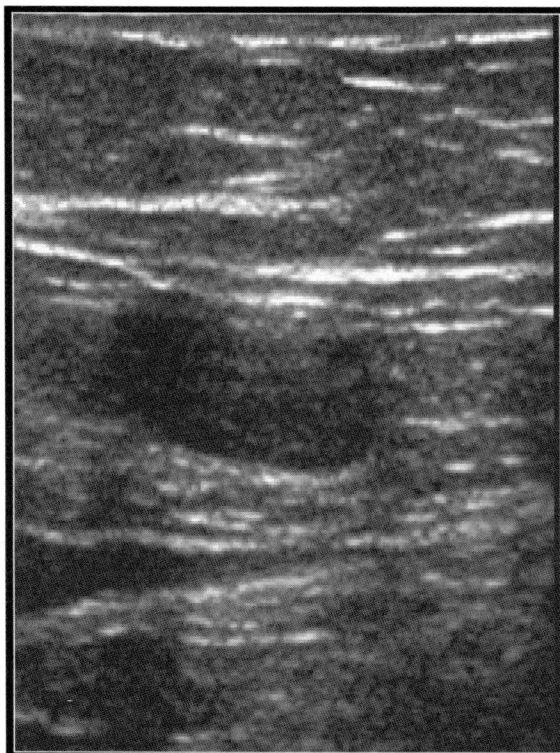

FIGURE 19–52 Although it happens less frequently than in metastatic disease, complete obliteration of the lymph node mediastinum can occasionally occur in severely inflamed nodes, especially those with necrotizing lymphadenitis.

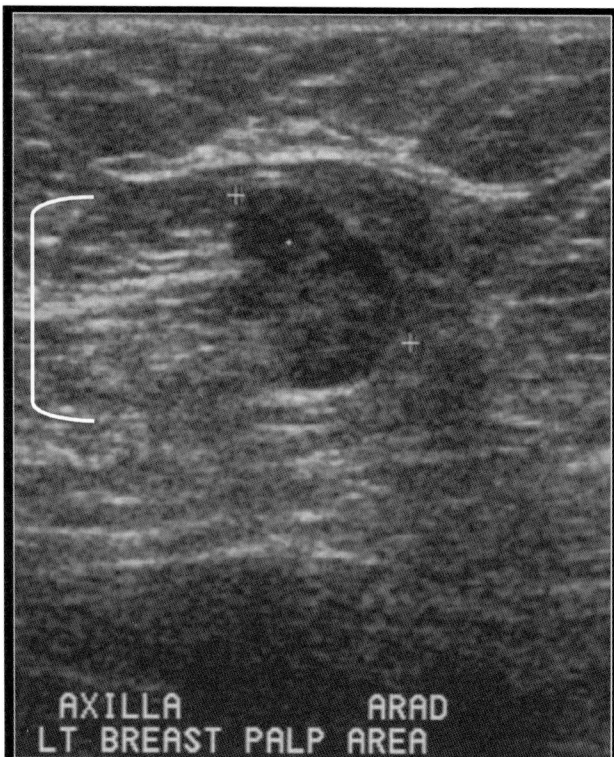

FIGURE 19–54 Some lymph nodes that are affected by perinodal invasion are frankly spiculated *(bracketed surface)*. Note that this node is also taller than wide because perinodal invasion fixes it to surrounding tissues, preventing sonographic compression from rotating it into the horizontal plane in which lymph nodes usually are oriented.

Relationship between Adjacent Lymph Nodes

Regional lymph nodes, such as the axillary nodes, occur in clusters. Frequently, it is possible to demonstrate multiple axillary lymph nodes in the same field of view during sonography. Metastatic involvement of lymph nodes tends to occur in a step-by-step process, one lymph node at a time. Thus, it is common for metastases to affect one axillary lymph node severely while either not affecting or only minimally affecting the immediately adjacent lymph node (Fig. 19–55). Inflammation, unlike metastatic disease, tends to affect all the lymph nodes in a regional chain at the same time. There can be slight asymmetry of involvement (Fig. 19–56), but not to such a degree that a grossly abnormal lymph node will appear immediately adjacent to a normal lymph node. Sonographic demonstration of an obviously abnormal lymph node immediately adjacent to a sonographically normal lymph node, therefore, strongly suggests the presence of metastatic disease rather than inflammation. We believe that this is one of the most specific findings for metastatic disease. It should be remembered, however, that severe neoplastic involvement can cause several immediately adjacent lymph nodes to be grossly ab-

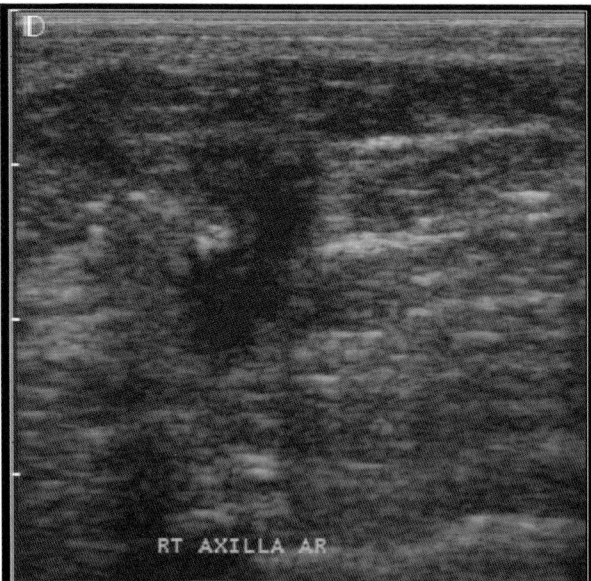

FIGURE 19–53 The loss of the outer thin, echogenic capsule, the taller-than-wide shape, and the presence of angular margins correctly suggest the presence of perinodal invasion in this case. Because of the perinodal invasion, the lymph node is fixed to surrounding tissues and cannot be rotated into a horizontally oriented plane by sonographic compression; hence, it appears taller than wide.

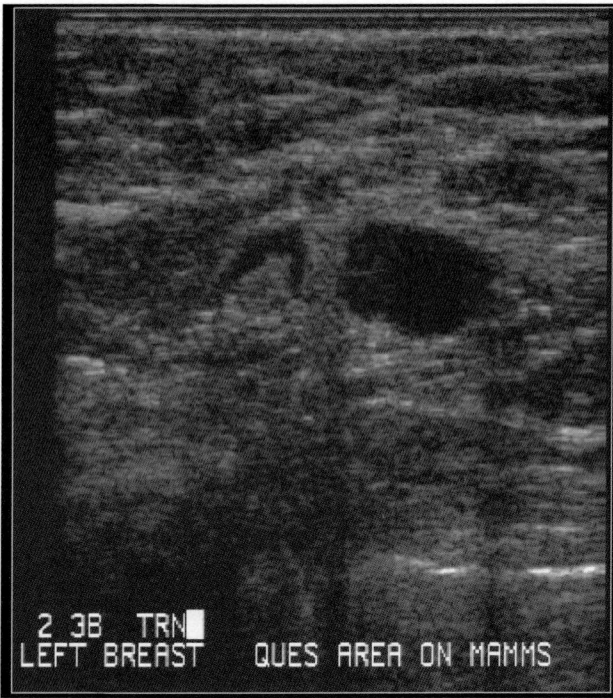

FIGURE 19–55 The presence of a sonographically grossly abnormal-appearing lymph node immediately adjacent to a normal-appearing lymph node strongly favors neoplasm over inflammation.

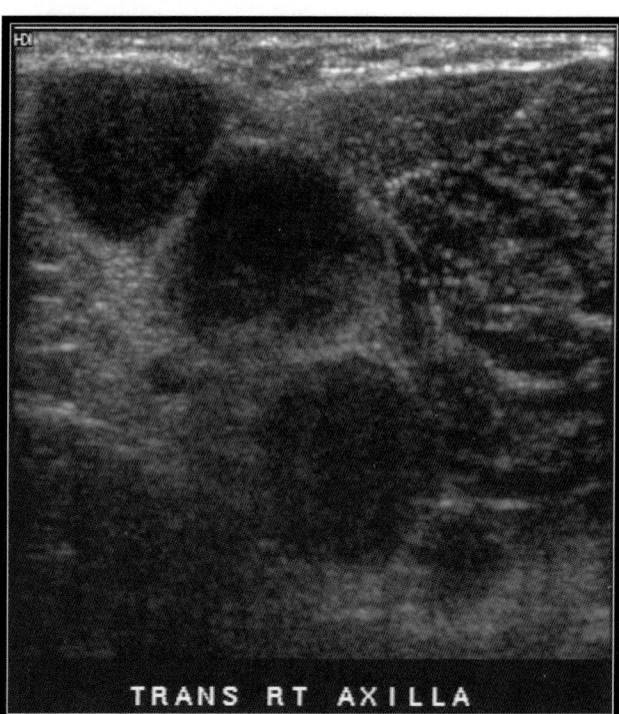

FIGURE 19–57 In severe neoplastic involvement, all of the regional lymph nodes may be abnormal. Thus, the negative predictive value of two or more grossly abnormal nodes lying adjacent to each other is less than the positive predictive value of adjacent normal and grossly abnormal nodes.

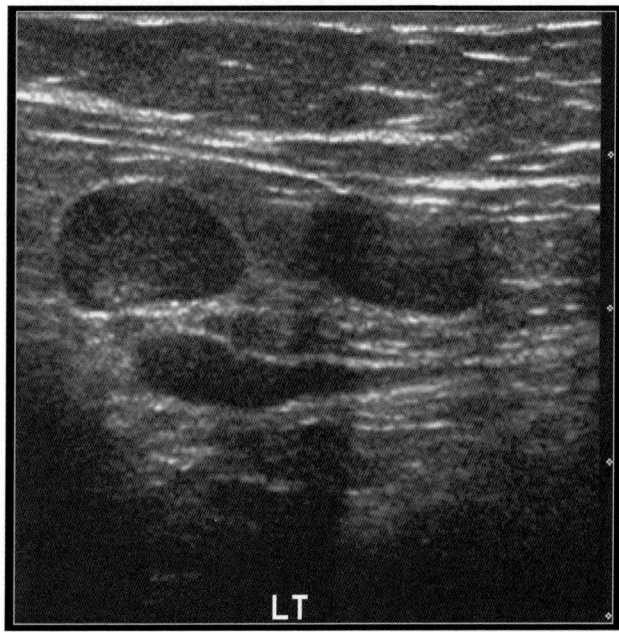

FIGURE 19–56 Inflammation tends to affect all of the lymph nodes in a chain, although the degree of abnormality may vary slightly in two adjacent nodes.

normal on sonography (Fig. 19–57). Thus, markedly asymmetric involvement of immediately adjacent lymph nodes is of greater positive predictor than is nearly equal involvement a negative predictor of metastatic disease.

Right-to-Left Symmetry or Asymmetry

Marked right-to-left asymmetry in the involvement of axillary lymph nodes favors metastatic disease over inflammation (Fig. 19–58). Viral lymphadenitis can be slightly asymmetric but is rarely truly unilateral (Fig. 19–59). Although unilateral involvement favors neoplasm over inflammation, it does not exclude inflammation or infection. Unilateral bacterial infection of the arm or breast (mastitis) can cause unilateral reactive lymphadenopathy that can be sonographically indistinguishable from neoplastic involvement.

Color Doppler Flow Patterns

Breast cancer metastases to lymph nodes are of the same histologic type as the primary tumor in 85% of cases. Thus, if the primary breast cancer is hypervascular, the lymph node metas-

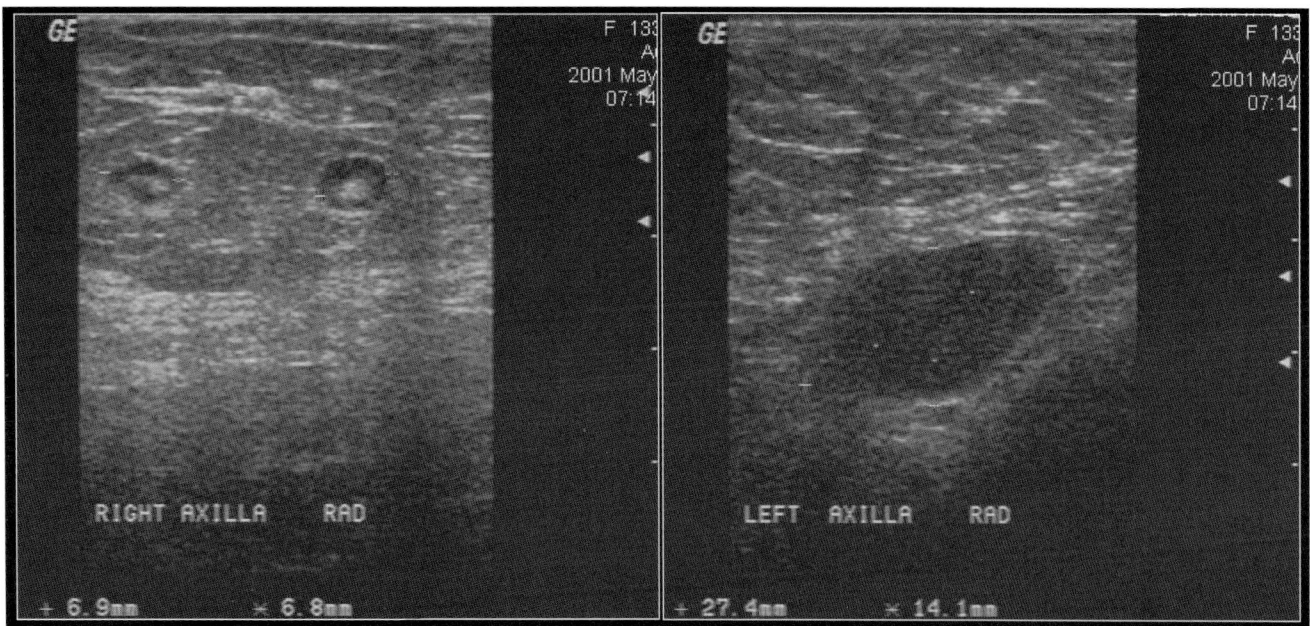

FIGURE 19–58 Right-to-left asymmetry favors neoplasm over inflammation unless there is a unilateral inflammatory process in the arm or breast. This finding would be of no help in trying to distinguish between mastitis with reactive nodes and inflammatory carcinoma with metastasis to axillary lymph nodes.

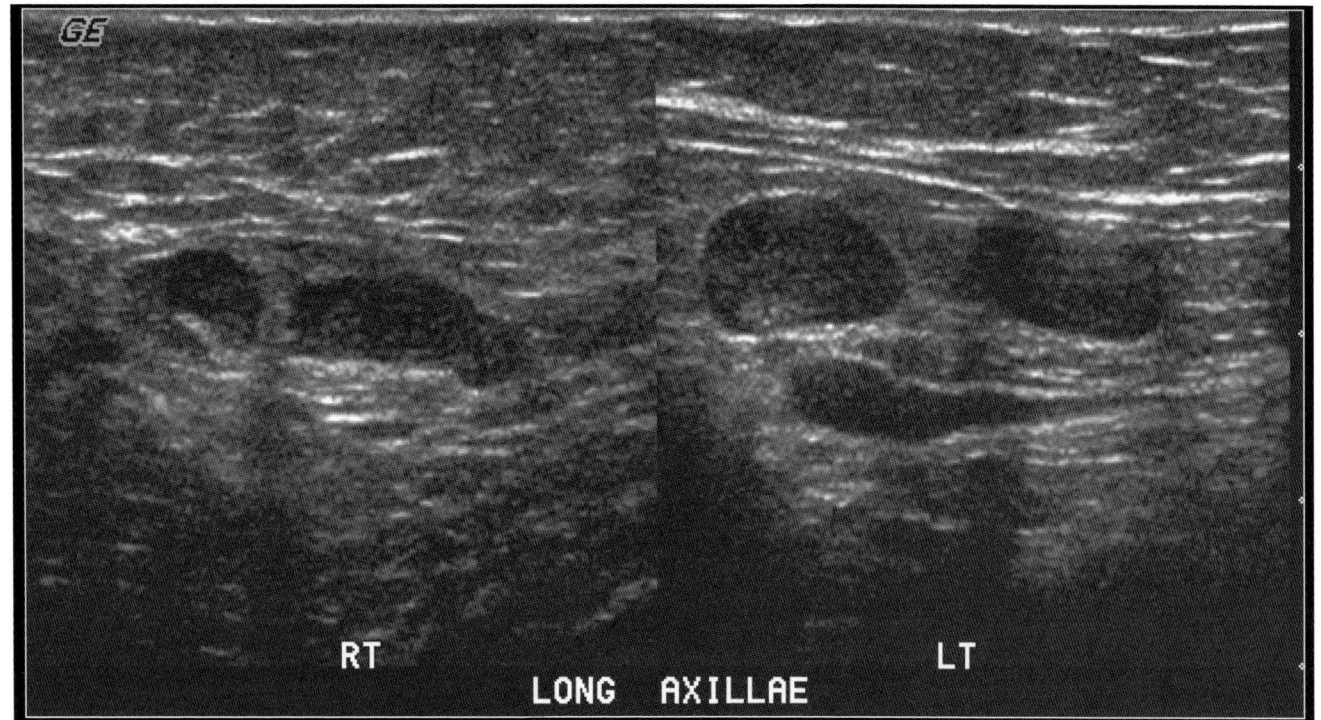

FIGURE 19–59 The most common cause of axillary lymphadenopathy is reaction to or inflammation by viral infection, which although slightly asymmetric, is usually bilateral.

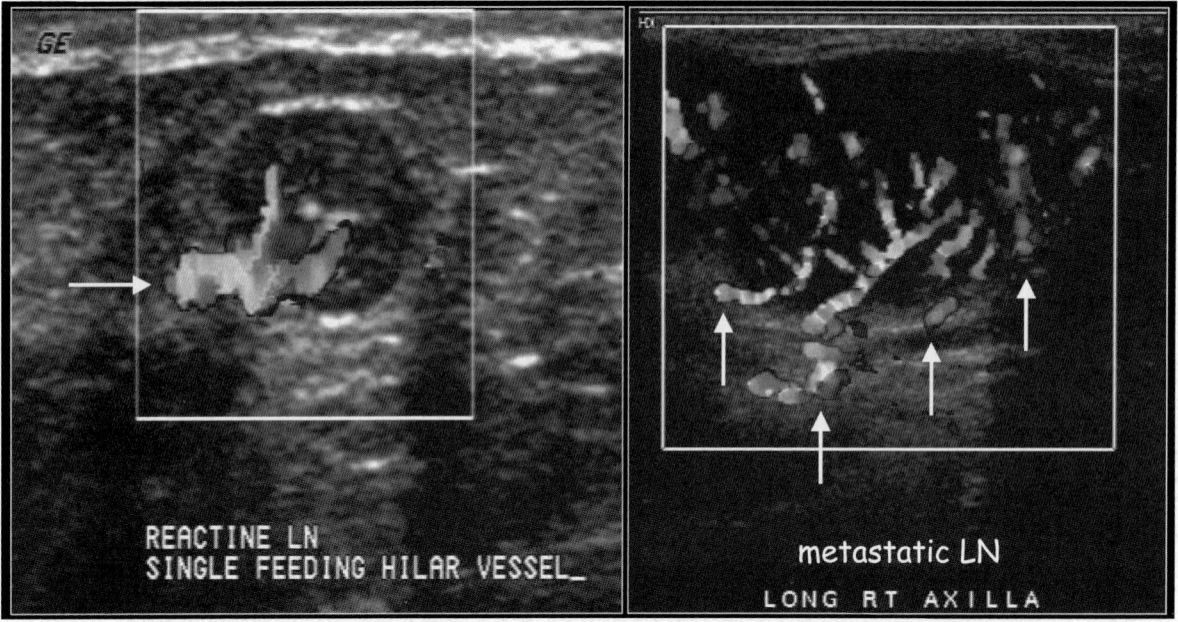

FIGURE 19–60 Enlarged reactive or inflamed lymph nodes are still usually fed by a dilated and enlarged single hilar artery **(left)**. Neoplasm-containing lymph nodes, on the other hand are often fed by multiple vessels **(right)**.

tasis will usually also be hypervascular (see color images in Chapter 20, Fig. 20–17). In cases in which lymph node metastases have vascularity that is demonstrable with color Doppler, the pattern of blood flow to metastases differs from the color Doppler pattern of inflamed, enlarged lymph nodes (Fig. 19–60). As noted earlier, all of the arterial supply of normal lymph nodes enters from the hilum, usually in a single artery. Inflammation causes vasodilation and increased flow through the normal hilar artery or arteries but does not lead to formation of new arteries. None of the blood flow to normal or inflamed or reactive lymph nodes enters the node through the capsule of the lymph node. Neoplasm within lymph nodes, on the other hand, can stimulate formation of new vessels. Thus, neoplastic lymph nodes, unlike inflamed nodes, often have multiple feeding vessels. Even more specific for metastatic diseases is the presence of transcapsular feeding vessels. Metastatic deposits that have lodged in the subcapsular sinuses can stimulate the formation of entirely new blood vessels that penetrate the capsule of the lymph node. Thus, demonstration of transcapsular vessels with color or power Doppler strongly favors metastatic disease (see the color images in Chapter 20, Fig. 20–21). As is always the case with Doppler, a positive result is of greater value than is a negative result. Some metastasis-containing lymph nodes may not have demonstrable flow. In severely enlarged and morphologically grossly abnormal lymph nodes in which the mediastinum of the lymph node is completely obliterated, it may not be possible to determine whether the feeding vessels enter through the hilar notch.

Pulsed Doppler Spectral Wave Flow Abnormalities

Because the histology of lymph node metastases is the same as the histology of the primary tumor in most cases, the pulsed Doppler spectral wave flow patterns of the primary tumor and its lymph node metastases also tend to be similar. The waveforms obtained by interrogating vessels on the interior of invasive breast carcinomas tend to have high systolic velocities with sharp systolic peaks. Diastolic flow, while present, tends to be increased less in velocity than is systolic flow, resulting in relatively high resistivity indices within the interior of the primary tumor. This pattern differs from the flow pattern in the periphery of the primary tumor, which tends to have lower systolic velocities, more rounded systolic peaks, and relatively high end-diastolic velocities and lower resistivity indices. The waveform of blood flow in the lymph node metastases is similar to the waveform obtained from the center of the primary tumor, but not to the waveform obtained from the periphery of the tumor. It has relatively high systolic peak velocities, sharp systolic peaks, and relatively low diastolic flow (Fig. 19–61). The waveform obtained from inflamed or reactive lymph nodes, on the other hand, differs from waveforms obtained from the center of the primary tumor and metastasis containing lymph nodes. Its peak systolic velocities are lower, the systolic peak is rounded, the diastolic flow is relatively higher, and the resistivity indices are relatively lower (Fig. 19–62). The waveform in inflamed nodes more

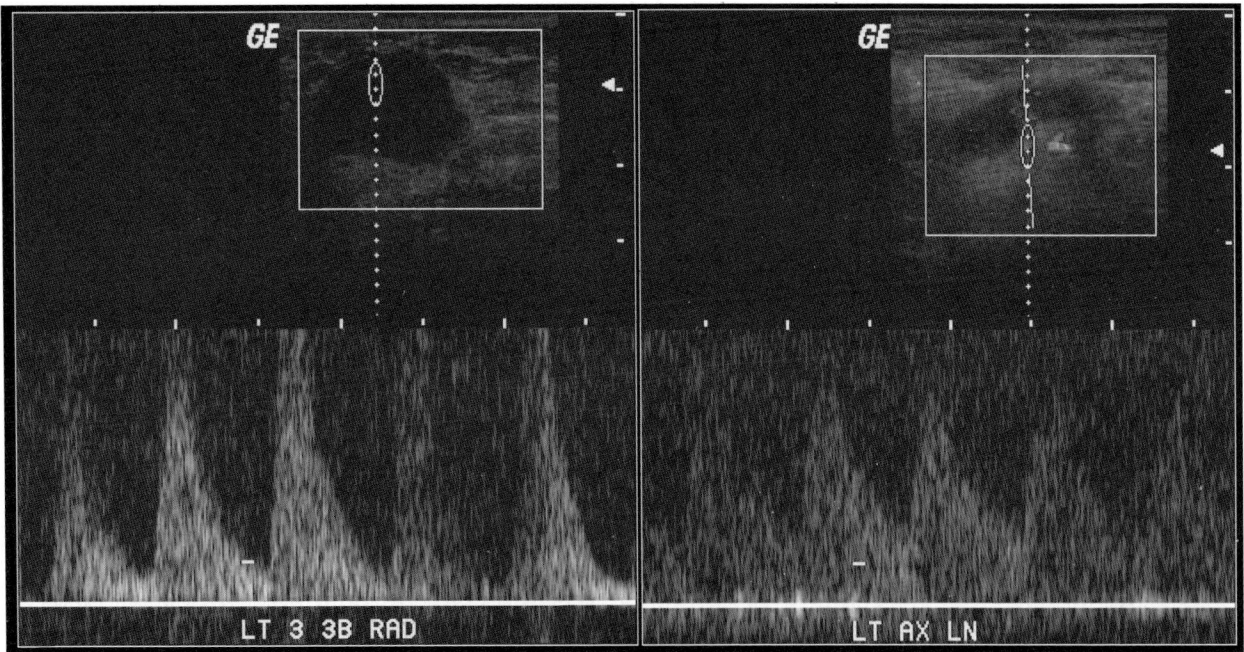

FIGURE 19–61 Not only do the color and power Doppler flow patterns within the metastasis-containing lymph node parallel those of the primary lesion, but so does the pulsed Doppler spectral waveform pattern. Most malignant tumors have high systolic velocities and relatively high resistivity indices in the center of the tumor (**left**). So do the lymph nodes that contain metastases from that primary (**right**).

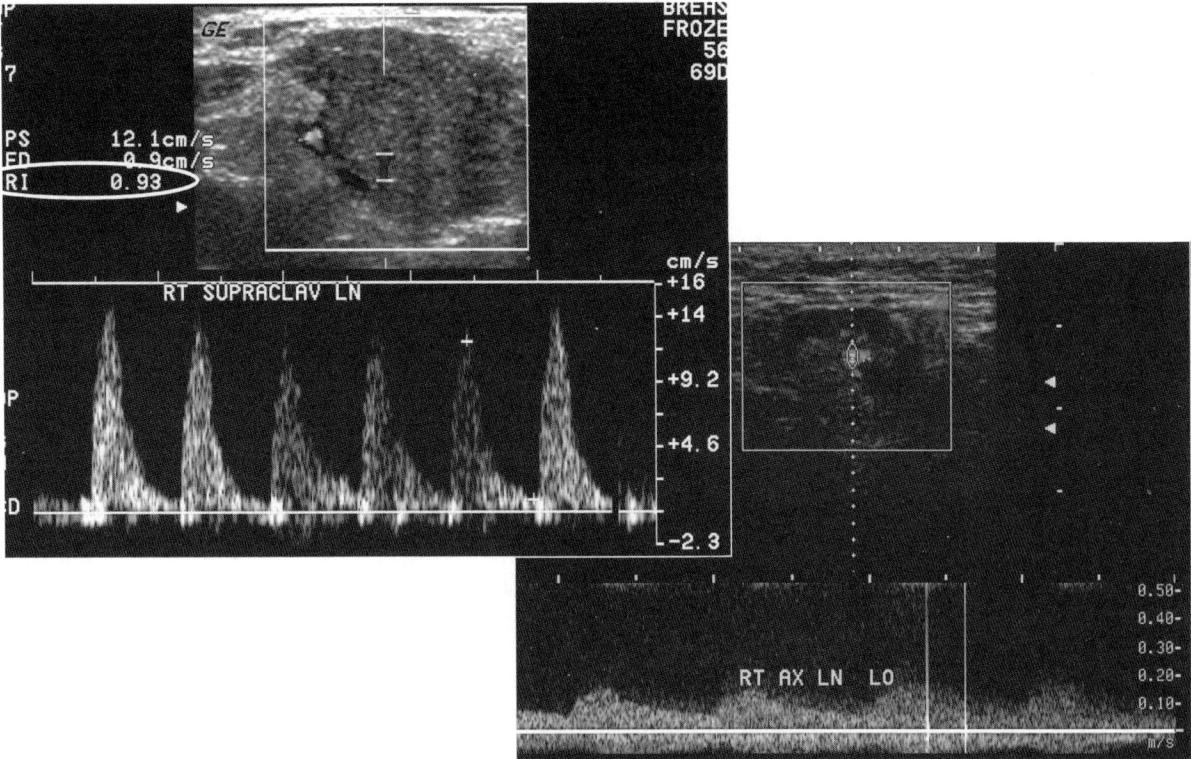

FIGURE 19–62 The pulsed Doppler spectral waveform in metastasis-containing lymph nodes differs from that of inflamed or reactive nodes. The node-bearing metastasis usually has a waveform characterized by high systolic velocities, sharp systolic peaks, and relatively high impedance (**upper left**). Reactive or inflamed nodes, on the other hand, have lower systolic velocities, more rounded systolic peaks, and lower impedance (**lower right**).

closely resembles the flow obtained from the periphery of primary tumor than it does the waveforms obtained from the center of the primary tumor.

WHY WE EVALUATE LYMPH NODES SONOGRAPHICALLY

Table 19–2 lists the reasons we evaluate lymph nodes sonographically.

Palpable Lumps, Mammographic Densities, Focal Pain, and Incidental Findings

During the process of assessing palpable lumps, mammographic abnormalities, or focal pain, it may be determined that the abnormality for which the sonogram was indicated is a lymph node. It is important to know whether the lymph node is normal. Normal intramammary lymph nodes are definitively benign, BIRADS 2, and the demonstration of a sonographically normal lymph node as the cause of a palpable lump, a mammographic abnormality, or focal pain obviates further workup, biopsy, and even follow-up. Similarly, normal lymph nodes may be found as incidental findings during sonographic evaluation of the breast could lead to unnecessary biopsies unless appropriately recognized as normal nodes. Intramammary lymph nodes are so common that one cannot assume a palpable lump is caused by a normal intramammary lymph node unless it is simultaneously palpated while being scanned (Fig. 19–63).

TABLE 19–2. WHY WE EVALUATE LYMPH NODES SONOGRAPHICALLY

The usual reasons
  Palpable lumps caused by lymph nodes
  Mammographic nodules caused by lymph nodes
  Focal pain caused by lymph nodes

Incidental mammographic findings

Assessing lymphatic uptake of silicone gel in patients with ruptured implants

Assessing extent of locoregional disease in cancer cases

Guiding needle biopsy of suspicious lymph nodes

Guiding sentinel lymph node procedures
  Guiding radionuclide injection
  Guiding needle localization of sentinel node
  Guiding large core directional vacuum-assisted biopsy of
    sentinel node

Second-look ultrasound after positive magnetic resonance imaging findings

Assessing arm swelling after cancer treatment

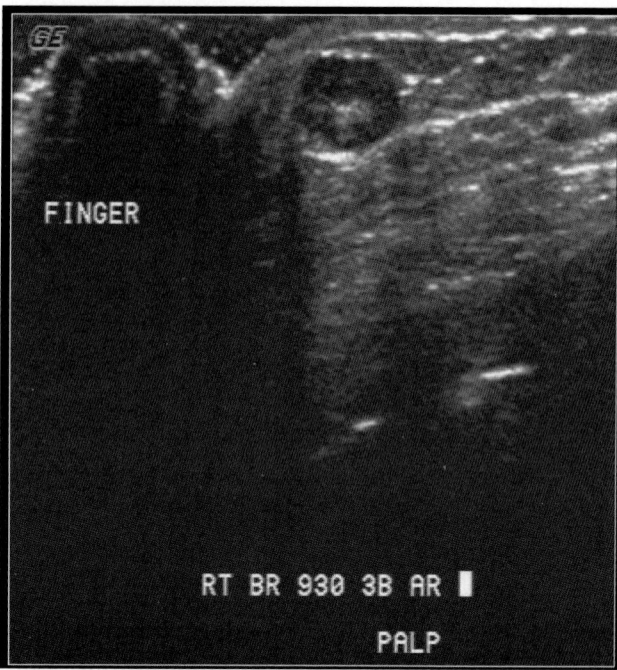

FIGURE 19–63 One of the most common presentations of breast-associated lymph nodes is as palpable lumps. Palpable lymph nodes are so common that one must palpate the node during scanning to make sure that it, and not some other lesion, is causing the palpable abnormality.

Assessing Lymphatic Uptake in Patients with Ruptured Silicone Gel Implants

The need for assessment of lymphatics in patients with ruptured silicone gel implants is controversial. It is likely that such assessment is necessary only in individuals who have extracapsular rupture of silicone gel implants and lupus-like signs and symptoms, and who are willing to undergo explantation. In such cases, detecting silicone gel–laden lymph nodes might require that involved lymph nodes be resected at the time of explantation in order to maximize the chances of recovery from the autoimmune symptoms. On the other hand, lymph node assessment is probably not necessary if the implants are intact, there is only intracapsular rupture, or there is extracapsular rupture but no evidence of autoimmune disease. Even if the patient has extracapsular rupture and autoimmune findings, lymph node assessment is probably necessary only if the patient is willing to undergo explantation.

Unlike metastases, which primarily involve the lymph node cortex, silicone gel accumulates first in the medullary sinuses, causing subtle, ill-defined, incoherent shadowing that arises from the lymph node mediastinum. As the amount of accumulated silicone gel increases, the hilum becomes more hyperechoic and the shadowing assumes the more classic "snowstorm" appearances of silicone granulomas. Eventually, even the cortex becomes hyperechoic and assumes the snowstorm appearance. Silicone can accumulate in intramammary lymph nodes that lie adjacent to the implant (Fig. 19–64) but may extend into axillary lymph nodes as well (Fig. 19–65).

Assessing Regional Lymph Node Involvement in Patients with Suspected Breast Cancer

Because lymph node status is such an important prognostic indicator in patients with breast cancer, assessment of lymph node status is also important. It is so important that, together with whole breast ultrasound, sonographic assessment of axillary lymph nodes is performed in all patients who have solid nodules that are characterized as BIRADS 4 or higher. The whole breast sonographic evaluation is performed to assess for extensive intraductal components, multifocal disease, and multicentric disease. The axillary assessment is designed to detect grossly abnormal lymph nodes. It is important to remember that sonographically normal lymph nodes can contain microscopic deposits of metastatic neoplasm. Therefore, the positive predictive value of demonstrating gross lymph node abnormalities will always be higher than the negative predictive value of demonstrating normal lymph nodes on sonography.

In cases in which there is a grossly abnormal axillary lymph node, ultrasound-guided large core needle biopsy of the node documenting suspected metastasis can make a sentinel node procedure superfluous. The patient can go straight to lumpectomy or mastectomy with formal axillary dissection. When sonographic assessment of axillary lymph nodes is negative or when ultrasound-guided biopsy of a sonographically abnormal lymph node is negative, a sentinel lymph node procedure may still be necessary. For this reason, only grossly abnormal axillary lymph nodes that have a high likelihood of containing metastatic disease are subjected to ultrasound-guided biopsy. Minimally abnormal lymph nodes that are as likely to be inflamed or reactive as they are to contain metastatic disease probably do not warrant ultrasound-guided biopsy. Our goals are to diagnose axillary lymph node metastasis accurately and to prevent unnecessary sentinel lymph node procedures. If we perform biopsy of borderline lymph nodes, there will be too many negative biopsies, and we will not be achieving our goal of avoiding unnecessary procedures.

The internal mammary lymph nodes can be assessed sonographically as well. However, the assessment is usually reserved for patients with proven breast cancer and is not used in all patients with BIRADS 4 findings. In cases in which the sonographic solid nodule is BIRADS 5, is located far medially, or is associated with multiple, grossly abnormal axillary lymph nodes, we assess the internal mammary lymph nodes before proving the presence of axillary lymph node metastases with ultrasound-guided biopsy.

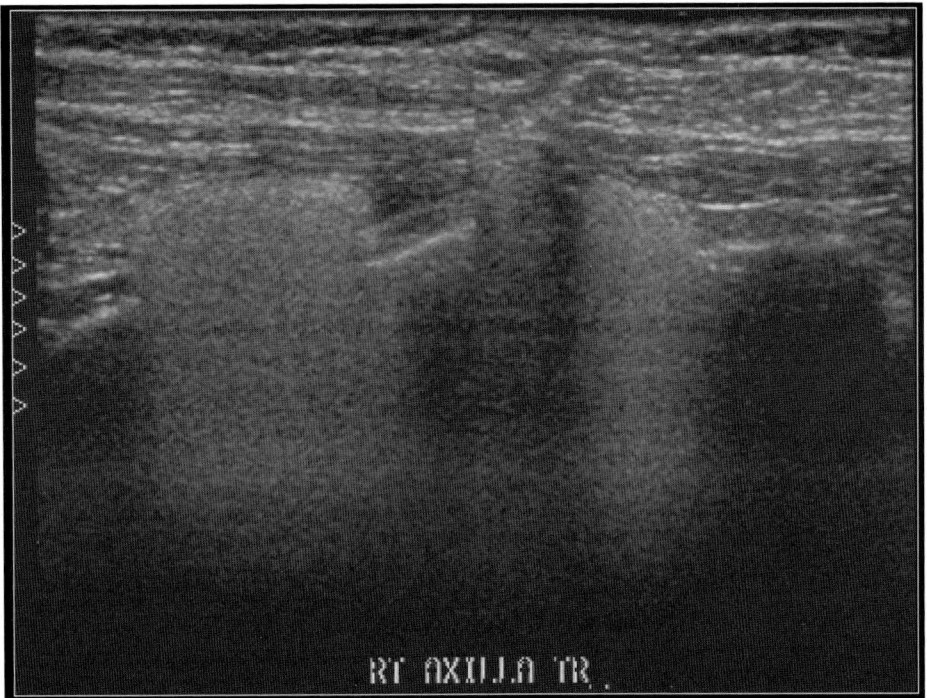

FIGURE 19–64 Intramammary lymph nodes that lie adjacent a ruptured silicone gel implant can accumulate silicone gel. This node has accumulated so much silicone gel that both the medullary and cortical sinuses are involved and hyperechoic, and the node has taken on the characteristics of a silicone granuloma, demonstrating the classic snowstorm appearance.

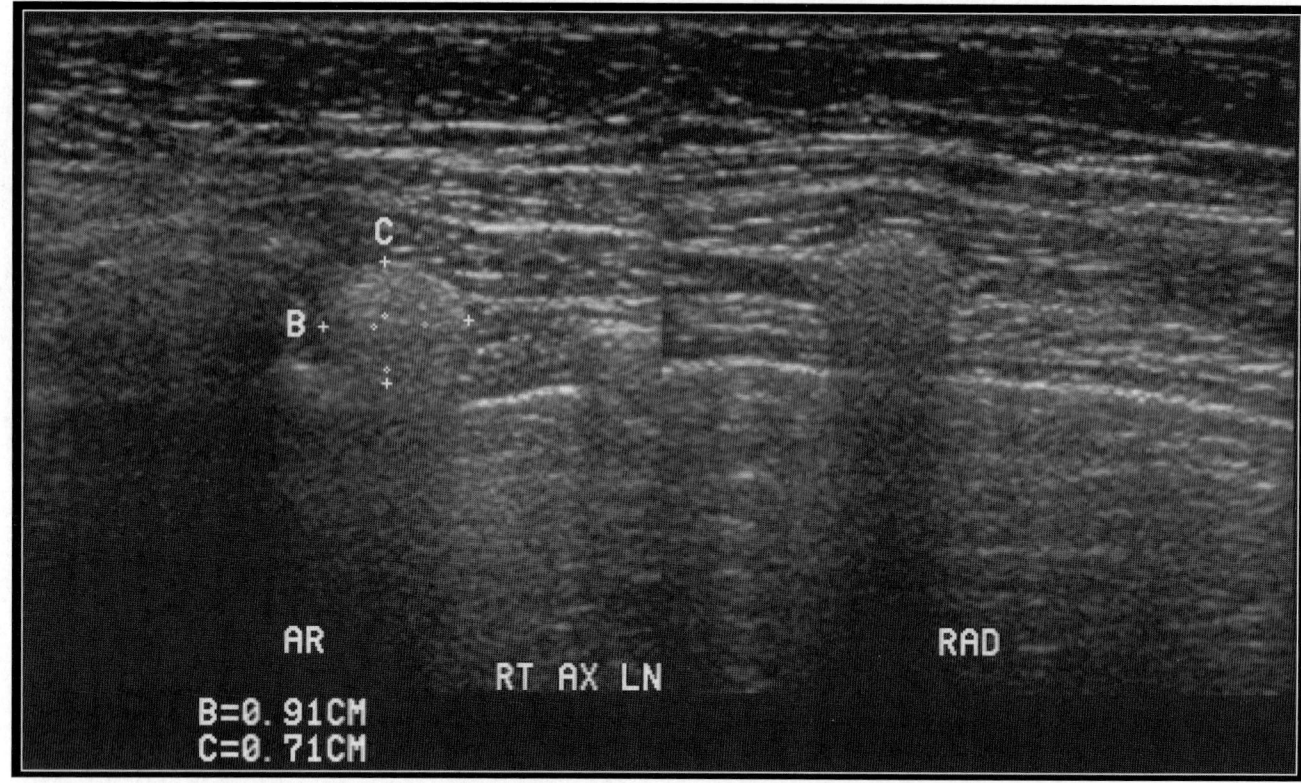

FIGURE 19–65 Silicone gel can accumulate in axillary lymph nodes as well as within intramammary lymph nodes that lie immediately adjacent to implants.

Guiding Biopsy of Suspicious Lymph Nodes

Ultrasound-guided biopsy of abnormal lymph nodes is a standard radiologic procedure in all parts of the body, including the axillary lymph nodes in patients with breast cancer. Ultrasound-guided biopsy can be performed when a grossly abnormal lymph node is detected during axillary assessment in a patient with a BIRADS 4 or 5 solid nodule that is also undergoing biopsy at the same sitting (Fig. 19–66). Lymph node biopsy can also be performed in patients in whom recurrent carcinoma is suspected and in patients with enlarged axillary lymph nodes and known lymphoma or nonbreast primary carcinomas such as melanoma.

Guiding Sentinel Lymph Node Procedures

Ultrasound can be used to guide injection of radionuclide for the sentinel lymph node procedure. We generally inject in the deep subcutaneous tissues overlying the primary nodule in four equal aliquots in positions just superior, just inferior, just lateral, and just medial to the primary lesion (12:00, 3:00, 6:00, and 9:00 positions relative to the lesion) (Fig. 19–67). For primary lesions that lie far peripherally in the upper outer quadrant, the lateral injection site can be avoided to prevent "shine-through" from obscuring the sentinel node. The need for precise targeting of the injection is controversial. Because the lymphatic drainage pattern of the breast is believed to be toward the skin, then to the periareolar area, and finally to the axilla, some believe that radionuclide does not need to be injected in the vicinity of the tumor under imaging guidance. Instead, they merely inject subdermally over the tumor or in the periareolar area.

In conjunction with marking of the skin overlying the sentinel node during radionuclide scanning and with a gamma probe, ultrasound can be used to guide needle localization of the sentinel lymph node if the sentinel node is sonographically visible. This makes finding the sentinel node easier for the surgeon and shortens the sentinel node surgical procedure. Localization of the sentinel node using ultrasound guidance is discussed in Chapter 17.

If the sentinel lymph node can be localized for surgical excision with ultrasound guidance, it could theoretically be removed using a large (11 gauge or larger) directional vacuum-assisted biopsy (DVAB). This is not an approved procedure at this time, but the details have been worked out already in the process of performing ultrasound-guided needle localizations of the sentinel lymph node. Using a coaxial system with a small gamma probe mounted on a small needle

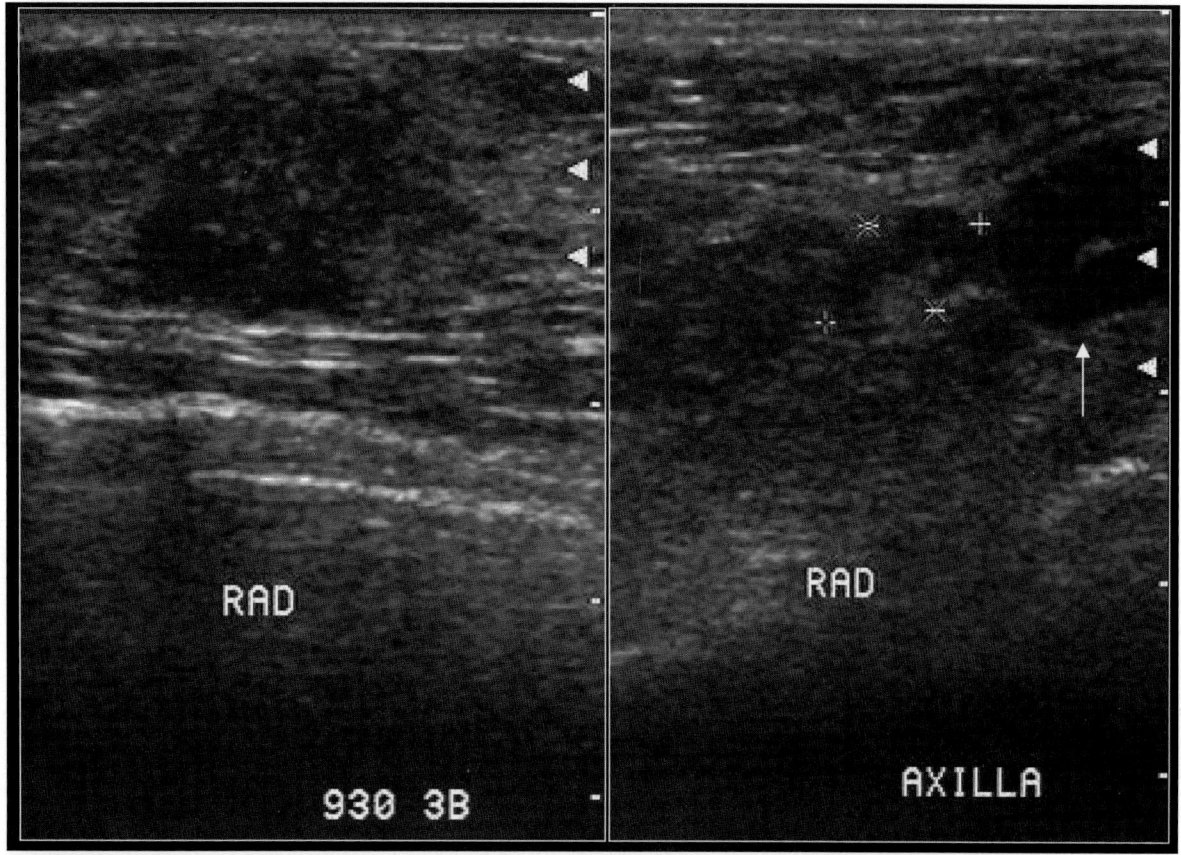

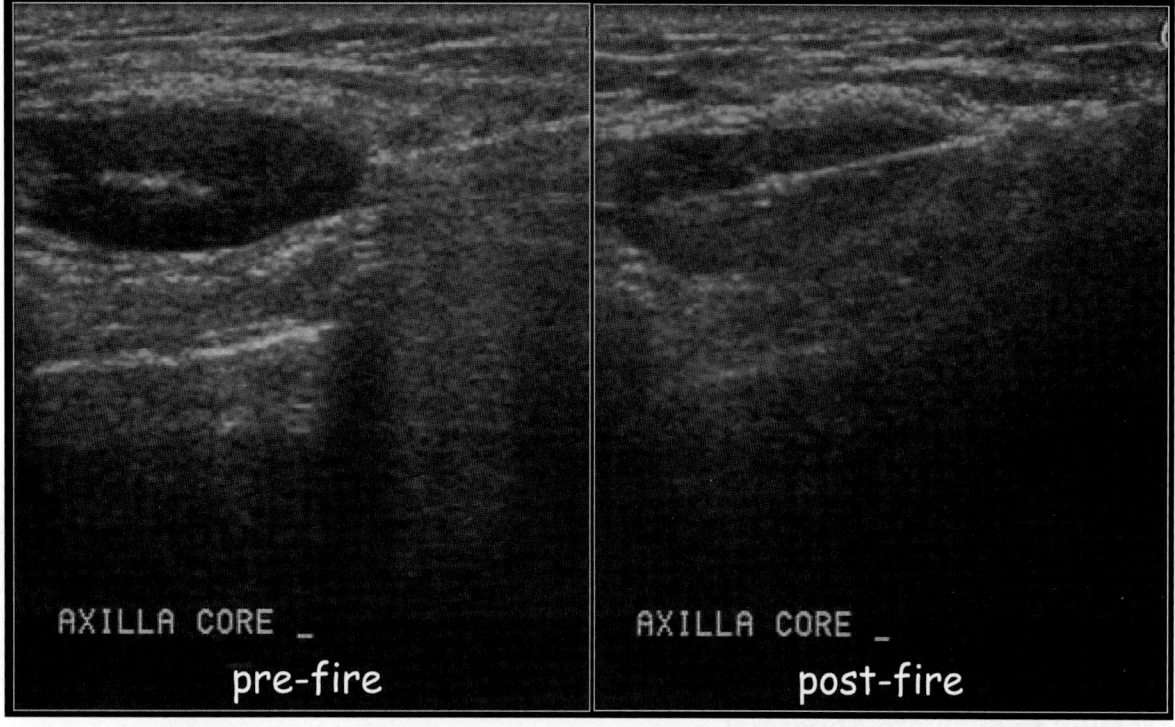

FIGURE 19–66 A: This solid breast nodule (**left**) has several suspicious features that require a BI-RADS 4b characterization. In patients with lesions such as this, one should scan the entire breast, looking for extensive intraductal components and multifocal or multicentric disease, and the axilla, looking for evidence of lymph node metastases. Axillary assessment (**right**) showed a grossly abnormal lymph node *(arrow)* adjacent to a sonographically normal lymph node, a finding that strongly favors metastasis as the cause of lymph node enlargement. **B:** Ultrasound-guided large core needle biopsy was performed at the same time that biopsy was performed on the primary lesion, confirming metastasis of intermediate-grade invasive ductal carcinoma to the abnormal-appearing lymph node and obviating sentinel node procedure. The patient underwent lumpectomy and level 1 and 2 axillary dissection in one procedure. (**left** = pre-fire; **right** = post-fire)

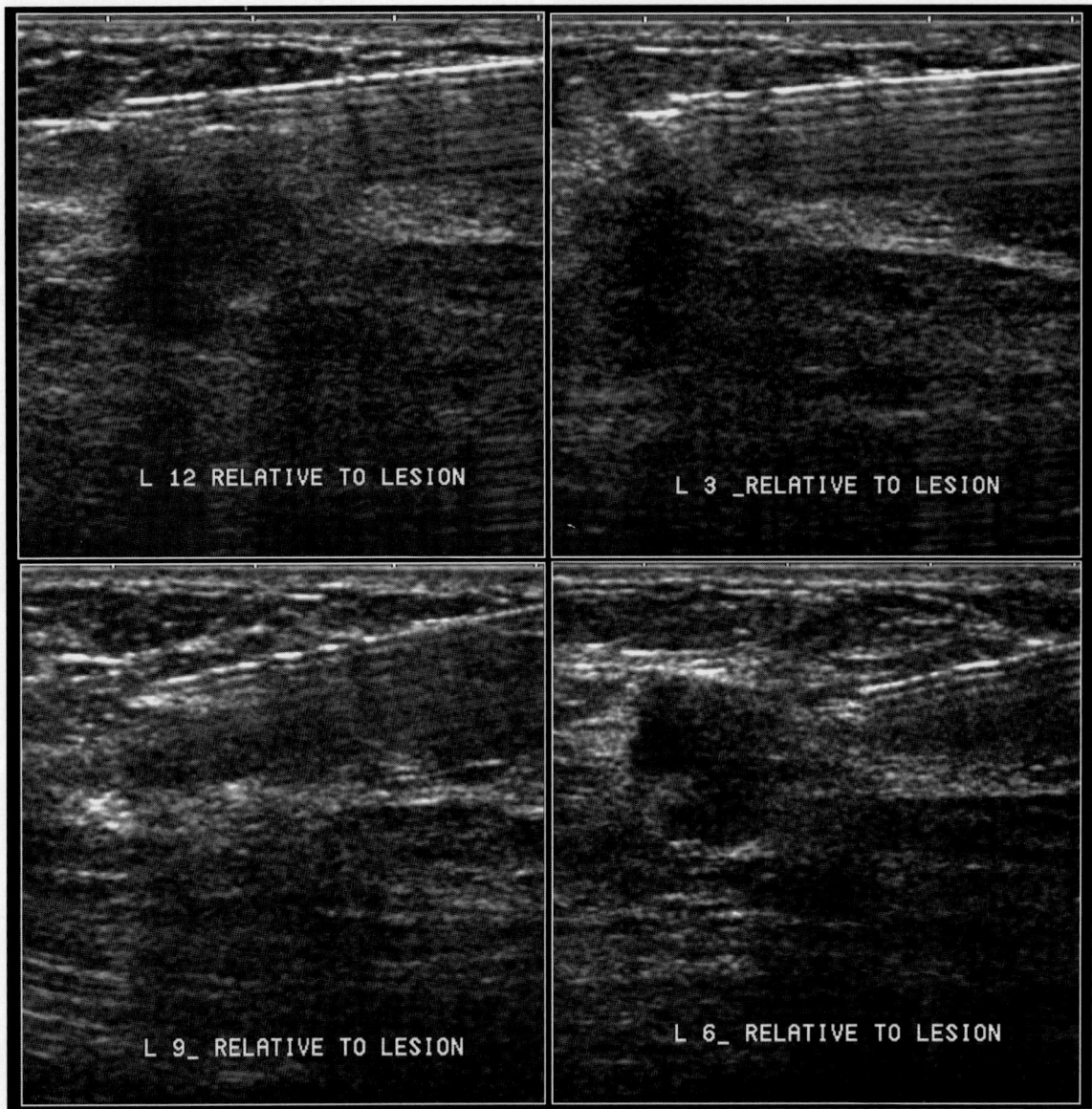

FIGURE 19–67 During ultrasound-guided injection of radionuclide for sentinel node procedure, technetium sulfur colloid is injected into the deep subcutaneous tissues that overly the primary lesions in the 12:00, 3:00, 6:00, and 9:00 positions relative to the lesion.

that fits inside the outer cannula could confirm the presence of appropriate levels of radioactivity within the sonographically visible suspected sentinel lymph node before DVAB.

Sonographic Assessment of Axillary Lymph Nodes during Second-Look Ultrasound to Evaluate Abnormal Magnetic Resonance Imaging Findings

Sonography can be used to assess lymph nodes that are suspected to be abnormal on MRI. Although contrast-enhanced high-spatial-resolution fat-suppression MRI sequences like rotating delivery excitation off-resonance (RODEO) appear to be more sensitive than ultrasound for ductal carcinoma *in situ* (DCIS) components and multifo-

cal and multicentric disease, it is not necessarily superior to ultrasound in detection of lymph node metastases. However, in some cases, MRI suggests the presence of lymph node metastasis. (A special contrast agent that improves the ability of MRI to assess lymph nodes is being investigated.) Sonography can be used to confirm the suspicions raised by MRI and to guide needle biopsy of such nodes.

Evaluation of Arm Swelling in Patients Already Treated for Breast Cancer

Sonography can be helpful in assessing the axilla in previously treated breast cancer patients who develop arm swelling. If the patient has undergone full axillary dissection, the swelling could be lymphedema related to removal

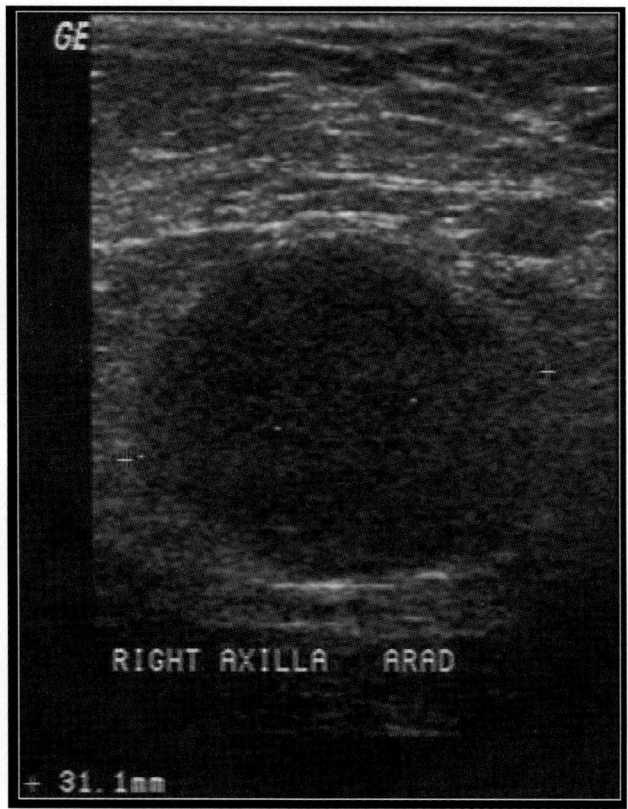

FIGURE 19–68 This patient had been treated for breast cancer with mastectomy, axillary dissection, and radiation 18 months earlier and now presented with recent onset of ipsilateral arm swelling. Sonography showed recurrent carcinoma within a lymph node that had not been detected or resected at the time of axillary dissection. Ultrasound-guided biopsy proved nodal recurrence.

of lymph tissue, and there may be no findings. Such patients might also have chronic seromas, hematomas, lymphoceles, or fat necrosis in the axilla, but they might also have recurrent carcinoma in previously undetected and unresected lymph nodes (Fig. 19–68). There might also be invasive tumor within the soft tissues of the axilla if there was perinodal invasion before lymphadenectomy. Ultrasound-guided biopsy can be performed to document the suspected recurrence.

SUMMARY

Understanding the range of normal and abnormal for lymph nodes is essential for the sonographer or sonologist who is performing breast ultrasound. A small but significant percentage of all palpable lumps and mammographic densities that are evaluated by ultrasound are caused by lymph nodes. Most of these are normal intramammary lymph nodes that are definitively benign in sonographic appearance and do not require any additional imaging

evaluation, biopsy, or short-interval follow-up. Some are reactive or inflamed nodes that are abnormally enlarged. Such nodes may benefit from short-interval follow-up and will return to normal sonographic appearances in a few weeks to months. Others have features that are suspicious for neoplasm and require biopsy.

Understanding the range of normal findings is also important in assessing possible lymph node involvement in patients who have primary solid breast nodules that are characterized as BIRADS 4 or 5. Accurate determination of local extent of disease is important in determining correct treatment, minimizing the number of surgeries necessary, and minimizing the risk for local recurrence. Assessment of regional lymph nodes is an important part of determining the extent of local disease. MRI appears to be the most efficacious method of determining local extent of disease, but ultrasound can be effective in a certain percentage of patients and is likely better than MRI for assessing lymph nodes. The role of ultrasound and its relationship to MRI are still evolving. Patients who present with palpable lumps or mammographic soft tissue densities or masses should undergo sonographic evaluation before staging MRI. If ultrasound shows a BIRADS 4 or 5 solid nodule within the breast that will require biopsy, it is useful to evaluate the axillary lymph nodes before ultrasound-guided biopsy of the primary breast nodule. If a grossly abnormal lymph node is found during assessment of the axilla, we believe that it should undergo biopsy with ultrasound guidance at the same time the primary nodule undergoes biopsy. If the lymph node that has undergone biopsy shows evidence of metastatic disease, a sentinel lymph node procedure will not be necessary, and the patient will need a formal axillary dissection. However, if the lymph node biopsy does not reveal metastasis, the sentinel lymph node procedure will still be necessary. Biopsy of minimally abnormal lymph nodes is probably not warranted in most cases because the percentage of biopsies revealing only reactive or inflamed nodes will be much higher. A negative ultrasound-guided needle biopsy cannot be relied on enough to determine whether the sentinel node will be negative. The sonographically mildly abnormal lymph node may not be the sentinel lymph node.

Even in patients who undergo stereotactic biopsy of calcifications and who are subsequently found to have abnormal-appearing lymph nodes on MRI, ultrasound will have a role in assessment of lymph nodes. MRI-guided biopsies are still not widely performed, and the economics of MRI-guided biopsies are very unfavorable compared with the economics of ultrasound-guided biopsies. Abnormal lymph nodes on MRI can be evaluated sonographically and can undergo ultrasound-guided biopsy if grossly abnormal.

Ultrasound can also play a role in the performance of sentinel lymph node procedures. It can be used to guide injection of radionuclide into the tissue around the tumor bed. It can also be used to localize the sentinel lymph node for surgical excision and in the future might even guide removal of the sentinel lymph node with minimally invasive needle techniques.

The internal mammary lymph nodes can be assessed sonographically. We routinely evaluate the internal mammary lymph nodes in patients with medial lesions, patients who have lesions that are near the chest wall, and patients with lesions in the lateral half of the breast that have gross and extensive axillary metastases. Our ability to detect abnormal internal mammary lymph nodes is actually ahead of our ability to deal with the knowledge that they are abnormal at this point. More advanced nonsurgical treatments of breast cancer such as immunotherapy might make knowledge about involvement of internal mammary lymph nodes more valuable in the future.

SUGGESTED READINGS

Asai S, Miyachi H, Suzuki K, et al. Ultrasonic differentiation between tuberculous lymphadenitis and malignant lymph nodes. *J Ultrasound Med* 2001;20:533–538.

Berg WA. Imaging the local extent of disease. *Semin Breast Dis* 2001;4:153–173.

Bruneton JN, Caramella E, Hery M, et al. Axillary lymph node metastases in breast cancer: preoperative detection with US. *Radiology* 1986;158:325–326.

Bruneton JN, Normand F, Balu-Maestro C, et al. Lymphomatous superficial lymph nodes: US detection. *Radiology* 1987;165:233–235.

Dershaw DD, Selland DLG, Tan LK, et al. Spiculated axillary adenopathy. *Radiology* 1996;201:439–442.

Eubank WB, Mankoff DA, Vesselle HJ, et al. Detection of locoregional and distant recurrences in breast cancer patients by using FDG PET. *Radiographics* 2002;22:5–17.

Glynne-Jones R., et al. A possible role for ultrasound of the axilla in staging primary breast cancer. *Clin Oncol (R Coll Radiol)* 1990; 2(1):35–38.

Gordon PB, Gilks B. Sonographic appearance of normal intramammary lymph nodes. *J Ultrasound Med* 1988;7:545–548.

Herrada J, Iyer RB, Atkinson EN, et al. Relative value of physical examination, mammography, and breast sonography in evaluating the size of the primary tumor and regional lymph node metastases in women receiving neoadjuvant chemotherapy for locally advanced breast carcinoma. *Clin Cancer Res* 1997;3:1565–1569.

Kuzo RS, Ben-Ami TE, Yousefzadeh DK, et al. Internal mammary compartment: window to the mediastinum. *Radiology* 1995;195: 187–192.

Liberman L, Cody HS, Hill AD, et al. Sentinel lymph node biopsy after percutaneous diagnosis of nonpalpable breast cancer. *Radiology* 1999;211:835–844.

Lindfors KK, Kopans DB, Googe PB, et al. Breast cancer metastasis to intramammary lymph nodes. *AJR Am J Roentgenol* 1986;146:614.

Meyer JE, et al. Mammographic appearance of normal intramammary lymph nodes in an atypical location. *AJR Am J Roentgenol* 1993;161:779–780.

Moriggl B, Steinlechner M. Ultrasono-anatomy for evaluation of the local lymphatic groups of the mamma. *Surg Radiol Anat* 1994; 16:77–85.

Newman LA, Kuerer HM, Fornage B, et al. Adverse prognostic significance of infraclavicular lymph nodes detected by ultrasonography in patients with locally advanced breast cancer. *Am J Surg* 2001;181:313–318.

Pamilo M, Martti S, Lavast EM. Real-time ultrasound, axillary mammography, and clinical examination in the detection of axillary lymph node metastases in breast cancer patients. *J Ultrasound Med* 1989;8:115–120.

Pamilo M, Sovia M, Lavast E. Real-time ultrasound, axillary mammography, and clinical examination in the detection of axillary lymph node metastases in breast cancer patients. *J Ultrasound Med* 1989;8:115–120.

Sciatarige JC, Hamper UM, Sheth S, et al. Parasternal sonography of the internal mammary vessels: technique, normal anatomy, and lymphadenopathy. *Radiology* 1989;172:453–457.

Sciatarige JC, et al. Internal mammary lymphadenopathy: imaging of a vital pathway in breast cancer. *Radiographics* 1990;10:857–870.

Shamiou KK. Intramammary lymph node in the lower outer quadrant detected mammographically [Letter]. *AJR Am J Roentgenol* 1992;159:899.

Svane G, Franzen S. Radiologic appearance of nonpalpable intramammary lymph nodes. *Acta Radiol* 1993;34:577–580.

Tateishi T, Machi J, Feleppa EJ, et al. In vitro B-mode ultrasonographic criteria for diagnosing axillary lymph node metastasis of breast cancer. *J Ultrasound Med* 1999;18:349–356.

Tschammler A, Ott G, Seelbach-Goebel B, et al. Lymphadenopathy: differentiation of benign from malignant disease—color Doppler US assessment of intranodal angioarchitexture. *Radiology* 1998; 208:117–123.

Vasallo P, Wernecke K, Roos N, et al. Differentiation of benign from malignant superficial lymphadenopathy: the role of high resolution US. *Radiology* 1992;183:215–220.

Walsh JS, Dixon JM, Chetty U, et al. Colour Doppler studies of axillary node metastases in breast carcinoma. *Clin Radiol* 1994;49: 189–191.

Yang WT, Ahuja A, Tang A, et al. Ultrasonographic demonstration of normal axillary lymph nodes: a learning curve. *J Ultrasound Med* 1995;14:823–827.

Yang WT, Ahuja A, Tang A, et al. High resolution sonographic detection of axillary lymph node metastases in breast cancer. *J Ultrasound Med* 1996;15:241–246.

Yang WT, Lam WW, Cheung H, et al. Sonographic, magnetic resonance imaging, and mammographic assessments of preoperative size of breast cancer. *J Ultrasound Med* 1997;16(12):791–797.

Yang WT, Metreweli C. Colour Doppler flow in normal axillary lymph nodes. *Br J Radiol* 1998;71:381–383.

20

DOPPLER EVALUATION OF THE BREAST

The physics and instrumentation of Doppler are similar to those of ultrasound with a few important differences. First, the sensitivity for detecting moving red blood cells is only about one hundredth the sensitivity of ultrasound for B-mode imaging of tissue interfaces. Second, most of our techniques in B-mode imaging are designed to scan tissue planes at a 90-degree angle of incidence. Doppler, on the other hand, is best done at angles of incidence near 0 degrees. Most machines allow each image pixel to display only gray scale information or color information. A setting called the *write priority* allows us to choose how gray a pixel can be before it can be overwritten with color. The breast is fairly echogenic; thus, displaying color Doppler or power Doppler in the breast requires a write priority setting toward the white end of the spectrum. Most ultrasound machines allow the color Doppler or power Doppler beam to be steered. Steering was developed to improve the angle of incidence in large peripheral vessels that lie nearly parallel to the transducer face, but at an angle of incidence nearly 90 degrees to the Doppler beam, the worst angle for Doppler. Steering reduces the angle of incidence to between 70 and 80 degrees. However, steering reduces sensitivity. Tumor vessels lie at all possible angles of incidence to the Doppler beam, and the strongest Doppler signals that we receive come from vessels that lie at 0 degrees to the beam. This will be true whether the beam is steered or not. Thus, there is little or no use for beam steering in the breast.

To maximize sensitivity, the beam should not be steered. If absolute velocities obtained from pulsed Doppler spectral analysis are used as cutoff values for benign versus malignant, angle correction should be used if a vessel is large enough and long enough to measure the angle of incidence. However, in many cases, the vessel being sampled is too small or too tortuous to allow angle correction. In such cases, it can be assumed that the highest velocities originate from small and unresolved vessels that lie at 0 de-

grees to the beam, that cosine theta is 1.0, and that angle correction is not necessary. Split-screen imaging is helpful when performing the power Doppler vocal fremitus maneuver. Split-screen color or power Doppler imaging is also useful for comparing amounts of blood flow in mirror-image locations on the right and left sides. Power Doppler is more sensitive to low levels of flow than is color Doppler and is also less angle sensitive than color Doppler, but cannot show direction of flow and cannot distinguish between arterial and venous flow without pulsed Doppler spectral analysis.

Power Doppler is also more sensitive to acoustic vibratory artifact than is color Doppler, which is useful when performing power Doppler vocal fremitus. Although performance differences between low-end and high-end machines may only be about 10% for imaging, the differences are much greater for Doppler. High-end ultrasound machines have much more sensitive Doppler than do low-end machines.

The most well-studied use for Doppler in breast ultrasound is characterizing breast lesions into benign and malignant categories. The basis for this is the need for tumors larger than a critical size to stimulate neovascularity in order to continue growing. However, the efficacy of Doppler for this purpose cannot be viewed in a vacuum. Instead, it must be compared with competitive imaging methods. In breast ultrasound, the efficacy of Doppler must be compared with the efficacy of the image, which is quite good. Frankly, Doppler is not as efficacious as is high-resolution real-time B-mode imaging for characterizing solid breast nodules. This is just as true with the more sensitive Doppler available today as it was with less sensitive Doppler available years ago because the quality of the B-mode image and our understanding of how to interpret imaging findings have advanced at least as fast as Doppler sensitivity has improved. Ultrasound contrast agents likely will contribute to improving Doppler sensitivity and efficacy, but even then may not be able to compete with real-time imaging for characterizing breast lesions. What Doppler is good at is determining the aggressiveness of a lesion. Lesions that develop enough neovascularity to be obviously positive on Doppler tend to be higher grade and larger than lesions that do not have demonstrable flow. Lesions with abundant flow on Doppler studies also tend to be associated with lymph node and hematogenous metastases more often than those that do not. Thus, the most appropriate roles for Doppler in breast diagnosis might be to determine which patients will benefit most from antiangiogenesis therapies and to monitor the success of such treatments.

Having stated that high-resolution real-time imaging is better than Doppler for characterizing breast lesions, one might falsely conclude we believe that Doppler is of little use in breast ultrasound. Nothing could be farther from the truth. At this time, we would never again consider the purchase of a machine for breast ultrasound that did not have color Doppler, power Doppler, and pulsed Doppler spectral analysis capabilities. Despite its current limitations in determining whether lesions are benign or malignant, it is valuable in determining the aggressiveness of sonographically suspicious lesions [Breast Imaging Reporting and Data System (BIRADS) category 4a or higher]. Additionally, Doppler is invaluable for numerous other niche applications within breast ultrasound that are listed in Table 20–1.

There are undoubtedly many other niche applications, as the uses are limited only by the imagination. All of these applications have been discussed and illustrated elsewhere in this book, and virtually every other chapter presents Doppler uses and findings. However, this chapter is intended to be a summary of those applications and to consolidate most of the color images in this book into one section.

DOPPLER CHARACTERIZATION OF BREAST LESIONS

After a malignant neoplasm achieves a certain size, simple diffusion becomes inadequate for feeding tumor cells with oxygen and nutrients and for carrying away waste products. At that point, the tumor must generate its own new blood vessels (or cease growing). To enable growth beyond this point, all malignant tumor cells have developed the capacity to elaborate and release angiogenesis factors. These factors stimulate the formation of new vessels (tumor neovascularity) to supply nutrients to and remove wastes from the tumor. The formation of neovascularity is typically most pronounced in the periphery of the tumor mass.

There is a complex interrelationship among angiogenesis, hyaluronic acid, and certain enzymes, particularly proteinases. Malignant nodules are composed of tumor

TABLE 20–1. USES OF DOPPLER IN BREAST DIAGNOSIS

Distinguishing between benign and malignant breast lesions

Determining aggressiveness of suspicious or malignant breast lesions

Assessing response to tumor therapy
Radiation
Chemotherapy
Antiangiogenesis
Immunotherapy

Assessing whether lymphadenopathy is caused by inflammation or metastatic breast carcinoma

Distinguishing solid nodules from complex cysts with low-level internal echoes

Distinguishing intracystic papilloma or carcinoma from papillary apocrine metaplasia

Determining whether internal echoes in complex cysts are subcellular particles or cells

Identifying necrotic debris that represents early abscess formation in patients with mastitis

Distinguishing between echogenic inspissated secretions or blood within a duct and ductal carcinoma *in situ* or papilloma

Demonstrating inflammatory hyperemia
In inflamed cysts
In puerperal mastitis
In the duct ectasia–periductal mastitis complex
In infected periimplant capsules

Identifying vascular landmarks, such as the internal mammary artery and vein, that facilitate identification of the internal mammary lymph nodes

Distinguishing fat necrosis and exuberant scar from recurrent tumor

Assessment of vascular conditions of the breast

Assessment of acoustic vibratory response to vocal fremitus

cells and extracellular matrix. In many cases, a large percentage of the mass is composed of extracellular matrix. The three main components of the extracellular matrix are hyaluronic acid, collagen, and fibroblasts. The extracellular matrix of tumors tends to have far more hyaluronic acid than does the extracellular matrix of normal tissues. In some cases, tumor cells directly synthesize hyaluronic acid, whereas in other cases, the tumor cells stimulate the fibroblasts in the extracellular matrix to synthesize hyaluronic acid. The presence of higher-than-normal amounts of hyaluronic acid facilitates the growth and spread of the tumor in several ways. First, it is extremely hydrated, facilitating the passage of nutrients into and wastes from tumor cells until the tumor reaches the critical size at which passive diffusion is no longer enough. Second, it offers structural support to the tumor. Third, it offers a path of low resistance for growth and motility of tumor cells. In fact, some hyaluronic acid molecules attach to and activate receptors on the tumor cell membranes attached to the intracellular myofibrils that create motility. Rather than being inert, hyaluronic acid is actively turned over. As much as one-fourth to one-third of the hyaluronic acid that surrounds tumor cells may be turned over daily. Most is pulled into the tumor cell at different receptors on the cell membranes and metabolized within the cells. However, enzymes within the extracellular matrix break down some. The breakdown products of hyaluronic acid, together with breakdown products of collagen, help stimulate tumor angiogenesis. Thus, hyaluronic acid facilitates tumor growth early on by enhancing passive diffusion and later by stimulating angiogenesis.

Detecting and characterizing breast cancer neovascularity is the goal of Doppler assessment of breast lesions. Blocking the development of these vessels is the goal of angiogenesis inhibitors.

Tumor vessels have several attributes that differ from those of normal blood vessels that can be evaluated with Doppler:

1. The number of vessels is increased. This could be shown as an increased number of vessels on color or power Doppler, as more rapid appearance and more intense contrast enhancement on computed tomography (CT) or magnetic resonance imaging (MRI) studies, or as more rapid and intense appearance of radionuclides such as technetium-99m (^{99m}Tc)-sestamibi.
2. The pattern of vessels usually is one of net of tumor vessels in the periphery of the tumor. This pattern would also theoretically be demonstrable by color and power Doppler if the sensitivity were good enough and by contrast-enhanced CT or MRI if the timing were quick enough and the resolution of the scanners good enough. Ultrasound contrast agents promise to improve the ability of ultrasound and Doppler to identify this peripheral vascular net.
3. There is often absence of normal capillary beds in tumor vessels. Instead of capillaries, the connections between arteries and veins are usually sinusoidal spaces with thin, nonmuscular or elastic walls or with no defined walls. This tends to cause higher-than-normal velocity flow and lower-than-normal impedance or resistance in comparison to normal blood vessels, which should be detectable on pulsed Doppler spectral analysis if the equipment is sensitive enough. It could also be shown as more rapid contrast enhancement or washout on CT or MRI scans or more rapid appearance and washout of radionuclide on vascular phases of radionuclide studies.
4. Because the walls of tumor vessels are not normal, they tend to be abnormally "leaky." They lack the basement membrane of normal capillaries. Particles that would be held tightly within the intravascular space by normal capillaries readily leak out of tumor vessels into the sur-

rounding extracellular space. Unfortunately, Doppler presently has no way to demonstrate this abnormal tumor vessel leakiness, even with current ultrasound contrast agents, which are too large to leak from the vessels. Contrast enhancement on CT or MRI, however, does show this. The persistent contrast enhancement that makes MRI so sensitive for breast malignancy is virtually entirely related to leakage of low-molecular-weight gadolinium from the vascular space into the extravascular space. In fact, contrast agents are currently being developed for MRI that target the hyaluronic acid that is so abundant within the extracellular matrix of malignant lesions.

Although it would appear that the ability of Doppler to demonstrate several different features of malignant neovascularity would make it ideal for accurately characterizing malignant nodules, there are significant limitations of the Doppler technique that must be kept in mind. As discussed in Chapter 12, breast cancer is very heterogeneous. The cellularity, amount of angiogenesis factors elaborated, and extent of tumor vascularity vary greatly from one malignant nodule to another. Highly cellular, circumscribed, and higher-grade malignant nodules develop enough neovascularity for even low-end ultrasound equipment to detect with color, power, or pulsed Doppler. In such cases, the absolute amount of Doppler-demonstrable vascularity of such lesions is usually obviously different from that of normal tissues and benign lesions (Fig. 20–1). Some special-type tumors, such as invasive papillary carcinoma, are also markedly hypervascular (Fig. 20–2).

However, many lower-grade, less cellular lesions, especially those whose volume is largely composed of extracellular matrix and desmoplastic tissue, generate significantly less of the angiogenesis factors and develop far less tumor neovascularity. In fact, they may stimulate so little neovascularity that even the best current ultrasound equipment is either unable to detect it or is unable to distinguish it from normal blood flow or blood flow to benign lesions such as fibroadenoma. Such lesions frequently have demonstrable flow within the tissues immediately surrounding the lesion but have no demonstrable internal flow (Fig. 20–3). Intermediate-grade lesions tend to have some internal flow, but much less than do high-grade lesions (Fig. 20–4). That all living tissues (including normal tissues and benign solid nodules such as fibroadenomas) have blood flow complicates things. Like cancers, the flow within fibroadenomas varies greatly. Fibroadenomas with cellular stroma (juvenile fibroadenomas) and some complex fibroadenomas often have more internal flow than the average low- or intermediate-grade carcinoma (Figs. 20–5 and 20–6). Lactating adenomas, greatly stimulated by the hormones of pregnancy, are among the most vascular of all lesions (Fig. 20–7). Fibroadenomas that have become hyalinized or fibrosclerotic, on the other hand, may have a small amount

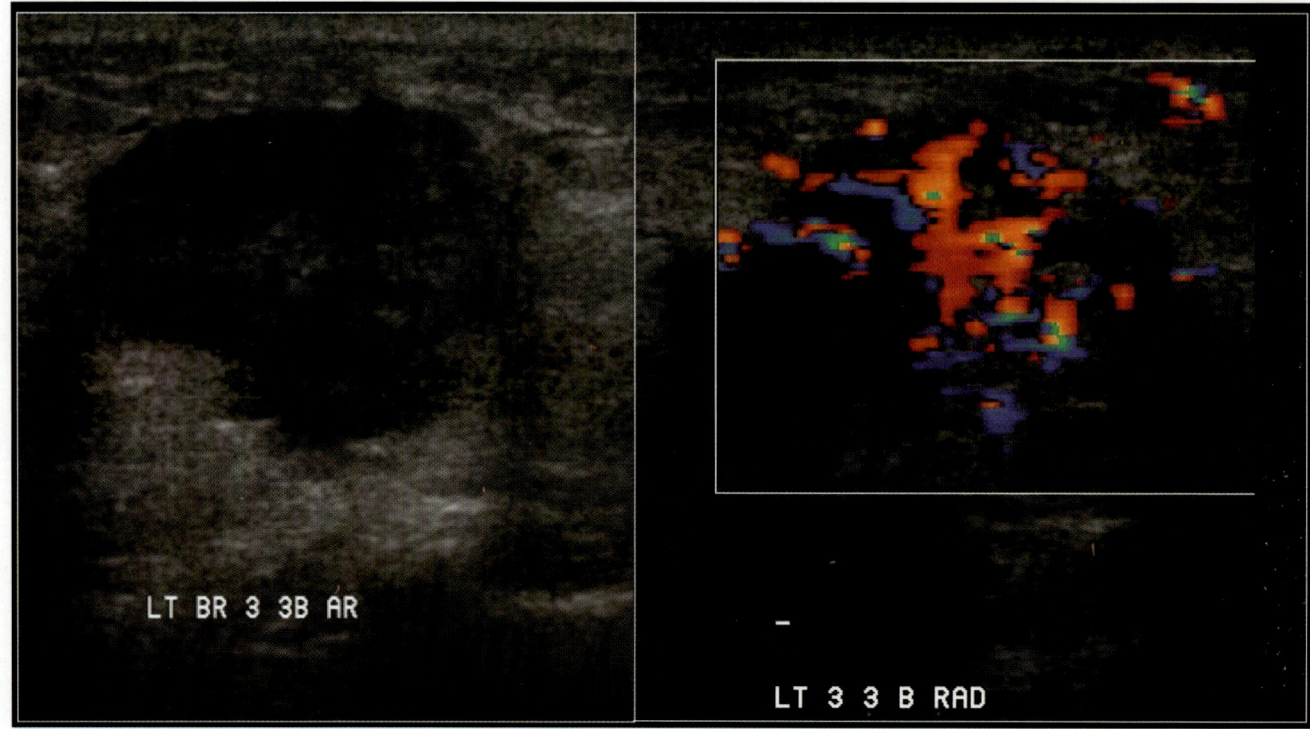

FIGURE 20–1 The hypervascularity of high-grade invasive not otherwise specified breast carcinomas tends to be very obvious on color Doppler evaluation.

of peripheral flow but generally have no demonstrable internal flow (Fig. 20–8).

Ultrasound contrast agents may or may not help improve sensitivity of Doppler in such lesions. Although ultrasound contrast will make flow within low-grade lesions

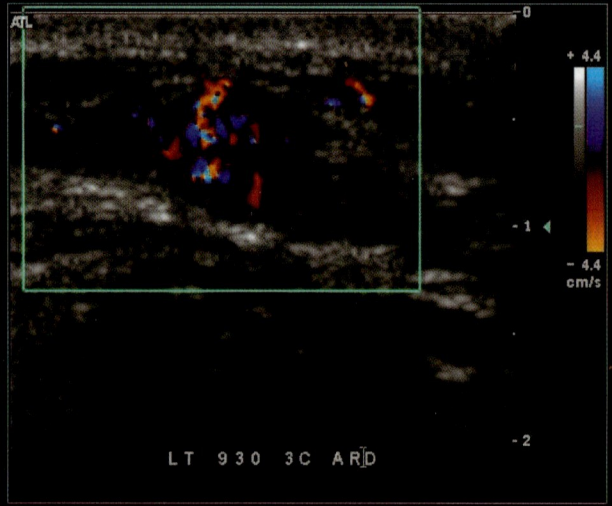

FIGURE 20–2. Some special-type tumors, such as this invasive papillary carcinoma, also tend to show obvious hypervascularity on color Doppler evaluation.

with little tumor neovascularity more readily detectable, the contrast will also make flow within normal tissue and benign lesions such as fibroadenomas more easily detectable. Thus, even with contrast, such paucicellular malignant lesions may not have perceptibly increased flow.

Similar limitations apply to the use of Doppler for demonstrating the pattern of a peripheral net of vessels around malignant tumors. The amount and density of peripheral vascularity varies greatly from lesion to lesion, and the ability of unaided Doppler to demonstrate it is still insufficient in the subgroup of breast tumors that is relatively paucicellular and in which the bulk of the tumor mass consists of desmoplasia. Once again, there is hope that further improvements in ultrasound equipment, combined with the use of ultrasound contrast agents, will improve Doppler's ability to demonstrate the typical peripheral vascular net of malignant tumors.

The use of Doppler for detection of abnormally high-velocity flow or abnormally low-impedance flow for definitive diagnosis of malignant lesions is also limited. There is considerable overlap among the maximum velocities of normal tissues, benign lesions, and malignant lesions. Furthermore, there is also considerable temporal variation in flow to normal tissues and benign lesions during the menstrual cycle or in patients who are undergoing hormone replacement therapy that could increase the overlap in blood flow between benign and malignant lesions in such

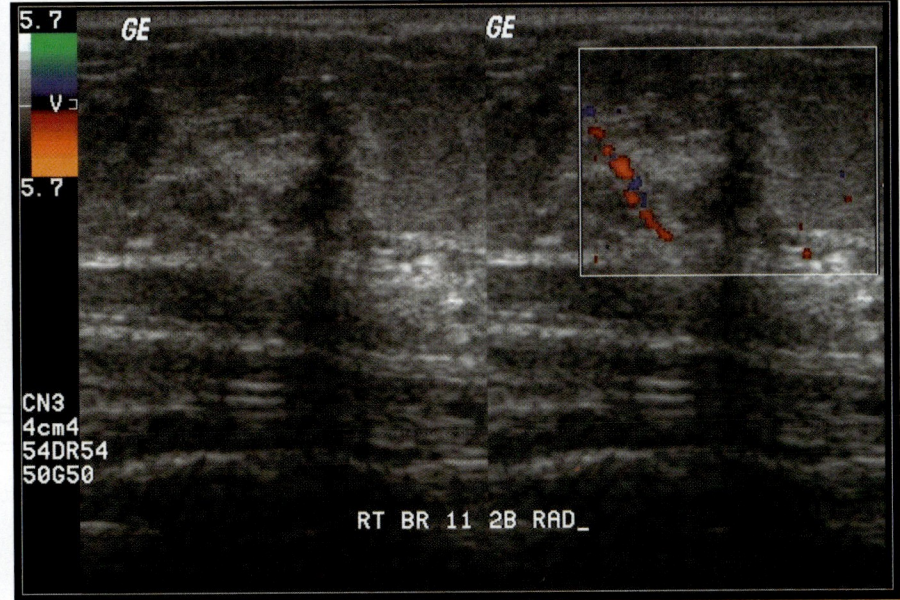

FIGURE 20–3 Low-grade invasive not otherwise specified carcinomas generally have little or no internal vascularity on color Doppler but often have demonstrable feeding vessels in the surrounding tissues.

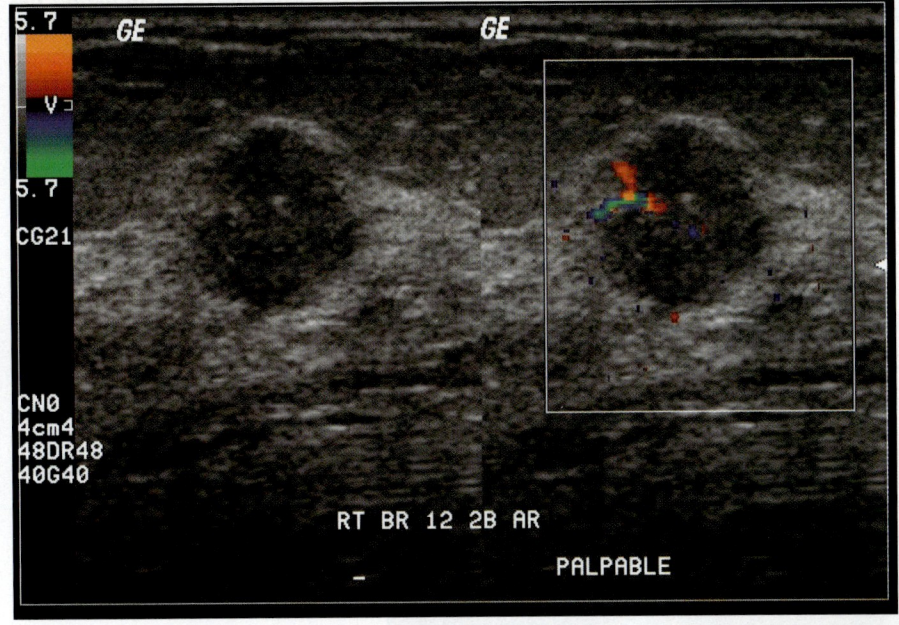

FIGURE 20–4 Intermediate-grade invasive not otherwise specified carcinomas have amounts of color Doppler–demonstrable flow that are intermediate between those of high-grade and low-grade lesions. Typically, a vessel or two are demonstrable within the substance of the nodule and another vessel or two on the periphery.

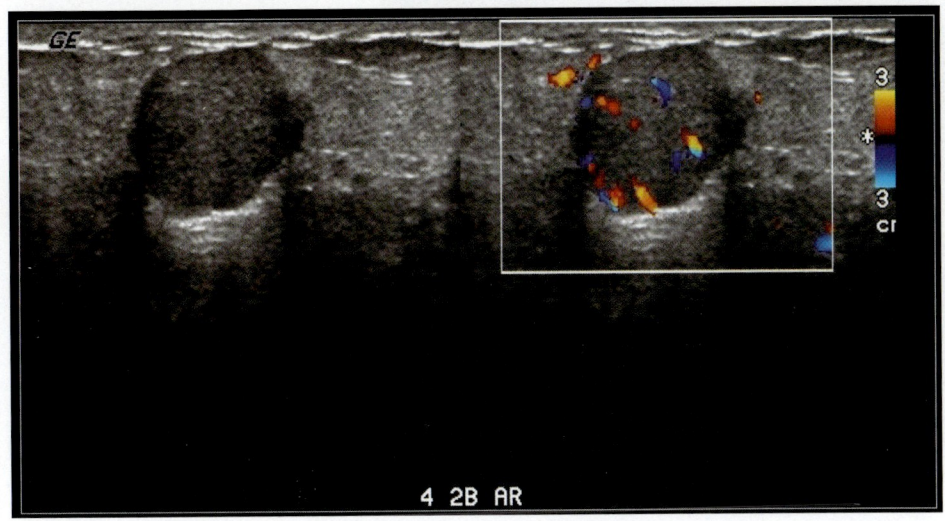

FIGURE 20–5 Some fibroadenomas that have cellular stroma have abundant internal vascularity that is demonstrable with Doppler.

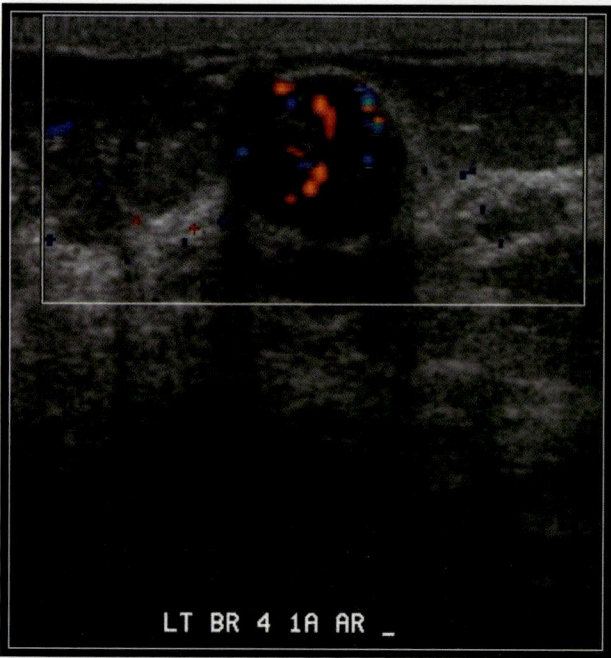

FIGURE 20–6 Some complex fibroadenomas, particularly those that contain adenosis, are hypervascular.

patients. Semi-quantitative measurements, such as peak systolic velocities and resistivity indices, will probably never achieve sufficient efficacy to enable us to use them alone in characterizing lesions as benign or malignant and in deciding whether to perform biopsy. Furthermore, this overlap in velocity and resistivity is an intrinsic feature that probably cannot be addressed by improvements in equipment or with the use of ultrasound contrast enhancement.

In our experience, one of the most reliable positive predictors of malignancy is a difference that exists in the pulsed Doppler spectral waveform patterns between vessels that lie within the substance of the tumor and those that lie on the periphery. In many malignant lesions, the waveforms obtained from the center of the lesion have high peak systolic velocities, sharp systolic peaks, early diastolic notches, relatively lower peak diastolic velocities, and higher measures of impedance such as systolic-to-diastolic ratios, resistivity indices, and pulsatility indices. On the other hand, the waveforms obtained from the periphery of the malignant nodule tend to have lower systolic velocities and more rounded systolic peaks, lack early diastolic notches, and have lower measurements of impedance (Fig. 20–9). In fibroadenomas, papillomas, and other benign lesions, the flow both centrally and peripherally tends to show lower systolic velocities with rounded systolic peaks, lack of early diastolic notches, and low measurements of impedance (Fig. 20–10). Thus, the difference in the waveform patterns between central and peripheral vessels is a strong positive predictor of malignancy, and flow patterns obtained from vessels within the center of a lesion that are similar to peripheral waveforms is a negative predictor for malignancy.

The literature as it pertains to peak systolic velocities and measurements of impedance in malignant lesions has been conflicting and very confusing. Some studies reported

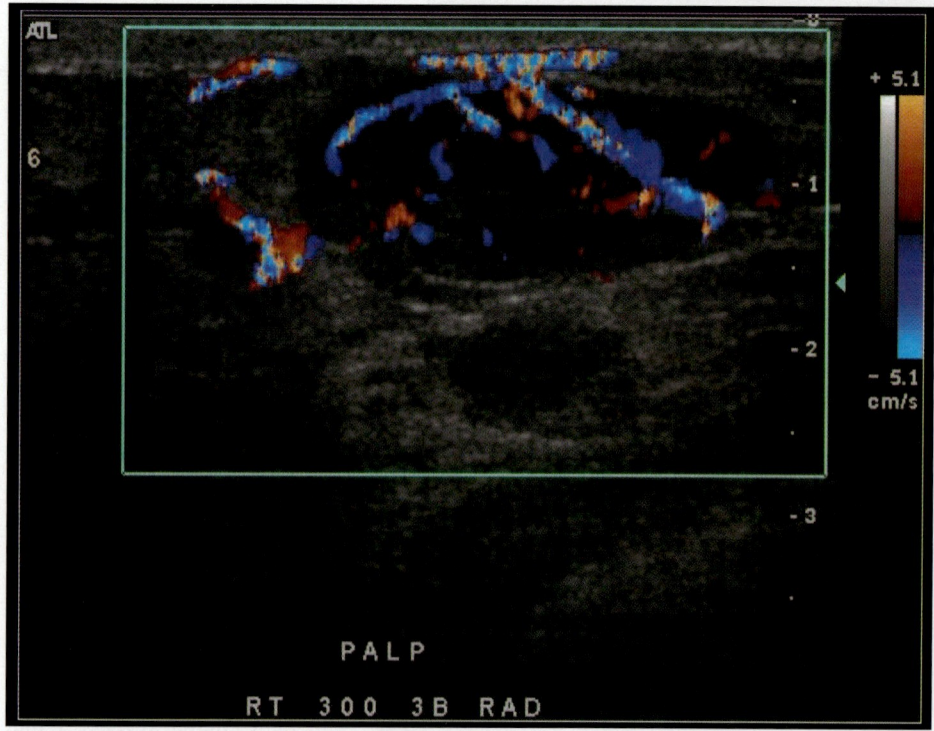

FIGURE 20–7 Lactating adenomas, stimulated by the hormones of pregnancy or lactation, typically appear very vascular on color Doppler evaluation.

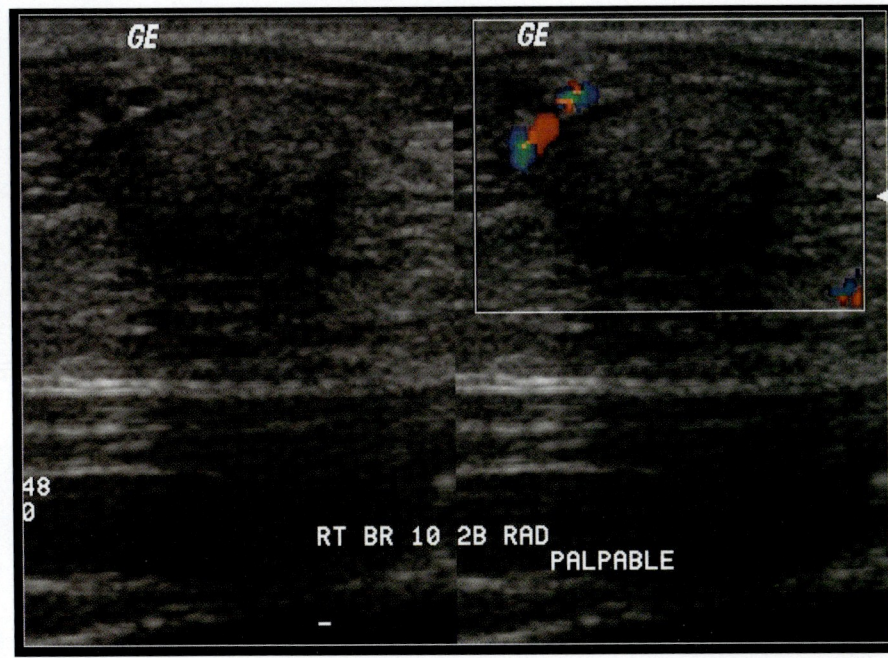

FIGURE 20–8 Hyalinized or sclerotic fibroadenomas typically have little or no internal flow that is demonstrable on color Doppler.

high peak systolic velocities and relatively high measurements of impedance in malignant lesions, whereas others reported lower systolic velocities and lower measurements of impedance in malignant lesions. We think these discrepant findings reflect differences in the location of tumor vessels that were interrogated. The reason for high resistance indices and high peak systolic velocities centrally within tumors is likely related to increased hydrostatic pressure within the extracellular matrix of such lesions. First, the extracellular matrix has large amounts of hyaluronic acid, a huge molecule that in three dimensions has innumerable

interstices that are highly hydrophilic. Thus, hyaluronic acid within the extracellular matrix actively pulls in water, increasing the hydrostatic pressure within the extracellular space. Second, the vessels within tumors are abnormally leaky, allowing large molecules that are normally held within the bloodstream to leak out into the extracellular space. Because tumors do not develop lymphatic vessels internally, there is no mechanism other than passive diffusion for removing these substances. Above a critical size, passive diffusion becomes inadequate for such purposes. Thus, in tumors above a certain size, substances (large proteins) that

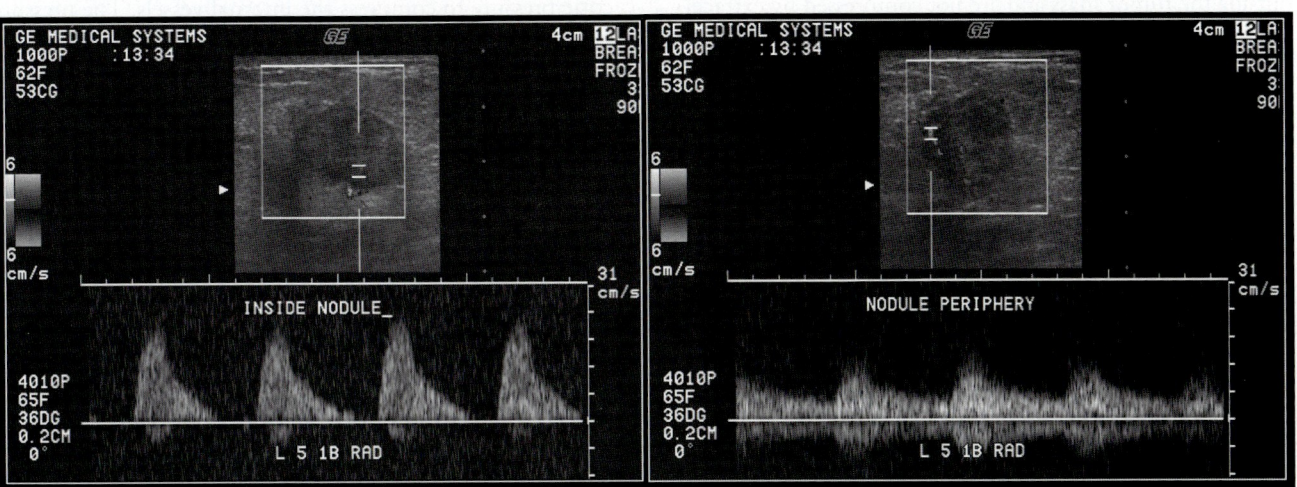

FIGURE 20–9 Pulsed Doppler waveforms vary with their location in many invasive breast carcinomas. Vessels on the surface of the node tend to have relatively low peak systolic velocities, rounded systolic peaks, and relatively high end-diastolic velocities and low resistivity indices (**right**). On the other hand, vessels deep within the nodule tend to have high systolic peak velocities, sharp systolic peaks, and relatively low end-diastolic velocities and high resistivity indices (**left**).

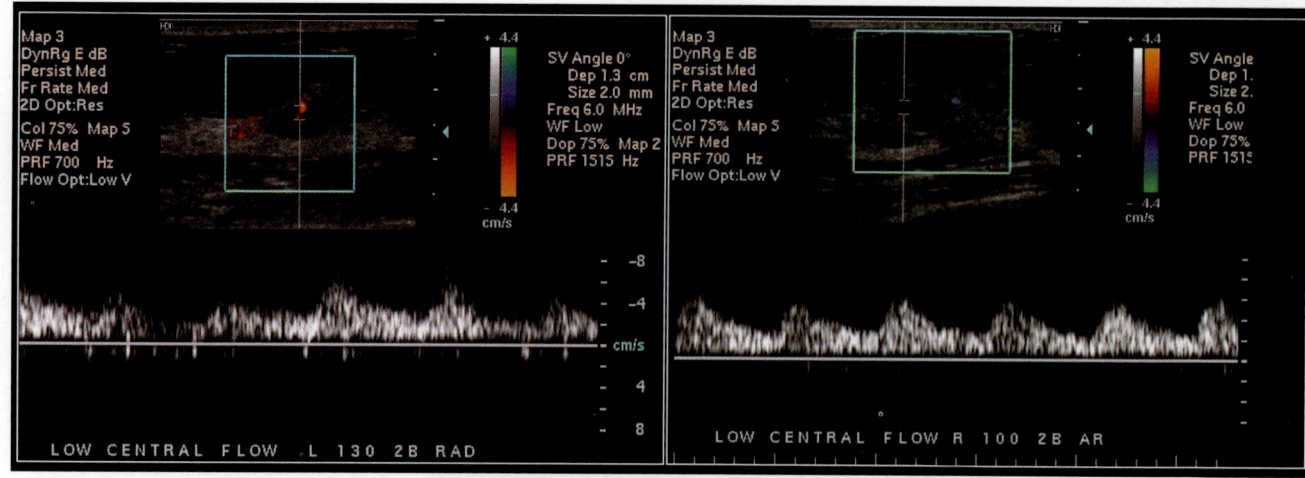

FIGURE 20–10 The waveforms obtained from the interior and periphery of fibroadenomas are similar to each other. Both have relatively low systolic peak velocities, rounded systolic peaks, and high end-diastolic velocities and low resistivity indices. Waveforms obtained from both the interior and surface of fibroadenomas resemble those obtained from surface vessels of malignant tumors. Only the waveforms obtained from the interior of malignant nodules have high peak systolic velocities, sharp systolic peaks, and high resistivity indices.

have leaked from the bloodstream into the extracellular matrix of the tumor continuously accumulate and are not removed, further increasing oncotic pressure within the extracellular matrix of the lesion. The combination of the highly hydrated hyaluronidase molecules and accumulated large protein molecules within the extracellular matrix near the center of tumors increases the oncotic pressure within the extracellular matrix so much that it extrinsically compresses the soft and pliable sinusoidal tumor vessels. Extrinsic compression of these sinusoids increases impedance to flow through them, explaining the higher measurements of impedance. Meanwhile, the veins that drain the lesion lie outside the tumor mass and are not compressed by extracellular matrix, maintaining very low impedance to outflow from the tumor. The high oncotic pressures within the tumor's extracellular matrix and the low pressures outside the tumor result in an increase pressure gradient that has the potential to increase flow velocities through the tumor. However, because the oncotic pressures within the extracellular matrix nearly equal diastolic pressures, very little flow can pass through the sinusoids during diastole. Thus, the increased velocities that result from the increased pressure gradient can manifest only during the systolic portion of the cardiac cycle, resulting in the increased systolic velocities and sharp systolic peaks noted within the center of tumors. Although one might expect flow in the periphery of the tumor to reflect indirectly the increased impedance within the tumor substance, most of the flow in the periphery never passes through the center of the tumor. Only a very small percentage of the flow actually passes through the center of the tumor. The tumor vessels in the periphery are not subject to such extrinsic compression by extracellular

matrix and therefore reflect mainly the low-impedance flow that occurs through uncompressed sinusoidal tumor vessels that lie in the peripheral tumor net.

Benign lesions such as fibroadenomas and papillomas have some hyaluronic acid in the extracellular matrix, but much less than malignant tumors. These benign lesions do not develop the abnormally leaky sinusoidal vessels that malignant lesions do; hence, protein molecules do not accumulate within the extracellular matrix to the degree that they do in malignant lesions. The net result is that benign lesions do not have as much extracellular matrix, and within the extracellular matrix that they do have, there is less oncotic pressure to compress the internal vessels. The pressure gradient between the center of the lesion and the draining veins is much less than diastolic blood pressures, resulting in lower-impedance flow and lower systolic velocities.

Unfortunately, the degree of compression pressure used during scanning can alter all of these relationships. For differences in spectral waveform patterns to have any predictive value at all, Doppler must be performed with as little compression pressure as possible. Using slightly too much compression pressure first compresses the draining veins, decreasing the pressure gradient between the tumor substance and draining veins and decreasing systolic velocities internally within malignant tumors. Using slightly too much compression pressure also increase impedance to flow through the peripheral vascular net, decreasing diastolic flow and measurements of impedance, and making the systolic peak sharper. Thus, using slightly too much compression pressure can obscure the differences in waveform patterns between the center and periphery in malignant lesions and between malignant and benign lesions. Using slightly more pressure can completely occlude venous outflow, reducing the pressure gradient to zero and stopping blood flow within the tumor. Arterial pressures can still force blood into the tumor for a short while, but once in, it cannot get out. Hemoglobin within the blood in the tumor substance rapidly becomes deoxygenated. Imaging techniques have actually been developed to exploit this phenomenon. By applying very light intermittent compression and scanning the breast lightly at wavelengths that are absorbed by deoxygenated hemoglobin, tumors can actually be displayed as absorptive areas on light scan. The spatial resolution of such techniques is very poor because light diffuses out equally in all directions, so that targeted diagnostic sonography will probably be necessary in conjunction with light scanning.

Although the waveform pattern differences between the center and periphery of malignant tumors discussed in the previous paragraph indirectly reflect the abnormal leakiness of tumor vessels, Doppler has little chance of improving its ability to demonstrate directly the abnormal leakiness of malignant vessels. Furthermore, current ultrasound contrast agents being developed will not improve this limitation for two reasons: (a) the agents currently being developed and evaluated are all high-molecular-weight substances specifically designed to stay within the intravascular space and are too large to leak out into the extracellular space of tumor vessels; and (b) Doppler is designed to detect moving particles. Ultrasound contrast agents, even if they did pass freely from the vascular space into the extravascular space of tumors, would be essentially stationary and therefore not detectable by Doppler. The agents used for contrast-enhanced MRI and radionuclide studies of the breast, gadolinium and ^{99m}Tc-sestamibi, on the other hand, are lower-molecular-weight substances that leak into the extracellular space, do not require movement for detection, and are readily detectable by their respective imaging modalities.

For Doppler to be competitive with MRI or nuclear medicine at demonstration of abnormally leaky vessels, two new ultrasound developments would be required. First, low-molecular-weight ultrasound contrast agents small enough to leak out of abnormal tumor vessels would have to be developed, and second, ultrasound equipment manufacturers would have to develop hardware and software algorithms for demonstrating stationary microbubbles. To our knowledge, there are no small low-molecular-weight ultrasound contrast agents being developed. However, stationary microbubbles can be detected by using high enough energy in the B-mode imaging beam to cause cavitation (bursting of the microbubble). We believe that, in the near future, Doppler will not be able to compete with either contrast-enhanced MRI or ^{99m}Tc-sestamibi for sensitivity in demonstrating abnormally leaky tumor vessels.

Finally, Doppler assessment of breast tumors should not be viewed as a stand-alone assessment of a lesion's risk for malignancy. It is best used in conjunction with the real-time B-mode image. Currently, high-frequency near-field B-mode imaging is quite effective in characterizing solid breast nodules, even in the absence of Doppler information. The most successful B-mode imaging algorithms all use multiple imaging findings. The published sensitivity of Doppler is competitive with the published sensitivity of most individual B-mode imaging findings but is less than that of algorithms using multiple imaging findings. Furthermore, the sensitivity of Doppler and the number of malignant findings on B-mode imaging vary with the type of breast tumor being imaged. Thus, depending on tumor type, the Doppler and imaging findings may be complementary.

At the spiculated end of the spectrum, lesions have relatively few tumor cells and a relatively large amount of desmoplasia. Doppler findings may be sparse or absent, but the B-mode imaging findings of such lesions are obviously malignant in almost all cases and do not offer a diagnostic challenge, even in the absence of Doppler findings.

At the circumscribed end of the malignant spectrum, however, the B-mode imaging findings suggesting malignancy may be fewer in number and subtler, increasing the risk for false-negative sonography. However, such circumscribed lesions are often highly cellular, high-grade, invasive ductal carcinomas. Because of their high neoplastic cellularity and high metabolic needs, such lesions generate a larger quantity of angiogenesis factors and have obviously increased vascularity that is readily demonstrable by Doppler. Thus, Doppler can be used in conjunction with a battery of multiple imaging findings to improve characterization of solid nodules even further, but at the present time, it should not be used as a stand-alone method of characterizing solid breast nodules.

Several different criteria have been used for distinguishing between benign and malignant lesions using Doppler. Many have used simple color or power Doppler assessments for increased vascularity, such as presence or absence of flow, number of vessels per unit area, or pattern of flow (e.g., the peripheral vascular net, number of feeding vessels, or eccentricity of flow within a lesion). Others have advocated semiquantitative pulsed Doppler spectral waveform analysis to assess the vascular shunting known to occur through tumor vessels. Pulsed Doppler criteria have included cutoffs above a certain peak systolic velocity or measurements of systolic-to-diastolic ratio, resistivity index, or pulsatility index below a certain level. Still others have compared velocities or measurements of resistivity within the center of the lesion to these same measurements in the periphery of the lesion. As noted earlier, carcinomas tend to have higher peak systolic velocity and higher resistivity indices centrally and lower peak systolic velocities and lower resistivity indices peripherally. Fibroadenomas and other benign etiologies of solid nodules, on the other hand, tend to have similar peak systolic velocities and resistivity indices centrally as they do in the periphery of the lesion.

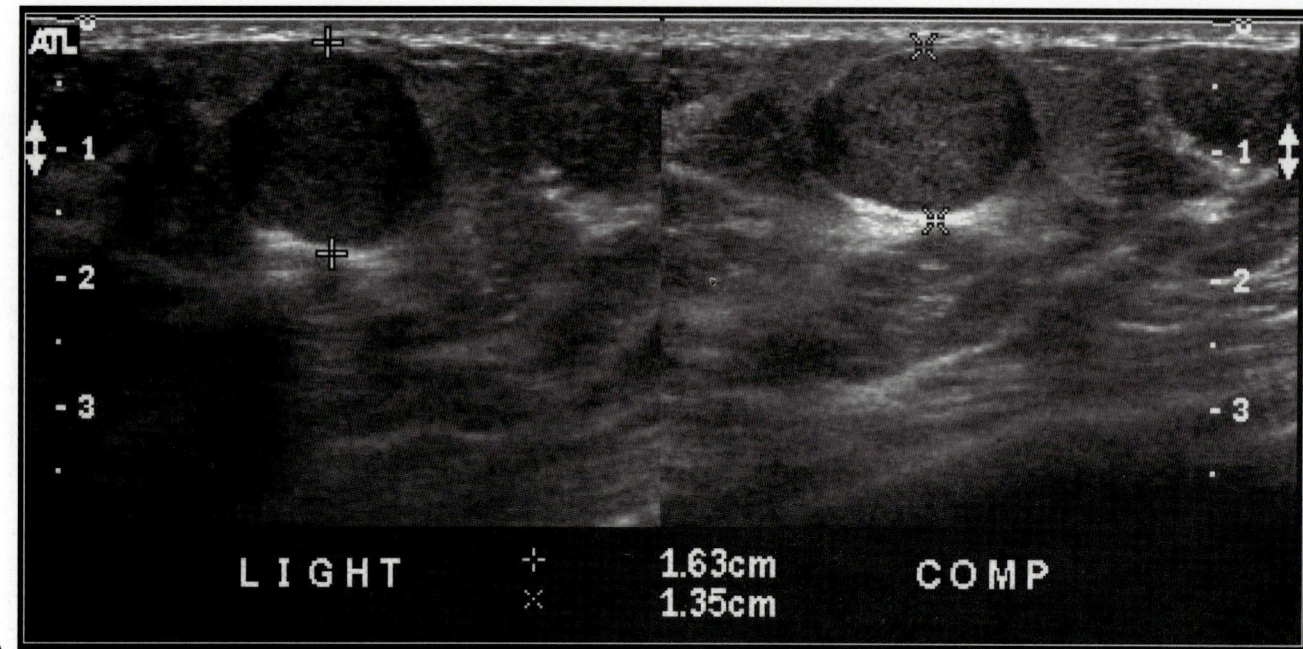

A

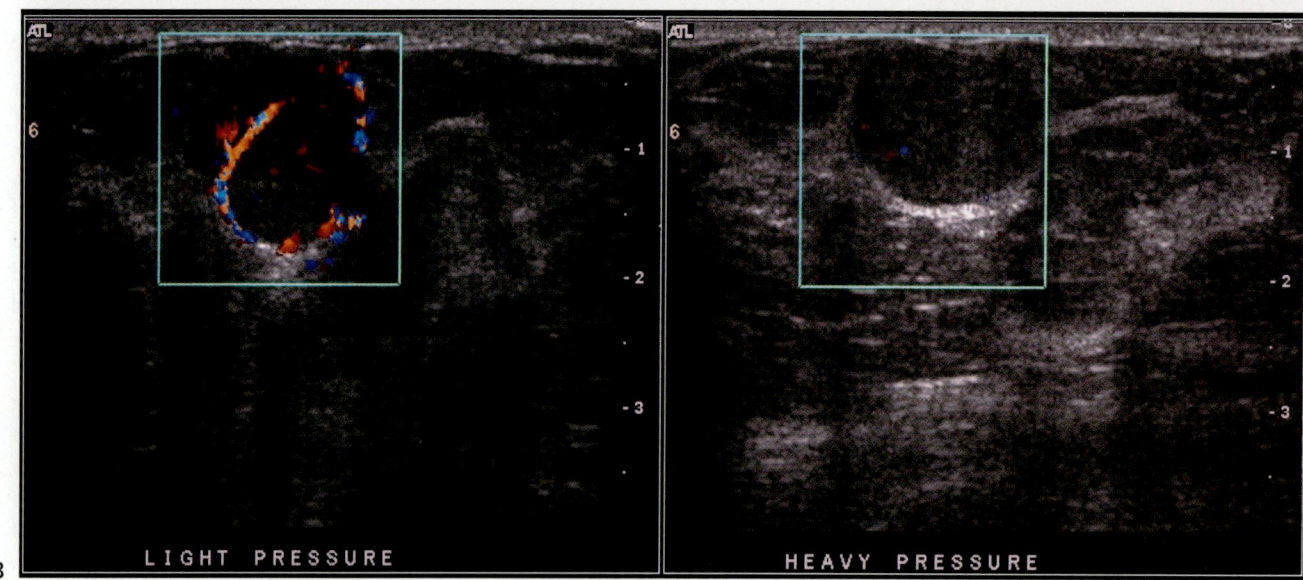

B

FIGURE 20–11 A: Many solid nodules, such as this fibroadenoma with cellular stroma, are partially compressible. **B:** If too much compression pressure is used during the color Doppler examination, vessels within and surrounding the nodule may be compressed or even completely collapsed, stopping blood flow (this nodule is a fibroadenoma that has cellular stroma).

The sensitivity for malignancy of these various Doppler criteria ranges from the mid-80s to low-90s percentile. Thus, Doppler sensitivities are good, but not great. However, the current feeling in the United States is that sensitivity and negative predictive value of 98% or greater (definition of BIRADS 3) is necessary to avoid biopsy on lesions believed to be benign. The few Doppler studies reporting sensitivities of 95% or greater included high per-

centages of large, advanced lesions (larger than 2 cm in diameter), in which the chance for long-term survival or cure is reduced and the contribution of Doppler findings to final outcome is minimized.

Additionally, few of these studies have emphasized enough the extreme sensitivity of flow within breast tumors to compression with the ultrasound transducer. Unfortunately, it is very easy to compress tumors inadver-

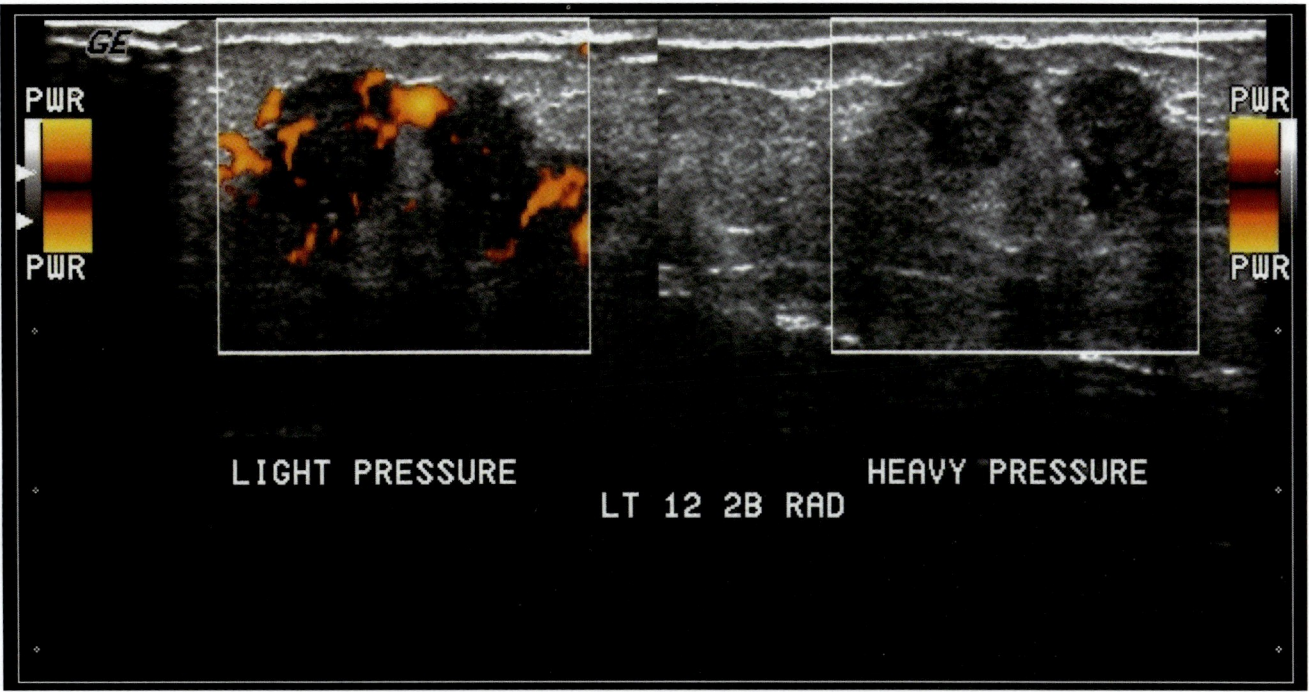

FIGURE 20–12 Scanning with too much compression pressure can obscure even the hypervascularity of malignant lesions (**right**). The image on the left, obtained with very little compression, shows abundant flow in the high nuclear-grade DCIS. When the weight of the arm is allowed to rest on the transducer (**right image**), however, internal flow ceases.

tantly between the hard transducer and firm chest wall. Excessive compression pressure can collapse the abnormal vascular spaces within and around the tumor, decreasing or even completely shutting off blood flow to the lesion. Inadvertent compression can greatly affect the Doppler assessment of flow to the tumor, regardless of the criteria being used, and lead to false-negative Doppler studies. This is especially true for highly cellular lesions that contain little desmoplasia and therefore are softer and more compressible than their lower-grade, more desmoplastic counterparts. We initially hoped that being able to stop flow with compression indicated that it was a benign lesion, but we quickly learned that blood flow to both benign and malignant lesions can be stopped by compressing vigorously (Figs. 20–11 and 20–12). The more cellular, less desmoplastic lesions are those most likely to have abundant blood flow demonstrable by Doppler if proper scan technique is used. It is absolutely essential that very little scan pressure be used with any form of Doppler to assess a breast lesion for tumor neovascularity. Whether the criteria used are presence or absence of flow, vessel density, color Doppler or power Doppler, or pulsed or abnormal peak systolic velocities or impedance indices on pulsed Doppler spectral analysis, excessive scan pressure can adversely affect the results. Simply allowing the weight of the arm to rest on the transducer is sufficient to alter the characteristics of the waveforms toward lower velocities and higher impedance

(Fig. 20–13). One must actually lift the transducer slightly while scanning so that it barely touches the skin in order to maximize the sensitivity of Doppler in the breast. Papillary breast lesions, such as invasive papillary carcinomas (Fig. 20–14) and benign intraductal papillomas (Fig. 20–15), are the softest of all breast lesions other than lipoma and are even more sensitive to compression pressure than are other lesions.

In our experience, presence or absence of flow, number of vessels per unit area, peak systolic velocities, and measurements of impedance have added little to the diagnosis of breast cancer. In cases in which the Doppler is abnormal, the B-mode imaging findings are always abnormal. Yet in many malignant lesions in which the B-mode image is highly suspicious, the Doppler findings are not.

In summary, we feel that Doppler is moderately sensitive for detection of malignancy. However, in our experience, the B-mode imaging findings are more sensitive for malignancy than Doppler. Thus, we believe that Doppler adds little to imaging findings in characterizing solid nodules. It usefulness in solid nodules lies in other areas.

Determining Aggressiveness of Suspicious or Malignant Breast Lesions

Despite the limitations of Doppler in characterizing lesions into benign and malignant categories, we believe that it is

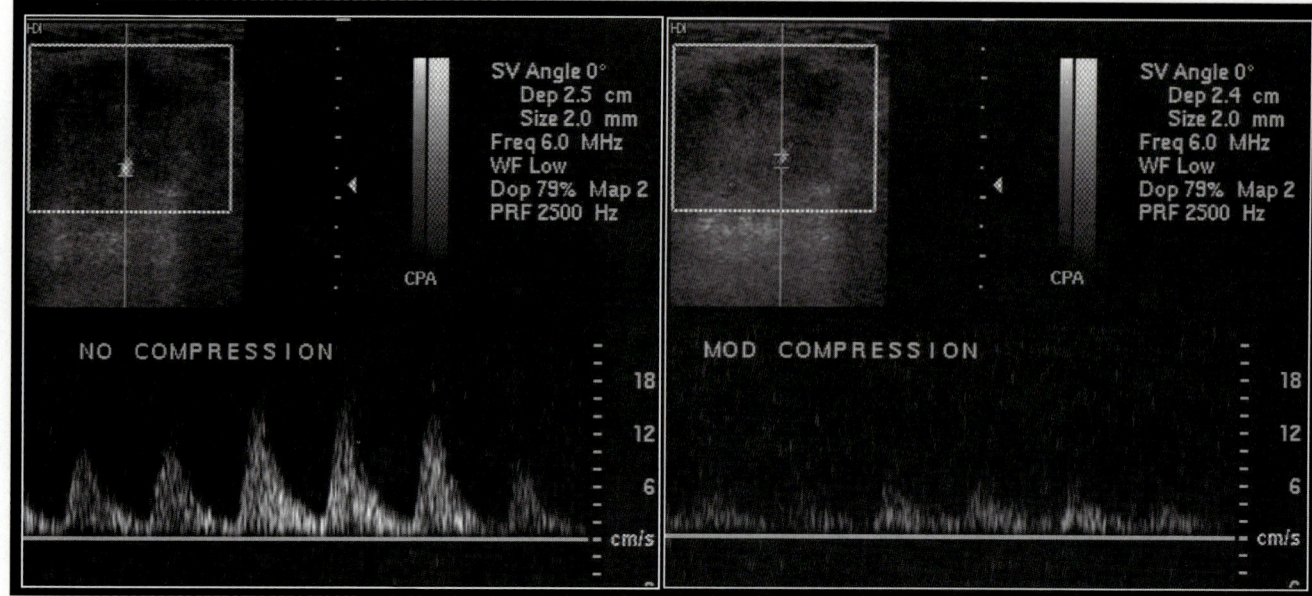

FIGURE 20–13 Using excessive compression pressure can alter pulsed Doppler spectral waveforms as well as the presence or absence of flow on color Doppler. Using too much pressure reduces both systolic and diastolic velocities but, as a percentage of original velocity, affects diastole to a greater extent than systole, increasing resistivity indices (**right**).

very useful in distinguishing "aggressive" from "nonaggressive" lesions. High-grade invasive breast carcinomas tend to have markedly increased flow compared with normal tissues for two reasons. First, they are highly cellular lesions that have high metabolic needs and elaborate abundant angiogenesis factors. Second, they incite an intense inflammatory response. The combination of high tumor neovascularity and inflammatory hyperemia contributes to easy detection of increased blood flow on color Doppler or power Doppler (Fig. 20–1). Such lesions grow more rapidly and metastasize to lymph nodes and hematogenously earlier and more extensively. Thus, Doppler readily

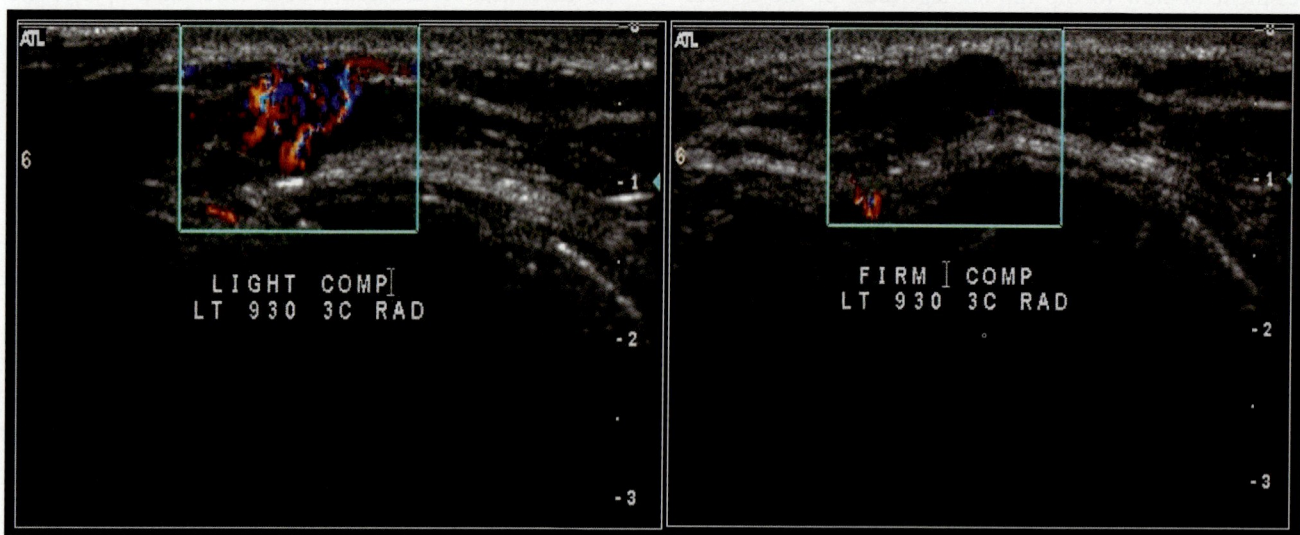

FIGURE 20–14 The softest and most easily compressed lesions in the breast are benign and malignant papillary lesions. Note that using too much compression pressure can completely shut off flow within this extremely vascular small invasive papillary carcinoma. To avoid inadvertently compressing such lesions, color Doppler should be done with the transducer barely keeping contact with the skin. Even minimal pressure can alter the flow in such soft and compressible lesions.

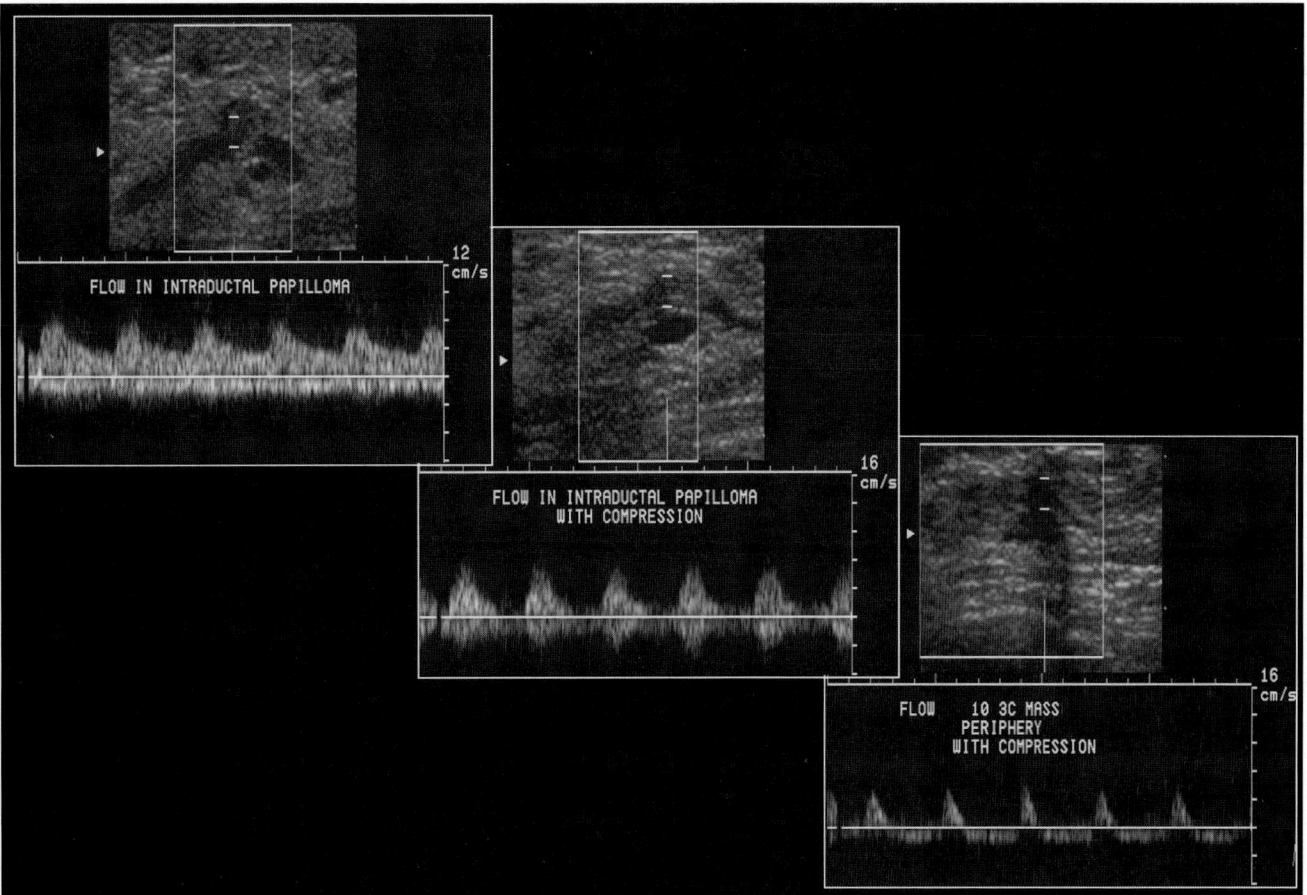

FIGURE 20–15 These pulsed Doppler spectral waveforms show the effect of only minimal amounts of compression pressure on a very soft and compressible benign intraductal papilloma. The **left** image shows the waveform obtained while actively lifting the transducer so that it barely maintains contact with the skin. The **middle** image was obtained with just the normal weight of the arm as contact pressure. Note that the velocities are lower and the resistivity higher. The lower **right** image shows the waveform obtained with very slight compression pressure. Note that the diastolic flow is reversed. With only slightly greater compression pressure, detectable flow within the lesion stopped completely.

detects lesions most likely to be locally aggressive as well as lethal as a result of distant spread.

Low-grade lesions are less cellular and stimulate a more desmoplastic than an inflammatory response. They have relatively little tumor neovascularity and essentially no inflammatory hyperemia (Fig. 20–3). Such lesions tend to grow slowly and to metastasize to lymph nodes distantly later and less extensively. Thus, lack of Doppler-demonstrable flow in such lesions indicates a less locally aggressive and less lethal tumor. Intermediate-grade lesions show intermediate Doppler findings (Fig. 20–4).

Doppler could be very helpful in determining how aggressive to be surgically, with respect to regional lymph node dissection, and in determining the need for and type of adjuvant nonsurgical therapy. Hypervascularity on Doppler might indicate the need for postoperative external radiation or brachytherapy, adjuvant chemotherapy, hormonal therapy, or antiangiogenesis therapy in addition to surgery.

Assessing Response to Tumor Therapy

If Doppler were used to help determine the need for radiation, chemotherapy, hormonal therapy, or antiangiogenesis therapy, it could also be used to monitor the response to treatment. We often use imaging and Doppler now to follow response to available chemotherapeutic agents. In some cases, vascularity decreases before there is a decrease in tumor volume (Fig. 20–16). Doppler could be especially useful in determining the effectiveness of antiangiogenesis therapy. In such cases, a favorable response would likely result in decreased blood nearly immediately, long before shrinkage of the tumor could be detected sonographically.

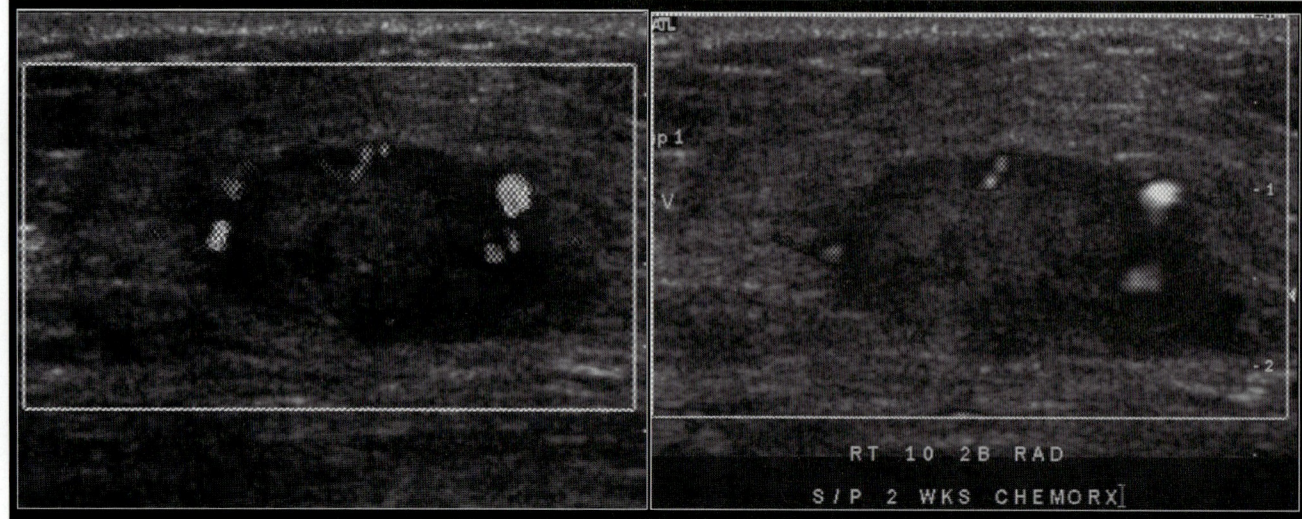

FIGURE 20–16 In lesions that respond well to chemotherapy tumor vascularity may decrease before the tumor decreases in size. The **left** image shows an intermediate-grade invasive not otherwise specified carcinoma before induction chemotherapy. The **right** image shows the lesion after 2 weeks of chemotherapy. The size of the lesion has not yet changed, but the number of visible blood vessels has decreased, suggesting that the lesion was responding favorably to chemotherapy, which was continued for another 4 weeks. At the end of 6 weeks of treatment, the lesion had decreased 75% in volume, and Doppler-demonstrable blood flow had ceased.

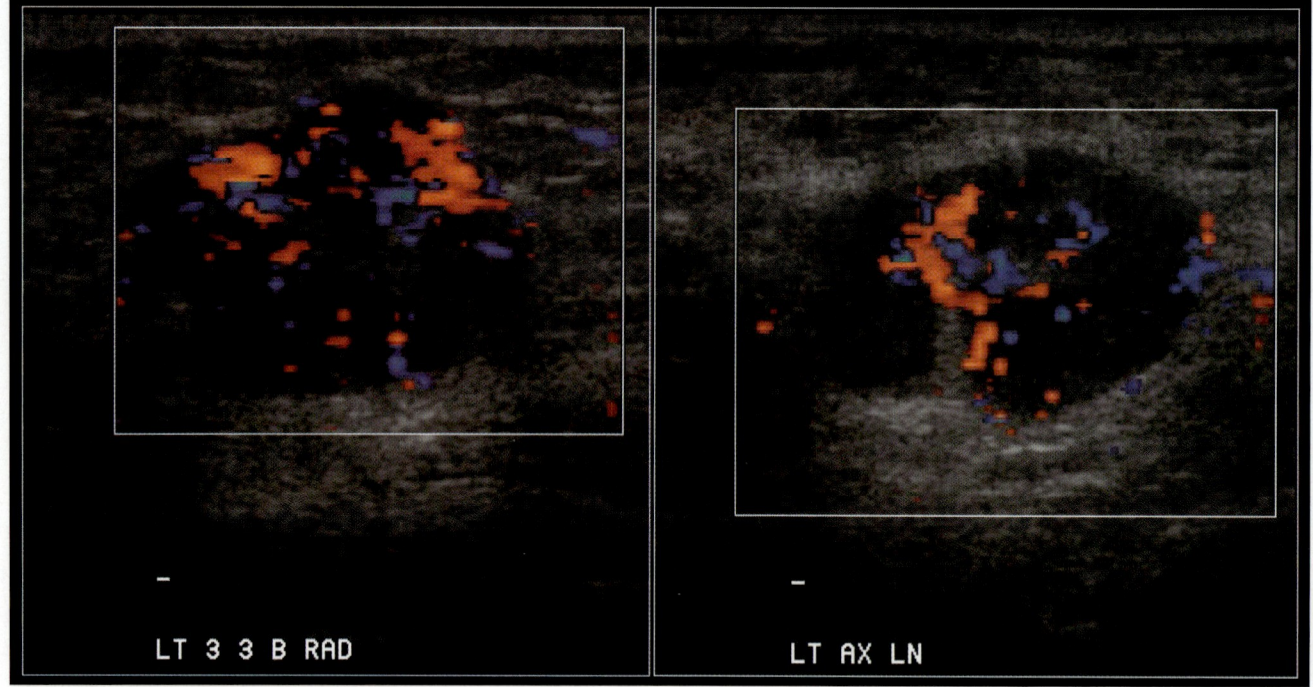

FIGURE 20–17 Because most lymph node metastases have histology that is identical to the primary lesion, the blood flow pattern in the metastatic lymph node (**right**) is usually nearly identical to the blood flow pattern in the primary carcinoma (**left**). This can be useful in trying to determine whether an enlarged lymph node is reactive or inflamed, or enlarged because of metastasis.

Assessing Whether Lymphadenopathy Is Caused by Inflammation or Metastatic Breast Carcinoma

We now routinely perform whole breast ultrasound and sonographic evaluation of axillary lymph nodes in patients who have solid nodules that are characterized into BIRADS 4b and 5 categories. We then perform ultrasound-guided large core needle biopsy in cases in which there are one or more grossly abnormal lymph nodes that are highly suspicious for metastatic disease. When no abnormal lymph nodes can be detected, the patient usually undergoes sentinel lymph node analysis, axillary dissection, or both. Sonographic assessment of axillary lymph nodes is plagued by three potential problems. First, microscopic lymph node metastases cannot be detected sonographically, resulting in false-negative findings. Second, some nodes that have gross disease will not be enlarged, again resulting in false-negative findings. Third, some enlarged lymph nodes are merely inflamed or reactive and do not contain metastasis. Such nodes will result in false-positive findings. There is no sonographic imaging or Doppler solution to the problem of micrometastases at the current time. However, Doppler may be very helpful in lymph nodes that are not enlarged but that have some morphologic abnormality and in cases in which the node is enlarged but has nonspecific sonographic features that could be caused by either inflammation or metastasis.

Most lymph node metastases from breast carcinoma have histology identical to that of the primary tumor. Thus, if the histology of the primary tumor is associated with hypervascularity, the lymph node metastases from that primary lesion will also be hypervascular (Fig. 20–17). Similarly, if the vessels in the center of the primary tumor have high peak systolic flows, sharp systolic peaks, and high resistivity indices, then the pulsed Doppler waveforms obtained from the metastasis-containing lymph node will have similar features in most cases (Fig. 20–18). This pattern of spectral waveform characteristics differs greatly from the waveform characteristics obtained from inflamed or reactive lymph nodes, for which the pulsed Doppler spectral waveforms tend to have lower systolic velocities, more rounded systolic peaks, and lower resistivity indices (Fig. 20–19). Unfortunately, some primary tumors either have no internal flow or have low, rounded systolic peaks similar to those seen in inflamed lymph nodes. In such cases, this finding will be ineffective. It is important to compare waveforms obtained within the interior of the primary tumor nodule to those obtained from the lymph node because flow in the periphery of most tumors is similar to that obtained from inflamed nodes.

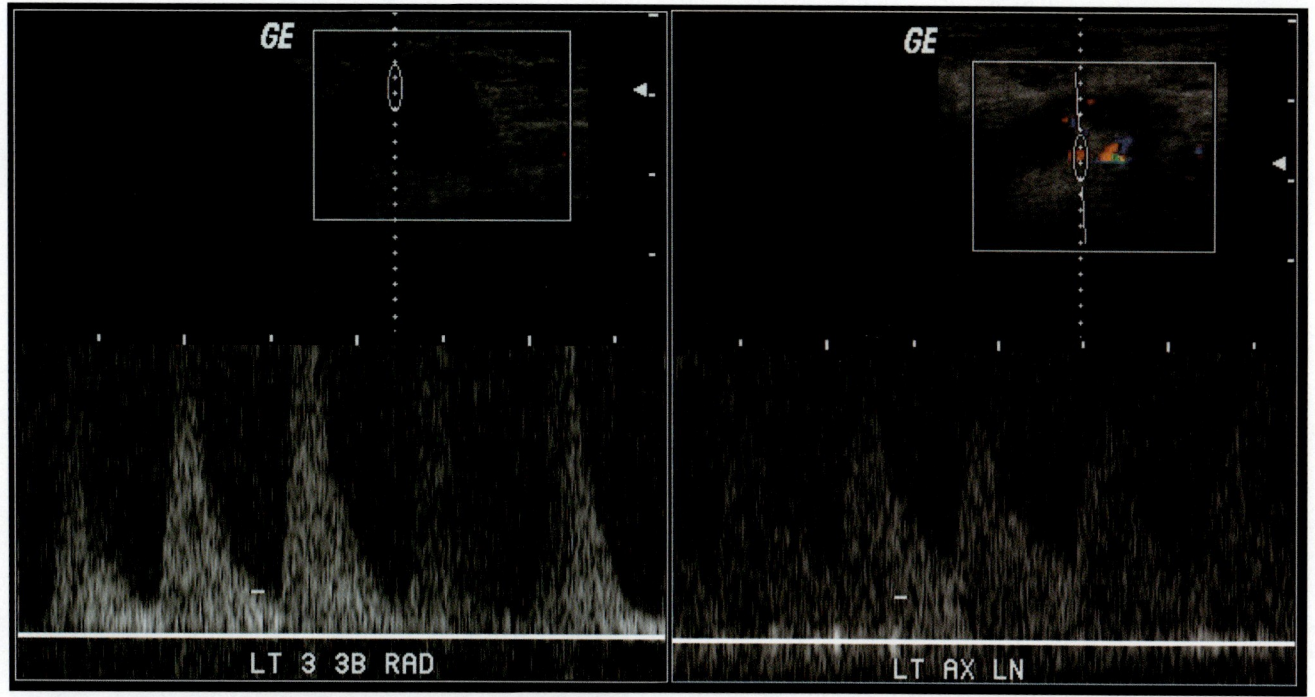

FIGURE 20–18 Not only do the color Doppler and power Doppler flow patterns within the metastasis-containing lymph node parallel those of the primary lesion, but so does the pulsed Doppler spectral waveform pattern. Most malignant tumors have high systolic velocities and relatively high resistivity indices in the center of the tumor (**left**). So do the lymph nodes that contain metastases from that primary lesion (**right**).

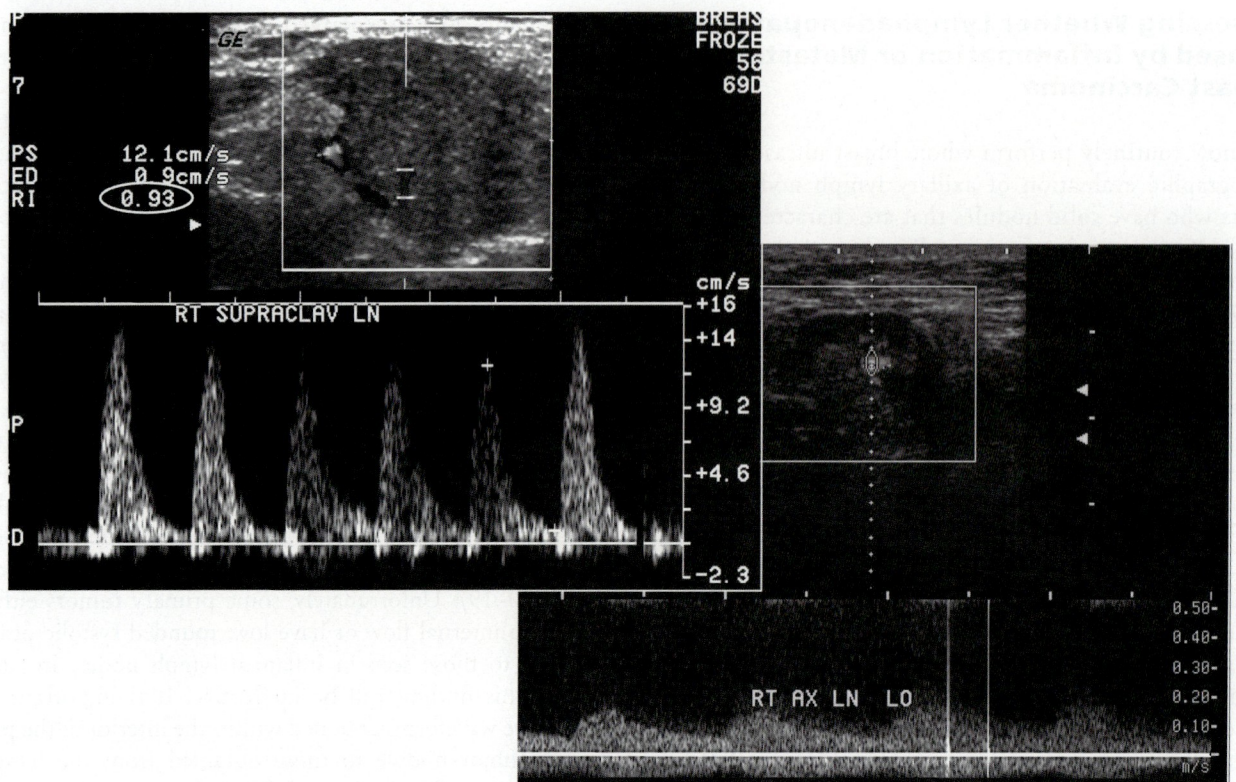

FIGURE 20–19 The pulsed Doppler spectral waveform in metastasis-containing lymph nodes differs from that of inflamed or reactive nodes. The node-bearing metastasis usually has a waveform characterized by high systolic velocities, sharp systolic peaks, and relatively high impedance (**upper left**). Reactive or inflamed nodes, on the other hand, have lower systolic velocities, more rounded systolic peaks, and lower impedance (**lower right**).

The most specific of all the Doppler findings for lymph node metastases is the presence of transcapsular feeding vessels. The vascular supply of normal lymph nodes enters and exits through the hilar notch. The normal lymph node has no vessels that traverse the lymph node capsule. In inflamed nodes, the normal hilar vessels enlarge and appear to arborize more extensively, but transcapsular feeding arteries do not develop (Fig. 20–20). Breast cancer metastases, on the other hand, tend to lodge in subcapsular and cortical sinusoids and can generate angiogenesis factor that lead to the formation of transcapsular feeding vessels (Fig. 20–21). Lymphoma may develop multiple feeding vessels, but these usually enter through the hilar notch, not through the capsule (Fig. 20–22). Thus, the presence of transcapsular feeding arteries suggests the presence of lymph node metastases.

Power Doppler is somewhat more sensitive than color Doppler and, in our experience, is better for demonstrating transcapsular vessels. In cases in which the lymph node is grossly abnormal, the mediastinum of the lymph node may be so compressed, displaced, and distorted that it cannot be identified. If the hilar area cannot be identified, this finding cannot be used. However, such nodes are usually so

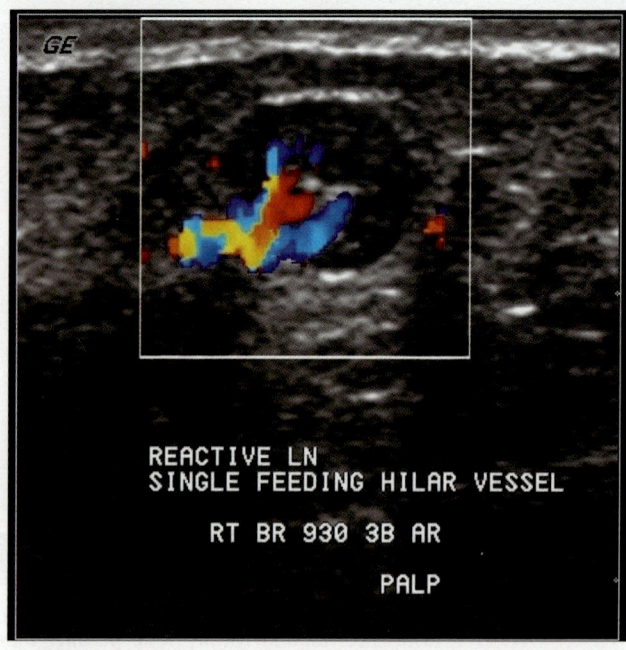

FIGURE 20–20 Lymph nodes that are enlarged because of inflammation do not develop neovascularity. The single hilar vessel may enlarge, but multiple vessels do not develop. In particular, there are no transcapsular vessels.

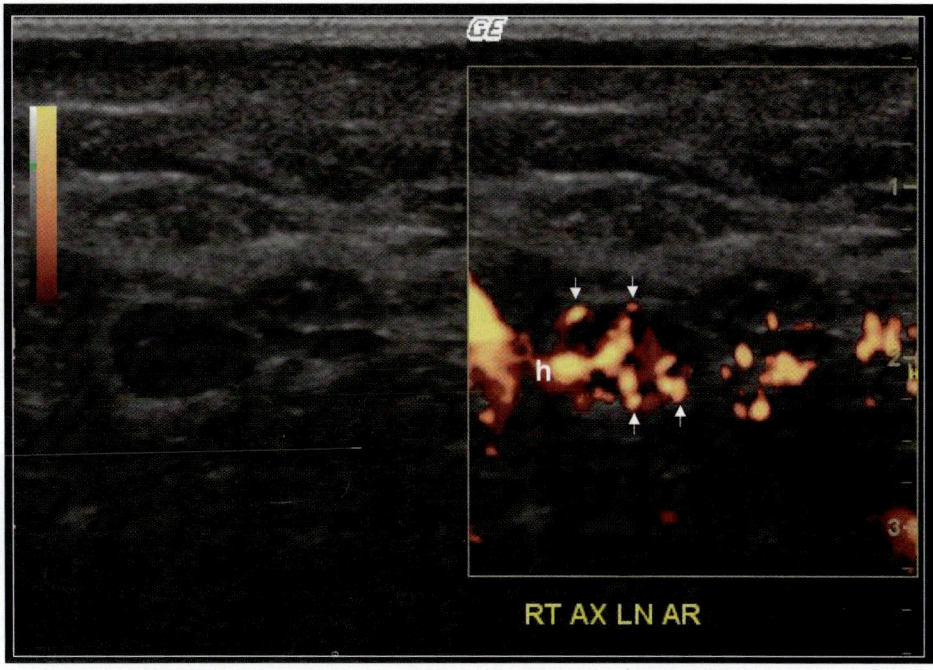

FIGURE 20–21 Even more specific for metastatic disease than multiple vessels is the presence of feeding arteries that enter the lymph node through a transcapsular route. Even lymphomas generally do not develop transcapsular feeders (*arrows* indicate transcapsular tumor vessels stimulated by subcapsular metastases). h, dilated hilar artery.

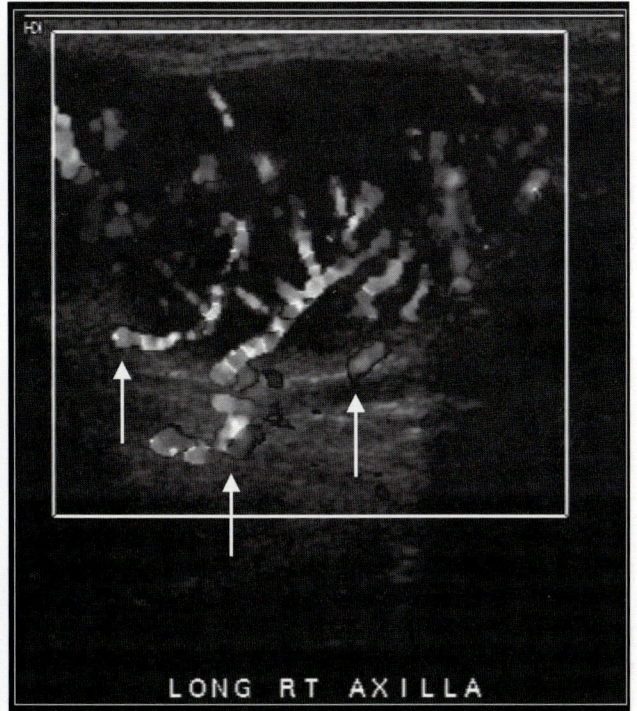

FIGURE 20–22 Lymphomatous lymph nodes may develop multiple feeding vessels, but they all tend to enter through the hilum. It is unusual for lymphomatous nodes to develop transcapsular feeding vessels.

grossly abnormal by imaging findings alone that Doppler is not necessary.

Distinguishing Solid Nodules from Complex Cysts with Low-Level Internal Echoes

About 3% of all lesions detected by sonography cannot be characterized with absolute certainty as being either cystic or solid. Fibroadenomas and complex cysts with diffuse low-level internal echogenicity are the lesions that make up most of this group. In some cases, the diffuse low-level echoes within cysts are artifactual. Technical advances, such as high-frequency coded harmonics and real-time compounding, can clear these artifactual echoes in many cases and are discussed in greater detail in Chapters 2 and 10. Other approaches are to attempt to aspirate or to assume all are solid and characterize all of these lesions as if they were solid nodules. Most will have BIRADS 3 characteristics. These approaches are discussed in Chapter 10. Color Doppler or power Doppler can be useful before attempting aspiration or assuming all that of these lesions are solid. Most complex cysts that have diffuse low-level echoes contain either echogenic fatty or proteinaceous fluid that require no blood flow or are filled with papillary apocrine metaplasia, which rarely develops a fibrovascular

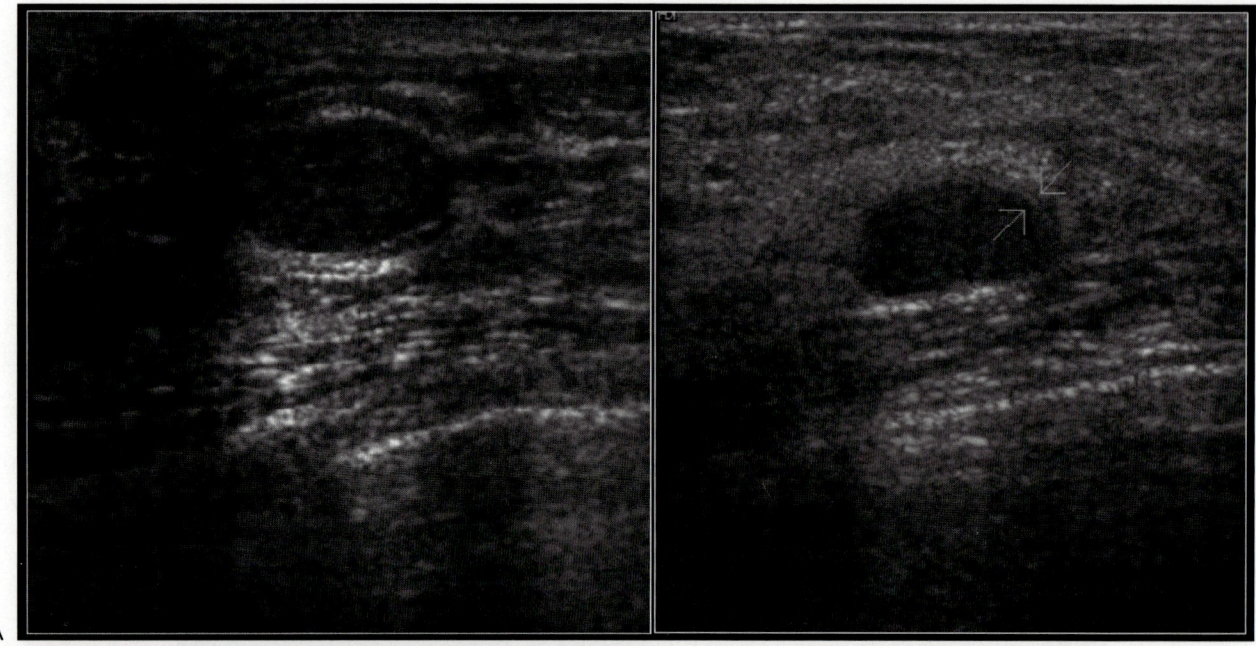

A

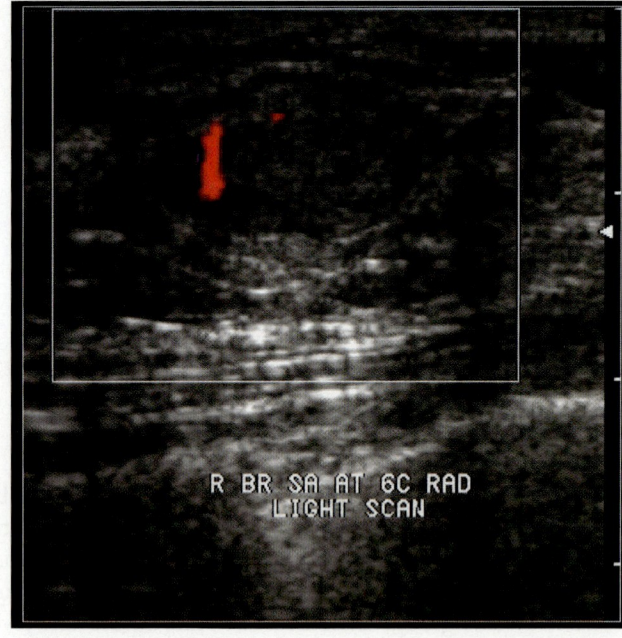

B

FIGURE 20–23 A: About 3% of breast lesions must be characterized as being indeterminate and cannot be determined to be cystic or solid. The lesion on the **left** is a well-transmitting fibroadenoma. The lesion on the **right** is cystic with echogenic secretions. They are sonographically indistinguishable. **B:** The lesion shown on the **left** in the image in part A had an internal blood vessel, indicating that it was solid. The lesion on the **right** had no internal blood flow and was aspirated completely.

stalk. Thus, demonstration of an internal vessel with color Doppler or power Doppler indicates that the lesion is either completely solid, such as a fibroadenoma (Fig. 20–23), or is an encysted papillary lesion that completely fills the cyst (Fig. 20–24).

Another group of lesions is classified as pseudocystic. These are solid lesions that are so homogeneous and so markedly hypoechoic that they appear nearly anechoic and can easily be mistaken for cysts. However, if color Doppler shows internal vascularity, the error of misclassifying these malignant solid nodules as cysts can be avoided. Medullary carcinoma, metastasis to intramammary lymph nodes, and

high-nuclear-grade ductal carcinoma *in situ* (DCIS) with a clinging pattern are the lesions most likely to present with a pseudocystic appearance (Figs. 20–22 and 20–25 to 20–27).

Distinguishing Intracystic Papilloma or Carcinoma from Papillary Apocrine Metaplasia

Some complex cysts contain mural nodules or thick, isoechoic septations or have eccentric isoechoic thickening of one wall. In most cases, such thickenings are caused by

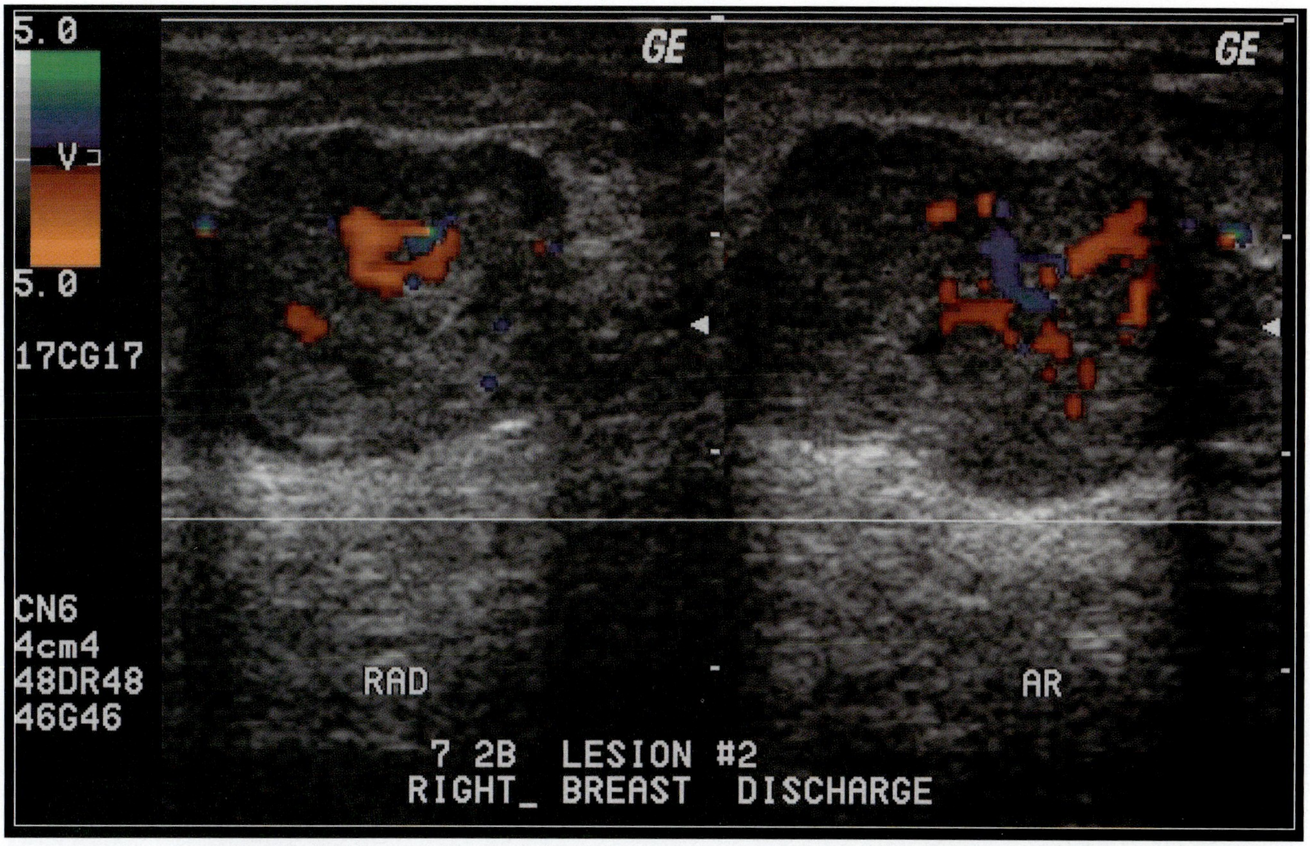

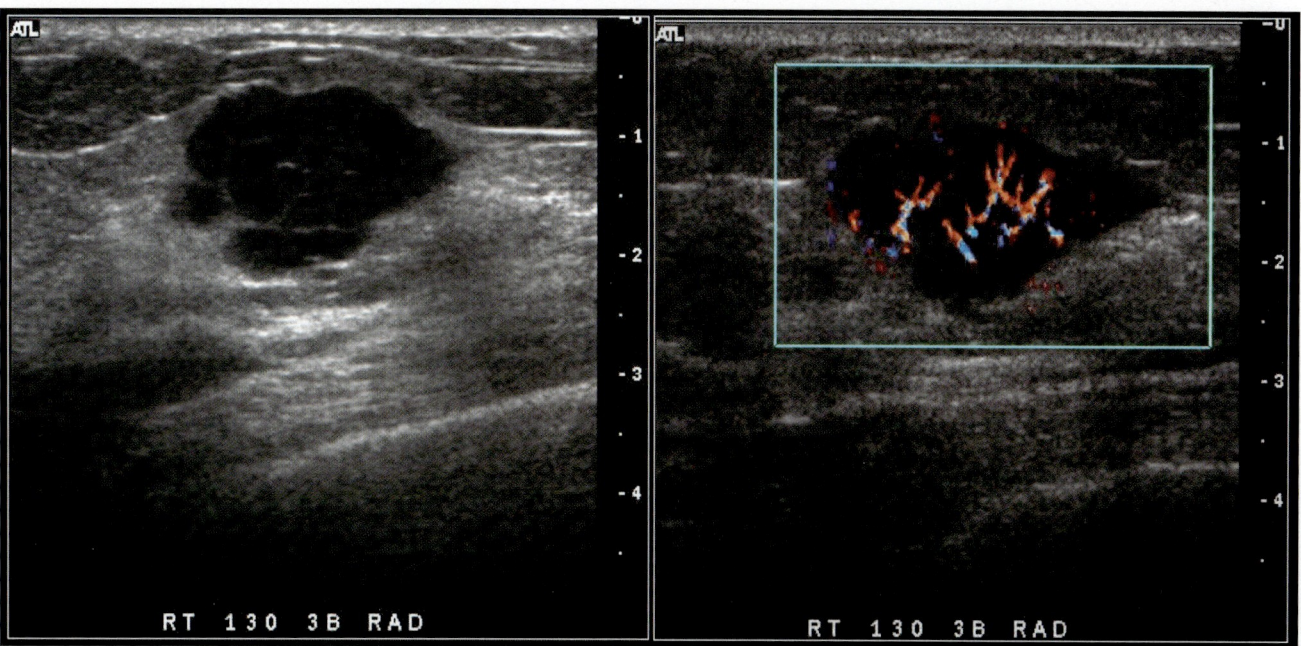

FIGURE 20–24 Color Doppler shows this highly vascular lesion to be solid rather than cystic. It is an encysted papilloma that completely fills the cyst.

FIGURE 20–25 Certain special-type tumors, such as this medullary carcinoma, are so hypoechoic that they are nearly anechoic and have a pseudocystic appearance. Color Doppler can be helpful in avoiding misdiagnosis of such lesions as clusters of cysts. Lymphoma of the breast, metaplastic carcinoma, and some high-grade invasive ductal carcinomas may also have a pseudocystic appearance.

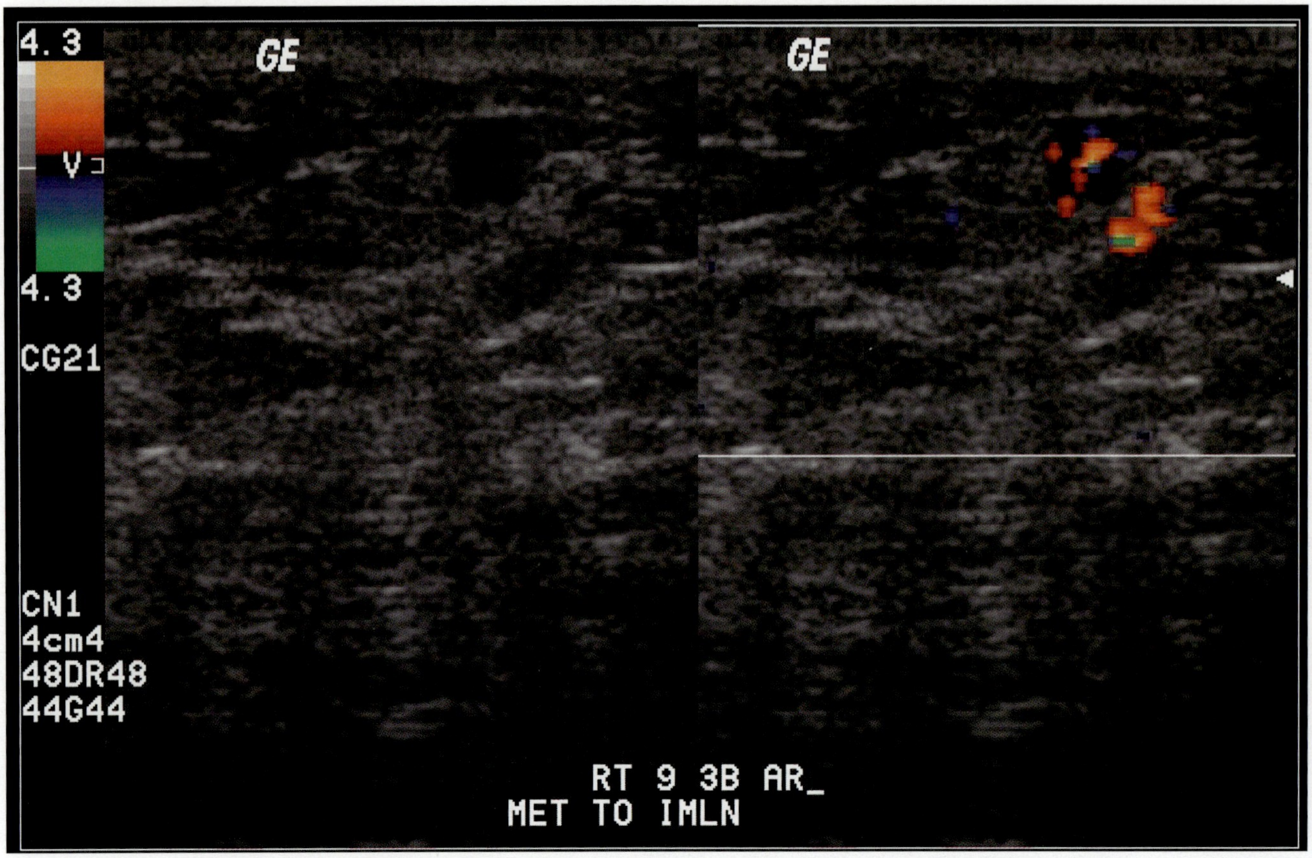

4.3
GE

V

4.3

CG21

CN1
4cm4
48DR48
44G44

GE

RT 9 3B AR_
MET TO IMLN

FIGURE 20–26 Metastases to intramammary lymph nodes are prone to be smaller than cutoff diameters for metastatic lymph nodes and to have a pseudocystic appearance. Color Doppler or power Doppler may be helpful in avoiding mischaracterization of such nodes as cysts.

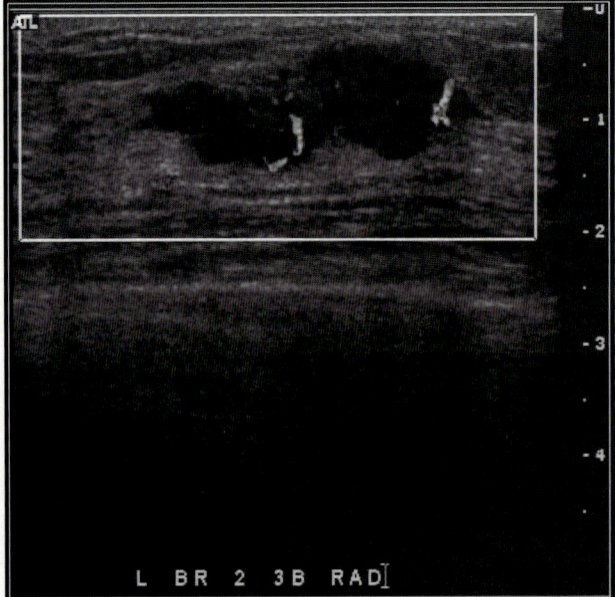

ATL

L BR 2 3B RAD

FIGURE 20–27 High-nuclear-grade ductal carcinoma *in situ* may have a pseudocystic appearance. Color Doppler can help avoid mischaracterizing such a lesion as cystic.

papillary apocrine metaplasia, part of the benign fibrocystic spectrum, but in a few cases, such findings may be caused by papillomas or intracystic carcinomas. With very few exceptions, papillary apocrine metaplasia does not develop a pronounced fibrovascular stalk that is demonstrable by Doppler (Fig. 20–28). On the other hand, intracystic papillomas and intracystic papillary carcinomas are among the most vascular of all breast lesions and have fibrovascular stalks that are readily demonstrable with color or power Doppler (Fig. 20–29). Thus, demonstration of a fibrovascular stalk indicates a very high probability of intracystic papilloma or carcinoma and the need for histologic evaluation. Occasionally, a fibrovascular stalk can be show within a mural nodule caused by papillary apocrine metaplasia, but this occurs rarely enough that all mural nodules with fibrovascular stalks must be assumed to be papillomas or papillary carcinomas until proved otherwise. Lack of a fibrovascular stalk favors papillary apocrine metaplasia over papillary lesions, but does not completely exclude intracystic papilloma or papillary carcinoma because hemorrhagic infarction of such lesions is a relatively common occurrence (Fig. 20–30). Interestingly, there can be a difference in the color Doppler or power

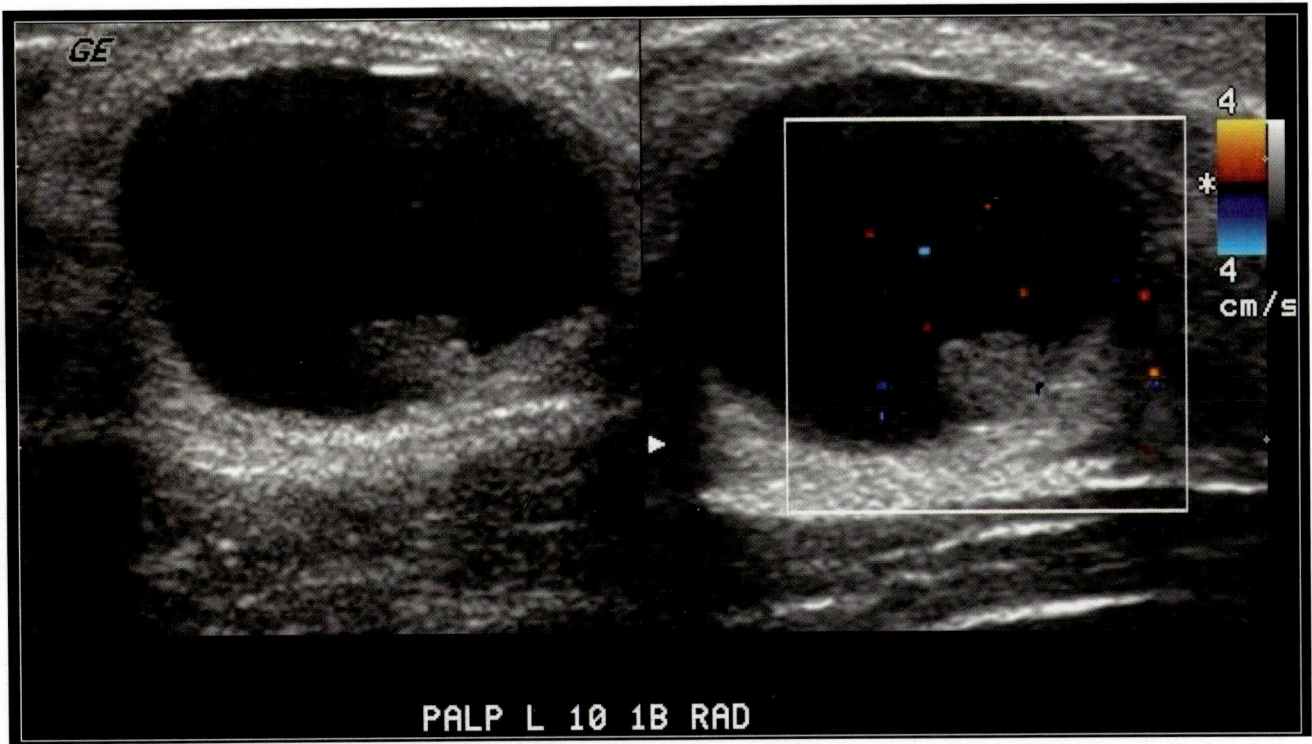

PALP L 10 1B RAD

FIGURE 20–28 Intracystic mural nodules caused by papillary apocrine metaplasia rarely develop a Doppler-demonstrable fibrovascular stalk.

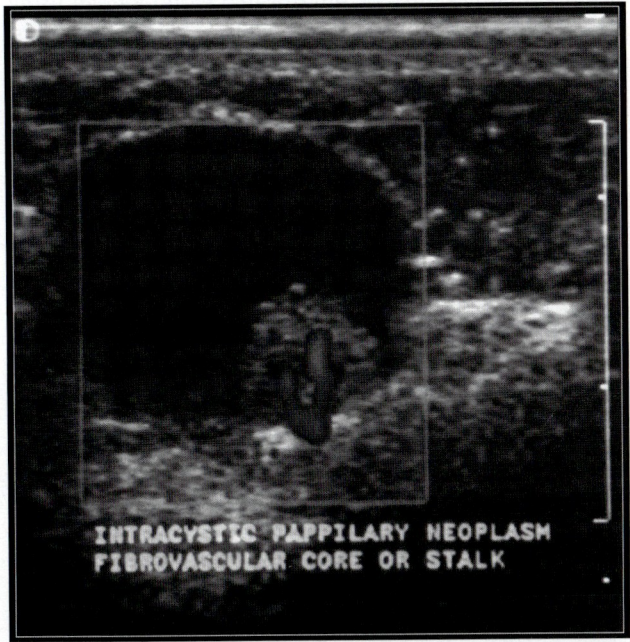

INTRACYSTIC PAPPILARY NEOPLASM
FIBROVASCULAR CORE OR STALK

FIGURE 20–29 A single artery usually feeds the vascular stalk of a benign intracystic papilloma.

Doppler flow pattern within the fibrovascular stalks of benign and malignant mural nodules. The invasion that occurs with malignant intracystic malignancies, unlike that in solid nodules, is mainly inward into the fibrovascular stalk. The tumor neovascularity that develops in such inwardly invading malignancies manifests as increasing numbers of new vessels within the fibrovascular stalk rather than within the typical peripheral vascular net. Thus, malignant mural nodules or eccentric wall thickenings tend to have multiple feeding vessels that can be shown with Doppler. Benign intracystic papillomas, on the other hand, tend to be fed by a single vessel within the stalk (Fig. 20–31).

In some cases, the echogenic lipid layer within cysts that contain fat–fluid levels or the debris or sludge layer in cysts with fluid–debris levels may simulate mural nodules or eccentric wall thickenings. Color Doppler or power Doppler may be very helpful in such cases. Obviously, there will be no Doppler-demonstrable flow to the unattached lipid level in cysts with fat–fluid levels or within tumefactive sludge in cysts with fluid–debris levels (Fig. 20–32). However, upright and decubitus positioning is usually adequate to prove mobility of internal echoes without the need for Doppler assessment but may require waiting as long as 5 minutes for the shift to occur. Demonstrating a vessel proves definitively that the internal echoes are not caused by mobile lipid material, sludge, or dependent debris.

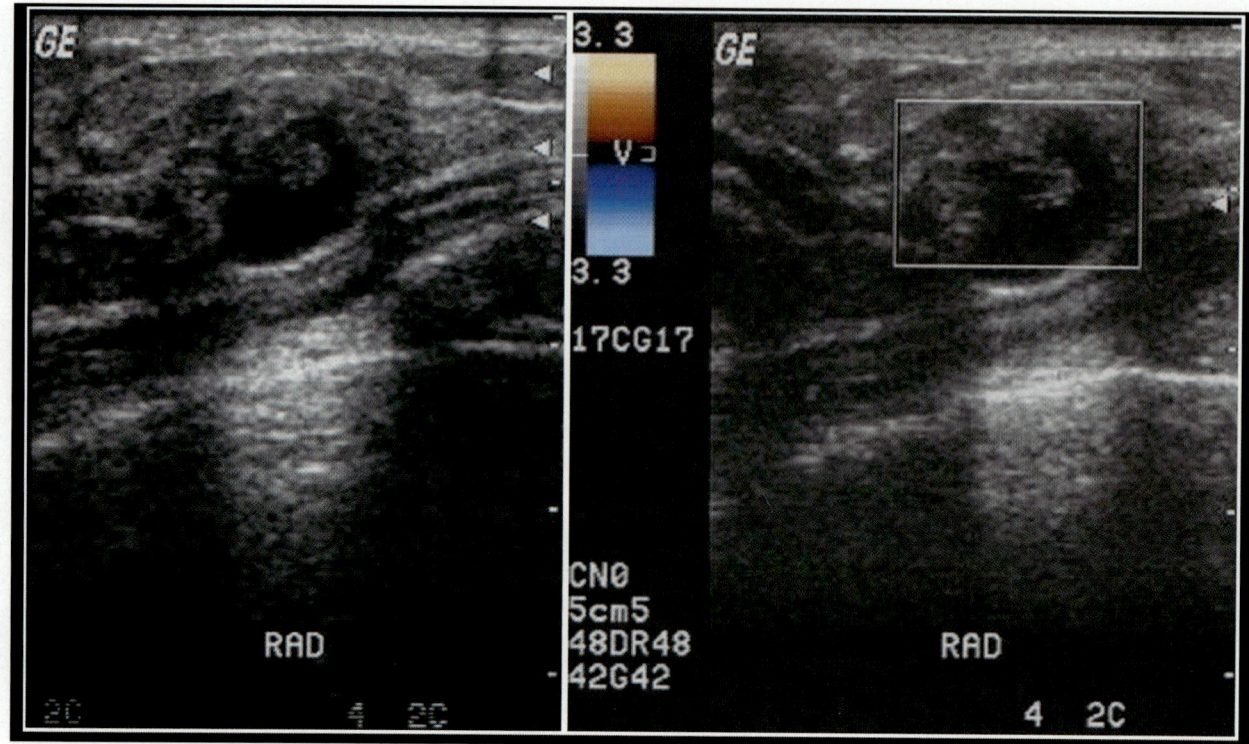

FIGURE 20–30 The absence of a Doppler-demonstrable vascular stalk is less valuable than its presence because intracystic papillomas (ICPs) frequently undergo hemorrhagic infarction. This infarcted ICP did not have a demonstrable vascular stalk.

Characterization of complex cysts is discussed and illustrated in greater detail in Chapter 10. The Doppler findings should be interpreted in light of the imaging findings. If there are suspicious imaging findings, the lesion should be characterized as BIRADS 4a or 4b and undergo biopsy regardless of the Doppler findings.

Complex breast cysts with eccentric wall thickenings or mural nodules must be interrogated with Doppler using a very light scan technique. Such lesions, like many others, are soft enough that inadvertent scan pressure can compress the lesion and decrease or occlude flow within the lesion, obscuring the presence of a fibrovascular stalk.

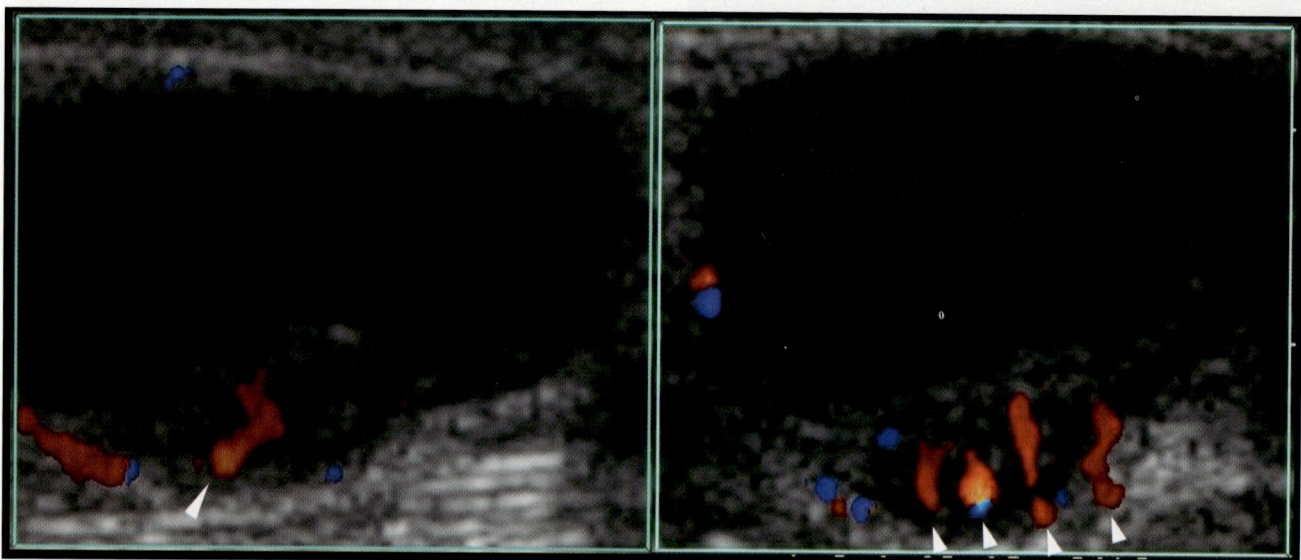

FIGURE 20–31 Benign intracystic papillomas tend to be fed by a single artery (**left**, *arrowhead*). Malignant intracystic malignancies tend to invade inwardly into the fibrovascular stalk and stimulate the formation of new vessels within the stalk. Thus, malignant intracystic mural nodules tend to be fed by multiple vessels (**right**, *arrowheads*).

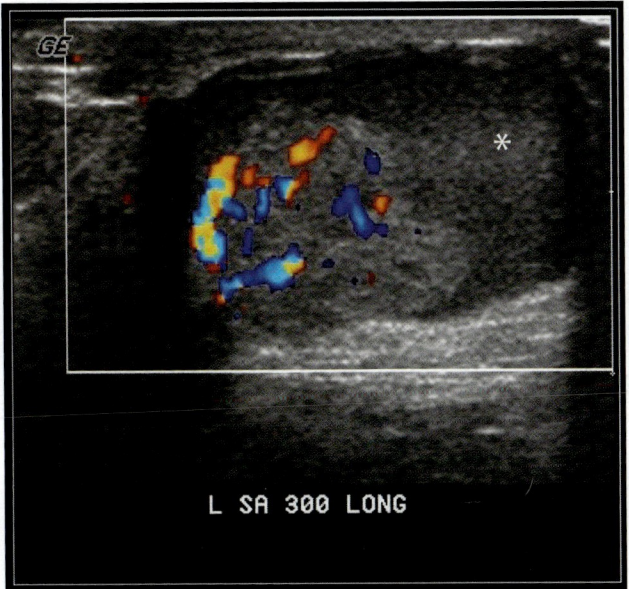

FIGURE 20–32 This intracystic papilloma has hemorrhaged into the cyst fluid, making the fluid almost as echogenic as the papillary lesion. Color Doppler shows multiple vessels within the mural nodule, but there are no vessels within the bloody cyst fluid.

Determining Whether Internal Echoes in Complex Cysts Are Subcellular Particles or Cells

Cysts that are characterized as complex by virtue of diffuse low-level internal echoes can also be further evaluated with color or power Doppler. The low-level internal echogenicity may be caused by small subcellular particles such as cholesterol crystals, cellular debris, and amorphous globs of protein or by complete cells such as red blood cells, white blood cells, epithelial cells, foamy macrophages, or apocrine metaplasia. Complex cysts in which intact cells cause the internal echoes are at slightly higher risk for infection or neoplasm. On the other hand, complex cysts whose internal echoes are caused by subcellular particles almost invariably represent uncomplicated fibrocystic change. Complete cells are too large and heavy to move by simply increasing transmit power of the ultrasound beam. Subcellular particles, such as cholesterol crystals, on the other hand, are small and light enough that in some cases they can be made to move simply by increasing the transmit power or by color or power Doppler beam if the transducer is held in a fixed position over the center of the cyst. The movement of such subcellular particles is termed *color streaking* (Fig. 20–33). In our experience, the presence of color streaking has been associated with benign uncomplicated fibrocystic change, and this has

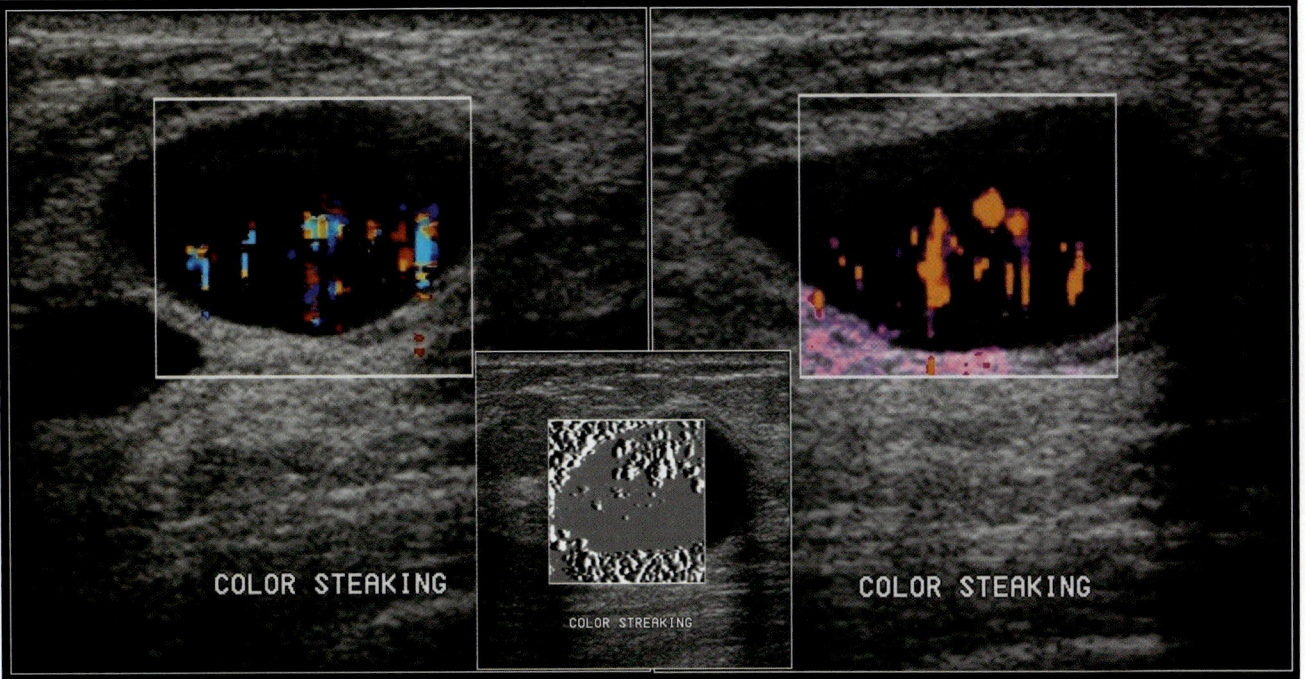

FIGURE 20–33 Internal echoes within the cyst are being moved posteriorly by the color Doppler beam **(left)** and the power Doppler beam **(middle and right)**, creating streaks of color in the anteroposterior direction. This phenomenon has been termed *color streaking*, a benign (BIRADS 2) finding in complex cysts. Particles that can be moved solely by the energy of the Doppler beam are usually subcellular particles, such as cholesterol crystals, that are a part of the fibrocystic spectrum.

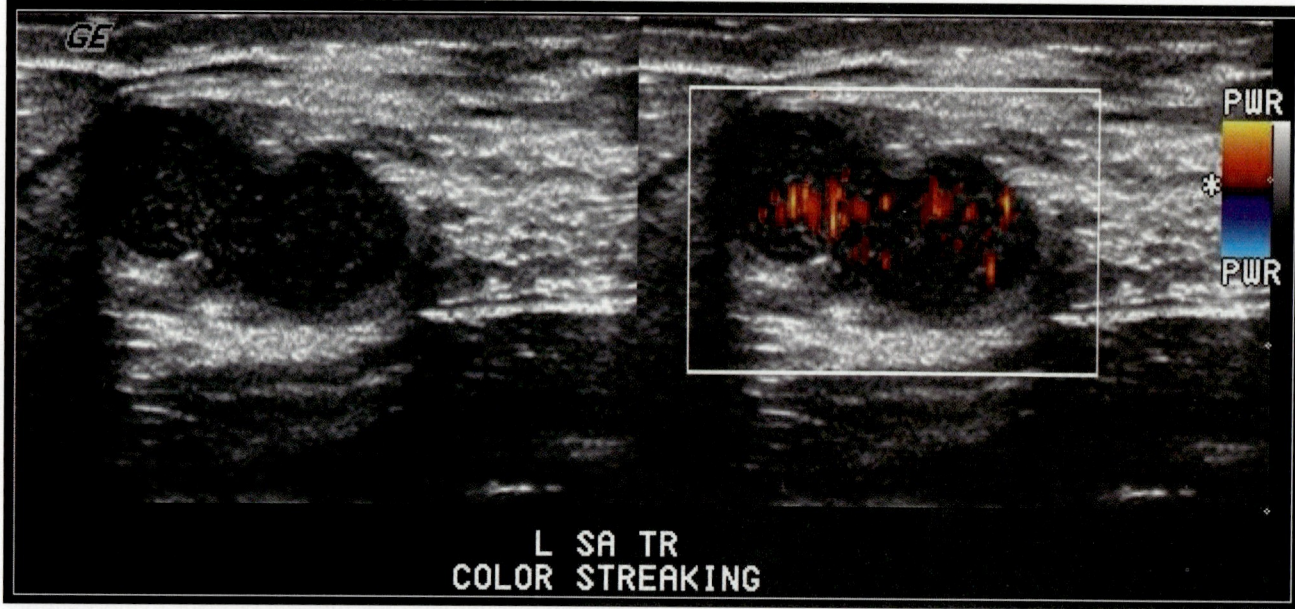

FIGURE 20–34 Color streaking and many other color Doppler findings can be best appreciated in split-screen simultaneous mode with the real-time image on one side and the Doppler image on the other. In this way, the imaging findings that correspond to color Doppler signals are not obscured by the color.

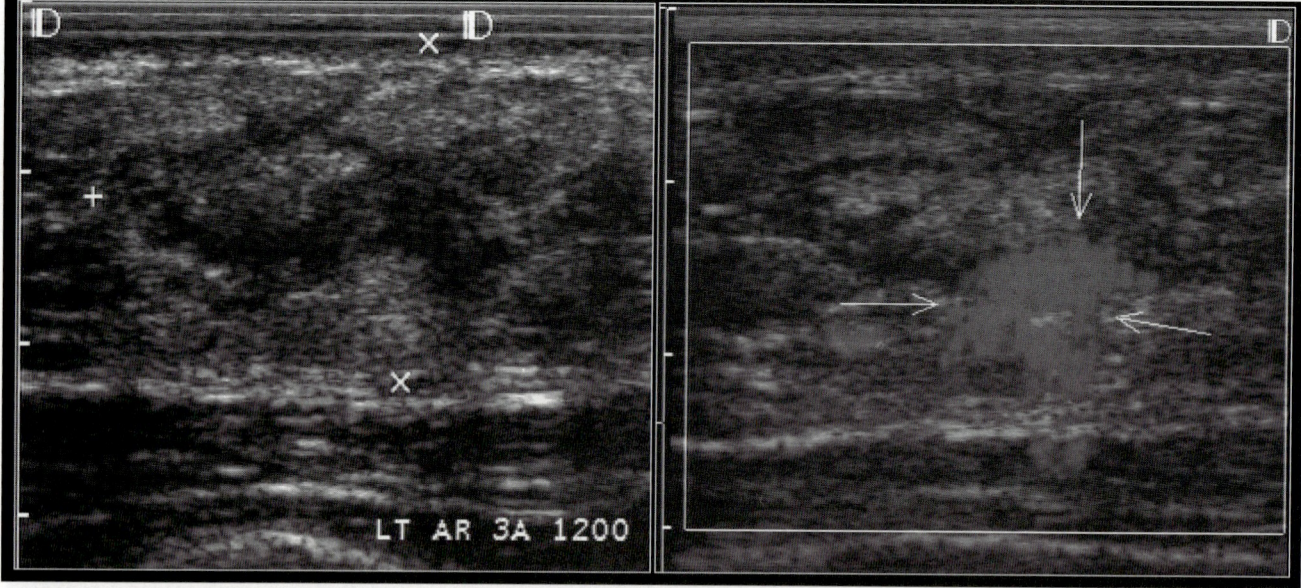

FIGURE 20–35 Abscesses that have a nonspecific pattern may be very difficult to identify early in the course of development. The area of liquefactive necrosis that will later become a well-defined abscess is usually slightly hypoechoic *(*)* with respect to surrounding breast tissues, but the margins remain ill defined until the abscess wall matures. Gentle ballottement of the inflamed area with the transducer may cause detached necrotic debris to slosh back and forth, defining the nascent abscess cavity. The movement to and fro, the color slosh, of necrotic tissue *(arrows)* can be documented on a single freeze-frame image with color or power Doppler. The necrotic tissue may be so close to that of surrounding viable tissue that it may no be identifiable on the image alone.

been confirmed by aspirating several of these cysts. The lack of color streaking does not indicate with certainty that the internal echoes are caused by complete cells. In some cases, the internal echoes are caused by gelatinized amorphous proteinaceous debris or lipid material that is too viscous to allow movement of particles.

Color streaking is best demonstrated, for purposes of obtaining a single hard-copy image, on split-screen images in simultaneous mode, with the B-mode image displayed on the left half of the screen, and the color Doppler or power Doppler image displayed on the right half of the screen (Fig. 20–34). Storing cine loops on a picture archiving and communications system (PACS) is an even better way to record color streaking.

Identifying Necrotic Debris that Represents Early Abscess Formation in Patients with Mastitis

In cases of acute puerperal or nonpuerperal mastitis, ultrasound is performed to determine whether an abscess has developed. Early in the course of abscess formation, tissue necrosis occurs. However, the necrotic tissue takes time to liquefy enough to be detectable as a fluid collection. The necrotic tissue may be detached and mobile but may appear to be solid on sonography. Gentle ballottement with

color or power Doppler may show a color swoosh as the necrotic tissue moves back and forth with compression and compression release, documenting necrosis before liquefaction has progressed enough to be identifiable on freeze-frame images (Fig. 20–35). Earlier detection of liquefaction enables early diagnostic aspiration for culture and sensitivity and in some cases may allow early therapeutic drainage.

Distinguishing between Echogenic Inspissated Secretions or Blood within a Duct and Ductal Carcinoma *In Situ* or Papilloma

In chronic duct ectasia, inspissated echogenic secretions can simulate the echogenicity of long intraductal papillary lesions such as papilloma or carcinoma. By ballottement of the duct, unattached echogenic secretions can be made to slosh back and forth within the duct. The secretions usually are pushed posteriorly during compression and return to a more anterior position during compression release. Although the motion of the echoes within the duct can be seen on the real-time B-mode image, color Doppler or power Doppler can be useful in demonstrating the movement on single or paired freeze-frame images (Fig. 20–36). The movement of echogenic secretions within the duct dur-

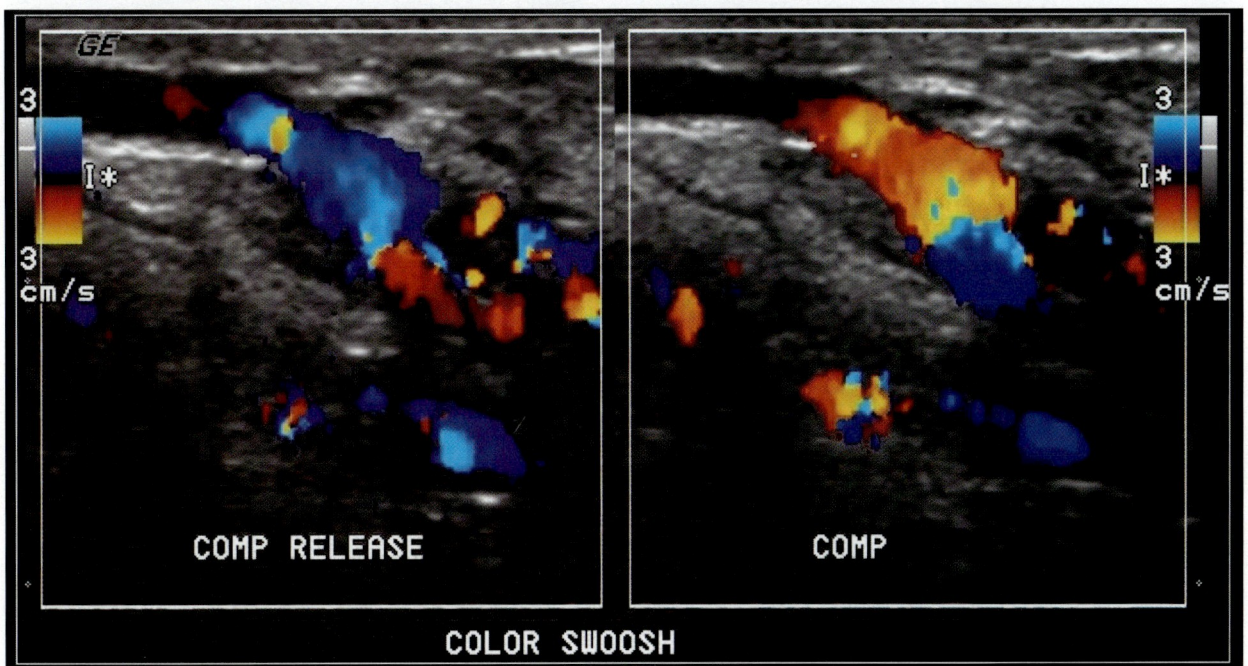

FIGURE 20–36 During ballottement, echogenic secretions move in one direction during compression and the opposite direction during compression release. Compression of the duct (**right**) forced secretions peripherally and deeper into the duct, resulting in a red signal with color Doppler. Compression release, on the other hand (**right**), resulted in secretions moving toward the nipple and superficially, resulting in a blue signal (**left**). The to-and-fro motion of echogenic secretions within the duct that are caused by ballottement is called the color swoosh.

ing ballottement (the color swoosh) generally can be demonstrated with duct ectasia but not when the echoes within the duct are caused by a long papilloma or DCIS. However, there are some caveats. The color swoosh should fill the entire duct before it is decided that there is only duct ectasia. Duct ectasia may be associated with papillomas or DCIS. In such cases, there may be echogenic secretions or blood within the duct in addition to the intraductal papillary lesion. However, in such cases, there will be a "defect" in the color signal generated by moving secretions that corresponds to the location of the papillary lesion. Additionally, in high-nuclear-grade DCIS, there may be extensive central necrosis, and the necrotic debris within the center of the tumor-filled ducts may give rise to a color swoosh. Such ducts often have extensive calcifications within the necrotic debris that helps prevent errors, however.

In some cases, communicating cysts cause nipple discharge. In such cases, ballottement of the cyst can cause secretions to swoosh back and forth within the duct into which the cyst drains, confirming the communication between the cyst and the duct in cases in which the duct may too small or tortuous to be certain of the communication with image alone (Fig. 20–37).

Similar to intracystic papillary lesions, benign and malignant intraductal papillomas are quite vascular, and frequently even very small intraductal papillomas have a vascular stalk that is demonstrable with color Doppler or power Doppler (Fig. 20–38). Very light and steady compression pressure should be used when interrogating an enlarged duct that contains echogenic material for two reasons. Light pressure is important because intraductal papillomas are among the softest and most compressible lesions in the breast, and using even slightly too much compression pressure can shut off flow to the papilloma, obscuring its fibrovascular stalk. Steady pressure is important because both benign and malignant intraductal papillary lesions often have associated echogenic secretions, necrosis, or blood within the duct lumen that can create a

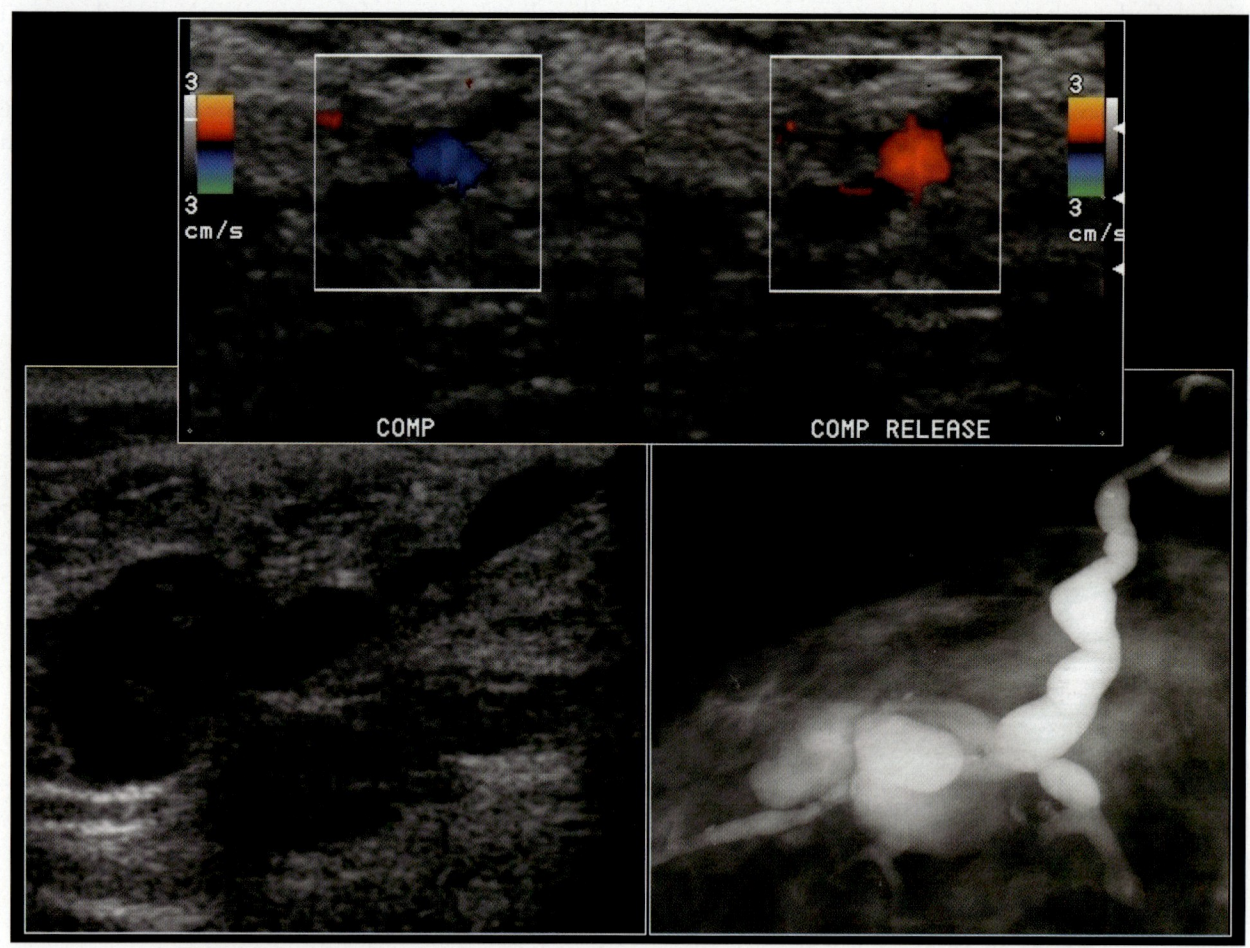

FIGURE 20–37 Ballottement of the communicating cyst with the transducer causes to-and-fro motion within the dilated draining duct that can be documented with color Doppler as the color swoosh. When the duct is tortuous, it can be difficult to confirm that it communicates with the cyst using B-mode imaging alone. Sonography was performed first, and the galactogram was later performed to confirm the sonographic findings.

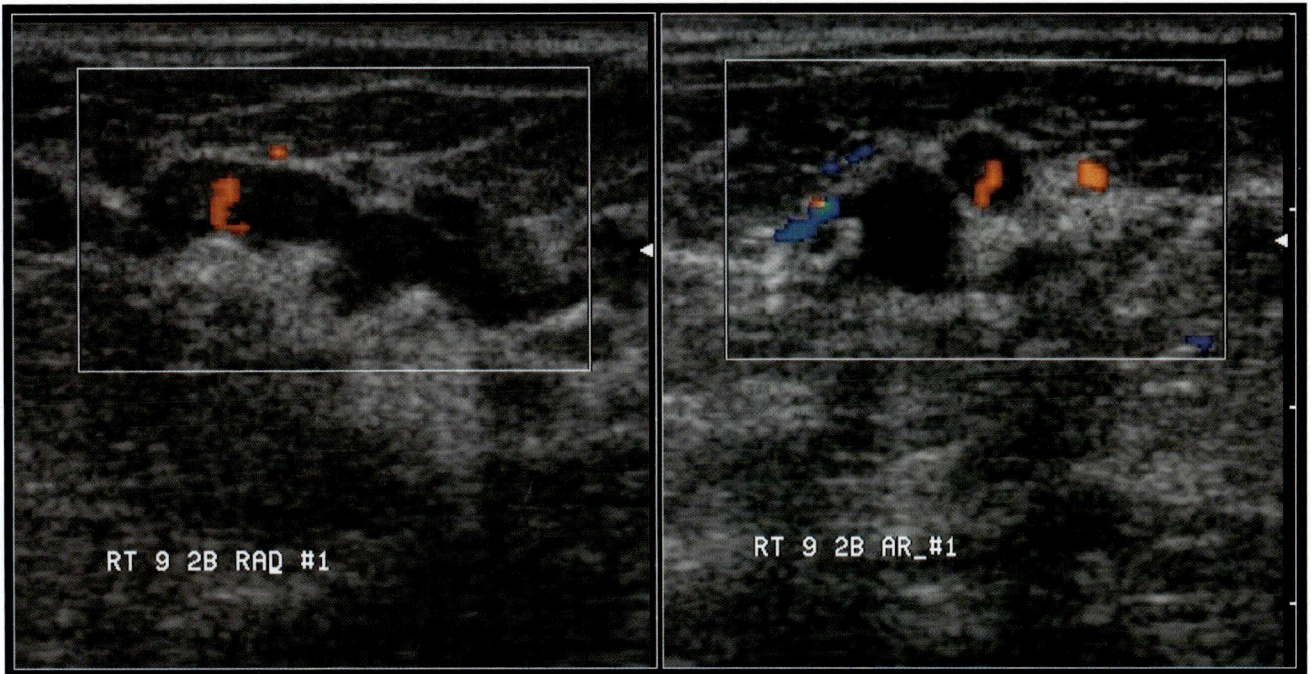

FIGURE 20–38 Even small intraductal papillomas often have easily demonstrable vascular stalks.

color swoosh if compression pressure is not kept absolutely constant and light. The color swoosh can completely obscure the fibrovascular stalk (Fig. 20–39). It must always be remembered that a positive Doppler study that demonstrates the presence of a fibrovascular stalk is more valuable than a negative Doppler study that does not show a stalk. Intraductal papillary lesions often undergo hemorrhagic infarction and hyalinization or fibrosis. Infracted or hyalinized papillary lesions will not have flow demonstrable by Doppler.

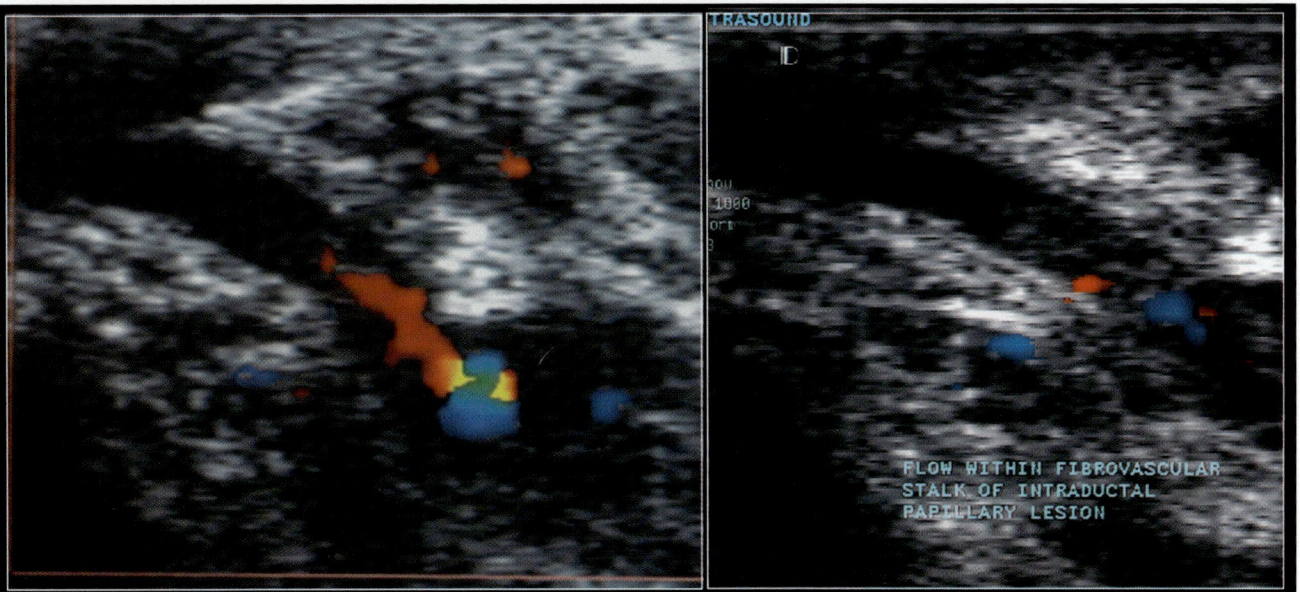

FIGURE 20–39 Color Doppler performed with steady, light scan pressure shows a fibrovascular stalk (**right**). Varying scan pressure causes a color swoosh of secretions to move over the surface of the papillary lesion, obscuring the vascular stalk (**right**). The color swoosh is typically most pronounced in the portion of lumen occupied by the papilloma because the lumen is narrowed there and velocities of fluid are the highest there. Thus, it is important to use steady, light scan pressure when seeking the presence of fibrovascular stalk.

Demonstrating Inflammatory Hyperemia

Infected and Acutely Inflamed Cysts

Doppler can be useful in evaluating thick-walled cysts for evidence of inflammation. The findings that suggest acute inflammation include relatively uniform isoechoic wall thickening, fluid–debris (pus) levels, and hyperemia within the thickened cyst wall. In most cases, all three findings are present (Fig. 20–40). Additionally, acutely inflamed cysts are usually tender. Noninflamed breast cysts typically have a thin, echogenic outer wall with no demonstrable flow within the wall on color Doppler. Circumferential thickening of the outer wall of complex cysts can also be caused by papillary apocrine metaplasia or fibrosis. Apocrine metaplasia does not cause hyperemia and generally does not develop a fibrovascular stalk and therefore rarely shows evidence of blood flow on Doppler evaluation. Cysts that have a thickened outer wall because of fibrosis cannot be distinguished from acutely inflamed cysts by real-time B-mode imaging along. The imaging appearance of cysts with thickened fibrotic walls is nearly identical to that of acutely inflamed cysts simply because fibrotic-walled cysts are simply healed inflamed cysts. Color Doppler can distinguish between the two because walls thickened by fibrosis have no Doppler-demonstrable hyperemia, whereas inflamed cysts do (Fig. 20–41). Interesting, there is an important and fairly consistent difference between the appearance of vessels in inflamed cysts and vessels supplying papillary growths that can cause wall thickenings—the orientation of the vessel. The vessels that we can identify in inflamed cysts supply the walls of the cyst and therefore have courses parallel to the cyst wall. On the other hand, the vessels that supply intracystic papillary lesions (papilloma or carcinoma) are merely passing through the cyst wall to supply intracystic lesions and therefore have courses that are perpendicular to the cyst wall (Fig. 20–42).

Unfortunately, once Doppler has helped demonstrate acute inflammation of the cyst wall, there is no way that using imaging, Doppler, or even aspiration with gross inspection of the aspirate can determine whether inflammation is bland or whether there is acute inflammation. In such cases, we send the aspirate for Gram stain and culture and tentatively treat the patient with antibiotics until the 72-hour culture results are available. We do not request cytologic evaluation of the fluid because the triad of findings indicates an inflammatory process, not neoplasm. Inflamed cysts are discussed in greater detail in Chapter 10.

Acute Puerperal Mastitis

Acute puerperal infection may manifest mainly as a superficial cellulitis or as acute infection of more deeply located breast tissues.

Superficial cellulitis usually spreads from an infection that begins in a cracked or fissured nipple and involves the nipple and periareolar skin and subcutaneous tissues. It

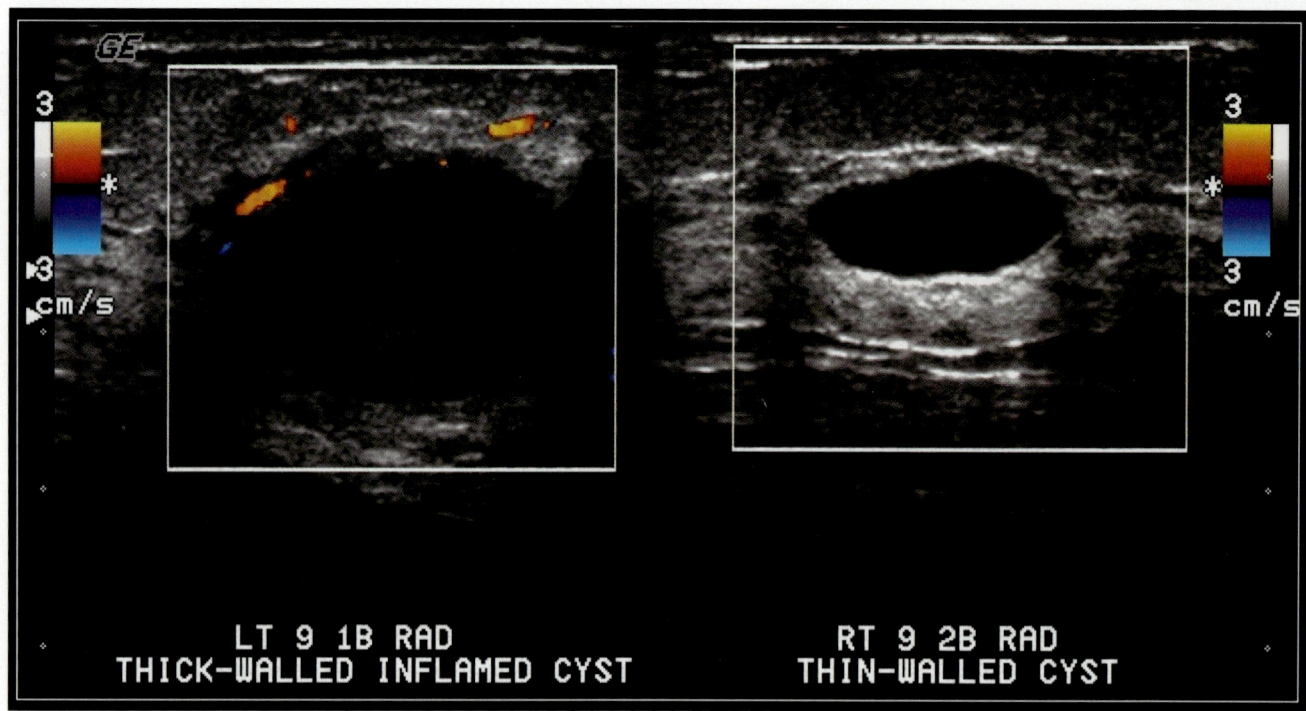

FIGURE 20–40 The walls of acutely inflamed cysts are hyperemic as well as thickened and isoechoic **(left)**. The walls of noninflamed cysts are thin and echogenic and have no demonstrable blood flow **(right)**.

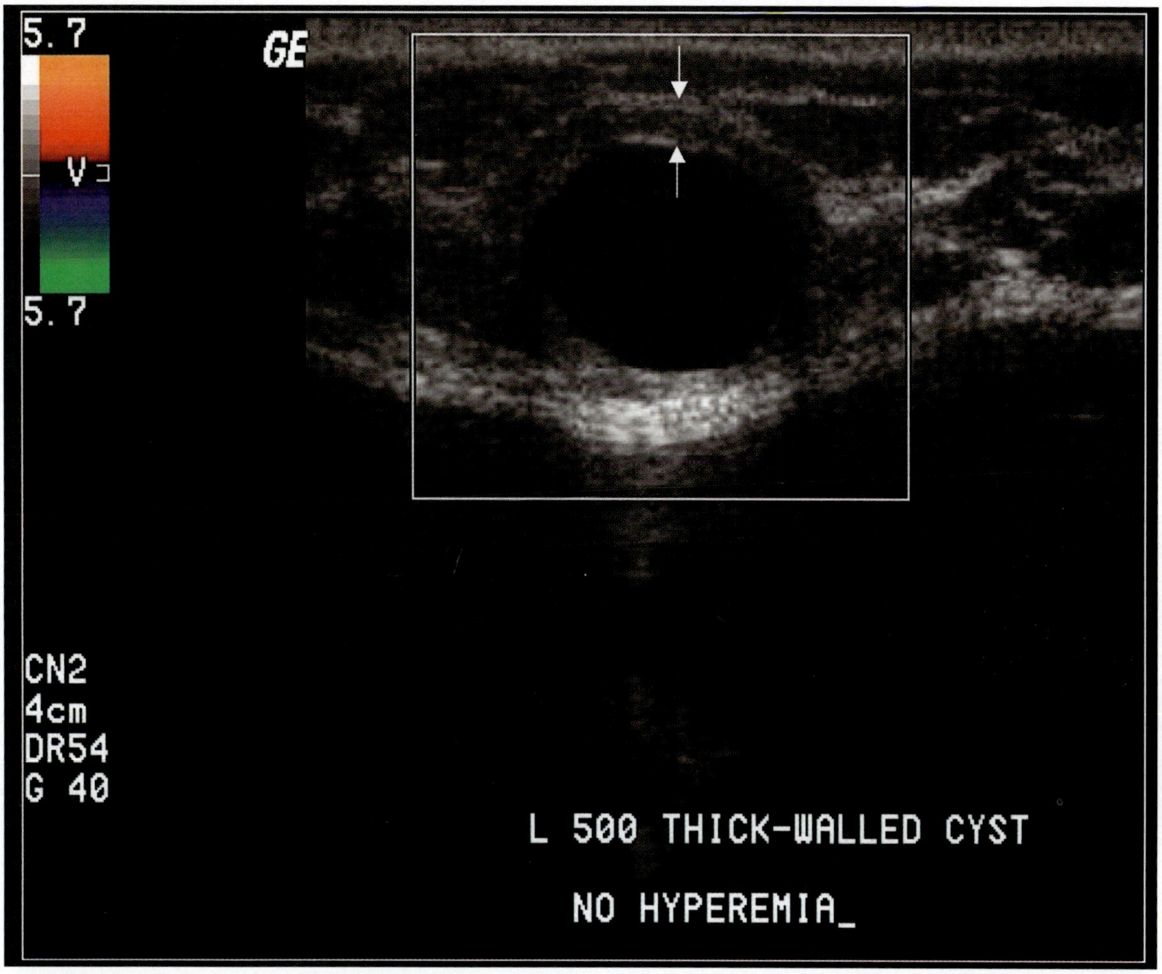

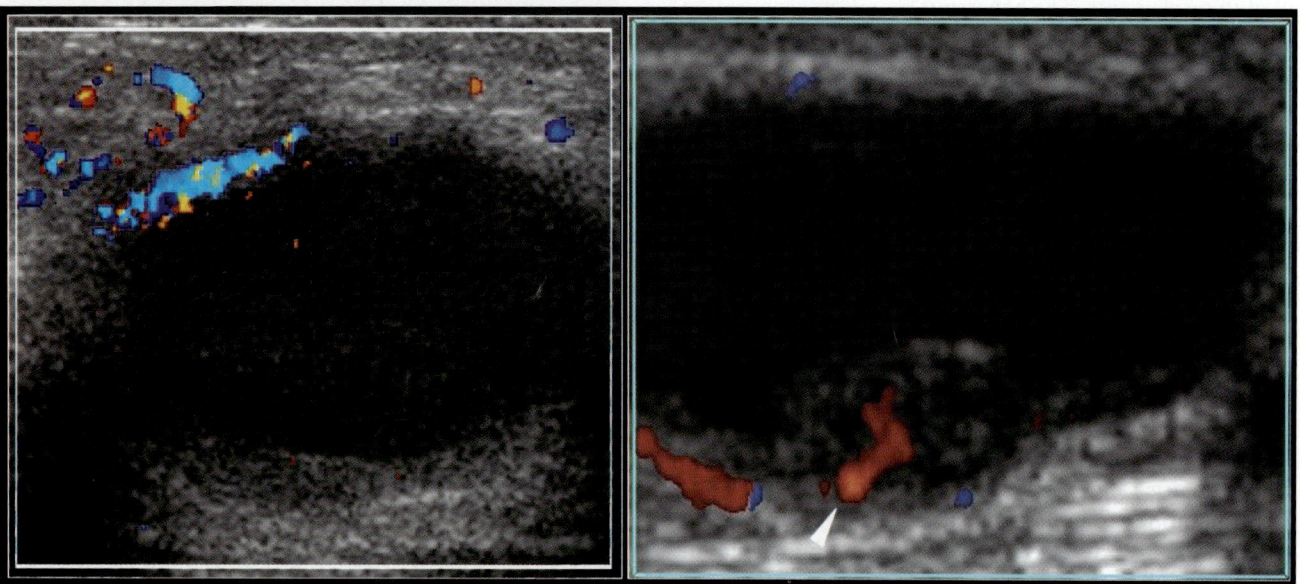

FIGURE 20–41 There is no Doppler-demonstrable blood flow in the two entities other than acute inflammation that cause uniform wall thickening—fibrosis and papillary apocrine metaplasia. The wall of this cyst is fibrotic. Fibrosis of the cyst wall is the healed end stage of an inflamed cyst, accounting for the remarkably similar imaging appearance. The presence or lack of hyperemia on color Doppler is the key to distinguishing between inflamed cysts and cysts with fibrotic walls.

FIGURE 20–42 The orientation of the vessels differs between inflamed cysts and intracystic pap-illary lesions. The demonstrable vessels in inflamed cysts course parallel to the inflamed cyst walls that they supply (**left**). On the other hand, the vessels that supply intracystic papillary le-sions are merely passing through the cyst wall to supply the papillary lesion on the inner surface of the wall (**right**), and therefore course perpendicular to the cyst wall.

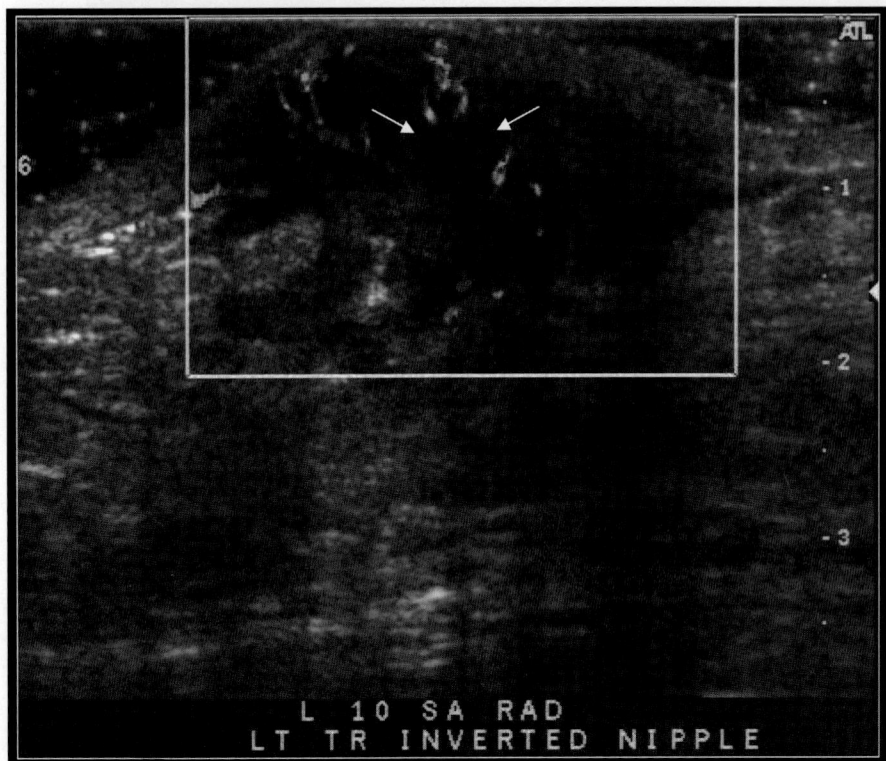

L 10 SA RAD
LT TR INVERTED NIPPLE

FIGURE 20–43 The superficial cellulite pattern usually arises from a fissure in the nipple and spreads to involve the entire nipple, periareolar skin, and subcutaneous tissues. The skin becomes thicker and less echogenic, the subcutaneous fat becomes hyperechoic, and the nipple becomes thicker and hyperemic. Microabscesses may develop within the nipple *(arrows)*.

may or may not be associated with infection of more deeply located breast tissues. Superficial cellulitis manifests as hyperechoic subcutaneous fat, thickened and mildly hypoechoic skin, thickened and mildly hypoechoic fibrous elements (including Cooper's ligaments), and hyperemia of all of these elements. The hyperemia manifests as increased numbers of vessels on color Doppler or power Doppler compared with the contralateral mirror-image location (Fig. 20–43) and with higher-velocity and lower-impedance flow on pulse Doppler spectral analysis than in the contralateral mirror-image location.

Infection of more deeply located breast tissues may present with peripheral or central patterns. The peripheral pattern is usually that of a secondarily infected galactocele. Usually, the wall of the infected galactocele is isoechoic and thickened and hyperemic, whereas an uninfected galactocele has a thin, echogenic wall without demonstrable blood flow. The inspissated milk within the galactocele varies in echogenicity. In some cases, the protein elements of milk will be denatured and appear as hyperechoic debris within the infected galactocele. It can be very difficult to distinguish an uninfected but tender galactocele from an infected galactocele and early abscess. Demonstrating hyperemia in the walls of the galactocele can help (Fig. 20–44), but in many cases, only aspiration helps.

The central pattern of puerperal mastitis, like the superficial cellulitis, is usually preceded by a crack or fissure

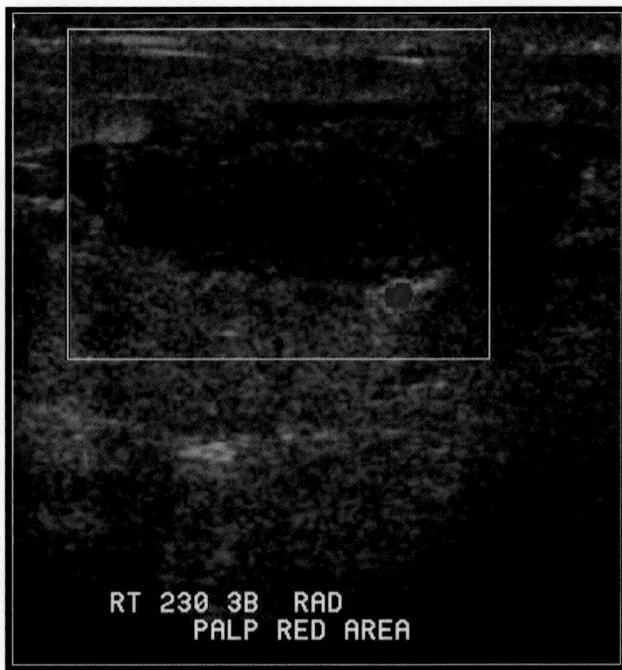

RT 230 3B RAD
PALP RED AREA

FIGURE 20–44 The peripheral deep pattern of puerperal mastitis reflects secondary infection of a preexisting galactocele. It can be very difficult to distinguish between a galactocele with inspissated milk and an abscess by imaging alone. The outer wall of abscesses tends to be thick and isoechoic, just like the wall of inflamed cysts. There is usually some hyperemia along the outer surface of the infected galactocele.

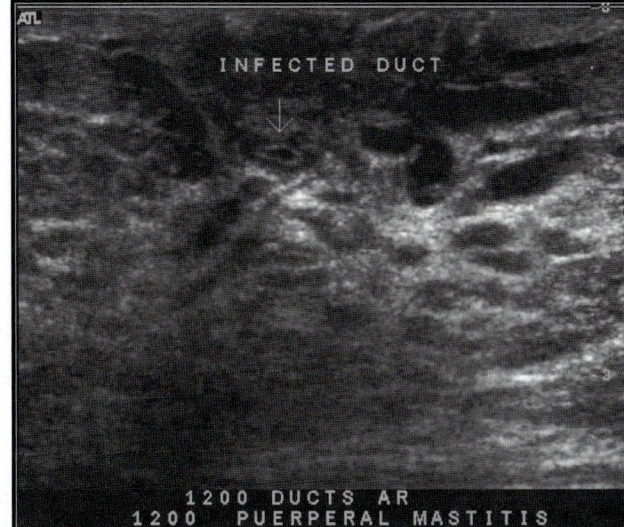

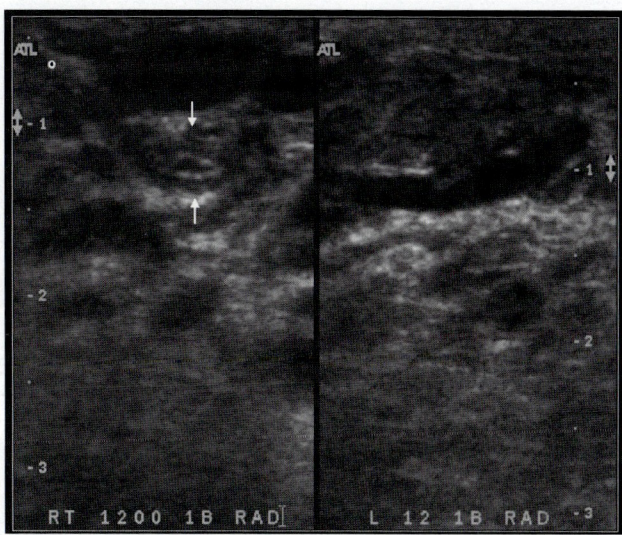

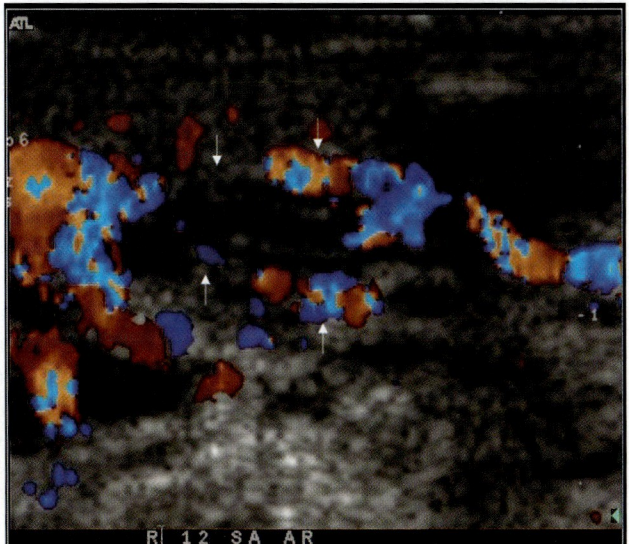

FIGURE 20–45 **A:** This patient with acute puerperal mastitis has one inflamed duct with isoechoic, thickened walls. The other ducts are filled with milk but have normal thin, echogenic walls. The mastitis in this patient began with a nipple fissure, which presumably obstructed the affected duct and allowed bacteria to enter it and infect it. Puerperal mastitis may involve one or more lobar ductal systems. **B:** These are split-screen short-axis images of an infected duct at the 10:30 position (**left**) and an uninfected duct at the 12:00 position (**right**) in the left breast. Note that the normal duct is only minimally dilated and has thin, echogenic walls (**right**, *arrows*). The normal duct is surrounded by isoechoic loose periductal stroma fibrous tissue. The infected duct (**left**) is abnormally dilated, contains echogenic, inspissated milk *(*)*, and has an abnormally thick and ill-defined wall *(arrows)*. **C:** The inflamed duct with the thickened wall and the tissues that surround it are markedly hyperemic.

in the nipple that leads directly to infection of the duct or first to obstruction of one or more lobar ducts and then secondary to infection of the duct. Like noninflamed cysts, noninflamed ducts have thin, echogenic walls on sonography and have no demonstrable flow to the duct walls. Similar to inflamed cysts, inflamed duct walls develop relatively uniform isoechoic wall thickening, debris within the lumen, and hyperemia of the duct walls (Fig. 20–45). In some cases, the proteinaceous elements of the milk will be denatured and form echogenic "plugs" within the center of the lumen (Fig. 20–46). With successful treatment of the infection, the hyperemia decreases first, the denatured proteinaceous elements of milk are resorbed, and finally, the wall thickening resolves (Fig. 20–47). Rupture of obstructed and acutely infected central ducts can lead to formation of the less common central abscess (Fig. 20–48).

Acute Periductal Mastitis in the Duct Ectasia–Periductal Mastitis Complex

Duct ectasia is a chronic inflammatory condition of the duct walls that leads to dilated, fluid-filled ducts. In some cases of chronic duct ectasia, the fluid within the ducts becomes thick, inspissated, and filled with lipid-rich inflammatory debris. The chronic inflammation weakens the duct walls enough that minor trauma so insignificant that the patient cannot remember it can cause rupture of the duct and leakage of the lipid-rich secretions into the surrounding tissues. The extravasated secretions cause an intense acute periductal chemical mastitis, a common cause of acute breast pain. Patients who present with acute pain caused by periductal mastitis often report previous episodes of pain in other parts of the breast. Sonography is frequently used to evaluate acute focal breast pain but too

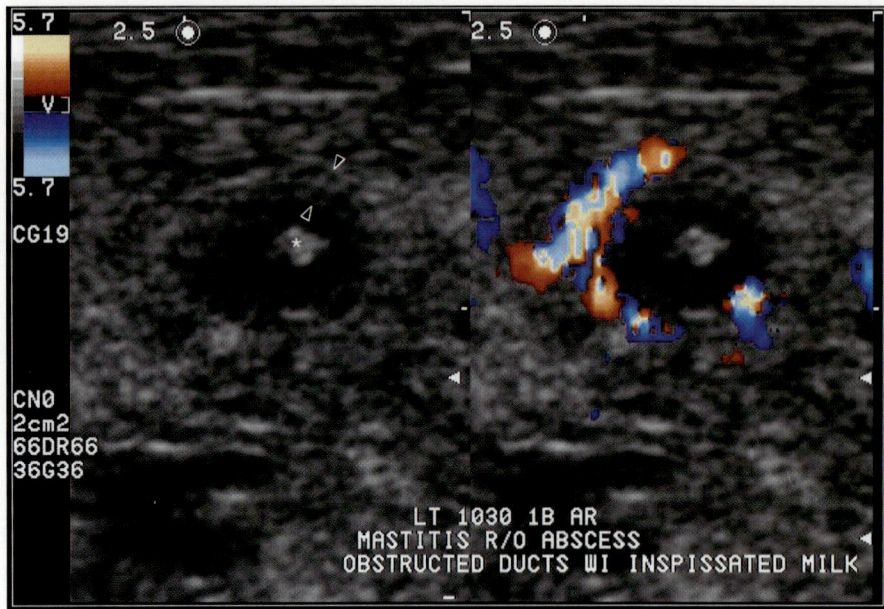

FIGURE 20–46 This is a split-screen image of an infected duct in a patient with acute puerperal mastitis showing simultaneous B-mode image (**left**) and color Doppler image (**right**). The duct is abnormally dilated, has abnormally thick and isoechoic walls (**left**, *between arrowheads*), and contains inspissated denatured hyperechoic milk *(*)*. Note the degree of inflammatory hyperemia present within the wall of the infected duct.

often is "negative," demonstrating no reason. However, in our experience, ultrasound with Doppler can often identify definitive findings of acute periductal mastitis. Similar to puerperal mastitis, acute periductal mastitis has peripheral and central patterns. The peripheral pattern arises from very small peripheral ducts that may be too small to show sonographic abnormalities other than mild ectasia. The key sonographic findings of periductal inflammation are hyperechogenicity of the inflamed periductal fat and hyperemia of the fat that may be seen as increased numbers of vessels or as higher-velocity flow with reduced impedance on pulsed Doppler spectral analysis (Fig. 20–49).

The central pattern involves ducts that are large enough to show classic findings of acute inflammation. Like uncomplicated cysts, normal ducts, and even ducts that are affected by chronic duct ectasia, have thin, echogenic walls and have no flow within the walls that can be demonstrated with color Doppler or power Doppler. But like acutely inflamed cysts, the walls of acutely inflamed ducts become uniformly thickened and isoechoic

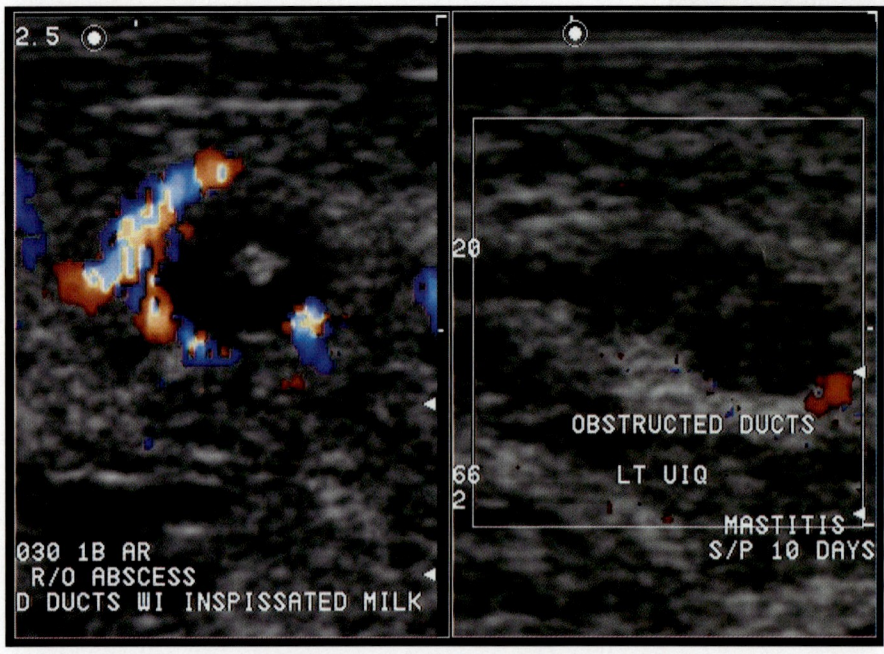

FIGURE 20–47 These are antiradial color Doppler images of a single infected duct the time of diagnosis (**left**) and after 10 days of antibiotic treatment (**right**). Not only did duct dilation and duct wall thickening decrease, and not only was the inspissated milk resorbed after antibiotic treatment, but also there is also a tremendous reduction in inflammatory hyperemia. In fact, the diminution in hyperemia precedes improvement in the imaging abnormalities, which take longer to resolve.

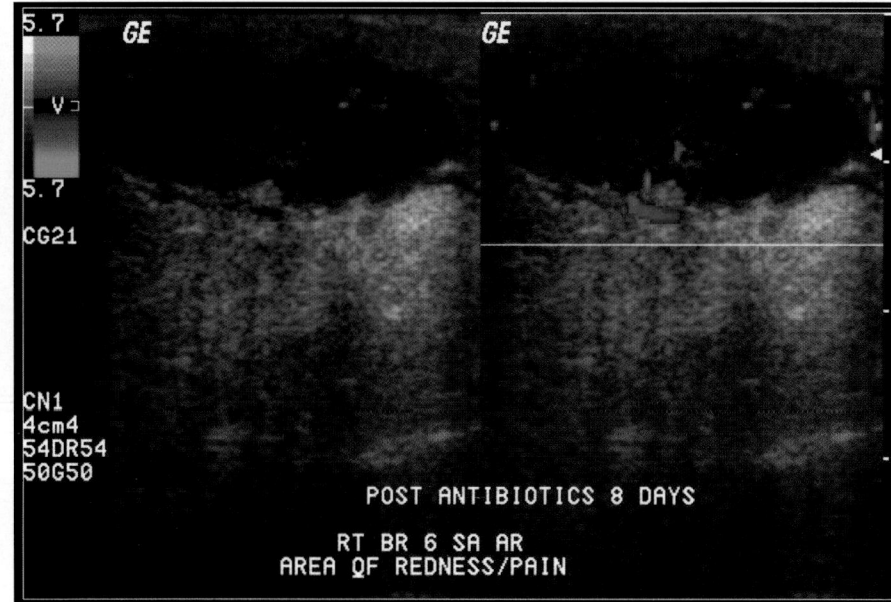

FIGURE 20–48 Central puerperal abscesses are usually the result of duct rupture. The wall of the infected, distended duct is weaker than normal and prone to rupture and release of infected milk into surrounding tissues, leading to abscess formation.

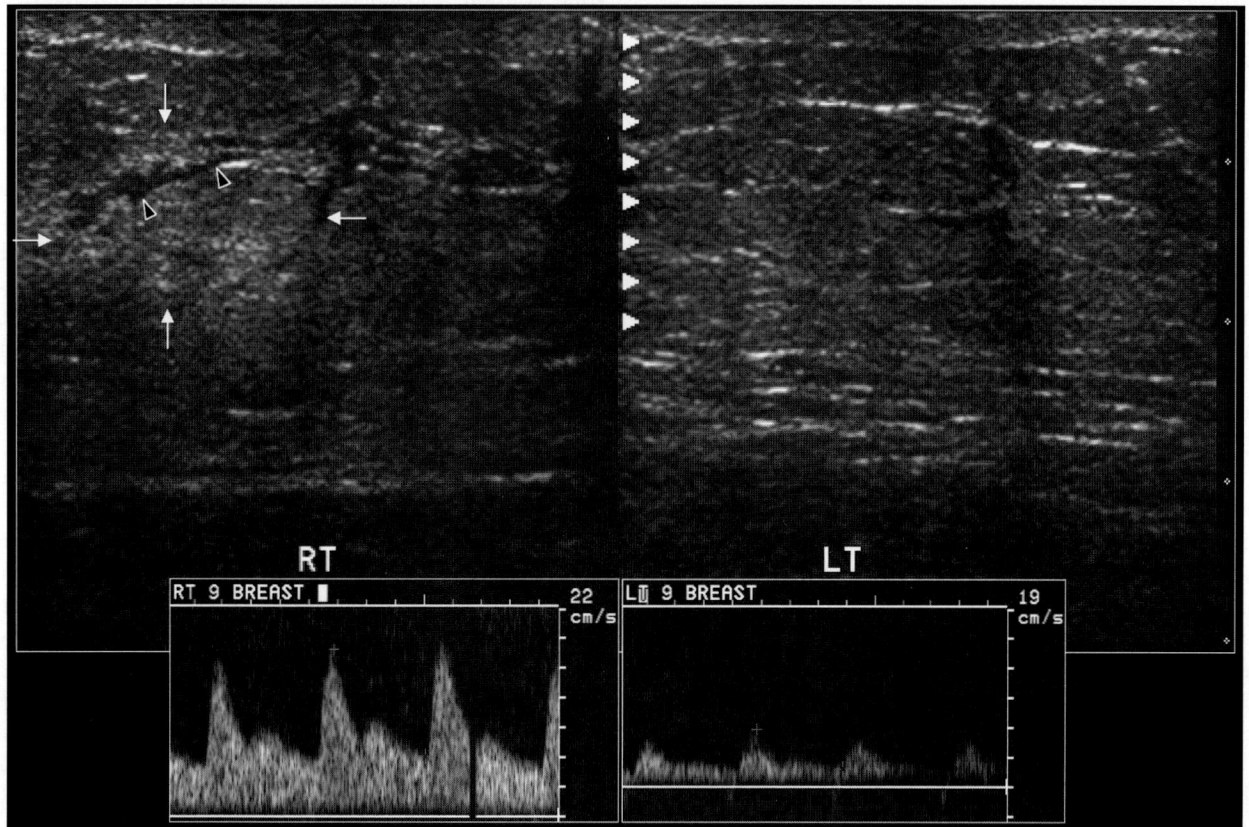

FIGURE 20–49 This figure illustrates focal acute periductal mastitis surrounding a small peripheral duct at the 9:00 position on the right. The patient presented with acute pain in the 9:00 position of the right breast. Split-screen mirror-image scanning of the lateral aspects of both breasts (left side location is mislabeled, should be 3:00) shows a focal area of hyperechoic fat *(arrows)* in the area of symptoms on the right, indicating acute edema. In the center of the edema is a mildly ectatic duct *(arrowheads)*. Color and power Doppler spectral analysis showed hyperemia within the edematous tissues. Note that the velocities are higher and the resistivity indices lower in the hyperemic area on the right side. The presence of focal edema and hyperemia around an ectatic duct indicates the presence of acute periductal mastitis.

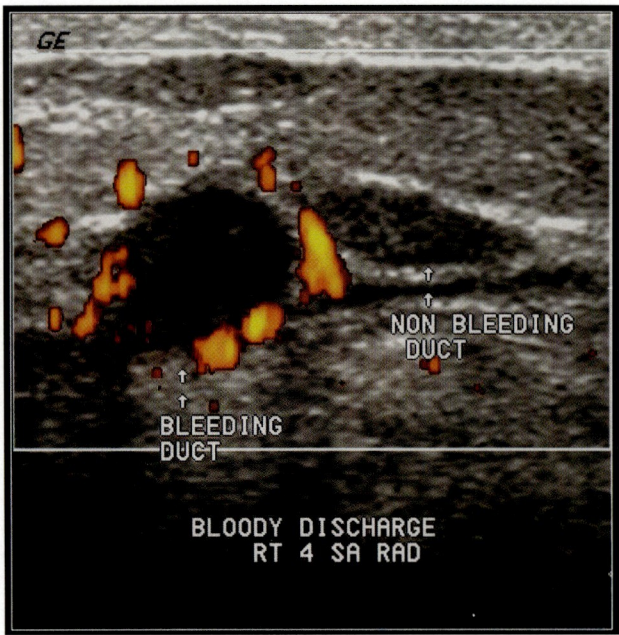

FIGURE 20–50 When a chronically ectatic duct becomes secondarily inflamed, it develops features that are very similar to those of inflamed cysts and infected ducts in puerperal mastitis. The duct walls become thickened and isoechoic and markedly hyperemic. Although duct ectasia may affect many lobar ducts, acute periductal mastitis tends to affect only one lobar ductal system at a time. Over time, multiple different ducts in different locations may become inflamed. Note that in this case, the inflamed duct is markedly hyperemic, but the adjacent duct is only slightly less distended and is not inflamed and hyperemic.

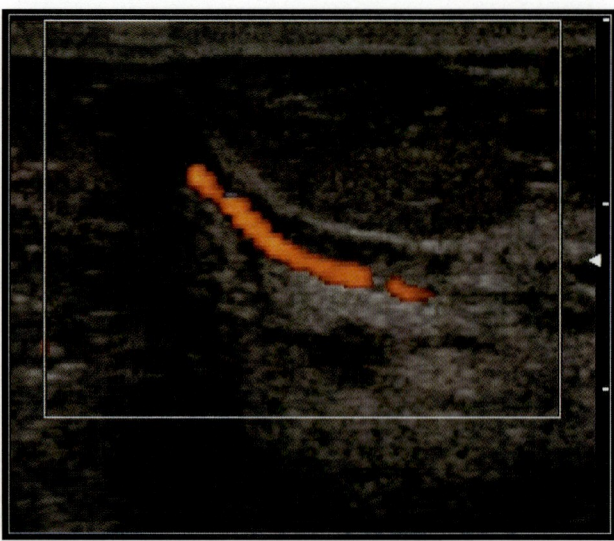

FIGURE 20–51 In acute periductal mastitis, hyperemia may be the dominant feature.

and also become hyperemic enough to have blood flow that is easily demonstrable with Doppler (Fig. 20–50). The hyperemia is often the dominant feature (Fig. 20–51). As the acute inflammation resolves spontaneously or during antibiotic treatment, the hyperemia resolves even before the duct wall thickening or debris within the duct resolves.

Chronic duct ectasia usually leads to bilaterally greenish, milky, or cheesy secretions and rarely causes frankly bloody secretions, but in the small percentage of patients with duct ectasia who do develop frankly bloody secretions, Doppler can usually show marked hyperemia within the duct wall (Fig. 20–52). Presumably, the epithelium overlying one of these dilated vessels ulcerates and causes bleeding. In such cases, the bloody discharge resolves when the inflammatory hyperemia resolves.

In patients with duct ectasia who present with acute pain or frankly bloody discharge, the sonographic and Doppler findings usually are far more specific than those of galactography (Fig. 20–53).

Interestingly, similar to the differences in blood vessel patterns that exist between inflamed cysts and cysts that contain papillary lesions, there is a difference in blood flow patterns between acute periductal mastitis and ducts

that contain vascular papillary lesions. The blood vessels that supply the inflamed duct wall in acute periductal mastitis course parallel to the thickened duct wall. The vascular stalk that supplies papillary lesions within the duct, however, courses perpendicular to the duct wall (Fig. 20–54). This assessment is generally best done in short axis at the base of the fibrovascular stalk. Papillary lesions can grow long distances down the duct, dragging their vascular stalks horizontally as they grow. Thus, some very elongated papillomas may have a horizontally oriented vascular stalk away from the point at which the stalk penetrates the duct wall that, at first glance, might be confused with the hyperemia seen in acutely inflamed ducts (Fig. 20–55). Even in such cases, there are subtle differences between the horizontally oriented vessels in acute periductal mastitis and the horizontal vascular stalks of papillary lesions.

When viewed in the long axis, the vascular stalk feeding an elongated intraductal papillary lesion will lie near the center of the papilloma within the lumen of the duct, whereas the dilated vessel supplying the inflamed duct will lie eccentrically within the thickened wall (Fig. 20–56).

Bacteria colonize the ectatic ducts in about 20% of patients with chronic duct ectasia. Duct rupture in such patients may lead to periductal abscess formation, usually in the periareolar area (Fig. 20–57).

Infected Periimplant Capsule

The fibrous capsule that surrounds all mammary implants is a normal structure that represents foreign body reaction to the implant. Frequently, there is also a periimplant effusion.

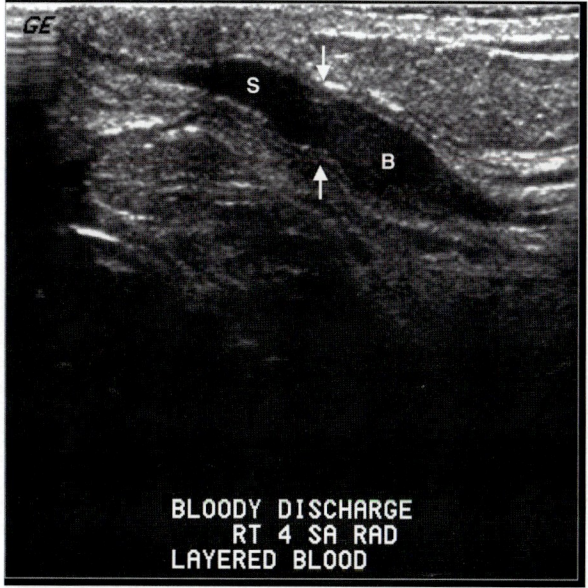

A

BLOODY DISCHARGE
RT 4 SA RAD
LAYERED BLOOD

FIGURE 20–52 A: Although duct ectasia usually causes milky or greenish nipple discharge, it can be a cause of acute frankly bloody secretions during episodes of acute periductal mastitis. This severely ectatic duct is the bleeding duct. Its wall is thickened and isoechoic, and the lumen contains a fluid–debris level *(arrows)*. The dependent debris is blood. S, secretions; B, blood. **B:** The acutely inflamed ectatic duct responsible for frankly bloody discharge is severely hyperemic. During acute episodes of periductal mastitis, the epithelium of the affected ducts may become ulcerated. If the epithelial ulceration erodes into one of the prominent vessels, brisk bleeding will ensue. Note that in the antiradial view, there are two very prominent vessels along the inner surface of the left side of the duct wall *(arrows)*. Because of the subepithelial location of these vessels, it is likely that mucosal ulceration has eroded one of them, resulting in the frankly bloody secretions.

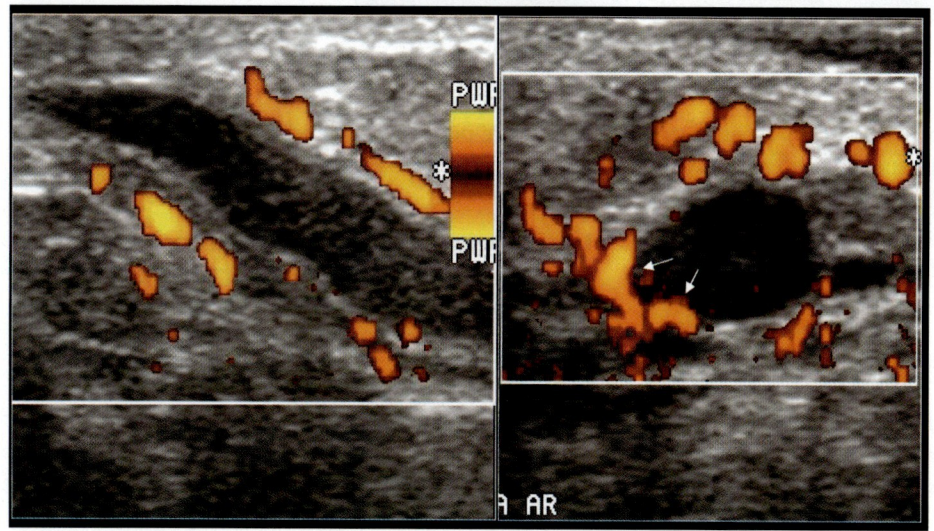

B

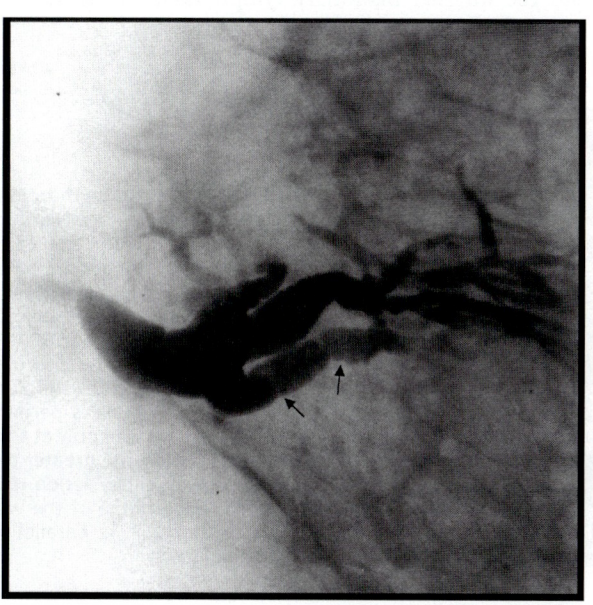

FIGURE 20–53 The galactogram shows no intraductal papillary lesion but shows blood filling one branch of the duct *(arrows)*. The layers could obscure an underlying intraductal papillary lesion (IPL). Sonography frequently reveals more in acutely bleeding or infected patients than does galactography.

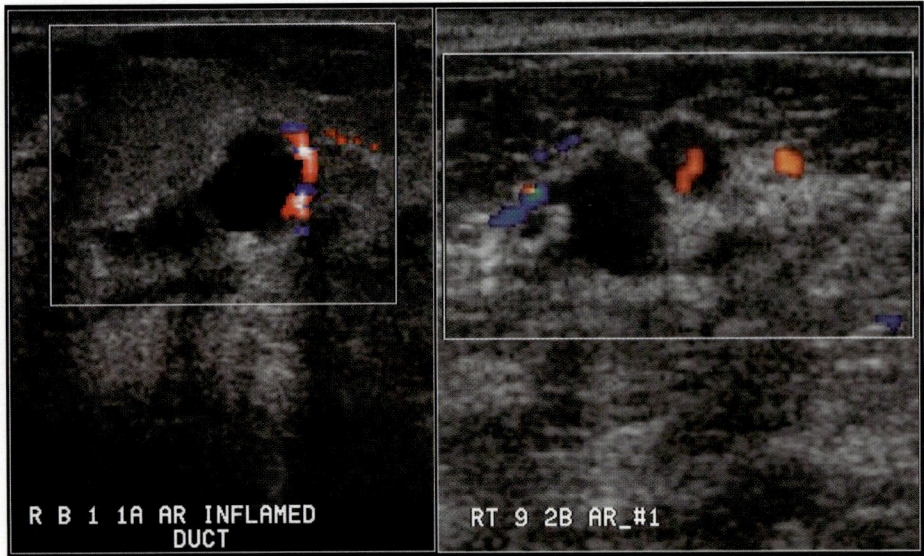

FIGURE 20–54 In a fashion that is analogous to complex cysts, the direction in which the prominent vessels course differs between inflamed ducts and those that contain isoechoic papillary lesions. The vessel supplying the inflamed duct wall lies parallel to the duct wall (**left**). The vessel supplying an intraductal papillary lesion merely passes through the duct wall to supply the papillary lesion and is oriented perpendicular to the duct wall (**right**).

The fibrous capsule around normal implants is usually visible sonographically as a thin, echogenic line and has no visible blood flow within it on color Doppler or power Doppler (Fig. 20–58). In patients who have capsular contracture, the capsule may become abnormally thickened and either isoechoic or hyperechoic, but like the normal capsule, thickened and contracted capsules do not have blood flow that is demonstrable with Doppler (Fig. 20–59). In rare cases, the capsule may become infected. This usually happens in the immediate postoperative period, but can occur as a late complication. The acutely infected capsule shows findings similar to the wall of an infected cyst or the wall of an acutely inflamed duct. It becomes thickened, isoechoic, and markedly hyperemic, and the effusion within the infected capsule develops fibrinous adhesions (Fig. 20–60).

The presence of Doppler demonstrable blood flow within the capsule, together with fibrinous adhesions within the periimplant effusion, is the key to differentiating infection from isolated capsular contracture.

Identifying Vascular Landmarks, such as the Internal Mammary Artery and Vein, that Facilitate Identification of the Internal Mammary Lymph Nodes

Color Doppler or power Doppler can show the position of the internal mammary vessels, which can be helpful in detecting the internal mammary lymph nodes that lie in a chain that is roughly parallel to the internal mammary vessels (Fig. 20–61).

Additionally, in some elderly patients, the internal mammary veins can be quite dilated and tortuous, making it difficult to distinguish segments of the tortuous veins from the internal mammary lymph nodes. Doppler can

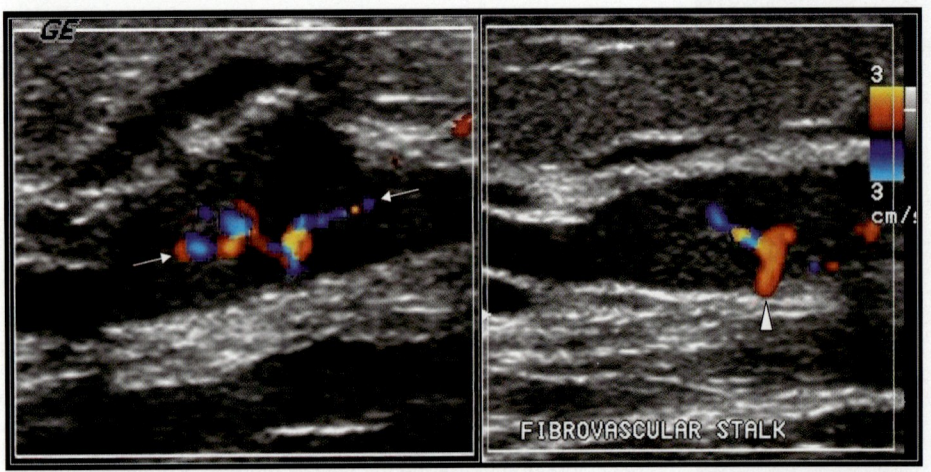

FIGURE 20–55 It can be more difficult to distinguish between inflammatory hyperemic vessels and those that supply long papillomas because both can be oriented with their long axes parallel to the long axis of the duct. In such cases, it is important to assess the vascular stalk where it penetrates the duct wall. The vascular stalk is perpendicular to the duct wall only at that point (*arrowhead*). The greater the length of the papillary lesion, the greater the percentage of the vascular stalk that will lie parallel to the duct walls.

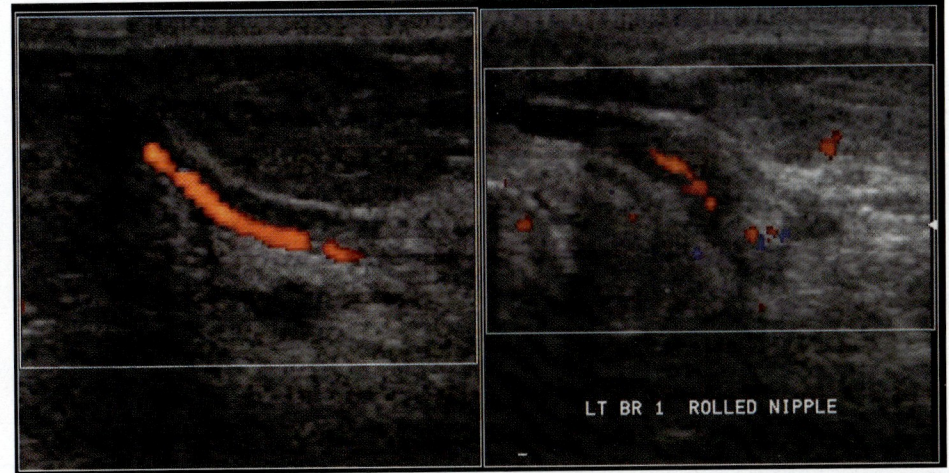

FIGURE 20–56 Radial views of an inflamed duct and a duct containing a long papilloma show subtle differences. The hyperemic vessel in an inflamed duct lies eccentrically along one wall of the duct (**left**). The vascular stalk of an elongated papilloma, on the other hand, lies parallel to the duct walls within the lumen of the duct (**right**).

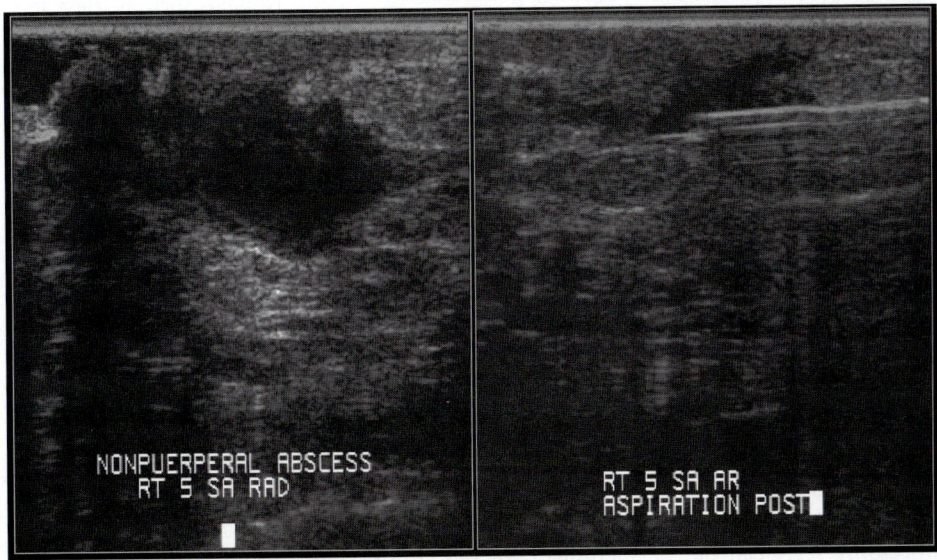

FIGURE 20–57 Rupture of an acutely inflamed ectatic duct is the most common cause of nonpuerperal periareolar abscesses in women older than 35 years of age. In younger women, it usually is a complication of congenital nipple inversion and squamous metaplasia.

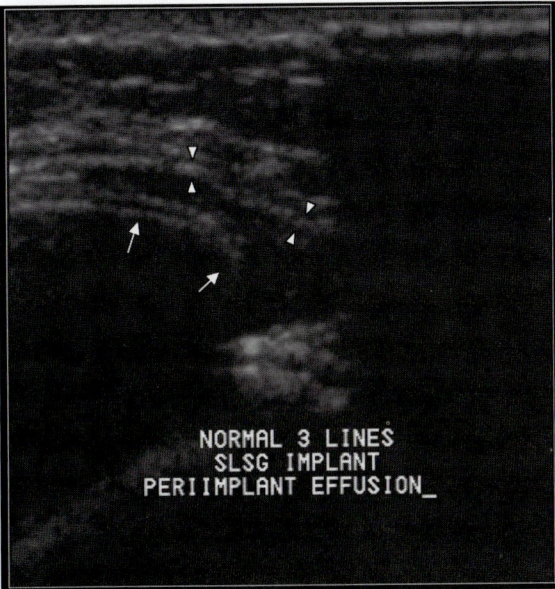

FIGURE 20–58 The fibrous capsule that surrounds all augmentation implants is normally thin and echogenic *(arrowheads)*, like the walls of normal ducts and uncomplicated cysts. The capsule is particularly well seen in this case because there is a periimplant effusion *(arrows indicate shell of implant)*.

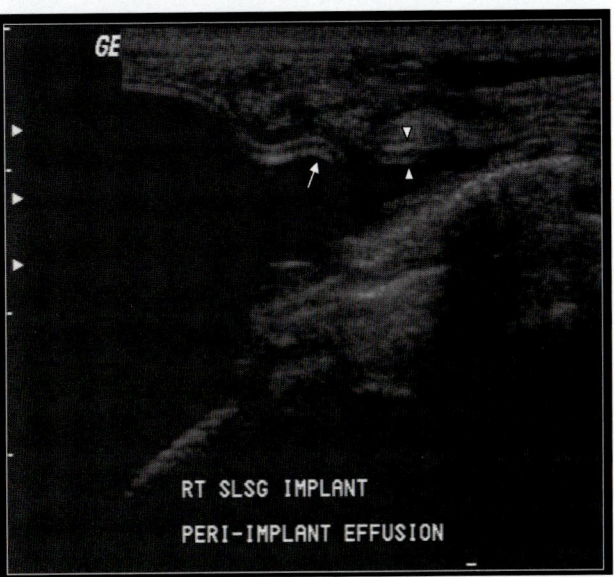

FIGURE 20–59 The periimplant capsule may be thickened and isoechoic in patients with capsular contracture but will not be hyperemic on color Doppler.

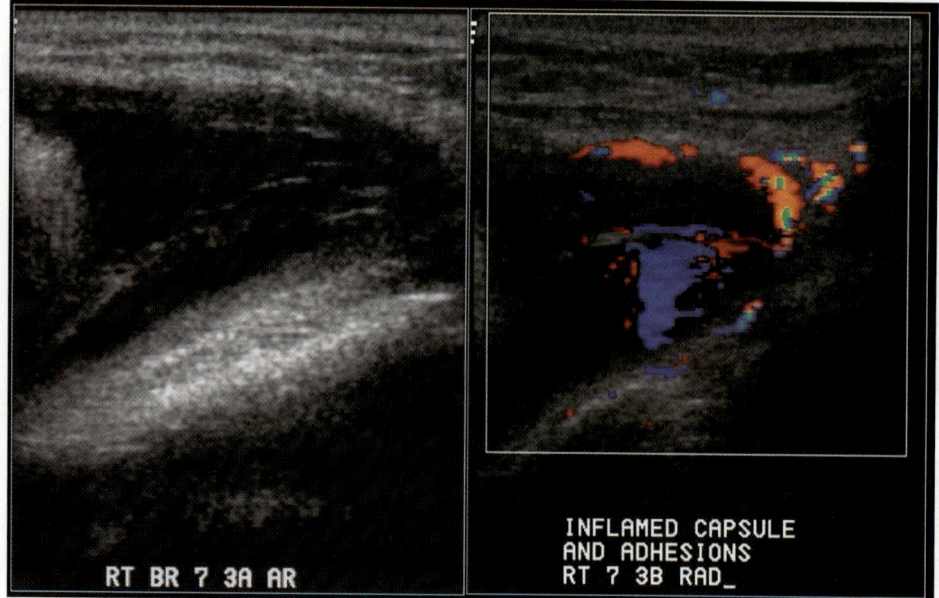

RT BR 7 3A AR

INFLAMED CAPSULE
AND ADHESIONS
RT 7 3B RAD_

FIGURE 20–60 In rare circumstances, what has been a normal periimplant effusion or seroma will become secondarily inflamed or infected years after implantation. In such cases, the fibrous periimplant capsule, normally represented by a thin, echogenic line, becomes abnormally thickened and isoechoic and also becomes hyperemic on color Doppler. The fluid, which did not contain adhesions earlier, will develop numerous fibrinous adhesions. Findings such as these indicate the need for aspiration, Gram stain, and culture. Unfortunately, once frank infection ensues, it usually cannot be cleared without removing the offending foreign body (i.e., explantation).

help to distinguish tortuous dilated veins from lymph nodes (Fig. 20–62).

Distinguishing Fat Necrosis and Exuberant Scar from Recurrent Tumor

Patients who have undergone conservative breast therapy, lumpectomy, or segmentectomy often require evaluation of the surgical site with ultrasound in addition to mammography to help distinguish between recurrent neoplasm and exuberant scar or fat necrosis. Lumpectomy scars can be very irregular and can have many sonographic and mammographic features that appear to be malignant. Early on, lumpectomy cavities may have some Doppler demonstrable blood flow within granulation tissue in the wall of the cavity that is part of the normal healing process, particularly if there is any associated inflammation or infection (Fig. 20–63). But after 6 months, it is very rare to see any demonstrable blood flow within the lumpectomy scar (Fig. 20–64). Additionally, fat necrosis by definition is avascular. Recurrent breast cancer, on the other hand, frequently has demonstrable blood flow (Fig. 20–65). Thus, the presence

(text continued on page 917)

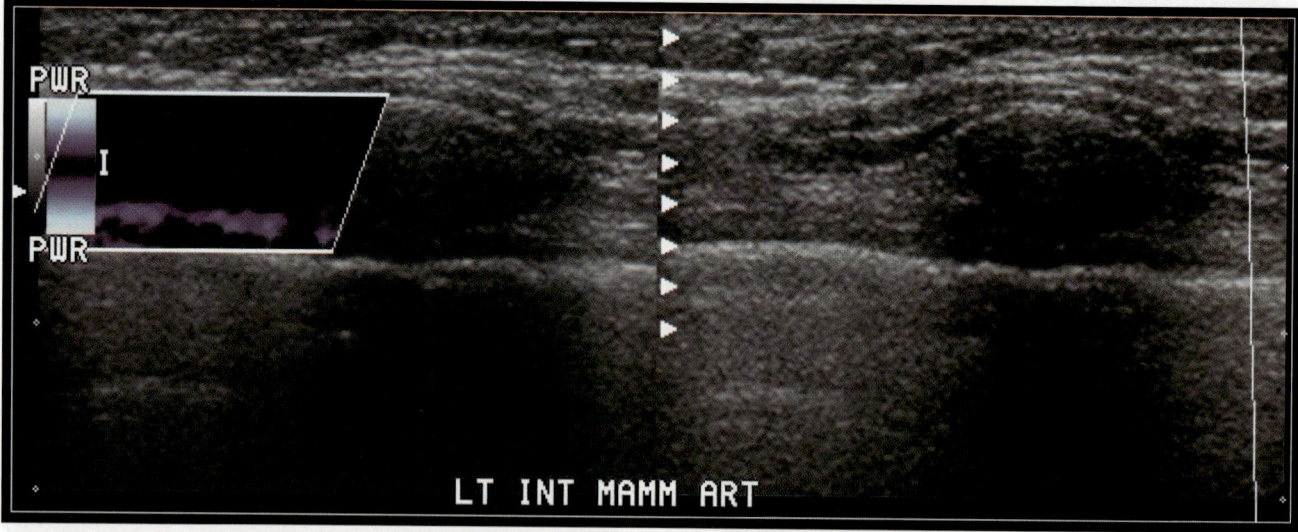

PWR

I

PWR

LT INT MAMM ART

FIGURE 20–61 Color Doppler or power Doppler may aid in finding internal mammary lymph nodes by identifying the course of the internal mammary artery and veins. The internal mammary lymph node chain lies parallel to the artery and vein.

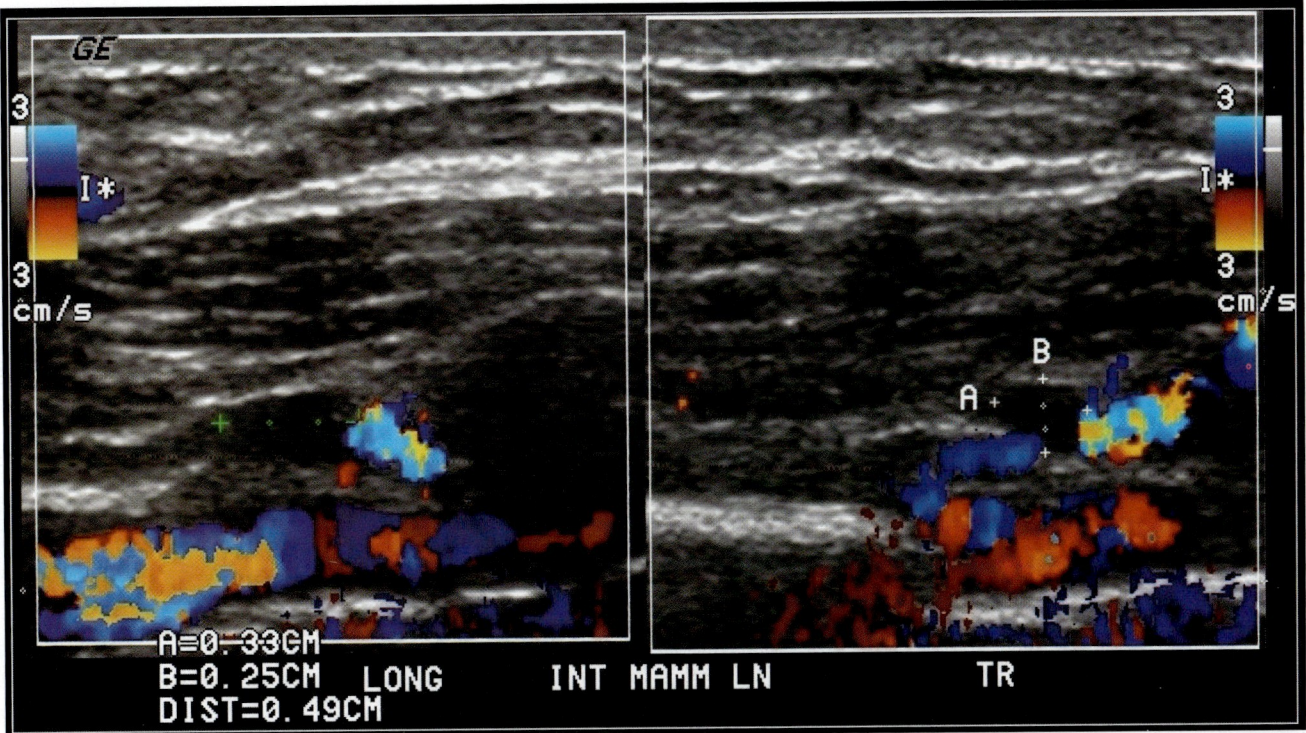

FIGURE 20–62 The internal mammary veins may be quite dilated and tortuous, particularly in elderly patients who have right heart failure. Note that the veins are about the same diameter as the internal mammary lymph nodes *(calipers)*. Without Doppler, it can be difficult to distinguish bends in a tortuous internal mammary vein from internal mammary lymph nodes.

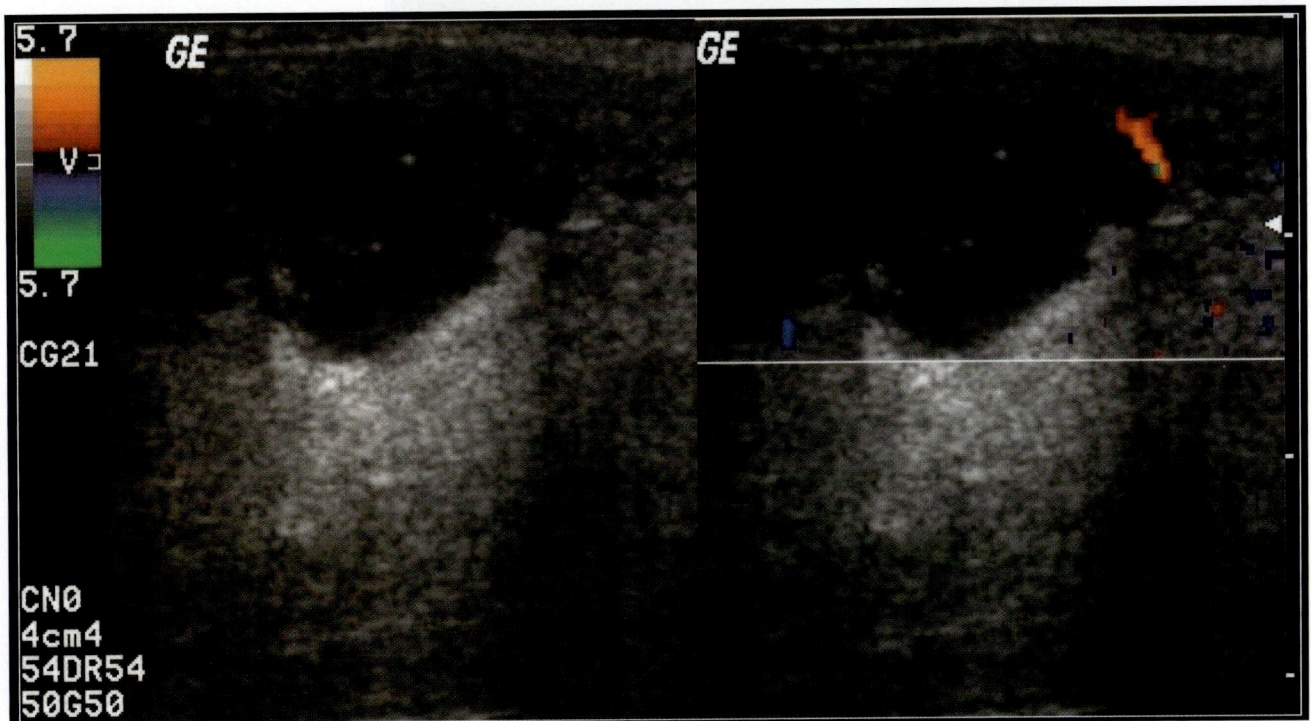

FIGURE 20–63 Granulation tissue in the walls of lumpectomy cavities may have demonstrable blood flow for about 6 months after surgery, particularly if there was any inflammation or infection in the perioperative period.

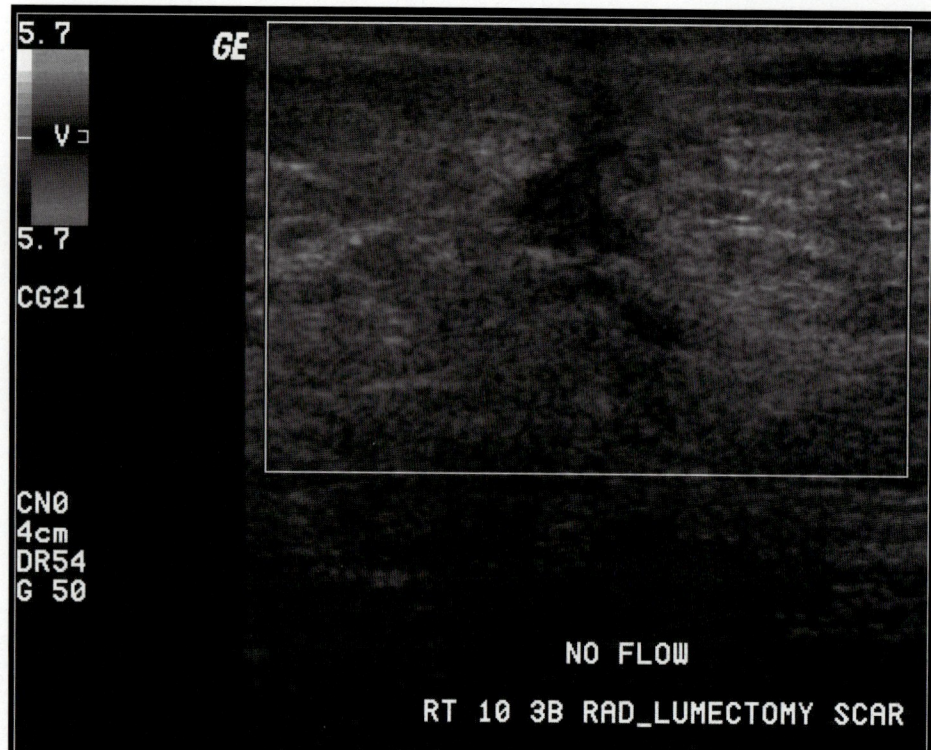

FIGURE 20–64 Six months or more after lumpectomy, the cavity or fat necrosis that develops within the cavity and its wells should not have any demonstrable flow on color Doppler. Doppler-demonstrable flow after 6 months is suspicious for recurrent tumor.

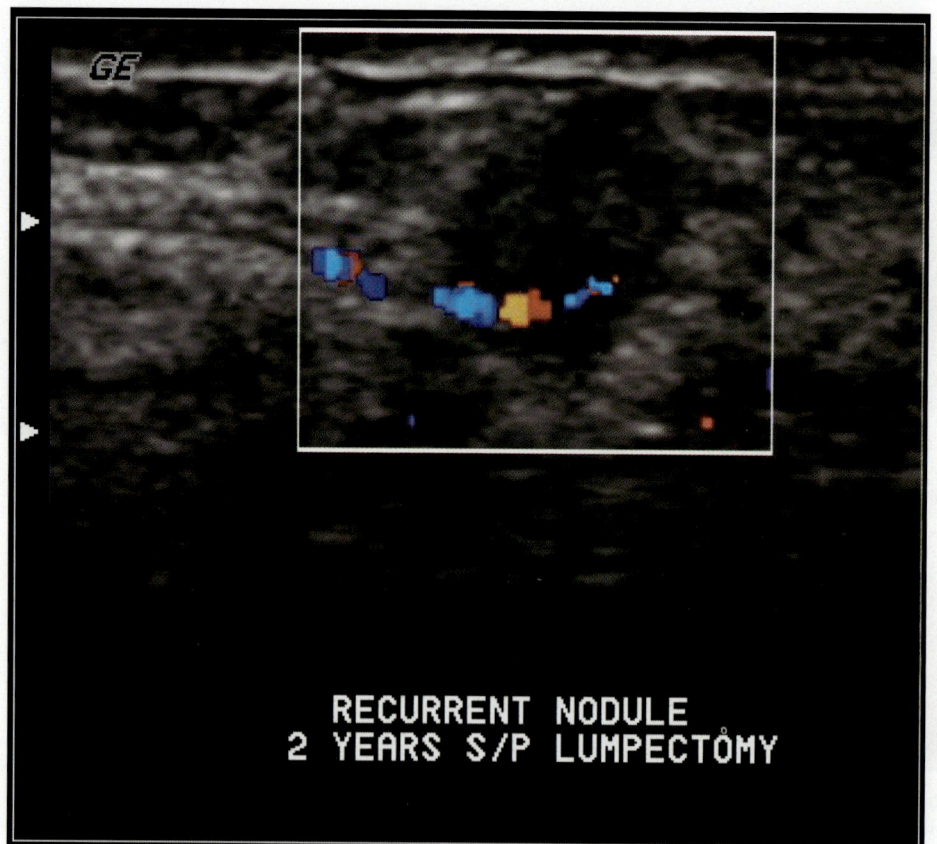

FIGURE 20–65 Most recurrent tumor nodes have demonstrable blood flow on color Doppler. Six months or more after lumpectomy, the presence of blood flow in the lumpectomy cavity or immediately surrounding tissues raises concerns about recurrent tumor.

of blood flow in a lumpectomy scar more than 6 months after surgery is worrisome for recurrent neoplasm and indicates the need for biopsy, whereas the lack of demonstrable blood flow favors exuberant scar or fat necrosis. Some recurrent tumor may not have demonstrable flow; thus, a positive study showing flow is a better positive predictor of recurrent cancer than lack of flow is a negative predictor.

Assessment of Vascular Conditions of the Breast

Doppler is essential for evaluating vascular conditions in the breast. These are conditions that are similar to vascular conditions elsewhere in the body but just happen to occur in the breast. The two most frequently encountered vascular conditions are superficial venous thrombosis and venous malformations. In infants and young children, lymphangiomas are also common residuals of fetal cystic hygromas. Superficial venous thrombosis, Mondor's disease, affects the subdermal veins through which much of the superficial venous drainage exits the breast. Spontaneous thrombosis can occur late in pregnancy (probably related to progesterone effect), after minor trauma (particularly seat-belt and air-bag injuries), and idiopathically. We cannot confirm the published data suggesting an increased risk for occult malignancy in patients who have Mondor's disease, but it is probably worth performing whole breast ultrasound in patients who present with superficial thrombosis just to be sure. The presenting symptom is a tender cord. Sonography shows a tortuous or beaded hypoechoic structure that has no demonstrable blood flow (Fig. 20–66) and is incompressible (Fig. 20–67).

Normal subdermal veins are thin walled, are completely collapsible with compression (Fig. 20–68), and have demonstrable flow with color Doppler or power Doppler (Fig. 20–69). Venous malformations and cavernous hemangiomas may be difficult to distinguish from each other. There is usually a cluster of dilated compressible veins (Fig. 20–70) interspersed with variable amounts of fibrous tissue (Fig. 20–71) that alter compressibility. Spontaneous thrombosis of a few venous channels is fairly common (Fig. 20–72), and chronically thrombosed channels may calcify, forming phleboliths (Fig. 20–73). The beaded appearance of small venous malformations and acutely thrombosed superficial veins in Mondor's disease make one wonder whether some cases of acute Mondor's disease actually represent spontaneous thrombosis of previously undiagnosed minimal venous malformations (Fig. 20–74).

(text continued on page 920)

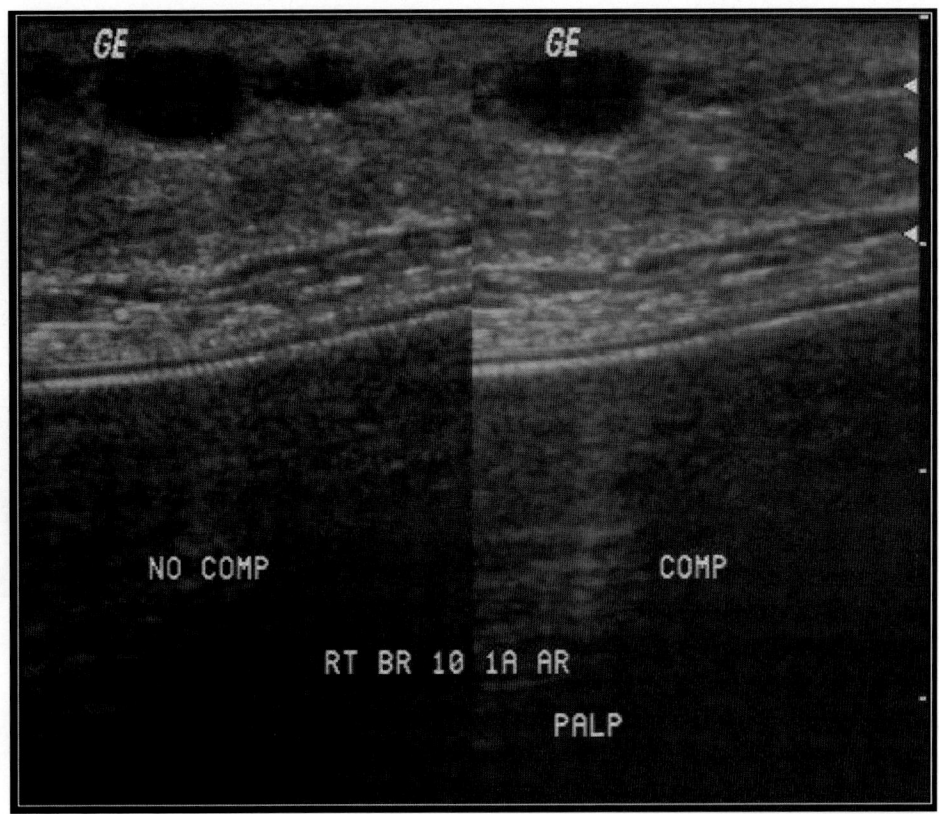

FIGURE 20–66 Split-screen images of an acutely thrombosed superficial breast vein (Mondor's disease) show it to be incompressible.

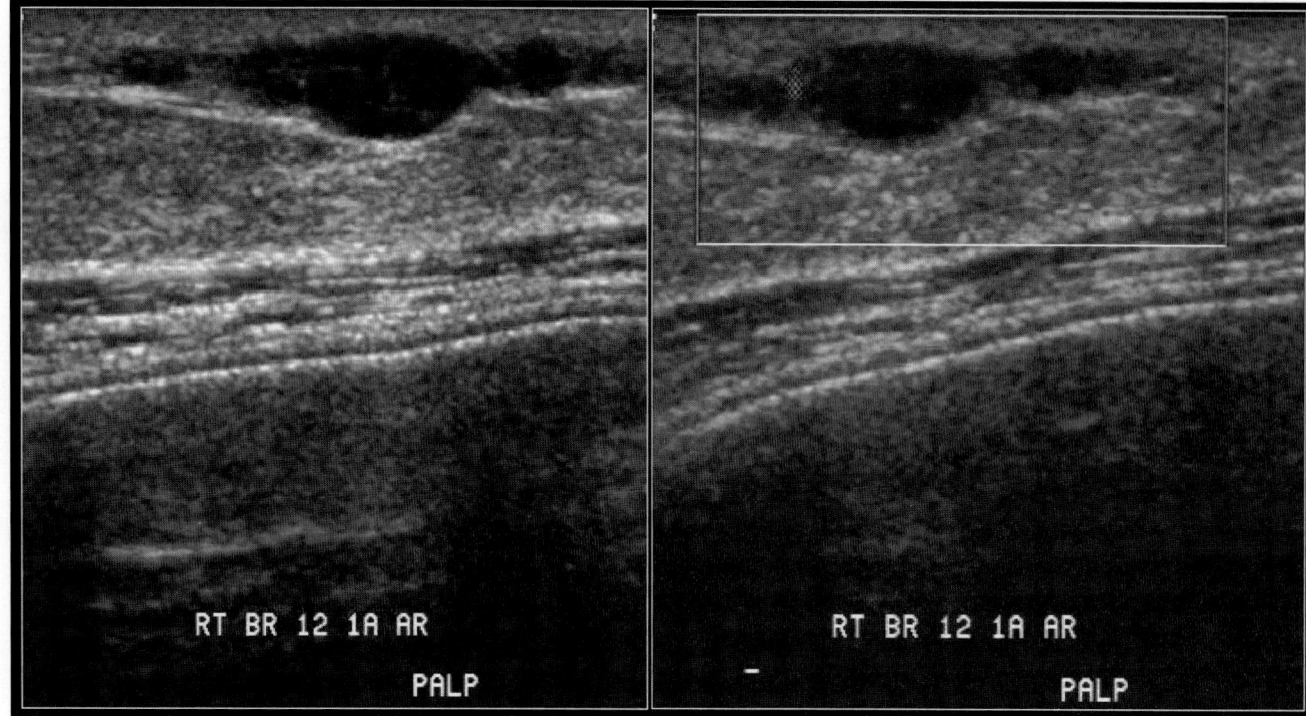

FIGURE 20–67 This acutely thrombosed superficial breast vein has no blood flow on color Doppler, indicating that the thrombus is completely occlusive.

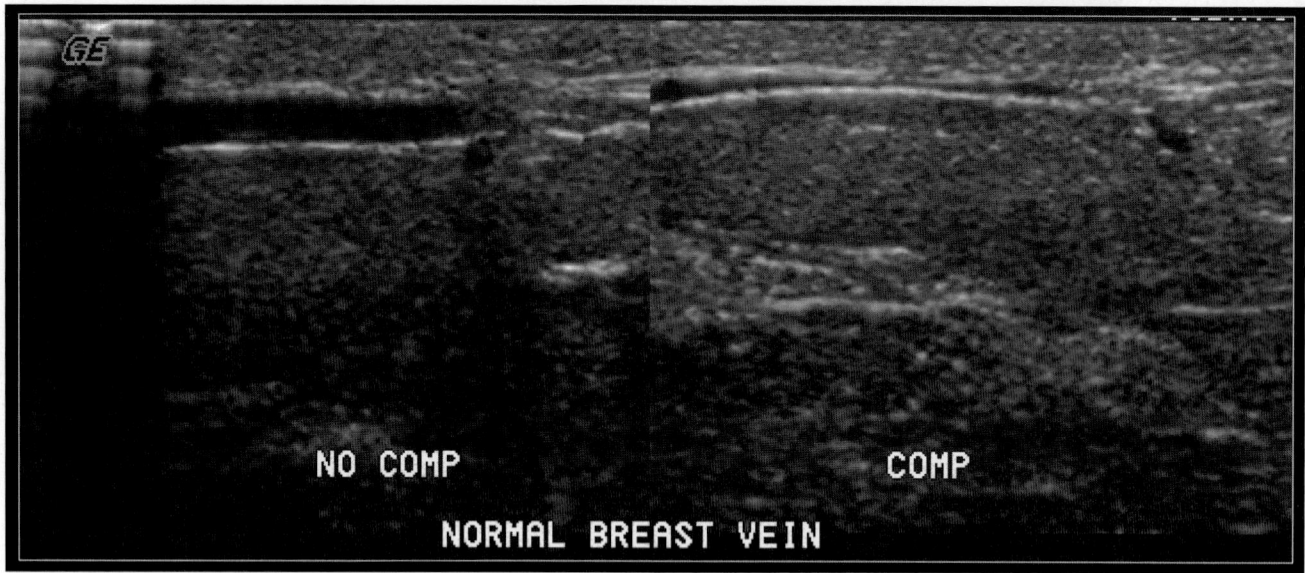

FIGURE 20–68 Normal breast veins course superficially through the subcutaneous fat, just deep to the skin (**left**), and are soft and completely collapsible with transducer compression (**right**).

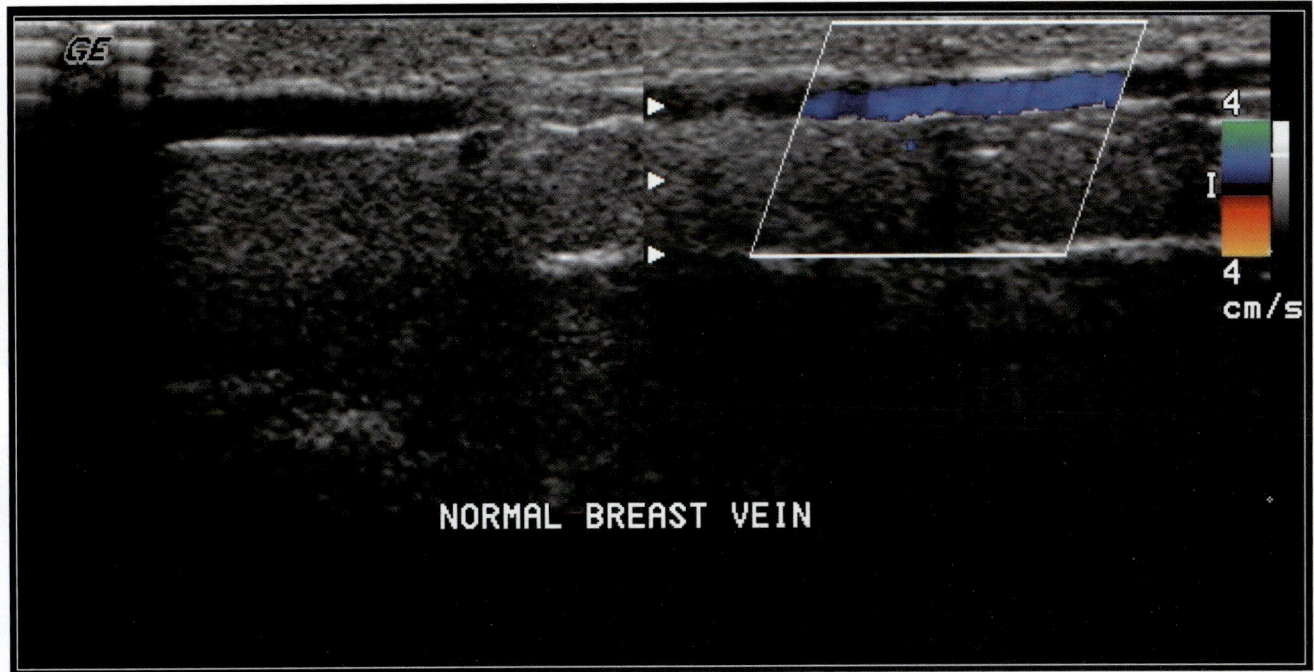

FIGURE 20–69 Blood flow is demonstrable in normal superficial breast veins with color or power Doppler using low wall filter, low velocity scale [pulse repetition frequency (PRF)], and adequate gain.

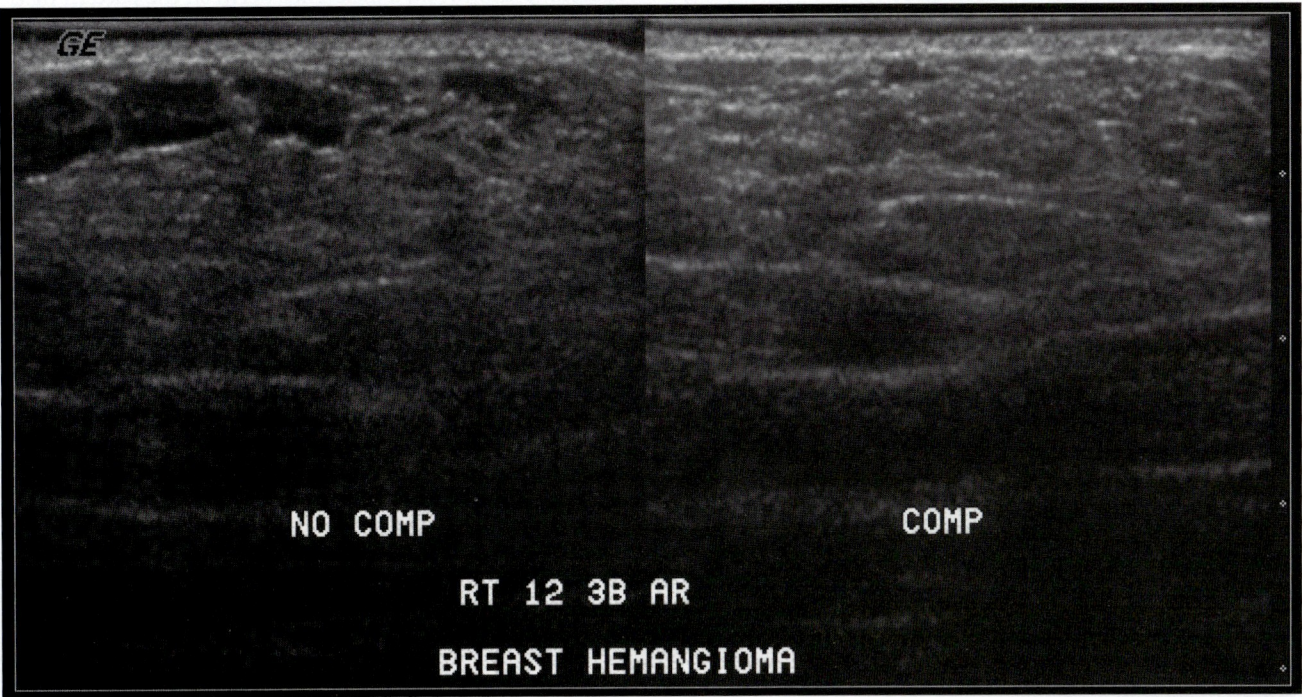

FIGURE 20–70 This superficial venous malformation, like a normal subdermal breast vein, is completely collapsible with transducer compression.

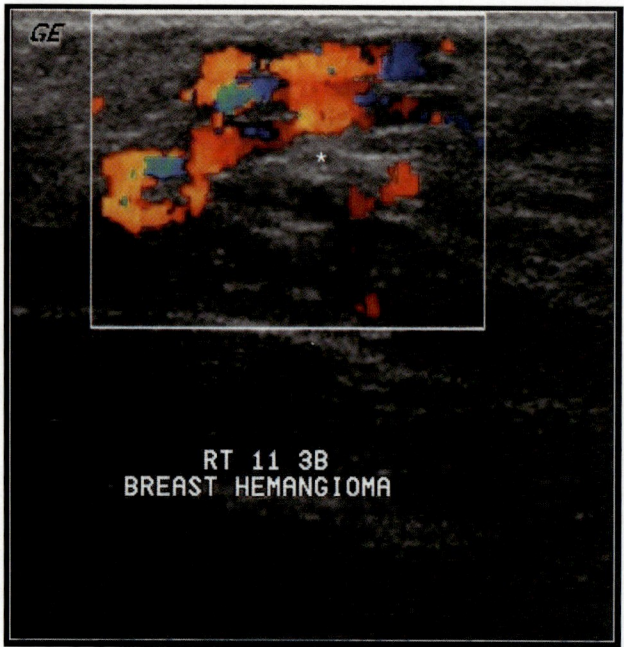

FIGURE 20–71 This venous malformation is composed of dilated venous channels and fibrous elements (*).

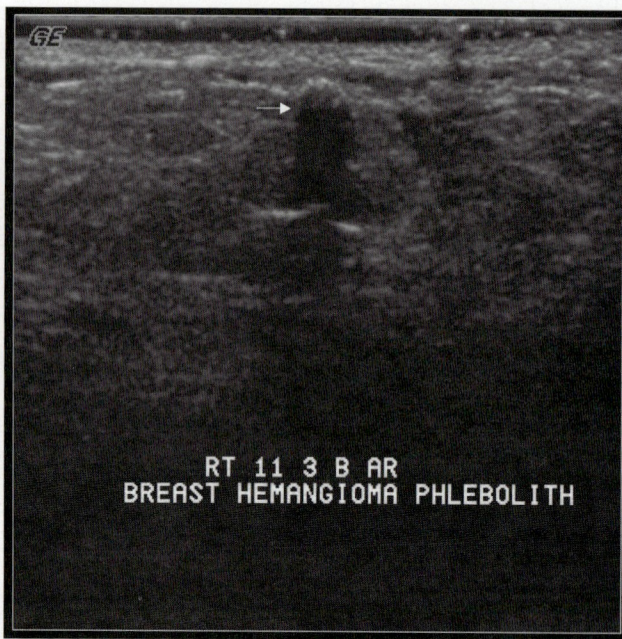

FIGURE 20–73 Chronically thrombosed venous channels in cavernous hemangiomas or venous malformations may calcify and form phleboliths.

Assessment of Acoustic Vibratory Response to Vocal Fremitus

Dr. Sohn of Germany first described Doppler vocal fremitus. He found that when a patient spoke during color Doppler examination, vibrations from the chest wall created color artifacts in normal tissue, but not within tumors. He also found a difference between the pattern of vibratory artifact defect caused by spiculated malignancies and circumscribed benign lesions. The vibratory artifact worked its way partway into the spiculated malignant nodules because of their infiltrating margins (Fig. 20–75) but

(text continued on page 923)

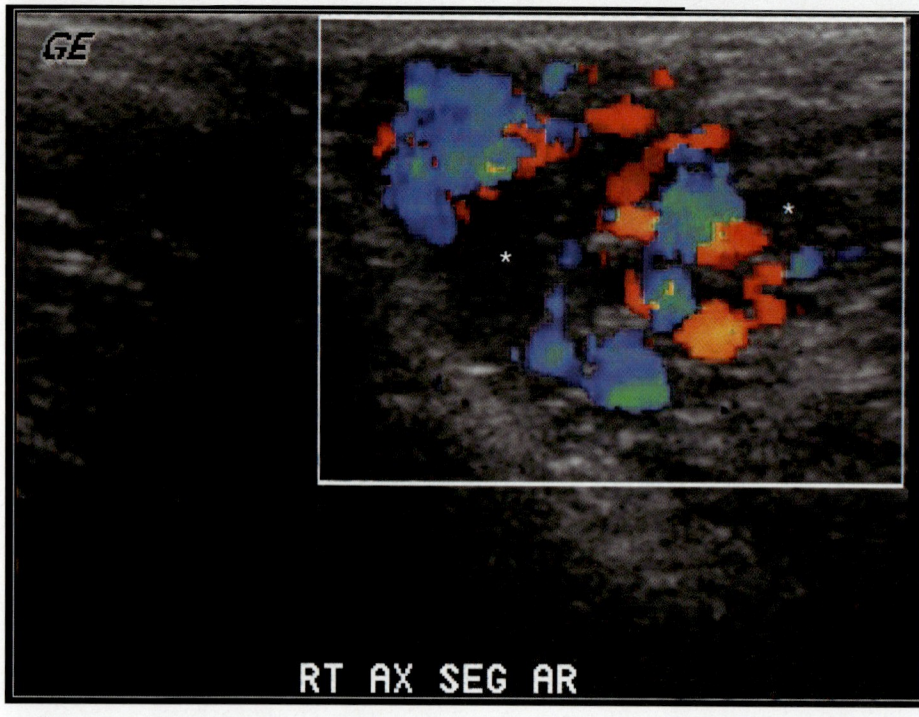

FIGURE 20–72 Venous malformations and cavernous hemangiomas frequently undergo spontaneous thrombosis in some channels with very slow flow (*).

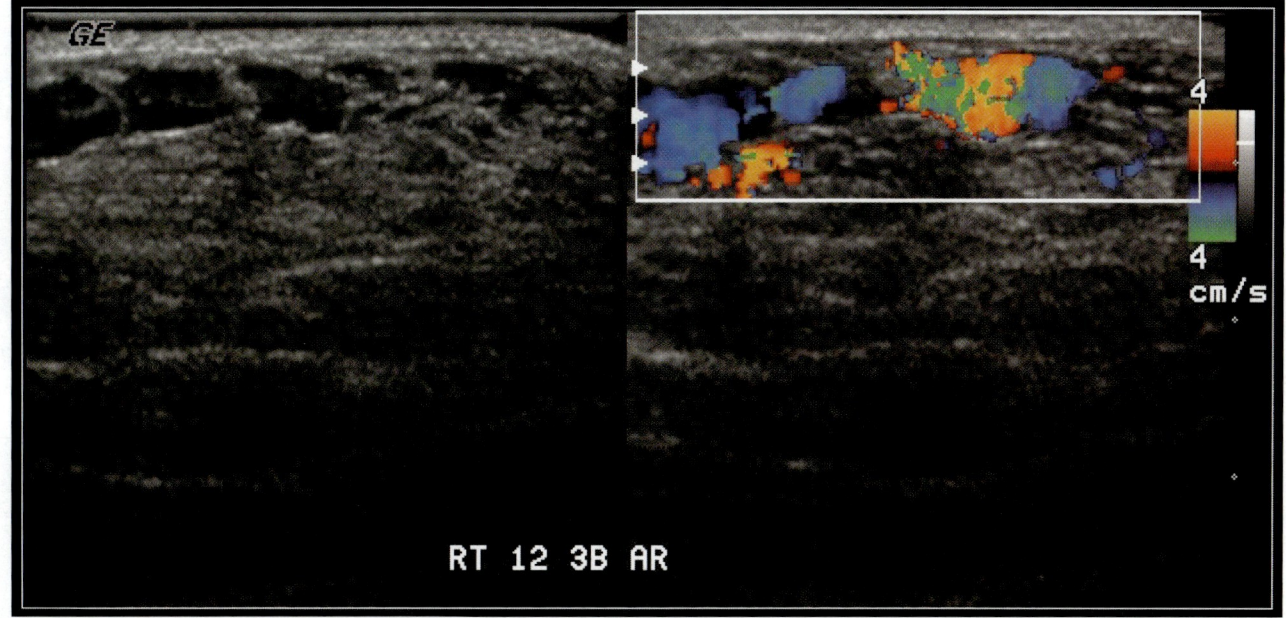

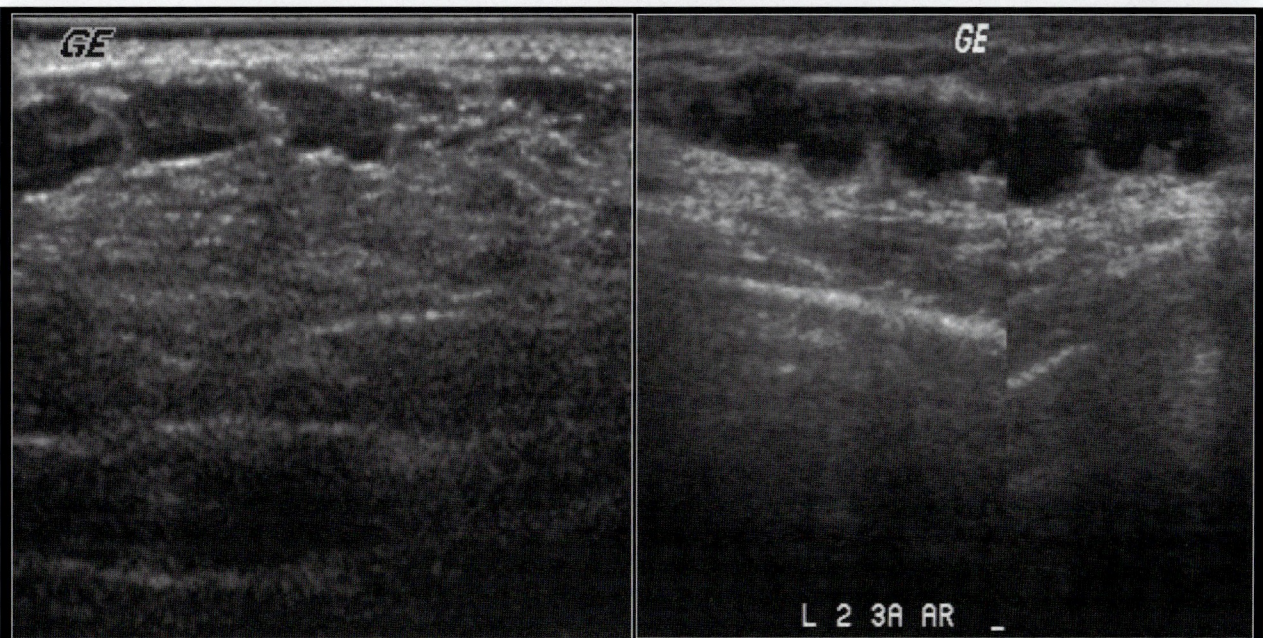

FIGURE 20–74 A: Color Doppler shows flow within an abnormal subdermal vein in a venous malformation. **B:** There is great similarity in the beaded appearance of malformed veins (**left**) and acutely thrombosed superficial veins (**right**). Normal subdermal veins are small and tubular and do not have a beaded appearance. The beaded appearance makes one wonder whether at least some cases of superficial thrombosis do not occur in malformed veins that were subclinical before thrombosis.

stopped abruptly at the margin of circumscribed benign lesions (Fig. 20–76). At the time Sohn believed that to be successful, Doppler vocal fremitus required a certain color Doppler algorithm [maximum entropy method (MEM)].

Independently, we noticed similar findings in patients with a wide variety of breast lesions. However, our findings have differed somewhat from those of Dr. Sohn. First, we

found that color Doppler was less effective than power Doppler. Furthermore, we found that a single color map, usually orange, worked better than multicolor maps available with both color Doppler and power Doppler. We found that color Doppler is less sensitive than power Doppler and that the multicolored maps available with color Doppler made the findings more difficult to interpret

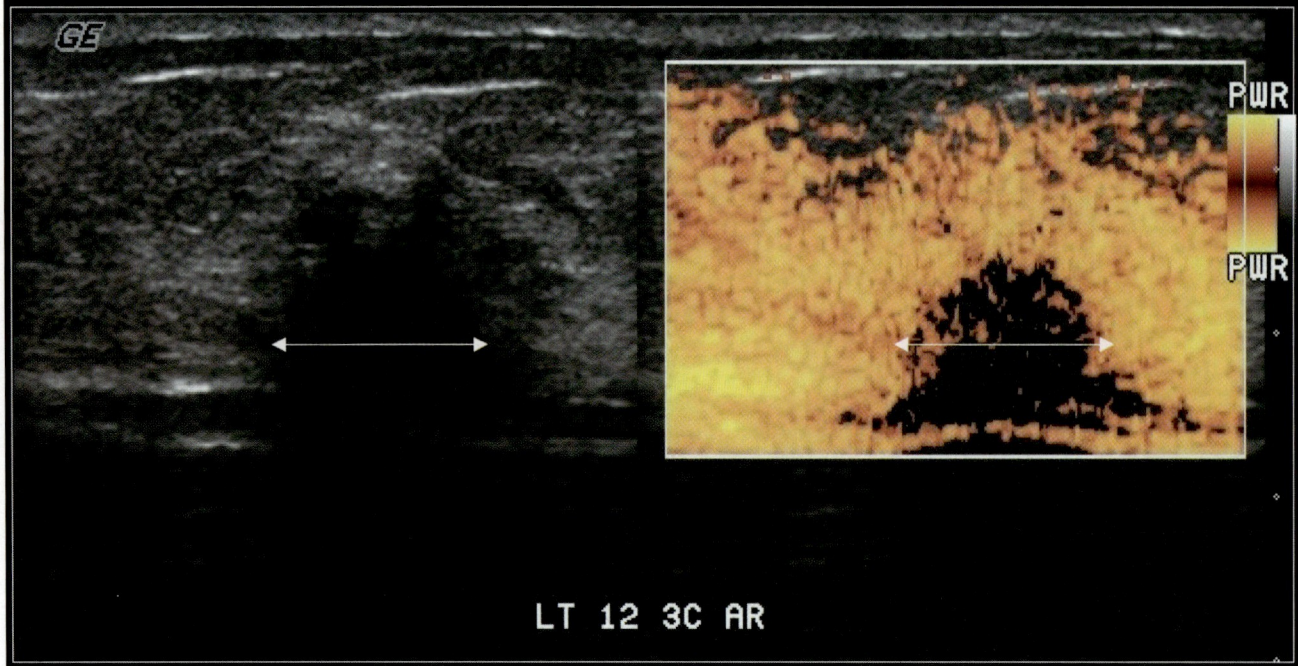

FIGURE 20–75 This split-screen simultaneous image shows the B-mode image on the left screen and the power Doppler fremitus image on the right. The acoustic vibratory artifact is orange, and the dark area that is not filled in with artifact, the acoustic vibratory defect, corresponds to the lesion. The image appears larger *(double-headed arrow)* on the B-mode image than is the vibratory defect, indicating that the edges of the lesion are infiltrating.

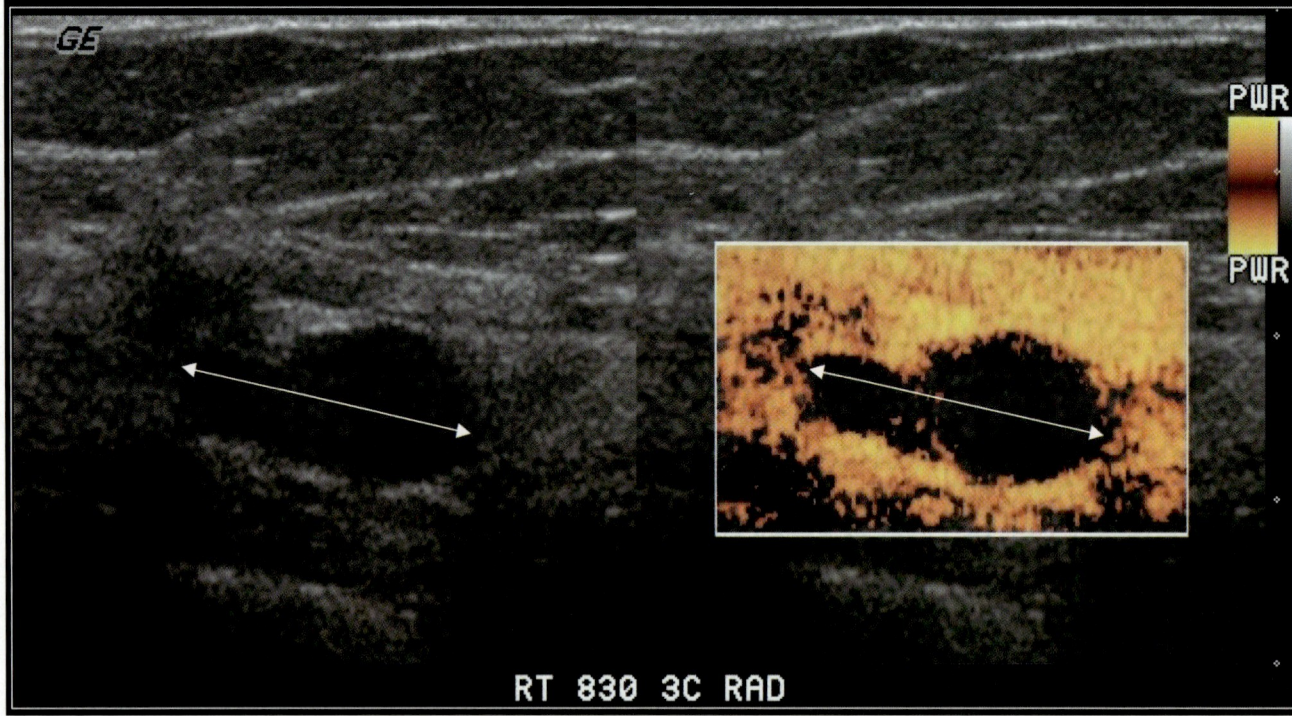

FIGURE 20–76 This bilobed circumscribed benign lesion causes a sharply circumscribed defect that is exactly the same size as the lesion on the B-mode image *(double-headed arrow)*, indicating that the margins are circumscribed and noninfiltrating.

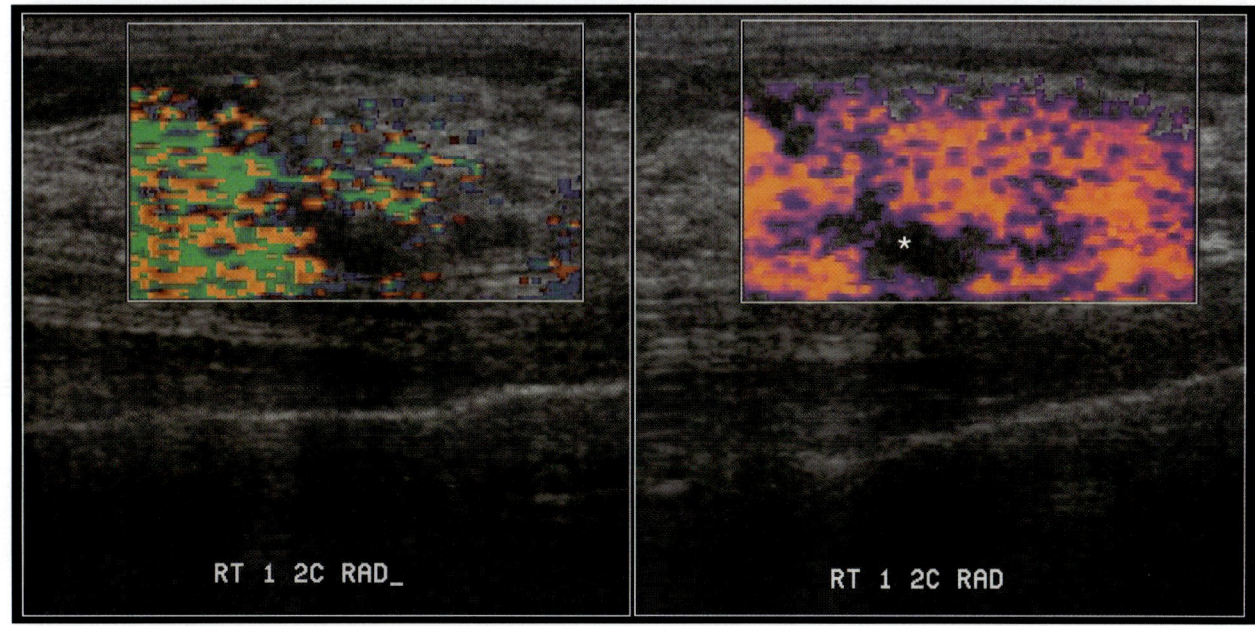

FIGURE 20–77 Color Doppler **(left)** is less effective than power Doppler **(right)** for assessing vocal fremitus because it is less sensitive and because the color maps tend to be multicolored and harder to interpret. Note that for similar settings of gain and pulse repetition frequency (PRF), there is more acoustic vibratory artifact with power Doppler that outlines the vibratory defect better *(*)*.

(Fig. 20–77). We do not find power Doppler vocal fremitus to be effective at distinguishing benign from malignant. Rather, we find it useful for distinguishing normal tissue from abnormal tissue. We find that invasive carcinomas (Fig. 20–75), fibroadenomas (Fig. 20–76), other benign solid nodules (Fig. 20–78), DCIS and simple cysts (Fig. 20–79), and various complex cysts (Fig. 20–80) can all cause acoustic vibratory defects. We do not find the pattern of the defect very useful in comparison to the image in distinguishing benign from malignant. We believe the

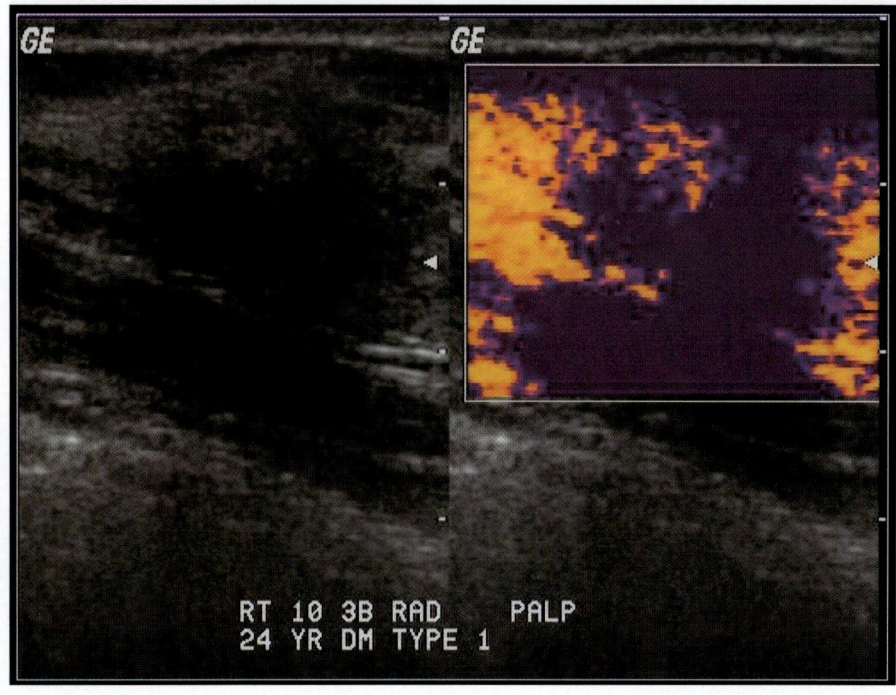

FIGURE 20–78 Benign lesions other than fibroadenomas can cause acoustic vibratory defects. This defect is caused by diabetic mastopathy.

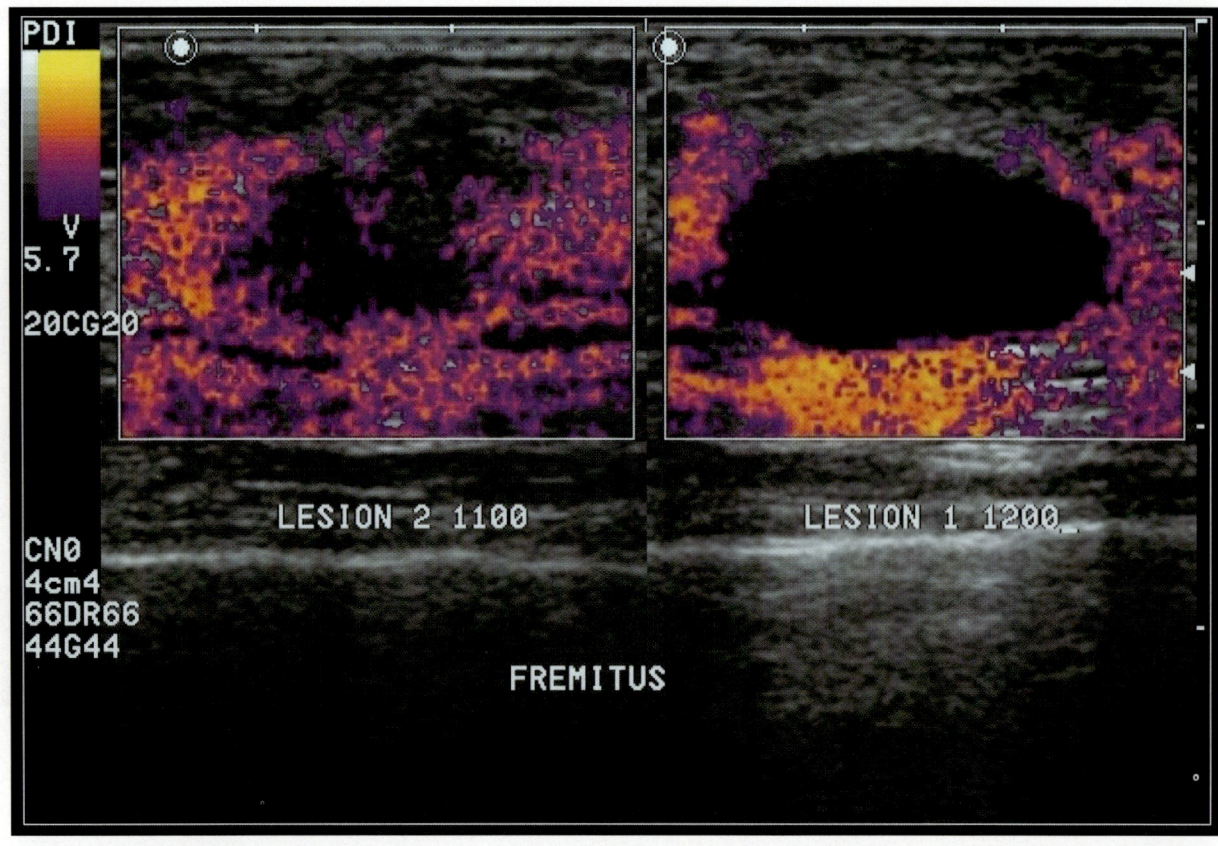

FIGURE 20–79 Pure ductal carcinoma *in situ* (**left**) and simple cysts (**right**) can also cause acoustic vibratory defects.

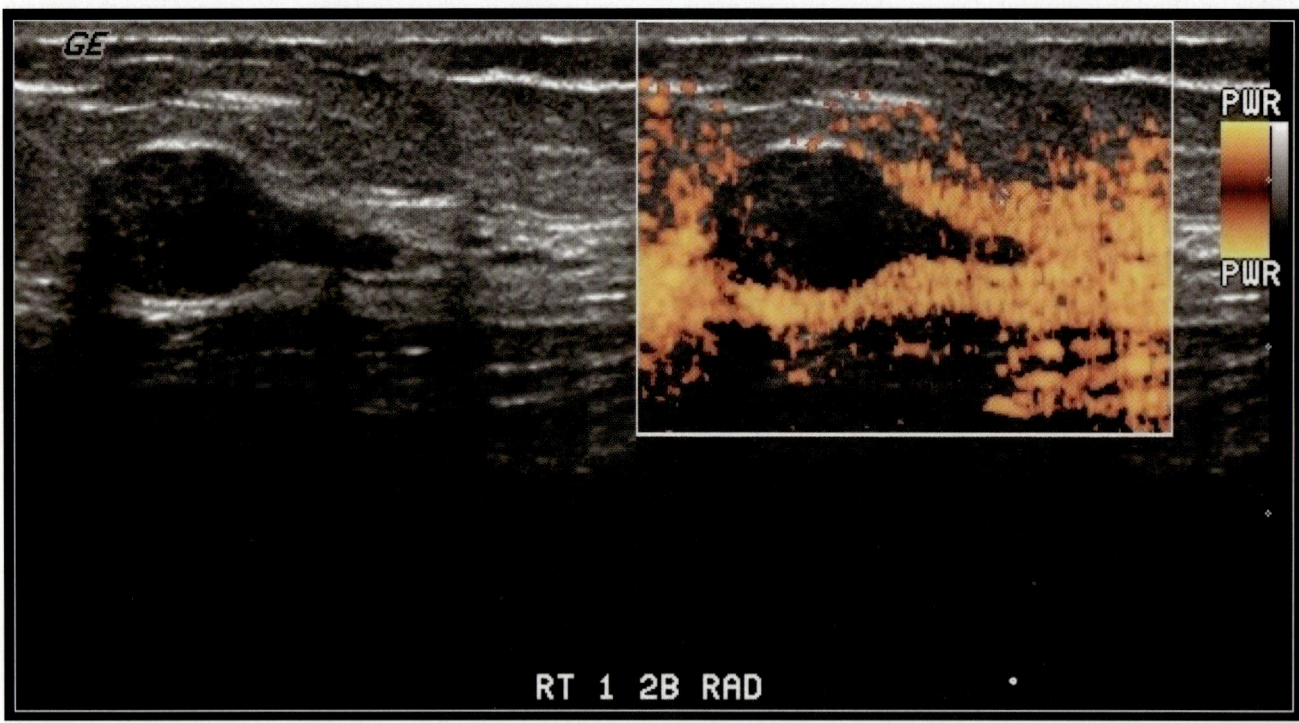

FIGURE 20–80 Complex cysts can cause acoustic vibratory defects.

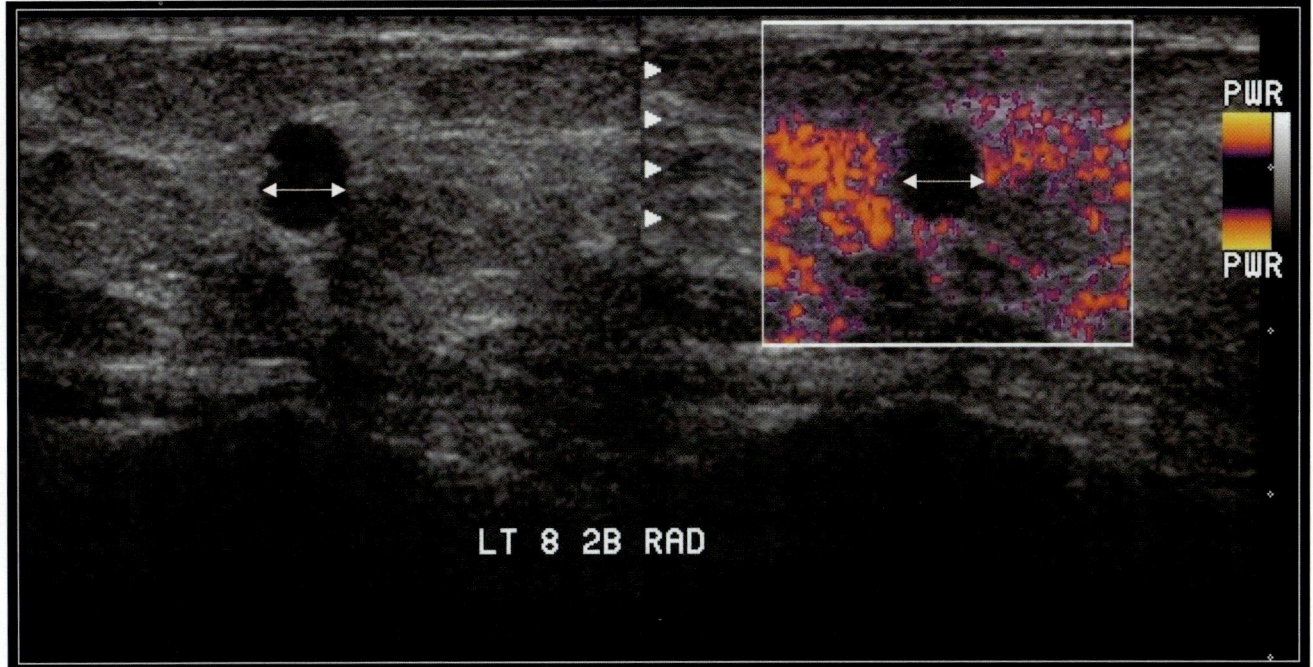

FIGURE 20–81 Circumscribed cancers cause sharply circumscribed acoustic vibratory defects that are the same size of the lesion on the B-mode image, just as benign circumscribed lesions such as cysts and fibroadenomas do. Thus, a circumscribed vibratory defect of the same size as the lesion on B-mode images indicates that the lesion is circumscribed, but not that it is benign.

findings described by Dr. Sohn do allow us to distinguish spiculated from nonspiculated lesions, but that is not at all the same as distinguishing benign from malignant. About one-third of breast carcinomas are circumscribed and cause acoustic vibratory defects very similar to those caused by circumscribed benign nodules such as fibroadenoma (Fig. 20–81).

Power Doppler vocal fremitus uses standard power Doppler pulse repetition frequency (PRF) of about 1,000 and default gain and write priority settings. The patient is asked to say something while the breast is being interrogated with power Doppler. A variety of different vocal stimuli can be used. The most effective maneuver is humming with a deep tone. Other stimuli include saying "99" or "eeee," or clearing the throat. The most effective maneuver varies from patient to patient, and in a small minority of patients, usually patients with chronic lung disease, none of the maneuvers is successful. All of these maneuvers generate vibrations that originate in the chest wall and progress outwardly, falling off proportional to the square of the distance from the chest wall. Additionally, vibrations are dampened by compression in tissues that lie just deep to the transducer face. For these reasons, power Doppler vocal fremitus is most useful in deeply seated lesions. Because of the variability in the effectiveness of the various vocal stimuli, some investigators are exploring mechanical devices to vibrate the breast tissues.

These mechanical devices have the theoretical advantage of supplying a vibratory stimulus that is more standardized and less variable from patient to patient. Additionally, vibrations at multiple frequencies can be assessed. Mechanical devices differ from vocal fremitus in that they generate vibrations from the skin surface inwardly rather than from the chest wall outwardly. They also would be expected to be more effective in evaluating superficially located lesions rather than more deeply located lesions than are shown better by vocal fremitus.

We find that split-screen images in simultaneous mode, with the real-time B-mode image on the left and the power Doppler image on the right, is the most effective way to assess acoustic vibratory artifact. It is not uncommon to have the transducer slide off the lesion of interest when the patient vocalizes forcefully. Thus, having the left image without overlain color can help us to make sure we do not slide off the lesion during the maneuver.

Normal breast tissues of different types vibrate differently from each other. The vibrating chest wall gives rise to the vibrations. It is dense and has fibers that are perpendicular to the direction of vibrations and vibrates intensely, creating abundant acoustic vibratory artifact and turning bright orange. Intensely echogenic interlobar fibrous tissue vibrates almost as well as does the chest wall (Fig. 20–82). It is compact tissue, with closely packed collagen fibers that lie roughly perpendicular to the vibrations. Fibers that are

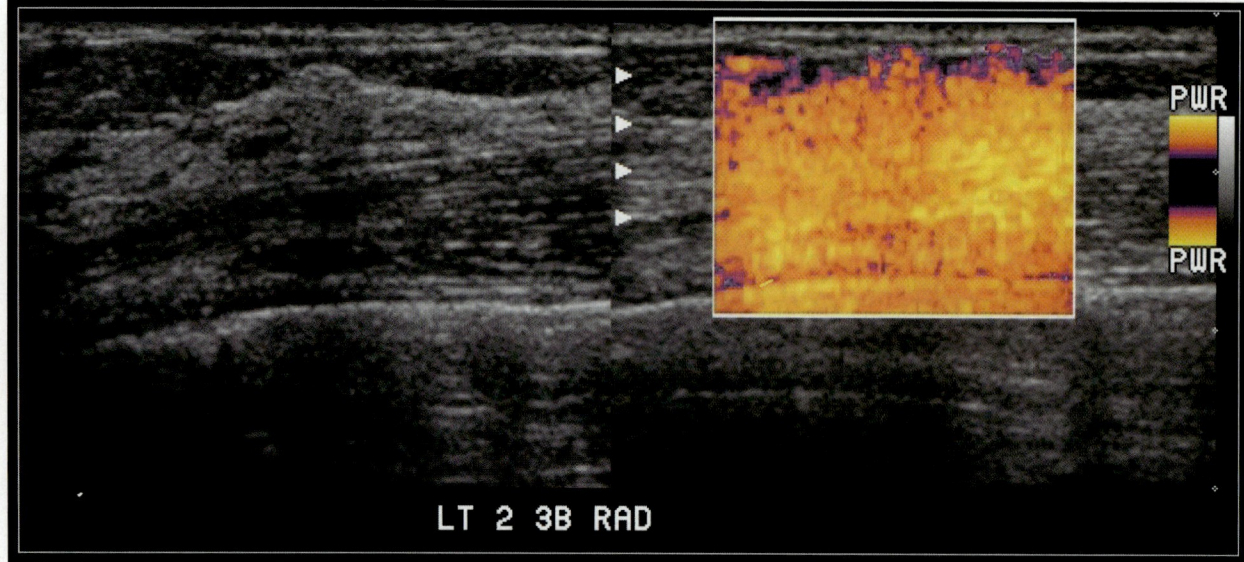

FIGURE 20–82 Chest wall and hyperechoic fibrous tissue vibrate the most intensely because they are the densest tissues in the chest and breast and because their fibers are roughly perpendicular to the direction in which the vibrations are being propagated, essentially forming a "stairway" for vibrations to climb out of the chest and into the breast. The more intense the vibration, the brighter the acoustic vibratory artifact is. Vibrations fall off with increasing distance from the chest wall and are also dampened in the tissues for a few millimeters deep to the transducer face.

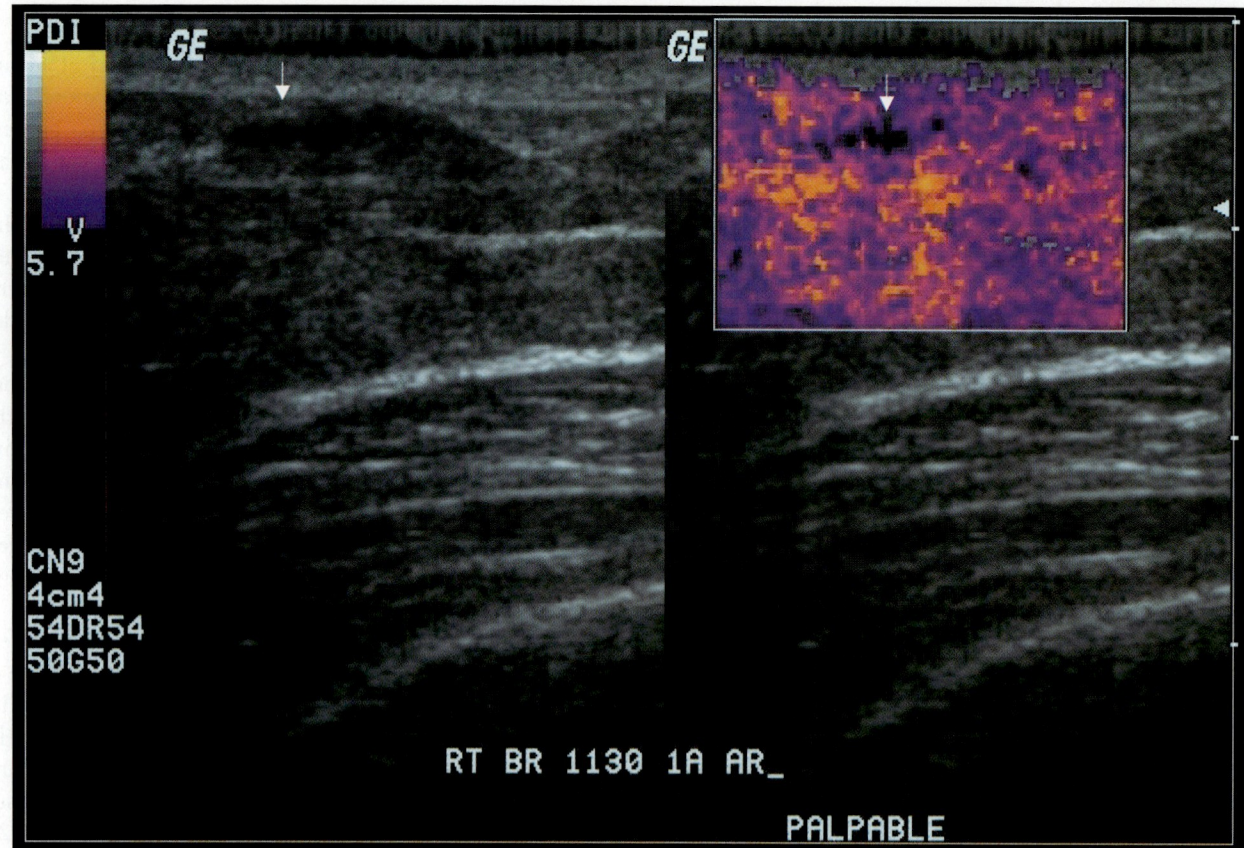

FIGURE 20–83 Isoechoic glandular tissue, such as the adenosis of pregnancy shown here, vibrates slightly less than does fibrous tissue, but more than does fat. The small defect anteriorly *(arrows)* represents a small galactocele.

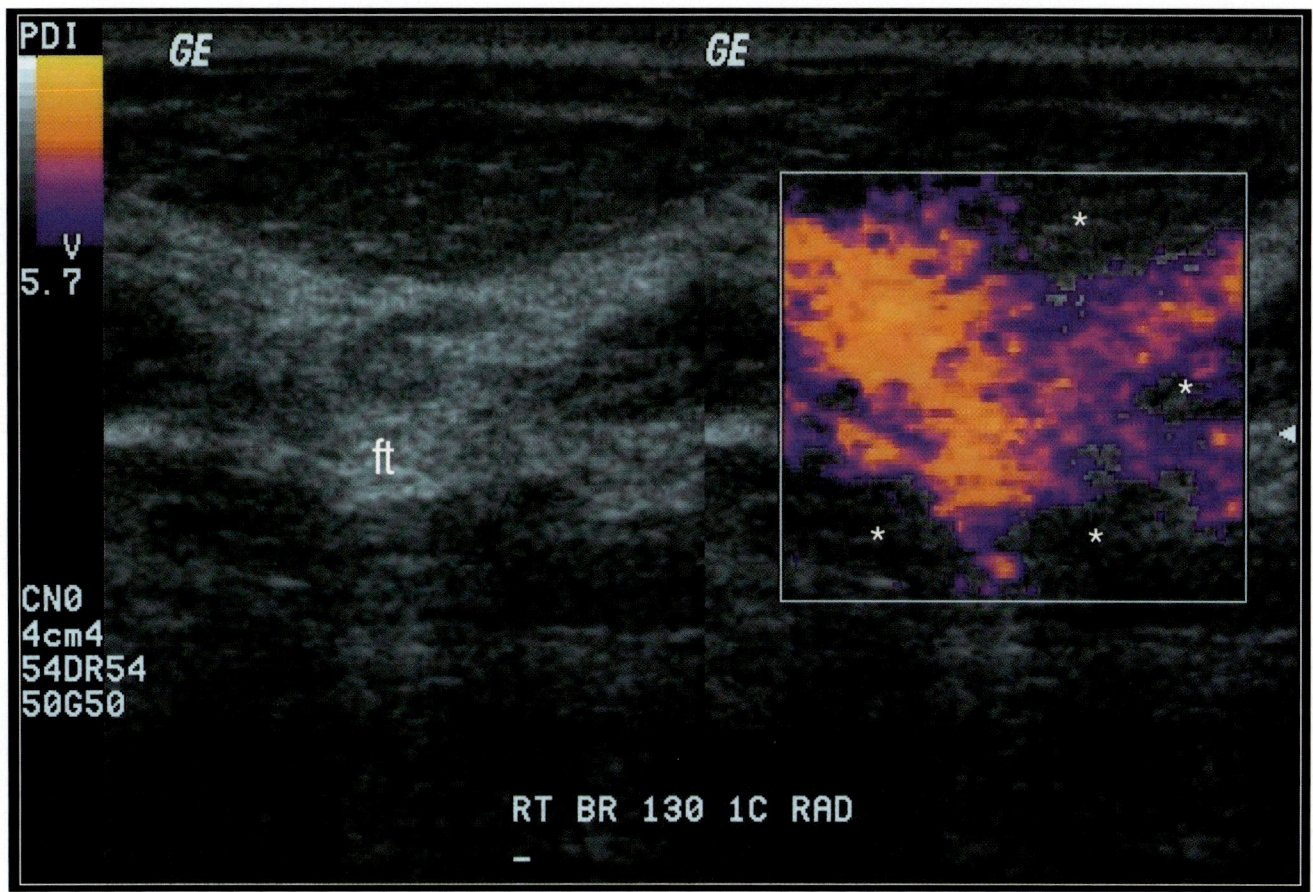

FIGURE 20–84 Fat *(*)* vibrates less than fibrous tissue *(ft)* and creates either no acoustic vibratory artifact or a weak one. Vibration artifact in fat can be increased by increasing gain, decreasing pulse repetition frequency, and compressing the breast more vigorously with the transducer.

oriented perpendicular to the vibrations essentially create a stairway for vibrations to climb out of the chest. Fibrous tissue vibrations create a bright orange artifact that is nearly as bright as the chest wall artifact (Fig. 20–82). Isoechoic glandular tissue vibrates almost as well as fibrous tissue but creates a slightly darker orange vibration (Fig. 20–83). Fat vibrates the least of normal tissues. It is the least dense and has widely spaced collagen fibers that are randomly oriented rather than being perpendicular to the axis of vibrations. In some cases, there is very little vibratory artifact within the fat at default power Doppler settings (Fig. 20–84). For this reason, it may be necessary to use a lower pulse repetition frequency (PRF) or higher gain settings when evaluating fat-surrounded lesions.

The effect of transducer scan pressure is also difficult to assess. In general, compression dampens vibrations and decreases fremitus. This is especially true closer to the skin, where compression dampens vibrations more. However, in some cases, compression may increase fremitus, especially in fatty tissue where sparse collagen fibers that are randomly distributed throughout the breast can be compressed into a pattern whereby they are closer together and more parallel and vibrate more intensely. The problem with using heavier compression is that it may also increase the vibration within real lesions, obscuring the vibratory defect they usually cause and resulting in false-negative findings (Fig. 20–85).

Despite its limitations in distinguishing benign from malignant lesions, we believe that power Doppler vocal fremitus has important niche uses. Table 20–2 lists the niche applications for which we find power Doppler vocal fremitus useful.

Distinguishing Isoechoic Glandular Tissue from Isoechoic Tumor

Acoustic vibratory artifact may help identify subtle isoechoic neoplasms that are identical in echogenicity to isoechoic glandular tissue. Individual lobules contain abundant hyaluronic acid, a huge and well-hydrated mol-

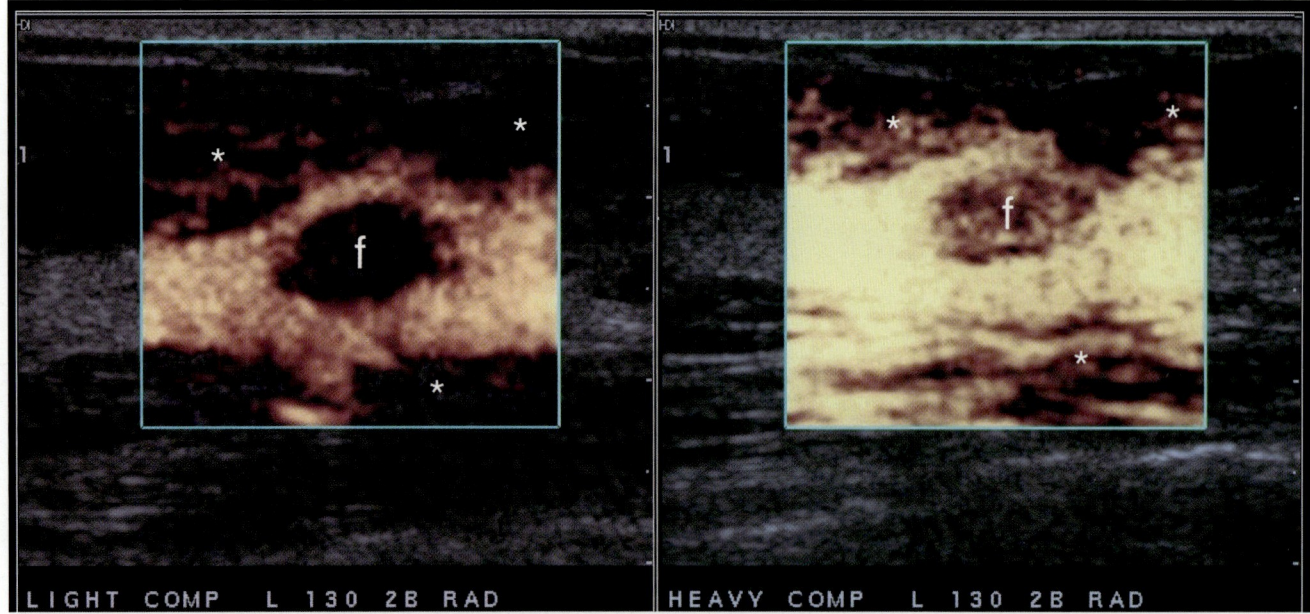

FIGURE 20–85 Compressing fat *(*)* with the transducer can make it denser and can make it vibrate more vigorously, except in the tissues immediately deep to the transducer, in which all vibrations are dampened. The problem with using greater compression is that it can make lesions that normally cause defects vibrate better, partially or completely obscuring them. Note that the defect from this fibroadenoma is partially filled with artifact when compressed too firmly. f, fibroadenoma.

ecule that is largely responsible for normal lobules being less echogenic than is interlobular stromal fibrous tissue. When lobules are diffusely physiologically enlarged by hormonal changes such as pregnancy or lactation, they may coalesce to form continuous sheets of isoechoic tissue. Because about half of malignant nodules are isoechoic with fat and glandular tissue, they may be more likely to be missed in an isoechoic glandular background than they would in a hyperechoic fibrous background. Normal acoustic vibratory artifact within isoechoic tissue is reassuring, suggesting that the tissue merely represents physiologically stimulated lobules, adenosis, or fibrocystic change (Fig. 20–86). On the other hand, the presence of an acoustic vibratory defect suggests the presence of a subtle isoechoic lesion that cannot be distinguished from glandular tissue by imaging alone. Diffusely infiltrating carcinomas such as classic invasive lobular carcinoma and intermediate-grade DCIS are the two malignant lesions that are most likely to masquerade as isoechoic glandular tissue (Fig. 20–87).

Distinguishing Fat Lobules from True Solid Nodules

Normal fat lobules are essentially normal isoechoic solid nodules that can be very difficult in certain cases to distinguish from circumscribed solid nodules such as fibroadenoma or colloid carcinoma. Fremitus can help make the distinction. Although fat vibrates much less than fibrous and glandular tissue, acoustic vibratory artifact can be shown within fat by lowering the PRF or raising the acoustic gain. With appropriate settings, fat will show more acoustic vibratory artifact than will equally isoechoic fibroadenomas or colloid carcinomas. Thus, demonstration of an acoustic vibratory defect within surrounding fat indicates the presence of a true solid nodule (Fig. 20–88), whereas vibration similar to surrounding fat strongly suggests that the structure is, indeed, merely a fat lobule (Fig. 20–89).

TABLE 20–2. NICHE APPLICATIONS FOR POWER DOPPLER VOCAL FREMITUS

Distinguishing isoechoic glandular tissue from isoechoic tumor

Distinguishing entrapped fat lobules from fibroadenomas

Assessing suspected artifactual acoustic shadowing

Assessing intracystic echoes to determine whether they are attached to the wall

Identifying multifocal carcinoma unsuspected from the image alone

Identifying internal mammary lymph nodes

(text continued on page 933)

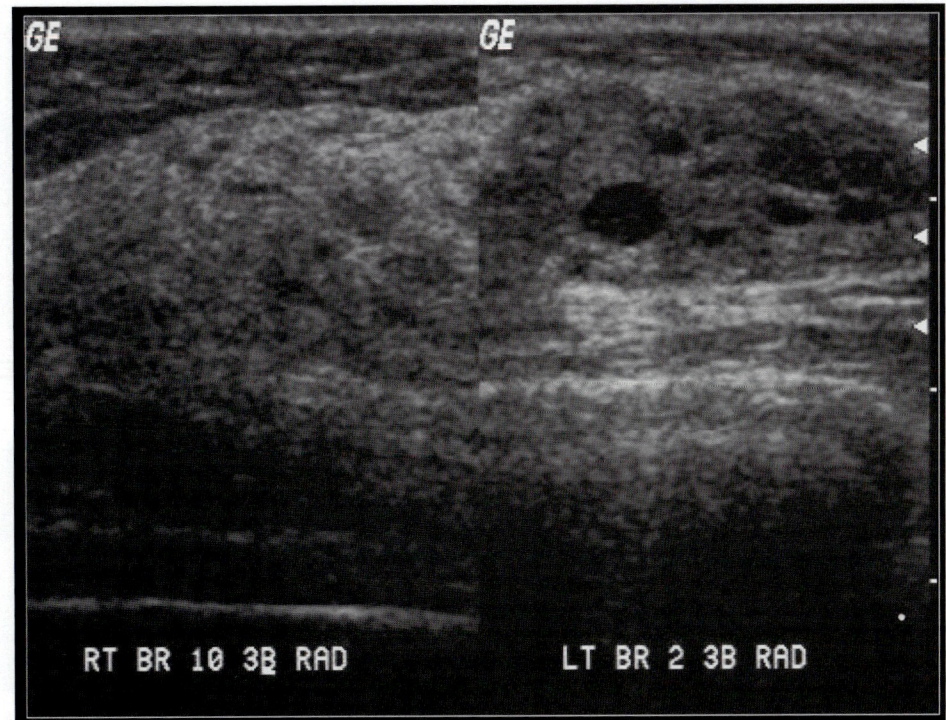

A

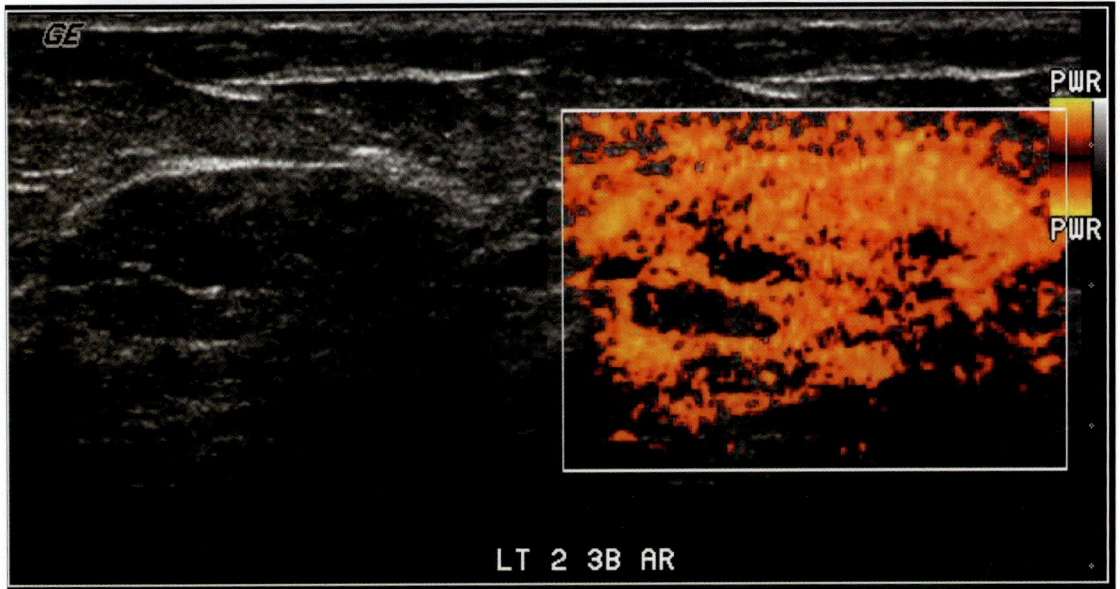

B

FIGURE 20–86 A: Split-screen images of the mirror-image locations in the upper outer quadrants show asymmetric isoechoic tissue or a lesion on the left. This isoechoic lesion containing cysts in the left breast could merely represent adenosis, adenosis containing an occult isoechoic lesion, or an isoechoic lesion based on the image alone. **B:** Power Doppler vocal fremitus shows normal vibration in the isoechoic tissue (except for the small cysts), indicating that it is normal isoechoic glandular tissue.

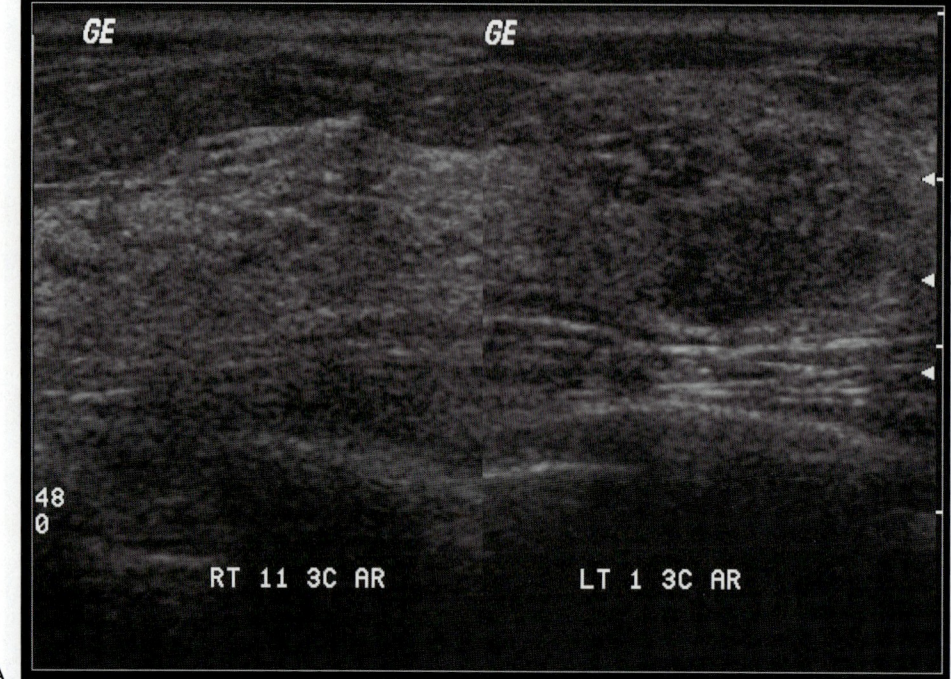

A

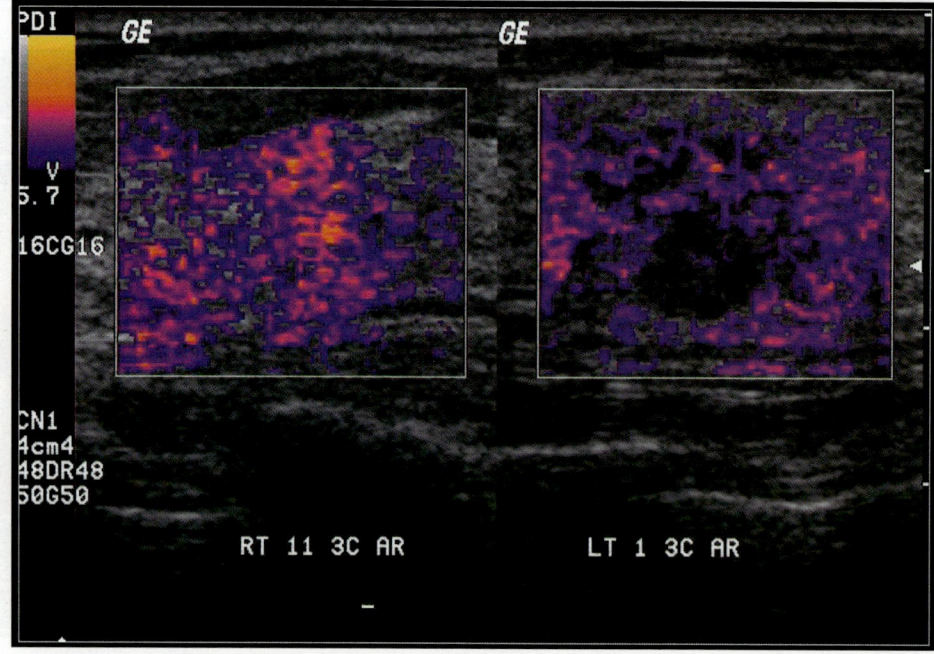

B

FIGURE 20–87 A: Split-screen images of the right and left upper outer quadrants show purely hyperechoic fibroductal tissues on the right and mixed isoechoic and hyperechoic tissue in the upper outer quadrant on the left side. As in the previous case, the isoechoic tissue on the left could represent glandular tissue, glandular tissue containing an occult isoechoic lesion, or an isoechoic lesion. Based on the image alone, we cannot be sure. **B:** Power Doppler fremitus in the same areas shown in Fig. 12.88A shows a defect in the power Doppler fremitus in the area of the isoechoic tissue on the left. That it vibrates differently from surrounding fibrous tissue increases the likelihood that there is occult neoplasm within the isoechoic area on the left. Biopsy revealed intermediate-nuclear-grade ductal carcinoma *in situ*.

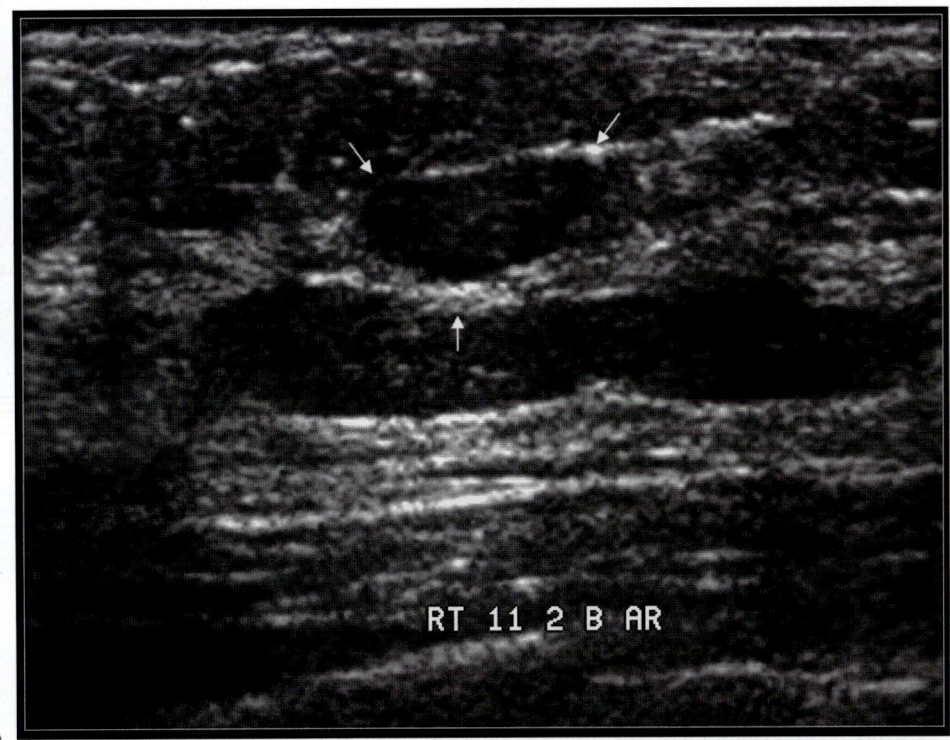

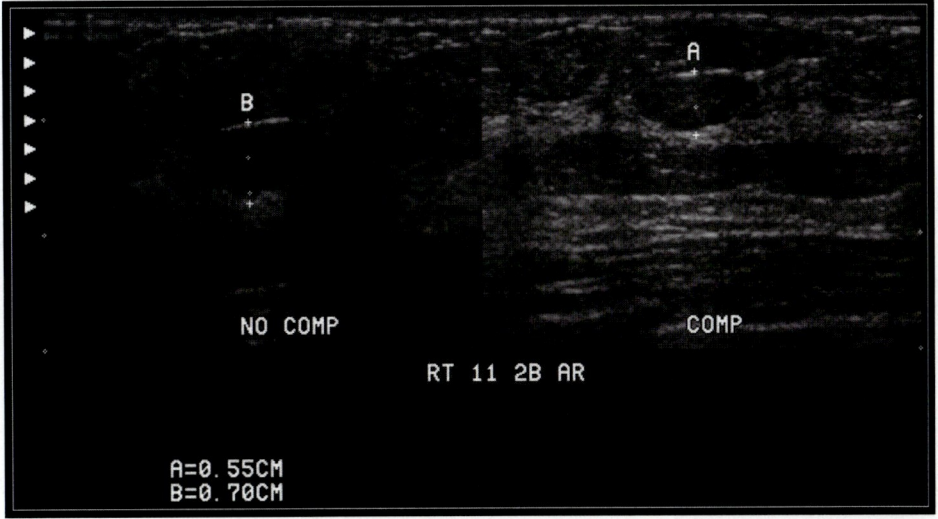

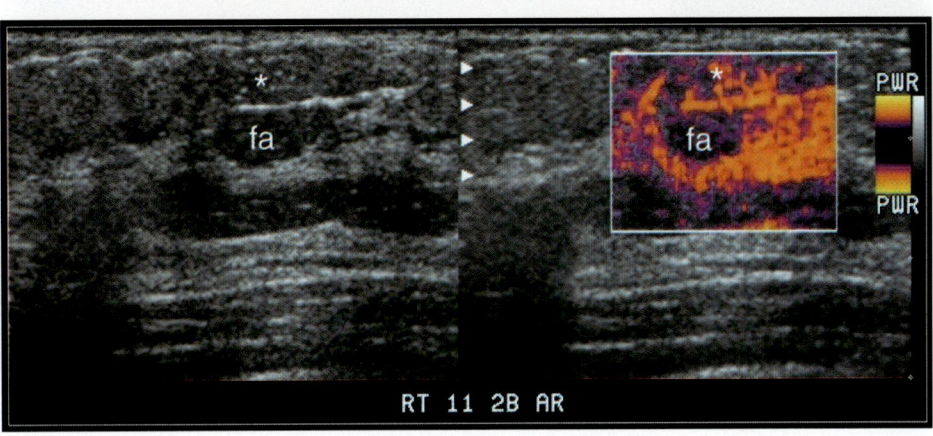

FIGURE 20–88 A: This isoechoic structure *(arrows)* could be a solid nodule but may merely be a fat lobule. Its echogenicity is identical to that of the fat that borders it anteriorly and posteriorly. **B:** Split-screen images with and without compression show this lesion to be compressible, but less compressible than the 30% that we expect of fat lobules. **C:** Power Doppler fremitus shows a defect in the vibratory artifact of fibrous tissue. This does not help because both fat and fibroadenomas will vibrate less than fibrous tissue. However, the area of interest also vibrates less than fat *(*)*, indicating that it is not a fat lobule, but a real solid nodule. The patient requested biopsy, which confirmed the impression from fremitus and imaging of fibroadenoma.

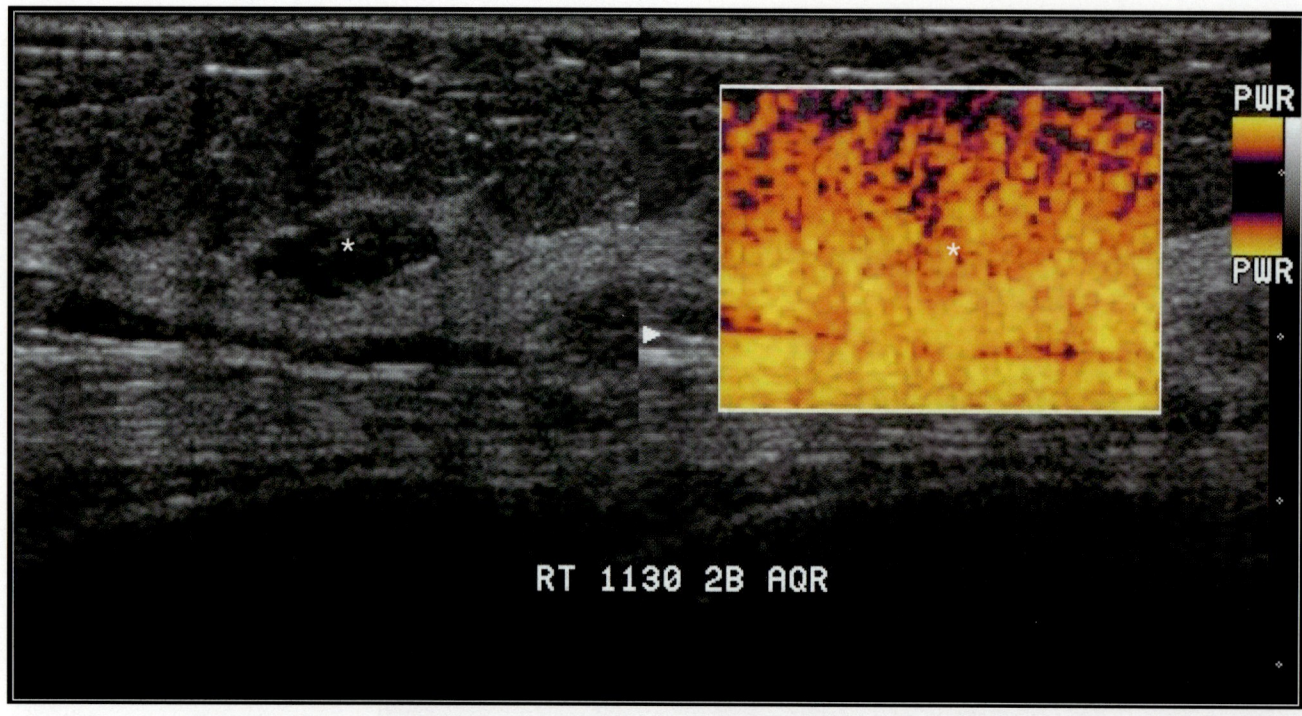

FIGURE 20–89 This structure *(*)* looks identical to the fibroadenoma shown in Fig. 20–88. However, it vibrates identically to surrounding fat, indicating that it is merely a fat lobule.

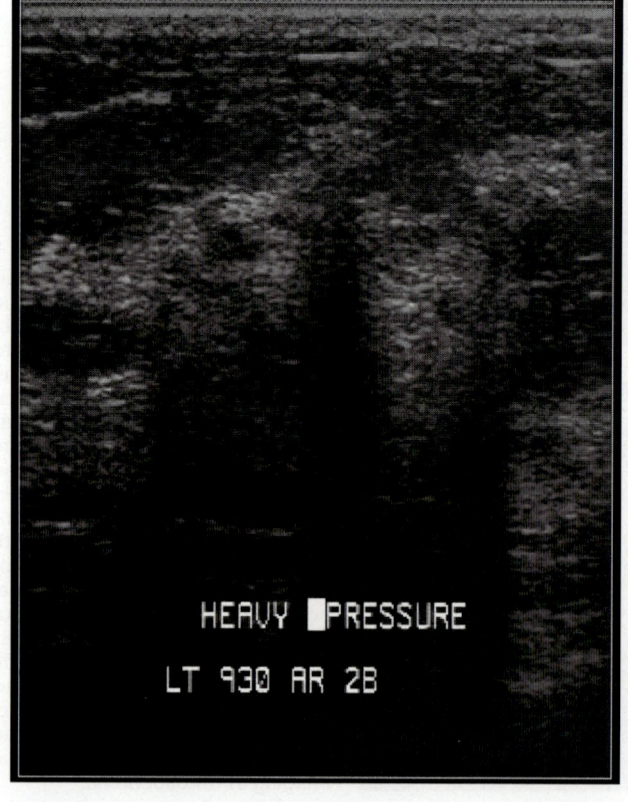

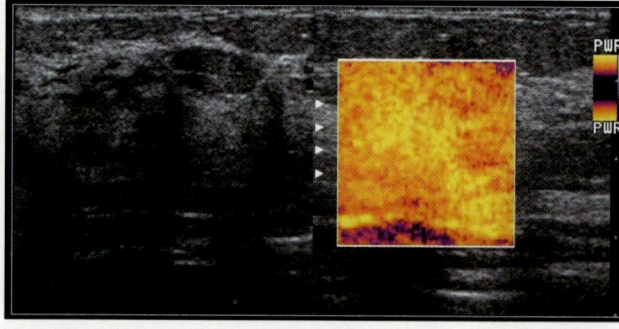

FIGURE 20–90 A: There is an area of intense acoustic shadowing within this fibroglandular ridge of tissue. It could be artifactual or could indicate the presence of a small malignant nodule that casts a dense acoustic shadow. Artifactual shadowing can usually be eradicated by compressing more vigorously, but in this case, the shadowing persisted despite heavy compression. **B:** Power Doppler fremitus shows normal vibration in the area of shadowing, suggesting that it was artifactual. Ultrasound-guided biopsy revealed only fibrosis.

Distinguishing Artifactual Critical Angle Shadowing from Absorptive Shadowing within Carcinomas

In some cases, artifactual shadowing may simulate the acoustic shadowing caused by malignant breast nodules. In most cases in which artifactual acoustic shadowing arises from steeply obliquely oriented tissue interfaces or Cooper's ligaments, the shadowing can be ablated simply by vigorously compressing the shadowing structure with the transducer. However, in some cases, the artifactual shadowing cannot be ablated, regardless of how much compression pressure is used. The persistent shadowing in such cases demands a BI-RADS 4a category and will lead to an unnecessary biopsy. Power Doppler fremitus can fill in the artifactual shadow with vibratory artifact, ablating it (Fig. 20–90). Intensely shadowing small malignant nodules, on the other hand, create a discrete defect within the vibratory artifact.

Identifying Multifocal Cancer that Was Initially Unsuspected on the Image Alone

During sonographic assessment of solid nodules, our attention is naturally focused on the primary lesion. Unfortunately, we focus so intensely on the primary nodule that we sometimes fail to notice additional nodules in the vicinity. Power Doppler vocal fremitus shows not only an acoustic vibratory defect caused by the primary lesion but also de-fects within the field of orange artifact for each of the additional lesions. Although these additional foci of tumor may be subtle on the image, they are quite obvious on vocal fremitus—black holes in the orange vibratory acoustic artifact of normal tissues (Fig. 20–91). We have found power Doppler vocal fremitus so consistent in showing additional foci that were unsuspected during imaging alone that we now use it routinely when a nodule with BIRADS 4a or higher characteristics is found (Fig. 20–92).

Determining whether Intracystic Echoes Are Attached to the Cyst Wall

Echogenic lipid layers in cysts that contain fat–fluid levels and debris levels in cyst that contain fluid–debris levels can simulate intracystic mural nodules. Upright or left lateral decubitus positioning usually enables us to distinguish between unattached echogenic lipids or debris and true mural nodules, but as much as 5 minutes may be required before the shift in lipids or debris is definitive. Power Doppler fremitus can shorten this process. Internal echoes that are attached to the cyst wall will transmit acoustic vibratory artifact to a degree similar to the surrounding tissues. On the other hand, unattached internal echoes will not (Fig. 20–93). Attached lesions that transmit vibrations include

(text continued on page 936)

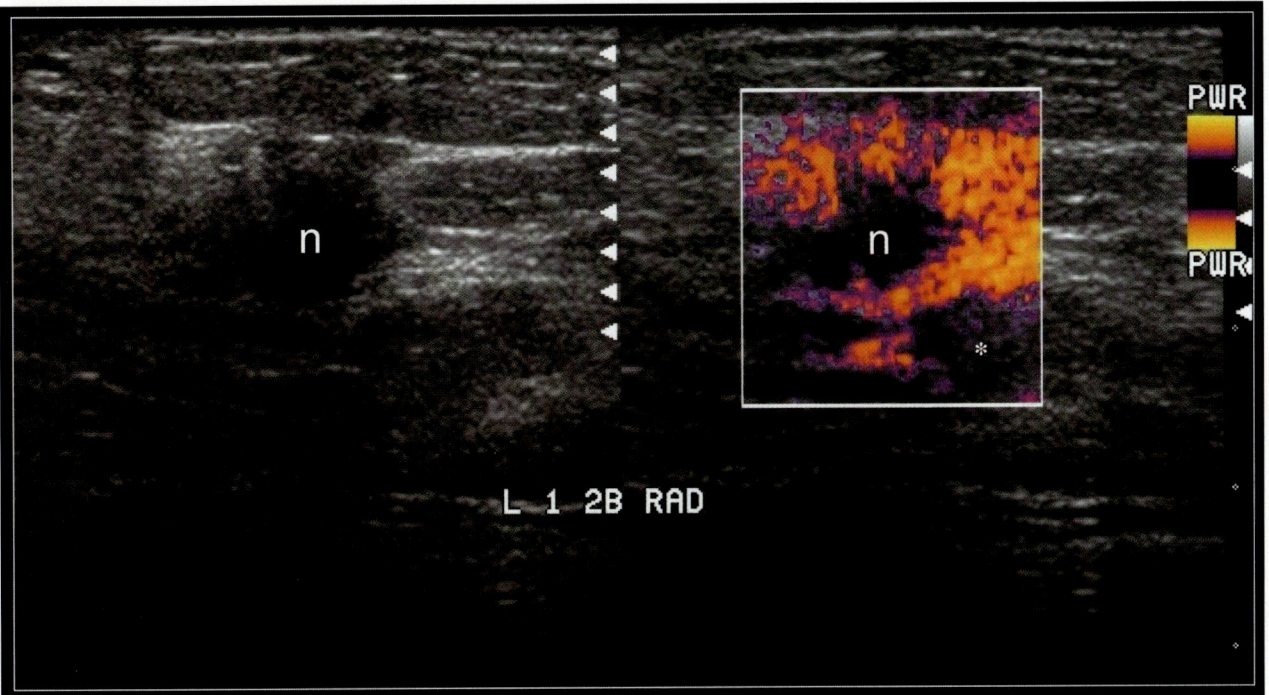

FIGURE 20–91 A: Power Doppler fremitus showed an acoustic vibratory defect corresponding to the hypoechoic angular nodule *(n)* shown in the **left** image. However, It suggested the possibility of a second lesion not seen on the B-mode image *(*)*. *(Continued.)*

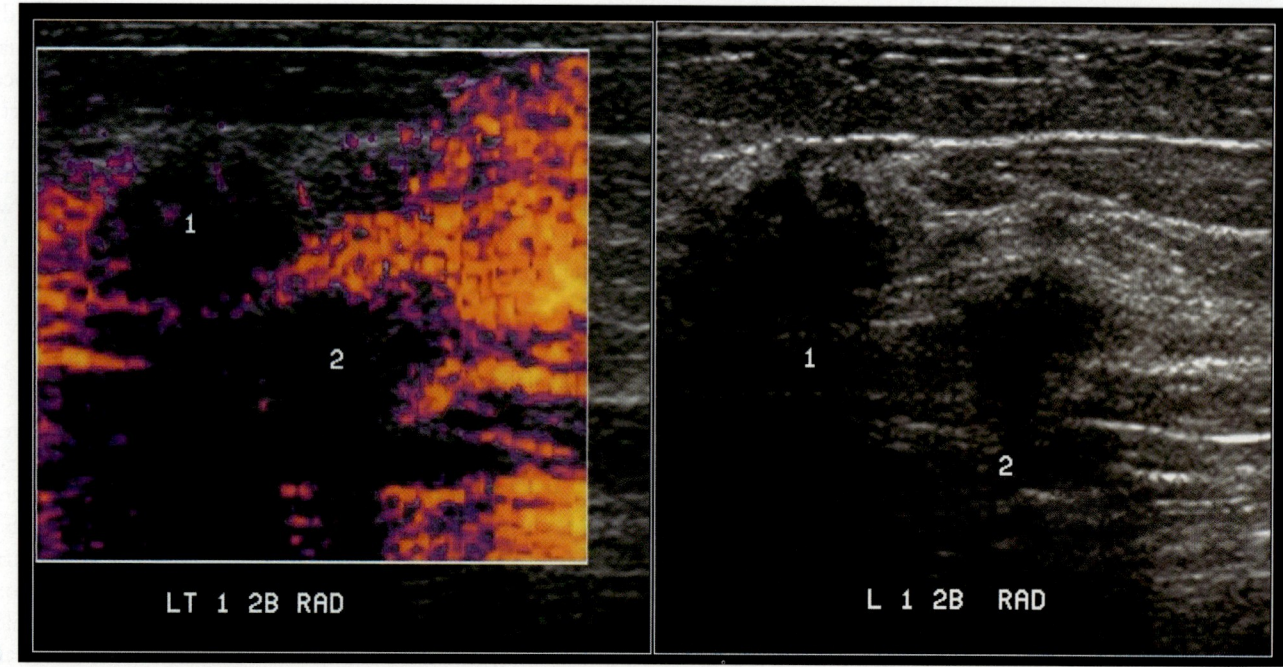

FIGURE 20–91 *(continued)* **B:** Enlarging the power Doppler box showed a second lesion that was initially missed on real-time imaging (**left**). After the second fremitus defect was noticed, the image was optimized, and the second lesion became obvious (**right**).

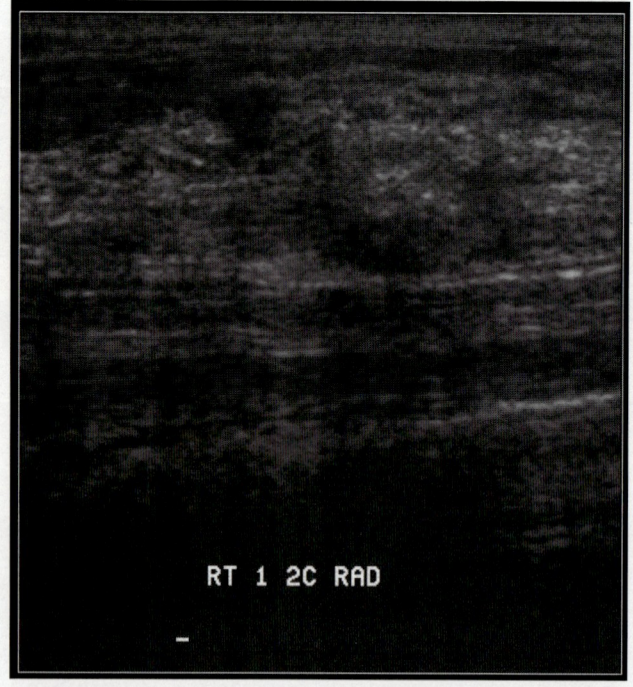

FIGURE 20–92 A: There are multiple foci of invasion present in this patient, but they are very subtle and uncertain based on sonographic image findings alone. (*Continued.*)

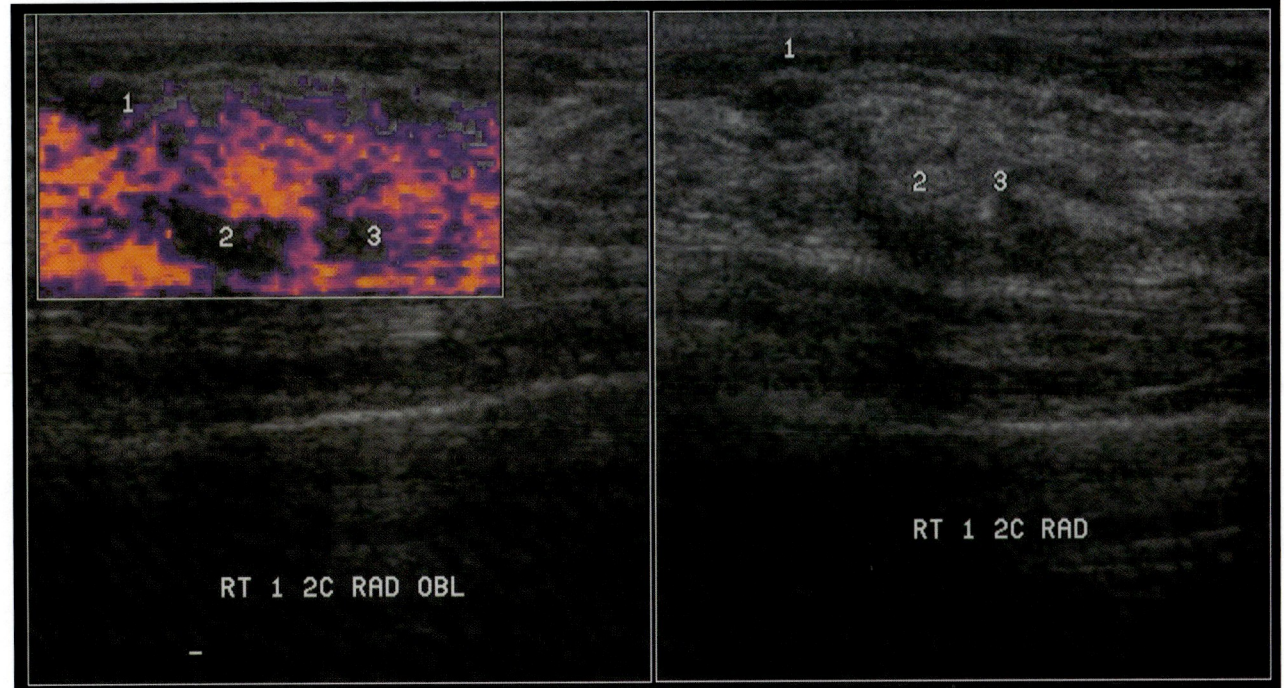

FIGURE 20–92 *(continued)* **B:** Power Doppler vocal fremitus clearly shows three different foci of abnormally decreased vibration within the breast. Adjusting imaging planes and imaging parameters after fremitus evaluation shows each of the three areas with absent fremitus is a separate focus of invasion. Power Doppler facilitates recognition of multifocal disease.

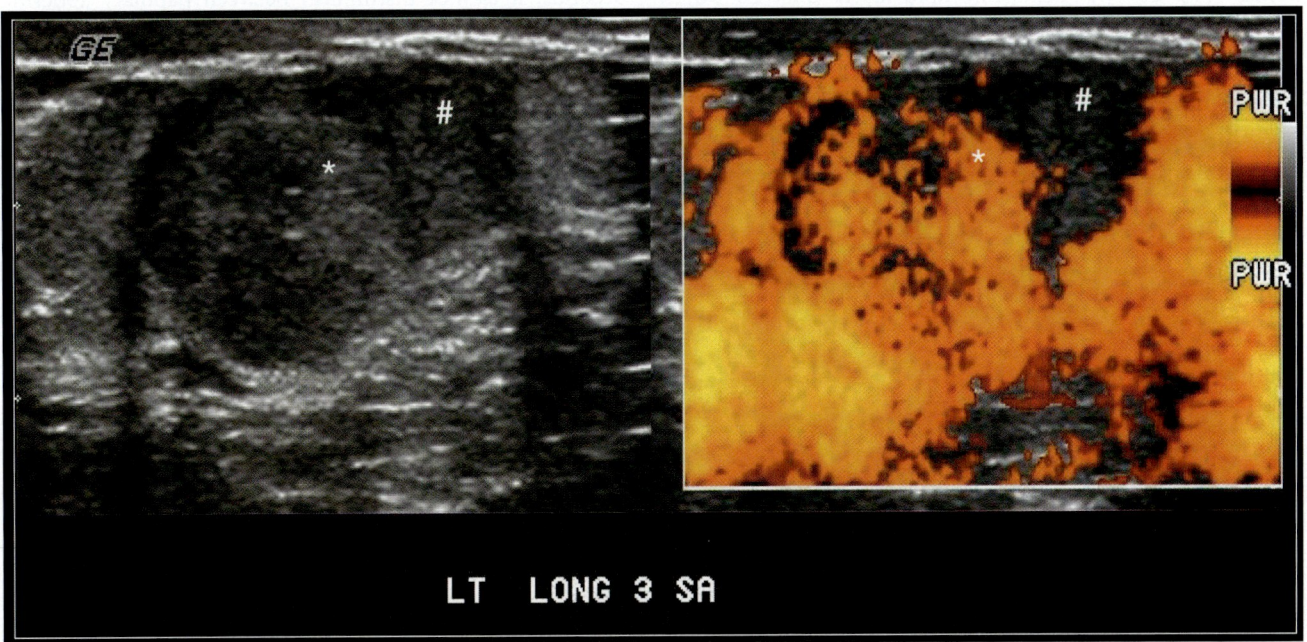

FIGURE 20–93 Intracystic invasive papillary carcinomas are prone to hemorrhagic infarction. In some cases, it can be difficult to distinguish the papillary lesion from clot of nearly equal echogenicity. Power Doppler fremitus can be useful in making this distinction because vibrations are readily transmitted into the attached papillary lesion *(*)*, but not into the unattached clot *(#)*.

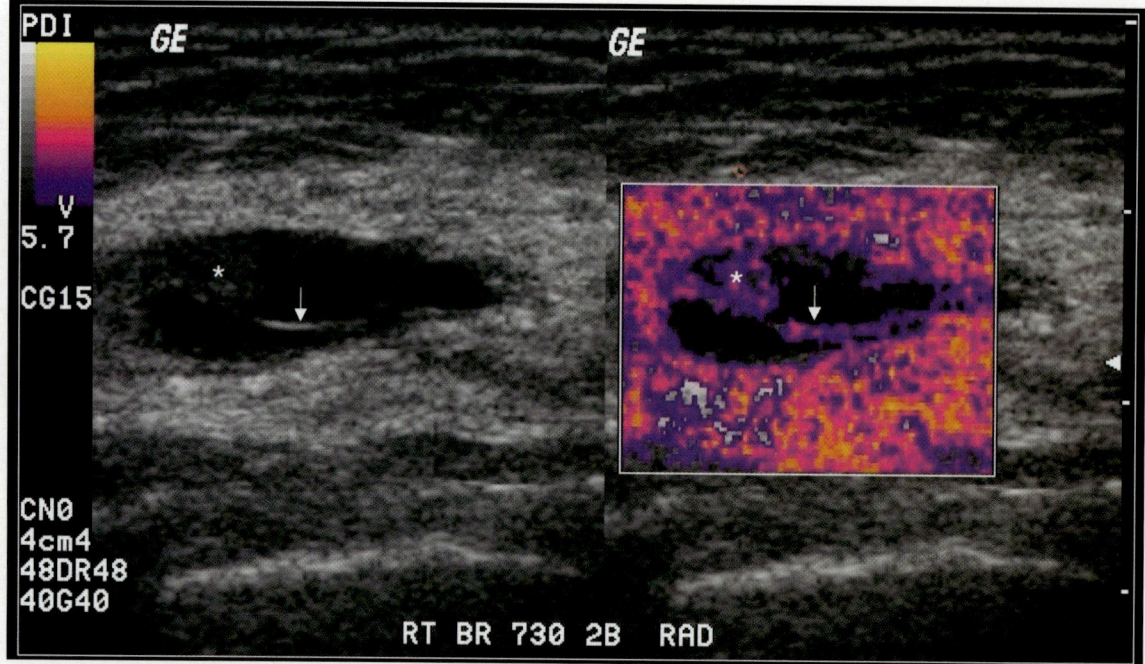

FIGURE 20–94 Power Doppler vocal fremitus demonstrates vibrations within mural nodules *(*)* and septations *(arrow)* that are attached to the cyst walls. This mural nodule was caused by papillary apocrine metaplasia, which is firmly attached to the cyst wall.

papillary apocrine metaplasia (Fig. 20–94), benign intracystic papillomas (Fig. 20–93), and intracystic papillary carcinomas (Fig. 20–95). Echogenic lipid layers (Fig. 20–96) and debris levels (Fig. 20–97) will not transmit acoustic vibratory artifact. Although fremitus allows distinction between attached and unattached internal echoes within a few seconds, it cannot distinguish between papillary apocrine metaplasia and true papillomas or carcinomas.

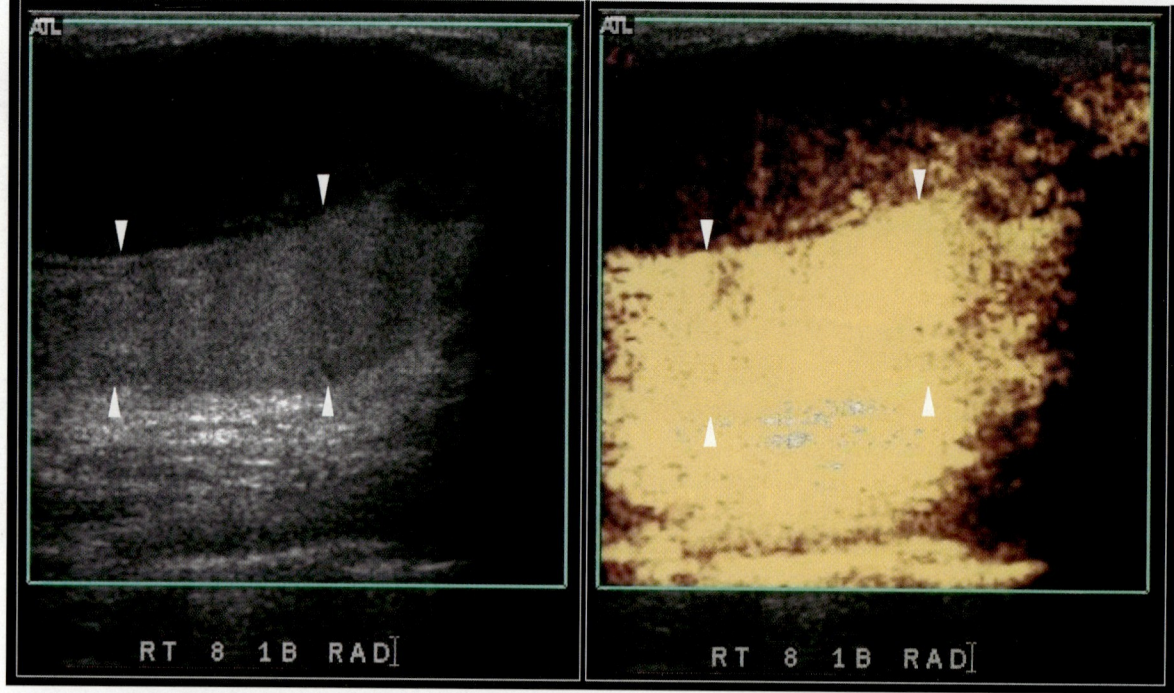

FIGURE 20–95 The echogenic structure on the dependent wall of the cyst has a configuration that simulates a debris level **(left)**. Power Doppler fremitus, however, shows intense vibration within the echogenic structure, indicating that it is attached to the cyst wall. Biopsy showed high-grade invasive carcinoma involving the posterior wall of the cyst.

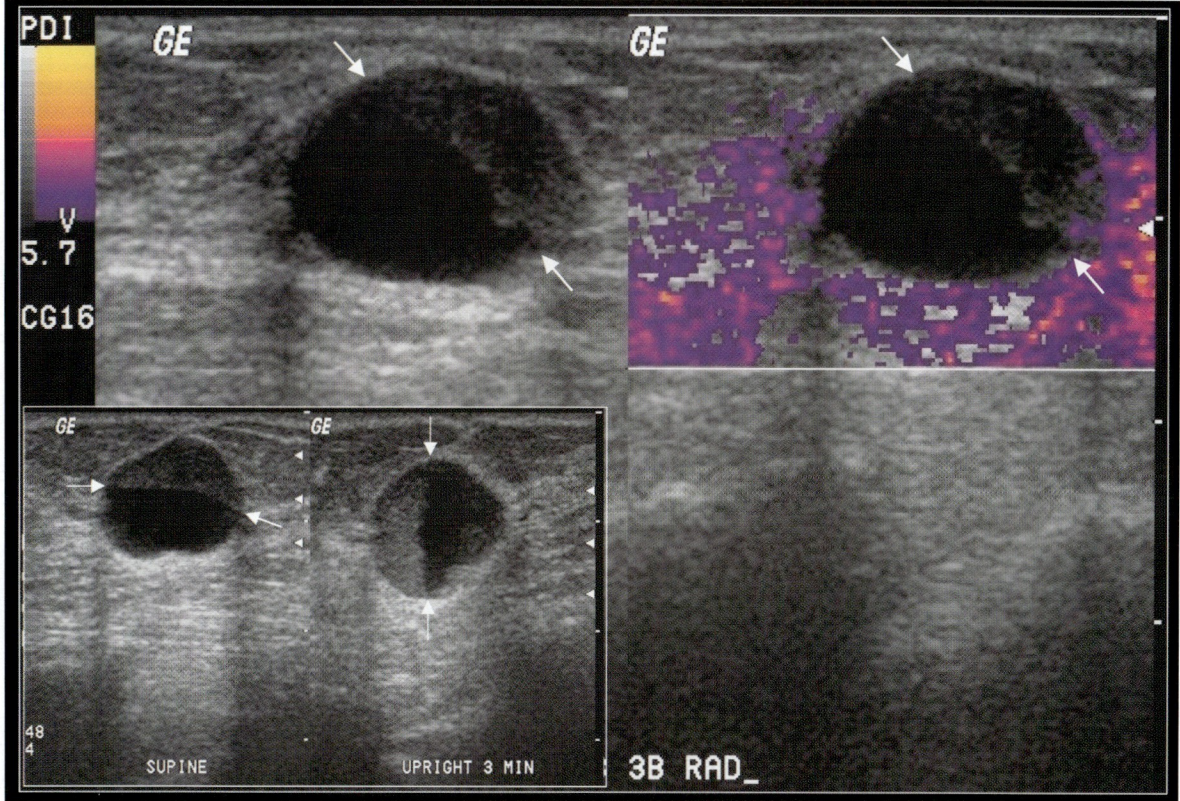

FIGURE 20–96 Power Doppler vocal fremitus will not cause vibrational artifact to pass into the echogenic lipid layer of a cyst that contains a fat–fluid level. Note that the echogenic lipid layer shifts to the nondependent superior portion of the cyst when the patient is moved from the supine to the upright position (**lower left,** *arrows*).

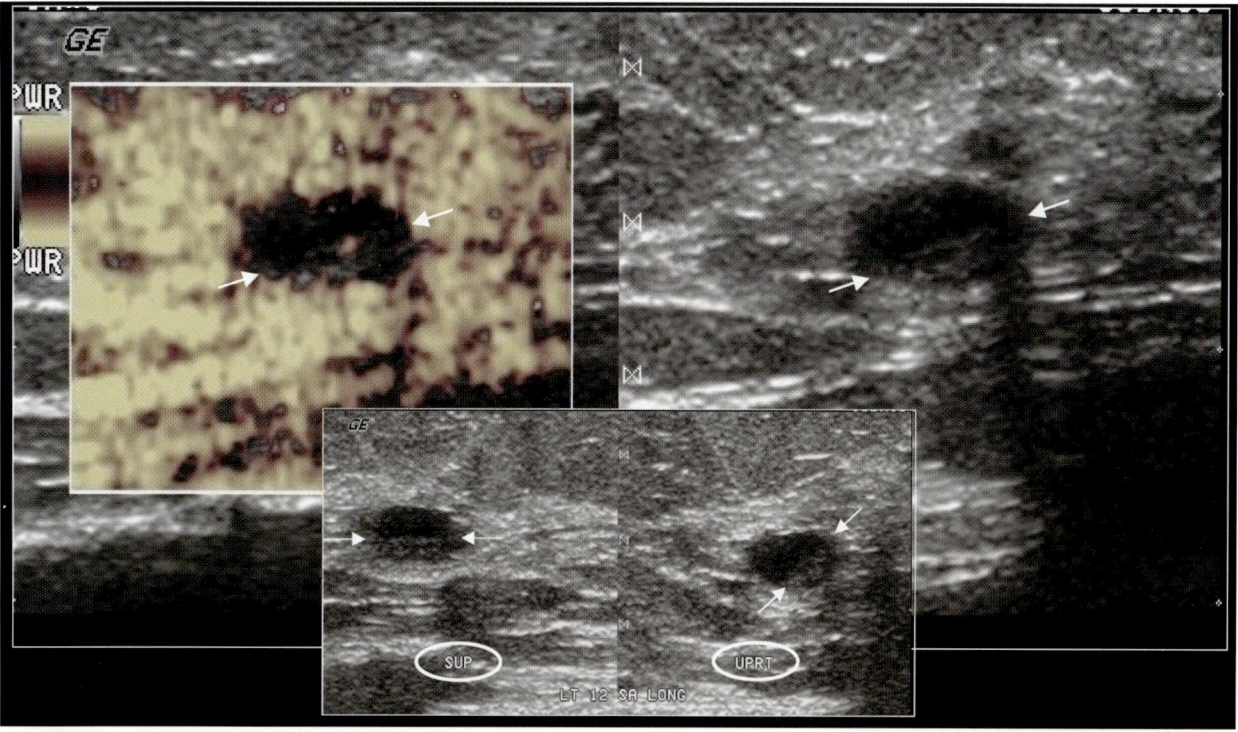

FIGURE 20–97 Power Doppler fremitus will not cause vibrational artifact within pseudonodules caused by sludge because it is not attached to the walls of the cyst. This inflamed cysts has a fluid–debris level that is demonstrated to shift to the dependent portion of the cyst on supine and upright views (**bottom center,** *arrows*). Note that the acoustic vibratory artifact does not enter the debris level (**upper left**).

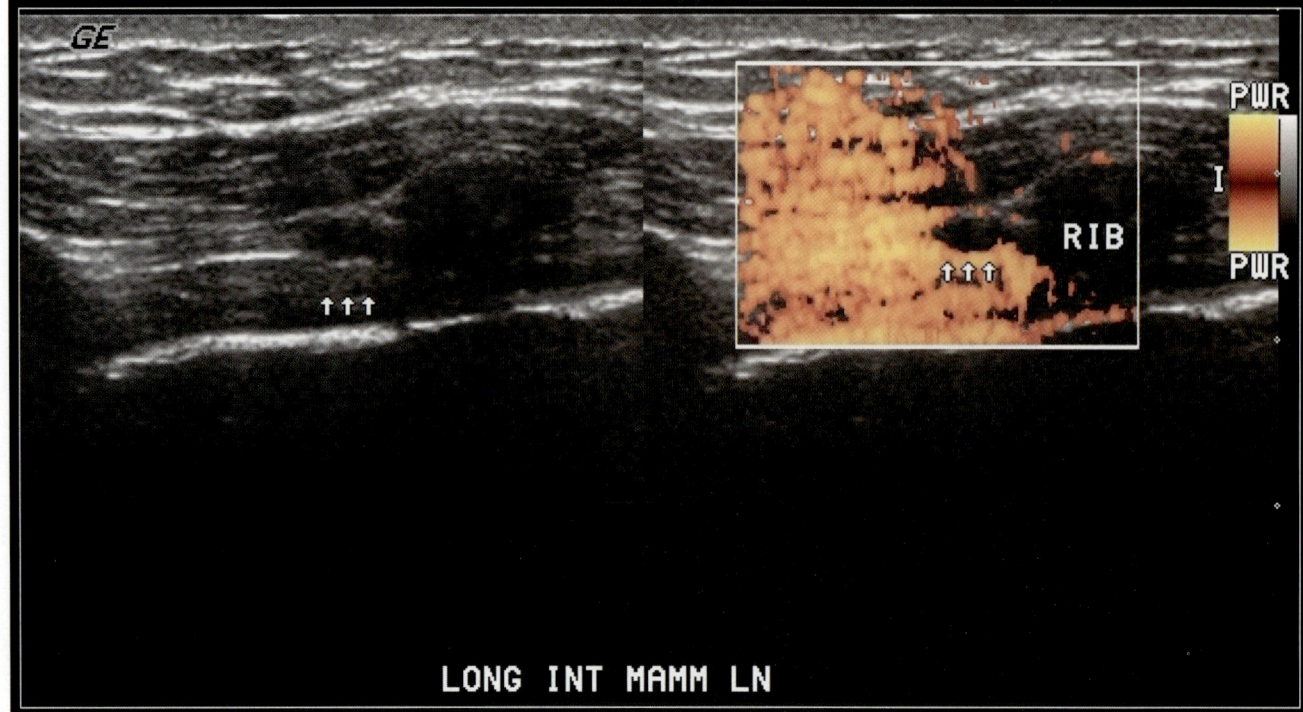

FIGURE 20–98 Internal mammary lymph nodes vibrate much less than the surrounding muscles and tendons in the chest wall during the power Doppler vocal fremitus maneuver, creating a defect in the acoustic vibratory artifact *(arrows).*

Identifying Internal Mammary Lymph Nodes

Internal mammary lymph nodes vibrate differently from the surrounding chest wall structures and can create a defect in the acoustic vibratory artifact if appropriate gain settings are used (Fig. 20–98). The vibrations within the chest wall are so intense and strong that it is sometimes necessary to increase the PRF slightly or to decrease gain slightly in order not to obscure the internal mammary lymph nodes.

CAUSES OF FALSE-NEGATIVE FINDINGS WITH POWER DOPPLER FREMITUS

Although the efficacy of power Doppler fremitus is unknown, we are developing a feeling for situations that may lead to false-negative fremitus assessments. Table 20–3 lists the causes of false-negative power Doppler fremitus examinations of which we are currently aware.

Using Too Much Gain or Using a Pulse Repetition Frequency that Is Too Low

Using too much gain or a PRF that is too low can obscure the acoustic vibratory defect caused by a malignant nodule. The acoustic vibratory artifact in fat should never be nearly as bright as chest wall or fibrous tissue. At appropriate gain

and PRF settings, fat should have only minimal vibratory artifact. If the vibratory artifact within fat is bright orange, either the gain is too high or the PRF is too low (Fig. 20–99).

Using Too Much Compression Pressure

The denser a tissue, the better and more rapidly it will transmit vibrations and sound, except immediately deep to the transducer for a few millimeters, where vibrations are dampened. Compressing tissues makes them denser and tends to align the internal interfaces parallel to each other and perpendicular to the chest wall, creating a "stairway"

TABLE 20–3. KNOWN CAUSES OF FALSE-NEGATIVE POWER DOPPLER FREMITUS

Using too much Doppler gain or a pulse repetition frequency that is too low

Using too much compression pressure

Calcifications

Fibrotic scars within tumor nodules

Lymph node medullary structures

Hyalinization of fibroadenomas

Radial scars that have little peripheral proliferative change

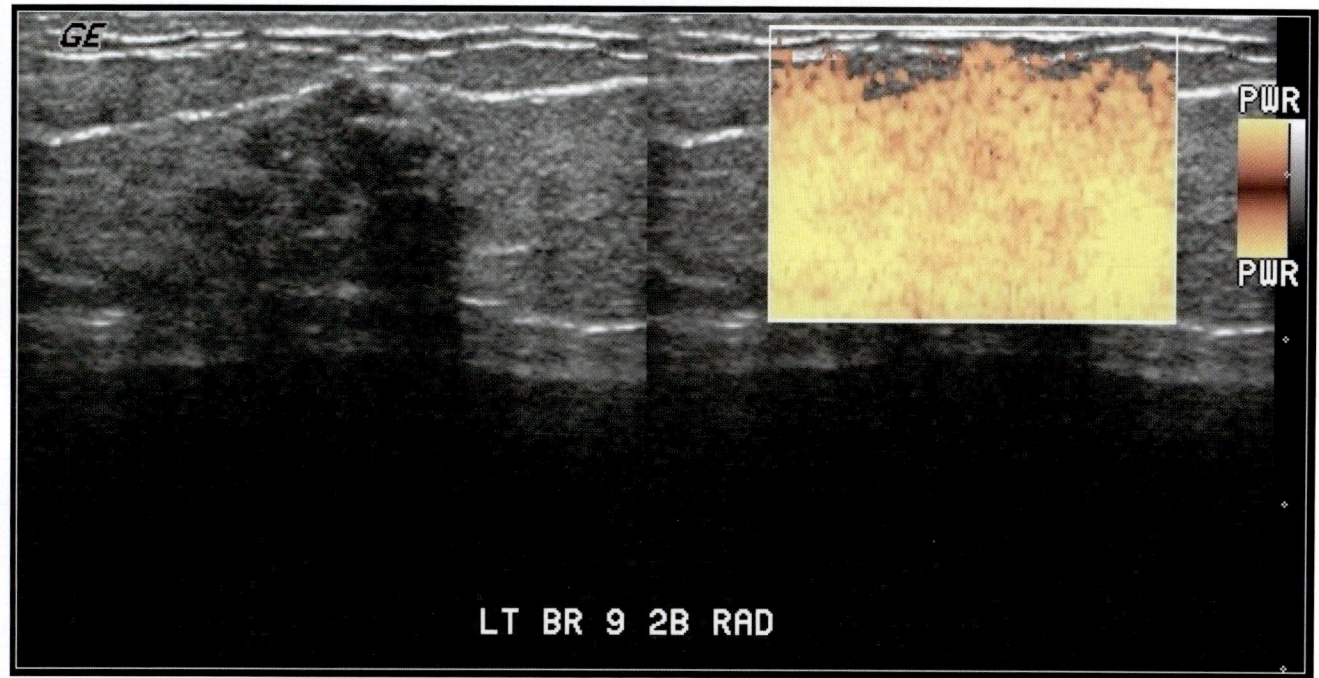

FIGURE 20–99 Power Doppler fremitus is falsely negative in this malignant nodule because the gain has been set too high. The vibratory artifact in the fat that surrounds this hypoechoic lesion is too bright, indicating excessive gain.

for vibrations to climb out of the chest wall. Thus, by compressing harder, the acoustic vibratory artifact in all tissues and lesions can be increased. This can increase the internal acoustic vibratory artifact within lesions enough to make them less apparent or even to obscure them (Fig. 20–85).

Calcifications

Calcifications are denser than any breast tissues and therefore vibrate more intensely. Lesions that contain only a few calcifications will have bright internal vibrations that likely will not obscure acoustic vibratory defect completely (Fig. 20–100). However, lesions that contain numerous calcifications may be completely obscured by the vibration of the internal calcifications. Thus, power Doppler fremitus will likely be of limited value in assessing lesions that contain multiple calcifications (Fig. 20–101).

Fibrotic Central Scars

Certain malignant nodules develop fibrotic central scars. Lesions that arise within preexisting radial scars and intermediate-grade invasive not otherwise specified carcinomas are most likely to do so. The fibrotic scar vibrates as intensely as does fibrous tissue, creating a bright orange artifact within the center of the lesion. When the central scar is small relative to the size of the lesion, it will not obscure the lesion's acoustic vibratory defect (Fig. 20–102). However, when the central scar is rela-

tively large, much of the lesion may be obscured by vibratory artifact. This may actually be of benefit in carcinomas that are undergoing chemotherapy because the lesion may become fibrotic rather than shrinking. In such cases, the development of a new vibratory artifact within a lesion suggests tumor necrosis and fibrosis of that part of the lesion (Fig. 20–103).

Echogenic Lymph Node Hila

Power Doppler vocal fremitus may be helpful in detecting lymph nodes. However, the echogenic portion of the lymph node mediastinum that represents the medullary cords and sinuses vibrates intensely. If the lymph node cortex is thin and the echogenic mediastinum is relatively large, most of the lymph node may be obscured by acoustic vibratory artifact (Fig. 20–104). Power Doppler vocal fremitus is much more effective at identifying abnormal lymph nodes than normal nodes.

Hyalinized Fibroadenomas

Fibroadenomas in which the stroma has become densely sclerotic or hyalinized vibrate more intensely than do fibroadenomas with myxoid or cellular stroma. They may vibrate nearly as much as fibrous tissue and may not show the acoustic vibratory defect expected of a fibroadenoma (Fig. 20–105).

(text continued on page 943)

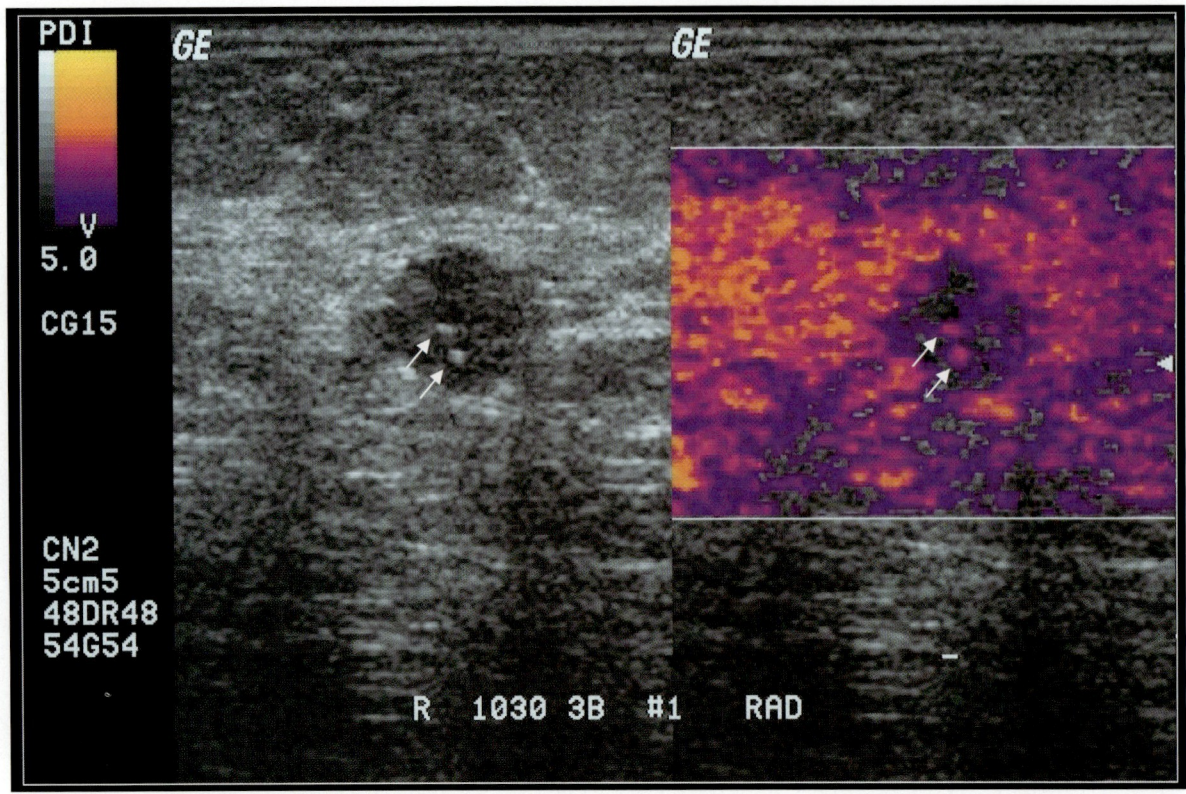

FIGURE 20–100 Calcifications are denser than any breast tissue and therefore vibrate more intensely, creating very bright artifacts. When there are only a few internal calcifications *(arrows)*, the acoustic vibratory defect of the carcinoma containing the calcifications will not be completely obscured.

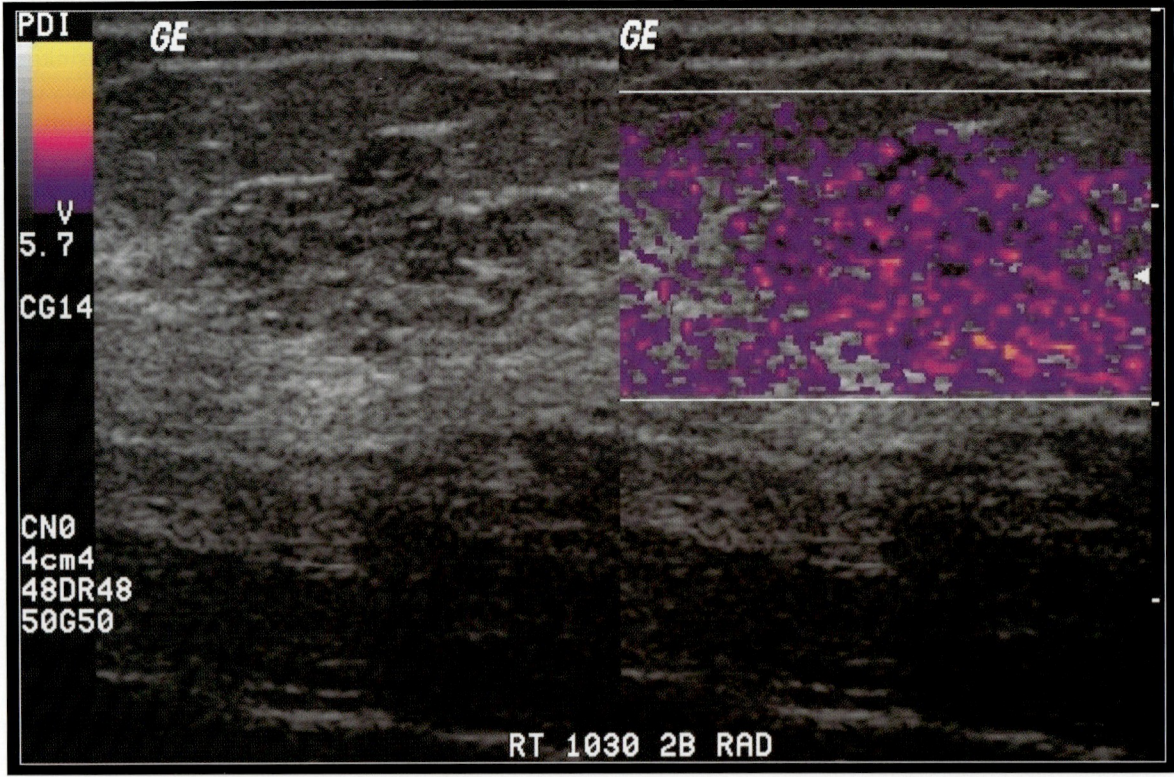

FIGURE 20–101 When calcifications within a lesion are numerous, their acoustic vibratory artifacts may completely obscure the lesion.

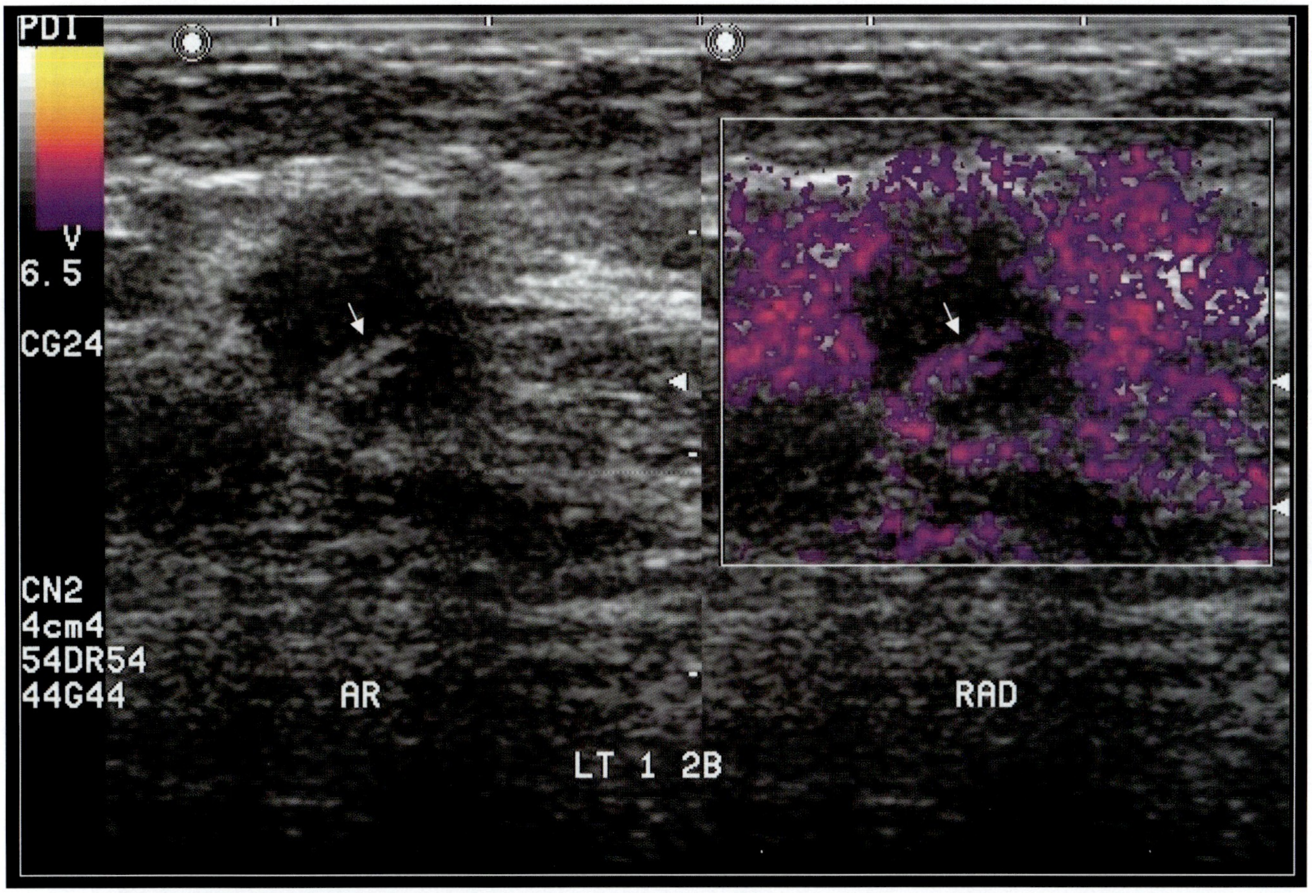

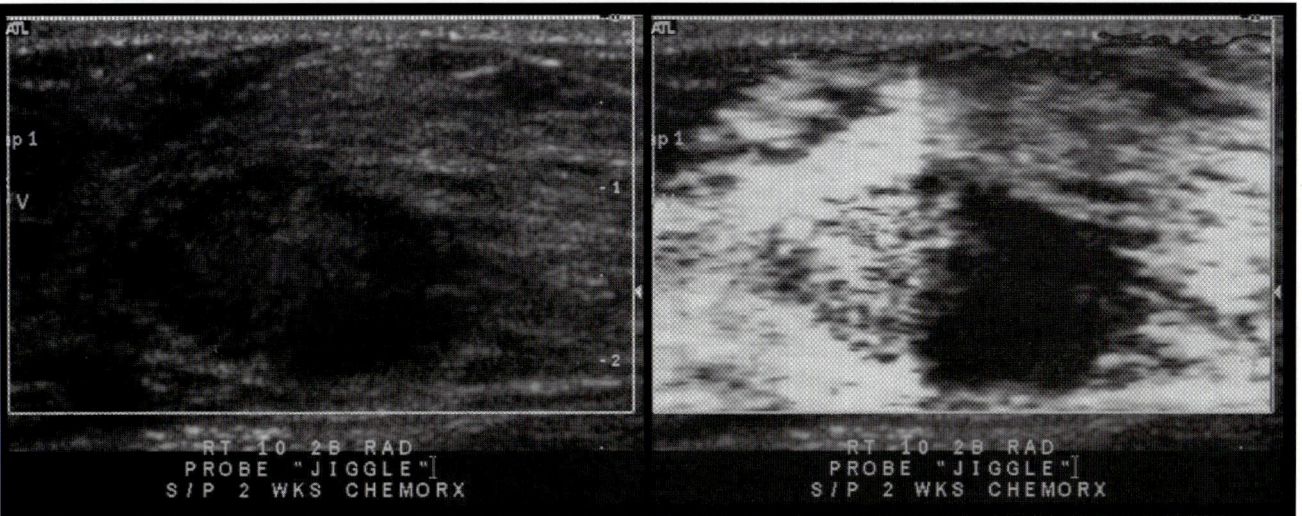

FIGURE 20–102 The fibrous scar *(arrow)* that forms within some malignant nodules will vibrate nearly as intensely as normal interlobular fibrous tissue.

FIGURE 20–103 This intermediate-grade invasive ductal carcinoma has undergone a trial of chemotherapy, and the left side of the lesion has undergone necrosis and fibrosis. Notice that the fibrotic part of the tumor that has been killed by chemotherapy vibrates, whereas the viable part does not. This may be helpful in assessing the response of a lesion to chemotherapy even in lesions that have not shrunk. Prior to chemotherapy the acoustic vibratory defect encompassed the entire lesion.

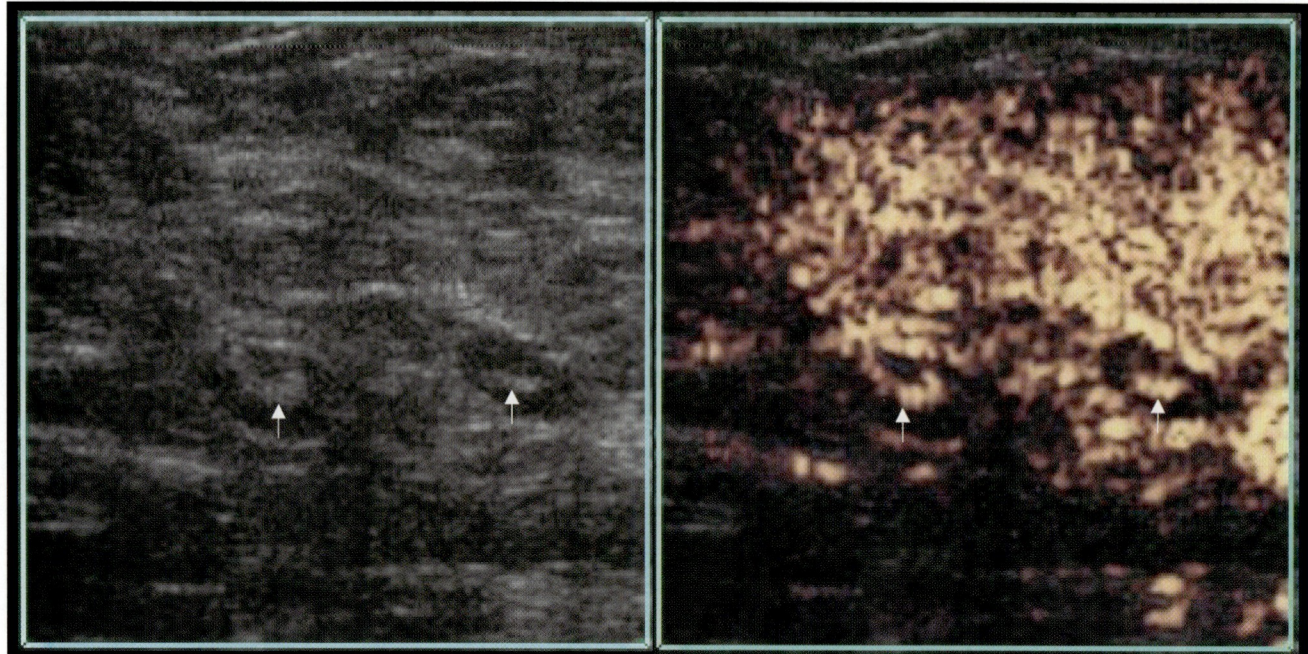

FIGURE 20–104 The medullary sinuses and medullary cords within the mediastinum of lymph nodes vibrate intensely *(arrows)*. If the echogenic portion that contains the medullary sinuses and cords is prominent in size, it may obscure the acoustic vibratory defect caused by normal lymph nodes. However, because the mediastinum is usually compressed in abnormal lymph nodes, its vibrations will not adversely affect the ability of power Doppler fremitus to detect an abnormal lymph node.

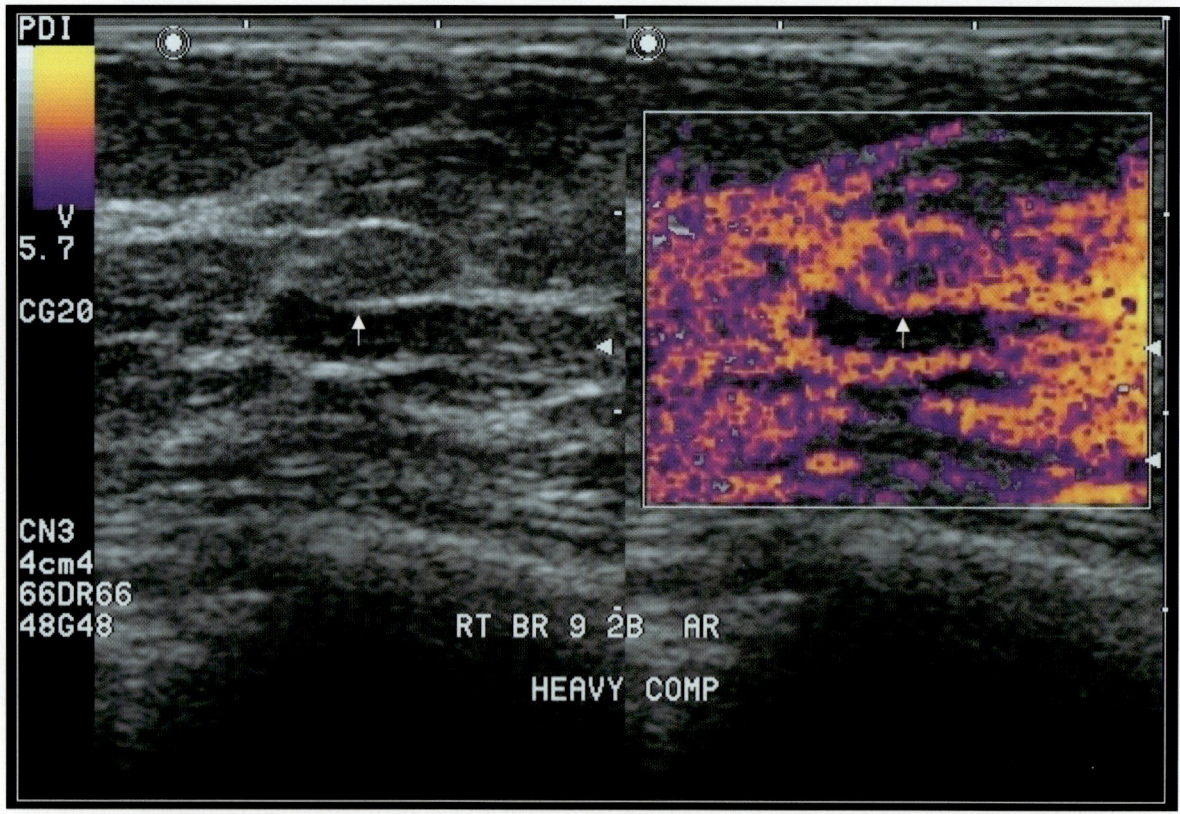

FIGURE 20–105 Hyalinized or sclerotic fibroadenomas *(arrow)* vibrate much more than fibroadenomas that have cellular or myxoid stoma and therefore may not cause an obvious acoustic vibratory defect.

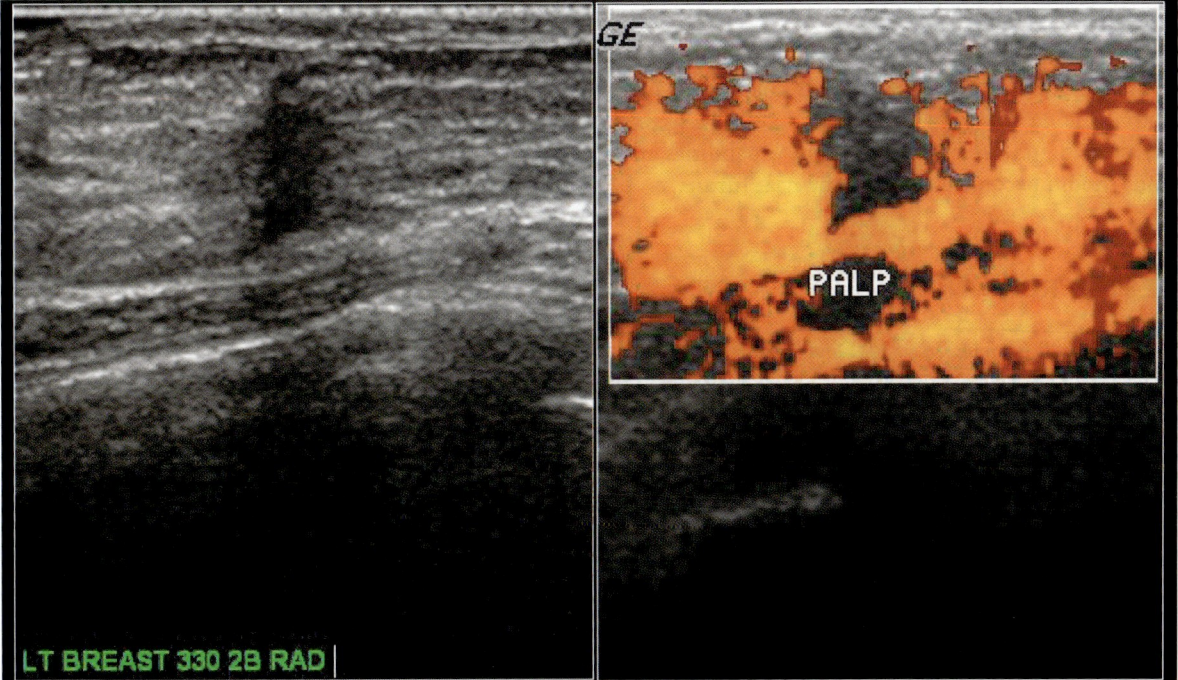

FIGURE 20–106 Radial scars are composed of a central fibroelastotic scar and variable amounts of peripheral proliferative change. Radial scars with abundant peripheral proliferative change cause an acoustic vibratory defect similar to defects caused by other solid nodules.

Radial Scars that Have Little Peripheral Proliferative Change

Radial scars are composed of central fibroelastotic scars and variable amounts of proliferative changes in the periphery. Radial scars that have abundant proliferative change in the periphery create acoustic vibratory defects similar to those of carcinoma and fibroadenomas (Fig. 20–106). On the other hand, radial scars that are composed primarily of central fibroelastotic scars and have very little peripheral proliferative changes may vibrate nearly as well as fibrous tissue and may cause little or no acoustic vibratory defect (Fig. 20–107).

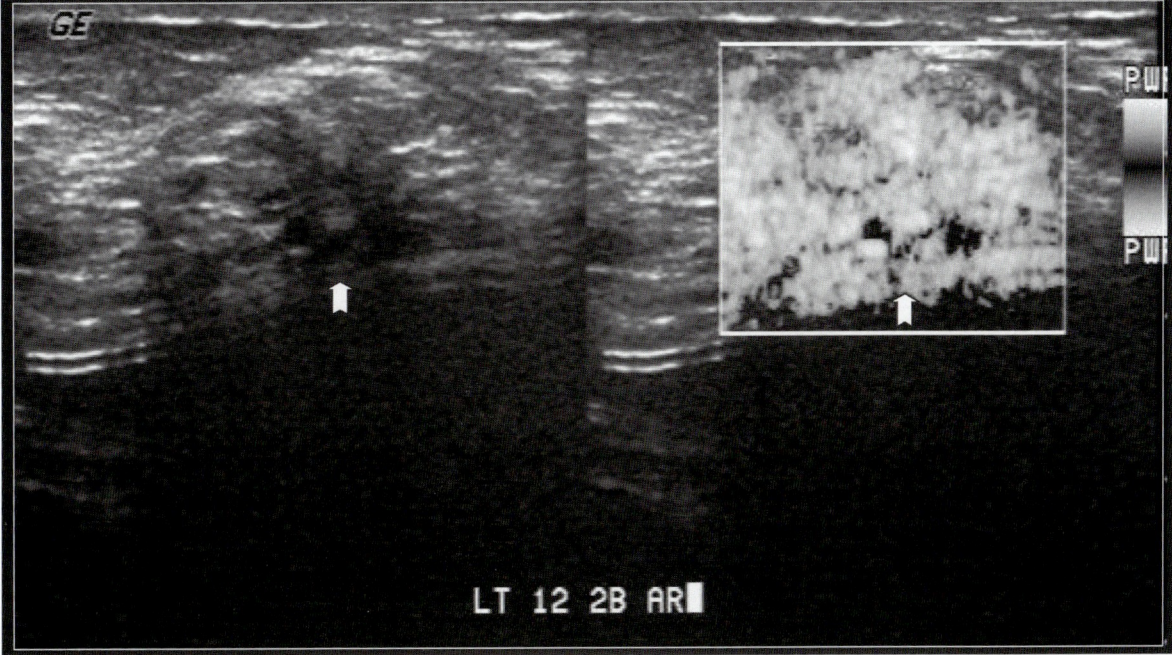

FIGURE 20–107 Radial scars that are composed primarily of central fibroelastotic scars, but have little proliferative change *(arrow)*, frequently do not cause a vibratory defect, especially if surrounded by fibrous tissues, because the central scar vibrates similarly to fibrous tissues.

Fremitus is still in an early phase of evaluation in comparison to B-mode imaging findings and other Doppler findings, and a better understanding of its capabilities and limitations should become evident in the near future.

SUGGESTED READINGS

Adler DD, Carson PL, Rubin JM, et al. Doppler ultrasound color flow imaging in the study of breast cancer: preliminary findings. *Ultrasound Med Biol* 1990;16:553–559.

Balu-Maestro C, Bruneton JN, Giudicelli T, et al. Color Doppler in breast tumor pathology. *J Radiol* 1991;72:579–583.

Berg WA, Chang BW, Dejong MR. Color Doppler flow mapping of abdominal wall perforating arteries for transverse rectus abdominis myocutaneous flap in breast reconstruction: method and preliminary results. *Radiology* 1994;192:447–450.

Birdwell RL, Ikeda DM, Jeffrey SS, et al. Preliminary experience with power Doppler imaging of solid breast masses. *AJR Am J Roentgenol* 1997;169(3):703–707.

Blohmer JU, Oellinger H, Schmidt C, et al. Comparison of various imaging methods with particular evaluation of color Doppler sonography for planning surgery for breast tumors. *Arch Gynecol Obstet* 1999;262(3–4):159–171.

Bohm-Velez M, Mendelson EB. Computed tomography, duplex Doppler ultrasound, and magnetic resonance imaging in evaluating the breast. *Semin Ultrasound CT MR* 1989;10(2):171–176.

Britton PD, Coulden RA. The use of duplex Doppler ultrasound in the diagnosis of breast cancer. *Clin Radiol* 1990;42:399–401.

Buadu LD, Murakami J, Murayama S, et al. Colour Doppler sonography of breast masses: a multiparameter analysis. *Clin Radiol* 1997;52(12):917–923.

Calliada F, Raieli G, Sala G, et al. Doppler color echo in the echographic evaluation of solid neoplasms of the breast: 5 years of experience. *Radiol Med* (Torino) 1994;87:28–35.

Campi R, Carlotto M, Gorreta L, et al. The role of color Doppler echography in the diagnosis of breast tumors. *Radiol Med* (Torino) 1990;79:182–184.

Carson PL, Adler DD, Fowlkes JB, et al. Enhanced color flow imaging of breast cancer vasculature: continuous wave Doppler and three-dimensional display. *J Ultrasound Med* 1992;11:377–385.

Carson PL, Fowlkes JB, Roubidoux MA, et al. 3-D color Doppler image quantification of breast masses. *Ultrasound Med Biol* 1998;24(7):945–952.

Carson PL, Moskalik AP, Govil A, et al. The 3D and 2D color flow display of breast masses. *Ultrasound Med Biol* 1997;23(6):837–849.

Caruso G, Cucciarre S, Lo Bello M, et al. Neoadjuvant intralesional chemotherapy for breast neoplasm in advanced stage: assessment of its efficacy with color Doppler. *Radiol Med* (Torino) 1995;89:613–618.

Chatterton BE, Spyropoulos P. Colour Doppler induced streaming: an indicator of the liquid nature of lesions. *Br J Radiol* 1998;71(852):1310–1312.

Choi HY, Kim HY, Baek SY, et al. Significance of resistive index in color Doppler ultrasonogram: differentiation between benign and malignant breast masses. *Clin Imaging* 1999;23:284–288.

Cosgrove DO, Bamber JC, Davey JB, et al. Color Doppler signals from breast tumors: work in progress. *Radiology* 1990;176:175–180.

Cosgrove DO, Kedar RP, Bamber JC, et al. Breast diseases: color Doppler US in differential diagnosis. *Radiology* 1993;189:99–104.

Cosgrove DO, Kedar RP, Bamber JC, et al. Breast diseases: color Doppler US in differential diagnosis [Comments]. *Radiology* 1994;189:99–104.

Cosgrove D, Eckersly R. Doppler indices in tumors: resolution or dilemma? [Comment on *Ultrasound Obstet Gynecol* 1997;10: 41–47, 48–53]. *Ultrasound Obstet Gynecol* 1997;10:9–11.

Daldrup H, Shames DM, Wendland M. Correlation of dynamic contrast-enhanced MR imaging with histologic tumor grade: comparison of macromolecular and small-molecular contrast media. *AJR Am J Roentgenol* 1998;171:67–78.

DeAlbertis P, Oliveri M, Quadri P, et al. Retrospective analysis of color Doppler ultrasonography and flowmetry findings in solid nodular pathology of the breast. *Radiol Med* (Torino) 1995;89: 28–35.

Delorme S, Zuna I, Huber S, et al. Colour Doppler sonography in breast tumours: an update. *Eur Radiol* 1998;8(2):189–193.

Dock W. Duplex sonography of mammary tumors: a prospective study of 75 patients. *J Ultrasound Med* 1993;12:79–82.

Dock W, Grabenwoger F, Metz V, et al. Tumor vascularization: assessment with duplex sonography. *Radiology* 1991;181:241–244.

Draghi F, Campani R. Power Doppler in breast diseases: preliminary results. *Radiol Med* (Torino) 1996;91:577–580.

Engin G, Acunas G, Acunas B. Granulomatous mastitis: gray-scale and color Doppler sonographic findings. *J Clin Ultrasound* 1999; 27(3):101–106.

Escolano E, Finck B, Allouch JM, et al. The value of color Doppler ultrasound in the diagnosis of breast tumors. *J Gynecol Obstet Biol Reprod* (Paris) 1992;21:868–876.

Ferrara KW, Zagar B, Sokil-Melgar J, et al. High resolution 3D color flow mapping: applied to the assessment of breast vasculature. *Ultrasound Med Biol* 1996;22(3):293–304.

Folkman J. *Angiogenesis-dependent imaging*. RSNA, Eugene P. Pendergrass New Horizons Lecture, 2001.

Fornage BD. Role of color Doppler imaging in differentiating between pseudocystic malignant tumors and fluid collections. *J Ultrasound Med* 1995;14:125–128.

Gembala RB, Hayward CS, Ball DS, et al. Color Doppler detection of a breast perilobular hemangioma. *J Ultrasound Med* 1993;12: 220–222.

Hayashi N, Miyamoto Y, Nakata N, et al. Breast masses: color Doppler, power Doppler, and spectral analysis findings. *J Clin Ultrasound* 1998;26(5):231–238.

Hollerweger A, Rettenbacher T, Macheiner P, et al. New signs of breast cancer: high resistance flow and variations in resistive indices evaluation by color Doppler sonography. *Ultrasound Med Biol* 1997;23(6):851–856.

Huber S, Delorme S, Knopp MV, et al. Breast tumors: computer-assisted quantitative assessment with color Doppler US. *Radiology* 1994;797–801.

Huber S, Helbich T, Kettenbach J, et al. Effects of a microbubble contrast agent on breast tumors: computer-assisted quantitative assessment with color Doppler US—early experience. *Radiology* 1998;208(2):485–489.

Jackson VP. Duplex sonography of the breast. *Ultrasound Med Biol* 1988;14[Suppl 1]:131–137.

Jellins J. Combining imaging and vascularity assessment of breast lesions. *Ultrasound Med Biol* 1988;[Suppl 1]:121–130.

Kedar RP, Cosgrove D, McCready VR, et al. Microbubble contrast agent for color Doppler US: effect on breast masses. Work in progress. *Radiology* 1996;198(3):679–686.

Kedar RP, Cosgrove DO, Smith IE, et al. Breast carcinoma: measurement of tumor response to primary medical therapy with color Doppler flow imaging. *Radiology* 1994;190:825–830.

Kiziltepe TT, Erden GA, Dingil G, et al. Breast metastasis from non-Hodgkin's lymphoma: evaluation with color Doppler sonography. *AJR Am J Roentgenol* 1996;167(6):1595–1596.

Kook SH, Park HW, Lee YR, et al. Evaluation of solid breast lesions with power Doppler sonography. *J Clin Ultrasound* 1999;27(5):231–237.

Kubek KA, Chan L, Frazier TG. Color Doppler flow as an indicator of nodal metastasis in solid breast masses. *J Ultrasound Med* 1996;15(12):835–841.

Kuijpers TJ, Obdeign AI, Kruyt RH, et al. Solid breast neoplasms: differential diagnosis with pulsed Doppler ultrasound. *Ultrasound Med Biol* 1994;20:517–520.

Lagalla R, Caruso G, Finazzo M. Monitoring treatment response with color and power Doppler. *Eur J Radiol* 1998;27[Suppl 2]:S149–56.

Lagalla R, Caruso G, Marasa L, et al. Angiogenetic capacity of breast neoplasms and correlation with color Doppler semiology. *Radiol Med* (Torino) 1994;88:392–395.

Lagalla R, Midiri M. Image quality control in breast ultrasound. *Eur J Radiol* 1998;27[Suppl 2]:S229–233.

Lee SK, Lee T, Su YG, et al. Evaluation of breast tumors with color Doppler imaging: a comparison with image-directed Doppler ultrasound. *J Clin Ultrasound* 1995;23:367–373.

Lee WJ, Chu JS, Chung MF, et al. The use of color Doppler in the diagnosis of occult breast cancer. *J Clin Ultrasound* 1995;23:192–194.

Lee WJ, Chu JS, Chang KJ, et al. Occult breast carcinoma—use of color Doppler in localization. *Breast Cancer Res Treat* 1996;37(3):299–302.

Lee WJ, Chu JS, Huang CS, et al. Breast cancer vascularity: color Doppler sonography and histopathology study. *Breast Cancer Res Treat* 1996;37(3):291–298.

Madjar H, Prompeler HJ, Sauerbrei W, et al. Color Doppler flow criteria of breast lesions. *Ultrasound Med Biol* 1994;20:849–858.

Madjar H, Sauerbrei W, Munch S, et al. Continuous-wave and pulsed Doppler studies of the breast: clinical results and effect of transducer frequency. *Ultrasound Med Biol* 1991;17:31–39.

Madjar H, Sauerbrei W, Prompeler HJ, et al. Color Doppler and duplex flow analysis for classification of breast lesions. *Gynecol Oncol* 1997;64(3):392–403.

Martinoli C, Pretolesi F, Crespi G, et al. Power Doppler sonography: clinical applications. *Eur J Radiol* 1998;27[Suppl 2]:S133–140.

McNichols MMJ, Mercer PM, Miller JC, et al. Color Doppler sonography in the evaluation of palpable breast masses. *AJR Am J Roentgenol* 1993;161:765–771.

Medl M, Peters-Engl C, Leodolter S. The use of color-coded Doppler sonography in the diagnosis of breast cancer. *Anticancer Res* (Greece) 1994;14:2249–2251.

Mehta TS, Raza S. Power Doppler sonography of breast cancer: does vascularity correlate with node status or lymphatic invasion? *AJR Am J Roentgenol* 1999;173:303–307.

Mehta TS, Raza S, Baum JK. Use of ultrasound in the evaluation of breast carcinoma. *Semin Ultrasound CT MR* 2000;21:297–307.

Meyer CR, Boes JL, Kim B, et al. Semiautomatic registration of volumetric ultrasound scans. *Ultrasound Med Biol* 1999;25(3):339–347.

Meyerowitz CB, Fleischer AC, Pickens DR, et al. Quantification of tumoral vascularity and flow with amplitude color Doppler sonography in an experimental model. *J Ultrasound Med* 1996;15:827–833.

Ozdemir A, Ozdemir H, Maral I, et al. Differential diagnosis of solid breast nodules: contribution of Doppler studies to mammography and gray scale. *J Ultrasound Med* 20:2001;1091–1101.

Peters-Engl C, Frank W, Leodolter S, et al. Tumor flow in malignant breast tumors measured by Doppler ultrasound: an independent predictor of survival. *Breast Cancer Res Treat* 1999;54(1):65–71.

Peters-Engl C, Medl M, Leodolter S. The use of color-coded and spectral Doppler ultrasound in the differentiation of benign and malignant breast lesions. *Br J Cancer* 1995;71:137–139.

Peters-Engl C, Medl M, Mirau M, et al. Color-coded and spectral Doppler flow in breast carcinomas—relationship with the tumor microvasculature. *Breast Cancer Res Treat* 1998;47(1):83–89.

Raza S, Baum JK. Solid breast lesions: evaluation with power Doppler US. *Radiology* 1997;203:164–168.

Rettenbacher T, Hollerweger A, Macheiner P, et al. Color Doppler sonography of normal breasts: detectability of arterial blood vessels and typical flow patterns. *Ultrasound Med Biol* 1998;24(9):1307–1311.

Rizzatto G, Chersevani R, Abbona M, et al. High-resolution sonography of breast carcinoma. *Eur J Radiol* 1997;24(1):11–19.

Rubin JM, Carson PL, Zlotecki RA, et al. Visualization of tumor vascularity in a rabbit VX2 carcinoma by Doppler flow mapping. *J Ultrasound Med* 1987;6:113–120.

Sahin-Akyar G, Sumer H. Color Doppler ultrasound and spectral analysis of tumor vessels in the differential diagnosis of solid breast masses. *Invest Radiol* 1996;31(2):72–79.

Sambrook M, Bamber JC, Minasian H, et al. Ultrasonic Doppler study of the hormonal response of blood flow in the normal human breast. *Ultrasound Med Biol* 1987;13:121–129.

Sauerbrei W, Madjar H, Prompeler HJ. Differentiation of benign and malignant breast tumors by logistic regression and a classification tree using Doppler flow signals. *Methods Inf Med* 1998;37(3):226–234.

Schelling M, Gnirs J, Braun M, et al. Optimized differential diagnosis of breast lesions by combined B-mode and color Doppler sonography. *Ultrasound Obstet Gynecol* 1997;10(1):48–53.

Schiller VL, Karlen L, Brenner RJ. Pseudoaneurysm of the breast: the use of color Doppler sonography. *AJR Am J Roentgenol* 1998;170(4):1112.

Schoenberger SG, Sutherland CM, Robinson AE. Breast neoplasms: duplex sonographic imaging as an adjunct in diagnosis. *Radiology* 1988;168:665–668.

Schroeder RJ, Maeurer J, Vogl TJ, et al. D-Galactose-based signal-enhanced color Doppler sonography of breast tumors and tumor-like lesions. *Invest Radiol* 1999;34(2):109–115.

Sohn C, Beldermann F, Bastert G. Sonographic blood flow measurements in malignant breast tumors: a potential new prognostic factor. *Surg Endosc* 1997;11(9):957–960.

Tonutti M, Bertolotto M, Cressa C, et al. Role of Doppler technique in the differential diagnosis of solid breast nodules. Personal experience. *Radiol Med* (Torino) 1997;93:56–60.

Van Dijke CF, Brasch RC, Roberts TPL, et al. Mammary carcinoma model: correlation of macromolecular contrast-enhanced MR imaging characterizations of tumor microvasculature and histologic capillary density. *Radiology* 1996;198:813–818.

Villena-Heinsen C, Konig J, von Tongelen B, et al. Validity of the minimal resistance index for discrimination between benign and malignant breast tumours. *Eur J Ultrasound* 1998;7(3):189–193.

Walsh JS, Dixon JM, Chetty U, et al. Colour Doppler studies of axillary node metastases in breast carcinoma. *Clin Radiol* 1994;49:189–191.

Weind KL, Maier CF, Rutt BK, et al. Invasive carcinomas and fibroadenomas of the breast: comparison of microvessel distributions—implications for imaging modalities. *Radiology* 1998;208(2):477–483.

Wilkens TH, Burke BJ, Cancelada DA, et al. Evaluation of palpable breast masses with color Doppler sonography and gray scale imaging. *J Ultrasound Med* 1998;17:109–115.

Wright IA, Pugh ND, Lyons K, et al. Power Doppler in breast tumours: a comparison with conventional colour Doppler imaging. *Eur J Ultrasound* 1998;7(3):175–181.

Yang WT, Metreweli C. Colour Doppler flow in normal axillary lymph nodes. *Br J Radiol* 1998;71(844):381–383.

Yang WT, Suen M, Metreweli C. Lactating adenoma of the breast: antepartum and postpartum sonographic and color Doppler imaging appearances with histopathologic correlation. *J Ultrasound Med* 1997;16(2):145–147.

Youssefzadeh S, Eibenberger K, Helbich T, et al. Use of resistance index for the diagnosis of breast tumours. *Clin Radiol* 1996; 51(6):418–420.

FALSE-NEGATIVE AND FALSE-POSITIVE BREAST SONOGRAPHIC EXAMINATIONS

There are two types of errors in breast ultrasound: false-negative and false-positive findings. False-negative findings result in a Breast Imaging Reporting and Data System (BIRADS) category assignment that is falsely low, and false-positive findings result in a BIRADS category assignment that is falsely high. The assignment of a falsely high or low BIRADS category can be the result of technical errors or interpretive errors, or it might simply be an unavoidable result of algorithms that are designed to minimize both missed carcinomas and biopsies of benign structures. The algorithms are based on receiver operating characteristics (ROC) curves. It is always possible to adjust an algorithm to avoid all false-negative results, but the cost is increased numbers of false-positive results. It is also possible to minimize false-positive findings and biopsies of benign structures, but the cost is increased numbers of false-negative findings and missed carcinomas. Diagnostic breast ultrasound algorithms attempt to reach a delicate balance between missed carcinomas and biopsies of benign structures. However, because the cost of a missed cancer (false-negative examination) is potentially much greater than the cost of a benign biopsy (false-positive examination), the algorithm is skewed toward avoiding missing the diagnosis of malignancy. Because we must err on the side of caution, false-positive examinations greatly outnumber false-negative examinations. Most false-positive and false-negative errors have been both discussed and illustrated in earlier chapters. We summarize the discussions in this chapter but refer to the original illustrations in the appropriate chapters rather than repeating them in this chapter.

FALSE-NEGATIVE EXAMINATIONS

Technical

Volume Averaging Artifact in the Near Field and Far Field

Volume Averaging in the Near Field. Even the most optimally focused near-field imaging probes commercially available have elevation plane (short-axis) focal points about 1.5 to 2 cm deep. Small breast lesions occasionally lie superficial to this focal point. If small near-field lesions (less than 1 cm in size and less than 1 cm deep) are smaller than the width of the ultrasound beam at that depth, adjacent soft normal soft tissues will be averaged with the small superficial lesion. The volume averaging artifact can alter the apparent echogenicity of a small, superficially located lesion enough to make it inapparent and indistinguishable from the surrounding normal soft tissues and therefore missed by routine ultrasound. Scanning such lesions with a thin standoff pad or a glob of acoustic gel can help prevent this type of error (see Chapter 2, Figs. 2–5 through 2–7).

Near-field volume averaging can also cause mischaracterization of lesions that are sonographically visible. Tiny hypoechoic carcinomas that are surrounded by thick, echogenic halos can falsely appear to be purely hypoechoic because of near-field volume averaging, and using an acoustic standoff can help prevent this type of error (see Chapter 12, Fig. 12–80).

Using a standoff pad in every patient is not practical and would not help the overall efficacy of ultrasound because other deeper lesions would then be scanned at depths below the optimal elevation plane focal zone of the transducer. Therefore, it is necessary to select patients for whom acoustic standoff will be more helpful than harmful. In general, palpable nodules that are pea sized or smaller must be very superficial to be palpable. Such lesions almost always benefit from the use of a standoff. Mammographic lesions that appear to be very superficial are also likely to benefit from the use of a standoff.

An alternative method of minimizing near-field volume averaging errors is to employ a 1.5-dimensional (1.5-D) array transducer that is capable of electronically focusing in the short axis. Such probes result in a narrower beam width and less volume averaging in the near field less than 1 cm deep, minimizing the effects of volume averaging artifact and reducing missed diagnoses of small near-

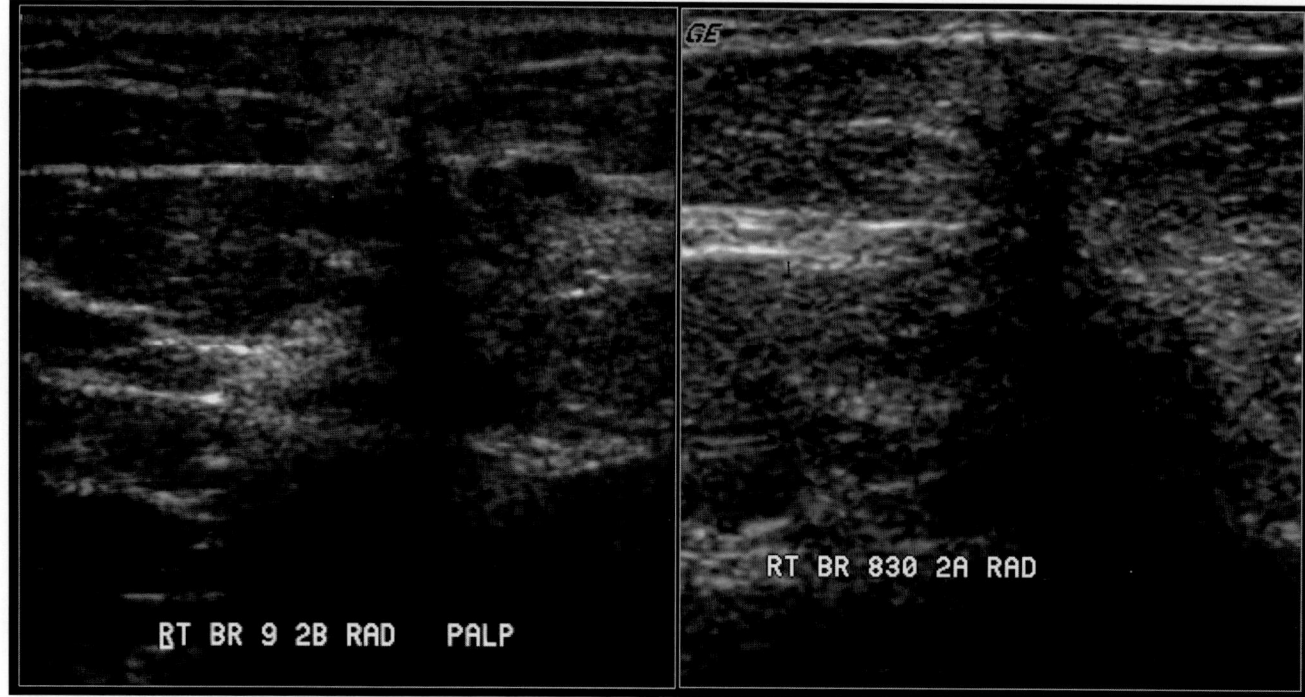

FIGURE 21–1 These images illustrate the value of a 1.5-D array transducer for characterizing palpable lesions that lie in the very near field (less than 8 mm deep). The **left** image, obtained using a conventional 1-D array, 12-MHz transducer, shows what appears to be a small focus of hyperechoic fibrous tissue causing some critical angle acoustic shadowing. The **right** image of the same lesion, obtained using a 1.5-D array, 12-MHz transducer, which allows electronic focusing in the short axis, shows the lump to be caused by a hypoechoic, multiangular mass.

field lesions (Fig. 21–1). The 1.5-D array transducers are especially important in evaluating patients with nipple discharge, in whom the duct must be shown all the way through the nipple to the duct orifice on the surface of the nipple. Demonstrating the intranipple portion of the duct requires performing the rolled-nipple maneuver. It is generally not possible to use an acoustic standoff while performing the rolled-nipple maneuver; thus, having the superior near-field focusing characteristics of a 1.5-D array transducer is very helpful in this subset of patients (Fig. 21–2).

Volume Averaging in the Far Field. Small breast lesions within very large breasts can lie deeper than the short-axis focal zone of 10- to 12-MHz transducers and, like near-field lesions, can be subject to beam-width or volume averaging artifact that causes them to be either missed or mischaracterized. Using a standoff in such patients will only make the volume averaging in the far field worse. Using greater compression pressure will reduce the depth of the lesion and minimize volume averaging in certain cases but in others will not be sufficient [macromastia, lactation, mastitis, inflammatory carcinoma (Fig. 21–3), large fibrous breasts, large irradiated breasts, and implants affected by capsular contracture].

In such cases, using a 5-MHz probe that has a deeper short-axis focal zone (3 to 4 cm) will be necessary to minimize far-field volume averaging.

Gain Too Low

Using a total gain setting that is too low or a time–gain curve that is too flat may make a markedly hypoechoic cancer appear to be anechoic, causing it to be misdiagnosed as a cyst. This is not usually a problem for experienced sonographers and sonologists but can be a problem for the novice, especially the mammographer who is just beginning to perform breast ultrasound.

There are several things that we can do to prevent such a misdiagnosis. First, there should be enhanced through-transmission through a cyst. Although a significant percentage of high-grade malignant solid breast malignancies also have enhanced through-transmission, and the presence of enhanced through-transmission does not exclude malignancy, the lack of through-transmission on a lesion thought to be cystic should make one suspicious that the lesion is really solid (see Chapter 10, Fig. 10–10). Second, such hypoechoic, pseudocystic solid malignancies rarely have the smooth spheroidal or elliptical shape or the thin echogenic

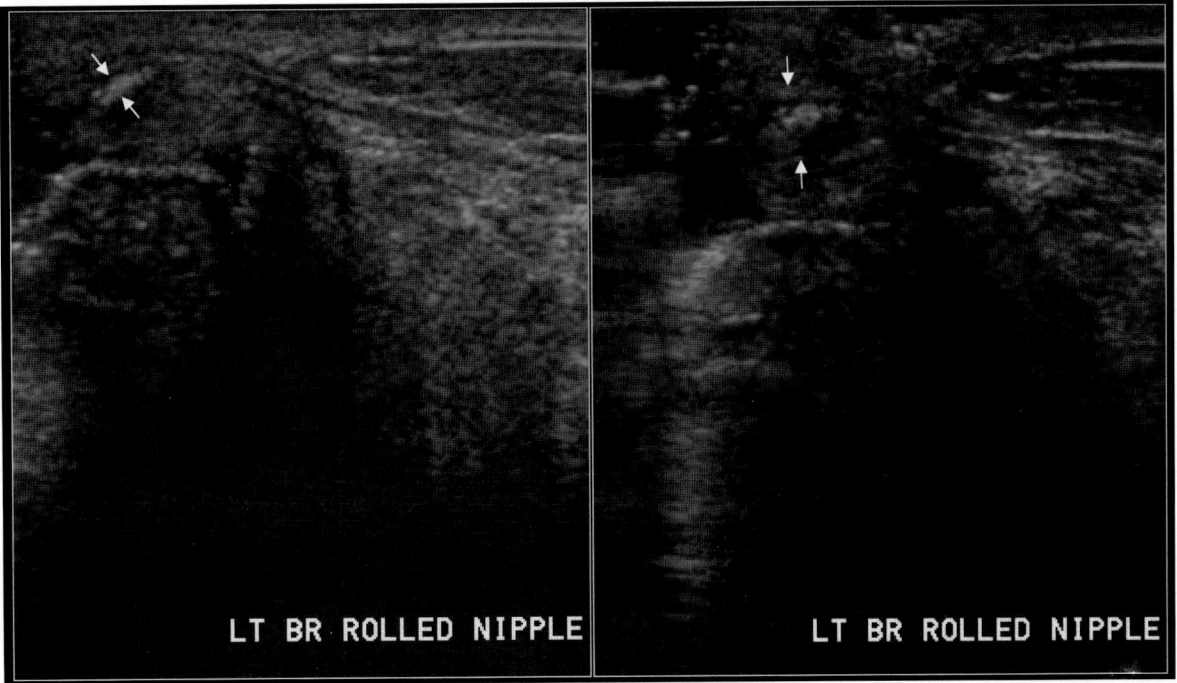

FIGURE 21–2 This faintly calcified nipple adenoma was barely visible using a conventional 12-MHz transducer and vigorous compression during the rolled nipple maneuver (**left**). The nipple adenoma and the expanded walls of the duct in which it lies are far better demonstrated using a 1.5-D array, 12-MHz transducer (**right**) and therefore much less likely to be missed sonographically.

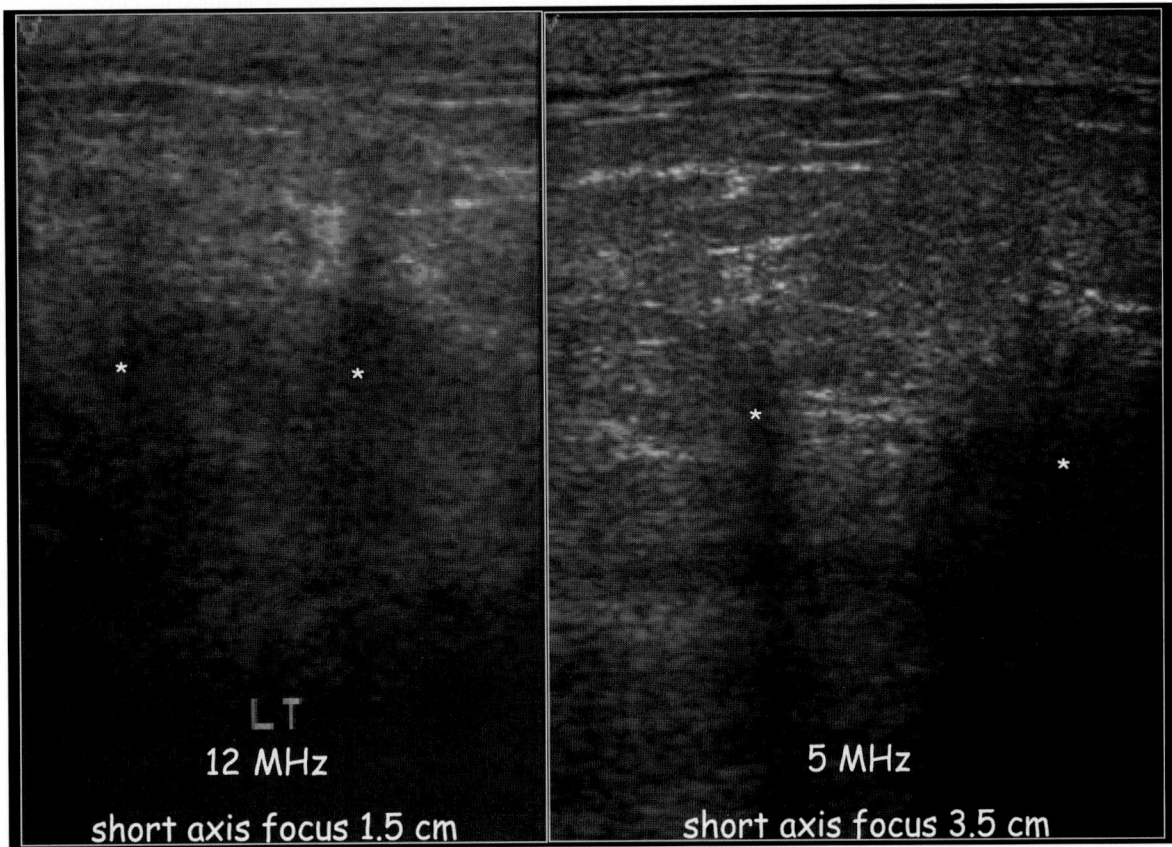

FIGURE 21–3 When the breasts are very large or very swollen, suboptimal penetration and far-field volume averaging may degrade images obtained with conventional 10- to 12-MHz transducers. The **left** image, obtained with a conventional 12 MHz transducer in this patient with inflammatory carcinoma, poorly shows a definitive cause because of poor penetration. The **right** image was obtained with a 5-MHz transducer and shows multifocal hypoechoic shadowing lesions. The 5-MHz transducer, focused at 3.5 cm in the short axis, too deeply focused for normal breast ultrasound, was more appropriate for the swollen condition of this patient's breast (histologic diagnosis is inflammatory carcinoma, multifocal intermediate-grade invasive ductal carcinoma).

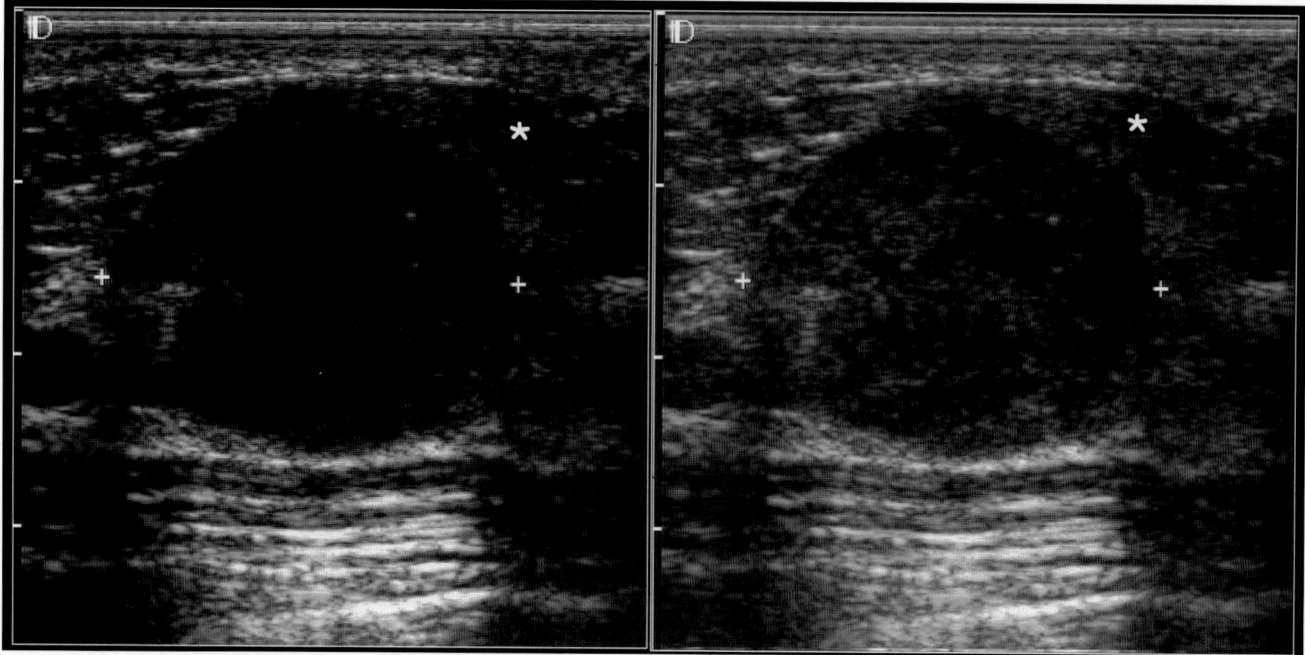

FIGURE 21–4 This high-grade invasive carcinoma has markedly enhanced through-transmission typical of high-grade lesions. The **left** image was obtained by an inexperienced sonographer with gain settings that were too low, causing the lesion to appear nearly anechoic and causing the sonographer to misinterpret the lesion as a cyst. Note that the fat surrounding the tumor appears to be black rather than a midlevel gray. The **right** image, obtained a few minutes later by a more experienced sonographer, shows the lesion to be solid. Note that the fat is appropriately displayed as isoechoic.

outer wall that cysts do. Additionally, the normal breast fat in cases in which this error has been made will appear black rather than the normal dark or medium gray. The appearance of "black fat" should be a clue that the gain settings were too low (Fig. 21–4; see also Chapter 10, Fig. 10–19). If fat appears too hypoechoic throughout the depth of field, the findings suggests too low a total gain setting. If the near-field fat is white, midfield fat is gray, and far-field fat is black, the time–gain curve has been set too flat or the transmit power too low. In such cases, it may be difficult to see the chest wall. If the chest wall is not visible, either the total gain setting was too low, the time–gain curve was too flat, or the transmit power was too low. Color Doppler may help. Some malignant nodules (medullary carcinoma, some high-grade invasive carcinomas, and lymphoma) are typically so hypoechoic that they are known to have a pseudocystic appearance. However, such lesions are generally quite vascular and often have an internal vessel that is demonstrable with color Doppler (see Chapter 10, Fig. 10–22, and Chapter 20, Fig. 20–25). Likewise, metastases to intramammary lymph nodes frequently have a pseudocystic appearance (see Chapter 20, Fig. 20–26). Of course, as is always the case, a positive Doppler is more useful than a negative Doppler. Many malignant nodules have demonstrable blood flow only in the periphery and are either necrotic centrally or primarily composed of extracellular matrix centrally. The demonstration of a central vessel indicates with certainty that the nodule is solid or is an encysted papillary lesion, but lack of flow does not indicate with certainty that the nodule is not malignant. The differential diagnosis for pseudocystic breast carcinomas includes (a) high-grade invasive ductal carcinoma; (b) medullary carcinoma; (c) high-nuclear-grade ductal carcinoma *in situ* (DCIS) with extensive comedonecrosis, which has a clustered microcystic appearance (see Chapter 10, Figs. 10–9 and 20–27); and (d) metastases to or lymphoma of intramammary lymph nodes and regional lymph nodes (Fig. 21–5).

Use of an improper probe for breast ultrasound can also result in this type of error. This is especially true of 5- or 3.5-MHz sector or curved linear probes, which have less contrast resolution than 7.5-MHz linear probes and make it more difficult to characterize lesions accurately as cystic or solid.

Inadequate Penetration

The chest wall should be demonstrated in all patients. If it cannot be demonstrated with the 10- to 12-MHz transducers usually used for breast ultrasound, the penetration is inadequate. Inadequate penetration is unusual with 10- to 12-MHz transducers in fundamental mode when patients are scanned in the supine or contralateral posterior

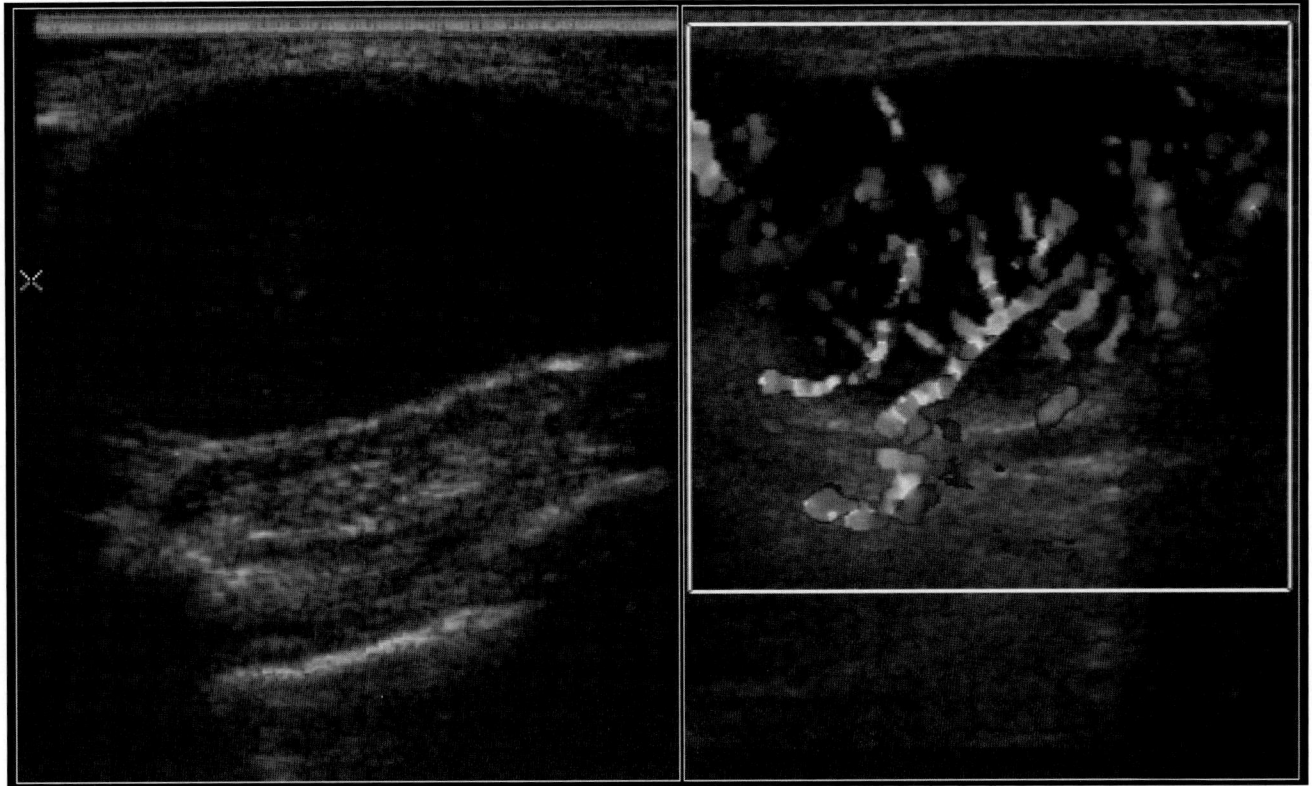

FIGURE 21–5 Lymphoma of the breast commonly presents with a pseudocystic appearance. Like the other pseudocystic malignant breast lesions, lymphomas typically have readily demonstrable internal blood flow with color or power Doppler.

oblique position, with the ipsilateral hand placed behind the head, and when some degree of compression is applied. To improve penetration, the total gain can be increased, the time–gain curve steepened, and the transmit power increased. Additionally, a swept wall filter can be used to select lower-frequency portions of the bandwidth. On some equipment, multiple scan parameters can be simultaneously present for patients who are large or transmit sound poorly. Additionally, using greater compression pressure while scanning the breast decreases the thickness of the breast and pushes the tissue planes into an orientation that minimizes critical angle shadowing (see Chapter 3, Fig. 3–5). Heavier compression is more useful for focused scanning than for surveying the whole breast.

In some cases, however, none of these adjustments will be enough to enable adequate penetration. This tends to occur in the same patient populations in which far-field volume averaging is a problem: those with breast thickness greater than 3.5 cm. Macromastia, lactation, mastitis, inflammatory carcinoma, edema due to radiation, lymphedema, and implants affected by capsular contracture are all conditions that increase the risk for inadequate penetration with 10- to 12-MHz transducers. When penetration is inadequate with 10- to 12-MHz transducers, a

5-MHz linear transducer may be necessary to demonstrate deeply located abscesses or malignant nodules (see Chapter 14, Fig. 14–119) or in women with implants who have capsular contracture.

The risk for inadequate penetration is increased to about 6% of cases when coded harmonics is used. Coded harmonics increases contrast resolution but decreases penetration. However, if penetration is inadequate with coded harmonics, fundamental imaging usually always allows adequate penetration to be achieved (see Chapter 2, Fig. 2–25). If a malignant lesion causes acoustic shadowing that obscures the posterior wall of the nodule and the retrotumoral breast tissues, and if the lesion is not too large, real-time compounding may facilitate demonstration of the back wall of the lesion and of the retrotumoral breast tissues better (see Chapter 2, Fig. 2–37).

Sonographer and Sonologist Observational Errors

Significant pathology may be missed by the sonographer or sonologist even though the transducer, technical settings, and acoustic standoff are appropriate. Observational errors occur for several reasons. First, during targeted examinations, the correct areas in the breast may not be scanned. Second, the echogenicity of the lesion mat be so nearly identical to the echogenicity of the background tissue that the lesion is not perceptible. Third, a normal structure may be so minimally enlarged that it cannot be distinguished from ducts and lobules in the vicinity that are normal or that contain benign fibrocystic change (FCC) or benign proliferative disorders.

The most common cause for such an error is a geographic miss. The person scanning simply does not scan the appropriate area of the breast. This can occur when the indication is evaluation of a mammographic abnormality that is visible only on one view. Geographic misses are rare when the indication is a palpable abnormality. It can be difficult to predict precisely the location of certain lesions during sonography from their positions on mammography because of movement and rotation of the breast that occurs in the upright position during mammographic compression. Mammographic lesions that are near the 12:00 or 6:00 position on the craniocaudal (CC) view seldom are difficult to locate by ultrasound. However, lesions that appear to be near the 3:00 or 9:00 position on the mediolateral oblique (MLO) view lie several centimeters higher or lower than where they appear to be on mammography (i.e., a lesion that appears to be at 1:00 to 2:00 on the mammogram may be at 4:00 dur-

ing ultrasound). Additionally, we are not usually certain exactly what degree of obliquity was used during the routine MLO view (anywhere between 30 and 60 degrees), adding to difficulties in locating lesions in the midbreast on MLO views. Sometimes obtaining a true mediolateral or lateral medial view will help us localize a lesion better. We scan a wedge of tissue around the suspected location of the mammographic lesion to minimize the chances of a geographic miss. For lesions near 6:00 or 12:00 on the CC view, scanning a 30-degree wedge of tissue will often suffice. For lesions that appear to be near 3:00 or 9:00 on mammography, scanning a 90-degree wedge of tissue will often be necessary.

Once a sonographically demonstrable structure is found that could explain the mammographic abnormality, a rigorous sonographic–mammographic correlation of size, shape, location, and surrounding tissue density is undertaken to make sure that the sonographic findings truly do explain the mammographic abnormality and that there are not really two separate abnormalities—a benign sonographic abnormality and a malignant mammographic abnormality.

Another reason for observational error is a lack of contrast between the lesion and the surrounding normal breast tissue. This would occur most commonly in a radiographically dense breast composed primarily of isoechoic glandu-

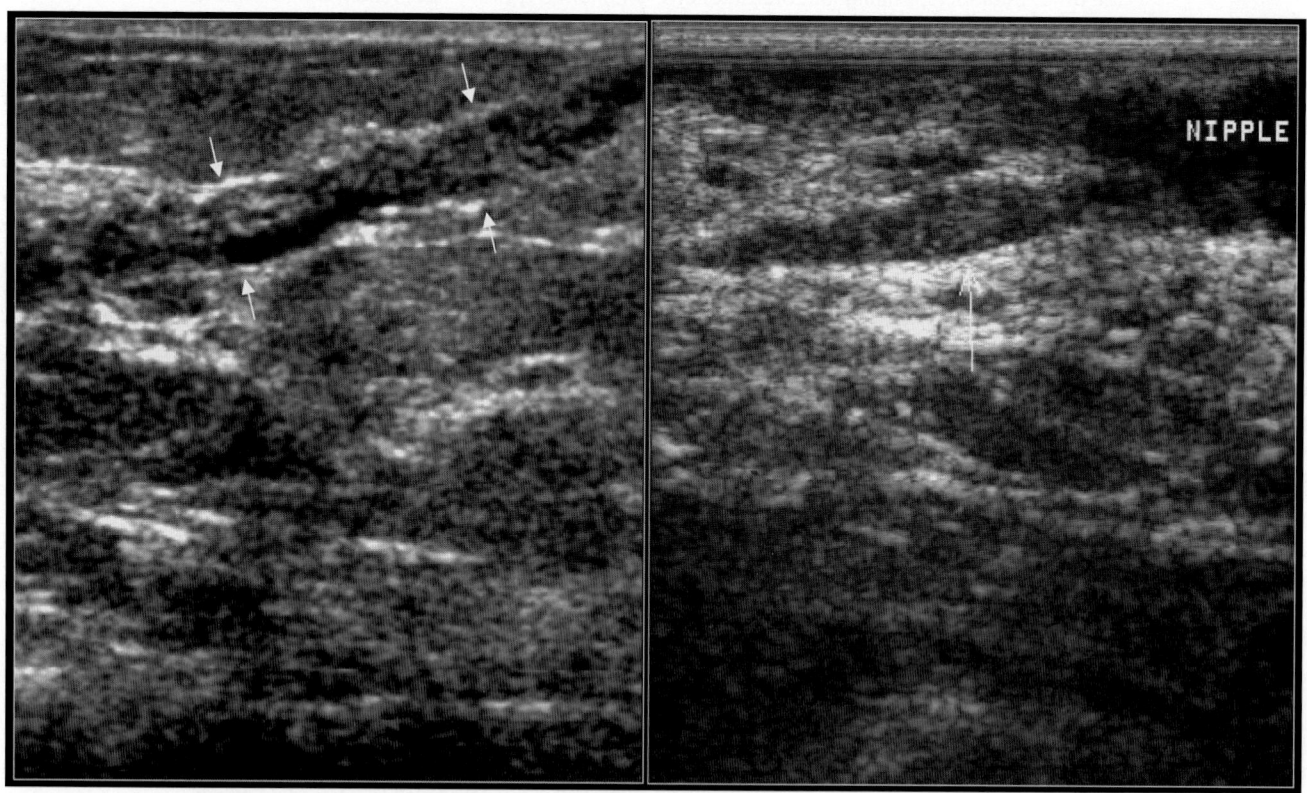

FIGURE 21–6 Enlarged central ducts that contain internal echoes can be a cause of false-negative and false-positive findings. It can be difficult to distinguish between ductal carcinoma *in situ* (**left**, *arrows*) and periductal fibrosis that represents the end stages of the duct ectasia–periductal mastitis complex (**right**, *arrow*).

lar tissue on ultrasound. Most fibroadenomas and about one-third of malignant solid nodules are nearly isoechoic or very mildly hypoechoic with respect to glandular tissue of the breast. In a dense breast composed primarily of isoechoic glandular elements, such nodules may be indistinguishable from surrounding glandular elements (see Chapter 4, Fig. 4–69). Such lesions may also be missed on the mammograms owing to surrounding dense tissue. The sensitivity of sonographically isoechoic nodules is lower in a background of isoechoic glandular elements than it is in a background of hyperechoic fibrous elements.

In other cases, a subtle isoechoic malignant lesion that is surrounded by hyperechoic fibrous tissue, and thus readily visible, might be mistaken for normal isoechoic glandular tissue surrounded by fibrous elements (see Chapter 12, Fig. 12–78). In many cases, subtle isoechoic malignant lesions vibrate differently from normal isoechoic glandular tissues. Thus, power Doppler fremitus can help distinguish between benign proliferative causes of isoechoic tissue and DCIS (see Chapter 20, Figs. 20–86 and 20–87).

Observational errors can occur when malignancies only minimally enlarge ducts or lobules to a degree that is indistinguishable from the enlargement caused by FCCs or benign proliferative disorders. Diffuse or focal enlargement of central ducts can be caused by benign large duct papillo-

mas, periductal fibrosis that represents the end stage of the ductal ectasia–periductal mastitis complex, or DCIS (Fig. 21–6). Enlargement of multiple smaller branch ducts can be caused by periductal fibrosis or DCIS (Fig. 21–7). Enlarged lobules may be caused by FCC, benign proliferative disorders, atypical duct or lobular hyperplasia, or DCIS (Fig. 21–8) or lobular carcinoma *in situ* (LCIS). There is no absolutely foolproof way of distinguishing between benign and malignant causes of ductal or lobular enlargement in every case. However, it is important to take the size of other ducts and lobules in the vicinity into account when deciding how suspicious mildly enlarged ducts and lobules are. Even though FCC and benign proliferative changes are not necessarily uniform in degree throughout the breasts, these benign processes usually diffusely affect all of the ducts or lobules. Thus, it is far more suspicious for malignancy or atypia if only one of a few lobules is focally involved than if all of the ducts or lobules in the breast of concern are enlarged (Fig. 21–9). Unfortunately, this is only a general rule because some aggressive cases of DCIS or extensive intraductal components of a mixed invasive and intraductal lesion may involve essentially all of the ducts and lobules in an entire quadrant of a breast (Fig. 21–10). Mild ductal or lobular enlargement is truly on the borderlands of

(text continued on page 956)

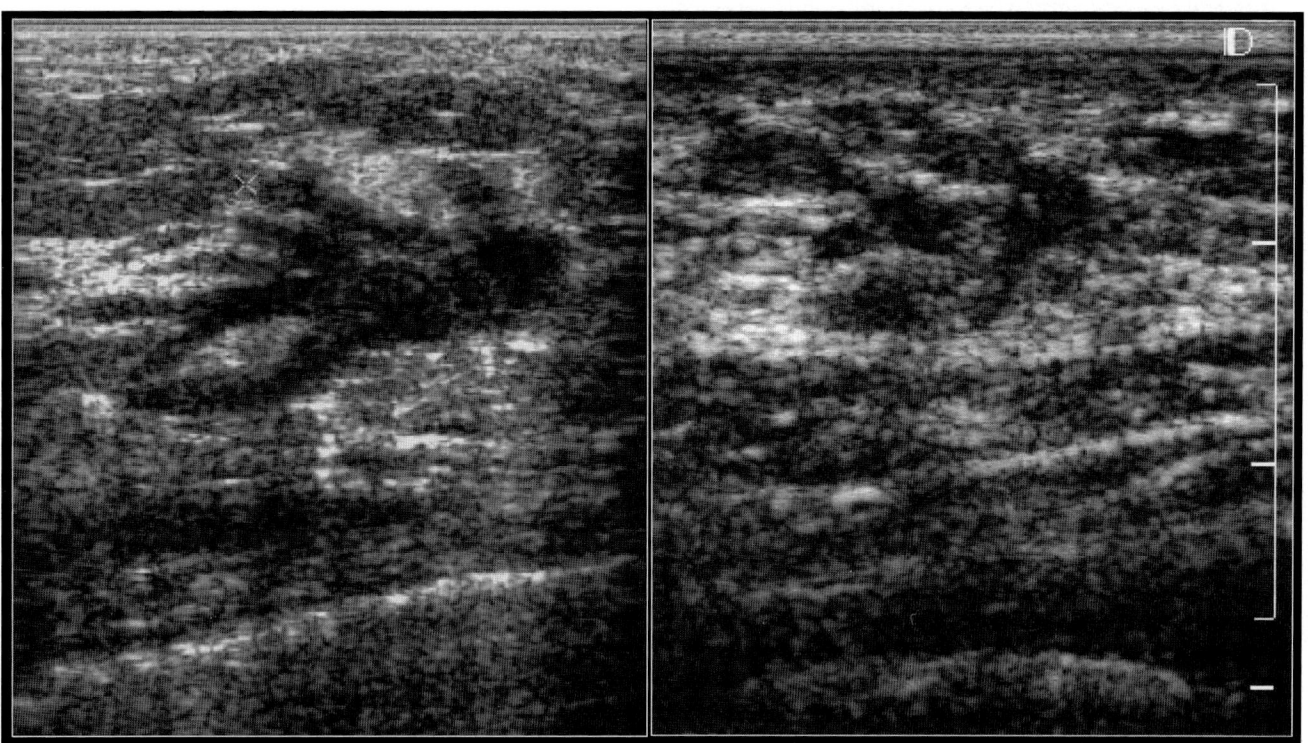

FIGURE 21–7 Similar to enlarged, echo-containing central ducts, enlarged echogenic branching peripheral ducts can be a cause of both false-positive and false-negative sonographic findings. It can be difficult to distinguish the enlarged, solid-appearing, branching ducts of ductal carcinoma *in situ* (**left**) from those of periductal fibrosis that represents the end stage of the duct ectasia periductal–mastitis complex (**right**).

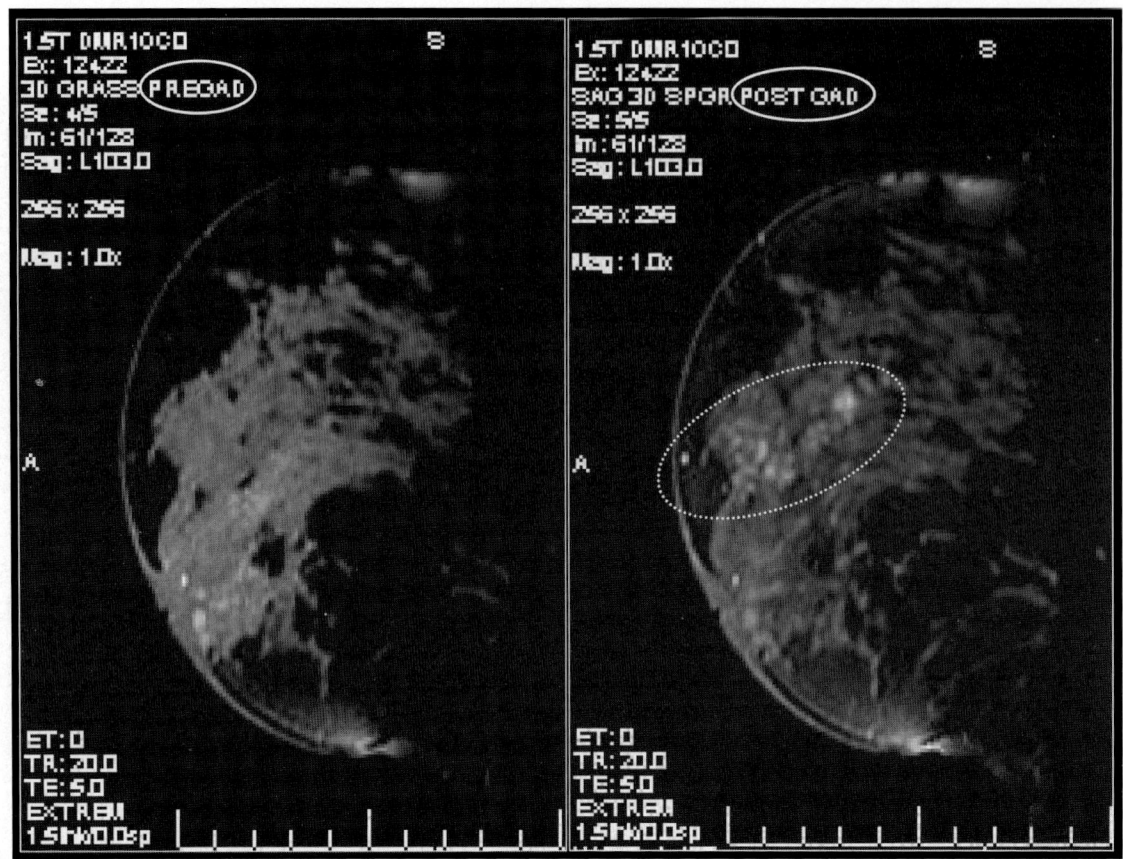

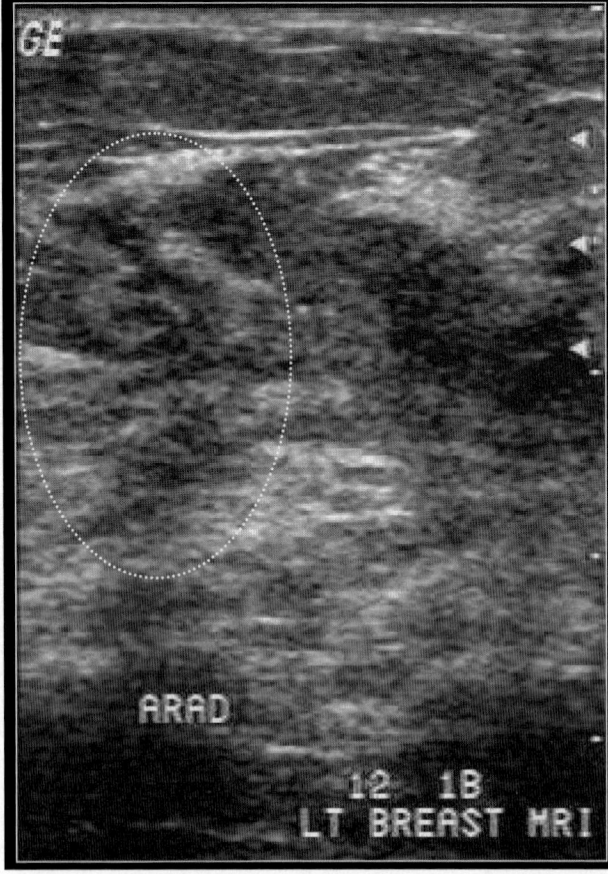

FIGURE 21–8 **A:** Magnetic resonance imaging (MRI) with rotating delivery excitation off-resonance (RODEO) before (**left**) and after (**right**) gadolinium shows a microlobulated enhancement in the upper central left breast suspicious for ductal carcinoma *in situ* (DCIS) *(dotted oval)*. **B:** Second-look sonography performed in the area of the microlobulated enhancement noted on MRI shows only nonspecific enlargement of terminal ductolobular units and distal ducts that could be caused by any of the fibrocystic or benign proliferative conditions, atypical ductal or lobular hyperplasia, or DCIS or lobular carcinoma *in situ*. However, because of enhancement on MRI and because the enlargement noted on ultrasound was mildly out of proportion to surrounding ducts and lobules, ultrasound-guided 11-gauge directional vacuum-assisted biopsy was performed and showed intermediate-grade DCIS.

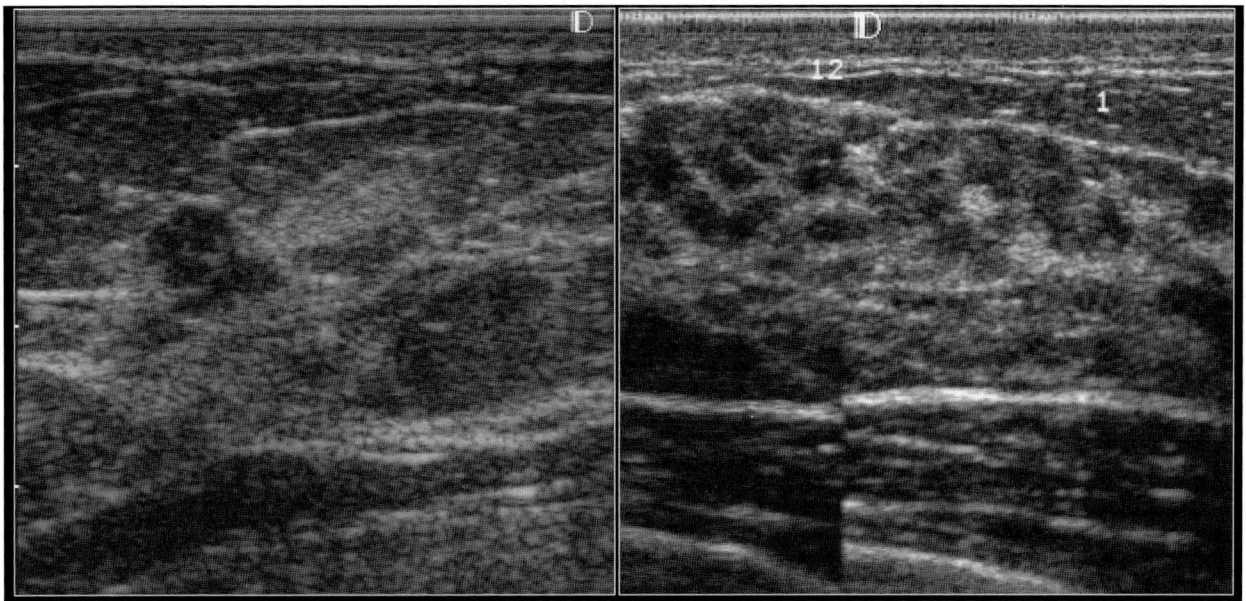

FIGURE 21-9 Mild enlargement of terminal ductolobular units (TDLUs) is nonspecific and most commonly represents some form of fibrocystic change or benign proliferative disorder. Therefore, mild enlargement of TDLUs must be interpreted in light of the prominence of the lobules elsewhere in the breasts. Focal enlargement of one TDLU or a cluster of TDLUs that is out of proportion to the surrounding lobules (**left**) should always be viewed with more suspicion than the case in which all of the lobules in both breasts are enlarged (**right**).

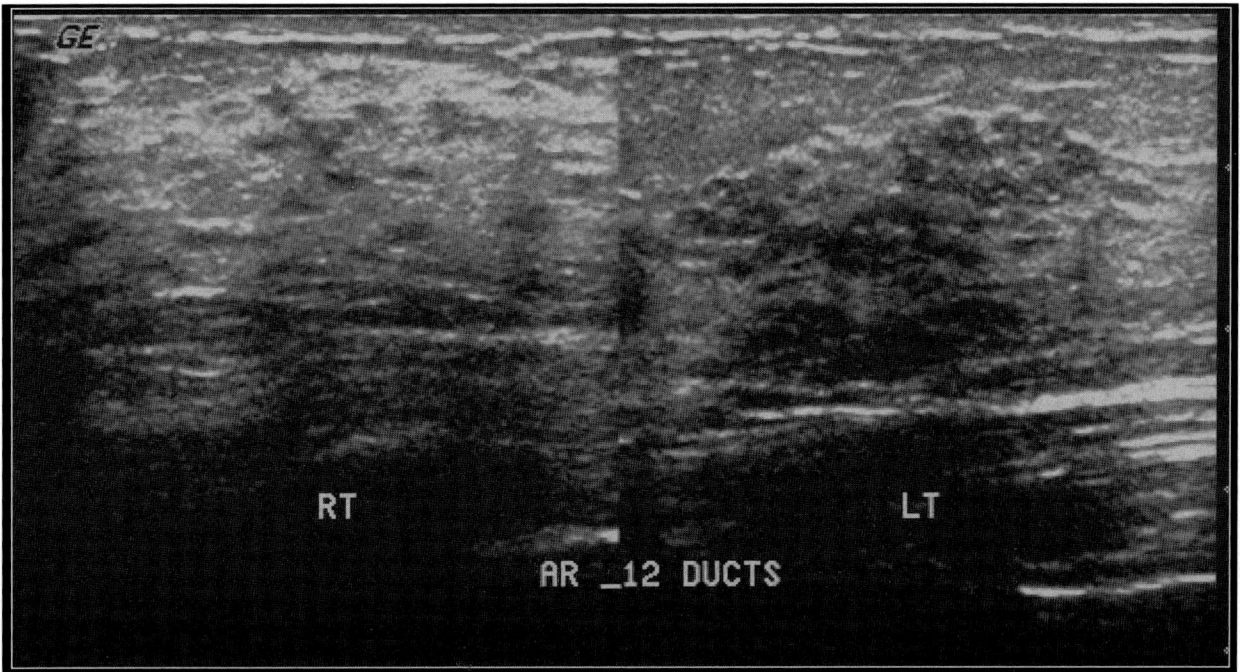

FIGURE 21-10 Although ductal carcinoma *in situ* (DCIS) typically causes focal enlargement of ducts and lobules, some particularly aggressive lesions can enlarge all of the lobules in an entire lobe. Split-screen images of the contralateral mirror-image location or of other quadrants in the ipsilateral breast may help to avoid misinterpreting such involvement as benign. Split-screen mirror-image scans of the 12:00 regions in this patient with a palpable lump show markedly asymmetric enlargement of ducts and lobules on the left (**right**) compared with the mirror-image contralateral location (**left**). Note also that the ducts and lobules on the left appear too numerous compared with the right side. High-nuclear-grade DCIS may form entirely new ducts, and this finding strongly suggests high-nuclear-grade DCIS, which biopsy subsequently proved.

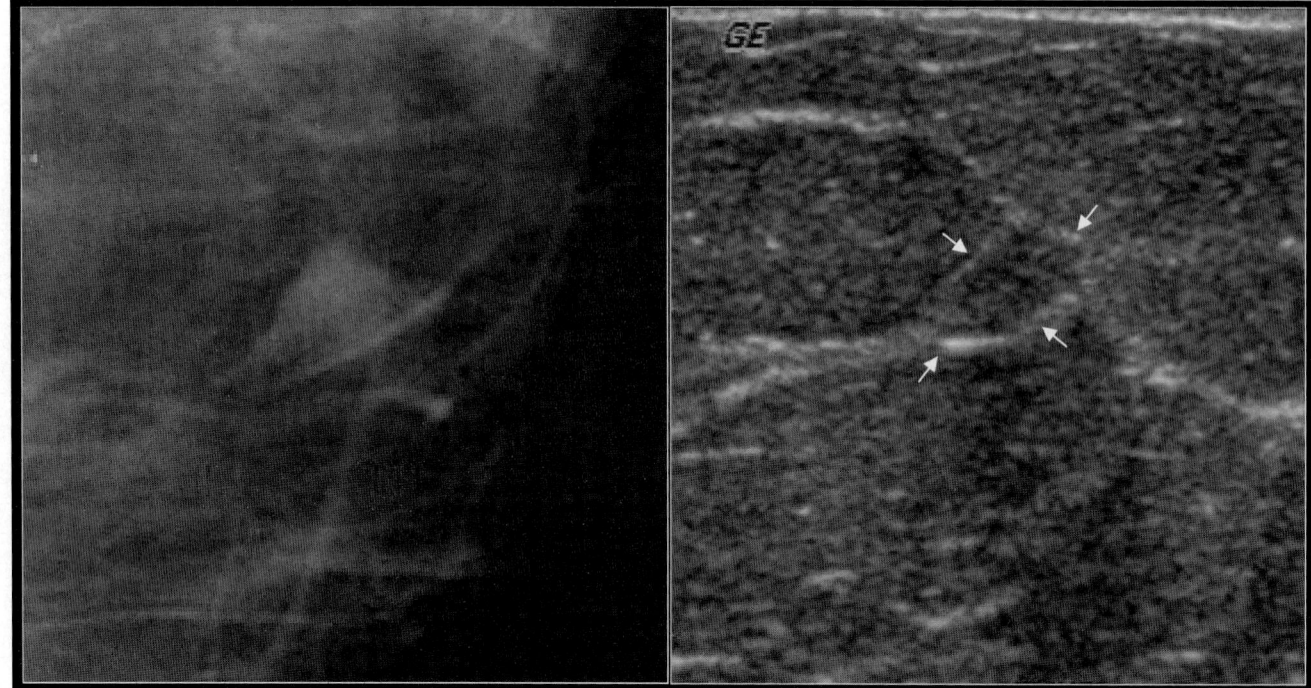

FIGURE 21–11 Some solid nodules that are isoechoic with fat are very difficult to demonstrate sonographically even though they are easily seen mammographically. In such cases, the best way to identify the nodule is to look for its hyperechoic capsule *(arrows)*.

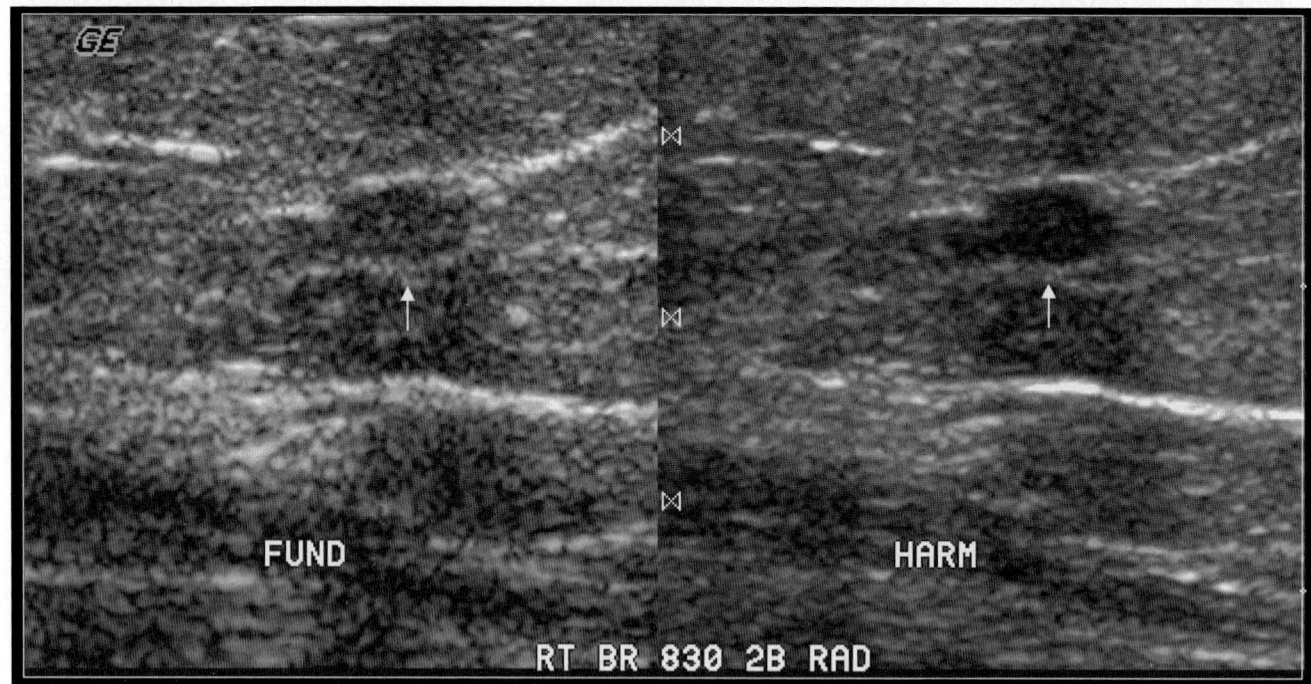

FIGURE 21–12 High-frequency coded harmonics helps identify nodules that are isoechoic with surrounding fat or glandular tissue and therefore difficult to identify with fundamental imaging **(left)** by suppressing speckle and other artifacts and making the nodule appear more hypoechoic in most cases **(right)**. Harmonics holds promise for reducing false-negative findings in patients who have subtle isoechoic solid nodules if used in all cases in which penetration is adequate.

normal—inhabited by the entire spectrum of breast pathology. Mild enlargement of ducts or lobules represents the inflection point of the ROC curve, the point at which the false-positive findings trouble us the most. Once the prominence of background ducts and lobules are taken into account, one must err on the side of caution in such cases, characterize the lesions as BIRADS 4, and recommend biopsy. The risk for a false negative finding is higher in cases in which ducts and lobules are focally enlarged than it is with discrete solid nodules that are characterized by a strict algorithmic approach using multiple findings.

Observational error can also sometimes occur when mammography shows a well-circumscribed nodule surrounded by fat that is isoechoic and therefore inconspicuous on sonography. Failure to demonstrate the cause of a discrete well-circumscribed isodense or hyperdense mammographic fat-surrounded nodule more than 5 mm in maximum diameter is strong indirect evidence that the nodule is an isoechoic solid nodule, not a cyst. The best way to identify such lesions is to look for the thin, echogenic capsule and surrounding landmarks such as Cooper's ligaments (Fig. 21–11; see also Chapter 6, Fig. 6–35). Coded harmonics might also be helpful because many nodules that appear to be isoechoic with fundamental imaging appear to

be hypoechoic when scanned with high-frequency coded harmonics (Fig. 21–12; see also Chapter 2, Fig. 2–19).

Malignant lesions that are well visualized mammographically, but isoechoic with fat and difficult to identify sonographically, include small colloid carcinomas, a small percentage of intermediate-grade invasive ductal carcinomas, and intermediate-nuclear-grade DCIS. Most large colloid carcinomas (>1.5 cm) demonstrate enhanced through-transmission. However, the lack of enhanced sound transmission in about half of colloid carcinomas less than 1.5 cm in maximum diameter makes their identification more difficult (Fig. 21–13). DCIS and intermediate-grade invasive not otherwise specified (NOS) carcinomas contain sonographically visible calcifications that prevent false-negative sonography in about 75% and 50% of cases, respectively (Figs. 21–14 and 21–15). However, calcifications do not help identify colloid carcinomas, which seldom contain calcifications.

Malignant Lesions Simulating Normal Structures

Some malignant nodules may escape detection by simulating normal solid components of the breast or definitively benign findings.

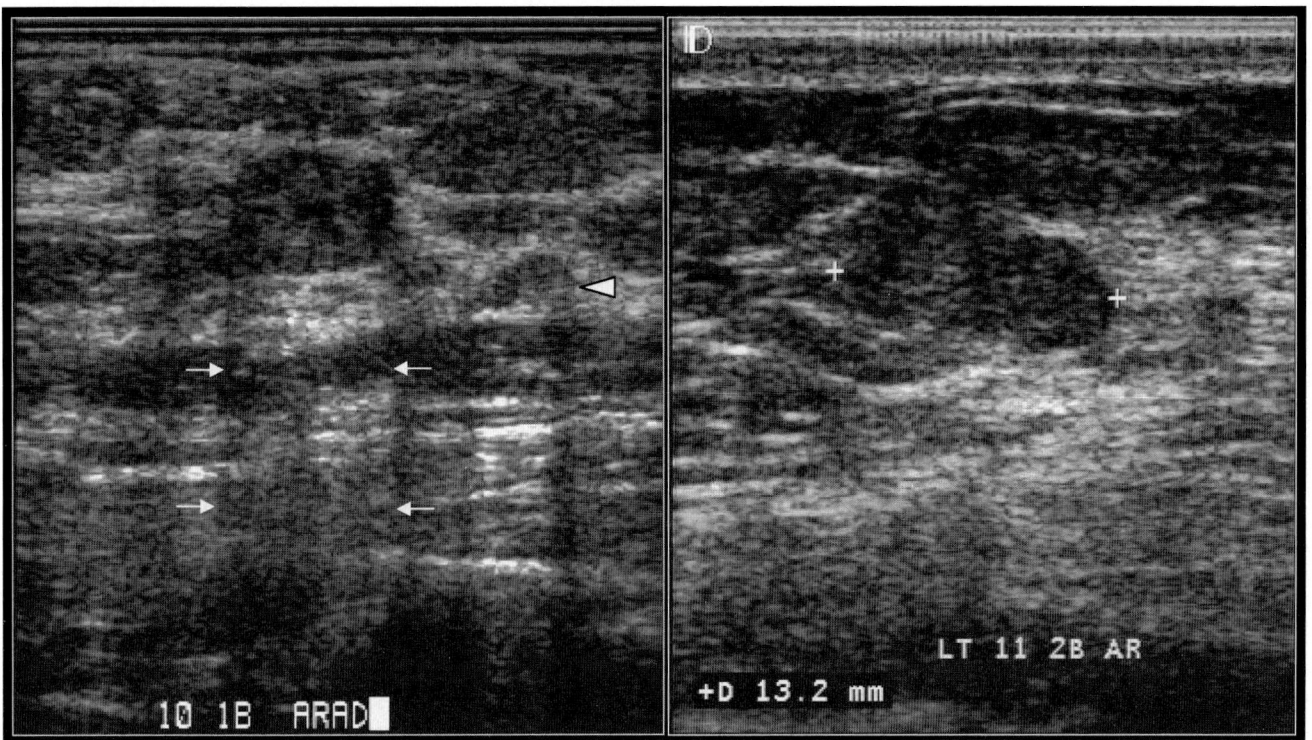

FIGURE 21–13 Colloid carcinomas are typically isoechoic to fat and glandular tissue and therefore difficult to identify. All colloid carcinomas larger than 1.5 cm in diameter and about half of smaller colloid carcinomas demonstrate enhanced though-transmission of sound, which can help distinguish them from surrounding fatty tissue (**left**, *arrows*). Note the second, smaller lesion that is distinguishable from fat only by its enhanced through-transmission (**left**, *arrowhead*). The chances of not identifying a small colloid carcinoma are higher if does not have enhanced through-transmission (**right**, *calipers*).

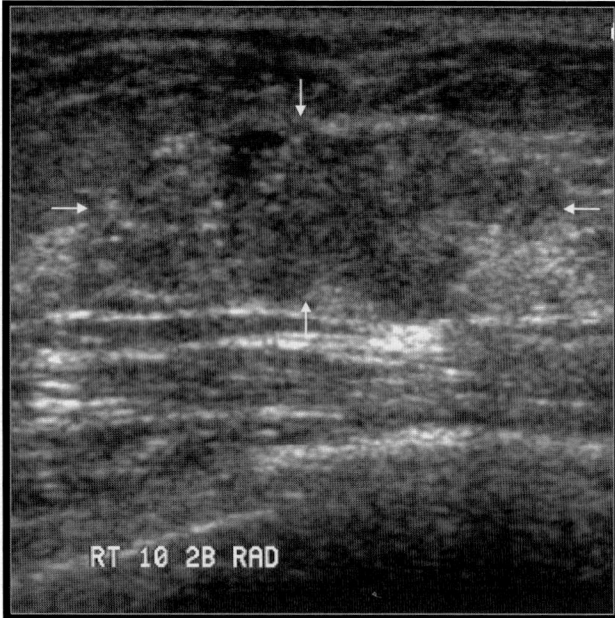

FIGURE 21–14 *Intermediate-nuclear-grade ductal carcinoma* in situ *(DCIS) is typically isoechoic and can be very difficult to distinguish from isoechoic glandular tissue and fat (arrows). However, calcifications occur in 75% of such cases, allowing identification on mammography. Sonography is capable of showing punctate echoes that do not shadow in about 80% of the cases in which mammography shows calcifications. Note that in this case, the calcifications are visible in the left half of the DICS, but not in the right half.*

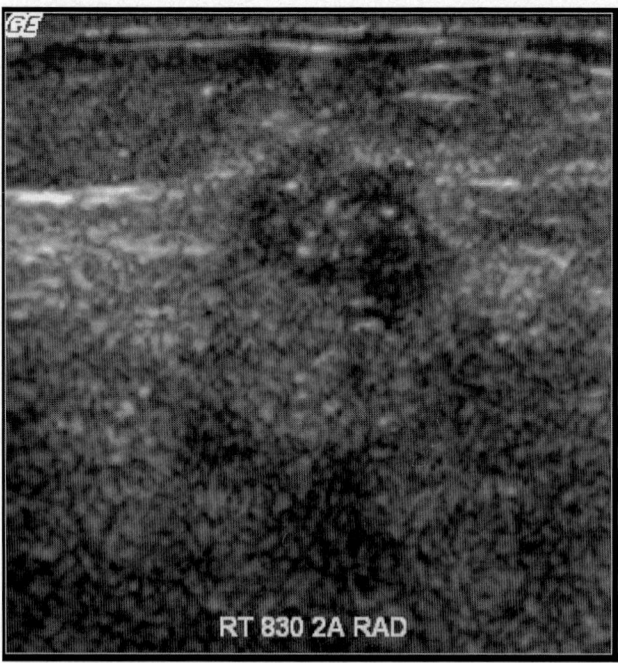

FIGURE 21–15 *Calcifications that lie within isoechoic solid malignant nodules can help to identify such lesions sonographically. Intermediate-grade invasive carcinoma is isoechoic in most cases and contains calcifications about half of the time. The calcifications make the nodule more apparent than it would be without calcifications.*

Circumscribed Ellipsoid or Gently Lobulated Lesions Simulating Fat Lobules

Fat lobules and lipomas can cause both false-negative and false-positive findings at sonography. Fat lobules can be falsely interpreted to represent solid nodules, leading to false-positive results. More important, malignant lesions can be misinterpreted as being fat lobules, leading to false-negative results. Because the relative cost of false-negative findings is much higher than the cost of false-positive findings, fat lobules are included in the section on false-negative examinations.

Most malignant solid breast nodules have obviously suspicious characteristics and are easily distinguishable from fat lobules or benign lipomas. However, a few malignant nodules, especially metastatic lesions, can simulate normal structures such as fat lobules. Fibroadenomas more commonly simulate fat lobules than do carcinomas. Both fibroadenomas and fat lobules tend to be well encapsulated, elliptically shaped or gently lobulated, and isoechoic and uniform in texture. Distinguishing between fat lobules and true solid pathologic nodules in the breast is most difficult when a fat lobule is completely or almost completely encompassed by echogenic fibrous tissue that separates it from other fat within the breast (entrapped fatty lobule).

There are techniques and findings that help to distinguish benign or malignant solid breast nodules from normal fat lobules or lipomas that are effective in most patients. Compression of the lesion is very useful. Fat lobules are soft and compressible to a greater degree than either fibroadenomas or malignant nodules in almost all cases. Fat lobules usually compress about 25% to 50%, depending on how much they are buttressed by firmer surrounding fibrous elements. Fat-surrounded isoechoic lipomas (see Chapter 3, Fig. 3–15) and fat lobules (see Chapter 4, Figs. 4–36 and 4–39) frequently compress more than 30%. Fat lobules or lipomas that are completely surrounded and buttressed by dense hyperechoic interlobular stromal fibrous tissue are generally slightly less compressible, usually in the range of 25% to 30% (Figs. 21–16). Additionally, hyperechoic lipomas have a higher fibrous content than do isoechoic lipomas and therefore are sometimes slightly less than 30% compressible (see Chapter 13, Fig. 13–70). Fibroadenomas, on the other hand, are less compressible. Fibroadenomas range from 0% to 25% compressible in most cases, depending on the cellularity of the stroma. Typical paucicellular fibroadenomas with sclerotic or hyalinized stroma are usually minimally compressible or incompressible, in the range of 0% to 15% (see Chapter 3, Fig. 3–13), but those with cellular or myxoid stroma may be as much as 20% to 25% compressible (Fig. 21–17). Most malignant nodules are completely incompressible (Fig. 21–18), but highly cellular circumscribed carcinomas can be 5% to 15% compressible (see Chapter 3, Fig. 3–14), similar in degree of compressibility to some fibroadenomas, but less compressible than

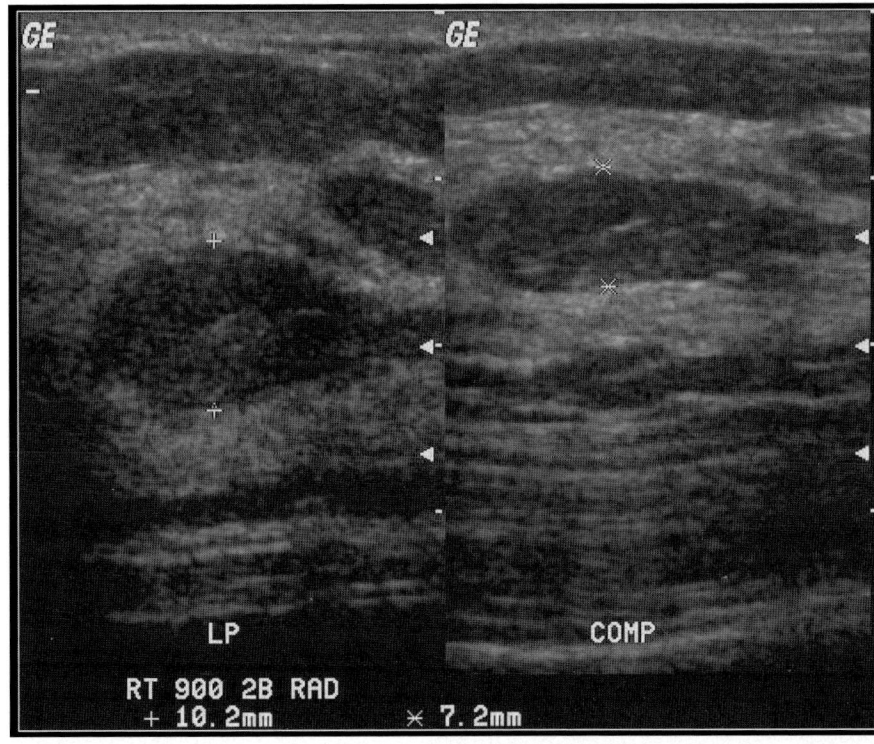

FIGURE 21–16 The surrounding tissues affect the compressibility of a structure. Fat lobules or lipomas that are completely encompassed in and buttressed by surrounding dense hyperechoic fibrous tissue are usually less compressible than are fat lobules or lipomas that are surrounded only by fat. Split-screen images with light compression (**left**) and heavy compression (**right**) show this fibrous-surrounded fat lobule to be less than 33% compressible.

fat lobules or lipomas. Malignant nodules that contain relatively little desmoplasia or cystic components or that have undergone liquefactive necrosis are those most likely to be mildly compressible. Such lesions include pure DCIS; special-type tumors such as papillary carcinoma, mucinous carcinoma, and medullary carcinoma; and high-grade invasive NOS carcinomas.

Compressibility is a useful method of distinguishing fat lobules or lipomas from more significant solid nodules.

However, in our experience, the compressibility of fibroadenomas and carcinomas overlaps too much for it to be useful in distinguishing between them.

The effect of compression on surrounding structures can also be assessed. Both fibroadenomas and malignant solid breast nodules compress and distort surrounding normal breast structures when compression is applied (Fig. 21–19; see also Chapter 3, Fig. 3–16, and Chapter 4, Fig. 4–37). On the other hand, even vigorous compression will

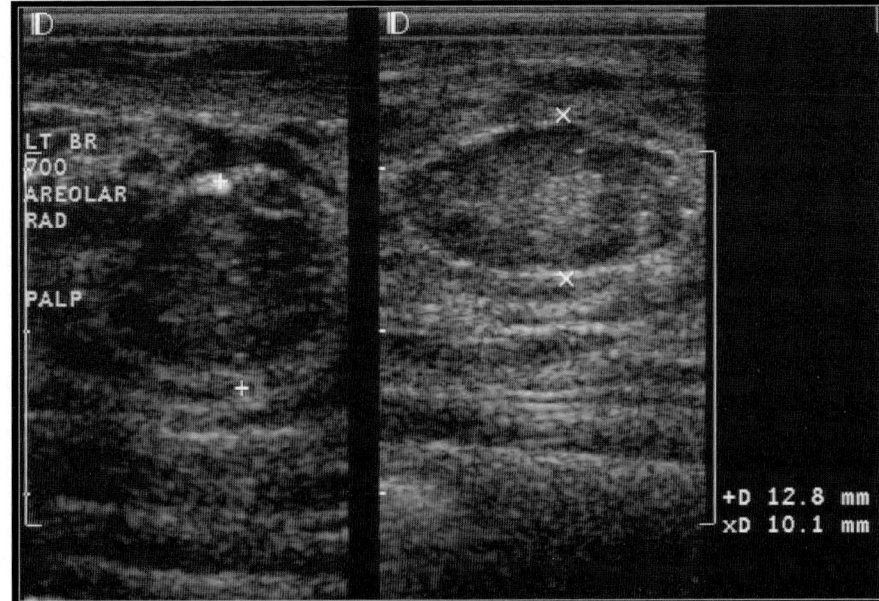

FIGURE 21–17 This myxoid fibroadenoma is 21% compressible. Highly cellular fibroadenomas or fibroadenomas with myxoid stroma can occasionally be compressed slightly more than 20% but will not compress the 30% or more that fat lobules or lipomas do.

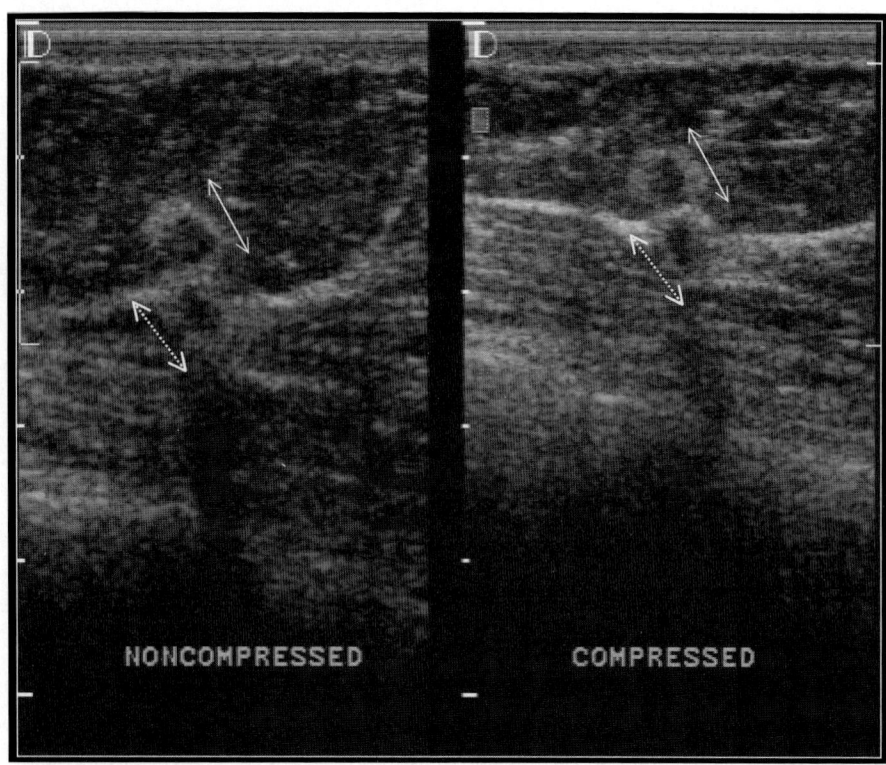

FIGURE 21–18 Like most carcinomas, these multifocal intermediate-grade invasive not otherwise specified carcinomas are incompressible. Although the individual nodules are incompressible, the compression has pushed the two nodules closer to each other.

alter the shape of a fat lobule, but the fat lobule will not indent or distort the surrounding structure (Fig. 21–20).

Fat lobules are rarely completely encompassed by fibroglandular elements. They usually communicate with

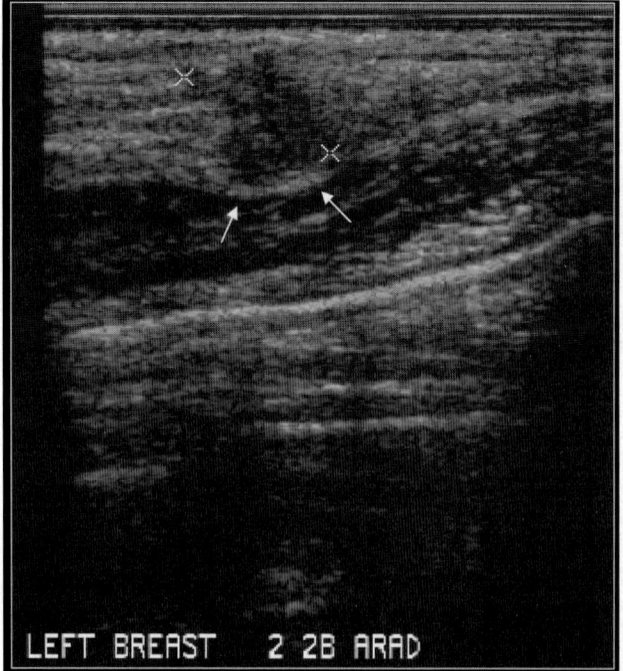

FIGURE 21–19 This carcinoma, like a fibroadenoma, will indent the pectoralis muscle when it is compressed with the transducer.

other fat lobules in the subcutaneous or retromammary fat zones (see Chapter 4, Fig. 4–35). Fibroadenomas and malignant solid nodules do not show such communication.

Finally, fat lobules often have a demonstrable thin, straight, well-circumscribed echogenic line within them, whose long axis is parallel to the skin (see Chapter 4, Fig. 4–38). This echogenic line represents a two-dimensional sheet, a fibrous septum that separates the fat lobule into smaller lobules. Normally, this septation is curved and makes a poor specular reflector. However, when the fat lobule is compressed, the septation straightens, becomes a better specular reflector, and is easier to identify (see Chapter 4, Fig. 4–39). Although there may be foci of increased echogenicity with both malignant breast nodules, the hyperechoic structure does not have the well-circumscribed linearity seen within fat lobules (see Chapter 14, Fig. 14–57). Occasional fibroadenomas contain fibrous septations (reported as nonenhancing fibrous septations in the magnetic resonance imaging literature) that can simulate the septation within fat lobules (see Chapter 4, Fig. 4–40). Microbubbles within the needle tract of solid nodules that are undergoing ultrasound-guided core needle biopsies can present as straight echogenic lines (see Chapter 4, Fig. 4–41). They are demonstrable only as an echogenic dot when scanned nearly perpendicular to the needle tract. The compressed hilum or mediastinum of abnormal lymph nodes can simulate the straight echogenic line seen within fat lobules in rare cases (see Chapter 19, Figs. 19–39, 19–47, and 19–48).

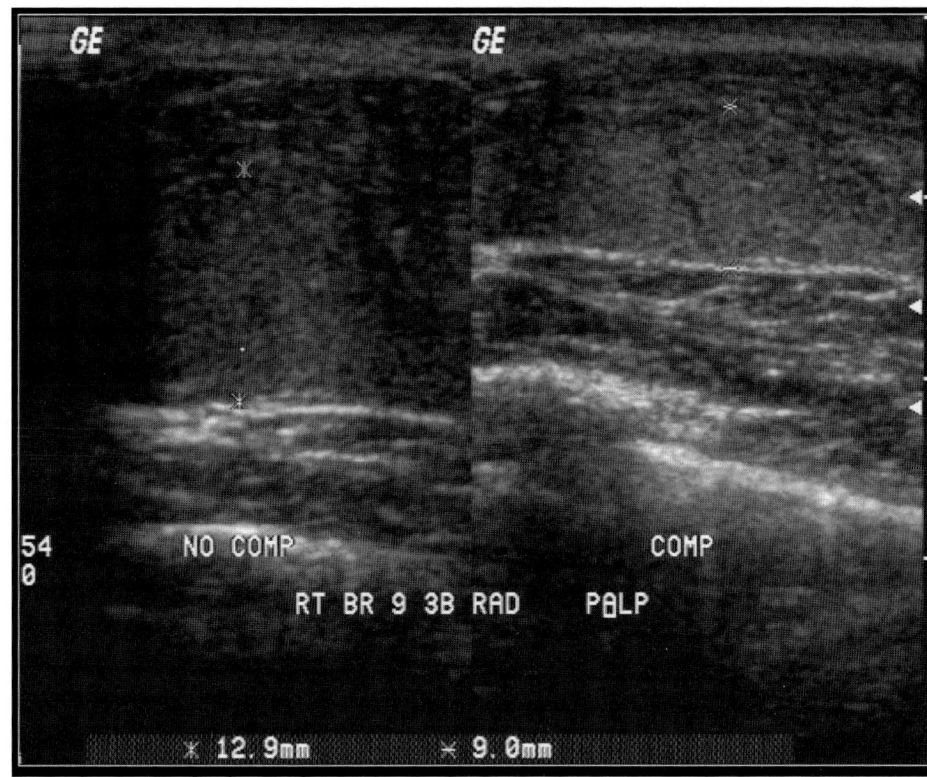

FIGURE 21–20 Fat lobules and lipomas are softer than the pectoralis muscle, regardless of how vigorously they are compressed, and therefore cannot induct the pectoris muscles during compressions.

Power Doppler fremitus can also be helpful in distinguishing between a solid breast nodule and an entrapped fatty lobule. True solid nodules such as fibroadenomas and carcinomas cause defects in the vibratory power Doppler artifact (see Chapter 20, Fig. 20–88), whereas fat-entrapped fatty lobules that simulate solid nodules generally do not (see Chapter 20, Fig. 20–89).

Echogenic Halo around Small Infiltrative Lesions Simulating Fibrous Tissue

Normal interlobular stromal fibrous tissue in the breast is intensely hyperechoic. Normal interlobular stromal fibrous tissue or focal fibrosis can cause both mammographic and palpable abnormalities in the breast. When sonography demonstrates hyperechoic tissue as the cause of a mammographic or palpable abnormality, the negative predictive value is nearly 100%. However, careful attention to detail is necessary to avoid false-negative results. Some very small, low-grade, infiltrating malignancies can have a small hypoechoic central nidus that is surrounded by an echogenic halo that is much larger than the central nidus. We have already discussed how near-field volume averaging can cause such a lesion to be mistaken for one that is purely hyperechoic. Errantly obtaining tangential images through the thick, echogenic halo and not demonstrating the hypoechoic central nidus can also falsely make such lesions appear to be purely hyperechoic (see Chapter 12, Fig. 12–81). To avoid making this mistake, it is important to scan the entire echogenic structure in three dimensions to make sure that there are no isoechoic or hypoechoic areas within the hyperechoic area larger than normal ducts or terminal ductolobular units (TDLUs). Only structures that are purely echogenic can be assumed to be normal fibrous tissue or focal fibrosis. Most women have at least some hyperechoic fibrous tissue, and simply showing that hyperechoic fibrous tissue exists in the same quadrant as the mammographic abnormality does not constitute adequate proof that the fibrous tissue is the cause of the mammographic density. Only if size, shape, location, and surrounding tissue density correspond can such a conclusion be made. Split-screen imaging of mirror-image right and left locations is helpful in confirming focal fibrous asymmetries (see Chapter 3, Fig. 3–12). For hyperechoic fibrous tissue to have a 100% negative predictive value, it should contain no isoechoic areas larger than normal ducts or 2 mm or smaller TDLUs.

Finally, some diffusely infiltrative lesions, such as infiltrating lobular carcinoma, can present as an ill-defined area of grayness within a larger area of hyperechoic fibrous tissue (see Chapter 14, Fig. 14–95). In other cases, an ill-defined peripheral zone of isoechoic tissue that represents diffuse infiltration at the edges of the lesion surrounds a discrete central hypoechoic nodule. Not recognizing that the peripheral isoechoic zone represents diffusely infiltrating components of the lesion can lead to underestimation of its true size (see Chapter 14, Fig. 14–93).

Shadowing from Malignancy Simulating Shadowing from Normal Breast Structures

Like fat lobules, acoustic shadowing can lead to both false-negative and false-positive sonography. If acoustic shadowing caused by critical angle phenomena arising from Cooper's ligaments or other obliquely oriented tissue planes is misinterpreted as being caused by breast carcinoma, a false-positive examination is the result. On the other hand, if acoustic shadowing that is caused by a desmoplastic breast carcinoma is misinterpreted as being artifactual, a false-negative examination can be the result. As is the case for fat lobules, the cost of false-negative diagnosis is much higher than the cost of false-positive diagnosis; hence, real versus artifactual shadowing is discussed in the false-negative examination section of this chapter.

Error can also occur in a breast that has areas of shadowing due to interfaces between fibrous tissue and fat lobules. Certain small, diffusely infiltrating lesions, such as infiltrating lobular carcinoma, can present with shadowing but no measurable discrete mass (Fig. 21–21). Analyzing the width of shadowing in orthogonal planes can be helpful. Most areas of shadowing due to normal breast structures are a result of sloping thin fibrous septae within the breast. Such septae shadow more intensely when the beam is parallel to their long axis. However, when the beam is perpendicular to the shadowing septum, there is only a very narrow linear shadow. Shadowing that arises from surgical scars, likewise, is narrow in the axis that is perpendicular to the scar (see Chapter 18, Fig. 18–25). Diffusely infiltrating malignancies, on the other hand, have wide shadows in both orthogonal planes (Fig. 21–22).

An additional method of evaluating areas of shadowing is to assess the effects of compression. Because shadowing due to normal fibrous septae within the breast is often due to the reflection and refraction from the oblique orientation of such tissue planes, angulating the transducer so that the angle of incidence is more nearly perpendicular to the shadowing structure can reduce or eradicate shadowing (see Chapter 3, Fig. 3–6). Using heavier compression pressure while scanning can also help. Compression of the breast with a linear probe pushes these shadowing tissue planes or Cooper's ligaments into planes that are more nearly parallel to the transducer face and more nearly perpendicular to the ultrasound beam, minimizing critical angle shadowing (see Chapter 3, Fig. 3–5). Shadowing that goes away with compression is usually due to normal breast structures. On the other hand, shadowing that has nearly equal dimensions in orthogonal planes and that does not go away with compression is more worrisome for malignancy. In some cases, artifactual acoustic shadowing is a byproduct of the very light scan pressure that is used to better demonstrate the thin, echogenic capsule around benign fibroadenomas (see Chapter 12, Fig. 12–92).

Power Doppler vocal fremitus can also be helpful in distinguishing between real and artifactual shadowing. The vibrations that create the typical power Doppler fremitus artifact tend to fill areas of artifactual shadowing all the way to the normal anatomic structure that creates the artifactual shadow (see Chapter 20, Fig. 20–90). On the other hand, power Doppler fremitus artifact fills the acoustic shadow only to the edges of the malignant nodule that is associated with the shadowing (Fig. 21–23).

Malignant Lesions Simulating Benign Lesions

Finally, there are numerous benign pathologic processes that affect the breast. There often is some overlap in the sonographic appearances of benign and malignant processes, causing both false-negative and false-positive diagnoses.

Circumscribed, Elliptically Shaped or Gently Lobulated Lesions Simulating Fibroadenoma

Lesions that had no suspicious features and met strict criteria for the BIRADS 3 category were, in fact, benign more than 99.5% of the time in the series presented in Chapter 11. This means that only about one-half of one percent of the time, lesions that meet strict criteria for BIRADS 3 category represent unusual malignancies. Lesions that

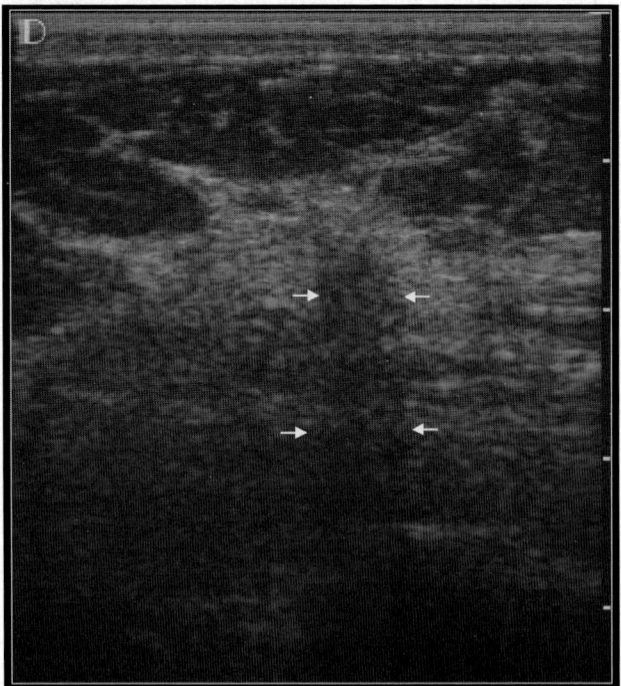

FIGURE 21–21 Certain breast malignancies, such as this small classic invasive lobular carcinoma, do not form a discrete mass and are detectable sonographically because they cause a focus of acoustic shadowing *(arrows)*.

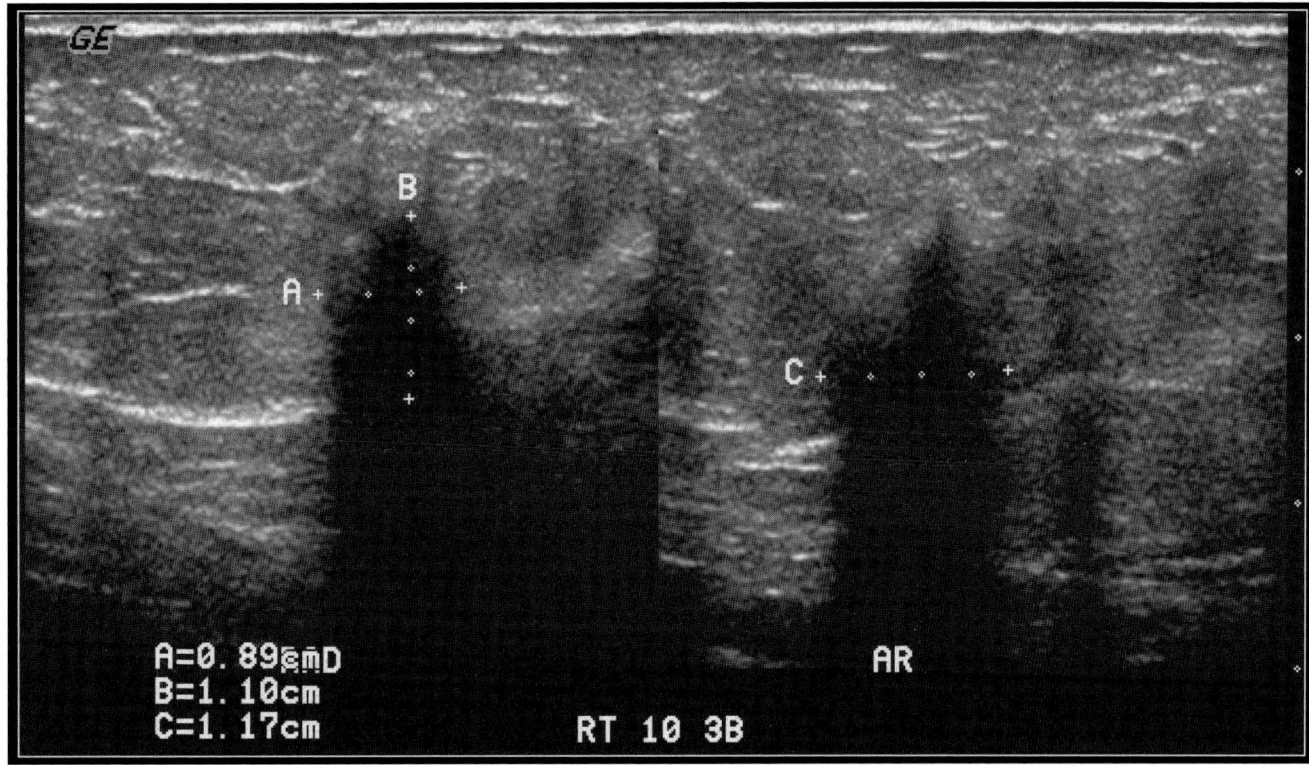

FIGURE 21–22 This invasive carcinoma has wide acoustic shadows in both radial and antiradial planes.

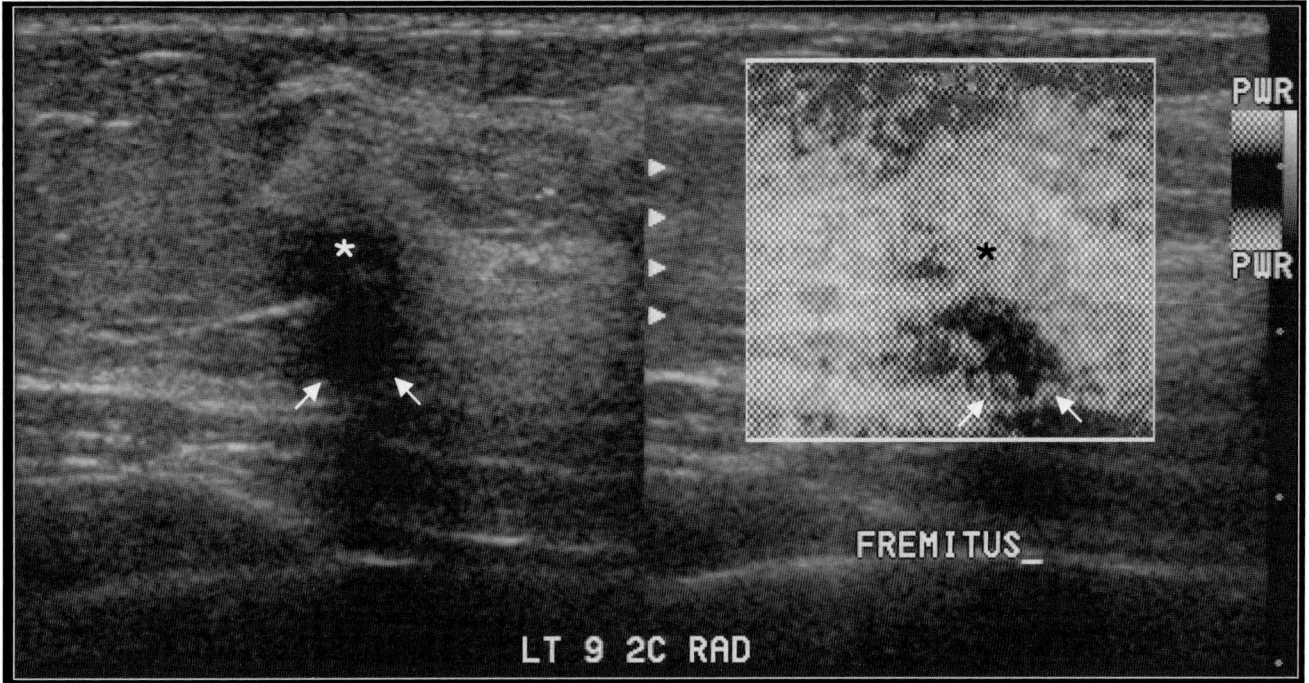

FIGURE 21–23 The **left** image shows an area of acoustic shadowing posterior to a collection of hyperechoic fibrous tissue that could not be ablated with vigorous compression pressure. The **right** image shows a defect in the acoustic vibratory power Doppler artifact *(arrows)*, indicating the presence of a lesion that was obscured by artifactual shadowing *(*)* that arose from the more superficially located fibrous elements.

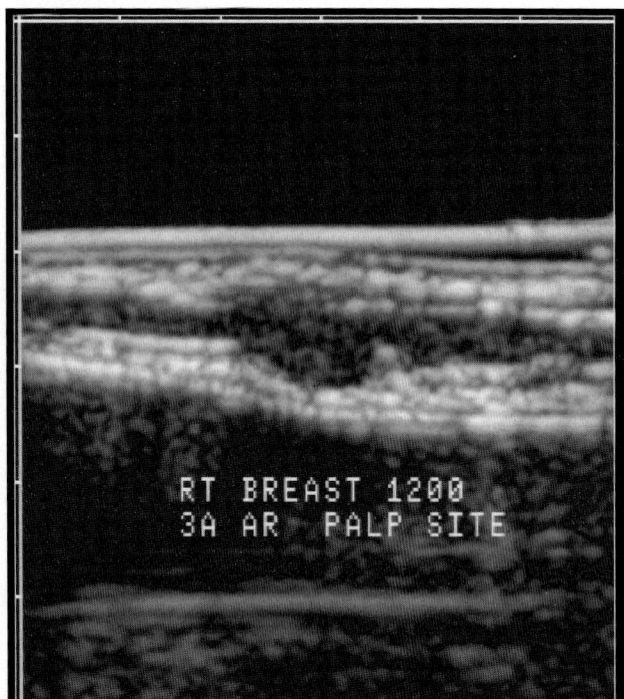

FIGURE 21–24 In less than 2% of cases, invasive not otherwise specified carcinomas might lack specific suspicious features. Such lesions might be mischaracterized as BIRADS 3, leading to false-negative sonography findings. This nodule lacks suspicious features and is ovoid in shape, but does not have the complete thin, echogenic capsule that is required for BIRADS 3 classification. Thus, it was mischaracterized. Note also that a standoff was required because of the extreme near-field location of the lesion.

simulate benign nodules usually lie at the circumscribed end of the malignant spectrum. Small infiltrating ductal carcinomas (Fig. 21–24); high-grade invasive NOS carcinomas (see Chapter 14, Fig. 14–43); metastatic lesions, especially to intramammary lymph nodes (see Chapter 20, Fig. 20–26); and special-type tumors that are well circumscribed, such as medullary carcinomas (Fig. 21–25; see also Chapter 14, Fig. 14–70) and colloid carcinomas (Fig. 21–26; see also Chapter 14, Fig. 14–74), are the lesions most likely to simulate BIRADS 3 nodules. Additionally, high-nuclear-grade DCIS with extensive necrosis can present as a cluster of microcysts that simulates benign fibrocystic change (FCC) (see Chapter 10, Fig. 10–9). Most of these lesions have at least one suspicious feature that will prevent false-negative findings if examined carefully and that will be detected and prevent error only if the algorithm presented in Chapter 11 is rigidly followed. Our data show that using gut-feeling characterization rather than a strict algorithmic approach results in at least 3% of malignant lesions being mischaracterized as BIRADS 3, probably benign.

Echogenic, Enlarged, Tumor-filled Ducts Simulating Ductal Ectasia with Inspissated Secretions

Dilated, fluid-filled mammary ducts are frequently encountered in the subareolar to periareolar location during the course of breast ultrasound. In most cases, these enlarged ducts are asymptomatic and are not associated with nipple discharge or findings of acute or chronic plasma cell mastitis and therefore should be considered variations of normal anatomy. However, the secretions within such dilated ducts can become inspissated and appear echogenic rather than anechoic on ultrasound. In such cases, it may be difficult to distinguish solid intraductal malignant tumor (DCIS or papilloma) from inspissated echogenic secretions. Intraductal tumor (DCIS) that causes echoes within a prominent duct might be assumed to represent inspissated secretions, lead-

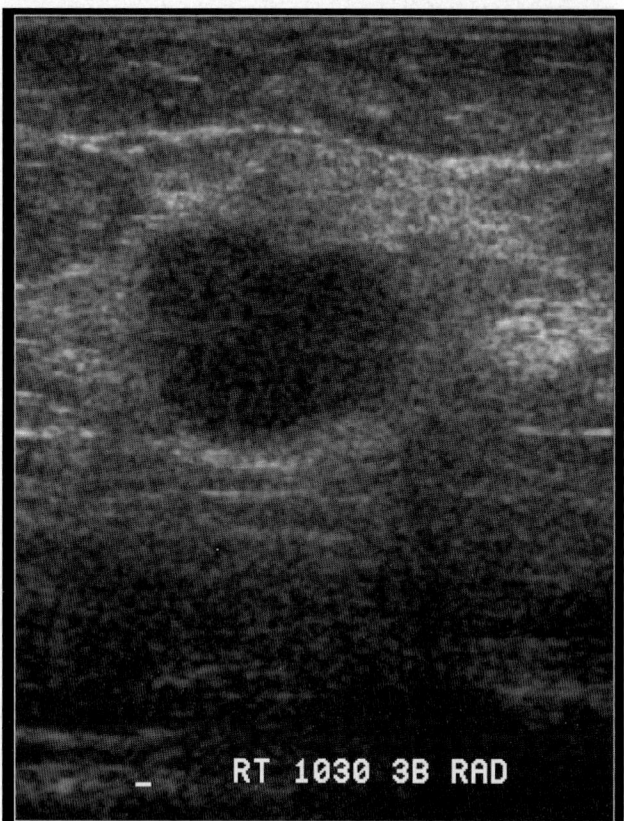

FIGURE 21–25 Medullary carcinomas are well-circumscribed lesions that are usually encompassed in a thin, echogenic capsule around most of their surface and are prone to mischaracterization as BIRADS 3 and sonographic false-negative diagnosis. It is essential to assess the entire surface area and volume of such lesions before concluding that there are no suspicious features. There are usually suspicious features such as angular margins, microlobulations, and a thick halo that affect one surface of medullary carcinomas. Errors in characterization of such lesions are most likely to occur when only two views of the lesion are obtained for interpretation.

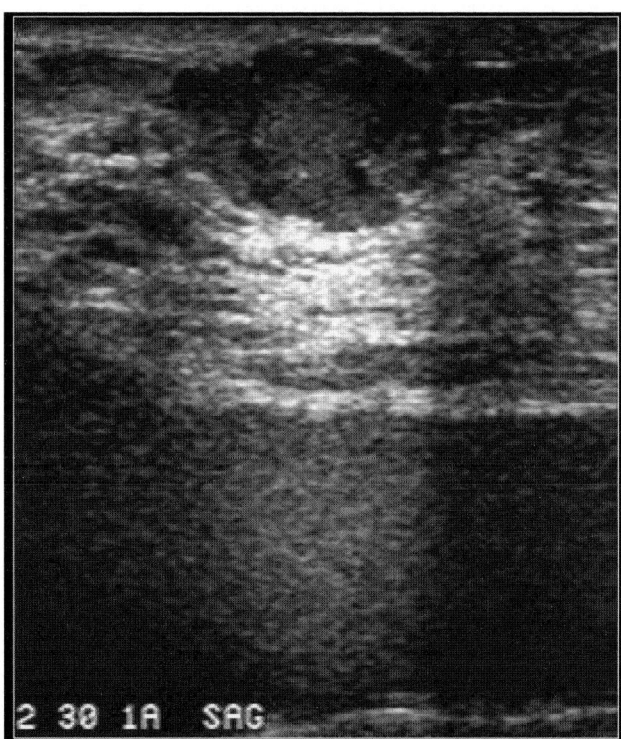

FIGURE 21–26 Similar to medullary carcinomas, colloid carcinomas can be well circumscribed and thinly encapsulated over most of their surfaces. As is the case with medullary carcinomas, at least one surface of the nodule usually has gross invasion that leads to suspicious findings; thus, it is important that the entire surface area and volume of the lesion be scanned before concluding that there are no suspicious features.

ing to a false-negative sonographic diagnosis. The echogenic secretions can be distributed evenly throughout the duct lumen, simulating DCIS or papilloma filling the entire duct (see Chapter 8, Fig. 8–42); a fluid–debris level, simulating a proximal intraductal papillary lesion (see Chapter 8, Fig. 8–34); or a fat–fluid level, simulating a distal intraductal papillary lesion (Fig. 21–27).

There are a few maneuvers that the sonographer or sonologist can use to help avoid this error. First, the duct can be balloted with the probe. Movement of the inspissated secretions back and forth within the duct can sometimes be demonstrated on real-time ultrasound during this maneuver (see Chapter 8, Figs. 8–22 and 8–35). Second, color Doppler can be used to document the movement of echogenic secretions with the ballottement maneuver in real time and can also be used to document such movement on a single hard-copy or soft-copy image. The secretions generally are forced posteriorly during the compression and return superficially when compression is eased (see Chapter 20, Fig. 20–36). Third, two-handed compression can be used to assess the compressibility of the echo-filled duct. Inspissated secretions, despite their

echogenicity, are compressible, and the duct caliber will usually decrease in size during this maneuver. A true intraductal papillary lesion, whether DCIS or papilloma, will usually be less compressible, preventing duct size from being decreased (see Chapter 8, Figs. 8–27, 8–65).

Finally, color Doppler may be useful in evaluating such ducts. True intraductal papillary lesions may have a demonstrable fibrovascular stalk (see Chapter 20, Fig. 20–38). Echogenic debris from ductal ectasia, whether due to high protein content, crystalline material, or floating foam cells, does not have a fibrovascular stalk. Flow within an enlarged echogenic duct strongly suggests the presence of a fibrovascular stalk and therefore a papillary lesion such as papilloma or carcinoma. Such lesions always require biopsy. On the other hand, lack of demonstrable flow is not helpful in excluding malignancy because papillary lesions may have too little flow to detect, and DCIS may not have a fibrovascular stalk. Care should be taken not to alter the degree of compression on the duct during color Doppler

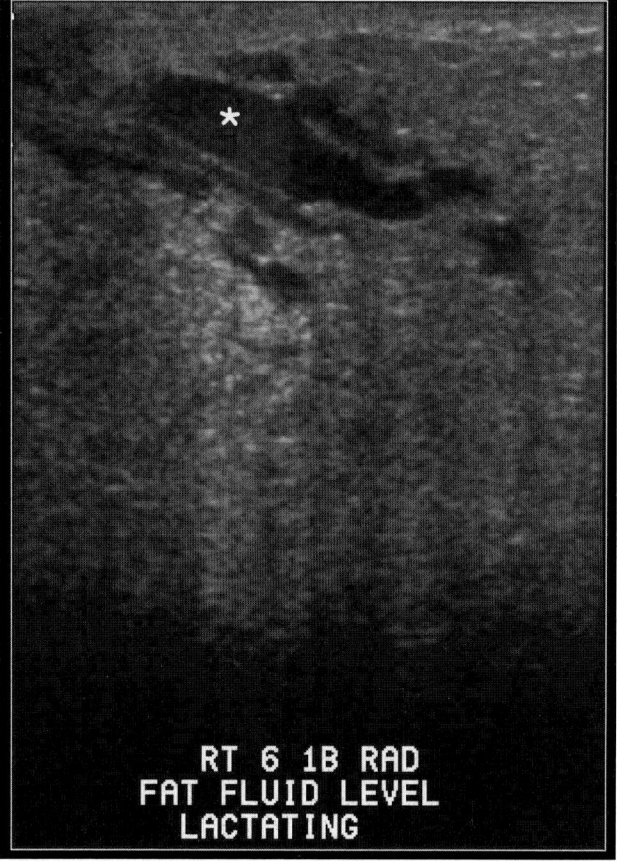

FIGURE 21–27 Similar to complex cysts, chronically ectatic ducts can contain fat–fluid levels that are difficult to distinguish from intraductal papillary lesions such as papilloma or ductal carcinoma *in situ*. The echogenic lipid layer floats in the nondependent portion of the duct *(*)*. Ballottement and two-handed compression may be helpful in making the distinction.

examination. Thick, echogenic debris within the duct that is moved by changes in the degree of compression can create a color Doppler signal that simulates blood flow (see Chapter 20, Fig. 20–39).

Intracystic Malignancy Simulating Papillary Apocrine Metaplasia in Fibrocystic Change

Intracystic malignancies are uncommon. Most of the intracystic solid material that is sonographically demonstrable is part of the spectrum of FCC. Papillary apocrine metaplasia, foamy macrophages (histiocytes), proteinaceous and lipid cell debris, cholesterol crystals, polymorphonuclear leukocytes, lymphocytes, red blood cells, and so forth, rather than malignant tumor cells, cause most of the echoes within cysts that cause them to be characterized as complex cysts. Unfortunately, in some cases, it can be difficult to determine whether intracystic contents are part of the fibrocystic spectrum or worrisome for malignancy. An intracystic malignancy or papilloma can be misinterpreted as merely representing papillary apocrine metaplasia, resulting in a false-negative sonographic diagnosis. Methods of evaluating such cysts are complex and are presented in detail in Chapter 11. In cases in which uncertainty exists, aspiration alone is not adequate because false-negative cytology is relatively common. Accurate diagnosis requires histology, which is most precisely obtained with ultrasound-guided 11-guage directional vacuum-assisted biopsy.

As is always the case when benign and malignant structures resemble each other, internal echoes within complex cysts can cause both false-negative and false-positive findings. The rare intracystic malignancy certainly might be mistaken for ubiquitous FCC, but far more frequently, FCC cannot be distinguished from intracystic malignancy, leading to false-positive results. For this reason, complex cysts are discussed in greater detail in the section on false-positive examinations.

Enlarged Terminal Ductolobular Units Filled with Low-Nuclear-Grade Ductal Carcinoma In Situ Simulating Adenosis or Fibrocystic Change

Sonographic equipment can demonstrate normal and abnormally enlarged TDLUs. Most pathologic processes in the breast, benign or malignant, can enlarge TDLUs. Apocrine metaplasia, microcysts, fibrosclerosis, adenosis, sclerosing adenosis, florid usual duct hyperplasia, atypical ductal hyperplasia, atypical lobular hyperplasia, and malignancy can all enlarge TDLUs. Malignant processes that enlarge TDLUs are usually *in situ*—either pure *in situ* or the *in situ* component of mixed invasive and *in situ* lesions. Invasive malignancies with *in situ* components usually create discrete nodules that enable us to distinguish them from surrounding lobules, preventing false-negative findings. However, pure DCIS or DCIS with microinva-

sion can present with enlargement of TDLUs as the only finding and can lead to false-negative diagnoses because of our inability to distinguish malignant from benign causes of lobular enlargement. Such lesions are usually low to intermediate nuclear grade. The degree of lobular enlargement caused by high-nuclear-grade DCIS is usually severe enough to distinguish involved TDLUs from surrounding TDLUs affected by benign changes.

Thus, we can readily identify individually enlarged TDLUs sonographically, but we cannot determine the histologic cause of enlargement. Being unable to determine the cause of lobular enlargement sonographically leads to mistakes that have been discussed earlier in the section on observational errors. In most cases, either a benign fibrocystic or a benign proliferative process causes enlargement of TDLUs. An atypical or a malignant process causes enlargement of TDLUs in only a minority of cases. When trying to determine the significance of prominent lobules, one must consider the size of the lobules in the surrounding areas and elsewhere in the breasts. In general, benign proliferative processes tend to enlarge all or most of the TDLUs in an area, whereas malignant or atypical processes tend to enlarge lobules more focally, involving only a single TDLU or a cluster of TDLUs (Fig. 21–9). However, involvement of TDLUs by benign proliferative processes can be focal and heterogeneous, and involvement by malignancy can be diffuse and extensive, involving entire lobes or quadrants. Diffuse lobular enlargement by extensive DCIS can simulate benign enlargement, leading to sonographic false-negative diagnosis. Split-screen imaging that allows comparison of lobular size with other quadrants of the same breast or with the mirror-image location in the contralateral breast may be helpful in determining whether the diffuse enlargement in the area of interest is out of proportion to the lobular enlargement caused by the background benign fibrocystic or benign proliferative changes (Fig. 21–10). The risk for falsely negatively misinterpreting lobular enlargement as benign is greatest when all of the lobules in the area of interest are grossly enlarged by benign fibrocystic or proliferative changes.

Intraductal Papillary Lesions Simulating Benign Papilloma

A malignant intraductal papillary lesion can be misinterpreted as being a benign papilloma, leading to a false-negative sonogram. Most intraductal papillary lesions are caused by benign large duct papillomas or papillary duct hyperplasia without atypia. However, in a small but significant percentage of cases, the intraductal papillary lesion is associated with atypia or DCIS. For this reason, until recently, we have recommended biopsy of all intraductal papillary lesions. We now further subdivide intraductal papillary lesions into BI-RADS 3 and BIRADS 4a or higher groups. We have found that intraductal papillary lesions that are nonexpansile, are

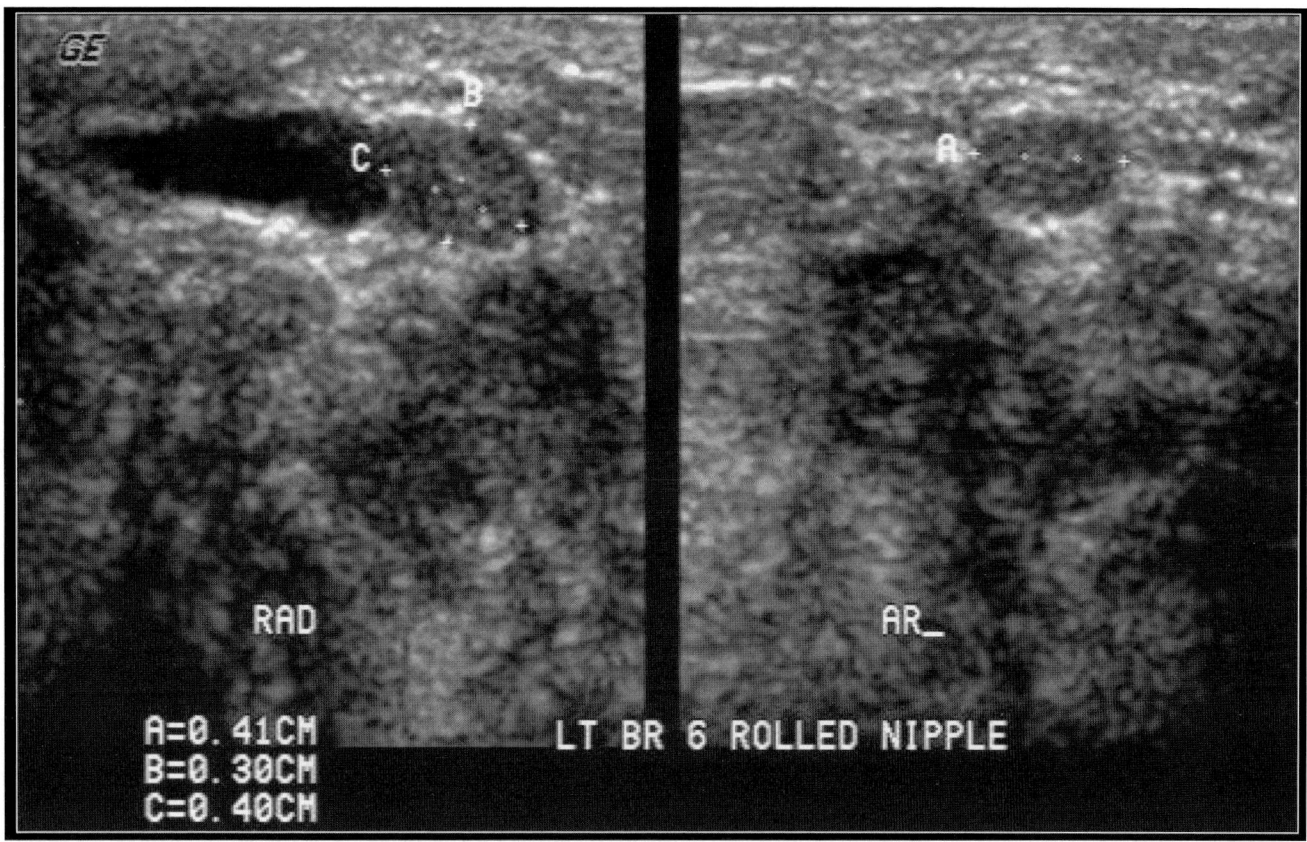

FIGURE 21–28 Small ovoid nonexpansile intraductal papillary lesions such as this are benign intraductal papillomas with 98% or greater certainty and thus qualify for BIRADS 3 characterization. Because such lesions often cause nipple discharge that the patient wants to be rid of, such lesions usually undergo biopsy despite the low risk for atypia or malignancy.

less than 1.5 cm in length, and do not affect branch ducts are benign in more than 98% of cases, thus qualifying for BI-RADS 3 characterization (Figs. 21–28). On the other hand, lesions that extend for more than 1.5 cm in length (see Chapter 8, Fig. 8–63), involve branch ducts (see Chapter 8, Figs. 8–28, 8–37, and 8–64), expand the duct (see Chapter 8, Fig. 8–65), or are peripheral in type, involving TDLUs (see Chapter 8, Figs. 8–66 and 8–67) have about a 6% risk for containing DCIS and a 7% risk for containing atypical ductal hyperplasia on their surface epithelium. Such lesions must be characterized as BIRADS 4a. Recognizing these findings is important to avoid false-negative characterization of intraductal papillary lesions as BIRADS 3 lesions. As a practical matter, patients who present with nipple discharge usually want the intraductal papillary lesion removed, so that nipple discharge stops, regardless of BIRADS category. Regardless of BIRADS category, we have found that 11-gauge directional vacuum-assisted biopsy (DVAB) of intraductal papillary lesions yields accurate diagnosis versus surgical in 100% of cases and unexpectedly leads to permanent cessation of nipple discharge in 90% of cases (see Chapter 8, Fig. 8–62).

Malignant Lesions that Do Not Create Sonographically Detectable Mass Effect

Some malignant breast lesions do not create a mass that can be detected by ultrasound. These include many cases of low-nuclear-grade DCIS, diffusely infiltrative lesions such as classic infiltrating lobular carcinoma, and some very small invasive malignancies.

Ductal Carcinoma In Situ

Although most cases of high-nuclear-grade DCIS can be readily detected sonographically, the percentage of cases of DCIS that can be sonographically detected decreases as the nuclear grade of the lesions decreases. Intermediate-nuclear-grade DCIS enlarges lobules and ducts to a lesser degree than does high-nuclear-grade DCIS, making it more difficult to distinguish from TDLU enlargement caused by FCC. Low-nuclear-grade DCIS often only minimally enlarges TDLUs or ducts, making it even more difficult to distinguish from underlying changes caused by FCC and benign proliferative changes. When low-nuclear-grade DCIS is sonographically

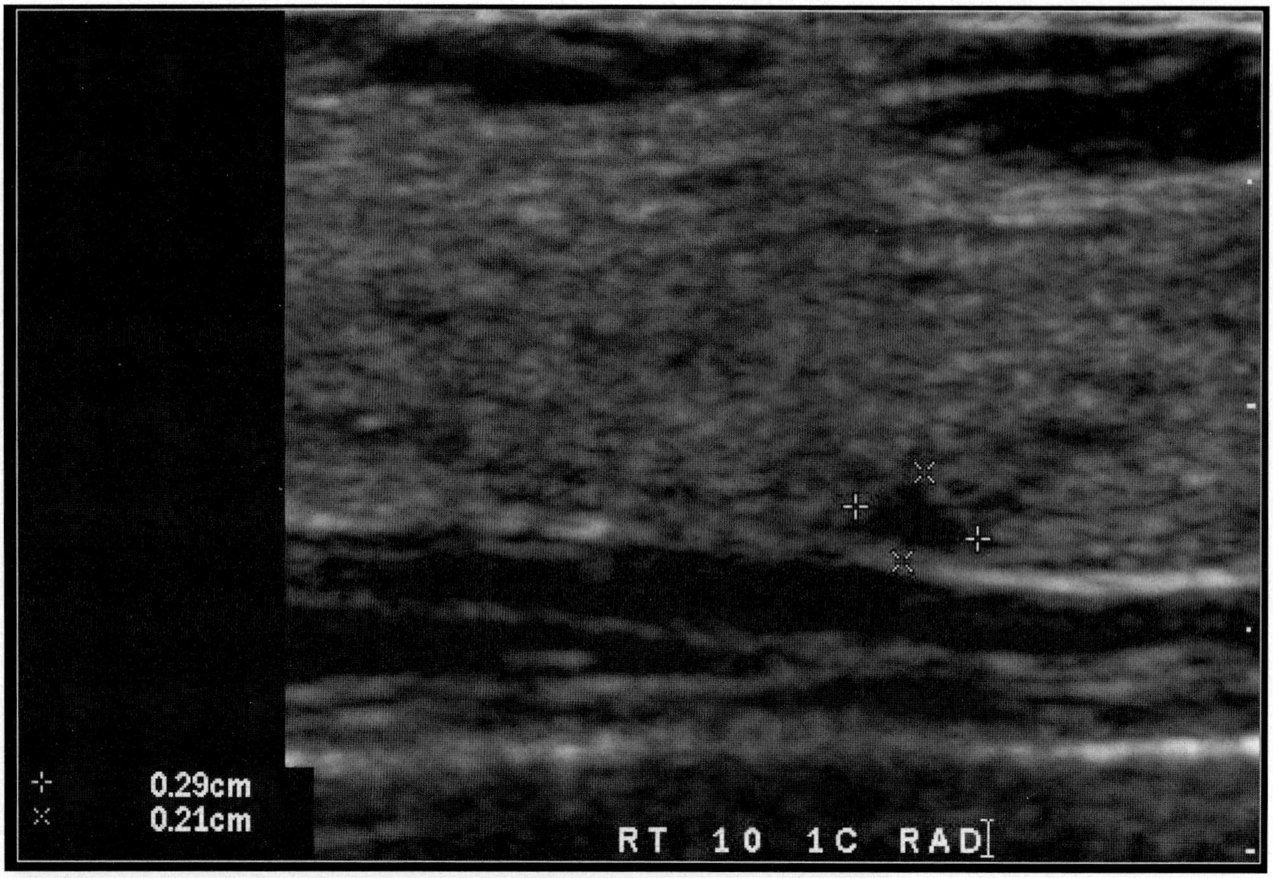

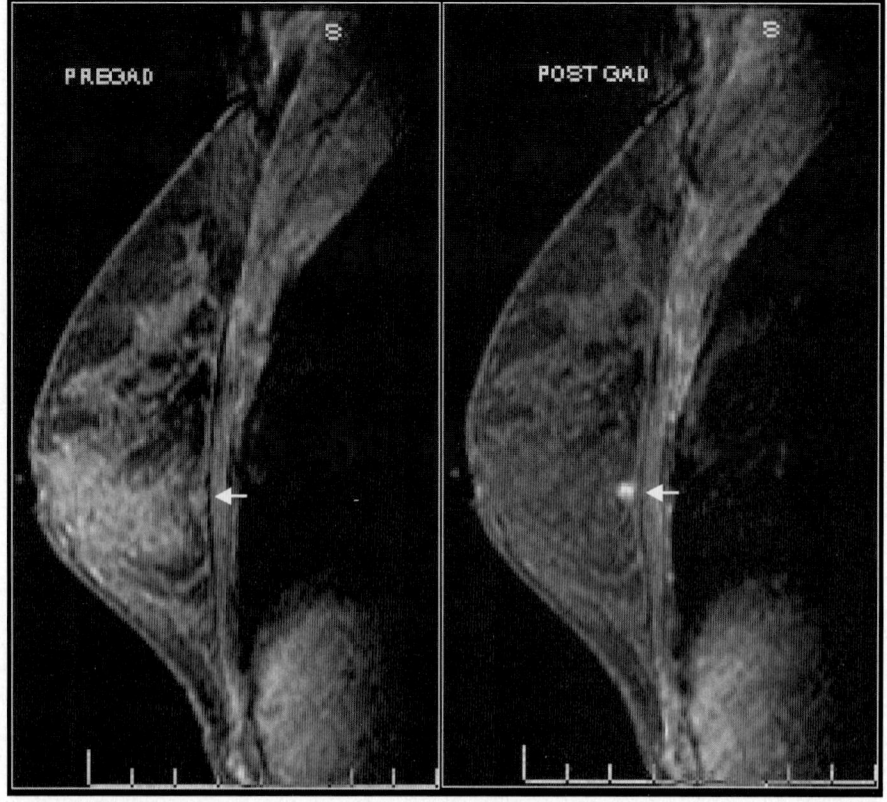

0.29cm
0.21cm

A

B

FIGURE 21–29 A: This 3-mm invasive lobular carcinoma was detected on secondary whole breast sonographic screening that was performed because of strong family history and very dense breast tissue on mammography. It is detectable because its hypoechogenicity contrasts with the surrounding hyperechoic fibrous tissue and because there are no other sonographically detectable lobules to confuse the issue. **B:** Images taken before (**left**) and after (**right**) gadolinium magnetic resonance imaging with RODEO sequence confirm the presence of an abnormally enhancing tiny nodule in the area earlier shown by ultrasound (*arrow*). The patient then underwent ultrasound-guided 11-gauge directional vacuum-assisted biopsy, which confirmed the diagnosis of a 3-mm invasive lobular carcinoma.

detectable, it usually has occurred within the surface epithelium of a preexisting benign lesion such as a papilloma (see Chapter 14, Fig. 14–15). Most cases of DCIS are diagnosed mammographically because of the presence of abnormal calcifications detected on routine screening mammography and have neither a palpable nor a mammographically or sonographically detectable mass associated with them. Although ultrasound can demonstrate some calcifications within breast masses, sonography is somewhat less sensitive than mammography for detecting the type of calcifications seen within most low- to intermediate-nuclear-grade DCIS that is not associated with a nodule or mass. Ultrasound, no matter how meticulously performed, will miss a larger percentage of low- to intermediate-nuclear-grade DCIS than will mammography. Breast cancers presenting with calcifications tend to be the earliest, smallest, and most curable of breast cancers; thus, their detection is paramount. Because ultrasound cannot detect these tumors with the efficacy of mammography, it cannot replace mammography in screening for them. Therefore, mammography is done before sonography in virtually all patients, with sonography reserved for evaluating palpable and nonspecific mammographic abnormalities.

Diffusely Infiltrative Lesions

Some breast malignancies, such as classic invasive lobular carcinoma, are prone to infiltrate into normal breast tissue without creating a mammographically or sonographically detectable mass and also tend not to develop mammographically detectable calcifications. In such cases, the only clues may be subtle areas of shadowing within echogenic fibrous tissue without a definite mass or a very subtle area of decreased echogenicity within hyperechoic fibrous elements (see Chapter 14, Figs. 14–93 and 14–95). Such findings may also be seen in FCC, however, and the changes are very subtle and easy to miss. Diffusely infiltrating lesions are a cause of observational errors.

Infiltrating Malignancies Smaller than 5 mm

Very small infiltrating malignancies that lie deeply within the breast or in the very near field and are subject to volume averaging can be missed sonographically. Using an acoustic standoff or 1.5-D array transducer can minimize near-field volume averaging and aid in detecting near-field lesions, but there are no easy techniques for improving detection of small far-field lesions. The size at which such lesions can be detected depends on the depth of the lesion, the echogenicity of surrounding tissues, and the size of TDLUs within the vicinity of the lesion. The deeper the lesion, the more isoechoic the surrounding tissues; and the larger the TDLUs, the more difficult it will be to identify a small cancer and to distinguish it from background changes of FCC and benign proliferative disorders. Homogeneously hyperechoic fibrous tissue breasts enhance the conspicuity of small hypoechoic malignant nodules (Fig. 21–29). Technical advances such as high-frequency coded harmonics and real-time compounding also facilitate detection of such small lesions, primarily by removing superimposed speckle artifact (Fig. 21–30).

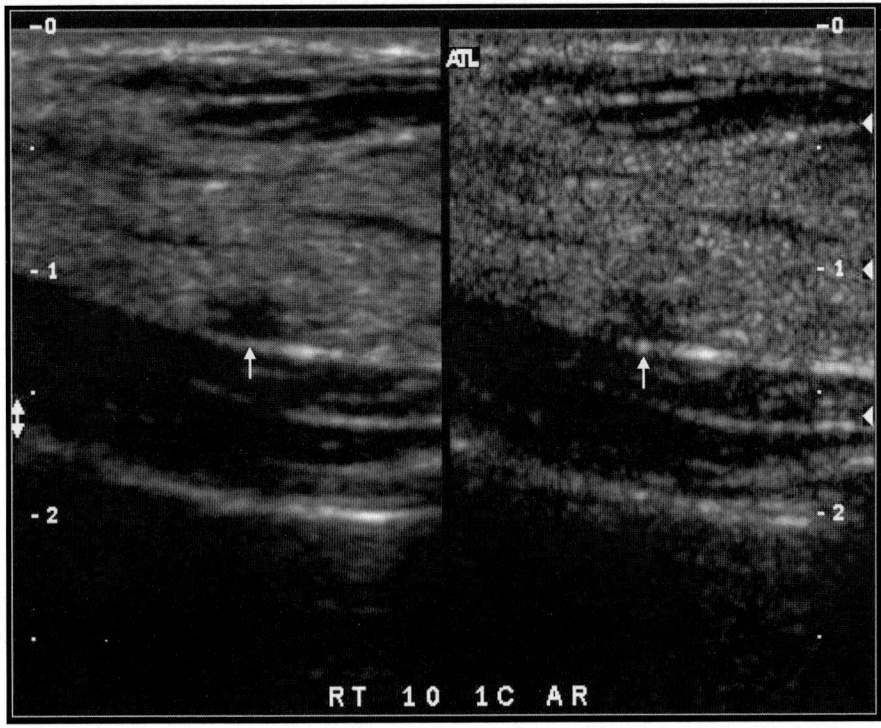

FIGURE 21–30 Real-time spatial compounding and high-frequency coded harmonics can be very helpful in detecting smaller lesions because they both suppress artifacts, particularly speckle artifact, that degrade the image. The **right** image shows conventional imaging of a 3-mm invasive lobular carcinoma, whereas the **left** image shows the same lesion using real-time compounding. Note that the lesion appears more hypoechoic, larger, and is better defined with real-time compounding.

FALSE-POSITIVE EXAMINATIONS

Technical

Near-Field and Far-Field Volume Averaging

Near-field and far-field volume averaging can be a cause of false-positive as well as false-negative sonographic evaluation. Solid normal surrounding tissues averaged in with cysts can make them appear complex cystic or solid and ill defined. As is the case for false-negative lesions, using a standoff will help minimize the presence of artifactual echoes within cysts caused by near-field volume averaging (see Chapter 2, Fig. 2–5). Electronic focusing in the short axis offered by 1.5-D array transducers also minimizes near-field volume averaging artifacts in both cystic and solid lesions and helps define the thin, echogenic capsule that surrounds benign nodules better (Fig. 21–31).

Filling in of Cysts with Artifactual Echoes

Simple cysts may have various types of artifactual echoes within them, making them appear complex cystic or solid, rather than simple cystic. Reverberation echoes, ring-down echoes, and side-lobe artifacts can appear within breast cysts. Reverberation and ring-down echoes tend to be parallel to the skin and involve the anterior part of the cyst (Fig. 21–32). Reverberation echoes are equally spaced and decrease in intensity with depth and are usually easy to distinguish from true intracystic lesions (see Chapter 10, Figs. 10–12 and 10–13). Reverberation echoes can be reduced by impedance matching. Side-lobe artifacts can be difficult to distinguish from true intracystic contents. Changing scan parameters will not necessarily ablate these artifactual echoes. Sometimes, changing the scan approach by rotation or angulation of the probe will help (Fig. 21–33). However, side-lobe artifacts in a given cyst may be unique to one machine, one probe, and one depth. Switching probes or scanning the patient on another type of machine will change the appearance of the cyst and make it apparent that it is a simple cyst (see Chapter 10, Figs. 10–11). There are enough real echoes in benign cysts to have to deal with. Every effort should be made to decrease artifactual echoes. High-frequency coded harmonics (see Chapter 2, Figs. 2–14 to 2–16) and real-time spatial compounding (see Chapter 2, Fig. 2–27) are two technical developments that can be initiated during real-time scanning with a simple button push that can rid cysts of all sorts of artifactual echoes in up to one-third of cases.

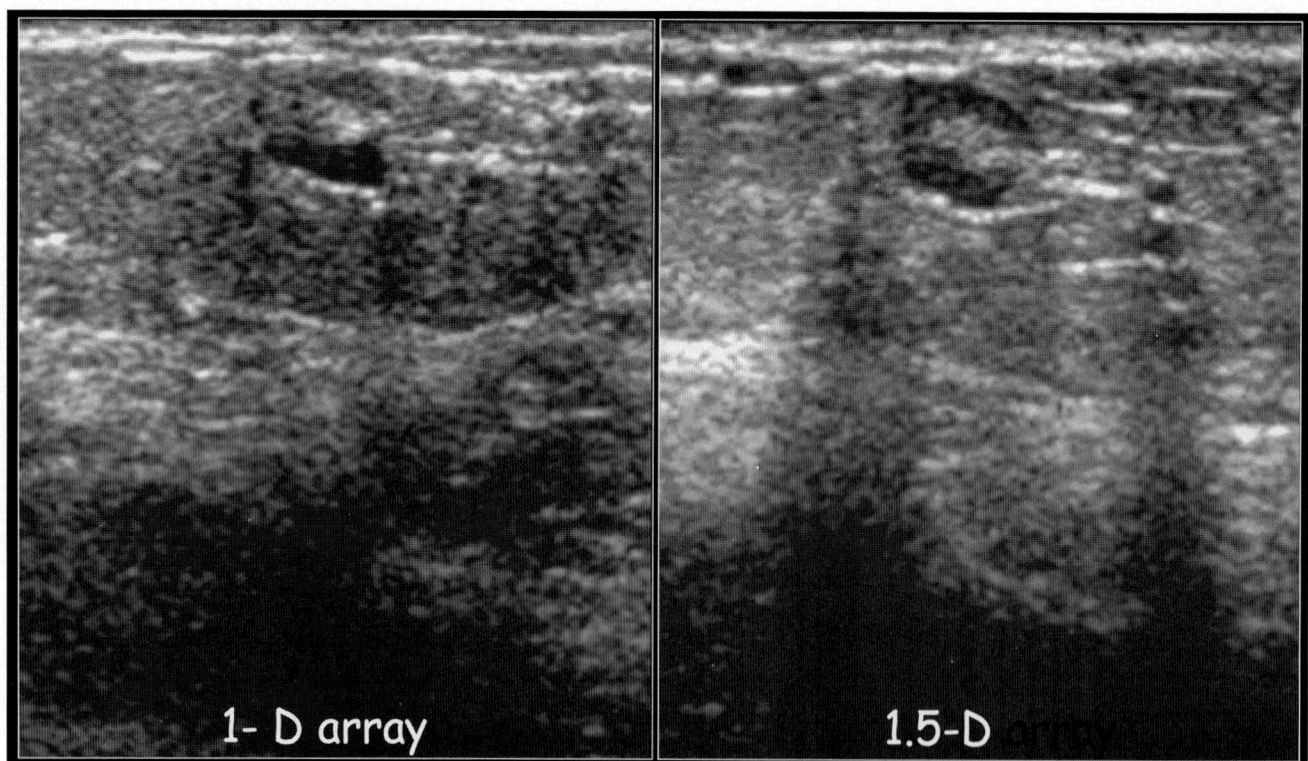

FIGURE 21–31 This superficially located intramammary lymph node does not have definitively benign characteristics when scanned with a conventional 1-D array, 12-MHz transducer because the superficial half of the lymph node is partially obscured by volume averaging artifact (**left image**). The **right** image of the lymph node was obtained with a 1.5-D array, 12-MHz transducer. The near-field volume averaging has been reduced, and the node now can be characterized as definitively benign, BIRADS 2.

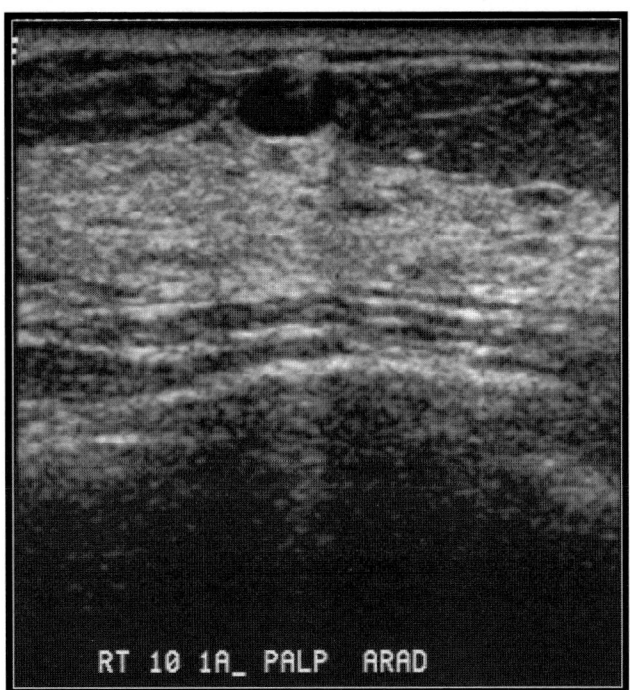

FIGURE 21–32 Reverberations in the near field of this superficial cyst can be mistaken for an intracystic papillary lesion, resulting in false-positive sonography findings.

Filling in of Ectatic Ducts with Artifactual Echoes

Reverberation, ring-down, and side-lobe artifacts may create artifactual echoes within an ectatic duct that simulate tumor within the duct. Compression and angulation of the transducer as well as coded harmonics and real-time compounding may also help minimize this problem (Fig. 21–34).

Shadowing Off Obliquely Oriented Fibrous Breast Structures

As noted in the section on false-negative examinations, shadowing can be a cause of both false-positive and false-negative sonograms. False-positive sonography occurs when artifactual shadowing, usually related to obliquely oriented tissue planes, simulates a shadowing carcinoma. As discussed earlier, artifactual shadowing arising from obliquely oriented normal structures can be reduced by altering the scan angle or compressing the breast more vigorously, whereas shadowing due to malignancy usually cannot (see Chapter 3, Figs. 3–5 and 3–6). Additionally, shadowing due to normal tissue planes and scars often appears linear when scanned orthogonal to the original scan plane (see Chapter 18, Fig. 18–25). Malignant shadowing, on the other hand, appears to be similar in size in the orthogonal and original scan planes, not linear in one plane (Fig. 21–22).

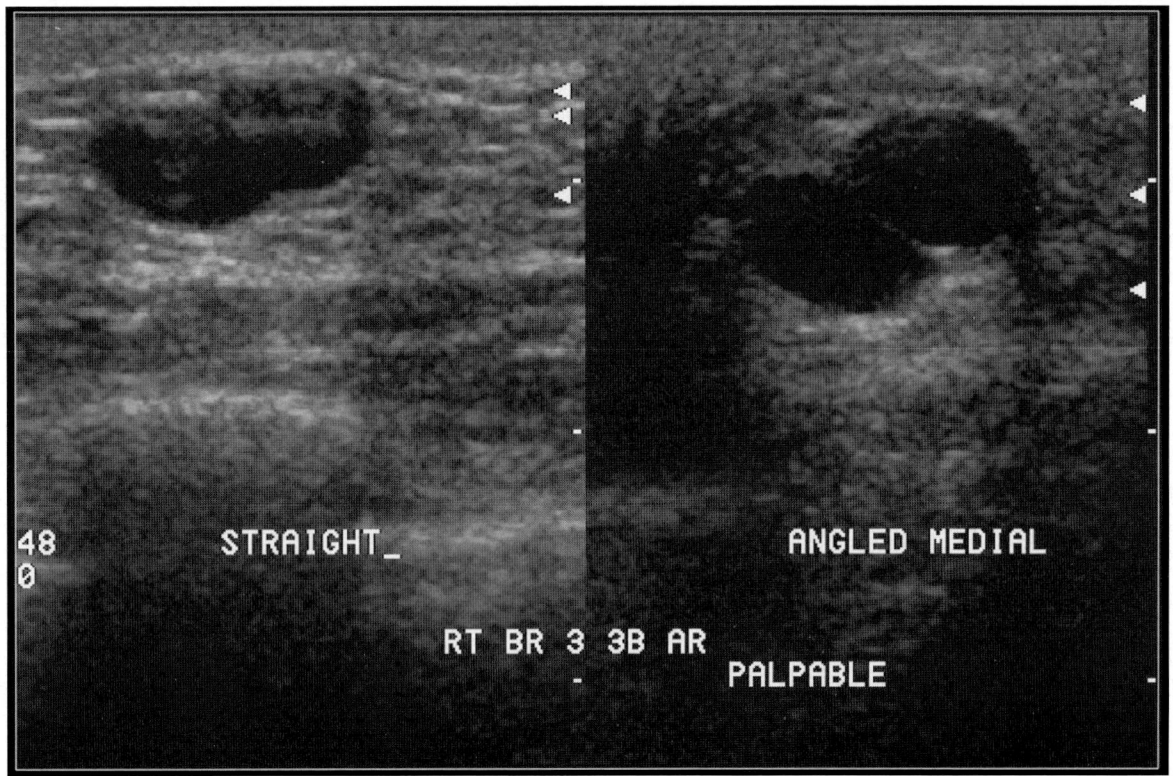

FIGURE 21–33 Scanning with less compression and changing the transducer angle to an oblique plane **(right)** can be helpful in minimizing reverberation echoes **(left)** that complicate characterization of cysts.

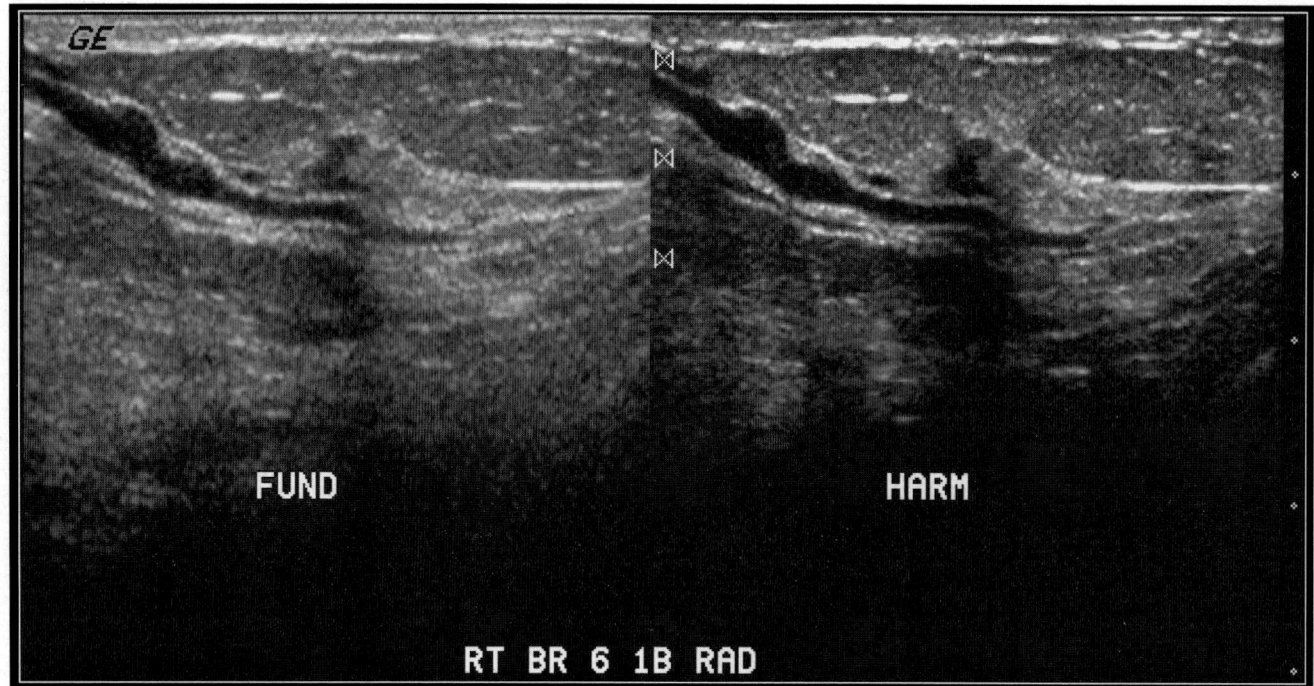

FIGURE 21–34 Coded harmonics can help minimize false-positive findings in patients with ectatic ducts by clearing artifacts from ectatic duct lumina. The **left** image, obtained with fundamental imaging, suggests the presence of echogenic fluid within the duct that could be caused by blood. The **right** image, obtained with coded harmonics, has cleared most of the internal echoes from the duct lumen.

Normal Structures Simulating Malignant Lesions

Fat Lobules Simulating Malignant Solid Nodules

As is case for many structures in the breast, fat lobules can be a cause of both false-positive and false-negative examinations. Fat lobules seldom simulate malignancy because their characteristics are benign. However, fat lobules may simulate a fibroadenoma, resulting in a false-positive upgrade of BIRADS category from BIRADS 1 or 2 to BIRADS 3. Alternatively, a true solid nodule such as a fibroadenoma may be mistaken for a fat lobule, resulting in a false-negative downgrade of BIRADS category to BIRADS 2 or 1. Methods of distinguishing between fat lobules and true solid nodules are discussed and illustrated in the section on false-negative examinations and in Chapter 4 (see Figs. 4–34 to 4–39).

Benign Lesions Simulating Malignant Lesions

Solid "Nodules"

Reactive Lymph Nodes. Most normal lymph nodes are definitively benign, BIRADS 2 sonographically. However, inflamed or reactive lymph nodes are frequently sonographically indistinguishable from lymph nodes bearing metastases, resulting in BIRADS categories of BIRADS 4a or higher and false-positive sonographic diagnoses. Sonographic distinction between inflamed or reactive lymph nodes and lymph nodes containing metastases or lymphoma is discussed and illustrated in detail in Chapter 19. Inflamed or reactive lymph nodes frequently return to a more normal appearance in a few weeks; thus, unless there is a compelling reason to perform immediate biopsy, short-interval follow-up in 2 or 3 months may be warranted. The key findings in distinguishing between benign and malignant causes of lymph node enlargement are the pattern of cortical enlargement and the blood flow pattern on color Doppler. Metastatic deposits tend to lodge in the subcapsular and cortical sinusoids of lymph nodes, resulting in eccentric cortical thickening and eccentric compression of the lymph node mediastinum, whereas benign causes of enlargement are more prone to thicken the cortex diffusely and symmetrically and to compress the mediastinum (Fig. 21–35; see also Chapter 19, Figs. 19–38, 19–39, 19–44, and 19–47). Additionally, malignant disease in nodes is more likely to make the shape of the lymph node rounder and to obliterate the mediastinum completely (see Chapter 19, Fig. 19–37). It is also typical

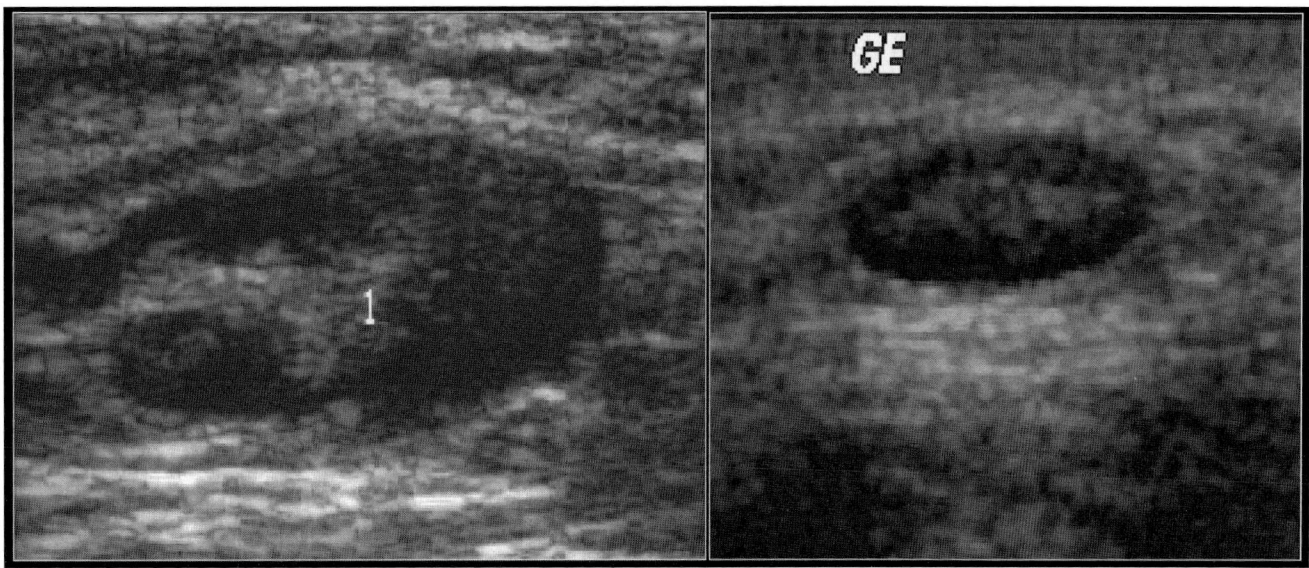

FIGURE 21–35 Inflamed or reactive lymph nodes can be difficult to distinguish from lymph nodes bearing malignancy and therefore can be a cause of false-positive sonography findings. Inflammatory changes in lymph nodes tend to affect the cortex uniformly, resulting in relatively uniform cortical thickening throughout the node and relatively uniform effects on the lymph node mediastinum **(right)**. Metastases to lymph nodes tend to affect the cortex asymmetrically, leading to asymmetric thickening and asymmetric compression of the lymph node mediastinum **(left)**.

of malignant involvement to distort the anatomy of one lymph node grossly while completely sparing the adjacent lymph node. Inflammatory lymphadenopathy has a greater tendency to affect all of the lymph nodes in the region of interest (see Chapter 19, Fig. 19–55). Metastatic deposits in the subcapsular and cortical sinuses tend to incite transcapsular neovascularity, whereas benign causes of lymph node enlargement tend to result in vasodilation and enlargement of normal hilar vessels and do not stimulate the formation of transcapsular vessels (see Chapter 20, Figs. 20–20 and 20–21).

Fibroadenomas. Although many fibroadenomas have a classically benign appearance consisting of an elliptically shaped, wider-than-tall appearance or a gently lobulated appearance with a thin, echogenic capsule, many others have malignant features that exclude them from benign classification. Some are multilobulated or even microlobulated (see Chapter 13, Fig. 13–6) or demonstrate duct extension (see Chapter 13, Fig. 13–11) or branch pattern (see Chapter 13, Fig. 13–12). Others, particularly those that have undergone infarction and become hyalinized, become adherent to surrounding tissues and develop angular margins (see Chapter 13, Fig. 13–10). Some do not have a demonstrable thin, echogenic capsule because fibrous tissue silhouettes the equally echogenic surrounding tissue (Fig. 21–36). Hyalinized fibroadenomas can cast suspicious acoustic shadows, even in the absence of typically benign mammographic calcifications (Fig. 21–37). Complex

fibroadenomas containing sclerosing adenosis have suspicious punctate internal calcifications (see Chapter 13, Fig. 13–32). Because the potential costs of false-negative diagnoses are so high, we must consider such lesions suspicious, classify them as BIRADS 4a or higher, and perform biopsy. Such cases must be considered false positive for malignancy, even though they are real lesions.

Enlarged Terminal Ductolobular Units Due to Fibrocystic Change, Adenosis, or Papillary Duct Hyperplasia. TDLUs that are enlarged out of proportion to surrounding TDLUs should be considered suspicious for neoplasm, especially in the postmenopausal age group. In many instances, such TDLUs are merely involved with adenosis, FCCs, or papillary duct hyperplasia (see Chapter 13, Fig. 13–93). Focal enlargement, however, is suspicious enough to justify biopsy of such areas.

Complex Cysts

As noted earlier, complex cysts can be a cause of both false-positive and false-negative examinations. Intracystic carcinomas can be mistaken for benign complex cysts, but far more often, benign complex cysts cannot be distinguished from intracystic carcinoma. Such complex cysts must be characterized as BIRADS 4a or higher, creating false-positive diagnoses. As is the case for ducts, several different entities that exist in benign cysts can create confusing internal echoes: papillary apocrine metaplasia, fat–fluid levels,

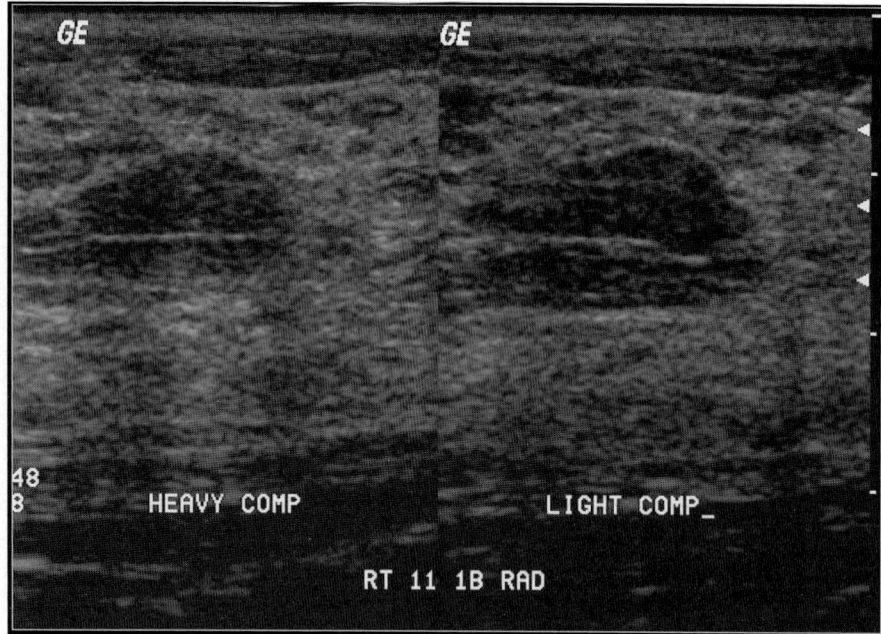

FIGURE 21–36 It can be difficult to identify a complete thin, echogenic capsule around a fibroadenoma that is surrounded by hyperechoic fibrous tissue. Note that the capsule is well demonstrated posteriorly, where it is outlined by isoechoic fat, but is poorly defined anteriorly, where hyperechoic fibrous tissue partially obscures it. Also, note that the capsule is better seen in the **right** image, which was obtained with light compression, than in the **left** image, which was obtained with greater compression.

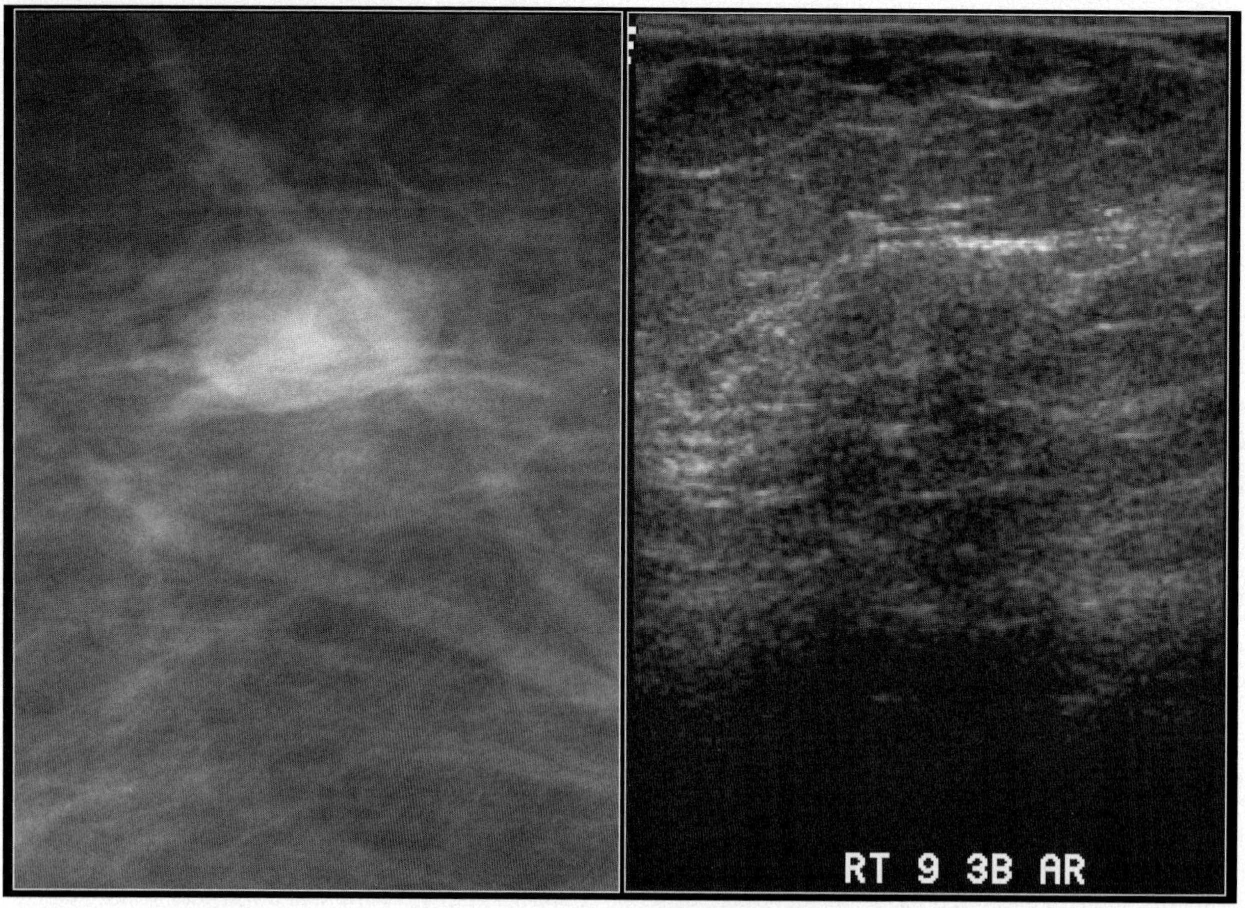

FIGURE 21–37 Only a very small percentage of fibroadenomas cause acoustic shadowing, and most of these contain coarse popcorn-type calcifications. An even smaller percentage of fibroadenomas, such as this one, cast acoustic shadows when there is no mammographically demonstrable calcium. Shadowing in such cases is related to the degree of hyalinization, requires a BIRADS 4a classification, and leads to biopsy, technically a false-positive sonogram.

tumefactive sludge, and volume averaged fibrosclerosis. Papillary apocrine metaplasia often grows in the form of mural nodules within cysts that are difficult to distinguish from mural nodules caused by intracystic papilloma or intracystic carcinoma. Methods of evaluating such complex cysts are discussed in much detail in Chapter 10, but in some cases, a distinction between a true intracystic papillary neoplasm and intracystic papillary apocrine metaplasia is not possible. In such cases, biopsy is necessary because aspiration alone is subject to too many false-negative cytology results.

In general, we are not able to characterize complex cysts sonographically as efficaciously as we can characterize solid nodules. The reason is that solid nodules tend to invade outwardly into surrounding tissues, affecting the surface characteristics that we rely so heavily on when characterizing breast lesions. Intracystic malignancies, on the other hand, tend to invade inwardly, into their fibrovascular stalks. The inward direction of invasion into the fibrovascular stalk tends not to affect the surface characteristics of the lesion, making surface characteristics much less useful in complex cysts than they are in solid nodules. The only point at which we can use surface characteristics to characterize complex cysts is at the point at which the mural nodule is attached to the outer cyst wall. Papillary apocrine metaplasia tends to be confined within the oval or circular shape of the cyst and is delimited outwardly by the thin, echogenic outer wall of the cyst. Intracystic papillomas and carcinomas, on the other hand, tend to have irregular attachments to the wall of the cyst, have angular or microlobulated borders, extend into ducts that course away from the cyst (usually toward the nipple), and lack the thin, echogenic outer cyst wall that delimits papillary apocrine metaplasia (see Chapter 10, Fig. 10–27). Intracystic papillomas and intracystic carcinomas are among the most vascular of all breast tumors and usually have an easily demonstrable vascular stalk, whereas papillary apocrine metaplasia, no matter how florid, seldom does (see Chapter 20, Fig. 20–29). Benign intracystic papillomas tend to be fed by a single arterial branch, whereas malignant intracystic lesions tend to form multiple feeding vessels (see Chapter 20, Fig. 20–31). This is a manifestation of the inward invasion into the fibrovascular stalk and tumor neoangiogenesis within the stalk.

Tumefactive sludge or pus within an inflamed cyst can simulate a mural nodule, but simply scanning while turning the patient into a left lateral decubitus position and having the patient sit upright can cause the sludge or pus to move to a newly dependent position within the cyst (see Chapter 10, Fig. 10–33), distinguishing it from an immobile mural nodule with absolute certainty (see Chapter 10, Figs. 10–32). It is important to allow enough time for this shift to occur. Sludge and pus are quite viscous and move very slowly. As long as 5 minutes may be necessary for completion of the shift to the newly dependent position

(see Chapter 10, Fig. 10–43). Tumefactive sludge and pus are frequently associated with inflammation that causes a fairly uniform isoechoic thickening of the outer wall of the cyst. The inflamed or infected cyst wall is also hyperemic, and the increased blood flow in the inflamed and thickened wall can readily be demonstrated with color Doppler. Interestingly, the orientation of the vessels within the walls of inflamed cysts differs from that of vessels in the walls of cystic malignancies. The vessels in inflamed cysts course parallel to the cyst wall, whereas the vessels that feed intracystic malignancies tend to course perpendicular to the cyst wall (see Chapter 20, Fig. 20–42).

The echogenic lipid layer in complex cysts with fat–fluid levels may also simulate mural nodules. However, similar to tumefactive sludge or pus, left lateral decubitus or upright positioning can cause a shift in position of the echogenic lipid layer to the newly nondependent part of the cyst (see Chapter 10, Fig. 10–69). Similar to tumefactive sludge, the contents of complex cysts with fat–fluid levels are viscous and may require as much as 5 minutes to shift completely to the newly nondependent position (see Chapter 10, Fig. 10–68).

Complex cysts that are completely filled with echogenic lipid material or papillary apocrine metaplasia can be indistinguishable from solid nodules (Fig. 21–37) unless color Doppler shows internal vessels, which indicate that the nodule is either solid or an intracystic lesion that completely fills a cyst (see Chapter 20, Fig. 20–5). In such cases, the only two choices available are to assume the lesions to be solid and to characterize them or to attempt to aspirate them. Unfortunately, it is also impossible to determine whether the contents of the cyst are papillary apocrine metaplasia, which is attached to the wall and cannot be aspirated, or echogenic lipid material, which can be aspirated completely. In lesions that cannot be aspirated, rocking the needle can help determine whether the lesion is a complex cyst filled with nonaspiratable papillary apocrine metaplasia or is solid. Although the papillary apocrine metaplasia is attached to the wall at multiple points, preventing its complete aspiration, the individual fronds and strands of apocrine metaplastic cells filling the cyst are thin, gracile, and weak, offering no resistance to the movement of the needle (see Chapter 10, Fig. 10–111). The position of the needle would remain fixed if the lesion were truly solid (see Chapter 10, Fig. 10–110). Rocking the needle within the cyst breaks some apocrine "snouts" loose and allows them to be aspirated and stained. This maneuver transforms a failed aspiration into a fine-needle aspiration biopsy, allowing confirmation of the diagnosis of papillary apocrine metaplasia and benign FCC.

Enlarged, Solid-appearing Ducts

Enlarged ducts filled with echoes are suspicious for DCIS. Ducts distended by DCIS can be mistaken for duct ectasia with inspissated secretions, creating false-negative diagnoses, but more commonly, ectatic ducts with inspissated secretions, blood, pus, or periductal fibrosis simulate DCIS, creating sonographic false-positive results. Because the cost of false-negative examinations is potentially so much greater than the cost of false-positive examinations in these situations, the sonographic techniques for distinguishing between benign ducts containing echogenic material and ducts that contain tumor were discussed and illustrated in the section on false-negative examinations.

Inspissated Secretions in Ductal Ectasia. Ductal ectasia is often associated with inspissated secretions and plasma cell mastitis. Inspissated secretions can become echogenic enough to have an isoechoic appearance nearly identical to that of intraductal tumor (see Chapter 8, Figs. 8–20, 8–42). Ectatic ducts, similar to complex cysts, may also contain tumefactive sludge (fluid–debris levels) (see Chapter 8, Fig. 8–34) and fat–fluid levels (Fig. 21–27) that simulate intraductal papillary lesions. In such cases, ballottement of the duct with the transducer may be helpful by demonstrating movement of the inspissated debris within the duct (see Chapter 8, Fig. 8–35) or by demonstrating compressibility or lack of compressibility of the duct (see Chapter 8, Fig. 8–27). Color Doppler can be useful in demonstrating the "color swoosh" of moving echogenic secretions and debris with the duct lumen (see Chapter 20, Fig. 20–36). Additionally, color Doppler may be useful because demonstration of blood flow in the solid material within the duct indicates the presence of a fibrovascular stalk within a true papillary lesion (papilloma or DCIS) (see Chapter 20, Fig. 20–38). Lack of demonstrable blood flow, however, does not exclude papilloma or DCIS.

Intraductal Papilloma or Papillary Duct Hyperplasia. Sonography is unable to distinguish between benign intraductal papillomas and intraductal malignancy in all cases. In most cases, the lesion represents benign large duct papilloma, but in a few cases, the lesion is an intraductal malignancy or contains changes of atypia. Nonexpansile, ovoid, small intraductal papillary lesions are benign with greater than 98% certainty and therefore qualify as BIRADS 3 lesions (Fig. 21–28). However, patients with nipple discharge usually want intraductal papillary lesions removed and nipple discharge to stop, regardless of the BIRADS category. We have found that the risk for an intraductal papillary lesion containing atypia or DCIS exceeds 2% and therefore requires a BIRADS 4a or higher classification if the lesion is expansile (see Chapter 8, Fig. 8–65), is longer than 1.5 cm (see Chapter 8, Fig. 8–63) and involves branch ducts (see Chapter 8, Figs. 8–28, 8–37, 8–64), or is peripheral in location and involves TDLUs (see Chapter 8, Figs. 8–66 and 8–67). Small intraductal papillary lesions can be accurately diagnosed with 11-gauge ultrasound-guided DVAB, and nipple discharge is permanently stopped in 90% of cases (see Chapter 8, Fig. 8–62).

Architectural Distortion and Shadowing

Sonography is subject to false-positive examination due to architectural distortion in many of the same disorders that cause false-positive mammograms.

Sclerosing Adenosis. Sclerosing adenosis can merely cause enlargement of TDLUs or large areas of isoechoic glandular tissue but sometimes can create solid nodules with angular margins and internal foci of hyperechogenicity that simulate invasive malignancy (see Chapter 13, Fig. 13–97). Sclerosing adenosis can also occur within fibroadenomas that are classified as complex. Complex fibroadenomas that contain sclerosing adenosis often contain ill-defined areas of hyperechogenicity or have angular or microlobulated borders (see Chapter 13, Figs. 13–35).

Fat Necrosis (Late Stage). Early phases of fat necrosis may appear as echogenic, edematous fat, or complex fluid collections representing hematoma or as lipid cysts. In later stages, the lipid cysts may calcify, having a typically benign appearance on mammography and even sonography. However, in some cases, late-stage fat necrosis will lead to severe fibrosis and scarring. Such lesions appear to be angular, markedly hypoechoic, and shadowing, simulating low-grade infiltrating ductal carcinoma, infiltrating lobular carcinoma, or tubular carcinoma (Fig. 21–36).

Biopsy Scar. Biopsy scars may, like fat necrosis, lead to angular, markedly hypoechoic, shadowing lesions that simulate malignancy. In fact, biopsy scars often also contain changes of fat necrosis. The degree of such scarring is related to the size of the lumpectomy and to the size of the hematoma associated with the resection. Scanning planes that are parallel and perpendicular to the scar may be helpful in confirming the nature of the lesion and excluding a recurrent mass. Scars tend to look much larger and more hypoechoic and to shadow more when the scan plane is parallel to the scar. When the scan plane is perpendicular to the scar, a thin, lucent, irregular obliquely oriented line, corresponding to the plane of incision, rather than a shadowing mass, is often seen in cases in which the lumpectomy cavity was sutured closed (see Chapter 18, Fig. 18–25).

Additionally, the appearance of the scar is related to whether or not the biopsy cavity was sutured closed or left open to accumulate blood and serum. In recent years, there has been a tendency to allow the lumpectomy cavity to remain open to minimize the indentation of the skin over the lumpectomy site. Leaving the cavity open, however, allows hematoma to develop in the lumpectomy cavity. This later progresses to fat necrosis and much larger scars on long-term follow-up. The sonographic appearance of the lumpectomy cavity that is left open is much more suspicious and much less specific than that of a primarily closed cavity (see Chapter 18, Figs. 18–26 and 18–27). Such areas of chronic fibrotic fat necrosis within the lumpectomy scar may be very difficult to distinguish from recurrent tumor.

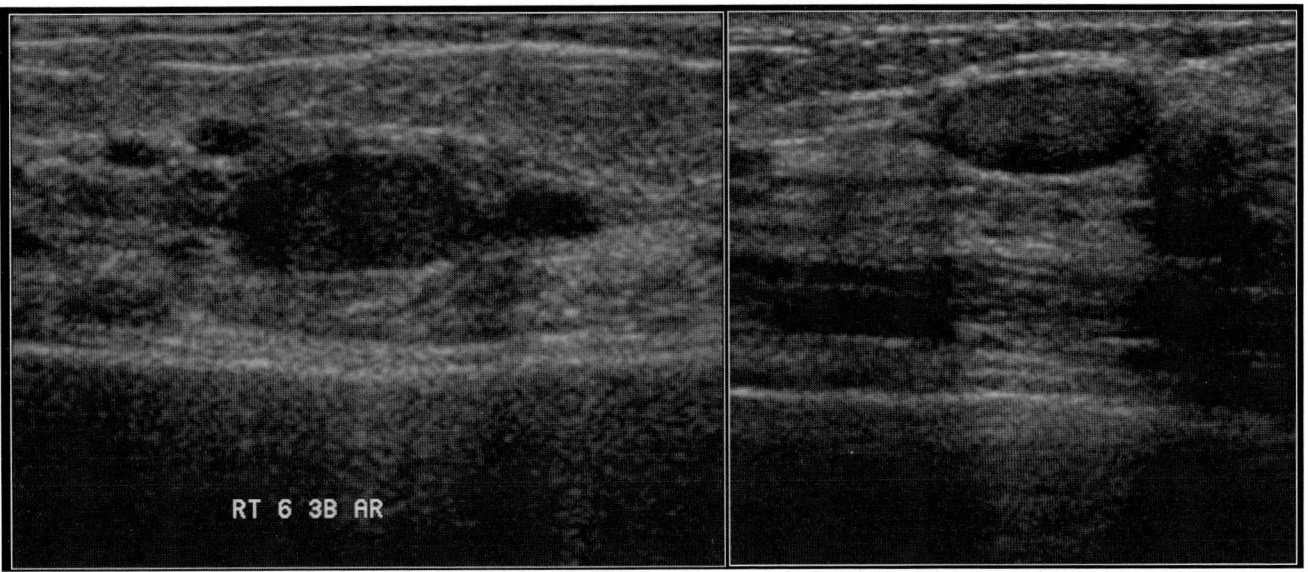

RT 6 3B AR

FIGURE 21–38 Cysts that are completely filled with either papillary apocrine metaplasia or echogenic lipid **(right)** can be sonographically indistinguishable from fibroadenomas **(left)**.

Radial Scar or Complex Sclerosing Lesion. Radial scars are sonographically demonstrable in some patients. Similar to their mammographic appearance, their sonographic appearance is suspicious. Their appearances vary, depending up the degree of proliferative changes in the periphery. When proliferative changes are florid, the lesions appear to be hypoechoic nodules with many suspicious features (see Chapter 15, Fig. 15–27). In some cases, the central scar is visible as an area of hyperechogenicity similar to the central scar sometimes seen in intermediate-grade invasive ductal carcinomas (see Chapter 15, Fig. 15–26). In cases in which peripheral proliferative changes are minor, the architectural distortion caused by the central scar dominates the appearance of the lesion (see Chapter 15, Fig. 15–25). The peripheral hypoechoic to isoechoic areas often represent FCC or adenosis but can represent atypical duct hyperplasia or tubular carcinoma in up to 15% of cases. Such an appearance strongly suggests malignancy, and biopsy is always required in these cases.

SUGGESTED READINGS

False-Negative Examinations

Bazzocchi M, Facecchia I, Zuiani C, et al. Diagnostic imaging of lobular carcinoma of the breast: mammographic, ultrasonographic, and MR findings. *Radiol Med* (Torino) 2000;100(6):436–443.

Butler RS, Venta LA, Wiley EL, et al. Sonographic evaluation of infiltrating lobular carcinoma. *AJR Am J Roentgenol* 1999;172(2):325–330.

Chopra S, Evans AJ, Pinder SE, et al. Pure mucinous breast cancer-mammographic and ultrasound findings. *Clin Radiol* 1996;51(6):421–424.

Dershaw DD, Moore MP, Liberman L, et al. Inflammatory breast carcinoma: mammographic findings. *Radiology* 1994;190(3):831–834.

Feig SA. Breast masses. Mammographic and sonographic evaluation. *Radiol Clin North Am* 1992;30(1):67–92.

Fornage BD. Role of color Doppler imaging in differentiating between pseudocystic malignant tumors and fluid collections. *J Ultrasound Med* 1995;14:125–128.

Hall FM. Sonography of the breast: controversies and opinions. *AJR Am J Roentgenol* 1997;169(6):1635–1636.

Harrison RL, Birtton P, Warren R, et al. Can we be sure about a radiological diagnosis of fat necrosis of the breast? *Clin Radiol* 2000;55:119–123.

Helvie MA, Paramagul C, Oberman HA, et al. Invasive lobular carcinoma. Imaging features and clinical detection. *Invest Radiol* 1993;28(3):202–207.

Heywang SH., et al. Advantages and pitfalls of ultrasound in the diagnosis of breast cancer. *JCU J Clin Ultrasound* 1985;13(8):525–532.

Hollingsworth AB, Taylor LD, Rhodes DC. Establishing a histologic basis for false negative mammograms. *Am J Surg* 1993;166:643–647.

Jackson VP. Management of solid breast nodules: what is the role of sonography? *Radiology* 1995;196(1):14–15.

Kopans DB. More on sonographic features in the differentiation of fibroadenoma and invasive ductal carcinoma. *AJR Am J Roentgenol* 1998;171(4):109–114.

Liberman L, et al. Benign and malignant phyllodes tumors: mammographic and sonographic findings. *Radiology* 1996;198(1):121–124.

Ma L, Fishell E, Wright B, et al. Case control study of factors associated with failure to detect breast cancer missed by mammography. *J Natl Cancer Inst* 1992;84:781–785.

Meyer JE, Amin E, Lindfors KK, et al. Medullary carcinoma of the breast: mammographic and US appearance. *Radiology* 1989;170:79–82.

Mendelson EB, Harris KM, Doshi N, Tobon H. Infiltrating lobular carcinoma: mammographic patterns with pathologic correlation. *AJR Am J Roentgenol* 1989;153:265–271.

Moss HA, Britton PD, Flower CD, et al. How reliable is modern breast imaging in differentiating benign from malignant breast lesions in the symptomatic population? *Clin Radiol* 1999;54(1): 676–682.

Ravichandran D, et al. Cystic carcinoma of the breast: a trap for the unwary. *Ann R Coll Surg Engl* 1995;77(2):123–126.

Reintgen D, et al. The anatomy of missed breast cancers. *Surg Oncol* 1993;2(1):65–75.

Sener SF, Candela FC, Paige ML, et al. Limitations of mammography in the identification of noninfiltrating carcinoma of the breast. *Surg Gynecol Obstet* 1988;167:135–140.

Sickles EA, Filly RA, Callen PW. Breast cancer detection with sonography and mammography: comparison using state–of-the-art equipment. *AJR Am J Roentgenol* 1983;140(5):843–845.

Skaane P, Skjorten F. Ultrasonographic evaluation of invasive lobular carcinoma. *Acta Radiol* 1999;40(4):369–375.

Smallwood JA, et al. The accuracy of ultrasound in the diagnosis of breast disease. *Ann R Coll Surg Engl* 1986;68(1):19–22.

Spencer GM, Rubens DJ, Roach DJ. Hypoechoic fat: a sonographic pitfall. *AJR Am J Roentgenol* 1995;164(5):1277–1280.

Stavros AT, et al. Solid breast nodules: use of sonography to distinguish between benign and malignant lesions. *Radiology* 1995; 196(1):123–134.

Vega A, Garijo F. Radial scar and tubular carcinoma: mammographic and sonographic findings. *Acta Radiol* 1993;34(1):43–47.

Wilson TE, Helvie MA, Oberman HA, Joynt LK. Pure and mixed mucinous carcinoma of the breast: pathologic basis for differences in mammographic appearance. *AJR Am J Roentgenol* 1999; 165:285–289.

False–Positive Examinations

Ciatto S, Morrone D, Bravetti P. Differential diagnosis of intracystic breast lesions in hemorrhagic cysts. *Radiol Med* (Torino) 1991; 81(5):592–596.

Cohen MA, Sferiazza SJ. Role of sonography in evaluation of radial scars of the breast. *AJR Am J Roentgenol* 2000;174(4):1075–1078.

Finlay ME, Liston JE, Lunt LG, et al. Assessment of the role of ultrasound in the differentiation of radial scars and stellate carcinoma of the breast. *Clin Radiol* 1994;49(1):52–55.

Garstin WI, et al. Fibrous mastopathy in insulin dependent diabetics. *Clin Radiol* 1991;44(2):89–91.

Gerlach B, Holzgreve W. Breast ultrasound in pre- and postoperative patients. *Ultrasound Q* 1995;13:27–40.

Jackson VP, et al. The spectrum of sonographic findings of fibroadenoma of the breast. *Invest Radiol* 1986;21(1):34–40.

Keen, M.E., et al., Benign breast lesions with malignant clinical and mammographic presentations. *Hum Pathol* 1985;16(11):1147–1152.

Kerlikowske K, et al. Positive predictive value of screening mammography by age and family history of breast cancer. *JAMA* 1993; 270(20):2444–2450.

Kimme-Smith C, et al. Ultrasound mammography: effects of focal zone placement. *Radiographics* 1985;5(6):955–969.

Kimme-Smith C, et al. Ultrasound artifacts affecting the diagnosis of breast masses. *Ultrasound Med Biol* 1988;1:203–210.

Mendelson EB. Imaging the post-surgical breast. *Semin Ultrasound CT MR* 1989;10:154–170.

Miller JA, Festa S, Goldstein M. Benign fat necrosis simulating bilateral breast malignancy after reduction mammoplasty. *South Med J* 1998;91:765–767.

Miller SD, McCollough ML, DeNapoli. Periductal mastitis. Masquerading as carcinoma. *Dermatol Surg* 1998;24:383–385.

Nussbaum SA, Feig SA, Capuzzi DM. Breast imaging case of the day. Fibroadenoma with microcalcification. *Radiographics* 1998; 18(1):243–245.

Omori LM, et al. Breast masses with mixed cystic–solid sonographic appearance. *J Clin Ultrasound* 1993;21(8):489–495.

Reynolds HE, Cramer HM. Cholesterol granuloma of the breast: a mimic of carcinoma. *Radiology* 1994;191(1):249–250.

Smith GL, et al. Cholesterol granuloma of the breast presenting as an intracystic papilloma. *Br J Radiol* 1997;70(839):1178–1179.

Sweeney DJ, Wylie EJ. Mammographic appearances of mammary duct ectasia that mimic carcinoma in a screening program. *Australas Radiol* 1995;39(1):18–23.

Tenekeci AN, et al. Sonographic pitfall in diagnosing breast cysts: pseudomural projections. *J Clin Ultrasound* 1998;26(3):181–182.

Wilhelmus JL, Schrodt GR, Mahaffey LM. Cholesterol granulomas of the breast. A lesion which clinically mimics carcinoma. *Am J Clin Pathol* 1982;77:592–597.

APPENDIX

The following textbooks were instrumental to my understanding of breast pathology and breast sonography, and I have read each of them "cover-to-cover" once and used them as references innumerable times. I would recommend them to anyone performing breast ultrasound.

The following breast pathology texts are excellent resources for understanding the histopathology of the breast:

1. Ahmed A. *Diagnostic breast pathology: a text and color atlas.* New York: Churchill Livingstone, 1992.
2. Bennington JL, Lagios M. The mammographically directed biopsy. In: *State of the art reviews.* Philadephia: Hanley & Belfus, 1992.
3. Ingleby H, Gershon-Cohen J. *Comparative anatomy, pathology, and roentgenology of the breast.* Philadelphia: University of Pennsylvania Press, 1960.
4. Page DL, Anderson TJ. *Diagnostic histopathology of the breast.* London: Churchill Livingstone, 1987.
5. Rosen PP, Oberman HA. *Atlas of tumor pathology: tumors of the mammary gland,* 3rd ed. Washington DC: AFIP, 1992.
6. Rosen PP. *Rosen's breast pathology,* 2nd ed. Philadelphia: Lippincott Williams & Wilkins, 2001.
7. Rosen PP. *Breast pathology: diagnosis by needle core biopsy.* Philadelphia: Lippincott Williams & Wilkins, 1999.
8. Tot T, Tabar L, Dean PB. *Practical breast pathology.* New York: Thieme, 2002..
9. Trojani M. *A color atlas of breast histopathology.* Philadelphia: JB Lippincott, 1991.

The following textbooks are excellent resources for clinical findings and surgical management in breast disease:

1. Bland, KI, Copeland EM 3rd. *The breast: comprehensive management of benign and malignant diseases,* 2nd ed. Philadelphia: WB Saunders, 1998.
2. Hughes LE, Mansel RE, Webster DJT. *Benign disorders of the breast: concepts and clinical management,* 2nd ed. Philadelphia: WB Saunders, 2000.
3. Silverstein MJ, Recht A, Lagios M. *Ductal carcinoma of the breast,* 2nd ed. Philadelphia: Lippincott Williams & Wilkins, 2002.

The following breast imaging and ultrasound textbooks have been helpful:

1. Barth V. *Atlas of diseases of the breast.* Stuttgart: Thieme Publishers, 1979.
2. Jellins J, Kobayashi T. *Ultrasonic examination of the breast.* Chichester, UK: John Wiley & Sons, 1983.
3. Teboul M, Halliwell M. *Atlas of ultrasound and ductal echography of the breast: the introduction of anatomic intelligence into breast imaging.* Cambridge: Blackwell Science, 1995.

INDEX

Page numbers followed by *f* indicate figures; page numbers followed by *t* indicate tables.